FOUNDATIONS OF RESPIRATORY CARE

FOUNDATIONS OF RESPIRATORY CARE

Edited by

David J. Pierson, M.D.
Professor
Division of Pulmonary and Critical Care Medicine
Department of Medicine
University of Washington School of Medicine
Medical Director
Department of Respiratory Care
Harborview Medical Center
Seattle, Washington

Robert M. Kacmarek, Ph.D., R.R.T.
Associate Professor
Department of Anesthesiology
Harvard Medical School
Director
Department of Respiratory Care
Massachusetts General Hospital
Boston, Massachusetts

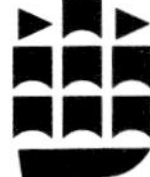

CHURCHILL LIVINGSTONE
New York, Edinburgh, London, Melbourne, Tokyo

Library of Congress Cataloging-in-Publication Data
Foundations of respiratory care / edited by David J. Pierson, Robert M. Kacmarek.
p. cm.
Includes bibliographical references and index.
ISBN 0-443-08509-9
1. Respiratory therapy. I. Pierson, David J. II. Kacmarek, Robert M.
[DNLM: 1. Respiratory Function Tests–methods. 2. Respiratory Mechanics–physiology. 3. Respiratory System–physiology. 4. Respiratory Tract Diseases–diagnosis. 5. Respiratory Tract Diseases–therapy. WF 140 F771]
RC735.I5F68 1992
616.2–dc20
DNLM/DLC
for Library of Congress 92-17459
CIP

Distributed in the United Kingdom by Churchill Livingstone, Robert Stevenson House, 1–3 Baxter's Place, Leith Walk, Edinburgh EH1 3AF, and by associated companies, branches, and representatives throughout the world.

Accurate indications, adverse reactions, and dosage schedules for drugs are provided in this book, but it is possible that they may change. The reader is urged to review the package information data of the manufacturers of the medications mentioned.

The Publishers have made every effort to trace the copyright holders for borrowed material. If they have inadvertently overlooked any, they will be pleased to make the necessary arrangements at the first opportunity.

Acquisitions Editor: *Avé McCracken*
Copy Editor: *Bridgett Dickinson*
Production Designer: *Patricia McFadden*
Production Supervisor: *Christina Hippeli*
Indexer: *Julia B. Figures*
Cover design: *Paul Moran*

Printed in the United States of America

First published in 1992 7 6 5 4 3 2 1

I dedicate this book to my family—Dona, Christine, and Erika—who sacrificed for it, and also to the Hosers at Harborview—past, present, and future—who inspired it.

David J. Pierson, M.D.

I dedicate this book to my wife Jan, to my children Darla, Robert, and Julia, to my parents Irene and George, to my sister Debbie and my brothers Bud, Mark, and Jeff, and to all the respiratory care practitioners who have challenged me to strive for excellence.

Robert M. Kacmarek, Ph.D., R.R.T.

Contributors

Steven H. Abman, M.D.
Associate Professor, Department of Pediatrics, University of Colorado Health Sciences Center; Co-Director, Department of Pediatrics, Special Care Nursery, The Children's Hospital, Denver, Colorado

Tammy H. Abuan, R.N.
Research Coordinator, Division of Pulmonary and Critical Care Medicine, Department of Medicine, University of Washington School of Medicine, Seattle, Washington

Joan Balik, R.R.T.
Assistant Director, Department of Respiratory Care, University of Colorado Health Sciences Center, Denver, Colorado

Richard K. Beauchamp, R.C.P.T., R.P.F.T.
Chief Technologist, Division of Pulmonary and Critical Care Medicine, Pulmonary Evaluation Laboratory, Henry Ford Hospital, Detroit, Michigan

Michael J. Bishop, M.D.
Professor of Anesthesiology, Adjunct Professor of Medicine, Division of Pulmonary and Critical Care Medicine, Department of Medicine, University of Washington School of Medicine; Associate Medical Director, Department of Respiratory Care, Harborview Medical Center, Seattle, Washington

Richard D. Branson, R.R.T.
Clinical Instructor, Department of Surgery, University of Cincinnati College of Medicine, Cincinnati, Ohio

John Butler, M.D.*
Professor, Division of Pulmonary and Critical Care Medicine, Department of Medicine, University of Washington School of Medicine; Attending Physician, University Affiliated Hospitals, Seattle, Washington

Paula Carvalho, M.D.
Acting Instructor, Department of Medicine, University of Washington School of Medicine, Seattle, Washington; Staff Physician, Department of Pulmonary and Critical Care Medicine, Medical Director, Sleep Laboratory, Veterans Affairs Medical Center, Boise, Idaho

Nirmal B. Charan, M.D.
Associate Professor, Department of Medicine, University of Washington School of Medicine, Seattle, Washington; Chief, Department of Pulmonary and Critical Care Medicine, Veterans Affairs Medical Center, Boise, Idaho

Robert L. Chatburn, R.R.T.
Director, Department of Respiratory Care, Rainbow Babies and Children's Hospital, Cleveland, Ohio

*Deceased.

Kent L. Christopher, M.D., R.R.T.
Assistant Clinical Professor, Department of Medicine, University of Colorado Health Sciences Center; Co-Director, The Institute for Transtracheal Oxygen Therapy, Denver, Colorado

Kimberly G. Clark, M.S.W.
Clinical Assistant Professor, University of Washington School of Social Work; President, Seattle International Association for Near Death Studies, Seattle, Washington

Bruce H. Culver, M.D.
Associate Professor, Department of Medicine, University of Washington School of Medicine; Chief of Medical Specialities, Department of Medicine, Pacific Medical Center, Seattle, Washington

Kenneth Davis, Jr., M.D.
Associate Professor, Department of Surgery, University of Cincinnati College of Medicine; Director, Division of Trauma and Critical Care, Department of Surgery, University of Cincinnati Medical Center, Cincinnati, Ohio

Juliann M. DiFiore, B.S.E.E.
Research Engineer, Department of Pediatrics, Rainbow Babies and Children's Hospital, Cleveland, Ohio

Eugene C. Fletcher, M.D.
Associate Professor, Department of Medicine, Baylor College of Medicine; Director, Department of Medicine, Pulmonary Physiology Sleep Laboratory, Veterans Administration Medical Center, Houston, Texas

Mary E. Gilmartin, R.N., R.R.T.
Clinical Nurse Specialist, Nursing Department, National Jewish Center for Immunology and Respiratory Medicine, Denver, Colorado

Robert J. Harwood, M.S.A., R.R.T.
Assistant Professor, Department of Cardiopulmonary Care Sciences, Respiratory Care Program, Georgia State University School of Allied Health Professions, College of Health Sciences, Atlanta, Georgia

Dean R. Hess, M.Ed., R.R.T.
Instructor, School of Respiratory Therapy, York College of Pennsylvania; Assistant Director, Department of Research, York Hospital, York, Pennsylvania

Thomas L. Higgins, M.D.
Director, Department of Cardiothoracic Anesthesia, Cardiothoracic Intensive Care Unit, Cleveland Clinic Hospital, Cleveland, Ohio

Jan V. Hirschmann, M.D.
Professor, Department of Medicine, University of Washington School of Medicine; Assistant Chief, Department of Medicine, Veterans Affairs Medical Center, Seattle, Washington

Leonard D. Hudson, M.D.
Professor and Head, Division of Pulmonary and Critical Care Medicine, Department of Medicine, University of Washington School of Medicine, Seattle, Washington

James M. Hurst, M.D.
Professor, Departments of Surgery and Anesthesia, University of Cincinnati College of Medicine; Director, Division of Trauma and Critical Care, Department of Surgery, University of Cincinnati Medical Center, Cincinnati, Ohio

David H. Ingbar, M.D.
Associate Professor, Division of Pulmonary and Critical Care Medicine, Department of Medicine, University of Minnesota Medical School—Minneapolis; Co-Director, Medical Intensive Care Unit, University of Minnesota Hospital and Clinic of the University of Minnesota Health Sciences Center, Minneapolis, Minnesota

Jay A. Johannigman, M.D.
Assistant Professor, Department of Surgery, Uniformed Services University of the Health Sciences, F. Edward Hébert School of Medicine, Bethesda, Maryland; Director of Surgical Critical Care, Department of Surgery, Wilford Hall United States Air Force Medical Center, San Antonio, Texas

Daniel J. Johnson, M.D.
Assistant Professor, Department of Surgery, University of Cincinnati College of Medicine; Medical Director, Department of Surgery, Trauma Service, University of Cincinnati Medical Center, Cincinnati, Ohio

Noel T. Johnson, D.O.
Medical Director, Departments of Pulmonary Diagnostic Services, Respiratory Care, and Sleep Disorders Center, Ballard Community Hospital, Seattle, Washington

Robert M. Kacmarek, Ph.D., R.R.T.
Associate Professor, Department of Anesthesiology, Harvard Medical School; Director, Department of Respiratory Care, Massachusetts General Hospital, Boston, Massachusetts

Colleen Kigin, M.S., M.P.A., P.T.
Associate in Anesthesia, Department of Anesthesia, Harvard Medical School; Director, Department of Physical Therapy Services, Massachusetts General Hospital, Boston, Massachusetts

Michael T. Kochansky, R.P.F.T.
Director of Pulmonary Diagnostics, Department of Pulmonary Services, York Hospital, York, Pennsylvania

Patricia B. Koff, M.Ed., R.R.T.
Development Coordinator, Department of Pulmonary Sciences, University of Colorado Health Sciences Center, Denver, Colorado

John M. Luce, M.D.
Associate Professor, Departments of Medicine and Anesthesia, University of California, San Francisco, School of Medicine; Associate Director, Medical-Surgical Intensive Care Unit, San Francisco General Hospital Medical Center, San Francisco, California

Thomas R. Martin, M.D.
Professsor of Medicine, Division of Pulmonary and Critical Care Medicine, Department of Medicine, University of Washington School of Medicine; Assistant Chief, Section of Pulmonary Critical Care Medicine, Veterans Affairs Medical Center, Seattle, Washington

Richard J. Maunder, M.D.
Clinical Associate Professor, Department of Medicine, University of Washington School of Medicine; Director, Critical Care Services, Swedish Hospital Medical Center, Seattle, Washington

Lynn Grose McHugh, M.N., R.N.
Critical Care Research Coordinator, Division of Pulmonary and Critical Care, Department of Medicine, Harborview Medical Center, Seattle, Washington

Eve Medvidofsky, R.R.T.
Supervisor, Department of Respiratory Care, Humana Hospital—Aurora, Aurora, Colorado

Pope L. Moseley, M.D., M.S.
Associate Professor, Division of Pulmonary Diseases, Departments of Internal Medicine and Exercise Sciences, University of Iowa College of Medicine; Attending Physician, Department of Internal Medicine, University of Iowa Hospitals and Clinics, Iowa City, Iowa

Janine Mundroff, M.S., R.D., C.N.S.D.
Trauma Dietician, Nutrition Support Service, York Hospital, York, Pennsylvania

Louise M. Nett, R.N., R.R.T.
Research Associate, Department of Clinical Research, Presbyterian/St. Luke's Center for Health Sciences Education, Denver, Colorado

David J. Pierson, M.D.
Professor, Division of Pulmonary and Critical Care Medicine, Department of Medicine, University of Washington School of Medicine; Medical Director, Department of Respiratory Care, Harborview Medical Center, Seattle, Washington

Thomas A. Raffin, M.D.
Associate Professor, Department of Medicine, Stanford University School of Medicine; Chief, Division of Pulmonary and Critical Care, Stanford Unviversity Medical Center; Co-Director, Stanford University Center for Biomedical Ethics, Stanford, California

Andrew L. Ries, M.D., M.P.H.
Associate Professor, Division of Pulmonary and Critical Care Medicine, Department of Medicine, University of California, San Diego, School of Medicine; Medical Director, Pulmonary Rehabilitation Program, University of California Medical Center, San Diego, California

Ray H. Ritz, R.R.T.
Assistant Director, Department of Respiratory Care, Massachusetts General Hospital, Boston, Massachusetts

Robert B. Schoene, M.D.
Associate Professor, Division of Pulmonary and Critical Care Medicine, Department of Medicine, University of Washington School of Medicine; Medical Director, Pulmonary Function and Exercise Laboratory, Harborview Medical Center, Seattle, Washington

David A. Schwartz, M.D.
Assistant Professor, Department of Medicine, University of Iowa College of Medicine; Director, Department of Occupational Medicine, University of Iowa Hospitals and Clinics, Iowa City, Iowa

Paul A. Selecky, M.D.
Associate Clinical Professor, Department of Medicine, University of California, Los Angeles, UCLA School of Medicine, Los Angeles, California; Medical Director, Pulmonary Department, Hoag Memorial Hospital Presbyterian, Newport Beach, California

Richard L. Sheldon, M.D.
Clinical Professor of Medicine, Department of Internal Medicine, Loma Linda University School of Medicine, Loma Linda, California

Charles B. Sherman, M.D., M.P.H.
Assistant Professor, Department of Medicine, Brown University School of Medicine; Director, Pulmonary Division, Miriam Hospital, Providence, Rhode Island

Justin P. Smith, M.D.
Visiting Scholar, Department of Chemistry, University of Washington School of Medicine; Diagnostic Radiologist, First Hill Diagnostic Imaging, Seattle, Washington

Michael G. Snow, R.P.F.T.
Manager, Division of Pulmonary Physiology and Research, Department of Respiratory Care, Pacific Medical Center, San Francisco, California

Kenneth P. Steinberg, M.D.
Senior Fellow, Division of Pulmonary and Critical Care Medicine, Department of Medicine, University of Washington School of Medicine; Medical Director, Respiratory Care Program, Seattle Community College, Seattle, Washington

James K. Stoller, M.D.
Head, Section of Respiratory Therapy, Department of Pulmonary and Critical Care Medicine, Cleveland Clinic Foundation, Cleveland, Ohio

Elizabeth Tarnell, M.D.
Pulmonologist, Dedham Medical Associates, Dedham, Massachusetts

Steven M. Weiss, M.D.
Senior Fellow, Division of Pulmonary and Critical Care Medicine, Department of Medicine, University of Washington School of Medicine, Seattle, Washington

Herbert P. Wiedemann, M.D.
Chairman, Department of Pulmonary and Critical Care Medicine, Cleveland Clinic Foundation, Cleveland, Ohio

Robert L. Wilkins, M.A., R.R.T.
Associate Professor, and Program Director, Department of Respiratory Therapy, Loma Linda University School of Allied Health Professions, Loma Linda, California

Preface

Is *Foundations of Respiratory Care* a book for physicians or for respiratory therapists? It is both. *Foundations of Respiratory Care* is intended to meet the needs of those who participate in the care of patients with respiratory illness. These needs are diverse but interrelated, and we believe that no previous text has succeeded in meeting all of them. Books written for physicians address pathophysiology and the clinical manifestations of disease, and may also describe general approaches to assessment and therapy. However, these texts routinely do not provide actual step-by-step instructions for the clinician at the bedside. On the other hand, respiratory therapy textbooks describe in detail the machines and procedures but not the scientific rationale behind their application (i.e., how disorders being managed affect the body and how the tests and treatments described may clarify or reverse these effects).

Respiratory care in the 1990s is a far cry from inhalation therapy, its ancestor of a generation ago. Modern assessment tools such as pulse oximeters and pulmonary artery catheters provide instant, direct measurement of physiology—within the body as it happens. Therapies used today, such as microprocessor-driven positive pressure ventilation and transtracheal oxygen administration, not only sustain patients who once would have died but also can themselves cause injury or death. Patient care using such therapies cannot be ordered effectively and safely by physicians who do not fully understand the operation and limitations of the devices, nor can it be carried out optimally by respiratory care practitioners who do not fully understand the physiologic derangements their use is designed to combat.

Respiratory care now demands the integration of pathophysiology, therapeutic rationale, and practical application. The first two are needed from the "doctor books" and the last from the "therapist books." *Foundations of Respiratory Care* provides this integration in a single source. It is thus both for physicians—who need to know the practical implications of the therapies they order—and for respiratory care practitioners—who need to know the pathophysiology underlying the therapies ordered. The five sections of *Foundations of Respiratory Care* discuss in turn normal structure and function, the physiologic derangements and clinical manifestations produced by disease, how these manifestations can be detected and quantified, overall goals and strategies for managing the disorders encountered in respiratory care, and finally—only after these foundations have been laid—the individual techniques and devices used in patient care.

Respiratory care is not only a complex array of physiology, machinery, and procedures. It is also the care of *people* with respiratory illness. This is what distinguishes clinicians from the research scientists, laboratory technicians, and engineers who also deal with respiratory disease. Physicians, respiratory care practitioners, nurses, and other clinicians work with people, not isolated organ systems, laboratory abnormalities, or lung-thorax-ventilator interfaces. This book pays much needed attention to this human side of respiratory care. It includes chapters on the psychosocial evaluation of patients with respiratory illness, taking into account such things as cultural influences on health beliefs and patient compliance, and the effects of the critical care environment on patients, their families and loved ones, and those who participate in their care.

Foundations of Respiratory Care seeks to integrate all these components into a coherent whole, and thus to be not only a "doctor book" and a "therapist book," but also a comprehensive resource for other health professionals who participate in the assessment and management of patients with disorders affecting the respiratory system.

David J. Pierson, M.D.
Robert M. Kacmarek, Ph.D., R.R.T.

Acknowledgments

Many people contributed to this book in addition to those listed as authors, and we would like to express our appreciation to the following people: to University of Washington colleagues Richard B. Goodman and Peter J. Kudenchuk for advice and editorial assistance on Chapters 18 and 77, respectively; to Harborview radiologists David P. Christie and Yoram Ben-Menachem for help with many of the radiographs; to Phyllis Wood, Andrew D. Blair, and Trudi Peek for their artistic skills; to Dona Pierson for help with the logo and long hours of proofreading; and to Gertrude Shaw, Pat Morin, and Margaret Nadler for secretarial assistance.

Charles B. Spearman played a substantial role in the original planning of this book, and we are grateful to him for this important input.

Special thanks are also due to many people at Churchill Livingstone—especially to Robert A. Hurley for somehow maintaining faith in this project for a very long time, and also to Avé McCracken, Carol Bader, and Bridgett Dickinson for their unflagging support and good cheer throughout the writing and editing of this book.

David J. Pierson, M.D.
Robert M. Kacmarek, Ph.D., R.R.T.

Contents

Introduction

Respiratory care encompasses a wide array of diseases, tests, and therapies, ranging from the commonplace to the exotic. *Foundations of Respiratory Care* does include the exotic, such as cyanide poisoning, extracorporeal membrane oxygenation, and artificial blood, but deals mainly with what clinicians encounter in day-to-day practice. The "bread and butter" of obstructive lung disease and acute respiratory failure, along with the tests and treatments used in managing them, comprise the core of the "curriculum" presented in this book. Although awareness of the diversity of pulmonary and critical care medicine is important, the clinician primarily needs a thorough familiarity with the most common and hence most important illnesses—what they do to the body, how they are manifested, how one identifies them and assesses their severity, and what the various approaches to therapy are intended to accomplish.

Foundations of Respiratory Care is not organized like other respiratory care texts. There is no chapter on chronic obstructive pulmonary disease (COPD) and none devoted to "monitoring" or "home care." These key topics are instead discussed throughout the text, much as they would be integrated into a medical school curriculum. For the kind of understanding we believe the reader should have, a disorder as important as COPD cannot be covered in a single chapter. Its clinical manifestations and prognosis (Chs. 22 and 24) do not truly make sense without an understanding of airflow obstruction (Ch. 21), which in turn cannot be mastered without a knowledge of the structure (Ch. 7) and mechanical function (Ch. 9) of the airways. Likewise, the safe and effective administration of therapies such as bronchodilators (Ch. 20), physical reconditioning (Ch. 96), and supplemental oxygen (Ch. 99) to patients with COPD requires an appreciation of the overall goals of management and the therapeutic strategies for each modality in COPD (Chs. 62 and 63).

We believe that for the practice of respiratory care to be rational, safe, and cost-effective it must be based on physiology, not memorized by rote or performed according to arbitrary protocol. Physiology and pathophysiology comprise the "bricks and mortar" out of which the *Foundations of Respiratory Care* are built. It is true that much of clinical practice remains empirical (based on experience rather than on rigorous scientific proof) and we have relied heavily on the experience and wisdom of the book's distinguished contributors. However, the approaches and regimens presented here are constructed logically and based wherever possible on established physiologic mechanisms.

Although most areas of medicine have adopted *le Système International d'Unites* (SI units), change has come slowly in respiratory care, particularly in the United States. For many of us this is at least partly because of the unwieldiness of dividing by 7.5 to convert millimeters of mercury (mmHg) to kilopascals (kPa). Throughout this book we have used the customary American units of measure, despite the technical incorrectness of this in international scientific parlance. To facilitate reference to SI units and other standards of measure we have provided conversion tables and nomograms in the Appendix.

David J. Pierson, M.D.
Robert M. Kacmarek, Ph.D., R.R.T.

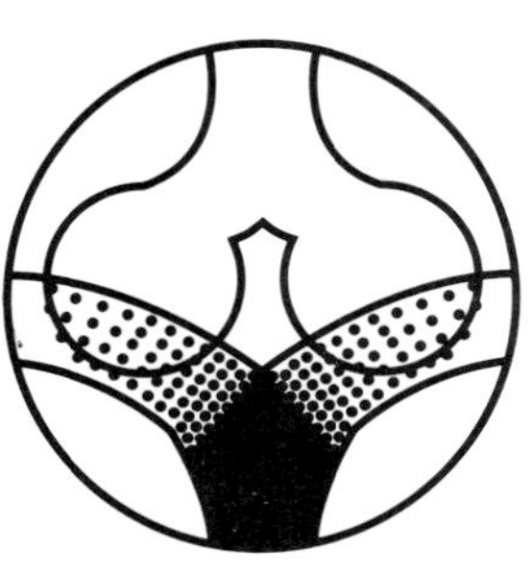

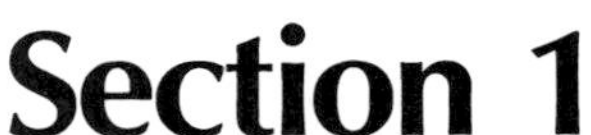

Section 1

Respiratory Structure and Function

Chapter 1

Chemical and Physical Background

Robert M. Kacmarek

CHAPTER OUTLINE

In order for the clinician to develop a sound understanding of the pathophysiology and treatment of disease, a thorough background in the related basic sciences is essential. Both chemistry and physics form the foundation upon which the concepts of respiratory care management are based. Much of the management of cardiopulmonary disease evolves about acid-base chemistry and fluid physics. This chapter is designed to present basic concepts in these areas. Although most topics included are presented in a detailed manner, a sound foundation in chemistry and physics is assumed. Those without basic skills in this area are referred to more fundamental texts.

SOLUTIONS

A solution is best defined as a homogeneous mixture of two substances, generally either two liquids or a liquid and a solid. Once mixed, the two are indistinguishable and occupy the complete volume of the solution in equal proportions. The substance being dissolved (the solid or the liquid in smallest volume) is referred to as the *solute*, while the substance in which the solute is dissolved is the *solvent*.[1] In most physiologic solutions water (H_2O) is the solvent. Addition of a solute creates an osmotic pressure, as is discussed later, and increases the boiling point while decreasing the melting point of the solvent. Qualitatively, a solution is classified as either (1) *dilute*, containing a small amount of solute per volume of solvent; (2) *saturated*, containing the maximum amount of solute per volume of solvent at a particular temperature (the higher the temperature, the more solute that can be dissolved per volume of solvent; or (3) *supersaturated*, containing a larger quantity of dissolved solute per volume of solvent than expected at a particular temperature. A supersaturated solution is formed by heating a solution to allow the excess solute to dissolve and then cooling it undisturbed, which allows the excess to stay in solution. Once the solution is physically disturbed, the excess precipitates (forms a solid at the bottom of the solution). A saturated solution is easily recognized by the presence of a precipitate. Most physiologic solutions are dilute. The quantitative relationship between the solvent and the solute may be expressed in many forms; the most common mathematical relationships used are defined below.

Volume and Gram Percent

Volume and gram percent are similar methods of expressing solute to solvent relationships based on quantity per 100 mL of solutions. A *volume percent* (Vol%) relationship is the number of milliliters of solute per 100 mL of solution.[2] For example

$$3.5 \text{ Vol\%} = 3.5 \text{ mL/100 mL solution}$$

$$6.2 \text{ Vol\%} = 6.2 \text{ mL/100 mL solution}$$

A *gram percent* (g%) relationship is the number of grams of solute per 100 mL of solution.[2] For example

$$20 \text{ g\%} = 20 \text{ g/100 mL solution}$$

$$5 \text{ g\%} = 5 \text{ g/100 mL solution}$$

Similar expressions are milliliters per deciliter (mL/dL) and grams per deciliter (g/dL). Since 1 dL equals 100 mL, 3.5 Vol% equals 3.5 mL/dL and 20 g% equals 20 g/dL.[2]

Ratio

A simple ratio between the quantity of solute and solvent expressed as the number of grams to the number of milliliters may be used to define the solution concentration.[3] For example

$$1{:}100 = 1 \text{ g to } 100 \text{ mL}$$

$$3{:}200 = 3 \text{ g to } 200 \text{ mL}$$

Problems regarding concentrations defined by ratios can be solved by simple proportionalities. For example, to find how many milligrams of solute are in 1 mL of a 3:200 solution:

$$3{:}200 = 3 \text{ g to } 200 \text{ ml}$$

$$3 \text{ g} = 3000 \text{ mg}$$

thus

$$\frac{3000 \text{ mg}}{200 \text{ ml}} = \frac{x}{1 \text{ ml}}$$

$$x = 15 \text{ mg}$$

Percent Weight to Volume

When solution concentration is expressed as percent weight to volume, the actual percentage listed represents the number of grams of solute per 100 mL of solution.[1] This method of defining the solute to solvent relationship is commonly used in pharmacology. For example

$$2.5\% \text{ W/V} = 2.5 \text{ g/100 mL}$$

$$1.0\% \text{ W/V} = 1.0 \text{ g/100 mL}$$

Proportionality relationships are also useful in solving percent weight to volume problems. For example, to find how many milligrams are in 0.5 mL of a 1.0% W/V solution:

$$1.0\% \text{ W/V} = 1 \text{ g/100 mL}$$

$$1 \text{ g} = 1000 \text{ mg}$$

thus

$$\frac{1000 \text{ mg}}{100 \text{ mL}} = \frac{x}{0.5 \text{ mL}}$$

$$x = 5 \text{ mg}$$

True Percent

Both the solute and solvent may be expressed in either weight or volume, which gives the quantity of solute as the actual percent by weight or volume of a given quantity of solution.[2] For example

$$10\% = 10 \text{ parts solute and } 90 \text{ parts solvent}$$

$$5\% = 5 \text{ parts solute and } 95 \text{ parts solvent}$$

Thus, to find how many grams of solute and solvent are in 500 g of a 3% solution:

$$\underset{(0.03)}{\text{Percent}} \times \underset{(500 \text{ g})}{\text{solution wt}} = \underset{(15 \text{ g})}{\text{solute wt}}$$

$$\underset{(500 \text{ g})}{\text{Solution wt}} - \underset{(15 \text{ g})}{\text{solute wt}} = \underset{(485 \text{ g})}{\text{solvent wt}}$$

The above defined expressions of solution concentrations are commonly used for physiologic solutions or pharmacologic agents. Three other relationships—molal, molar, and normal concentrations—are used mostly in laboratories to express the concentrations of reagents and are defined in standard chemistry texts.[4]

Dilution Calculations

During the administration of aerosolized drugs it is not uncommon to dilute a given agent with water to obtain a less concentrated solution for delivery. In order to determine the final concentration formed after dilution, the following proportional relationship is commonly used:

$$(\text{conc A})(\text{vol A}) = (\text{conc B})(\text{vol B}) \qquad (1)$$

where A is the condition before dilution and B is the condition after dilution. For example, what is the final concentration of a solution formed by addition of 3 mL of H_2O to 1.0 mL of a 1.0% W/V solution?

$$\underset{(1.0\ \text{mL})}{\text{Vol A}}\ \underset{(1.0\%\ \text{W/V})}{\text{conc A}} = \underset{(4\ \text{mL})}{\text{Vol B}}\ \underset{(x)}{\text{conc B}}$$

$$x = 0.25\%\ \text{W/V}$$

EQUIVALENT WEIGHTS

The concentration of many electrolytes may be expressed in units of chemical reactivity, that is, in terms of the quantity of the substance that will react completely with a predictable quantity of another substance. Equivalent weights are one method of expressing chemical reactivity.[5] One equivalent weight of a substance reacts completely with one equivalent weight of another substance, providing the two react chemically. Specifically, an equivalent weight is defined as the amount of a substance that will react completely with 1 mol of hydrogen ion or hydroxyl ion (OH^-) or of any monovalent substance.[2] Since equivalent weights are expressions of units of chemical reactivity, the quantity equal to one equivalent weight is based on the chemical nature and/or reactivity of the substance. For atoms and free radicals, the equivalent weight is equal to the atomic or molecular weight divided by the absolute value of the valence of the substance. For example, for calcium ion (Ca^{2+}) and bicarbonate ion (HCO_3^-):

Ca^{2+}, atomic weight 20 g

$$\frac{20}{2}\ \text{g} = 10\ \text{g/equivalent weight}$$

HCO_3^-, molecular weight 61 g

$$\frac{61\ \text{g}}{1} = 61\ \text{g/equivalent weight}$$

For acids, equivalent weights are determined by dividing the molecular weight of the acid by the number of H^+ ions replaceable in a chemical reaction. For example, for sulfuric acid (H_2SO_4) and carbonic acid (H_2CO_3):

H_2SO_4, molecular weight 98 g, replaceable $H^+ = 2$

$$\frac{98\ \text{g}}{2} = 49\ \text{g/equivalent wt}$$

H_2CO_3, molecular weight 62 g, replaceable $H^+ = 1$

$$\frac{62}{1} = 62\ \text{g/equivalent wt}$$

The equivalent weight of a base is determined in a similar manner by dividing the molecular weight by the number of replaceable OH^- ions. Thus, for calcium hydroxide [$Ca(OH)_2$] and magnesium hydroxide [$Mg(OH)_2$]:

$Ca(OH)_2$, molecular weight 74 g, replaceable $OH^- = 2$

$$\frac{74\ \text{g}}{2} = 37\ \text{g/equivalent wt}$$

$Mg(OH)_2$, molecular weight 58.3 g, replaceable $OH^- = 2$

$$\frac{58.3}{2} = 29.15\ \text{g/equivalent wt}$$

Finally, for salts the equivalent weight is equal to the molecular weight divided by the total positive or negative charge in the molecule. Thus, for sodium chloride (NaCl) and aluminum fluoride (AlF_3):

NaCl, molecular weight 58.5 g, total positive (or negative) charge = 1

$$\frac{58.5\ \text{g}}{1} = 58.5\ \text{g/equivalent wt}$$

AlF_3, molecular weight 84 g, total positive (or negative) charge = 3

$$\frac{84\ \text{g}}{3} = 28\ \text{g/equivalent wt}$$

Normally, the equivalent weight is expressed in grams as the gram equivalent weight (GEW) or in milligrams as the milliequivalent weight (mEq).[6] Numerically these are related by a factor of 1000—that is, 1 GEW of sodium (Na^+) is 23 g and 1 mEq of Na^+ is 23 mg, but 1000 mEq of Na^+ is needed to equal 1 GEW of Na^+.

Equivalent weights are used clinically to quantify the volume of electrolytes administered or the volume of acid or base administered to correct acid/base deficiencies.[7] For example: If a severe metabolic acidosis resulted in a deficiency of 15 mEq of base per liter of extracellular fluid (see Ch. 47), what quantity of HCO_3^- would be necessary to reverse the acidosis? Since the acidosis is expressed in milliequivalents, a quantity of base equivalent to the deficit caused by the acidosis should neutralize the excess acid and return the acid/base balance to normal. Assuming the extracellular fluid volume is 20 L, the total body deficit of base is

$$(20\ \text{L})\ (15\ \text{mEq/L}) = 300\ \text{mEq}$$

Thus, administration of 300 mEq of HCO_3^- would neutralize the deficit.

$$(300\ \text{mEq}\ HCO_3^-)\ (61\ \text{mg/mEq}) = 18{,}300\ \text{mg}\ HCO_3^-$$

or 18.3 g of HCO_3^- is required to completely reverse the metabolic acidosis.

OSMOSIS

Osmosis is the movement of water from an area of high concentration to an area of low concentration of water through a membrane semipermeable only to water. Figure

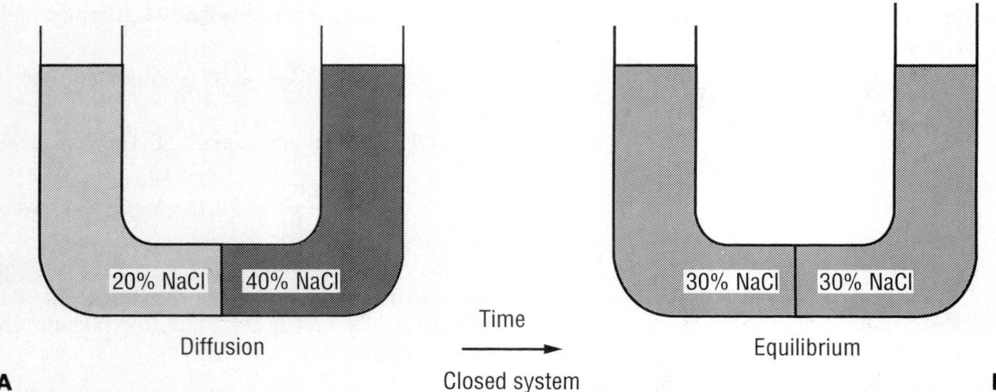

Figure 1-1. **(A)** Diffusion across a membrane permeable to both water and NaCl. **(B)** Since both the solvent and the solute diffuse, at equilibrium the concentration and volume of solution on each side of the membrane is equal. (From Wojciechowski,[4] with permission.)

1-1 illustrates the effect of separating two solutions of differing concentrations of water by a membrane permeable to both water and solute, while Figure 1-2 illustrates the effect of replacing the permeable membrane with one selectively permeable only to water. Since both the solute and water can move across the membrane in Figure 1-1, not only are the final concentrations of these solutions equal after the movement of both water and solute, but the volumes of the two solutions are also equal. This occurs because the membrane essentially allows the two solutions to act as one—water and solute move freely back and forth across the membrane as if it did not exist. However, in Figure 1-2 the semipermeable membrane allows only water to move, with the quantity of solute on each side of the membrane remaining constant. Thus, at equilibrium the concentration of water and solute is the same on each side of the membrane, but the volume of each solution differs. In fact, if pure water were placed on one side of a semipermeable membrane and a solution of specific concentration on the other, virtually all the water would move by osmosis through the membrane into the side with the solution. This occurs because equilibration of water concentration on each side of the membrane is impossible because the solute is kept in one compartment.

Movement of water by osmosis results from potential pressure differences between water and a solution.[8] This potential pressure difference is termed the *osmotic pressure* of the solution. The osmotic pressure of pure water is always zero, but the osmotic pressure of a solution is directly related to the quantity of particles dissolved in the solution. The greater the number of dissolved particles, the greater the osmotic pressure of the solution. As depicted in Figure 1-3, osmotic pressure is the force drawing water into the solution. In order for osmosis to be stopped, a force equal to the osmotic pressure must be applied. Normally, hydrostatic pressure (the pressure due to the weight of water) is the force opposing osmosis. As illustrated in Figure 1-4, osmosis can be prevented if the hydrostatic pressure of a solution equals its osmotic pressure.

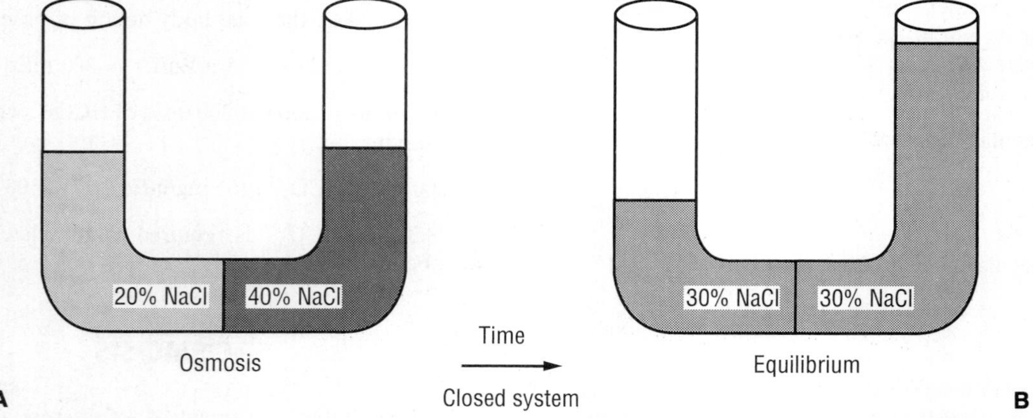

Figure 1-2. **(A)** Osmosis across a membrane permeable only to water. **(B)** Since only water diffuses, at equilibrium the concentration of solution on each side of the membrane is equal, but solution volumes differ. (From Wojciechowski,[4] with permission.)

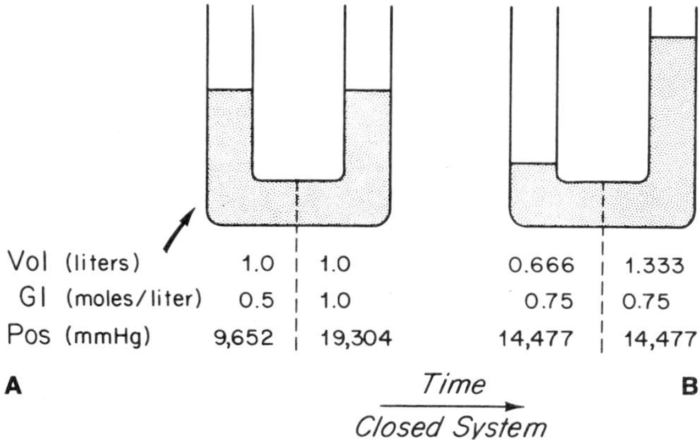

Figure 1-3. Two solutions separated by a semipermeable membrane (water only). **(A)** As a result of different osmotic pressures, a total potential pressure gradient favoring water movement from the left to the right is established. Any solution with particles of 1 mol/L of solution creates an osmotic pressure (P_{os}) of 19,304 mmHg within the solution. Thus, the osmotic pressure gradient causing movement is 9,652 mmHg (19,304 mmHg − 9652 mmHg). **(B)** At equilibrium, the concentration of glucose (Gl) and the osmotic pressure are equal on both sides of the membrane; however, the volume on the left side has decreased by 0.33 L, and the volume on the right side has increased by 0.33 L.

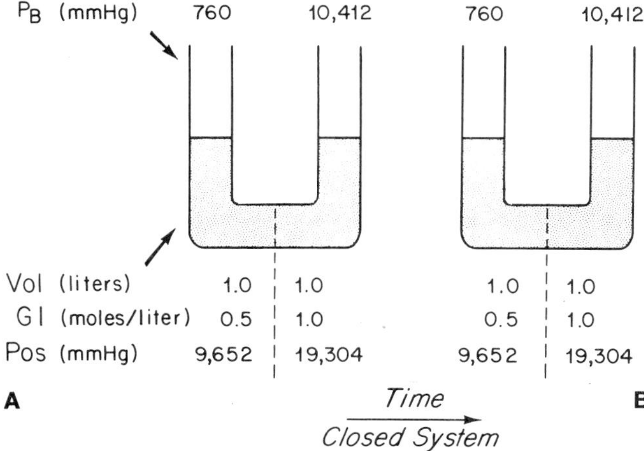

Figure 1-4. Two solutions separated by membrane permeable only to water. **(A)** An osmotic pressure (P_{os}) gradient exists between the two glucose solutions (Gl), which is equal to 9652 mmHg (19,304 mmHg − 9652 mmHg). However, a barometric pressure (P_b) difference also equal to 9652 mmHg (10,412 mmHg − 760 mmHg) exists. Thus, the P_b gradient on the left side counteracts the effect of the P_{os} gradient. **(B)** At equilibrium *no* movement has occurred because no total pressure gradient exists between the two sides of the system.

Both osmotic and hydrostatic pressure occur in all body fluids. Hydrostatic pressure is dependent on compartment fluid pressures (e.g., pulmonary or systemic blood pressure), while osmotic pressure is dependent on all dissolved substances. However, most dissolved particles are capable of moving freely across body membranes, the major exception being proteins. The osmotic pressure established in a given compartment as a result of protein is termed *colloid osmotic pressure* or *oncotic pressure*.

Starling's Law of Fluid Exchange

Fluid movement across capillaries is characterized by Starling's law of fluid exchange:

$$Q = k\,[(P_{cap} - P_{is}) - \sigma\,(\pi_{cap} - \pi_{is})] \qquad (2)$$

where Q is net fluid movement across the capillary, k is the capillary filtration coefficient (the permeability characteristic of the membrane), P_{cap} is capillary hydrostatic pressure, P_{is} is interstitial hydrostatic pressure, π_{cap} is capillary (plasma) colloid osmotic pressure, π_{is} is interstitial colloid osmotic pressure, and σ is the reflection coefficient (the membrane's ability to prevent the passage of protein).

Normally, as a result of the interaction of these forces, fluid moves from the capillary into the interstitium on the arterial side and from the interstitium into the capillary on the venous side. However, the net movement of fluid is into the interstitium from all capillaries as a result of a slight pressure gradient favoring fluid leaving the capillary[9] (Table 1-1). In general, the capillary hydrostatic pressure, the interstitial colloid osmotic pressure, and the interstitial hydrostatic pressure favor movement into the interstitium.[2] The interstitial hydrostatic pressure is normally subatmospheric, while the capillary colloid osmotic pressure maintains fluid within the capillary. As may be noted from Table 1-1, there is a difference in the level of these four forces in the pulmonary and in the systemic capillary bed, primarily, because of a difference in pulmonary versus systemic vascular resistance and blood pressure and a variation in capillary permeabilities. Since the pulmonary capillaries are more permeable than systemic capillaries, the pulmonary interstitial colloid osmotic pressure is higher than the systemic colloid osmotic pressure.

As should be readily apparent, a change in any of these five variables may greatly alter fluid balance at a given capillary bed. Edema can be caused by an increase in capillary hydrostatic pressure or a decrease in capillary colloid osmotic pressure, as well as by an alteration in capillary permeability.[10] Clinically, maintenance of normal equilibrium at capillary membranes is essential to ensure alveolar–capillary integrity and to prevent specific gas exchange abnormalities.

KINETIC THEORY OF GASES

The kinetic theory of gases accounts for the behavior of dilute gases under temperature and pressure conditions not

Table 1-1. Forces Interacting at Body Capillaries[a]

	Systemic Capillaries					Pulmonary Capillaries				
	P_{cap}	P_{is}	π_{cap}	π_{is}	Diff	P_{cap}	P_{is}	π_{cap}	π_{is}	Diff
Arterial side	25	−7	28	4.5	+8.5	12	−17	28	4.5	+5
Venous side	9	−7	28	4.5	−7.5	2	−17	28	4.5	−4
Net	17	−7	28	4.5	+0.5	7	−17	28	4.5	+0

P_{cap}, capillary hydrostatic pressure; P_{is}, interstitial hydrostatic pressure; π_{cap}, capillary colloid osmotic pressure; π_{is}, interstitial colloid osmotic pressure; Diff, pressure differential (*negative* values favor fluid movement *into* and *positive* values favor fluid movement *out of* the capillary); Net, mean values across the total capillary network.

[a] π_{cap} is the only force keeping fluid within the capillary. The sum of P_{cap}, P_{is}, and π_{is} is the total force moving fluid out of the capillary.

involving a change of state. All molecules of a gas are in constant random motion, experiencing collisions with the environment and collisions and near collisions with each other; provided heat is not lost to the environment, their interactions are elastic.[4] The motion of gas molecules is a result of their kinetic energy, which is directly related to the system temperature—the higher the temperature, the greater the kinetic energy, and the greater the kinetic energy, the greater the velocity of gas movement, the frequency of collisions with the environment, and thus the pressure exerted by the gas.[4]

Opposing the kinetic energy of gases are weak intermolecular attraction forces, which generally do not affect molecular motion until conditions exist favoring a change to a less active state (solid or liquid). The kinetic theory of gases forms the basis for the ideal behavior of gases (see discussion of ideal gas laws, below).

Avogadro's Law

Before discussing the ideal gas laws, a brief discussion of Avogadro's law and density is necessary as background. Essentially, Avogadro's law states that one gram-atomic-, one gram-molecular-, or one gram-ionic-weight of a substance contains 6.02×10^{23} particles of that substance; this mass of a substance is referred to as a *mole* of the substance. Furthermore, 1 mole of a gas at 0°C and 760 mmHg, the conditions referred to as standard temperature and pressure (STP) (Table 1-2), occupies a volume of about 22.4 L.[3] However, some variations exist regarding this volume, depending on the physical and chemical properties of a given gas (e.g., for carbon dioxide [CO_2] it is 22.3 L). In addition, equal numbers or fractions of moles of different gases at a specific temperature and pressure occupy the same volume and contain the same number of particles.

Table 1-2. Standard Definitions

	Temperature	Pressure	H_2O Vapor
STPD	0°C	760 mmHg	Zero
STPS	0°C	760 mmHg	Saturated
ATPD	Atmospheric	Atmospheric	Zero
ATPS	Atmospheric	Atmospheric	Saturated
BTPS	37°C	Atmospheric	Saturated

S, standard; P, pressure; A, atmospheric; D, dry; B, body; S, saturated; T, temperature.

Density

Density (D) is an expression of the mass (M) of an object per unit volume (V):

$$D = M/V \tag{3}$$

and is usually expressed in grams per liter. The determination of the density of liquids and solids is generally straightforward; however, since the volume of gases is dependent on temperature and pressure, gas densities must be determined under standard conditions (STP), in which the volume is assumed to be 22.4 L. To calculate the density of a gas, the gram-molecular-weight (GMW) of the gas is divided by 22.4 L.

$$D = \frac{\text{GMW}}{22.4\ \text{L}}$$

For example, to find the density of oxygen (O_2):

$$\text{GMW } O_2 = 32\ \text{g}$$

$$1.43\ \text{g/L} = \frac{32\ \text{g}}{22.4\ \text{L}}$$

The specific gravity of a substance is the ratio between the density of a substance and the density of a standard. For solids and liquids the standard is water, whereas for gases O_2 is frequently used as the standard. For example, to find the specific gravity (SG) of mercury (Hg), whose density (D) is 13.6 g/cm^3:

$$\text{D of Hg} = 13.6\ \text{g/cm}^3$$

$$\text{D of } H_2O = 1\ \text{g/cm}^3$$

$$\text{SG of Hg} = 13.6{:}1, \text{ or } 13.6$$

Gas Pressure

Pressure is defined as force applied per unit area, expressed, for example, in grams per square centimeter or pounds per square inch (psi). For gases, pressure is directly dependent on system temperature owing to its effect on kinetic energy and on the gravitational attraction of the earth. Thus, the force exerted by gases is greatest at the earth's surface and decreases with altitude.[2] In fact, in spite of the constancy of O_2 concentration up to an altitude of about 50 miles, the density of the atmosphere markedly decreases, as does the total force exerted by the atmosphere and its component gases (Table 1-3), as altitude increases.

Gas pressure is frequently expressed as the height of a column of fluid (e.g., mmHg or ft of H_2O). The use of these expressions is based on the principle that the barometric pressure (P_b) is equal to the height of a column of fluid housed in a vacuum when exposed to atmospheric pressure multiplied by the fluid's density.[4] Thus, pressure expressed in millimeters can be converted to true pressure by multiplying it by the density of Hg (13.6 g/cm^3). The pressure exerted by an individual gas in a mixture is referred to as the partial pressure of the gas (e.g., PO_2, PCO_2) and is usually expressed in millimeters of Hg.

The Ideal Gas Laws

The ideal gas laws describe mathematically the relationship among pressure (P), volume (V), temperature (T), and amount (n) of a dilute gas at temperatures well above the boiling point of the corresponding liquid. Throughout the use of the gas laws, temperature is expressed in kelvins (K) that is, on the absolute temperature scale, in order to enhance mathematical simplicity.

According to the ideal gas laws, the product of pressure and volume divided by the product of temperature and the number of moles of gas yields a constant (R), referred to as the Boltzmann constant:

$$R = \frac{PV}{nT} \qquad (4)$$

or

$$PV = nRT$$

where the Boltzmann constant equals 82.1 mL $\times$ atm/mol $\times$ K or 62.3 L $\times$ mmHg/mol $\times$ K.[1] The ideal gas law equation includes within it all the relationships defined by the other gas laws.

Boyle's law states that the pressure and volume of a gas system vary inversely if the temperature and amount of gas in the system are constant

$$PV = nRT \qquad (5)$$

where nRT equals a constant. Charles law states that the volume and temperature of a gas system vary directly if the pressure and amount of gas in the system are constant:

$$\frac{V}{T} = \frac{nR}{P} \qquad (6)$$

where nR/P equals a constant. Gay-Lussac's law states that pressure and temperature of a gas system vary directly if the volume and amount of gas in the system are constant

$$\frac{P}{T} = \frac{nR}{V} \qquad (7)$$

where nR/V equals a constant. The combined gas law states that the product of pressure and volume varies inversely with the system temperature if the amount of gas in the system is constant

$$\frac{PV}{T} = nR \qquad (8)$$

where nR equals a constant.

Table 1-3. Altitude and Depth Comparisons

Feet	psi	mmHg	PO_2	% O_2 Equiv	Density
50,000	1.69	87.4	18.3	2.41	0.190
40,000	2.72	140.6	29.4	3.87	0.306
30,000	4.36	225.7	47.3	6.22	0.467
20,000	6.76	348.8	73.1	9.62	0.666
15,000	8.29	428.6	89.8	11.82	0.786
10,000	10.11	522.9	109.5	14.41	0.922
5,000	12.23	623.3	132.5	17.43	1.08
Above sea level					
0	14.70	760.0	159.6	20.95	1.25
Below sea level					
33	29.4	1520.0	318.0	41.90	2.50
66	44.1	2280.0	477.0	62.85	3.75
99	58.8	3040.0	636.0	83.80	5.00
132	73.5	3800.0	795.0	104.75	6.25

(Modified from Dittmer and Greve,[20] with permission.)

Each of these five relationships (Equations 4 to 8) can be modified and used to mathematically determine how variables within a single system change when individual variables are altered. Specifically

$$\frac{P_1V_1}{n_1T_1} = \frac{P_2V_2}{n_2T_2} \quad \text{Ideal gas law} \tag{9}$$

$$P_1V_1 = P_2V_2 \quad \text{Boyle's law} \tag{10}$$

$$\frac{V_2}{T_1} = \frac{V_2}{T_2} \quad \text{Charles law} \tag{11}$$

$$\frac{P_1}{T_1} = \frac{P_2}{T_2} \quad \text{Gay-Lussac's law} \tag{12}$$

$$\frac{P_1V_1}{T} = \frac{P_2V_2}{T_2} \quad \text{Combined gas law} \tag{13}$$

where the left sides of the above equations indicate original conditions of the gas system and the right sides indicate final conditions. Of these five relationships, Boyle's and Charles laws are used most frequently. Boyle's law provides the basis for body plethysmographic total thoracic gas volume determinations,[11] Charles law allows for correction of gas volumes from STP to body temperature and pressure saturated (BTPS)[12]; and Gay-Lussac's law is used in temperature corrections for blood gas data.[13]

All gases common to respiratory physiology conform to the ideal gas laws except water vapor. Since normal body temperature is below the boiling point of water, water vapor is not an ideal gas. The quantity of water vapor present in a gas is dependent on temperature and on the amount of water vapor available. Thus, in order to perform calculations involving gas volumes containing H_2O vapor, the system's original and final pressures must first be corrected for the water vapor pressure. For example, if the original system pressure is 1000 mmHg and the gas is saturated with water vapor at 37°C, the total pressure of all gases except water vapor is

$$\text{Total pressure} - H_2O \text{ vapor pressure} = \text{corrected pressure}$$

$$1000 \text{ mmHg} - 47 \text{ mmHg} = 953 \text{ mmHg}$$

Whenever greater precision is required, the system pressure read from a barometer should also be corrected for the expansion of Hg at the system temperature.

Let us apply these considerations to a physiologic problem: If the volume of gas exhaled during a forced vital capacity maneuver is equal to 2500 mL at 20°C and a barometric pressure of 740 mmHg dry, what is the patient's actual vital capacity at BTPS and the same barometric pressure?

$P_1 = 740$ mmHg $\qquad P_2 = 740$ mmHg

$PH_2O = 0 \qquad PH_2O = 47$ mmHg

$P_{1c} = 740$ mmHg $\qquad P_{2c} = 693$ mmHg

$t_1 = 20°C \qquad t_2 = 37°C$

$T_1 = 20°C + 273 = 293K \qquad T_2 = 37°C + 273 = 310K$

$V_1 = 2500$ mL $\qquad V_2 = —$

Since BTPS is body temperature and pressure saturated, the final pressure P_2 must be corrected for saturation with water vapor at 37°C. The combined gas law is used to solve this problem because all three (P, V, T) variables are altered. Thus

$$\frac{P_{1c}\,V_1}{T_1} = \frac{P_{2c}\,V_2}{T_2}$$

P_{1c} and P_{2c} indicate pressure corrections for water vapor. Rearranging this equation, we can solve for the unknown V_2:

$$V_2 = \frac{(P_{1c})\,(V_1)\,(T_2)}{(T_1)\,(P_{2c})}$$

$$V_2 = \frac{(740 \text{ mmHg})\,(2500 \text{ mL})\,(310K)}{(293K)\,(693 \text{ mmHg})}$$

$$V_2 = 2825 \text{ mL}$$

Humidity

Since water vapor is not an ideal gas and the boiling point of water is much higher (100°C) than atmospheric temperature, the water vapor content of the atmosphere is variable. Temperature and available water for evaporation are the two factors affecting water vapor content.[2] As temperature increases, molecules of water gain kinetic energy and a larger number gain sufficient energy to enter the gaseous state, increasing water vapor content. It should be noted that water vapor exerts a partial pressure, as do other gases, but at the expense of all other gases; that is, if the water vapor pressure is increasing because of increasing temperature, the partial pressure of all other gases in a system will decrease if the system's total pressure is to remain constant.[3] At the point at which water begins to boil, the water vapor pressure over the boiling liquid must equal the atmospheric pressure, thus all other gases will have been eliminated from the system.

Water vapor content is expressed in two ways, as absolute and relative humidity. Absolute humidity is an expression of the actual amount of water vapor present, usually listed as weight of water per unit volume air (e.g., mg/L, g/m^3) or as the partial pressure of water (mmHg). On the other hand, relative humidity (RH) is the relationship between the actual water vapor content and the maximum possible water vapor content at a given temperature:

$$RH = \frac{\text{content}}{\text{capacity}}\,(100) \tag{14}$$

where content is actual water vapor present and capacity is maximum possible water vapor content.

Let us consider a problem: At 37°C the maximum absolute

Table 1-4. Water Vapor Pressure and Content at Various Temperatures

Temp (°C)	PH_2O (mmHg)[a]
20	17.5
21	18.7
22	19.8
23	21.1
24	22.4
25	23.8
26	25.2
27	26.7
28	28.3
29	30.0
30	31.8
31	33.7
32	35.7
33	37.7
34	39.9
35	42.2
36	44.6
37	47.0
38	49.8
39	52.5
40	55.4
41	58.4
42	61.6

[a] Data from Lide.[21]

humidity is 43.8 mg/L. What is the RH at 37°C if the actual water vapor content is 22 mg/L?

$$RH = \frac{\text{content}}{\text{capacity}}$$

$$50.2\% = \frac{22 \text{ mg/L}}{43.8 \text{ mg/L}} (100)$$

Since both actual and maximum water vapor content are affected by temperature (Table 1-4), a change in temperature can affect relative humidity. If, in the above problem, temperature were to decrease, the RH would increase because capacity would decrease. If temperature continued to decrease until capacity fell below actual content, condensation (rain) would form.

Normally, the nose, nasal pharynx, and oral pharynx humidify inspired gas, so that by the time gas reaches the carina, it is 100 percent saturated with water vapor at body temperature. If the upper airway is bypassed (artificial airways), a humidity deficit is established (water vapor leaves the lung as a result of humidification of inspired gas). Under these conditions, supplemental water vapor must be added to inspired gas to prevent this deficit. Water vapor is normally provided by a heated aerosol or heated humidifying system.

Dalton's Law of Partial Pressures

Dalton's law states that the sum of the individual partial pressures of the gases in a mixture is equal to the total pressure of the mixture, the pressure of each gas being proportional to its fractional concentration.[13] Thus

$$P_p = (P_b)\,(\text{conc}) \qquad (15)$$

where P_p is the partial pressure of a gas, P_b is barometric pressure or total system pressure, and conc is the fractional concentration of the gas inspired. For example, if the P_b is 760 mmHg and the inspired oxygen fraction ($F_{I}O_2$) is 0.21, what is the PO_2?

$$PO_2 = (P_b)\,(\text{conc})$$

$$159.6 \text{ mmHg} = (760 \text{ mmHg})\,(0.21)$$

Rearranging Equation 15 allows for the calculation of the concentration of a specific gas in a mixture if the barometric pressure and the partial pressure of the gas are known:

$$\text{conc} = \frac{P_p}{P_b} \qquad (16)$$

Since water vapor concentration is affected by temperature, it does not follow Dalton's law under normal atmospheric conditions. Thus, when determining the partial pressure of a gas containing water vapor, the P_b must be corrected for the water vapor present before the P_p is calculated.

$$P_p = (P_b - PH_2O)\,(\text{conc}) \qquad (17)$$

For example, if the P_b is 750 mmHg, the PH_2O is 40 mmHg, and the $F_{I}O_2$ is 0.5, what is the PO_2?

$$P_p = (P_b - PH_2O)\,(\text{conc})$$

$$350 \text{ mmHg} = (740 \text{ mmHg} - 40 \text{ mmHg})\,(0.5)$$

As noted above, the PO_2 of the atmosphere is 159.6 mmHg (dry). As atmospheric gas enters the lung, it becomes saturated with water vapor; thus, by the time it reaches the carina, PO_2 has decreased to 149.7 mmHg.

$$149.7 \text{ mmHg} = (760 \text{ mmHg} - 47 \text{ mmHg})\,(0.21)$$

PH_2O at 37°C saturated is 47 mmHg. Dalton's law provides the basis for the ideal alveolar gas equation (see Ch. 47).

DIFFUSION

Diffusion is the movement of a substance from a region of high concentration to a region of low concentration. As gases diffuse, they distribute themselves throughout a container as if they occupied the total container. That is, once equilibration has occurred, each gas will occupy the container as if no other gas is present.

Numerous factors affect the rate of diffusion of a gas through another gas and can be best summarized in the following equation[2]:

$$\text{Diffusion rate} = \frac{(\text{pressure})\,(\text{temperature})\,(\text{cross-sectional area})}{(\text{molecular weight})\,(\text{distance})} \qquad (18)$$

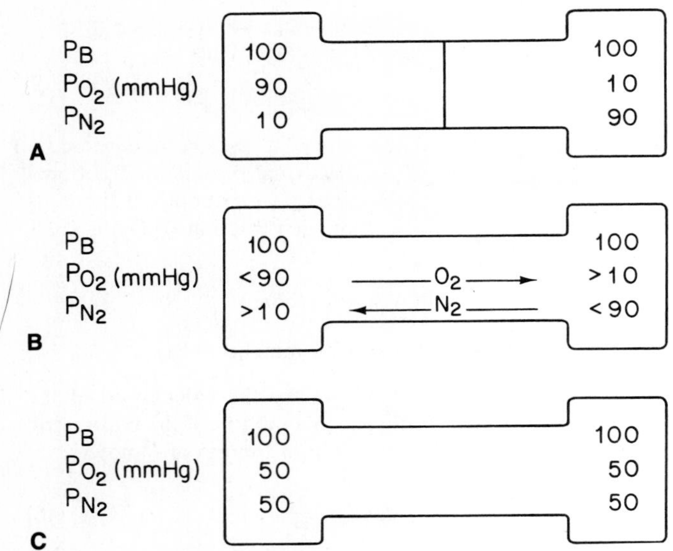

Figure 1-5. Diffusion of two gases. **(A)** The system is separated into two parts in which the P_b is equal but PO_2 and PN_2 differ. **(B)** When the two systems are allowed to communicate, O_2 and nitrogen (N_2) diffuse as a result of partial pressure gradients. **(C)** Diffusion continues until the partial pressures of N_2 and O_2 are equal throughout the system. During this process the P_b in each part of the system is constant.

As the concentration gradient (pressure) increases, the force moving the molecules increases, accelerating the rate of diffusion. In the context of diffusion, the term *pressure gradient* refers to the *partial* pressure differences that drive the diffusion of a specific gas, not to differences in the total system pressure (Fig. 1-5). Total system pressure differences account for convection (i.e., gross gas volume movement), while partial pressure differences account for diffusion. Temperature also relates directly to the kinetic energy of the gas. The cross-sectional area of the container represents the area of communication for the two gases; the greater this area, the greater the diffusion rate. Molecular weight (MW) and distance both indirectly affect rate of diffusion, since large gas molecules diffuse slowly, and the greater the distance the gas must diffuse, the longer the time required for equilibration.

In the lung, convection accounts for gas movement to about the terminal bronchiole level, and diffusion is the primary mechanism for gas movement at the lung parenchymal level.[14] Since temperature, pressure, distance, and molecular weight of gases are constant during normal breathing, the factor most affecting diffusion in the lung is cross-sectional area. Secretions, bronchospasm, and mucosal edema all decrease cross-sectional area, thereby slowing diffusion.

In order for gas to diffuse across the alveolar capillary membrane, it must first dissolve in a liquid, the plasma. Henry's law defines those factors affecting gas solubility. It states that the amount of a gas that can dissolve in a liquid is directly related to the partial pressure of the gas and indirectly related to the temperature of the system.[4] In addition, the amount of gas that can dissolve in a liquid is dependent on the chemical nature of the gas; that is, an ionic or a highly polar compound (e.g., CO_2) dissolves to a greater extent in an ionic solution (plasma) than does a nonpolar molecule (e.g., O_2). As a result, the solubility coefficients for O_2 and CO_2 in plasma at 37°C and 760 mmHg pressure of the respective gases are

O_2: 0.023 mL of O_2/mL of blood

CO_2: 0.510 mL of CO_2/mL of blood

As noted, CO_2 is over 20 times as soluble as O_2 in plasma.

Once dissolved, gases must diffuse through the liquid. Graham's law states that the rate of diffusion of a gas through a liquid is indirectly related to the square root of the gram molecular weight of the gas.[4]

When considering diffusion into and through the alveolar-capillary membrane, both Henry's and Graham's laws must be taken into account. The rate of diffusion of CO_2 compared with O_2 is expressed as follows:

$$\frac{CO_2}{O_2} = \frac{(\text{sol coef } CO_2)\ (\text{GMW } O_2)}{(\text{sol coef } O_2)\ (\text{GMW } CO_2)}$$

$$\frac{CO_2}{O_2} = \frac{(0.510)\ (5.66)}{(0.023)\ (6.66)} \tag{19}$$

$$\frac{CO_2}{O_2} = \frac{19}{1}$$

Equation 19 would seem to indicate that CO_2 would diffuse across the alveolar-capillary membrane 19 times as fast as O_2. This would only be true if all other conditions—specifically, partial pressure gradients—were equal for O_2 and CO_2. However, the gradient is about 6 mmHg for CO_2 and 60 mmHg for O_2 (see Fig. 1-7). As a result, under normal physiologic conditions O_2 equilibrates in about 0.23 seconds and CO_2 in about 0.25 seconds[14] (Table 1-5). However, disruption of the normal processes at the lung parenchymal and alveolar-capillary membrane level usually results primarily in an alteration in the diffusion of O_2 long before CO_2 is affected because of the chemical conditions favoring CO_2 movement.

ELASTANCE AND COMPLIANCE

Most tissue has properties that allow it to be distorted without permanently altering its shape. This characteristic

Table 1-5. Partial Pressure Gradients and Diffusion Times Across the Alveolar-Capillary Membrane

Venous Blood	Alveolus	Gradient	Equilibration Time
46 mmHg	40 mmHg	6 mmHg	0.25 s
40 mmHg	100 mmHg	60 mmHg	0.23 s

is referred to as *elastance* (E), the ability of a distorted object to return to its original shape. The inverse of elastance is *compliance* (C), the ease with which an object can be distorted

$$C = \frac{1}{E} \quad (20)$$

Obviously, a system that readily returns to original shape requires a large force to distort it, whereas one that does not recoil easily requires a minimum distortion force.

Hooke's law defines essential components of elastance/compliance.[15] It states that an elastic body stretches equal units of length or volume for each unit of weight or force applied to it. This relationship holds until the elastic limit of the system is reached (Fig. 1-6). Beyond this limit, each unit of weight or force produces smaller and smaller changes in length or volume. In the case of a true spring, exceeding the elastic limit results in permanent distortion.

Elastance is mathematically expressed as a change in pressure per unit change in volume

$$E = \frac{\Delta P}{V} \quad (21)$$

and compliance is expressed as a change in volume per unit change in pressure:

$$C = \frac{V}{\Delta P} \quad (22)$$

In addition to tissue elasticity, surface tension must be considered when discussing the elastic properties of the total lung-thoracic system and the lung itself.

SURFACE TENSION

The force that exists at the interface between a liquid and a gas or between two liquids, referred to as *surface tension*[4] (Fig. 1-7), develops as a result of like molecules being attracted to each other but not to the molecules of the other substance. Thus, a barrier (interface) is established that requires force to break. Essentially, surface tension causes the molecules of a substance to tend to move away from the interface so as to occupy the smallest volume possible. Surface tension is usually expressed in dynes per centimeter and varies inversely with temperature.[15]

LaPlace's law defines the relationship among surface tension, pressure, and the radii of various structures. Specifically, the pressure (P) in dynes per square centimeter as a

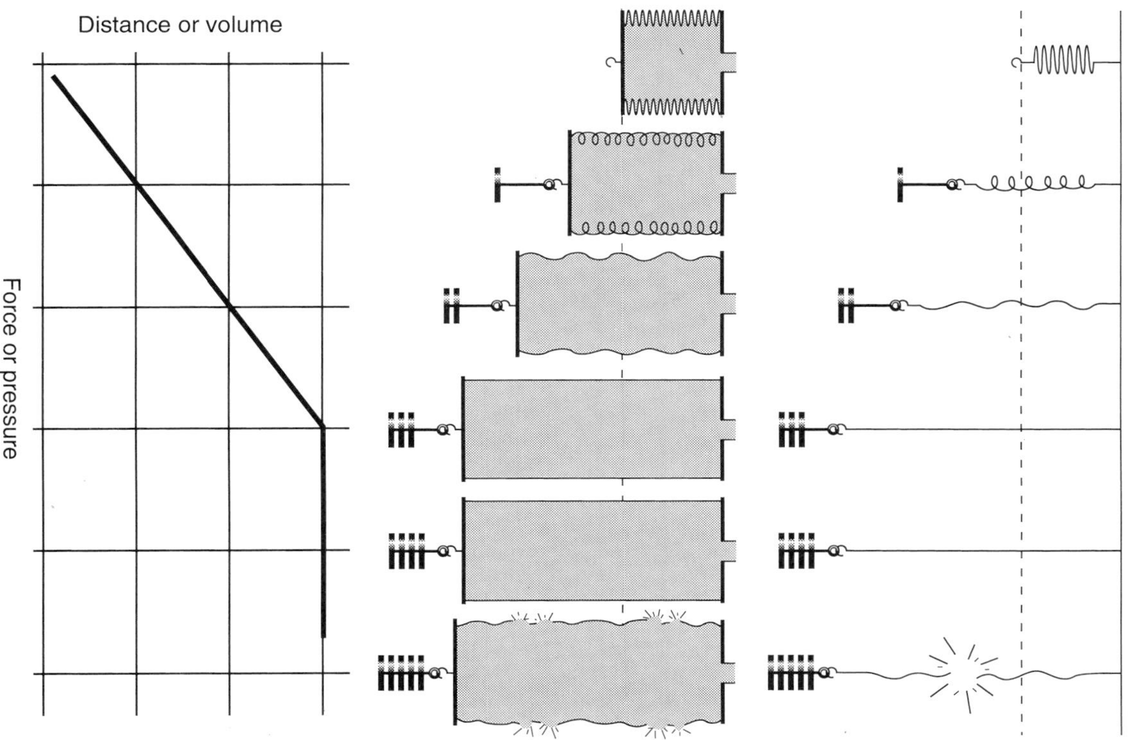

Figure 1-6. Hooke's law applied to a spring and to the lungs. For an elastic structure, the increase in length (or volume) varies directly with the increase in force (or pressure) until the elastic limit is reached. This linear relationship applies equally to normal lungs over the physiologic range. (From Comroe,[19] with permission.)

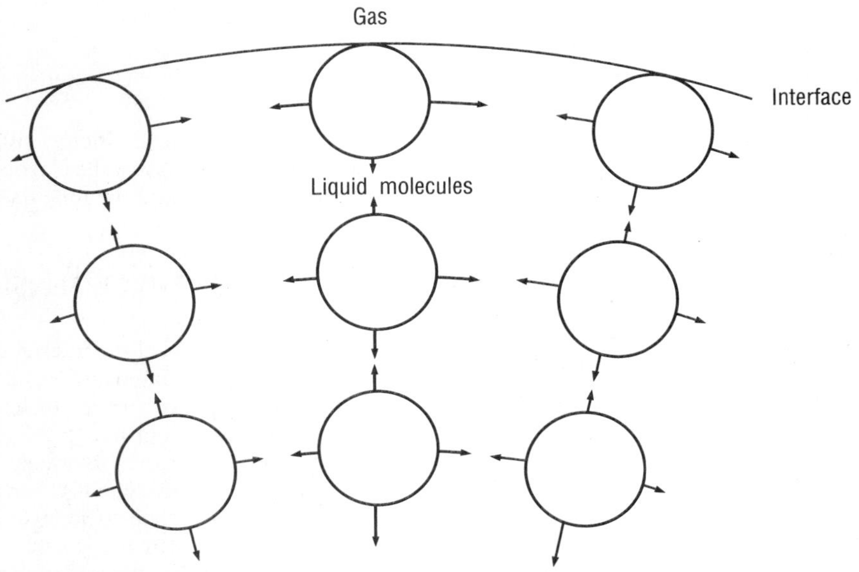

Gas
Interface
Liquid molecules

Figure 1-7. The surface tension in a drop of liquid is shown by the action of the molecules of the liquid, which are mutually attracted to each other (arrows) but can move about randomly in a state of equilibrium. Mass attraction can pull the molecules of the outermost layer inward only, creating a centrally directed force, surface tension, which tends to contract the liquid into a sphere. Thus, the pressure within the drop is raised above atmospheric. (From Spearman et al.,[1] with permission.)

result of surface tension (ST) in dynes per centimeter is equal to the surface tension of the liquid multiplied by the sum of the reciprocals of the radii (r) of curvature in centimeters:

$$P = ST\left(\frac{1}{r_1} + \frac{1}{r_2} + \cdots + \frac{1}{r_n}\right) \qquad (23)$$

When LaPlace's law is applied to a drop we obtain

$$P = \frac{2ST}{r} \qquad (24)$$

Since a drop can be considered a perfect sphere, so that the radii of curvature in the vertical plane and in the horizontal plane are equal, only one radius is considered. If LaPlace's law is applied to a bubble, Equation 24 still applies.

$$P = \frac{4ST}{r} \qquad (25)$$

Here, two interfaces exist, one on the outer and one on the inner surface of the bubble; this corresponds to a total of four radii, but since the bubble film is only angstroms thick, all radii are considered equal (Equation 25). If LaPlace's law is applied to a long cylinder (e.g., a blood vessel), Equation 24 still applies; however, only the cross-sectional radius is considered.

$$P = \frac{ST}{r} \qquad (26)$$

Since the length is so great and its reciprocal so small, length is normally disregarded (Equation 26).

In all the above relationships, it is important to note that the pressure resulting from the surface tension is indirectly related to the radius. That is, the pressure inside a sphere or cylinder due to surface tension is greater the smaller the sphere.[1] Figure 1-8 illustrates this phenomenon. The two bubbles have equal surface tension; however, A has a smaller radius than B. Thus, if the two are allowed to communicate, the gas from A enters B, with A eventually collapsing. This phenomenon can occur in the lung, where small alveoli can empty into large alveoli if the surface tension of smaller alveoli is not modified by a naturally occurring surfactant. Surfactants are chemicals (Fig. 1-9) that interfere with the intermolecular attraction at the interface of the two substances. Essentially, molecules of the surfactant are distributed between molecules of the fluid at the interface, preventing attraction. Soaps and detergents are common surfactants. Surfactants "make water wetter." They allow liquids to exist in smaller unit volumes.

As a structure increases or decreases in volume, it must pass its *critical volume*, below which the effects of surface tension are so great that the structure will collapse. In general, the force required to expand a sphere (bubble) increases as the volume approaches the critical volume and decreases once the system's volume exceeds the critical volume[2] (Fig. 1-10).

FLUID DYNAMICS

Those specific aspects of the dynamics of gas flow that are essential to the function of a clinician are discussed below. First, a distinction must be made between velocity and flow. *Velocity* is the speed of movement between two

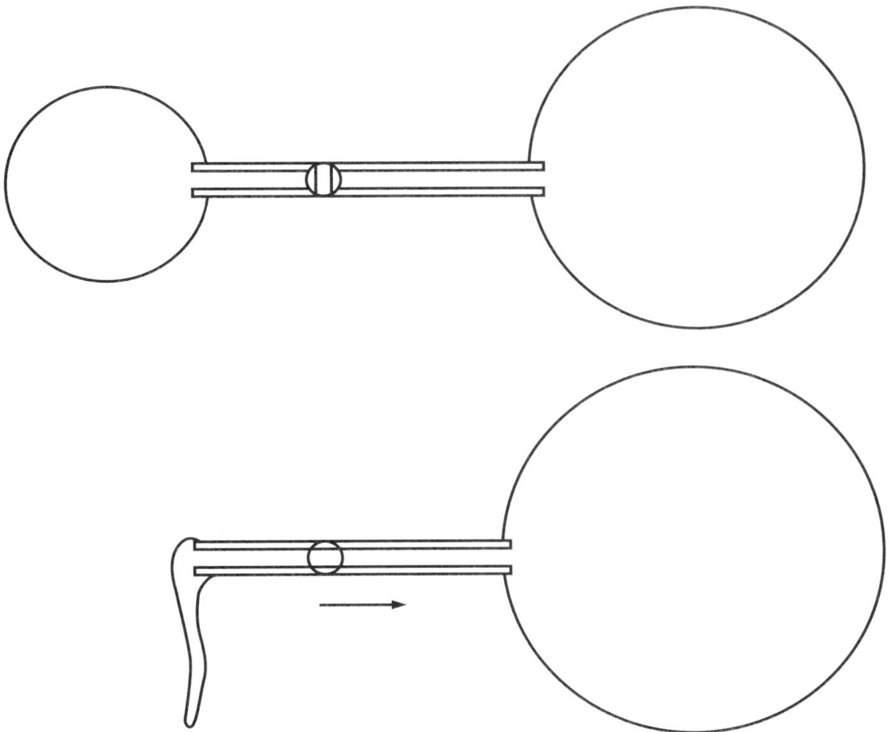

Figure 1-8. When bubbles of different sizes but with the same surface tension, are allowed to communicate, the greater pressure in the smaller bubble causes it to empty into the larger bubble. (From Spearman et al.,[1] with permission.)

points, usually expressed as miles per hour or centimeters per second, while *flow* is the volume of fluid passing a single point per unit time, usually expressed in liters per minute (L/min). The two are related, but may vary directly or indirectly with each other, depending on the system. If the structure of a continuously flowing system is fixed, then flow and velocity are normally directly related.

A general overall relationship that provides the basis for many of the laws to follow is the law of continuity, which states that at a specific flow rate the product of the cross-sectional area of a system and the velocity of gas movement is constant.[16] Figure 1-11 illustrates this relationship; as noted, the velocity at point A and B differ because the cross-sectional area differs. Velocity and cross-sectional area are inversely related. This occurs because the total flow entering a fixed system must also exit it, thus a given volume of gas must move through the narrow sections of the system more rapidly than through the larger sections.

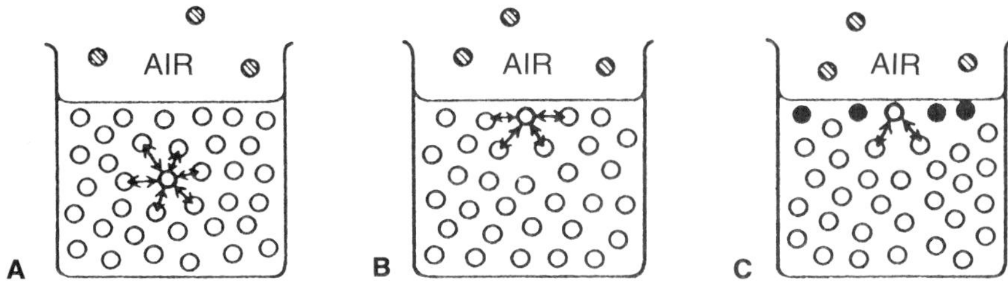

Figure 1-9. (**A**) Intermolecular attraction among molecules in the center of a given volume. (**B**) Intermolecular attraction among molecules at the surface of a liquid, establishing a surface tension. (**C**) Surface-active particles (black circles) interfere with the molecular attraction among molecules at the surface of the liquid. (From Comroe,[15] with permission.)

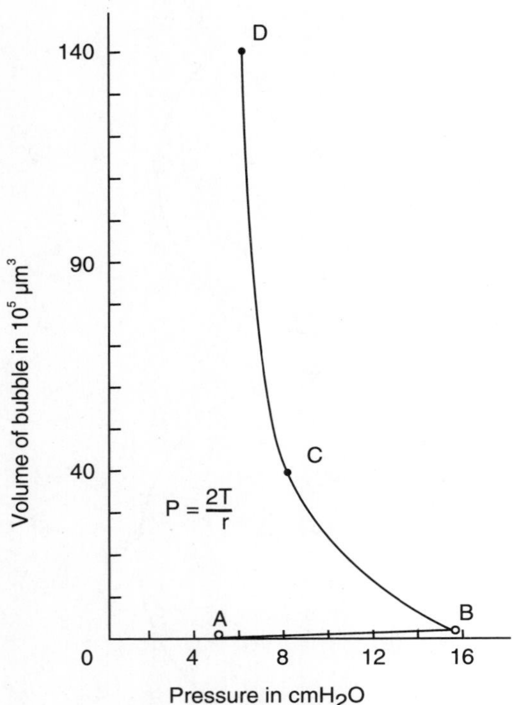

Figure 1-10. Pressure-volume curve of a bubble. Large pressure changes are required to cause a small volume change at volumes below the critical value. Once the critical volume is exceeded, less and less pressure is required to increase the bubble's volume. A, minimal volume providing shape; B, critical volume; C and D, decreased pressure is necessary to maintain a given volume as the radius of the sphere increases. (From Kacmarek et al.,[2] with permission.)

Resistance to Gas Flow

Resistance is essentially the frictional force inhibiting flow through a system and is dependent on the physical structure of the system. Essentially, the smaller the cross-sectional area and the longer the system, the greater the resistance to flow.[17] In mathematical terms, resistance (R) is equal to change in pressure (P) divided by flow ($\dot{V}$):

$$R = \frac{\Delta P}{\dot{V}} \tag{27}$$

That is, for a particular system the flow and the pressure gradient across the system are directly related—the greater

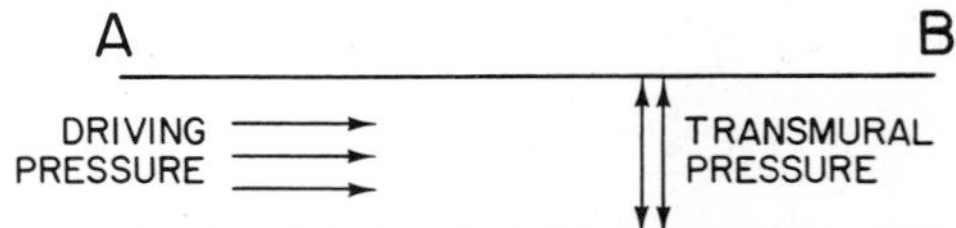

Figure 1-12. Driving pressure, the force necessary to maintain flow, is the difference in pressure across a system: pressure at A − pressure at B. Transmural pressure is the force exerted on the lateral wall of a system. In a given system actual transmural pressure may vary, depending on the structure of the system, even though the driving pressure is constant.

the flow, the greater the pressure gradient necessary. When evaluating the pressure gradient, it is important to remember that the driving pressure is involved, not the transmural pressure (i.e., the pressure against the lateral wall of the system) (Fig. 1-12). In a continuous flow system, driving pressure (P) must increase as flow increases, but transmural pressure may change in any direction, depending on the system structure and the point of measurement (see the Bernoulli effect, discussed below).

In the respiratory system resistance to flow is greatest in the upper airways and actually diminishes as gas proceeds deeper into the respiratory tract as a result of the continually increasing cross-sectional area of the tracheobronchial tree.[14,16] However, any factor that decreases the lumen of a particular airway increases the resistance to gas flow across the airway (e.g., partial airway obstruction by foreign bodies, secretions, mucosal edema, and bronchospasm).

Conductance is the inverse of resistance and is the capability of a system to maintain flow. That is, a system with high resistance has low conductance. Mathematically, conductance is equal to flow divided by change in pressure.

$$\text{Conductance} = \frac{\dot{V}}{\Delta P} \tag{28}$$

Resistance is expressed in either centimeters of water per liter per minute or centimeters of water per liter per second, whereas conductance is given in liters per minute per centimeter of water or liters per second per centimeter of water.

Types of Flow

Essentially, gas flow is of two types, laminar and turbulent (Fig. 1-13). Laminar flow is smooth, even, and nontumbling, proceeding with a conical front. That is, the molecules at

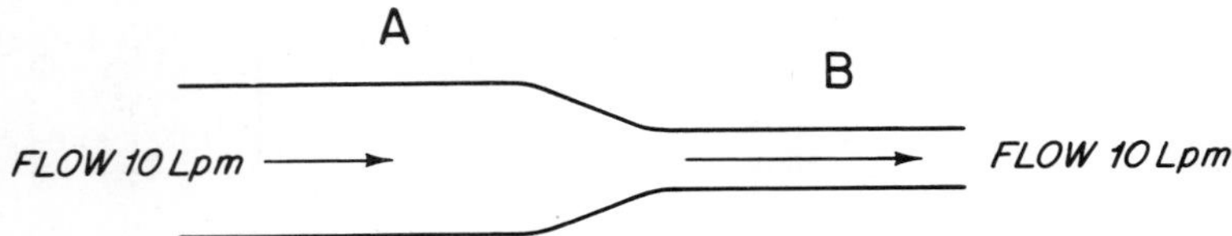

Figure 1-11. Representation of the law of continuity. Since the cross-sectional area A is greater than B and the flow is constant, the velocity at B must be greater than the velocity at A. However, the product of velocity and cross-sectional area is constant at both A and B.

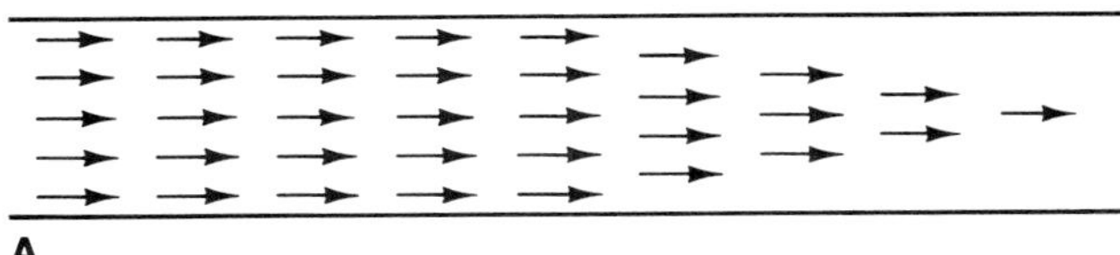

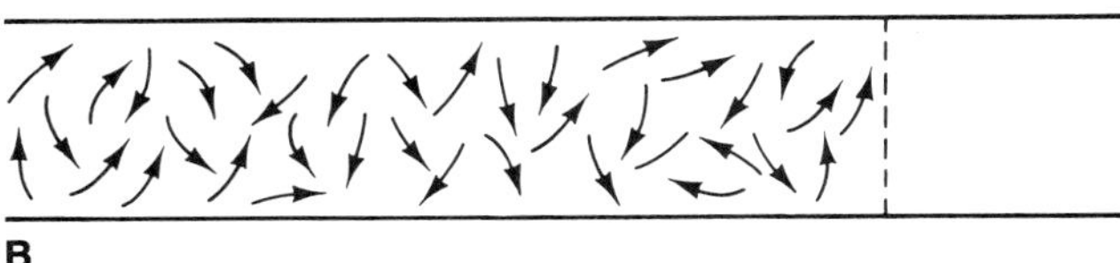

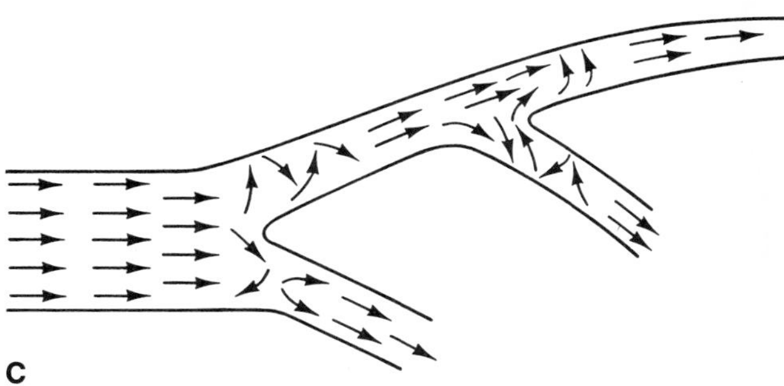

Figure 1-13. **(A)** In laminar flow, movement is smooth, there is no tumbling of gas molecules, and all molecules proceed in a direct path. Resistance is indirectly related to flow rate. **(B)** In turbulent flow, movement is rough and tumbling, with no direct path followed by any molecules. Resistance is indirectly related to flow rate squared. **(C)** In tracheobronchial flow, a combination of laminar and turbulent flow, flow becomes turbulent at bifurcations or points where direction changes.

the center of the gas stream move with greater velocity than those at the periphery, and only those at the periphery experience the resistance drag of the system. In this situation R is equal to $\Delta P/\dot{V}$.

Turbulent flow exhibits a rough, tumbling pattern that proceeds with a blunt front. All molecules proceed at the same velocity and all encounter the sides of the system. As a result, the effects of resistance to flow are increased. In fact, during turbulent flow resistance is related to $\dot{V}^2$.

$$R = \frac{\Delta P}{\dot{V}^2} \quad (29)$$

Thus, a much larger pressure gradient is required to maintain turbulent than laminar flow.

For example, if system resistance is 10 $cmH_2O/L/min$, we may calculate the pressure gradient necessary to maintain 10 L/min flow in a laminar and in a turbulent manner.

For laminar flow

$$R = \frac{\Delta P}{\dot{V}}$$

$$10\ cmH_2O/L/min = \frac{x}{10\ L/min}$$

$$x = 100\ cmH_2O$$

For turbulent flow

$$R = \frac{\Delta P}{\dot{V}^2}$$

$$10\ cmH_2O/L/min = \frac{x}{10^2\ L/min}$$

$$x = 1000\ cmH_2O$$

Tracheobronchial (transitional) flow, the type of flow occurring in the larger airways of the respiratory tract because of the branching and continually decreasing lumen, involves both laminar and turbulent flow. At points where branching or a change in lumen diameter occurs, flow is turbulent; however, in straight sections of the airway, flow is laminar.

The type of flow occurring in a system can be predicted by the Reynolds number (Re). This is a dimensionless number based on the diameter of the system, the velocity of gas flow, and the density and viscosity of the flowing gas:

$$Re = \frac{(\text{diameter})\ (\text{velocity})\ (\text{density})}{\text{viscosity}} \quad (30)$$

An Re of 2000 or greater indicates that turbulent flow is present, while a value less than 2000 indicates laminar flow.[16]

Theoretically, the Re takes into consideration the tendency of a fluid to tumble as it flows. Less dense but more viscous gases (helium [He]) have less tendency to flow in a turbulent manner, all other factors being equal. The least obviously apparent factor in the relationship is diameter. Normally, the smaller the diameter, the greater the velocity of gas flow. However, small diameters favor laminar flow, while high velocity favors turbulent flow. Turbulent flow is more likely to occur in large diameter systems because there is more room for gas molecules to tumble over each other, whereas in narrow systems gas is more likely to follow a direct path. Viscosity (discussed later) is based on the adhesive forces holding molecules of a fluid together. As a result the more viscous a fluid, the greater the tendency to maintain a given path when flowing. This phenomenon is best illustrated by comparing water with syrup. Syrup is much more viscous than water and it is almost impossible to force it to flow in a turbulent manner.

Bernoulli Effect

The Bernoulli effect is an extension of the law of continuity. Essentially, it states that as a gas moves through a continuous flow system, the transmural pressure is inversely related to the velocity of the gas. That is, as the velocity increases, the transmural pressure decreases (Fig. 1-14); this occurs under conditions of a constant driving pressure and flow.[1,2] The Bernoulli effect is explained by the law of conservation of energy, which states that energy can be neither

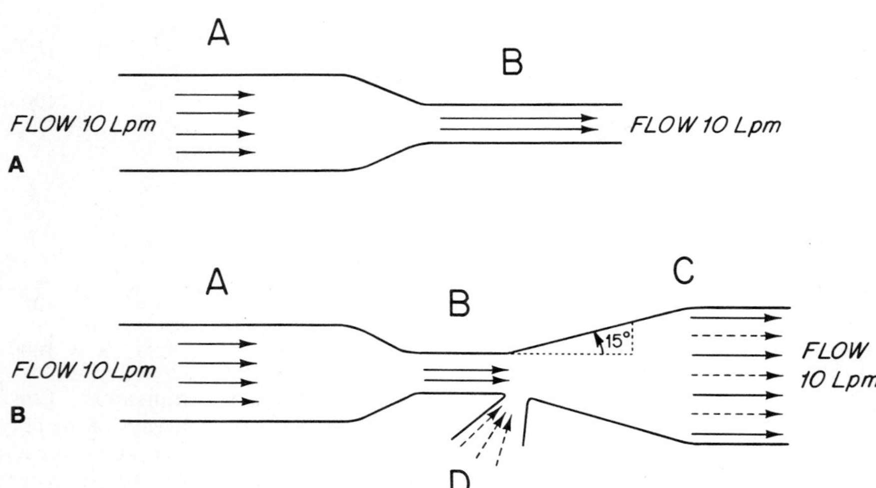

Figure 1-14. **(A)** The Bernoulli effect. The velocity at B is greater than at A, while the transmural pressure is greater at A than at B as a result of the law of conservation of energy. **(B)** The Venturi effect. At B the transmural pressure is subatmospheric because of the increased kinetic energy. A second gas is entrained at D. If the angle of divergence distal to the stenosis is not greater than 15 degrees, the transmural pressures at C and A are equal (see text for details).

created nor destroyed—it simply changes form. Basically, in a continuous flow, non-gravity-dependent gas system, energy exists in two forms, kinetic energy and transmural pressure energy. The latter can be expressed as an active force against the lateral wall (P_{trans}), while kinetic energy (KE) is given by

$$KE = 0.5\ (D)\ (Vel)^2 \quad (31)$$

where D is density and Vel is velocity. Thus, the total energy at any point in a continuous flow system is

$$\text{Total energy} = 0.5\ (D)\ (Vel)^2 + P_{trans} \quad (32)$$

As gas moves through a system with a decreasing diameter, the velocity of the gas must increase, and as a result the transmural pressure must decrease (Equation 30). However, if the original diameter is then restored, velocity and transmural pressure return to their original levels. The extent to which velocity and transmural pressure change is affected by density. The less dense the gas, the less alteration in transmural pressure for a given change in velocity as the gas moves through a constriction (stenosis).

The *Venturi principle* is a modification of the Bernoulli effect to allow for entrainment of a second fluid. If the lumen of any tube is decreased beyond a specific level and a constant flow of gas is maintained, the transmural pressure at the narrowest point becomes subatmospheric. This occurs because the kinetic energy of the system is markedly increased by the high velocity required to pass the constriction, as shown by Equation 30. The Venturi principle further indicates that if the angle of divergence of the system distal to the constriction does not exceed 15 degrees, the transmural pressure existing proximal to it can be restored.[1] The cross-sectional area of the system must also be increased to accommodate the second fluid entrained as a result of the subatmospheric transmural pressure.

Venturi systems can be designed to entrain a second gas or liquid and create an aerosol. If a second gas is entrained to establish a specific F_IO_2 (source gas O_2, entrained gas air) the volume entrained per liter of source gas is dependent on the extent of stenosis at the point of entrainment or the size of the entrainment port. The smaller the stenosis or the larger the entrainment port, the greater the volume of secondary gas entrained (Table 1-6).

Back pressure at the output port of a Venturi system decreases the level of entrainment by decreasing the flow and velocity of the source gas, thus increasing the transmural pressure. If a Venturi system is used to establish an F_IO_2, back pressure results in an increase in the delivered F_IO_2.

Table 1-6. Entrainment Ratios in Venturi and Jet Mixing Systems

F_IO_2	Entrainment Ratio	Source Gas Flow[a]	Entrained Gas[a]	Total Flow[a]
0.24	1:25	4	100	100
0.28	1:10	4	40	44
0.31	1:7	6	42	48
0.35	1:5	8	40	48
0.40	1:3	12	36	48
0.50	1:1.7	12	20.4	32.4
0.60	1:1	12	12	24
0.70	1:0.6	12	7.2	19.2

[a] All flows in liters per minute.

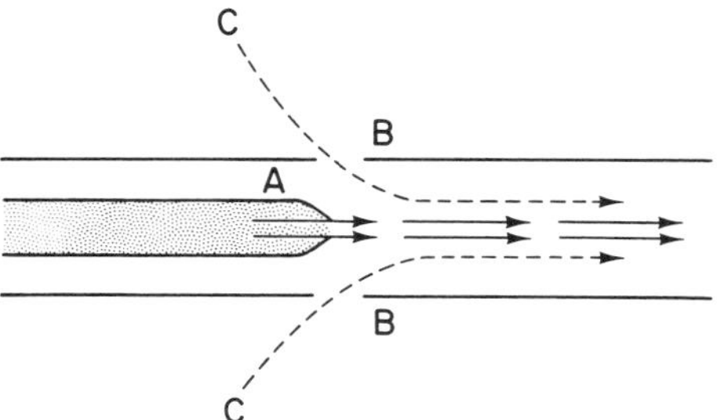

Figure 1-15. Jet mixing results from the shearing force of a rapid flow of gas A on a relatively stationary gas C. The velocity of the stationary gas is thus increased, resulting in gas entrainment at point B.

Jet Mixing

A variation of the Venturi entrainment phenomenon is jet mixing (Fig. 1-15), in which a constant flow of gas from a small orifice jet is used to entrain a second gas.[18] In this situation no pressure gradient is established between the jet flow and the ambient environment. Entrainment is a result of the viscous shearing force developed between a dynamic and a stationary fluid, resulting in a decrease in the velocity of the dynamic fluid and an increase in that of the stationary fluid. A similar phenomenon is noted when standing near a speeding train. As the train passes, the shearing force created increases the velocity of air near the train, drawing the adjacent air mass to the train. Like Venturi systems, jet mixing systems entrain a second gas at a specific ratio of source gas to entrained gas (Table 1-5). In addition, back pressure reduces the entrainment ratio, resulting in a higher F_{IO_2}. Most air entrainment and aerosol generating systems used in respiratory care actually use jet mixing and are not true Venturi devices.[18]

Poiseuille's Law

The viscosity of a fluid, or its ability to resist deformity, is defined by Poiseuille's law.[14] In general, the viscosity of liquids decreases with increasing temperature but that of gases increases with increasing temperature. Specifically, Poiseuille's law states that the viscosity (μ) of a fluid is equal to the product of the pressure change (ΔP) across a cylinder of specific length (l), π, and the radius of the cylinder to the fourth power (r^4), divided by 8 l times the flow ($\dot{V}$) established.

$$\mu = \frac{(\Delta P)\ (\pi)\ (r^4)}{(8\ l)\ (\dot{V})} \qquad (33)$$

If Poiseuille's law is rearranged so that all variables that remain constant for gas flow through a given system occur on one side of the equation, the following results:

$$\frac{(\mu)\ (8\ l)}{\pi} = \frac{(\Delta P)\ (r^4)}{\dot{V}} \qquad (34)$$

The right side of Equation 32 identifies the relationship between pressure, flow, and the radius of a gas flow system. If the radius is decreased by half, the resistance to gas flow increases 16-fold, so that to maintain a given flow would require pressure to increase 16-fold.

Although Poiseuille's law can only be properly applied to continuous, nonpulsatile, laminar, flow of a homogeneous fluid through a single cylinder, it does define relationships that help to predict behavior in the clinical setting and demonstrates the effect of change in radius on resistance, pressure, and flow.

WORK

Classically, *work* (W) is defined as force (F) times distance (d).

$$W = (F)\ (d) \qquad (35)$$

From a pulmonary perspective, force can be replaced by pressure and distance by volume. Thus, the clinician can look at work of breathing (WOB) as pressure times volume.

$$WOB = PV \qquad (36)$$

It is important to realize that work does not necessarily represent the actual effort, since no work is done unless movement occurs, regardless of effort. In spite of this, work of breathing has become the primary approach used to express patient effort.

Work of breathing is expressed in units of joules per liter or kilogram-meters per liter (1 j is equal to 10 kg-m). Work per unit time is referred to as *power* and expressed in units of joules per minute or kilogram-meters per minute. The actual measurement of pulmonary work is discussed in Chapter 52.

References

1. Spearman CB, Sheldon RL, Egan DF: Egan's Fundamentals of Respiratory Therapy. 4th Ed. CV Mosby, St. Louis, 1982
2. Kacmarek RM, Mack C, Dimas S: Essentials of Respiratory Care. 3rd Ed. Year Book Medical Publishers, Chicago, 1990
3. Brooks S: Integrated Basic Sciences. 4th Ed. CV Mosby, St. Louis, 1979
4. Wojciechowski WV: Respiratory Care Sciences. John Wiley & Sons, New York, 1985
5. Filley G: Acid-Base and Blood Gas Regulations. Lea & Febiger, Philadelphia, 1971
6. Shapiro BR, Harrison RA, Walton JR: Clinical Application of Arterial Blood Gases. 3rd Ed. Year Book Medical Publishers, Chicago, 1982
7. Cohen JJ, Kassirer JP: Acid/Base. Little Brown, Boston, 1982
8. Guyton A: Basic Human Physiology: Normal Function and

Mechanisms of Disease. 2nd Ed. WB Saunders, Philadelphia, 1977
9. Smith J, Kampine J: Circulatory Physiology. The Essentials. Williams & Wilkins, Baltimore, 1980
10. Little RC, Little WC: Physiology of the Heart and Circulation. Year Book Medical Publishers, Chicago, 1989
11. Ruppel G: Manual of Pulmonary Function Testing. 4th Ed. CV Mosby, St. Louis, 1987
12. Cherniack RN: Pulmonary Function Testing. WB Saunders, Philadelphia, 1977
13. Davenport HW: The ABC's of Acid-Base Chemistry. 7th Ed. University of Chicago Press, 1977
14. West JB: Respiratory Physiology—The Essentials. 4th Ed. Williams & Wilkins, Baltimore, 1990
15. Comroe JH Jr: Physiology of Respiration. 2nd Ed. Year Book Medical Publishers, Chicago, 1974
16. Murray JF: The Normal Lung, 2nd Ed. WB Saunders, Philadelphia, 1984
17. Foster RE, Dubois AB, Briscoe WA, Fisher AB: The Lung: Physiologic Basis of Pulmonary Function Tests. 3rd Ed. Year Book Medical Publishers, Chicago, 1986
18. Scacci R: Air entrainment masks: Jet mixing is how they work; the Bernoulli and Venturi principles is how they don't. Respir Care 1979;24:928–934
19. Comroe JH Jr: The Lung. 2nd Ed. Year Book Medical Publishers, Chicago, 1962
20. Dittmer DS, Greve RM (eds): Handbook of Respiration. WB Saunders, Philadelphia, 1958
21. Lide DR (ed): Handbook of Chemistry and Physics. 71st Ed. Chemical Rubber Publishing Co., Boca Raton, FL, 1990

Chapter 2

Overview of Respiratory Processes and Needs

David J. Pierson

CHAPTER OUTLINE

DEFINITIONS OF RESPIRATION

Respiratory care, as presented in this book, is an extension of physiology. Instead of a collection of empirically derived maneuvers to be learned by rote, clinical practice ought to be a logical system based naturally on an understanding of how the cardiorespiratory system works and how disease causes it to malfunction. To help lay a foundation for that system, this chapter presents an overview of what respiration is and what the basic functions of the respiratory system are.

A definition of respiration can be either coarse or fine. On the "macro" scale it is simply the act of breathing: "In with the good air and out with the bad air." To make sense physiologically, however, more than this is needed. The two primary elements are provision of sufficient quantities of O_2 and adequate removal of CO_2 from the lungs and hence from all the body's respiring tissues. Webster's dictionary offers a good, physiologically based definition[1]:

> Respiration: the physical and chemical processes by which an organism supplies its cells and tissues with the oxygen needed for metabolism and relieves them of the carbon dioxide formed in energy-producing reactions.

Although the human respiratory apparatus has several additional purposes, its primary ones, and the primary components of the respiratory process, are ventilation of the alveoli, oxygenation of the blood, and delivery of O_2 to the respiring tissues of the body. Each of these components in turn has two elements: alveolar ventilation serves both to remove CO_2 and to deliver O_2 to the gas exchange surface; blood oxygenation involves both the partial pressure of O_2 in the arterial system (PaO_2) and arterial O_2 content (CaO_2); and provision of O_2 to the tissues requires both its delivery to them and their subsequent use of this basic respiratory fuel (Table 2-1). Much of respiratory care is devoted to the assessment and manipulation of these elements.

OXYGEN AND THE "RESPIRATORY ENGINE"

Respiration may be thought of as the running of an engine. Fuel for the engine consists of sugars, formed out of more

Table 2-1. Basic Components of Respiration

Alveolar ventilation	
CO_2 removal:	Physical movement of CO_2 from the alveoli, which it has reached by diffusion from venous blood in the pulmonary capillaries, to the atmosphere via the conducting airways
Alveolar oxygenation:	Physical movement of inspired O_2 into the alveoli, from which it can diffuse across the alveolar-capillary membrane into the blood
Blood oxygenation	
Arterial O_2 tension:	Pressure exerted by the O_2 present in blood after it leaves the lungs (expressed in mmHg, torr, or kilopascals [kPa])
Arterial O_2 content:	Actual amount of O_2 present, in mL/dL of blood, after leaving the lungs but before any O_2 is consumed by the body
Tissue oxygenation	
O_2 transport:	Physical movement of the O_2 contained in arterial blood to the tissues, where it can be used (expressed in mL/min)
Tissue O_2 utilization:	Intracellular uptake and metabolic consumption of O_2 by a specific tissue bed or by the entire body (expressed in mL/min)

complex carbohydrates broken down by intracellular "mini-engines," the mitochondria, into their component parts. The sugars are in turn broken down into CO_2 and H^+ ions. The latter are then "burned" by the mini-engines along with molecules of O_2, to produce energy in the form of high-energy phosphate compounds such as adenosine triphosphate (ATP), with water as a by-product. The energy in ATP is the primary output of the respiratory engine, and it enables the cell—and hence the body—to carry out all its other functions.

Operation of this respiratory engine depends ultimately on the sun, since it is solar energy that enables green plants to produce the O_2 required. This grand "sun-to-mitochondrion" cycle is shown schematically in Figure 2-1.[2] Plants use the sun's energy to produce O_2 by means of photosynthesis, and also to make fruit and other plant-derived foods. We eat the fruit, which provides the carbohydrates to be broken down into simple sugars and then into H_2O and H^+ ions; we breathe in O_2, which combines with the H^+ ions and releases energy (ATP) to operate the machinery of the body. We excrete the waste products of this operation, CO_2 and H_2O, which ultimately return to the plants as fuel for the manufacture of more O_2 and more fruit.

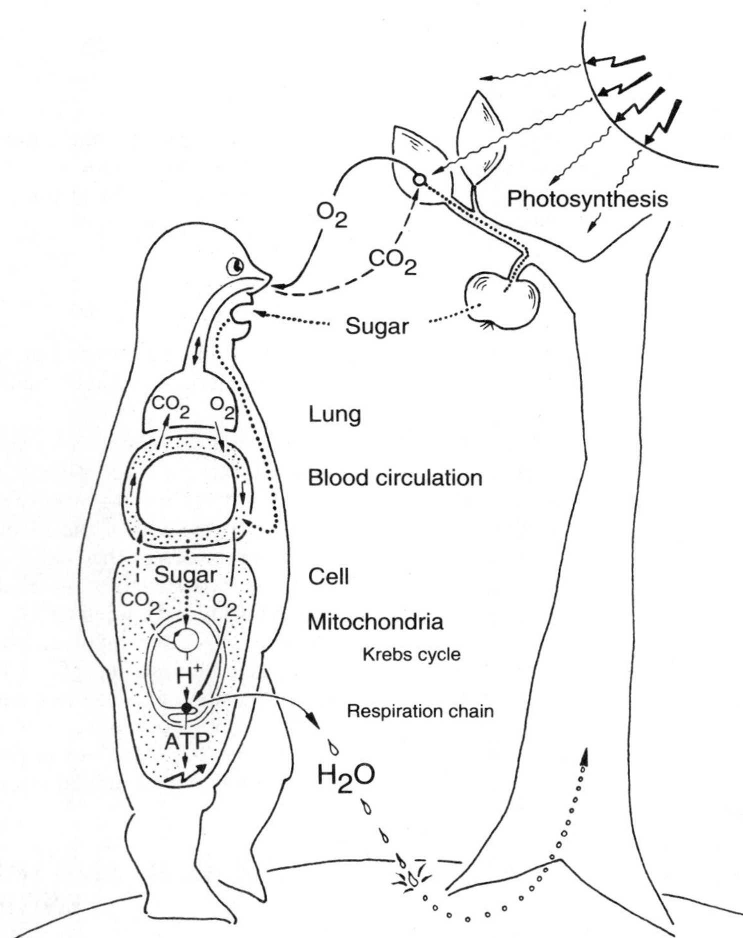

Figure 2-1. How the body's "respiratory engine" is fueled by O_2 and sugars from the foods we eat; its source is ultimately the sun's energy. (From Weibel,[2] with permission.)

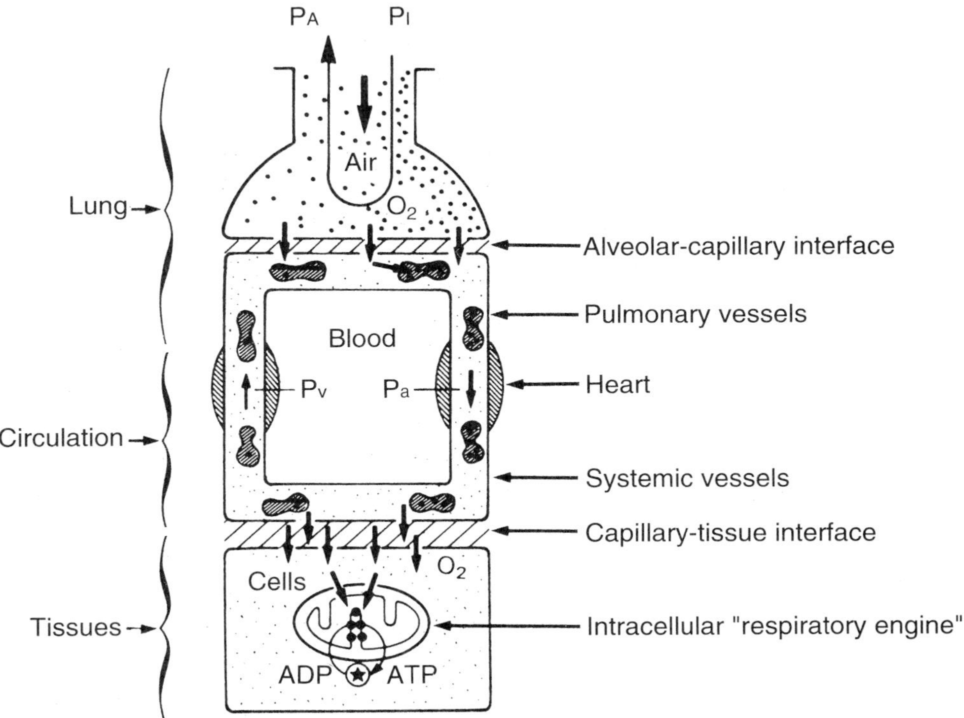

Figure 2-2. The pathway for O_2, from outside air to ultimate consumption within the mitochondria of cells. PA, alveolar O_2 tension; PI, inspired (e.g., room air) O_2 tension; Pa, arterial O_2 tension; Pv, venous O_2 tension; ADP, adenosine diphosphate; ATP, adenosine triphosphate. (Adapted from Taylor and Weibel,[4] with permission.)

All animals are faced with the same basic challenge for respiration: to get enough O_2 into their tissues and to remove the CO_2 produced when this O_2 is used. Because CO_2 diffuses into and out of tissues more readily than does O_2, in most instances providing an adequate O_2 supply is the primary task.

There are several basic adaptations, or strategies, for increasing access of an organism's tissues to O_2.[3] These include increasing the total surface area of the body exposed to O_2, renewing the respiratory medium (e.g., air) by causing it to flow over or through parts of the body, and more effectively moving the O_2 extracted from the medium to the body's tissues. Means for more effective delivery of O_2 to the tissues include physically carrying it from gas-exchange surface to tissues and increasing the quantity that can be carried in a given volume of blood; in humans these objectives are met by the circulatory system (see Ch. 8) and by the O_2-carrying function of hemoglobin (see Ch. 11).

Figure 2-2 shows the path of O_2 in humans from the outside air to the mitochondria, site of the "respiratory engine."[4] Oxygen at ambient pressure (inspired PO_2 or PIO_2) is drawn into the alveoli. Water vapor is added, somewhat reducing the PIO_2 to the level present in the alveoli (PAO_2). The O_2 then diffuses across the alveolar-capillary membrane into hemoglobin contained in red blood cells and is transported via arteries and systemic capillaries to the tissues. Moving down the O_2 pressure gradient from capillary to tissue and then intracellularly into the mitochondria, the O_2 is used to convert adenosine diphosphate (ADP) into the higher-energy ATP. Deoxygenated hemoglobin returns via the venous system to the lungs, where more O_2 is added and the process is repeated.

RESPIRATORY ADAPTATIONS IN OTHER SPECIES

A detailed discussion of the evolution of breathing mechanisms in nonhuman animals is beyond the scope of this book. However, the clinician who sees beauty in the human respiratory system's design and efficiency cannot help being intrigued by the different but no less elegant means by which other creatures meet the same basic needs. Maintaining access to O_2, and to a lesser extent ridding the tissues of CO_2, are challenges every organism has had to meet, whatever its size, diet, habits, or environment. Figure 2-3 diagrams the eight fundamental approaches taken by animals to meet these challenges, and Table 2-2 gives a brief description of each, along with some familiar examples of creatures that use them. Several reviews,[5] books on comparative respiratory physiology,[6–10] and a chapter in a major respiratory

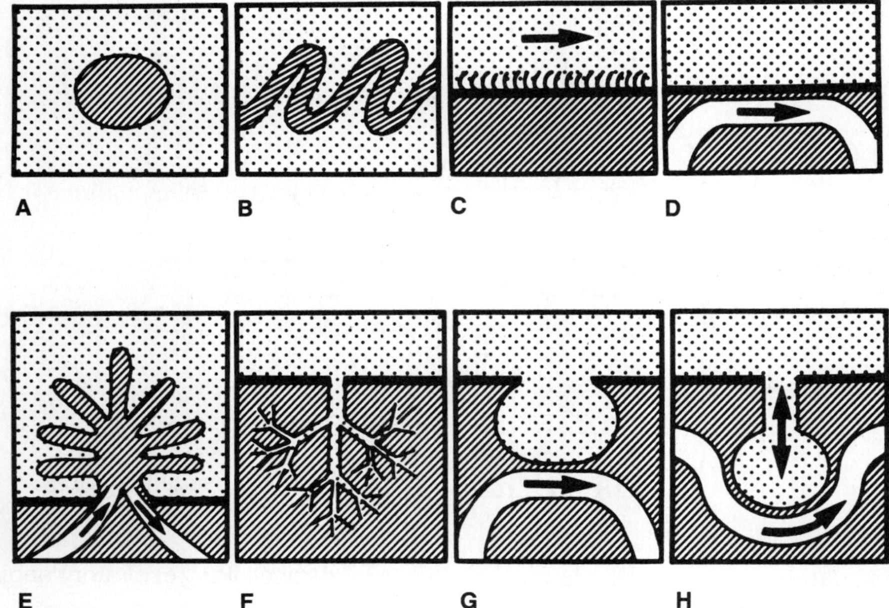

Figure 2-3. Basic types of respiratory apparatus in animals: **(A & B)** diffusion alone; **(C)** diffusion plus convection; **(D)** diffusion plus perfusion; **(E)** gill; **(F)** tracheal system of insects; **(G)** lung (unventilated); **(H)** lung (ventilated). For further explanation see Table 2-2. Hatched area represents body tissues of organism; heavy solid line represents its integument or skin; stippled area represents the respiratory medium, whether water (in Figs. A–C, E, and sometimes H) or air (in Figs. D, F, G, and H). Arrows indicate the direction of flowing respiratory medium or blood within vessels. (Modified from Pierson,[3] with permission.)

Table 2-2. Basic Types of Respiratory Mechanism in Animals

Breathing Mechanism	Strategy	Respiratory Medium	Examples
Diffusion only	Small size (<1 mm); no structural modifications	Water	Protozoans
	Large body surface area but body thickness <1 mm	Water	Flatworms
Diffusion plus convection	Short diffusion path plus renewal of medium by ciliary beating	Water	Sponges; corals
Diffusion plus perfusion	Extensive capillary flow to skin, with circulation to deeper tissues	Air	Earthworms
Gill	Evagination of high-surface area, vascular tissue out of body into medium (''lung turned inside out'')	Water (air)	Mollusks; crustaceans; fishes; tadpoles
Trachea	Many branching air-filled tubes (capillaries) with diffusion from outside medium directly into respiring tissues	Air	Insects
Lung (unventilated)	Invagination of vascular tissue into body	Air	Land snails; slugs; spiders
Lung (ventilated)	Invagination of vascular tissue into body, plus tidal renewal of medium	Water Air	Sea cucumbers; amphibians; reptiles; birds; mammals

(Modified from Pierson,[3] with permission.)

Table 2-3. Determinants and Assessment of the Basic Components of Respiration

Main Function	Physiologic Components	Physiologic Determinants[a]	Clinical Assessment[a]
Alveolar ventilation	CO_2 removal	Load (how much CO_2 is produced: $\dot{V}CO_2$) Efficiency (dead space ventilation: V_D/V_T)	$PaCO_2$
	Alveolar oxygenation	Alveolar gas equation	$PaCO_2$; $P(A\text{-}a)O_2$
Blood oxygenation	Arterial O_2 tension	P_IO_2; $\dot{V}_A$; matching of $\dot{V}_A$ and $\dot{Q}$; R→L shunt; (diffusion limitation)	PaO_2
	Arterial O_2 content	SaO_2; quantity and function of available hemoglobin; PaO_2	SaO_2; Hb; (PaO_2)
Tissue oxygenation	O_2 transport	CaO_2; cardiac output	CaO_2; $\dot{Q}_T$
	Tissue O_2 utilization	Delivery of O_2 to tissues; ability of tissues to use available O_2	$\dot{V}O_2$

$PaCO_2$, partial pressure of CO_2 in arterial blood; $\dot{V}CO_2$, CO_2 production; V_D/V_T, dead space/tidal volume ratio; $P(A\text{-}a)O_2$, alveolar-arterial O_2 partial pressure difference; P_IO_2, partial pressure of inspired O_2; $\dot{V}_A$, alveolar ventilation; PaO_2, partial pressure of O_2 in arterial blood; $\dot{Q}$, blood flow (perfusion); SaO_2, oxyhemoglobin saturation in arterial blood; Hb, hemoglobin concentration; CaO_2, arterial O_2 content; $\dot{Q}_T$, cardiac output; $\dot{V}O_2$, O_2 consumption.

[a] Concepts, measurement, and applications of these are developed in subsequent chapters in Sections I, II, and III of this book.

medicine text,[11] plus an excellent volume on animal physiology in general,[12] are available for readers who would like to explore this subject further.

BASIC DETERMINANTS AND ASSESSMENT OF HUMAN RESPIRATION

For mammals in general and humans in particular, the three primary respiratory components described earlier—alveolar ventilation, oxygenation of the blood, and tissue oxygenation—take place as defined in Table 2-1. Table 2-3 elaborates on these components for purposes of respiratory care by expressing them in clinical terms. In later chapters much attention will be paid to the physiologic determinants of each of the six components listed, as well as to the ways they become deranged by disease and the means clinicians have for assessing them.

A generation ago, clinicians managing critically ill patients focused their attention primarily on PO_2 and PCO_2, assuming that these measurements alone adequately gauged the function of the respiratory system and hence the patient's condition. In part this was because PaO_2 and $PaCO_2$ measurements were easy to obtain, but there also tended to be incomplete appreciation of the importance of *tissue* oxygenation as opposed to oxygenation measurable in the blood. Respiratory care today integrates all the components shown in Table 2-3 and can assess directly how well the needs of each are being met.

Table 2-4. Major Functions of the Respiratory System

Function	Importance	Main Chapters in Which Discussed
Oxygenation	Provision of adequate O_2 to tissues to maintain metabolic needs	10, 11
Ventilation	Provision of O_2 to gas exchange surface of lung; removal of CO_2 as waste product of body's metabolism; acid-base regulation	9, 10, 12, 13
Lung inflation	Maintenance of adequate expansion of lung tissue to prevent atelectasis, ensure normal gas exchange, and maintain cellular and metabolic function	5, 9, 18
Maintenance of airway patency	Maintenance of adequate ventilation; clearance of secretions and foreign bodies; prevention of atelectasis; avoidance of and response to infection	4, 7, 9
Prevention against the environment	Filtering and humidification of inspired air; cellular and humoral immunity; avoidance of and response to infection	17
Metabolic functions	Synthesis, activation, transformation, and/or degradation of vasoactive substances, hormones, and other molecules; maintenance of lung inflation through surfactant production; uptake and metabolism of drugs	18, 20

ADDITIONAL FUNCTIONS OF THE RESPIRATORY SYSTEM

While primary attention is often rightly focused on respiration per se, as detailed in Tables 2-1 and 2-3, the human respiratory system has several other basic functions of major concern in respiratory care. These include maintaining adequate lung inflation, keeping the main airways patent, protecting the lower respiratory tract against injurious agents in the inspired air, and carrying out various metabolic processes. These functions and summaries of their importance are listed in Table 2-4, along with the chapters in which they are discussed.

References

1. Webster's Third New International Dictionary. Merriam-Webster, Springfield, MA, 1981, p. 1934
2. Weibel ER: The Pathway for Oxygen. Structure and Function in the Mammalian Respiratory System. Harvard University Press, Cambridge, MA, 1984, p. 2
3. Pierson DJ: The evolution of breathing: 3. Viable solutions: Types of respiratory apparatus in animals. Respir Care 1982; 27:267–270
4. Taylor CR, Weibel ER: Design of the mammalian respiratory system. I. Problem and strategy. Respir Physiol 1981;44:1–10
5. Pierson DJ: The evolution of breathing. (Series) Respir Care 1982;27:51–54, 160–163, 267–270, 569–599, 963–970, 1063–1069, 1392–1396, and 1983;28:195–202
6. Wood SC, Lenfant C (eds): Lung Biology in Health and Disease. Vol. 13. Evolution of Respiratory Processes: A Comparative Approach. Marcel Dekker, New York, 1979
7. Dejours P: Principles of comparative respiratory physiology. 2nd Ed. Elsevier North-Holland Biomedical Press, New York, 1981
8. Randall DJ, Burggren WW, Farrell AP, Haswell MS: The evolution of air breathing in vertebrates. Cambridge University Press, Cambridge, 1981
9. Jones JD: Comparative Physiology of Respiration. Edward Arnold (Publishers) Ltd., London, 1972
10. Krogh A: The Comparative Physiology of Respiratory Mechanisms. University of Pennsylvania Press, Philadelphia, 1941
11. Tenney SM: A comparative survey of the design of respiratory systems for gas exchange. pp. 282–297. In Fishman AP (ed): Pulmonary Diseases and Disorders. McGraw-Hill, New York, 1980
12. Schmidt-Nielsen K: Animal Physiology: Adaptation and Environment. 2nd Ed. Cambridge University Press, New York, 1979

Chapter 3

Embryology and Growth of the Respiratory System

Robert J. Harwood

CHAPTER OUTLINE

Lung development begins at 24 days' gestation and continues up to about 8 years of age. Although the lung does not function to provide gas exchange while in utero, it is actively developing in preparation for extrauterine life, which requires that the lung be ready to change from a liquid-filled organ to an air-filled organ and to accommodate gas exchange.

Clinicians who provide care to newborns must have an understanding of fetal pulmonary development to ensure appropriate care. A premature infant requires immediate attention because of underdevelopment of the lung and potential inability to maintain gas exchange. Understanding the development of the fetus enhances management skills and reduces the risk of morbidity and mortality. This chapter discusses fetal development, with particular attention to lung maturation and circulatory adjustments.

LUNG MATURATION

Within the first 12 days following fertilization of the egg (zygote) and implantation into the wall of the uterus, the three primary germ layers—ectoderm, mesoderm, and endoderm—develop. These give rise to all organs and tissues of the body: the ectoderm develops into the brain and the structures of the central nervous system; the mesoderm develops into the vasculature, bones, muscles, and connecting tissue; and the endoderm gives rise to the other major organs, namely, heart, liver, and lungs. The actual development of the lung is divided into four distinct periods.[1]

Embryonic Period

The embryonic period begins with fertilization and continues through week 5. The esophagus and laryngotracheal groove develop early in this period, and the latter deepens and forms a pouch at 24 days. The pouch, which is blind-ended, is considered the first lung bud (Fig. 3-1); it divides quickly, forming two buds over the next few days. From this division the right and left main stem bronchus develop.[2]

Pseudoglandular Period

The pseudoglandular period, extending from week 5 to week 16, is the second stage of lung development. During

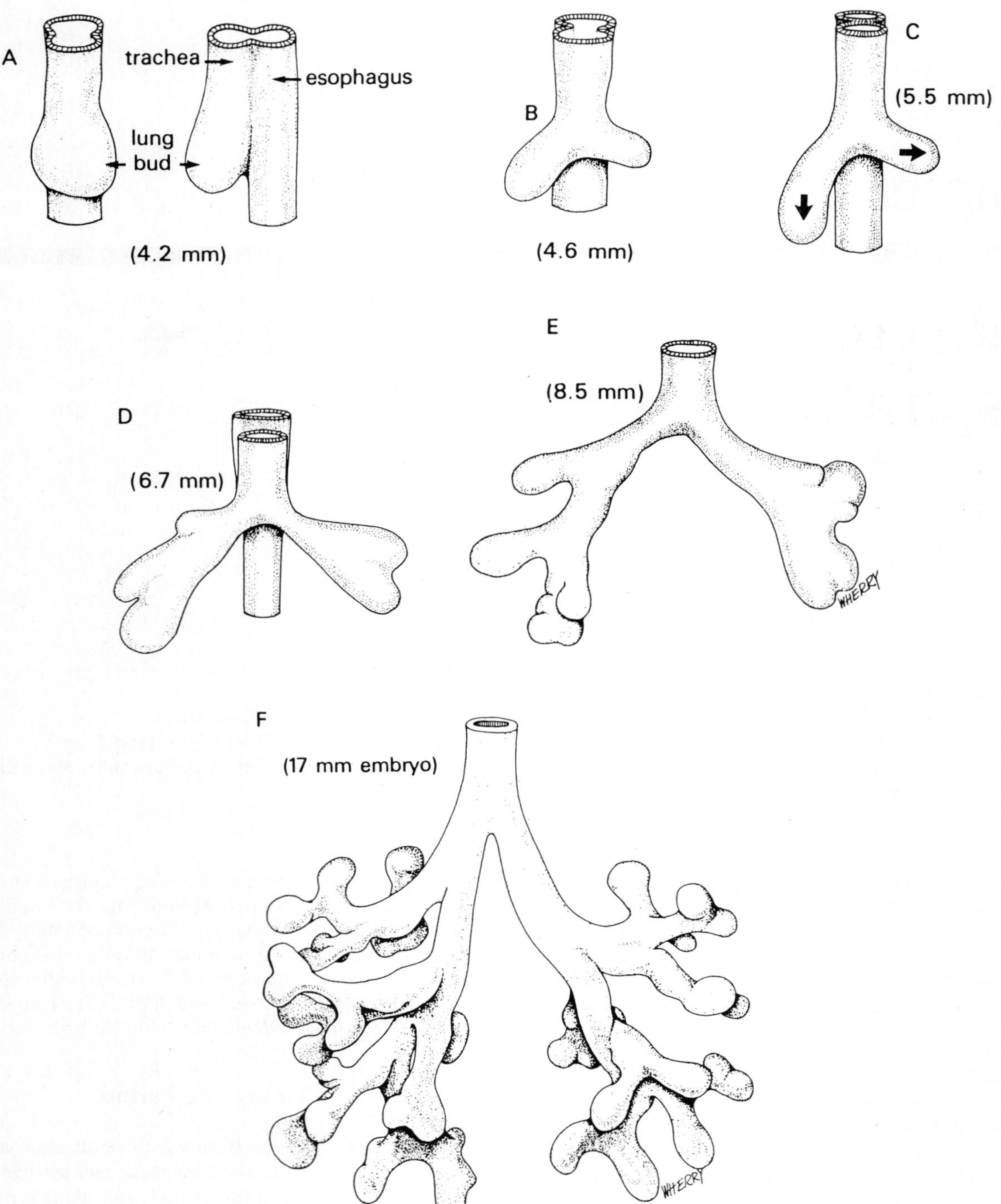

Figure 3-1. Lung development of the fetus during the embryonic and pseudoglandular period (see text for details). (**A**) 26 days (4.2 mm); (**B**) 28 days (4.6 mm); (**C**) 30 days (5.5 mm); (**D**) 32 days (6.7 mm); (**E**) 34 days (8.5 mm); (**F**) 38–40 days (17 mm embryo). (From Fraser and Pare,[22] with permission.)

this stage the conducting airways develop. Mucous glands, goblet cells and pseudostratified ciliated columnar epithelium line the airways by the end of this period. Segmental, subsegmental, and preacinar airways develop, all with blind endings during this period.[2,3]

Canalicular Period

The third period of development, the canalicular period, extends from week 17 to week 24. Enlargement of the lung and glandular structures continues, and respiratory bronchioles begin to arise from terminal bronchioles in this period. Each respiratory bronchiole contains an alveolar duct and sac. Pulmonary capillaries develop and begin to surround the rudimentary air sacs. Toward the end of this period, type I and type II alveolar pneumocytes first appear. Breathing movements of the fetus have been detected as early as 11 to 12 weeks' gestation.[4–6]

Terminal Sac Period

The fourth development period of lung maturation is the terminal sac period, extending from 24 weeks' gestation to birth (at 38 to 40 weeks). During this period primitive alveoli start to develop from alveolar ducts. Pulmonary blood vessels further develop and become intimately associated with alveoli. Fetal lungs now represent 2 to 3 percent of the total body weight. At 26 to 28 weeks, the normal developing fetus weighs approximately 1000 g.[1]

The cells forming the alveoli change from cuboidal to squamous at the beginning of this period. As the lung matures, the number of alveoli increases and the thickness of the alveolar wall decreases in preparation for gas exchange. At birth there are approximately 24 million to 75 million alveoli, and the surface area available for gas exchange is approximately 2.8 m^2. By 8 years of age the surface area available for gas exchange has increased to 70 m^2, and the number of alveoli has increased to about 300 million (Table 3-1).[2]

Table 3-1. Chronologic Development of the Lungs

Development Period	Structural Development
Embryonic (fertilization to 5 weeks)	Primitive lung bud Trachea Main stem bronchus
Pseudoglandular (5–16 weeks)	Pulmonary artery/vein Conducting airways Mucous glands, goblet cells Lung lobes Diaphragm
Canalicular (17–24 weeks)	Respiratory bronchioles Alveolar ducts Type I, II alveolar pneumocytes Pulmonary vasculature proliferation Surfactant synthesis begins
Terminal sac (25 weeks to birth)	Increased surfactant production Alveoli increase to 24 million at birth, surface area 2.8 m^2
Postnatal growth (birth to 8 years of age)	Alveoli increase to 300 million, surface area increases to 70 m^2

LUNG FLUID

By day 70 of gestation the lung begins secreting fluid from the capillary endothelium and alveolar epithelium. This fluid is necessary for continued lung growth and establishes the functional residual capacity (FRC). Lung fluid is composed primarily of H_2O, Na, potassium (K), Cl^-, and HCO_3^- and has a pH of 6.27, while the amniotic fluid has a pH of 7.02.[7] Lung fluid is secreted at a rate of 2 to 3 mL/h/kg body weight, and its secretion increases throughout gestational development. At term, the lung fluid volume approximates the FRC of the lung (25 to 30 mL/kg).[1] Lung fluid is distributed throughout the tracheobronchial tree; some is swallowed, and a portion moves out of the lungs and mixes with amniotic fluid. Breathing movements are thought to assist in the movement of fluid from the lungs. Surfactant is present in the lung fluid after 24 weeks' gestation. Since lung fluid mixes with amniotic fluid, the presence of surfactant can be determined by amniocentesis.[8]

Surfactant

Surfactant is a surface-active substance that is synthesized and stored in the lamellar inclusion bodies of the type II alveolar pneumocytes and released into alveoli after 24 weeks' gestation. Surfactant reduces surface tension and stabilizes lung volumes and is composed of a complex mixture of protein and phospholipids. Two phospholipids, lecithin and sphingomyelin, have been identified as the major components of surfactant. Together, these substances give surfactant its ability to reduce surface tension.[8]

Lung maturation is determined by sampling amniotic fluid and determining the ratio of lecithin to sphingomyelin. The concentrations of both these phospholipids vary during gestational development[2] (Fig. 3-2). Early in gestation, between 18 and 24 weeks, sphingomyelin and lecithin concentrations remain at fairly constant low levels. Production of lecithin increases after 24 weeks and surges at 34 weeks, indicating lung maturity (ability to maintain gas exchange). The lecithin/sphingomyelin (L/S) ratio has been demonstrated to indicate the maturity of the lung and the probability of the development of respiratory distress syndrome (RDS) and hyaline membrane disease (HMD). An L/S ratio of 2:1 indicates lung maturity, with a very low probability of these disorders; an L/S ratio of 1:1.5 indicates a transitional lung, with an increased probability of RDS and HMD; and an L/S ratio of 1:1 or lower is associated with a high incidence of RDS and HMD. Newborns with L/S ratios of 1:1 or lower

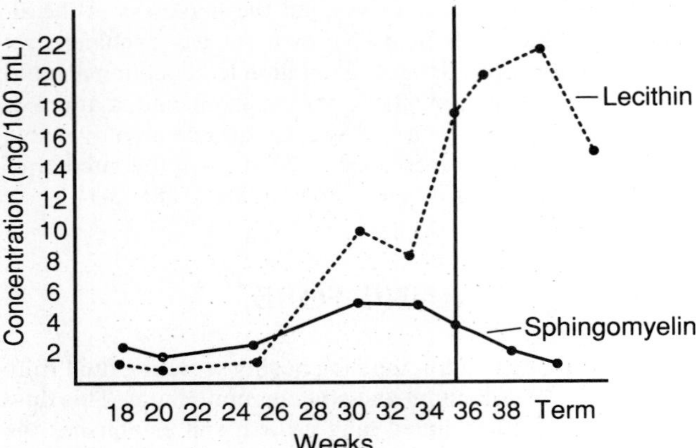

Figure 3-2. Lecithin (dotted line) and sphingomyelin (solid line) concentrations plotted against gestational age. (From Gluck et al.,[23] with permission.)

have decreased lung compliance, increased work of breathing, and increased O_2 consumption, and normally require mechanical ventilation.[9]

PULMONARY VESSELS

The right and left pulmonary arteries start to develop at approximately 26 days' gestation. They arise from the aortic sac and grow caudally within the lung. Pulmonary vasculature continues to proliferate along with the growth of the lung and becomes most abundant at 26 to 28 weeks.

In early gestation (prior to 26 to 28 weeks) only a small portion of the cardiac output (approximately 3 percent) enters the lung. Local pulmonary hypoxia and acidosis constrict the smooth muscle of the pulmonary vasculature, increasing pulmonary vasculature resistance and thereby limiting the portion of the cardiac output entering the lung. As the number and size of the pulmonary capillaries increase, the percentage of the cardiac output perfusing the lung increases to approximately 7 to 10 percent at term.

During birth, there is a sudden change in the resistance of the pulmonary vasculature. As the PO_2 increases and the pH normalizes, the pulmonary vascular resistance decreases, allowing greater blood flow to the lungs. An asphyxiated newborn presenting with hypoxemia maintains an increased pulmonary vascular resistance, which prevents blood from flowing into the lungs.[2,9,10]

AMNIOTIC FLUID

During gestation the fetus develops within the amniotic fluid, the amount of which ranges from 30 mL in early gestation to approximately 1 L at term. Amniotic fluid surrounds the fetus, protecting it from trauma, allowing movement, providing a heat regulating environment, ensuring biochemical homeostasis, and assisting in provision of nutritional requirements. The amniotic fluid consists primarily of water, a small portion of the volume being occupied by carbohydrates, cholesterol, phospholipids, proteins, and enzymes. The fetus regularly swallows a small portion of the amniotic fluid and absorbs it via the gastrointestinal tract. Amniotic fluid is completely replaced every 3 hours by exchange between the placenta, tracheobronchial tree, umbilical cord, fetal skin, and fetal urine. Analysis of amniotic fluid by amniocentesis can determine (1) fetal maturity, (2) genetic abnormalities, (3) Rh isoimmunization, and (4) fetal status.[7,11]

PLACENTA

The placenta is a highly vascular organ, which provides communication between the fetus and the mother by delivering O_2 and nutrients to the fetus and removing metabolic wastes (e.g., CO_2). The placenta is attached to the uterine fundus of the mother and to the fetus by the umbilical cord, which contains two arteries and one vein[12] (Fig. 3-3). Blood entering the placenta by the two umbilical arteries is routed to anchoring villi, which are immersed in maternal capillary complexes within the intervillous space. Maternal blood enters the placenta through the endometrial arteries and is forced into the intervillous space by hydrostatic pressure gradients. Exchange of O_2 and CO_2 occurs between these two blood supplies, which are essentially separated by the thin placental tissue. Maternal blood entering the placenta has a PO_2 of 100 mmHg, while fetal blood enters with a PO_2 of 17 mmHg. Diffusion of O_2 into fetal blood raises its PO_2 to approximately 29 mmHg and increases its O_2 saturation to about 80 percent. Maternal blood leaves the placenta by way of the endometrial veins and reenters the maternal circulation. Fetal blood leaves the placenta by the umbilical vein.[13]

Although the PO_2 of the blood entering the fetus is relatively low, the saturation of hemoglobin with O_2 (SaO_2) is high because of fetal hemoglobin (HbF). Unlike adult hemoglobin (HbA), HbF has no beta chains but contains two gamma chains. The absence of beta chains prevents 2,3-diphosphoglycerate (2,3-DPG) from attaching to the hemoglobin molecule, thereby increasing the affinity of hemoglobin for O_2. The oxyhemoglobin dissociation curve of the fetus is thus shifted to the left of the normal adult curve (Fig. 3-4). At birth HbF represents 77 to 85 percent of the total hemoglobin present, but within 8 to 11 months, it is totally converted to HbA.[14,15]

FETAL CIRCULATION

As shown in Figure 3-5, blood leaves the placenta by one umbilical vein, with a PaO_2 of 29 mmHg and an SaO_2 of 80 percent. On leaving the placenta, the arterialized blood is routed to the kidney, where a portion of it enters via the portal sinus. The rest of this blood enters the inferior vena cava (IVC) by way of the ductus venosus. Blood within the

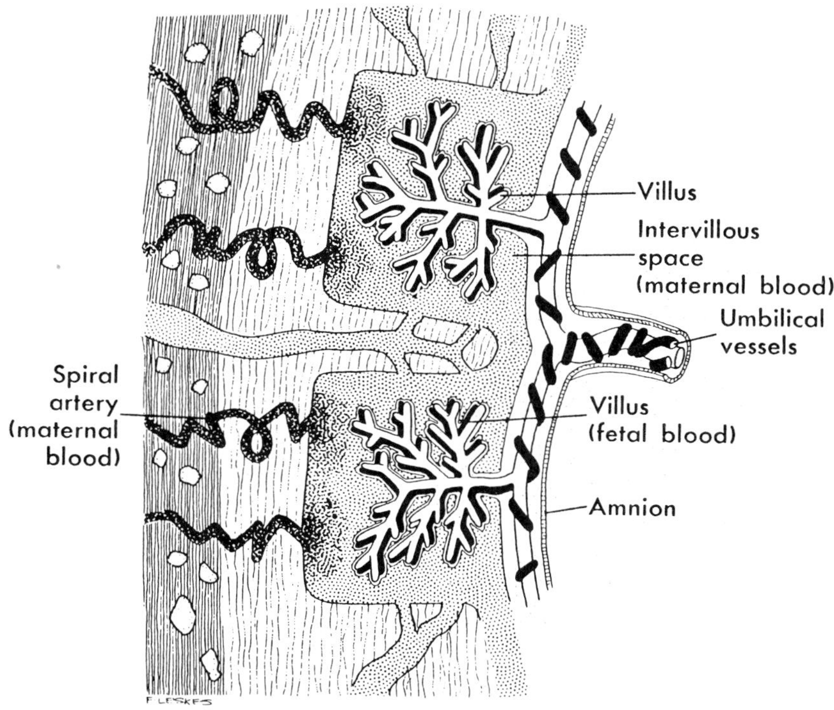

Figure 3-3. Placental blood flow. (From Korones,[10] with permission.)

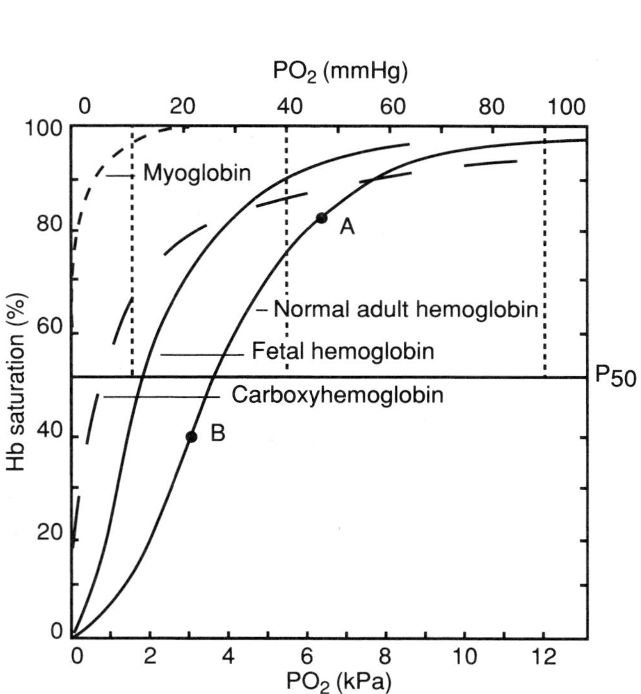

Figure 3-4. Dissociation curves for fetal hemoglobin and adult hemoglobin. The fetal curve is shifted to the left of the adult curve because of the composition of fetal hemoglobin (see text for details). Carboxyhemoglobin and myoglobin curves are also identified. (From Martin and Youtsey,[14] with permission.)

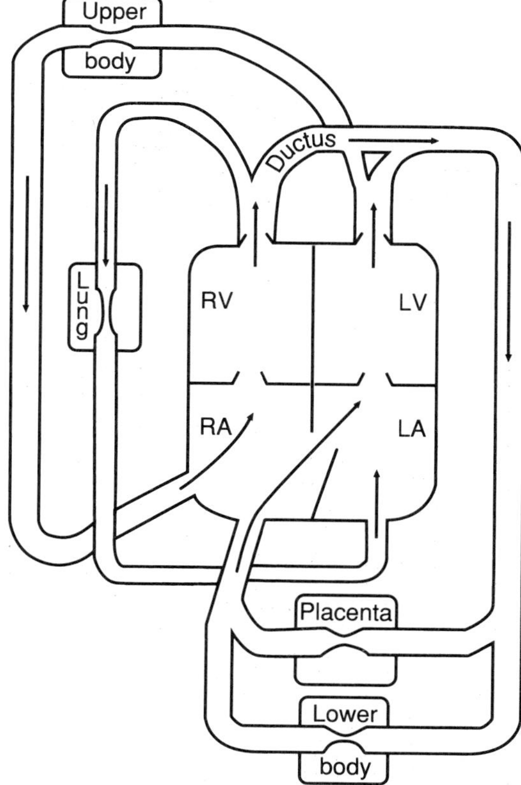

Figure 3-5. Fetal circulation. Note the presence of the ductus arteriosus coming off the pulmonary artery and foramen ovale between the right and left atrium. RA, right atrium; LA, left atrium; RV, right ventricle; LV, left ventricle. (From Lough et al.,[24] with permission.)

IVC before the attachment of the ductus venosus is unoxygenated, since it is returning from the lower extremities of the fetus. Mixing of these two blood supplies drops the SaO_2 to approximately 67 percent.

Upon entering the right atrium, the bloodstream is directed to the lower portion of the septum secundum, called the *crista dividens,* which is located within the intra-atrial septum. As the blood reaches the crista dividens, a portion enters the left atrium through the foramen ovale, an opening within the intra-atrial septum, causing a right-to-left shunt. The blood entering the left heart has a higher saturation (67 percent) than the portion that remains in the right heart (62 percent).

After entering the left atrium, blood moves into the left ventricle and out via the aorta. Here, a portion of the blood enters the subclavian, common carotid, and brachiocephalic arteries, which deliver it to the upper half of the fetus. Blood diverted back into the right atrium mixes with blood returning from the upper half of the fetus. The venous return has an SaO_2 of approximately 50 percent, and when mixed with blood entering from the IVC, it lowers the SaO_2 of that blood to approximately 62 percent. Blood then continues into the right ventricle and is pumped out via the pulmonary artery. Here, a small portion of blood enters the lungs by way of the right and left pulmonary arteries. Since no gas exchange occurs in utero, the lung has little need for blood other than to support its nutritional needs.

As the fetus grows, a greater portion of the cardiac output perfuses the lungs. Blood not entering the lungs continues through the ductus arteriosus (a vascular communication between the pulmonary artery and aorta), which remains open as a result of the hypoxemia, acidosis, and prostaglandin E_1 and E_2 levels in the fetus. This right-to-left shunt allows blood to reenter the systemic circulation without perfusing the lung and eventually to return to the placenta via the two umbilical arteries. Blood entering the placenta has a PO_2 of approximately 17 mmHg.[1,3,16]

INITIATION OF THE FIRST BREATH

As the process of birth begins, the warm, acidic, hypoxemic environment within which the fetus has developed begins to change rapidly. Uterine contractions move the fetus down the birth canal. With these contractions blood flow from the placenta decreases, causing fetal blood gas values to change. Generally, the PO_2 decreases below prelabor levels and the pH becomes more acidic. The small amount of blood that is perfusing the lungs is further reduced by vasoconstriction of the pulmonary vasculature in response to the imposed acidosis and hypoxemia.

As the chest is presented during birth, it is compressed, forcing lung fluid out of the upper airway and conducting airways, preparing the lung to receive its first breath. As the chest moves out of the vaginal opening, it recoils, thereby introducing the first breath into the lungs. For successive breaths, respiratory muscles must begin to contract to generate the inspiratory force needed to bring air into the lungs and overcome the effects of surface tension. The increase in respiratory muscle tone is believed to result from sympathetic and catecholamine stimulation (by release of epinephrine and norepinephrine) and increased sensitivity of the chemoreceptors to the changes in PaO_2 and $PaCO_2$.[17]

The first breath of the newborn generates a pleural pressure between -40 cmH_2O and -100 cmH_2O (Fig. 3-6). This pressure change causes a volume of 20 to 30 mL of air to enter the lung, some of which immediately establishes the FRC. The lung fluid remaining in the alveoli is removed by drainage via the pulmonary capillaries and lymphatics. Air begins to replace the lung fluid, and within a short time air completely replaces fluid, providing the newborn with an FRC equal to 25 to 30 mL/kg body weight. Subsequent breaths provide consistent tidal volumes with minimal intrapleural pressure changes as a result of the establishment of the FRC. Within a few hours after birth, respirations become rhythmic and tidal volumes of about 4 to 6 mL/kg body weight are established.[18]

CIRCULATORY ADJUSTMENTS AFTER BIRTH

As shown in Figure 3-7, a number of circulatory adjustments occur following birth. When the umbilical cord is clamped and cut, the umbilical arteries and vein constrict as does the ductus venosus, which closes functionally within 24 hours and anatomically within 3 to 7 days to become the ligamentum venosum. The foramen ovale closes functionally

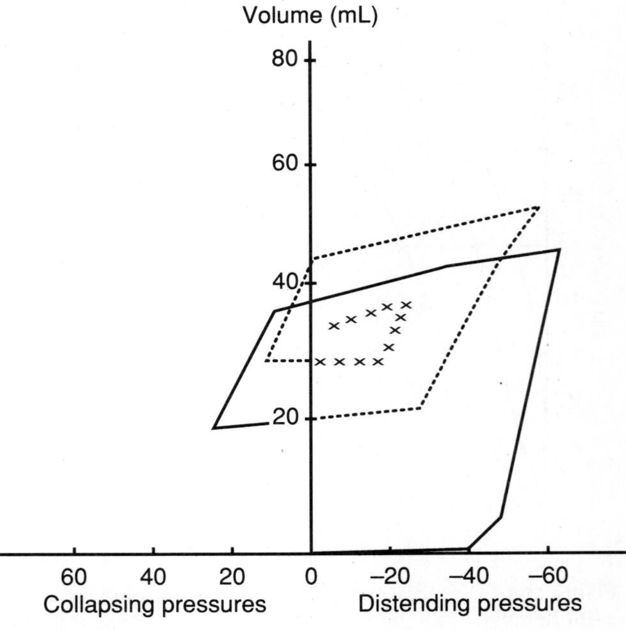

Figure 3-6. Relationship between distending pressures and collapsing pressures of the newborn's first (solid line), second (dotted line), and third (xxx) breaths. (From Avery and Fletcher,[25] with permission.)

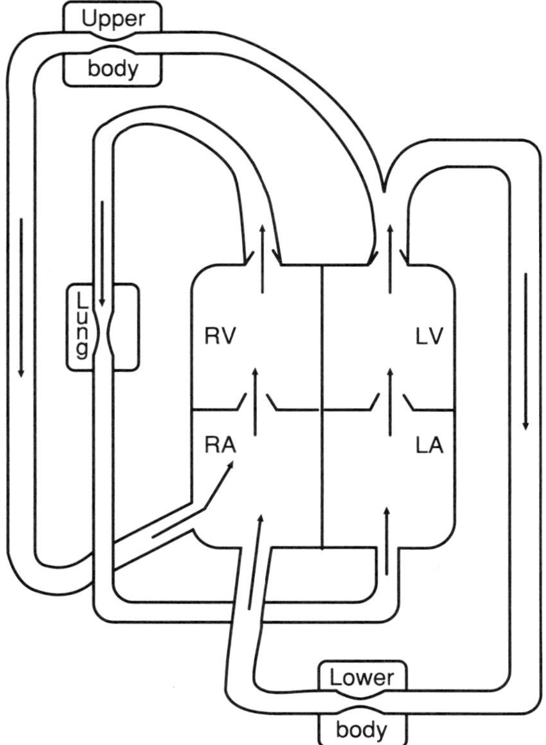

Figure 3-7. Normal newborn circulation. Note that the ductus arteriosus and foramen ovale are no longer present, indicating that these structures have closed. (From Lough et al.,[24] with permission.)

after the first few breaths as a result of intracardiac pressure changes, left ventricular pressure now being greater than right ventricular pressure.[16]

With the first breath and removal of lung fluid, gas exchange between the alveoli and pulmonary capillaries occurs. As the PaO_2 increases with each successive breath, pulmonary vascular resistance falls and blood flow into the lungs increases. In addition to the local PaO_2-mediated response of the pulmonary vasculature, vasculature tone is also affected by pH and PCO_2. Alkalosis, hypocarbia, and hyperoxia reduce pulmonary vascular resistance, whereas, conversely, acidosis, hypercarbia, and hypoxemia increase it. Recruitment of small unperfused capillaries also helps to reduce pulmonary vascular resistance by increasing the cross-sectional area of the pulmonary circulatory system.[19,20]

With the increase of pulmonary blood flow, pulmonary venous return to the left atrium increases, thereby increasing left atrial pressure. When left atrial pressure is greater than right atrial pressure, the foramen ovale closes. This is a functional closure, which can reopen if right atrial pressure becomes greater than left atrial pressure. An example of this change in atrial pressures is seen in the newborn who demonstrates persistent pulmonary hypertension. The increased pulmonary vascular resistance from hypoxemia causes right ventricular pressure to increase, thereby reducing pulmonary venous return to the left atrium. As a result, the foramen ovale opens, creating a right-to-left shunt, which results in further hypoxemia. Administration of O_2 helps to reduce the pulmonary vascular resistance, which allows pulmonary venous return to increase, with restoration of the left atrial pressures and closure of the foramen ovale. In the normally developing newborn, the foramen ovale permanently closes in approximately 3 months.

Throughout gestational development the ductus arteriosus remains open because of low PO_2, acidosis, prostaglandin E_1 and E_2 levels, and a constant blood flow through this vessel. Following birth, constriction of the ductus occurs as the PO_2 increases, levels of prostaglandins are reduced metabolically, intrauterine acidosis is eliminated, and blood flow through the ductus is decreased. The ductus arteriosus may, however, reopen if the newborn becomes hypoxic, which causes blood flow to bypass the lungs and enter the aorta, again resulting in a right-to-left shunt. Administration of O_2 and the prostaglandin synthetase inhibitor indomethacin have been successful in closing the ductus arteriosus. A newborn presenting with asphyxia, hypoxemia, and acidosis could have both a patent ductus arteriosus and a patent foramen ovale from failure of the cardiopulmonary system to adjust normally to birth.[21]

References

1. Moore K: The Developing Human. Clinically Oriented Embryology. 4th Ed. WB Saunders, Philadelphia, 1988
2. Murray J: The Normal Lung. 2nd Ed. WB Saunders, Philadelphia, 1986
3. Carlo W, Chatburn E: Neonatal Respiratory Care. 2nd Ed. Year Book Medical Publishers, Chicago, 1988
4. Stang LB: Neonatal Respiration. Physiological and Clinical Studies. Blackwell Scientific Publications, Oxford, 1977
5. Waggener T: Development of respiratory control: Fetal breathing movements. Respir Care 1984;29:811–815
6. Presswell J, Goodrick C: Perinatal respiration: Cultivating baby's breath. Respir Ther 1982;2:77–81
7. Beard R, Nathonielsz P: Fetal Physiology and Medicine. 2nd Ed. Marcel Dekker, New York, 1984
8. Clark A: Human surfactant as prophylactic treatment of respiratory distress syndrome in newborns. Res Resources Reporter 1988;12:1–15
9. Avery G: Neonatology, Pathophysiology and Management of the Newborn. 3rd Ed. JB Lippincott, Philadelphia, 1987
10. Korones S: High-Risk Newborn Infants: The Basis for Intensive Care Nursing. 4th Ed. CV Mosby, St. Louis, 1986
11. Malvihill SJ, Stone MM, Debas HT, Fonkalrud FW: The role of amniotic fluid in fetal nutrition. J Pediatr Surg 1985;20:668–672
12. Longo L, Bartels H: Respiratory gas exchange and blood flow in the placenta. Proceedings of a Symposium with the Twenty-fifth International Congress of Physiological Sciences, U.S. Department of Health & Human Services, National Institutes of Health, DHEW Publication No. 73-361, 1972
13. Goodwin J, Godden J, Chance G: Perinatal Medicine. The Basic Science Underlying Clinical Practice. Williams & Wilkins, Baltimore, 1976
14. Martin D, Youtsey J: Respiratory Anatomy and Physiology. CV Mosby, St. Louis, 1988
15. Wimberley P: Fetal Hemoglobin 2,3-Diphosphoglycerate and Oxygen Transport in the Newborn Premature Infant. Depart-

ment of Clinical Hematology, University College Hospital Medical School of London, London, 1982
16. Aloan C: Respiratory Care of the Newborn: A Clinical Manual. JB Lippincott, Philadelphia, 1987
17. Copper R, Goldenberg R: Catecholamine secretion in fetal adaptation to stress. J Obstet Gynecol Neonatal Nurs 1990;19:223–226
18. Barch M: The newborn, not just a little person. Respir Ther 1985;15:47–49
19. Anderson J, Martin R, Fanaroff A: Neonatal respiratory control and apnea of prematurity. Perinatology-Neonatology 1983;6:65–70
20. Thibeault D, Gregory G: Neonatal Pulmonary Care. 2nd Ed. Appleton-Century Crofts, East Norwalk, CT, 1986
21. Thalji AA, Carr I, Yeh TF et al: Pharmokinetics of intravenous administered indomethacin in premature infants. J Pediatr 1980;97:995
22. Fraser R, Pare JA: Organ Physiology: Structure and Function of the Lung. 2nd Ed. WB Saunders, Philadelphia, 1977
23. Gluck L, Kulovich MV, Borer RC Jr et al: Diagnosis of the respiratory syndrome by amniocentesis. Am J Obstet Gynecol 1971;109:440–445
24. Lough M, Doershuk C, Stern L: Pediatric Respiratory Therapy, 2nd Ed. Year Book Medical Publishers, Chicago, 1982
25. Avery ME, Fletcher B: The Lung and Its Disorders in the Newborn Infant. 4th Ed. WB Saunders, Philadelphia, 1981

Chapter 4

The Upper Airway

Michael J. Bishop

CHAPTER OUTLINE

Diseases of the upper airway may either mimic or produce lower airway disease. The stridor of laryngeal obstruction may be confused with asthma, or an infection of the paranasal sinuses may lead to a chronic cough.

The upper, or extrathoracic, airway extends from the nares and mouth to the thoracic inlet and includes the pharynx and the larynx (Fig. 4-1). The airway serves both as a passive conduit for ventilatory gases and as an active guard for the lower airways and lungs. The upper airway also conditions the gases passing through it by warming and humidifying them. In humans the upper airway has developed the remarkable ability to vary tone and pitch, providing us with an ability to communicate with sound at a level of complexity exceeding that of other animals.

In the normal subject the upper airway provides a substantial fraction of the total resistance to gas flow. Resistive work constitutes approximately 20 percent of the work of breathing, and thus the work needed to overcome upper airway resistance normally is small. However, the passages of the airway, described in detail below, are soft and compliant and deform easily. Their resistance can increase manyfold to the point at which they prohibit gas flow.

The volume of the extrathoracic airways averages 75 mL. While this is only a small fraction of the normal tidal volume, it may constitute a significant fraction of an inspired breath in patients with severe restrictive disease.[1] Since an 8-mm diameter endotracheal tube has an internal volume of approximately 12 to 15 mL, endotracheal intubation greatly reduces wasted ventilation, although it increases resistance to airflow.

SUPRAGLOTTIC ANATOMY

Nose and Nasopharynx

The nose's central location in the face makes it a prominent feature of physiognomy. However the nose's prominence is not limited to the face alone. It has played a key role in literary works as diverse as *Cyrano de Bergerac* and *Pinocchio*, and the livelihood of cartoonists and caricaturists depends on their ability to capture an entertaining perspective of this vital organ.

The nose plays a key role in the respiratory system as the usual portal of entry for inspired gases. The anterior nares are relatively narrow in cross section and therefore have a relatively high resistance.

Although the nose provides approximately half of the total resistance of a normal respiratory system, this is a small price to pay for the conditioning features that the nose provides. The lateral wall of the nose has three overhanging structures called turbinates, which are covered by mucosa (Fig. 4-2). As air enters the nares, the narrow opening and the turbinates lead to turbulent flow, which increases impaction of

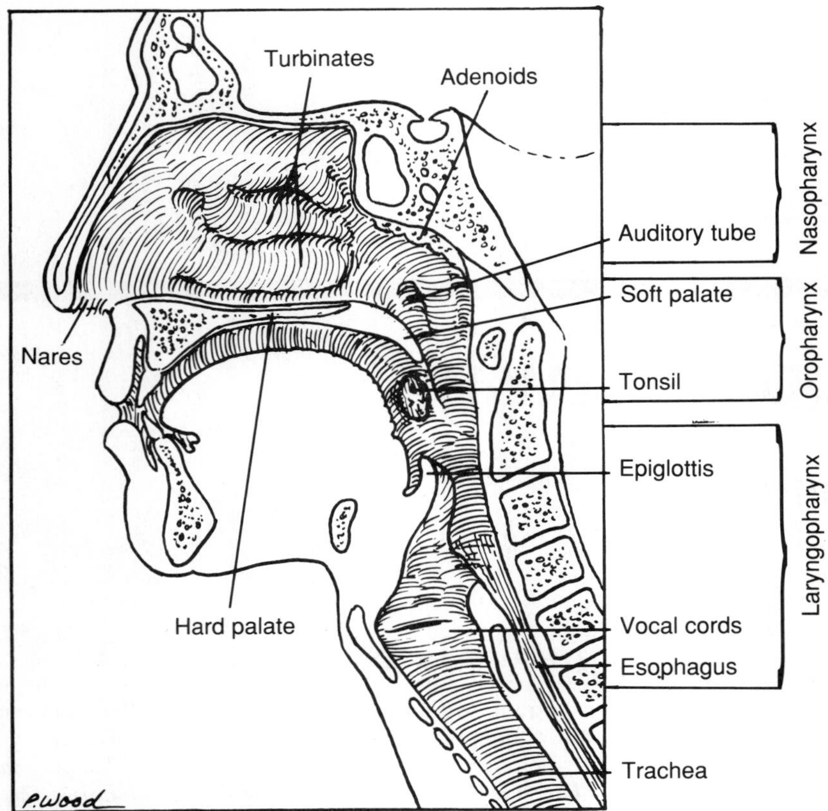

Figure 4-1. A sagittal view of the upper airway.

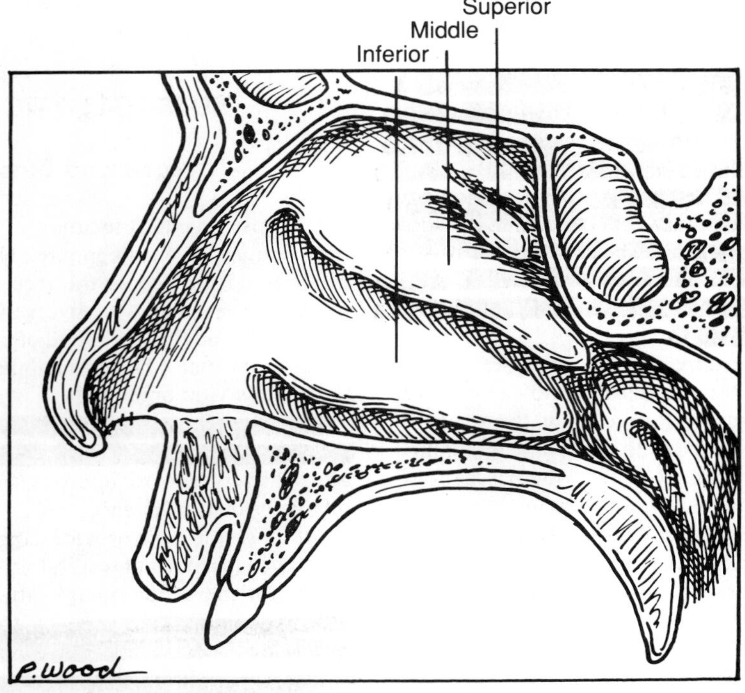

Figure 4-2. The nasal turbinates. Note that these are easily traumatized during nasal instrumentation.

particles greater than 5 μm in diameter and prevents them from reaching the lower respiratory tract. The generous blood flow to the nasal mucosa also results in rapid warming and humidification of the inspired gases.

However, this ample blood flow may at times be detrimental. The mucosa is easily engorged during infections, allergic reactions, pregnancy, and hypothyroidism, following the use of topical vasoconstrictors, and even in the absence of an apparent stimulus in patients with nonspecific rhinitis. Furthermore, the vascularity of the tissue makes it highly susceptible to bleeding following trauma, whether external from an errant fist or internal as in attempted nasal intubation for placement of a nasotracheal, nasogastric, or suction catheter.

The key respiratory structures of the nose include the anterior orifices, the turbinates, and the nasal septum. The septum frequently is not midline, and one nostril may be substantially larger than the other. An important clinical consideration arising from this asymmetry is the need to have the patient sniff through one nostril at a time to determine if one appears to be partially occluded. This simple clinical test will often make introduction of a catheter or airway much easier for both the patient and the operator. The turbinates increase the turbulence of airflow and increase the mucosal surface area, thereby contributing to conditioning of the inspired air. Underneath each turbinate lies a meatus for a paranasal sinus. Occlusion of the meatus leads to fluid accumulation in the sinus, which has a high potential for infection. Indwelling nasal tubes cause infection routinely, and sinusitis must be suspected in the febrile patient with a nasogastric or nasotracheal tube.

The floor of the nose leading to the nasopharynx lies in the same plane as the nasal orifices. When introducing catheters into the nose, it is important to follow this plane by lifting the tip of the nose and placing the catheter straight back rather than pointing it toward the top of the head (Fig. 4-3).

The two nasal passages join posteriorly in the nasopharynx. The nasopharynx contains prominent lymphatic tissue called *adenoids*, which are especially prominent in children but atrophy after puberty. Nasal intubation in children carries the risk of displacing an adenoid and causing possible hemorrhage or obstruction of the endotracheal tube.

The ability of the nose to condition air makes it the preferred route for normal inspiration. However, peak flow through the nose is limited to 1.5 to 2 L/s. If more effort is exerted in attempts to reach higher flows, the negative pressures generated tend to lead to collapse of the passages. At the normal resting inspiratory flows of 0.5 L/s, nasal breathing is ideal, but the higher flows required during exercise or with severe respiratory impairment lead to breathing through the lower-resistance oral route.

Mouth

During rapid inspiration the oral cavity is wide open, providing a large-diameter airway. This airway is much larger than the nasal airway, but its lower surface area/volume ratio results in less complete conditioning of the airway and less upper airway impaction of inspired particles.

The teeth and alveolar ridge are important because of their

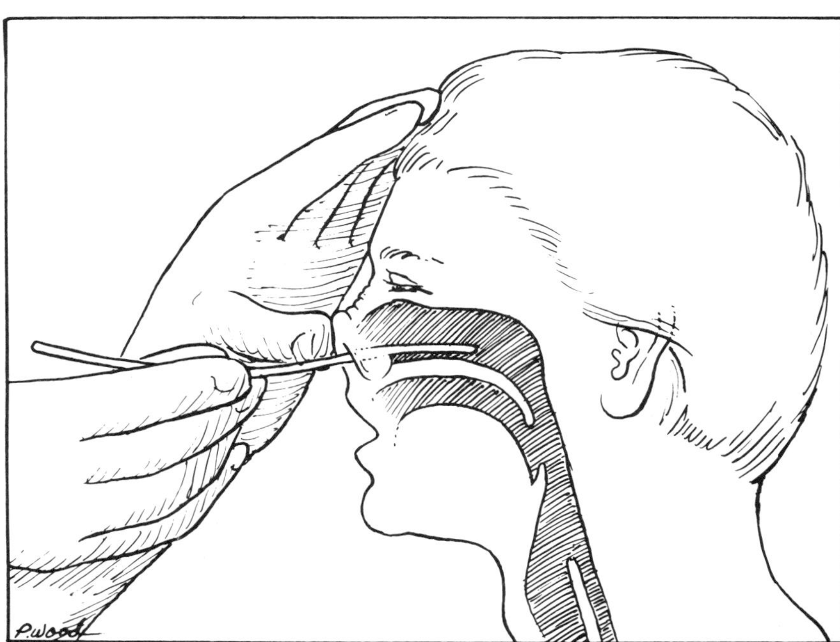

Figure 4-3. Insertion of a catheter into the nose. Note the importance of going in parallel to the floor of the nose.

role in the shape of the face. In the edentulous patient, fitting a mask to the face is often difficult. The cheeks collapse into the oral cavity and an inadequate seal results, making positive pressure ventilation ineffective. The experienced clinician learns to pull the cheeks up to the mask to provide a seal. Masks with large inflatable rims often provide a better seal in such patients. The teeth provide no respiratory function, but their integrity should be assessed for several reasons. Patients with inadequate dentition are more likely to aspirate large pieces of food, with resulting airway obstruction. In the patient with facial trauma, missing teeth may fall into the pharynx, or, in less fortunate patients, may be aspirated and lodge in the lower airways. A final reason for assessing dentition is the risk that a therapeutic maneuver such as insertion of an endotracheal tube may lead to breakage or extraction of an already damaged tooth. Detection of such damage in advance should lead to consideration of an alternate procedure.

The roof of the mouth is formed by the hard palate anteriorly and the soft palate posteriorly. The uvula is suspended from the soft palate and is primarily of interest as a landmark for the midline during direct laryngoscopy and endotracheal intubation. However, in rare circumstances it can become markedly inflamed and contribute to airway obstruction.

The lower margin of the airway is provided by the tongue, which is attached to the mandible and the hyoid bone and is composed of muscle. Its role in airway obstruction in the unconscious patient remains controversial (see discussion of tongue and soft tissue problems). Because of its attachments, the tongue can be moved forward by forward traction on the mandible. This is best achieved in the supine patient by placing the fingers bilaterally along the ramus of the mandible and providing steady upward traction (see Ch. 72).

The lateral margins of the dorsal part of the mouth are formed by the lymphatic tissue containing the tonsils. These are of little consequence to respiration in normal subjects but can lead to acute obstruction when swollen. In rare cases chronic enlargement of the oral and pharyngeal lymphoid tissue may lead to chronic airway obstruction and right heart failure.[2]

Pharynx

The cone-shaped pharynx includes the nasopharynx and the oropharynx, which join to form the hypopharynx (Fig. 4-4). The pharynx is surrounded by constrictor muscles, which support the esophagus and larynx and aid in swallow-

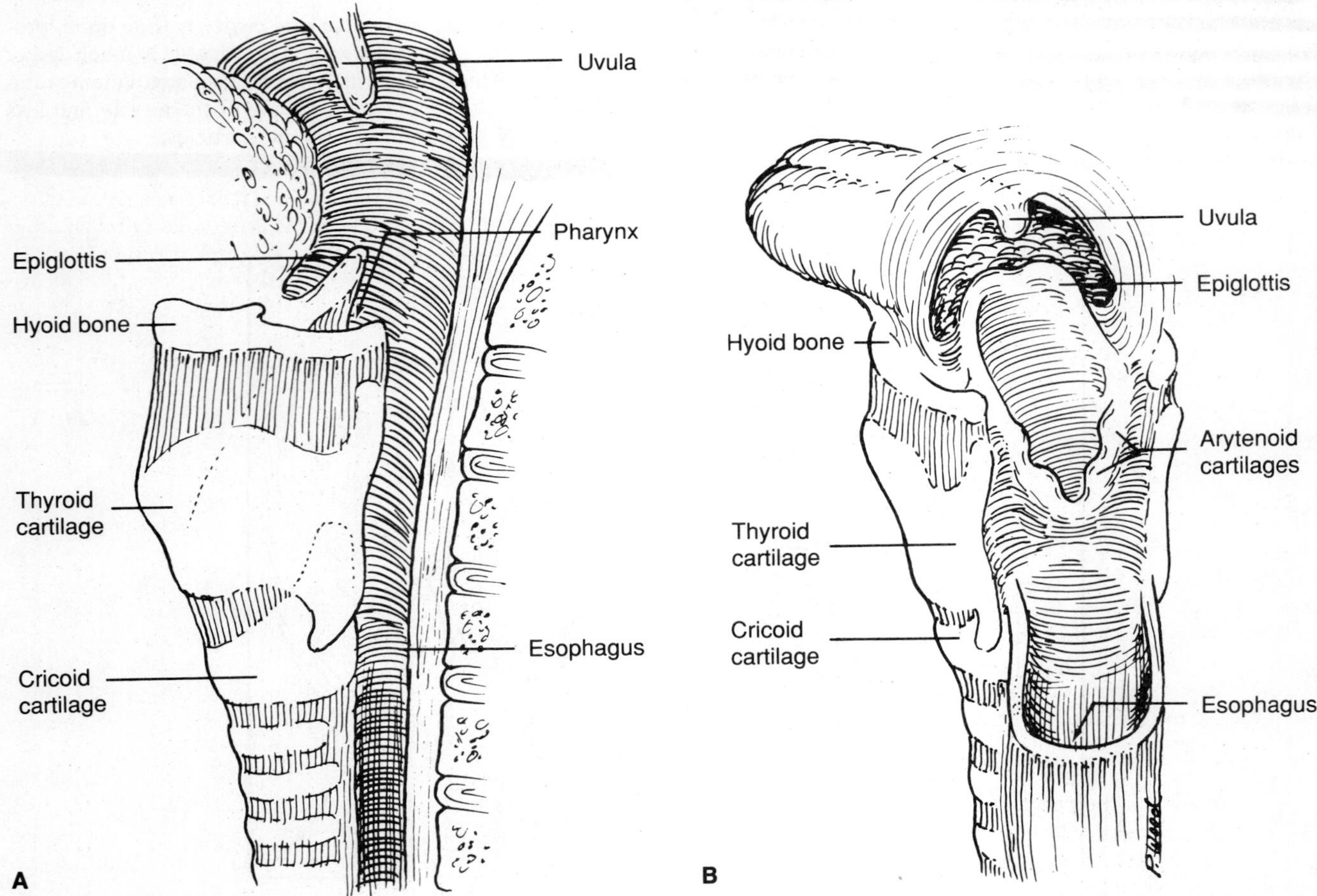

Figure 4-4. (**A**) Lateral and (**B**) posterior oblique views of the pharynx and larynx, including the laryngeal skeleton.

ing. The walls of the pharynx are relatively soft and compliant, allowing the lumen to increase during rapid inspiration. Their compliance can also easily lead to decreases in luminal diameter when swelling from inflammatory processes or trauma occurs in the neck.

In the pharynx the digestive and respiratory tracts share a lumen. The pharynx continues posteriorly to form the esophagus whereas anteriorly it ends in a series of pouches or fossae surrounding the larynx. The epiglottis forms the posterior wall of the anterior pouch, which is called the *vallecula* and is an important landmark in endotracheal intubation. Laterally the pharynx ends in the *pyriform fossae*, which are shaped so as to direct boluses of food posteriorly, away from the larynx and toward the esophagus.

LARYNGEAL ANATOMY

Cartilaginous Skeleton and Relation to Bony Skeleton

The skeleton of the larynx consists of a series of cartilages (Fig. 4-4), which extend between the fourth and the sixth cervical vertebrae. The main body of the larynx consists of the thyroid cartilage (known colloquially as the Adam's apple) anteriorly and the cricoid cartilage posteriorly. The cricoid cartilage forms a complete ring, which is much wider posteriorly than anteriorly. By placing two fingers over the thyroid cartilage and moving them down the neck, one will encounter a brief depression followed by another hard prominence, only a few millimeters in width at this point, which is the anterior portion of the cricoid. The depression is the cricothyroid membrane.

Because the cricoid forms a complete ring, the airway that it encloses is fixed in diameter. This makes the mucosa covering the cricoid especially susceptible to pressure-induced injury, since it can be trapped between an endotracheal tube cuff and the stiff cartilage. For this reason, it is important to pass the cuff below the level of the cricoid to avoid mucosal damage with its sequelae of scarring and stenosis.

The cricothyroid membrane is a key anatomic structure that should be readily identifiable by all medical personnel involved in emergency care. As it has little soft tissue in front of it, the cricothyroid membrane is easily identifiable and provides ready access to the airway in case of obstruction higher in the respiratory tract. Although it feels relatively narrow, the space is more than ample to permit fitting of a small catheter, which can deliver life-preserving fresh gas. In addition, the space will expand to accommodate small tracheostomy tubes. When an emergency airway must be opened surgically, it should be via the cricothyroid membrane rather than the cervical trachea, which is deeper and surrounded by more vascular tissues.

The leaf-shaped epiglottic cartilage is attached to the posterior surface of the thyroid cartilage, with the main body of the epiglottis lying rostral to it. The epiglottis helps to direct food away from the larynx by sitting almost tent-like over the laryngeal aperture. When the trachea moves down during inspiration, the epiglottis is pulled forward, opening the larynx.[3] During swallowing the trachea moves up and the epiglottis is forced back over the larynx. However, this role of the epiglottis in protecting the airway is part of a complex mechanism, since the airway is still adequately protected even after surgical removal of the epiglottis.

Anteriorly, the epiglottis is attached to the hyoid bone by the hyoepiglottic ligament. This anatomic feature facilitates endotracheal intubation since anterior traction can be applied to the hyoid by a laryngoscope blade placed in the vallecula. This pulls the epiglottis forward from its usual position overhanging the laryngeal opening, permitting the operator to see the vocal cords.

The arytenoid cartilages sit posteriorly atop the cricoid cartilage. These small, delicate, paired cartilages are critical to movement of the vocal cords. An arm of each cartilage forms the posterior third of each vocal cord, and the cricoarytenoid joint permits rotation and sliding of the arytenoids to abduct the vocal cords. Damage to these joints can result in immobile or poorly mobile cords and consequent respiratory difficulties.[4]

The true vocal cords appear white when viewed on direct laryngoscopy and are attached anteriorly to the thyroid cartilage and posteriorly to the arytenoids. Knowing this relationship enables the clinician to intubate the larynx in cases in which the arytenoids can be seen but the cords are hidden by the epiglottis.

Functional Anatomy of the Larynx

During normal respiration the larynx descends, causing the epiglottis to be pulled forward. The vocal cords are actively abducted from the midline, and the resistance across the larynx becomes small.

During swallowing the trachea and larynx rise and the epiglottis folds back over the laryngeal inlet. If the epiglottis is fixed by tumor, inflammation, or scarring, normal swallowing may be difficult and may place the patient at risk for aspiration. Protection against aspiration is also provided by closure of the cords by the laryngeal muscles.

A *cough* consists of the generation of a high pressure within the thorax followed by a sudden release of the pressure, resulting in a high airflow. In order to generate the necessary pressures of more than 100 cmH_2O, the glottis must close extremely tightly. This closure requires more than just the apposition of the vocal cords—the aryepiglottic folds fold inward and the thyroid and hyoid move together, leading to a sphincteric closure of the airway.

When the supraglottic or glottic area is stimulated, reflex laryngeal closure, termed *laryngospasm*, may occur. Severe stridor or even total obstruction may provide frightening moments for the clinician. Laryngospasm occurs because of an abnormal prolongation of the glottic closure reflex described above and sometimes requires administration of paralyzing drugs to permit ventilation.[5]

THE ABNORMAL UPPER AIRWAY

A wide variety of pathologic conditions obstruct the upper airway or make access for endotracheal intubation difficult.[6–8] The following overview briefly describes various conditions that may obstruct the airway.

Face

Facial swelling caused by trauma or burns can be severe enough to obstruct the airway. With massive facial trauma or obvious severe burns, prophylactic intubation before maximum swelling may be life-saving or at least may avoid the need for a tracheotomy.

Abnormalities of the upper airway may be produced by a variety of congenital syndromes, including large tongues, small jaws, and short necks. The clinician must examine the patient before attempting endotracheal intubation and must recognize that patients with unusual facial features may require special consideration.

Tongue and Soft Tissue Problems

Obstruction Associated with Altered Mental Status

Altered mental status is undoubtedly the most common cause of airway obstruction. Muscle tone normally helps to maintain an open airway, and loss of that tone associated with change in mental state contributes to partial or complete airway closure.

The precise cause of airway obstruction during altered mental states remains controversial. The traditional concept that the tongue falls back and occludes the pharynx[9] has come under scrutiny.[10] Fiberoptic observation of the airway in anesthetized patients has demonstrated that the epiglottis falls back to the posterior pharynx resulting in closure. Whichever view is correct, the remedy is the same. Extension of the neck and forward traction on the mandible will pull the tongue forward, and the epiglottis will move forward as the hyoid bone moves anteriorly.

Pharyngeal artificial airways inserted through the nose or mouth also will relieve obstruction in the unconscious patient (Fig. 4-5). Whether the improved airway results from the tongue being held away from the posterior pharyngeal wall or from the epiglottis being moved forward remains unclear.

Other Causes of Obstruction

Increased soft tissue in the obese patient increases the likelihood of airway obstruction. Neck trauma, like facial trauma, rapidly leads to swelling, which may occlude the pharyngeal airway. Still another source of obstruction is Ludwig's angina, a circumferential infection in the pharynx producing an often lethal occlusion of the airway. Such infections often arise from a tooth abscess that has spread.

Epiglottitis

Epiglottitis, an infectious process affecting the whole supraglottic larynx (and probably more appropriately termed *supraglottitis*), occurs primarily in children but also may de-

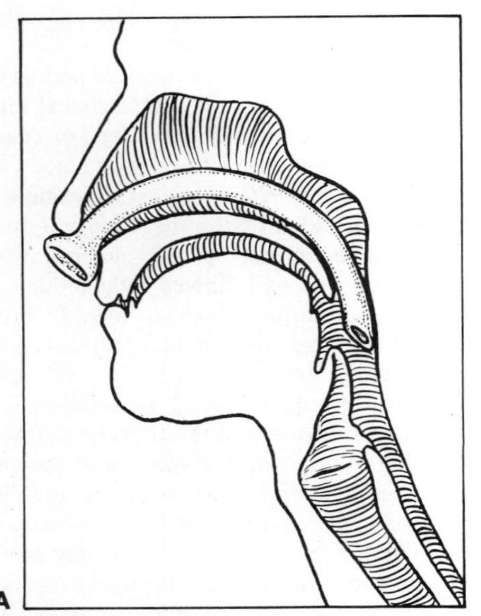

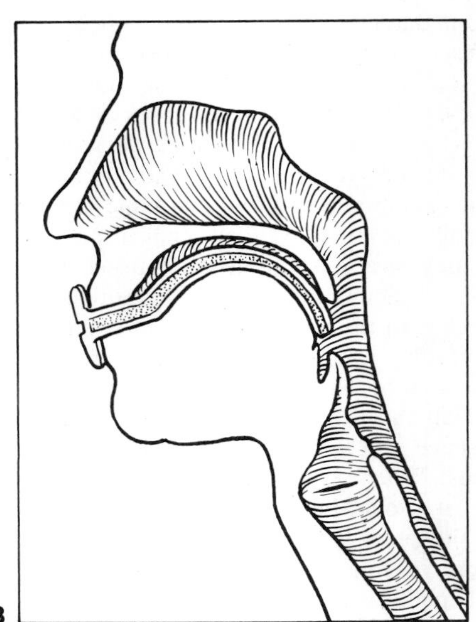

Figure 4-5. **(A)** Nasal and **(B)** oral artificial airways in place. These improve the airway by separating the tongue and epiglottis from the posterior pharyngeal wall.

velop in adults. Patients first complain of pain on swallowing because the inflamed epiglottis cannot fold down when the trachea is elevated. If an artificial airway is not established, the inflammation may lead to complete airway obstruction.[11,12]

References

1. Nunn JF, Campbell EJM, Peckett BW: Anatomical subdivisions of the volume of respiratory dead space and effect of position of the jaw. J Appl Physiol 1959;14:160–162
2. Sofer S, Weinhouse E, Tal A et al: Cor pulmonale due to adenoidal or tonsillar hypertrophy or both in children. Chest 1988;93:119–122
3. Fink BR, Demarest RJ: Laryngeal Biomechanics. Harvard University Press, Cambridge, MA, 1978
4. Castella X, Gilabert J, Perez C: Arytenoid dislocation after tracheal intubation: An unusual cause of acute respiratory failure? Anesthesiology 1991;75:613–615
5. Sasaki CT, Isaacson G: Dynamic anatomy of the larynx. Probl Anesth 1988;2:163–174
6. Sharar SR, Bishop MJ: Complications of tracheal intubation. Intensive Care Med 1992 (in press)
7. Murrin KR: Intubation procedure and causes of difficult intubation. pp. 75–89. In Latto IP, Rosen M (eds): Difficulties in Tracheal Intubation. Baillière Tindall, London, 1984
8. Quartararo C, Bishop MJ: Complications of tracheal intubation: Prevention and treatment. Semin Anesthesia 1990;9:119–127
9. Safar P, Escarraga LA, Chang F: Upper airway obstruction in the unconscious patient. J Appl Physiol 1959;14:760–764
10. Boidin MP: Airway patency in the unconscious patient. Br J Anaesth 1985;57:306–310
11. Bishop MJ: Epiglottitis in the adult. Anesthesiology 1981;55:701–702
12. Mayo Smith MF, Hirsch PJ, Wodzinski SF, Schiffman FJ: Acute epiglottitis in adults. N Engl J Med 1986;314:1133–1139

Chapter 5

The Thorax and Ventilatory Muscles: The Respiratory Pump

Robert M. Kacmarek

CHAPTER OUTLINE

The primary function of the cardiopulmonary system is gas exchange—the delivery of O_2 to cells and the removal of CO_2 from the body. Breathing is a central aspect of this system and is best defined as the rhythmic movement of gas into and out of the lungs. This is accomplished by the respiratory pump produced by the interrelationship of the lungs and thorax, along with the diaphragm and the muscles of the thorax, abdominal wall, and neck. This chapter discusses on a macro scale the process of breathing. Details of gas distribution within the lung and actual gas exchange are found in Chapters 9 and 10, respectively.

ANATOMIC RELATIONSHIP OF THE LUNGS AND THORAX

The lungs are essentially suspended in the thoracic cavity, being attached at their hila to the mainstem bronchi but otherwise free to move within the thorax. Lining the exterior of the lungs is a thin connective tissue sheath, the visceral pleura. A similar sheath, the parietal pleura, lines the inside of the thoracic cavity (Fig. 5-1). These two sheaths are in direct contact with each other, separated only by a thin film of serous fluid. As a result the lungs and thoracic cage can slide across each other unimpeded during breathing. Since the tendency of the lungs is to deflate and that of the thorax is to inflate at resting exhalation, a negative pressure exists between the two pleurae. The relationship of the lungs and thorax is similar to that of two microscope slides separated by a thin film of water with opposing forces attempting to pull them apart. The adhesion of the film keeps them together, yet allows them to freely slide over each other. Thus, as the muscles of the chest wall and diaphragm contract, expanding the thoracic cavity, a greater negative intrapleural pressure is created, distending the lungs. This decreases the pressure in the lungs from atmospheric at functional residual capacity (FRC) to subatmospheric during inspiration and causes air to enter the lungs. With relaxation of the muscles of inspiration, the lungs and thoracic cage recoil to their resting positions, increasing both intrapleural and intrapulmonary pressure and resulting in exhalation.

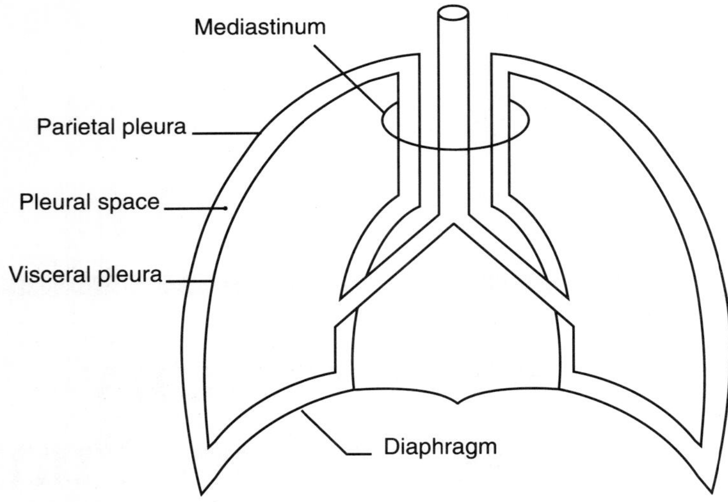

Figure 5-1. The pleurae (visceral and parietal), along with the diaphragm and the mediastinum. The visceral pleura encapsulates the entire lung. The parietal pleura covers the chest wall and the diaphragm. (From Scanlon et al.,[1] with permission.)

At FRC, the pressure in the intrapulmonary space is atmospheric, while the pressure in the pleural space is about -5 cmH_2O. With normal inspiration, the intrapleural pressure drops to about -9 cmH_2O and the intrapulmonary pressure to about -3 cmH_2O. At the end of inspiration, the intrapleural pressure is at its most negative; however, the intrapulmonary pressure returns to atmospheric as flow into the lung stops. During exhalation, intrapleural pressures return to their resting level of -5 cmH_2O and intrapulmonary pressures first increase to about $+3$ cmH_2O and then return to atmospheric as exhalation ends. In addition to these changes, intra-abdominal pressure is altered during breathing by the movement of the diaphragm (see below). At FRC intra-abdominal pressure is atmospheric, while during inspiration it becomes positive, about $+3$ cmH_2O, but returns to atmospheric at end exhalation.

PRESSURE GRADIENTS IN THE CHEST

Based on the pressure changes discussed above, a number of different pressure gradients have been defined to describe forces moving the thoracic cage during breathing (Table 5-1). Three specific compartments have been defined: intrapulmonary, intra-abdominal, and intrapleural. The atmosphere also exerts a force on the thoracic cage. Four distinct pressure gradients are commonly used: transairway pressure, defined as the difference between intrapulmonary pressure (P_{pul}) and atmospheric pressure, is zero when gas flow is zero, becoming negative during inspiration and positive during expiration. Transpulmonary pressure is the difference between P_{pul} and intrapleural pressure (P_{pl}); transthoracic pressure is the difference between atmospheric pressure (P_{atm}) and P_{pl}; and transdiaphragmatic pressure is the dif-

Table 5-1. Pressure Gradients Defining Gas Movement

Pressure Gradient	Definition	FRC Value[a]	Change during Inspiration	End Inspiration Value[a]	Change during Exhalation	End Exhalation Value[a]
Transairway	$P_{pul} - P_{atm}$	0	Negative	0	Positive	0
Transpulmonary	$P_{pul} - P_{pl}$	+5	More positive	+9	Less positive	+5
Transthoracic	$P_{atm} - P_{pl}$	+5	More positive	+9	Less positive	+5
Transdiaphragmatic	$P_{pl} - P_{ab}$	0	More positive	−10	Less positive	0

P_{pul}, intrapulmonary pressure; P_{pl}, intrapleural pressure; P_{ab}, intra-abdominal pressure; P_{atm}, atmospheric pressure.
[a] All numbers represent average values during resting breathing in the upright position.

ference between P_{pl} and the intra-abdominal pressure (P_{ab}). The transpulmonary, transthoracic, and transdiaphragmatic pressures are all positive at FRC and become more positive during inspiration, returning to their FRC levels during exhalation.

THE THORACIC CAGE

The thorax is shaped like a truncated cone, being narrowest at the level of ribs 1 and 2 and widest at the level of ribs 8 and 9. The chest is somewhat compressed from the anteroposterior perspective, appearing elliptical instead of circular in profile. The thoracic cage is composed of 12 pairs of ribs and the sternum. The orientation of these ribs varies considerably—the two uppermost ribs (ribs 1 and 2) face downward, but as the lower ribs are successively viewed, the orientation shifts, so that ribs 10 to 12 face somewhat upward. Pairs 1 to 6 on either side of the sternum articulate directly with the sternum anteriorly; pairs 7 to 10 articulate anteriorly with the rib above them; and pairs 11 and 12 are considered floating ribs with no anterior articulation. All ribs articulate posteriorly with the vertebral column.

Movement of the rib cage varies, depending on the rib pairs involved. Generally, three movements have been described: the "pump handle" movement, the "bucket handle" movement, and the "caliper" movement (Fig. 5-2). The pump handle movement is a result of rotation of the rib at its spinal articulation, resulting in a forward and upward but only slightly lateral movement. This occurs in ribs whose orientation is downward, being noted primarily in rib pairs 1 to 6, and to a decreasing extent with successively lower ribs. The bucket handle movement is a lateral and upward movement of the rib with lesser forward movement. This movement occurs primarily at rib pairs 7 through 10, but is also present in the upper ribs. The caliper movement is a lateral and backward movement in rib pairs 11 and 12, which occurs primarily because of a lack of anterior articulation and muscular fixation. As a result, the anteroposterior diameter is greatest in the upper chest, whereas the transverse diameter is greatest at the lower ribs.

CHEST WALL MOVEMENT DURING BREATHING

During quiet breathing a distinct inspiratory pattern is noticeable. First the abdomen protrudes, next the lower lateral chest wall expands, and finally, the anterior upper chest wall expands. This movement is the result of a coordinated contraction of the muscles of inspiration. The abdomen protrudes as a result of contraction of the diaphragm, while lateral chest wall movement is a combined effect of diaphragmatic contraction and intercostal muscle contraction, and upper chest wall movement is primarily a result of the intercostal and scalene muscle movement. Exhalation is essentially a passive maneuver. Relaxation of the inspiratory muscles allows the lungs and thorax to recoil to their resting positions.

THE VENTILATORY MUSCLES

Inspiration is accomplished under normal resting condition by contraction of the diaphragm, scalene muscles, and parasternal intercostal muscles. Of these, the diaphragm is most important. During increased ventilatory demand, additional muscles of the neck, chest wall, and back are recruited. As a group these are referred to as *accessory muscles of inspiration*. Exhalation, on the other hand, is gen-

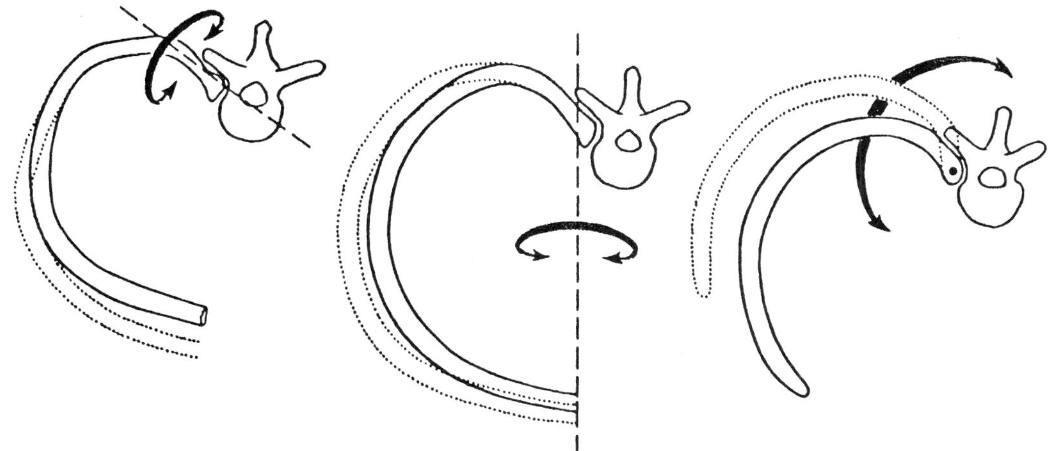

Figure 5-2. Scheme of axes and direction of movement of **(A)** upper ribs ("pump handle" movement); **(B)** lower ribs ("bucket handle" movement); **(C)** floating ribs ("caliper" movement). Inspiratory positions are indicated by broken lines. (From Osmond,[2] with permission.)

erally a passive maneuver accomplished by the recoil of lung and chest wall. During increased ventilatory demand the accessory muscles of expiration, the internal intercostals, and the abdominal wall muscles are recruited.

Diaphragm

The diaphragm is a thin musculotendinous sheet that forms the floor of the thoracic cavity. It is formed by two separate muscles (costal and crural) joined by a central tendon. The costal portion originates from the inner surfaces of ribs 7 to 12 and the sternum. Its fibers run parallel to the long axis of the body and directly opposed to the inner surface of the rib cage (Fig. 5-3). The crural portion originates primarily from the first three lumbar vertebral bodies. The costal and crural portions insert on the central tendon, which forms most of the dome of the diagram. In the standing position at FRC, the dome is located at the eighth thoracic vertebra on the right and at the ninth on the left. During contraction it is primarily the costal portion that shortens, decreasing the length of the zone of apposition (Fig. 5-4). Contraction of the diaphragm results in an increased transpulmonary pressure gradient and an increased transdiaphragmatic pressure gradient, as well as an increase in the transverse lower rib diameter and the superior-inferior thoracic volume. During tidal breathing, the diaphragm moves about 1.0 to 1.7 cm and may descend as much as 10 cm during a vital capacity inspiration. As a result, the abdominal cavity is compressed, the intra-abdominal pressure increased, and the abdomen is forced to protrude (Fig. 5-5). The presence of the zone of apposition ensures costal contraction and results in lateral rib cage expansion. At greater and greater lung volumes the zone of apposition becomes smaller and smaller. This causes the costal fibers to orient radially rather than axially and causes costal contraction to result in a decrease in lateral chest wall dimensions or an expiratory movement. This can become a major problem in patients with chronic airflow limitation, an increased FRC, and a flattened diaphragm. Also, as costal fiber length decreases, the muscle position shifts to one corresponding to a less advantageous portion of its length-tension curve, which results in a decreased transdiaphragmatic pressure gradient for a given neural stimulation (see Ch. 52). The diaphragm is innervated by the phrenic nerve, which originates at cervical vertebrae C3–C5.

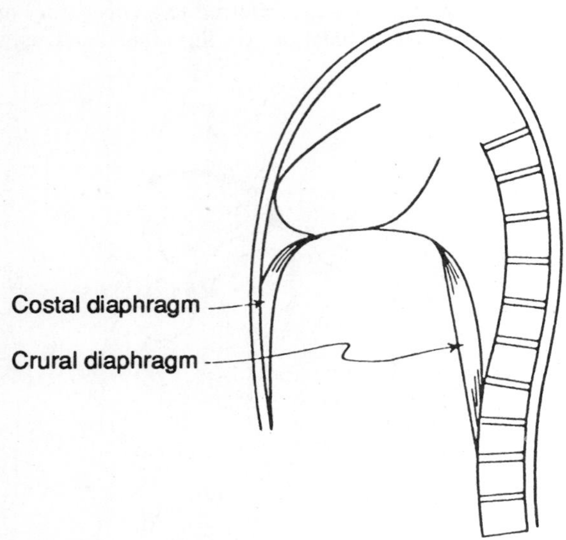

Figure 5-3. Anatomic representation of the costal and crural diaphragm. Both aspects of the diaphragm insert on the diaphragm's central tendon, which makes up most of the actual dome of the diaphragm. (From Macklem et al.,[3] with permission.)

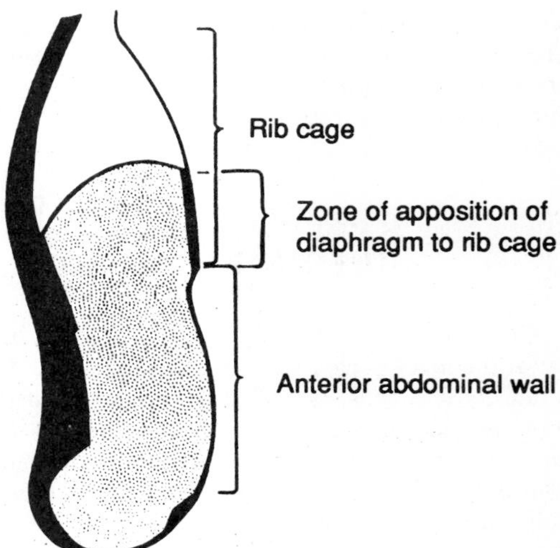

Figure 5-4. Schematic diagram of the major components of the body surface that displace volumes during breathing. The zone of apposition of the diaphragm to the rib cage covers a variable fraction of the rib cage's surface area. At residual volume, the zone of apposition covers half of the rib cage surface area. With increasing lung volume, the zone of apposition decreases. (From Mead et al.,[4] with permission.)

Intercostal Muscles

Between all ribs are located both external and internal intercostal muscles (Fig. 5-6). The internal muscle is actually two separate muscles, the parasternal intercostal muscle and the interosseous or the internal intercostal muscle. The external intercostal muscle runs obliquely downward and forward from upper rib to lower rib. Its insertion on the lower rib is thus further from the vertebral column than its origin on the upper rib. As a result, contraction tends to lift the lower rib, expanding thoracic volume. Both the parasternal and the interosseous intercostal muscles are located between adjacent costal cartilages, but since the upper insertion of the parasternal muscles is also on the sternum, contraction of the parasternal results in rib cage expansion, whereas con-

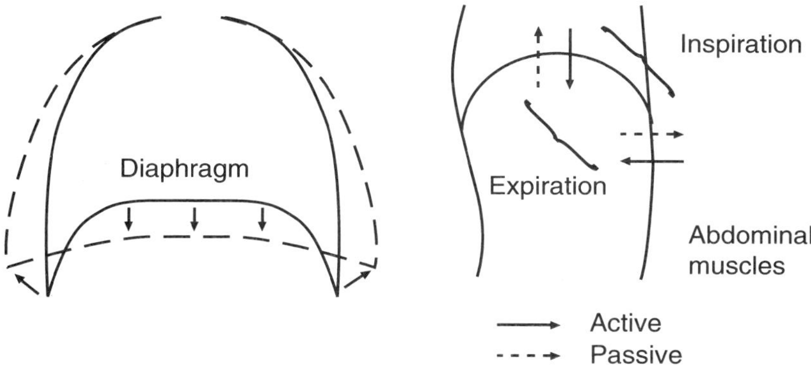

Figure 5-5. On inspiration, the dome-shaped diaphragm contracts, forcing the abdominal contents downward and forward, and the rib cage is lifted. Both movements increase the volume of the thorax. On forced expiration, the abdominal muscles contract and push the diaphragm upward. (From West et al.,[5] with permission.)

traction of the interosseous internal intercostal muscle results in rib cage compression. The parasternal muscles are active during quiet breathing, and the external and interosseous internal intercostal muscles are considered accessory muscles of ventilation. The external intercostal muscles become active during forced inspiration, and the interosseous internal intercostal muscles become active during forced expiration.

Scalene Muscles

Three sets of scalene muscles—anterior, medius, and posterior (Fig. 5-6)—arise from the lower five cervical vertebrae and insert on the first and second ribs. All are active during normal inspiration, raising both the first two ribs and the sternum. Some consider these to be accessory muscles of inspiration; however, recent data suggest they are active during normal breathing.

Sternomastoid Muscles

The sternomastoid muscles originate on the manubrium sterni and the medial third of the clavicle and insert onto the mastoid process and the occipital bone. Their action is inspiratory during stressed breathing, lifting the upper ribs and expanding the thorax. These muscles become very promi-

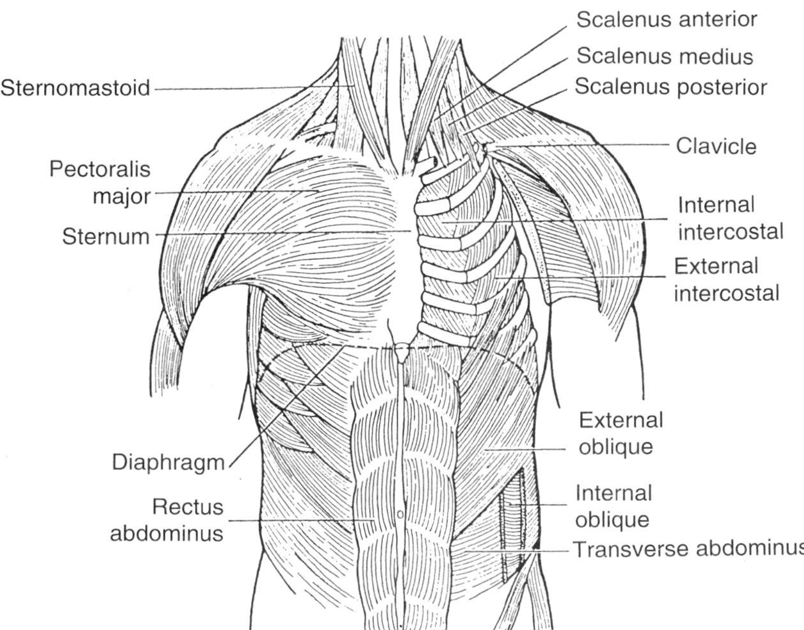

Figure 5-6. Schematic illustration of the major primary and accessory muscles of ventilation. See text for details. (From Scanlon et al.,[1] with permission.)

nent, as thick bands lateral to the larynx, during significant respiratory distress.

Abdominal Muscles

Four muscle groups make up the abdominal wall: the rectus abdominis, the internal oblique, the external oblique, and the transverse abdominis (Fig. 5-6). All of these function as accessory muscles of exhalation. As a group, their contraction results in a decrease in lower rib cage diameter and a compression of abdominal contents, forcing the diaphragm upward. During severe respiratory distress they also function as accessory muscles of inspiration by decreasing end-expiratory volume below its resting level. As a result, relaxation of the abdominals during inspiration allows re-establishment of resting end-expiratory volume and provides an inspiratory boost; thus, some of the inspiratory work is shifted to the accessory muscles of expiration.

Accessory Muscles of the Chest and Back

The pectoralis major and minor (Fig. 5-6), the serratus muscles, and the latissimus dorsi (Fig. 5-7) can all function as accessory muscles of ventilation during forced breathing. The pectoralis group and the serratus anterior assist in lifting the upper chest wall, while the actions of the latissimus dorsi, serratus posterior superior, and serratus posterior inferior during forced breathing are controversial. It would appear that they assist in stabilizing the spinal column during forced breathing and may play a role during expiration.

COORDINATED ACTIONS OF THE VENTILATORY MUSCLES DURING BREATHING

With different breathing patterns the various ventilatory muscle groups interact, combining their individual actions according to changing demands for depth and forcefulness of inhalation and exhalation. Quiet, tidal breathing involves mainly the diaphragm. Forcible exhalation against an obstruction, or performance of a maximal forced expiratory maneuver for spirometry, may activate all the expiratory muscles listed in Table 5-2; to hold one's breath at full inspiration with the glottis open requires near maximal contraction of all the corresponding inspiratory muscles. Precise, coordinated interaction of the ventilatory muscles is required for such voluntary acts as speaking, singing, and

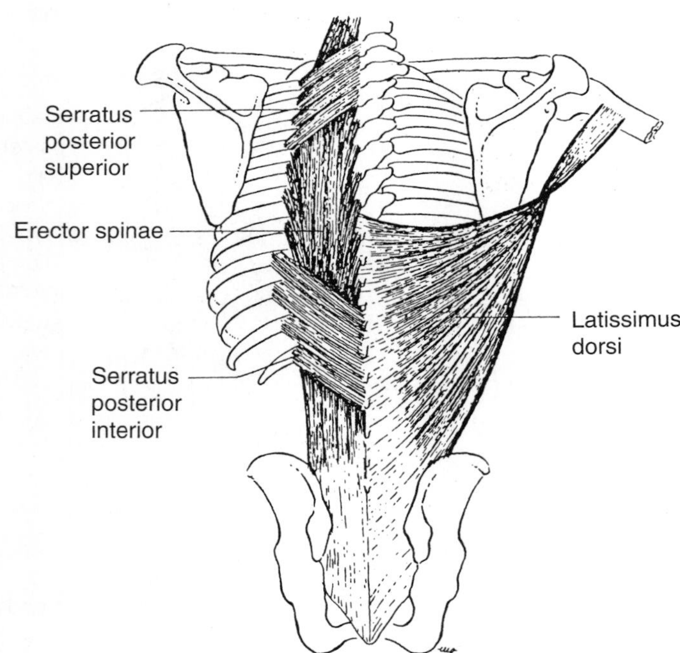

Figure 5-7. Schematic illustration of the muscles of the back that play a controversial role in ventilation. (From Osmond,[2] with permission.)

Table 5-2. Muscles of Breathing

Muscle(s)	Phase	Use	Origin	Insertion	Action
Costal diaphragm	Inspiration	Normal	Inner surface of ribs 7–12 and sternum	Central tendon	Increases superior-inferior lung volume; lower lateral rib cage expansion
Crural diaphragm	Inspiration	Normal	First 3 lumbar vertebrae	Central tendon	Increases superior-inferior lung volume; lateral rib cage expansion
Parasternal intercostal	Inspiration	Normal	Costal cartilage	Costal cartilage, sternum	Lift ribs and sternum
Interosseous internal intercostal	Expiration	Accessory	Costal cartilage	Costal cartilage	Pull ribs downward
External intercostal	Inspiration	Accessory	Upper ribs	Lower ribs	Lift ribs forward and upward
Scalene, medius and anterior	Inspiration	Normal	Lower 5 vertebrae	1st and 2nd ribs	Lift 1st and 2nd ribs and sternum
Sternomastoid	Inspiration	Accessory	Manubrium sterni and clavicle	Mastoid process and occipital bone	Lift upper ribs
External oblique	Expiratory	Accessory	Lower 8 ribs above the costal margins	Iliac crest and inguinal ligament	Constrict and compress diaphragm
Internal oblique	Expiratory	Accessory	Lumbar fascia, iliac crest, inguinal ligament	Costal margin, pubis	Constrict and compresses diaphragm
Transverse abdominis	Expiratory	Accessory	Costal margin	Midline aponeurosis of the rectus sheath	Constricts and compresses diaphragm
Rectus abdominis	Expiratory	Accessory	Costal cartilage of ribs 5–7	Pubis	Constricts and compresses diaphragm
Pectoralis major	Inspiration	Accessory	Clavicle	Sternum, costal cartilage	Lifts upper chest wall
Pectoralis minor	Inspiration	Accessory	Ribs 3–5, near costal cartilage	Scapula	Lifts upper chest wall
Latissimus dorsi	Expiratory (controversial)	Accessory	Lumbar and sacral vertebrae	Humerus	Stabilizes back and vertebral column
Serratus anterior	Expiratory	Accessory	8 upper ribs	Scapula	Stabilizes back and vertebral column
Serratus, posterior superior	Expiratory	Accessory	Cervical and dorsal vertebrae	Ribs 2–5	Stabilizes back and vertebral column
Serratus, posterior inferior	Expiratory	Accessory	Dorsal and lumbar vertebrae	Ribs 9–12	Stabilizes back and vertebral column

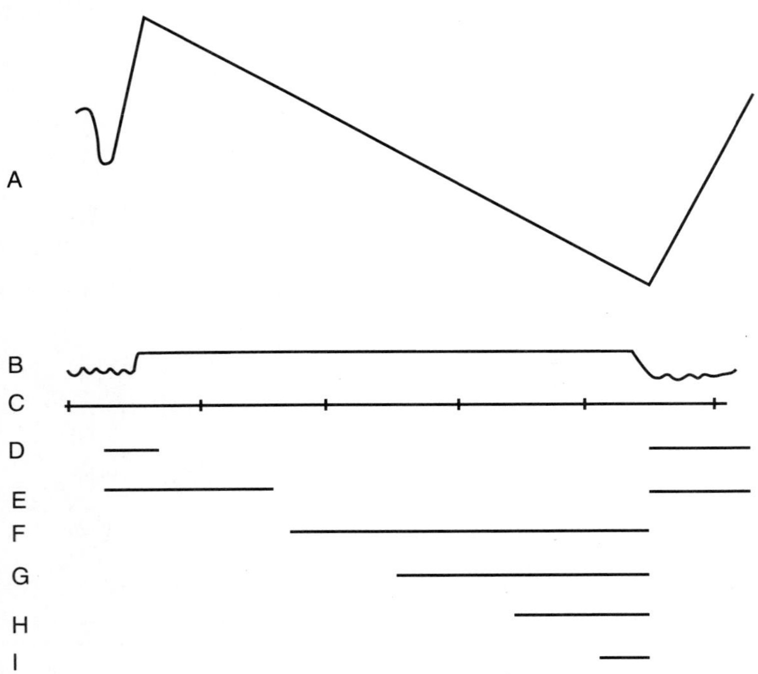

Figure 5-8. Simultaneously recorded pressure and volume events, plus electromyographic activity, during the production of a continuous tone by a singer, starting at full inspiration and continuing to the lowest possible lung volume. The different ventilatory muscles become active at different stages in the maneuver. A, lung volume; B, subglottic pressure; C, time in 10-second intervals; D–I, electromyographic activity of different muscle groups (inspiratory: D, diaphragm; E, external intercostal muscles; expiratory: F, internal intercostal muscles; G, external oblique muscles; H, rectus abdominus; I, latissimus dorsi). (From Proctor,[6] as adapted from Ladefoged,[7] with permission.)

wind instrument playing, as illustrated by Figure 5-8, which represents a subject taking a maximal inspiration and then singing a single continuous tone for as long as possible. Control of the air escaping from the lungs is accomplished at first by the inspiratory muscles and then by first one followed by progressively larger numbers of the expiratory muscles in order to maintain a constant airflow and subglottic pressure as lung volume progressively decreases. Similarly coordinated actions of the different ventilatory muscle groups are used during pulmonary function testing, breathing retraining, and other aspects of respiratory care.

References

1. Scanlan CL, Spearman CB, Sheldon RL: Egan's Fundamentals of Respiratory Therapy. 5th Ed. CV Mosby, St. Louis, 1989
2. Osmond DG: Functional anatomy of the chest wall. pp. 208–235. In Roussos C, Macklem PT (eds): The Thorax, Part A. Marcel Dekker, New York, 1985
3. Macklem PT, Macklem DM, DeTroyer A: A model of inspiratory muscle mechanics. J Appl Physiol 1983;55:547–557
4. Mead J, Smith JC, Loring SH: Volume displacement of the chest wall and its mechanical significance. pp. 260–281. In Roussos C, Macklem PT (eds): The Thorax, Part A. Marcel Dekker, New York, 1985
5. West JB: Respiratory Physiology—The Essentials. 4th Ed. Williams & Wilkins, Baltimore, 1990
6. Proctor DF: Modifications of breathing for phonation. pp. 597–604. In Macklem PT, Mead J (eds): The Respiratory System. Vol. 3. Mechanics of Breathing, Part 2. American Physiological Society, Bethesda, 1986
7. Ladefoged P: Three Areas of Experimental Phonetics. Oxford University Press, London, 1967

Chapter 6

The Pleura and Pleural Space

David J. Pierson

CHAPTER OUTLINE

The *pleurae* are the serous membranes that cover the outside surface of the lungs and line the thoracic cavity, enabling the lungs to move freely during breathing, coughing, and other activities. Between them lies the *pleural space* or *pleural cavity*. These structures are important in respiratory care because of the frequency with which they are affected by disease, trauma, diagnostic procedures, or therapy. Several general sources provide more information on the pleural space and its disorders than can be presented here.[1–3]

ANATOMY

The normal pleura[4] is a smooth, glistening, semitransparent membrane made up of a single layer of mesothelial cells, along with blood vessels, lymphatics, and connective tissue. It is divided into the *visceral* and *parietal* pleurae. The parietal pleura lines the chest cavity, covering the mediastinum, the diaphragm, and the structures of the chest wall. It is supplied with sensory nerve fibers and is thus the source of pain originating from the pleura. The visceral pleura lines the lungs themselves, including the interlobar fissures, and lacks pain fibers. At the lung hilum the two pleural surfaces join.

Laterally where the diaphragm meets the rib cage and especially far posteriorly, the pleural cavity extends inferiorly (caudal) to the rest of the diaphragm into the costophrenic recesses or sulci. During normal breathing the tips of these recesses contain only the two pleural surfaces and a little fluid, but during maximum inspiration, as for example during sighing or coughing, the lung moves downward into them.

Normally the amount of pleural fluid is very small—a few milliliters at most—although a substantial volume of liquid moves through the pleural space each day. In humans the two pleural cavities are separate, so that an accumulation of air or liquid on one side does not generally cross into the other; this is not the case in dogs and some other mammals, in which the right and left pleural cavities are continuous.

PHYSIOLOGY

The pressures and fluid dynamics of the pleural space[5–7] are complex topics that continue to be the focus of research.[8] However, conceptual understanding of these functions is crucial to the physiologic approaches to assessment and management presented in this book.

A primary function of the pleural space is to maintain effective coupling between the visceral and parietal pleurae in order to keep the lungs inflated. If the thorax is opened at operation or autopsy, the chest wall springs outward and the lung collapses. Under normal conditions the lung and chest wall coexist in a state of tension, the lung attempting to become smaller and the chest wall attempting to become larger,

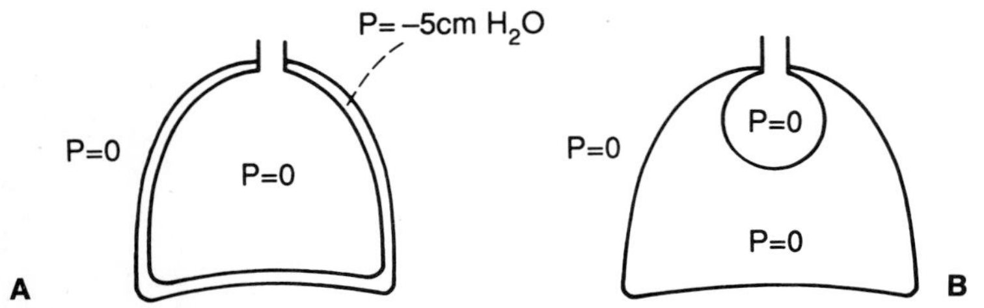

Figure 6-1. The lung's tendency to recoil to a smaller volume is countered by that of the chest wall to expand. **(A)** At the normal end-expiratory resting lung volume (functional residual capacity), the pressures in both lung and surrounding air are zero, but their opposing recoil forces generate a pressure in the pleural space of approximately -5 cmH_2O. **(B)** If air were allowed to enter the pleural cavity freely, the seal between visceral and parietal pleural surfaces would be lost, and both lung and chest wall would assume their "natural" resting volumes. In this instance (total pneumothorax) all three pressures would be zero.

as discussed further in Chapter 9. This tension results in a negative pressure in the pleural space with respect to that in the alveoli. At normal resting end-expiratory lung volume, or functional residual capacity (FRC), at which alveolar pressure is zero, pleural pressure is about -5 cmH_2O.[9,10]

During inspiration pleural pressure becomes more negative, thereby transmitting the force generated by the diaphragm and chest wall muscles to the lung. Because there is normally no source of air entry into the pleural space, the lungs must also expand when the respiratory muscles expand the thorax, being sucked open because of the close coupling of the visceral and parietal pleural surfaces. If air were permitted to enter the pleural space, both the negative pleural pressure and the coupling between the two pleural surfaces would be lost, and the lung and chest wall would each move independently toward their natural resting states. This concept is illustrated in Figure 6-1.

Another primary function of the pleural space is to lubricate the lung surfaces[6] by maintaining a continuous fluid layer to cover them. Fluid is elaborated from both the parietal and visceral pleural membranes, each of which is supplied by systemic vessels (in the case of the visceral pleura,

Table 6-1. Potential Mechanisms for Accumulation of Pleural Fluid

Mechanism	Explanation	Clinical Examples
Increased hydrostatic pressure in microvascular circulation	At parietal surface Increased systemic venous pressure	Right-sided heart failure
	At visceral surface Increased pulmonary venous pressure (e.g., increased pulmonary capillary wedge pressure)	Left-sided heart failure
	Combination of both	Combined left- and right-sided heart failure
Decreased osmotic pressure in microvascular circulation	Increased tendency for pleural interstitial fluid to move into pleural space (relatively infrequent clinically because of large functional reserve of parietal pleural lymphatics)	Nephrotic syndrome; severe malnutrition
Decreased pressure in pleural space	Increased negativity of pleural space pressure; increased tendency for pleural interstitial fluid to move into pleural space; decreased tendency for this fluid to be absorbed	Collapse (atelectasis) of one entire lung
Increased microvascular permeability	Decrease in physical integrity of capillary walls due to release of inflammatory mediators, with increased leakage of liquid and proteins across lung and pleural microvessels	Effusion association with pneumonia (parapneumonic effusion)
Impaired lymphatic drainage from pleural space	Blockage anywhere from tiny lymphatic stomata on pleural surface to mediastinal lymph nodes, with loss of normal lymphatic drainage (main mechanism for removal of pleural fluid)	Malignant effusion; effusion associated with mediastinal fibrosis
Movement of fluid from peritoneal space	Passage of ascitic fluid via diaphragmatic lymphatics or through defects in diaphragm into pleural space	Hepatic failure (e.g., alcoholic cirrhosis) with massive ascites

(Adapted from Pierson,[2] with permission.)

Table 6-2. Disorders of the Pleura and Pleural Space

Air in the pleural space
Pneumothorax: Presence of air in the pleural space

Tension pneumothorax: Accumulation of pleural air under sufficient positive pressure to cause adverse physiologic effects (e.g., hypotension)

Bronchopleural fistula: Communication between the airways and the pleural space, occurring either spontaneously or as a result of therapy or diagnostic procedure

Hemo-, hydro-, or pyopneumothorax: Presence of both air and liquid in pleural cavity (see below)

Fluid accumulation in the pleural space
Pleural effusion: Accumulation of fluid in the pleural space, more precisely designated by one or more of the following terms if the necessary information is available

Transudate: Pleural fluid that accumulates because of systemic rather than local pleural factors, such as increased hydrostatic pressure, decreased osmotic forces, or decreased pressure in the pleural cavity (see Table 6-1); transudates have low concentrations of proteins and cells and resemble a filtrate of plasma

Exudate: Pleural fluid that accumulates as a result of local pleural factors, primarily inflammation; exudates have a high protein concentration and other characteristics of inflammatory fluid

Hydrothorax: Another term (literally, "water in the chest") for pleural effusion, particularly when it is not described by one of the following terms

Hemothorax: Pleural fluid that is grossly bloody

Chylothorax: Lymph (chyle) in the pleural space, generally from lymphatic disruption by trauma or malignancy

Malignant effusion: Accumulation of pleural fluid caused by cancer

Parapneumonic effusion: Pleural effusion occurring in association with pneumonia

Thoracic empyema (pyothorax): Condition (literally, "pus in the pleural space") present if the fluid is frankly purulent, if Gram stain or culture is positive for infectious organisms, or if the leukocyte count in the fluid is very high (e.g., >50,000–100,000 cells/mL)

Increased pleural tissue
Plaque: Localized thickening of parietal pleura over chest wall or diaphragm, often calcified, usually caused by asbestos exposure

Diffuse thickening (fibrothorax): Generalized pleural thickening, either unilateral (e.g., following trauma or empyema) or bilateral (e.g., related to abestos exposure)

Localized mass: May be either malignant (mesothelioma or metastatic carcinoma, both usually with associated effusion) or benign (numerous uncommon causes)

via the bronchial circulation). Absorption of pleural fluid is principally (approximately 90 percent[8]) by lymphatics, which also absorb particles, large proteins, and cells. The remainder is absorbed via convection across the pleural mesothelium into the lung and chest wall.

The pleural cavity remains one of the body's "potential spaces" of negligible volume so long as the formation and absorption of pleural fluid are equal. Elaboration and elimination of pleural fluid are affected by the Frank-Starling principle, which relates hydrostatic pressure with oncotic pressure and membrane permeability, as discussed in Chapter 1. If the rate of fluid production increases beyond a certain limit or if its absorption is reduced, fluid will accumulate in the pleural space. Potential mechanisms by which this may occur are shown in Table 6-1, along with clinical examples of each.

DISORDERS OF THE PLEURA AND PLEURAL SPACE

Pleural disease causes predictable manifestations, depending on the derangements it causes in normal structure and function.[1–3,9] Irritation of sensory fibers in the parietal pleura typically produces *pleuritic chest pain*, which is sharp, stabbing, usually unilateral, and worsened by inhaling deeply, coughing, or otherwise moving the chest. Pleural disease also commonly causes *dyspnea* due to its restrictive effect on pulmonary mechanics, whether from pain or from alterations in lung and chest wall compliance.

Disorders of the pleura can be categorized into those caused by air in the chest, by an accumulation of pleural fluid, or by an increase in solid tissue in the pleural space (Table 6-2). All produce a restrictive-type functional abnormality, as described more fully in Chapter 21. Some of the specific diseases affecting the pleura are discussed in Chapter 23, and the management of pleural air and fluid is covered in Chapter 92.

References

1. Light RW: Pleural Diseases. 2nd Ed. Lea & Febiger, Philadelphia, 1990
2. Sahn SA: State of the art: The pleura. Am Rev Respir Dis 1988;138:184–234
3. Pierson DJ: Disorders of the pleura, mediastinum, and diaphragm. pp. 1111–1116. In Wilson JD, Braunwald E, Fauci AS et al (eds): Harrison's Principles of Internal Medicine. 12th Ed. McGraw-Hill, New York, 1990
4. Wang NS: Anatomy and physiology of the pleural space. Clin Chest Med 1985;6:3–16
5. Staub NC, Wiener-Kronish JP, Albertine KH: Liquid transport through the pleura: Physiology of normal liquid and solute exchange in the pleural space. pp. 169–193. In Chretein J, Bignon J, Hirsh A (eds): The Pleura in Health and Disease. Marcel Dekker, New York, 1985
6. Lai-Fook SJ: Mechanics of the pleural space: Fundamental concepts. Lung 1987;165:249–267
7. Hills BA: The pleural interface. Thorax 1985;40:1–8
8. Broaddus VC, Wiener-Kronish JP, Berthiaume Y, Staub NC: Removal of pleural liquid and protein by lymphatics in awake sheep. J Appl Physiol 1988;64:384–390
9. Culver BH (ed): The Respiratory System: Syllabus for Human Biology 541. Lecture Notes. University of Washington, Seattle, 1991
10. West JB: Respiratory Physiology: The Essentials. 3rd Ed. Williams & Wilkins, Baltimore, 1985

Chapter 7

The Lungs and Airways

Robert L. Wilkins
David J. Pierson

CHAPTER OUTLINE

The primary function of the airways and lungs is gas exchange between the blood and the environment. During ventilation air will come into contact with many different tissues, which direct and prepare the inhaled gas for presentation to the terminal gas exchange units. A solid understanding of the structures related to gas exchange is essential to the understanding of respiratory function in health and disease. To this end the gross and microscopic anatomy of the intrapulmonary airways and lungs is described in this chapter. The references at the end of the chapter provide more detailed descriptions of pulmonary anatomy.[1–8]

ANATOMY OF THE INTRAPULMONARY AIRWAYS

Organization of the Airways

The tracheobronchial tree (Fig. 7-1), which takes on the appearance of an inverted tree, contains three types of airways: cartilaginous airways, membranous bronchioles, and gas exchange ducts. While all three serve to conduct gas, only the last also serves a dual purpose of conduction and gas exchange. The cartilaginous airways include the trachea, primary bronchi (right and left main stem bronchi), lobar bronchi, segmental bronchi, subsegmental bronchi, and approximately five generations of small bronchi (Fig. 7-2). The primary bronchi, as well as the trachea, contain horseshoe-shaped rings of cartilage in their walls to provide structural support, but here the cartilaginous rings are more complete and regular than in the trachea. Distal to the primary bronchi the cartilage becomes progressively scarcer and more irregular in shape.

It is important to note that the larger bronchi ventilate very specific sections of the lung and precisely match specific lobes and segments (Fig. 7-3). Because of this, the larger bronchi are called *lobar* and *segmental* bronchi accordingly. This matching is the result of embryologic development (see Ch. 3). Each lobe and segment has a specific name, as shown in Figure 7-3. Familiarity with the topographic location of the lobes and segments can be of clinical value during the localization of physical examination findings and in the application of chest physical therapy to specific sections of the lung. As seen in Figure 7-3, the right lung has three lobes, upper, middle, and lower. The left lung has only two lobes, the upper and lower. Although the left lung does not have

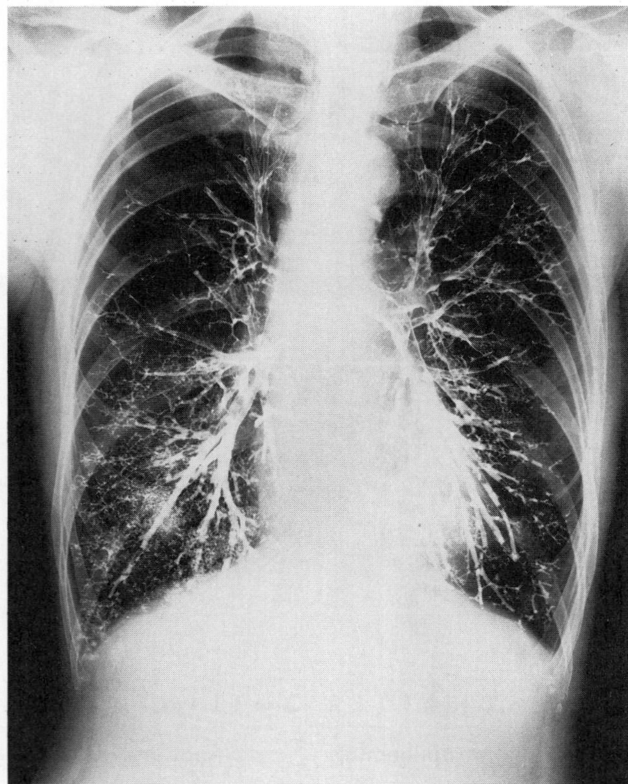

Figure 7-1. Normal bronchogram of both lungs, outlining the tracheobronchial tree.

a middle lobe, the lower, anterior portion of the left upper lobe (the lingula) is analogous to the right middle lobe.

The membranous bronchioles are very small in diameter (1 mm or less) and length and do not contain cartilage in their walls (Table 7-1). While these airways are numerous, they contribute very little to the anatomic dead space and airway resistance. Most of the airway resistance and most of the anatomic dead space reside in the cartilaginous bronchi, trachea, and upper airways. The membranous bronchioles consist of eight generations of airways, including the primary, secondary, terminal, and respiratory bronchioles.

The respiratory bronchioles give way to the first generation of gas exchange ducts, called the *alveolar ducts*, of which there are five generations. The alveolar ducts are connected to tightly packed alveolar sacs. A discussion of the gas exchange units at the microscopic level is presented in Chapter 10.

Microscopic Anatomy of the Intrapulmonary Airways

The larger intrapulmonary airways are lined with ciliated pseudostratified columnar cells, which extend distally into the respiratory bronchioles. Mixed with the ciliated cells are secretory and basal cells. All three types of cells rest on a basement membrane, overlying the *lamina propria*, a loose network of fibers containing smooth muscle and other cells, a rich capillary network, and unmyelinated nerves. The thickness of the epithelial lining gradually decreases as the airways decrease in diameter, so that in the terminal bronchiole the mucosa is composed of low, ciliated cells that are more cuboidal than columnar. At the point of transition to the gas exchange region, the epithelium abruptly becomes very thin (Fig. 7-4).

Two types of mucus-secreting cells are present in the intrapulmonary airways, epithelial mucous cells and epithelial serous cells. Mucus-secreting cells are also called *goblet cells* when they are enlarged by the accumulation of mucus (Fig. 7-5). Mucus-secreting cells are more commonly identified in the larger airways, decreasing in number as the airways become smaller and normally disappearing at the terminal bronchioles. In the airways of smokers, mucous cells are more numerous and are more frequently found in the distal airways.[9]

Lining the respiratory tract is a mucus blanket, which serves to protect the airway walls. This mucus blanket is 10 to 20 μm thick and is made up of two layers, a top layer of

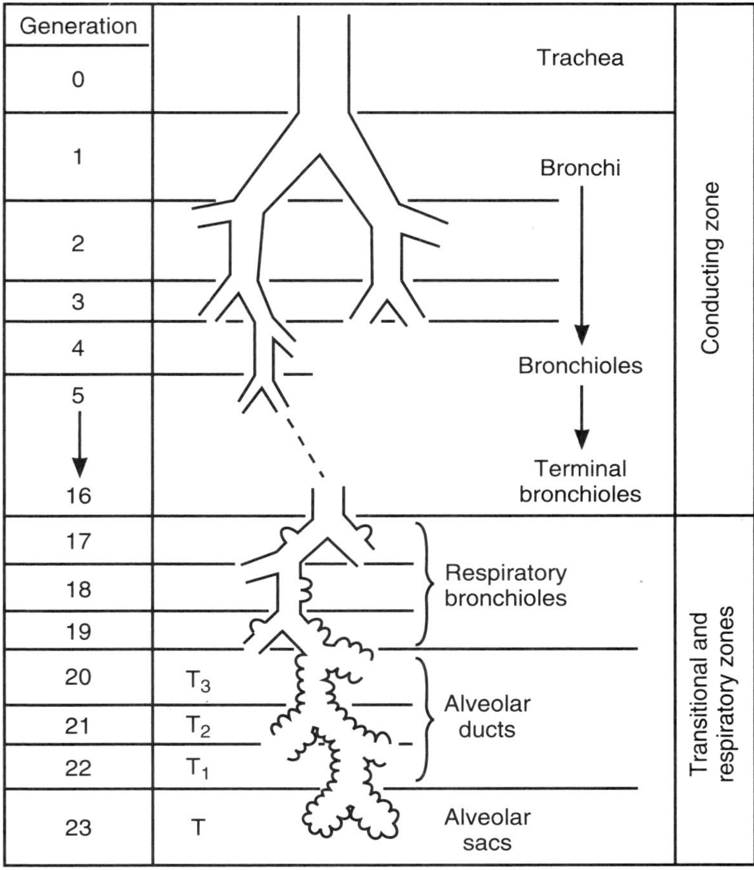

Figure 7-2. Airway branching in the human lung by regularized dichotomy from the trachea (generation 0) to alveolar ducts and sacs (generations 20–23), according to scheme of Weibel.[21] The first 16 generations are strictly conducting, and transitional airways lead into the respiratory zone containing alveoli. (Data from Weibel.[21])

gel and a lower layer of *sol*. The gel layer is made up of hydrated mucus, while the underlying sol layer is less viscous. The mucus blanket, which is capable of trapping inhaled particles of dust and debris, is gradually moved towards the larynx by the coordinated sweeping action of the cilia (Fig. 7-6). Healthy ciliary function will move the mucus toward the larynx at a rate of 20 mm/min.[10] This cleansing mechanism prevents the respiratory tract from harboring bacteria and debris and delivers a steady flow of mucus toward the pharynx. In most cases the mucus delivered to the larynx is swallowed and goes unnoticed. A more detailed discussion of lung defense mechanisms is presented in Chapter 17.

In the trachea and large bronchi a band of smooth muscle is present within the opening of the U-shaped cartilage on the posterior side of the airway. Moving peripherally as the cartilaginous rings are replaced with plates, the smooth muscle begins to become a more dominant part of the airway wall. In the medium and small bronchi the smooth muscle has a helical orientation, with fibers spiraling in many directions and crisscrossing the walls. The bands of muscle are not uniform, some areas having a greater thickness than others. Owing to the crisscross design of the smooth muscle at this point, contraction of the muscles will shorten the airways as well as reduce their diameter.[2]

ANATOMY OF THE LUNGS

Gross Anatomy

The normal lungs at end exhalation are approximately 24 cm in height and weigh 900 to 1000 g. The right lung is slightly larger and wider but shorter than the left lung (Fig. 7-7). This

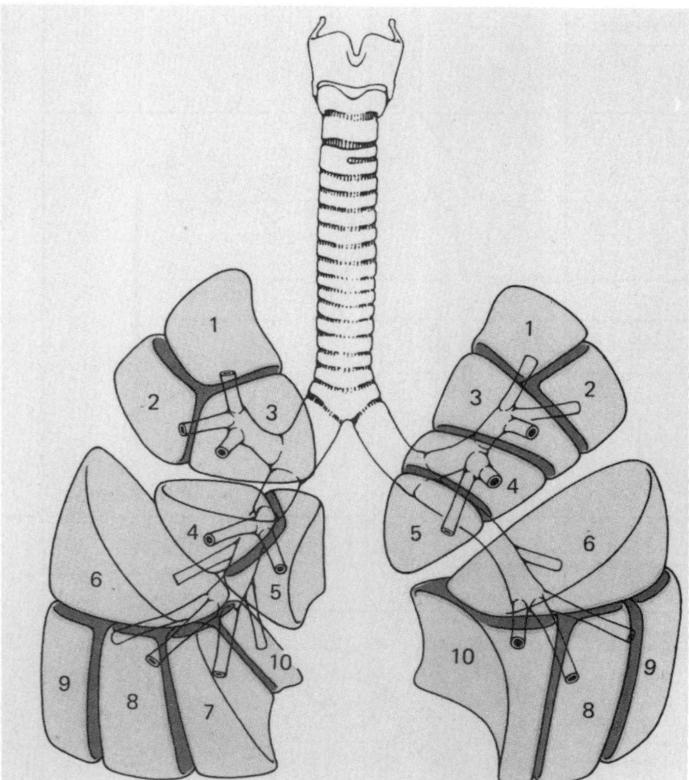

Figure 7-3. Bronchopulmonary segments of the lungs. Left and right upper lobes: 1, apical; 2, posterior; 3, anterior; 4, superior lingular; and 5, inferior lingular segments. Right middle lobe: 4, lateral; and 5, medial segments. Lower lobes: 6, superior (apical); 7, medial basal; 8, anterior basal; 9, lateral basal; and 10, posterior basal segments. The medial basal segment 7 is absent in the left lung. (*Note*: The lungs are represented as slightly turned inward in order to display part of the lateral face. (From Weibel and Taylor,[1] with permission.)

is partly due to the position of the pericardium, which is notched into the medial surface of the left lung. The apex of the lungs extend approximately 2 cm above the medial third of the clavicles. The inferior margin of the lungs is dome-shaped, rests on the diaphragm, and varies with breathing. At rest the anterior diaphragmatic margin does not extend to the limits of the pleural margins but is located at about the sixth anterior rib at the midclavicular line of the anterior chest.

After birth, the lungs are spongy masses of tissue, which will float because of the many air-filled alveoli. The density of the lungs varies with the amount of air contained within. At the end of a passive exhalation, the adult lungs contain approximately 2.5 L of gas and have a density of 0.30 g/mL. At total lung capacity, the lungs contain about 6 L and have a density of 0.14 g/mL. The density of the lung is not uniformly the same throughout all lung regions. The peripheral lung tissue is less dense than the regions around the hilum, and the top of the lung is less dense than the lower lung fields.

On the surface of both lungs a deep interlobular fissure, known as the *oblique* or *major fissure* is visible (Fig. 7-7). The right lung also has a *horizontal* or *minor fissure*. The oblique fissure extends from the inferior border of the lung, at the midclavicular line on the anterior chest, laterally and upward to near the apex and dorsally to about the third thoracic vertebra. In the right lung, the oblique fissure separates the middle lobe from the lower lobe anteriorly and divides the upper lobe from the lower laterally and posteriorly. In the left lung the oblique fissure serves to separate the upper lobe from the lower.

Generation	Name	Diameter (cm)	Length (cm)	No. per Generation	Histologic Notes
0	Trachea	1.8	12	1	Wealth of goblet cells
1	Primary bronchi	1.2	4.8	2	Right larger than left
2	Lobar bronchi	0.8	0.9	5	3 right, 2 left
3	Segmental bronchi	0.6	0.8	19	10 right; 8 left
4	Subsegmental bronchi	0.5	1.3	20	
5 ↓	Small bronchi	0.4	1.1	40	Still have cartilage; many cell types as well as respiratory epithelium
10		0.1	0.5	1020	
11 ↓	Bronchioles, primary and secondary	0.1 0.1	0.4	2050	No cartilage; smooth muscle, cilia, goblet cells present
13			0.3	8190	
14 ↓	Terminal bronchioles	0.1	0.2	16,380	No goblet cells; smooth muscle, cilia, and cuboidal cells
15		0.1	0.2	32,770	
16 ↓	Respiratory bronchioles	0.1	0.2	65,540	No smooth muscle; cilia, cuboidal cells; cilia disappear
18		0.1	0.1	262,140	
19 ↓	Alveolar ducts	0.05	0.1	524,290	No cilia; cuboidal cells
23		0.04	0.05	8,390,000	
24	Alveoli[a]	244	238	300,000,000	

Table 7-1. Subdivisions of the Respiratory Tree

[a] Alveolar dimensions given in micrometers.
(From Weibel,[21] with permission.)

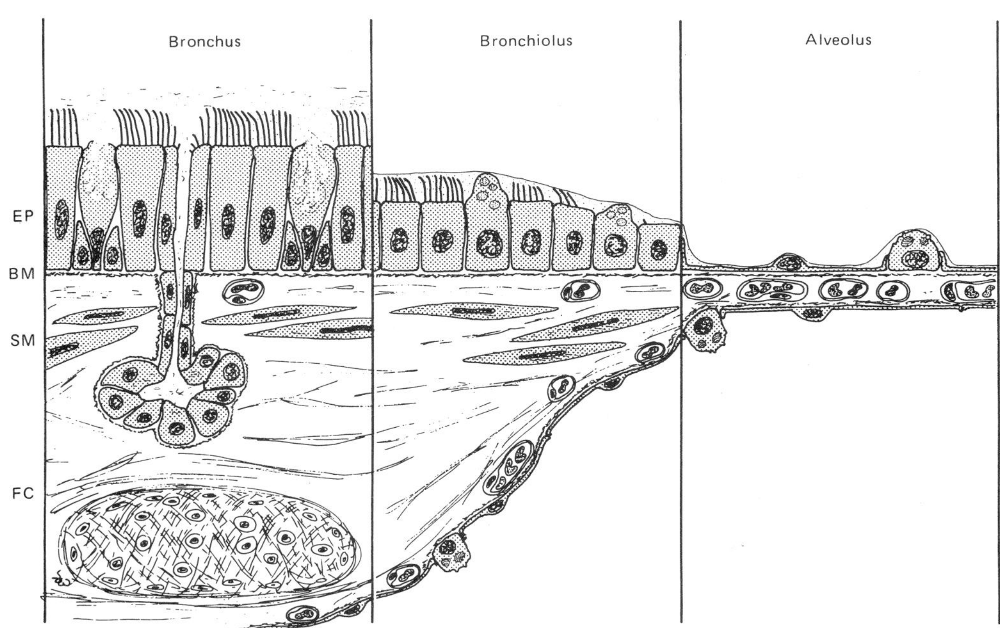

Figure 7-4. Airway wall structure at the three principal levels. The epithelial layer (EP) gradually becomes thinner, changing from pseudostratified to cuboidal and then to squamous in structure, but retains its organization as a mosaic of lining and secretory cells. The smooth muscle layer (SM) disappears in the alveoli. The fibrous coat (FC) contains cartilage only in bronchi and gradually becomes thinner as the alveolus is approached. BM, basement membrane. (From Weibel and Taylor,[1] with permission.)

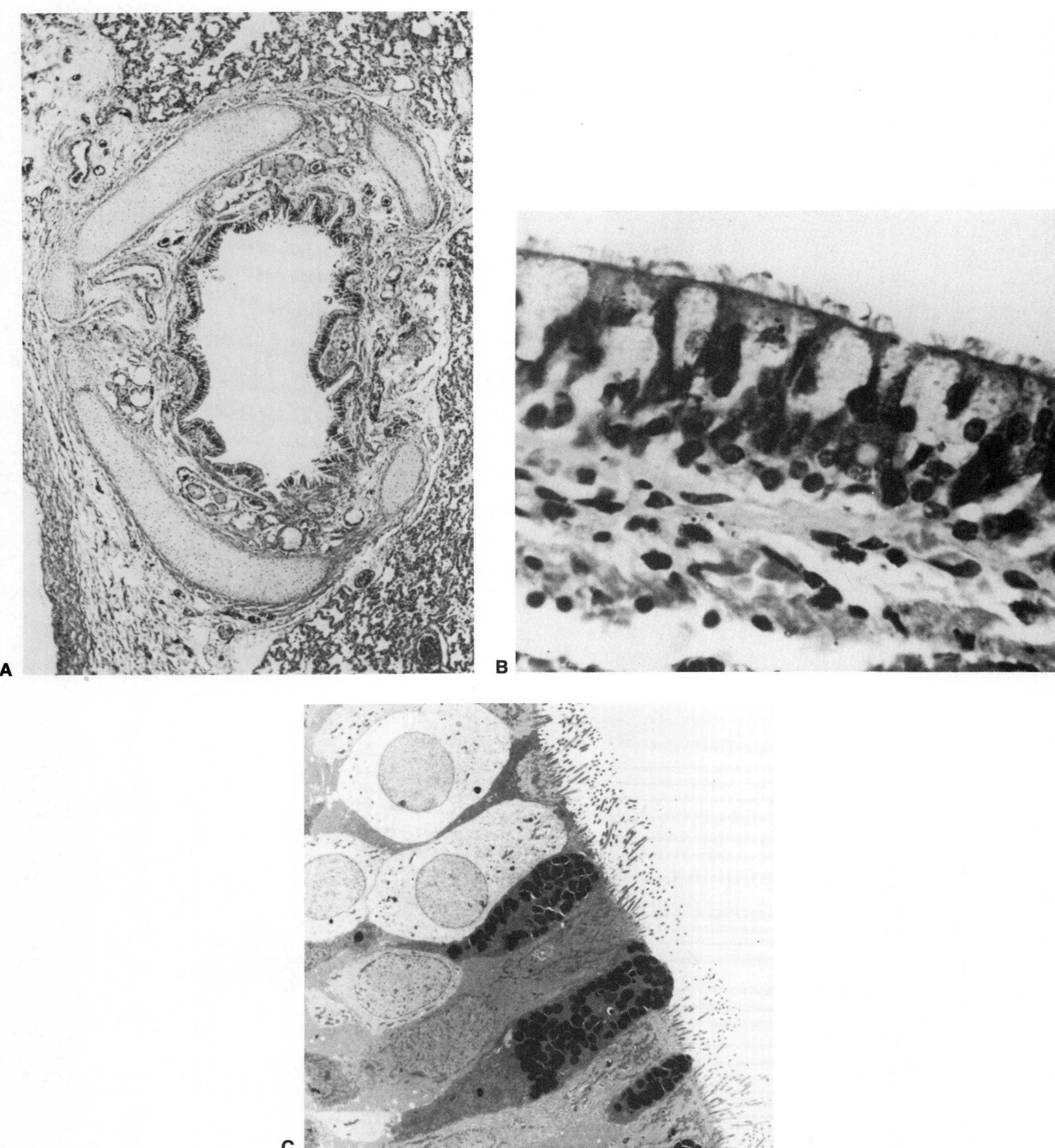

Figure 7-5. **(A)** Cross section through an intrapulmonary bronchus, showing cartilages incompletely encircling the lumen. (× 150.) **(B)** Light photomicrograph of normal bronchial mucosa, composed of columnar ciliated cells, goblet cells, and basal cells. (H&E, × 350.) **(C)** Electron micrograph of normal human bronchial mucosa at high power, showing ciliated cells interspersed with goblet cells. (Fig. A from Kuhn[23] and Figs. B & C from Dunnill,[24] with permission.)

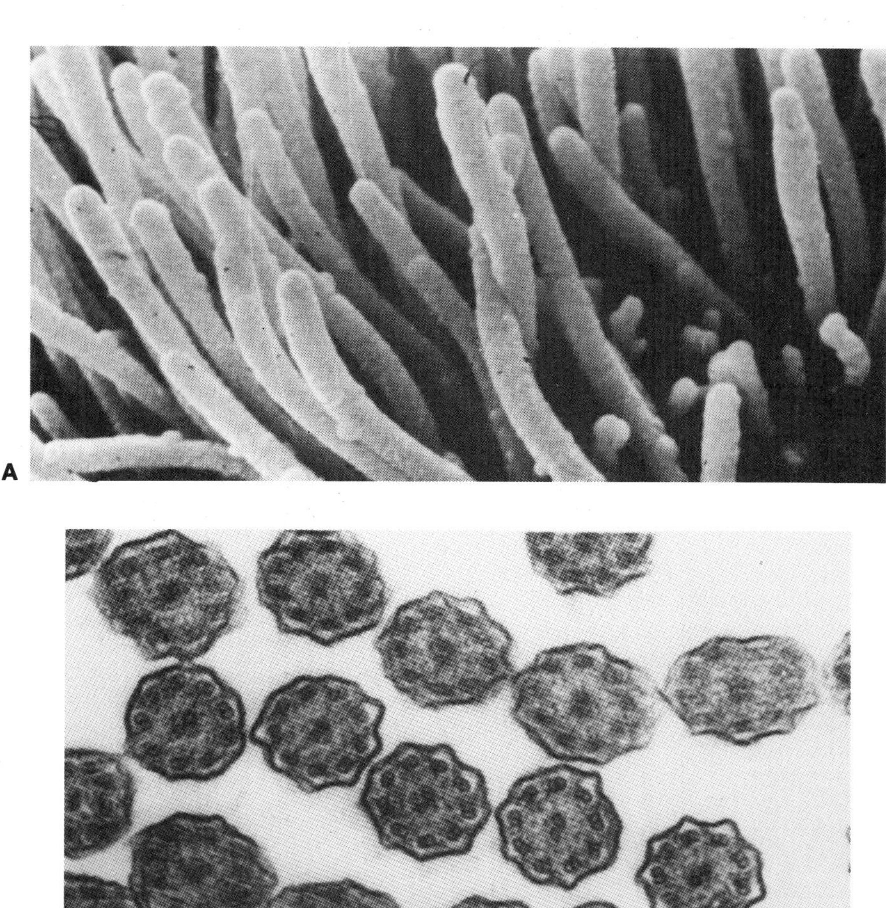

Figure 7-6. (**A**) Scanning electron micrograph of cilia. (**B**) Transmission electron micrograph showing normal cilia in cross section. ($\times$ 65,000.) (From Dunnill,[24] with permission.)

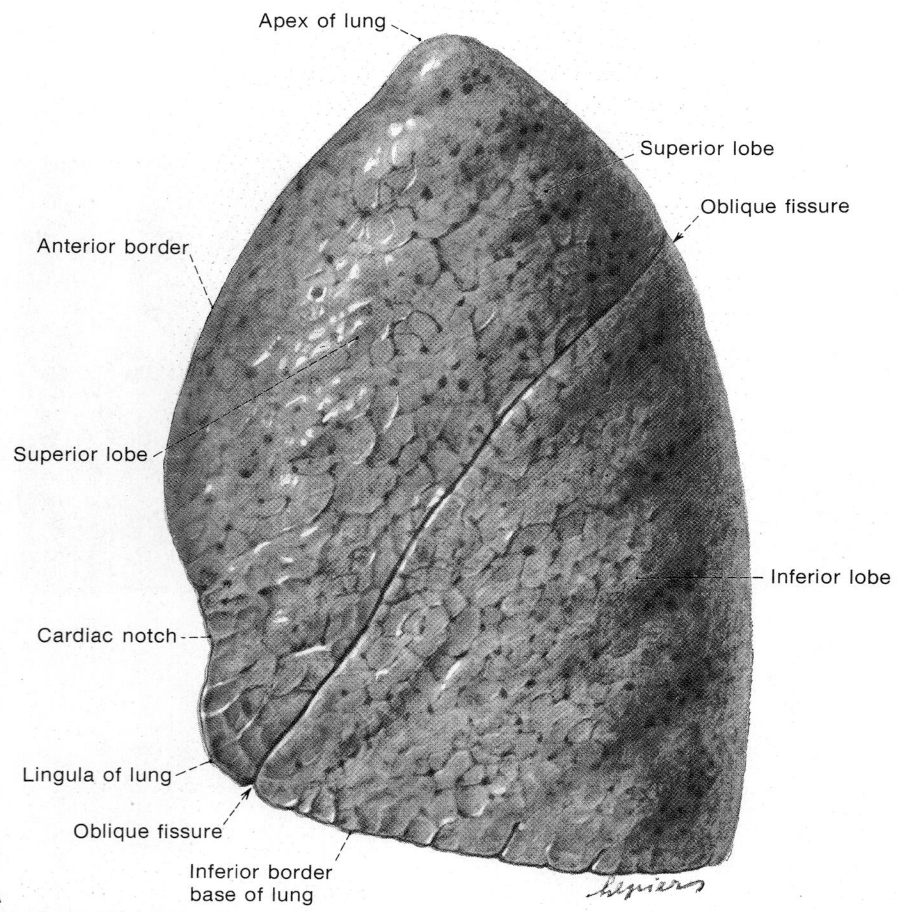

Figure 7-7. Gross photograph of normal lung, showing costal view of **(A)** left and **(B)** right lung. (From Montgomery,[4] with permission.)

Microscopic Anatomy

The process of gas exchange occurs in the *terminal respiratory units* of the lungs. Each of these units, also called *acinus*, is made up of all the alveolar ducts and alveoli that stem from the most proximal or first respiratory bronchiole (Fig. 7-8). An acinus can also be defined as consisting of all structures distal to the end of a terminal bronchiole. Each acinus is believed to contain about 100 alveolar ducts and 2000 tightly packed alveoli.[6] At the end of a passive exhalation this unit is approximately 5 mm in diameter and has a volume of 0.02 mL. Each lung of a healthy adult contains approximately 150,000 terminal respiratory units, from which it is estimated that approximately 300 million alveoli are present in the adult respiratory system. This number varies directly with the height of the individual.[2]

Since it is believed that the average neonate has 50 million alveoli,[11] the majority of the gas exchange units are developed after birth. The age at which alveolar multiplication stops is controversial[12]; however, one careful study has reported this age as about 8 years.[13]

Although the typical lung model depicts round alveoli, this depiction is not accurate; in reality the alveolus is a complex geometric structure with flat walls and sharp curvature at the junction between walls (Fig. 7-9). This complex design is believed to be responsible for the large surface area for gas exchange, which is in the range of 40 to 100 m^2, the average being 70 m^2.

Two routes for collateral movement of gas within the lung have been described. Pores 5 to 10 μm wide have been identified in the interalveolar septa; these are referred to as the *pores of Kohn* (Fig. 7-10). It has been theorized that gas can circulate from one alveolus to another through these tiny openings. However, Takaro et al.[14] have suggested more recently that the majority of the pores are covered with a film of surfactant, which would indicate that the pores probably contribute very little to collateral ventilation. Other authors have suggested that the pores may allow the equalization of pressures among alveoli and serve as a route for macrophages to travel from one alveolus to another. Another source of collateral ventilation is the *canals of Lambert*, which are approximately 30 μm in diameter and allow intra-acinar collateral ventilation.

The alveolar wall is made up primarily of two types of epithelial cells: type I or *squamous pneumocytes*, and type II or *granular pneumocytes*. Type I cells make up about 40

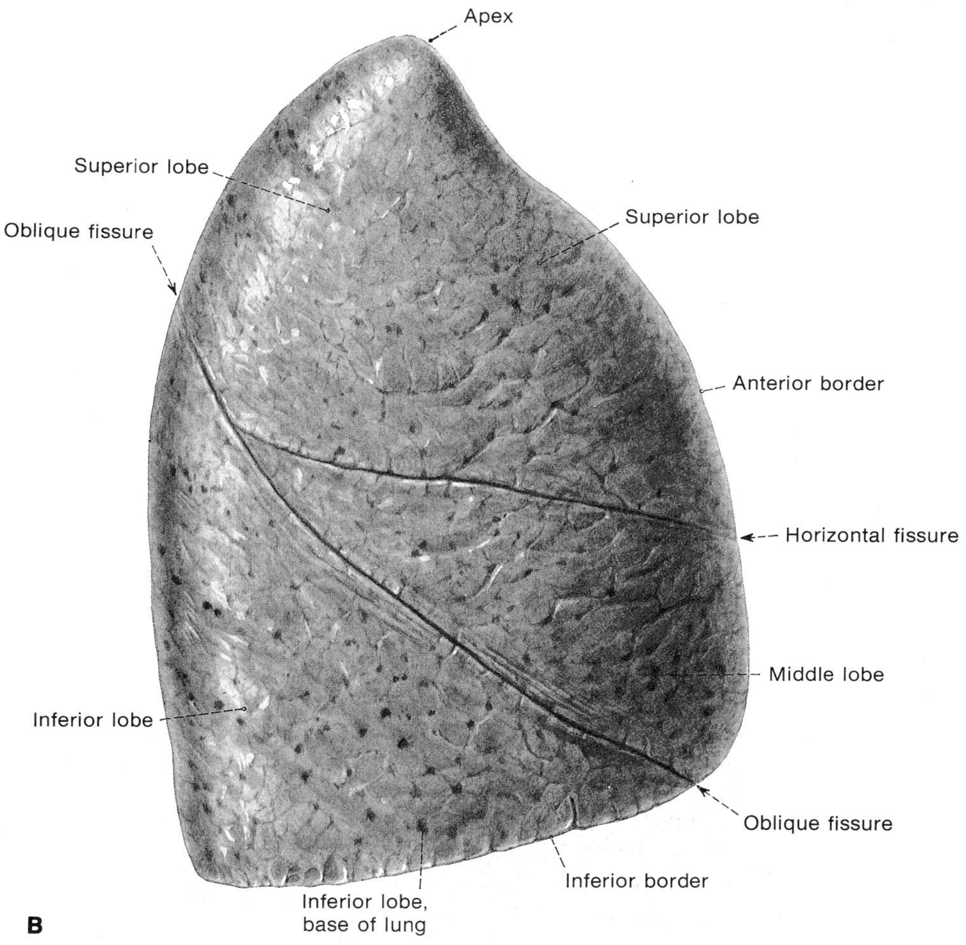

Figure 7-7. (*Continued*). **(B)**

percent of the alveolar epithelial cells but cover more than 90 percent of the alveolar surface. This is due to their extremely thin nature, which also leaves them more susceptible to injury. Type II cells are more numerous, but because of their cuboidal shape they occupy only 7 percent of the alveolar surface (Fig. 7-11). Type II cells fulfill an essential function by producing surfactant, which plays an important role in lowering surface tension within the alveolar lining and thereby reducing the tendency for alveolar collapse. This layer of surfactant represents a barrier, although minimal, to the diffusion of gas. Type II cells are readily identified under the electron microscope because of their brush microvilli.

Once O_2 diffuses across the alveolar epithelium, it encounters the interstitial space and the cells within it. Next O_2 must cross the capillary endothelium and its basement membrane. At this point the O_2 molecules have crossed the *alveolar-capillary* membrane and are presented to the red blood cells (Fig. 7-12). The alveolar-capillary membrane is only about 1 μm thick in healthy individuals and normally represents only a minimal obstacle to gas diffusion. Respiratory disease may increase the membrane thickness or reduce the surface area available for gas exchange.

PULMONARY LYMPHATICS

Many organs within the body contain lymphatic tissue, but the lung is more richly supplied than any other organ. The lymphatic system, made up of many channels and lymph nodes, serves two very important functions. First, the lymphatic system assists in the fluid homeostasis needed for proper lung function. This is accomplished through the maintenance of low protein concentration in the interstitial tissue. The lymphatic channels remove protein molecules, which, if allowed to accumulate, would increase the colloid oncotic pressure of the interstitial tissues, leading to pulmonary edema. Second, the pulmonary lymphatic system plays a role in respiratory defense mechanisms. While most inhaled toxins and particulate matter are removed by the mucociliary escalator, some are removed by the lymphatic tissue.

Interstitial fluid that flows into the lymphatic channels is referred to as *lymph*. Lymph is created by the normal process of fluid and protein movement from the pulmonary capillaries into the interstitial tissues. While most of the fluid is reabsorbed by the capillaries, the protein molecules and some of the fluid are not. The lymphatic channels have the

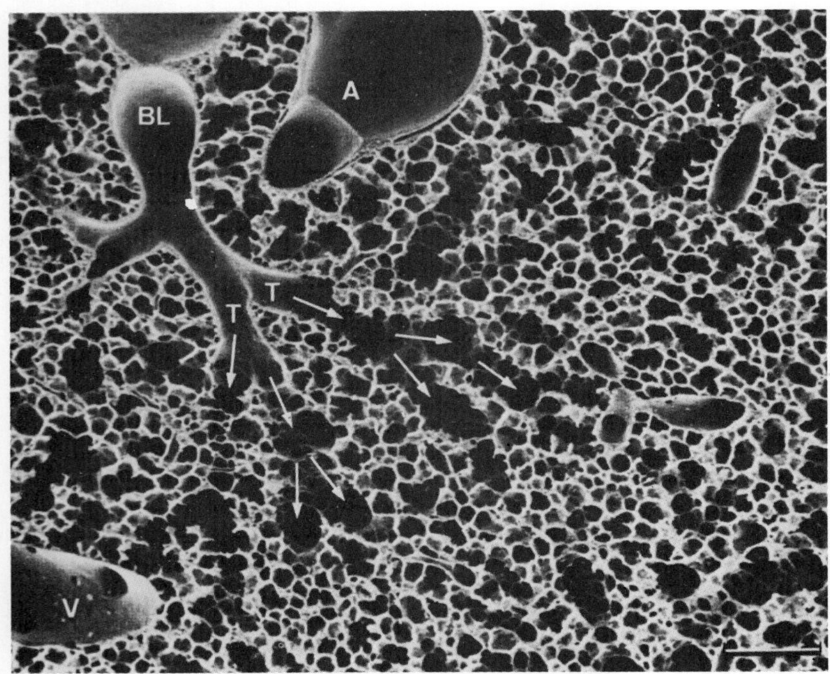

Figure 7-8. Scanning electron micrograph of lung, showing branching of small peripheral bronchiole (BL) into terminal bronchioles (T), from where the airways continue into respiratory bronchioles and alveolar ducts (arrows). Note the location of the pulmonary artery (A) and vein (V). (From Weibel,[22] with permission.)

Table 7-2. Characteristics of the Three Pulmonary Vagal Sensory Receptors

Receptor	Location	Fiber Type	Stimulus	Response
Pulmonary stretch, slowly adapting	Associated with smooth muscle of intrapulmonary airways	Medullated	1. Lung inflation 2. Increased transpulmonary pressure	1. Hering-Breuer inflation reflex 2. Bronchodilation 3. Increased heart rate 4. Decreased peripheral vascular resistance
Irritant, rapidly adapting	Epithelium of (mainly) extrapulmonary airways	Medullated	1. Irritants 2. Mechanical stimulation 3. Anaphylaxis 4. Lung inflation or deflation 5. Hyperpnea 6. Pulmonary congestion	1. Bronchoconstriction 2. Hyperpnea 3. Expiratory constriction of larynx 4. Cough 5. Mucous secretion
C-fibers Pulmonary (type J) Bronchial	 Alveolar wall Airways and blood vessels	Nonmedullated	1. Increased interstitial volume (congestion) 2. Chemical injury 3. Microembolism	1. Rapid shallow breathing 2. Laryngeal and tracheobronchial constriction 3. Bradycardia 4. Spinal reflex inhibition 5. Mucous secretion

(From Murray,[2] with permission.)

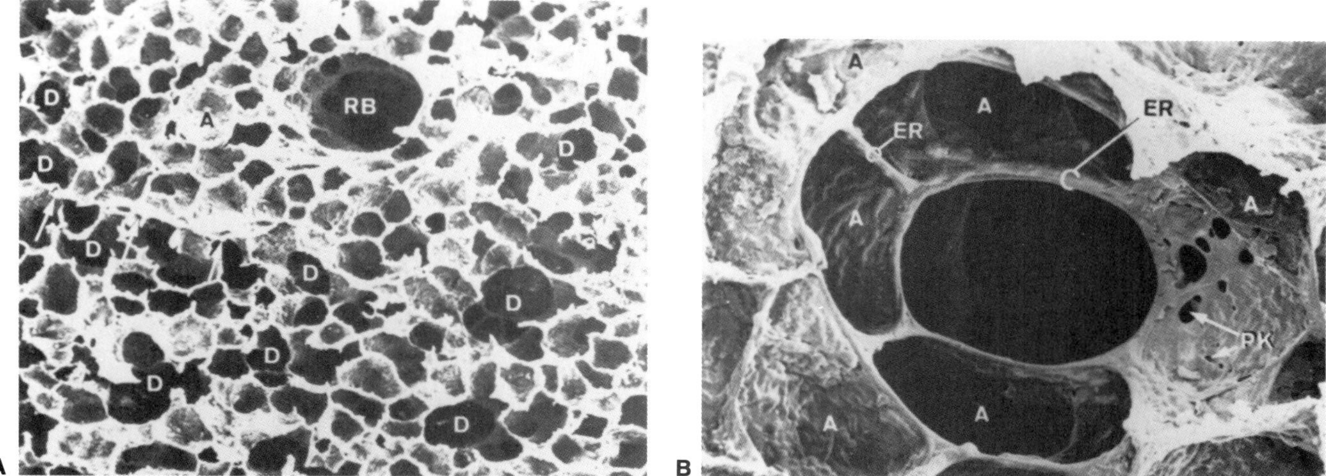

Figure 7-9. **(A)** Scanning electron micrograph (SEM) of a slice of normal human lung parenchyma. It shows a small respiratory bronchiole (RB) and several alveolar ducts (D) surrounded by alveoli (A). Arrows indicate an interlobular septum. (× 55.) **(B)** Larger magnification SEM of gas exchange parenchyma, showing an alveolar duct with adjacent alveoli (A). The free edge of alveolar septa is reinforced by thick bundles of connective tissue, which form the entrance rings (ER). Pores of Kohn (PK) of varying size are present between alveoli. (× 235.) (From Gehr et al.,[25] with permission.)

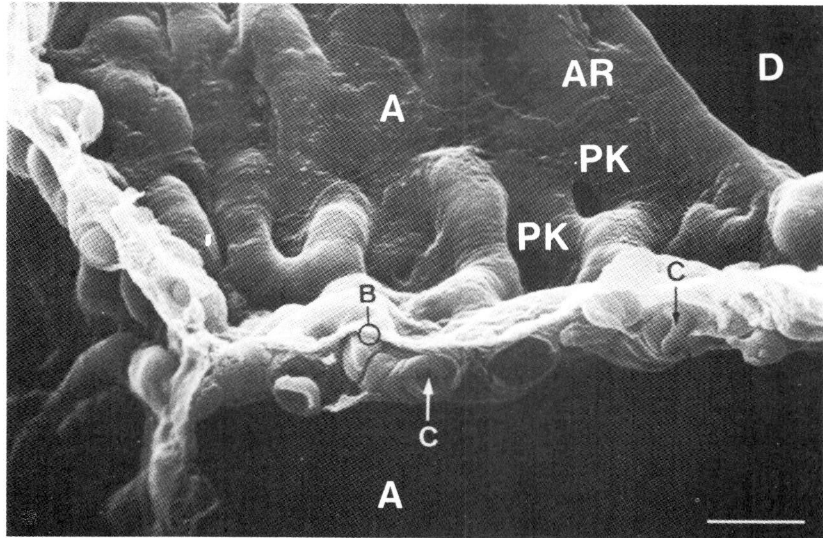

Figure 7-10. Scanning electron micrograph of lung parenchyma showing the very thin tissue barrier between the blood and air. The capillary blood (C) is separated from the air by a tissue barrier (B). Above, below, and to the left of the barrier are alveoli, and an alveolar duct is shown at the upper right. PK, pore of Kohn; D, duct; AR, alveolar entrance ring; C, capillary; A, alveolus. (Scale marker, 10 μm.) (From Weibel,[22] with permission.)

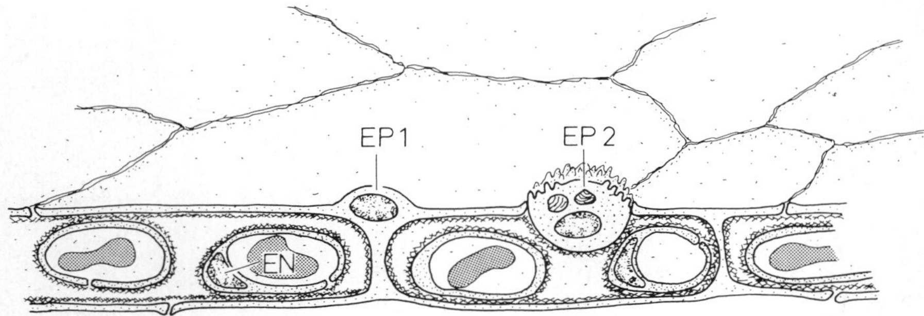

Figure 7-11. Diagram of the alveolar wall showing the complexity of a type I epithelial cell (EP 1) and its relation to a type II cell (EP 2) and an endothelial cell (EN). (From Weibel,[22] with permission.)

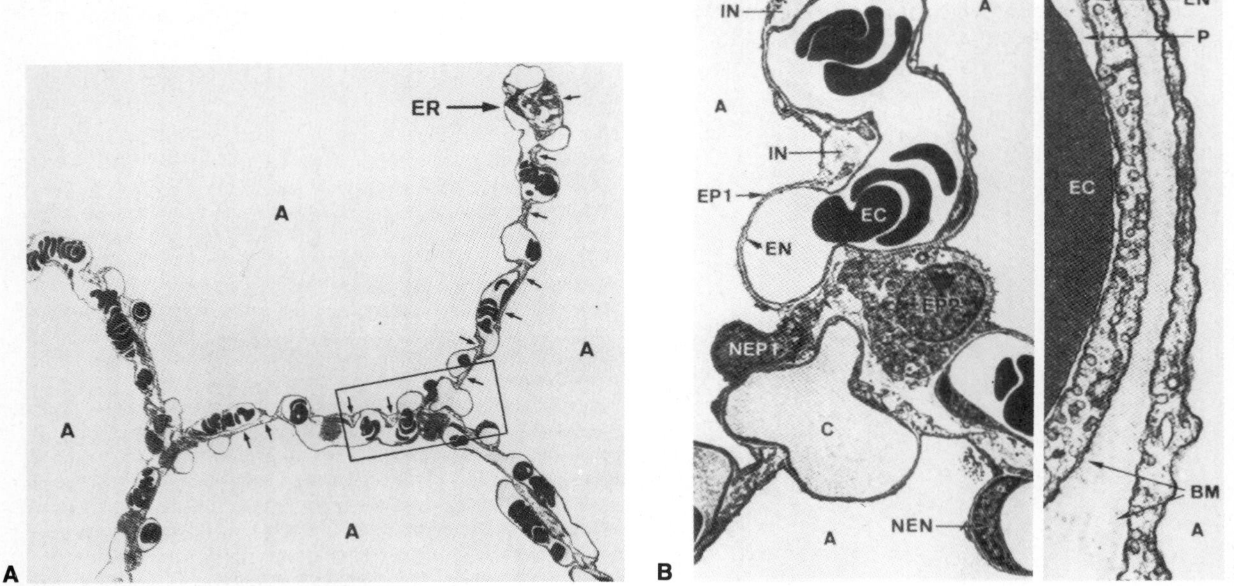

Figure 7-12. Transmission electron micrographs of normal alveolar septa seen in increasing magnification. **(A)** Capillaries mostly in a single layer are seen twisting around the connective tissue framework (arrows) between the alveoli (A). At upper right a reinforced entrance ring (ER) is seen. (× 595.) The area marked with a rectangle is seen at higher magnification in Figure B. **(B)** Higher magnification (× 3375) of the rectangle in Figure A, seen in mirror image and rotated 90 degrees clockwise. Alveolar capillaries (C) contain erythrocytes (EC) and are bound by endothelial cells (EN), one with a nucleus (NEN). Types I and II epithelial cells (EP1 and EP2, respectively) with nuclei (NEP1) are shown. The type II epithelial cell, which produces surfactant, is typically situated in a "niche." In places the interstitial space (IN) is widened. **(C)** Very high power view (× 43,110) of air-blood barrier, with interstitial space reduced to fused basement membranes (BM). Only a thin film of plasma (P) lies between the erythrocyte (EC) and the alveolar-capillary membrane. (From Gehr et al.,[25] with permission.)

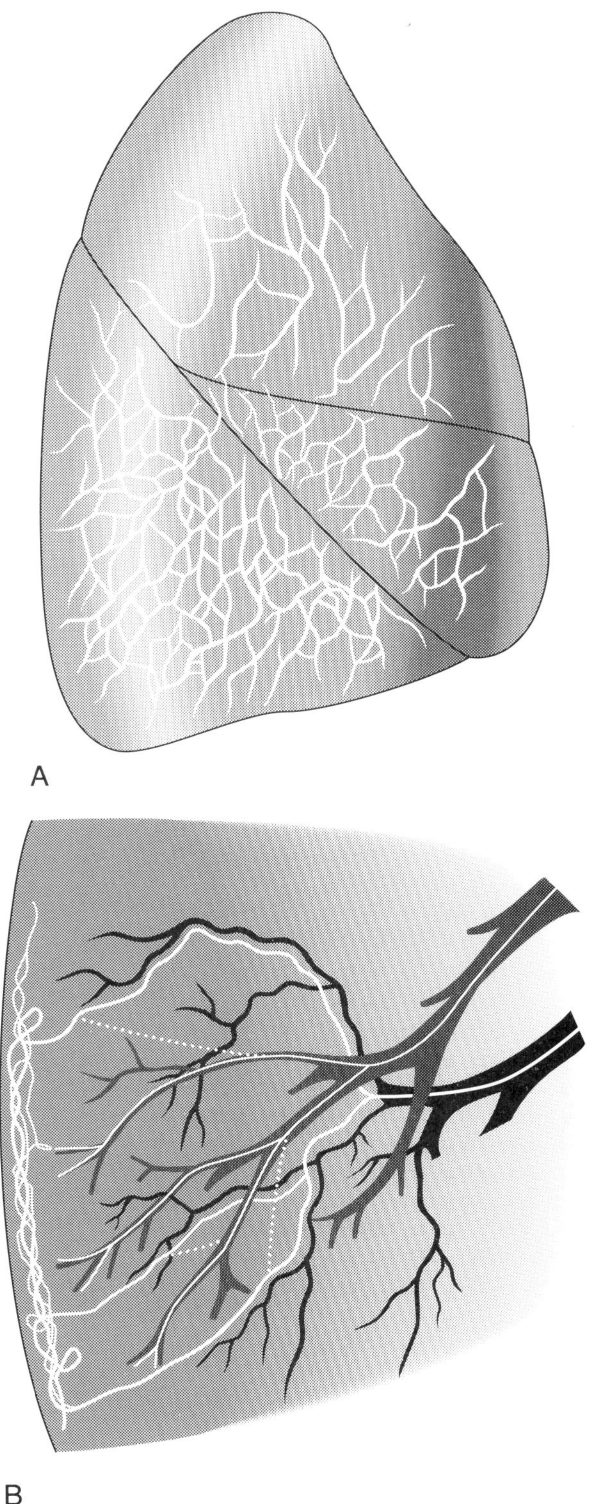

Figure 7-13. Lymphatic drainage of the pleura and lungs. **(A)** Drawing of the lateral aspect of the right lung shows the pleural lymphatics to be much more numerous over the lower half. **(B)** In a coronal section through the midportion of the lung, lymphatic channels from the pleura enter the lung at the interlobular septa and extend medially to the hilum along venous radicals (dark shaded vessels); lymphatic channels originating in the peripheral parenchyma extend medially in the bronchovascular bundles (light shaded vessels). Communicating lymphatics (dotted lines) extend between the peribronchial and perivenous lymphatics. (From Fraser et al.,[8] with permission.)

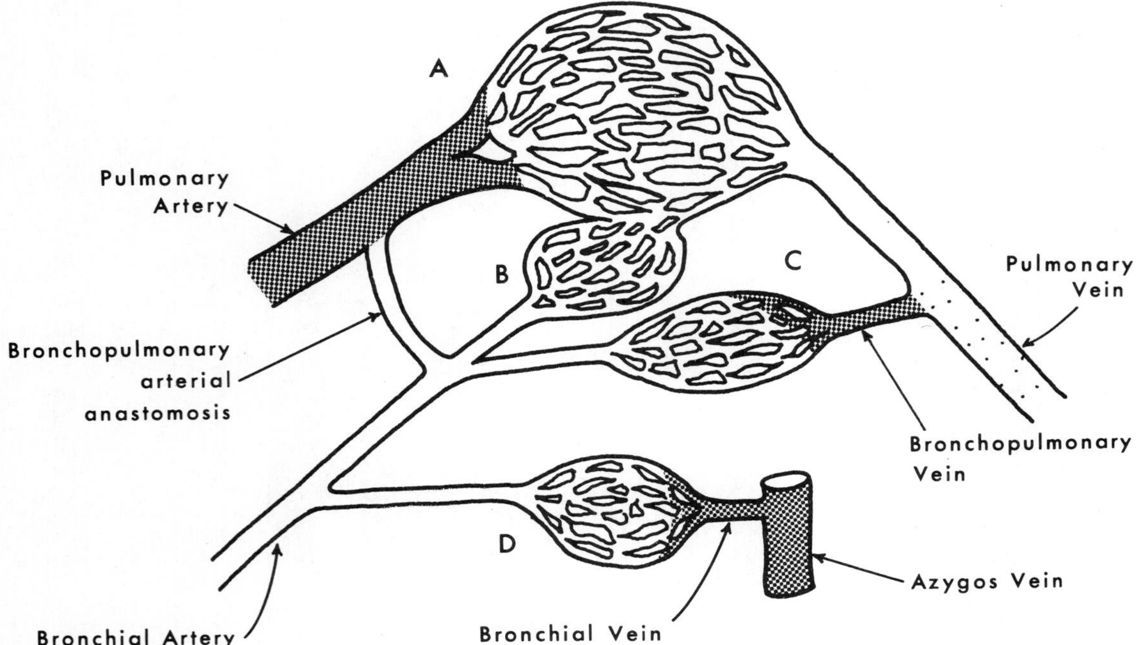

Figure 7-14. Schematic representation of the relationships between the bronchial and pulmonary circulations. The pulmonary artery supplies the pulmonary capillary network A. The bronchial artery supplies the capillary networks B, C, and D. Network B represents the bronchial capillary supply to bronchioles that anastomose with pulmonary capillaries; it drains through pulmonary veins. Network C represents the bronchial capillary supply to most bronchi; these vessels form bronchopulmonary veins, which empty into pulmonary veins. Network D represents the bronchial capillary supply to lobar and segmental bronchi; these vessels form true bronchial veins, which drain into the azygos, hemiazygos, or intercostal veins. Shaded areas represent blood of low O_2 content. (From Murray,[2] with permission.)

responsibility of moving the lymph back into the systemic veins by way of the thoracic or right lymphatic duct. The healthy lung is believed to be able to increase lymphatic flow 10-fold. Any factor that decreases the movement of lymph (e.g., elevated central venous pressures or blocked lymphatic channels) will encourage pulmonary edema.

The lymphatic channels possess valves that promote unidirectional flow of the lymph toward the hilum. The valves occur every few millimeters along the larger channels and are even more closely spaced in the smaller channels. Movement of lymph within the channels occurs when the vessels are compressed by any of several different effects, including muscle contraction, arterial pulsations, and the passive movement of body parts. Contraction of the smooth muscles within the walls of the lymphatic channels has been shown to move lymph in animal studies.[15]

The pulmonary lymphatic system has been subdivided into two parts on the basis of location, the superficial plexus and the deep plexus. The superficial plexus is well developed in humans and is located in the visceral pleura (Fig. 7-13). It is responsible for keeping the pleural lining free from excess fluid accumulation. The deep plexus is located in the connective tissue surrounding the airways and blood vessels of the lung. The lymphatic channels of the deep plexus extend peripherally to the respiratory bronchioles but do not invade the alveolar walls. The lymphatic channels located around the airways and blood vessels have been referred to as *juxta-alveolar lymphatics* to indicate their close proximity to the alveolar sacs. It has been estimated that the juxta-alveolar channels are no more than 1 mm away from the alveolar-capillary membrane.[2]

The lymph is directed toward the trachea by way of the main lymphatic channels located along the bronchial tree. Along the trachea lymph moves through the right and left mediastinal lymph channels, which drain into the right and left subclavian veins, respectively. Located intermittently throughout the lymphatic channels are lymph nodes, which serve as filters for the lymph and also serve as depositories for the filtrate to protect the blood and the entire body from dissemination of the foreign matter.

INNERVATION OF THE LUNGS

The human lung is innervated with afferent and efferent pathways of the autonomic nervous system. The afferent, or sensory, pathways originate in the epithelium of the bronchial walls, submucosa, interalveolar septa, and smooth muscle. These are parasympathetic fibers, which transmit signals to the nervous system via the vagus nerves. Three groups of vagal sensory fibers have been identified in the lungs: the pulmonary stretch receptors, the irritant receptors, and the C-fiber receptors. These receptors and their respective characteristics are described in Table 7-2.

The efferent, or motor, pathways reach the lungs through the sympathetic and parasympathetic nervous systems. The sympathetic fibers terminate in the airway walls, vascular smooth muscle, and submucosal glands. Stimulation of these fibers causes bronchial smooth muscle relaxation, constriction of pulmonary arteries, and diminished glandular secretion. The parasympathetic fibers are also present in the airways, but their presence and effect on pulmonary circulation has been difficult to document. Stimulation of parasympathetic fibers has been shown to cause airway constriction and increased glandular secretion, but no physiologically important changes in pulmonary circulation have been demonstrated.[16]

BRONCHIAL CIRCULATION

The metabolic needs of the airways are supplied by the bronchial arteries, which arise from the aorta or the upper intercostal arteries[17] and accompany the bronchial tree down to the terminal bronchioles. Structures distal to the terminal bronchioles are believed to obtain their nutrients from the mixed venous blood of the pulmonary circulation. Since lung transplant patients do not require bronchial arteries for survival, this circulation is supplementary. Normally the bronchial circulation represents only 1 to 2 percent of the cardiac output; however, in certain lung diseases (e.g., bronchiectasis or carcinoma) it may be significantly increased.[18] In such cases, the bronchial circulation may be the source of hemoptysis.[18]

A portion of the venous blood from the capillaries of the bronchial circulation returns to the right side of the heart by way of the azygos, hemiazygos, or intercostal veins (Fig. 7-14). The remainder of the venous blood returns to the left heart through the pulmonary vein by one of two routes: (1) bronchial artery plexuses deep in the lung that anastomose with capillaries from the pulmonary arteries; or (2) the bronchopulmonary veins, which empty directly into the pulmonary vein. Since this venous blood, termed *venous admixture*, is poorly oxygenated, it lowers the oxygenation status of the arterialized blood. The exact amount of the bronchial circulation that contributes to venous admixture in humans is not known; however, on the basis of animal studies, it is believed to be the major portion.[18–20]

References

1. Weibel ER, Taylor CR: Design and structure of the human lung. pp. 11–57. In Fishman AP (ed): Pulmonary Diseases and Disorders. 2nd Ed. McGraw-Hill, New York, 1988
2. Murray JF: The Normal Lung. 2nd Ed. WB Saunders, Philadelphia, 1986
3. Martin DE, Youtsey JW: Respiratory Anatomy and Physiology. CV Mosby, St. Louis, 1988
4. Montgomery RL: Basic Anatomy for the Allied Health Professions. Urban & Schwarzenberg, Baltimore, 1981, pp. 367–387
5. Netter FH: The CIBA Collection of Medical Illustrations. Vol. 7. The Respiratory System. CIBA-Geigy Corp., Summit, NJ, 1979
6. Staub NC, Albertine KH: The structure of the lungs relative to their principal function. pp. 12–36. In Murray JF, Nadel JA (eds): Textbook of Respiratory Medicine. WB Saunders, Philadelphia, 1988
7. Williams PL, Warwick R, Dyson M, Bannister LH: Gray's Anatomy. 37th Ed. Churchill Livingstone, Edinburgh, 1989, pp. 1248–1285
8. Fraser RG, Pare JAP, Pare PD et al: Diagnosis of Diseases of the Chest. 3rd Ed. WB Saunders, Philadelphia, 1988, pp. 1–155, 176–203
9. Cosio MG, Hale KA, Neiwoehner DE: Morphologic and morphometric effects of prolonged cigarette smoking on the airways. Am Rev Respir Dis 1980;122:265–271
10. Santa Cruz R, Landa J, Hirsch J, Sackner MA: Tracheal mucous velocity in normal man and patients with obstructive lung disease: effects of terbutaline. Am Rev Respir Dis 1974;109:458–463
11. Langston C, Kida K, Reed M, Thurlbeck WM: Human lung growth in late gestation and in the neonate. Am Rev Respir Dis 1984;129:607–613
12. Agnus GE, Thurlbeck WM: Number of alveoli in the human lung. J Appl Physiol 1972;32:483–485
13. Dunhill MS: Postnatal growth of the lung. Thorax 1962;17:329–333
14. Takaro T, Price HP, Parra SC: Ultrastructural studies of apertures in the interalveolar septum of the adult human lung. Am Rev Respir Dis 1979;119:425–434
15. Reddy NP, Staub NC: Intrinsic propulsive activity of thoracic duct perfused in anesthetized dogs. Microvasc Res 1981;21:183–192
16. Widdicombe JG, Sterling GM: The autonomic nervous system and breathing. Arch Intern Med 1970;126:311–329
17. Cauldwell EW, Siekert RG, Lininger RE, Anson BJ: An anatomic study of 150 human cadavers. Surg Gynecol Obstet 1948; 86:395–412
18. Charan NB: The bronchial circulatory system: Structure, function, and importance. Respir Care 1984;29:1226–1235
19. Deffebach ME, Charan NB, Lakshminarayan S, Butler J: The bronchial circulation (state of the art). Am Rev Respir Dis 1987; 135:463–481
20. Murray JF: Disorders of the pulmonary circulation: General principles and diagnostic approach. pp. 1271–1298. In Murray JF, Nadel JA (eds): Textbook of Respiratory Medicine. WB Saunders, Philadelphia, 1988
21. Weibel ER: Morphometry of the Human Lung. Springer-Verlag, Berlin, 1973
22. Weibel ER: The Pathway for Oxygen, Harvard University Press, Cambridge, MA, 1984
23. Kuhn C III: Normal anatomy and histology. pp. 11–50. In Thurlbeck WM (ed): Pathology of the Lung. Thieme, New York, 1988
24. Dunnill MS: Pulmonary Pathology. 2nd Ed. Churchill Livingstone, New York, 1987
25. Gehr P, Bachofen M, Weibel ER: The normal human lung: Ultrastructure and morphometric estimation of diffusion capacity. Respir Physiol 1978;32:121–140

Chapter 8

The Heart and Blood Vessels

Robert L. Wilkins
David J. Pierson

CHAPTER OUTLINE

The process of respiration is dependent on an adequate uptake of O_2 by the lung and its distribution throughout the body. The cardiovascular system provides the pipeline between the source of O_2 uptake and the tissues in which O_2 is utilized to create energy. For this reason it has been said that the purpose of the circulatory system is to support respiration. This chapter describes the anatomy and physiology of the cardiovascular system, with emphasis on information pertinent to the provision of respiratory care to patients. The references provide a more detailed description of cardiac anatomy and physiology.[1–8]

ANATOMY OF THE PERICARDIUM AND HEART

Pericardium

Just as the lungs are contained within the pleural lining, the heart is surrounded by the *pericardium*. This sac-like structure consists of a thin lining with two layers, the *fibrous* and the *serous pericardium* (Fig. 8-1). The tough, outer, fibrous layer is connected to the diaphragm inferiorly by a wide area of fibers attached to the central tendon; it is also attached anteriorly to the sternum, laterally to the pleura, and posteriorly to the vertebral column. Whereas the fibrous pericardium is pierced by the great vessels of the heart, the serous pericardium is a closed sac with two components, the *inner* or *visceral layer*, which covers the entire surface of the heart, and the *outer* or *parietal layer*, which lines the inner surface of the fibrous pericardium.

The potential space between the inner and outer layers of the serous pericardium, known as the *pericardial cavity*, is analogous to the pleural cavity between the visceral and parietal pleurae, and like the pleural space, it normally contains only a small amount of fluid. This *pericardial fluid* minimizes the friction between the heart and the pericardial sac as the heart contracts and relaxes. As a result of disease or injury the pericardial sac may fill with an excessive amount of blood or other fluid. Rapid accumulation of fluid, such as may occur with pericardial injury or infection, may produce serious impairment of cardiac function (acute pericardial tamponade); more slowly accumulating effusions tend to have less physiologic impact even when they are large.

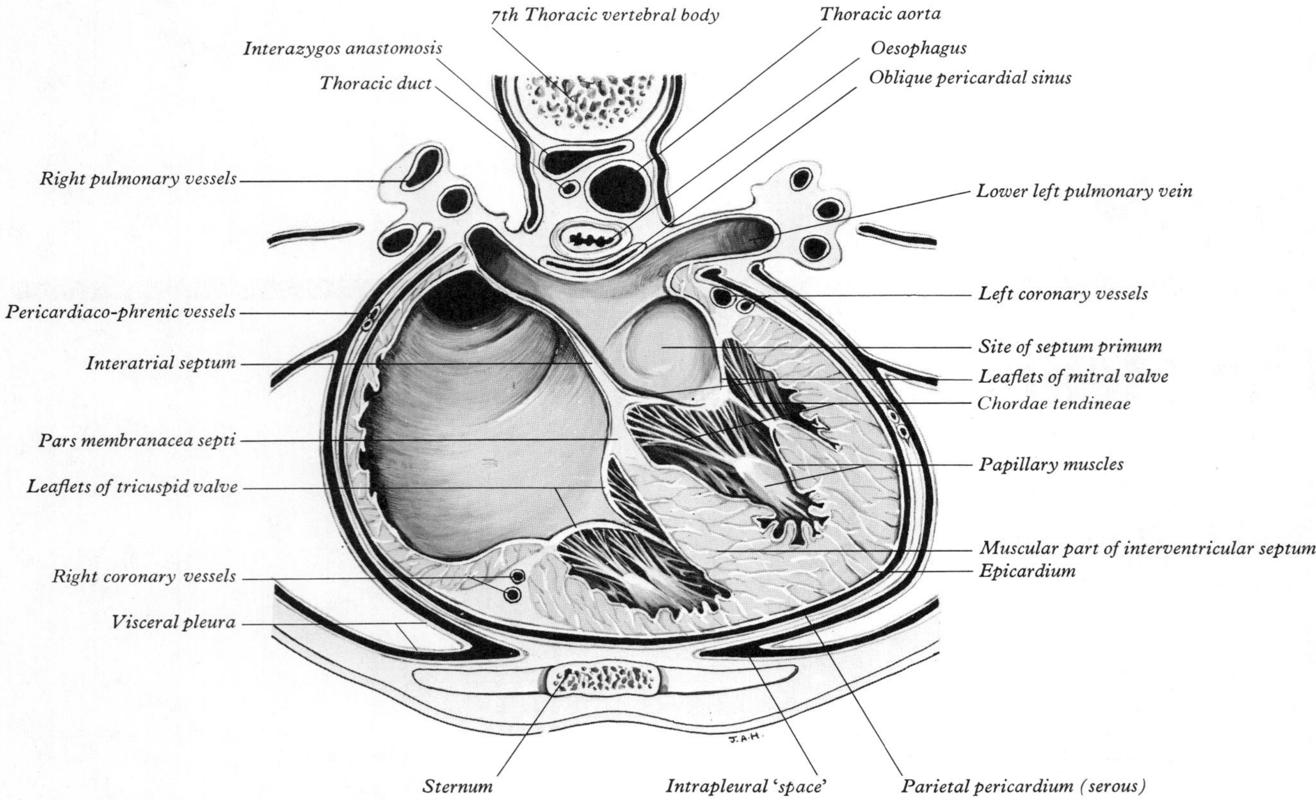

Figure 8-1. Transverse section through the heart, pericardium, and related structures at the level of the seventh thoracic vertebra. This view shows how the heart is enveloped within the pericardium and positioned between the sternum and the vertebral column (viewed from below). (From Williams et al.,[8] with permission.)

Heart Chambers

The heart is a muscular organ containing four chambers (Fig. 8-2). The upper chambers are called the right and left *atria* and the lower chambers are referred to as the right and left *ventricles*. The atria are small, thin-walled chambers, which represent the venous portion of the heart and are separated by the *interatrial septum*. Each atrium is made up of two parts, a smaller portion called the *auricle* and a smooth-walled portion constituting the principal part of the chamber. The auricle is a blind pocket lined by small ridges termed *pectinate muscles*. The smooth-walled portion of the atrium serves to temporarily store blood before it passes into the ventricle.

The ventricles, which are larger chambers than the atria, have thicker, more muscular walls and represent the arterial portion of the heart. They have the primary responsibility for moving blood throughout the lungs and the rest of the body and are separated by the *interventricular septum*. The left ventricle receives blood from the left atrium and ejects it into the aorta. The right ventricle receives blood from the right atrium and pumps it into the pulmonary artery.

In clinical practice the terms *right heart* and *left heart* are commonly used. This is because the human heart has two separate pumps, each with its own function (Fig. 8-3). The right heart, consisting of the right atrium and right ventricle, serves to receive the deoxygenated venous blood from the body and to pump it into the pulmonary circulation for oxygenation. The left heart, made up of the left atrium and left ventricle, receives the oxygenated blood from the lungs and pumps it throughout the body via the arterial system.

Although they are connected, it is necessary that the chambers and vessels of the two circulatory systems be kept separate because of the different pressures that they require. As Figure 8-3 shows, the cardiovascular system is actually two circuits arranged in series and sharing different chambers of the same pump. To perfuse the body's tissues the systemic circuit requires high pressures and thick-walled, narrow-gauge vessels; however, the delicate gas exchange surfaces of the pulmonary circuit could not withstand such pressures. Therefore, the pulmonary system is composed of low-pressure, thinner-walled vessels of greater cross-sectional area.

Heart Valves

Heart valves are responsible for preventing back flow of blood as the heart contracts and relaxes in order to circulate blood. Abnormalities in one or more of the heart valves can

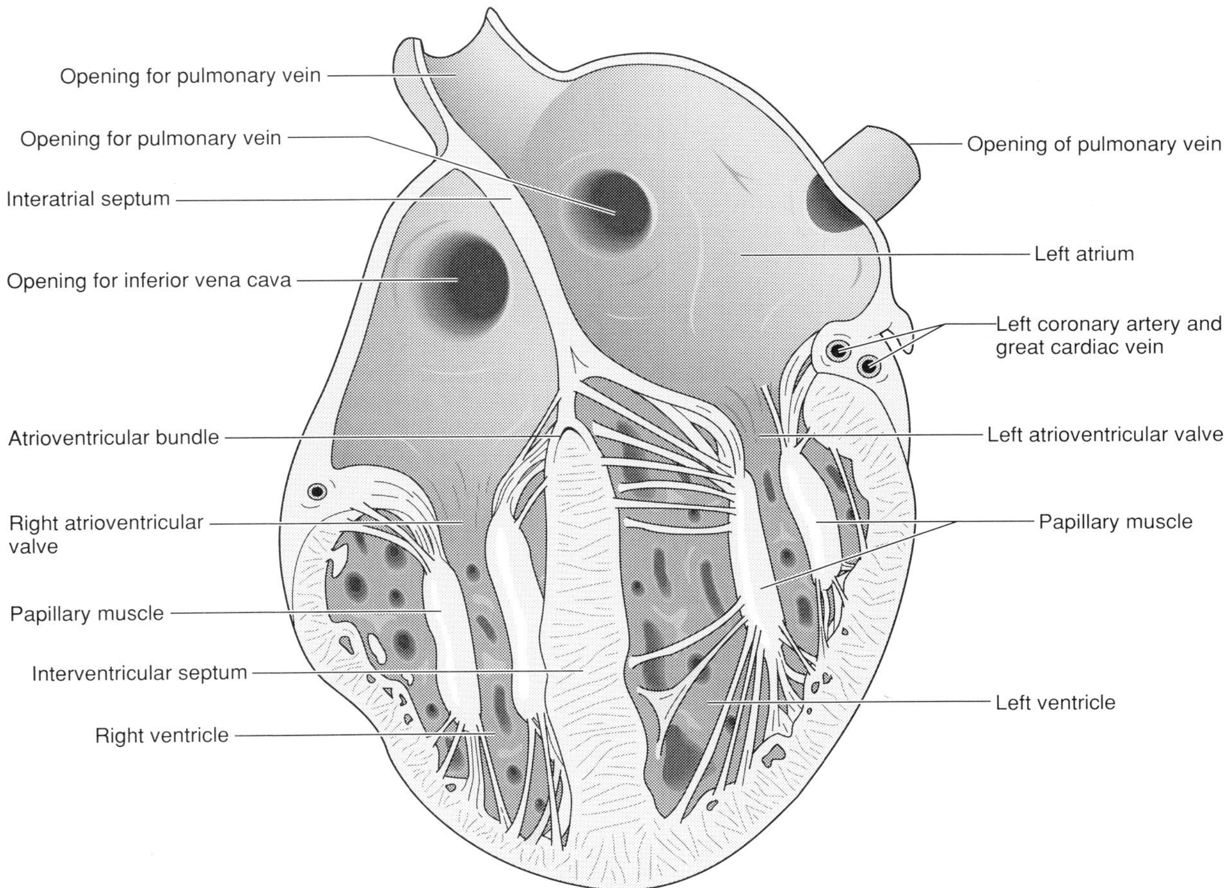

Figure 8-2. Cross-sectional view of the heart chambers. Note the thickness of the left ventricular wall as compared with the right. (From Staubesand,[11] with permission.)

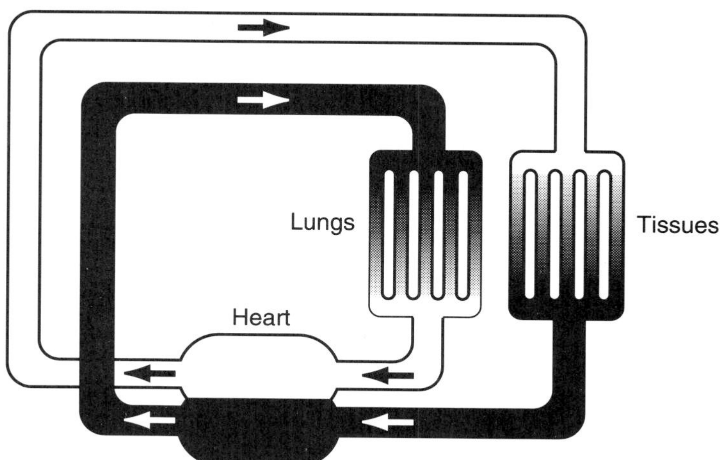

Figure 8-3. Schematic diagram of the human circulatory system. Separation of the blood into right and left circuits allows the pressures in them to be markedly different—low in the pulmonary circuit with its high-area, delicate, diffusing surface, and high in the high-velocity, narrow-gauge systemic circuit. The two circuits are in series, and the blood is pumped twice in each complete circulation. White represents oxygenated and black deoxygenated blood. (From Pierson,[6] with permission.)

interfere with the unidirectional flow of blood and lead to circulatory failure. There are four heart valves, two *atrioventricular* (AV) valves (located between the atria and the ventricles) and two *semilunar* valves. The *mitral* or bicuspid valve is the atrioventricular valve located between the left atrium and ventricle (Figs. 8-1 and 8-2); it is called *bicuspid* because it has two cusps, which fit tightly together when the valve is closed. The other AV valve, known as the *tricuspid* valve because it has three cusps, is located between the right atrium and ventricle. The cusps of the AV valves are composed of fibrous tissue, which is thick centrally and thin laterally.

The ventricular surface of the cusps is attached to *chordae tendinae*, which are thin, strong fibrous cords (Figs. 8-1 and 8-2), connected to papillary muscles attached to the wall of the ventricle. The chordae tendinae and papillary muscles serve to anchor the flaps of the AV valves during ventricular contraction and prevent back flow of blood into the atria. If the flaps were not anchored, they would invert into the atria when pressure in the ventricles increases. During ventricular relaxation the flaps of the AV valves hang down to allow movement of blood from the atria into the ventricles.

The semilunar valves have also been referred to as the *arterial* valves because they open into the roots of the two large arteries stemming from the ventricles. The valve located at the opening of the pulmonary artery is referred to as the *pulmonic* valve and the valve located at the opening of the aorta is called the *aortic* valve (Fig. 8-4). Each semilunar valve has three cusps, which when closed prevent back flow of blood into the ventricles when the ventricles are relaxed. Normally, during ventricular contraction the semilunar valves open widely and their cusps flatten against the walls of the artery as blood rushes by. Passage of blood through the heart is normally silent except for the closing of the valves. However, when one or more valves become stenotic (unable to open completely) or regurgitant (unable to close completely), turbulence is created, which is audible through a stethoscope as a *murmur*.

Heart Wall

The wall of the heart consists of three layers. The outer layer is the *epicardium*, which is the visceral layer of the serous pericardium (Fig. 8-1). The middle layer is the *myocardium*, which is made up of muscle fibers that are arranged in a spiral manner to allow more effective compression of the heart during contraction (see discussion of the physiology of heart muscle under Cardiac Output). The myocardium is thickest around the ventricles and much thinner around the atria. Normally, the wall of the left ventricle is significantly thicker than that of the right ventricle (Figs. 8-1 and 8-2) owing to the larger work load imposed on the left ventricle, which is responsible for pumping blood at high pressure throughout the entire body. The third or inner layer of the heart wall is a very thin, smooth membrane, which resembles squamous epithelium and is referred to as the *endocardium*.

Conduction System of the Heart

In order for the heart to circulate blood effectively, it is important for the atria and ventricles to contract in a coordinated manner. The conduction system of the heart is responsible for initiating and spreading electrical stimuli throughout the heart muscle to coordinate contraction of the various parts of the heart during each cycle. This role of the conduction system is important because when its function is abnormal, patients may experience serious consequences, such as inadequate cardiac output and death.

Normally the electrical stimulus that begins the cardiac cycle comes from the *sinoatrial* (SA) node, which also is referred to as the *pacemaker* of the heart (Fig. 8-5). This node, which is a collection of special cells that have the ability to depolarize spontaneously, is located in the wall of the right atrium. Once the SA node depolarizes, a wave of elec-

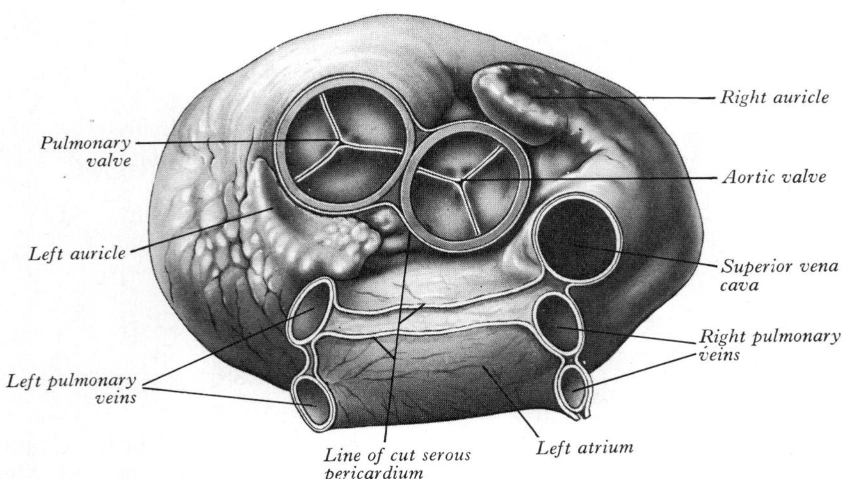

Figure 8-4. View from above the heart, showing the pulmonic ('pulmonary' in figure) and aortic valves. (From Williams et al.,[8] with permission.)

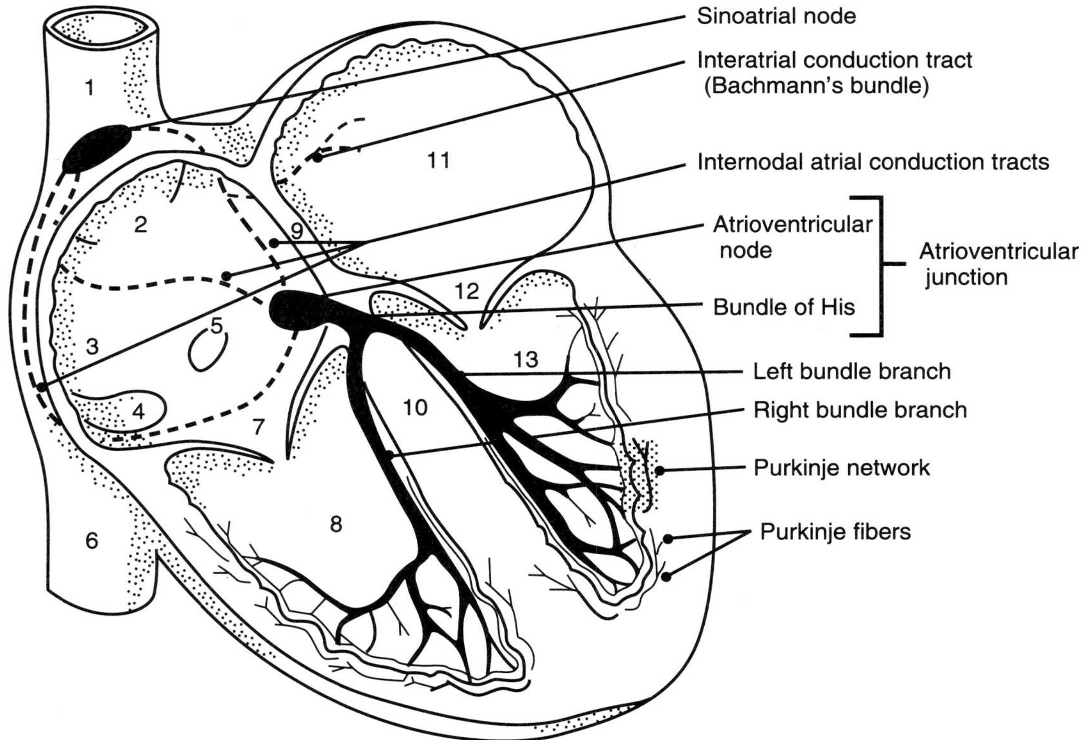

Figure 8-5. Conduction system of the heart. 1, Superior vena cava; 2, inlet of the superior vena cava; 3, right atrium; 4, inlet of the inferior vena cava; 5, coronary sinus; 6, inferior vena cava; 7, tricuspid valve; 8, right ventricle; 9, interatrial septum; 10, interventricular septum; 11, left atrium; 12, mitral valve; 13, left ventricle. (From Huszar,[12] with permission.)

trical activity spreads over the atria to initiate contraction. The electrical activity of the atria is recorded on the electrocardiogram (ECG) as the P wave.

Located at the junction between the atria and the ventricles is the *atrioventricular* node. This node also consists of special cells with the ability to depolarize spontaneously; normally, however, the AV node does not depolarize as rapidly as the SA node. The AV node normally responds to the electrical activity of the atria and depolarizes according to the pace set by the SA node. Once the AV node depolarizes, the electrical impulses move into the *bundle of His* and then travel down the respective sides of the interventricular septum through the right and left bundle branches, from which they are transmitted throughout the myocardium by way of the *Purkinje fibers*. These fibers are tiny finger-like projections that cannot be seen grossly because they are located within the cardiac muscle. The electrical activity of the ventricles that corresponds with ventricular contraction is seen as the QRS complex on the ECG.

Coronary Circulation

The heart muscle must receive a constant supply of oxygenated blood in order to pump blood effectively. This is achieved through the coronary circulation, which consists of the left and right *coronary arteries* and their branches (Fig. 8-6). The right and left coronary arteries arise from the respective sinuses of the ascending aorta. The right coronary artery passes between the pulmonary trunk and the right atrium to the dorsal aspect of the heart, where it anastomoses with the left coronary artery. The two main branches of the right coronary artery are known as the *marginal* and the *posterior interventricular* branches. The left coronary artery passes between the pulmonary trunk and the left atrium and soon branches into the *anterior interventricular* and *circumflex* branches. The former spans toward the apex of the heart while the latter courses along the dorsal surface.

PHYSIOLOGY OF THE HEART

The Cardiac Cycle

The cardiac cycle is a series of events that occurs during a single heart beat. The cycle begins with contraction of the atria, which serves to add blood volume to the ventricles. After the atria contract, they relax and the ventricles begin to contract. As the pressure in the ventricles builds, the AV

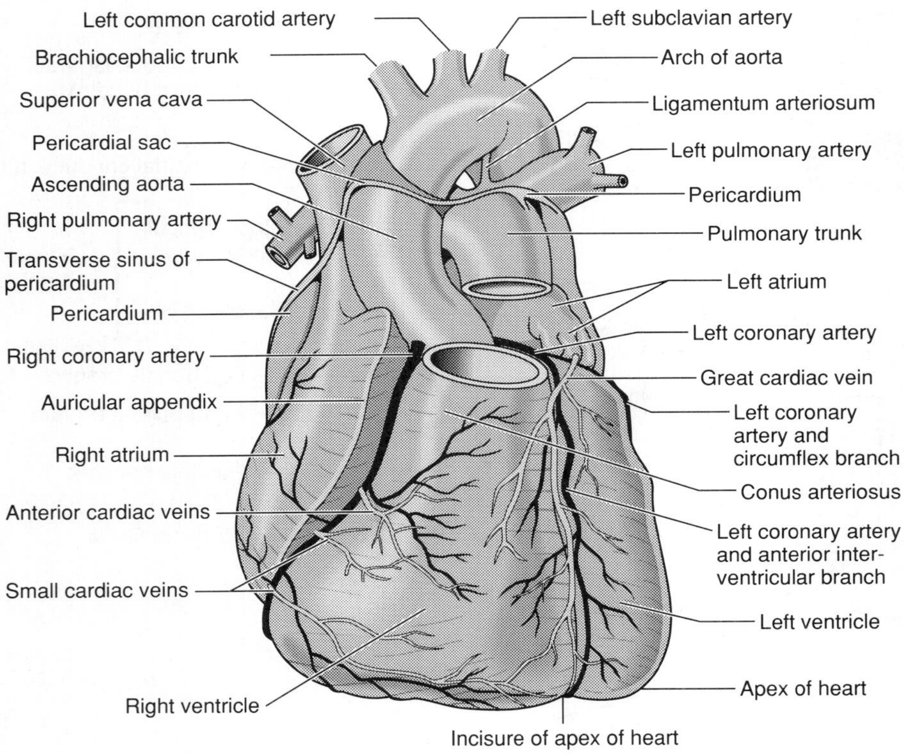

Figure 8-6. Coronary circulation of the heart. (From Staubesand,[11] with permission.)

valves close and the semilunar valves open. It is the closing of the AV valves that creates the first heart sound (S_1).

The ventricles squeeze most of their contents into the arteries and then relax. The amount of blood ejected by each ventricle during contraction is known as the *stroke volume*, which normally amounts to 60 to 130 mL in each beat. The fraction of the ventricular end diastolic volume that is ejected during systole is known as the *ejection fraction*, which normally is approximately 65 to 70 percent. As the ventricles relax, the pressure within decreases, the AV valves open, and the semilunar valves close when the pressure in the arteries exceeds that in the relaxing ventricles. Closure of the semilunar valves creates the second heart sound (S_2).

The process of heart contraction is also referred to as *systole*. Even though this term could apply to atrial or ventricular contraction, in the clinical setting it is most often used to refer to ventricular contraction. *Diastole* is the relaxation of the heart and also is most often used in reference to ventricular relaxation.

Cardiac Output

The volume of blood pumped by each ventricle per minute is referred to as the *cardiac output*. It is a product of heart rate and stroke volume and normally is 4 to 8 L/min for an adult at rest. Since the normal cardiac output varies with the size of the individual, it is useful to describe the cardiac output in relation to the patient's body surface area. This results in the use of a *cardiac index*, which is the cardiac output divided by the patient's body surface area and is reported in liters per minute per square meter. Normal cardiac index is 2.5 to 4.0 $L/min/m^2$.

As demonstrated in Figure 8-7, stroke volume is a function of three factors: (1) preload, the amount of stretch on the ventricular muscle prior to systole; (2) afterload, the tension that the ventricular muscle must create during contraction; and (3) contractility, the ability of the heart muscle to shorten rapidly during contraction.[9]

Preload

According to *Starling's law*, cardiac muscle will contract in direct proportion to the amount by which it is stretched prior to systole, within physiologic limits (Fig. 8-8). The volume of blood filling the ventricle before each contraction, known as the end diastolic volume (EDV), determines the degree of myocardial stretch and therefore provides a true picture of preload.

It is possible for preload to be inadequate, adequate, or excessive. When a patient has insufficient circulating blood volume, as with hemorrhage, the filling volume of the ventricles will be inadequate and preload will be abnormally low. In such cases the stretch on heart muscle prior to contraction is minimal and the subsequent stroke volume is reduced. By contrast, ventricular filling in patients with congestive heart

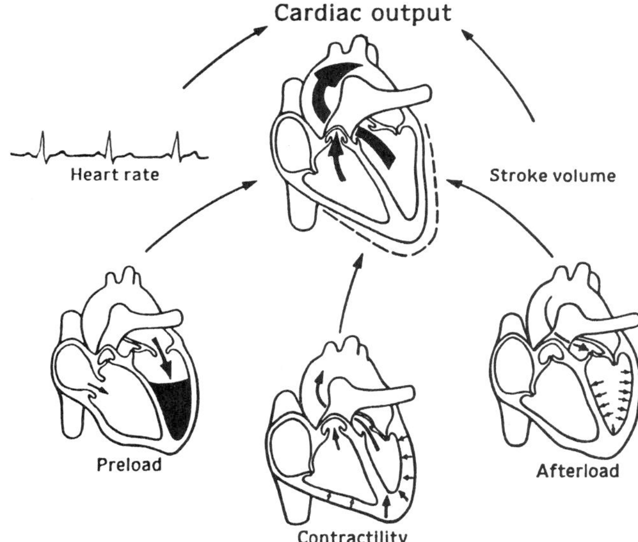

Figure 8-7. Factors affecting stroke volume and cardiac output. (From Krider,[9] with permission.)

Table 8-1. Normal Hemodynamic Values

Parameter	Abbreviation	Normal Value
Arterial pressure	BP	120/80 mmHg
Mean arterial pressure	MAP	80–100 mmHg
Central venous pressure	CVP	<6 mmHg; <12 CmH_2O
Right atrial pressure	RAP	2–6 mmHg
Right ventricular pressure	RVP	20–30/0–5 mmHg
Pulmonary artery pressure	PAP	20–30/6–15 mmHg
Pulmonary capillary wedge pressure	PCWP, PAOP	4–12 mmHg
Left atrial pressure	LAP	4–12 mmHg
Left ventricular pressure	LVP	100–140/0–5 mmHg
Systemic vascular resistance	SVR	900–1400 dyne/s/cm^{-5}
Pulmonary vascular resistance	PVR	110–250 dyne/s/cm^{-5}

failure is excessive and exceeds the physiologic limits of the myocardium. This contributes to a diminished stroke volume as the heart muscle is "overstretched" and cannot contract effectively (Fig. 8-8).

In clinical practice it is very difficult to measure EDV, and as a result the end diastolic pressure is used to evaluate ventricular filling or preload. For the right ventricle, preload is assessed by measuring central venous pressure (CVP), which is the blood pressure in the right atrium or in the vena cava, by which the venous blood is returned to the heart from the venous system. Since the tricuspid valve is open during diastole, CVP can reflect right ventricular filling pressure or preload for the right ventricle. Normal values for CVP and other hemodynamic measurements are listed in Table 8.1.

To assess the filling pressures for the left side of the heart, a pulmonary artery catheter is most frequently used. This catheter has a small balloon near the tip, which assists the physician in positioning the catheter in the pulmonary artery. Once the catheter enters the pulmonary artery, it will continue to float downstream until the balloon wedges into a smaller branch of the pulmonary circulation. When the catheter wedges, the tip is now able to measure left heart filling pressures. During diastole the mitral valve is open, and the

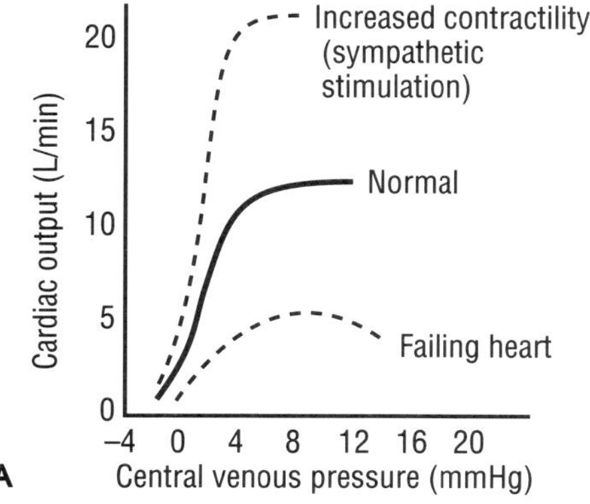

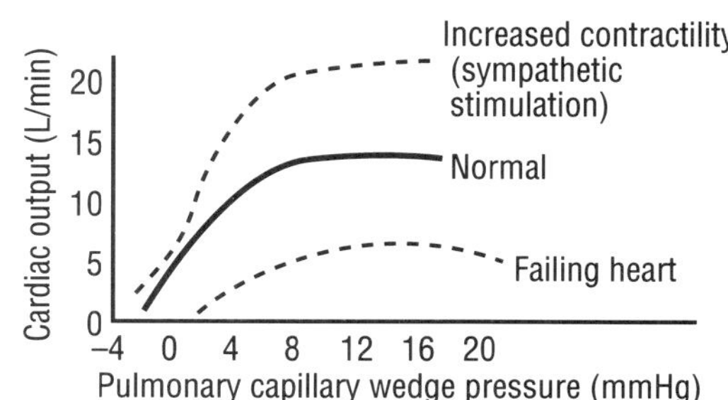

Figure 8-8. Ventricular function curves for the (**A**) right and (**B**) left ventricles. Note that the filling pressures are used to represent end diastolic volume. The upstroke of the curve for normal ventricles initially shows a rapid increase in output for a small change in end diastolic pressure, but the curve then plateaus, with little change in output for large changes in filling pressure. Dashed curves show change in output for a given pressure occurring with altered contractility from sympathetic stimulation and heart failure. (From Krider,[9] with permission.)

wedge pressure measured by the pulmonary artery catheter reflects the left ventricular end diastolic pressure (LVEDP), which is used to evaluate preload for the left ventricle. (Ch. 50 provides a more detailed discussion of the pulmonary artery catheter.)

Afterload

As the ventricles contract and attempt to eject blood into the arteries, a certain degree of resistance will be encountered. This resistance to ventricular ejection, the major factor determining afterload, has two components, tension in the ventricular wall and peripheral resistance. Factors such as interventricular pressure increases and distention of the ventricles will increase the tension in the ventricular wall and thereby increase afterload. Narrowing of the arteries will increase peripheral vascular resistance and will also increase afterload. Whenever afterload increases, the stroke volume is likely to decrease and cardiac output may fall.

It should be noted that afterload is primarily estimated in clinical practice by the measurement of vascular resistance. Afterload is determined for the left ventricle by evaluating the peripheral vascular resistance and for the right ventricle by assessing pulmonary vascular resistance. Normal values for these measurements are listed in Table 8-1.

Afterload for the left ventricle can be reduced by use of vasodilators, which will cause the peripheral arteries to dilate, thereby reducing the peripheral vascular resistance and often resulting in an increase in stroke volume. If the vasodilation is excessive, however, blood may tend to pool peripherally and not return to the heart efficiently, and this decreased venous return may cause the preload and stroke volume to fall.

Contractility

Optimal preload and afterload do not guarantee an adequate stroke volume, since the ability of the heart muscle to contract and move blood is equally important. Contractility cannot be measured directly but is estimated by use of hemodynamic parameters such as stroke volume and by a process of elimination. For example, when preload and afterload have been evaluated and optimized with treatment and yet the stroke volume remains low, inadequate contractility should be considered.

The ability of the myocardium to contract forcefully is referred to as the *inotropic* status of the heart. Factors that increase contractility are said to have a positive inotropic effect and those that decrease contractility are said to have a negative inotropic effect. Medications that stimulate the beta-adrenergic system (see Ch. 20) often have a positive inotropic effect and improve stroke volume. While the increase in stroke volume is often beneficial to the patient's overall tissue oxygenation status, it will result in an increase in myocardial O_2 consumption. This can be a serious consequence, especially in patients with coronary artery disease. Myocardial ischemia and certain medications such as beta-blockers are examples of factors that will have a negative inotropic effect, a potential benefit of which is reduction of myocardial O_2 consumption.

Innervation of the Heart

The heart is supplied with fibers from the sympathetic and parasympathetic nervous systems. The sympathetic fibers, which extend to the SA and AV nodes and the myocardium, act to increase the rate and force of myocardial contraction and are activated by various factors, including exercise, hypoxemia, certain medications, and stress. The increase in heart rate typically increases cardiac output; however, if the rate is excessively fast, the filling time for the ventricles will not be adequate, and output may fall. Moreover, increases in heart rate decrease the duration of the diastolic phase, which in turn decreases coronary blood flow. Since approximately 75 percent of coronary blood flow occurs during diastole,[7] significant increases in heart rate not only increase myocardial O_2 demand but also reduce perfusion of the heart.

The parasympathetic fibers, which are contained in the vagus nerve, are found primarily in the SA and AV nodes and act to slow heart rate and to inhibit AV conduction. Since few parasympathetic fibers are found in the ventricular myocardium, stimulation of the vagus nerve has little effect on contractility.

SYSTEMIC ARTERIES

The systemic arteries serve to carry oxygenated blood throughout the body. They have three layers of tissue: an inner coat of endothelium, a middle layer of smooth muscle fibers, and an outer layer of elastic tissue. The smooth muscle layer is partially replaced with elastic tissue in the large arteries and gradually decreases in thickness as the diameter of the arteries diminishes. The smallest arteries, termed *arterioles*, supply the capillary networks of the tissues.

Aorta

The left ventricle ejects oxygenated blood into a large artery, the *aorta*, which has several different sections named according to their location. The first section, the *ascending* aorta, is of greater diameter than the rest of the aorta and is relatively short. The next section is the *arch* of the aorta, located in the superior mediastinum (Fig. 8-9). In the arch of the aorta the direction changes from upward toward the head to downward toward the feet. Just distal to the arch of the aorta is the *descending* aorta, which is initially located in the posterior mediastinum to the left of the spine but assumes a slightly more ventral position as it pierces the aortic opening of the diaphragm. Below the diaphragm the aorta is known as the *abdominal* aorta.

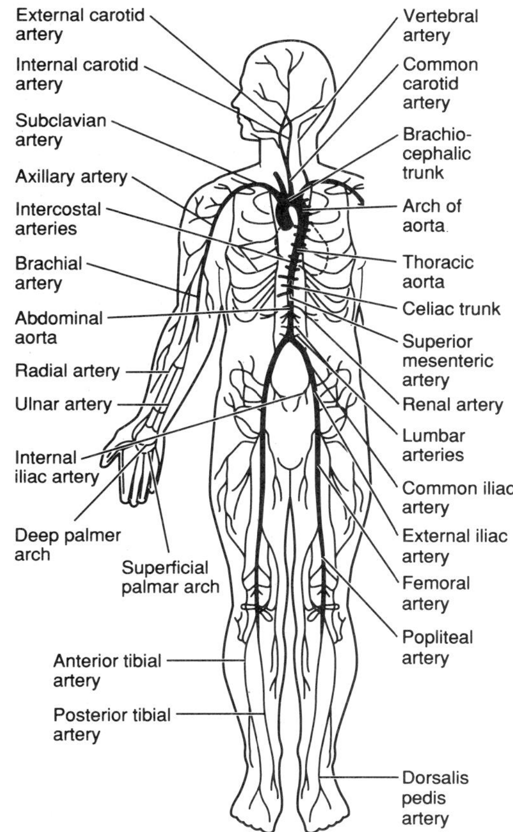

Figure 8-9. Major arteries of the body. (From Staubesand,[11] with permission.)

Aortic Branches

The arch of the aorta gives rise to the *brachiocephalic, left common carotid*, and *left subclavian* arteries (Fig. 8-9). The brachiocephalic artery arises from the right part of the aortic arch and travels superiorly 4 to 5 cm before it divides into the *right subclavian* and *right common carotid* arteries. The right and left common carotid arteries are located in the lower neck region and are situated deep to the sternocleidomastoid muscles. The common carotid arteries are rather large in diameter and are useful in evaluations when a central pulse is desired. As the common carotid arteries transcend superiorly, they divide into the *internal* and *external carotid* arteries at the level of the superior margin of the thyroid cartilage. The carotid arteries provide the major route for oxygenated blood to travel to the head while the subclavian arteries supply the neck and upper limbs.

Arteries of the Upper Limbs

The subclavian artery gives way to the *axillary* artery at the outer border of the first rib. The axillary artery extends to the lower border of the teres major muscle, where it becomes the *brachial* artery (Fig. 8-9), which courses the length of the humerus in the upper arm. The brachial artery extends to a point just past the elbow, where it divides into the *radial* and *ulnar* arteries, which run the length of the forearm to the wrist.

Arteries of the Lower Limbs

The abdominal aorta branches into the left and right *common iliac* arteries at the level of the fourth lumbar vertebra. The common iliac divides into the *internal* and *external* iliac arteries at the level of the lumbosacral articulation. The internal iliac enters the pelvic region while the external iliac artery courses beneath the inguinal ligament and becomes the *femoral* artery (Fig. 8-9), which begins in the thigh and spans the length of the femoral bone to the posterior knee region. At this point the femoral artery becomes the *popliteal* artery, which divides into the posterior and anterior *tibial* arteries in the upper portion of the calf region. The anterior tibial artery courses in the anterior part of the lower leg from the knee to the level of the ankle, where it becomes the *dorsalis pedis* artery, which courses in the dorsum of the foot.

SYSTEMIC VEINS

Systemic veins serve to carry deoxygenated blood back to the right side of the heart, where it is pumped into the pulmonary circulation for oxygenation. The structure of systemic veins is similar to that of systemic arteries; however, the walls of the veins are thinner, since the smooth muscle and elastic connective tissue are not as prevalent as in the arteries. Because of their ability to stretch, veins can accommodate large amounts of blood. Veins, unlike arteries, are frequently supplied with valves, which function to maintain a one-way blood flow.

The veins of the head, neck, and arms drain into the *superior vena cava*. This major vein, formed by the union of the right and left *brachiocephalic veins*, is short and empties into the right atrium. The *inferior vena cava* also empties into the right atrium and receives the venous blood from the structures inferior to the diaphragm. It is much longer than the superior vena cava, extending from the right atrium to the lower abdominal region. It is beyond the scope of this text to describe the details of the venous system; however, the interested reader is referred to several texts providing more complete information about all aspects of the circulatory system.[1–8]

PULMONARY CIRCULATION

Venous blood is ejected from the right ventricle into the *pulmonary trunk* (pulmonary outflow tract), which is the

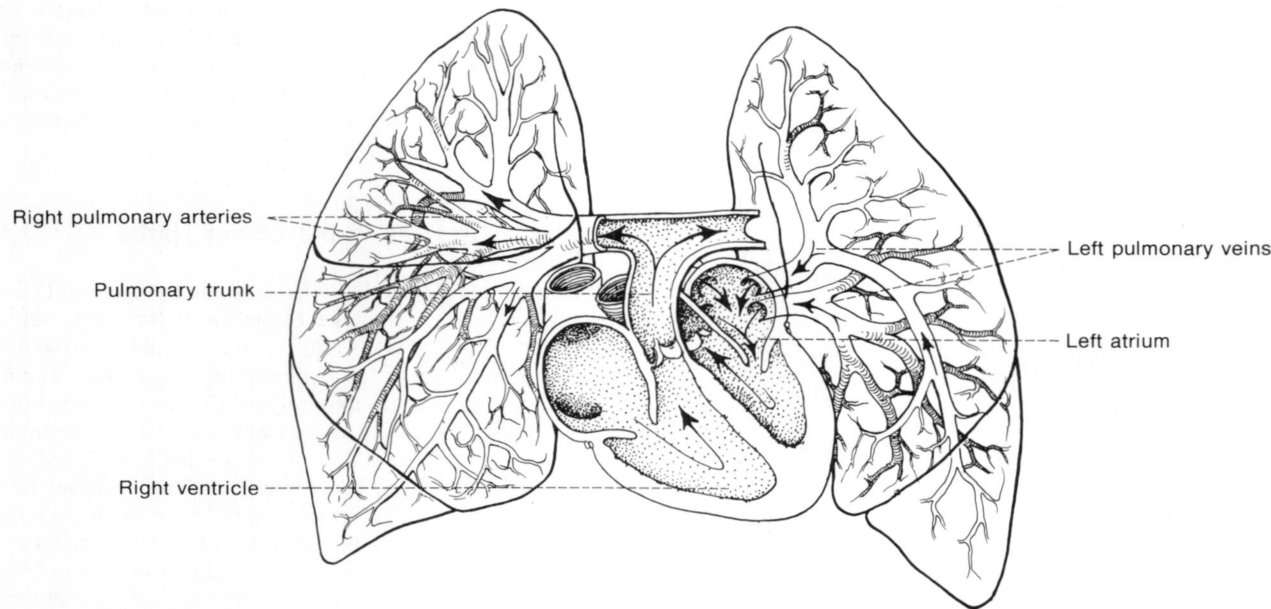

Figure 8-10. Schematic representation of the pulmonary circulation. Note how blood flows from the right ventricle into the pulmonary arteries and returns to the left atrium through the pulmonary vein. (From Montgomery,[1] with permission.)

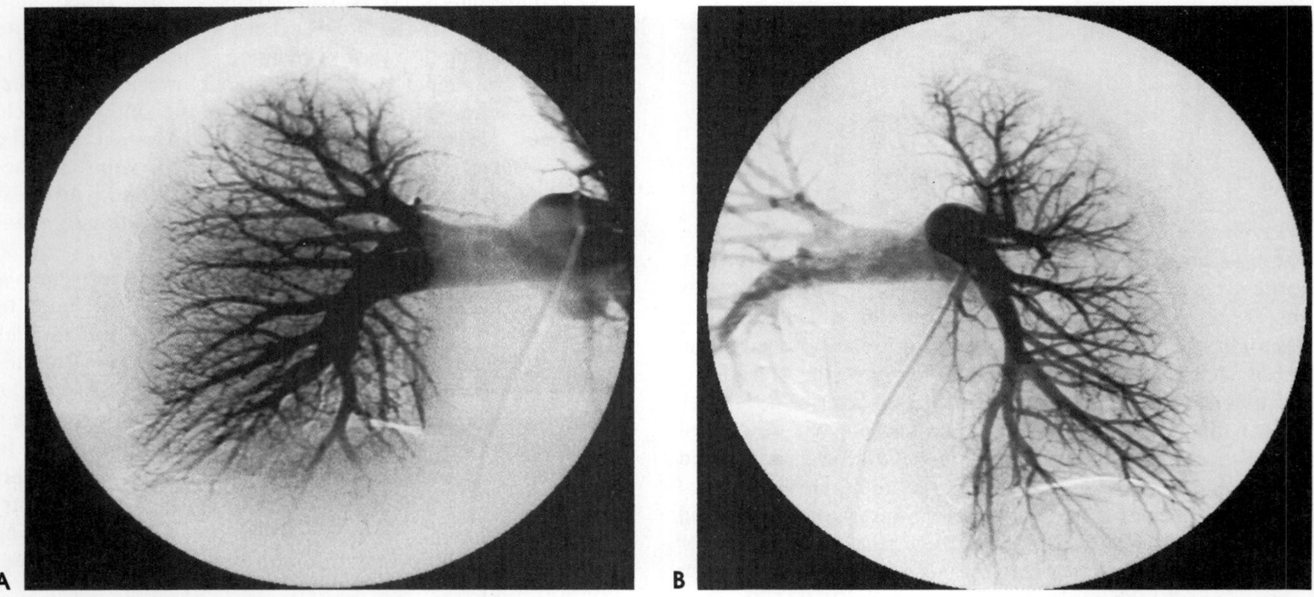

Figure 8-11. The normal pulmonary arterial tree, as seen via digital subtraction angiography. (**A**) Right lung, (**B**) left lung.

largest and the initial vessel of the pulmonary circulation (Figs. 8-10 and 8-11). This main artery soon divides into the right and left *pulmonary arteries*, which carry the blood to the right and left lungs, respectively, where the pulmonary capillaries allow gas exchange to take place. The capillaries link the pulmonary arteries with the *pulmonary veins*, which carry the oxygenated blood back to the left side of the heart. There are four pulmonary veins, two from each lung, which converge at the left atrium.

It is worth noting that the oxygenation status of pulmonary arterial and pulmonary venous blood is the reverse of that in the systemic circuit. Pulmonary arteries contain deoxygenated blood and are usually depicted as blue on anatomic charts, while pulmonary veins contain fully oxygenated blood and are shown in red.

The blood volume of the pulmonary circulation is small in comparison with that of the systemic circulation. Normally the lungs contain about 12 percent of the total blood volume, or about 600 mL of blood.[10] Under certain conditions, as in left heart failure, the amount of blood in the pulmonary circulation can increase significantly. In right heart failure the opposite occurs, with the blood volume of the lungs decreasing and the systemic volume increasing.

Normally the pulmonary circulation is a low-pressure system, normal systolic pulmonary artery pressure being 20 to 30 mmHg, diastolic 6 to 15 mmHg, and mean between 10 and 20 mmHg (Table 8-1). Left heart failure and factors that increase the pulmonary vascular resistance, such as hypoxia, cause pulmonary artery pressure to increase, whereas pulmonary artery pressures may actually decrease with right heart failure.

References

1. Montgomery RL: Basic anatomy for the Allied Health Professions. Urban & Schwarzenberg, Baltimore, 1981, pp. 275–345
2. Marieb EN: Essentials of Human Anatomy and Physiology. 2nd Ed. Benjamin Cummings, Menlo Park, CA, 1988
3. Memmler RL, Wood DL: Structure and Function of the Human Body. 4th Ed. JB Lippincott, Philadelphia, 1987
4. Lindner HH: Clinical Anatomy. Appleton & Lange, East Norwalk, CT, 1989
5. McClintic JR: Human Anatomy. CV Mosby, St. Louis, 1983
6. Pierson DJ: The evolution of breathing: There and back again: The respiratory advantages of a circulatory system. Respir Care 1982;27:569–579
7. Daily EK, Schroeder JP: Techniques in Bedside Hemodynamic Monitoring. 3rd Ed. CV Mosby, St. Louis, 1989
8. Williams PL, Warwick R, Dyson M, Bannister LH: Gray's Anatomy. 37th Ed. Churchill Livingstone, Edinburgh, 1989
9. Krider SJ: Cardiac output assessment. pp. 213–230. In Wilkins RL, Sheldon RL, Krider SJ (eds): Clinical Assessment in Respiratory Care. 2nd Ed. CV Mosby, St. Louis, 1990
10. Guyton AC: Textbook of Medical Physiology. 7th Ed. WB Saunders, Philadelphia, 1986
11. Staubesand J (ed): Sobotta: Atlas of Human Anatomy. Vol. 2. 11th English Ed. Urban & Schwarzenburg, Munich, 1990
12. Huszar RH: Basic Dysrhythmias: Interpretation and Management. CV Mosby, St. Louis, 1988

Chapter 9

Mechanics of Ventilation

Bruce H. Culver

CHAPTER OUTLINE

Movement of air in and out of the lungs is fundamental to the process of ventilation. The properties of the lung and chest associated with this movement are considered the "mechanics" of ventilation and are central to understanding both normal and abnormal lung function. They include the static properties of volume, elastic recoil, and compliance, and the dynamic properties of airflow, resistance, and work. Many of the laboratory tests used clinically to assess lung disease are measurements of these mechanical properties.

This chapter begins with a definition of the subdivisions of lung volume, then considers the elastic properties of the lungs, including surface tension, which contribute to understanding the interrelationship of lung, chest wall, and pleural space forces during ventilation. It summarizes the factors determining resistance to airflow and discusses the special dynamics of forced expiratory maneuvers as used in spirometry testing. Additional discussion of respiratory mechanics can be found in pertinent chapters of pulmonary texts,[1–4] with more detailed reviews of primary sources available in two recent compendiums.[5,6]

LUNG VOLUMES

The total gas-containing capacity of the lungs can be divided into a series of volumes,[7,8] as shown in Figure 9-1 and described in Table 9-1. The greatest amount of air that can be held in the lungs at full inspiration is the *total lung capacity* (TLC). After a complete forced exhalation the lungs are not empty but contain a *residual volume* (RV). The difference between TLC and RV and thus the greatest volume of air that can be inhaled or exhaled is the *vital capacity* (VC). This has been an important clinical measurement of lung function since the development of the spirometer in the 1840s.[9] It can be affected by factors that limit either the expansion or the emptying of the lung. A normal breath has a *tidal volume* (V_T or TV) that is only a small portion of the VC (about 10 percent) and even during strenuous exercise the V_T increases only to 50 to 60 percent of the VC. At the end of each tidal exhalation the lungs return to a resting position, which is normally about one-third of the way between RV and TLC. The volume contained in the lungs at this end-tidal position is the *functional residual capacity* (FRC).

THE LUNG–CHEST WALL SYSTEM

Understanding the process of normal breathing, special maneuvers such as coughing, and the effects of positive-pressure ventilators, requires knowledge of the mechanical properties of the thorax. The three forces primarily involved

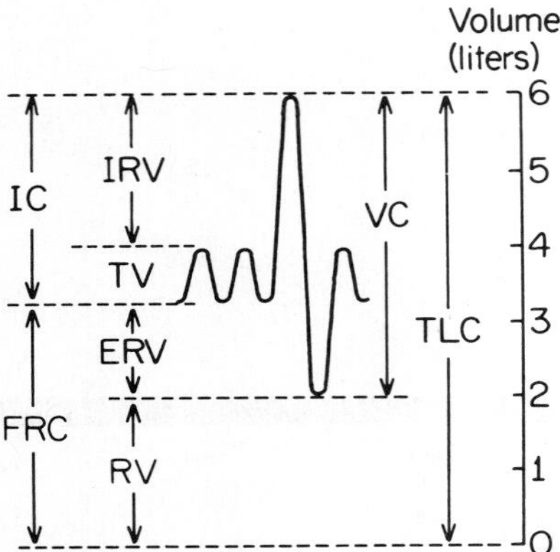

Figure 9-1. The normal spirogram and subdivisions of lung volume. See Table 9-1 for definitions. The volume scale would be appropriate only for an individual of a particular height and age. (From Culver,[7] with permission.)

are the elastic recoil properties of the lung, the elastic recoil properties of the chest, and the muscular efforts of chest wall, diaphragm, and abdomen. These result in changes in lung (and thorax) volume, in alveolar pressure, and in intrapleural pressure. This becomes clearer if the components are first considered separately.

Elastic Structures

The recoil tendency of a spring can be expressed in terms of an unstressed or resting length and a length-tension relationship. Similarly, the relevant properties of expandable volumetric structures are the unstressed volume and the relationship between volume and the transmural pressure required to achieve that volume. By convention, transmural pressures are expressed as the difference between the pressure inside and that outside the structure ($P_{in} - P_{out}$). It is sometimes convenient to think of this as the *distending pressure* required to achieve a certain volume, but it is also the *recoil pressure,* reflecting the tendency of the structure to return to its unstressed volume (defined as the point at which transmural pressure is zero). A positive recoil pressure indicates a tendency to become smaller. A structure distorted to a volume below its unstressed volume will have a negative recoil pressure, indicating its tendency to become larger. Some hypothetical expandable structures and their relationship of volume to transmural pressure are shown in Figure 9-2. Most will have an S shape, with a midrange in which volume increases readily with pressure, a flattened upper portion in which further distension is limited, and if volume can be made less than the unstressed volume, a flattened lower portion in which further reduction is limited. The unstressed volume may be relatively low (Fig. 9-2A), or relatively high (Fig. 9-2B) in the volume range.

Table 9-1. Subdivisions of Lung Volume

Volume[a]
Residual volume (RV): The volume of air that remains in the lungs after a maximal expiratory effort
Expiratory reserve volume (ERV): The volume of air that could be actively exhaled after a passive exhalation to the resting end-expiratory position has been completed
Tidal volume (VT or TV): The volume of air inspired (and expired) with each breath
Inspiratory reserve volume (IRV): The volume of air that could be actively inhaled after a tidal inhalation to the end-inspiratory position has been completed
Capacities[a]
Functional residual capacity (FRC): The volume of air that remains in the lungs after a passive tidal expiration (i.e., at the end-expiratory position)
Inspiratory capacity (IC): The maximum volume of air that can be inhaled from the resting end-expiratory position
Vital capacity (VC): The maximum volume of air that can be actively exhaled after a maximal inspiratory effort
Total lung capacity (TLC): The volume of air contained in the lungs at the end of a maximum inspiration

[a] By convention the term *volume* is applied to the smallest subdivisions that do not overlap and the term *capacity* is used for combinations of these.

Elastic Properties of the Lung

The lungs are elastic structures with a tendency to recoil to a small *unstressed volume* (usually slightly less than RV).[10] Maintaining any lung volume larger than this requires the presence of a force acting to distend the lungs. This force is the difference between the alveolar pressure (P_{alv}) and the intrapleural pressure surrounding the lungs, often more simply referred to as pleural pressure (P_{pl}). The elastic properties of the lungs and their tendency to recoil can be represented by plotting lung volume against the distending (or recoil) pressure (Fig. 9-3). It does not matter whether this is an excised lung being blown up by a pump, an in vivo lung inflated by a ventilator, or the more physiologic normal lung inflated by expanding the chest (creating a more negative pleural pressure); in each case the curve of volume versus the pressure difference ($P_{alv} - P_{pl}$) is the same.

The slope of this pressure-volume curve represents the *compliance* of the lungs:

$$C_L = \frac{\Delta V}{\Delta P}$$

The compliance decreases as the lungs near the limit of their distensibility at TLC. Compliance is usually measured just above FRC in the tidal breathing range. Since it is normally expressed in absolute volume units (e.g., L/cmH_2O) compliance is strongly dependent on lung size. A single lung, for example, will have only half the volume change for the same pressure change as two lungs. A small child's normal lung compliance would be considerably lower than an adult's. For this reason, compliance is often divided by lung volume to give the volume independent *specific compliance.*

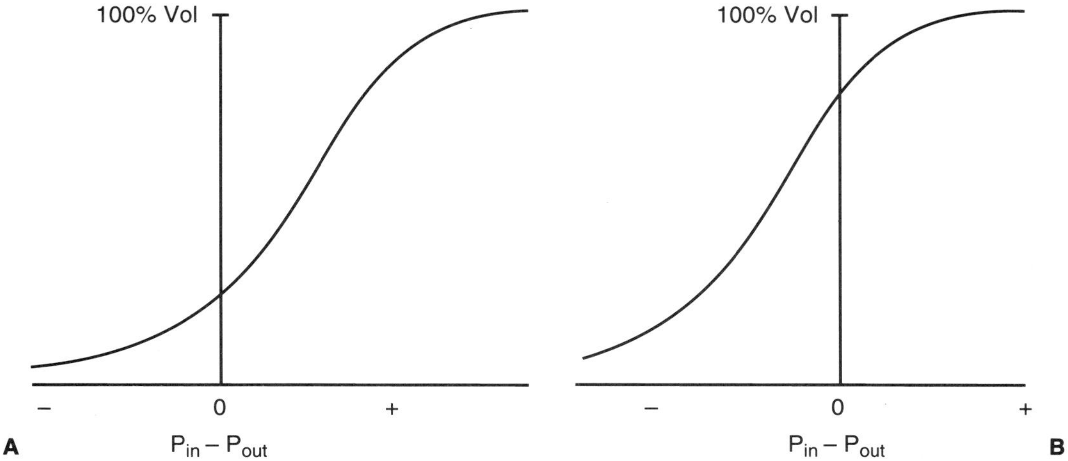

Figure 9-2. Two hypothetical expandable structures and their relationship of volume to transmural pressure ($P_{in} - P_{out}$). **(A)** Relatively low unstressed volume (e.g., an inner tube); **(B)** relatively high unstressed volume (e.g., a tubeless tire).

Elastic Properties of the Chest Wall

The chest wall has elastic properties that can be expressed in the same way as those of the lung. Figure 9-4 shows a plot of volume versus recoil pressure for the relaxed chest wall (solid line) as well as the curve for the lung. The unstressed volume of the chest wall (where recoil pressure is zero) is normally quite high, above the usual tidal breathing range. When the chest wall is "distorted" to a smaller volume, it tries to recoil outward, and when expanded above its unstressed volume, it recoils inward. Recoil pressure for the relaxed chest wall ($P_{in} - P_{out}$) is $P_{pl} - P_{atm}$ (atmospheric pressure) or simply P_{pl}, since P_{atm} is taken to be zero.

The compliance of the chest wall is similar to that of the lungs in the midrange of volume, but at TLC the chest remains as distensible as it is at FRC. This suggests that it is the lungs rather than the chest wall that normally limit further volume expansion at TLC.

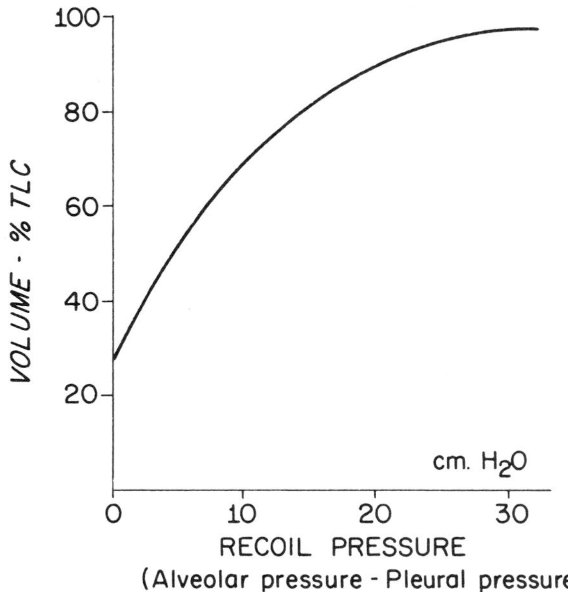

Figure 9-3. The normal pressure-volume curve of the lung as obtained during a very slow expiration from total lung capacity. (From Culver,[7] with permission.)

Lung and Chest Wall: The Respiratory System

In the intact thorax the lungs and the chest wall move together. The muscular effort required to inspire a volume of air or the pressure that must be developed by a ventilator to achieve the same volume change is determined by the pressure-volume curve of the combined respiratory system,[11] shown by the dashed line in Figure 9-4. The lungs and chest wall normally contain the same volume of air, so that only points on the same horizontal line in Figure 9-4 can coexist. Since both the lungs and the chest wall are expanded together, the distending pressure for the respiratory system will be the sum of the distending pressures required by the lungs and chest wall. The transmural pressure for the respiratory system ($P_{in} - P_{out}$) is $P_{alv} - P_{atm}$, which can be seen to equal the sum of ($P_{alv} - P_{pl}$) + ($P_{pl} - P_{atm}$). The flatter slope of the dashed line in Figure 9-4 shows that a greater pressure change is required to add volume to the total respiratory system than to either of its components alone; thus the compliance of the respiratory system is lower than that of either lungs or chest wall at the same volume. This is often confusing, as it may seem that adding the chest wall

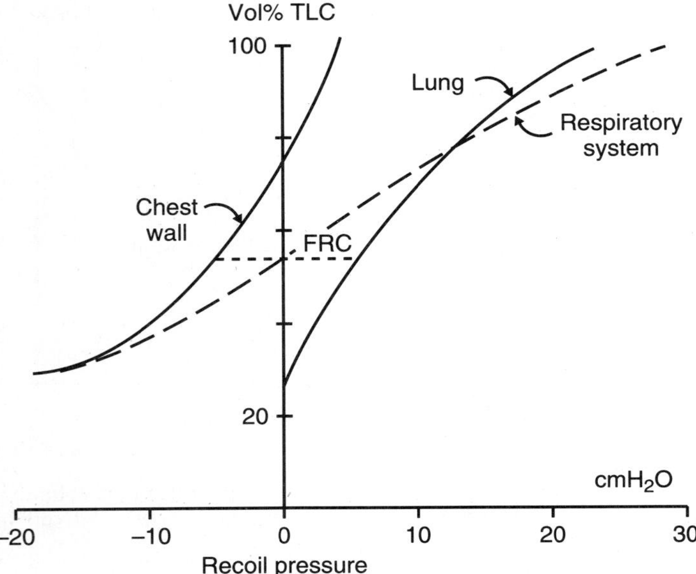

Figure 9-4. The pressure-volume curves of the relaxed chest wall, the lungs, and the combined respiratory system. (From Culver,[7] with permission.)

with its outward recoil should help the lung expand. Note, however, that as the system is inflated above FRC, the outward recoil of the chest wall diminishes, and its contribution to lung inflation must be replaced by added muscle force or ventilator pressure. If one measures the V_T passively delivered to a relaxed patient on mechanical ventilation and divides this by the airway pressure required to hold this volume in the chest (minus any end-expiratory airway pressure), the result is the compliance of the respiratory system (C_{RS}), often expressed in milliliters per centimeter of water.

The third mechanical factor, muscle force, is not considered in this diagram. Thus the pressure difference across the lung, which has no muscle, can always be taken from its curve, but the pressure across the chest wall (and diaphragm) may reflect muscle tension and will only be described by this curve during complete relaxation. Similarly, the curve for the respiratory system shows the pressure that would be measured by a manometer held tightly in the mouth after a subject had inhaled or exhaled to a particular volume and then relaxed all muscle effort.

At the resting end-tidal position of the respiratory system (FRC) no active muscular forces are applied and P_{alv} equals P_{atm} (distending pressure is zero). The lung is distended above its unstressed volume and the chest wall is held below its unstressed volume. The FRC is the volume at which the opposing tendencies of the lungs to recoil inward and the chest wall to recoil outward are evenly balanced. Any change in the unstressed volume or the compliance of either lungs or chest wall would result in a new FRC. For example, obesity shifts the chest wall curve to the right (less outward recoil) and so tends to reduce the FRC. Emphysema increases lung compliance and unstressed volume and so tends to increase FRC.

The opposing forces of lung and chest wall create a subatmospheric (negative) pressure in the intrapleural space at FRC (Fig. 9-5). Since the lungs and chest wall are not directly linked, it is actually the intrapleural pressure that opposes both lung recoil and chest wall recoil. Intrapleural pressure must therefore have the same magnitude as each of these recoil forces. It is normally about -5 cmH_2O at FRC.

EVENTS OF THE RESPIRATORY CYCLE

Inspiration is an active process. Contraction of the inspiratory muscles (primarily the intercostals and the diaphragm) changes the balance of forces on the lung. The expanding thorax creates a more negative intrapleural pressure, which expands the lungs. The alveolar pressure becomes negative with respect to the atmosphere and air flows into the lungs, as shown in Figure 9-6. This process continues until lung volume reaches a point at which lung recoil pressure is increased to balance the combined muscular and elastic forces of the chest wall. At this point alveolar pressure becomes zero and the inspiratory flow stops because there is no longer a pressure gradient along the airways.

During normal breathing expiration is a passive process. The inspiratory muscles relax, and the balance of forces is again shifted. With expiration the alveolar pressure becomes positive and the air moves from alveoli through the airways to the outside atmosphere. (Since the chest wall is still below its unstressed volume, it still has a small outward recoil

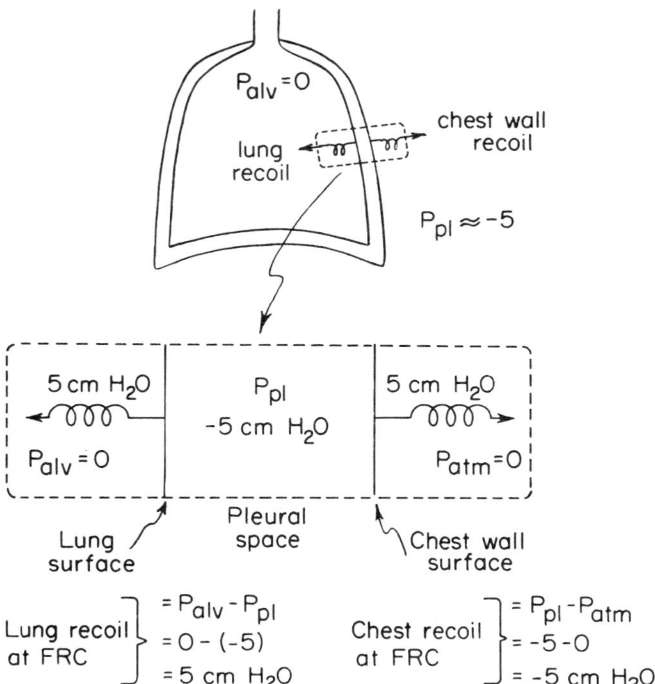

Figure 9-5. The balance of respiratory system pressures and forces creates a negative intrapleural pressure at FRC. (From Culver,[7] with permission.)

force, and pleural pressure will be negative.) This process continues until the lung reaches a volume at which the forces are again balanced and alveolar pressure is zero. During active expiration this process can be assisted by contraction of the expiratory muscles (intercostal and abdominal wall muscles), making pleural pressure positive.

RESPIRATORY MUSCLE EFFORT

The maximum inspiratory and expiratory pressures measure the maximal efforts of the respiratory muscles[12] (Fig. 9-7). That is, if one were to try to inhale against a closed pressure manometer, the negative pressure that can be generated at the mouth is about 100 cmH_2O at a low lung volume. It becomes progressively less at higher lung volumes until at TLC no negative pressure can be generated, which indicates that no more air can be drawn into the chest. Maximum expiratory pressures are somewhat greater, 150 to 200 cmH_2O at high lung volume, and fall to zero at RV.

EFFECT OF SURFACE TENSION

At the surface of a liquid the intermolecular forces are not balanced by the more widely spaced molecules of the gas phase, which creates *surface tension*. The surface tension

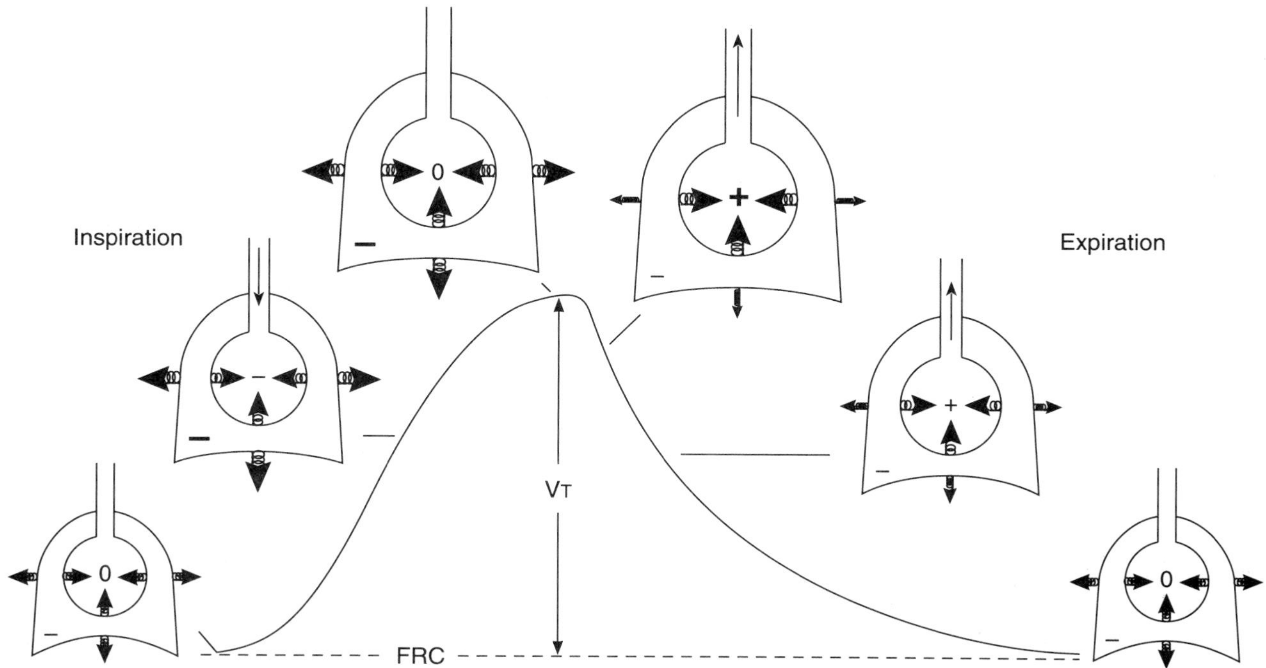

Figure 9-6. Spontaneous inspiration of the V_T is generated by the addition of muscle force to create a more negative intrapleural pressure. With relaxation of muscles at end inspiration, only the diminished outward recoil of the chest wall remains to oppose the increased lung recoil that drives passive expiration.

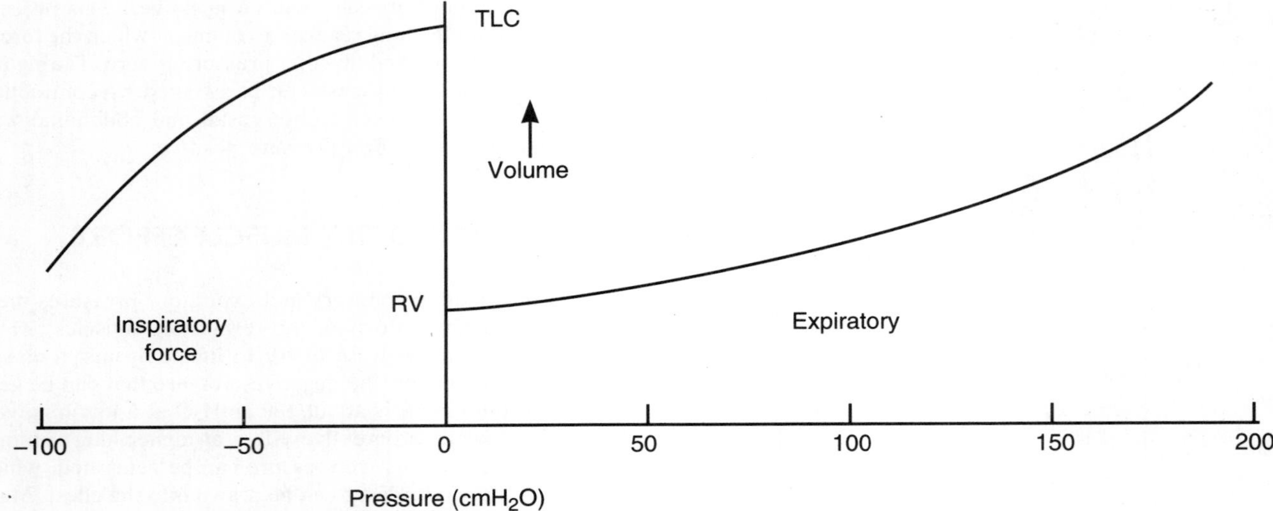

Figure 9-7. The normal maximum inspiratory and expiratory forces generated by the diaphragm, chest wall, and abdominal and accessory muscles. (From Culver,[7] with permission.)

of the air-liquid interface lining the alveoli makes an important contribution to the elastic properties of the lung shown by the pressure-volume curve. If a lung is filled with liquid, these surface forces are abolished and the resultant pressure-volume curve (Fig. 9-8) reflects only the tissue properties of the lung.[13] The curve of the liquid-filled lung is shifted to the left, showing that the lung can be distended with much less pressure than when air-filled. The air-filled lung, in addition to requiring greater pressure, demonstrates marked *hysteresis;* that is, the pressure-volume curve during inflation is different from that during deflation.

Although there is surface tension in the air-filled lung, it is much lower and behaves differently from what would be expected in an air-filled lung with a saline-covered surface.

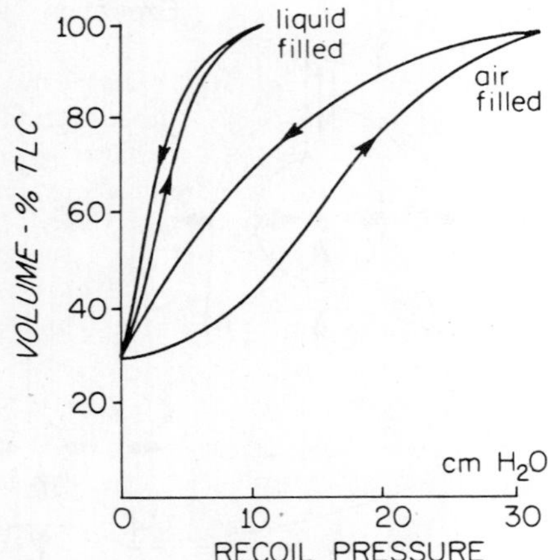

Figure 9-8. Pressure-volume curves obtained on inflation and deflation of a normal air-filled lung and the same lung when filled with liquid to eliminate the forces due to surface tension. (From Culver,[7] with permission.)

The deflation curve for the air-filled lung approaches that for the liquid-filled lung at low lung volume, this shows that the pressure due to surface forces becomes small, whereas the pressure due to a constant surface tension should increase as alveoli become smaller. Laplace's law relates the pressure (P) within a sphere to wall tension (T) and radius (r): $P = 2T/r$. If the surface tension remained constant as r decreased (smaller alveoli), the pressure due to surface tension would rise.

This situation is avoided in the lung by the presence of a unique surface lining material, *surfactant,* which not only reduces surface tension (as would a detergent) but does so in a volume-dependent manner.[14] The molecules are oriented with their polar ends in the water and their hydrophobic ends, which tend to repel one another, on the surface. As lung volume and surface area decrease, the lining layer is compressed and the increased repelling force of these molecules opposes the intermolecular attraction of water molecules, so that net surface tension decreases until it is nearly abolished at the RV. As an important consequence, the work needed to expand the lungs is greatly reduced. Surfactant also helps to maintain the stability of small alveoli.[15] If pressure increased in smaller alveoli, they would quickly empty into larger (lower-pressure) alveoli and would require great forces to reopen. Surfactant allows interconnecting alveoli of different sizes to coexist at the same pressure. The inward-directed force of surface tension in the curved alveoli lowers interstitial pressure in the adjacent tissue, tending to draw fluid from the capillaries. By lowering surface tension, surfactant helps to prevent lung edema.

INTERDEPENDENCE IN THE LUNG

Since the lung parenchyma is made up of interconnected alveolar walls, interstitial tissues, and fibers, a local distortion will be opposed by the surrounding tissue. That is, if we try to collapse a small zone of alveoli within a lobe, the surrounding tissue will be stretched and thus will tend to pull it back open. This property is termed *structural interdependence.*[10] It, along with surfactant and the presence of collateral air pathways, helps to prevent the collapse of alveoli (atelectasis) even when small bronchioles become plugged. Since the bronchi and blood vessels travel through the lung parenchyma, they too are affected by the surrounding tissue. As the lung expands, the caliber of these channels will also be increased.

DYNAMICS OF VENTILATION

Flow Resistance

Air flow between the atmosphere and alveolar gas is dependent on driving pressure and airway resistance. The normal airway resistance (RAW) during quiet breathing (or a panting maneuver, as it is usually measured clinically) is less than 2 $cmH_2O/L/s$). Flow rate ($\dot{V}$) is given by

$$\dot{V} = \frac{\Delta P}{R} = \frac{P_{atm} - P_{alv}}{R_{aw}}$$

and airflow resistance (R) is affected by: (1) viscosity of air; (2) length of airways (R is directly proportional to length); and (3) caliber of airways (R is proportional to $1/r^4$). Thus a doubling of length would double resistance but a halving of caliber would cause a 16-fold increase in resistance. Airways have an initial caliber determined by their anatomic location in the bronchial tree, but this is further modified by lung volume, bronchial muscle contraction, mucous secretions, and the instantaneous pressure across the airway wall. All these factors except the last are similar during both inspiration and expiration. During inspiration (Fig. 9-9A) the intrathoracic pressure surrounding airways is more negative than the intra-airway pressure, so that airways tend to be distended. With forced expiratory efforts (Fig. 9-9B) the pleural pressure becomes positive and greater than intra-airway pressure. Since their cartilaginous structure is incomplete, airways are compressed under such forces, reducing the caliber of the lumen. This dynamic compression of airways is a cause of flow limitation during forced expiration.[16,17]

Maximum airflow rates are evaluated by having the subject take a full inspiration (to TLC) and then blow the air out as forcefully and completely (to RV) as possible.[18–21] From a spirometer one can record this *forced expiratory spirogram* as volume versus time[22] (Fig. 9-10A), or if the flow rate is also measured, one can record the same information as a *maximum expiratory flow volume* curve[23–25] (Fig. 9-10B). A remarkable feature of this maneuver is that the maximum flow rate for any volume, except the highest lung volumes near the beginning of the exhalation, is achieved with submaximal effort and cannot be exceeded with further effort. This effect, demonstrated in Figure 9-11, results from the dynamic compression noted above. Since this compression begins when intra-airway pressure falls below pleural pressure, the *effective* driving pressure becomes $P_{alv} - P_{pl}$ (30 − 25 = 5 in Fig. 9-9B). This is the same as the elastic recoil pressure of the lung and is a function of lung volume (Fig. 9-3), not effort.

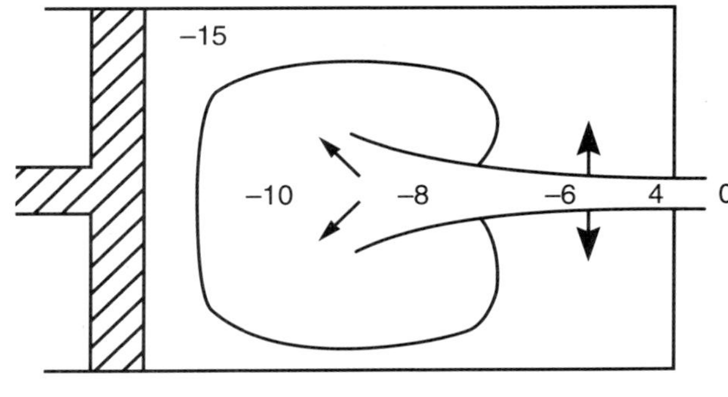

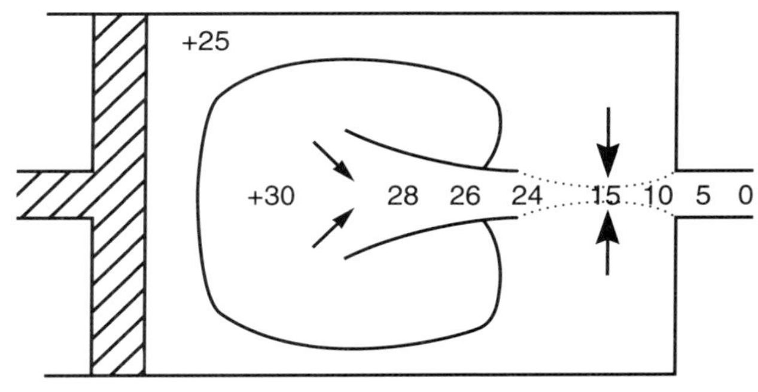

Figure 9-9. **(A)** Inspiration. Intrathoracic airways tend to be distended by a negative extramural pressure, which lowers airway resistance. During a relaxed expiration there is less distension and a slightly higher resistance. **(B)** Forced expiration. Intrathoracic airways are compressed by an extramural pressure that exceeds the intraluminal pressure in central airways. The effective driving pressure becomes $P_{alv} - P_{pl}$ (30 − 25 = 5 in the example shown). If a greater expiratory effort were made, for example, by raising pleural pressure to +50 cmH_2O at the same lung volume, the alveolar pressure would be +55 and the effective driving pressure (55 − 50 = 5) and resultant flow rate would remain unchanged. (From Culver,[7] with permission.)

This mechanism may have its major physiologic significance in normal subjects during a cough. Although overall airflow rate (in liters per second) out of the lungs is not increased by the high pleural and alveolar pressures generated, the *velocity* (in meters per second) of air particle motion through the narrowed major airways is greatly increased, aiding in the removal of secretions and foreign material.

Work of Breathing

The muscle effort required to raise lung volume above the FRC during inspiration is a form of work. Part of this is the

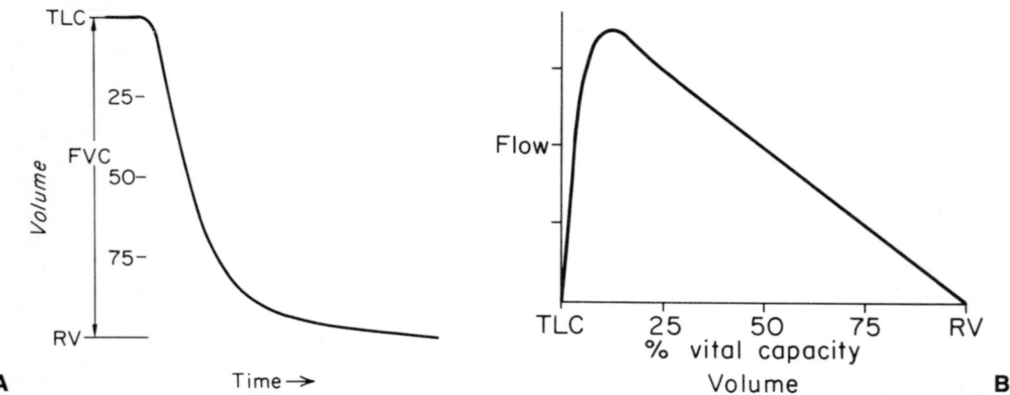

Figure 9-10. The forced vital capacity maneuver can be displayed as (**A**) an expiratory spirogram or (**B**) as a flow-volume curve. Volume axes typically show percent of vital capacity expired for the spirogram but, unlike the example above, show percent of vital capacity remaining for the flow-volume curve. (From Culver,[7] with permission.)

elastic work used to stretch the tissues and surface lining of the lung; another part is the *frictional work* required to overcome airflow resistance in the airways. The elastic work stored in stretched alveolar walls on inspiration then provides the energy needed to push air out during the subsequent passive exhalation. With active expiratory efforts, additional muscle work is done on expiration as well. When tidal breathing is done at a low lung volume, airways are narrower and resistance (and thus frictional work) markedly increased (R is proportional to $1/r^4$). At high lung volumes the muscles must do more elastic work to stretch the lungs. The combined elastic and frictional work tends to be at a minimum near the normal FRC.[26] The lung volume at which tidal breathing occurs may change rapidly, or may change chronically, if either the elastic or the frictional contributions to work of breathing change.

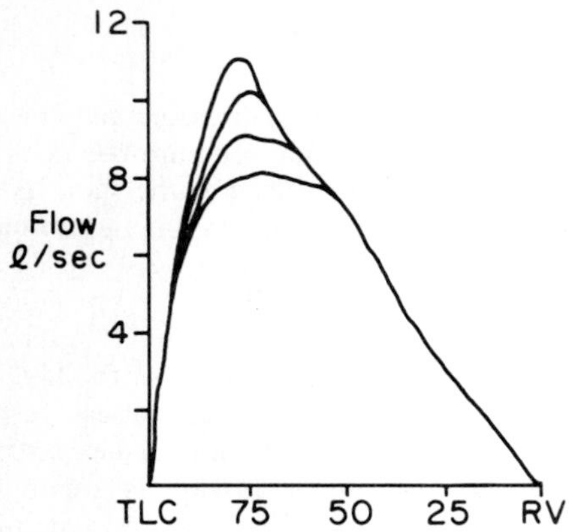

Figure 9-11. The top curve represents a maximum expiratory effort, and the lower curves show the flow resulting from progressively less effort. At lower lung volumes the maximum flow rate is relatively independent of effort. (From Culver,[7] with permission.)

The narrowed airways present in obstructive lung disease increase frictional work, and the volume for least work shifts up. The accompanying shift of the resting tidal breathing range to a higher volume occurs progressively with chronic obstructive disease. A further increase in end-expiratory lung volume can occur rapidly in an asthma attack[27] or when respiratory frequency increases with exercise. In these circumstances expiratory time may be insufficient to allow full exhalation of the tidal breath to the usual FRC. Transiently, inspiratory volume will exceed expiratory volume and both end-inspiratory and end-expiratory lung volumes will increase. As this occurs, the accompanying increases in elastic recoil pressure and airway caliber will allow expiratory flow rate to increase until the full V_T can again be exhaled in the time allowed. Since exhalation does not continue to equilibration with atmosphere, the alveolar pressure will still be positive when the next breath is initiated. Respiratory muscles must do additional work to reduce alveolar and airway pressure below zero before inspiratory flow can begin.[28] This will contribute to dyspnea and fatigue. The same process of "air trapping" is common when patients with severe airflow obstruction receive mechanical ventilation, in which case the increase in positive end-expiratory pressure (PEEP) is termed *auto-PEEP* and may have important consequences[29] (see Ch. 84).

Restrictive disease processes reduce lung compliance, requiring the muscles to generate more force to stretch the lung. The elastic work required to breathe at any lung volume is higher, and this decreases the volume for least work. In addition to breathing from a lower FRC, these patients tend to conserve work by breathing with a smaller V_T and at a correspondingly higher rate.[26]

Normally the energy consumed by breathing is very small. In metabolic terms it requires less than 1 mL/min of O_2 consumption for 1 L/min of ventilation or only about 1 to 2 percent of our total body O_2 consumption at rest. With severe airway obstruction the energy cost of breathing becomes much higher.[30]

Distribution of Ventilation

The incoming air of each tidal breath is not distributed evenly to all alveoli in the lung.[31] Earlier in this chapter pleural pressure is described as if it were the same throughout the chest, but in fact there is a vertical gradient of several centimeters of H_2O due to gravity and the configuration of the chest and diaphragm. At FRC the -5 cmH_2O value represents an average value at midlevel, but the pressure outside the lung might be -8 cmH_2O near the apices and only -2 cmH_2O near the bases. Since alveoli throughout the lung have similar maximum volume and pressure-volume relationships and since alveolar pressure is everywhere the same, those airspaces near the top of the lung are held at larger volume (distending pressure of 8 cmH_2O) than those near the bottom (distending pressure of 2 cmH_2O).[32] This places the lower alveoli on a steeper (more compliant) portion of their pressure-volume curve. In addition, the proximity of the basal alveoli to the motion of the diaphragm exposes them to a greater increase in distending pressure with inspiration. These two factors combine to give the lower portion of the normal lung a relatively greater tidal expansion and thus a greater proportion of the tidal ventilation than the apices.

A second consequence of the higher pleural pressure in the basal portions of the lung is that the distending pressure of the small airways is also less. At RV airways may become closed,[33] and the basal portions of the lung will reach this "closing volume" first, while higher portions of the lung are still partially distended. Thus a patient breathing at very low lung volumes, near RV (e.g., an obese patient), may have basal airway closure and consequently little ventilation to the lung bases.[34–37]

In summary, respiratory units in the basal portion of the lung contain less gas but receive more ventilation as long as they remain open. However, they are more susceptible to airway closure and loss of ventilation at low lung volume.

References

1. Bates DV: Respiratory Function in Disease. 3rd Ed. WB Saunders, Philadelphia, 1989
2. Murray JF: The Normal Lung. 2nd Ed. WB Saunders, Philadelphia, 1986
3. Murray JF, Nadel JA (eds): Textbook of Respiratory Medicine. Vol. 1. WB Saunders, Philadelphia, 1988
4. West JB: Respiratory Physiology—The Essentials. 4th Ed. Williams & Wilkins, Baltimore, 1990
5. Crystal RG, West JB (eds): The Lung: Scientific Foundations. Vol. 1. Raven Press, New York, 1991
6. Macklem PT, Mead J (eds): Handbook of Physiology. Section 3: The Respiratory System, Vol. 3 (parts 1 and 2). Mechanics of Breathing. American Physiological Society, Bethesda, 1986
7. Culver BH: Mechanics of ventilation. p. 11. In Culver BH (ed): The Respiratory System. Syllabus for Human Biology. University of Washington Health Sciences Academic Services, Seattle, WA, 1990
8. Pappenheimer JR, Comroe JH, Cournand A et al: Standardization of definitions and symbols in respiratory physiology. Fed Proc 1950;9:602–615
9. Hutchinson J: On the capacity of the lungs, and on the respiratory movements, with the view of establishing a precise and easy method of detecting disease by the spirometer. Lancet 1846;1:630–632
10. Hoppin FG Jr, Hildebrandt J: Mechanical properties of the lung. pp. 83–162. In West JB (ed): Bioengineering Aspects of the Lung. Vol. 3. Lung Biology, Health, Disease Series. Marcel Dekker, New York, 1977
11. Rahn H, Otis AB, Chadwich LE, Fenn WO: The pressure-volume diagram of the thorax and lung. Am J Physiol 1946;146:161–178
12. Cook DC, Mead J, Orzalesi MM: Static volume-pressure characteristics of the respiratory system during maximal efforts. J Appl Physiol 1964;19:1016–1022
13. Bachofen H, Hildebrandt J, Bachofen M: Pressure-volume curves of air- and liquid-filled excised lungs—surface tension in situ. J Appl Physiol 1970;29:422–431
14. Dobbs LG: Pulmonary surfactant. Annu Rev Med 1989;40:431–446
15. Clements JA, Hustead RF, Johnson RP, Gribetz I: Pulmonary surface tension and alveolar stability. J Appl Physiol 1961; 16:444–450
16. Mead J, Turner JM, Macklem PT, Little JB: Significance of the relationship between lung recoil and maximum expiratory flow. J Appl Physiol 1967;22:95–108
17. Pride NB, Permutt S, Riley RL, Bromberger-Barnea B: Determinants of maximum expiratory flow from the lungs. J Appl Physiol 1967;23:646–662
18. American Thoracic Society: Standardization of spirometry—1987 update. Am Rev Respir Dis 1987;136:1285–1298
19. Morris AH, Kanner RE, Crapo RO, Gardner RM (eds): Clinical Pulmonary Function Testing: A Manual of Uniform Laboratory Procedures. 2nd Ed. Intermountain Thoracic Society, 1984
20. Enright PL, Hyatt RE: Office Spirometry: A Practical Guide to the Selection and Use of Spirometers. Lea & Febiger, Philadelphia, 1987
21. Crapo RO, Morris AH, Gardner RM: Reference spirometric values using techniques and equipment that meet ATS recommendations. Am Rev Respir Dis 1981;123:659–664
22. Gaensler EA: Analysis of the ventilatory defect by timed capacity measurements. Am Rev Respir Dis 1951;64:256–278
23. Knudson RJ, Lebowitz MD, Holberg CJ, Burrows B: Changes in the normal expiratory flow-volume curve with growth and aging. Am Rev Respir Dis 1983;127:725–734
24. Black LF, Offord K, Hyatt RE: Variability in the maximal expiratory flow volume curve in asymptomatic smokers and in nonsmokers. Am Rev Respir Dis 1974;110:282–292
25. Culver BH: Pulmonary function testing. pp. 1992–1999. In Kelley WN (ed): Textbook of Internal Medicine. JB Lippincott, Philadelphia, 1989
26. Bates JHT, Milic-Emili J: Breathing patterns and the concepts of minimum respiratory work and minimum effort. pp. 243–249. In von Euler C, Lagercrantz H (eds): Neurobiology of the Control of Breathing. Raven Press, New York, 1986
27. Woolcock AJ, Rebuck AS, Cade JF, Read J: Lung volume changes in asthma measured concurrently by two methods. Am Rev Respir Dis 1971;104:703–709
28. Milic-Emili J, Gottfried SB, Rossi A: Intrinsic PEEP and its ramifications in patients with respiratory failure. pp. 141–148. In Grassino A, Fracchia C, Rampulla C, Zocchi L (eds): Respiratory Muscles in COPD. Springer-Verlag, Berlin, 1988
29. Pepe PE, Marini JJ: Occult positive end-expiratory pressure in mechanically ventilated patients with airflow obstruction. Am Rev Respir Dis 1982;126:166–170
30. Field S, Kelly S, Macklem PT: The oxygen cost of breathing in patients with cardiorespiratory disease. Am Rev Respir Dis 1982;126:9–13
31. Crawford ABH, Makowska M, Engel LA: Effect of tidal volume on ventilation maldistribution. Respir Physiol 1986;66:11–25
32. Glazier JB, Hughes JMB, Maloney JE, West JB: Vertical gra-

dient of alveolar size in lungs of dogs frozen intact. J Appl Physiol 1967;23:694–705

33. Leith DE, Mead J: Mechanisms determining residual volume of the lungs in normal subjects. J Appl Physiol 1967;23:221–227
34. Leblanc P, Raff F, Milic-Emili J: Effects of age and body position on airway closure in man. J Appl Physiol 1970;28:448–451
35. Engel LA, Grassino A, Anthonisen NR: Demonstration of airway closure in man. J Appl Physiol 1975;38:1117–1125
36. Craig DB, Wahba WM, Don HF et al: "Closing volume" and its relationship to gas exchange in seated and supine positions. J Appl Physiol 1971;31:717–721
37. Crawford ABH, Cotton DJ, Paiva M, Engel LA: Effect of airway closure on ventilation distribution. J Appl Physiol 1989;66:2511–2515

Chapter 10

Perfusion, Ventilation, and Gas Exchange

John Butler

CHAPTER OUTLINE

Previous chapters have given an overview of respiratory processes and described the chest as a bellows for the inhalation and exhalation of gas, with the heart functioning as a pump to perfuse the lungs with blood. This chapter discusses the main function of the lungs, which depends on both these mechanisms, ventilation and perfusion, to oxygenate the blood and eliminate CO_2. Although some of the concepts considered in this chapter are difficult to understand, they are important as the basis for much of our work. If they are known, it is very unlikely that serious mistakes will be made in the care of patients even when something unexpected happens.

The three functions brought together in this chapter are discussed in more detail by J. B. West in Chapters 3, 4, and 5 of the third edition of his book *Respiratory Physiology: The Essentials*[1] and in Chapter 15 (by E. Weibel) of *Pulmonary Diseases and Disorders*,[2] (edited by A. P. Fishman).

PERFUSION

Although the function of the heart and blood vessels has been considered in Chapter 8, some features of the pulmonary circulation are reconsidered here because of their importance in gas exchange. Certain aspects of lung blood flow appear incomprehensible in an organ developed to exchange gas between the atmosphere and the blood. For instance, the matching of ventilation to perfusion, even in the normal lung, is far from exact.[3] However, in pondering these aberrations one should remember that the pulmonary circulation is designed to provide other functions as well. These include filtering out particles that might otherwise embolize the brain or heart; altering chemicals that regulate many functions of the body (e.g., converting angiotensin I to angiotensin II and thereby affecting blood pressure); aiding the heart in propelling blood around the body; and acting as a radiator to get rid of excess heat generated by exercise.

Anatomy

The pulmonary vessels divide into branches, as does a tree, finally forming thin sheets of blood like leaves in the alveolar walls. These alveolar microvessels are the capillaries, and gases can pass easily across their walls in and out of the blood. Most gas exchange takes place via these alveolar vessels. It is sometimes claimed that the alveolar capillaries always function as separate tubes, but the flow of

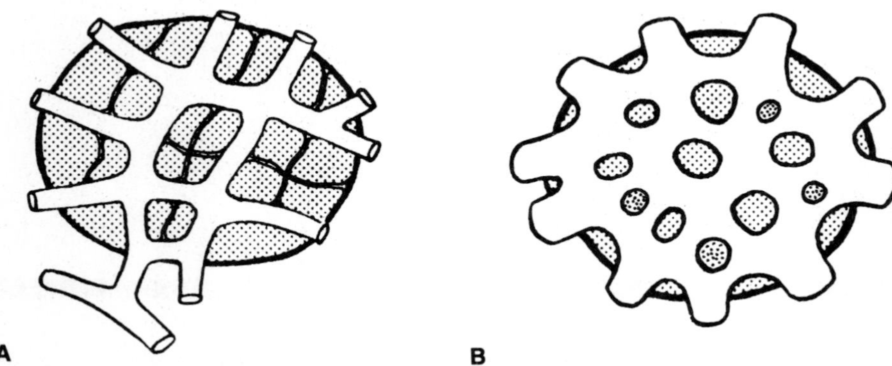

Figure 10-1. **(A)** The normal cardiac output requires only a portion of the alveolar capillary tubes. **(B)** These vessels are distended and other vessels recruited to simulate a sheet of blood when transmural pressures rise.

blood in the alveolar wall has also been likened to that of a sheet of blood. In this latter model the movement of the red blood cells (RBCs) may be compared to that of cars in an underground parking garage, the roof of which is separated from the floor by posts[4] (Figs. 10-1 and 10-2). This "sheet flow" is theoretically more efficient for gas exchange and perfusion, but less well adapted for filtering particles and chemical conversion of blood components by the endothelial cells lining the walls. Blood flow into the pulmonary capillaries is pulsatile, distending them with each systole, so the adjacent alveolar gas is churned and mixed.

The arteries and veins (extra-alveolar vessels) leading to and from those in the alveolar walls, although sturdier than the capillaries, are much more delicate and narrow than those in the systemic circulation. Because they are so elastic, their caliber depends on the pressure difference between the inside and the outside, called the *transmural pressure*. The outside (extramural) pressure drops and stretches the vessel

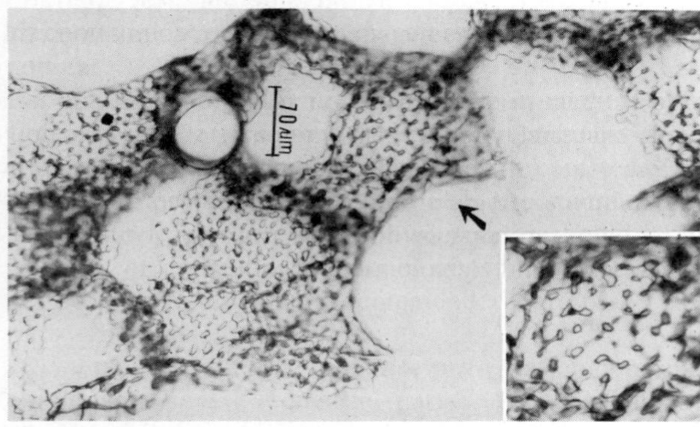

Figure 10-2. Actual photomicrograph of distended, fully recruited alveolar vessels, showing the resemblance to a sheet with posts. The posts are formed by alveolar tissue extending between alveoli through the sheet. (Arrow indicates portion of photomicrograph enlarged in insert.) (Courtesy of Sidney S. Sobin.)

open as lung volume increases; the reverse occurs on lung deflation[5] (Fig. 10-3). The intravascular pressure depends on the impetus given by the heart and does not change much with lung volume. The resistance to blood flow through the pulmonary circulation, which determines the pressure difference between the pulmonary artery and the left atrium necessary for unit flow (driving pressure), increases as the vessel becomes longer or narrower. The resistance of the extra-alveolar vessels decreases as lung volume increases because the widening has more effect in reducing resistance than the lengthening has in increasing it. By contrast, the alveolar vessels narrow as lung volume increases,[6] because the extramural pressure reflects the pressure in the alveolus that does not fall, but the vessels do lengthen. This causes an increase in resistance, which overshadows the drops in the extra-alveolar vessel resistance. The overall effect, therefore, is a reduction in flow as the volume of the lung increases. This can be an important cause of restriction of pulmonary blood flow leading to a fall in cardiac output with positive end-expiratory pressure (PEEP). When chronic, as in chronic obstructive pulmonary disease (COPD), lung distension leads to right ventricular enlargement and hypertrophy (cor pulmonale). Local overdistension in COPD, particularly emphysema, leads to such stretching of alveolar vessels that only the corner vessels remain open. This can lead to a fall in capillary blood volume and in diffusing capacity (see under Diffusion). The resistance also increases if the viscosity of the blood increases, as happens, for instance, when there is a severe excess of RBCs (polycythemia). An excess of RBCs is common in hypoxemia, a condition in which excess erythropoietin (RBC formation factor) is generated in the kidneys.

Unfortunately the pulmonary vascular resistance (PVR), which is the calculated resistance of the whole pulmonary circulation, cannot be used to assess vasodilation or vasoconstriction because it is not constant. PVR falls with increasing flow, probably because the increased intravascular pressures recruit new vessels and distend the vessels already open. A positive intravascular pressure is necessary to open

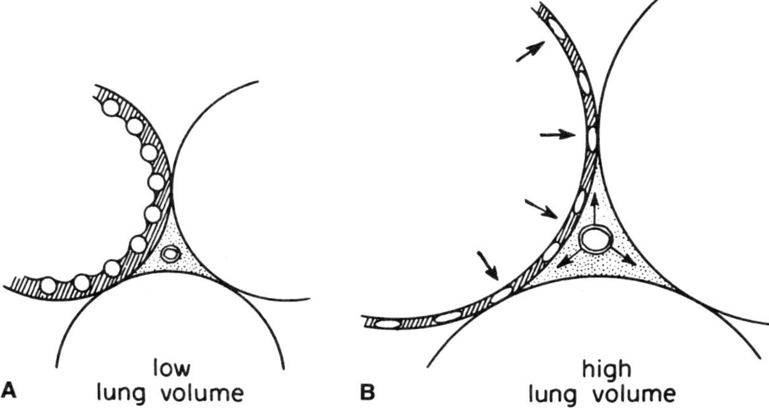

Figure 10-3. (**A & B**) Effect of lung volume on the pulmonary vasculature. At high lung volume (Fig. B) the alveolar microvessels are stretched and compressed. However, extra alveolar vessels between air spaces are expanded. At low lung volumes (Fig. A) these changes are reversed.

the vessels before flow can start. Thus the assessment of a vasoactive effect requires a change in driving pressure at the same flow rate (Fig. 10-4).

The regional distribution of blood flow in the lung depends on gravity, anatomy, and the effect of hypoxic vasoconstriction. Since gravity causes blood to fall to the bottom of the air-filled lung, in the upright lung the lower lobes' vessels are more distended and thus have higher flow. Conceptually, the upright lung can be divided into four zones by this gravitational effect[7] (Figs. 10-5 and 10-6). In the uppermost zone, zone 1, there is no perfusion through the alveolar wall capillaries because the average pulmonary artery pressure cannot drive the blood up that high, although blood can still be siphoned through vessels held open in the corners of the alveoli. In the next zone, zone 2, the driving pressure is the pressure difference between the pulmonary artery and the alveolus, so that flow is uninfluenced by changes of left atrial pressure. This is because the alveolar pressure causes collapse of the alveolar vessels when it exceeds the left atrial pressure. However, when flow ceases, pressure within the alveolar vessels increases to the pulmonary artery pressure, and the vessels reopen. Thus they remain open with a "flow-limiting segment" at their downstream end, which prevents an increase in flow however negative left atrial pressure may become.[8] Below this is zone 3, in which flow is determined by the difference between pulmonary artery and left atrial pressure, since both these pressures are higher than the alveolar pressure. Below this is zone 4, in which the pressure outside the vessels is more positive at the unstretched bottom of the lung. This reduces transmural expanding pressure and narrows the vessel, reducing the blood flow.

Anatomy, as well as gravity, determines the distribution of blood flow in the pulmonary circulation. The central parts of the lung are served by shorter and wider vessels, so that the flow rate in these regions is higher and the time for a blood cell to pass from artery to vein is shorter than at the lung periphery. These two effects, gravity and anatomy, are largely responsible for the increased flow and for the increased blood volume and radiographic density in the central and basal regions of the lung. Hydrostatic edema, due to abnormal transudation through the vessel walls, also occurs here. Radiographically, vascular markings are lacking in the

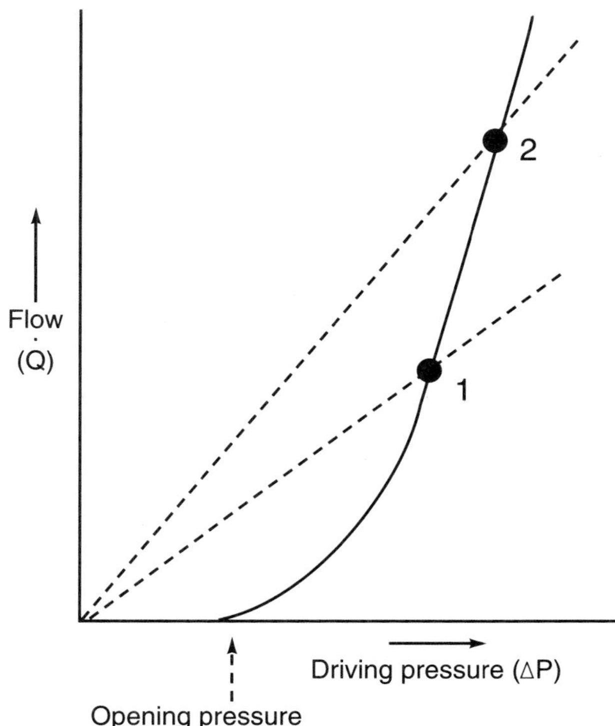

Figure 10-4. The relation of pulmonary blood flow to driving pressure between pulmonary artery and left atrium is non-linear. Note that resistance or driving pressure per unit flow ($\Delta P/\dot{Q}$) is higher at a lower (1) than at a faster (2) flow rate.

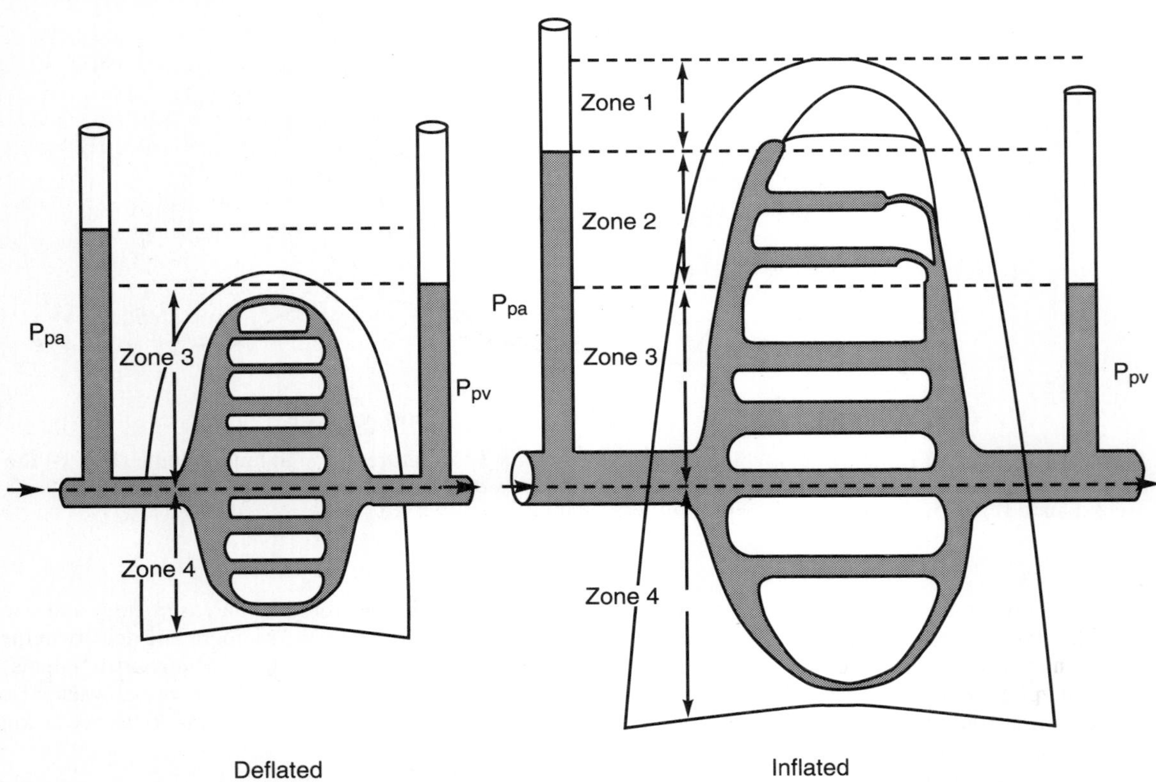

Figure 10-5. Zones of perfusion in the lungs determined by the relationship of pulmonary arterial pressure to alveolar and left atrial pressures. In zone 1 there is no flow, pulmonary arterial pressure (P_{pa}) being insufficient to perfuse alveolar vessels (except those held open in the corners of alveoli). In zone 2 the driving pressure determining flow is the difference between pulmonary artery pressure and alveolar pressure. In zone 3, flow is determined by driving pressure between pulmonary artery and pulmonary vein, and in zone 4 flow is determined by the same driving pressure in unstretched lung. P_{pv}, pulmonary venous pressure.

upper zones of the upright lung under normal conditions. These become more visible when pulmonary artery pressure rises in exercise or disease.

Hypoxic vasoconstriction is a powerful mechanism altering this gravity- and anatomy-dependent distribution of perfusion in favor of one matching the distribution of ventilation[9,10] (Fig. 10-7). Hypoxic vasoconstriction is a narrowing, by hypoxia, of the extra-alveolar small arterial vessels. These vessels are very thin and yet have enough muscle in their walls (because they are so thin) to narrow their cal-

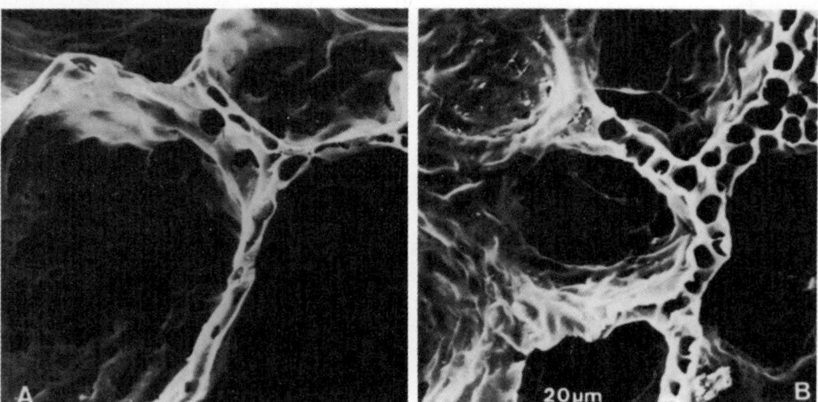

Figure 10-6. Scanning electron micrographs of alveolar walls of rabbit lungs fixed under **(A)** zone 2 and **(B)** zone 3 conditions of perfusion. Note that capillaries are wide in zone 3 and slit-like in zone 2, except for corner capillaries, which are wide in both zones. (From Bachofen et al.,[17] with permission.)

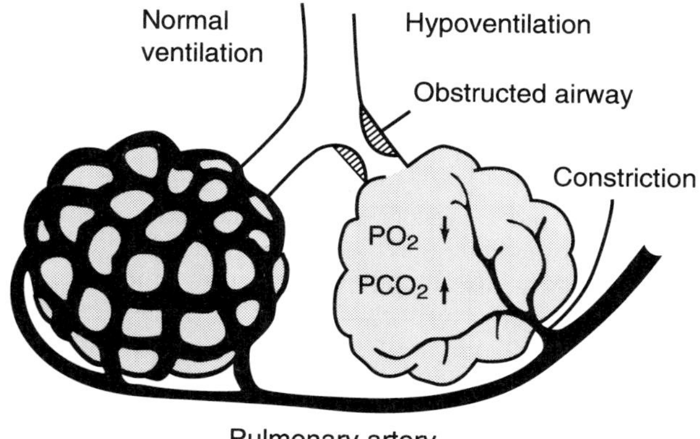

Figure 10-7. Hypoxic vasoconstriction (right) reduces blood flow to poorly ventilated regions, thus improving $\dot{V}/\dot{Q}$ matching.

iber and thus profoundly influence the distribution of blood flow. It is *alveolar hypoxia* that triggers this reaction through mechanisms that appear to depend on the integrity of the endothelial lining cells of the blood vessels. Intravascular hypoxia (e.g., hypoxia of pulmonary artery blood on exercise) does not cause hypoxic vasoconstriction.

Since the alveolar O_2 concentration (C_AO_2) depends on the amount of O_2 brought into the alveolus (ventilation) as compared with the amount of O_2 absorbed from the alveolus (perfusion), a low C_AO_2 occurs when ventilation is inadequate for the perfusion. This low C_AO_2 reduces perfusion by causing hypoxic vasoconstriction of the vessels serving the region. Perfect hypoxic vasoconstriction should lead to perfect matching of ventilation and perfusion. However, this does not occur in the normal lung and is even less likely to occur in the diseased lung, in which factors such as endotoxemia and metabolites from the liver blunt the hypoxic vasoconstrictive response.[12]

Hypoxic vasoconstriction can be a powerful force toward restoring normality of the blood gases in a lung afflicted by regional disease. Unfortunately, when widespread disease is present causing overall hypoxia due to underventilation, the hypoxic vasoconstriction throughout the lungs restricts blood flow and increases pulmonary artery pressure. Under these conditions the underventilating patients develop cor pulmonale and eventually right heart failure with edema; their cyanosis and dropsical swelling has led to the term "blue bloater." By contrast, patients with COPD who do not hypoventilate but who puff hard to maintain normal gas exchange do not suffer overall hypoxic vasoconstriction and cardiac afflictions; they are known as "pink puffers."

Pulmonary Edema

Pulmonary edema (Fig. 10-8) may be either hydrostatic or exudative.

Hydrostatic Edema

It is likely that a continuous transudation of fluid from both extra-alveolar arterioles and upstream alveolar capillary vessels occurs normally. The fluid conveys nutrients to the lung tissues and is reabsorbed downstream at the venular end of

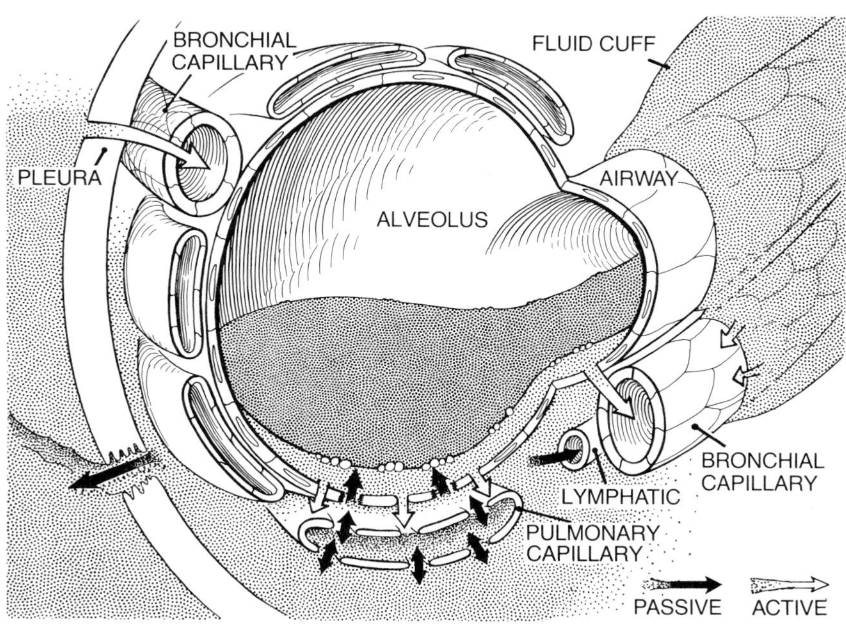

Figure 10-8. Mechanisms of pulmonary edema. Fluid leaks from the pulmonary vessels and is actively and passively reabsorbed into the pulmonary, bronchial, and lymphatic vessels. Stippled region denotes fluid in interstitium and in alveolus.

the capillaries. This fluid passes through the permeable vascular endothelium into the interstitium beneath the impermeable airway epithelium. When the intravascular pressure is increased, the outward fluid flux increases. This outward movement is normally balanced by an inward-directed osmotic pressure gradient (oncotic pressure) resulting from the high intravascular protein content relative to that in the extravascular space.[12]

An increase in intravascular pressures, due to exercise or to a reclining position for instance, does not usually produce evident pulmonary edema because of simple compensatory mechanisms. If excess fluid does accumulate in the tight "sandwich" of the alveolar wall, local pressures rise, impeding further outflow. Similarly, the outflow of nonproteinaceous fluid dilutes the local tissue protein around the vessel while increasing the protein concentration within the vessel. This tends to suck fluid back. However, should excess fluid filter into the alveolar walls in diseases in which pulmonary capillary pressure is persistently high (e.g., left heart failure) or plasma protein is low (e.g., cirrhosis, nephrosis, overhydration), it is sucked out into the interstitium around the bronchovascular bundles, where it forms cuffs. It then moves toward the hilum along a negative pressure gradient. En route it is absorbed into the lymphatics and into the capillaries of the bronchial circulation, which forms a network in the region where the fluid cuffs form.

These mechanisms help to keep fluid away from the alveoli so that it does not interfere with gas exchange. However, should the transudation become overwhelming, fluid starts to leak into the alveoli, presumably because its accumulation underneath stretches open the cell junctions of the epithelium. Once in the airspaces it may still be reabsorbed by the alveolar epithelial cells and, if normality is restored, into the pulmonary capillaries again, or it may move up along the bronchial epithelium, through which it can be actively reabsorbed into the bronchial circulation. Should the fluid continue to accumulate, its presence may be life-threatening because of airway obstruction. However, it can be coughed up, and large amounts of fluid can be cleared by this "last-ditch" mechanism for preventing asphyxia.

Exudative Edema

The high-protein edema fluid of an exudate usually forms as a result of vascular damage (from ischemia or toxic injury) or inflammation. In severe left heart failure rises in intravascular pressures may be such that vessels are bruised and torn, and the edema, initially a transudate, may become protein-rich and even be bloodstained. The inflammatory response is a local active reaction to an initial cell damage. Both the primary injury and the inflammatory types of exudative edema can occur as a local or a widespread lesion. When they occur in the widespread, patchy fashion of the adult respiratory distress syndrome (ARDS), such inflammatory edema can be impossible to differentiate radiographically from hydrostatic edema. However, exudative, particularly inflammatory, edema is more disruptive of normal clearance mechanisms; thus its effects on gas exchange are more profound. It never clears quickly with diuretics, as does the transudative edema of left heart failure, overhydration, or low plasma protein states.

Hydrostatic edema is more marked in the dependent regions because of the vascular distension caused by gravity. In a patient who habitually lies in the lateral decubitus position, the lower lung may be relatively flooded. Improvement can occur after the patient turns onto the other side because the edema redistributes itself. Placing the patient in the prone position (if possible) allows the well perfused and ventilated lower lobes to lose their fluid to the less important anterior parts of the lung.

VENTILATION

Anatomy

The airways are analogous to the pulmonary vessels in that they are tree-like, with extra-alveolar conducting bronchi leading to gas exchange zones in the respiratory bronchioles and alveoli[2] (Fig. 10-9). The "hollow trunk" of the tree is the trachea, and in the conducting airways the total cross-sectional diameter of all the branches that follow the third or fourth bifurcation increases like the flare of a trumpet, although the diameters of the individual airways become

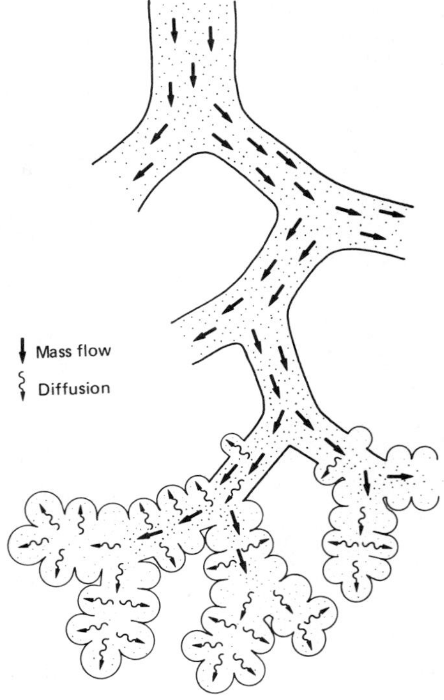

Figure 10-9. O_2 molecules reach alveoli by a combination of mass airflow and molecular diffusion. The importance of diffusion increases toward the alveoli. (From Pedley et al.,[13] with permission.)

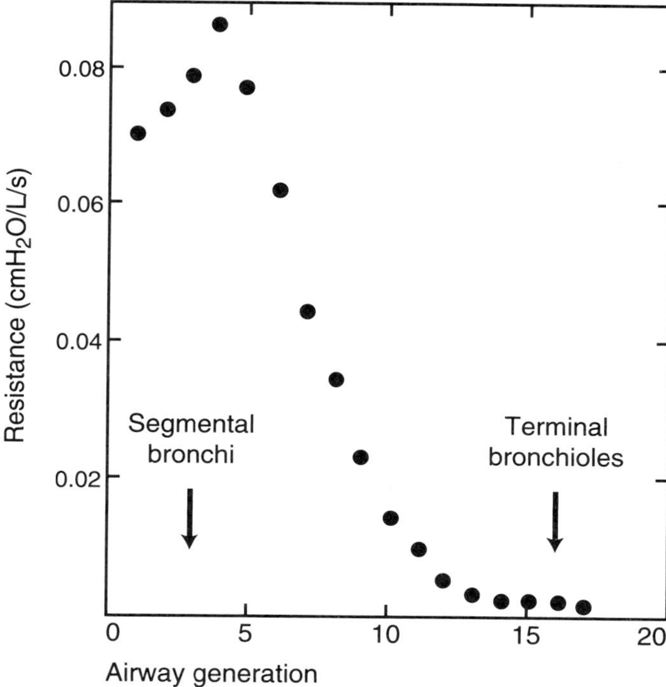

Figure 10-10. Airway resistance is located mainly in the conducting airways and falls rapidly as the total cross section of all the airways increases toward the alveoli. (From Fishman,[18] with permission.)

smaller.[13] Because of this, airflow resistance, again defined as the driving pressure per unit flow, is highest where the cross section is smallest—namely, in the segmental bronchi at about the third generation of the branches—and lowest in the alveolar duct region (Fig. 10-10).

As with the extra-alveolar vasculature, the resistance in the conducting airways depends on the transmural pressure. The transmural distending pressure increases at high lung volumes. It is higher at the top of the lungs because here the weight of the lung stretches the airways open; the upright, cone-shaped lungs hang down from the top, where they are "vacuum-sealed" to the chest wall. After reaching the alveoli, the gas can also move sideways through the pores of Kohn, the small openings between alveoli. The extent of this "collateral" ventilation is normally small but increases with age, at higher lung volumes, and when the pores are abnormally large in COPD, particularly with severe emphysema.

Gas Exchange

Regional volume change during breathing varies in different parts of the lung. It is less at the top of the lung, where the alveoli are tensely stretched open, than at the bottom, where they are more relaxed and are directly moved by the diaphragm.[14] The posterior lower lobes, where most gas exchange takes place, are not as well ventilated in the supine position as in the prone position because of the anatomic relationships.

Total ventilation, measured in liters per minute, has two components, gas exchange ventilation and wasted ventilation.[1] Gas exchange ventilation (also called *alveolar ventilation*) contacts the perfusing blood, whereas wasted ventilation (also called *dead space ventilation*) does not. Each inhaled tidal volume (V_T) is distributed to gas-exchanging and non-gas-exchanging regions. Dead space ventilation consists of the gas going to the conducting airways (anatomic dead space) plus that going to the alveolar regions that are not perfused (alveolar dead space). Actually the alveolar dead space equals the gas going to completely nonperfused alveoli plus that going to partly perfused alveoli, which act "as if" a lesser volume were going to completely nonperfused units (Fig. 10-11). Alveolar dead space gas comes normally from unperfused alveoli at the top of the lung and, in disease, from alveoli cut off from pulmonary perfusion by vascular obstructions of large vessels, such as pulmonary emboli.

The anatomic dead space in the conducting airways may be gauged, after inhalation of a pure gas such as O_2, from the volume of the pure gas that is exhaled before the mixed alveolar gas appears at the lips. The total physiologic dead space (made up of anatomic and alveolar dead space) is usually given as a percentage of tidal volume [(V_D/V_T)%]. It is derived from

$$V_D/V_T = (PaCO_2 - P_ECO_2)/PaCO_2 \qquad (1)$$

where $PaCO_2$ equals arterial PCO_2 (in millimeters of Hg) and P_ECO_2 equals mixed exhaled PCO_2 (in millimeters of Hg).

Although this relationship will not be rigorously derived, it may be appreciated empirically (Fig. 10-12). $PaCO_2$ always equals the alveolar CO_2 pressure (P_ACO_2) owing to the ex-

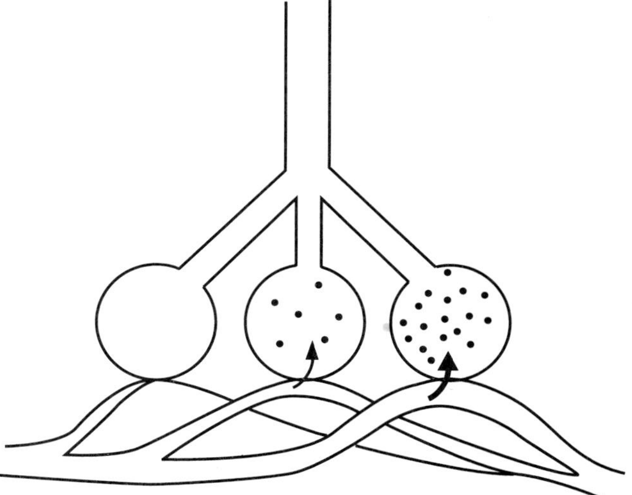

Figure 10-11. Gas from alveoli with no perfusion, reduced perfusion, and normal perfusion contributes to the concentration of CO_2 in the mixed exhaled air. Arrows indicate CO_2 excretion.

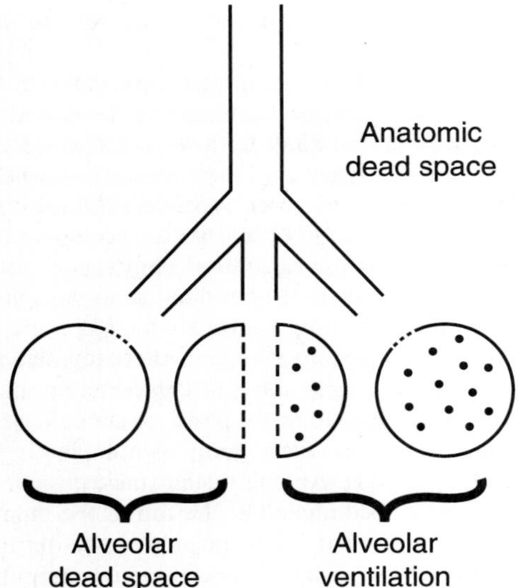

Figure 10-12. Subdivision of total ventilation into wasted ventilation (from anatomic dead space and alveolar dead space with no perfusion) and effective alveolar ventilation with ideal perfusion.

tremely diffusible nature of CO_2, and therefore $PaCO_2$ can be used to evaluate the difference between P_ACO_2 and P_ECO_2, which is diluted by the dead space gas containing no CO_2. Thus, the greater the difference between P_ACO_2 and P_ECO_2, the larger the dead space. This difference is standardized for the volume of ventilation by dividing it by P_ACO_2 (or its equivalent, $PaCO_2$). Normally dead space makes up no more than one-third of each V_T, and during exercise this fraction drops to about one-tenth because of better perfusion of the upper parts of the lung. In lung diseases such as COPD, in which regions of overdistension have hardly any pulmonary blood flow, the wasted ventilation is over half and typically makes up about two-thirds of each breath, a debilitating inefficiency.

Carbon Dioxide Excretion

In the long term the amount of CO_2 excreted is equivalent to the CO_2 produced by metabolism, but in the short term it varies with the ventilation.

$$\dot{V}CO_2 = (\dot{V}_A)(F_ACO_2) \quad (2)$$

where $\dot{V}CO_2$ is CO_2 excretion, $\dot{V}_A$ is alveolar ventilation, and F_ACO_2 is fraction of CO_2 in the alveoli. P_ACO_2 is derived by multiplying F_ACO_2 by $(P_b - PH_2O)$, where P_b is barometric pressure and PH_2O is water vapor pressure (always 47 mmHg when fully humidified at body temperature).

$PaCO_2$ always equals P_ACO_2, always drops with increasing alveolar ventilation (hyperventilation causes hypocarbia), and always rises with decreasing ventilation (hypoventilation causes hypercarbia). These relationships can keep the arterial pH constant via the variation of P_ACO_2 with ventilation. This is regulated by the chemosensors at the base of the brain and to some extent by the chemosensors in the carotid arteries in the neck.

These pH sensors are up-regulated by hypoxia or stimulants and down-regulated by narcotics, which characteristically lead to underventilation and a rise of $PaCO_2$. This regulatory mechanism is abolished when a patient is mechanically ventilated at a fixed ventilation volume. It should be noted that the correct setting of the ventilator is that which maintains blood pH at 7.4. When total ventilatory volumes are fixed, $PaCO_2$ increases and pH decreases if there is an increase in dead space, which could be due to maldistribution of ventilation because of airway obstruction or to maldistribution of perfusion because of vascular shunts. It is also possible that $PaCO_2$ rises because the metabolic generation of CO_2 is increased as a result of an acidosis (including the lactic acidosis occurring when poor blood flow leads to anaerobic metabolism) because of the buffering that releases CO_2 from the HCO_3^- in the blood. The output of CO_2 also rises if metabolism is suddenly increased by fever or by excess catacholamines or other metabolically active agents or if excess HCO_3^- is given therapeutically.

Oxygen Uptake

The uptake of O_2 from the alveoli by the blood reduces the concentration delivered by ventilation. In contrast to CO_2, which is present only in the exhaled gas, O_2 is present in both the inhaled and the exhaled gas.

$$\dot{V}O_2 = \dot{V}_A(F_IO_2 - F_AO_2) \quad (3)$$

where $\dot{V}O_2$ is O_2 uptake, $\dot{V}_A$ is alveolar ventilation, F_IO_2 is inhaled O_2 fraction, and F_AO_2 is alveolar O_2 fraction.

Let us see if we can calculate P_AO_2, on which PaO_2 obviously depends. In the long term the ratio $\dot{V}CO_2/\dot{V}O_2$ (respiratory exchange ratio) equals 0.8, the same value as the respiratory quotient for the metabolism of the body. However, in the short term one can briefly increase ventilation as more CO_2 is excreted, and the respiratory exchange ratio (R) can be made equal to 1, although the respiratory quotient (RQ) of the body remains 0.8. In this case, when CO_2 excretion equals O_2 uptake

$$\dot{V}_A(F_IO_2 - F_AO_2) = \dot{V}_A(F_ACO_2 - F_ICO_2) \quad (4)$$

or

$$P_IO_2 - P_AO_2 = P_ACO_2 - P_ICO_2 \quad (5)$$

where P_AO_2 is alveolar O_2 pressure, P_IO_2 is inhaled O_2 pressure (about 150 mmHg at sea level), and P_ACO_2 is alveolar CO_2 pressure (equal to $PaCO_2$).

Since P_ICO_2 is zero, then from Equation 5,

$$P_AO_2 = P_IO_2 - P_ACO_2 \quad (6)$$

and therefore

$$P_AO_2 = P_IO_2 - PaCO_2 \text{ when } R = 1 \quad (7)$$

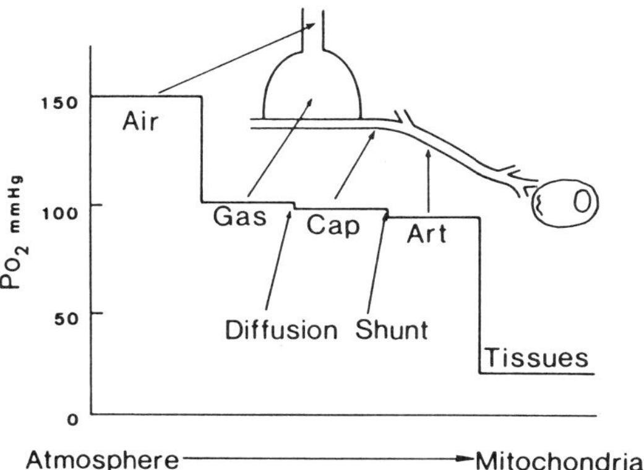

Figure 10-13. O_2 transfer from air to tissues, showing relative depression of PO_2 caused by ventilation, diffusion, and shunt. Cap, pulmonary capillaries; Art, systemic arterial blood. (From West,[1] with permission.)

However, when R = 0.8 (long term), this is modified to the notorious *alveolar gas equation* to derive the P_AO_2:

$$P_AO_2 = P_IO_2 - \frac{PaCO_2}{0.8} \tag{8}$$

Note that solution of the alveolar gas equation requires the measurement of R (or the assumption that R = 0.8) and of $PaCO_2$.

The alveolar gas equation is important because it allows the calculation of the difference between alveolar and arterial O_2 pressure [$P(A\text{-}a)O_2$] when the PaO_2 has been found to be too low. This difference is used to distinguish underventilation, which does not affect it, from the other causes of hypoxemia, which increase it. $P(A\text{-}a)O_2$ for air breathing at sea level is normally about 15 mmHg and should not exceed 30 mmHg.

There are three possible causes of an increase in $P(A\text{-}a)O_2$: reduced O_2 diffusion in exceptional conditions, increase in the anatomic shunt, and mismatching of ventilation with perfusion. The last cause is by far the most important.

Diffusion

The rate of O_2 diffusion from the alveolus into the blood (Fig. 10-13) depends on the pressure gradient between alveolar and blood O_2.

$$D_L = \dot{V}/P_A - P_c$$

where D_L is diffusing capacity (in milliliters per minute per millimeters of Hg pressure difference), $\dot{V}$ is the volume of gas diffusing per minute; P_A is alveolar gas pressure, and P_c is capillary gas pressure.

It increases with the amount of blood (corrected for anemia), and the surface area of the alveoli through which the O_2 diffuses.[15] It decreases with the thickness of the tissues separating the alveolar gas from the RBC.

Carbon monoxide (CO) rather than O_2 is used for measuring diffusing capacity in the pulmonary function laboratory because there is no backpressure from CO in the pulmonary capillary blood (as opposed to the variable backpressure from O_2) and there is a simple relation between D_LCO and D_LO_2.

A decrease in D_L does *not* cause measurable hypoxemia during air breathing at sea level since the RBC spends so much time exposed to the alveolar gas (0.75 seconds) as compared with the time necessary for full oxygenation (0.10 to 0.25 seconds).

Theoretically there could be a slight measurable increase in $P(A\text{-}a)O_2$ due to reduction of D_L below one-third of its predicted value. This could occur during exercise if the time of RBC exposure decreases, or at high altitude when the difference between alveolar and capillary PO_2 at low atmospheric pressure is markedly reduced. Hypoxemia due to poor diffusion is never a problem if supplemental O_2 is given and thus the P_AO_2 (the driving pressure) is increased.

Although a reduced D_L is not the cause of hypoxemia, it is useful in showing a loss of capillary blood volume due to vasculitis, emphysema, or an inflammation or thickening of the alveolar wall (alveolitis).

Shunt

The total shunt flow (Fig. 10-14) is made up of the anatomic shunt plus the venous admixture from mismatching of ventilation and perfusion. An *anatomic shunt* is defined as a blood flow through the lungs that does not contact any alveolar gas. A small anatomic shunt is normally present. It equals the sum of the bronchial blood flow, which drains into the pulmonary veins after giving up its O_2 to the lung tissues, and the blood flow through the thebesian (coronary)

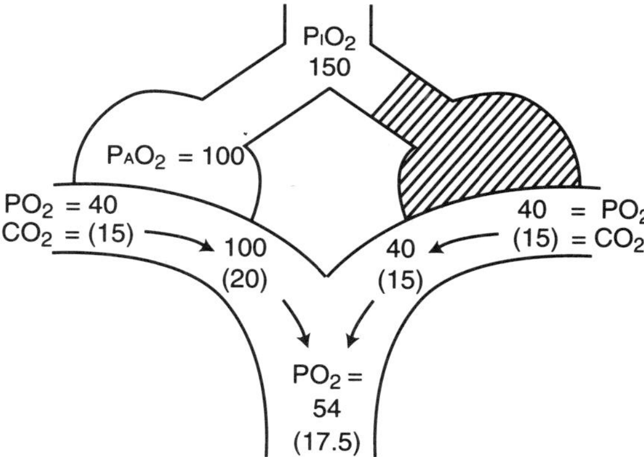

Figure 10-14. Shunt: 50 percent of the cardiac output is not exposed to the alveolar gas (right). The systemic arteriovenous O_2 difference has been halved from 5 to 2.5 mL/100 mL owing to a doubling of cardiac output in response to the hypoxemia. The systemic venous O_2 content (15 mL/100 mL) and therefore the PaO_2 is higher than if output had remained unchanged. CO_2, O_2 content.

veins in the heart, which drains into the left ventricle after giving up its O_2 to the myocardium. The *venous admixture* is defined as the unsaturated lung blood flow resulting from ventilation to perfusion mismatching that is not due to an anatomic shunt (see below). A small amount of such mismatching is normal. It is calculated as equivalent to a smaller amount of mixed systemic venous flow acting as if it were passing through an anatomic shunt.

A test of the size of the anatomic shunt is to measure PaO_2 during the breathing of 100 percent O_2 for long enough to wash out all the alveolar nitrogen (N_2); often more than one-half hour in patients with COPD. Because all the N_2 is washed out of even very poorly ventilated alveoli, all the remaining gas is CO_2 (P_ACO_2 = 40 mmHg) and H_2O vapor (P_AH_2O = 47 mmHg); the hypoxic effect of any mismatching of ventilation to perfusion is lost. By assuming that the difference in O_2 content between the arterial and mixed venous blood remains the same (i.e., the cardiac output does not change), the approximate amount of the anatomic shunt can be gauged during 100 percent O_2 breathing by the following rule-of-thumb: each 20 mmHg decrement of PaO_2 below about 670 mmHg (P_b equals 760 mmHg minus P_ACO_2 and P_AH_2O) represents about 1 percent of shunt. It should be noted that this is only true during O_2 breathing because then, on the uppermost part of the oxyhemoglobin dissociation curve, dissolved O_2 is linearly related to O_2 pressure. Normally up to 5 percent of true anatomic shunt is present, bringing the normal PaO_2 during 100 percent O_2 breathing down to about 570 mmHg.

Although PCO_2 is higher in the mixed venous blood than in the arterial blood, and this high CO_2 blood traverses the shunt, it is interesting that the $PaCO_2$ does not increase in the presence of an anatomic shunt. This is because the chemoreceptors are stimulated by a rise in $PaCO_2$ to increase ventilation, so that sufficient CO_2 is washed out of the blood perfusing the alveoli to restore the $PaCO_2$ to normal. It is, of course, of little use to treat hypoxemia due to anatomic shunt by increasing the inhaled O_2 concentration, although a very small amount of extra O_2 (0.003 mL/100 mL/mmHg) is thereby dissolved in the nonshunted blood. It should be remembered that, except over brief periods, high O_2 concentrations burn the airspaces (O_2 toxicity) and favor atelectasis.[16]

VENTILATION TO PERFUSION RELATIONSHIPS

The ventilation/perfusion ratio ($\dot{V}/\dot{Q}$) is normally different in different parts of the lung, and $\dot{V}$ and $\dot{Q}$ may be grossly different in lung regions affected by disease (Figs. 10-15 and 10-16). Normally $\dot{V}/\dot{Q}$ is high at the top of the lung and low at the bottom. Total $\dot{V}$ and total $\dot{Q}$ are higher at the bottom of the lung than at the top, but the effect of gravity in increasing blood flow overwhelms the anatomic mechanisms directing $\dot{V}$ to the bottom of the lungs. Hypoxic vasoconstriction of the pulmonary arterioles, because it responds to P_AO_2 and because P_AO_2 depends on alveolar $\dot{V}/\dot{Q}$, is a sensitive regulator matching regional $\dot{Q}$ to $\dot{V}$.

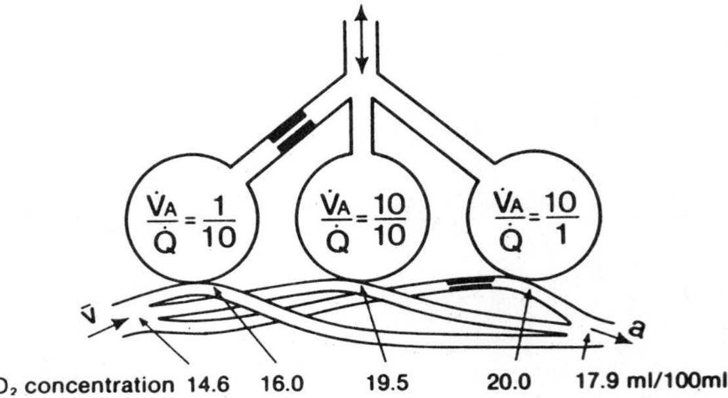

Figure 10-15. The depression of PaO_2 due to mismatching of ventilation and perfusion. The lung units with high $\dot{V}_A/\dot{Q}$ add relatively little O_2 to the blood as compared with the decrement caused by the units with low $\dot{V}_A/\dot{Q}$. (From West,[1] with permission.)

Just as overall underventilation of the lung in relation to its perfusion leads to arterial hypoxemia, so does regional underventilation in relation to the regional blood flow. This is because pulmonary capillary blood hypoxia in one region cannot be corrected by relative overventilation in other regions. Such overventilation does not add a "makeup" volume of O_2 because this blood is already carrying its full O_2 load in accordance with the oxyhemoglobin dissociation curve. It is interesting that the same does not hold true for CO_2, the excretion of which *is* made up by overventilation of other regions, because dissolved CO_2 concentration varies directly with PCO_2. The hypoxemia from regional underventilation is worsened because more blood flows through the regions that are relatively overperfused relative to ventilation (low $\dot{V}/\dot{Q}$). The corollary of this is that more exhaled

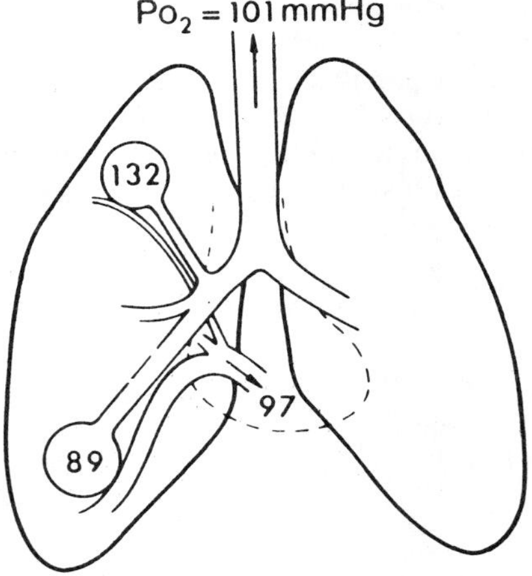

Figure 10-16. Depression of PaO_2 by ventilation/perfusion inequality. This diagram of the upright lung shows only two groups of alveoli at the apex and base. The relative sizes of the airways and blood vessels indicate their relative ventilation and blood flow. Because most of the blood comes from the poorly oxygenated base, depression of the blood PO_2 is inevitable. (From West,[1] with permission.)

gas comes from regions that are relatively overventilated relative to perfusion (high $\dot{V}/\dot{Q}$).

At the low extreme, where ventilation is absent, the lowest $\dot{V}/\dot{Q}$ equals the anatomic shunt. At the other extreme, where there is no flow but ventilation persists, the unperfused alveoli constitute alveolar dead space. Because underventilation in one region is not made up by overventilation in another, an abnormal spread of the disparities of regional $\dot{V}$ to $\dot{Q}$ also leads to hypoxemia.

The effects of low $\dot{V}/\dot{Q}$ and a wide spread of $\dot{V}/\dot{Q}$ in causing hypoxemia in lung disease are easily treated by adding O_2 to the inhaled air. This is particularly good news because $\dot{V}/\dot{Q}$ mismatching is the commonest cause of hypoxemia in lung disease, and addition of the low concentrations of O_2 that readily overcome $\dot{V}/\dot{Q}$ mismatching does not entail risk of O_2 toxicity. Toxic concentrations of O_2 can also sometimes be avoided in severe, widespread diseases such as ARDS which cause shunt and very bad $\dot{V}/\dot{Q}$ mismatching, by increasing lung volume with PEEP. The addition of PEEP reduces the atelectasis and shunt, making O_2 more effective so that concentrations below the toxic level can be used. A benefit for mechanically ventilated patients is that additional O_2, which might depress ventilation in hypoxemic patients with COPD or obesity, is no problem because their ventilation can be regulated to normalize blood pH.

The distribution of pulmonary blood flow to different regions is unequal because it depends on anatomy and on the pressures within the pulmonary vessels that are influenced by gravity. The pressures outside the vessels also vary with lung volume. The bellows function of the chest depends on the chest wall muscles, especially the diaphragm, in relation to the mechanical properties of the lungs, particularly the resistance to airflow. Considerable regional inequality of ventilation is normally present owing to the anatomy of the lung.

Because $\dot{V}$ and $\dot{Q}$ are matched by anatomic factors and hypoxic vasoconstriction, there is normally much less than the expected inequality of regional $\dot{V}/\dot{Q}$ in the upright lung. However PaO_2, which depends on the $\dot{V}/\dot{Q}$ relations throughout the lung, is not well maintained when the lung is diseased. Nevertheless, it can usually be restored to normal levels by modest additions of O_2 to the inhaled gas.

References

1. West JB: Respiratory Physiology: The Essentials. 3rd Ed. 1985, pp. 11–66
2. Weibel ER: Design and structure of the human lung. pp. 224–271. In Fishman AP (ed): Pulmonary Diseases and Disorders. McGraw-Hill, New York, 1980
3. West JB: Ventilation/Blood Flow and Gas Exchange. 3rd Ed. Blackwell, Oxford, 1977
4. Fung YC, Sobin SS: Theory of sheet flow in lung alveoli. J Appl Physiol 1969;16:472–488
5. Culver BH, Butler J: Mechanical influences on the pulmonary circulation. Annu Rev Respir Physiol 1980;42:187–198
6. Howell JBL, Permutt S, Proctor F, Riley RL: Effect of inflation of the lung on different parts of the pulmonary vascular bed. J Appl Physiol 1961;16:71–76
7. West JB, Dollery CT, Naimark A: Distributions of blood flow in isolated lung: Relation to vascular and alveolar pressures. J Appl Physiol 1964;19:713–724
8. Permutt S, Riley RL: Hemodynamics of collapsible vessels with tone: The vascular waterfall. J Appl Physiol 1963;18:924–932
9. von Euler US, Liljestrand G: Observations on the pulmonary arterial blood pressure in the cat. Acta Physiol Scand 1946; 12:307–320
10. Harris P, Heath D: The Human Pulmonary Circulation. 2nd Ed. E & S Livingstone, Edinburgh, 1978
11. Fishman AP: The enigma of hypoxic pulmonary vasoconstriction. In Fishman AP (ed): The Pulmonary Circulation: Normal and Abnormal. University of Pennsylvania Press, Philadelphia, 1990
12. Starling EH: On the absorption of fluid from the connective tissue spaces. J Physiol (Lond) 1896;19:312–326
13. Pedley TJ, Schroter RC, Sudlow MF: Gas flow and mixing in the airways. In West JB (ed): Bioengineering Aspects of the Lung. Marcel Dekker, New York, 1977
14. Milic-Emili J, Henderson JAM, Dolovich MB et al: Regional distribution of inspired gas in the lung. J Appl Physiol 1966; 21:749–759
15. Wagner PD: Diffusion and chemical reaction in pulmonary gas exchange. Physiol Rev 1979;57:257–312
16. Dantzker DR, Wagner PD, West JB: Instability of lung units with low $\dot{V}/\dot{Q}$ ratios during O_2 breathing. J Appl Physiol 1975; 38:886–895
17. Bachofen H, Weber J, Wangensteen D, Weibel ER: Morphometric estimates of diffusing capacity in lungs fixed under zone II and zone III conditions. Respir Physiol 1983;41–52
18. Fishman AP: In Fishman AP (ed): Structure and Function in Pulmonary Diseases and Disorders. 2nd Ed. McGraw-Hill, New York, 1988

Chapter 11

Oxygen Carriage, Transport, and Utilization

Robert M. Kacmarek

CHAPTER OUTLINE

O_2 is essential for the preservation of life. Sufficient quantities of O_2 must be delivered to tissues to ensure cellular function; in fact, tissue death is normally a result of its insufficient availability. It enters the body at the lungs, is carried in the blood, and is used at the tissue level, specifically by the mitochondria of cells during aerobic metabolism. The processes involved in the carriage, transport, and utilization of O_2 are covered in this chapter. Specifics regarding movement across the alveolar-capillary membrane are covered in Chapters 1 and 10.

CARRIAGE OF OXYGEN

The blood carries O_2 in two distinct compartments: plasma, in which it is physically dissolved, and hemoglobin (Hb), to which it is chemically attached. Although by far the greatest part of the O_2 carried is chemically attached to the hemoglobin, the quantity physically dissolved has a direct effect on the quantity bound to hemoglobin (Fig. 11-1).

Quantity Physically Dissolved in Plasma

Since the O_2 molecule is covalent and plasma is a polar solution, O_2 dissolves poorly in plasma.[1] According to the Bunsen solubility coefficient for O_2, only 0.023 mL of O_2 can be dissolved in 1 mL of plasma for every 760 mmHg PO_2 at 37°C.[2] Normally, the quantity of O_2 carried in the blood is expressed in volume percent or milliliter per deciliter and since the normal arterial O_2 partial pressure (PaO_2) is about 100 mmHg, the Bunsen solubility coefficient is modified for mathematical simplicity. That is, if 0.023 is divided by 760, the coefficient can be rewritten as

$$0.00003 \text{ mL } O_2/\text{mL plasma/mmHg } PO_2 \qquad (1)$$

Converting this to the number of milliliters of O_2 physically dissolved in 100 mL of blood (multiplying by a factor of 100) results in

$$0.003 \text{ mL } O_2/100 \text{ mL plasma/mmHg } PO_2 \qquad (2)$$

This factor is used to determine the quantity of O_2 physically

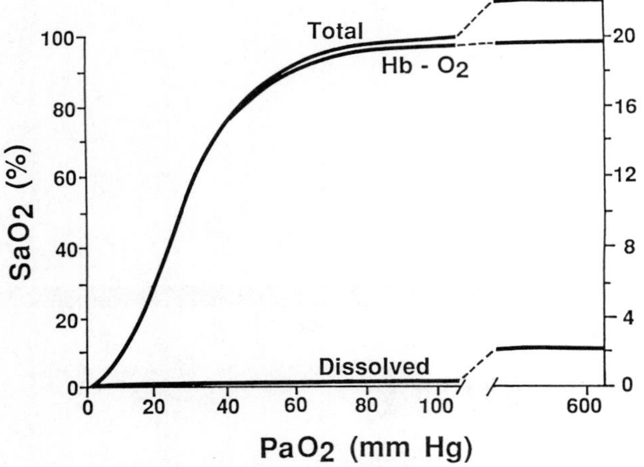

Figure 11-1. The oxyhemoglobin dissociation curve, showing the contribution of chemically bound and dissolved O_2 to the total O_2 content. Note that most of the O_2 by far is O_2 chemically bound to hemoglobin.

dissolved in plasma by multiplying it by the actual PO_2 in the blood:

$$(PO_2\ \text{mmHg})(0.003) = \text{mL } O_2 \text{ physically dissolved per 100 mL of plasma or Vol\%} \quad (3)$$

However, this factor accounts for only a small fraction of the quantity of O_2 carried in the blood.

Quantity Chemically Attracted to Hemoglobin

The hemoglobin molecule is a large (molecular weight 64,500), highly complex molecule capable of altering its physical shape, depending on the extent of its chemical reaction with O_2 and other substances (Figs. 11-2 and 11-3). Each hemoglobin molecule is composed of four *heme* units (porphyrin rings each containing a central iron atom) and four polypeptide chains, referred to as the *globin* portion of the molecule.[3] Each chain is twisted and folded into a "basket" in which a heme unit sits. Normally, the polypeptide chains are of specific amino acid configuration, resulting in two chain types, alpha and beta. Each hemoglobin molecule contains two chains of each type. The four chains are attached to each other (alpha to beta, beta to alpha, etc.), forming the total molecule. The iron atom in each heme unit is attached via four covalent bonds to the four pyrrole rings and has one bond to the globin chain and one bond available to bind O_2.[4,5] In addition, the porphyrin rings of each heme contain amino groups $R\text{-}NH_2$ to which CO_2 can attach, as well as terminal R-NH groups available for buffering of H^+ ion.[6]

Since O_2 attaches at each of the four iron atoms in the hemoglobin molecule, 4 gram molecular weights (GMWs) of O_2 (4 mol) can combine with 1 GMW of hemoglobin.

$$\frac{64{,}500 \text{ g Hb}}{4 \text{ mol } O_2} = 16{,}125 \text{ g Hb/mol } O_2 \quad (4)$$

That is, 1 mol of O_2 can combine maximally with 16,125 g of Hb, and since 1 GMW of O_2 at STP (standard temperature and pressure) occupies a volume of 22.4 L

$$\frac{22{,}400 \text{ mL } O_2}{16{,}125 \text{ g Hb}} = 1.34 \text{ mL } O_2\text{/g Hb} \quad (5)$$

Thus, at 100 percent saturation of hemoglobin with O_2 at STP, 1.34 mL of O_2 can be carried chemically attached to each gram of hemoglobin. A factor of 1.39 mL O_2/g Hb is used by some authors.[2,4,7] This value is derived by converting 1.34 mL of O_2 at STP to its volume at BTPS (body temperature and pressure, saturated). The 1.39 value is more accurate, but convention has entrenched the 1.34 mL factor, which is used throughout this book.

The actual volume of O_2 carried in the blood chemically combined with hemoglobin can be determined by multiplying hemoglobin content by saturation of hemoglobin with O_2 in arterial blood (SaO_2) and by the 1.34 mL O_2/g Hb factor:

$$(HB)(SaO_2)(1.34) = \text{Vol\% of } O_2 \text{ attached to Hb} \quad (6)$$

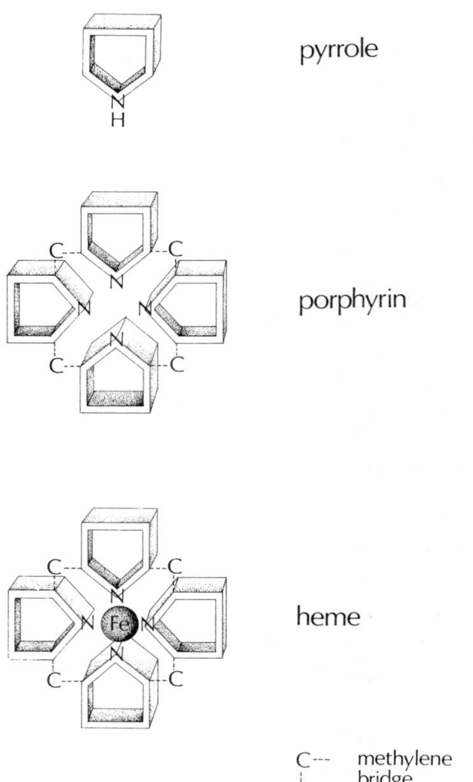

Figure 11-2. The basic structure of each heme consists of four pyrrole rings bound together to form a porphyrin unit, which contains a central iron atom. (From Shapiro et al.,[5] with permission.)

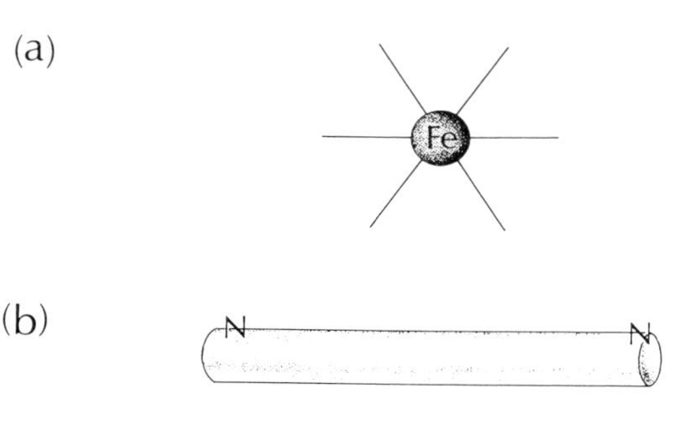

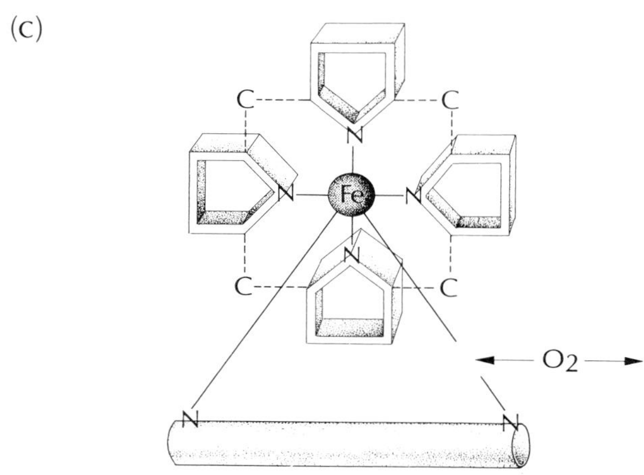

Figure 11-3. (A) The Fe^{2+} ion with six potential valence bonds. **(B)** Schematic representation of a polypeptide chain with two imidazole nitrogens that are capable of forming covalent bonds with the Fe^{2+} ion. A protein molecule containing two alpha and two beta polypeptide chains is known as a globin molecule. **(C)** Heme molecule attached to a polypeptide chain. Four heme molecules attached to the four polypeptide chains of a globin molecule constitute the hemoglobin molecule. (From Shapiro et al.,[5] with permission.)

Hemoglobin chemically attached to O_2 is referred to as *oxyhemoglobin* (HbO_2), while *reduced hemoglobin* (HHb) is hemoglobin that has not reacted with O_2. As Hb combines with O_2 to form HbO_2, the complex takes on a negative charge and as a result forms a salt with K^+, $KHbO_2$. As the K^+ combines with Hb, Cl^- moves from the red blood cell (RBC) into the plasma, and a HCO_3^- (bicarbonate) ion enters the RBC. When O_2 is released at the tissue level, K^+ is also released and the Hb becomes better able to buffer H^+, forming HHb. In addition, Cl^- moves back into the RBC as HCO_3^- leaves. See Chapter 12 for more details. As noted in Chapters 13 and 47, hemoglobin is a major body buffer.

Total Oxygen Content

The total quantity of O_2 carried in the blood is the sum of the O_2 carried in physical solution and that chemically bound to hemoglobin. O_2 content (in volume percent) may be calculated as follows:

$$O_2 \text{ Vol\%} = (PO_2)(0.003) + (Hb)(SaO_2)(1.34) \qquad (7)$$

Assuming an Hb content of 15 g, normal O_2 content equals about 20.5 Vol%. Alterations in PO_2, Hb content, and SaO_2 will all affect O_2 content (Table 11-1 and Fig. 11-4).

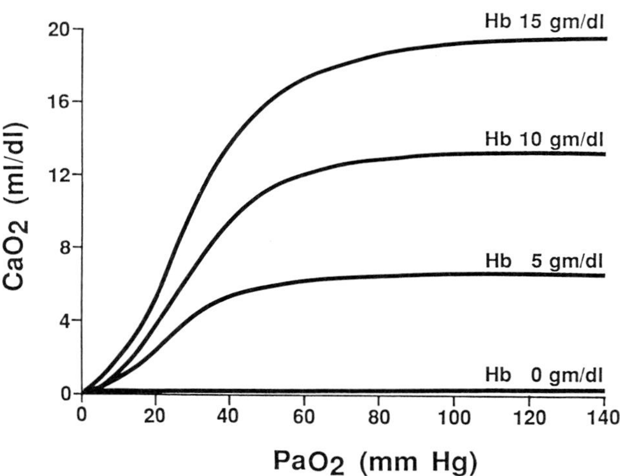

Figure 11-4. The relationship between O_2 content and PaO_2 as affected by difference in hemoglobin levels. Note that a decrease in hemoglobin content has a more dramatic effect on O_2 content than a decrease in PaO_2.

Oxyhemoglobin Dissociation Curve

The spatial orientation of the hemoglobin molecule is variable, depending on the number of O_2 atoms attached to each molecule. This results in a large variation in the affinity of hemoglobin for O_2. Figures 11-1, 11-4, and 11-5 depict the oxyhemoglobin dissociation curve, the sigmoidal shape of which illustrates the varying affinity of hemoglobin for O_2. The oxyhemoglobin dissociation curve can be considered to consist of three sections. In section 1, at very low to 25 percent SaO_2, the spatial configuration of the molecule is partially "closed" and as a result, a relatively large PO_2 change is required to load the molecule (a PO_2 of 20 mmHg

Table 11-1. Effect of PO_2, Hb, and SaO_2 on O_2 Content (CaO_2)[a]

PO_2 (mmHg)	Hb (g%)	SaO_2 (%)	CaO_2 (Vol%)
100	15	98	20.0
75	15	94	19.3
50	15	84	17.0
100	10	98	13.4
100	5	98	6.9

[a] A decrease in Hb has a greater effect on O_2 content than a decrease in PO_2.

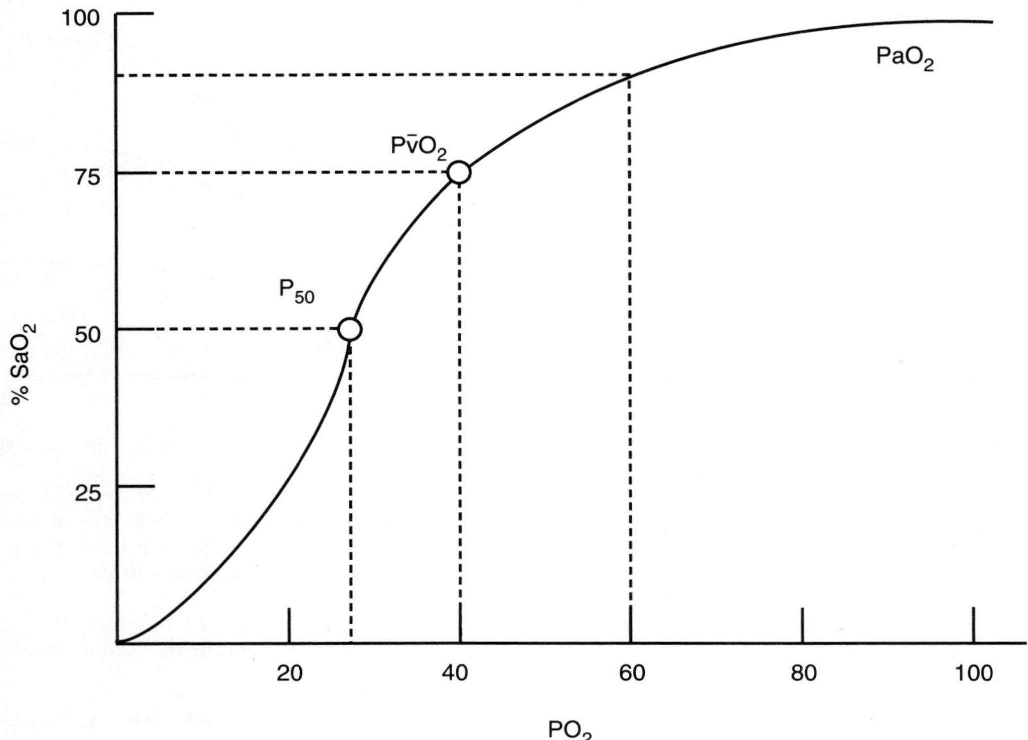

Figure 11-5. The partial pressure at which hemoglobin is 50 percent saturated is 27 mmHg (P_{50}). Normal mixed venous PO_2 ($P\bar{v}O_2$) of 40 mmHg and 75 percent oxyhemoglobin saturation are also indicated. A PO_2 of 60 mmHg results in 90 percent saturation of the hemoglobin, whereas the normal PaO_2 of 97 mmHg results in 97 percent saturation of the hemoglobin. (From Shapiro et al.,[5] with permission.)

results in an SaO_2 of 25 percent). In section 2, the middle percent saturation range (25 to 90 percent SaO_2), the molecule has "opened up" and has a high affinity for O_2, so that a small PO_2 change (from 20 to 60 mmHg) causes SaO_2 to increase from 25 to 90 percent. Section 3, corresponding to the last 10 percent SaO_2, represents the lowest affinity of hemoglobin for O_2; since a PO_2 of about 150 mmHg is required for 100 percent saturation, a PO_2 increase of 90 mmHg (from 60 to 150 mmHg) is necessary to increase SaO_2 from 90 to 100 percent. Clinically, severe hypoxemia is defined as a PO_2 in the 40 to 60 mmHg range.[8] Providing sufficient F_IO_2 to maintain PO_2 slightly above 60 mmHg normally ensures at least 90 percent plus SaO_2. To increase the SaO_2 to its normal level of 98 percent frequently requires costly increases in F_IO_2 with little physiologic gain in O_2 content, provided that hemoglobin content is normal. In critically ill patients, a PO_2 of 60 mmHg, with its corresponding 90 percent saturation, is a frequent goal of therapy to correct hypoxemia.[9]

The overall shape and position of the curve (Fig. 11-6) is affected by many factors, the total effect of which can be summarized by the P_{50} value, defined as the PO_2 at which hemoglobin is 50 percent saturated with O_2. The normal P_{50} value is 27 mmHg; an increase above this value indicates a shift in the oxyhemoglobin dissociation curve to the right and downward, corresponding to a decreased affinity of hemoglobin for O_2. This normally occurs at the peripheral tissue level, allowing for greater unloading of O_2 from the hemoglobin. On the other hand, a shift to the left and upward indicates an increased affinity of hemoglobin for O_2, which normally occurs at the pulmonary capillary bed. This phenomenon is explained by the *allosteric* property of the hemoglobin molecule. Allosteric substances have multiple binding sites, one primary and the rest secondary, with binding at secondary sites capable of affecting binding at the primary site. The following alter the affinity of hemoglobin for O_2 by affecting the secondary sites: PCO_2, molar H^+ ion concentration ($[H^+]$) temperature, 2,3-diphosphoglycerate (2,3-DPG), CO, and abnormal forms of hemoglobin[10] (Table 11-2 and Fig. 11-6). Three abnormal hemoglobins deserve special mention: fetal hemoglobin (HbF), methemoglobin (MetHb), and carboxyhemoglobin (HbCO). Fetal hemoglobin, which accounts for about 85 percent of the hemoglobin in the full-term infant,[11] contains two gamma chains instead of the normal two beta chains. As a result, the affinity of hemoglobin for O_2 is markedly increased, with the oxyhemoglobin dissociation curve shifted to the left. After birth 3 to 6 months are required for all HbF to be converted to normal Hb. In methemoglobin, the iron atoms exist in the ferric (Fe^{3+}) state instead of the ferrous (Fe^{2+}) state. Methemoglobin is formed in some individuals after the administration of certain pharmacologic agents, primarily nitrates. It also

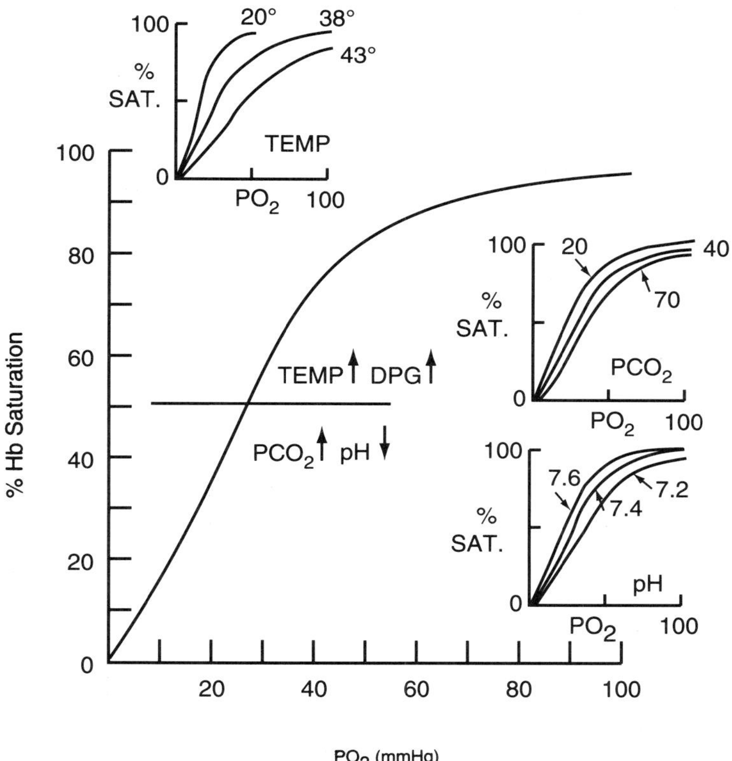

Figure 11-6. Shifting of the oxyhemoglobin dissociation curve caused by pH, PCO_2, temperature, and 2,3-DPG. (From West,[2] with permission.)

shifts the oxyhemoglobin curve to the left and upward. HbCO contains CO which binds at the same site as does O_2, but hemoglobin has 200 to 250 times as great an affinity for CO as for O_2. CO is the major substance capable of reducing hemoglobin's carrying capacity for O_2.

The Bohr Effect

Normal physiologic shifting of the oxyhemoglobin dissociation curve is summarized as the *Bohr effect.*[12] (As mentioned earlier, the curve shifts to the left at the lung and to the right at peripheral tissue.) The Bohr effect is defined as the effect of CO_2 or $[H^+]$ has on the uptake and release of O_2 from the hemoglobin molecule. Although this effect is relatively mild, it does account for the decreased O_2 affinity of hemoglobin at peripheral tissue and its increased affinity at the lung.

Table 11-2. Factors Affecting Hb Affinity for O_2

Increased Affinity
Decreased PCO_2
Decreased $[H^+]$ or increased pH
Decreased temperature
Decreased 2,3-DPG
Carboxyhemoglobin
Fetal hemoglobin
Methemoglobin
Decreased Affinity
Increased PCO_2
Increased $[H^+]$ or decreased pH
Increased temperature
Increased 2,3-DPG

OXYGEN TRANSPORT

The importance of carrying sufficient quantities of O_2 in the blood cannot be overstated. However, in order for peripheral tissue to consume O_2, the O_2 must be transported to the tissue, and transportation requires adequate cardiac output. An inadequate cardiac output can result in tissue hypoxia in spite of adequate O_2 content. The total O_2 transported to peripheral tissue is equal to O_2 content times cardiac output times a factor of 10:

$$\begin{aligned}(O_2 \text{ content})(\text{cardiac output})(10) &= O_2 \text{ transport} \\ (20 \text{ Vol\%})(5 \text{ L/min})(10) &= 1000 \text{ mL/min}\end{aligned} \tag{8}$$

Assuming a hemoglobin content of 15 g, 97 percent SaO_2, a PO_2 of 100 mmHg, and a cardiac output of 5 L/min, 1000 mL/min of O_2 is delivered to peripheral tissue.[13] A decrease in any of the above variables could result in a decrease in

Table 11-3. Effect of Cardiac Output and O_2 Content on Oxygen Transport[a]

CaO_2 (Vol%)	Cardiac Output (L/min)	O_2 Transport (mL/min)
20	5	1000
15	5	750
10	5	500
20	10	2000
20	2.5	500
15	10	1500
15	2.5	375
10	10	1000
10	2.5	250

[a] Reductions in both CaO_2 and cardiac output can affect O_2 transport. Marked reductions in O_2 transport occur if CaO_2 and cardiac output are simultaneously reduced.

available O_2. Whenever therapy to improve oxygenation is evaluated, appropriate assessment of cardiovascular capabilities must be made, as an increase in O_2 content at the expense of cardiac output may actually result in decreased O_2 transport (Table 11-3).

OXYGEN UTILIZATION

The final step in the oxygenation process is tissue utilization. The primary role of O_2 is to function as the final electron acceptor in the electron transport chain within the mitochondria of the cell (see Ch. 49). The actual chemical reaction accounting for about 90 percent of the O_2 consumed is

$$\tfrac{1}{2}\,O_2 + 2H^+ \rightarrow H_2O \qquad (9)$$

As simple as this reaction may seem, it is vital in the production of adenosine triphosphate (ATP), a high-energy phosphate compound essential to the performance of bodily functions. In the presence of sufficient O_2 normal glucose metabolism follows an aerobic pathway, resulting in the net production of 38 mol of ATP for every mole of glucose. However, in the absence of O_2, the primary metabolic pathway for glucose metabolism is glycolysis, which produces a net of 2 mol of ATP for 1 mol of glucose. O_2 consumption is generally listed as about 250 mL/min.[8] However, as with most metabolic processes, the amount of O_2 consumed is dependent on body weight. As a general rule, O_2 consumption is equal to about 3.0 to 3.5 mL O_2/kg body wt/min. (See Ch. 51 for details regarding metabolism.)

HYPOXIA

Lack of O_2 at the tissue level is referred to as *hypoxia*. Many have categorized hypoxia by the mechanistic problem causing it. Essentially, four processes are necessary for proper tissue oxygenation: (1) movement of O_2 across the alveolar capillary membrane; (2) carriage of O_2 in the blood; (3) transport of O_2 to the tissue; and (4) consumption of O_2 by the tissue.[2] Pathophysiologic problems at any of these levels result in hypoxia. Hypoxia resulting from pulmonary gas exchange deficiencies is termed *hypoxic hypoxia*; that due to inadequate O_2-carrying capacity is *anemic* hypoxia; that resulting from inadequate transport is *stagnant* hypoxia; and that resulting from inability of tissue to use O_2 is *histotoxic* hypoxia. Therapy for hypoxia should always be directed toward resolving the actual cause of the hypoxia.

References

1. Bauman R, Bartels H, Bauer C: Blood oxygen transport. pp. 147–172. In Handbook of Physiology: Section 3, The Respiratory System. Vol. 4: Gas Exchange. American Physiological Society, Bethesda, 1987
2. West J: Respiratory Physiology: The Essentials. 3rd Ed. Williams & Wilkins, Baltimore, 1985
3. Pierson DJ: The evolution of breathing: 5. Oxygen-carrying pigments: Respiratory mass transit. Respir Care 1982;27:963–970
4. Comroe JH: Physiology of Respiration. 2nd Ed. Year Book Medical Publishers, Chicago, 1974
5. Shapiro BA, Harrison RA, Walton JR: Clinical Application of Arterial Blood Gases. 3rd Ed. Year Book Medical Publishers, Chicago, 1982
6. Davenport HW: ABC's of Acid Base Chemistry. 6th Ed. University of Chicago Press, Chicago, 1974
7. Cohen JJ, Kassirer JP: Acid/Base. Little Brown, Boston, 1982
8. Shapiro BA, Harrison RA, Kacmarek RM, Cane R: Clinical Application of Respiratory Care. 3rd Ed. Year Book Medical Publishers, Chicago, 1985
9. Kacmarek RM: In-hospital administration of oxygen. pp. 1–9. In Kacmarek RM, Stoller J (eds): Current Respiratory Care. BC Decker, Toronto, 1988
10. Jones RT, Shih TB: Hemoglobin variants with altered oxygen affinity. Hemoglobin 1980;4:143–261
11. Battaglia FC, Bowes W, McGaughey HR et al: The effect of fetal exchange transfusions with adult blood upon fetal oxygenation. Pediatr Res 1969;3:60–65
12. Murray JF: The Normal Lung. 2nd Ed. WB Saunders, Philadelphia, 1984
13. Snyder JV, Pinsky MR: Oxygen Transport in the Critically Ill. Year Book Medical Publishers, Chicago, 1987

Chapter 12

Carbon Dioxide Production, Carriage, and Transport

Robert M. Kacmarek

CHAPTER OUTLINE

The by-products of normal metabolism are primarily CO_2 and water, water being excreted by the kidney while CO_2 is excreted by the lungs (see Ch. 2, Fig. 2-1). The CO_2 produced originates primarily in the mitochondria of the cell during aerobic metabolism, diffuses into the blood, and is carried to the lung and exhaled. This chapter details the mechanism associated with CO_2 homeostasis, addressing production, carriage, and transport, beginning with the formation of CO_2 by the cell and progressing to its delivery to the lung. This approach is directly opposite to that followed with O_2 in Chapter 11, primarily because CO_2 originates in the cell. Specifics regarding diffusion of CO_2 across the alveolar-capillary membrane are covered in Chapters 1 and 10.

PRODUCTION OF CARBON DIOXIDE

CO_2 is primarily produced during the metabolism of glucose. For each glucose molecule metabolized, six CO_2 molecules are formed:

$$C_6H_{12}O_6 + 6O_2 \rightarrow 6CO_2 + 6H_2O \qquad (1)$$

In addition, large quantities of CO_2 are formed in the conversion of carbohydrates to fats (see Ch. 51). The *respiratory quotient* (RQ) for the metabolism of glucose (or carbohydrates in general) is 1.0 (i.e., six CO_2 molecules are produced and six O_2 molecules consumed for each glucose molecule metabolized). The RQ is defined as follows:

$$RQ = \frac{\dot{V}CO_2}{\dot{V}O_2} \qquad (2)$$

where $\dot{V}CO_2$ is the volume of CO_2 produced and $\dot{V}O_2$ is the volume of O_2 consumed per unit time. For the other major classes of nutrients the RQ differs from 1.0; it is 0.8 for protein and 0.7 for fat. As a result, the average human RQ is about 0.85. For conversion of carbohydrates to fats the RQ is greater than 8.0.

Overall, total CO_2 production is based on body size, metabolic rate, and diet. In general, it varies from 120 to 280 mL/min in the adult and can be estimated as about 2.4 mL/kg/min.[1]

CARRIAGE OF CARBON DIOXIDE IN THE BLOOD

CO_2 is carried both in the plasma and in the red blood cells (RBCs). In both compartments CO_2 is dissolved as PCO_2, attached to protein, and converted to HCO_3^- (Fig. 12-1).

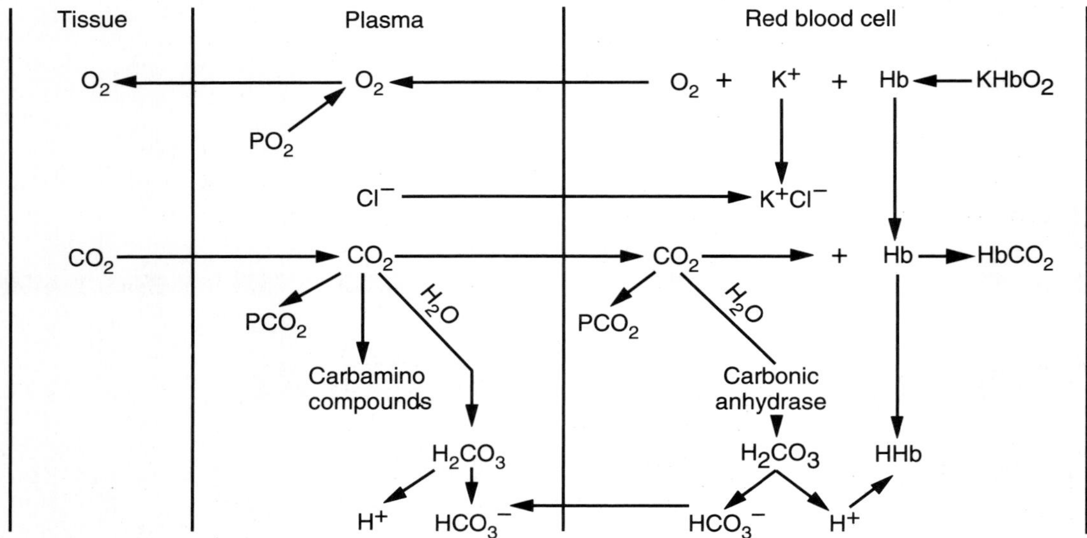

Figure 12-1. Overall scheme of O_2 and CO_2 transport in the blood. See text and Chapter 10 for details. (From Kacmarek et al.,[1] with permission.)

Carriage in the Plasma

As CO_2 diffuses into the blood from peripheral tissue, it physically dissolves in the plasma as PCO_2. However, by far the greatest amount of CO_2 in the plasma is carried as HCO_3^-. As CO_2 dissolves, it reacts with water to form H_2CO_3, which in turn dissociates to form H^+ and HCO_3^-.

$$CO_2 + H_2O \rightleftharpoons H_2CO_3 \rightleftharpoons H^+ + HCO_3^- \quad (3)$$

Equation 3 represents a reversible reaction; in the peripheral tissue CO_2 enters the blood, pushing the equilibrium to the right to form more HCO_3^-. However, as blood moves to the lungs and CO_2 begins to be exhaled, the equilibrium shifts to the left to convert more HCO_3^- to CO_2, which is exhaled.[2] The H^+ formed is buffered in the venous blood, which accounts for venous blood being more acidic (7.35) than arterial blood (7.40).

The pressure of dissolved CO_2, expressed in millimeters of Hg, is related by a factor of 0.0301 to the H_2CO_3 level expressed in millequivalents per liter (mEq/L) or millimoles per liter (mmol/L),[3]

$$(PCO_2 \text{ mmHg})(0.0301) = H_2CO_3 \text{ mEq/L or mmol/L} \quad (4)$$

This factor is used to determine total CO_2 levels (dissolved CO_2 plus HCO_3^-) and in calculations involving the buffering capacity of HCO_3^-/H_2CO_3 in the blood (Ch. 45).

Finally, CO_2 is attached to plasma proteins to form terminal carbamino compounds ($NHCOO^-$ groups) by reaction of CO_2 with terminal amino (NH_2) groups[4]:

$$R\text{—}N\begin{matrix}/H\\ \backslash H\end{matrix} + CO_2 \rightleftharpoons R\text{—}N\begin{matrix}/H\\ \backslash COO^-\end{matrix} + H^+ \quad (5)$$

(R indicates the remainder of the protein). The H^+ formed is buffered by the blood and is in part responsible for the acidity of venous blood. This reaction is reversible, the equilibrium being shifted to the right at peripheral tissue and to the left at the lung.

Carriage in the Red Blood Cells

CO_2 is carried in the RBCs in a manner similar to that in the plasma. The PCO_2 in plasma and in the RBCs is in equilibrium. CO_2 is also carried as HCO_3^-; however, the rate of the reaction of CO_2 with H_2O is greatly increased by the enzyme carbonic anhydrase (CA).[5]

$$CO_2 + H_2O \xrightarrow{CA} H_2CO_3 \rightleftharpoons H^+ + HCO_3^- \quad (6)$$

Carbonic anhydrase is located in the RBC but does not exist free in the plasma. As a result of its presence, large quantities of HCO_3^- are produced by the RBC, most of which diffuses into the plasma. As this occurs, Cl^- moves into the RBC to maintain electrostatic equilibrium. This process is called the *chloride shift* or the *Hamburger phenomenon*. The Cl^- that diffuses into the RBC associates with the K^+ released from the hemoglobin molecule as it gives up O_2 to the tissue and buffers H^+ (Fig. 12-1).

CO_2 also reacts with the terminal NH_2 groups of the hemoglobin molecule in the same manner as it reacts with plasma protein (Equation 5), and the H^+ released from the reactions forming HCO_3^- and R-$NHCOO^-$ must be buffered.[6] The primary buffers in the RBC are the imidazole groups on the hemoglobin molecule; however, the ability of these groups to buffer is dependent on the oxyhemoglobin saturation. With O_2 bound to the heme, the imidazole groups are poor buffers, but when O_2 is not attached, they are good buffers. This is a result of the formation of R-NH_3^+ com-

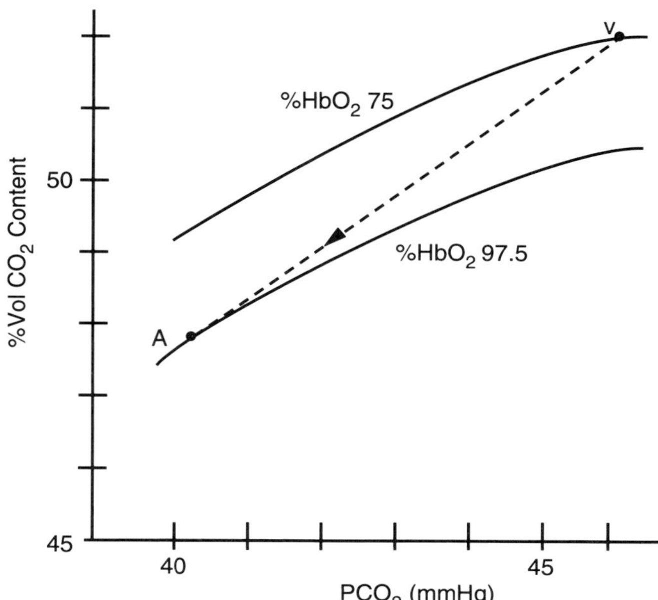

Figure 12-2. Effect of oxyhemoglobin saturation on the volume of CO_2 carried in the blood. The capacity of blood for CO_2 is decreased as oxyhemoglobin saturation is increased (Haldane effect). The arrow from V to A depicts change of CO_2 content from venous to arterial blood. (From Kacmarek et al.,[1] with permission.)

plexes by R-NH_2 groups reacting with H^+ as O_2 attaches to the heme; these complexes react poorly with CO_2.

THE HALDANE EFFECT

The effect of oxyhemoglobin saturation on the pickup and release of CO_2 is referred to as the *Haldane effect* (Fig. 12-2). Since hemoglobin becomes oxygenated at the lung, more of the R-NH_2 groups form R-NH_3^+ complexes, inhibiting CO_2 binding and enhancing CO_2 release, while at the peripheral tissue the opposite occurs. As O_2 is released by the hemoglobin, the R-NH_3^+ complexes form R-NH_2 groups, which react readily with CO_2. This shifting of the CO_2–hemoglobin reaction curve (Fig. 12-2) allows for the carriage and release of 4 Vol% CO_2 during the normal venous to arterial change in PCO_2 (46 to 40 mmHg).

QUANTITATIVE DISTRIBUTION OF CARBON DIOXIDE

The greatest amount (90 percent) of CO_2 carried in the blood is in the form of HCO_3^-, although it should be remembered that most of this HCO_3^- is actually formed by the kidney (see Ch. 13). About 5 percent is carried as PCO_2 and the remaining 5 percent as carbamino compounds. Of the CO_2 exhaled, about 60 percent is carried as HCO_3^-, 30 percent as carbamino compounds, and 10 percent as PCO_2.[2]

References

1. Kacmarek RM, Mack C, Dimas S: The Essentials of Respiratory Care. 3rd Ed. Year Book Medical Publishers, Chicago, 1990
2. West J: Respiratory Physiology: The Essentials. 3rd Ed. Williams & Wilkins, Baltimore, 1985
3. Davenport HW: ABC's of Acid Base Chemistry. 6th Ed. University of Chicago Press, Chicago, 1974
4. Comroe JH: Physiology of Respiration 2nd Ed. Year Book Medical Publishers, Chicago, 1974
5. Shapiro BA, Harrison RA, Walton JR: Clinical Application of Arterial Blood Gases. 3rd Ed. Year Book Medical Publishers, Chicago, 1982
6. Klocke RA: Carbon dioxide transport. pp. 173–198. In The Handbook of Physiology: Section 3, The Respiratory System. Vol. 4: Gas Exchange. American Physiological Society, Bethesda, 1987

Chapter 13

Water, Solute, and Acid-Base Balance

John M. Luce

CHAPTER OUTLINE

It is thought that the earliest vertebrates inhabited a salt water environment, the composition of which was similar to that of their own *extracellular fluid* (ECF).[1] These animals could ingest the sea around them without disturbing their internal environment, and they could easily excrete waste products by flushing them through their skin. However, when these early vertebrates migrated into streams, they were required to develop an impermeable body covering to prevent fatal dilution with fresh water. Later vertebrates moved into the land, where they had to maintain their internal salt water milieu within a dry external environment. This necessitated the evolution of kidneys that could concentrate water and salt and excrete nitrogenous wastes into a highly concentrated urine. Today, human kidneys work in concert with other organs to guarantee the body's water, solute, and acid-base balance. Appreciation of how this balance is preserved is essential in understanding how perturbations of the balance can threaten life.

DISTRIBUTION OF WATER AND SOLUTES

Body fluids contain water and dissolved substances called solutes. Water makes up 40 to 80 percent of the total weight of the human body, depending on an individual's amount of lean tissue; because lean tissue holds more water than does fat, young, muscular individuals have the greatest amount of water for a given weight. Assuming an average 60 percent water content, a 70-kg adult has 42 L of total body water.

The body's normal solutes include electrolytes; sugars, such as glucose; and urea, a product of protein metabolism, which is toxic in high concentrations. The *electrolytes* consist of cations (positively charged ions) such as Na^+ and K^+ and anions (negatively charged ions) such as Cl^- and HCO_3^-. In solution these electrolytes are capable of carrying an electrical current. When combined chemically as salts, their electrical charges, which reflect their valences, are balanced, so that they do not carry a net charge. The electrolyte concentration of body fluids is expressed in terms of milliequivalents per liter of solution, usually aqueous. (A milliequivalent is one one-thousandth of the molecular weight of a substance in grams divided by its valence.) Electrolyte concentrations also may be expressed as millimoles per liter (a millimole being one one-thousandth of the molecular weight of a substance).[2]

The semipermeable membranes that surround body cells allow free passage of water molecules but are relatively impermeable to the passage of solutes and large molecules such as albumin. When a solute to which a membrane is impermeable is placed on one side of a membrane, water flows to the side on which the solute is more concentrated until the original concentration difference, or gradient, no longer exists. The power of this gradient to attract water is proportional to the number of particles in solution. It is called osmolality and is expressed in milliosmoles per kilogram of water (mOsm/kg H_2O).

Electrolytes are the most numerous and therefore the most osmotically active particles in the body. They are distributed proportionally within and outside of cells because of the permeability of the cell membranes and because the electrolytes are actively transported across the membranes by ion pumps to maintain the electrical milieu inside and outside the cells. Na^+ is the major cation and Cl^- and HCO_3^- the major anions in ECF. Their counterparts in *intracellular fluid* (ICF) are K^+ and anionic proteins. Although K^+ may move out of cells in the presence of increased extracellular acid or alpha-adrenergic stimulation, its concentration in the ECF is miniscule compared with that in the ICF. By contrast, more than 95 percent of total body Na^+ is extracellular.

The fluid spaces of the body, ECF and ICF, are also called body compartments. The extracellular compartment contains the *interstitial space,* which consists of lymphatics, connective tissue, and bone, and the *intravascular space,* which is filled with blood (Fig. 13-1). Blood from which red and white blood cells have been separated is called *plasma; serum* is plasma from which platelets and clotting factors have been removed. Since water passes freely across cell membranes, the amount in one compartment or the other depends primarily on their concentrations of electrolytes. Normally, two-thirds of body water is found within cells, and is therefore neither interstitial nor intravascular, and the remaining one-third is extracellular. In a 70-kg individual two-thirds of the 42 L total body water, 28 L, is in the form of ICF, and one-third, or 14 L, is in the form of ECF. Blood makes up one-third of ECF volume, so intravascular volume amounts to approximately 5 L and interstitial volume 9 L. Because the normal hematocrit is 40 to 45 percent, plasma volume is approximately 3 L. At the same time, the total volume of formal blood elements, mainly red blood cells, is 2 L.[2,3]

WATER MOVEMENT BETWEEN BODY COMPARTMENTS

Water content in the two body compartments will be altered if the concentration of electrolytes within the compartments changes. Thus, when Na^+ is added to the ECF, it attracts water osmotically from the intracellular compartment in proportion to the amount of Na^+ added. This results

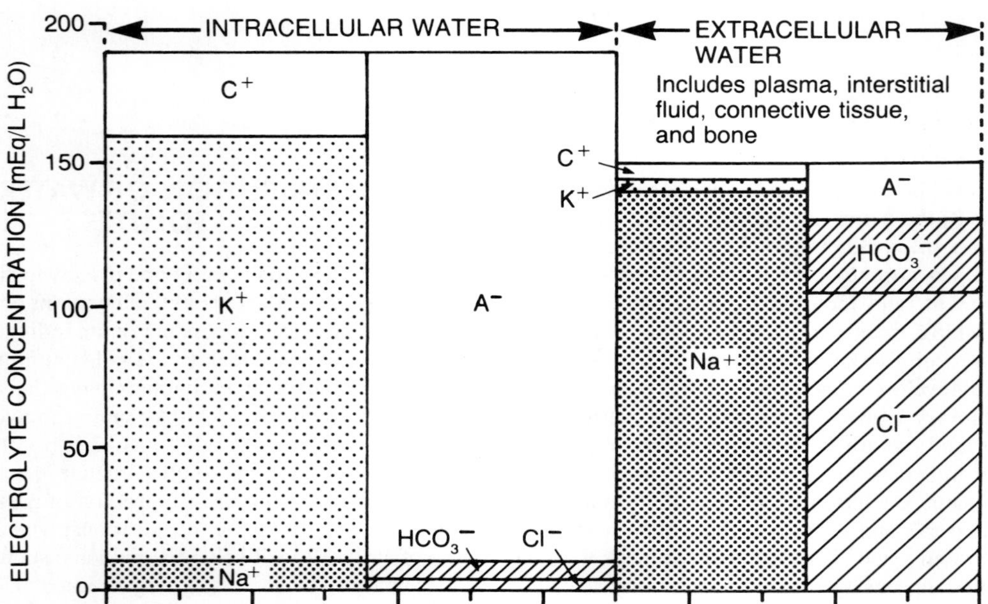

Figure 13-1. Electrolyte concentration in milliequivalents per liter of water in the body's two major aqueous compartments. C^+, unmeasured cations; A^-, unmeasured anions. (From Luce et al.,[2] with permission.)

in an increase in ECF volume at the expense of the ICF. Preservation of ECF volume is essential because the ECF includes the intravascular fluid, that is, the blood necessary for organ perfusion. Indeed, the body defends ECF volume over osmolality in most instances, as will be discussed.

The process just described is that of water movement between body compartments. Another important process is that of water movement within one compartment, the ECF. This compartment contains the interstitial and the intravascular spaces, which are separated by the walls or membranes of the blood vessels, including capillaries. Normally the capillary membranes are freely permeable to water and small solutes. The concentrations of water and Na^+ within the interstitial and intravascular spaces therefore are the same, and if water or Na^+ is added to the ECF, it will equilibrate across the capillaries. However, the capillary membranes normally are not permeable to albumin or other macromolecules. These molecules (proteins) are present in much smaller quantities in plasma than are Na^+ and other solutes, and they contribute comparatively little to ECF osmolality. However, because they normally are restricted to the intravascular space, they may exert a pressure of 30 mmHg or greater inside the capillaries that contain them.

The pressure exerted by albumin and other macromolecules is called *oncotic pressure* to distinguish it from the *osmotic pressure* generated by electrolytes. Oncotic pressure is important because it tends to draw water from the interstitial to the intravascular space, thereby maintaining the volume of plasma, which is 95 percent water. The oncotic pressure in turn is offset by the hydrostatic pressure of water within the capillaries, which tends to drive water out. The capillaries are surrounded by the interstitium, which exerts oncotic and hydrostatic pressure of its own. Normally the interstitial oncotic pressure is weaker than the intravascular oncotic pressure because fewer protein molecules are found in the interstitial space. Interstitial hydrostatic pressure also tends to be lower than hydrostatic pressure in the intravascular space.

The flux of fluid in and out of a given capillary obviously depends on a balance between these various pressures.[4] This flux is summarized in the modified Starling equation

$$F = k(P_{cap} - P_{is}) - \sigma(\pi_{cap} - \pi_{is}) \quad (1)$$

where F is the net flux of the capillary; k is a permeability factor describing how readily water traverses the capillary membrane; P_{cap} is capillary hydrostatic pressure; P_{is} is interstitial hydrostatic pressure; σ is a reflection coefficient describing how well the capillary membrane keeps proteins on one side; π_{cap} is capillary oncotic pressure; and π_{is} is interstitial oncotic pressure (see Ch. 1, Equation 2). Assuming that capillary membrane integrity is intact and k and σ stay constant, water normally passes out of the capillary at its arteriolar end, where P_{cap} is higher than π_{cap}, and reenters the capillary at its venular end, where the situation is reversed (Fig. 13-2).

The net effect of the Starling forces, as mentioned earlier, is to keep water within the intravascular space and thereby maintain blood volume. Nevertheless, because water is constantly flowing into and out of capillaries, body tissues that contain capillaries—which most tissues do—are never truly dry. Furthermore, an unbalancing of the Starling forces, as would occur with greatly increased P_{cap}, greatly decreased π_{cap}, or increased k, can greatly increase fluid flow out of a capillary and into the interstitial space. Extravascular interstitial fluid of this sort is called *edema*. P_{cap} can be increased when total body Na^+ and ECF volumes are increased, as occurs in congestive heart failure, in which left ventricular function is inadequate. Conversely, π_{cap} decreases in cirrhosis, in which albumin synthesis is impaired; and in nephrosis, in which albumin leaks from the kidneys into the urine. Increased capillary permeability is seen in diseases, such as the adult respiratory distress syndrome (ARDS), that are characterized by disruption of capillary membrane integrity.

Because the capillary membrane is permeable to water and small solutes but not to protein when P_{cap} or π_{cap} only is affected, the edema fluid that collects outside the capillary has a low specific gravity and protein concentration as compared with that of plasma. This fluid, called a *transudate*, generally looks thin and clear. However, when the permeability constant k is altered, the capillary membrane allows the passage of protein as well as water and small solutes, so that the edema has a high specific gravity and a protein concentration similar to that of plasma. This fluid, called an *exudate*, generally looks thick and more opaque. Although differentiating transudates from exudates is sometimes difficult, the distinction between the two types of edema assists the clinician in determining how the fluid was formed.[5]

Pulmonary edema is fluid that collects in the interstitium or the alveolar air space in the lung. Normally P_{cap} in the pulmonary capillaries is about 10 mmHg; this is exceeded by π_{cap}, so there is a net flux of water into the capillaries, which keeps the interstitium and air spaces relatively dry. However, P_{cap} may increase when pressure rises in the left ventricle during congestive heart failure or when left atrial pressure rises independently, as in mitral stenosis. When P_{cap} greatly exceeds π_{cap}, transudation out of the capillaries begins. The opposite situation is seen in ARDS, in which damage to the pulmonary capillary membrane allows the exudation of water and protein regardless of P_{cap} or π_{cap}. When this happens, the pressure of proteins in the interstitial space reverses the previous oncotic gradient (π_{cap} greater than π_{is}) and draws even more water from the capillaries. If interstitial lymphatics located around the bronchi and the branches of the pulmonary artery cannot drain the water, it floods the alveolar air spaces and worsens gas exchange.[6–8]

Edema in the pleural space is called *pleural effusion*. The pleural space normally contains a small amount of fluid, which lubricates the parietal pleura on the inside of the chest wall and the visceral pleura that envelops the lungs. This fluid probably comes from capillaries in both the parietal and visceral pleurae. Pleural effusions can collect if parietal pleural P_{cap} increases, if π_{cap} decreases, if lymphatic drainage is compromised, or if the pleural capillaries are inflamed. Large transudative effusions are common in congestive heart

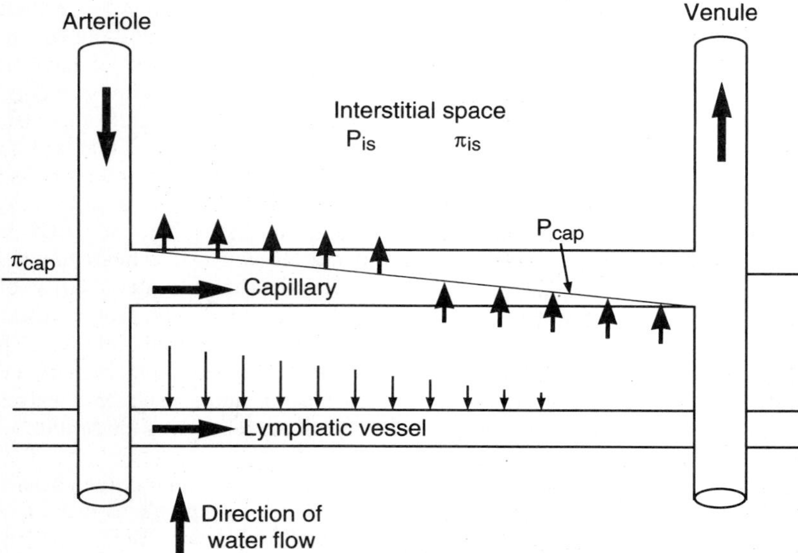

Figure 13-2. Water flow across a capillary and the pressures responsible for this flow. Interstitial hydrostatic (P_{is}) and oncotic (π_{is}) pressures and capillary oncotic (π_{cap}) pressure are assumed to remain constant, as is capillary permeability. However, capillary hydrostatic pressure (P_{cap}) decreases from arteriole to venule. Water therefore leaves the capillary at its arteriolar end and reenters at the venular end. Excess extravascular water is removed by lymphatic vessels located at or near the capillary. Unbalancing of the forces (as with increased P_{cap}, decreased π_{cap}, or increased capillary permeability) or damage to the lymphatics would increase the flux of fluid out of the capillary. (From Luce et al.,[2] with permission.)

failure and also occur in cirrhosis and nephrosis. Exudative pleural effusions accumulate most commonly in pneumonia and in carcinomatous involvement of the pleura.[2,5,9]

Peripheral edema is the name given to fluid that collects in the interstitial spaces of dependent regions of the body, such as the ankles of ambulatory patients and the presacral area of patients in bed. It also tends to accumulate in the periorbital and scrotal regions when π_{cap} is low. When present in the abdomen, where it collects in the peritoneal cavity, the edema is termed *ascites*. A condition called *anasarca* exists if the entire body is swollen with fluid. Peripheral edema may result primarily or in part from a low π_{cap}, as is the case in cirrhosis or nephrosis, or from a high P_{cap}, as is the case in congestive heart failure. Obstruction of the large veins of the leg or the inferior vena cava in the abdomen will also cause peripheral edema owing to the increased venous pressure in those areas.

The generalized edema seen in congestive heart failure, cirrhosis, and nephrosis is a sign that both total body Na^+ and water are increased.[7] Even though the ECF volume may be increased to begin with in the first two of these disorders, the kidneys detect that circulating blood volume is inadequate, either because cardiac output is low in congestive heart failure or because arterial vasodilation causes decreased vascular filling in cirrhosis. Circulating blood volume is truly reduced in nephrosis because albumin is lost in the urine. Because the kidneys sense that blood volume is inadequate in all three conditions, they tend to limit urinary Na^+ excretion, as is discussed further. Water also is retained to preserve volume and osmolality within the ECF.[10–12]

ESTIMATION OF EXTRACELLULAR FLUID VOLUME

As stressed throughout this chapter, ECF volume depends on the amount of Na^+ in the ECF because that electrolyte attracts water osmotically. Therefore, Na^+ excess causes ECF volume excess, and Na^+ depletion causes ECF volume depletion. Assuming that it is not due to local venous obstruction, peripheral edema is an indication that ECF volume has been increased by the addition of Na^+ and water to the ECF. It is estimated that the interstitial space in which edema forms, which is two-thirds of the normal ECF volume, must be expanded by approximately 5 L of water for peripheral edema to be clinically evident. Since two-thirds of total body water is contained in the ICF and only one-third is in the ECF, it follows that more than 15 L of water must be added to the body for edema to become manifest in patients with generalized edematous disorders. The same patients also have distension of the internal jugular veins when they sit at a 45-degree angle, a sign that their intravascular space is expanded.

Depletion of ECF volume results in the opposite of edema, a shrinkage of the interstitial space. This results in wrinkled skin, sunken eyeballs, and other manifestations of dehydration. The decreased intravascular volume that is also observed is reflected in a lack of jugular venous distension and in orthostatic changes in blood pressure and pulse. Normally, when people change from a reclining to a sitting position or when they stand, systolic blood pressure and pulse change little and diastolic blood pressure increases by 5 to 10 mmHg. However, if intravascular volume is reduced by about 10 percent, pulse will rise by 10 beats/min and diastolic pressure will fall by 10 mmHg; the systolic pressure also may fall slightly. Orthostatic changes of these sorts can also occur in patients who are bedridden or who lack autonomic nervous system tone, and therefore signs of interstitial as well as intravascular volume inadequacy often must be sought.

Unfortunately for clinicians, ECF volume status cannot always be determined by physical examination, especially in patients whose Na^+ status varies from day to day. Because of this, daily records of weight gain or loss and Na^+ and water intake and outflow are useful in such patients. The urinary concentration of Na^+ also serves as a guide for estimating ECF volume, assuming that it is not altered by diuretics or other agents. This is because the kidneys retain Na^+ when their perfusion is reduced, as will be discussed, and excrete urine with a concentration of Na^+ that usually is less than 10 mEq/L.

Some patients also require direct measurement of intravascular and intracardiac pressures. Right atrial pressure, also called central venous pressure (CVP), can be measured by a catheter placed in the superior vena cava. The CVP may be used as a reflection of left atrial and left ventricular end-diastolic pressures in patients in whom right- and left-sided pressures are likely to be equal. Although a low CVP almost invariably reflects low left atrial pressure and therefore signifies hypovolemia, the CVP may be much higher than the left atrial pressure in patients with disorders that affect primarily the right side of the heart, such as right ventricular infarction or pulmonary embolism. As a result, clinicians may choose to measure the pulmonary artery wedge pressure or occlusion pressure with a flow-directed pulmonary artery (Swan-Ganz) catheter.

In this approach a catheter with an inflatable balloon just proximal to the distal tip is carried by the flow of blood into a branch of the pulmonary artery until it "wedges" there, so that the branch is momentarily occluded and blood flow in it and in the downstream pulmonary vein ceases. The pressure that is then sensed by the catheter tip, called the *pulmonary artery wedge* or *occlusion pressure,* will be that transmitted back through the pulmonary veins from the left atrium. When the mitral valve is open and the left ventricle is filling with blood, the left atrial pressure is the same as the left ventricular end-diastolic pressure. Thus, the wedge pressure provides a good estimate of left-ventricular end-diastolic pressure and, by implication, end-diastolic volume.[13]

ESTIMATION OF EXTRACELLULAR FLUID OSMOLALITY

Because Na^+ is the major ECF cation and must be balanced by Cl^- and HCO_3^- for the ECF to remain electrically neutral, ECF osmolality can be approximated by doubling the plasma or serum Na^+ concentration and adding the smaller contribution of other solutes. Thus

$$\text{Osmolality} = [(2)\ (\text{Na}^+ \text{ concentration})] + \left(\frac{\text{glucose concentration}}{18}\right) + \left(\frac{\text{BUN}}{2.8}\right)$$

where BUN is blood urea nitrogen. The normal serum Na^+ concentration is 140 mEq/L; the glucose concentration is approximately 100 mg/dL, and the BUN is around 10 mg/dL. Normal serum osmolality therefore is about 285 mOsm/kg H_2O, with a range of 280 to 295. *Hypo-osmolality* or *hyperosmolality* exist when the osmolality lies outside the normal range.

Osmolality also can be measured in the laboratory by the freezing point depression and change in water vapor methods. If the measured osmolality exceeds the estimated osmolality, an *osmolar gap* is said to exist, and the clinician should be alerted to the presence of other unmeasured osmoles.[14] These might come from alcohols such as ethanol (osmolar contribution equals ethanol concentration in milligrams per deciliter divided by 4.6); mannitol or glycerol, which are given intravenously to patients with cerebral edema or glaucoma (osmolar contribution equals mannitol concentration in milligrams per deciliter divided by 9); or sorbitol, a sugar contained in certain medications. The clinical use of the osmolar gap is discussed further in Chapter 28.

CONCEPT OF TONICITY

As noted earlier, solutes such as Na^+ exert their osmotic effect because they stay on one side or the other of cell membranes owing to their molecular size or electrical charge or because of active cellular pumping mechanisms. These solutes are called *impermeant* because of their normally fixed location in one body compartment. The term *tonicity* is used to describe the osmotic equivalence of fluids that contain impermeant solutes. *Isotonic* fluids have the same osmolality as serum or plasma; hypertonic fluids have higher osmolality. Table 13-1 lists the tonicity of commonly used intravenous fluid preparations. *Hypotonicity* results when the concentration of ECF solutes, in most cases Na^+, decreases and causes net ICF volume excess. On the other hand, *hypertonicity* occurs when ECF solutes increase and cause net ICF volume depletion.

Most solutes that cause hypertonicity, including Na^+, glucose, mannitol, glycerol, and sorbitol, also cause *hyperosmolarity*. Because of this clinicians may assume that hypertonicity and hyperosmolarity are the same. However, the terms are not always interchangeable. For example, high lev-

Table 13-1. Intravenous Solutions and Additives Used to Maintain Water and Solute Balance

Solution	Tonicity			Glucose Concentration (mEq/L or per Ampule)	Electrolyte Concentration (mEq/L or per Ampule)					
	Hypotonic	Isotonic	Hypertonic		Na^+	Ca^{2+}	K^+	Cl^-	HCO_3^-	Lactate
5% D/W[a]	x			50						
10% D/W	x			100						
20% D/W			x	200						
50% D/W			x	500						
5% D/0.45% NaCl	x			50	77			77		
5% D/0.9% NaCl		x		50	154			154		
0.45% NaCl	x				77			77		
0.9% NaCl		x			154			154		
3% NaCl			x		513			513		
Ringer's solution		x			148	4	4	156		
Ringer's lactate		x			130	3	4	109		28
7.5% NaHCO3			x		44 in 50-mL ampule				44 in 50-mL ampule	
25% mannitol			x	12.5 g/50 mL/ ampule						
50% glucose			x	25 g in 50-mL ampule						

[a] D, dextrose; W, water.
(From Luce et al.,[2] with permission.)

els of urea or ethanol raise serum or plasma osmolality but do not cause hypertonicity because they produce no lasting osmotic gradient across cell membranes and therefore do not cause water to shift between body compartments. Clinicians cannot differentiate hyperosmolality and hypertonicity by measuring plasma osmolality because both the freezing point depression and the change in water vapor method depend on colligative properties and cannot detect whether a solute is impermeant. Thus, tonicity must be calculated by adding the contribution of each impermeant solute in ECF or by subtracting from the measured osmolality in milliosmoles per kilogram water the osmotic contribution of urea or ethanol.[15]

The physiologic result of ECF hypotonicity is a relative increase in ICF volume. This increase, which is the same as cell swelling and intracellular cerebral edema, can cause a syndrome of central nervous system (CNS) depression, which is called *water intoxication*. At the same time, because the brain is encased in rigid skull, cerebral edema can lead to an increase in intracranial pressure (ICP), which can further depress consciousness and precipitate shifts of brain tissue. Intracranial pressure is measured in several disease states characterized by cerebral edema (see Ch. 93).

On the other hand, ECF hypertonicity produces ICF dehydration and cell crenation within the CNS. When hypertonicity develops abruptly, the shrunken brain actually may tear away from its supporting structures and result in fatal hemorrhage. Alternatively, if the hypertonicity develops more slowly, brain cells appear to protect their volume by generating new intracellular solutes, called *idiogenic osmoles,* which limit the movement of water from the CNS. The source of these solutes is not known, nor is it certain that they are produced by a true homeostatic mechanism and are not the result of hypertonic damage. Furthermore, the formation of idiogenic osmoles may be problematic in that they can draw water into the CNS and cause isotonic water intoxication if plasma hypertonicity is corrected too rapidly by administration of hypotonic fluids.[15]

PRESERVATION OF EXTRACELLULAR FLUID VOLUME

The previous discussion of cerebral cell swelling and crenation emphasizes the clinical consequences of changes in volume and osmolality within the ECF. Given these consequences, it is not surprising that the body has developed complicated mechanisms to preserve ECF volume and osmolality. These mechanisms usually work in concert, so that volume and osmolality are both protected. Nevertheless, the potential adverse effects of intravascular volume loss and hypoperfusion of vital organs are so severe that ECF volume is defended to the detriment of osmolality in certain circumstances.[3] It is therefore preferable to discuss preservation of volume and of osmolality separately and in sequence according to the body's apparent priorities.

The body loses fixed amounts of water and solutes each day. For example, to rid the body of urea and other metabolic waste products, the kidneys daily excrete 1500 mL of water containing 50 mEq Na^+, 40 mEq K^+, and 90 mEq Cl^-. Approximately 1000 mL of water is lost through the skin as sweat and through the lungs as water vapor. This amount can rise markedly as the ambient temperature increases, particularly if the air is poorly humidified. Water also leaves the body in stool and gastrointestinal fluids, which vary in their solute content (Table 13-2). To preserve ECF volume and maintain osmolality, the body either must compensate for these inevitable losses by increasing its intake of water

Table 13-2. Daily Volumes and Concentrations of Major Solutes in Body Fluids

	Average Volume (L/d)	Electrolyte Concentration (mEq/L)				
		Na^+	K^+	H^+	Cl^-	HCO_3^-
Saliva	1.5	30[a] (20–50)[b]	20 (16–23)	— —	31 (20–50)	15 (10–20)
Gastric juice	2.5	50 (30–90)	10 (5–10)	90 —	110 (50–130)	0 —
Bile	0.5	140 (120–170)	5 (5–10)	— —	105 (80–120)	40 (30–50)
Pancreatic juice	0.7	140 (110–150)	5 (5–10)	— —	60 (50–100)	90 (70–110)
Small intestine	1.5	120 (70–160)	5 (0–5)	— —	110 (70–130)	35 (20–40)
Diarrhea	1.0–10	130 (120–140)	10 (5–15)	— —	95 (90–100)	20 (15–30)
Sweat	0–3	50 (20–100)	5 (0–15)	— —	50 (20–100)	0 —

[a] Mean.
[b] Range.
(From Luce JM et al.,[2] with permission.)

and solutes, especially Na^+, or must invoke mechanisms to conserve them.[2]

The need for conservation is even more pronounced during disease. Vomiting and diarrhea can deplete the body of solutes and water in short order, and water losses in febrile patients who sweat and increase their minute ventilation can be quite severe. In addition, nasogastric tubes and other devices may drain off large quantities of body fluids and electrolytes. Finally, surgical blood loss or traumatic hemorrhage may suddenly threaten ECF volume. The body responds to these and other threats through what has been called the *integrated volume response*. This important process represents an extension of normal protective mechanisms and involves the autonomic nervous system as well as the kidneys[3] (Fig. 13-3).

Extreme alterations in effective ECF volume are sensed both by low-pressure baroreceptors in the left atrium and thoracic veins and by high-pressure baroreceptors in the ca-

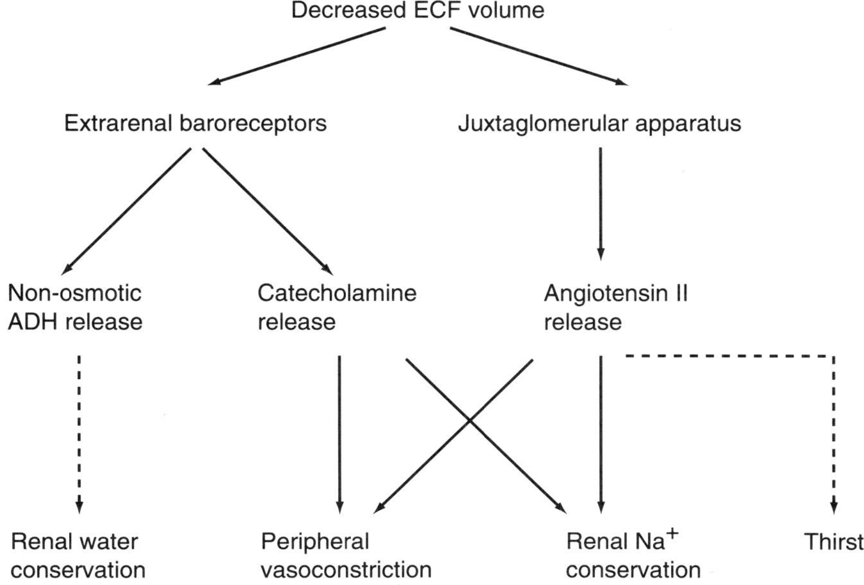

Figure 13-3. Integrated volume responses to a decrease in ECF volume. See text for further explanations. ADH, antidiuretic hormone. (Adapted from Andreoli,[3] with permission.)

rotid body and aortic arch. Activation of these baroreceptors results in increased autonomic nervous system activity and catecholamine release into the bloodstream. The combination of autonomic nervous system activity and catecholamine release raises blood pressure by increasing arteriolar resistance and heart rate and by decreasing venous capacitance. The increase in arteriolar resistance decreases P_{cap} throughout the body, favoring fluid movement from the interstitial space into the capillaries; this movement may be reflected by a fall in the hematocrit. At the same time, the autonomic stimulation causes increased Na^+ retention by direct action on renal epithelial cells. This, in combination with the effects of aldosterone (discussed below), decreases the urinary Na^+ concentration.[3,10,11]

A second aspect of the integrated volume response is the release of antidiuretic hormone (ADH), also called vasopressin, by the pituitary gland. Release of ADH normally occurs because of hypertonicity and is thought to be due to osmotic dehydration of osmoreceptor cells in the hypothalamus, as will be discussed. However, in the case of ECF volume depletion, ADH release is stimulated by the autonomic nervous system and operates independently of osmotic regulation. In fact, bleeding patients may conserve so much water to preserve ECF volume that they develop dilutional hypotonicity in the process.[15]

While these events are occurring, the juxtaglomerular apparatus in the kidneys is prompted by autonomic nervous system stimulation, reduction of blood pressure, and perhaps other mechanisms to release the hormone renin into the circulation. Renin release in turn stimulates production of angiotensin II, which enhances peripheral vasoconstriction, induces aldosterone secretion by the kidneys, and stimulates thirst. Aldosterone prompts the kidneys to retain Na^+ in exchange for K^+ and H^+, which tends to cause hypokalemia and metabolic alkalosis, as discussed below. At the same time thirst prompts patients to increase their water intake even to the point of ECF hypotonicity.

The kidneys respond to slight Na^+ and ECF volume depletion by increasing Na^+ absorption in the proximal tubules without changing the rate of glomerular filtration. Aldosterone, which is released as depletion becomes more severe, promotes increased Na^+ reabsorption in the distal tubule. Finally, when volume depletion becomes still more severe, the vasoconstriction induced by angiotensin II and circulating catecholamines reduces renal blood flow, glomerular filtration, and renal Na^+ excretion to the point that almost no Na^+ is excreted. At this point renal ischemia and a potentially irreversible decline in kidney function may occur.[3,10,11]

PRESERVATION OF EXTRACELLULAR FLUID OSMOLALITY

Although preservation of ECF volume is paramount, as has been stressed, the body also attempts to maintain ECF osmolality within the range of 280 to 295 mOsm/kg H_2O through a process called osmoregulation. This process also serves to keep the Na^+ concentration of the ECF constant because Na^+ is the most abundant and osmotically active solute in the ECF. At the same time, because cell membranes are permeable to water, and ECF osmolality and Na^+ concentration are kept constant, the solute/water ratio in all body compartments is kept constant. Osmoregulation therefore should be thought of as a way to regulate water balance in the body.[3]

Water balance is regulated by the activation or inhibition of ADH release from the posterior pituitary gland and by the stimulation or nonstimulation of thirst (Fig. 13-4). The release of ADH is due to the osmotic dehydration of osmoreceptor cells in the hypothalamus that prompt the pituitary to release ADH, whereas the osmotic dehydration of cells in the hypothalamic thirst centers stimulates thirst by unknown mechanisms. This dehydration can be achieved only by impermeant solutes such as Na^+ and not by urea or ethanol. In addition, Na^+ is a more potent impermeant solute than glucose in causing ADH release.[15]

When the osmolality of the ECF rises above 298 mOsm/kg H_2O and hypertonicity is present, the pituitary is maximally stimulated to release ADH. The ADH in turn acts on the kidneys to promote maximum urinary concentration, so that they excrete as little as 300 mL of urine per day with an osmolality of between 800 and 1000 mOsm/kg H_2O as the osmolality of the ECF is corrected. Renal concentrating mechanisms cannot go further, but the thirst centers also are stimulated when the ECF osmolality exceeds 290 mOsm/kg H_2O. Thirst is actually more important than urinary concentration in preventing dehydration.

In contrast to the situation with hypertonicity, ADH release by the pituitary will be totally inhibited if the osmolality of the ECF falls below 280 mOsm/kg H_2O (i.e., if hypotonicity develops) assuming that ECF volume is normal. As a result of the lack of ADH, the kidneys will daily excrete up to 18 L of dilute urine with an osmolality as low as 50 mOsm/kg H_2O. The thirst mechanism will be shut off when the osmolality is low, so that water will not normally be drunk and ECF osmolality will be corrected.[15]

POTASSIUM BALANCE

So far this chapter has focused on the body's regulation of Na^+, the major extracellular solute, and water because disorders of ECF volume and tonicity are common in clinical practice. However, disorders of K^+ balance also occur. These disorders do not involve problems in ECF volume or tonicity because K^+ is found for the most part in the ICF, but instead, they depend on alterations in the ratio of K^+ concentrations in the ICF and ECF and the effects of these alterations on excitable tissues.[3]

The extracellular concentration of K^+ normally ranges between 3.5 and 5.5 mEq/L. In a 70-kg person whose ECF volume is 14 L, the amount of extracellular K^+ would be 50 to 75 mEq, representing only 2 percent of total body K^+; the other 98 percent, which amounts to 3400 mEq, is found in the ICF, primarily in skeletal muscle. The usual daily level of K^+ intake, including that in food and that which results from cellular breakdown, is 100 mEq. Thus, to maintain K^+

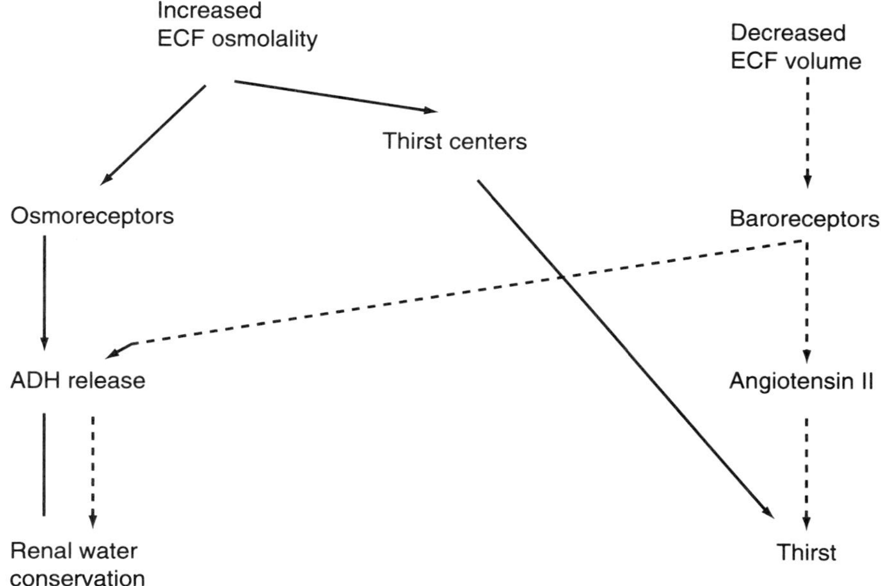

Figure 13-4. Integrated defense of increased ECF osmolality and decreased ECF volume. See text for further explanation. (Adapted from Andreoli,[3] with permission.)

balance, the body must excrete 100 mEq of K^+ per day. Normally only small amounts of the solute are excreted by the skin and gastrointestinal tract, although the gut may excrete up to 40 mEq of K^+ each day in the presence of renal failure. For the most part, then, K^+ excretion is handled by the kidneys.[16]

Excretion of Na^+ by the kidneys involves filtration, partial absorption by the tubules, and the appearance of nonabsorbed Na^+ in the urine. By contrast, K^+ excretion involves primarily tubular secretion, which is enhanced by Na^+ delivery to the tubules, increased ECF alkalinity, the presence of unresorbable anions such as phosphate and sulfate in tubular flow, and, especially, the presence of the hormone aldosterone, which causes an exchange of Na^+ for K^+ and H^+ in defense of ECF volume. Thus, while the body can virtually eliminate Na^+ excretion when ECF volume is depleted, at least 10 to 15 mEq/L of K^+ will be excreted.[16]

Although K^+ is correctly considered an intracellular solute, its distribution within the body can be altered by a number of processes. As noted earlier, increased ECF acidity, hypertonic fluids, and alpha-adrenergic stimulation all increase the K^+ concentration of ECF. Conversely, insulin, aldosterone, and beta-adrenergic stimulation increase cellular K^+ uptake.[17,18] A a general rule, a reduction of plasma pH by 0.1 unit raises the plasma K^+ concentration by 0.6 mEq/L, whereas a 0.1 pH unit increase causes a similar decline in the K^+ concentration. The changes in pH may be caused by either metabolic or respiratory processes, as discussed below.

Although changes in K^+ concentration cause many physiologic alterations, the most pronounced are seen in excitable tissues such as the heart and muscles. At rest, the cells of these tissues are more permeable to K^+ than to Na^+. The interior of the cell is electrically negative compared with the ECF, and the voltage is dependent on the K^+ ratio of ICF/ECF. During depolarization the cell membranes become more permeable to Na^+ than to K^+, and the intracellular flux of Na^+ causes the cell interior to become electrically negative and produces an action potential. During repolarization of the cell, the cell membranes again become more permeable to K^+ than to Na^+, and the extracellular flux of K^+ restores the electrical negativity of the cell interior.[3,16,19]

Increases in the K^+ concentration of the ECF reduce the K^+ ratio of ICF/ECF and thereby partially depolarize the cells at rest. In addition, the increased K^+ concentration of the ECF, which is called *hyperkalemia,* increases the K^+ permeability of cells. The end result is that tissues such as skeletal muscle and the heart become depolarized at rest and then become resistant to excitation. On the other hand, a decrease in the K^+ concentration of the ECF, which is called *hypokalemia,* increases the K^+ ratio of ICF/ECF and initially hyperpolarizes cells. Hypokalemia also decreases the K^+ permeability of cells, which prolongs repolarization. The end result is that the heart becomes more subject to disturbances of electrical rhythm and the muscles become paralyzed.[3,16,20,21]

ACID-BASE PHYSIOLOGY

When the body is in normal acid-base balance, its ICF and ECF are neither excessively acidic nor excessively alkaline. Acid-base status may be quantified in terms of either the serum or the plasma concentration of H^+ or of pH (the negative logarithm of H^+ concentration). Use of this logarithmic scale not only is conventional but also allows relatively small changes in units to express large changes in the availability of H^+. The pH of systemic arterial blood is ideally 7.4, a value slightly more alkaline than that of water, the pH of which is 7.0. Normally the arterial pH ranges from 7.35 to 7.45. The widest range of pH values compatible with life is 6.8 to 7.8, an interval of 1 pH unit.[2,3]

Acids are defined as substances that donate H^+, whereas bases are substances that accept H^+. In the reaction HA $\leftrightarrow$ $H^+ + A^-$, HA is the acid and A^- is its conjugate base. The strength of the acid HA depends on its degree of dissociation (i.e., the extent to which it forms H^+ and A^-). The tendency of an acid to dissociate in water is quantified by the Henderson-Hasselbalch equation:

$$pH = pK + \log \frac{\text{base concentration}}{\text{acid concentration}} \quad (2)$$

where pK is a constant that reflects the strength of a given acid. The combination of a weak acid or base and its salt is a buffer, which is a substance that resists change in H^+ concentration upon addition of a stronger acid or base.

The H_2CO_3/HCO_3^- buffering system is the major buffering system in ECF. H_2CO_3 is formed by the hydration of CO_2 in the presence of the enzyme carbonic anhydrase (CA) by the reaction

$$CO_2 + H_2O \overset{CA}{\longleftrightarrow} H_2CO_3 \longleftrightarrow H^+ + HCO_3^- \quad (3)$$

H_2CO_3 is a weak acid from a chemical standpoint because its dissociation into H^+ and HCO_3^- is limited as compared with strong acids such as hydrochloric acid (HCl). The Henderson-Hasselbalch equation for carbonic acid is

$$pH = 6.1 + \log \frac{HCO_3^- \text{ concentration}}{CO_2 \text{ concentration}} \quad (4)$$

Since the CO_2 concentration is linearly related to the partial pressure of CO_2 in systemic arterial blood ($PaCO_2$) by a solubility constant, the equation can be rewritten:

$$pH = 6.1 + \log \frac{HCO_3^- \text{ concentration}}{(0.3)(PaCO_2)} \quad (5)$$

This equation is useful in assessing acid-base status, first because its components can be measured in an arterial blood gas sample, and second because the $PaCO_2$ reflects the respiratory component of the acid-base balance and the HCO_3^- concentration reflects the metabolic component.[2,3]

The usefulness of the HCO_3^- concentration can be seen in the following example of H_2CO_3/HCO_3^- buffering. If HCl is added to a solution containing sodium bicarbonate ($NaHCO_3$) in ECF, the following reaction takes place:

$$\begin{array}{c} CO_2 + H_2O \\ \updownarrow \scriptstyle{CA} \\ HCl + NaHCO_3 \longleftrightarrow H_2CO_3 + NaCl \\ \updownarrow \\ H^+ + HCO_3^- \end{array} \quad (6)$$

The H^+ produced by dissociation of H_2CO_3 is less than that which might result from direct dissociation of HCl, first because H_2CO_3 ionizes less than HCl, and second because H_2CO_3 also forms CO_2, which escapes from the body through the lungs. The respiratory contribution of CO_2 is assumed to be held constant in the equation, so that all the CO_2 comes directly from H_2CO_3. In fact, the ready escape of CO_2 drives the reaction so much farther toward the CO_2 side that very little H^+ is ultimately produced. That which is produced reacts with HCO_3^-, whose concentration can be used as an index of metabolic alterations in acid-base status.[2]

Strictly speaking, the use of a change in HCO_3^- concentration as a reflection of the amount of H^+ added to or subtracted from a solution is valid only when H_2CO_3 and its salts are the only buffers in the solution. Yet many noncarbonic buffers exist inside and outside the ECF. For example, hemoglobin, which exists within red blood cells as a weak acid and its K^+ salt, shares in the extracellular buffering of an unstable acid or alkali load. Because of this, the change in HCO_3^- concentration of ECF does not precisely equal the amount of metabolic base or acid added, as it would in a pure H_2CO_3 solution, but is slightly smaller, around 1 mEq/L per 0.1 pH unit.

This slight difference is incorporated in the term base excess or deficit, which describes the change in all ECF buffers, including HCO_3^-. The base excess or deficit can be calculated from arterial blood gas data or measured directly in serum or plasma, and it is included in arterial blood gas analysis at many medical centers. Nevertheless, this practice adds little to an understanding of acid-base physiology and is not essential for clinical purposes. Because of this the concept of base excess is not pursued further in this chapter.

VOLATILE AND NONVOLATILE ACID PRODUCTION AND ELIMINATION

Although the previous discussion has illustrated how the H_2CO_3/HCO_3^- buffer system is used to buffer exogenous acids added to the body, the system is most often called on to buffer endogenous acid. The largest source of endogenous acid is the oxidation of nutrients, in particular carbohydrates and fats, to CO_2 and H_2O during cellular respiration. For example, glucose ($C_6H_{12}O_6$) is oxidized by $6O_2$ in the following reaction:

$$C_6H_{12}O_6 + 6O_2 \rightarrow 6CO_2 + 6H_2O \quad (7)$$

The CO_2 formed in this reaction is in turn hydrated within red blood cells in this fashion:

$$CO_2 + H_2O \longleftrightarrow H_2CO_3 \longleftrightarrow H^+ + HCO_3^- \quad (8)$$

The H^+ formed in this reaction is buffered by hemoglobin, whereas the HCO_3^- leaves red blood cells in exchange for Cl^-. Then, as the red blood cells enter the pulmonary circulation from the systemic circulation, HCO_3^- reenters the cells and combines with the H^+ to form H_2CO_3, which dissociates to CO_2 and H_2O again. CO_2 then diffuses out of the red blood cells and across the alveolar-capillary membrane, and is ventilated from the body by the lungs.[2,3]

Because the CO_2 produced by cellular respiration ($\dot{V}CO_2$) is a source of H_2CO_3 and ultimately H^+ and because the CO_2 is a gas that can be excreted through the lungs, it is considered to be a volatile acid. Approximately 22,000 mmol of CO_2 is produced each day by a 70-kg adult, so the rate of volatile acid production is 22,000 mEq of H^+ daily. Although fluctuations in $\dot{V}CO_2$ occur as a result of exercise, food intake, and other factors, the rate of cellular metabolism is relatively constant. The rate of CO_2 removal, which is called the *alveolar ventilation* ($\dot{V}_A$), also is constant in normal persons, so that the ratio $\dot{V}CO_2/\dot{V}_A$ is constant and $PaCO_2$ remains at 40 mmHg (range 35 to 45 mmHg).[3,23]

$\dot{V}_A$ and $PaCO_2$ are regulated primarily by respiratory control centers in the brain stem that sense changes in the pH of cerebrospinal fluid (CSF). The changes occur promptly in response to increases or decreases in $PaCO_2$, because CO_2 readily crosses the blood-brain barrier and combines with H_2O to form H_2CO_3 and ultimately H^+. Increases or decreases in the H^+ and HCO_3^- concentrations in blood, which result from alterations in the amount of nonvolatile acid in the body, also change the pH of CSF, but they do so more slowly than does the CO_2 level because the blood-brain barrier is relatively impermeable to electrically charged ions. Thus, $\dot{V}_A$ is stimulated by increases and depressed by decreases in volatile and nonvolatile acids. Changes in $\dot{V}_A$ due to changes in volatile acid help to rid the body of CO_2 and avoid respiratory acid-base disturbances, whereas changes in $\dot{V}_A$ due to changes in nonvolatile acid help the body to compensate for metabolic acid-base disturbances.[2,3]

The body's nonvolatile acids result primarily from the cellular metabolism of sulfur-containing amino acids such as cysteine and methionine, which results in production of H_2SO_4. Thus, the rate of nonvolatile acid production is related to dietary protein intake as well as to endogenous protein catabolism. Other nonvolatile acids produced by the body are phosphoric acid, which results from the oxidation of phosphate-containing proteins; uric acid, which comes from the breakdown of nucleic proteins; and lactic acid and ketoacids, which are generated by the incomplete oxidation of carbohydrate and fat.

In health, the rate of nonvolatile acid production is approximately 1 mEq/kg body weight/d. The acid in turn is buffered by the H_2CO_3/HCO_3^- system, so that the body's supply of HCO_3^- is reduced. This reduction would reach dangerously low levels were it not for the excretion of H^+ by the kidneys, which occurs primarily in the distal nephron segments, where H^+ is excreted either as acids (e.g., H_2SO_4), or as ammonia. At the same time and in amounts equal to the H^+ excretion, HCO_3^- is regenerated for the body acid. Because these processes are accompanied by Na^+ absorption,[3,28] they therefore enhance Na^+ absorption (e.g., increased delivery of Na^+ to the kidneys or an increase in the level of aldosterone) also enhance renal H^+ excretion, as noted earlier. Excretion of H^+ also is enhanced by K^+ deficiency and by increased acidity of the blood; conversely, it is diminished by increased alkalinity, K^+ excess, falling levels of aldosterone, and impaired Na^+ delivery to the kidneys.

In addition to regenerating HCO_3^- during the excretion of H^+, the kidneys also must reabsorb the bulk of the HCO_3^- that passes through them in the bloodstream each day. This is accomplished in the more proximal part of the nephron, where Na^+ also is routinely absorbed. Since renal Na^+ absorption is increased by decreases in ECF and by rising aldosterone levels, it follows that HCO_3^- reabsorption also increases in this condition, just as HCO_3^- is reabsorbed less avidly when the intravascular volume is augmented. Renal reabsorption of HCO_3^- also is influenced by $PaCO_2$; high $PaCO_2$ favors HCO_3^- retention, whereas low $PaCO_2$ influences the kidneys to excrete HCO_3^- into the urine.[3]

ESTIMATION OF ACID-BASE BALANCE

The relative acidity of blood with a pH of 7.35 or lower is called *acidemia,* whereas the relative alkalinity of blood with a pH of 7.45 or higher is called *alkalemia*. These terms are preferable to the words *acidosis* and *alkalosis,* which describe the processes through which acidemia and alkalemia occur. Respiratory acidosis and alkalosis are disturbances in the production or elimination of volatile acid. *Respiratory acidosis* results from an increase in $PaCO_2$ occurring because the $\dot{V}CO_2/\dot{V}_A$ ratio increases; the increase in $PaCO_2$ is called *hypoventilation* because $\dot{V}_A$ is decreased relative to $\dot{V}CO_2$. On the other hand, *respiratory alkalosis* results from a decrease in $PaCO_2$ due to a decrease in the $\dot{V}CO_2/\dot{V}_A$ ratio; because $\dot{V}_A$ is increased relative to $\dot{V}CO_2$, the decrease in $PaCO_2$ is called *hyperventilation*.[2,24,25]

Metabolic acidosis and alkalosis are disturbances in the production or elimination of nonvolatile acid. *Metabolic acidosis* results from a decrease in HCO_3^- that occurs because HCO_3^- is lost from or H^+ is added to the body. The HCO_3^- may be lost in diarrhea fluid or because the kidney malfunctions and either wastes HCO_3^- or fails to regenerate it; alternatively, H^+ may enter the body in the form of HCl. Metabolic acidosis may be divided into one of two types, depending on whether an anion gap is present. As noted earlier, the body's electrolytes consist of cations, especially Na^+ and K^+, and anions such as Cl^-, HCO_3^-, and small amounts of phosphate, sulfate, and other metabolic salts. Normally, the cations and anions must be equal for the serum or plasma to be electrically neutral. However, a 10 mEq/L difference between $Na^+ - (Cl^- + HCO_3^-)$ is usually reported in samples sent to the laboratory because phosphates, sulfates, and other anions are not measured.

Although HCO_3^- is generally reduced in all forms of metabolic acidosis, the concentration of Cl^- increases when an endogenous acid such as HCl is added to the body, and the anion difference or gap does not increase. However, when some unmeasured anions are added, the fall in HCO_3^- is not balanced by a rise in Cl^-, and Na^+; the sum of Cl^- and HCO_3^- will then exceed 10 mEq/L, indicating the presence of an anion gap (Fig. 13-5). Some of the unmeasured anions responsible for an anion gap include lactic acid and ace-

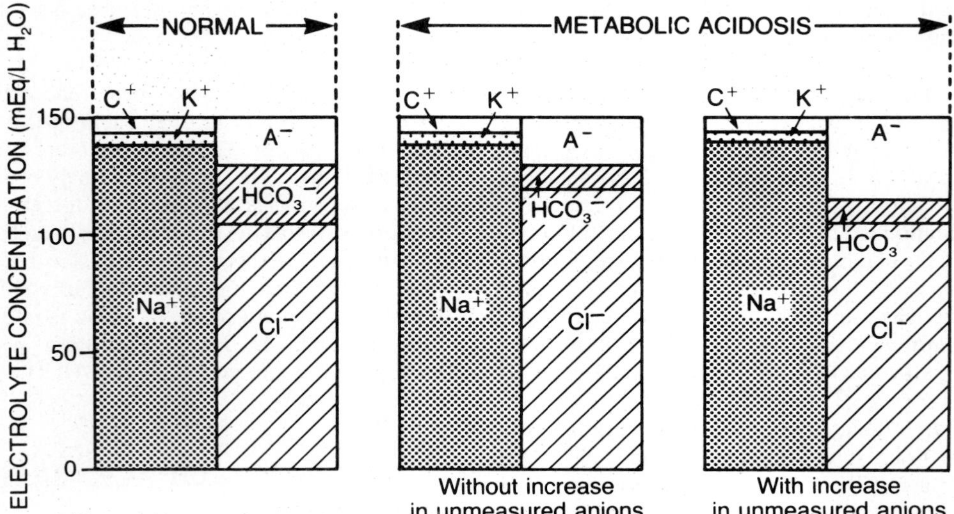

Figure 13-5. Electrolyte concentration in milliequivalents per liter of water under normal conditions and during metabolic acidosis, with or without an increase in unmeasured anions. C^+, unmeasured cations; A^-, unmeasured anions. (From Luce et al.,[2] with permission.)

tate.[26,27] These and the disorders that cause them are discussed in Chapter 28.

In contrast to metabolic acidosis, *metabolic alkalosis* results from an increase in HCO_3^- that occurs because H^+ is lost or HCO_3^- is added to the body. In this case, H^+ may be lost through protracted vomiting or through renal exchange of Na^+ or H^+ when increased amounts of aldosterone are present; HCO_3^- retention usually occurs because of ECF volume contraction and increased delivery of Na^+ to the kidney. Since total body Cl^- stores are reduced, the urinary concentration of Cl^- should be low. Alternately, HCO_3^- can be retained in states of severe K^+ depletion and hyperaldosteronism; in this case, the urinary Cl^- concentration should be high. These and other aspects of metabolic alkalosis are discussed further in Chapter 28.

PRESERVATION OF ACID-BASE BALANCE

Regardless of the processes that underlie it, excess acidity of body fluids (e.g., increased H^+ and low pH) generally depresses organ function. This is especially true of the heart, which pumps less effectively. Cardiac rhythm disturbances, or dysrhythmias, also may develop. Vascular smooth muscle relaxes in the presence of H^+, so blood vessels dilate and become less responsive to drugs, such as epinephrine, that would otherwise alter their caliber. In acidemia of a respiratory nature, the high CO_2 concentration further dilates cerebral blood vessels and increases blood flow through them. Excess alkalinity (e.g., decreased H^+ and high pH) also depresses organ function, but in addition it may lead to a neuromuscular excitability that can precipitate severe cardiac dysrhythmias. Given these possible consequences, it is fortunate that the body defends itself against acid-base imbalance in several ways.

The body's initial defense against acidemia involves the H_2CO_3/HCO_3^- and noncarbonic buffers described previously and takes minutes to occur. In the second defense, which is called *secondary compensation* and occurs over hours or days, the ratio of HCO_3^- concentration to $PaCO_2$ as expressed in the Henderson-Hasselbalch equation for the dissociation of H_2CO_3 is brought toward normal by altering whichever of the two variables was unchanged primarily. Thus, a metabolic acidosis that causes a decrease in HCO_3^- will be compensated by a respiratory alkalosis that causes a decrease in $PaCO_2$, and vice versa.

Changes in HCO_3^- concentration not resulting from H_2CO_3/HCO_3^- and noncarbonic buffering are controlled by the kidneys, which excrete or retain HCO_3^-, whereas the lungs control $PaCO_2$. Because of this, the Henderson-Hasselbalch equation for H_2CO_3 can be rewritten as

$$pH = pK + \frac{\text{kidneys}}{\text{lungs}} \quad (9)$$

to conceptualize how secondary compensation occurs. The $PaCO_2$ can change quickly if the respiratory control center is stimulated. However, the relatively slow process of renal HCO_3^- adjustment accounts for the time required for secondary metabolic compensation. Neither form of compensation is usually complete, so the pH may not return exactly to normal. Nevertheless, secondary compensation is a vital defense against acid-base imbalance that must be called on if corrections of the primary abnormalities in production and elimination of volatile and nonvolatile acid cannot occur.[2,24,25]

DISORDERS OF ACID-BASE, WATER, AND SOLUTE BALANCE

Disorders of acid-base balance occur commonly in clinical medicine. Frequently these disorders are accompanied by disorders of water and solute balance. As a result, analysis of arterial blood gas values of pH, $PaCO_2$, and PaO_2 and of serum electrolyte values of Na^+, K^+, Cl^-, and HCO_3^- concentrations is often essential in managing patients, especially those who are critically ill. Such analysis is discussed more fully in Chapter 28.

References

1. Schrier RW, Berl T: Disorders of water metabolism. pp. 1–44. In Schrier RW (ed): Renal and Electrolyte Disorders. Little Brown, Boston, 1976
2. Luce JM, Tyler ML, Pierson DJ: Intensive Respiratory Care. WB Saunders, Philadelphia, 1984, pp. 22–48
3. Andreoli TE: Disorders of fluid volume, electrolyte, and acid-base balance. pp. 515–554. In Wyngaarden JB, Smith LH (eds): Cecil's Textbook of Medicine. 17th Ed. WB Saunders, Philadelphia, 1985
4. Staub NC: Pulmonary edema. Physiol Rev 1974;54:678–811
5. Light RW, Macgregor MI, Luchsinger PC, Ball WC: Pleural effusions: The diagnostic separation of transudates and exudates. Ann Intern Med 1972;77:507–513
6. Luce JM: Adult respiratory distress syndrome. pp. 253–260. In Cherniack RM (ed): Current Therapy of Respiratory Disease. 2nd Ed. BC Decker, Toronto, 1986
7. Staub NC: The pathogenesis of pulmonary edema. Prog Cardiovasc Dis 1980;23:53–79
8. Hudson LD: Causes of the adult respiratory distress syndrome—clinical recognition. Clin Chest Med 1982;3:195–222
9. Broaddus VC, Staub NC: Pleural liquid and protein turnover in health and disease. Semin Respir Med 1987;9:7–12
10. Schrier RW: Pathogenesis of sodium and water retention in high-output and low-output cardiac failure, nephrotic syndrome, cirrhosis, and pregnancy. Part 1. N Engl J Med 1988;319:1065–1072
11. Schrier RW: Pathogenesis of sodium and water retention in high-output and low-output cardiac failure, nephrotic syndrome, cirrhosis, and pregnancy. Part 2. N Engl J Med 1988;319:1127–1134
12. Schrier RW: Renal sodium excretion, edematous disorders, and diuretic use. pp. 45–77. In Schrier RW (ed): Renal and Electrolyte Disorders. Little Brown, Boston, 1976
13. O'Quin R, Marini JJ: Pulmonary artery occlusion pressure: Clinical physiology, measurement and interpretation. Am Rev Respir Dis 1983;127:319–325
14. Smithline N, Gardner KD: Gaps—anionic and osmolal. JAMA 1976;236:1594–1597
15. Feig PU, McCurdy DK: The hypertonic state. N Engl J Med 1977;297:1444–1454
16. Gabow P: Disorders of potassium metabolism. pp. 143–165. In Schrier RW (ed): Renal and Electrolyte Disorders. Little Brown, Boston 1976
17. Cox M, Sterns RH, Singer I: The defense against hyperkalemia: The rules of insulin and aldosterone. N Engl J Med 1984;299:525–532
18. Brown MJ, Brown DC, Murphy MB: Hypokalemia from $beta_2$-receptor stimulation by circulating epinephrine. N Engl J Med 1978;309:1414–1419
19. Knochel JP: Neuromuscular manifestations of electrolyte disorders. Am J Med 1982;72:521–535
20. Ott SM: Hyperkalemia. pp. 302–306. In Luce JM, Pierson DJ (eds): Critical Care Medicine. WB Saunders, Philadelphia, 1988
21. Ott SM: Hypokalemia. pp. 307–315. In Luce JM, Pierson DJ (eds): Critical Care Medicine. WB Saunders, Philadelphia, 1988
22. Ott SM, Luce JM: Acid-base disturbances. pp. 271–284. In Luce JM, Pierson DJ (eds): Critical Care Medicine. WB Saunders, Philadelphia, 1988
23. Narins RG, Jones ER, Stom MC et al: Diagnostic strategies in disorders of fluid, electrolyte, and acid-base homeostasis. Am J Med 1982;76:496–515
24. McCurdy DK: Mixed metabolic and respiratory acid-base disturbances: Diagnosis and treatment. Chest, Suppl. 1972;35S–44S
25. Narins RG, Emmett M: Simple and mixed acid-base disorders: A practical approach. Medicine (Baltimore) 1980;59:161–187
26. Emmett M, Narins RG: Clinical use of the anion gap. Medicine (Baltimore) 1977;56:38–54
27. Gabow PA, Kaehny WD, Fennessey PV et al: Diagnostic importance of an increased serum anion gap. N Engl J Med 1980;303:854–858

Chapter 14

Regulation of Ventilation

Robert B. Schoene

CHAPTER OUTLINE

In humans, breathing is a precisely regulated, instantaneous event. It is unfortunate that a more thorough understanding and appreciation of breathing in health and disease is not the required standard for clinicians.

In day-to-day clinical practice, alterations in chemical stimuli, such as hypoxia and hypercarbia, and in mechanical stimuli, such as resistive or elastic loading, can make a great difference in a patient's emotional and functional status. By returning some of these stimuli to a more normal level, the clinician can greatly improve patients' perception of their disease and thereby their daily activities. The primary purpose of this chapter is to review the normal mechanisms of the control of ventilation and the clinical methods by which ventilatory drives can be assessed.

PHYSIOLOGY

Successful ventilation is defined as the body's maintenance of metabolic homeostasis during waking, sleep, rest, and exercise. A complex interaction of chemical and neurologic events is required to maintain this homeostasis. The main chemical stimuli are pH, partial pressure of O_2 (PO_2), and partial pressure of CO_2 (PCO_2), all of which can be quantitated precisely with clinical techniques. Less quantifiable but equally important as regulators of ventilation are mechanical factors.

Chemical Stimuli

Hypoxia

The sensing of a low PO_2 in the blood is an elegantly evolved characteristic, which protects the body from asphyxia. The PO_2 is sensed at the peripheral chemoreceptor, the carotid body, which is located at the bifurcation of the internal and external carotid arteries.[1] This highly metabolic organ is minute but is exquisitely sensitive to decreases in PO_2. Nerve impulses from the carotid body to the brain course along the carotid sinus nerve and effect a neuromuscular response that results in an increase in ventilation, the purpose of which is to protect and maintain arterial PO_2 (PaO_2).[2–4] There appears to be a functional relationship between oxyhemoglobin dissociation and the hypoxic ventilatory response. Specifically, the hyperbolic shape of the ventilatory response to hypoxia (Fig. 14-1A) correlates with the existence of a PO_2 level (approximately 60 mmHg) at which the oxyhemoglobin dissociation curve becomes quite steep and O_2 saturation (SaO_2) and subsequently O_2 content in the arterial blood drops more precipitously with decrease

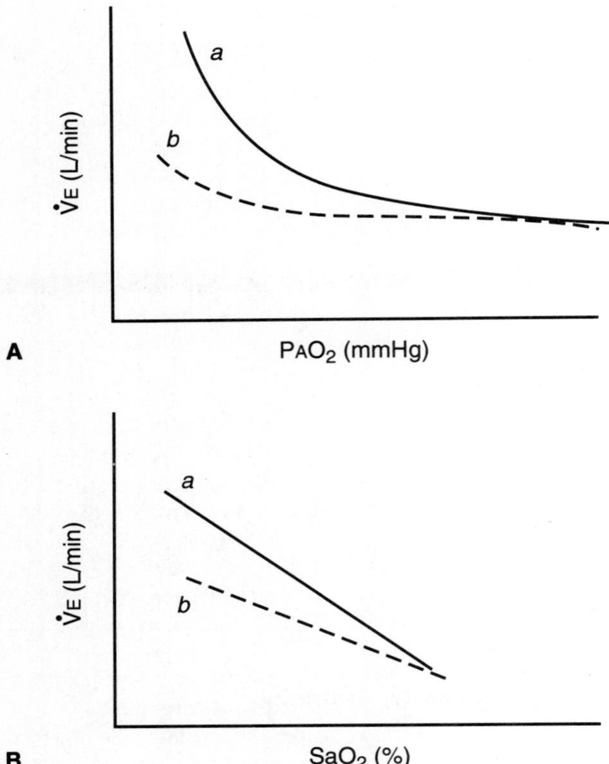

Figure 14-1. Hypoxic ventilatory response (HVR). **(A)** HVR expressed as the intensity of the response ($\dot{V}_E$) in liters per minute plotted against partial pressure of alveolar O_2 (P_{AO_2}), which resulted in a hyperbolic relationship; a being a greater response than b. **(B)** HVR expressed as $\dot{V}_E$ in liters per minute plotted against SaO_2, in percent; slope a being greater than slope b.

in PO_2 (Fig. 11-1). The nature of this response, therefore, is to maintain an adequate content of O_2 in the blood. The carotid body is sensitive only to PO_2 and not to SaO_2. Therefore, at PO_2 levels at which the saturation is above 90 percent, hypoxic chemosensitivity acts as a subtle overseer of ventilation, whereas when the PO_2 drops below 60 mmHg, ventilation is stimulated to a much greater degree to protect the blood and tissue oxygenation.

Carbon Dioxide and pH

The sensing of PCO_2 takes place primarily at the central chemosensors, which are located on the ventral surface of the medulla near the choroid plexus in the brain stem.[5,6] This site contributes about 80 percent of the CO_2 sensing, approximately 20 percent being mediated by the carotid body. The rise and fall in CO_2 that is related to ventilation effects a change in extracellular H^+ concentration, which is probably the stimulus for ventilation at the central chemosensors. In normal individuals the stimulus from rising PCO_2 is much more potent than that from hypoxia.[7] An interpretation of this relationship may be that on a breath-to-breath basis the maintenance of eucapnia and thus acid-base status is more critical to the survival of an organism than is correction of a modest drop in oxygenation.

While hypoxia and CO_2 are discrete and quantifiable stimuli to ventilation,[8] alterations in acid-base status play an important role in overall ventilatory regulation. Resting ventilation and chemosensitivity are increased by acidosis and blunted by alkalosis.[9–11]

Mechanoreceptors

A less well understood and quantifiable aspect of breathing control has to do with mechanical alterations. Mechanoreception is independent of chemoreception, but in all states of health and disease there is an important and undeniable interaction between the two processes.[12,13] Both resistive[14–16] and elastic[17,18] loading affect breathing response. Inspiratory resistive loading, if it is severe enough, may result in a decrease in ventilatory response to PCO_2 but an increase in the actual neural output for respiration. On the other hand, expiratory resistance, such as that due to obstructive airway disease, does not result in an increase in ventilatory drive. Because of a change in end-expiratory volume with respiratory loading, the difference in load perception may be secondary to stretch receptor sensing.

Elastic loading can be defined as parenchymal or extraparenchymal restriction on ventilation. Although specific disease entities are discussed at length later, interstitial lung disease exemplifies intraparenchymal elastic loading, whereas ankylosing spondylitis, which restricts the thorax by fixation of the rib cage, illustrates extraparenchymal elastic loading. Elastic loading results in an increase in respiratory drive, with a decrease in tidal volume and an increase in respiratory frequency.

Exercise

The control of ventilation during exercise is not fully understood. It is generally accepted that a large percentage of the ventilatory response to exercise is dictated by an increase in metabolic rate, reflected in O_2 and CO_2 consumption and production ($\dot{V}O_2$ and $\dot{V}CO_2$), respectively.[19–24] Alveolar ventilation ($\dot{V}_A$) closely tracks $\dot{V}CO_2$. On the other hand, at the onset of exercise as well as during the highest levels of exhaustive work, not all ventilation can be accounted for by an increase in metabolic rate.[25,26] The abrupt onset of exercise does not allow enough time for the metabolic by-products of exercise to circulate to the chemosensors; therefore, there is believed to be some neuronal input from the exercising limbs that acts immediately on the neural output for ventilation. At the highest levels of exercise above the ventilatory or anaerobic threshold, at which time a metabolic (lactic) acidosis is increasing, other factors contribute to the steeper increase in exercise ventilation (see Ch. 15).

The nature of these factors and of their quantitative contribution to these high levels of ventilation is not understood.

MEASUREMENT OF VENTILATORY SENSITIVITY AND RESPONSE

A distinction must be made between the ventilatory response and the ventilatory drive to various stimuli. The ventilatory response is in fact just that—either the overall inspired or expired ventilation ($\dot{V}_I$ or $\dot{V}_E$), which is the sum of alveolar ventilation ($\dot{V}_A$) and dead space ventilation ($\dot{V}_D$). On the other hand, the response is measured as the gain in ventilation from a resting state to a stimulated state (e.g., the change in ventilation from a PO_2 of 100 mmHg to a PO_2 of 40 mmHg). The ventilatory response can be further broken down to ventilatory pattern, which is $\dot{V}_E$ = tidal volume (V_T) × respiratory frequency (f). In exercise in healthy individuals, ventilatory stimulation results first in an increase in V_T that is disproportionately great as compared with the more linear response of increased respiratory frequency (see Ch. 15). The ventilatory response is further defined by the respiratory duty cycle, which is merely a description of the timing of ventilation. The components that define this relationship are respiratory flow (V_T/T_I) and inspiratory time (T_I in relation to total breathing (T_I/T_{TOT}). The equation that defines the duty cycle is therefore: [$\dot{V}_E = V_T/T_I \times T_I/T_{TOT}$].

Ventilatory Response

In the normal individual the measured ventilatory response is usually a valid reflection of the ventilatory drive. Pathologic states such as altered lung mechanics can change the relationship between response and drive. The next section discusses the measurement of ventilatory response and drive.

Hypoxic Ventilatory Response

The hypoxic ventilatory response (HVR) can be measured by a number of different techniques,[4,28–30] although all response tests must be initiated only after the subject has been ascertained to be at rest. This may require the subject to remain for 10 to 15 minutes or longer in a seated or supine position. A constant end-tidal CO_2 is the best indicator of a resting state. It is also important to know whether the patient has been fasting or is receiving any medication, since the ventilatory drive is affected by food ingestion and by some medications. Ventilation is measured with the subject breathing through a tightly fitting mask or a mouthpiece with nose clips.

The HVR test can then be begun with the subject breathing a hyperoxic mix in order to put the carotid body in a "resting state." The subject should be monitored with an electrocardiogram (ECG) and breath-by-breath measurements of end-tidal gases and ventilation, and ventilation should be visible either on an oscilloscope or a strip chart recorder. A rapidly responding oximeter (preferably on the ear) should be used to monitor O_2 saturation.

The most common techniques for measuring HVR use a gradual hypoxic test,[4,28,29] which in normal subjects should decrease SaO_2 to 20 percent below ambient saturation and which should take anywhere from 7 to 12 minutes. If the test is prolonged, a well-described hypoxic ventilatory depression occurs at approximately 20 minutes after sustained hypoxia.[31–36] Since the ventilatory response to hypoxia results in respiratory alkalosis, which may then blunt the ventilatory response, most tests employ an isocapnic technique, which involves titrating the end-tidal CO_2 to the same level that was present during the hyperoxic restful breathing.[4] This technique usually dictates the addition of CO_2 at the mouth to maintain isocapnia. The poikilocapnic technique is sometimes used; this allows the subject to ventilate naturally, resulting in respiratory alkalosis.[37]

Progressive hypoxia is usually attained by diluting a reservoir balloon filled with hyperoxic gas to a point that allows the saturation to fall to the predetermined level. A rebreathing technique carried out in a closed system with an in-line CO_2 scrubber represents another approach.[29] Other techniques employ pulse breaths of nitrogen, which result in acute desaturation for one to three breaths and a subsequent ventilatory response.[30] This technique is based on the assumption that the hypoxic stimulus occurs quickly without alteration of CO_2 so that attempts to maintain isocapnia are not necessary.

Quantitation of the HVR involves plotting $\dot{V}_E$ on the ordinate and either partial pressure of end-tidal O_2 ($P_{ET}O_2$) (in millimeters of Hg) or SaO_2 (in percent) on the abscissa (Fig. 14-1). The relationship of $\dot{V}_E$ to $P_{ET}O_2$ is a hyperbolic one and can be described mathematically by the equation

$$\dot{V}_E = \dot{V}_0 + A/(P_{ET}O_2 - 32),$$

where $\dot{V}_0$ is the asymptote for ventilation and A is the hyperbolic shape parameter, which is proportional to the hypoxic response. Another valid technique is to plot ventilation versus SaO_2, which results in a linear relationship, the slope of which is inversely proportional to the strength of the HVR.

Hypercapnic Ventilatory Response

The hypercapnic ventilatory response (HCVR) can also be measured by a progressive or steady-state technique. The most common approach is a rebreathing technique in which the subject is placed in a closed circuit with a hyperoxic gas mix in a balloon with a volume approximately 2 L greater than the subject's vital capacity (VC).[7] CO_2 progressively accumulates with rebreathing, and ventilation increases with the CO_2 stimulus. The measurement of ventilation is begun when PCO_2 approximates the PCO_2 in the pulmonary capillaries (which at sea level is about 46 mmHg) and should be continued until $P_{ET}CO_2$ is approximately 60 mmHg or $\dot{V}_E$ is between 30 and 40 L/min. This portion of the ventilatory response is linear and is expressed as

$$\dot{V}_E = S\,(P_{ET}CO_2 - B)$$

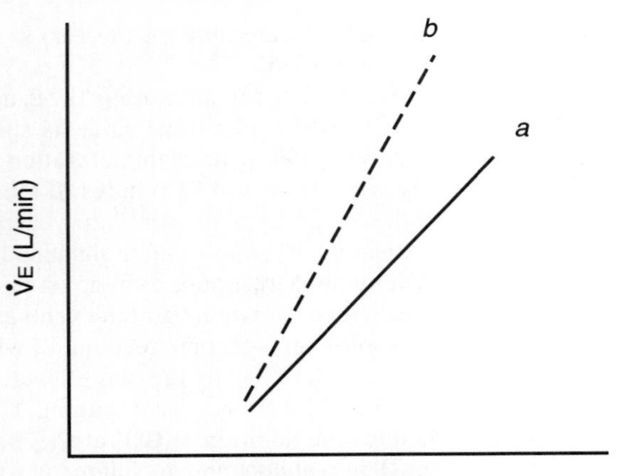

Figure 14-2. Hypercapnic ventilatory response (HCVR) expressed as ventilation ($\dot{V}_E$) in liters per minute versus P_{ACO_2}, which is a linear relationship, slope a showing a lower response than slope b.

where S is the slope of $\dot{V}_E/P_{ETCO_2}$ and B is the x-axis intercept[8] (Fig. 14-2). The slope is used to quantitate HCVR and can be calculated as a linear regression.

Ventilatory Drive

As mentioned above, in healthy individuals the ventilatory response correlates well with ventilatory drive because normal lung mechanics allow the lungs to respond instantaneously and appropriately to ventilatory drive. In patients with mechanical dysfunction of the lungs, the lungs cannot respond appropriately to the afferent signals from the central nervous system. A number of techniques are available to gain some insight into ventilatory drives, but most are difficult to carry out accurately and for practical purposes are not clinically very useful.

Mouth Occlusion Pressure

Mouth occlusion pressure ($P_{0.1}$) is the pressure in centimeters of H_2O generated at the mouth during the first 100 ms (0.10 second) of inspiration upon a closed airway.[38–40] The plot of $P_{0.1}$ versus time is linear up to about 150 ms, during which time the subject is unaware of the occlusion. In normal humans the $P_{0.1}$ correlates well with the ventilatory response to various stimuli and with diaphragmatic electromyographic (EMG) responses. The maneuver must be done with a constant functional residual capacity (FRC) since changes in lung volume affect the shape of the diaphragm and thus the length versus tension relationship of the diaphragmatic muscle. The $P_{0.1}$ is independent of airflow, and in a number of studies in which the ventilatory result was impaired during ongoing ventilatory stimuli, the $P_{0.1}$ continued to increase.[41,42]

Diaphragmatic Electromyogram

The EMG of the diaphragm (EMG_{di}) also correlates highly with the ventilatory drive and is a direct reflection of phrenic nerve output.[44–46] Its clinical utility, however, is questionable, since measurements have been difficult to reproduce and may involve a number of muscle groups other than the diaphragm. Diaphragmatic EMG measurements therefore are probably not clinically very useful.

ALTERATIONS OF VENTILATORY DRIVES

A number of endogenous and exogenous influences may affect ventilatory drive and need to be taken into consid-

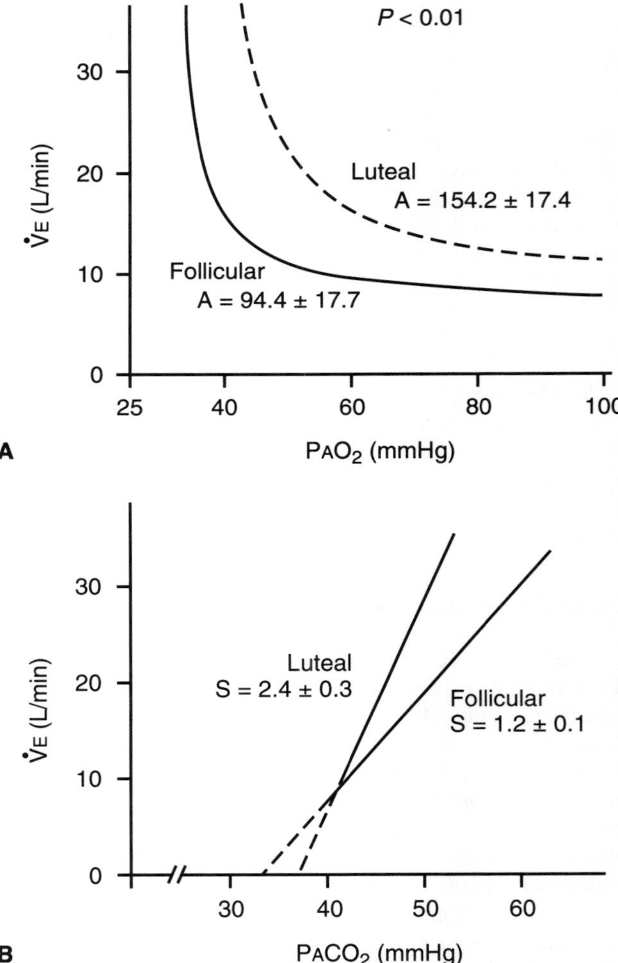

Figure 14-3. The effect of progesterone flux during the menstrual cycle on (**A**) hypoxic and (**B**) hypercapnic ventilatory responses. A is a mathematical expression describing the hypoxic ventilatory response; S represents the hypercapnic ventilatory response in liters per minute per millimeter of Hg. (From Schoene et al.,[47] with permission.)

eration in the interpretation of ventilatory responses. In healthy individuals both hormonal fluctuations and changes in metabolic rate may play an important role in altering ventilatory drive. For instance, progesterone, which fluctuates during the menstrual cycle and pregnancy, is a potent ventilatory stimulant. Progesterone, which increases substantially during the luteal phase of the menstrual cycle and during pregnancy, stimulates ventilation[47] (Fig. 14-3). Therapeutic use of progesterone can be an effective respiratory stimulant in some patients who hypoventilate.[48]

Pathologic states of hyper- and hypothyroidism affect metabolism, and since ventilatory responses track $\dot{V}CO_2$, ventilatory drive and ventilation will be either stimulated or blunted, respectively. Fever and hypothermia also involve alterations of the metabolic rate such that drive is altered accordingly. Various states of starvation also blunt ventilatory drives.

A number of medications alter either the metabolic rate or the ventilatory drive itself, and therefore it is important for the clinician to take a careful history. As mentioned, progesterone increases ventilatory drive, as do a number of other stimulants, including amphetamines, theophylline, cocaine, tricyclic antidepressants, thyroid supplements, and caffeine. On the other hand, sedatives and depressants, such as alcohol, benzodiazepines, barbiturates, opiates, dopamine, and phenothiazines, can suppress ventilation.

The purpose of this chapter has been to review the regulation and measurement of breathing (see Ch. 25 for a discussion of some of the disorders of ventilation regulation that are seen in clinical practice).

References

1. McDonald DM: Peripheral chemoreceptors: Structure-function relationships of the carotid body. pp. 105–319. In Hornbein TF (ed): Regulation of Breathing. Part 1. Marcel Dekker, New York, 1981
2. Biscoe TJ, Purbes MJ, Samson SR: The frequency of nerve impulses in single carotid body chemoreceptor afferent fibres recorded *in vivo* with intact circulation. J Physiol (Lond) 1970; 208:121–131
3. Lahiri S, DeLaney RG: Relationship between carotid chemoreceptor activity and ventilation in the cat. Respir Physiol 1975; 24:267–286
4. Weil JV, Byrne-Quinn E, Sodal IE et al: Hypoxic ventilatory response in normal man. J Clin Invest 1970;49:1061–1072
5. Bledsoe SW, Hornbein TF: Central chemosensors in the regulation of their chemical environment. pp. 347–428. In Hornbein TF (ed): Regulation of Breathing. Part 1. Marcel Dekker, New York, 1981
6. Loeschcke HH: Central chemoreceptors. pp. 41–77. In Pallot DJ (ed): Control of Respiration. Oxford University Press, New York, 1983
7. Reed DJC: A clinical method for assessing the ventilatory response to carbon dioxide. Australas Ann Med 1967;1620–1632
8. Hirschman CA, McCullough RE, Weil JV: Normal values for hypoxic and hypercapnic ventilatory drives in man. J Appl Physiol 1975;38:1095–1098
9. Pavlin E, Hornbein TF: Distribution of [H^+] and [HCO_3^-] between CSF and blood during metabolic acidosis in dogs. Am J Physiol 1975;228:1134–1140
10. Pavlin E, Hornbein TF: Distribution of [H^+] and [HCO_3^-] between CSF and blood during metabolic alkalosis in dogs. Am J Physiol 1975;228:1141–1144
11. Pavlin E, Hornbein TF: Distribution of [H^+] and [HCO_3^-] during respiratory acidosis in dogs. Am J Physiol 1975;228:1145–1148
12. Widdicombe JG: Nervous receptors in the respiratory tract and lungs. pp. 429–472. In Hornbein TF (ed): Regulation of Breathing. Part I. Marcel Dekker, New York, 1981
13. Iscoe S: Pulmonary stretch receptor discharge patterns in eupnea, hypercapnia and hypoxia. J Appl Physiol 1982;53:346–354
14. Freedman S, Campbell EJM: The ability of normal subjects to tolerate added inspiratory loads. Respir Physiol 1970;10:213–235
15. Hill AR, Caiser DL, Lu JG, Rochester DF: Steady-state response of conscious man to small expiratory resistive loads. Respir Physiol 1985;61:369–381
16. Martin J, Aubier M, Engell A: Effects of inspiratory loading and respiratory muscle activity during expiration. Am Rev Respir Dis 1982;125:352–358
17. Green M, Mead J, Sears TA: Effects of loading on respiratory muscle control on man. pp. 73–80. In Pengelly LD, Rebuck AS, Campbell EJM (ed): Loaded Breathing; Proceedings of an International Symposium on the Effects of Mechanical Loads on Breathing. Hamilton, Ont. April 1973. Churchill Livingstone, Edinburgh, 1974
18. Altose MD, McCaulley WC, Kelsen SG, Cherniack NS: The effects of hypercapnia and inspiratory flow resistive loading and respiratory activity in COPD. J Clin Invest 1977;59:500–507
19. Whipp BJ: The rate constant for the kinetics of oxygen uptake during light exercise. J Appl Physiol 1971;30:261–263
20. Whipp BJ, Wasserman K: Oxygen uptake kinetics for various intensities of constant load work. J Appl Physiol 1972;33:351–356
21. Whipp BJ, Mahler M: Dynamics of pulmonary gas exchange during exercise. pp. 33–96. In West JB (ed): Pulmonary Gas Exchange. Academic Press, New York, 1980
22. Wasserman K, Whipp BJ, Casaburi R et al: CO_2 flow to the lungs and ventilatory control. pp. 105–135. In Dempsey JA, Reed CE (eds): Muscular Exercise and the Lung. University of Wisconsin Press, Madison, 1977
23. Sutton JR, Jones NL: Control of pulmonary ventilation during exercise and mediators in the blood: CO_2 and hydrogen ion. Med Sci Sports Exerc 1979;11:198–203
24. Wasserman KH, Whipp BJ: Coupling of ventilation to pulmonary gas exchange during non-steady state work in man. J Appl Physiol 1983;54:587–593
25. Kao FF, Michel CC, Mei SJ, Li WK: Somatic effluent influences on respiration. Ann NY Acad Sci 1963;109:696–710
26. Eldridge FL, Milhorn DE, Waldrop TG: Exercise hyperpnia in locomotion; parallel activation of the hypothalamus. Science 1981;211:844–846
27. Kao FF: An experimental study of a pathway involved in exercise hyperpnea employing cross-circulation techniques. pp. 461–462. In Cunningham DJC, Lloyd BB (eds): The Regulation of Human Respiration. Blackwell Scientific Publications, Oxford, 1963
28. Lourenco RV: Assessment of respiratory control in humans. Am Rev Respir Dis 1977;115:1–5
29. Rebuck AS, Campbell EJM: A clinical method for assessing the ventilatory response to hypoxia. Am Rev Respir Dis 1974; 109:345–350
30. Edelman NH, Epstein PE, Lahiri S, Cherniack NS: Ventilatory responses to transient hypoxia and hypercapnia in man. Respir Physiol 1973;17:302–314
31. Cherniack NS, Edelman NH, Lahiri S: Hypoxia and hypercapnia as respiratory stimulants and depressants. Respir Physiol 1970;11:113–126
32. Morrill CG, Meyer JR, Weil JV: Hypoxic ventilatory depression in dogs. J Appl Physiol 1975;38:143–146
33. Weiskopf RB, Gabel RA: Depression of ventilation during hypoxia in man. J Appl Physiol 1975;39:911–915

34. Easton PA, Slykerman AN, Anthonisen NR: Ventilatory response to sustained hypoxia in normal adults. J Appl Physiol 1986;61:906–911
35. Easton PA, Anthonisen NR: Ventilatory response to sustained hypoxia after pretreatment with aminophylline. J Appl Physiol 1988;64:1445–1450
36. Suzuki A, Nishimura M, Yamamoto H et al: No effect of brain blood flow on ventilatory depression during sustained hypoxia. J Appl Physiol 1989;66:1674–1678
37. Moore LG, Huang SY, McCullough RE et al: Variable inhibition by falling CO_2 of hypoxic ventilatory response in humans. J Appl Physiol 1984;656:207–210
38. Whitelaw WH, Derenne JP, Milic-Emili J: Occlusion pressure as a measure of respiratory center output in conscious man. Respir Physiol 1975;23:181–199
39. Lopata M, Evanich MJ, Lourenco RV: Relationship between mouth occlusion pressure and electrical activity in the diaphragm: Effects of flow resistive loading. Am Rev Respir Dis 1977;116:449–455
40. Cherniack NS, Lederer DH, Altose MD, Kelsen SG: Occlusion pressure as a technique in evaluating respiratory control. Chest, suppl. 1976;70:137S–141S
41. Lopata M, Lafata J, Evanich MJ, Lourenco RV: Effects of flow resistance loading on mouth occlusion pressure during CO_2 rebreathing. Am Rev Respir Dis 1977;115:73–81
42. Holle RHO, Schoene RB, Pavlin EG: Effect of respiratory muscle weakness on $P_{0.1}$ induced by partial curarization. J Appl Physiol 1984;57:1150–1157
43. Grassino AE, Derrene JP, Almirall J et al: Configuration of the chest wall and occlusion pressure in awake humans. J Appl Physiol 1981;50:134–142
44. Lourenco RV, Mueller EP: Quantification of electrical activity of the human diaphragm. J Appl Physiol 1967;22:598–600
45. Sharp JT, Druz W, Danon J, Kim MJ: Respiratory muscle function and the use of respiratory muscle EMG in the evaluation of respiratory regulation. Chest, suppl. 1976;70:150S–153S
46. Gribben HR, Pride NB, Bye PT et al: Electrical activation of the diaphragm during stimulated breathing in patients with severe chronic airflow limitation and CO_2 retention. Chest, suppl. 1984;85:51S–54S
47. Schoene RB, Robertson HT, Pierson DJ, Peterson AP: Respiratory drives and exercise in the menstrual cycles of athletic and non-athletic women. J Appl Physiol 1981;50:1300–1305
48. Sutton FD, Zwillich CW, Creagh CE et al: Progesterone for outpatient treatment of pickwickian syndrome. Ann Intern Med 1975;83:476–479

Chapter 15

Physiology of Exercise

Robert B. Schoene

CHAPTER OUTLINE

With interest growing in clinical exercise testing to evaluate dyspnea and to determine impairment and disability, there is an even greater need for understanding of basic exercise physiology. The purpose of this chapter is to lay a foundation that will allow the reader to evaluate the information in Chapter 49 (i.e., to understand an abnormal physiologic response to physical work, the clinician must understand how to administer a test and how to interpret the normal response).

An intact and integrated cardiovascular and pulmonary system is necessary to obtain and deliver O_2 and dispose of CO_2, the metabolic by-product of exercise. It is important from a metabolic standpoint to think of exercise merely as an immoderate form of rest. In other words, all the normal factors involved in resting O_2 consumption and CO_2 production are accentuated, as exercise imposes a greater metabolic stress. A reasonably thorough evaluation of each of the systems necessary to carry out the task of exercise can be undertaken in humans by relatively noninvasive techniques. In this way, the clinician can evaluate the cardiopulmonary response with a high degree of accuracy and diagnostic capabilities (see Ch. 49). Several excellent reviews are available.[1–5]

METABOLIC RATE

With increasing work, O_2 consumption ($\dot{V}O_2$) and CO_2 production ($\dot{V}CO_2$) increase.[6] At low and moderate work loads the response is linear with respect to work. At higher work loads, above the so-called ventilatory or anaerobic threshold, $\dot{V}CO_2$ increases disproportionately to $\dot{V}O_2$ (Fig. 15-1). The ratio of $\dot{V}CO_2$ to $\dot{V}O_2$, called the *respiratory exchange ratio* (R), can be measured with inhaled and exhaled air. The ratio depends on the foods used as the fuel substrate and the level of work. For instance, with a normal diet R at rest is approximately 0.80. A higher carbohydrate diet results in more molecules of CO_2 being produced per molecule of carbohydrate consumed, so that R at rest may be as high as 0.85 or 0.90. On the other hand, a diet high in fats or proteins or a starvation state shifts R to a lower value, such as 0.70 or 0.75. Since these values are measured on exhaled gas, *voluntary* hyperventilation for a short time results in high CO_2 production for a given metabolic rate, so that R may be abnormally high and not an accurate reflection of true cellular metabolic rate.

$\dot{V}O_2$ and $\dot{V}CO_2$ at rest in a normal-size adult is usually between 200 and 250 mL/min. This resting metabolic rate is called a *met*, and work capability can be measured in factors of mets, with the resting metabolic rate as the baseline. The gross values of $\dot{V}O_2$ and $\dot{V}CO_2$ can be corrected for body weight, and they would then be expressed in milliliters per kilogram per minute. Normal values are usually based on age and sex,[7–11] so that when they are corrected for body weight, they can give the clinician a reasonable understanding of the range in normal subjects. $\dot{V}O_2$, especially when corrected for body weight, is a good standard for aerobic fitness, and some accomplished athletes have maximum $\dot{V}O_2$

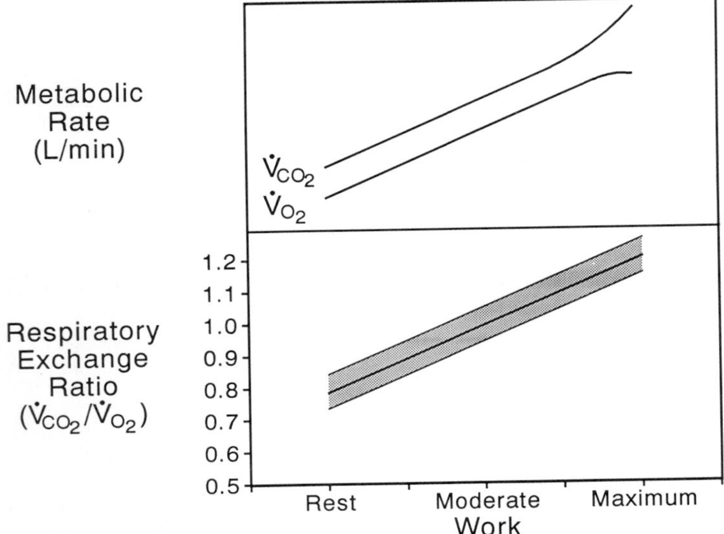

Figure 15-1. Metabolic response and respiratory exchange ratio (R) during incremental exercise to exhaustion: $\dot{V}O_2$ and $\dot{V}CO_2$ rise in parallel during moderate levels of work, but $\dot{V}CO_2$ increases disproportionately to $\dot{V}O_2$ at high levels of work. This relationship is reflected in R ($\dot{V}CO_2/\dot{V}O_2$), which, depending on dietary intake, starts at approximately 0.8 and rises to 1.2 at exhaustive exercise.

levels that are almost double the normal range. The ability to consume this much O_2 is only in small part (10 to 15 percent) secondary to training; thus, the ability to achieve these extremely high levels is largely inborn.

VENTILATION

Intact lungs are necessary to obtain O_2 and excrete CO_2 at moderate and high levels of work, although this task can also be achieved with mildly impaired lungs.[12] During exercise testing, expired ventilation ($\dot{V}_E$) is measured (in liters per minute). $\dot{V}_E$ is composed of alveolar ventilation ($\dot{V}_A$), which is the gas exchange portion of $\dot{V}_E$, and dead space ventilation ($\dot{V}_D$): $\dot{V}_E = \dot{V}_A + \dot{V}_D$ (Fig. 15-2A). $\dot{V}_E$ increases with increasing work load and metabolic rate and is proportional to $\dot{V}CO_2$ throughout exercise.[13] Thus, $\dot{V}_E$ increases linearly with work until the ventilatory or anaerobic threshold is reached, at which time the slope of the ventilation versus work plot becomes steeper.[14–16]

Ventilation is a product of respiratory frequency (f) and tidal volume (V_T): [$\dot{V}_E = f \times V_T$] (Fig. 15-2B). In order to achieve increased levels of ventilation, the normal response consists of a more rapid increase in V_T, which then plateaus, while f increases more linearly and in proportion to work until very high work loads, at which time f increases at a steeper rate.

Another important measure of the ventilatory response to exercise is the ventilatory equivalent ($\dot{V}_E/\dot{V}O_2$) (Fig. 15-2C). This parameter, expressed as a ratio, can be defined as the amount of ventilation dedicated to any given metabolic rate. Since the units of measure (liters per minute) for both the numerator and denominator cancel, the ventilatory equivalent is expressed as a pure number. Its normal value is usually in the mid-twenties range but can be in the high teens or low twenties in individuals with normally blunted ventilatory responses. The more common finding in the clinical arena is that of a high ventilatory equivalent, which is secondary to either increased ventilatory drive and/or increased dead space ventilation (see Ch. 49).

In normal subjects V_D decreases with increasing work load[13] (Fig. 15-2D). This observation is secondary to a disproportionately greater recruitment of the pulmonary microvasculature by the increased cardiac output and, perfusion of the lung, especially at the apices, as compared with an increase in ventilation. The proportion of V_D is easily determined from the Bohr dead space equation:

$$V_D/V_T = (PaCO_2 - P_ECO_2)/PaCO_2$$

where $PaCO_2$ is arterial CO_2 partial pressure and P_ECO_2 is the CO_2 partial pressure in expired air. Accurate measurement of V_D/V_T requires arterial blood, and its value in normal subjects varies from approximately 0.40 at rest to 0.10 during high levels of exercise. An intact pulmonary vascular system is necessary for this decrease in V_D/V_T to occur.

GAS EXCHANGE

The transfer of O_2 from air to blood and the excretion of CO_2 from blood to air take place at the pulmonary alveolar-capillary interface. The transfer of O_2 and CO_2 takes place with great ease in normal individuals even at extreme levels

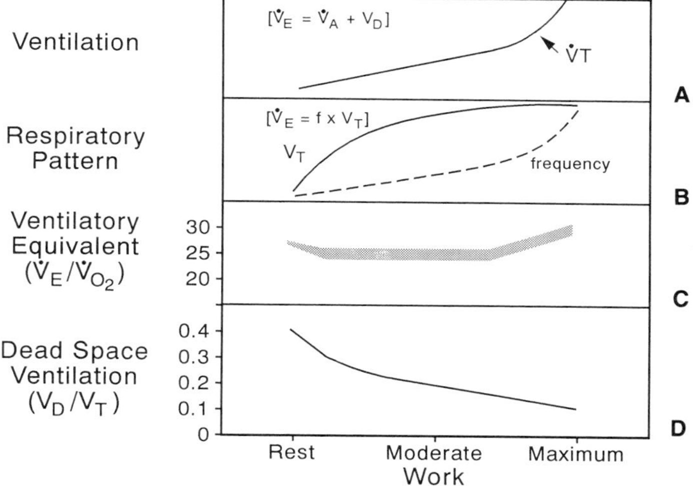

Figure 15-2. Ventilatory response to incremental exercise. **(A)** Minute ventilation, which is the sum of $\dot{V}_A$ and $\dot{V}_D$, rises with increasing work during moderate levels of exercise but increases at a more rapid rate once the individual reaches the ventilatory threshold ($\dot{V}T$). **(B)** Ventilation is the product of respiratory frequency (f) and tidal volume (V_T). Increases in V_T occur early and at a steeper slope and then plateau near the end of exhaustive work, while f increases linearly throughout exercise until the exhaustive phase, at which point it rises more rapidly. **(C)** Ventilatory equivalent ($\dot{V}_E/\dot{V}O_2$), the amount of ventilation dedicated to any given metabolic rate, can be affected by respiratory drive and dead space ventilation. **(D)** $\dot{V}_D$ decreases during exercise when perfusion increases to the areas of the lung that were previously underperfused or nonperfused.

of exercise. At sea level the ventilatory response and the facility with which O_2 is obtained from the air are adequate to prevent a decrease in SaO_2 (Fig. 15-3A). During low and moderate levels of exercise the alveolar partial pressures of O_2 (P_AO_2) and that of CO_2 (P_ACO_2) remain constant (Fig. 15-3B). At high levels of work, above the anaerobic or ventilatory threshold, hyperventilation ensues and P_AO_2 and P_ACO_2 increase and decrease by several millimeters of Hg, respectively. Since CO_2 is so soluble and diffusible, this decrease in P_ACO_2 is reflected also in a decrease in $PaCO_2$. On the other hand, O_2 is not as soluble or diffusible, and the alveolar-arterial oxygen difference [$P(A\text{-}a)O_2$] increases even in normal subjects. In normal persons at sea level, however, the PaO_2 still should remain in the mid-90 mmHg

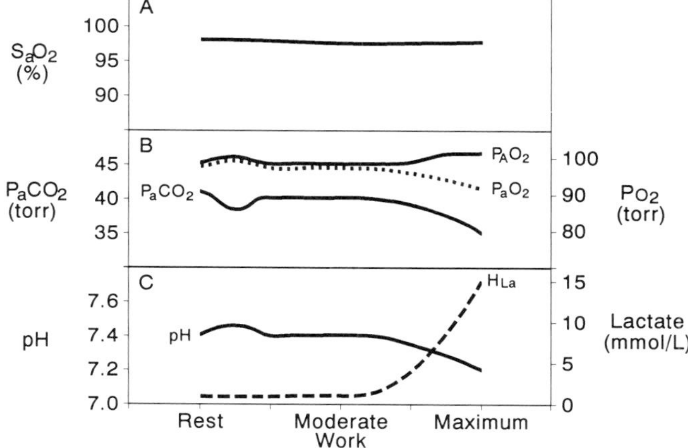

Figure 15-3. Arterial blood gases and acid-base status during incremental exercise. **(A)** In normal subjects at sea level, SaO_2 does not decrease. **(B)** During moderate levels of work P_AO_2 and PaO_2 maintain a constant relationship, with $P(A\text{-}a)O_2$ increasing at high levels of work. PCO_2 in humans is regulated precisely until the hyperventilatory phase of high levels of work sets in to compensate for the metabolic acidosis. **(C)** Arterial pH remains constant during exercise until higher levels, at which time pH drops as a reflection of the metabolic acidosis, which is marked by the increase in lactic acid concentration.

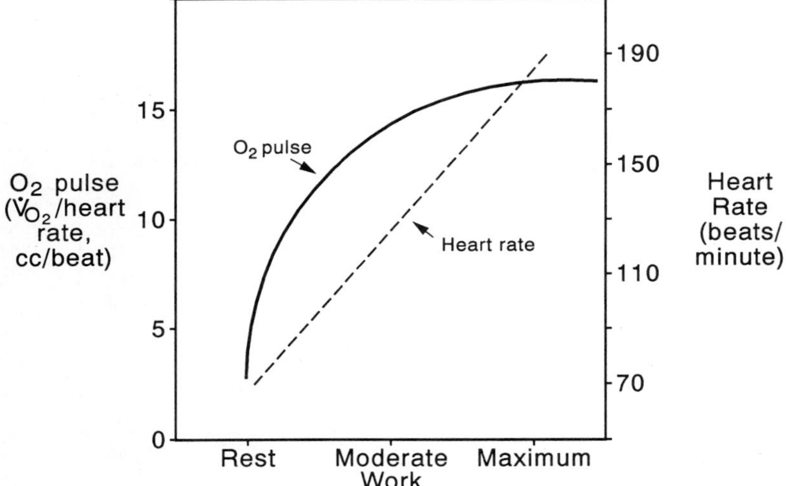

Figure 15-4. Cardiac response during incremental work. Cardiac output is equal to the product of stroke volume and heart rate. An indirect measurement of stroke volume is the O_2 pulse, which increases steeply early during incremental exercise and then plateaus at higher levels of work. The heart rate increases linearly throughout exercise, the maximum heart rate being determined in part by age.

range.[14] Blood pH reflects the finely tuned regulation of gas exchange and ventilatory control during moderate levels of work, but it drops as the metabolic acidosis from increased lactate production and/or decreased lactate uptake overwhelms the lungs' ability to excrete higher levels of CO_2 (Fig. 15-3C).

CARDIAC RESPONSE

An intact cardiac response is necessary to deliver O_2 to the tissues. Cardiac output ($\dot{Q}T$), expressed in liters per minute, increases linearly with work and is the product of stroke volume (SV) times heart rate [$\dot{Q}T = SV \times$ heart rate][15] (Fig. 15-4). Actual measurement of cardiac output is invasive and difficult in the clinical exercise laboratory, but heart rate can be accurately measured while stroke volume can be inferred from the O_2 pulse ($\dot{V}O_2$/heart rate). Heart rate increases linearly with work, and the predicted maximum heart rate can be approximated from the patient's age (220 bpm − age). The O_2 pulse reflects the degree of O_2 consumption per heart beat, and its maximum values are based on age and body size. Stroke volume at first increases rapidly with an increase in work but plateaus as the level of work becomes still higher. Systolic blood pressure increases with higher levels of exercise, while diastolic pressure stays the same or decreases slightly.

VENTILATORY OR ANAEROBIC THRESHOLD

As mentioned above, at higher levels of work there is a disproportionate increase in $\dot{V}CO_2$ with respect to $\dot{V}O_2$ (Figs. 15-1 and 15-2A). This phenomenon occurs presumably because the O_2 supply to the exercising tissues becomes inadequate for the increasing metabolic demand at high levels of work. The term *anaerobic threshold* implies that the tissues are functioning under anaerobic metabolism while the term *ventilatory threshold* is merely descriptive of the increased slope of the ventilation versus work relationship and the increase in $\dot{V}_A$ that occurs at this point.[16,17] A metabolic acidosis can be documented in the blood by a decrease in pH, a decrease in base excess, and an increase in lactic acid concentration.[14] In most clinical situations it is important to determine these values in arterial blood as a means by which to document the effort or extent of exercise as well as to calculate V_D/V_T. The increase in lactic acid is secondary to an increase in lactate production as well as to the overwhelming of the lactate-metabolizing ability of the muscle and liver.

References

1. Wasserman K, Whipp BJ: Exercise physiology in health and disease. Am Rev Respir Dis 1975;112:219–249
2. Jones NL: Exercise testing in pulmonary evaluation: Rationale, methods, and the normal respiratory response to exercise. N Engl J Med 1975;293:541–544
3. Astrand PO, Rodahl K: Textbook of Work Physiology. 3rd Ed. McGraw-Hill, New York, 1980
4. Jones NL, Campbell EJM: Clinical Exercise Testing. 2nd Ed. WB Saunders, Philadelphia, 1982
5. Wasserman K, Hansen JE, Sue DY, Whipp BJ: Principles of Exercise Testing and Interpretation. Lea & Febiger, Philadelphia, 1987
6. Hansen JE, Sue DY, Wasserman K: Predicted values for clinical exercise testing. Am Rev Respir Dis 1984;129:S49–S55
7. Whipp BJ, Wasserman K: Oxygen update kinetics for various intensities of constant load work. J Appl Physiol 1972;323:351–356

8. Sue DY, Hansen JE: Normal values in adults during exercise testing. Clin Chest Med 1984;5:87–89
9. Drinkwater BL, Horvath SM, Well CL: Aerobic power of females, ages 10 to 68. J Gerontol 1975;30:385–394
10. Bruce RA, Kusumi F, Hosmer D: Maximal oxygen uptake in normographic assessment of functional aerobic impairment in cardiovascular disease. Am Heart J 1973;85:546–562
11. Astrand I, Astrand PO, Hallback I, Kilborn A: Reduction in maximal oxygen uptake with age. J Appl Physiol 1973;35:649–654
12. Wasserman K: Breathing during exercise. N Engl J Med 1978; 298:780–785
13. Jones NL, McHardy CJR, Naimark A: Physiological dead space and alveolar-arterial gas pressure differences during exercises. Clin Sci 1966;31:19–29
14. Young IH, Woolcock AJ: Changes in arterial blood gas tensions during unsteady state exercise. J Appl Physiol 1978;44:93–96
15. Weissman ML, Jones PW, Oren A et al: Cardiac output increase in gas exchange at the start of exercise. J Appl Physiol 1982; 52:236–244
16. Wasserman K: The anaerobic threshold measurement to evaluate exercise performance. Am Rev Respir Dis 1984;129:S35–S40
17. Beaver WL, Wasserman K, Whipp BJ: Improved detection of the lactate threshold during exercise using a log-log transformation. J Appl Physiol 1985;59:1936–1940

Chapter 16

Adaptation and Maladaptation to High Altitude

Robert B. Schoene

CHAPTER OUTLINE

Acute ascent and chronic habitation at high altitude can lead to a number of diseases whose underlying problem is lack of O_2. As one ascends, the fraction of O_2 in the atmosphere remains constant while the barometric pressure (P_b) decreases. The amount of O_2 that is available to the body is therefore correspondingly decreased. For instance, at 14,000 ft the barometric pressure is about 450 mmHg and the inspired partial pressure of oxygen (P_IO_2) is approximately 80 mmHg, as opposed to 150 mmHg at sea level (Table 16-1). Consequently, the body is required to make adaptations that will optimize the delivery of O_2 to the cells in this hypoxic environment. The adaptations that take place at high altitude are not dissimilar to those that a person with hypoxic cardiac or pulmonary disease undergoes to compensate for a failure to transport O_2 in one or more steps from the air to the cell.

The purpose of this chapter is twofold: (1) to describe briefly the adaptations that the body undergoes to achieve a viable level of O_2 to the cells as O_2 travels from the atmosphere to the lung into the blood, where circulation to the cells and their mitochondria takes place; and (2) to describe the clinical diseases of both acute ascent to, and chronic habitation at, high altitude. More extensive reviews of both these topics are available.[1,2]

ADAPTATION TO HIGH ALTITUDE

A number of important steps take place in the body as O_2 travels from the air to the cell. The first step is an increase in alveolar ventilation ($\dot{V}_A$), which is mediated in large part by the peripheral chemoreceptor, the carotid body.[3–5] Although this response differs between individuals and may contribute to varying degrees of success or failure in adaptation to high altitude, $\dot{V}_A$ increases immediately and continues to do so for at least 2 weeks at any given altitude. The higher one ascends, the longer it takes for the ventilatory adaptation to be complete, and at some extreme altitudes it may never be complete. At extreme altitude (higher than 26,000 ft) the ventilatory response can be quite great, and alveolar O_2 partial pressure (P_AO_2) in this environment is defended at approximately 30 mmHg, which can result in a P_ACO_2 as low as 10 mmHg.[6,7] The increase in $\dot{V}_A$ results in a higher P_AO_2 and subsequently in higher arterial O_2 content.

In the adult lung, acute ascent does not result in any morphologic changes, so that optimization of O_2 transfer from the air to the blood must take place over the same surface area for gas exchange that exists at sea level. The hypoxic pulmonary vasoconstriction that occurs from global

Table 16-1. Respiratory Alterations during a Simulated 40-Day Ascent of Mount Everest[a]

Altitude (ft)	Barometric Pressure (mmHg)	P_IO_2 (mmHg)	Minute Ventilation (L/min)	pH	$PaCO_2$ (mmHg)	PaO_2 (mmHg)	SaO_2 (%)
0	760	150	11.0	7.43	33.9	99.3	97.6
15,000	429	80	14.6	7.46	25.0	52.4	84.8
20,000	347	63	20.9	7.50	20.0	41.1	75.2
26,500	282	49	36.6	7.53	12.5	36.6	67.8
29,029	240	43	42.3	7.56	11.2	30.3	58.0

P_IO_2, inspired O_2 pressure; $PaCO_2$, arterial CO_2 tension; PaO_2, arterial O_2 tension; SaO_2, arterial O_2 saturation.
[a] Mean data measured in seven healthy subjects participating in "Operation Everest II."
(Modified from Sutton et al.,[49] with permission.)

alveolar hypoxia, along with the modest accompanying increase in cardiac output, results fortuitously in better ventilation/perfusion ($\dot{V}/\dot{Q}$) matching.[8–10] Lifelong habitation, on the other hand, does result in larger lung volumes and a greater surface area for gas exchange, which is reflected in an increase in diffusion capacity.[11–16]

In contrast to the situation at sea level, at high altitude there is a true diffusion limitation to O_2 at the lung, which is accentuated with exercise.[7,17–20] This limitation occurs because of (1) the decrease in driving pressure of O_2 from the air to the blood; and (2) a decrease in transit time of the red blood cell across the capillary secondary to an increase in cardiac output from exercise, with resulting failure of full equilibration of O_2 from the air to capillary blood.

The hematologic adaptations to high altitude begin immediately but take 1 week or more for their effects to be realized. There is an immediate rise in erythropoietin, which stimulates the production of red blood cells.[21] The increase in hematocrit, which is apparent in the first few days, is also a reflection in part of the water diuresis that occurs early and persists during a person's stay at high altitude, while the subsequent increase in hemoglobin concentration is secondary to the erythropoietin stimulation. At modest altitude (perhaps below 12,000 ft) there is a rightward shift of the oxyhemoglobin dissociation curve, which facilitates the unloading of O_2 from the hemoglobin molecule to the peripheral tissues.[22] At much higher altitudes, however, the dissociation curve is shifted to the left, which improves loading of O_2 to the red blood cell at the lung, where the diffusion gradient is very low. This leftward shift is a result of the marked respiratory alkalosis that occurs at extremely high altitude.[23]

There is much less agreement as to what happens at the peripheral tissues during high altitude adaptation. There is probably a decrease in muscle cell size, which decreases the radial diffusion distance for O_2 from the blood across the cell membrane to the mitochondria. Additionally, there may be an increase in both mitochondrial and capillary density as well as optimization of the enzymes of oxidative phosphorylation, all of which result in improved O_2 availability and utilization of O_2 at the mitochondria.[24–27] All these adaptations are beneficial to the high altitude visitor or dweller, but as in all biologic adaptations, there is marked variation between individuals, and some of the adaptations either primarily or secondarily become maladaptations, leading to high altitude illnesses (see Table 16-2).

HIGH ALTITUDE ILLNESSES

Acute Mountain Sickness

All altitude illnesses are caused by decreased O_2 delivery to the cells. The organ that is probably affected initially is the brain, for many of the symptoms of early altitude illness can be attributed to depression of the central nervous system secondary to mild cerebral edema. This initial form of altitude illness is called acute mountain sickness (AMS) and is usually a benign, self-limited disorder, which can, however, be debilitating and aggravating for the sojourner.[2,28,29] Rapid ascent without time for adequate acclimatization is the main predisposing factor. Symptoms can begin at altitudes as low as 8000 ft but are much more common (40 to 60 percent) above 10,000 ft.

Symptoms of AMS include one or all of the following: headache, lethargy, insomnia, loss of appetite, nausea and vomiting, and mild shortness of breath. These symptoms may be accompanied by tachycardia, which usually subsides with acclimatization, and mild tachypnea. The symptoms of AMS abate in 1 to 2 days with rest and no further ascent. Mild analgesics are adequate for the headache, which can also be quite severe (Table 16-2).

The most important step for avoiding altitude illness is to ascend slowly and enjoy the scenery. Once above 8000 ft, which is where most recreational sites for sports such as skiing and hiking are located, the ascent should not be faster than 1000 to 2000 ft/d. The higher one goes, the less should be the altitude gain each day. Another approach is to climb higher but to sleep at a lower altitude, which anecdotally seems to optimize acclimatization and help the sojourner to avoid altitude illness. Many individuals on vacation at high altitude, particularly skiers who come from sea level and ski at 8000 to 10,000 ft, have symptoms of altitude illness for the first several days of their stay, which are often thought to be due to alcoholic hangover.

Table 16-2. High Altitude Illnesses

	Acute Mountain Sickness (AMS)	High Altitude Pulmonary Edema (HAPE)	High Altitude Cerebral Edema (HACE)	Chronic Mountain Sickness (CMS)
Location	Above 8000 ft	Usually above 10,000 ft	Above 12,000 ft	Above 10,000 ft
Time	1–2 days after ascent	3–4 days after ascent, or possibly later	4–7 days after ascent, or possibly later	Months, years, generations
Symptoms	Headache, lethargy, sleep disturbances, anorexia, nausea, vomiting	Dyspnea at rest, weakness, cough, can progress to production of pink, frothy sputum	Severe headache, confusion, hallucinations	Lethargy, decreased exercise capacity
Signs	Mild tachycardia, possible mild peripheral edema	Tachycardia, tachypnea, low-grade fever, cyanosis	Ataxia, focal neurologic or visual signs, retinal hemorrhage	Plethora, peripheral edema, conjunctival injection
Laboratory findings	Possible mild arterial O_2 desaturation	Moderate to severe arterial O_2 desaturation, relative hypoventilation	Moderate arterial O_2 desaturation	Polycythemia, severe arterial O_2 desaturation, relative hypercapnia
Treatment	Rest at same altitude, hydration, mild analgesics; usually ascent can continue in 1–2 days; prophylaxis and treatment with acetazolamide (250 mg bid)	Immediate descent,[a] O_2 if available, acetazolamide and dexamethasone (4 mg q6h) (both unproven but possibly effective), hyperbaric therapy if available and descent impossible	Descent,[a] dexamethasone (8 mg bolus, 4 mg q6h), hyperbaric therapy if descent impossible	Descent, O_2, respiratory stimulants (acetazolamide, progesterone), phlebotomy

[a] Descent must not be delayed to implement other modalities.

Pharmacologic prophylaxis with either acetazolamide or dexamethasone is effective. A number of studies have shown acetazolamide to be very effective in reducing the incidence of AMS in individuals who ascend rapidly.[29,30] This carbonic anhydrase inhibitor acts in a number of different ways, including stimulation of ventilation, prevention of periodic breathing and O_2 desaturation at night,[31] and rapid development of a metabolic acidosis secondary to excretion of HCO_3^- at the renal tubules.[32] The drug is also a mild diuretic. All responses to acetazolamide resemble normal acclimatization but occur more rapidly, and any one or all of these mechanisms may facilitate acclimatization to high altitude.

Acetazolamide may even be taken when early signs of altitude illness appear rather than prior to ascent. The dosage that has been shown to be effective is either 500 mg in a sustained-release preparation or 250 mg tid, although lower doses such as 250 or 125 mg bid are probably effective. Some side effects, such as tingling in the extremities, mild diuresis, nausea, and a metallic taste to carbonated beverages, prevent acetazolamide from being the ideal drug, but all the side effects are self-limited and benign. Prophylaxis should probably be reserved for those individuals who have a history of AMS on several occasions, and slow ascent should be prescribed as the first line of defense. The drug can be taken for the first several days at altitude and then tapered accordingly.

Dexamethasone at high doses of 4 mg PO qid has also been shown to be effective in preventing altitude illness and has been claimed to have fewer side effects.[33–35] However, the potency of this drug, which may act by the mechanism of decreasing leak from the microvasculature into the tissues, makes it less than ideal. Additionally, it probably does not facilitate acclimatization, so that if the drug is stopped, subjects may again become sick. Dexamethasone should be reserved for use in rescue situations and in severe forms of altitude illness, in which the beneficial effects of the drug may improve symptoms sufficiently that victims can become ambulatory and assist in their own descent.

High Altitude Cerebral and Pulmonary Edema

The more severe forms of altitude illness, high altitude cerebral edema (HACE) and high altitude pulmonary edema (HAPE), often occur together in varying degrees. Both are secondary to leak of fluid from the microvasculature into the lung and brain, and both can be fatal. HAPE and HACE usually occur at higher altitudes (above 12,000 ft). All sojourners to these altitudes should be aware of the symptoms, since early intervention, which primarily includes descent, can prevent potential disasters.

HAPE occurs in 1 to 3 percent of individuals ascending to 14,000 ft or higher and is marked by tachypnea, dry cough, lethargy, and marked dyspnea. The symptoms can progress to a cough productive of pink frothy sputum and be accompanied by the signs of tachycardia and tachypnea. Physical examination reveals crackles, usually beginning in the right middle lobe area and becoming diffuse, and the victims are usually cyanotic. Many of the subjects have a low-grade fever, which is the reason that before 1960 HAPE was thought to be pneumonia. The symptoms can progress and are potentially fatal.[36–38] Bronchoscopic evaluation of the edema fluid obtained by bronchoalveolar lavage shows that it is very high in protein and additionally has a high content of cells, primarily alveolar microphages.[39,40]

If the patient is still ambulatory once HAPE has been recognized, descent is mandatory to avoid progression of the disease and possibly death. If trauma or bad weather prevents descent a temporizing measure may be taken by the use of a lightweight, portable continuous positive air pressure (CPAP) mask with 5 to 10 cmH_2O pressure, which is used in the expiratory positive airway pressure (EPAP) mode since compressed air to maintain the CPAP mode is not available in the field setting.[41] If O_2 is available, it should be given at 3 to 4 L/min flow, but none of these measures should delay descent. Good studies of drug intervention have not been made, but azetazolamide and dexamethasone may be beneficial both for prophylaxis and treatment. Diuretics, cardiac glycosides, morphine, and aminophylline do not have any beneficial effect and may in fact be dangerous. It has recently been suggested that the calcium channel blocker nifedipine may improve gas exchange and prevent HAPE in some individuals, but further work is necessary before it can be recommended as treatment.[42]

HACE often occurs in conjunction with HAPE, and the pulmonary or cerebral symptomatology varies. HACE usually occurs at a higher altitude and may have a subtle onset. However, the symptoms may progress rapidly to coma and death. Severe headache, unrelieved by analgesics, confusion, ataxia, and asymmetric localizing neurologic signs may all occur.[43,44] If any of these signs is present, descent must be undertaken immediately to prevent progression of the disease.

Prevention is still the best treatment, and as in other altitude illnesses, slow ascent is the watchword of the day. However, once the symptoms of HACE have appeared, descent must be effected. If trauma or weather prevents descent, O_2 is helpful but is usually not available. Dexamethasone in doses of 4 mg every 6 hours is indicated in this situation.

Chronic Mountain Sickness

Millions of individuals live at altitudes above 9000 ft, where they are subject to the development of chronic mountain sickness (CMS), also known as Monge's disease.[45–47] There appear to be some geographic differences in the incidence of the disease; thus, although it is not uncommon in the Andes and in the Rocky Mountains of the United States, it is very unusual in the natives of the Himalayan and the Tibetan plateau. This difference may reflect the time that these populations have lived at high altitude and some evolutionary adaptive processes that have taken place. For instance, the Himalayan native population has existed in this region for 1 million to 2 million years, while the other high altitude native populations have been at their respective locations for perhaps only 30,000 years.

The disease is primarily secondary to a lack of O_2, which has led to maladaptation. Patients are inordinately hypoxemic and relatively hypercapnic and have marked pulmonary hypertension and polycythemia. Right heart failure is common, and mental slowing often accompanies the clinical syndrome.

Of course, descent is the best cure, but often this is very impractical for individuals who live in high towns or villages where family and traditions bind them. Several temporizing measures may be undertaken, however, which may help stave off the inexorable course of the disease. First, respiratory stimulants, particularly acetazolamide or medroxyprogesterone acetate, may be helpful in decreasing the nocturnal periodic breathing and arterial O_2 desaturation that occur.[48] This may minimize the chronic, ravaging manifestations of severe hypoxemia at night as well as improve ventilation and oxygenation during the day. Second, phlebotomy may be helpful to decrease the polycythemia and the pulmonary hypertension and optimize perfusion to the peripheral tissues. Often the hematocrit may be as high as 75 percent, and careful, graded phlebotomy to hematocrits in the high 40 percent range may be quite helpful and last for a number of weeks or months. Third, if O_2 is available, its administration is also beneficial, but it is often unavailable or logistically impossible to obtain, particularly in remote high altitude habitations.

References

1. Schoene RB, Hornbein TF: High altitude adaptation. pp. 196–220. In Murray JF, Nadel JA (eds): Textbook of Respiratory Medicine. WB Saunders, Philadelphia, 1988
2. Hackett PH, Hornbein TF: Disorders of high altitude. pp. 1646–1663. In Murray JF, Nadel JA (eds): Textbook of Respiratory Medicine. WB Saunders, Philadelphia, 1988
3. Boycott AE, Haldane JS: The effects of low atmospheric pressure on respiration. J Physiol 1908;37:355–377
4. Rahn H, Otis AB: Man's respiratory response during and after acclimatization to high altitude. Am J Physiol 1946;157:445–559
5. Lahiri S, Edelmann H, Cherniack NS, Fishman AP: Role of carotid chemoreflex in respiratory acclimatization to hypoxia in goat and sheep. Respir Physiol 1981;46:367–382
6. West JB, Hackett PH, Maret KH et al: Pulmonary gas exchange on the summit of Mt. Everest. J Appl Physiol 1983;55:678–687
7. Wagner PD, Sutton JR, Lees JT et al: Operation Everest II: Pulmonary gas exchange during a simulated ascent of Mt. Everest. J Appl Physiol 1987;63:2348–2359
8. Fishman AP: Hypoxia in the pulmonary circulation: How and where it acts. Circ Res 1976;38:221–231
9. Dawson A: Regional pulmonary blood flow in sitting and supine man during and after acute hypoxia. J Clin Invest 1969;48:301–310.
10. Haab P, Held DR, Ernst H, Fahri LE: Ventilation-perfusion relationships during high altitude adaptation. J Appl Physiol 1969;26:77–81
11. Hurtado A: Respiratory adaptations in the Indian natives of the Peruvian Andes. Am J Phys Anthropol 1932;17:137–161
12. Frisancho AR, Vilasquez T, Sanchez J: Influence of develop-

mental adaptation on lung function at high altitude. Hum Biol 1973;45:583–594
13. Huang SY, Ning XH, Zhou ZN et al: Ventilatory function and adaptation to high altitude: Studies in Tibet. pp. 173–177. In West JB, Lahiri S (eds): High Altitude and Man. American Physiological Society, Bethesda, 1984
14. Dempsey JA, Reddun WG, Birmbaum ML et al: Effects of acute through life-long hypoxic exposure on exercise pulmonary gas exchange. Respir Physiol 1971;13:62–89
15. Vincent J, Hellot MF, Vargas E et al: Pulmonary gas exchange, diffusing capacity in natives and newcomers of high altitude. Respir Physiol 1978;34:219–231
16. Remmers JE, Mithoefer JC: The carbon monoxide diffusing capacity in permanent residents at high altitude. Respir Physiol 1969;6:233–244
17. Gale GE, Torre-Bueno JR, Moon RE et al: Ventilation-perfusion inequality in normal humans during exercise at sea level and simulated altitude. J Appl Physiol 1985;58:958–988
18. West JB, Boyer SJ, Graber DJ et al: Maximal exercise at extreme altitudes on Mt. Everest. J Appl Physiol 1983;55:688–702
19. Wagner PD, Gayle GE, Moon RE et al: Pulmonary gas exchange in humans exercising at sea level in simulated altitude. J Appl Physiol 1986;61:280–287
20. West JB, Lahiri S, Gill MB et al: Arterial oxygen saturation during exercise at high altitude. J Appl Physiol 1962;17:617–621
21. Abbrecht PH, Littell JK: Plasma erythropoiethin in men and mice during acclimatization to different altitudes. J Appl Physiol 1972;32:54–58
22. Cymerman A, Maher JT, Cruz JC et al: Increased 2,3-diphosphoglycerate during normocapnic hypobaric hypoxia. Aviat Space Environ Med 1976;47:1069–1072
23. Winslow RM, Samaha M, West JB: Red cell function at extreme altitude on Mt. Everest. J Appl Physiol 1984;56:109–116
24. Banchero N: Capillary density of skeletal muscle in dogs exposed to simulated altitude. Proc Soc Exp Biol Med 1975; 148:435–439
25. Tenney SM, Ou LC: Physiological evidence for increased tissue capillarity in rats acclimatized to high altitude. Respir Physiol 1970;8:137–150
26. Ou LC, Tenney SM: Properties of mitochondria from hearts of cattle acclimatized to high altitude. Respir Physiol 1970;8:151–159
27. Terrados N, Jansson E, Sylven C, Kaijser L: Is hypoxia a stimulus for synthesis of oxidative enzymes and myoglobin? J Appl Physiol 1990;68:2369–2372
28. Singh I, Khannap K, Srivastava MC et al: Acute mountain sickness. N Engl J Med 1969;280:175–182
29. Hackett PH, Rennie ID, Levine HD: Incidence, importance, and prophylaxis of acute mountain sickness. Lancet 1976;2:1149–1155
30. Larsen EB, Roach RC, Schoene RB, Hornbein TF: Acute mountain sickness and acetazolamide: Clinical efficacy and effect on ventilation. JAMA 1982;248:328–331
31. Sutton JR, Houston CS, Mansell AL et al: Effect of acetazolamide on hypoxemia during sleep at high altitude. N Engl J Med 1979;301:1329–1332
32. Maren TH: Carbonic anhydrase: Chemistry, physiology, and inhibition. Physiol Rev 1967;47:595–781
33. Hackett PH, Roach RC, Wood RA et al: Dexamethasone for prevention and treatment of acute mountain sickness. Aviat Space Environ Med 1988;59:950–954
34. Ellsworth AJ, Larsen EB: Randomized trial of dexamethasone and acetazolamide for acute mountain sickness prophylaxis. Am J Med 1987;83:1024–1030
35. Johnson TS, Rock PB, Fulcoc S et al: Prevention of acute mountain sickness by dexamethasone. N Engl J Med 1984;310:683–685
36. Houston CS: Acute pulmonary edema of high altitude. N Engl J Med 1960;363:478–480
37. Hultgren HN, Marticorena AE: High altitude pulmonary edema: Epidemiologic observations in Peru. Chest 1978;74:372–376
38. Schoene RB: Pulmonary edema at high altitude: Review, pathophysiology, and update. Clin Chest Med 1985;6:491–507
39. Schoene RB, Hackett PH, Henderson WR et al: High altitude pulmonary edema: Characteristics of lung lavage fluid. JAMA 1986;256:63–69
40. Schoene RB, Swenson ER, Pizzo CJ et al: The lung at high altitude: Bronchoalveolar lavage in acute mountain sickness and pulmonary edema. J Appl Physiol 1988;64:2605–2613
41. Schoene RB, Roach RC, Hackett PH et al: Effect of expiratory positive airway pressure on high altitude pulmonary edema and exercise at 4400 m on Mount McKinley. Chest 1985;87:330–333
42. Bartsch P, Maggiorini M, Ritter M et al: Prevention of high altitude pulmonary edema by nifedipine. N Engl J Med 1991;325:1284–1289
43. Hamilton AJ, Cymerman A, Black PM: High altitude cerebral edema. Neurosurgery 1986;19:841–849
44. Houston CS, Dickinson JD: Cerebral form of high altitude illness. Lancet 1975;2:758–761
45. Monge-M C, Monge-C C: High Altitude Diseases: Mechanism and Management. Charles C Thomas, Springfield, IL, 1966
46. Winslow RM, Monge CC: Hypoxia, Polycythemia, and Chronic Mountain Sickness. Johns Hopkins University Press, Baltimore, 1987
47. Kryger MH, Grover RF: Chronic mountain sickness. Semin Respir Med 1983;5:164–168
48. Kryger M, McCullough RE, Collins D et al: Treatment of excessive polycythemia of high altitude with respiratory stimulant drugs. Am Rev Respir Dis 1978;117:455–461
49. Sutton JR, Reeves JT, Wagner PD et al: Operation Everest II: Oxygen transport during exercise at extreme simulated altitude. J Appl Physiol 1988;64:1309–1321

Chapter 17

Defense Mechanisms and Immune Reactions in the Respiratory System

Thomas R. Martin

CHAPTER OUTLINE

The gas exchange surface of the lungs is the largest surface area of the body that is in contact with the outside environment. The integrity of this surface is critical to our survival. Its defense against gases and particulates in inspired air poses a formidable challenge, and a complex system of defense mechanisms has evolved for its protection. Many of the therapies used in respiratory care are designed to augment the defense of the lungs in patients with acute and chronic lung disease. Paradoxically, many of the treatments that are used in critically ill patients inadvertently impair defense mechanisms in the lungs, particularly defenses against inspired bacteria. This chapter describes the important defense mechanisms of the lungs and illustrates the ways in which these defenses are strengthened and weakened by modern therapies.

GENERAL CONSIDERATIONS

Important Anatomic Relationships

The airspace of the lungs begins at the glottis, the thumb-sized opening between the true vocal folds. Beyond the trachea, the conducting airways branch more than 16 times to reach the respiratory bronchioles and alveolar spaces.[1] The cross-sectional area of the airspaces increases exponentially with each generation of airways. The trachea is smaller in cross section than the handle of a tennis racket, and the surface area of the entire bronchial tree is about the size of the face of a standard tennis racket. By contrast, the alveolar surface is about the size of a tennis court. These anatomic relationships suggest an important principle about airflow rates in the lungs: airflow is fastest in the glottis and trachea and falls progressively as the branching airways subtend a larger and larger cross-sectional area.[2] In the respiratory bronchioles and on the alveolar surface there is probably little actual airflow; instead, most of the movement of gases and very small particles occurs by diffusion in the gas exchange parenchyma of the lungs. Therefore, shearing forces between flowing air and the airway walls are greatest in the trachea and proximal airways and fall steadily toward the terminal bronchioles. This means that the greatest propulsive forces for mucus and particles that deposit along the airway walls occur in the trachea and the proximal bronchi. Conversely, in the terminal bronchioles and on the alveolar surface, gas movement occurs principally by diffusion, and particles that deposit on this very large surface must be removed from the lungs by different mechanisms.

Interplay between Physical Factors, Soluble Factors, and Cellular Factors in the Defense of the Lungs

Each day over 10,000 L of air enters the lungs during the course of quiet breathing. This large volume of air contains inorganic particles, exhaust gases, and infectious and allergenic particles. The defense of the lungs against the many types of particulates and vapors in the inspired air involves a coordinated interplay of physical factors in the nasopharynx and conducting airways, soluble factors in respiratory tract fluids, and phagocytes in the distal airways and gas exchange parenchyma. In addition, local defense mechanisms in the lungs are reinforced by the systemic immune system. Signals generated in the lungs recruit circulating neutrophils, monocytes, and lymphocytes into the lungs to participate in local immune reactions. In addition, immunoglobulins, complement, and other plasma components exude into the lungs when the permeability of the lung vasculature is altered by inflammatory reactions.

Methods for Studying Defense Mechanisms in the Respiratory Tract

A variety of techniques are used to study defense mechanisms in the lungs. To study local defense mechanisms in the nasopharynx, mucosal washings and biopsies are obtained to sample mucosal secretions and tissue. Secretions can be analyzed for the presence of antibody and antibacterial proteins. Biopsies provide tissue for study by light and electron microscopy for the analysis of cellular, glandular, and ciliary morphology.

Defense mechanisms in the conducting airways can be studied by measuring the clearance of radiolabeled aerosols of particles or liquids.[3] This method has provided insight into the mechanisms by which cough and the mucociliary escalator contribute to particle clearance in the conducting airways.

Cells and fluids from the gas exchange parenchyma can be sampled by the technique of bronchoalveolar lavage.[4–7] A fiberoptic bronchoscope is passed into the lower airway and advanced into a subsegmental orifice. Aliquots of sterile saline are instilled through the bronchoscope and aspirated under gentle suction. The lavage fluid can be analyzed for cellular content of specific proteins, including immunoglobulins, complement, and plasma proteins that have leaked into the airspaces. Bronchoalveolar lavage can be performed safely in normal volunteers, in patients with chronic lung diseases, and in critically ill patients on mechanical ventilators in intensive care units. Bronchoalveolar lavage has contributed a great deal to our understanding of the composition of normal airspace fluids and of the events that occur during inflammatory processes in a variety of diseases.

DEFENSE MECHANISMS IN THE UPPER AIRWAYS

The major defense mechanisms in the nasopharynx include the physical factors governing particle deposition, the soluble constituents of mucosal fluid, the nasal mucociliary system, and the lymphoid tissue in the posterior nasopharynx.

Physical Factors in the Nasopharynx

The physical factors governing the likelihood that inhaled particles and gases will deposit in the nasopharynx include the size and mass of inhaled particles, the flow rate of inspired air, the solubility of gases in water, and the pattern of breathing (i.e., via the nose or the mouth). Three physical forces govern the deposition of inhaled particles in the nasopharynx and conducting airways, namely inertial impaction, sedimentation, and diffusion.[8] Inertial impaction is the most important of these factors in the nasopharynx. In a suspension of inhaled particles, larger particles (e.g., more than 10 μm in diameter) account for most of the mass inhaled because mass is a function of particle volume. However, the greatest number of suspended particles are small particles with relatively little mass (e.g., less than 1 to 3 μm in diameter). Particles larger than about 10 μm in diameter deposit in the posterior nasopharynx by inertial impaction because their large angular momentum carries them in a straight line, out of the bending airstream in the posterior nasopharynx, and they deposit against the posterior tracheal wall.

Because momentum is the product of mass and velocity,

higher airflow rates increase the deposition of larger particles in the upper airway. This process is most efficient during nasal breathing because of the more angular path of inspired air in the nasal turbinates (Fig. 17-1). Essentially all particles larger than 10 μm in aerodynamic diameter deposit in the upper airway during quiet nasal breathing. This helps explain why many pollens such as ragweed, which have particle sizes of up to 100 μm, cause predominantly nasal symptoms. Mouth breathing reduces this deposition efficiency by up to 50 percent, providing a greater opportunity for large particles to enter the lower airway (Fig. 17-2). Particles less than 10 μm in aerodynamic diameter pass through the upper airway in the inspired airstream and enter the lower airway to deposit on either the airway walls or the alveolar surface.

A large collection of lymphoid tissue, Waldeyer's ring, surrounds the region of greatest particle deposition in the posterior nasopharynx.[9] Waldeyer's ring consists of the tonsils on the lateral pharyngeal walls and the adenoids on the posterior pharyngeal wall. The surface of this specialized lymphoid tissue consists of a very thin epithelium, which allows particles to penetrate easily into the subepithelial lymphoid tissue, where particles can be inactivated by the cooperation of macrophages and lymphocytes.

In contrast to the site of deposition of particles, which is governed by size, the depth of penetration of inhaled gases is governed by water solubility.[10] The more water-soluble a gas, the more proximally it is retained. For example, sulfur oxides produced as atmospheric pollutants are very water-soluble and deposit almost entirely in the nasopharynx. Oxides of nitrogen, such as nitrogen dioxide (NO_2), a major component of photochemical smog, are less soluble and more likely to reach the lower airways. Ozone (O_3) is relatively insoluble in water and is the most likely to reach the peripheral airways and alveolar spaces.[11] Gases also may enter the lung dissolved in fine aqueous aerosols or absorbed on the surface of suspended particles. In this case, they will cause local effects wherever the particles are deposited.

Soluble Factors in the Nasopharynx

The major soluble defensive factor in the nasopharynx is IgA, a secretory immunoglobulin.[12] IgA is a "boundary immunoglobulin" because it is the major secretory immunoglobulin in the upper airways, gut mucosa, tears, and breast milk. It is also the predominant immunoglobulin in the nasopharynx and salivary secretions. The concentration of IgA exceeds that of IgG in nasal washings by about threefold. Most of the IgA exists in dimeric form in nasal and airway secretions, two molecules of IgA being connected via the heavy chains by a protein called the *J chain*. A second glycoprotein, termed the *secretory component*, also joins the

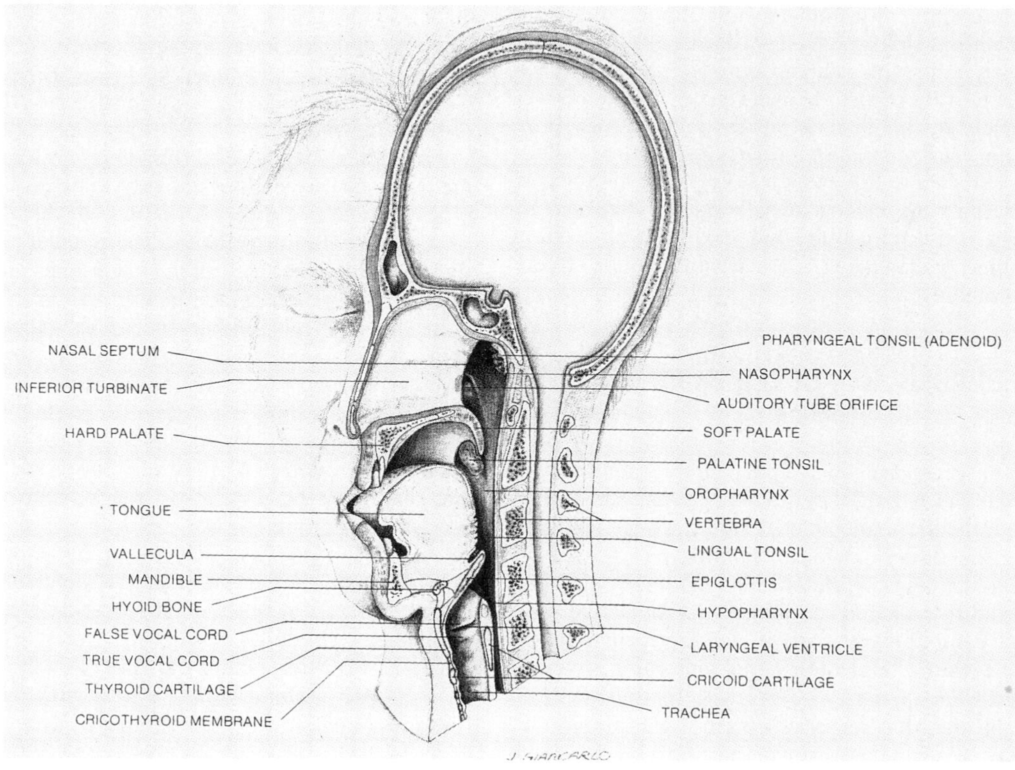

Figure 17-1. Side view of the nasopharynx showing the oral and nasal air passages. The tonsils are located in the region in which particle deposition is greatest due to inertial impaction. (From Appelbaum and Bruce,[75] with permission.)

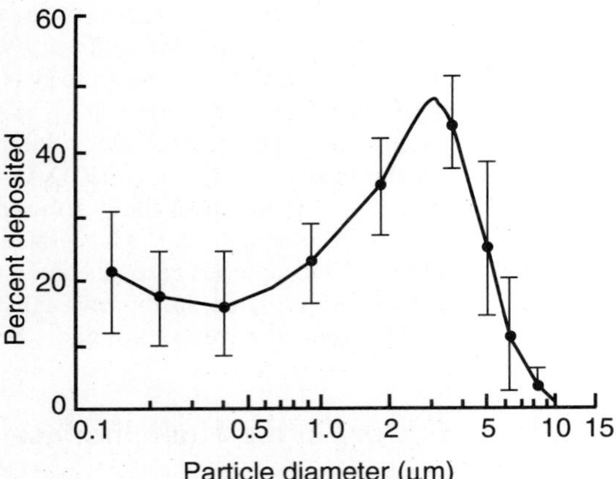

Figure 17-2. Particle deposition in the lower airways during mouth breathing. Particle diameter is plotted on the x axis against deposition on the y axis. Larger particles (> 10 μm) do not reach the lower airways because they are deposited in the nose and mouth. Deposition is maximal for particles 2 to 3 μm in aerodynamic size. (From Lippman,[74] with permission.)

heavy chains of the two IgA molecules and may serve as an anchor for dimeric IgA in epithelial cell membranes. The two isotypes of IgA, IgA_1 and IgA_2, are both present in upper airway secretions. IgA binds inhaled antigens, neutralizes viruses, and interferes with the adhesion of bacteria to the respiratory mucosa. Unlike IgG, IgA does not fix complement and does not function as an opsonin to promote phagocytosis of particles by neutrophils and macrophages. Some bacterial species, including most strains of *Streptococcus pneumoniae* and *Haemophilus influenzae*, produce an IgA protease that can cleave IgA, which suggests a role for IgA protease in the pathogenesis of these bacterial infections in the lungs.[13] The secretory peptide that joins the heavy chains of two IgA molecules makes IgA less sensitive to the effects of bacterial proteases.

Clinical Relevance of Upper Airway Defenses

The most important aspect of upper airway defenses in critically ill patients is that they are very often eliminated by modern therapeutic maneuvers. Upper airway defenses constitute the first line of defense, limiting penetration of particulates into the lungs. The placement of an endotracheal tube bypasses all these defenses and permits the delivery of aerosols directly into the lower airways. Endotracheal tubes also bypass the glottis, eliminating this important physical barrier to the lower airways. Studies with methylene blue dye have established that secretions often drain around the outside of endotracheal tubes through the glottis directly into the lower airway, thus providing organisms in the pharynx direct access to the lower airways. Endotracheal tubes therefore eliminate the normal barriers in the upper airway that limit particle penetration into the lungs. In addition, they eliminate the neutralizing effects of IgA in nasopharyngeal fluids. This places an important responsibility on the providers of respiratory care to ensure that the aerosols generated in the inspiratory circuits of mechanical ventilators are not contaminated with bacteria or other foreign material.

DEFENSE MECHANISMS IN THE CONDUCTING AIRWAYS

In the conducting airways (Fig. 17-3), two defensive factors limit the penetration of particles that pass through the upper airway, namely, physical forces that favor particle deposition and airway reflexes that narrow airway diameter and stimulate cough. Once particles enter the conducting airways, they are cleared by the mucociliary system. In addition, soluble substances in airway fluids help to limit the toxicity of inspired particles and to inactivate infective agents.

Physical Factors in the Conducting Airways

In contrast to larger particles with greater momentum, particles of about 5 to 10 μm in diameter pass through the nasopharynx and deposit predominantly in the conducting airways by sedimentation under the force of gravity.[8] These particles fall on the ciliated surfaces of the conducting airways, and the mucociliary system carries them up and out of the airways.

Particles less than 1 μm in diameter are very likely to enter the lower airway but are unlikely to deposit on the surfaces of the conducting airways because of their small mass and slow sedimentation velocity. These small particles are carried into the distal airspaces of the lungs, where their deposition is governed predominantly by diffusion (i.e., by random collisions with other suspended particles, gas molecules, and alveolar walls). In the terminal airways and alveolar spaces, where airflow is extremely slow, the likelihood of deposition is greatest for particles approximately 2 μm in diameter, which have a deposition efficiency of about 40 percent, that is, 40 percent of the particles of this size that enter the respiratory tree would be expected to deposit in the terminal airways and in the alveoli. Therefore, in contrast to pollens, (100 μm in diameter) which deposit predominantly in the nasopharynx, aerosolized bacteria (of diameter 1 μm or less) are much more likely to reach the airspaces of the lungs, especially if they are inhaled in fine aerosols. If bacteria enter the lower airway in a larger bolus of aspirated oropharyngeal secretions, they will deposit more proximally in the conducting airways.

As in the oropharynx, the water solubility of gases determines the extent to which the gases penetrate the lower airways. As noted earlier, the less water-soluble gases such as O_3 penetrate to the alveolar surface, whereas the more sol-

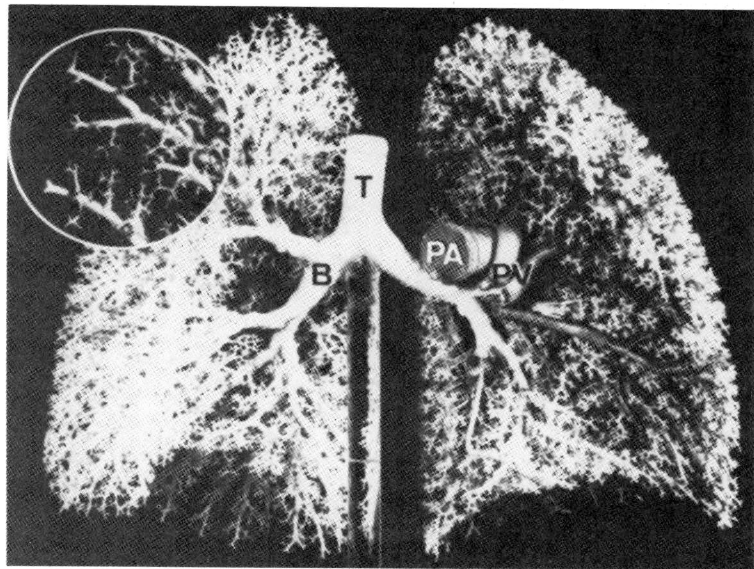

Figure 17-3. Bronchial tree cast. T, trachea; B, main bronchus; PA, pulmonary artery; PV, pulmonary vein. (From Weibel,[1] with permission.)

uble gases dissolve in the fluids of the more proximal airways, where they produce their effects.

Airway Reflexes

Clinicians usually think of cough and bronchoconstriction as symptoms that require treatment, but they also are very important defensive mechanisms in the lung.[14] Cough is one of the most important means of clearing the lower airway, and efforts to improve cough are often crucial to the prevention of pneumonia in critically ill patients. The cough reflex is vagally mediated and begins when irritant receptors are triggered in the airway.[15] The cricopharyngeal muscles constrict, closing the glottis; the diaphragm and intercostal muscles then contract forcefully, which rapidly raises intrathoracic pressure, causing the glottis to open suddenly and air to be expelled forcefully from the thorax at very high speeds. The shearing force generated along the airway walls propels mucus upward out of the chest and into the environment. In experimental studies that measured the clearance of radiolabeled aerosols, cough was much more effective in removing particles from the lower airways than chest percussion, incentive spirometry, or intermittent positive pressure breathing.[14]

Bronchoconstriction also serves a defensive function. Like the cough reflex, bronchoconstriction can be triggered by vagally mediated impulses from irritant receptors in the airways.[14,16] The resulting contraction of smooth muscle that spirals around the medium and small airways decreases airway caliber, and this reduction in airway cross-sectional area limits the penetration of inhaled particles into the distal lung units. Airflow is speeded in the narrowed airways, which helps to move mucus and trapped particles upward during exhalation. Although bronchoconstriction is a normal defensive mechanism in the airways, the bronchoconstriction response is exaggerated in all patients with clinical asthma and in many patients with obstructive airways disease and results in clinical symptoms.

Mucociliary System

The mucociliary system moves inhaled particles that deposit on the conducting airways upward toward the glottis. This complex system consists of ciliated columnar epithelial cells lining the surface of the airways, specialized mucus-producing goblet cells interspersed among the ciliated epithelial cells, and serous and goblet cells in submucosal glands (Fig. 17-4).[17] Goblet cells and ciliated epithelial cells decrease in number toward the periphery of the airways and are scarce in the respiratory bronchioles. In normal subjects who do not smoke, the turnover of ciliated epithelial cells is very slow, on the order of months. In the large and medium-sized airways, differentiating basal epithelial cells replace the surface epithelial cells. The luminal surface of each ciliated cell contains up to 200 cilia, each of which contains nine pairs of filaments arranged circumferentially around one central pair (Fig. 17-5). Small dynein arms act as hooks to bridge each pair of filaments.[18–20] Cilia bend when pairs of filaments slide along each other in an energy-dependent process that requires adenosine triphosphate (ATP). Cilia beat with a rapid stroke that is directed toward the larynx and a slower caudal recovery stroke. Ciliary beat frequencies exceeding 1000 bpm have been recorded experimentally.[17] The motion of adjacent cilia is coordinated so that waves of ciliary motion move toward the larynx. The cilia are surrounded by an aqueous layer of periciliary fluid that is se-

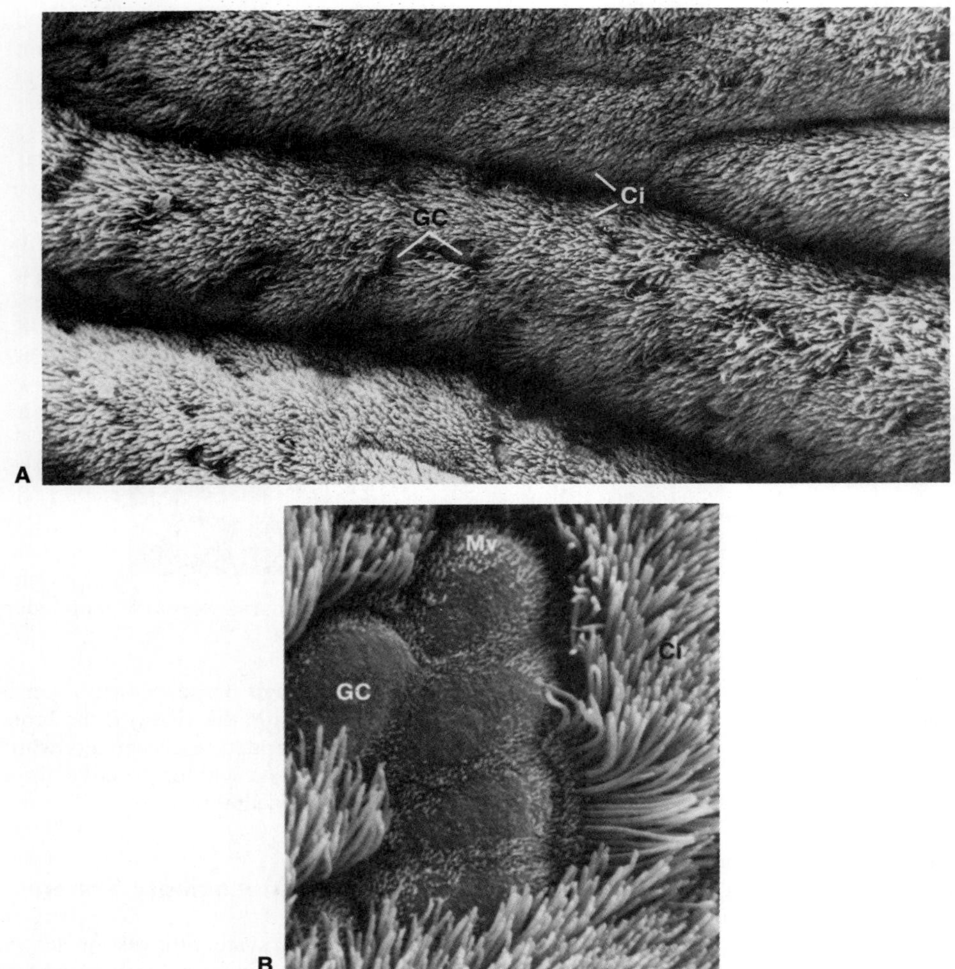

Figure 17-4. Normal ciliated bronchial mucosa as seen in scanning electron micrographs. (**A**) Continuous "shag carpet" surface consisting of cilia (CI) interspersed with occasional mucus-producing goblet cells (GC). The folded appearance results from incomplete distension of the specimen during fixation. (**B**) Higher-power view showing delicate filamentous nature of cilia along with several goblet cells (GC) from which mucus has been removed. (From Kessel and Kardon,[76] with permission.)

creted by the active transport of chloride and the passive movement of water across the epithelium into the airway lumen. The depth of this periciliary layer is probably critical for optimal mucus transport.[21] The ciliary tips are thought to make contact with mucus floating on the periciliary fluid during the fast stroke and then to bend below the mucus during the recovery stroke. This facilitates unidirectional movement of mucus toward the larynx.

Mucus is produced in goblet cells and submucosal glands and extruded onto the surface of the airways.[22] Although it was originally thought that mucus covered the conducting airways in a continuous blanket, it is clear from experimental observations and theoretical calculations that the mucus layer is not continuous in normal humans and animals. Rather, mucus coalesces into flakes, which float on the periciliary layer. Mucus consists of tangles of complex mucopolysaccharide polymers connected by hydrogen bonds. Disulfide bonds were originally thought to connect the mucus polymers, but this would result in very inelastic properties. It now is clear that hydrogen bonding accounts for most of the three-dimensional structure of mucus. Mucus has viscoelastic properties, so that when stretched it contracts, facilitating movement up the airway by ciliary activity. As mucus moves upward along the airway surfaces, eddies form at airway branch points, where clearance is slower. This provides an interesting correlation with the finding that neoplasia occurs more commonly at or near airway branchings.

The state of hydration of the mucus and the ionic concentration of the airway secretions are important factors that influence the viscosity of mucus.[23] Patients with cystic fibrosis have abnormally thick and tenacious airway secretions, which contain increased concentrations of Cl^- and Na^+.[24] These patients have mutations in a critical gene that codes for a protein that functions in the regulation of Cl^-

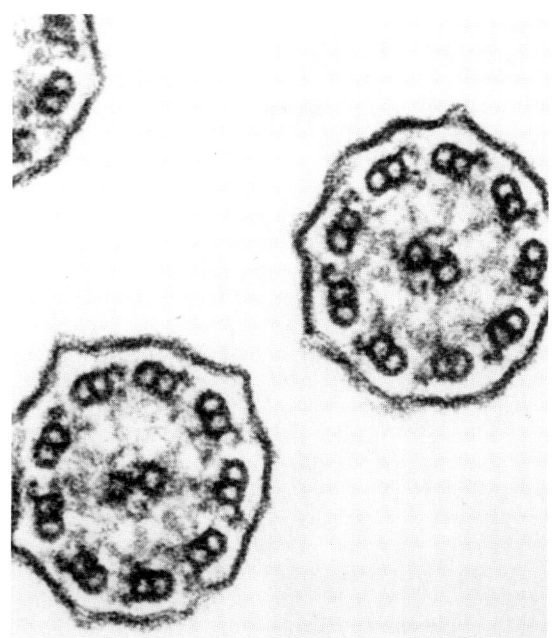

Figure 17-5. Electron micrograph of airway cilia in cross section showing the microtubules and dyneian arms extending between adjacent outer pairs of microtubules. (From Corrin,[77] with permission.)

secretion through Cl^- channels in airway epithelial cell membranes.[25] This impairs the movement of water into the airway lumen and results in thick airway secretions and impaired mucociliary clearance.

Mucociliary transport rates are fastest in the trachea and slowest in the peripheral airways[18]: the half-time for clearance of 5 to 6 μm particles is about 3 minutes in the trachea, 30 minutes in medium-sized airways, and hours to months in distal airways approaching the alveolar surface. Mucociliary transport is slowed by drying of the airway, which presumably leads to thicker mucus and altered composition of the periciliary fluid. Chronic exposure to cigarette smoke also slows mucociliary transport. This is relevant for patients with chronic bronchitis, who have reduced mucociliary transport rates. Environmental pollutants such as SO_2, NO_2, and O_3 all slow mucociliary transport rates in animals when inhaled in high concentrations (e.g., 5 ppm or greater).[10] The effects of these agents at the lower concentrations present in atmospheric pollution, especially in individuals without lung disease, remains a subject of debate.

The activity of the mucociliary system is regulated by neurohumoral stimuli.[16,26] Sensory and motor nerve fibers are present in the mucosa and submucosa of large airways, ending near the bases of ciliated epithelial cells and mucous glands. Alpha- and beta-adrenergic and peptidergic receptors all have been identified by using histochemical methods. Substance P and vasoactive intestinal peptide (VIP) appear to be the predominant peptidergic transmitters in the airway mucosa.

Neurohumoral stimuli alter mucociliary transport, secretion by serous and by mucous glands, and the anatomy of mucous glands.[27] Direct stimulation of vagal and adrenergic nerves increases mucous gland secretion and water transport into the airway lumen in humans and animals and increases mucociliary transport. Whether the increase in mucociliary transport is a direct effect or is a consequence of the increased load of secretions is uncertain. Similarly, alpha- and beta-adrenergic stimulation, cholinergic stimulation, and substance P all increase both mucus secretion by submucosal glands and water movement across the tracheal epithelium. In animals alpha-adrenergic stimuli cause watery mucous gland secretions of low viscosity and produce histologic evidence of serous cell secretion. Beta-adrenergic agonists result in mucous gland secretions that are lower in volume and higher in protein content and viscosity and produce histologic evidence of mucous cell depletion.

Ciliary beating is stimulated by cholinergic and beta-adrenergic agonists, but alpha-adrenergic agonists seem to have little direct effect on ciliary activity.[21] Atropine reduces ciliary activity in vivo and slows net mucociliary transport, but the basal rate of secretion is not affected. Interestingly, ipratropium bromide, an anticholinergic bronchodilator agent in widespread clinical use, has no effect on either ciliary beating or mucociliary transport at clinically used doses.

These experimental observations correctly predict that a number of different drugs commonly used in the treatment of critically ill patients alter mucociliary function.[27] In addition to adrenergic and cholinergic agents, methylxanthines stimulate ciliary beating and mucociliary transport, presumably by increasing intracellular cyclic adenosine monophosphate (cAMP) levels. Narcotic agents, including codeine, depress ciliary beat frequency and mucociliary transport in animals. Ethanol depresses mucus transport in direct relation to blood alcohol concentration. Barbiturates used as general anesthetics slow tracheal mucus transport rates in a variety of animal models. Topical anesthetics such as cocaine, tetracaine, and lidocaine all have concentration-dependent depressive effects on ciliary beating.

Although mucolytic agents and expectorants are widely available in over-the-counter medications, their usefulness in improving mucociliary transport remains uncertain (see Ch. 20). Clinical reports suggest that oral guaifenesin and bromhexine may slightly improve mucociliary clearance of inhaled particles in patients with chronic bronchitis, but they have little effect in normal subjects.

Substances in Airway Fluids

Immunoglobulins and other proteins present in airway secretions have important defensive functions in conducting airways. Unlike the nasopharynx, in which IgA is the predominant immunoglobulin, the concentrations of IgA and IgG are about equal in the fluid lining the large airways. The proportion of IgG increases distally in the conducting airways and the concentration of IgG exceeds that of IgA about fourfold at the alveolar level.

In the lower airway and the alveolar surface, IgG is the major immunoglobulin.[28] Each of the four isotypes of IgG is present in bronchoalveolar lavage specimens from humans. The function of IgG differs from that of IgA in important ways. IgG fixes complement and opsonizes bacteria, which increases the efficiency of phagocytosis by macrophages and neutrophils. IgG can be produced locally in the lung parenchyma by B lymphocytes recruited to the lung during humoral immune responses. Prior immunization of the lungs with an antigen results in the local production by lymphocytes of antigen-specific IgG molecules following rechallenge with the immunizing antigen.[29] Deficiencies of IgG subclasses IgG_2 and IgG_4, usually occurring together with IgA deficiency, are associated with recurrent respiratory tract infections and bronchiectasis.

Normally only trace amounts of IgM are found in airway fluids, but the concentration of IgM rises during inflammatory responses in the lung, either by local production or by exudation from the plasma into the lung. In the airway mucosa and submucosa, IgE is found bound to the surface of mast cells and basophils in the tissue.[30] When antigens penetrate the respiratory epithelium, they bind to several molecules of IgE on the mast cell surface. This "bridging" of adjacent IgE molecules triggers the secretion of mast cell granules and the release of histamine and other potent inflammatory mediators into the submucosa. These mediators increase epithelial permeability, cause bronchoconstriction, and recruit inflammatory cells into the airway walls.

Lysozyme and lactoferrin are two additional antibacterial proteins that are present in airway secretions. Lysozymes, a group of hydrolytic enzymes that lyse bacteria by attacking cell wall mucopolysaccharides,[31] are present in tears and in the secretions of airway submucosal glands. Lactoferrin is a 90,000-dalton Fe-binding protein, which is found in airway secretions and is also a constituent of neutrophil-specific granules.[32] Although lactoferrin has little direct antibacterial effect, it may serve to limit the availability of iron for bacterial metabolism. In addition, iron bound to lactoferrin may play a role in the generation of toxic oxygen species such as the hydroxyl radical from hydrogen peroxide (H_2O_2) and molecular O_2.

DEFENSE MECHANISMS OF THE ALVEOLAR MEMBRANE

Structure of the Alveolar Surface

The alveolar membrane provides the closest interface between blood and the outside environment. This thin epithelial layer lies beyond the mucociliary defenses of the conducting airways, and a different system of defenses has evolved to protect it. Although alveolar fluids contain soluble factors that can inactivate some bacteria and inhaled particles, resident and recruited phagocytes play the major role in the defense of the alveolar surface against infection.

Most of the thin alveolar surface is covered by type I pneumocytes, which are flattened epithelial cells that adhere to a basement membrane scaffold[17,33] (Fig. 17-6). Capillary endothelial cells are anchored to the other side of this scaffold, providing for very close contact between blood and air. Type II pneumocytes are specialized epithelial cells found in the corners of alveoli.[17,34] They differentiate into type I pneumocytes during repair processes in the lung. They also produce surfactant, a mixture of lipids that reduces surface tension and decreases the tendency of alveoli and terminal bronchioles to collapse at low lung volumes. Surfactant lipids are bactericidal toward some bacteria, particularly gram-positive organisms present in oral secretions.[35] Gram-negative organisms are resistant to the effects of surfactant but can be injured by one or more partially characterized peptides present in alveolar fluids.[19] Surfactant also has some opsonic properties, as it promotes the phagocytosis of *Staphylococcus aureus* by alveolar macrophages in vitro. Surfactant may also help to reduce the toxicity of inhaled particles by coating the particles and altering their surface composition or charge. In the case of crystalline silica, which is highly toxic, this change in surface chemistry minimizes the interactions between the particles and biologic membranes and greatly reduces toxicity.[36]

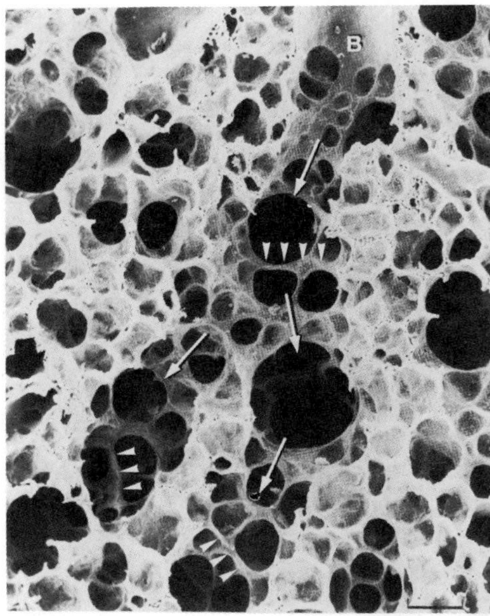

Figure 17-6. Scanning electron micrograph of lung parenchyma showing interconnecting airspaces. Arrows indicate alveolar ducts. Arrowheads highlight network of axial support structures in walls of alveolar ducts. B, terminal bronchiole. Scale marker = 100 μm. (From Weibel and Bachofen,[78] with permission.)

The predominant immunoglobulin in bronchoalveolar fluids is IgG,[7] although IgM accumulates during inflammatory reactions. Complement components also are present, which along with IgG serve as opsonins for inhaled particles, promoting phagocytosis by macrophages and neutrophils.

Role of the Alveolar Macrophage

In the normal lung, a few alveolar macrophages (less than one in each alveolus) are present on the alveolar surface[7] (Fig. 17-7). Alveolar macrophages are relatively long-lived

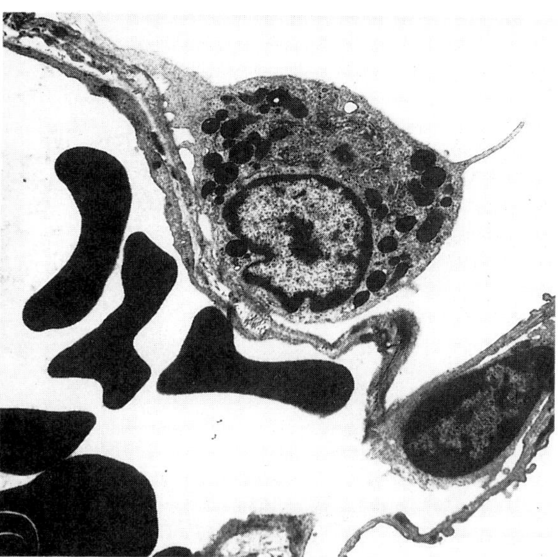

Figure 17-7. Transmission electron micrograph of an alveolar macrophage in an airspace. The electron dense structures are erythrocytes in a blood vessel. The alveolar wall is a thin unicellular structure. The alveolar macrophage adheres to the type I pneumocyte that makes up the alveolar wall in this region. A capillary containing several erythrocytes is seen in the lower left. (From Corrin,[77] with permission.)

cells and are derived predominantly from bone marrow precursors, although they have a limited capacity to replicate locally in the alveoli during inflammatory processes. Following bone marrow transplantation, most of the recoverable macrophages in bronchoalveolar lavage fluids have the donor phenotype by about 3 months. Alveolar macrophages leave the lung either by ascending the mucociliary pathway or by penetrating the epithelium and migrating to regional lymph nodes.

Alveolar macrophages are active phagocytes and can ingest inorganic mineral particulates and bacteria.[37,38] In addition, they also can ingest erythrocytes, other leukocytes, and various inflammatory products. Alveolar macrophages have been called the primary defenders of the alveolar spaces, and this is undoubtedly true for inorganic particulates that reach the alveolar surface. Inhaled mineral particles that reach the respiratory bronchioles and alveolar surface are ingested rapidly by alveolar macrophages and persist for months in macrophages recovered by bronchoalveolar lavage. Indeed, in one study the clearance half-time for inhaled respirable radioactive volcanic ash in rodents was determined as 39 days.[39]

In contrast to mineral particles, bacteria are ingested and killed much more slowly by alveolar macrophages than by circulating neutrophils and monocytes. The rate at which alveolar macrophages ingest bacteria varies with the bacterial species. For example, *Staphylococcus epidermidis* is ingested and killed rapidly in vitro, whereas *S. aureus*, most gram-negative rods, and organisms that stimulate cell-mediated immune responses (e.g., *Mycobacterium tuberculosis, Legionella pneumophila,* and *Listeria monocytogenes*) are phagocytosed poorly. Alveolar macrophages have surface receptors for complement and the Fc fragment of immunoglobulins. Opsonization of bacteria with complement and specific IgG markedly improves the rate of phagocytosis. During phagocytosis, alveolar macrophages undergo a respiratory burst and produce superoxide anion (O_2^-) and H_2O_2, but the amount produced is much less than that produced by neutrophils unless the macrophages have been activated by immunologic stimuli. In contrast to blood neutrophils and monocytes, alveolar macrophages lack myeloperoxidase, an enzyme that catalyzes the conversion of H_2O_2 and Cl^- or iodide ion (I^-) to hypohalous acids, which are powerful reducing agents. Therefore alveolar macrophages have a more limited range of toxic oxygen metabolites than neutrophils. Organisms coated experimentally with peroxidase are killed faster by alveolar macrophages, indicating that alveolar macrophages can use exogenous peroxidase to augment bacterial killing.[40]

Studies measuring the clearance of inhaled or injected bacteria in rodents have shown that alveolar macrophages do not function as the sole antibacterial defenders of the alveolar spaces. Rather, the type of phagocyte response depends on the bacterial species,[41] the inhaled bacterial dose, and possibly the method of inoculation. When low numbers of *S. aureus* organisms are inhaled, they are cleared rapidly, and the clearance correlates with their ingestion by alveolar macrophages. When the inhaled dose is higher, neutrophils are recruited into the alveolar spaces and ingest the organisms. Gram-negative organisms such as *Klebsiella pneumoniae* and *Pseudomonas aeruginosa* are not cleared in animals depleted of neutrophils[41] and are phagocytosed poorly by alveolar macrophages in vivo. Similarly, the recruitment of lymphocytes and activated macrophages is important for organisms cleared by cell-mediated immune mechanisms. Thus, the alveolar macrophage functions as a first-line defender of the alveolar spaces, but the recruitment of systemic phagocytes and lymphocytes into the lung also is a crucial component of lung antibacterial defenses.

Enzymes and Other Products of Alveolar Macrophages

Alveolar macrophages contain large amounts of three different general types of enzymes that may be important in inflammatory responses in the lung, namely, lysozyme, acid hydrolases, and neutral proteases.[38] Lysozyme is a major secretory protein that attacks disaccharides in bacterial cell walls. Gram-negative bacteria that have thick outer lipid coats protecting their cell walls are not affected by lysozyme. Acid hydrolases function primarily intracellularly, but they also can be released during phagocytosis, and in an acid environment they can degrade collagen and basement membrane constituents. The major neutral proteases include elastase, collagenase, and plasminogen activator. Alveolar macrophage elastase differs from neutrophil elastase in that it is a metalloprotease, and it is much less active than neutrophil elastase against elastin substrates.[42] Furthermore, alveolar macrophage elastase is not inhibited by alpha-1-antitrypsin, the major serum antiproteinase that neutralizes neutrophil elastase. Neutrophil elastase can be identified in alveolar macrophages under some conditions; however, because alveolar macrophages have surface receptors for neutrophil elastase they can take up and then later release active neutrophil elastase when stimulated. This allows alveolar macrophages to sequester inflammatory products but also provides a mechanism for their subsequent release.

Like other macrophages, alveolar macrophages synthesize and release a variety of lipid and protein products that can initiate and modulate inflammatory reactions in the lung. During phagocytosis alveolar macrophages release leukotriene B_4, a lipoxygenase product of membrane arachidonic acid that stimulates the directed migration (chemotaxis) of neutrophils[43] and to a lesser extent of monocytes. Leukotriene B_4 in the airspaces recruits neutrophils from the capillaries into the airspaces, expanding the phagocyte population with cells that have more potent microbicidal activity.[44] Leukotriene B_4 also attracts fibroblasts, which may be important in repair processes. In response to bacterial endotoxin, alveolar macrophages also produce a potent chemotactic peptide, interleukin-8 (IL-8), which attracts neutrophils from the bloodstream into the lungs.[45–47]

Alveolar macrophages produce a number of proteins that are important in inflammatory responses. Among these products are interleukin-1 (IL-1), tumor necrosis factor (TNF-alpha), IL-8, several different growth factors, and procoagulants. IL-1 is a chemotactic factor for lymphocytes and initiates the proliferation of responsive T lymphocytes. It also causes fever and stimulates the synthesis of acute-phase reactants in the liver.[48] TNF-alpha, also known as *cachectin*, is produced by alveolar macrophages activated by endotoxin. TNF-alpha was originally found to cause necrosis of tumor cells, but when injected into living animals it causes intense ischemia of the bowel followed by shock.[49] TNF-alpha interrupts intermediary metabolism by reducing the activity of lipoprotein lipase in cell membranes. Like IL-1, TNF-alpha causes fever and the production of acute-phase proteins by the liver. Activation of alveolar macrophages increases the production of TNF-alpha and IL-1. Increased production of TNF-alpha by alveolar macrophages has been reported in patients with sarcoidosis. Alveolar macrophages also produce large amounts of platelet-derived growth factor (PDGF), a growth factor originally found in platelets that stimulates fibroblast proliferation.[50,51] Alveolar macrophages from patients with idiopathic pulmonary fibrosis have been found to produce large amounts of PDGF, which suggests that alveolar macrophage products may contribute to the ongoing fibrosis in this disorder.[52]

Other Phagocytic Cells of the Lung Parenchyma

Although the alveolar macrophage is the phagocytic cell of first contact in the lungs, neutrophils and lymphocytes recruited from the blood and systemic lymphoid tissue also have important roles in the defense of the alveolar membrane against infection. Neutrophils migrate into the lungs in response to signals from alveolar macrophages (e.g., leukotriene B_4 and IL-8) bacterial peptides, and activated complement components, of which C5a is the most potent. As noted previously, neutrophils are much more potent microbicidal cells than are alveolar macrophages because of the large amounts of reactive oxygen species (e.g., O_2^-, H_2O_2, and hydroxyl radical) that they produce during the respiratory burst stimulated by phagocytosis. Neutrophils are a typical feature of the pathology of lung bacterial infections, and animals depleted of neutrophils fail to clear aerosolized gram-negative organisms from the lungs.[41] In patients with granulocytopenia the lungs are a common site of bacterial infection.

GENERATION OF IMMUNE REACTIONS IN THE LUNGS

Immune reactions are either nonspecific or specific. Nonspecific immune reactions involve the interaction of foreign particles with pre-existing defensive mechanisms that are not specific for that particular type of particle. Specific immune reactions involve the generation of antibodies and/or cells that recognize and respond to the specific foreign particle.

Nonspecific Immune Reactions

Nonspecific immune, or defensive, reactions involve the interactions of inhaled particles with soluble factors in airway fluids and alveolar macrophages. This includes the neutralization of viruses by IgA in airway secretions and the phagocytosis of inorganic particles in urban air by alveolar macrophages if they reach the gas exchange parenchyma of the lungs. Bacteria that reach the gas exchange parenchyma are opsonized by IgG in alveolar fluid, which facilitates the recognition and uptake of the bacteria by alveolar macrophages. Bacterial peptides, complement fragment C5a, and signals from alveolar macrophages, including leukotriene B_4 and IL-8, recruit additional white blood cells from the bloodstream into the lungs. In the airspace these recruited phagocytes ingest the opsonized bacteria that evade alveolar macrophages. Although the recruitment of phagocytes from the bloodstream expands the phagocyte population in the lungs and enhances the elimination of invading microorganisms, this response usually is not specific for the organism that initiates it.

Specific Immune Reactions

Specific immune reactions involve the participation of lymphocytes and macrophages that cooperate to eliminate or inactivate the infective agent. Two major types of specific immune responses occur in the lungs, humoral and cellular (Fig. 17-8). It is unlikely that these responses occur primarily

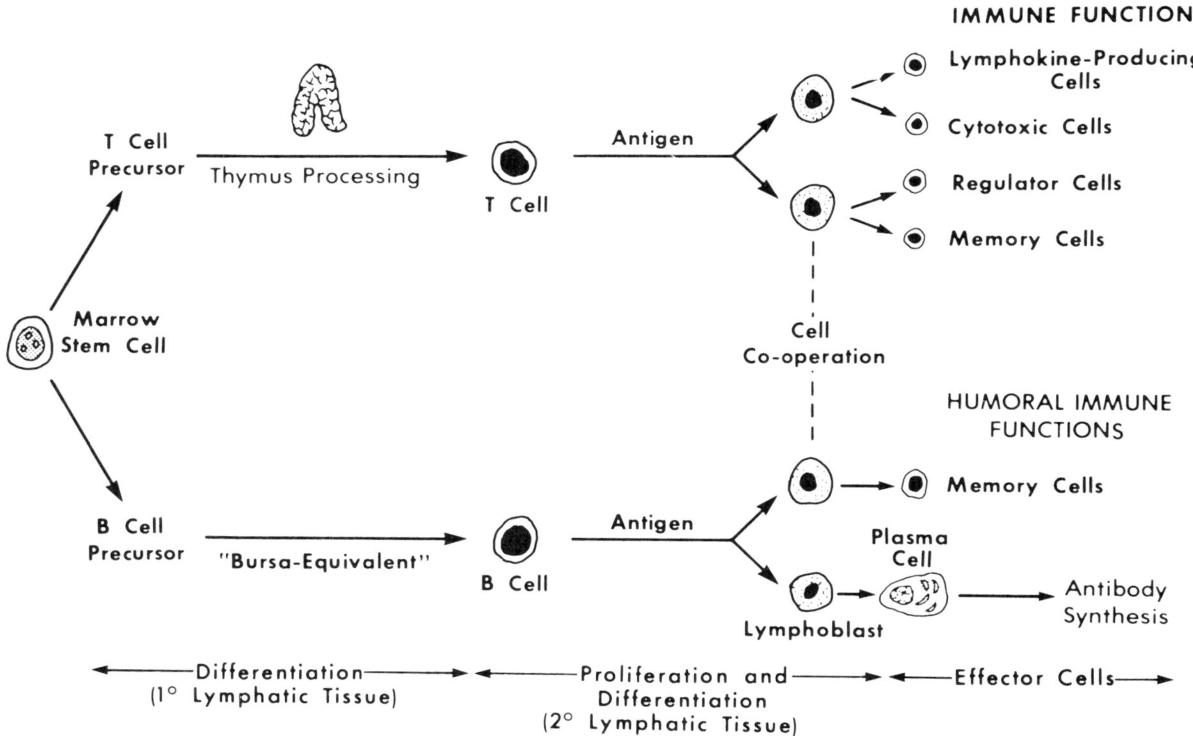

Figure 17-8. Diagram of the humoral and cell-mediated immune systems. Marrow stem cells give rise to T cell and B cell precursors. Following antigen stimulation, T cells differentiate into effector cells of cell mediated immunity. B cells differentiate into plasma cells that produce specific antibodies. (From Kaltreider,[29] with permission.)

in the lung parenchyma in response to inhaled antigens; rather, they require the cooperation of alveolar macrophages and lymphocytes in regional and systemic lymphoid tissue. As noted earlier, alveolar macrophages are found in the airspaces of the lungs, and one of their functions is to recognize foreign antigens and present them to responsive lymphocytes. Lymphoid tissue is scant in the lung parenchyma, but it occurs in lymph nodes in the drainage pathways from the gas exchange parenchyma and airways of the lungs. Lymph nodes are complex collections of B lymphocytes, T lymphocytes, and macrophages. Foreign antigens in the airspaces penetrate the airway epithelium and travel in the lymph fluid to lymph nodes, where they are recognized by macrophages or other accessory cells. Alternatively, foreign particles in the airspace may be taken up by alveolar macrophages, which can migrate through the airway or alveolar walls to reach the regional lymph nodes.

Humoral Immune Responses

Humoral immune responses involve the activation of specific B lymphocytes to produce antibodies directed at antigens on the surface of the particle (e.g., bacterial, viral, fungal) that initiated the response in the lungs[53] (Fig. 17-9). These antibodies bind to the surface of the infective agent and promote the destruction of the foreign particle. For example, IgG antibodies fix complement and facilitate phagocytosis by neutrophils and macrophages. In addition, complement fixation on the surface of bacteria can lyse the organisms via a cascade of reactions that lead to disruption of the surface of the organism.

Humoral immune responses occur in two stages, an initial or priming response and a secondary or specific response.[29] The initial response results in the generation of clones of specific B cells that make antibodies specific for the initial antigen. This initial response occurs in regional and systemic lymphoid tissue, and antibody-forming cells do not accumulate in the lung parenchyma. However, when the antigen is introduced again into the lungs, these specific antibody-forming cells are recruited into the lungs and become localized to the site in which the specific antigen is located. This results in local production of high concentrations of specific antibody, which favors elimination of the primary antigen. This humoral response pattern in the lungs was originally identified in mice, but it is also characteristic of responses in dogs and primates. Thus, the system provides for an initial sensitization followed by localization of the immune response to the site of antigen deposition.

Clinical examples of humoral immune responses in the

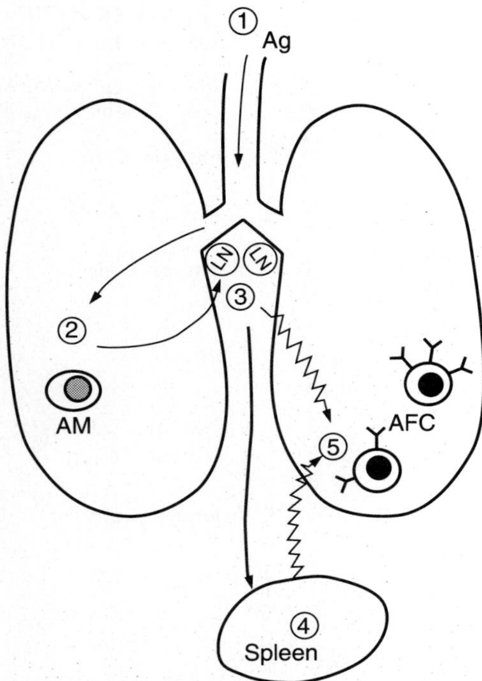

Figure 17-9. Induction of humoral immune responses in the lungs. Following entry of antigen (Ag) into the airspaces (1,2), antigen is transported to the regional lymph nodes (LN) in the lungs and the systemic lymphoid system (3,4), where specific antibody-forming cells (AFC) mature. When the antigen is reintroduced in the lungs, the specific antibody forming cells accumulate in the lungs at the site of the antigen (5).

lungs include the responses to vaccines, such as the influenza and pneumococcal vaccine. Vaccination stimulates the production of specific IgG antibodies by responding B cells in systemic lymphoid tissue. These antibodies circulate and are probably represented in the lung parenchymal fluids that contain IgG as the predominant antibody. Anti-influenzal IgG binds to inhaled influenza viruses and minimizes the chance that the viruses can penetrate epithelial cells in the airways and cause disease. Although the humoral response to the influenza vaccine is sustained, the virus changes antigenically from year to year and revaccination is required to maintain specific immunity. The pneumococcal vaccine stimulates the production of circulating IgG antibodies directed at antigenic determinants on the capsule of the pneumococcus. These antibodies bind to the capsule and thus promote rapid phagocytosis of the organisms by neutrophils in the lungs and facilitate the clearance of circulating organisms by the reticuloendothelial system. The specific humoral immune response to pneumococci is highly efficient in facilitating clearance of the organism, particularly in patients with compromised immune systems or absent spleens. Most patients with chronic obstructive pulmonary disease (COPD) have some pre-existing antibody to pneumococci. Although the pneumococcal vaccine causes a rise in titer of antipneumococcal IgG in the circulation, it has been difficult to prove that this offers these patients significant protection from pneumococcal pneumonia.[54–56]

Cellular Immune Responses

Cellular immune responses involve the participation of macrophages that recognize a specific foreign antigen and of T-helper lymphocytes, which produce proteins that activate macrophages to eliminate the original antigen[29] (Fig. 17-10). Two clinical examples of cellular immune responses in the lungs include the immune reactions involved in tuberculosis and legionellosis (Legionnaire's disease). In cellular immune reactions the invading organism evades ingestion and killing by neutrophils for poorly understood reasons. Initially, the organisms that reach the airspaces proliferate in the lungs, often inside alveolar macrophages. The alveolar macrophages digest some of the intracellular organisms, and in a process called *antigen processing and presentation* some of the partially digested bacterial proteins are combined with macrophage proteins and transported to the surface of the macrophage.[57] These bacterial protein fragments on the surface of the macrophages are recognized by T-helper lymphocytes, which bind to the macrophage. At the same time the macrophage produces IL-1, which stimulates the responding T cells to begin proliferation. These T cells in turn produce a second protein called interleukin-2 (IL-2), which markedly enhances lymphocyte proliferation. This process leads to an expansion of the lymphocyte population in the lung parenchyma. The proliferating lymphocytes produce interferon-gamma (IFN-gamma), which activates macrophages, increasing their microbicidal activity so that they become able to eliminate the invading organisms or at least to limit their intracellular proliferation. A successful cell-mediated immune response eliminates some organisms (e.g., *Legionella*) from the lungs, whereas with other pathogens (e.g., *M. tuberculosis*) the cell-mediated immune response prevents the proliferation of the organisms but may fail to eliminate all of them from the original focus of infection.

The exact locations in the lungs at which the various stages of the cell-mediated immune response occur remains uncertain. As noted previously, under normal circumstances few lymphocytes are found in the lung parenchyma. Furthermore, normal alveolar macrophages from humans are relatively poor antigen-presenting cells,[58] although they are capable of presenting antigen in vitro when the ratio of alveolar macrophages to lymphocytes is optimal.[59] In comparison, interstitial and lymph node dendritic cells isolated from human lung mincings are very effective antigen-presenting cells.[60] Therefore, it seems likely that, as with humoral responses, the regional lymphoid tissue is an important site for the initiation of cellular immune responses. The recruitment of activated macrophages and T-helper cells into the lungs is probably an important step in the development of cell-

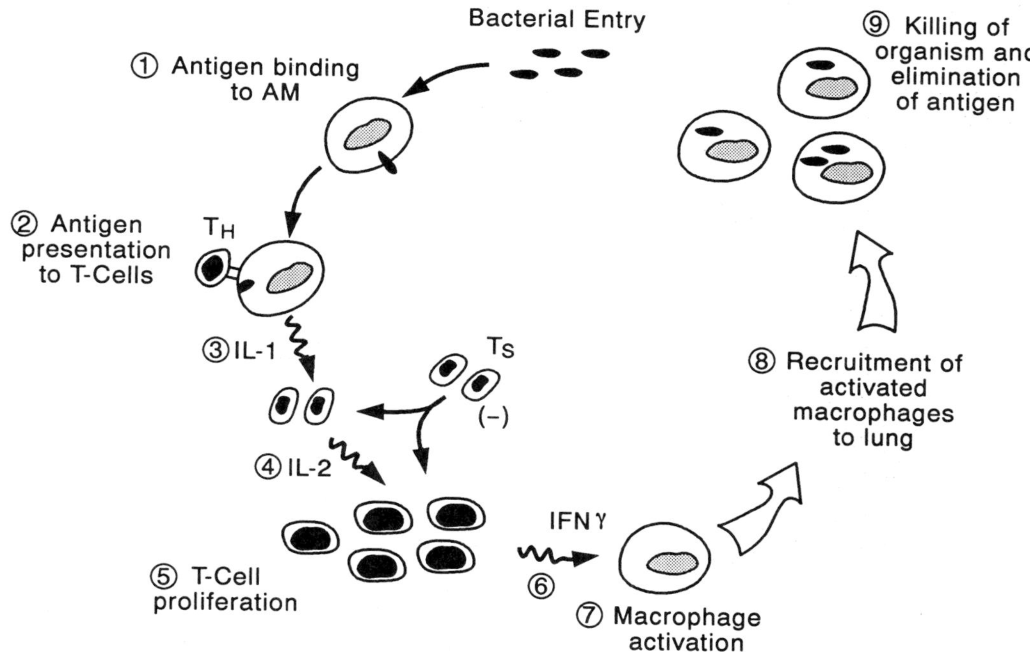

Figure 17-10. Induction of cell-mediated immune responses in the lungs. Following the entry of the bacterial or antigenic stimulus into the lungs, the material is taken up and processed by responding macrophages in the airspaces and regional lymphoid tissue (1). These macrophages present the antigen to responsive T lymphocytes (2), which proliferate (3–5) and release gamma interferon (6), which activates additional macrophages (7). In a successful cell-mediated immune response, these activated macrophages are capable of eliminating the antigen or killing the initial organism that stimulated the immune response (8,9).

mediated immune responses. Following experimental infection with organisms that stimulate cell-mediated immune responses, activated macrophages and T-helper cells accumulate in the lung parenchyma.

Misdirected Immune Reactions in the Lungs

Immune reactions that may occur in the lungs in response to unidentified stimuli can destroy normal lung tissue, causing clinical diseases in the lungs.[13] Both humoral and cell-mediated processes can occur, and sometimes the immune reactions are a mixture of both types of reactions. In still other cases the immune system is involved but the reaction does not fit the classical categories. Well-known clinical examples of misdirected immune reactions in the lungs include Goodpasture's syndrome, sarcoidosis, different types of vasculitis, eosinophilic pneumonia, and idiopathic interstitial fibrosis, among many others. Some evidence suggests that intrinsic asthma in adults also should be included on this list.

Goodpasture's syndrome is an example of a misdirected humoral reaction in which antibodies formed against an unknown antigen cross-react with determinants on the basement membrane of the lung microvasculature and the renal glomerulus.[61,62] The antibodies can be identified by immunofluorescence binding in a linear pattern to the basement membrane of capillaries in the lungs. Complement activation occurs, and neutrophils are attracted to the sites of antibody deposition. Toxic products released from the neutrophils, including proteases and oxidants, damage the microvasculature of the lungs and the kidneys. This damage causes hemoptysis and hematuria and can lead to pulmonary and renal insufficiency. Treatment is very difficult, but attempts to remove the circulating antibodies by plasmapheresis have sometimes been successful.

Sarcoidosis is an example of an idiopathic cell-mediated immune reaction in the lungs that destroys lung tissue.[63–65] Lymphocytes and macrophages accumulate and form granulomas in the lung parenchyma. The lymphocytes recovered by bronchoalveolar lavage spontaneously proliferate in tissue culture and release IL-2 and IFN-gamma, and alveolar macrophages are activated and spontaneously release IL-1 and TNF-alpha. Efforts to identify the antigen that initiates the immune response in sarcoidosis have so far been unsuccessful. In some patients with sarcoidosis, immunosuppression with corticosteroids or methotrexate helps to control the disease. Although these agents have many effects, their antiproliferative effects on lymphocytes may explain their beneficial effects in sarcoidosis.

Vasculitis reactions (angiitis) involve inflammatory reactions that occur in and around blood vessels.[66–69] Although several different types of vasculitis occur, all involve blood vessel destruction. In the lungs this results in pulmonary infiltrates and hemoptysis. Allergic angiitis involves small vessels throughout the body, with lesions that appear to be similar in age, as if the process began at the same time. Humoral immunity with antibody formation directed at unknown antigens may contribute to this form of vasculitis. Immune complex vasculitis is another form of vasculitis in which misdirected humoral immunity is important. Antigen-antibody complexes formed in the circulation deposit in the microvasculature, causing local inflammation with destruction of small vessels. Granulomatous vasculitis, including Wegener's granulomatosis, is a destructive granulomatous reaction centered around small and medium-sized blood vessels in different organ systems. A limited form of Wegener's granulomatosis involves only the lungs and the kidneys and has a relatively good prognosis. This form of vasculitis appears to involve misdirected cell-mediated immunity, and treatment with immunosuppressive agents such as cyclophosphamide is often very successful.[67]

Idiopathic pulmonary fibrosis is a disease of unknown etiology characterized by increased numbers of alveolar macrophages in the airspaces and relentless proliferation of fibrous tissue in the lungs.[70,71] A number of hypotheses have been proposed to explain this disorder, yet none explains all the clinical data. Almost all patients with idiopathic pulmonary fibrosis have increased numbers of alveolar macrophages in bronchoalveolar lavage fluid. Some patients also have increased numbers of lymphocytes, and others have increased numbers of neutrophils or eosinophils. The alveolar macrophages from many of these patients appear to be activated in that they spontaneously release growth factors for fibroblasts and inflammatory cytokines. The production of growth factors could contribute to the proliferation of fibroblasts and the deposition of collagen in the lungs. Alveolar macrophages from some of these patients release large amounts of TNF-alpha when stimulated with endotoxin. Circulating immune complexes have been identified in the blood of some patients, suggesting that humoral immunity may be involved in the pathogenesis of this disorder in some cases.[72] These observations do not suggest an easy classification for the immune abnormality in idiopathic pulmonary fibrosis.

CLINICAL RELEVANCE OF HOST DEFENSES AND IMMUNE REACTIONS IN RESPIRATORY CARE

One of the most important roles of the clinician is to help in the defense of the lungs against infection through efforts to improve cough and mucociliary clearance and efforts to ensure that the aerosols used in respiratory care are not contaminated inadvertently with infectious agents. As noted earlier, a forceful cough is the most effective means of clearing the conducting airways. Studies measuring the clearance of inhaled radioactive particles have shown that particle clearance is much more rapid during a period of forceful coughing than with intermittent positive-pressure breathing (IPPB), exercise, or incentive spirometry. Cough is only effective in clearing the larger conducting airways, and effective clearance depends on the mucociliary system to move particles that deposit more peripherally up into the larger airways, where they can be cleared by cough. The crucial step in the generation of an effective cough is contraction of the respiratory muscles with the glottis closed, causing a sudden increase in intrathoracic pressure. When the glottis opens, the pressure gradient drives air from the airways upward at high velocity, generating high shear forces along the airway walls. Patients with weak respiratory muscles or inability to close the glottis completely are unable to generate high intrathoracic pressures, and the effectiveness of their cough is greatly diminished. Cough is greatly impaired in patients with COPD, in whom the airways are obstructed by secretions and collapse during exhalation because of loss of the normal elastic recoil forces of the lungs.

Clinicians encounter patients with diminished cough in intensive care units and also on the hospital wards. Intubated patients and those with tracheostomies or tracheal stomas following laryngectomy are typical examples of patients who cannot close the glottis. Respiratory muscle weakness occurs in patients with neuromuscular disease. Patients with thoracic or upper abdominal pain (e.g., following surgery) voluntarily fail to use ventilatory muscles effectively unless their pain is managed effectively. Patients with acute exacerbations of COPD often cough repeatedly, but luminal obstruction and early airway closure limit the effectiveness of their cough.

As noted earlier, many of the medications used in the treatment of patients in intensive care units interfere with effective cough and mucociliary clearance.[27,73] Although analgesics make it easier for patients to cough, narcotic analgesics suppress the cough reflex and reduce the patient's desire to cough. Narcotics also impair mucociliary clearance, reducing the rate at which debris from the peripheral airways is transported into the central airways, where cough is effective. Beta-agonist bronchodilators have the opposite effect, increasing mucociliary activity. The predominant effect in a patient receiving many different medications is usually impossible to predict with confidence.

The first important challenge to the clinician is to encourage effective coughing. This is best done in regular visits to the bedside and often can be combined with deep breathing exercises and chest physiotherapy. Although patients can be told to cough by any medical personnel, the respiratory care practitioner usually has the best training and the greatest interest in seeing that patients cough effectively.

The second important challenge to the clinician is to ensure that the aerosols used in respiratory care are not inadvertently contaminated with bacteria or fungi. Endotracheal intubation bypasses all the defense mechanisms of the upper airways, allowing aerosolized material direct access to the lower airways. Careful attention to the use of in-line filters and careful technique in mixing bronchodilator solutions are essential. In addition, small volumes of oropharyngeal secretions often pass down into the lower airway through the glottis around the outside of the endotracheal tube. This provides a route by which bacteria in the oropharynx can colonize the lower airway without entering the ventilator circuit.

References

1. Weibel ER: Design of airways and blood vessels considered as branching trees. pp. 711–720. In Crystal RG, West JB (eds): The Lung. Scientific Foundations. Raven Press, New York, 1991
2. Chang HK, Menon AS: Airflow dynamics in the human airways. pp. 77–122. In Moren F, Newhouse MT, Dolovitch MB (eds): Aerosols in Medicine. Principles, Diagnosis and Therapy. Elsevier, Amsterdam, 1985
3. Moren F, Newhouse MT, Dolovitch MB (eds): Aerosols in Medicine. Principles, Diagnosis and Therapy. Elsevier, Amsterdam, 1985
4. Helmers RA, Hunninghake GW: Bronchoalveolar lavage in the nonimmunocompromised patient. Chest 1989;96:1184–1190
5. Reynolds HY: Bronchoalveolar lavage. Am Rev Respir Dis 1987;135:250–263
6. Goldstein RA, Rohatgi PK, Bergofsky EH et al: Clinical role of bronchoalveolar lavage in adults with pulmonary disease. Am Rev Respir Dis 1990;142:481–486
7. The BAL Cooperative Group Steering Committee: Bronchoalveolar lavage constituents in healthy individuals, idiopathic pulmonary fibrosis and selected comparison groups. Am Rev Respir Dis 1990;141:S169–S202
8. Brain JD, Valberg PA, Sneddon S: Mechanisms of aerosol deposition and clearance. pp. 123–147. In Moren F, Newhouse MT, Dolovitch MB (eds): Aerosols in Medicine. Principles, Diagnosis and Therapy. Elsevier, Amsterdam, 1985
9. Jeffrey PK, Corrin B: Structural analysis of the respiratory tract. pp. 1–27. In Bienenstock J (ed): Immunology of the Lung and Upper Respiratory Tract. McGraw-Hill, New York, 1984
10. Schlesinger RB: The interaction of inhaled toxicants with respiratory tract clearance mechanisms. CRC Crit Rev Toxicol 1990;20:257–286
11. Lippmann M: Effects of ozone on respiratory function and structure. Annu Rev Public Health 1989;10:49–67
12. Brandtzaeg P: Immune functions of human nasal mucosa and tonsils in health and disease. pp. 28–95. In Bienenstock J (ed): Immunology of the Lung and Upper Respiratory Tract. McGraw-Hill, New York, 1984
13. Reynolds HY: Lung inflammation: Normal host defense or a complication of some diseases? Annu Rev Med 1987;38:295–323
14. Fuller RW, Jackson DM: The physiology and treatment of cough. Thorax 1990;45:425–430
15. Karlsson JA, Sant'Ambrogio G, Widdicombe J: Afferent neural pathways in cough and reflex bronchoconstriction. J Appl Physiol 1988;65:1007–1023
16. Barnes PJ: Neural control of human airways in health and disease. Am Rev Respir Dis 1986;134:1289–1314
17. Weibel ER: Lung cell biology. pp. 47–91. In Fishman AP, Fisher AB (eds): Handbook of Physiology. Section 3: The Respiratory System. American Physiological Society, Bethesda, 1985
18. Satir P, Sleigh MA: The physiology of cilia and mucociliary interactions. Annu Rev Physiol 1990;52:137–155
19. Lee RMKW, Forrest JB: Structure and function of cilia. pp. 169–181. In Crystal RG, West JB (eds): The Lung. Scientific Foundations. Raven Press, New York, 1991
20. Satir P, Dirksen ER: Function-structure correlations in cilia from mammalian respiratory tract. pp. 473–494. In Fishman AP, Fisher AB (eds): Handbook of Physiology. Section 3: The Respiratory System. American Physiological Society, Bethesda, 1985
21. Sleigh M: Mucus propulsion. pp. 189–196. In Crystal RG, West JB (eds): The Lung. Scientific Foundations. Raven Press, New York, 1991
22. Wu R, Carlson DM: Structure and function of mucins. pp. 183–188. In Crystal RG, West JB (eds): The Lung. Scientific Foundations. Raven Press, New York, 1991
23. Yeates DB: Mucus rheology. pp. 197–203. In Crystal RG, West JB (eds): The Lung. Scientific Foundations. Raven Press, New York, 1991
24. Welsh MJ: Abnormal chloride and sodium channel function in cystic fibrosis. pp. 2073–2082. In Crystal RG, West JB (eds): The Lung. Scientific Foundations. Raven Press, New York, 1991
25. Riordan JR, Rommens JM, Kerem B et al: Identification of the cystic fibrosis gene: Cloning and characterization of complementary DNA. Science 1989;245:1066–1073
26. Forrest JB: Lower airway: Structure and function. pp. 21–52. In Moren F, Newhouse MT, Dolovitch MB (eds): Aerosols in Medicine. Principles, Diagnosis and Therapy. Elsevier, Amsterdam, 1985
27. Nadel JA, Widdicombe JH, Peatfield AC: Regulation of airway secretions, ion transport, and water movement. pp. 419–445. In Fishman AP, Fisher AB (eds): Handbook of Physiology. American Physiological Society; 1986
28. Young KR Jr, Reynolds HY: Bronchoalveolar washings: Proteins and cells from normal lungs. pp. 157–173. In Bienenstock J (ed): Immunology of the Lung and Upper Respiratory Tract. McGraw-Hill, New York, 1984
29. Kaltreider HB: Local immunity. pp. 191–215. In Bienenstock J (ed): Immunology of the Lung and Upper Respiratory Tract. McGraw-Hill, New York, 1984
30. Casale TB, Kaliner M: Allergic reactions in the respiratory tract. pp. 326–344. In Bienenstock J (ed): Immunology of the Lung and Upper Respiratory Tract. McGraw-Hill, New York, 1984
31. Hinman LM, Stevens CA, Matthay RA, Gee JBL: Elastase and lysozyme activities in human alveolar macrophages. Am Rev Respir Dis 1980;121:263–271
32. Lehr RI, Ganz T: Antimicrobial polypeptides of human neutrophils. Blood 1990;76:2169–2181
33. Schneeberger EE: Alveolar type I cells. pp. 229–234. In Crystal RG, West JB (eds): The Lung. Scientific Foundations. Raven Press, New York, 1991
34. Mason RJ, Williams MC: Alveolar type II cells. pp. 235–246. In Crystal RG, West JB (eds): The Lung. Scientific Foundations. Raven Press, New York, 1991
35. Coonrod JD, Lester RL, Hsu LC: Characterization of the extracellular bactericidal factors of rat alveolar lining material. J Clin Invest 1984;74:1269–1279
36. Wallace WE Jr, Vallyathan V, Keane MJ, Robinson V: In vitro biologic effects of native and surface-modified silica and kaolin. J Toxicol Environ Health 1985;16:415–424
37. Brain JD: Macrophages in the respiratory tract. pp. 447–471. In Fishman AP, Fisher AB (eds): Handbook of Physiology. Section 3: The Respiratory System. American Physiological Society, Bethesda, 1985
38. Fels AO: The alveolar macrophage. J Appl Physiol 1986;60:353–369
39. Wehner AP, Wilerson CL, Stevens DL: Lung clearance of neutron activated volcanic ash in the rat. Environ Res 1984;35:211–217
40. Ramsey PG, Martin TR, Chi EY, Klebanoff SJ: Arming of mononuclear phagocytes by eosinophil peroxidase bound to *Staphylococcus aureus*. J Immunol 1982;128:415–420
41. Rehm SR, Gross GN, Pierce AK: Early bacterial clearance from murine lungs. Species-dependent phagocyte response. J Clin Invest 1980;66:194–199
42. Chapman HA Jr, Stone OL: Comparison of live human neutrophil and alveolar macrophage elastolytic activity in vitro. J Clin Invest 1984;74:1693–1700
43. Martin TR, Raugi G, Merritt TL, Henderson WR: Relative contribution of leukotriene B4 to the neutrophil chemotactic activity

produced by the resident human alveolar macrophage. J Clin Invest 1987;80:1114–1124
44. Martin TR, Pistorese BP, Chi EY et al: Effects of leukotriene B4 in the human lung. Recruitment of neutrophils into the alveolar spaces without a change in protein permeability. J Clin Invest 1989;84:1609–1619
45. Baggiolini M, Walz A, Kunkel SL: Neutrophil-activating peptide-1/interleukin 8, a novel cytokine that activates neutrophils. J Clin Invest 1989;84:1045–1049
46. Sylvester I, Rankin JA, Yoshimura T et al: Secretion of neutrophil attractant/activation protein (NAP-1) by lipopolysaccharide-stimulated lung macrophages determined by both enzyme-linked immunosorbent assay and N-terminal sequence analysis. Am Rev Respir Dis 1990;141:683–688
47. Goodman RB, Forsgren J, Chi EY, Martin TR: Identification of two neutrophil chemotactic peptides produced by porcine alveolar macrophages. J Biol Chem 1991;266:8455–8463
48. Dinarello CA: Biology of interleukin 1. FASEB J 1988;2:108–115
49. Beutler B, Cerami AA: Cachectin: More than a tumor necrosis factor. N Engl J Med 1987;316:379–385
50. Shimokado K, Raines EW, Madtes DK et al: A significant part of macrophage-derived growth factor consists of at least two forms of PDGF. Cell 1985;43:277–286
51. Mornex JF, Martinet Y, Yamauchi K et al: Spontaneous expression of the c-sis gene and release of a platelet-derived growth factorlike molecule by human alveolar macrophages. J Clin Invest 1986;78:61–66
52. Martinet Y, Rom WN, Grotendorst GR et al: Exaggerated spontaneous release of platelet-derived growth factor by alveolar macrophages from patients with idiopathic pulmonary fibrosis. N Engl J Med 1987;317:202–209
53. Willoughby WF, Willoughby JB: Antigen handling. pp. 174–190. In Bienenstock J (ed): Immunology of Lung and Upper Respiratory Tract. McGraw-Hill, New York, 1984
54. Leads from the MMWR: Recommendations of the Immunization Practices Advisory Committee. Pneumococcal polysaccharide vaccine. JAMA 1989;261:1265–1267
55. LaForce FM: Pneumococcal vaccine. Semin Respir Infect 1989;4:293–298
56. Spika JS, Fedson DS, Facklam RR: Pneumococcal vaccination. Controversies and opportunities. Infect Dis Clin North Am 1990;4:11–27
57. Unanue ER: Macrophages, antigen-presenting cells and the phenomena of antigen handling and presentation. pp. 95–116. In Paul WE (ed): Fundamental Immunology. Raven Press, New York, 1989
58. Lipscomb MF, Lyons CR, Nunez G: Human alveolar macrophages: HLA-DR-positive macrophages that are poor stimulators of a primary mixed leukocyte reaction. J Immunol 1986;136:497–504
59. Rich EA, Tweardy DJ, Fujiwara H, Ellner JJ: Spectrum of immunoregulatory functions and properties of human alveolar macrophages. Am Rev Respir Dis 1987;136:258–265
60. Weissler JC, Lyons CR, Lipscomb MF, Toews GB: Human pulmonary macrophages. Functional comparison of cells obtained from whole lung and by bronchoalveolar lavage. Am Rev Respir Dis 1986;133:473–477
61. Leatherman JW: Alveolar hemorrhage syndromes: Diffuse microvascular lung hemorrhage in immune and idiopathic disorders. Medicine (Baltimore) 1984;63:343–361
62. Albelda SM: Diffuse pulmonary hemorrhage: A review and classification. Radiology 1985;154:289–297
63. Sharma OP: Sarcoidosis: Clinical Management. Butterworths, London, 1984
64. Crystal RG, Roberts W, Hunninghake GW: Pulmonary sarcoidosis: A disease characterized and perpetuated by activated lung T-lymphocytes. Ann Intern Med 1981;94:73–94
65. Rochat T, Hunninghake GW: Sarcoidosis. pp. 229–238. In Schwartz MI, King TE (eds): Interstitial Lung Disease. BC Decker, Philadelphia, 1988
66. Leavitt RY, Fauci AS: Pulmonary vasculitis. Am Rev Respir Dis 1986;134:149–166
67. Fauci AS: Wegener's granulomatosis: Prospective clinical and therapeutic experience with 85 patients for 21 years. Ann Intern Med 1983;98:76–85
68. Fauci AS: Lymphomatoid granulomatosis. Prospective clinical and therapeutic experience over 10 years. N Engl J Med 1982;306:68–74
69. Churg A: Pulmonary angiitis and granulomatosis revisited. Hum Pathol 1983;14:868–883
70. King TE: Idiopathic pulmonary fibrosis. pp. 139–169. In Schwarz MI, King TE (eds): Interstitial Lung Disease. Philadelphia: BC Decker, 1988
71. Crystal RG, Bitterman PB, Rennard SI et al: Interstitial lung disease of unknown cause. N Engl J Med 1984;310:154–235, 166–244
72. Dreisin RB, Schwarz MI, Theofilopoulos AN, Stanford RE: Circulating immune complexes in the idiopathic interstitial pneumonias. N Engl J Med 1978;298:353–357
73. Irwin RS, Curley FJ, Pratter MR: The effects of drugs on cough. Eur J Respir Dis 1987;153:173–181
74. Lippman M: Regional deposition of particles in the human respiratory tract. pp. 212–232. In Lee D (ed): Handbook of Physiology. Section 9. Reactions to Environmental Agents. American Physiological Society, Bethesda, 1977
75. Applebaum EL, Bruce DL: Tracheal Intubation. WB Saunders, Philadelphia, 1976
76. Kessel RG, Kardon RH: Tissues and Organs: A Text-Atlas of Scanning Electron Microscopy. WH Freeman, New York, 1979
77. Corrin B (ed): The lungs. In Symmers W St C (General ed): Systemic Pathology. Vol. 5. 3rd Ed. Churchill Livingstone, Edinburgh, 1990
78. Weibel ER, Bachofen H: The fiber scaffold of lung parenchyma. pp. 787–794. In Crystal RG, West JB (eds): The Lung. Scientific Foundations. Raven Press, New York, 1991

Chapter 18

Metabolic Functions of the Lung

David J. Pierson

CHAPTER OUTLINE

Pulmonary research in cellular and molecular biology has led to an increasing understanding of the lung's metabolic and endocrine functions. (Reference books,[1] symposium issues,[2] and an entire volume of the *Handbook of Physiology*[3] bear witness to the volume of data accumulating in this area. Concise reviews of the lung's metabolic functions, which are both more accessible and less unwieldy for the clinician, are also available.[4–8]) While pulmonary biochemistry and subcellular organelle function might seem irrelevant to the practice of respiratory care, much of what is being discovered is in fact clinically important. Examples include new concepts in the pathophysiology and in the management of asthma, pulmonary fibrosis, neonatal respiratory distress syndrome, and acute lung injury as typified by the adult respiratory distress syndrome (ARDS).

Table 18-1 summarizes the most important metabolic functions of the lung. To provide the clinician with an introduction to what will surely soon be a burgeoning body of information, this chapter gives a brief conceptual overview of several of these areas.

CELLS OF THE LUNG

More than 40 distinct populations of cells occur in the lung,[4,9] although the functions of only some of these are thoroughly understood. The principal types of lung cells are listed in Table 18-2. Airway mucosal cells include goblet and serous cells, which produce glycoproteins, lipids, and other components of mucus. Once it has been constituted by the addition of water and salts, airway mucus is moved toward the pharynx (along with foreign materials and cellular debris) by the action of cilia, which are present on airway columnar epithelial cells (see Ch. 17 and Fig. 17-4).

The most abundant cells of the parenchyma are endothelial cells (which account for 30 percent of all parenchymal cells), alveolar type I (8 percent) and type II (16 percent) pneumocytes, interstitial cells (36 percent), and alveolar macrophages (10 percent).[10] Ninety-three percent of the lung's alveolar surface is comprised of type I pneumocytes, which are very thin cells lining the alveolar walls; the remaining 7

Table 18-1. Principal Metabolic Functions of the Lung

Oxygen utilization and energy production
Synthesis and release of hormones and other biologically active substances
Activation and metabolism of drugs and hormones
Hypoxic pulmonary vasoconstriction
Synthesis, storage, and release of surfactant
Maintenance of lung structure
Modulation of lung injury and repair

percent is made up primarily of type II cells, which are less differentiated and more metabolically active than their type I counterparts.[10]

Among the most metabolically active of the cell types shown in Table 18-2 are the endothelial cells lining the lung's vascular surfaces.[6,9] A person's entire blood volume comes into contact with the pulmonary endothelial surface, so that this "organ" is ideally situated for controlling and processing vasoactive substances and for other aspects of metabolic regulation. An example of this is the role of pulmonary endothelial cells in the renin-angiotensin system, which helps to regulate systemic blood pressure. When sensors in the kidney detect low blood pressure or low blood sodium concentration, the kidney releases renin, an enzyme that produces the peptide angiotensin I from its carrier protein in the circulating blood; angiotensin I is converted by angiotensin-converting enzyme in lung endothelial cells to the more active angiotensin II, which has a direct pressor effect and also causes the adrenal cortex to release aldosterone, conserving sodium through renal tubular absorption.[6] The result is a combination of vasoconstriction and volume expansion, thereby restoring blood pressure. Table 18-3 lists some of the other functions now known to be carried out by pulmonary vascular endothelial cells, and the reader is referred to more detailed discussions for further information on the function of these complex cells.[5,7–9]

Table 18-2. Types of Lung Cells

Cells that are part of the lung structure
Airway cells
Alveolar macrophages
Ciliated epithelial cells
Goblet cells
Serous cells
Smooth muscle cells
Chondrocytes
Lung parenchymal cells
Endothelial cells
Type I epithelial cells
Type II epithelial cells
Nonciliated bronchiolar epithelial (Clara) cells
Lung endocrine (APUD) cells
Interstitial cells (e.g., fibroblasts)
Interstitial macrophages
Circulating blood cells that are active in the lung
Neutrophils (polymorphonuclear leukocytes)
Lymphocytes
Eosinophils
Basophils
Monocytes

Table 18-3. Metabolic Functions of Pulmonary Endothelial Cells

Cleared from the bloodstream
Adenine nucleotides
Adenosine
Angiotensin I[a]
Bradykinin
Heparin
Insulin
Norepinephrine
Prostaglandins E and F
Serotonin
Released into the bloodstream
Adenosine
Angiotensin II
Lipids
Prostaglandins
Unaffected by the endothelium
Angiotensin II
Epinephrine
Prostaglandin A
Synthesized by the endothelium
Adenosine triphosphate (ATP)
Elastin
Prostaglandin A
Endothelium-derived hyperpolarizing factor (EDHF)
Endothelium-derived relaxing factor (EDRF)
Interleukin-1
Leukotriene B_4
Platelet-activating factor
Prostacyclin
von Willebrand factor

[a] Converted by the endothelium to angiotensin II.

Another important parenchymal cell population is a poorly understood group of hormone-producing cells that occur singly or in small aggregations called *neuroepithelial bodies*.[6,9] These cells are collectively referred to as *APUD* cells (for their cytochemical functions of *a*mine and amine *p*recursor *u*ptake and *d*ecarboxylation). They are part of a farflung collection of similar cells occurring throughout the body and resemble endocrine cells of the pituitary, pancreas, and thyroid gland. The APUD cell is believed to be the cell of origin for small cell (oat cell) lung carcinoma.

OXYGEN UTILIZATION AND ENERGY PRODUCTION BY THE LUNG

Unique among the major organs, the lung receives O_2 from several sources—from the bronchial arteries, from the pulmonary circulation, and also directly from the inspired air. These and other factors make the precise measurement of the lung's O_2 utilization and energy production difficult. However, available data indicate that the lung's O_2 consumption, while less than that of very active tissues such as the myocardium, kidney, and brain, is about the same as that of resting skeletal muscle and portions of the gut.[4]

The lung relies heavily for its metabolic functions on the consumption of energy-producing substrates such as glucose, amino acids, and lactate. Surfactant synthesis and other functions to be described below require a continuous supply of metabolic "fuel" via the pulmonary circulation, especially since relatively little energy is stored in the form of glycogen and other reserves in pulmonary tissue. The lung's reserves of lipids, important in the metabolism of type II pneumocytes and other very active cells, are somewhat larger.

PRODUCTION, STORAGE, AND DISTRIBUTION OF SURFACTANT

The alveoli and respiratory bronchioles would collapse and normal gas exchange would be impossible if it were not for the presence of surfactant, a complex mixture of phospholipids, proteins, and other substances that lines the surface of the terminal respiratory units and markedly reduces surface tension. Maturation of the lung's surfactant-producing apparatus is a primary determinant of whether a fetus is of sufficient gestational development to survive outside the uterus (see Ch. 3).

Surfactant is produced mainly by the type II cells of the alveolar epithelium via an intricate, extensively studied process,[11,12] which is shown schematically in Figure 18-1. The production and function of surfactant are influenced by numerous factors, one of which is a requirement for regular stretching of the pulmonary parenchyma; interference with this process is the primary reason for progressive microatelectasis and increasing alveolar-arterial O_2 partial pressure difference [$P(A\text{-}a)O_2$] during anesthesia or mechanical ventilation if insufficient tidal volumes are used. The lung's high lipid content (10 to 20 percent of its dry weight[7]) and extensive lipid metabolism as compared with other organs are due primarily to the production and processing of surfactant.

MAINTENANCE OF LUNG STRUCTURE

For the lung's structural integrity to be maintained, a complex balance of protein synthesis and breakdown (proteolysis) must exist in the lung throughout fetal development, postnatal growth, and adult life. This balance is influenced by growth factors and various other messengers, which act on an array of receptors on lung cells to up-regulate or down-

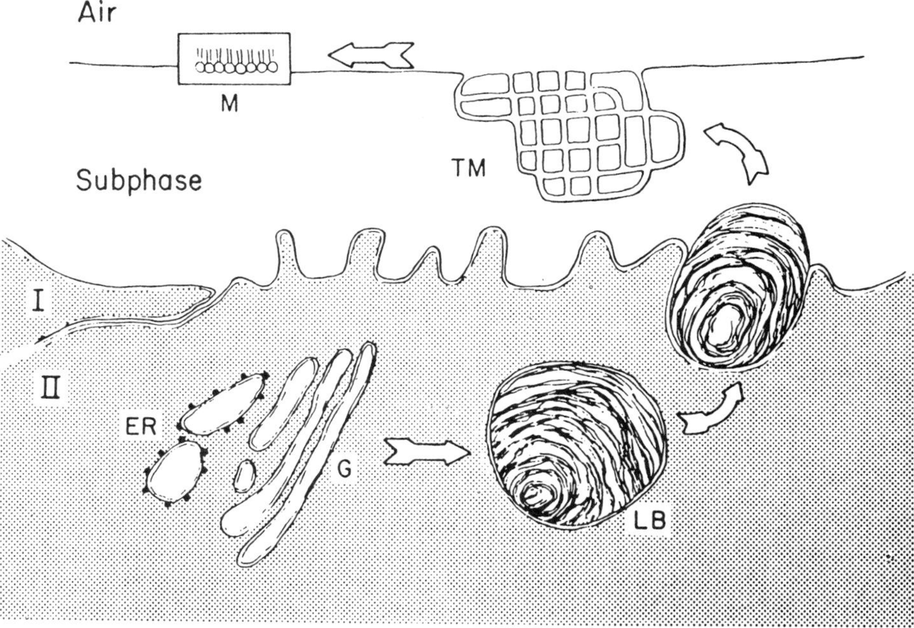

Figure 18-1. Diagrammatic representation of the formation, storage, and deployment of pulmonary surfactant. Synthesis of surfactant occurs within the alveolar type II epithelial cell (II), where it begins in the endoplasmic reticulum (ER), passes to the Golgi apparatus (G), and is then moved to the lamellar bodies (LB), in which it is stored. These lamellar bodies later migrate to the apical surface of the cell and are ejected into the alveolar subphase, where they expand into tubular myelin (TM). The material constituting the tubular myelin then spreads as a monolayer (M) at the alveolar air-liquid interface, where it exerts its surface tension-lowering effects. (From Goerke,[11] with permission.)

Table 18-4. Actions of the Main Arachidonic Acid Metabolites on the Lung

Metabolite	Chemotaxis	Vasoactivity	Bronchospasm	Increased Vascular Permeability
Leukotriene B_4	++	—	—	+(?)
Sulfidopeptide leukotrienes (C_4, D_4, and E_4)[a]	—	Vasospasm	++	+
Thromboxane	—	Vasospasm	(?)	—
Prostaglandins I_2 and E_2	—	Vasodilation	—	—
Prostaglandins F_2 and D_2	—	Vasodilation	+	—
Platelet-activating factor	++	Vasospasm	++	++

[a] Also called slow-reacting substance of anaphylaxis (SRS-A).

regulate production and breakdown of the huge number of different proteins made by the lung. Important among these proteins are those comprising connective tissue, such as collagen and elastin, the two most abundant proteins in human lungs. Collagen and elastin form most of the connective tissue network that supports the lungs and establishes physiologic attributes such as elasticity and distensibility (e.g., compliance).[4] Many of the lung's cells, as listed in Table 18-2, synthesize proteins. The five types of collagen found in the lung are produced to varying extents by endothelial cells, types I and II pneumocytes, and mesenchymal cells (including smooth muscle cells and chondroblasts).[4]

Maintenance of the balance between protein synthesis and proteolysis is crucial for normal structural integrity in the lung. Weakening and breakdown of lung connective tissues is believed to be a main mechanism of emphysema, while overproduction of connective tissue and/or failure of normal breakdown are hallmarks of diseases producing pulmonary fibrosis.

MODULATION OF LUNG INJURY AND REPAIR

The years since the late 1980s have seen near exponential growth in knowledge about the lung's defenses against injury, the processes set into motion when injury occurs, and the mechanisms of both normal and abnormal lung repair in response to injury.[1,2,7,13,14] Areas of continuing interest for respiratory care, in which clinical management will surely be altered by future discoveries, include the modulation of airway inflammation and bronchoconstriction (as in asthma, now considered primarily an inflammatory disorder) and the mediators of acute lung injury (as in ARDS, in which modifying the cascade of mediator-driven events leading to severe respiratory failure may eventually improve prognosis).

Present knowledge indicates that a key to initiation of the pulmonary response to injury is the alveolar macrophage, which serves as a "sentinel cell" in the lung. When some injury occurs, macrophages release substances (chemoattractants) that draw neutrophils and other cells to the area or that stimulate nearby cells to produce other substances (cytokines) or to take other action (e.g., phagocytosis). Chemoattractants, cytokines, and other vasoactive substances involved in lung injury and repair have been studied extensively, especially with respect to their biochemistry and synthesis; how they influence the evolution and repair of lung injury and how they may be manipulated therapeutically are important areas for further study during the 1990s.

Arachidonic acid, an essential fatty acid abundant in cell membranes, serves as the substrate for several metabolic pathways leading to the production of substances important in the modulation of lung injury and repair. Arachidonic acid metabolites, produced by neutrophils, macrophages, and other lung cells, serve as powerful mediators of several cellular processes, including chemotaxis (the attraction of other cells to an area of injury), vasoactivity (causing either spasm or dilatation of pulmonary blood vessels), bronchospasm, and increased vascular permeability. Two important pathways by which arachidonic acid is transformed into biologically active substances are the cyclooxygenase pathway, products of which include the *prostaglandins* and *thromboxane*, and the 5-lipoxygenase pathway, which leads to the production of substances called *leukotrienes*.[14] These and most other known arachidonic acid products are known as *eicosanoids*[13]; an important one that is not an eicosanoid is *platelet-activating factor*. The main pulmonary effects of these arachidonic acid metabolites, as illustrated by several important examples, are summarized in Table 18-4.

Research in the cellular and molecular biology of lung metabolism is expanding so rapidly that any brief summary is sure to be outdated within months. However, the topics touched on briefly here are certain to remain important and to have increasing clinical application even as whole new areas emerge and expand. Respiratory care will remain practical and focused at the bedside, but in the near future it will also be increasingly influenced by advances in the basic science of lung function and metabolism.

References

1. Massaro D (ed): Lung Cell Biology. In Lenfant C (Series ed): Lung Biology in Health and Disease. Marcel Dekker, New York, 1989
2. Metabolic functions of the lungs. Clin Chest Med 1989;10:1–125
3. Fishman AP, Fisher AB (eds): Circulatory and Nonrespiratory Functions. Vol. 1. In Fishman AP (Section ed): Handbook of Physiology. Section 3. The Respiratory System. American Physiological Society, Bethesda, 1985
4. Murray JF: The Normal Lung. 2nd Ed. WB Saunders, Philadelphia, 1986, pp. 283–312

5. Block ER, Stalcup SA: Metabolic functions of the lung. Of what clinical significance? Chest 1982;81:215–223
6. Hyers TM: Metabolic functions of the lung. pp. 1855–1857. In Kelley WN (ed): Textbook of Internal Medicine. JB Lippincott, Philadelphia, 1989
7. Voelkel NF: Metabolic functions of the lungs. pp. 1692–1694. In Kelley WN (ed): Textbook of Internal Medicine. 2nd Ed. JB Lippincott, Philadelphia, 1992
8. Fishman AP, Pietra GG: Handling of vasoactive materials by the lung. N Engl J Med 1974;291:884–890, 953–959
9. Gail DB, Lenfant CJM: Cells of the lung: Biology and clinical implications. Am Rev Respir Dis 1983;127:366–387
10. Crapo JD, Barry BE, Gehr P et al: Cell number and cell characteristics in the normal human lung. Am Rev Respir Dis 1982; 125:740–745
11. Goerke J: Lung surfactant. Biochim Biophys Acta 1974; 344:241–261
12. Wright JR, Hawgood S: Pulmonary surfactant metabolism. Clin Chest Med 1989;10:83–93
13. Voelkel NF, Stenmark KR, Westcott JY, Chang S-W: Lung eicosanoid metabolism. Clin Chest Med 1989;10:95–106
14. Lewis RA, Austen KF, Soberman RJ: Leukotrienes and other products of the 5-lipoxygenase pathway: Biochemistry and relation to pathobiology in human diseases. N Engl J Med 1990; 323:645–655

Chapter 19

Effects of Aging on the Respiratory System

David J. Pierson

CHAPTER OUTLINE

Most chronic lung disease, and hence much of respiratory care, involves individuals who are middle-aged or older and whose respiratory function is affected by aging as well as by disease. It is therefore important for the clinician to understand the effects of "normal" aging on the respiratory system so that these may be clearly distinguished from pathologic changes. This chapter summarizes the changes in respiratory structure and function that occur when healthy people grow older; for more comprehensive discussions the reader is referred to several excellent reviews.[1–6]

MORPHOLOGIC ALTERATIONS IN THE THORAX, LUNGS, AND AIRWAYS

An increase in the anteroposterior diameter of the chest, especially in its upper portion, is normal in old age and does not necessarily signify the presence of emphysema.[4,6,7] The lung itself becomes more rounded, its upper zones expanding and those at the bases losing volume.[7] There is a progressive enlargement of the respiratory bronchioles and alveolar ducts and an increase in the average distance between interalveolar septae; alveolar wall tissue gradually and progressively diminishes as alveolar shape becomes less complex.[5] At the same time the pores of Kohn progressively enlarge,[8] and elastic tissue and bronchiolar muscle become less prominent.[5]

These changes are suggestive of emphysema, and in fact diagnosis of this disease becomes in a sense more quantitative than qualitative in the lungs of the very old. However, physiologically the morphologic alterations described here are of less clinical importance than those occurring in the chest wall and respiratory muscles. The misleading term "senile emphysema," with its implication of disabling lung destruction due solely to the aging process, is fortunately much less commonly used than in the past. Individuals with clinically significant emphysema have anatomic changes much more extensive than those seen in otherwise healthy (even if barrel-chested) elderly persons.

CHANGES IN RESPIRATORY FUNCTION

Mechanics of Ventilation

Table 19-1 lists the main changes in respiratory function that occur with aging, along with their most important clinical manifestations. With increasing age the chest wall becomes stiffer as the spine, the ribs, and their articulations become less mobile. At the same time the lungs themselves lose elastic recoil and become more compliant[1,9] (Fig. 19-1A). These changes cause a progressive decrease in vital capacity (to about 75 percent of a person's original maximum value by age 70)[1] and a corresponding increase in residual volume (RV), so that total lung capacity (TLC) remains about the same (Fig. 19-1B).

The forced expiratory volume in the first second (FEV_1) also declines progressively with age, roughly in proportion to the decline in forced vital capacity (FVC), so that the FEV_1/FVC ratio declines only slightly. Average yearly losses in FEV_1 for healthy men and women are approximately 30 and 23 mL/yr, respectively[1] (Fig. 19-1C), although recent studies have cast doubt on whether this rate of loss is the same throughout adult life[2,10,11] (Fig. 19-1D). With advancing age there is an increase in respiratory rate; in one study 82 healthy individuals with a mean age of 84 years had resting respiratory rates of 16 to 25 breaths per minute.[12] The increase in breathing frequency is accompanied by a decrease in tidal volume (V_T) such that arterial CO_2 partial pressure ($PaCO_2$) does not change.

Perfusion, Ventilation, and Gas Exchange

Because of the changes in lung elastic recoil and airway caliber, the distribution of ventilation changes with increasing age. An important consequence of this is an increase in closing volume (that lung volume at which some airways in dependent regions of the lung close, such that their alveoli receive no ventilation),[13] with a concomitant increase in the mismatching of ventilation and perfusion. Closing capacity (CC), which equals closing volume (CV) plus RV, increases with age so as to exceed functional residual capacity (FRC) in the upright position by about age 65 and in the supine position at age 40 to 45 years[14] (Fig. 19-1E). These changes, along with slight drops in cardiac output and mixed venous O_2 content ($C\bar{v}O_2$) with age, produce a progressive increase in the alveolar-arterial O_2 partial pressure difference [$P(A\text{-}a)O_2$]: arterial PO_2 (PaO_2) decreases approximately 4 mmHg per decade in later life[15] (Fig. 19-1F). In one study a group of 24 healthy subjects over age 60 (mean age, 71 years) had a PaO_2 of 74 ± 4.4 mmHg (mean ± 1 SD).[15] This is the source of the mnemonic "70 at 70" for an absolute lower limit of normal PaO_2; most healthy elderly persons, however, have PaO_2 values well above 70 mmHg at sea level.

Less uniform ventilation/perfusion matching also leads to an increase in physiologic dead space and a slight compensatory increase in resting minute ventilation, although these are of no clinical significance. $PaCO_2$ and pH remain unchanged with advancing age.[15,16] The previously mentioned progressive loss in alveolar surface area results in a decline

Table 19-1. Changes in Respiratory Function with Aging

Function	Mechanism	Clinical Manifestation
Mechanics of ventilation	Loss of lung elastic recoil; decreased chest wall compliance	↓ VC; ↑ RV; no change in TLC; ↓ expiratory flow rates
	Decreased respiratory muscle mass and strength	↓ Maximal inspiratory and expiratory force
Perfusion, ventilation, and gas exchange	Decreased uniformity of ventilation, with small airway closure during tidal breathing, especially while supine; ↓ cardiac output; ↓ $C\bar{v}O_2$	↑ $P(A\text{-}a)O_2$; ↓ PaO_2; no change in $PaCO_2$ or pH
	Increased physiologic dead space	None (slightly ↑ $\dot{V}_E$)
	Decreased alveolar surface area	↓ DLCO
Exercised capacity	Decreased aerobic work capacity of skeletal muscle; deconditioning	↓ Maximum $\dot{V}O_2$
	Decreased efficiency of ventilation	↑ $\dot{V}_E$/L $\dot{V}O_2$
Regulation of ventilation	Decreased responsiveness of central and peripheral chemoreceptors	↓ $\dot{V}_E$ and $P_{0.1}$ responses to hypoxia and hypercapnia
Sleep and breathing	Decreased ventilatory drive	↑ Frequency of apneas, hypopneas, and desaturation episodes during sleep
	Decreased upper airway muscle tone	Snoring; ↑ incidence of obstructive sleep apnea
	Decreased arousal and cough reflexes	↑ Susceptibility to aspiration and pneumonia
Lung defense mechanisms	Decreased upper airway function; decreased mucociliary clearance	↑ Susceptibility to aspiration and pneumonia
	Decreased humoral and cellular immunity	↑ Susceptibility to infection; ↓ clinical response to infection

$\dot{V}_E$, expired minute ventilation; DLCO, diffusing capacity for carbon monoxide; $\dot{V}O_2$, O_2 consumption; $P_{0.1}$, mouth occlusion pressure; $C\bar{v}O_2$, mixed venous O_2 content; $P(A\text{-}a)O_2$, alveolar-arterial PO_2 difference.

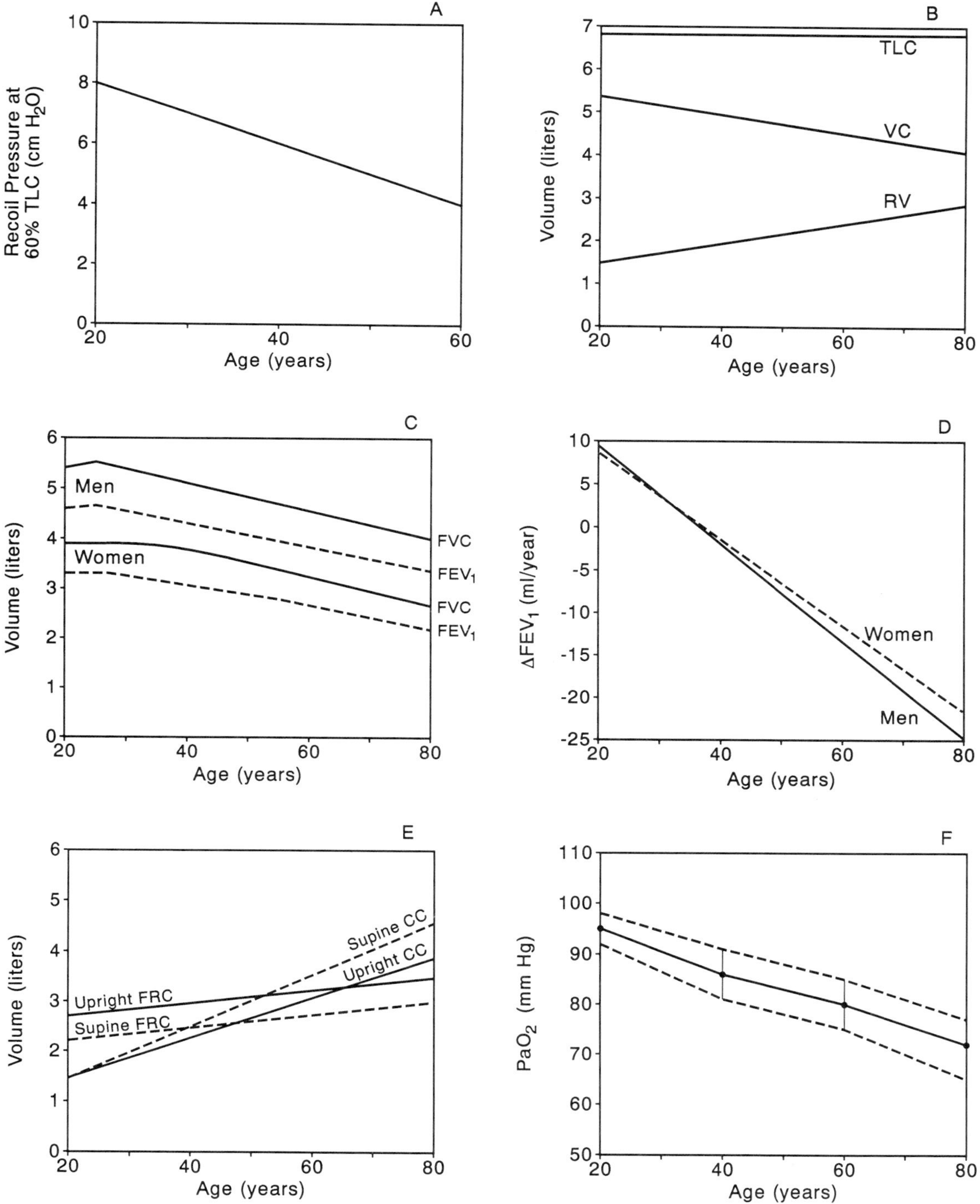

Figure 19-1. Representative changes in respiratory function with age. Curves show mean or generalized changes, and there may be considerable variation among individuals. Note the varying age scales on the horizontal axes. **(A)** Changes in lung elastic recoil with age. (Adapted from Murray,[1] with permission, with data from Turner et al.[9]) **(B)** Changes in static lung volumes with age. TLC, total lung capacity; VC, vital capacity, RV, residual volume. **(C)** Changes in FVC (solid lines) and FEV_1 (dashed lines) with age in men and women. (Adapted from Burrows et al.,[10] with permission.) **(D)** Changes in the rate of loss of FEV_1 with age in men (solid line) and women (dashed line). (Adapted from Burrows et al.,[11] with permission.) **(E)** Changes in CC (defined as RV plus CV) and in FRC with age. Solid lines, upright posture; dashed lines, supine posture. **(F)** Changes in PaO_2 (at sea level) with increasing age. Dashed lines represent ±2 SD from the mean for the subjects studied. (Adapted from Sorbini et al.,[15] with permission.)

in pulmonary diffusing capacity,[17] although this does not contribute to the drop in PaO_2 with increasing age.

Exercise Capacity

Maximum exercise capability declines 5 to 10 percent per decade once a person's optimal age for performance has passed.[18,19] The deterioration is apparently due to a decrease in the aerobic work capacity of skeletal muscle rather than to limitation by gas exchange, ventilation, or cardiac function.[19] A reduction in muscle mass in later years, along with physical deconditioning associated with a more sedentary life-style, likely accounts for this phenomenon.[1,20] With increasing age there is an increase in the O_2 ventilation equivalent (ventilation per liter of O_2 consumed),[21] consistent with the increase in physiologic dead space mentioned earlier.

Regulation of Ventilation

Both central and peripheral chemoreceptors are affected by age. Ventilatory,[22] occlusion pressure,[23] and heart rate responses to hypoxia and hypercapnia diminish in old age, by perhaps 50 percent in comparison with those of subjects in their twenties.[22] Although direct confirmation is lacking, this loss of ventilatory drive could contribute to the severity and duration of gas exchange disturbances in elderly persons with acute or chronic pulmonary disorders.

Sleep and Breathing

As summarized in Table 19-1, several alterations in the sleep of older persons could also contribute to the incidence and severity of illness. Diminished ventilatory drives and loss of upper airway tone in comparison with those present during wakefulness predispose to apneas, hypopneas, and nocturnal desaturation, and less active cough and arousal reflexes increase the likelihood of aspiration during sleep. These sleep disturbances tend to become more common with age.

Lung Defense Mechanisms

Elderly persons have increased susceptibility to infections of all kinds and tend to have more severe illnesses when infected.[24] The incidence of malignancies also increases with age,[25] which is further evidence of a relaxation of host defenses. Mucociliary clearance becomes less effective, accounting in part for the increased susceptibility of elderly patients to atelectasis and pneumonia following anesthesia and surgery.

As the lymphatic system atrophies progressively during later life, humoral immunity declines. Specific antibody production decreases progressively in old age, rendering immunizing agents such as pneumococcal vaccine desirable but relatively ineffective. Cell-mediated immunity also deteriorates, for although the T lymphocytes of elderly persons may be normal or even increased in number, both in blood and in bronchoalveolar lavage fluid,[26] fewer of them appear capable of responding to new stimuli. A loss of cellular immunity is also shown by the absence of skin test reactivity to tuberculin and other antigens in many elderly individuals.

References

1. Murray JF: The normal lung. 2nd Ed. WB Saunders, Philadelphia, 1986, pp. 339–360
2. Knudson RJ: Aging of the respiratory system. Curr Pulmonol 1989;10:1–24
3. Bates DV: Respiratory Function in Disease. 3rd Ed. WB Saunders, Philadelphia, 1989, pp. 81–86
4. Brody JS, Thurlbeck WM: Development, growth, and aging of the lung. pp. 355–386. In Macklem PT, Mead J (eds): Handbook of Physiology. Section 3: The Respiratory System. Vol. 3. Mechanics of Breathing, Part 1. American Physiological Society, Bethesda, 1986
5. Thurlbeck WM: Growth, aging, and adaptation. pp. 37–46. In Murray JF, Nadel JA (eds): Textbook of Respiratory Medicine. WB Saunders, Philadelphia, 1988
6. King TE Jr, Schwarz MI: Pulmonary function and disease in the elderly. pp. 124–148. In Schrier RW (ed): Clinical Internal Medicine in the Aged. WB Saunders, Philadelphia, 1982
7. Beeckman P, Demedts M, Clarysse I, Vanclooster R: Radiographic evaluation of the influence of age and smoking on thoracic and regional pulmonary dimensions. Lung 1983;16:39–46
8. Pump KK: Emphysema and its relation to age. Am Rev Respir Dis 1976;114:5–13
9. Turner JM, Mead J, Wohl MD: Elasticity of human lungs in relation to age. J Appl Physiol 1968;25:664–671
10. Burrows B, Cline MG, Knudson RJ et al: A descriptive analysis of the growth and decline of the FVC and FEV_1. Chest 1983; 83:717–724
11. Burrows B, Lebowitz MD, Camilli AE, Knudson RJ: Longitudinal changes in forced expiratory volume in one second in adults. Am Rev Respir Dis 1986;133:974–980
12. McFadden JP, Price RC, Eastwood HD, Briggs RS: Raised respiratory rate in elderly patients: A valuable physical sign. Br Med J 1982;284:626–627
13. Holland J, Milic-Emili J, Macklem PT, Bates DV: Regional distribution of pulmonary ventilation and perfusion in elderly subjects. J Clin Invest 1968;47:81–92
14. Leblanc P, Ruff F, Milic-Emili J: Effects of age and body position on "airway closure" in man. J Appl Physiol 1970;28:448–451
15. Sorbini CA, Grassi V, Solinas E, Muiesan G: Arterial oxygen tension in relation to age in healthy subjects. Respiration 1968; 25:3–13
16. Amaducci S, Mandelli V, Morpugo M, Rampulla C: Aging, cigarette smoking, and respiratory function. Bull Eur Physiopathol Respir 1977;13:523–532
17. Georges R, Saumon G, Loiseau A: The relationship of age to pulmonary membrane conductance and capillary blood volume. Am Rev Respir Dis 1978;117:1069–1078
18. Bottiger LE: Regular decline in physical working capacity with age. Br Med J 1978;3:270–271
19. Rodeheffer RJ, Gerstenblith G, Becker LC et al: Exercise cardiac output is maintained with advancing age in healthy human subjects: Cardiac dilation and increased stroke volume compensate for diminished heart rate. Circulation 1984;69:203–213

20. Hossack KF, Bruce RA: Maximal cardiac function in sedentary normal men and women: Comparison of age-related changes. J Appl Physiol 1982;53:799–804
21. Patrick JM, Bassey EJ, Fentem PH: The rising ventilatory cost of bicycle exercise in the seventh decade: A longitudinal study of nine healthy men. Clin Sci 1983;65:521–526
22. Kronenberg RS, Drage CW: Attenuation of the ventilatory and heart rate responses to hypoxia and hypercapnia with aging in normal men. J Clin Invest 1973;52:1812–1819
23. Peterson DD, Pack AI, Silage DA, Fishman AP: Effects of aging on ventilatory and occlusion pressure responses to hypoxia and hypercapnia. Am Rev Respir Dis 1981;124:387–391
24. Goldstein S: The biology of aging. N Engl J Med 1971;285:1120–1129
25. Newell GR, Spitz MR, Sider JG: Cancer and age. Semin Oncol 1989;16:3–9
26. The BAL Cooperative Group Steering Committee: Bronchoalveolar lavage constituents in healthy individuals, idiopathic pulmonary fibrosis, and selected comparison groups. Am Rev Respir Dis 1990;141(5,pt 2):S169–S202

Chapter 20

Drugs Used in Respiratory Care

David J. Pierson

CHAPTER OUTLINE

Much of respiratory care has to do with drugs—their administration, the assessment of their therapeutic effects, and the detection and quantitation of adverse effects resulting from their use. A basic working knowledge of respiratory pharmacology is therefore essential for the clinician. This chapter provides an introduction to the drugs used in respiratory care (Table 20-1). It identifies the main categories of agents used in the management of respiratory disease, describes their actions and available preparations, summarizes the indications and contraindications for their use, identifies their principal adverse effects, and indicates how their clinical efficacy can be assessed and monitored. Even for the most important drugs, space limitations prohibit coverage in detail; for others, only brief mention is possible. For more in-depth information the reader is referred to comprehensive sources on drugs in general[1–4] and to texts,[5–8] chapters,[9,10] and symposium issues[11,12] on respiratory pharmacology in particular.

Prior to a discussion of each category of drug used in respiratory care, it is necessary to summarize several important general concepts about the effects and clinical use of these agents.

GENERAL CONCEPTS

Principles of Drug Use in Respiratory Care

Several general concepts apply to all the drugs discussed in this chapter. The clinician should always choose preparations with specific, known modes of action. Whenever possible, drug dosages should be individualized for each patient, as determined by weight, age, organ function, and/or functional status rather than by a fixed "cookbook" dosing schedule. Administration should be tailored to the patient's schedule and life-style. Fixed-dose proprietary drug com-

Table 20-1. Drugs Used in Respiratory Care

Group	Description	Examples
Beta-2-agonist bronchodilators	Sympathomimetic agents that dilate bronchi by stimulating adenyl cyclase and thus increasing cAMP	Albuterol Terbutaline
Anticholinergics	Agents that block acetylcholine-mediated bronchoconstriction via the parasympathetic nervous system	Ipratropium Atropine
Corticosteroids	Adrenocortical glucocorticoid hormones and synthetic analogs with potent anti-inflammatory and other effects	Prednisone Beclomethasone
Methylxanthines	Bronchodilators related to xanthine that also affect respiratory muscle function, cardiac rhythm, and a variety of other functions	Theophylline Aminophylline
"Mast cell stabilizers"	Antiasthma agents intended to prevent release of mediators in response to certain stimuli and hence to provide prophylaxis against acute attacks	Cromolyn Ketotifen
Mucolytics and expectorants	Symptomatic therapies that promote the clearance of respiratory secretions from the lung	Acetylcysteine Postassium iodide
Respiratory stimulants	Centrally and/or peripherally acting agents that increase the drive to breathe and, in patients who are capable of it, augment alveolar ventilation	Doxapram Progesterone
Respiratory depressants	Centrally acting drugs that decrease central ventilatory drives	Morphine Diazepam
Other/miscellaneous	Antitussives	Codeine Lidocaine
	Replacements for congenitally or developmentally deficient normal substances	Alpha-1-antitrypsin Surfactant
	Specialized antimicrobial agents given by inhalation	Pentamidine Ribavirin
	"Steroid-sparing" agents used in severe asthma	Troleandomycin Methotrexate
	Adjuvant agents used in smoking cessation	Nicotine gum Transdermal nicotine

binations should be used cautiously if at all, particularly in seriously ill or unstable patients, since the individual quantities of their component agents are unlikely to be optimum doses for a given person. Some assessment of a drug's effects, good and bad, should always be made, whether precise and objective or purely subjective. This assessment should be repeated at appropriate intervals as dictated by the clinical stability of the patient and the duration of treatment.

Within a given category of drugs the clinician usually has a choice of agents, sometimes with varying clinical effectiveness but almost always with varying costs to the patient. The cost aspect of drug therapy must always be kept in mind, and whenever possible the least expensive effective preparation should be selected.

Routes of Administration

An agent can often be given by numerous routes, and its effectiveness and toxicity may vary accordingly. Oral administration (e.g., tablets, capsules, or elixirs) has the advantages of convenience, gradual (timed) release, and, at least sometimes, lower cost than other routes; its disadvantages include unpredictable absorption, nonspecificity of effects for the respiratory tract, and gastrointestinal side effects. Inhalation (e.g., liquid or powder aerosols) puts the drug directly onto its presumed site of action but may be cumbersome and more expensive than the oral route. Respiratory drugs may be injected intravenously, intramuscularly, or subcutaneously; they may be instilled into the nose or directly into the trachea; they may be given under the tongue or inserted into the rectum. Finally, although this route is not yet common in respiratory care, drugs can be administered through the skin by means of ointments or drug-impregnated patches.

For an agent acting on the airways, inhalation is more effective and produces fewer side effects than other routes. This is especially true with inhalation versus oral administration,[13] as illustrated in Figure 20-1, which shows changes in FEV_1 (forced expiratory volume in 1 second) produced in eight adult asthmatic patients by different doses of the beta-agonist bronchodilator albuterol given in aerosol versus tablet form. On average, it took 18 mg of the oral preparation to produce as much bronchodilation as 0.6 mg by inhalation; because of the dosage necessary to achieve this much effect by the oral route, patients experienced considerably more side effects.

Whenever a drug is available in aerosol form, this route should be used if possible, especially with beta-agonist bronchodilators and anticholinergics. Some agents such as cromolyn are available only in inhaled form. Corticosteroids are also effective by the inhaled route in some instances. Unfortunately, other mainstay respiratory drugs such as theophylline and most antibiotics cannot be administered directly to the airways.

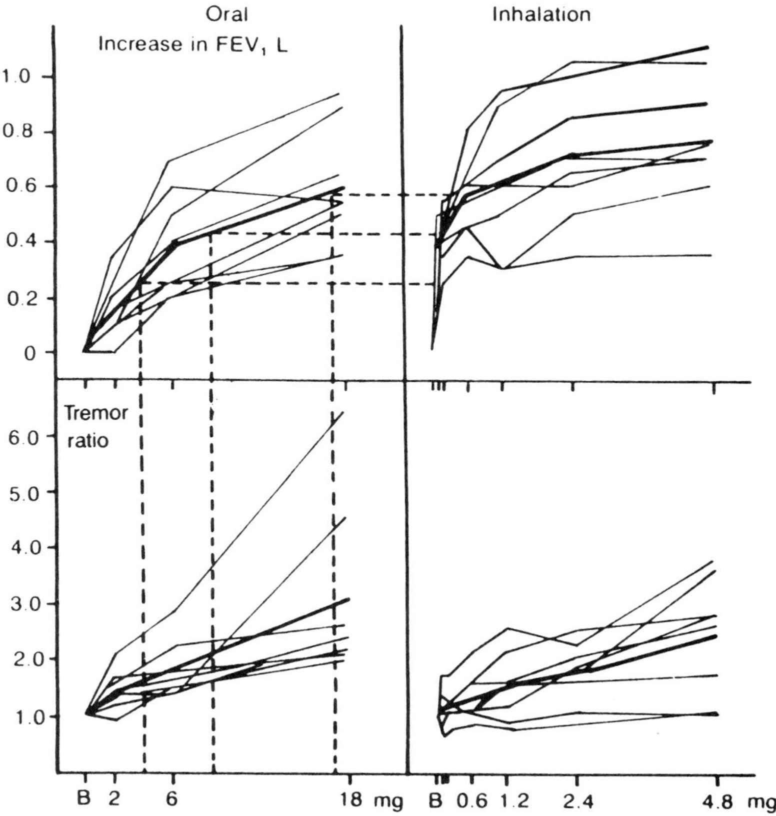

Figure 20-1. The therapeutic effect (increase in FEV_1) and side effects (tremor) produced by oral versus inhaled albuterol in the same patients illustrate the advantages of the inhaled route for bronchodilators. Each thin line represents the dose-response curve for an individual patient; the thick lines show mean dose-response curves for the eight adult asthmatic patients. The horizontal axes show increasing doses of drug, and dashed lines show the amount of tremor produced at each of three degrees of improvement in FEV_1. See text for further explanation. (From Larsson and Svedmyr,[13] with permission.)

Types of Adverse Effects from Drugs

Although the introduction of a new drug is often accompanied by claims of improved therapeutic efficacy and freedom from adverse effects, in time the accumulation of clinical experience generally proves the latter, at least, not to be the case. Adverse effects can be of several types; they may be *side effects* or normal pharmacologic actions of the drug other than those desired, as with the tremor produced by beta-2-agonist stimulation of skeletal muscle. *Toxicity* is a dose-related adverse effect observed in most people if enough drug is given, for example, cardiac arrhythmias with isoproterenol or nausea and vomiting with theophylline.

Allergy to a drug, such as a rash or an asthmatic reaction to penicillin, is a specific antigen-antibody reaction in previously exposed, susceptible individuals. An extreme, potentially fatal form of allergic reaction is *anaphylaxis*, characterized by respiratory distress and cardiovascular collapse. *Idiosyncrasy* is a rare, paradoxical reaction to a specific drug, such as the bronchospasm produced by isoproterenol and other beta-agonist bronchodilators. *Tachyphylaxis*, another clinically uncommon phenomenon, is a diminution in the therapeutic effectiveness of a drug on repeated (usually prolonged) use, as may be seen with oral ephedrine.

BETA-AGONIST BRONCHODILATORS

Identification and Actions

The beta-adrenergic bronchodilators, also called beta-2 agonists or beta-2 adrenoceptor stimulants, constitute the most important class of antiasthma drugs.[10,14–16] They are sympathomimetics (i.e., agents that mimic the actions of the natural mediators of the sympathetic nervous system, and most are analogues of the naturally occurring substances epinephrine, norepinephrine, and dopamine.

Sympathomimetics act by stimulating receptors in the bronchi as well as in other organs. There appear to be different receptors in different tissues, whose stimulation produces sufficiently different effects to classify them into three

Table 20-2. Effects of Adrenergic Receptor Stimulation

Tissue or Function	Alpha Response	Beta-1 Response	Beta-2 Response
Airway smooth muscle	–	–	Bronchodilation
Blood vessels	Vasoconstriction	–	Vasodilation
Blood pressure	↑	– or ↑	– or ↓
Heart rate	– or ↓	↑ ↑ ; ectopy	Little effect
Skeletal muscle	–	–	Tremor
Central nervous system	?	?	Anxiety; insomnia
Gut	Sphincter constriction	Decreased motility	–
Uterine smooth muscle	–	–	Relaxation

distinct groups—alpha, beta-1, and beta-2 receptors (Table 20-2). One can infer from Table 20-2 that an ideal bronchodilator would stimulate beta-2 receptors without affecting alpha or beta-1 receptors; furthermore, it would stimulate only bronchial beta-2 receptors and not act on those in skeletal, cardiac, or vascular smooth muscle. However, although billions of dollars worth of pharmaceutical research since the mid-1960s has produced definite advances, no drug completely meets these criteria.

Activation of bronchial beta-2 receptors stimulates the enzyme adenyl cyclase, which in turn increases intracellular production of cyclic 3′,5′-adenosine monophosphate (cAMP) from adenosine triphosphate (ATP),[17] as shown schematically in Figure 20-2. An increase in cAMP causes bronchial smooth muscle relaxation. Although beta-2 receptor stimulation causes little change in bronchial caliber in the normal person, dramatic bronchodilation may occur when there is abnormal bronchoconstriction, as in asthma.

Available Preparations

Figure 20-3 shows the chemical structures of eight representative beta-2-agonist bronchodilators. Among the agents shown, epinephrine, isoproterenol, and isoetharine are chemically classified as catecholamines; metaproterenol and terbutaline are resorcinols; and albuterol (known as *salbutamol* outside the United States) is a saligenin. Bitolterol, a so-called prodrug, must be hydrolyzed in the body to its active catecholamine form. The newest American beta-2 ag-

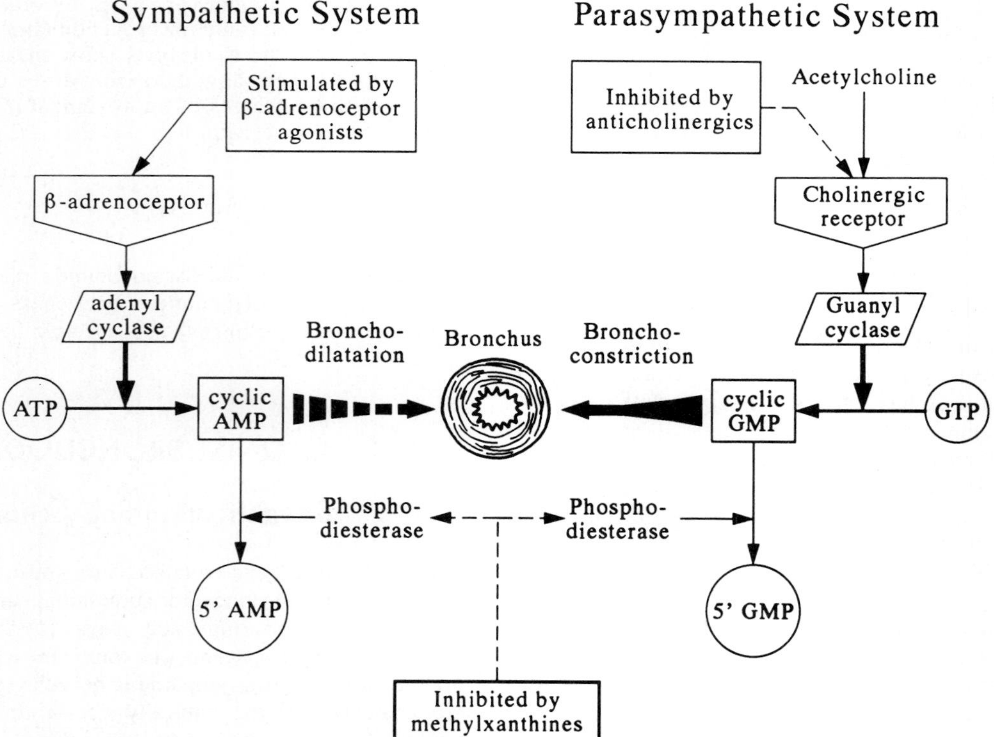

Figure 20-2. Schematic representation of the sites of action of the three main groups of bronchodilating drugs. (From Shenfield,[17] with permission.)

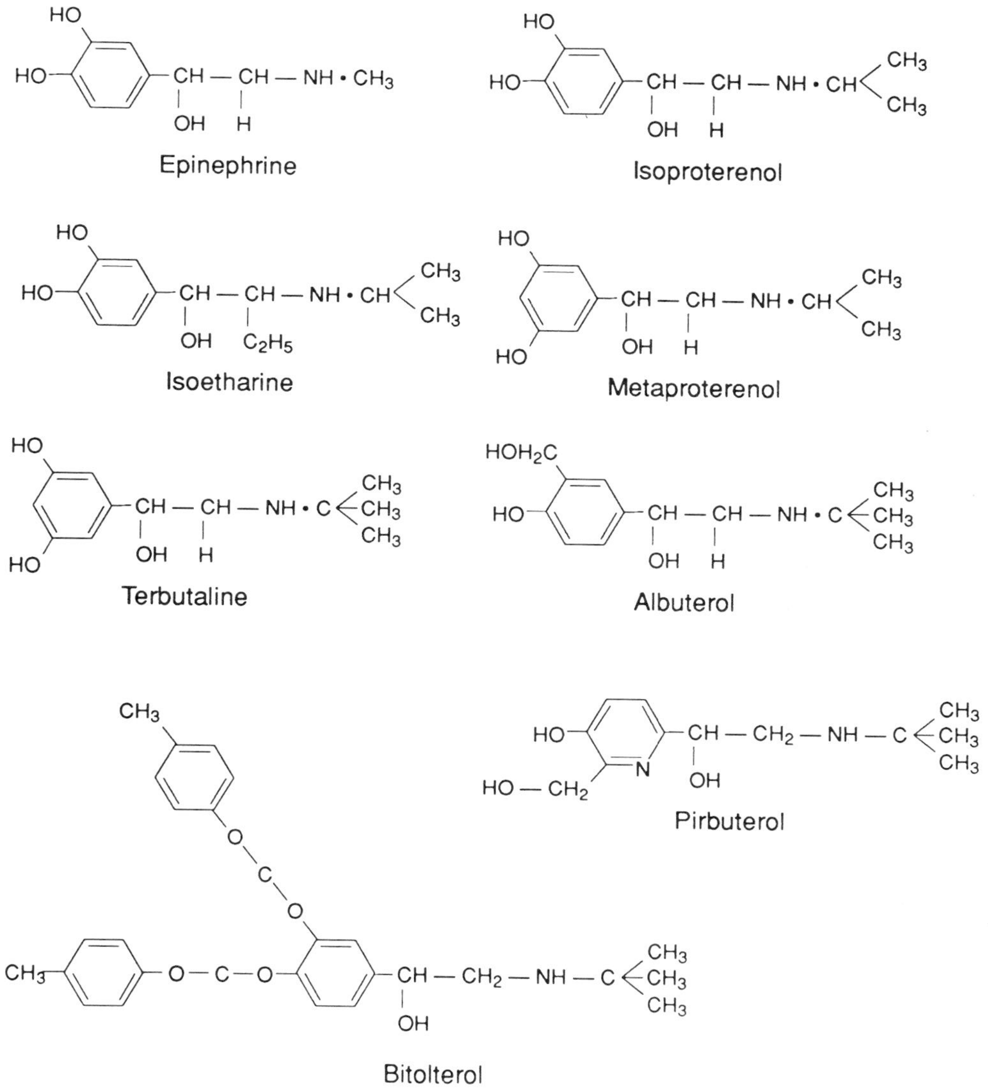

Epinephrine

Isoproterenol

Isoetharine

Metaproterenol

Terbutaline

Albuterol

Pirbuterol

Bitolterol

Figure 20-3. Chemical structures of eight representative beta-agonist bronchodilators.

onist is pirbuterol, which belongs to the pyridine class of chemical compounds.

Dozens of other agents have been tried clinically as bronchodilators. Table 20-3 lists those beta agonists currently available in North America for inhalational use. In general terms, those higher in the table are more rapid in onset, have a shorter duration of effect, and are less beta-2 specific than those below them.

Epinephrine and isoproterenol are nonselective: epinephrine stimulates all three types of receptors about equally, while isoproterenol is beta-selective but has equal beta-1 and beta-2 effects. Both are potent bronchodilators but must be used cautiously in patients over age 40 or in those with hypertension or other cardiovascular disease because of their propensity to cause hypertension, tachycardia, and dysrhythmias. A curious paradox of government regulation allows epinephrine, the most potentially hazardous of inhaled bronchodilators, to be purchased without prescription,[4] while the others (all safer than epinephrine) require a physician's prescription.[3]

Isoetharine and metaproterenol are more beta-2 selective than epinephrine and isoproterenol but in general are less specifically selective, and for most patients do not last as long, as those agents listed beneath them in Table 20-3. The last five drugs in the table are the most beta-2-selective bronchodilators currently available. According to a number of published studies, bitolterol, pirbuterol, and fenoterol may have longer durations of therapeutic effect than albuterol and terbutaline, although there is much variation among individuals. All five drugs are more effective and safer to use than any bronchodilators available around 1970, and choosing among them is more a matter of personal preference than of consistent objective differences in either peak effect or duration.

Table 20-3. Beta-Agonist Bronchodilators for Aerosol Administration

Drug	Brand Names	Relative Beta-2 Selectivity	MDI Dose per Activation (mg)[a]	Nebulizer Solution Dose (mg)[b]	Usual Duration of Effect (h)[c]
Epinephrine	Bronkaid, Primatene, etc.	–	0.16–0.25	NA	0.5–1.5
Isoproterenol	Isuprel, Nedihaler-iso, etc.	–	0.08–0.14	2.5	1–2
Isoetharine	Bronkometer, Bronkosol	+	0.34	2.5–5.0	2–4
Metaproterenol	Alupent, Metaprel	+	0.65	10–15	2–4
Albuterol	Proventil, Ventolin	++	0.09	2.5	4–6
Terbutaline	Brethaire, Brethine	++	0.20	0.25–0.50[d]	4–6
Bitolterol	Tornalate	++	0.37	NA	4–6+
Pirbuterol	Maxair	++	0.20	NA	4–6+
Fenoterol[e]	Berotec	++	0.20	NA	4–6+

[a] Usual dose 2 activations.
[b] Nebulized in 2 to 3 mL total volume.
[c] Varies among individuals.
[d] Not approved for this indication in the United States.
[e] Available in Canada and Europe but not in the United States.

All the drugs shown in Table 20-3 are available in aerosol form via propellant-powered metered-dose inhalers (MDIs). However, planned restrictions on the use of chlorofluorocarbon propellants, including a proposed worldwide ban by the year 2000, are prompting development of different methods of airway administration. Albuterol is currently available in capsules containing the drug in powdered form; the capsule is inserted into a hand-held device, which releases the powder for the patient to inhale. Other approaches to propellant-free inhalation of these drugs can be expected soon.

Although aerosol administration is the mainstay of therapy, several beta agonists are available for use by other routes. Three agents listed in Table 20-3 may be obtained in tablet form: metaproterenol (10 and 20 mg), albuterol (2 and 4 mg), and terbutaline (2.5 and 5 mg). These doses are all 5 to 10 times those delivered by one puff from an MDI; this and their systemic route of administration guarantee more adverse effects than when the same drugs are taken by inhalation, even if several puffs are used. Albuterol is available in slow-release tablets, which extend the duration of action, and albuterol and metaproterenol are also available in liquid form for easier dosing in pediatric patients.

Ephedrine, an orally administered bronchodilator in use for thousands of years, resembles epinephrine but is a phenylalkylamine alkaloid rather than a catecholamine.[5] It is relatively ineffective and has numerous side effects. Ephedrine has some use in younger patients with mild asthma and is a constituent of several fixed-combination antiasthma preparations, but it is less appropriate for older individuals or those with moderate or severe disease.

Beta-agonist bronchodilators may also be given intravenously (albuterol and isoproterenol, which, however, are not approved for this route of administration in the United States) or subcutaneously (epinephrine and terbutaline). Continuous intravenous infusion of albuterol has been used in Europe for refractory status asthmaticus,[18] although the advantages of this over aerosol delivery are doubtful[16,18] and the drug must be administered with great care. Subcutaneous epinephrine and terbutaline are useful in short-term emergency treatment of acute bronchospasm, particularly in younger patients.[14,16]

The search for more powerful, more beta-2-specific, longer-acting sympathomimetic drugs continues, and new agents will likely be introduced before the year 2000. Agents that look promising at the time of writing (1992) include broxaterol, formoterol, procaterol, and salmeterol; others are sure to appear, in the literature if not in the local pharmacy.

Indications and Administration

Beta-agonist bronchodilators are indicated as primary treatment for the clinical manifestations of asthma, namely, wheezing, dyspnea, cough, and chest tightness. While they have little effect on the underlying disease process, they are the most effective agents available for symptom control. Although the potential for improvement tends to be less in other obstructive disorders such as chronic obstructive pulmonary disease (COPD) and cystic fibrosis, beta agonists are also an important component of comprehensive management in these conditions.

In addition to treating symptoms that are already present, the beta agonists are valuable prophylactically in settings in which the development of bronchospasm can be predicted in advance. These agents can prevent or attenuate symptoms when used 10 to 20 minutes before strenuous exercise or exposure to cold air, allergens, or emotionally stressful situations.

Aerosol

The inhalation route is preferable to all others whenever it can be used.[18,19] In the past, administration has tended to be via MDI for intermittent or mild symptoms and via nebulizer for more frequent or severe manifestations. The doses used for nebulization tended to be much larger than that which could be delivered in two puffs of an MDI, and clinicians and patients alike concluded that the former was more effective. However, numerous studies have shown no significant difference between the two delivery methods when physiologic assessment of effect is used.[20]

Because nebulization is cumbersome and more expensive and because the drugs used today are essentially free from adverse effects when given by inhalation, a reasonable initial approach is to use larger doses via MDI than the two puffs traditionally recommended (Fig. 20-1). Although the U.S. Food and Drug Administration still recommends only one or two puffs per dose, this is far less than what is routinely used in many parts of the world.[18] The addition of a spacer device can improve the response for many patients.[18,19,21–23] When one of the more beta-2-specific agents listed in Table 20-3 is used, a reasonable dosing sequence might be the following, proceeding down the list if the previous maneuver is clinically ineffective:

1. MDI two puffs
2. MDI three to six puffs over several minutes (as many as 10 to 20 puffs may be required in sicker patients and may safely be given under appropriate medical supervision[18])
3. MDI as above, with spacer device
4. Administration as solution via nebulizer

Some clinicians prefer that patients take one or two puffs initially and then wait a few minutes for the airways to "open up" so that subsequent puffs will deliver the drug more effectively to more distal airways. Patients are instructed to repeat this sequence as many times as necessary to achieve the greatest bronchodilation possible.

Individuals vary in their responses to different beta agonists. This variation applies to onset and duration of action and also to adverse effects. For this reason there is no single "best" drug among those listed in Table 20-3, and trying different agents may be worthwhile, especially for patients with severe symptoms.

Subcutaneous

Either epinephrine or terbutaline may effectively be given subcutaneously for emergency treatment of acute severe bronchospasm. The dose of epinephrine is 0.3 to 0.5 mg, which can be repeated every 15 to 30 minutes up to a maximum of 1.0 mg in 2 hours or 2.0 mg in 24 hours; subcutaneous terbutaline is given in doses of 0.25 to 0.35 mg, repeated in 20 to 30 minutes if necessary to a maximum dosage of 0.5 mg in 4 hours or 1.0 mg in 24 hours.[14] This route should generally be restricted to younger patients and those without cardiovascular disease.

Oral

There is probably no advantage to be gained from oral administration if adequate inhaled doses can be given, and even at higher aerosol doses adverse effects are less than with oral dosing. If the oral route is used, the smaller dose of albuterol, metaproterenol, or terbutaline should be tried, initially twice a day, and subsequently increased if needed. Tremor may be bothersome for many patients, although it usually becomes less troublesome with time.

Contraindications, Adverse Effects, and Monitoring

Beta agonists are generally not indicated in pulmonary disorders other than those producing an obstructive defect, such as asthma and COPD. Individual agents should not be used in those rare patients who have previously manifested allergic or idiosyncratic reactions to them. Ephedrine is contraindicated in hypertension, cardiac disease, glaucoma, prostatic hypertrophy, and other conditions predisposing to urinary retention.

The adverse effects of epinephrine and ephedrine are due to stimulation of alpha- and beta-1 receptors in the central nervous and cardiovascular systems, and include restlessness, headache, tremor, palpitations, insomnia, and weakness. More beta-2-specific agents produce dose-related side effects by stimulating both beta-1 and beta-2 receptors; palpitations, tachycardia, and tremor are the most frequent of these. Tremor, especially prominent with oral administration, is produced not in the central nervous system but by direct stimulation of beta-2 receptors in skeletal muscle.

Currently available agents, such as the last five shown in Table 20-3, are remarkably safe even at much higher inhaled doses than traditionally recommended. Beta-agonist aerosols (primarily isoproterenol at very high doses) were implicated in a rash of fatalities in Britain in the mid-1960s; whether members of the current generation of inhaled bronchodilators have played any role in a possible recent worldwide increase in asthma deaths has not been established.

Efficacy should ideally be monitored by using objective, physiologic measurements such as FEV_1 or peak flow rate. This is especially important in patients with severe, constant functional impairment. For many patients with less disabling symptoms, the subjective effects of these drugs are sufficient for monitoring. Side effects are likewise generally tracked by the patient's subjective report. Blood levels are not available for routine clinical use.

ANTICHOLINERGIC BRONCHODILATORS

Identification and Actions

Anticholinergic agents inhibit the action of the natural neurotransmitter acetylcholine at the cholinergic receptor sites of the parasympathetic postganglionic system[24,25] (Fig. 20-2). Such drugs counteract the effects of muscarine (an alkaloid found in poisonous mushrooms), the classic stimulator of the cholinergic nervous system, and are thus also known as antimuscarinic agents.

Muscarinic receptors are found in smooth muscle (in the bronchi, the heart, and the intestine), in secretory glands (e.g., sweat, salivary, and tear glands, plus mucus-secreting glands of the respiratory and gastrointestinal tracts), and in the muscles of the iris and of ocular accommodation. Stimulation of these receptors thus produces smooth muscle contraction, glandular secretion, and pupillary constriction. Blockade of the muscarinic receptors by anticholinergic agents produces the opposites of these: smooth muscle relaxation (i.e., bronchodilation), drying of secretions, pupillary dilation (mydriasis), and paralysis of accommodation (cycloplegia).

Except for bronchodilation, all these effects are undesirable, at least with respect to the treatment of airway obstruction. The ideal anticholinergic bronchodilator would therefore affect only airway smooth muscle; it should be inhaled directly onto its site of action, should not penetrate to the bronchial mucous glands (which derive their innervation from nerves deep to the mucosa), and should not be systemically absorbed. Of the two agents used as bronchodilators in the United States, atropine and ipratropium bromide (Fig. 20-4), the latter meets these requirements very well.

While beta-agonist bronchodilators exert a prominent effect on distal bronchioles, anticholinergics preferentially act on the more proximal airways, which are more richly supplied with muscarinic receptors. These agents tend therefore to have a relatively greater effect in bronchitis and in bronchospasm of reflex origin, than in asthma.[25] Although the absolute improvement in FEV_1 tends to be greater in asthma because of its greater degree of reversibility, patients with bronchitis and emphysema (i.e., COPD) generally experience a proportionately greater improvement with anticholinergic agents than they do with beta agonists.

The onset of the therapeutic effect is often more gradual with these drugs than with the beta agonists. Peak improvement in airflow occurs at 30 to 90 minutes, and the duration of effect for most patients is about the same as with the newer adrenergic agents. Anticholinergics are generally less effective in allergic and exercise-induced asthma than in bronchospasm with a prominent emotional component.[24] They also tend to be less successful prophylactically than the beta agonists.

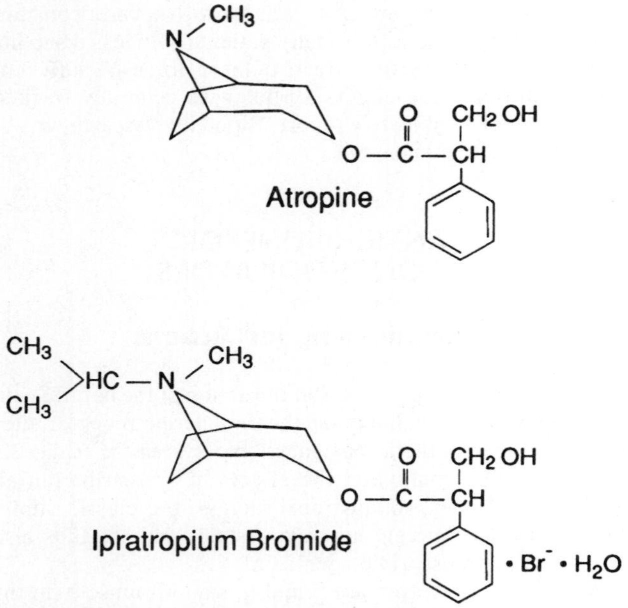

Figure 20-4. Chemical structures of atropine and ipratropium bromide, two anticholinergic bronchodilators.

Available Preparations

Atropine, a tertiary ammonium compound, has been used as a bronchodilator in Europe since about 1960. It must be nebulized from solution, since it cannot be sufficiently concentrated for use in an MDI. Being readily absorbed through the bronchial mucosa, inhaled atropine may produce drying of secretions, along with tachycardia and other systemic effects, although these are tolerated by many patients. Atropine given systemically is valuable in anesthesia; it is also used in pulmonary medicine to prevent vasovagal attacks and to deliberately reduce airway secretions during bronchoscopy and other procedures.

The quaternary ammonium compounds have been developed more recently and are virtually free of systemic effects when administered topically to the airway. Ipratropium bromide (Atrovent), which is available in Europe in inhalant solution but in the United States only by MDI, is the only member of this group used as an aerosol in this country. Atropine methonitrate is similar and has been used as an aerosol bronchodilator. A more recently developed drug, oxitropium, has effects like those of ipratropium but a longer duration of action; it and other analogues may be introduced in the United States in the future. Glycopyrrolate is a quaternary ammonium compound used orally and parenterally as a premedication for bronchoscopy to reduce airway secretions.

Indications and Administration

Ipratropium bromide is a first-line drug for use along with beta-2 agonists in COPD and may be more effective than the latter in this condition.[26] It is a second-line drug in asthma in that fewer patients respond to it than to beta agonists; only one-third to one-half generally report clinically important improvement. Therapeutic responses to ipratropium and to beta agonists correlate poorly in individual patients, particularly those with COPD. Improvement in FEV_1 following inhaled beta agonist should thus not be used to predict which patients will respond to anticholinergics. Atropine and ipratropium can be given concomitantly with beta agonists and methylxanthines and in fact may provide a synergistic effect. In some countries ipratropium is available along with a beta-2 agonist in the same MDI canister.

The delivered dose of ipratropium bromide is 0.02 mg per MDI activation, and the usual starting dose for adults is two puffs every 4 to 6 hours. Two to three times this amount may safely be administered if needed. Atropine is administered via nebulizer at a dose of 0.02 mg/kg (1 to 2 mg for most adult patients) in a total volume of 2 to 3 mL every 4 to 6 hours. As a premedication for bronchoscopy, thoracentesis, etc., 0.6 to 0.8 mg of atropine is injected subcutaneously or intramuscularly 30 to 60 minutes before the procedure begins.

Contraindications and Adverse Effects

Atropine should not be used in nonpulmonary disorders exacerbated by blockade of parasympathetic innervation, such as angle-closure glaucoma, gastric outlet obstruction, or prostatic hypertrophy or other causes of bladder outlet obstruction. There are essentially no contraindications to ipratropium.

Systemically administered atropine produces tachycardia, dry mouth, pupillary dilation, and blurring of near vision even in the usual therapeutic dosages. Inspissation of secretions can be a significant problem for patients with respiratory disease. These effects can also occur with aerosols, particularly with prolonged use. Urinary retention may occur, especially with higher doses and in elderly men. Atropine overdose produces the classic manifestations of antimuscarinic poisoning, namely, diffuse cutaneous vasodilation, thirst, agitation, and delirium ("red as a beet, hot as a pistol, dry as a bone, and mad as a hatter").

Patients taking ipratropium occasionally complain of dryness of the mouth and throat and may find the drug's bitter taste disagreeable. However, the dose required to produce systemic side effects is some 100-fold greater than that usually given by inhalation.[27] Tachyphylaxis to anticholinergic bronchodilators has not been reported.

CORTICOSTEROIDS

Identification and Actions

Steroid hormones isolated from the adrenal cortex (adrenocorticoids)[28,29] were first introduced into clinical medicine in the early 1940s. Both naturally occurring and synthetic agents are derivatives of hydrocortisone, sharing a common four-ring, 21-carbon structure (Fig. 20-5). The actions of adrenocorticoids fall into three groups: androgenic, mineralocorticoid, and glucocorticoid. Only the last of these is desirable in treating pulmonary disorders.

Glucocorticoids are not bronchodilators but exert an anti-inflammatory effect through mechanisms that remain incompletely understood. They have several known effects on disorders characterized by an inappropriately severe immune or inflammatory response,[28,30] including

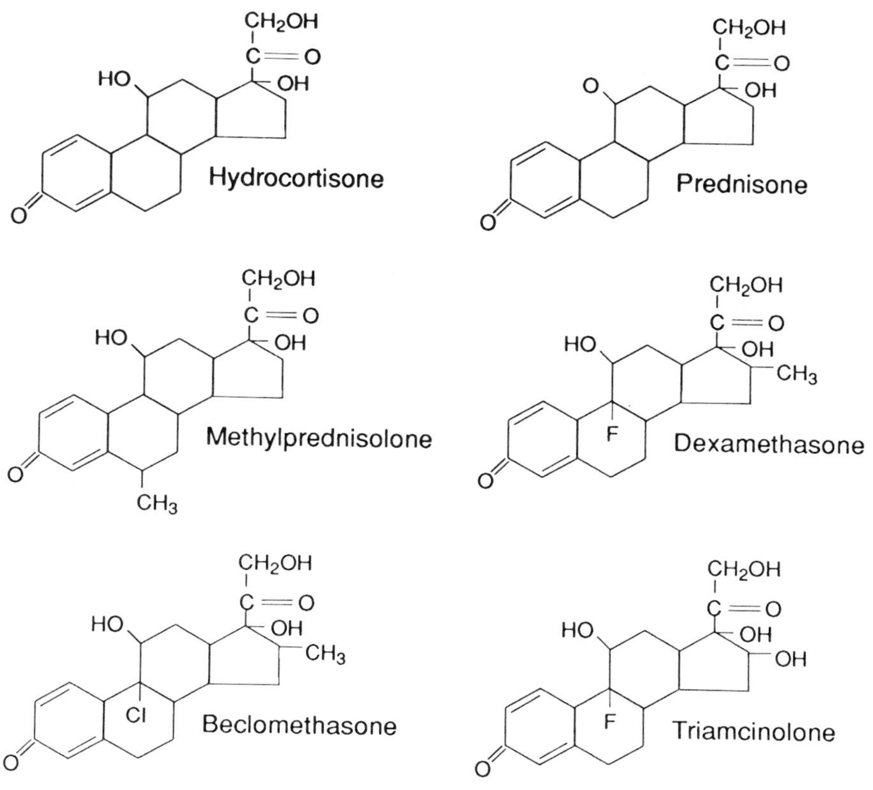

Figure 20-5. Chemical structures of six representative corticosteroid drugs used in the treatment of respiratory disease.

Inhibition of arachidonic acid conversion pathways

Suppression of IgE binding by receptors on cell surfaces

Enhancement of responsiveness of beta-2 receptors to bronchodilators

Inhibition of release of several mediators of inflammation

Reduction of abnormal mucus production

Modification of entry of calcium ions into cells, thus decreasing airway reactivity

Through these and presumably other mechanisms, corticosteroids diminish the exudation and migration of inflammatory cells, protect cell membranes against damage by a variety of agents, and reduce edema.

Available Preparations

Figure 20-5 shows the chemical structure of six representative glucocorticoids used in the management of respiratory disease.

Drugs Used Systemically

Available preparations vary according to relative anti-inflammatory potency, and are listed in Table 20-4 in order of increasing strength on a per weight basis. They also vary in duration of activity after a single dose; although serum half-life varies from 1 hour for prednisone to about 5 hours for triamcinolone, their effective biologic half-lives are much longer. This accounts for both their powerful anti-inflammatory effect and their propensity to exert undesirable hormonal and other effects on the body.

Prednisone is the drug most often used in the United States for oral administration; in Europe and elsewhere, prednisolone is more prevalent. Prednisone is converted to prednisolone in the liver. For short-term parenteral therapy methylprednisolone sodium succinate (Solu-Medrol) is most often used. *Hydrocortisone* is an effective alternative, although correspondingly larger doses must be used.

Drugs Used by Inhalation

Glucocorticoids with high potency and low systemic absorption have become a mainstay in controlling the inflammatory component of asthma.[22] Three preparations are available in the United States: beclomethasone diproprionate (Beclovent, Vanceril), flunisolide (AeroBid), and triamcinolone acetonide (Azmacort). All three are available by MDI, delivering 0.042, 0.25, and 0.10 mg per actuation, respectively. Although poorly absorbed from the bronchial mucosa, all three agents can produce detectable systemic effects when used in sufficiently high dosage; usual maximal recommended doses (16 inhalations per 24 hours for beclomethasone or triamcinolone, 8 for flunisolide) are roughly equivalent to 10 mg prednisone daily.

Corticotropin (adrenocorticotropic hormone [ACTH]) stimulates endogenous secretion of glucocorticoids and was formerly used in parenteral therapy of severe asthma. Because it has pronounced mineralocorticoid as well as androgenic effects and because the clinical response produced is erratic, it is no longer indicated in respiratory disease.

Indications and Administration

Corticosteroids are valuable in the management of asthma, both in prophylaxis and in treatment of acute attacks. Some patients with severe impairment require systemic doses for long-term administration. Short-term administration of corticosteroids is beneficial in acute exacerbations of COPD; perhaps 10 to 20 percent of patients with severe, disabling disease will also benefit in the long term, although the degree of improvement must be weighed against the high incidence of serious adverse effects (see Ch. 62). Other pulmonary diseases such as sarcoidosis, idiopathic pulmonary fibrosis, and hypersensitivity pneumonitis are often treated with systemic corticosteroids; clinical responses tend to vary, and the efficacy of these agents remains unproven in these conditions. Steroids do not help in aspiration pneumonia, smoke inhalation, or the adult respiratory distress syndrome (ARDS).

The use of these agents in obstructive airways disease (asthma and COPD) owes more to empiricism than to hard scientific data. Outpatients are generally treated orally and

Table 20-4. Corticosteroid Drugs Used Systemically in Treating Respiratory Diseases

Drug	Brand Names	Route of Administration	Equivalent Potency[a] (approx)	Equipotent Dose (mg) (approx)	Physiologic Half-life (h)
Hydrocortisone	Solu-Cortef, etc.	IV	1	20	8–12
Prednisone	Deltasone, etc.	Oral	4	5	12–30
Prednisolone	Prednisolone	Oral	4	5	12–30
Methylprednisolone	Medrol, Solu-medrol	Oral, IV	5	4	15–30
Triamcinolone	Aristocort, etc.	Oral, IM[b]	5	4	18–48
Dexamethasone	Decadron	Oral, IM, IV[b]	25	0.75	36–54
Betamethasone	Celestone	Oral, IM, IV	25	0.75	36–54

[a] glucocorticoid potency, with hydrocortisone arbitrarily designated as 1.
[b] Also available in aerosol form (inappropriate for systemic use).

hospitalized patients intravenously; much larger doses, given more often, are commonly used for inpatients. More precise guidelines than those presented below are unlikely to be forthcoming soon, owing to the difficulty of performing adequate clinical studies pertinent to these aspects of management. However, it is important to distinguish *short-term* from *long-term* steroid therapy. Short-term systemic administration of even high doses of these agents tends to be benign and can generally be undertaken empirically. By contrast, long-term oral therapy is fraught with enough serious adverse effects that objective documentation of efficacy and repeated attempts to discontinue it are warranted. *Inhaled* steroids, although expensive and bothersome to use for prolonged periods, have a low incidence of side effects and are gaining more importance in the long-term management of asthma. However, inhaled corticosteroids are ineffective in the management of an acute asthmatic attack and are probably not clinically useful in COPD.

Status Asthmaticus

Corticosteroids should be administered empirically and immediately to status asthmaticus patients. Commonly used initial doses for adults are intravenous methylprednisolone 80 to 1000 mg or hydrocortisone 400 to 2000 mg/24 h, usually in four divided doses. Tapering should follow over several days once clinical improvement occurs.

Acute Asthma

Patients with acute asthma, who do not respond to intensive bronchodilator therapy, or who have required steroids in the past for similar episodes, should be given prednisone or prednisolone, 20 to 40 mg immediately and then daily for several days, tapering over several more days once the attack has subsided.

Chronic Severe Asthma

For chronic severe asthma, the lowest morning dose of prednisone or prednisolone that maintains remission should be used, and an attempt should be made to switch to alternate-day therapy and/or an inhaled steroid as soon as possible. High doses of an inhaled agent (e.g., beclomethasone four puffs qid, triamcinolone four puffs tid or qid, or flunisolide four puffs bid) should be tried in an attempt to discontinue oral steroids. Oral candidiasis (thrush), which is common with these higher doses, is much less frequent when a spacer device is used.

COPD with Acute Exacerbation

For hospitalized COPD patients with acute exacerbation, methylprednisolone 2 mg/kg/24 h IV in four divided doses should be given for several days,[31] followed by tapering over 3 to 5 additional days. For most outpatients, prednisone or prednisolone, 40 to 60 mg every morning for 3 to 5 days followed by tapering over an equivalent period, is effective.[32]

Stable, Disabling COPD

For patients with stable but disabling COPD, steroid therapy for more than 1 to 2 weeks requires objective documentation of efficacy because of the likelihood of long-term side effects. Bronchodilator and other therapy should first be optimized (see Ch. 62), and baseline spirometry then obtained. Prednisone or prednisolone, 20 to 40 mg every morning for 2 to 4 weeks (with continuation of all other therapy), should be followed by repeat spirometry. The drug should be tapered over 5 to 10 days and discontinued unless a substantial improvement (e.g., 30 percent increase in FEV_1) has occurred, in which case an attempt should be made to decrease the dose to the lowest alternate-day or daily amount that maintains the improvement.[32]

Contraindications, Adverse Effects, and Monitoring

Systemically administered corticosteroids are contraindicated whenever acceptable disease control can be achieved with other therapy. For patients who have had disabling adverse effects (e.g., psychosis, vertebral fractures), optimal control of airway obstruction with corticosteroids may not be clinically feasible. A rare patient manifests allergy or idiosyncrasy to these agents, in which case they should not be used.

Acute effects of steroid use include euphoria and a sense of well-being. Restlessness, insomnia, and frank psychosis can occur within a few days after systemic therapy is begun, as can hyperglycemia, peptic ulceration, and upper gastrointestinal bleeding. However, these short-term effects are relatively uncommon, unlike the situation with prolonged administration. Table 20-5[5] lists the principal adverse effects of corticosteroid use, the majority of which occur with long-term, systemic administration. The main complication of use of inhaled steroids is oral candidiasis, but its incidence may be reduced through the use of spacer devices.

Although short-term systemic steroids are commonly used empirically without physiologic monitoring, the use of serial peak expiratory flow or FEV_1 measurements in this setting is common in Europe and should be more widely employed in the United States. Physiologic measurements are mandatory in long-term systemic administration of corticosteroids.

METHYLXANTHINES

Identification and Actions

Theophylline and related methylxanthine compounds (Table 20-6 and Fig. 20-6) have been mainstays in the therapy of asthma and COPD for many years.[33,34] They still play an important role in these conditions, but their toxicity, the expense and inconvenience of establishing appropriate blood levels, and the introduction of more effective inhalational

Table 20-5. Complications of Corticosteroid Therapy

Site	Minor Adverse Effects	Major Adverse Effects
Skin	Acne, hirsutism, facial erythema, panniculitis	Loss of subcutaneous tissue; poor wound healing
Vascular	Petechiae, bruising	Vasculitis, thrombosis, thromboembolism
Appearance	Fat deposition on face, back of neck, trunk	Stunting of growth in children
Central nervous system	Euphoria, insomnia, restlessness	Psychosis, personality change
Cardiovascular	Sodium retention (edema, nocturia)	Hypertension, heart failure
Metabolic	Electrolyte disturbance, calcium loss, alkalosis, negative nitrogen balance, hyperlipidemia	Diabetogenic effect
Musculoskeletal	Weakness (due to myopathy, hypokalemia, wasting), osteoporosis	Fractures (especially vertebrae), aseptic necrosis
Endocrine	Menstrual disorders, menopausal symptoms	Suppression of hypothalamic-pituitary-adrenal axis
Gastrointestinal	Gastritis, esophagitis, increased appetite	Increased risk of peptic ulceration, large bowel perforation, pancreatitis
Ocular	Exophthalmos	Cataract, benign intracranial hypertension
Immunologic	Suppression of skin responses to antigenic tests	Impaired response to infection, opportunistic infections

(Adapted from Ziment,[5] with permission.)

agents have relegated them to second- or third-line therapy in most instances.[35]

The methylxanthines are inhibitors of the enzyme phosphodiesterase and have long been believed to act by the mechanism shown in Figure 20-2. However, the clinical importance of this mechanism has been called into doubt, and it must be admitted that we do not really know how these drugs work.[35,36] The methylxanthines have numerous effects in addition to bronchodilation: they render the diaphragm more efficient and resistant to fatigue,[37,38] stimulate ventilatory drives and other central nervous system functions, modify the sensation of dyspnea,[39,40] stimulate the heart,[39] and act as diuretics. Patients with COPD whose airflow obstruction does not improve with the use of theophylline may nonetheless report greater exercise tolerance and decreased dyspnea, although these effects are inconsistent and unexplained.[35]

Table 20-6. Methylxanthine Bronchodilators

Agent	Brand Name	Equivalent Dosage (by weight) to Anhydrous Theophylline
Theophylline, anhydrous	(many)	100
Aminophylline (theophylline ethylenediamine)	(many)	80
Dyphylline (dihydroxypropyl theophylline)	Dilor; Lufyllin	70
Oxtryphilline (choline theophyllinate)	Choledyl	64
Theophylline calcium salicylate	Quadrinal[a]	50
Theophylline sodium glycinate	Asbron G[a]	50

[a] Fixed-combination product also containing other agents.

All the agents listed in Table 20-6 are metabolized by the liver to theophylline, the active agent. When administering preparations other than anhydrous theophylline, the clinician should keep in mind their therapeutic equivalencies (shown in Table 20-6).

Available Preparations

Theophylline and the other methylxanthines are not suitable for aerosol administration. All the agents in Table 20-6 are available in oral preparations, most of them in both rapid-release and sustained-release forms and some as elixirs. Theophylline is also available in 24-hour preparations, which permit once per day dosing in some patients and better control of nocturnal symptoms in others. Aminophylline is commonly used intravenously; and dyphylline is also available in an injectable preparation. Rectal aminophylline is seldom used in the United States today, although this route of administration remains in more common use in some other countries.

Theophylline is a common constituent of fixed-dose antiasthma preparations, some of them available without prescription. Table 20-7 lists those combinations currently sold in the United States.

Indications and Administration

Parenteral therapy with aminophylline consists of two phases, an initial loading dose (to establish a therapeutic level of theophylline in the patient's serum), and a subsequent continuous infusion (to maintain the serum level in the

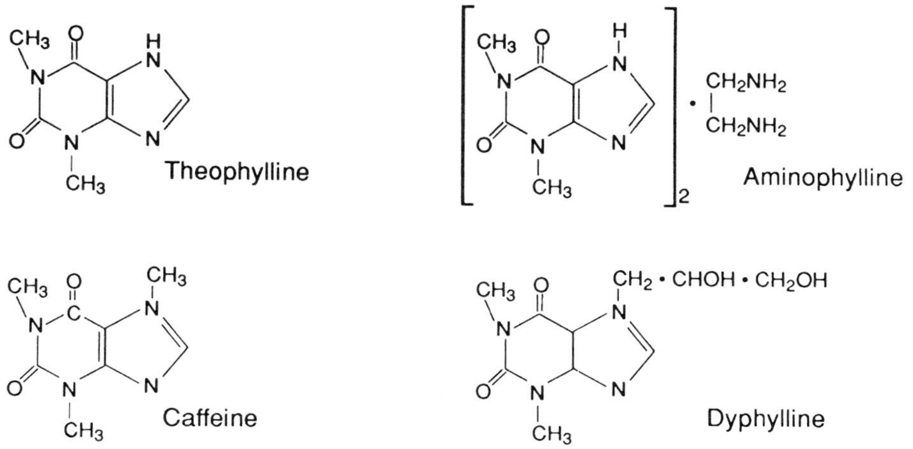

Figure 20-6. Chemical structures of theophylline and three other familiar methylxanthine compounds.

desired range).[33] Table 20-8 summarizes current recommendations for intravenous loading and maintenance therapy. The maintenance infusion rates shown are considerably less than those advocated in the past and even so will be excessive for some patients. Because methylxanthines are metabolized by the liver, any degree of hepatic dysfunction will markedly reduce the clearance and hence raise the serum levels of these drugs. In all instances blood theophylline should be measured soon after loading and frequently thereafter as long as parenteral therapy is continued.

Conversion from intravenous aminophylline to oral anhydrous theophylline once a stable daily requirement has been established can be accomplished by using an aminophylline theophylline ratio of 1.2:1.0.

Table 20-7. Methylxanthine-Containing, Fixed-Combination Bronchodilator Preparations Available in Tablet or Capsule Form in the United States

Brand	Theophylline (or Equivalent)	Ephedrine	Guaifenesin	Other Agents
Asbron G	150	—	100	—
Bronkaid[a]	100	24[b]	100	—
Bronkotabs[c]	100	24[b]	100	Phenobarbital 8 mg
Dilor-G	140[d]	—	200	—
Marax	130	25[b]	—	Hydroxyzine HCl 10 mg
Mudrane	100[e]	16[f]	—	Phenobarbital 8 mg Potassium iodide 195 mg
Mudrane-2	100[e]	—	—	Potassium iodide 195 mg
Mudrane GG	100[e]	16[f]	100	Phenobarbital 8 mg
Mudrane GG-2	100[e]	—	100	—
Primatene[a]	130	24[f]	—	—
Primatene P formula[c]	130	24[f]	—	Phenobarbital 8 mg
Primatene M formula[g]	130	24[f]	—	Pyrilamine maleate 16.6 mg
Quadrinal	65[h]	24[f]	—	Phenobarbital 24 mg Potassium iodide 320 mg
Quibron	150	—	90	—
Quibron-300	300	—	180	—
Slo-Phylline GG	150	—	90	—
Tedral SA	180[i]	48[f,j]	—	Phenobarbital 25 mg

[a] Available without prescription.
[b] As ephedrine sulfate.
[c] Available without prescription in states in which this is legal for phenobarbital.
[d] As dyphylline 200 mg.
[e] As aminophylline 130 mg.
[f] As ephedrine HCl.
[g] Available without prescription in states in which phenobarbital is prescription-only.
[h] As theophylline calcium salicylate 130 mg.
[i] 90 mg in immediate-release form, 90 mg in sustained-release form.
[j] 16 mg in immediate-release form, 32 mg in sustained-release form.

Table 20-8. Guidelines for Intravenous Administration of Aminophylline

Clinical Setting	Initial Loading Dose (mg/kg) Administered over 30 min[a]
Patient not receiving theophylline	6.0[b]
Patient receiving theophylline; serum level considered subtherapeutic	3.0[c]
Patient receiving theophylline; serum level excessive, therapeutic, or unknown	No loading dose

Patient Description	Initial Maintenance Infusion Rate (mg/kg/h)[d]
Child 1–16 yr	0.8
Young adult smoker	0.6
Young adult nonsmoker (e.g., asthma)	0.5
Older adult (e.g., COPD without cor pulmonale)	0.4
Patient with cor pulmonale, congestive heart failure, or liver disease	0.2

[a] Calculated on the basis of estimated ideal body weight for obese patients; serum level measured 30 min following completion of loading dose.

[b] Intended to achieve serum level of 10–12 μg/mL.

[c] Intended to raise serum level by 5–6 μg/mL.

[d] Recheck serum level 6–12 hours after infusion begins and then periodically as long as patient is receiving IV aminophylline.

Combination antiasthma preparations (Table 20-7) offer apparent convenience, but their fixed doses of multiple agents increase the likelihood of adverse reactions, with little chance that any of their components will be in optimum quantity for a given patient. These products should not be used by patients with moderate or severe asthma (e.g., those with daily symptoms), and combinations containing ephedrine should be avoided by middle-aged and older persons.

Adverse Effects and Monitoring

Theophylline's therapeutic index (the ratio of its therapeutic to its toxic serum levels) is narrow and highly variable among different patients. When it is given in the usual therapeutic range (serum level 10 to 20 μg/mL), many patients experience nausea, vomiting, bloating, vague abdominal discomfort, irritability, and insomnia. Some individuals develop these side effects even at subtherapeutic blood levels. Other, more serious adverse effects include cardiac arrhythmias (extrasystoles, tachycardia) and convulsions; these generally occur only at blood levels above 30 μg/mL in otherwise healthy persons but can develop even in the therapeutic range in those with underlying cardiac disease or seizure disorder. Numerous other adverse effects may also occur with theophylline.[5,33,41]

Serum levels should be checked intermittently in any patient regularly receiving methylxanthine therapy, both to ensure sufficient dosage and to guard against serious toxicity. Blood levels do not correlate perfectly with adverse effects, however, and patients should be queried at intervals for development of subtle symptoms such as vague gastrointestinal discomfort and insomnia.

CROMOLYN

A chromone derivative, cromolyn sodium (known as disodium cromoglycate in Europe) is an inhalational agent used prophylactically to prevent bronchospasm.[42,43] It is not a bronchodilator and has no role in the treatment of acute asthma. It appears to work by "stabilizing" airway mast cells and thus preventing them from degranulating (and releasing histamine and other mediators of bronchoconstriction) in response to antigen or osmotic challenge. Regulation of intracellular calcium flux also seems to be involved.

Cromolyn (Intal) is available in several preparations. The original and most widely used of these is a dry powder contained in gelatin capsules, which are punctured in a special device (Spinhaler turbo-inhaler) that allows the drug to be inhaled over several breaths. The drug is also marketed in an MDI and in solution for nebulization; nasal and ophthalmic forms are available as well.

Cromolyn is especially helpful in allergic, "extrinsic" asthma, particularly in younger patients, and can enable some steroid-dependent individuals to discontinue these more dangerous drugs. It is also effective for many patients in preventing exercise-induced bronchospasm. Older, "intrinsic" asthmatics respond less consistently, and cromolyn is not effective in COPD.

Except in purely exercise-induced asthma, a trial of several weeks is necessary to determine whether a given patient will respond to cromolyn. The drug must be taken regularly in order to maintain its prophylactic effect, although many patients can go from a four times daily to a twice daily regimen after 2 to 3 weeks.

Cromolyn is largely free from adverse effects, although a rare individual manifests allergy to the preparation. The powder form not infrequently causes throat irritation; some patients also experience cough and bronchospasm, which can be prevented by prior or concomitant inhalation of a beta agonist.

MUCOLYTICS AND EXPECTORANTS

Mucolytic agents alter the characteristics of airway secretions; expectorants cause an increase in the amount of fluid in the respiratory tract. Together these agents are known as *mucokinetics*, a term coined and popularized by Ziment[5,44,45] and defined as symptomatic therapies that promote the clearance of respiratory secretions from the lung. Mucokinetic therapies have been used for thousands of years and are still highly regarded worldwide by physicians and

Table 20-9. Agents That Affect Airway Mucus

Type of Agent	Action	Examples
Hydrating agent	Adds water to respiratory secretions	Water; hypotonic saline
Bronchorrheic	Topical irritant, stimulating secretion of free water into airways	Hypertonic saline
Detergent	Decreases adhesiveness of mucus to airways through surfactant effect	Sodium bicarbonate
Mucolytic	Breaks up mucoproteins and DNA molecules into smaller units	Acetylcysteine
Mucotropic	Stimulates bronchial mucus glands	Potassium iodide; iodinated glycerol
Ciliary stimulator	Increases mucociliary clearance	Beta-2 agonists; corticosteroids; theophylline
Expectorant	Stimulates bronchial mucus glands through vagal reflex	Guaifenesin; ipecac; terpin hydrate

patients alike.[46] However, they have long been eyed skeptically by the American medical community, largely because of a lack of objective documentation of their efficacy.[47] Widespread administration of these agents via intermittent positive pressure breathing (IPPB) and other apparatus during the 1960s and 1970s helped to give respiratory therapy a reputation for being unscientific and unnecessary.

The main types of mucokinetic agents are listed and defined in Table 20-9. There is no question that these preparations have the effects listed. What continues to stimulate controversy, however, is the difficulty of detecting and interpreting their effects clinically. Meaningful studies of the characteristics and quantity of secretions in patients with airway disease are exceedingly difficult to carry out. In addition, the meaning of any differences shown by such studies is hard to evaluate: increased sputum expectoration might signify either improved clearance or additional irritation or inflammation—the former desirable, the latter undesirable. Likewise, a decrease in sputum expectoration could have either good or bad implications. As Ziment himself admits, "although we can classify [these] agents on the basis of their apparent primary physiologic effects, there is little proof that any class of mucokinetic medication is of clinical benefit."[45]

Acetylcysteine (Mucomyst) has numerous actions in addition to being a mucolytic: it is an antidote for acetaminophen overdose and certain other poisonings and may eventually prove beneficial in protecting tissues from oxidant and free-radical injury.[48] Acetylcysteine quickly liquefies mucus in vitro and can be effective when instilled directly onto mucus plugs or inspissated secretions during bronchoscopy. It is most commonly used, however, as an aerosol, and clinical efficacy in this application has never been demonstrated convincingly in large studies.[45,49] An oral form of the drug, which may be more effective, is not available in the United States.

Iodides, such as potassium iodide and iodinated glycerol, are used in cystic fibrosis, chronic bronchitis, and other conditions in which raising secretions is difficult. Like the other agents described, they have not been unequivocally proved to work, although many patients believe they are effective. However, unlike acetylcysteine, guaifenesin, and the agents discussed below, which are generally free from significant side effects, iodides cause adverse effects in as many as half of all patients.[47] These may consist only of a metallic taste, increased salivation, coryza, acne, or headache, but more serious problems such as urticaria, angioedema, serum sickness, and thrombotic thrombocytopenic purpura also occur.

Sodium bicarbonate, which acts as a detergent in the airways, can be instilled directly into the airways or nebulized as a 2 to 10 percent solution. This can be of significant benefit in intubated or tracheostomized patients with thick, inspissated secretions. Bicarbonate solution is inexpensive and generally free from side effects. Hypertonic saline (3 to 5 percent NaCl) also facilitates sputum expectoration and is currently the preferred agent for sputum induction in diagnosing *Pneumocystis carinii* pneumonia in patients with the acquired immunodeficiency syndrome (AIDS).[50] Plain *water* has long been touted as an effective hydrating agent for secretions, although its effects have been as difficult to prove as those of other mucokinetics.[49] Aerosolized water stimulates cough, particularly when it is delivered via devices such as ultrasonic nebulizers, but it is unclear what else it accomplishes. It is important for patients with airway disease to drink enough water to avoid dehydration, but it is likewise uncertain whether consuming additional fluids benefits mucus clearance.

Probably the most effective mucokinetic agents for the clinician in the United States are already used for other reasons in these patients. Beta agonists, theophylline, and the corticosteroids all improve ciliary beating and facilitate mucociliary clearance.[45] However, use of these drugs for these effects in patients whose airway function does not improve (e.g., as measured by FEV_1 or peak flow) is fraught with the same vagaries as administration of the agents discussed above.

RESPIRATORY STIMULANTS

Drugs that increase the drive to breathe do so either by stimulating the central respiratory centers in the brain stem or by peripherally affecting the carotid and/or aortic chemoreceptors.[51,52] Table 20-10 shows the major respiratory stimulant drugs, which represent a wide variety of agents. All have in common the ability to augment the urge to

Table 20-10. Drugs That Stimulate Ventilatory Drives

Drug	Type	Site of Action	Clinical Uses
Doxapram (Dopram)	Analeptic	Peripheral; central	May be useful in post-anesthetic arousal
Acetazolamide (Diamox)	Carbonic anhydrase inhibitor	Central	Altitude illness; central sleep apnea; primary hypoventilation
Progesterone (Provera)	Progestational hormone	Central	Primary hypoventilation; sleep apnea (?); COPD (?)
Almitrine[a]	Piperazine derivative	Peripheral chemoreceptors	Hypoxemic COPD (possible alternative to home O_2)
Theophylline	Methylxanthine	Central (?); peripheral (?); respiratory muscles (?)	Not specifically indicated as a respiratory stimulant
Protriptyline (Vivactil)	Tricyclic	Central	Sleep apnea
Naloxone (Narcan)	Opiate antagonist	Central	To counteract opiate-induced hypoventilation

[a] Used in Europe but not available in the United States.

breathe. Their use thus has theoretical value in conditions characterized by hypoventilation in patients whose peripheral breathing apparatus (efferent nerves, muscles, thorax, airways, and lungs) is intact. However, stimulating the ventilatory drives of individuals who are incapable of increasing their ventilation (e.g., because of paralysis, muscle weakness, or airway obstruction) could only be expected to increase respiratory distress without augmenting the end result. Thus, although some of the drugs in this category are quite effective, they are useful in only a few clinical circumstances.

Doxapram is given by continuous intravenous infusion and must be monitored carefully. It has limited use today in hastening postanesthetic awakening. In the past some clinicians also used it in COPD and other patients with impending acute respiratory failure as a means of avoiding intubation and mechanical ventilation.[51] However, neither doxapram nor any other respiratory stimulant has been shown in controlled studies to affect this or any other aspect of acute respiratory failure, and the drug should not be used in this way.

Progesterone is useful in chronic alveolar hypoventilation of central origin (e.g., the pickwickian syndrome), and also in some forms of sleep apnea.[53] It may also be useful in patients with COPD and chronic CO_2 retention whose airflow limitation is not so severe as to prevent them from breathing more; selecting appropriate patients is difficult, however. The drug is given orally (Provera, 20 mg tid), and 1 to 2 weeks' use may be necessary to see a clinical effect. Its long-term side effects include diminished libido and impotence in men and vaginal bleeding in women.

Almitrine bismesylate stimulates ventilation and also appears to modify the matching of pulmonary ventilation and perfusion in such a way that PaO_2 (arterial partial pressure of O_2) is raised even when PCO_2 (partial pressure of CO_2) does not change. It has been studied in Europe as a possible alternative to long-term O_2 therapy in patients with chronic hypoxemia; while it is effective, adverse effects from prolonged use may limit its future role.[54]

Protriptyline, a nonsedating tricyclic antidepressant, also has respiratory stimulant properties, which make it useful in treating depression in patients with severe COPD. In addition, preliminary evidence suggests that this drug may be effective in raising PaO_2 and decreasing $PaCO_2$ in patients with chronic hypoventilation, both during the day and while asleep.[55] Like almitrine, however, protriptyline may prove unacceptably toxic for routine long-term use for this purpose.

Theophylline appears to have both central and peripheral stimulatory effects in addition to augmenting the contractility of the diaphragm.[34,35,39] The contributions of these and other mechanisms to the modest increase in overall ventilation produced by the methylxanthines are uncertain. At present, a role for these agents as respiratory stimulants apart from their use as bronchodilators has not been firmly established.

RESPIRATORY DEPRESSANTS

Any centrally acting agent that sedates or calms a patient will also diminish the drive to breathe.[52] While this effect is inconsequential (or even helpful) in stable patients in the chronic setting, it can precipitate life-threatening hypoventilation in those who are acutely unstable. Respiratory depression is encountered most often with opiates (morphine, meperidine [Demerol], codeine, etc), used for systemic analgesia and as premedication for surgical procedures, and benzodiazepines (diazepam [Valium], midazolam [Versed], triazolam [Halcion], etc) and other agents used for anxiolysis, sedation, and hypnosis. Although it is less widely appreciated, alcohol and even mild sleeping aids such as diphenhydramine (Benadryl) can cause hypoventilation, especially in hypoxemic, acutely unstable patients.

In properly selected patients, respiratory depressants can be used effectively in the treatment of dyspnea.[56] Hydrocodone, oxycodone, dihydrocodeine, and other analogues of the opiate codeine can ameliorate disabling dyspnea in clinically stable patients with COPD, pulmonary fibrosis, and other disorders; this therapy must be undertaken cautiously and with careful patient supervision. Benzodiazepines have also been tried as therapy for dyspnea but with inconsistent results.

ANTITUSSIVES

In most instances cough is a helpful physiologic phenomenon that should not be eliminated. Drugs to suppress cough should be used to enable the patient to remove airway secretions while not being kept awake coughing because of airway irritation or reflex.[47]

Antitussives act either centrally (by raising the threshold necessary to stimulate the cough center) or peripherally (by reducing local irritation in the airways). The best centrally acting agents are narcotics, of which codeine and hydrocodone are the most effective preparations. The dose required to suppress cough (e.g., 10 to 20 mg codeine or 5 to 10 mg of hydrocodone every 4 to 6 hours for adult patients) is generally less than that necessary for pain relief. Constipation is the chief adverse effect, especially with repeated administration. Dextromethorphan is the most widely used non-narcotic centrally acting antitussive, and is available in numerous preparations. The usual dose is 10 to 20 mg every 4 hours or 30 mg every 6 to 8 hours; nausea, dizziness, and slight drowsiness are occasionally reported as side effects.

Agents acting in the airway to suppress the cough reflex include topical anesthetics, demulcents, and expectorants. Lidocaine and other "caine" drugs such as cocaine and tetracaine are very effective when applied topically to the airways via aerosol or by instillation and are a mainstay of preanesthesia for bronchoscopy, endotracheal intubation, and other procedures. Demulcents are compounds of high molecular weight that dissolve to form syrup-like fluids, which soothe inflamed mucosal surfaces by coating them.[5] In addition to traditional home antitussives, such as honey and sugar syrup, demulcents are used in a wide variety of proprietary cough syrups and lozenges and include methylcellulose, propylene glycol, glycerin, and agar.[47] The effectiveness of expectorants such as guaifenesin as cough suppressants is unproven, although they are commonly employed for this purpose.

OTHER DRUGS OF IMPORTANCE IN RESPIRATORY CARE

Alpha-1-antitrypsin has recently been introduced as specific replacement therapy for homozygous alpha-1-antitrypsin deficiency, a cause of precocious emphysema.[57,58] Exceedingly expensive, and presumably required lifelong, this drug can raise serum and aleveolar fluid alpha-1-antitrypsin levels, but its effect on the progression of the lung disease is yet unknown. It is given by IV infusion, 60 mg/kg, once each week. Three forms of surfactant (bovine, human, and synthetic) have been studied as replacement therapy for respiratory distress syndrome. Initial experience with surfactant replacement in neonates is promising,[59] although for several reasons the outlook may be less bright in ARDS.[60]

Pentamidine (Pentam), an antimicrobial agent used in the treatment of *Pneumocystis carinii* pneumonia in patients with AIDS and other forms of severe immunosuppression, is administered by aerosol both for prophylaxis and for treatment of established disease.[61,62] When given by inhalation, this drug is considerably less toxic to the patient than in its intravenous form; however, whether repeated low-level exposure to pentamidine poses a health risk to patients or caregivers remains to be established.[18]

Ribavirin (Virasole) is a synthetic nucleoside antiviral agent used in treating severe respiratory syncytial virus (RSV) pulmonary infections in infants.[63] Technical aspects of this drug's administration are important because of its propensity to deposit on ventilator circuitry and other apparatus if not handled properly.[64,65] As with pentamidine, there is concern but conflicting evidence for a health risk to those administering ribavirin.[18]

Several drugs are used in severe asthma for their steroid-sparing effects. One such agent is troleandomycin (TAO), a macrolide antibiotic related to erythromycin, which permits the daily dose of prednisolone (but not prednisone) to be reduced, often by 50 percent or more, without loss of anti-inflammatory effect. It is controversial, however, whether this effect is of clinical importance for most patients, and it may be that both the therapeutic and the adverse effects of the corticosteroid are simply "turbocharged" by TAO, so that lower doses exert the same systemic effect.[66]

Methotrexate, and potentially other anticancer drugs, have been reported to have a long-term steroid-sparing effect in severe chronic asthma.[67] This appears to be true for at least some patients, although recent data cast doubt on the initial claims.[68] Further studies are clearly needed before these potentially hazardous agents can be recommended routinely for use in asthma.[69]

Nedocromil (Tilade), an inhaled drug used in Europe, has prophylactic effects similar to those of cromolyn in both allergen- and non-allergen-induced bronchoconstriction.[70] Ketotifen (Zaditen) is an antihistamine effective orally in prophylaxis against acute asthma, also producing effects similar to those of cromolyn. Although clinical studies to date are inconclusive, ketotifen could have a place in the future management of asthma and airway hyperreactivity.

The calcium channel blockers, a group of drugs that includes verapamil, nifedipine, and diltiazem among others, are used in treatment of cardiac arrhythmias, angina pectoris, and hypertension. On theoretical grounds they should also be effective in asthma, as calcium ion flux is known to be important to the function of smooth muscle cells, mast cells, neutrophils, and mucus-secreting cells. Although some studies have demonstrated modest antibronchospasm activity, thus far this important class of therapeutic agents has been disappointing in asthma management.[71,72]

Beta blockers, also important drugs in the management of cardiovascular disease, are important in respiratory care because of their opposite effects to the beta-2 agonists. Propanolol and the other beta blockers can precipitate or worsen bronchospasm in both asthma and COPD, sometimes fatally, and their use should be avoided if possible in patients with these conditions. Several agents have been promoted as cardiac-specific, with less propensity to worsen airflow obstruction, but none so far is completely without airway effects. Even topically applied beta blockers, such as timolol and others used in treatment of glaucoma, can precipitate life-threatening bronchospasm in susceptible individuals.

Nicotine substitution using Nicotine gum (Nicorette) is used as an adjunct in smoking cessation therapy in a manner analogous to methadone maintenance in individuals being treated for heroin addiction.[73,74] The preparation contains nicotine bound to an ion-exchange resin in a gum base and is available in 2 mg and (outside the United States) 4 mg doses. As described in Chapter 102, the gum must be used as part of a multifaceted program involving behavior modification and must be chewed in prescribed fashion (rather than ad lib as with ordinary chewing gum) in order to be maximally effective.[74] Dependency on the gum occurs in a small but significant minority of patients.

References

1. Gilman AG, Rall TW, Nies AS, Taylor P (eds): Goodman and Gilman's The Pharmacological Basis of Therapeutics. 8th Ed. Pergamon Press, New York, 1990
2. U.S. Pharmacopeial Convention, Inc.: USP DI. Drug Information for the Health Care Professional. U.S. Pharmacopeial Convention, Rockville, MD, 12th Ed., 1992
3. PDR: Physician's Desk Reference. Medical Economics Co., Oradell, NJ, 1992 (published yearly)
4. PDR: Physician's Desk Reference for Nonprescription Drugs. Medical Economics Co., Oradell, NJ, 1992 (published yearly)
5. Ziment I: Respiratory Pharmacology and Therapeutics. WB Saunders, Philadelphia, 1978
6. Cherniack RM (ed): Drugs for the Respiratory System. Grune & Stratton, Orlando, FL, 1986
7. Chernow B (ed): Essentials of Critical Care Pharmacology. Williams & Wilkins, Baltimore, 1989
8. Maunder RJ (ed): Drugs in the Intensive Care Unit. WB Saunders, Philadelphia, (in press)
9. Ziment I: Drugs used in respiratory therapy. pp. 411–448. In Burton GG, Hodgkin JE, Ward J (eds): Respiratory Care: A Guide to Clinical Practice. 3rd Ed. JB Lippincott, Philadelphia, 1991
10. Seligman M: Bronchodilators. pp. 207–221. In Chernow B (ed): Essentials of Critical Care Pharmacology. Williams & Wilkins, Baltimore, 1989
11. Ziment I, Popa VT (eds): Respiratory pharmacology. Clin Chest Med 1986;7:313–518
12. Witek TJ Jr, Schachter EN (eds): Advances in Respiratory Care Pharmacology. Probl Respir Care. 1988;1:1–153
13. Larsson S, Svedmyr N: Bronchodilating effect and side effects of beta$_2$-adrenoceptor stimulants by different modes of administration (tablets, metered aerosol, and combinations thereof). Am Rev Respir Dis 1977;116:861–869
14. Popa VT: Beta-adrenergic drugs. Clin Chest Med 1986;7:313–329
15. McFadden ER Jr: Inhaled aerosol bronchodilators. Williams & Wilkins, Baltimore, 1986
16. Swedish Society of Chest Medicine: High-dose inhaled versus intravenous salbutamol combined with theophylline in severe acute asthma. Eur Respir J 1990;3:163–170
17. Shenfield GM: Combination bronchodilator therapy. Drugs 1982;24:414–439
18. Consensus Conference on Aerosol Delivery. Respir Care 1991;36:914–1044
19. Sackner MA, Kim CS: Auxiliary MDI aerosol delivery systems. Chest, suppl. 1985; 88:161s–170s
20. Tashkin DP: Dosing strategies for bronchodilator aerosol delivery. Respir Care, 1991;36:977–988
21. Summer W, Elston R, Tharpe L, et al: Aerosol bronchodilator delivery methods. Arch Intern Med 1989;149:618–623
22. Konig P: Inhaled corticosteroids—their present and future role in the management of asthma. J Allergy Clin Immunol 1988;82:297–306
23. Newman SP: Delivery of therapeutic aerosols. Prob Respir Care 1988;1:53–82
24. Ziment I, Au JP: Anticholinergic agents. Clin Chest Med 1986;7:355–366
25. Gross NJ, Skorodin MS: Anticholinergic, antimuscarinic bronchodilators. Am Rev Respir Dis 1984;129:856–870
26. Gross NJ: Ipratropium bromide. N Engl J Med 1988;319:486–494
27. Engelhardt A: Pharmacology and toxicity of Atrovent. Scand J Respir Dis, suppl. 1979;103:110–115
28. Ziment I: Steroids. Clin Chest Med 1986;7:341–354
29. Chang S-W, King TE: Corticosteroids. pp. 77–138. In Cherniack RM (ed): Drugs for the Respiratory System. Grune & Stratton, Orlando, FL, 1986
30. Morris HG: Mechanisms of glucocorticoid action in pulmonary diseases. Chest, suppl. 1985;88:133s–141s
31. Albert RK, Martin TR, Lewis SW: Controlled clinical trial of methylprednisolone in patients with chronic bronchitis and acute respiratory insufficiency. Ann Intern Med 1980;92:753–758
32. Pierson DJ: Chronic obstructive pulmonary disease and bronchiectasis. pp. 97–106. In Rakel RE (ed): Conn's Current Therapy. WB Saunders, Philadelphia, 1985
33. Cummiskey J, Popa VT: Theophyllines—a review. J Asthma 1984;21:243–257
34. Jenne JW (ed): Rationale for the use of theophylline in COPD: Bronchodilation and beyond. Chest, suppl. 1987;92:1s–51s
35. Hill NS: The use of theophylline in "irreversible" chronic obstructive pulmonary disease. An update. Arch Intern Med 1988;148:2579–2584
36. Krzanowski JJ, Polson JB: Mechanisms of action of methylxanthines in asthma. J Allergy Clin Immunol 1988;82:143–145
37. Aubier M: Pharmacology of the respiratory muscles. Clin Chest Med 1988;9:311–324
38. Decramer M, Janssens S: Theophylline and the respiratory muscles. Eur Respir J 1989;2:399–401
39. Matthay RA, Mahler DA: Theophylline improves global cardiac function and reduces dyspnea in chronic obstructive lung disease. J Allergy Clin Immunol 1986;78:793–799
40. Stark RD: Dyspnoea: Assessment and pharmacological manipulation. Eur Respir J 1988;1:280–287
41. Albert S: Aminophylline toxicity. Pediatr Clin North Am 1987;34:61–73
42. Falliers CJ, Tinkelman DG: Alternative drug therapy for asthma. Clin Chest Med 1986;7:383–391
43. Murphy S, Kelly HW: Cromolyn sodium: A review of mechanisms and clinical use in asthma. Drug Intell Clin Pharm 1987;21:22–35
44. Ziment I: Hydration, humidification, and mucokinetic therapy. pp. 756–775. In Weiss EB, Segal MS, Stein M (eds): Bronchial asthma: Mechanisms and Therapeutics. 2nd Ed. Little Brown, Boston, 1985
45. Ziment, I: Agents that affect respiratory mucus. Problems Respir Care 1988;1:15–41
46. Braga PC, Allegra L (eds): Drugs in Bronchial Mucology. Raven Press, New York, 1989
47. Cott GR: Drug therapy in the management of cough. pp. 165–190. In Cherniack RM (ed): Drugs for the Respiratory System. Grune & Stratton, Orlando, FL, 1986
48. Ziment I: Acetylcysteine: A drug that is much more than a mucokinetic. Biomed Pharmacother 1988;42:513–520

49. Wanner A, Rao A: Clinical indications for and effects of bland, mucolytic, and antimicrobial aerosols. Am Rev Respir Dis, suppl. 1980;122:79–87
50. Leigh TR, Parsons P, Hume C et al: Sputum induction for diagnosis of *Pneumocystis carinii* pneumonia. Lancet 1989;2:205–206
51. Pierson DJ: Respiratory stimulants: Review of the literature and assessment of current status. Respir Care 1973;18:549–554
52. Altose MD, Hudgel DW: The pharmacology of respiratory depressants and stimulants. Clin Chest Med 1986;7:481–494
53. Mathewson HS: Drug therapy for obstructive sleep apnea. Respir Care 1986;31:717–719
54. Watanabe S, Kanner RE, Cutillo AG et al: Long-term effect of almitrine bismesylate in patients with hypoxemic chronic obstructive pulmonary disease. Am Rev Respir Dis 1989;140:1269–1273
55. Series F, Cormier Y: Effects of protryptyline on diurnal and nocturnal oxygenation in patients with chronic obstructive pulmonary disease. Ann Intern Med 1990;113:507–511
56. Woodcock AA, Gross ER, Gellert A et al: Effects of dihydrocodeine, alcohol, and caffeine on breathlessness and exercise tolerance in patients with chronic obstructive lung disease and normal blood gases. N Engl J Med 1981;305:1611–1616
57. Crystal RG, Brantly ML, Hubbard RC et al: The alpha 1-antitrypsin gene and its mutations: Clinical consequences and strategies for therapy. Chest 1989;95:196–208
58. Hubbard RC, Crystal RG: Augmentation therapy of alpha$_1$-antitrypsin deficiency. Eur Respir J, suppl. 1990;3:44s–52s
59. Merritt TA, Hallman M: Surfactant replacement. A new era with many challenges for neonatal medicine. Am J Dis Child 1988;142:1333–1339
60. Einhorning G: Surfactant replacement in adult respiratory distress syndrome. Am Rev Respir Dis 1989;140:281–283
61. Armstrong D, Bernard E: Aerosol pentamidine. Ann Intern Med 1988;109:852–854
62. Corkery KJ, Luce JM, Montgomery AB: Aerosolized pentamidine for treatment and prophylaxis of *Pneumocystis carinii* pneumonia: An update. Respir Care 1988;33:676–685
63. Rodriguez WJ, Parrott RH: Ribavirin aerosol treatment of serious respiratory syncytial virus infections in infants. Infect Dis Clin North Am 1987;1:425–439
64. Demers RR, Parker J, Frankel LR, Smith DW: Administration of ribavirin to neonatal and pediatric patients during mechanical ventilation. Respir Care 1986;31:1188–1195
65. Byron PR, Phillips EM, Kuhn R: Ribavirin administration by inhalation: Aerosol-generation factors controlling drug delivery to the lung. Respir Care 1988;33:1011–1019
66. Harris R, German D: The incidence of corticosteroid side effects in chronic steroid-dependent asthmatics on TAO (troleandomycin) and methylprednisolone. Ann Allergy 1989;63:110–111
67. Mullarkey MF, Lammert JK, Blumenstein BA: Long-term methotrexate treatment in corticosteroid-dependent asthma. Ann Intern Med 1990;112:577–581
68. Erzurum SC, Leff JA, Cochran JE et al: Lack of benefit of methotrexate in severe, steroid-dependent asthma: A double-blind, placebo-controlled study. Ann Intern Med 1991;114:353–360
69. Cott GR, Cherniack RM: Steroids and "steroid-sparing" agents in asthma. N Engl J Med 1988;318:634–636
70. Rocchiccioli KM, Riley PA: Clinical pharmacology of nedocromil sodium. Drugs, suppl. 1989;37:123–126
71. Mathewson HS: Anti-asthmatic properties of calcium antagonists. Respir Care 1987;30:779–781
72. Townley RG, Cheng J, Bewtra AK et al: The role of calcium channel blockers in reactive airway disease. Ann NY Acad Sci 1988;522:732–746
73. Benowitz NL: Drug therapy. Pharmacologic aspects of cigarette smoking and nicotine addiction. N Engl J Med 1988;319:1318–1330
74. Nett LM, Dingus SM: Smoking cessation techniques. pp. 107–116. In Kacmarek RM, Stoller JK (eds): Current Respiratory Care. BC Decker, Philadelphia, 1988

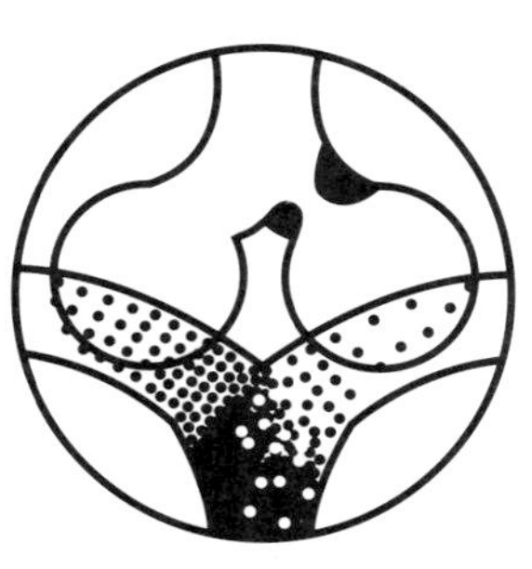

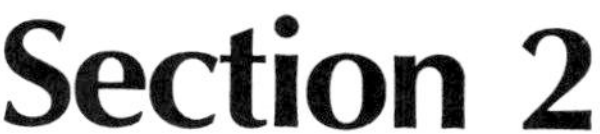

Section 2

Pathophysiology: How Disease Affects the Cardiorespiratory System

Chapter 21

Types of Respiratory Dysfunction in Disease

David J. Pierson

CHAPTER OUTLINE

Diseases were originally described and classified from the outside—according to the patient's symptoms and external appearance and what an examiner could detect by using the hands and a few simple instruments. Later diseases were described from the inside, according to pathologic changes in tissue that had been removed from the body, usually after the patient had died. With this change in approach, our knowledge of the structural effects of disease expanded greatly, although generally there was little that could be done to alter its course or modify its manifestations.

Parallel with the explosion of medical knowledge in the twentieth century has come the ability to detect and measure the *functional* impact of disease on the body during life, enabling clinicians to base treatment on pathophysiology rather than on trial and error.[1–5] This emphasis on pathophysiology rather than on empiricism constitutes one of the main foundations of respiratory care on which this book is based; it considers diseases in terms of how they affect cardiorespiratory function, and wherever possible it addresses therapy in terms of ways to reverse or counteract these functional effects.

The current age of molecular biology is providing increasing understanding of the ultimate mechanisms of disease[6] and will produce ever more specific treatments to prevent or reverse these. For the foreseeable future, however, a pathophysiologic approach to respiratory care will be indispensable for dealing with individuals already affected by disabling cardiopulmonary disease.[7,8]

BASIC PATTERNS OF RESPIRATORY DYSFUNCTION

Diseases affecting the respiratory system cause four basic types of dysfunction: obstruction, restriction, vascular impairment, and disordered ventilatory control (Table 21-1).

Airway obstruction produces reduced airflow, usually on expiration. The obstruction can be localized or generalized. Generalized lower airway obstruction reduces the elastic recoil of the lungs, which tend to enlarge, trapping air peripherally. Disorders producing pulmonary restriction cause an opposite effect: they increase elastic recoil and hence the tendency of the lungs to retract and collapse, resulting in reduced lung volumes. Figure 21-1 shows the characteristic pressure-volume changes in generalized obstructive versus restrictive pulmonary diseases, as exemplified by emphysema and pulmonary fibrosis, respectively.[1]

Table 21-1. Primary Characteristics of the Four Basic Forms of Respiratory Dysfunction in Disease[a]

Type of Defect	Description	Defining Functional Abnormality	Other Characteristics
Obstructive	Reduced airflow on expiration (tendency of lungs to enlarge)	$\downarrow$ FEV_1/FVC	$\uparrow$ RV $\uparrow$ FRC $\uparrow$ TLC
Restrictive	Increased lung elastic recoil (tendency of lungs to collapse)	$\downarrow$ TLC	$\downarrow$ VC with normal FEV_1/FVC
Vascular	Loss of pulmonary capillary surface area	$\downarrow$ DLCO	$\uparrow$ VD/VT
Control	Reduced sensitivity or central response to usual breathing stimuli	$\downarrow$ HVR and/or $\downarrow$ HCVR	$\downarrow$ PaO_2 $\uparrow$ $PaCO_2$

PaO_2, arterial O_2 partial pressure; $PaCO_2$, arterial CO_2 partial pressure; VD, dead space; VT, tidal volume; HVR, ventilatory response to hypoxia; HCVR, ventilatory response to hypercapnia.

[a] These are the typical or commonest findings, although variations do occur (e.g., inspiratory obstruction or increased ventilatory drive).

Pulmonary vascular disorders affect perfusion of gas exchange units and other lung tissues. Many obstructive and restrictive disorders have prominent vascular components, although some diseases affect only the circulation. Vascular disorders reduce the available capillary surface area in the lung and hence increase the amount of ventilation that is wasted (dead space). Disorders of ventilatory control affect the "thermostat" that regulates breathing according to need; most commonly this results in insufficient ventilation, either constantly, during sleep, or under stress by disease or the environment.

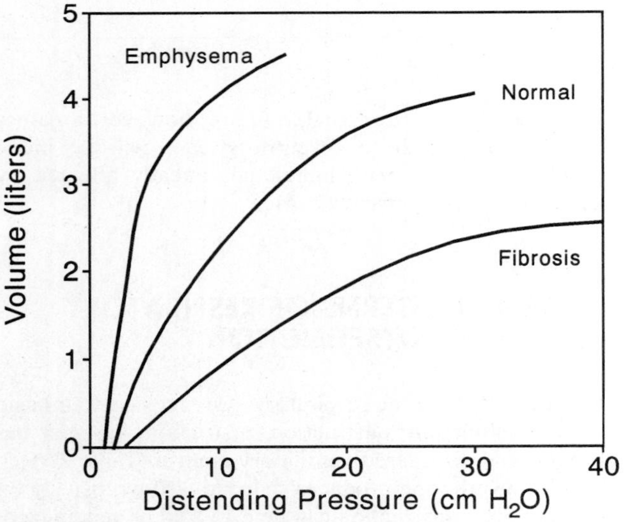

Figure 21-1. Representative pressure-volume curves for the lungs of a normal adult as compared with those of patients with obstructive and restrictive lung diseases, illustrated by emphysema and pulmonary fibrosis, respectively. The emphysematous lungs are larger and easier to distend (more compliant) than normal, while those of the patient with fibrosis are contracted and require higher pressures to inflate (e.g., their compliance is lower than normal). (Adapted from Murray,[1] with permission.)

All known diseases produce their respiratory effects via these four basic processes, any one of which may occur in isolation and be severe enough to be fatal. Each may be congenital or acquired. Their presence and severity may change with time or in response to therapy, and two or more may coexist in a given patient. In such instances, correct application of the assessment techniques described in Section 3 of this book can assist in detecting and quantifying the contributions of each.

AIRFLOW OBSTRUCTION

Generalized Lower Airway Obstruction

As described in Chapter 9, functional residual capacity (FRC) may be thought of either as the volume at which the static recoil forces of the lung and chest wall are balanced, or as that degree of end-expiratory tidal lung inflation at which the work of breathing is least.[8] The effects of expiratory airflow obstruction on FRC may be understood conceptually by using the second of these definitions and by separating the work of breathing into elastic and frictional components, as shown in Figure 21-2. The elastic component is the work necessary to stretch the tissues and surface lining of the lung, as well as the overlying chest wall; the frictional component is that work necessary to overcome airflow resistance in the conducting airways.

In airflow obstruction (Fig. 21-2B), as typified by chronic obstructive pulmonary disease (COPD) or asthma, elastic work remains about the same but airway narrowing (because of bronchospasm, mucosal edema, and/or secretions) increases the frictional component. The position of least work is thus at a higher lung volume than normal, and FRC is increased.

It would be natural to reason that increased effort would compensate for increased airway resistance and that by simply blowing harder a patient could overcome an obstructive ventilatory defect. However, this is not the case. Increasing the driving pressure of exhalation increases airflow only up

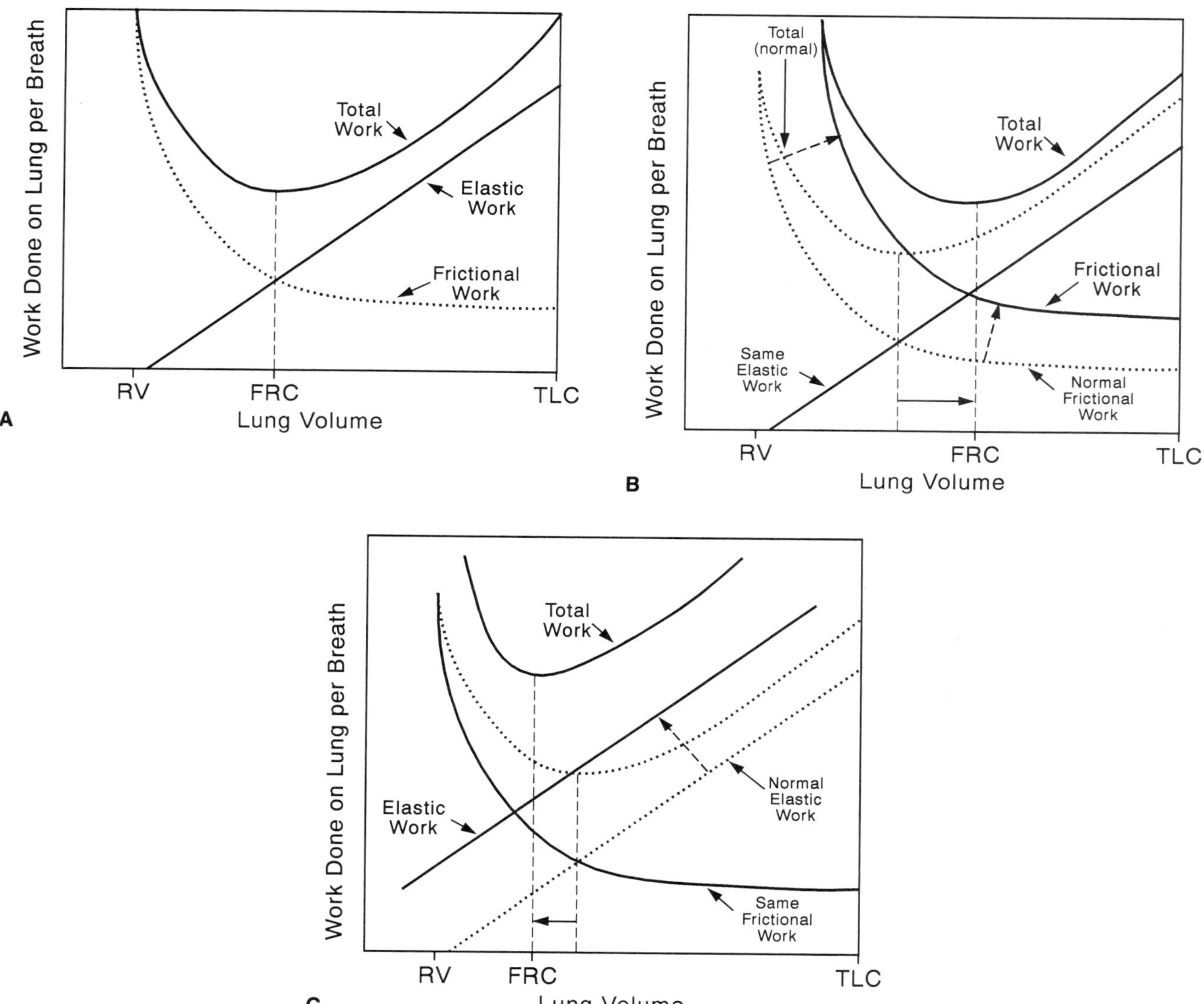

Figure 21-2. (**A**) Normal; (**B**) airflow obstruction; (**C**) pulmonary restriction. Effects of airflow obstruction and pulmonary restriction on the work of breathing, as determined by changes in its frictional and elastic components in comparison with the normal pattern. These diagrams illustrate the definition of FRC in terms of work rather than of volume: FRC is the resting end-expiratory lung volume at which the least work is required to inflate the lungs. In obstruction (e.g., bronchospasm, airway collapse), the increased work necessary to overcome frictional resistance to expiration results in a greater than normal FRC. By contrast, restrictive disorders increase the elastic forces that must be overcome to inflate the lungs, so that the position of least work is at a lower than normal lung volume. (Adapted from Culver,[8] with permission.)

to a certain point, beyond which the airways collapse and no further increase in flow is possible, as illustrated in Figure 21-3.[9]

Airflow obstruction is detected clinically by comparing two functions measured during a timed forced expiratory maneuver, namely, the forced expiratory volume in the first second (FEV_1) and the forced vital capacity (FVC). The tracing made during such a maneuver, a plot of exhaled volume versus time, is called a *forced expiratory spirogram*[8] (Figure 21-4). Normal individuals can forcibly exhale at least three-quarters of their vital capacity (VC) in the first second, regardless of age, height, or sex, the primary determinants of a person's lung volumes. If the ratio FEV_1/FVC is less than 0.70 to 0.75, clinically significant airflow obstruction is present. Lesser degrees of obstruction, as in disease confined to the small airways, may be detectable only by using additional tests, although, as discussed in Chapter 22, the clinical importance of such obstruction is debatable.

Figure 21-5 illustrates the appearance of spirograms in the presence of airflow obstruction and pulmonary restriction in

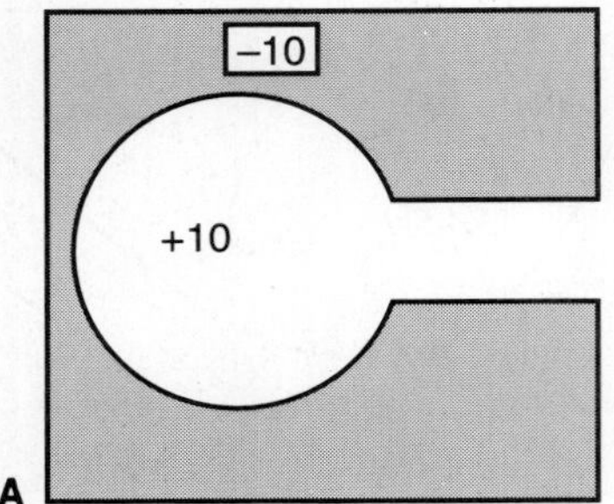

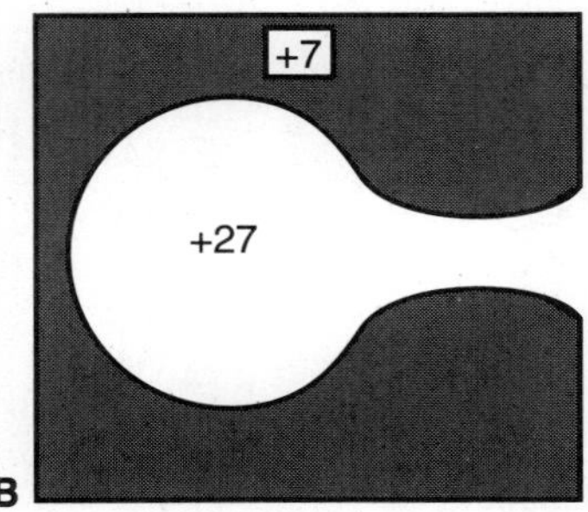

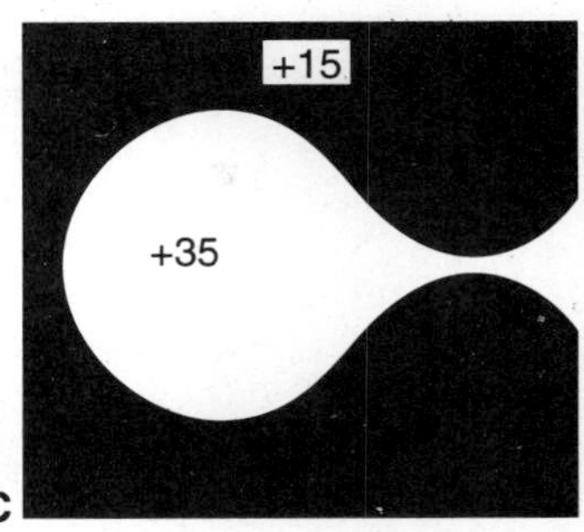

Figure 21-3. Schematic demonstration of why blowing harder does not necessarily increase airflow in the presence of an obstructive defect. The lung volume in each case is the same. Although increasing expiratory force raises the pressure that is driving air out of the alveoli, it also increases the pressure around the conducting airways and tends to collapse them. These effects tend to offset each other, so that above a certain point no increase in expiratory airflow can occur despite increased effort. (**A**) Passive exhalation (Vol = X, flow = Y); (**B**) Moderate effort (Vol = X, flow = 2Y); (**C**) Maximal effort (Vol = X, flow = 2Y). (From Marini,[9] with permission.)

comparison with normal tracings. The arrangement of the tracings in Figures 21-5A and B demonstrates the importance of using FEV_1/FVC rather than the absolute value of FEV_1 in detecting airflow obstruction, and of considering airflow obstruction in ascribing a low FVC to pulmonary restriction. The results of a forced expiratory maneuver can also be displayed in terms of flow versus volume (flow-volume loops), as shown in Figure 21-6.

Reduced lung elastic recoil and increased expiratory work of breathing in the presence of generalized lower airway obstruction both lead to air trapping and hyperinflation. These phenomena are illustrated by increases in residual volume

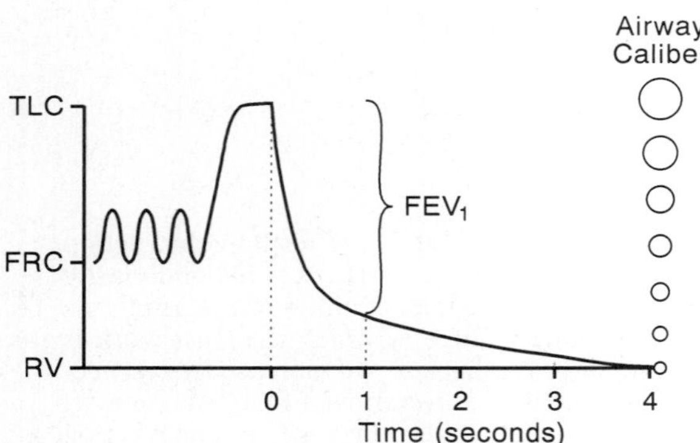

Figure 21-4. Normal spirogram: tracing of exhaled volume versus time during a forced expiratory maneuver. Exhalation begins at total lung capacity (TLC) and ends at residual volume (RV). Despite continued maximal effort, the flow rate decreases progressively as lung volume decreases, reflecting both smaller airway caliber (far right) and decreasing lung elastic recoil driving force. Time is measured from the moment the expiratory maneuver begins. Several measures of expiratory airflow can be made from the spirogram (see Ch. 46), but the most important in terms of identifying airflow obstruction is the FEV_1; obstruction is present whenever the ratio of FEV_1 to FVC is less than normal. (Adapted from Culver,[8] with permission.)

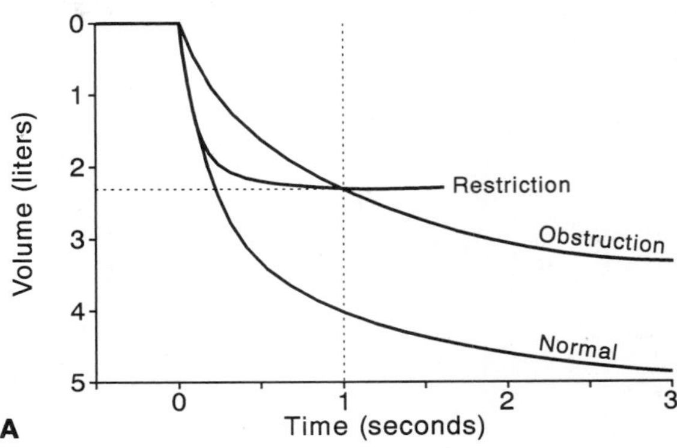

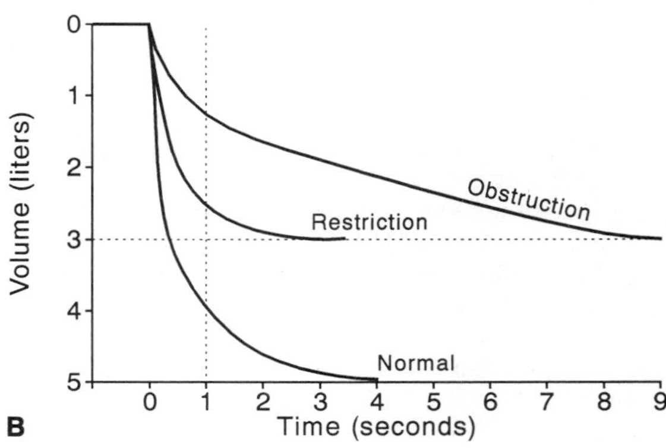

Figure 21-5. Representative spirograms showing obstructive and restrictive patterns in comparison with normal tracings. (**A**) Both abnormal tracings have FEV_1 values that are markedly reduced, but only one indicates obstruction (reduced FEV_1/FVC ratio, or $FEV_1\%$). (**B**) Similarly, although both abnormal tracings have the same FVC, only the one with the normal FEV_1/FVC ratio is consistent with a restrictive defect; air trapping rather than pulmonary restriction limits FVC in the obstructive tracing. (Note the different time scales in Figs. A and B.)

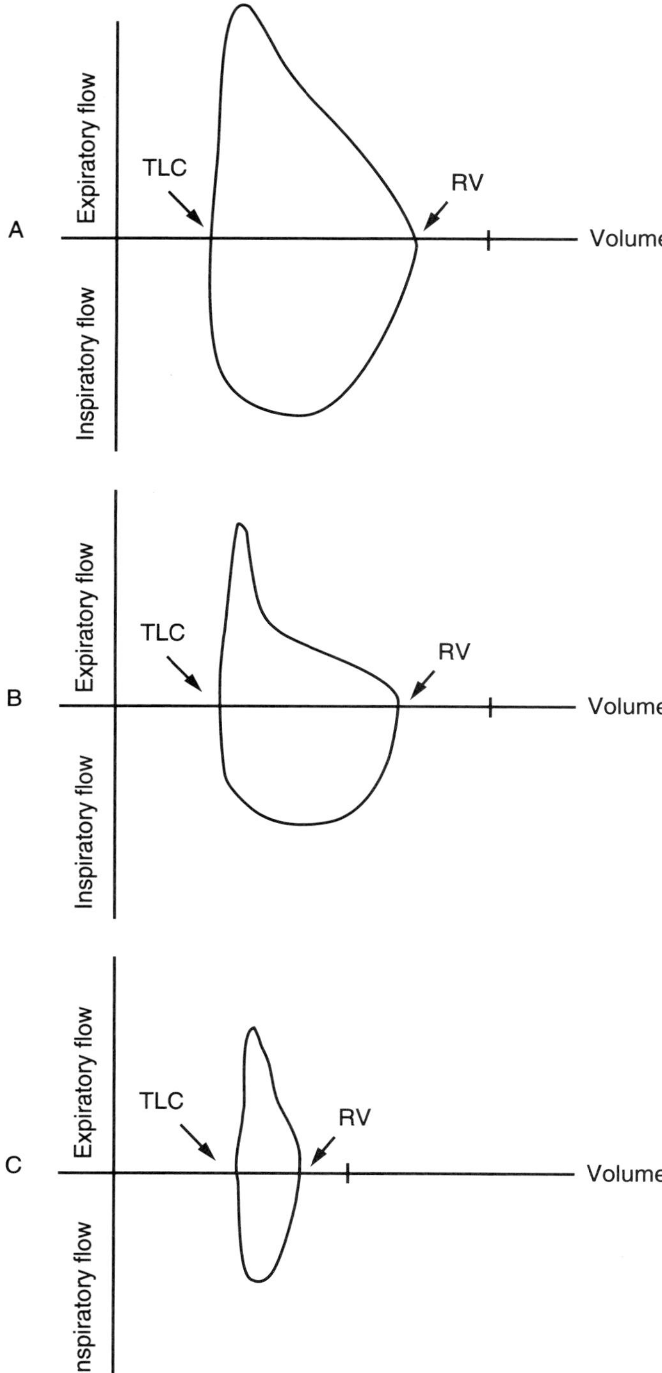

Figure 21-6. (**A**) Normal; (**B**) obstruction; (**C**) restriction. Flow-volume loops in severe generalized lower airway obstruction (e.g., COPD) and in severe pulmonary restriction (e.g., pulmonary fibrosis) as compared with a normal tracing. Expiration is impaired more than inspiration in lower airway obstruction; patients with predominantly emphysema may have little or no inspiratory obstruction, whereas those with bronchospasm and airway inflammation (e.g., asthma or COPD with prominent bronchitic component) will have greater reductions in inspiratory flow.

(RV) and total lung capacity (TLC), as well as in FRC, as measured by helium dilution or other techniques (Fig. 21-7).

Localized Lower Airway Obstruction

A tumor, stricture, or foreign body in a lobar or segmental bronchus may cause obstruction to airflow into and out of that portion of lung by the mechanisms discussed above. However, the clinical and physiologic effects of this would be slight in view of the relatively small amount of lung involved unless there were numerous such lesions. If a localized lesion obstructed the bronchus completely, physiologic tests would show restriction rather than obstruction because the affected lung tissue would no longer communicate with the major airways. Similarly, unless body plethysmography is used, a localized bulla or other intrapulmonary air collection communicating poorly with the main airways may produce a defect that is restrictive rather than obstructive.

Upper Airway Obstruction

Lesions causing obstruction to airflow in the upper airways (that is, proximal to the right and left mainstem bronchi) produce different effects depending on whether they lie inside or outside the thoracic cage.[10,11] Causes of extrathoracic upper airway obstruction include croup, acute epiglottitis, bilateral vocal cord paralysis, angioedema, adenotonsillar hypertrophy, and tumors proximal to the thoracic outlet. These and other lesions of the airway outside the chest produce obstruction that worsens during inspiration, when airway pressure becomes negative.

The opposite effect occurs with lesions producing a variable intrathoracic upper airway obstruction, such as tracheomalacia or a tumor of the lower trachea: positive pressure surrounding the trachea during forced exhalation increases

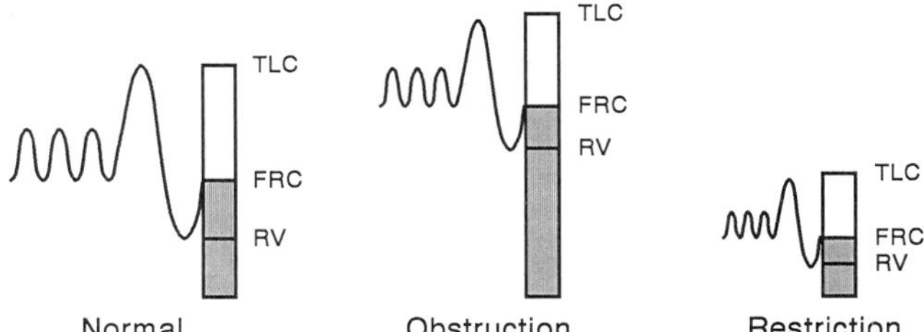

Figure 21-7. Effects of obstructive and restrictive disorders on lung volumes. The spirometric tracings indicate slow, unforced maneuvers, in contrast to those in Figures 21-4 and 21-5. Obstructive disorders such as emphysema and asthma tend to trap air in the lungs, increasing TLC, FRC, and RV; diseases producing pulmonary restriction, such as pulmonary fibrosis and severe obesity, tend to reduce the various lung compartments below normal. The boxes show static lung volumes; these should be compared with the dynamic effects shown in Figure 21-2.

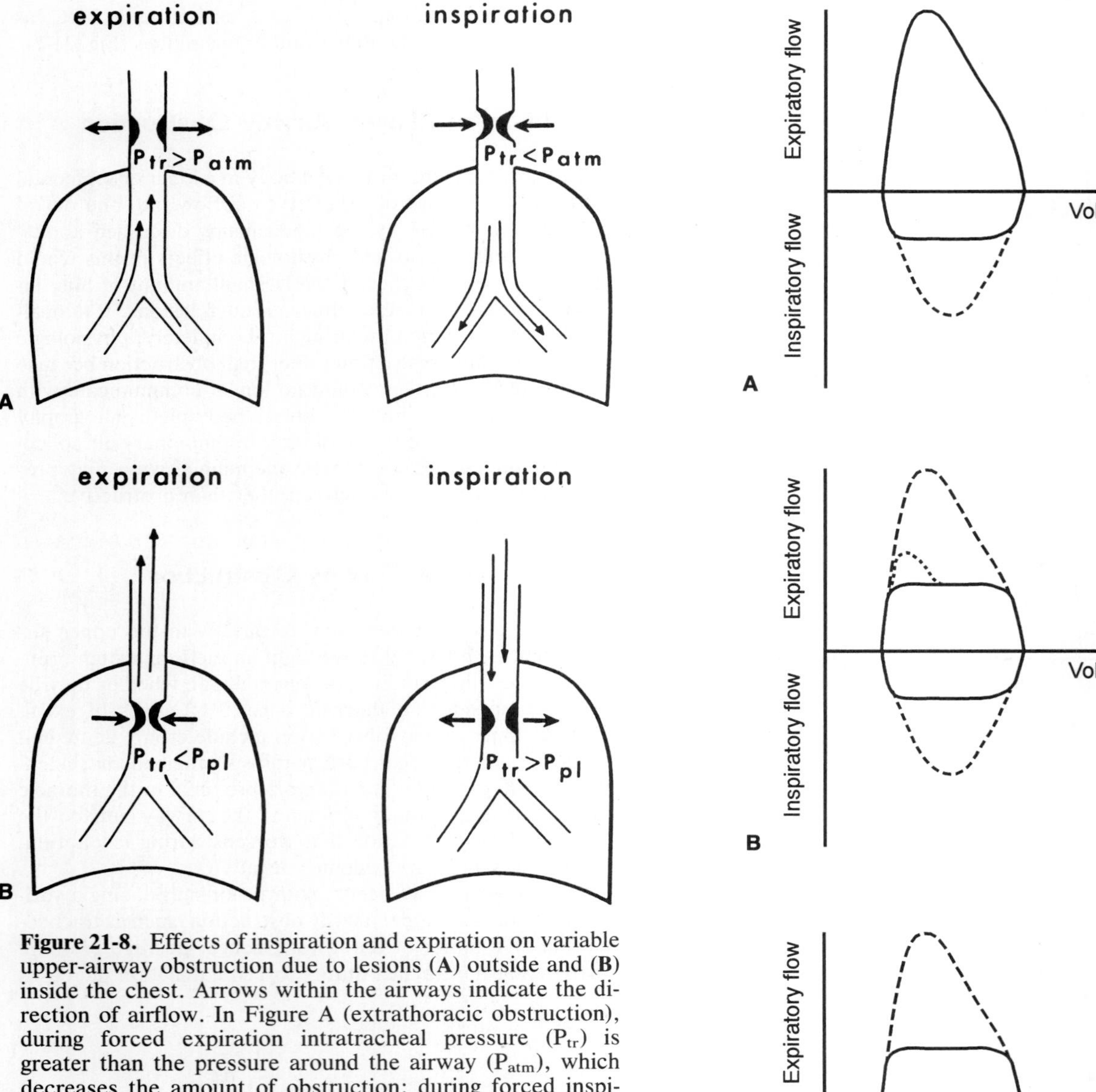

Figure 21-8. Effects of inspiration and expiration on variable upper-airway obstruction due to lesions (**A**) outside and (**B**) inside the chest. Arrows within the airways indicate the direction of airflow. In Figure A (extrathoracic obstruction), during forced expiration intratracheal pressure (P_{tr}) is greater than the pressure around the airway (P_{atm}), which decreases the amount of obstruction; during forced inspiration, when the surrounding atmospheric pressure is greater than that in the trachea, the obstruction increases. In Figure B (intrathoracic obstruction), the situation is reversed: forced expiration increases pleural pressure (P_{pl}) above intratracheal pressure, increasing the obstruction, while negative P_{pl} during inspiration, now exceeded by P_{tr}, tends to pull the trachea open and to decrease the obstruction. (From Kryger et al.,[11] with permission.)

the tendency of the airway to collapse. These effects are diagrammed in Figure 21-8. Lesions such as tracheal stenosis and goiter can produce upper airway obstruction of fixed degree that does not vary with the respiratory cycle.

The different forms of upper airway obstruction produce characteristic patterns of abnormality on the flow-volume loop,[10,11] as shown in Figure 21-9.

Figure 21-9. Representative flow-volume loops in different types of upper airway obstruction. (**A**) Variable extrathoracic obstruction (inspiration impaired more than expiration); (**B**) fixed upper airway obstruction, either intra- or extrathoracic (obstruction approximately the same during inspiration and expiration); (**C**) variable intrathoracic obstruction (expiration impaired more than inspiration). Broken lines indicate expected normal flows.

PULMONARY RESTRICTION

Restrictive disease processes reduce lung compliance and thus require the respiratory muscles to generate more force to stretch the lung. As a result of the increases in elastic recoil and the work required to expand the lung normally, lung volumes are reduced[8] (Figs. 21-1, 21-2, and 21-7).

A restrictive defect is present by definition whenever TLC is reduced below the normal range. Such a defect can be transient or long-standing and can be produced by a wide variety of disease processes, including disorders of the lung itself—either generalized, as in pulmonary fibrosis or pulmonary edema, or localized, as in lung cancer or lobar pneumonia—and disorders of the tissues surrounding the lungs or responsible for their normal expansion. Examples are pleural effusion, kyphoscoliosis, and muscle splinting due to pain following upper abdominal surgery.

While a reduced FVC without airflow obstruction is presumptive evidence for pulmonary restriction, the "gold standard" defining this type of disorder is a lower than normal TLC. Thus, identification and quantification of restrictive defects requires assessment beyond simple spirometry. Chapter 45 describes the different techniques by which TLC can be measured in the laboratory. Most disorders producing acute respiratory failure are predominantly restrictive in effect, so that accurate quantification of FRC or TLC would be highly desirable in the intensive care unit. Unfortunately, although such methods are available, they are too cumbersome and time-consuming for routine use in patient care.[12]

PULMONARY VASCULAR DISORDERS

Some diseases, such as emphysema or asbestosis, affect the pulmonary circulation as part of a generalized process involving air spaces, interstitium, and blood vessels. In other disorders, such as primary pulmonary hypertension and acute pulmonary thromboembolism, the blood vessels may be the only tissues affected, at least initially. In still other conditions, such as chronic hypoxic cor pulmonale, the pulmonary vessels and right ventricle are "innocent bystanders," whose pathologic changes are secondary effects of disease primarily affecting other tissues.

Pulmonary vascular disease per se causes no change in airflow or lung volumes, although secondary effects may occur, such as bronchospasm produced by the release of vasoactive mediators from the clot in pulmonary thromboembolism. The main physiologic effect of pulmonary vascular disease is a reduction in available capillary surface area, reflected in a reduction in the diffusing capacity for carbon monoxide (D_LCO) and in an increase in dead space ventilation. Hypoxemia is commonly observed in pulmonary vascular disorders and is believed to be caused by ventilation/perfusion mismatching, but the mechanism(s) for this are unclear.

DISORDERS OF VENTILATORY CONTROL

Patients without obstructive, restrictive, or vascular disease may nonetheless die from respiratory failure because of an insufficient drive to breathe. A familiar example is overdose with heroin or another respiratory depressant drug; the sudden infant death syndrome (SIDS) may be another. Chronic respiratory failure, with secondary disease of the pulmonary circulation, is a defining characteristic of the primary alveolar hypoventilation syndrome and certain other rare neurologic conditions. Patients with these disorders have in common a severe maladjustment in respiratory regulation—they simply do not breathe when they should or as much as they should.

Chapter 14 describes the components of the normal ventilatory control system. This system may malfunction in any of several places, including the peripheral sensing of hypoxia or hypercapnia, central activation in response to these stimuli, and central output to the ventilatory apparatus. Although abnormal hyperventilation and dyspnea out of proportion to physiologic stimuli are occasionally encountered by the clinician, disordered ventilatory control is more often characterized by the absence of dyspnea in the face of stimuli that should produce this symptom.

Unlike the situation with the other three basic forms of respiratory dysfunction, there is no simple, constant laboratory marker for disorders of respiratory control. Patients with such disorders typically hypoventilate inappropriately, as in failing to demonstrate hypocapnia in response to hypoxemia, although their arterial blood gases may be normal when measured in the laboratory. Tests of hypoxic and hypercapnic ventilatory response, as described in Chapters 14 and 66, can detect and quantitate disordered ventilatory control but are too complicated for routine clinical use. Sleep disorders involve abnormal respiratory regulation, although affected individuals are usually normal if tested while awake. The assessment of breathing during sleep is discussed in Chapter 55.

CLINICAL-PHYSIOLOGIC CORRELATIONS

Consideration of the physiologic categories described in this chapter facilitates logical thinking and a rational approach to assessment and management of patients with respiratory disease. Identification of the dominant type of dysfunction is especially important for patients with vague or inconsistent complaints or in whom initial evaluation does not produce a clear diagnosis.

Table 21-2 summarizes the expected findings on laboratory investigation in patients with obstructive, restrictive, vascular, and ventilatory control disorders. More than one type of dysfunction may be produced by a single disease. Examples are emphysema, which reduces airflow and diffusing capacity in roughly equal proportion, and sarcoidosis, which

Table 21-2. Physiologic and Clinical Effects of the Four Primary Categories of Respiratory Disorders

Effect	Clinical Assessment	Expected Changes from Normal: Obstruction	Restriction	Vascular	Control
Lung volumes	TLC	0 or ↑	↓↓	0	0
	FRC	↑	↓	0	0
	RV	↑↑	↓	0	0
	VC	0 or ↓	↓	0	0
Lung/thorax compliance	CL; CSTAT	↑	↓	0	0
Airflow	FEV_1	↓	0 or ↓	0	0
	FEV_1/FVC	↓↓	0 or ↑	0	0
	FEF_{25-75}	↓	0	0	0
Gas exchange	PaO_2	0 or ↓	0 or ↓	0 or ↓	↓
	$PaCO_2$	0 or ↑	0 or ↓	0 or ↓	↑
Pulmonary vascular bed	DLCO	0 or ↓	↓	↓↓	0
Minute ventilation	$\dot{V}_E$	0 or ↑ or ↓	0 or ↑	↑	↓
Inefficiency of ventilation	V_D/V_T	↑	0	↑↑	0
Response to hypoxia and/or hypercapnia	HVR/HCVR	0 or ↓	0 or ↑	0 or ↑	↓↓
Dyspnea	History	↑	↑	↑	0

↑, increase; ↓, decrease; ↑↑ or ↓↓, characteristic change; CL, lung compliance; CSTAT, static compliance; FEF_{25-75}, forced expiratory flow from 25–75% of FVC; $\dot{V}_E$, expired minute ventilation.

Table 21-3. Examples of Typical Findings in Patients with the Four Primary Types of Respiratory Dysfunction

Disorder	FEV_1 (% pred)	FEV_1/FVC (%)	TLC (% pred)	PaO_2 (mmHg)	$PaCO_2$ (mmHg)	DLCO (% pred)
Obstructive						
Asthma, asymptomatic	90	70	100	80	40	100–120
Asthma, moderate attack	50	50	110	58	32	[a]
Asthma, severe attack	30	30	130	50	46	[a]
COPD, mild, stable	60	60	100	80	40	70
COPD, moderate, stable	50	50	110	80	40	60
COPD, severe, stable						
Type A[b]	30	30	130	65	40	40
Type B[c]	30	30	120	53	55[d]	60
COPD, acute exacerbation	20	20	140	45	65[e]	[a]
Restrictive						
Idiopathic pulmonary fibrosis, moderate	60	90	60	80	35	55
Idiopathic pulmonary fibrosis, severe	45	100	45	50	30	30
Vascular						
Primary pulmonary hypertension	90	80	90	75	35	30
Ventilatory control						
Primary alveolar hypoventilation	90	80	90	50	60	100

[a] Should not be attempted during acute exacerbation.

[b] Predominantly emphysema in clinical picture—dyspnea severe, sputum minimal, hypoxemia mild to none (''pink puffer'').

[c] Predominantly chronic bronchitis in clinical picture—dyspnea moderate to absent, sputum prominent, hypoxemia moderate to severe (''blue bloater'').

[d] With normal arterial pH.

[e] With acute respiratory acidosis (e.g., arterial pH 7.25).

may produce airflow obstruction as well as restriction and vascular impairment. Patients may have more than one disease, but even in this more difficult situation a physiologic approach to assessment is beneficial. An example is the patient with both heavy asbestos exposure and a long smoking history, who may have COPD (obstructive disease), parenchymal asbestosis (restrictive and vascular disease), or both in a characteristic pattern.[13]

As examples of actual findings in patients with each of the dysfunction patterns discussed in this chapter, Table 21-3 gives typical results for spirometry, TLC, arterial blood gas analysis, and DLCO for individuals with common disorders in each category. The chapters that follow provide clinical descriptions of the main diseases encountered in respiratory care, categorized according to their primary physiologic abnormality.

References

1. Murray JF: The Normal Lung. 2nd Ed. WB Saunders, Philadelphia, 1986
2. West JB: Pulmonary Pathophysiology—the Essentials. 2nd Ed. Williams & Wilkins, Baltimore, 1982
3. Bates DV: Respiratory Function in Disease. 3rd Ed. WB Saunders, Philadelphia, 1989
4. Pride NB, Green M: Abnormalities of respiratory mechanics. pp. 669–688. In Scadding JG, Cumming G, Thurlbeck WM (eds): Scientific Foundations of Respiratory Medicine. WB Saunders, Philadelphia, 1981
5. Pride NB, Macklem PT: Lung mechanics in disease. pp. 659–692. In Macklem PT, Mead J (eds): Handbook of Physiology, Section 3: The Respiratory System. Vol. 3: Mechanics of Breathing, Part 2. American Physiological Society, Bethesda, 1986
6. Crystal RG, West JB, Barnes PJ et al (eds): The Lung. Scientific Foundations. Raven Press, New York, 1991
7. Luce JM, Tyler ML, Pierson DJ: Intensive Respiratory Care. 2nd Ed. WB Saunders, Philadelphia, 1992
8. Culver BH (ed): Syllabus: Human Biology 541—The Respiratory System. University of Washington School of Medicine, Health Sciences Academic Services, Seattle, 1992
9. Marini JJ: Respiratory Medicine and Intensive Care for the House Officer. Williams & Wilkins, Baltimore, 1981
10. Miller RD, Hyatt RE: Evaluation of obstructing lesions of the trachea and larynx by flow-volume loops. Am Rev Respir Dis 1973;108:475–481
11. Kryger MH, Bode F, Antic R, Anthonisen N: Diagnosis of obstruction of the upper and central airways. Am J Med 1976;61:85–93
12. Pierson DJ: Measuring and monitoring lung volumes outside the pulmonary function laboratory. Respir Care 1990;35:660–668
13. Barnhart S, Hudson LD, Mason SE et al: Total lung capacity. An insensitive measure of impairment in patients with asbestosis and chronic obstructive pulmonary disease? Chest 1988;93:299–302

Chapter 22

Disorders Producing Airflow Obstruction

Noel T. Johnson
David J. Pierson

CHAPTER OUTLINE

Obstructive lung diseases all have the common pathophysiologic features of reduced airflow and narrowed airways. The physiologic changes that occur in these diseases are described in Chapter 21. Briefly, the narrowed airways lead to increased airway resistance, requiring more work to breathe. These changes result most commonly in obstruction to expiratory airflow. Hence, mention of airflow obstruction in this chapter refers to expiratory obstruction unless otherwise noted. Airflow obstruction also occurs most commonly through generalized changes in lower airways and airspaces. This generalized or diffuse type of airflow obstruction is the primary focus of this chapter. Upper airway obstruction is covered in Chapter 21.

As discussed in Chapter 19, a gradual loss of lung elastic recoil with aging leads to progressively diminished airflow.[1] This normal aging process, although physiologically detectable, does not become clinically problematic because it develops so slowly that normal persons succumb to other illnesses long before symptoms of airflow obstruction develop. Obstructive lung disease occurs when this normal aging process is substantially accelerated. As a group, the obstructive diseases comprise the bulk of clinical respiratory disease.

Although obstructive lung diseases share certain pathophysiologic mechanisms, they are distinguished from each other by the nature of the predominant damaging process (pathology) and the course of the illness (natural history). They are commonly grouped into categories reflecting these distinctions (Table 22-1). These categories include chronic obstructive pulmonary disease (COPD), asthma, bronchiectasis, cystic fibrosis, bullous lung disease, and focal lower airway obstruction. The interrelationships among the most common of these disorders are depicted in Figure 22-1.

Table 22-1. Diseases and Conditions Producing an Obstructive Pattern of Pulmonary Dysfunction

Upper airway obstruction
- Extrathoracic
  - Variable: croup; laryngeal paralysis
  - Fixed: stenosis of cervical trachea; goiter
- Intrathoracic
  - Variable: tracheomalacia; tracheal tumor
  - Fixed: stenosis of intrathoracic trachea

Lower airway obstruction
- Generalized
  - Primary feature of disease: COPD (emphysema, chronic bronchitis, asthmatic component); asthma; cystic fibrosis; diffuse bronchiectasis; small airways disease
  - Secondary or (usually) minor feature of disease: sarcoidosis; post-ARDS; bronchiolitis
- Localized
  - Extrinsic bronchial compression: neoplasm; enlarged lymph nodes
  - Partially occluding endobronchial obstruction: neoplasm (carcinoma, adenoma); foreign body (tooth, food); mucoid impaction; endobronchial granuloma (tuberculosis, sarcoidosis)
  - Bronchomalacia
  - Right middle lobe syndrome

ARDS, adult respiratory distress syndrome; COPD, chronic obstructive pulmonary disease.

CHRONIC OBSTRUCTIVE PULMONARY DISEASE

Definitions and Diagnosis

Patients with COPD have symptomatic airflow obstruction that is unremitting (chronic), although symptoms and the degree of obstruction may periodically wax and wane. Other terms such as chronic obstructive lung disease (COLD) and chronic airflow obstruction (CAO) have been proposed to describe this illness but the term COPD has endured in the mainstream medical vernacular.[2]

As its name implies, COPD is defined as a disorder with airflow obstruction that is chronic (e.g., that persists at least 3 months).[2] In fact, most patients with COPD have had symptoms for years when the diagnosis is made. Specifically excluded from this definition are localized disease of the upper airways, bronchiectasis, and cystic fibrosis. Demonstration of airflow obstruction is readily accomplished by spirometry (see Figs. 21-5 to 21-7). There may be a bronchospastic component to COPD, as revealed by improved airflow rates following administration of bronchodilators. Figure 22-2 shows volume-time and flow-volume tracings from spirometry before and after inhalation of aerosolized bronchodilator by a patient with moderately severe airflow obstruction and nearly complete reversibility. Care must be taken to avoid making an empirical diagnosis of COPD without spirometry. Other pulmonary diseases may present with similar symptoms and thus be misdiagnosed. An erroneous empirical diagnosis of COPD may delay proper diagnosis and treatment, to the detriment of patient care.

Within the broad category of COPD three discrete disorders that contribute to the airflow obstruction are recognized: emphysema, chronic bronchitis, and a reversible, or asthmatic component (Table 22-1). In general, all three are present to a viable degree in a given patient (Fig. 22-1). However, one disorder may predominate in an individual, leading to distinct clinical features as discussed below.

Epidemiology and Etiology

More than 10 million people in the United States have COPD, and when combined with asthma, this disorder is the major cause of pulmonary disability.[2] The true incidence is unknown because this figure includes only reported cases and in all likelihood underestimates the incidence substantially.

Death rates from COPD have been slowly rising since 1960, and a disproportionate number occur in the winter months of December through February. Large state-to-state variations occur in the United States. In addition to inconsistencies in reporting, age differences, migration, climate, and pollution may contribute to this variation. Age, male sex, white race, lower socioeconomic status, and population density are all associated with increased incidence of illness and/or death from COPD[3]; differences in smoking behavior likely account for most of these increases.

Cigarette smoking is by far the most important cause of COPD, although only a minority of smokers develop this illness. There are several other less common etiologic factors (see Ch. 38). Outdoor air pollution has long been known to cause respiratory symptoms and to be associated with reduced levels of pulmonary function; indoor air pollution has been increasingly recognized and may be a causative factor in respiratory disease as well. Exposure to occupational dusts and fumes of many types is linked to the occurrence of chronic bronchitis and emphysema. Gold, fluorspar, coal, flax, cotton, foundry, and furnace dust have all been implicated in this respect. Less is known about COPD following inhalation of fumes. A notable exception is the association between cadmium fume inhalation and emphysema.[4]

Heredity also plays a role in the development of COPD. Symptoms of bronchitis and indices of pulmonary function correlate more closely with those of relatives than with nonfamily members. In addition, diminished levels of alpha-1-antitrypsin (also called alpha-1-antiprotease) are found in a very small number of people with severe emphysema. This deficiency, which permits the development of early emphysema and increases susceptibility to the damaging effects of cigarette smoke, has been elegantly characterized as a hereditary disorder and traced to a number of specific deficient phenotypes of the responsible gene.[5]

Emphysema in patients with alpha-1-antitrypsin deficiency has a different anatomic pattern from that seen in other individuals. It generally presents with the radiologic findings of pulmonary oligemia (diminished vascular markings), predominantly in the lung bases. While this pattern may be seen in emphysematous patients with normal alpha-

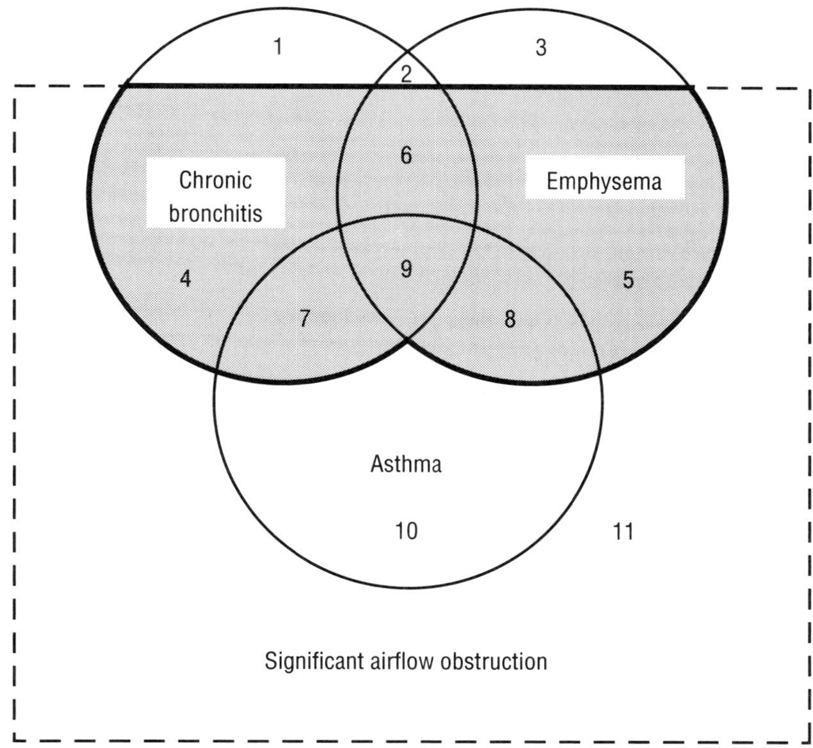

Figure 22-1. Relationships among the main clinical types of obstructive lung disease, depicted in the form of a nonproportional Venn diagram. Included in the rectangle are all patients with significant airflow obstruction. The circles represent the pathophysiologically distinct entities of chronic bronchitis, emphysema, and asthma and the shaded portions of the three circles together represent the spectrum of chronic obstructive pulmonary disease (COPD). Note that there are patients with chronic bronchitis and/or emphysema who do not manifest clinically significant airflow obstruction (groups 1–3). COPD is the aggregate of groups 4–9, illustrating the wide clinical spectrum of this syndrome. Group 10 represents individuals with intermittent, acute airflow obstruction that is completely reversible, either spontaneously or in response to therapy. Cystic fibrosis, bronchiectasis, and all other causes of airflow obstruction are incorporated into group 11. (Adapted from Snider,[46] with permission.)

1-antitrypsin levels, most of such individuals exhibit disease primarily in the upper lung fields.

A syndrome of severe precocious emphysema resembling alpha-1-antitrypsin deficiency has recently been described in long-time intravenous users of the stimulant drug methylphenidate (Ritalin).[6,7] The pathogenesis of emphysema in these patients is unknown.

Pathophysiology

The physiologic abnormalities and symptoms of COPD result from three distinct disorders: emphysema, chronic bronchitis, and asthma. These disorders may be present singly or in combination in any given patient with COPD.

Emphysema

Emphysema is permanent abnormal enlargement of the airspaces distal to the terminal bronchioles. There is destruction (nonuniformity of enlargement) of the airspace walls without fibrosis (thickening)[8] (Figs. 22-3 and 22-4). Severe cases may be recognized with the naked eye at autopsy or in surgical specimens. Less severe cases require microscopy. The presence of emphysema correlates with airflow obstruction, but not all emphysematous lungs manifest airflow obstruction.[9] These changes in lung structure result in a loss of gas exchange membrane surface area (alveoli juxtaposed with capillaries), which may be reflected as a decrease in CO diffusing capacity (DLCO) (see Table 21-3). These changes also result in a loss of elastic recoil, one of

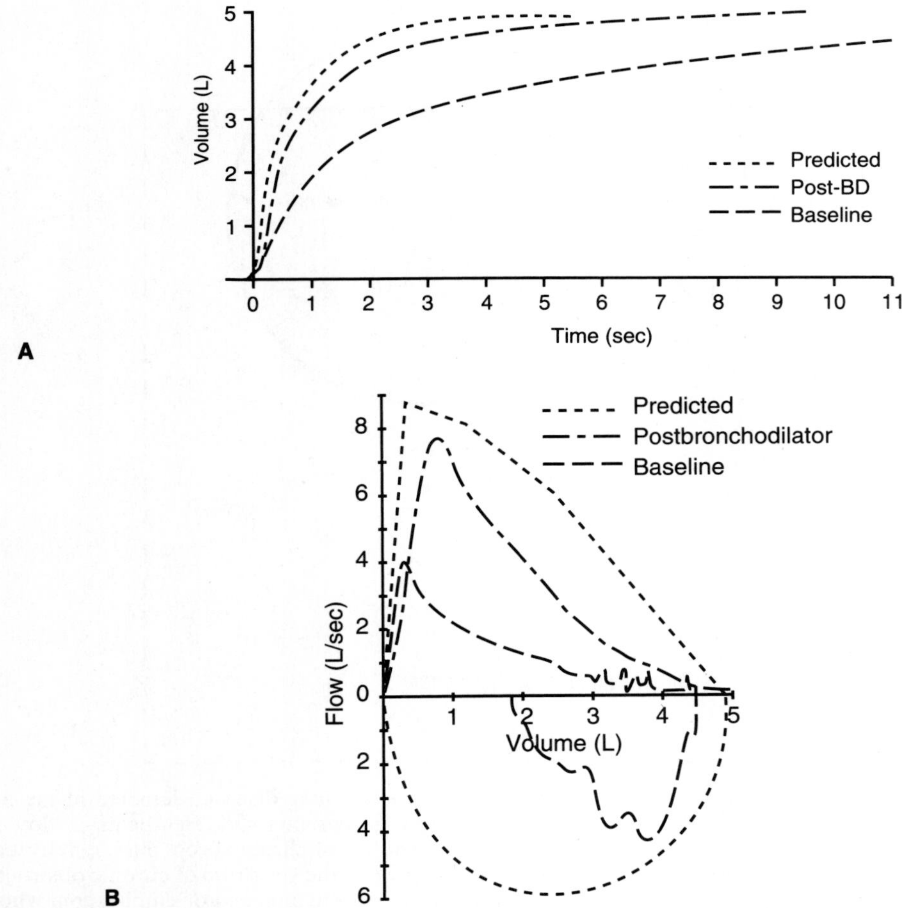

Figure 22-2. Spirometry (**A**) in a patient with COPD and (**B**) showing marked reversibility following inhalation of bronchodilator. In Figure A (volume-time tracing), the patient continues forcibly exhaling for 11 seconds and stops because of dyspnea even though airflow continues. The initial forced expiratory volume in the first second (FEV_1) is 2.0 L (53 percent of predicted for this patient). After bronchodilator use, exhalation is virtually complete after 8 seconds and the FEV_1 is 3.3 L (85 percent of predicted). In Figure B (expiratory flow-volume tracing) the dramatic improvement in airflow following bronchodilator inhalation is shown.

the forces that drives passive exhalation. In addition, the enlarged airspaces result in a loss of the tethering effect exerted on the airways by the intact pulmonary parenchyma, so that airways become more prone to collapse.

Chronic Bronchitis

Chronic bronchitis is defined clinically by a history of productive cough occurring on most days for at least 3 months per year for at least 2 successive years, in the absence of tuberculosis, abscesses, tumors, and bronchiectasis.[10] Microscopically, mucous glands enlarge and goblet cells become more numerous in the large airways. The epithelial wall becomes thicker with these changes, encroaching on the lumen. The wall thickness may be increased by edema as well, and there may be airway muscle enlargement. Accumulation of mucus in small airway lumina combines with wall thickening to narrow airways. Neither the symptoms of cough and mucus hypersecretion nor the finding of mucous gland hyperplasia, however, has been convincingly and independently linked to the presence of airflow obstruction.[2] In addition, chronic bronchitis has little impact on the lung's capillary surface area and hence little effect on the DLCO.

Peripheral (Small Airways) Disease

Peripheral (small airways) disease is detectable microscopically as inflammation of the terminal and respiratory bronchioles (infiltration of white blood cells). Fibrosis (thickening) of the airway walls is noted in association with airway narrowing, and goblet cell metaplasia (change of one form of tissue into another) of the bronchiolar epithelium takes place. These changes also correlate with airflow obstruction in COPD.[11]

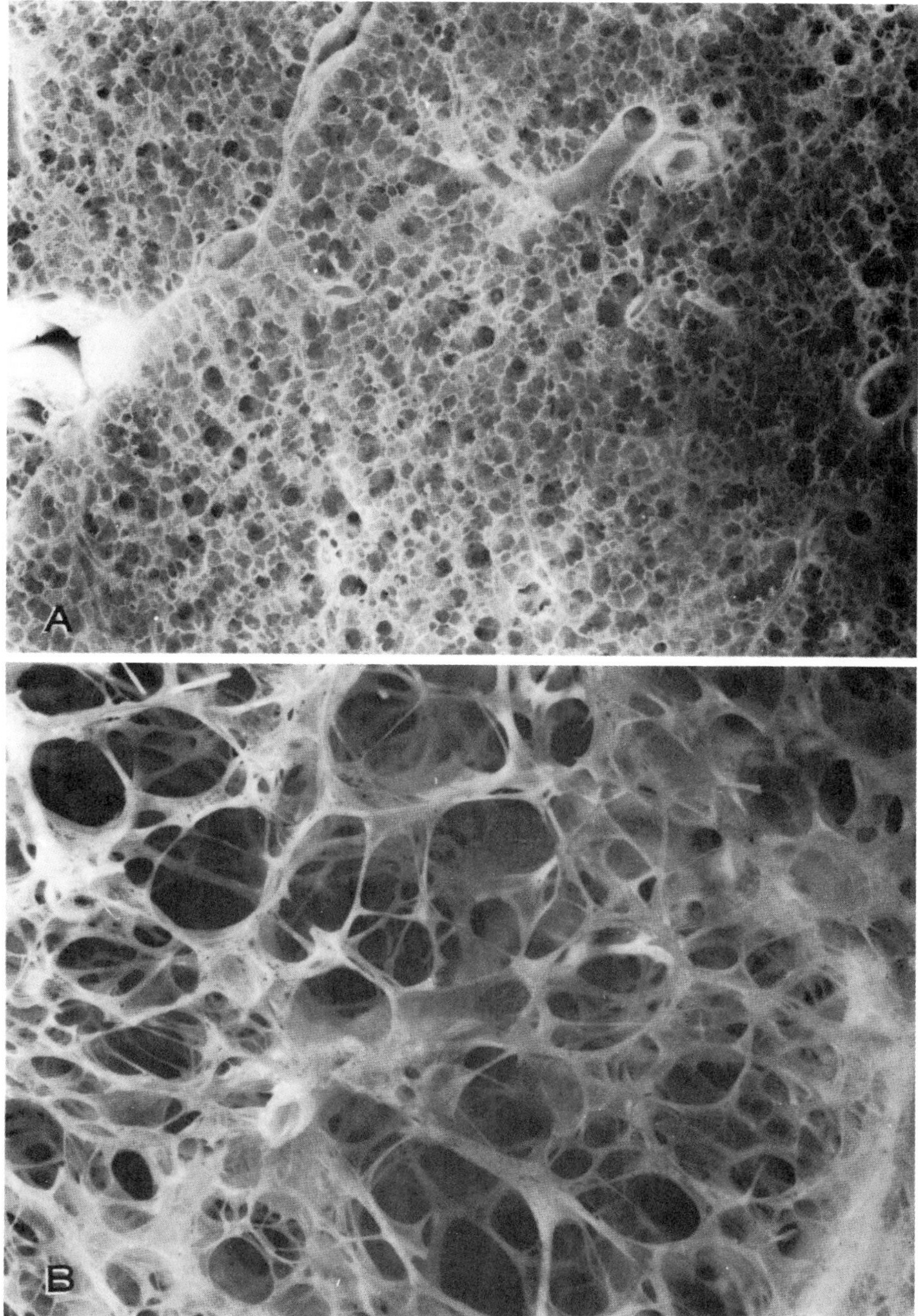

Figure 22-3. Overall appearance of slices of normal and emphysematous lungs. (**A**) normal; (**B**) panlobular emphysema. Both specimens have been impregnated with barium sulfate and magnified ×14. (From Heard BE: Pathology of Chronic Bronchitis and Emphysema. Churchill, London, 1969, with permission.)

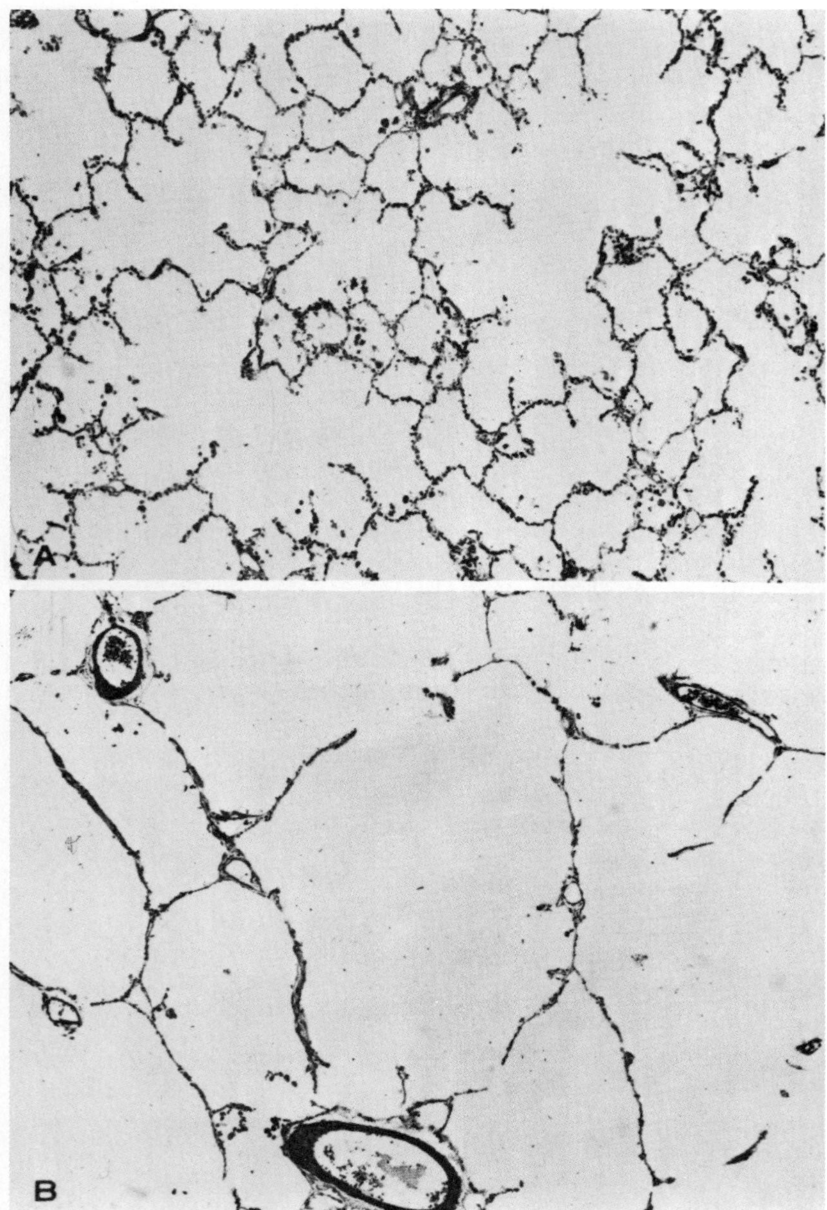

Figure 22-4. Microscopic appearance of emphysematous lung. **(A)** normal; **(B)** showing loss of alveolar walls and consequent enlargement of airspaces. Figure A and B enlarged to the same degree (×90). (From Heard BE: Pathology of Chronic Bronchitis and Emphysema. Churchill, London, 1969, with permission.)

Asthma

Asthma in the setting of COPD is defined physiologically as the component of the syndrome that produces day-to-day variation in symptoms and/or airflow obstruction or that improves with bronchodilators and other asthma therapies. Because asthma's effects involve predominantly functional changes in the airways rather than anatomic changes as in emphysema, this component of COPD does not reduce the DLCO.

Clinical Presentation

COPD most commonly presents in middle age or later. Dyspnea is almost invariably present, although it may not be the chief complaint, and may occur at rest, in paroxysms at night, on lying down, or with specific activities (e.g., eating, talking, walking). COPD patients with severe dyspnea, mild hypoxemia, and no CO_2 retention or cor pulmonale (type A COPD) have been called "pink puffers," a term descriptive of their characteristic hue and breathless appearance. COPD patients with severe hypoxemia, CO_2 retention, cor pulmonale, cough, and relatively little dyspnea (type B COPD) have been called "blue bloaters," which describes their cyanotic hue and tendency to develop edema[12] (Fig. 22-5). The variance in hypoxemia and CO_2 retention in these two clinical types has been ascribed to differences in ventilation/perfusion ($\dot{V}/\dot{Q}$) matching and ventilatory drive, respectively. Worse $\dot{V}/\dot{Q}$ mismatching results in more profound hypoxemia, whereas diminished ventilatory drive results in a higher CO_2 partial pressure (PCO_2). Patients with type B COPD tend to have more evidence of chronic bronchitis on microscopic examination of the lungs, while both types tend to have significant emphysema. In practice, these patient types represent two extremes in a broad spectrum of COPD patients. Most patients fall somewhere in between.

When patients with airflow obstruction become tachypneic, for whatever reason (e.g., dyspnea, fever, anxiety), dynamic air trapping may occur because of incomplete exhalation prior to the following inhalation in consecutive breaths. This phenomenon has been well described in patients receiving mechanical ventilation, in whom it is said to cause auto-PEEP (positive end-expiratory pressure), and also is seen in COPD patients not receiving such ventilation. The dynamic air trapping leads to an increased sensation of dyspnea, and a vicious cycle is begun. This is illustrated by the tidal volume tracings plotted as a function of time in Figure 22-6. Dynamic air trapping has been found to be present to some degree in a majority of stable, severe COPD patients and is positively correlated with arterial PCO_2 ($PaCO_2$) and negatively correlated with forced expiratory volume in 1 second (FEV_1); that is, this phenomenon is more likely to be significant in those with lower FEV_1 and higher $PaCO_2$.[13] Other clinical manifestations of COPD include cough, sputum production, wheezing, and recurrent respiratory infections.

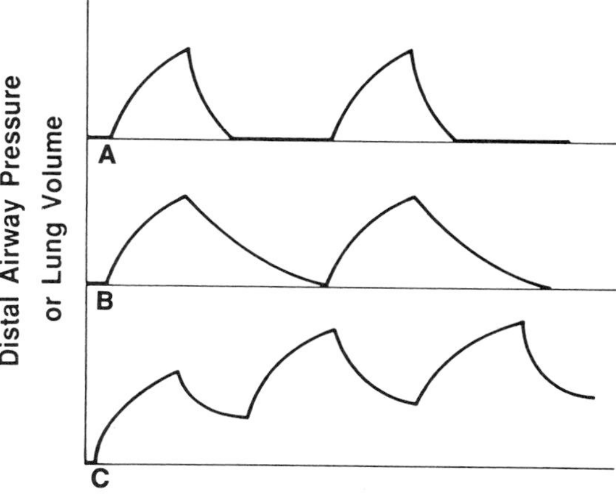

Figure 22-6. Development of dynamic air trapping in airflow obstruction. **(A)** Normal—no expiratory airflow obstruction. **(B)** Airflow obstruction present but exhalation complete prior to next breath. **(C)** Airflow obstruction with incomplete exhalation prior to succeeding inhalation, resulting in air trapping and hyperinflation. If pressure were measured in the periphery at the lung, it would remain positive at end-exhalation (auto-PEEP).

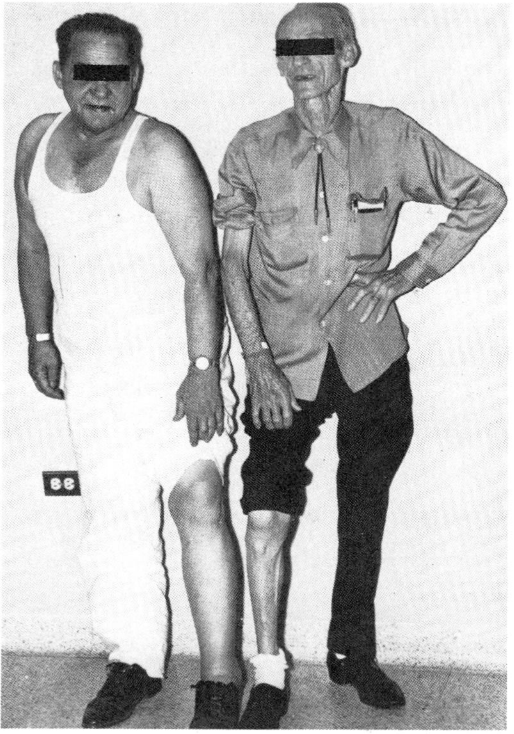

Figure 22-5. Two patients with severe, disabling COPD. The man on the right has severe dyspnea, relatively normal oxygenation, no CO_2 retention, and a clinical picture dominated by emphysema (type A, or "pink puffer," COPD). The man on the left, with equally severe airflow obstruction, has relatively little dyspnea, severe hypoxemia, chronic hypercapnia, cor pulmonale, and a clinical picture dominated by chronic bronchitis (type B, or "blue bloater," COPD). (From Petty,[12] with permission; photograph courtesy of Dr. Thomas L. Petty.)

Physical examination of the patient with COPD is generally more remarkable as airflow obstruction becomes more severe. Early on, there may be wheezes on forced exhalation only. As obstruction becomes more severe, and particularly during acute exacerbations, patients talk in short sentences (conversational dyspnea), may purse their lips to exhale, and may show evidence of accessory ventilatory muscle recruitment (prominent sternocleidomastoid muscles). As obstruction becomes more severe, the most effective ventilatory pressure shifts from the diaphragm to the rib cage inspiratory muscles and the expiratory muscles. Costal or supraclavicular retractions suggest increased work of breathing,[14] and there may be an exaggerated inspiratory fall in blood pressure (pulsus paradoxus). Lung auscultation may reveal wheezes during tidal breathing, and/or lung sounds may be diminished. The expiratory phase is typically prolonged. Persistent, early inspiratory crackles may be heard at the lung bases.

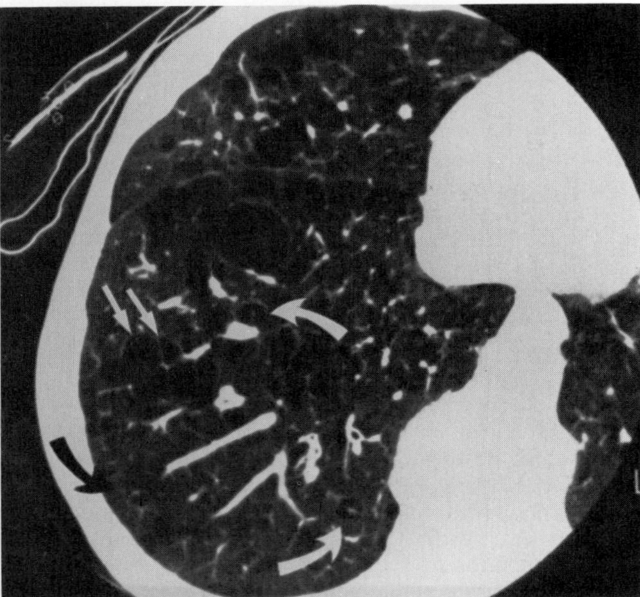

Figure 22-7. High-resolution computed tomographic (HRCT) image of the chest (right lower lobe) in a patient with emphysema. There are well-defined zones of diminished lung density, without definable walls. Instead, these spaces typically are delimited peripherally by interlobular veins, which are particularly well seen along the course of large central veins (small straight arrows). Occasionally, when sectioned tangentially, central or core lobular vessels can be identified as well (large curved arrows). (From Naidich et al.,[48] with permission.)

Pulmonary function tests are critically important in the diagnosis of COPD. All other laboratory tests are adjunctive and provide confirmatory evidence or uncover complications (e.g., pneumonia, lung tumors). The major finding is reduced expiratory flow rates. As noted in Chapter 21, the inability to exhale roughly three-fourths of one's forced vital capacity (FVC) in 1 second (FEV_1/FVC ratio less than 0.75) defines airflow obstruction. Pulmonary function patterns of obstructive diseases are compared with other patterns in Figures 21-1 to 21-3.

Chest radiographs are neither highly sensitive nor specific in the diagnosis of COPD, although several concurrent changes are commonly seen. Patients with advanced cases may show signs of hyperinflation, but this may be indistinguishable from that found in asthma. Regional hyperlucency (or vascular attenuation) suggests advanced emphysema. A benefit to patient management may accrue, however, when these studies reveal intercurrent illness such as pneumonia, pleural effusion, or lung tumors that have escaped detection on physical examination.

Thin-section (1.5-mm) computed tomography (CT) of the chest demonstrates emphysema in some cases (Fig. 22-7) but misses most lesions less than 0.5 cm.[15] It is not sensitive for the earliest lesions of emphysema, and its clinical role in COPD is uncertain.

Arterial blood gas levels may or may not be abnormal. The degree of hypoxemia generally reflects the degree of $\dot{V}/\dot{Q}$ mismatching, while the degree of hypercapnia reflects the strength of the respiratory drive (except in the presence of very severe airflow obstruction). The electrocardiogram (ECG) may show evidence of right heart enlargement. Low levels of alpha-1-antitrypsin may be found in the smoker between 30 and 45 years of age with symptomatic emphysema.[5]

Natural History and Prognosis

As noted above, the FEV_1 declines progressively in the normal aging lung, with an average loss of 20 to 30 mL/yr after the age of 30 years,[16] but 15 to 20 percent of cigarette smokers have an accelerated rate of decline and may lose as much as 60 to 80 mL/yr. However, as shown in Figure 22-8, smokers with COPD may be able to modify this rate of loss by smoking cessation.[17]

Along with decline in lung function, patients with COPD are subject to premature death.[18] The clinical index most closely related to survival is the FEV_1.[19] The relationship between FEV_1 and survival in COPD[20] is graphically illustrated in Figure 22-9; diminished FEV_1 is associated with shorter survival.[21]

Patients with chronic hypoxemia, with or without cor pulmonale, have a lower survival rate than would be expected for the severity of their airflow obstruction. As discussed in Chapters 24 and 63, this excessive mortality can be reduced or eliminated through the appropriate administration of long-term O_2 therapy.

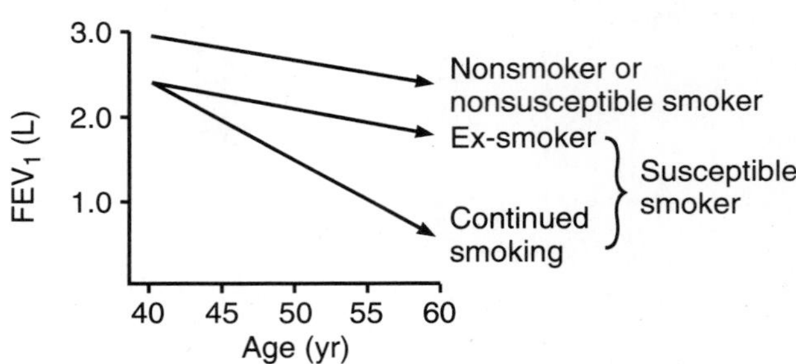

Figure 22-8. Effect of smoking cessation on the rate of loss of lung function among individuals susceptible to chronic airflow obstruction. Normal lifelong nonsmokers (and the 80 to 85 percent of smokers who are not susceptible to developing COPD) lose FEV_1 at the rate of 20 to 30 mL/yr. Patients susceptible to COPD (about 15 to 20 percent of smokers) lose FEV_1 at 60 to 80 mL/yr. For a "susceptible" smoking individual who stops at age 40, despite the lung function already lost, the rate of further loss would revert to that of the nonsmoker; this could make the difference between disability and early death from airflow obstruction versus no significant interference with life-style. (Modified from Fletcher et al.,[17] with permission.)

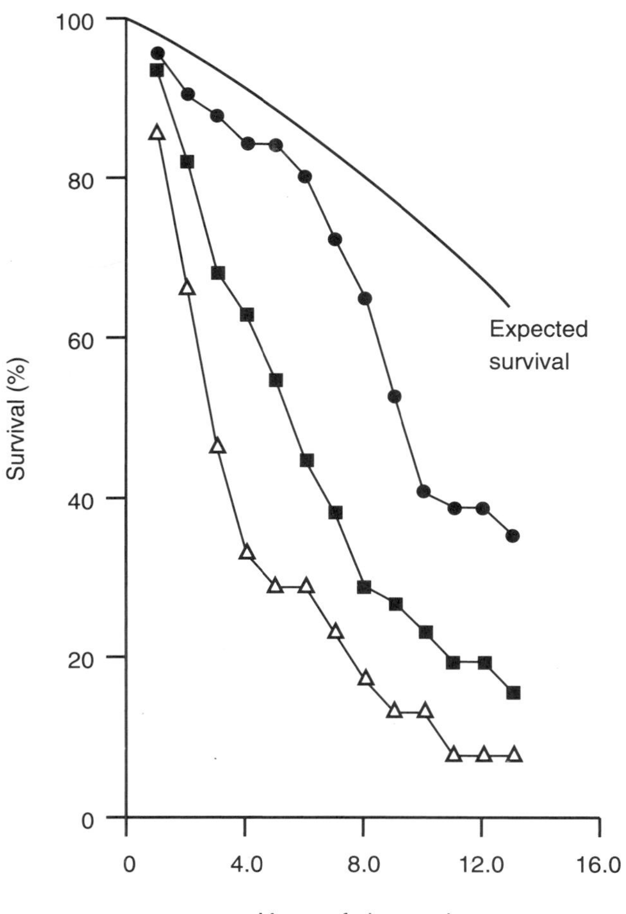

Figure 22-9. Survival among patients with COPD according to the severity of their airflow obstruction as measured by FEV_1 at the time of entry into a longitudinal study. Dots indicate patients with initial FEV_1 more than 1.25 L; squares, 0.75 to 1.25 L; and triangles, less than 0.75 L. The curved line at the top of the plot indicates the expected actuarial survival for U.S. residents of the same age. (From Diener and Burrows,[20] with permission.)

ASTHMA

Definitions and Diagnosis

Asthma is an obstructive lung disease in which the tracheobronchial tree has an increased responsiveness to various stimuli.[2] While the normal tracheobronchial tree responds to various stimuli to a small degree, asthma is distinguished by an exaggerated responsiveness, which results in generalized fluctuating airway narrowing and obstruction. Another, more traditional definition for asthma is *episodic wheezing dyspnea*, although this definition is not broad enough to include all cases.

Airflow obstruction in asthma may occur or worsen after exposure to specific (allergens) or nonspecific (e.g., methacholine) stimuli. Airflow obstruction may spontaneously improve with recovery from stimuli or following use of medications (e.g., beta-adrenergic agonists or corticosteroids). Exacerbations may be followed by symptom-free intervals, or the illness may be chronic, with fluctuations in the severity of symptoms. Because the airflow obstruction in asthma may be chronic, the distinction from COPD may at times become blurred. This distinction assumes greatest importance when specific stimuli can be identified and avoided, with resulting amelioration of asthmatic symptoms.

Asthma is suspected clinically when cough, wheeze, or shortness of breath follows exposure to various air conditions (dusts, fumes, cold air) or exertion, especially when preceded by an asymptomatic period. The diagnosis is confirmed when spirometry reveals airflow obstruction that can be reversed with bronchodilators (Fig. 22-2). Occasionally in acute, severe asthma, airflow obstruction may not improve following bronchodilator use.

If spirometry does not show airflow obstruction, inhalation challenge testing may demonstrate hyperreactive airways. This is demonstrated by using one of various inhaled provocative substances (e.g., methacholine or histamine) in a serial and incremental manner. Serial spirometry with successive inhalations will demonstrate an abnormal degree of airflow obstruction in the course of testing a patient with asthma. Inhalation challenge testing is discussed in greater detail in Chapter 56.

Epidemiology and Etiology

The true incidence and prevalence of asthma are unknown, but it is estimated that the disorder affects approximately 4 percent of the U.S. population (10 million individuals).[22] Asthma accounts for at least 2000 deaths annually in the United States. Unlike COPD, asthma may develop in early childhood as well as later in life. Also unlike COPD, childhood onset asthma may remit with advancing age.

Asthma patients have been categorized into extrinsic and intrinsic types. Extrinsic asthma patients characteristically present in childhood and have identifiable allergic stimuli. They may have elevated serum levels of immunoglobulin E (IgE) and family histories of allergy. Patients with intrinsic asthma characteristically present following childhood, have no family history of allergy, and have normal IgE levels. Characteristics of extrinsic and intrinsic asthma tend to occur so commonly in the same individual, however, that this distinction has limited usefulness. It is useful, however, to identify a number of factors that are commonly implicated in causing an asthma attack. These asthma triggers are tabulated in Table 22-2 and discussed below.

Airborne allergens may precipitate or worsen asthma in one-third to one-half of patients. Common airborne allergens include pollens and animal dander, but there are many others. Ingested allergens provoke asthma less frequently. Patients become sensitized to an allergen only after sufficient length and intensity of exposure. Following sensitization,

Table 22-2. Asthma Triggers

Allergens	
Respiratory tract infections	Ingested substances
Physical exertion	Emotional stress
Air pollution	Occupational exposures

however, only small amounts of the allergen are required to provoke asthma.[23]

Allergens are thought to be processed in the peripheral lymphoid tissue. Simply stated, the allergen (called an *antigen* while in the body) causes B lymphocytes to proliferate and differentiate into IgE-secreting B lymphocytes and plasma cells. This antigen-specific IgE combines with IgE receptors on mast cells and basophils throughout the body. Repeat exposure to the allergen/antigen is recognized by these specific IgE molecules on the mast cells and basophils and results in granule release from the mast cells and basophils. The granules contain chemical mediators, which orchestrate the inflammatory response in the airways.

The inflammatory response commonly occurs in two phases. An early phase, which occurs within minutes and lasts up to 1 hour, is brought about by the mediators of immediate hypersensitivity, the action of which is thought to involve the smooth muscle of the bronchial tree and bronchial vessels, resulting in bronchospasm and vasospasm. A second phase (late phase) occurs in up to half of patients. This more severe obstructive response develops several hours after the initial exposure and is more refractory to beta-adrenergic agonists. This late phase is thought to result from the chemotactic mediators and the cells that they recruit. A more detailed review of the inflammatory response in asthma can be found elsewhere.[24,25]

Infections of the respiratory tract, most frequently viral upper respiratory illnesses, commonly provoke asthma. Infection causes epithelial cell damage and triggers an inflammatory response, which results in an increased sensitivity to nonspecific stimuli, a condition that persists long after the initial infection occurs.[26]

Physical exertion can trigger asthma. This exercise-induced asthma is particularly troublesome for younger patients who regularly participate in athletics. Symptoms generally ensue following rather than during exertion. Such episodes generally are not protracted and remit spontaneously. Low temperatures and low humidity of the ambient air during exercise magnify the severity of obstruction manifested during such episodes.[27]

Air pollution, such as that caused by sulfur dioxide (SO_2), ozone (O_3), and nitrogen dioxide (NO_2), can trigger asthma as well. This trigger becomes significant in heavily industrialized areas, especially when atmospheric conditions permit pollutants to accumulate in high concentrations. When atmospheric conditions change to produce cold and damp weather, asthma attacks also tend to increase.

Ingested substances may induce asthma by a variety of mechanisms, which are largely unknown. Aspirin and other nonsteroidal anti-inflammatory agents may trigger airflow obstruction in 10 percent of asthma patients.[28] This response can be inhibited by giving a daily desensitizing dose of the offending medication. Patients with aspirin sensitivity may also react adversely to ingestion of tartrazine, a yellow food dye formerly also found in some medications. Sulfites, used extensively as preservatives in the food and pharmaceutical industries, may also induce asthma. Sulfite-induced asthma may be suspected when an attack occurs directly following the ingestion of food or beverages. Beta-adrenergic blocking drugs such as propranolol, used in treating hypertension, cardiac arrhythmias, and glaucoma, also may cause exacerbation of asthma. This problem may occur less commonly with the beta-1-selective types, but any beta-blocker can exacerbate asthma. Occasionally even the small doses used in ophthalmic preparations are sufficient to aggravate symptoms.

The ability of emotional stress to worsen asthma has long been noted.[29] This may play some role in up to half of all asthma patients through vagal afferent pathways. The exact contribution of psychic stress to each asthmatic attack is difficult to quantitate, and stress is probably seldom the sole trigger.

A variety of asthma triggers exist in the workplace as a result of the materials used. Asthma of this type is called *occupational asthma* (see Ch. 38). These occupational triggers can be grouped into general categories: organic dusts, metal salts, pharmaceuticals, industrial chemicals and plastics, enzymes, and animal proteins. Workers who handle certain of these materials generally have a higher incidence of asthma than that found in the general population. They may exhibit a characteristic pattern of work-related exacerbations and remissions while away from the workplace. An extensive detailed review of occupational asthma can be found elsewhere.[30]

Pathophysiology

Regardless of the precise nature of triggering factors in an asthmatic event, the end result is airway narrowing. This narrowing results from swelling of the bronchial wall, increased mucus volume in the airway lumen, and circumferential contraction of bronchial smooth muscle. The contribution to airway narrowing or occlusion afforded by each of these factors may vary from patient to patient and may depend on the combination of triggering factors involved.

The bronchial wall is swollen by increased water, infiltrating leukocytes, and mucosal gland enlargement. Mucus volume likely increases owing to accelerated production of mucus and the thickened nature of this mucus. These aberrations combine to overcome the normal primary and secondary bronchial clearance mechanisms, namely the ciliary transport of mucus and cough, respectively. Bronchial smooth muscle tone is regulated by both cholinergic and adrenergic influences. The bronchi are innervated by the vagus nerve and have alpha- and beta-adrenergic receptors as well. Untoward perturbations in the balance of activity in the system results in an abnormal increase in bronchial smooth muscle tone, constricting the airway lumen. This stimulus-response coupling via the adrenergic and cholinergic pathways in asthma is shown graphically in Figure 20-2.

Some airways may become totally occluded by these factors, thereby eliminating ventilation from subtended alveoli. Others may close early in expiration (i.e., at high lung volumes), limiting ventilation in these regions. Reduced flow rates and hyperinflation characterize the abnormalities in pulmonary function. FVC, peak expiratory flow rate, FEV_1, and FEV_1/FVC are reduced, while functional residual capacity (FRC) and residual volume (RV) are elevated. More detailed discussion of these abnormalities of pulmonary function may be found in Chapter 21.

Because the airflow obstruction is nonuniform, albeit diffuse, certain areas of the lung are underventilated and others overventilated relative to perfusion (blood flow), producing $\dot{V}/\dot{Q}$ mismatch. Areas of very high $\dot{V}/\dot{Q}$ (physiologic dead space) result in hypercapnia, whereas those of low $\dot{V}/\dot{Q}$ result in hypoxemia. Chapter 10 provides a more detailed discussion of abnormalities of ventilation and perfusion.

These regional differences in ventilation and perfusion are summed in the pulmonary veins and reflected in arterial blood gas values. Early in an attack patients are hypoxemic and/or the alveolar-arterial O_2 partial pressure difference $[P(A\text{-}a)O_2]$ is increased. The PCO_2 is reduced initially, with an elevation of arterial pH (acute respiratory alkalosis), but it may rise later if the duration and severity of the attack stress the ventilatory muscles to the point of fatigue. Metabolic acidosis may supervene at the point at which O_2 delivery becomes compromised as a result of hypoxemia.

Clinical Presentation

The cardinal symptoms of asthma are wheezing, dyspnea, cough, and phlegm production. These symptoms often worsen following exertion, at night, or following exposure to specific triggers, as discussed above. Symptomatology is characteristically intermittent, and symptomatic periods may be separated by long symptom-free intervals.

Tachypnea is common during an acute asthma attack, with the respiratory rate usually exceeding 20 breaths per minute. Findings on auscultation of the lungs will usually consist of wheezing and rhonchi but will vary depending on the severity of obstruction. While wheezing is the hallmark auscultatory finding in asthma, in mild airflow obstruction a forced exhalation may be required to provoke wheezing. When airflow obstruction is severe, breath sounds may be diminished because of severely limited tidal ventilation, and wheezing may not be apparent. As such, auscultatory findings in asthma may not be counted on to reliably indicate severity of obstruction. Patients may show evidence of use of accessory ventilatory muscles and may be diaphoretic.

An exaggerated inspiratory fall in systemic arterial blood pressure (pulsus paradoxus) may be noted and generally parallels the degree of obstruction.[31] Sinus tachycardia is usually present in an acute attack, and ventricular premature beats may be detected at increased frequency. Other reversible ECG abnormalities may be present, including enlarged P-waves (P-pulmonale), right axis deviation, right bundle branch block, right ventricular strain pattern, and clockwise rotation. There are no radiologic findings specific to asthma. Radiographs of the chest, taken generally to exclude other causes of diffuse wheezing or to exclude an intercurrent pneumonia, may show signs of hyperinflation but also may be normal.

Natural History and Prognosis

Of patients with childhood onset of asthma, half or more are symptom-free 20 years later, whereas, those with later onset are less likely to attain remission of the illness.[32] Intermittent rather than chronic symptoms are also associated with improved prognosis in both children and adults. Asthma deaths in children occur most often in the 8- to 18-year-old range,[33] and most adult fatalities occur after the age of 30 years.[34,35] Although it is uncertain and a subject of current controversy, fatality rates in asthma appear to be increasing.[36,37] Whether this is due to natural variation, effects of global pollution, some aspect of medical management (such as bronchodilator therapy), or other factors remains to be established.

BRONCHIECTASIS

Bronchiectasis is an abnormal, permanent dilation of bronchi.[38] In diffuse and severe cases it is associated with airflow obstruction. The permanent nature of bronchiectasis is in contradistinction to the dilation that is present temporarily during and following limited lower respiratory infections and/or with atelectasis (pseudobronchiectasis). The mechanism of temporary or pseudobronchiectasis is unknown, but destruction of muscular and elastic components of the bronchial wall accompany the dilation in permanent bronchiectasis.

Epidemiology and Etiology

The prevalence of bronchiectasis in the United States is unknown, but this condition is much less common than COPD or asthma. Its incidence is declining in the United States, as demonstrated by a dramatic decrease since the early 1940s in hospital admissions for the purpose of diagnosing or treating it.[39]

Infection of the bronchial tree is a common thread, which probably links all types of bronchiectasis. Bronchiectasis may thus be considered to be largely a complication of necrotizing lower respiratory infection. Bronchiectasis may complicate lower respiratory infection in otherwise normal individuals or may complicate infections in patients with abnormal bronchial trees.

In otherwise normal individuals, bacterial infection with *Mycobacterium tuberculosis, Bordetella pertussis, Staphylococcus aureus, Pseudomonas aeruginosa, Haemophilus influenzae, Klebsiella* spp., and anaerobic bacteria have been implicated as possible causes of bronchiectasis. Viral infections (measles, influenza, herpes simplex, and adenovirus) and fungal infection with *Histoplasma* have been implicated as well.

A variety of bronchial disorders also predispose to the development of lower respiratory infection and bronchiectasis. These disorders include bronchial obstruction, congenital anatomic defects, immunodeficiency states, and hereditary and other functional abnormalities of the bronchus, as well as inhalation and aspiration injuries. More detailed reviews of these disorders can be found elsewhere.[38,40]

Pathophysiology

As noted above, infection appears to be closely linked to the development of bronchiectasis. Inflammatory consequences of infection are associated with destructive changes, chiefly in the medium-sized and smaller bronchi. Bronchial lumina are dilated and replete with thick mucus, and fibrotic tissue may replace bronchial smooth muscle and cartilage. This dilation impedes the normal mucus clearance mechanisms. A number of distinct radiographic patterns can be identified; these are tabulated in Table 22-3. Bronchial arteries may be enlarged to triple their normal size.

Pulmonary function findings depend on the extent and distribution of the bronchiectatic process. Pulmonary function may be normal in limited focal bronchiectasis. Where the process is diffuse, an obstructive pattern may emerge, with reductions in FVC, FEV_1, and FEV_1/FVC and an increase in RV. In advanced cases with extensive fibrosis and atelectasis, a combined restrictive and obstructive pattern may be noted (an obstructive pattern with reduced total lung capacity). Hypoxemia develops in extensive cases; cor pulmonale may ensue with chronic hypoxemia. Hypercapnia may supervene as airflow obstruction worsens.

Table 22-3. Characteristics of Types of Bronchiectasis

Cylindrical bronchiectasis
Regularly outlined bronchi
Not greatly increased diameters peripherally
Abrupt ending of the bronchiectatic segment
Varicose bronchiectasis
Greater bronchial dilatation than in cylindrical bronchiectasis
Irregular outlines caused by local restrictions
Bulbous terminations
Saccular (cystic) bronchiectasis
Ballooned outline
Cystic spaces may be present and may contain air-fluid levels
Follicular bronchiectasis
Defined by histologic criteria only
Lymphoid follicles and nodes in the walls of bronchi and bronchioles and adjacent pulmonary parenchyma
Occurs in setting of collagen vascular disease and immunodeficiency syndromes
Congenital bronchial cysts or congenital (bronchial) cystic disease
Cysts are filled with mucus and lined by respiratory epithelium
May mimic bronchiectasis
Central congenital cysts
Peripheral congenital cysts
Intralobar bronchopulmonary sequestration
Pseudobronchiectasis
Reversible; follows acute pneumonia or obstruction

Clinical Presentation

The cardinal symptom of bronchiectasis is cough with expectoration. In extensive disease the sputum is copious, purulent, thickened, and usually foul-smelling. In limited, focal disease intermittent hemoptysis may be the only symptom. In extensive disease infectious exacerbations may be accompanied by fever. Inspiratory crackles may be heard over involved areas, and rhonchi and wheezes may be present. Clubbing of the fingers, dyspnea, and weight loss may occur in advanced cases.

Plain radiographs of the chest are usually abnormal in symptomatic patients but are not usually diagnostic of bronchiectasis. Rather, focal areas of increased lung markings, "tram" lines, and "ring" shadows support the diagnosis when present.[38] Bronchography is the most sensitive method for detection of the type and extent of bronchiectasis.[41] Thin-section CT of the chest shows promise in identifying most clinically significant bronchiectasis and is less invasive than bronchography.[42] Figure 22-10 depicts the plain radiographic, bronchographic, and computed tomographic appearance of bronchiectasis.

Natural History

The natural history of bronchiectasis has in all likelihood changed substantially since the advent of antibiotics. However, its prevalence has diminished such that the natural history and prognosis are difficult to evaluate. Prognosis can be surmised to depend on the severity of the underlying predisposing factors, as well as on the rapidity and success with which infectious aspects are treated and bronchial damage thereby limited. Patients with childhood-onset bronchiectasis and no underlying predisposing factors generally improve in their adolescent years and stabilize. Patients with focal bronchiectasis and recurrent hemoptysis may require regional lung resection for control, and a "cure" may be effected in these cases.

CYSTIC FIBROSIS

Cystic fibrosis is an inherited illness whose effects are fomented by an abnormal secretory process, resulting in abnormal products of secretion.[43,44] These secretory products include mucus and are relatively dehydrated and thickened as compared with normal secretions. The thick secretions become problematic to varying degrees in given patients. They generally lead to obstructive complications in organs

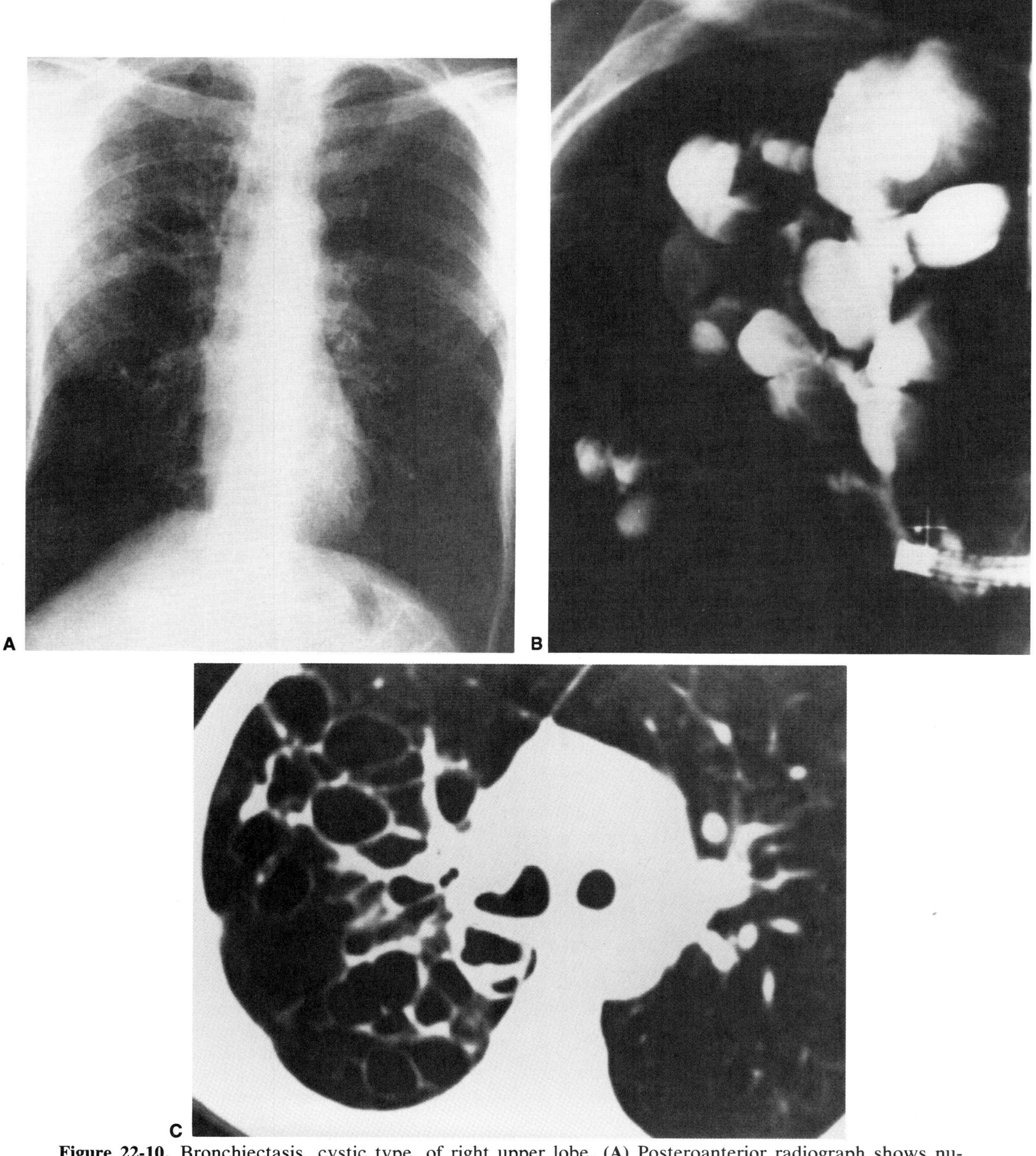

Figure 22-10. Bronchiectasis, cystic type, of right upper lobe. (**A**) Posteroanterior radiograph shows numerous cystic spaces and increased interstitial markings in the right upper lobe. (**B**) Coned-down fluoroscopic spot film taken during fiberoptic bronchoscopy (note bronchoscope at lower right) after injection of contrast material, which fills the bronchiectatic spaces in the apical segment of the right upper lobe. (**C**) Enlargement of CT section through the right upper lobe. The dilated bronchi have the configuration of a cluster of grapes, and a few air-fluid levels are visible medially. (From Naidich et al.,[48] with permission.)

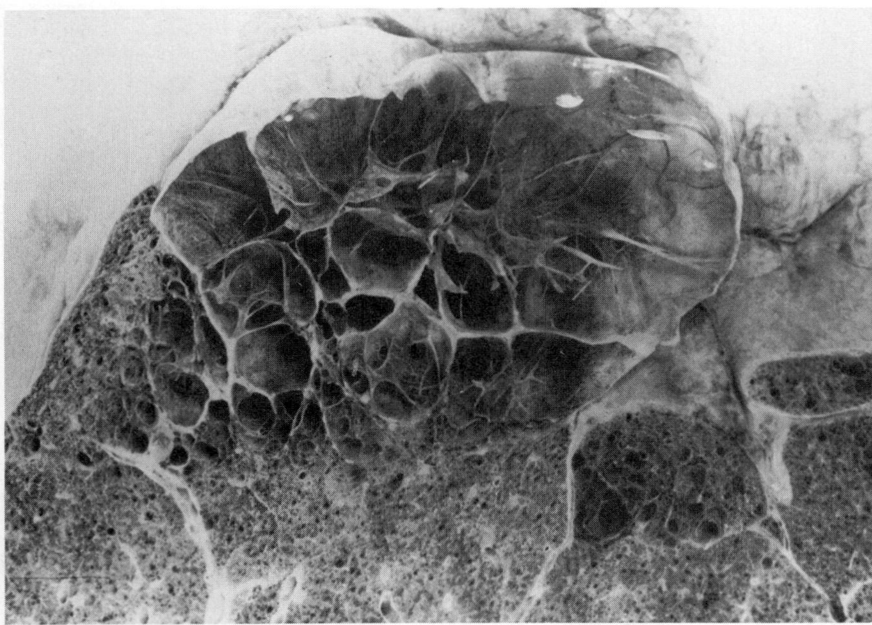

Figure 22-11. Cut surface of a lung showing bullous disease in the upper lobe. The pulmonary parenchyma beneath the bullae is normal. (From Dunnill,[45] with permission.)

in which transport of secretory products is critically linked to function. These organs include the lung, biliary tree, pancreatic tree, colon, epididymis, and fallopian tubes.

Diffuse bronchitis and bronchiectasis are common complications of cystic fibrosis, and airflow obstruction commonly accompanies these processes. As in other forms of bronchiectasis, a restrictive pattern may emerge in pulmonary function testing of cystic fibrosis patients as a result of atelectasis and scarring.

As improved methods have emerged for caring for the many complications of cystic fibrosis (notably the infectious complications in the lung), the prognosis has improved. Over half of those diagnosed with cystic fibrosis survive beyond 10 years.[43] As a result, adults with cystic fibrosis are more commonly encountered.

BULLOUS LUNG DISEASE

Bullous lung disease is characterized by the existence of extremely large airspaces within the lung parenchyma, called *bullae*. A bulla arises from fusion of multiple areas of emphysematous enlargement or from the ball valve effect of a bronchus on the subtended lung tissue. Bullae occur most often in the upper lobes[45] (Fig. 22-11) and are of three commonly recognized types. Type I bullae have narrow necks, thin walls, and an empty interior. In type II bullae, which arise in the subpleural areas, the neck consists of panacinar emphysematous lung tissue while the interior consists of emphysematous lung. Type III bullae have extremely broad necks and consist of slightly hyperinflated lung.

Clinical manifestations associated with bullous lung disease vary.[46] If the bullae are simply a focal exaggeration of a generalized process in diffusely emphysematous lung, symptoms will likely depend on the degree of airflow obstruction. If the bullae represent aberrations in an otherwise normal lung, the patient may be asymptomatic or may experience symptoms that depend on the extent to which surrounding lung tissue is compressed. These airspace enlargements may be complicated by hemorrhage, pneumothorax, or infection.

SMALL AIRWAYS DISEASE

The detection and significance of small airways obstruction[47] have been topics of considerable interest since the early 1970s. Abnormalities in the single breath N_2 test and the maximum expiratory flow-volume curve using gases of different densities indicate dysfunction in the small airways (less than 2 mm in diameter) and were thought to be the harbinger of COPD. After much study, however, these tests have not been found to be reliable predictors of COPD.[47] The mean forced expiratory flow between 25 and 75 percent of FVC (FEF_{25-75}) has such high variability within and between individuals, resulting in an extremely broad range of normal values, that this determination has not proved very useful for this purpose either. These tests are not only poor predictors of incipient COPD but also do not provide an adequate explanation for dyspnea when an abnormal value is found in the face of a normal FEV_1, FVC, and FEV_1/FVC.

CONDITIONS CAUSING LOCALIZED LOWER AIRWAY OBSTRUCTION

Occasionally, a focal obstruction of one or more of the larger airways may develop and cause airflow obstruction. Common causes of such obstruction of the lower airways are listed in Table 22-1. Neoplastic or granulomatous lesions may initially cause obstruction by partially occluding the lumen of a bronchus. However, as these lesions enlarge and completely block the lumen, a restrictive pattern supervenes.

References

1. Klocke RA: Influence of aging on the lung. pp. 432–444. In Finch CE, Hayflick I (eds): Handbook of the Biology of Aging. Van Nostrand Reinhold, New York, 1977
2. American Thoracic Society: Standards for the diagnosis and care of patients with chronic obstructive pulmonary disease (COPD) and asthma. Am Rev Respir Dis 1987;136:225–244
3. Higgins ITT: Epidemiology of bronchitis and emphysema. pp. 1237–1246. In Fishman AP (ed): Pulmonary Diseases and Disorders. McGraw-Hill, New York, 1988
4. Morgan WKC, Seaton A: Occupational Lung Diseases. 2nd Ed. WB Saunders, Philadelphia, 1984
5. Buist AS, Burrows B, Cohen A et al: Guidelines for the approach to the patient with severe alpha-1-antitrypsin deficiency. Am Rev Respir Dis 1989;140:1494–1497
6. Sherman CE, Hudson LD, Pierson DJ: Severe precocious emphysema in intravenous methylphenidate (Ritalin) abusers. Chest 1987;92:1085–1087
7. Schmidt RA, Glenny RW, Godwin JD, et al: Panlobar emphysema in young intravenous Ritalin[R] abusers. Am Rev Respir Dis 1991;143:649–656
8. National Heart, Lung, and Blood Institute, Division of Lung Diseases: Workshop report. The definition of emphysema. Am Rev Respir Dis 1985;132:182–185
9. Nagai A, West WW, Thurlbeck WM: The National Institutes of Health intermittent positive-pressure breathing trial: Pathology studies. II: Correlation between morphologic findings, clinical findings and evidence of expiratory-airflow obstruction. Am Rev Respir Dis 1985;132:946–953
10. American Thoracic Society: Chronic bronchitis, asthma, and pulmonary emphysema. Am Rev Respir Dis 1962;85:762–768
11. Thurlbeck WM: Chronic airflow obstruction in lung disease. pp. 350–444. In Bennington JL (ed): Major Problems in Pathology. Vol. 5. WB Saunders, Philadelphia, 1976
12. Petty TL: Definitions, clinical assessment, and risk factors. pp. 1–30. In Petty TL (ed): Chronic Obstructive Pulmonary Disease. 2nd Ed. Marcel Dekker, New York, 1985
13. Haluszka J, Chartrano DA, Grassino AE, Milic-Emili J: Intrinsic PEEP and arterial PCO_2 in stable patients with chronic obstructive pulmonary disease. Am Rev Respir Dis 1990;141:1194–1197
14. Martinez FJ, Couser JI, Celli BR: Factors influencing ventilatory muscle recruitment in patients with chronic airflow obstruction. Am Rev Respir Dis 1990;142:276–282
15. Miller RR, Muller NL, Vedal S et al: Limitations of computed tomography in the assessment of emphysema. Am Rev Respir Dis 1989;139:980–983
16. Speizer FE, Tager IB: Epidemiology of chronic mucous hypersecretion and obstructive airways disease. Epidemiol Rev 1979;1:124–142
17. Fletcher C, Peto R, Tinker C, Speizer FE: The Natural History of Chronic Bronchitis and Emphysema. Oxford University Press, Oxford, 1976
18. Burrows B, Earle RH: Course and prognosis of chronic obstructive pulmonary disease. N Engl J Med 1969;280:397–404
19. Kanner RE, Renzetti AD: Predictions of spirometric changes and mortality in the obstructive airway disorders. Chest, suppl. 1984;85:15–17
20. Diener CF, Burrows B: Further observations on the course and prognosis of chronic obstructive lung disease. Am Rev Respir Dis 1975;111:719–724
21. Traver GA, Cline MG, Burrows B: Predictions of mortality in COPD: A 15-year follow-up study. Am Rev Respir Dis 1979; 119:895–902
22. Lenfant C, Hurd S: National asthma education program. Chest 1990;98:226–227
23. Barnes PJ: Pathogenesis of asthma. J R Soc Med 1983;76:580–586
24. Barnes PJ: A new approach to the treatment of asthma. N Engl J Med 1989;321:1517–1527
25. Djukanovic R, Roche WR, Wilson JW et al: Mucosal inflammation in asthma. Am Rev Respir Dis 1990;142:434–457
26. Ellis EF: Role of infection in asthma. Adv Asthma Allergy Pulmon Dis 1977;4:28–33
27. McFadden ER, Lenner KA, Strohl KP: Postexertional airway rewarming and thermally induced asthma. J Clin Invest 1986; 78:18–25
28. Samter M, Beers RF: Intolerance to aspirin. Ann Intern Med 1968;975–983
29. Kelly E, Zeller B: Asthma and the psychiatrist. J Psychosom Res 1969;13:377–395
30. Pepys J: Occupational asthma: Review of present clinical and immunological status. J Allergy Clin Immunol 1980;66:179–185
31. Knowles GK, Clark TJH: Pulsus paradoxus as a valuable sign indicating severity of asthma. Lancet 1973;2:1356–1359
32. Ogilvie AG: Asthma: A study in prognosis of 1000 patients. Thorax 1962;17:183–189
33. Strunk RC, Mrazek DA, Fuhrmann GSW, LeBrecque JF: Physiologic and psychological characteristics associated with deaths due to asthma in childhood. JAMA 1985;254:1193–1198
34. Benatar SR: Fatal asthma. N Engl J Med 1986;314:423–428
35. Alexander HL: A historical account of death from asthma. J Allergy 1963;34:305–313
36. Buist AS: Is asthma mortality increasing? Chest 1988;93:449–450
37. Whitelaw WA: Asthma deaths. Chest 1991;99:1507–1510
38. Luce JM: Bronchiectasis. pp. 1107–1125. In Murray JF, Nadel JA (eds): Textbook of Respiratory Medicine. WB Saunders, Philadelphia, 1988
39. Field CE: Bronchiectasis. Third report on a follow-up study of medical and surgical cases from childhood. Arch Dis Child 1969; 45:551–561
40. Crofton J: Diagnosis and treatment of bronchiectasis. Br Med J 1966;1:721–723
41. Reid L: Reduction in bronchial subdivision in bronchiectasis. Thorax 1950;5:233–247
42. Silverman PM, Godwin JD: CT/bronchographic correlations in bronchiectasis. J Comput Assist Tomogr 1987;11:52–56
43. Cystic fibrosis. Semin Respir Med 1985;6:243–333
44. Davis PB: Cystic fibrosis. pp. 1732–1735. In Kelley WN (ed): Textbook of Internal Medicine. 2nd Ed. JB Lippincott, Philadelphia, 1992
45. Dunnill MS: Pulmonary Pathology. Churchill Livingstone, Edinburgh, 1987, p. 115
46. Snider GL: Chronic bronchitis and emphysema. pp. 1069–1106. In Murray JF, Nadel JA (eds): Textbook of Respiratory Medicine. WB Saunders, Philadelphia, 1988
47. Buist AS: Tests of small airways function. Respir Care 1989; 34:446–454
48. Naidich DP, Zerhouni EA, Siegel SS: Computed tomography and magnetic resonance of the thorax. 2nd Ed. Raven Press, New York, 1991

Chapter 23

Restrictive Disorders

Noel T. Johnson
David J. Pierson

CHAPTER OUTLINE

Restrictive pulmonary disorders are those that prevent normal lung inflation, an effect that may be caused by a wide variety of conditions. These disorders exert their restrictive effect either by alteration of the lung tissue itself or by functional and structural alterations of the tissues and organs surrounding the lungs. Regardless of the mechanism, all are characterized by reduced lung volumes. Reductions in vital capacity, functional residual capacity, residual volume, and total lung capacity (as described more fully in Ch. 21) may all be seen. Some of the more common disease processes causing pulmonary restriction are tabulated in Table 23-1.

The clinical manifestations and physiologic consequences of these disorders are protean and in most instances are proportional to the degree of the restrictive impairment. Most of the clinical manifestations and physiologic consequences derive from the reduction in functional gas exchanging tissue (i.e., in the alveolar-capillary surface area available for gas exchange). Dyspnea and cough are common complaints, hypoxemia is frequently observed, and the diffusing capacity for carbon monoxide (D_{LCO}) may be reduced. In addition, stimulation of irritant and J receptors by changes in the lung interstitium may play a role in producing the hyperventilation frequently seen in patients with restrictive lung disease.[1]

PULMONARY DISORDERS PRODUCING A RESTRICTIVE PATTERN

Generalized Pulmonary Processes

Diffuse processes affect the lung parenchyma ubiquitously, although regional variations occur. They are characterized by diffusely increased lung markings on the chest radiograph. Patients usually complain of dyspnea, and inspiratory crackles and tachypnea may be present.

Idiopathic Pulmonary Fibrosis

Idiopathic pulmonary fibrosis (IPF), a condition of unknown cause producing progressive breathlessness and often accompanied by a nonproductive cough,[2] has been estimated to occur in 3 to 5 individuals per 100,000 population.[3] It is characterized on the chest radiograph by a generalized increase in lung markings, usually predominating in the lower lung zones,[4] (Fig. 23-1A). High-resolution computed tomographic (HRCT) images of lung tissue in IPF (Fig. 23-1B) demonstrate the generalized increase in solid tissue through-

Table 23-1. Diseases Producing a Restrictive Pattern of Pulmonary Dysfunction

Pulmonary disorders
- Generalized processes (see Table 23-2)
  - Idiopathic pulmonary fibrosis
  - Sarcoidosis
  - *Pneumocystis carinii* pneumonia
  - Cardiogenic pulmonary edema
  - Adult respiratory distress syndrome
  - Pneumoconioses
- Localized processes
  - Parenchymal neoplasms (e.g., lung cancer)
  - Lobar pneumonia
  - Lung abscess
  - Lung resection
  - Large bullae
  - Atelectasis
  - Radiation fibrosis
  - Focal, postinfectious scarring (e.g., tuberculosis)

Extrapulmonary disorders
- Vascular processes
  - Cardiomegaly (e.g., dilated cardiomyopathy)
  - Dilated vessels (e.g., aortic aneurism)
- Pleural processes
  - Pleuritic pain (pleurisy)
  - Pleural effusion
  - Pneumothorax
  - Masses (e.g., malignant mesothelioma)
  - Diffuse pleural thickening
- Pericardial processes
  - Pericardial effusion (e.g., with uremia or malignancy)
  - Pericardial malignancies
  - Pericardial cysts
- Mediastinal processes
  - Massive lymph node enlargement (e.g., metastatic malignancy, lymphoma, sarcoidosis, tuberculosis)
  - Thymoma
  - Thyroid enlargement (substernal goiter)
  - Pneumomediastinum
  - Mediastinitis (histoplasmosis; post-cardiac surgery)
  - Dilated esophagus (e.g., achalasia, large hiatus hernia)
- Thoracic cage/abdominal wall abnormalities
  - Kyphoscoliosis
  - Pectus excavatum
  - Obesity
  - Body casts, bandages, corsets
  - Thoracoplasty
- Neuromuscular disorders
  - High spinal cord lesions
  - Diaphragmatic paralysis
  - Poliomyelitis; Guillain-Barré syndrome; botulism; myasthenia gravis
  - Pharmacologic paralysis (pancuronium, curare)
  - Pain-related splinting following upper abdominal surgery

out the lung and show a reticular pattern and often evidence of honeycombing of the pulmonary parenchyma. The pulmonary function pattern is restrictive, and the DLCO is typically decreased (see Table 21-3). Patients typically present with dyspnea and may have a nonproductive cough. The physical examination usually reveals inspiratory crackles, predominantly in the lung bases. Finger clubbing is also common.

IPF is thought to be caused by the inflammatory response of the lung to an injury that cannot be identified (Fig. 23-2). By definition, known causes of interstitial lung disease have been excluded. The tissue reaction in IPF is a common response of the lung to several types of lung injury.[5] The injury and reaction are of sufficient magnitude to prevent re-establishment of normal interstitial architecture. The collagen and mesenchymal cell deposits in the interstitial matrix are long-lived and refractory to normal physiologic repair mechanisms.[6]

IPF may occur at any age but most commonly presents in the fourth and fifth decades.[7] A male predominance has been found, and there is an inferential, if not established, relationship with cigarette smoking.[8] There is only a 50 percent 5-year survival rate even with treatment.[5] Established fibrosis itself is untreatable, but if the inflammatory process is active, its course and the progression of the disease may be modulated by use of corticosteroids and immunosuppressant drugs such as cyclophosphamide.

Sarcoidosis

Sarcoidosis is a multisystem disease, which commonly and prominently affects the lung.[9,10] Estimates of its incidence vary widely among countries, ranging to as high as 64 per 100,000 in Sweden; a female predominance has been reported, and in the United States blacks are more likely to be affected than whites.

Sarcoidosis is an inflammatory process of unknown cause, characterized by formation of granulomas in affected tissues. These granulomas typically do not show a central necrosis, as do the typical granulomas in tuberculosis or other granulomatous infections, but similar granulomas are found in many other diseases of specific known cause. These causes must be excluded in order to verify the diagnosis of sarcoidosis. Bronchoalveolar lavage often reveals an increased proportion of lymphocytes and/or an elevated T-helper/T-suppressor lymphocyte ratio.[11] Inflammation and the subsequent repair process lead to fibrosis, and if the inflammatory process is sustained, the ensuing fibrosis may result in impaired function of the lung and/or other target organs (e.g., eyes, heart, nerves). This is typically manifested in the lung by a restrictive pattern and a decreased DLCO.

Sarcoidosis presents most commonly in the second and third decades of life. It may be discovered incidentally as an abnormality on the chest radiograph of a patient without symptoms or physical findings referable to the chest. Patients may also present with cough, wheezing, or dyspnea on exertion. Most frequently, physical examination of the lung is normal. Various skin lesions occur, including erythema nodosum (nodular reddened areas), subcutaneous granulomas, and lupus pernio (bluish papules). Systemic symptoms such as weight loss and fatigue occur infrequently. Serum angiotensin-converting enzyme may be ele-

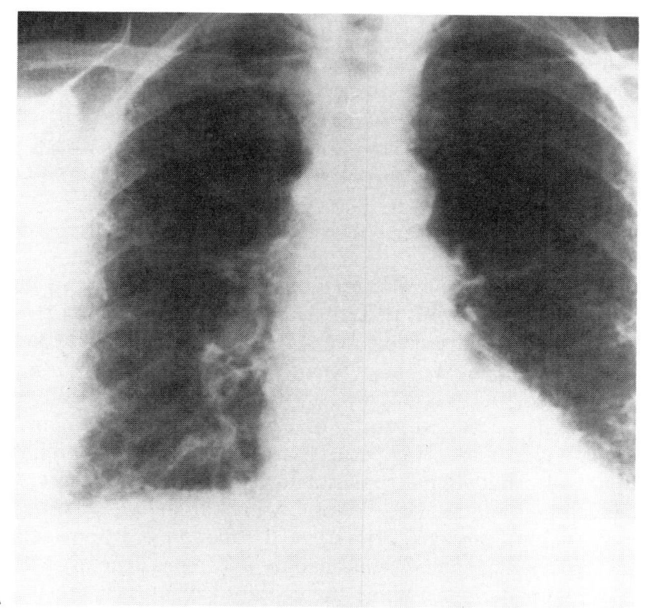

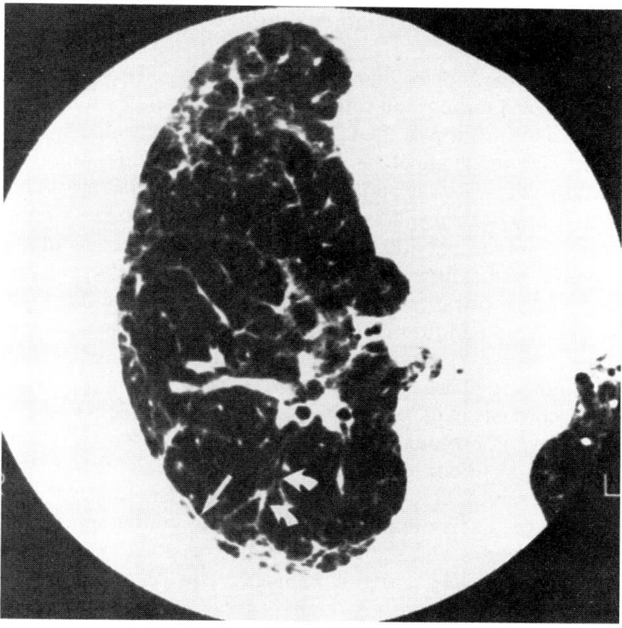

Figure 23-1. (**A**) Chest radiograph of a patient with IPF. There is a nonspecific pattern of increased linear densities especially prominent peripherally and in the lung bases. (**B**) HRCT image through the right lower lobe of the same patient. The pattern consists of medium-sized reticular elements, mainly involving the periphery, as well as subpleural lines (straight arrow). Central secondary pulmonary lobules are easily seen (curved arrows). There are changes of early honeycombing along the mediastinal (left-hand) border. (From Naidich et al.,[43] with permission.)

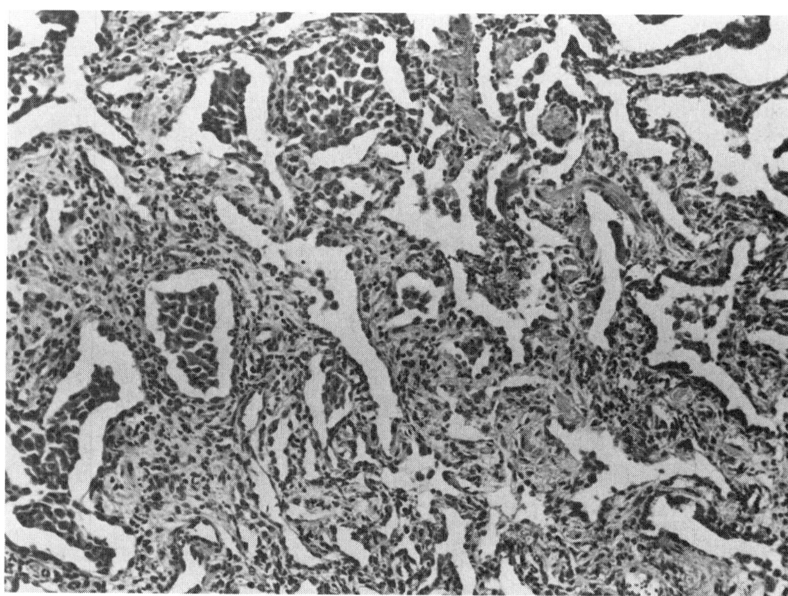

Figure 23-2. Histologic picture in IPF. This section shows changes typical of usual interstitial pneumonitis (UIP). The septa are widened by dense fibrosis and a mild chronic inflammatory cell infiltrate. Alveolar capillaries are diminished in number. Clusters of macrophages are seen in the airspaces. (H&E, × 150.) (From Katzenstein and Askin,[44] with permission.)

vated, but this test is neither sensitive nor specific for this disorder.

The appearance of bilateral hilar lymph node enlargement on the chest radiograph suggests the diagnosis of sarcoidosis. Diffuse infiltration of the lung parenchyma may also be seen. The following staging classification of chest radiographic appearance has been proposed to identify progression.[12] A normal chest radiograph is designated stage 0; bilateral hilar node enlargement indicates stage 1; the presence of pulmonary infiltrations along with hilar adenopathy indicates stage 2A; infiltrations without the adenopathy is designated stage 2B; and additional radiographic features suggesting extensive fibrosis, such as hilar retraction and/or honeycombing, indicate stage 3.

Sarcoidosis is usually self-limited,[9,10] but in some patients its course is prolonged and devastating. In such cases therapy with systemic corticosteroids is undertaken, but it is a challenge to decide which patients will benefit from treatment. This decision is based on a global patient evaluation, which includes an assessment of disease activity as well as evidence for target organ damage. The onus of deciding whether to undertake treatment is greatest when there is evidence of disease activity (e.g., lymphocytes in bronchoalveolar lavage fluid) as well as evidence of organ damage (e.g., progressively reduced lung volume measurements and/or reduced D_{LCO}). Regardless of the decision, patients must be followed with clinical indices (e.g., pulmonary function studies) to determine the course of the disease or the response to therapy.

Pneumocystis carinii Pneumonia

Pneumocystis carinii pneumonia (PCP) is a lung infection caused by a microorganism variously believed to be a protozoan or a fungus.[13,14] Otherwise healthy persons virtually never develop PCP; instead, it is a disorder confined to immunosuppressed individuals, particularly those with the acquired immunodeficiency syndrome (AIDS). It is spread by airborne transmission and presumed to be acquired by the respiratory route. The risk of infection increases as the degree of immunosuppression increases. Groups at increased risk for PCP include premature infants, the malnourished, patients undergoing chemotherapy (including treatment with corticosteroids), those with disorders of cellular immunity, and those with AIDS. AIDS accounts for the preponderance of cases of PCP in the United States today.

The organism is found in the alveolar spaces of the lung, attaching to and injuring the lining cells. The lung responds with the appearance of lymphocytes and macrophages in the interstitial spaces as well as the exudation of proteinaceous material into the alveolar spaces.

The symptoms of PCP commonly include a nonproductive cough and dyspnea, with fever and night sweats usually present. Patients are generally tachypneic and may have inspiratory crackles but commonly have normal auscultatory findings. The chest radiograph almost always demonstrates a diffuse increase in lung markings although other patterns may be encountered. The pulmonary function pattern is often restrictive and the D_{LCO} typically decreased.

Pneumocystis organisms cannot be cultured in the laboratory, but the diagnosis can be made by analysis of sputum with Giemsa or silver methenamine stains and identification of the organism by its characteristic appearance. Vigorous sputum induction with hypertonic saline may be sufficient for these purposes,[15] although bronchoscopic lavage is the standard diagnostic procedure. Open lung biopsy, formerly the "gold standard" of diagnosis, is rarely required now owing to the success of these less morbid diagnostic procedures.

Well over half of all patients with PCP will survive the illness if treated with effective medications, although two-thirds of survivors who have AIDS have persistent organisms on bronchoscopic evaluation following therapy. The prognosis for survivors varies with the degree to which the underlying condition can be reversed. Patients with simple malnutrition may be expected to annul their risk of recurrence with nutritional repletion, but PCP may be expected to recur in patients with inexorably progressive AIDS if they survive long enough. Primary and secondary prophylactic therapy, with inhaled pentamadine and more recently with oral regimens, can reduce the recurrence rates in those at risk for recurrence.[16]

Other Disorders

Other disorders producing a restrictive pattern of pulmonary dysfunction as a result of generalized lung involvement include the adult respiratory distress syndrome (see Ch. 35), the pneumoconioses (see Ch. 38 and Table 44-9), many of the drug-induced pulmonary diseases (see Ch. 39), and others listed in Table 23-2.

Localized Pulmonary Processes

Focal pulmonary processes cause a restrictive pattern of pulmonary dysfunction by interdicting the ability of that portion of the lung to stay inflated, the degree of ventilatory restriction being generally proportional to the amount of lung tissue involved. These processes may exert their effect on the airway, alveolar structure, and/or insterstitium. Some examples of such focal processes are listed in Table 23-1.

Obstruction of the larger airways results in a restrictive (rather than obstructive) pattern once it becomes complete.

Table 23-2. Some Diffuse Lung Diseases Causing a Restrictive Pattern

Idiopathic pulmonary fibrosis
Drug-induced interstitial lung disease
Interstitial lung disease associated with collagen-vascular disease
Interstitial lung disease associated with ankylosing spondylitis
Histiocytosis X
Sarcoidosis
Adult respiratory distress syndrome
Pneumocystis carinii pneumonia
Viral pneumonias (e.g., cytomegalovirus, varicella)
Pneumoconioses (e.g., asbestosis, silicosis)
Hypersensitivity pneumonitis (e.g., pigeon fancier's disease)
Pneumonoultramicroscopicsilicovolcanoconiosis

Tumors, retained foreign bodies, and bronchiectasis (by causing loss of bronchial structural support) may all compromise the airway and limit ventilation therein. Subtended lung tissue is depleted of gas via diffusion of the gas into the bloodstream, while alveolar surfactant stability is lost owing to the lack of periodic expansion. Atelectasis occurs in such regions, with attendant loss of lung volume. In essence, the effect is the same as if the postobstructive segment had been resected; a similar pattern is seen after lung resection.

Focal atelectasis for other reasons[17] (e.g., mucus plugging, postoperative splinting, pulmonary infarction) will similarly cause loss of lung volume attended by a restrictive pattern. Focal pneumonia with its alveolar exudate results in sharply reduced ventilation in the involved lobes and thus in reduced lung volume.

Lung abscesses are large collections of pus within the lung parenchyma. Necrotizing infections result in focal loss of the normal lung structure and produce an abnormally large fluid collection, which necessarily excludes air. Such abnormal fluid collections result in loss of lung volume and if large enough may produce a restrictive pattern on pulmonary function testing. Enormous tumors of the lung may obliterate lung parenchyma in a like manner, resulting in loss of lung volume and a restrictive pattern. Table 23-3 lists tumors found in the chest and capable of causing ventilatory restriction.[18]

Focal scarring as the result of inflammation, which may be seen in postradiation fibrosis or following severe pneumonia, also produces a restrictive pattern. Pulmonary tuberculosis often results in extensive scarring, especially in the apical regions of the lung.

Lung bullae are abnormally large airspaces within the lung parenchyma (see Fig. 22-12). As such airspaces expand, the surrounding lung tissue tends to collapse (atelectasis) owing to loss of normal tethering forces. In this way there is a loss of functional lung tissue due to atelectasis although actual lung volume may remain normal. Because these airspaces communicate poorly with the central airways, commonly used lung volume measurements, such as those obtained by the He dilution method, will indicate a smaller lung volume. Lung volumes determined plethysmographically (with the body box), however, are likely to be accurate, as this method does not depend on the communication of pulmonary airspaces (see Ch. 45).

Table 23-3. Neoplasms of the Chest

Primary lung tumors
- Adenocarcinoma
- Squamous cell carcinoma
- Large cell carcinoma
- Small cell (oat cell) carcinoma
- Bronchoalveolar cell carcinoma
- Benign tumors (e.g., hamartoma, bronchial adenoma, pseudotumor)

Metastatic tumors to lung parenchyma

Pleural tumors
- Mesothelioma (malignant; benign)
- Metastatic carcinoma

Mediastinal tumors
- Thymoma
- Teratoma
- Lymphoma
- Germ cell tumor

EXTRAPULMONARY PROCESSES PRODUCING A RESTRICTIVE PATTERN

Extrapulmonary restrictive processes exert their effect by encroachment on the space in the chest cavity normally accorded to the lungs as a result of functional or structural abnormalities in the organs or structures juxtaposed to the lung.

Vascular Disorders

Disorders of the heart and great vessels that result in considerable enlargement may cause pulmonary restriction. In advanced cases of left ventricular dysfunction, the heart commonly becomes widely dilated and may displace a significant amount of lung tissue. Aneurysmal dilation of the aorta may cause left main-stem bronchial compression and lead to atelectasis.

Pleural, Pericardial, and Mediastinal Disorders

Pleural processes that encroach on the lung include morphologic changes in the pleural membrane itself as well as enlargement of the pleural space (the potential space between the visceral and parietal pleura).

Malignant mesotheliomas most commonly arise in the pleural cavity and are relatively rare (2.2 cases per 1,000,000 in the United States and England).[19] The incidence of this malignancy is closely but not exclusively linked with past exposure to asbestos. The lead time between exposure and development of mesothelioma ranges from 20 to 40 or even 50 years, and the usual presenting age is between 50 and 70 years. The tumor may grow to encase the lung (Fig. 23-3), resulting in contraction of the chest cage. Patients commonly present with chest pain and dyspnea, and chest radiographs demonstrate a thickened pleura and typically a pleural effusion. Median survival after diagnosis is less than 1 year, and there is no known treatment that consistently prolongs life. Palliative treatments aimed at control of the pleural effusion, such as chemical pleurodesis and pleurectomy, are effective in achieving this limited goal but probably do not prolong survival.[20]

Benign fibrous mesotheliomas are rare focal pleural tumors, which rarely invade neighboring structures.[10] Patients may have cough, chest pain, or dyspnea, but half of them are asymptomatic. The tumors appear radiographically as focal chest masses at the lung periphery, although an occasional tumor may grow so large as to fill the entire ipsilateral chest cavity. In 90 percent of cases, such tumors may be removed without recurrence.[21]

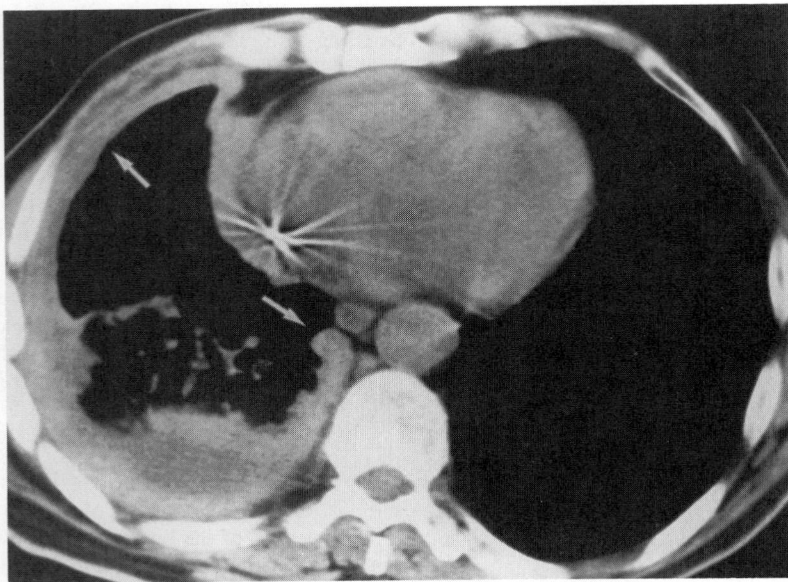

Figure 23-3. Extrapulmonary restriction caused by diffuse pleural malignancy (malignant mesothelioma). There is a circumferential rind of thickened, nodular pleura surrounding the lung (arrows). (From Naidich et al.,[43] with permission.)

Metastatic tumors of the pleura most commonly exert their restrictive effect by the development of pleural effusions rather than by an encroaching mass. Adenocarcinoma of the breast is the most common cause of malignant pleural effusion; other malignancies that commonly cause this complication include carcinomas of the lung and gastrointestinal tract.

Fibrothorax results from deposition of a dense fibrous tissue following severe pleural inflammation, such as is seen in an empyema or hemothorax. Focal deposition of this scar tissue most commonly occurs in the area of prior inflammation. In asbestos-induced fibrothorax, commonly found in asbestos-exposed patients who have developed pleural effusion, the deposition is usually bilateral. The chest radiograph reveals uniform pleural thickening in the involved area, frequently with calcification along the medial aspect. This pleural thickening may result in a pattern of pulmonary restriction. In severe cases with bilateral involvement, respiratory failure may develop.[22]

Both liquid (hydrothorax/pleural effusion [see Fig. 57-15]) and air (pneumothorax [see Fig. 57-16]) in the pleural space may cause a pattern of pulmonary restriction, which is proportional to the amount of pleural space occupied. Pericardial effusion and neoplasms arising from the pericardium can also lead to restriction, as can mediastinal enlargement, such as that caused by lymph nodes or tumors (Table 23-3 and Fig. 57-21B).

Disorders of the Ventilatory Pump

The respiratory pump (Ch. 5) can be thought of as an engine, which consists of relatively stiff outer casing (the chest wall); two pumping cylinders/chambers (the two separate pleural cavities); two main pumping pistons (the two hemidiaphragm muscles) as well as some auxiliary pumps (the accessory muscles of respiration); and a timed driving system (the brain stem respiratory center). The driving or triggering system is wired to the pumping mechanism through peripheral nerves. In addition to the baseline respiratory rhythm signal from the brain stem, the respiratory rhythm may be altered by input received from upper airway, tracheobronchial, and chest wall receptors, from the cerebral cortex, and from peripheral arterial and central nervous system chemoreceptors.

Disorders of the Chest Wall

Damage to or dysfunction in any of the components of this intricate pump will result in diminished ventilatory excursion and ultimately in a pattern of pulmonary restriction. Disorders of the thoracic cage and abdominal wall (the outer casing of the pump) restrict ventilation by physically reducing the upper limits of thoracic inflation. If these disorders are progressive and become severe, respiratory failure can occur.

Kyphoscoliosis

Kyphoscoliosis is an exaggerated curvature of the thoracic spine, giving the appearance of a hump in the back (see Fig. 44-7). A variety of disease processes are associated with the development of scoliosis and/or kyphoscoliosis, but in 80 percent of cases the cause is unknown.[23] Figure 23-4 shows

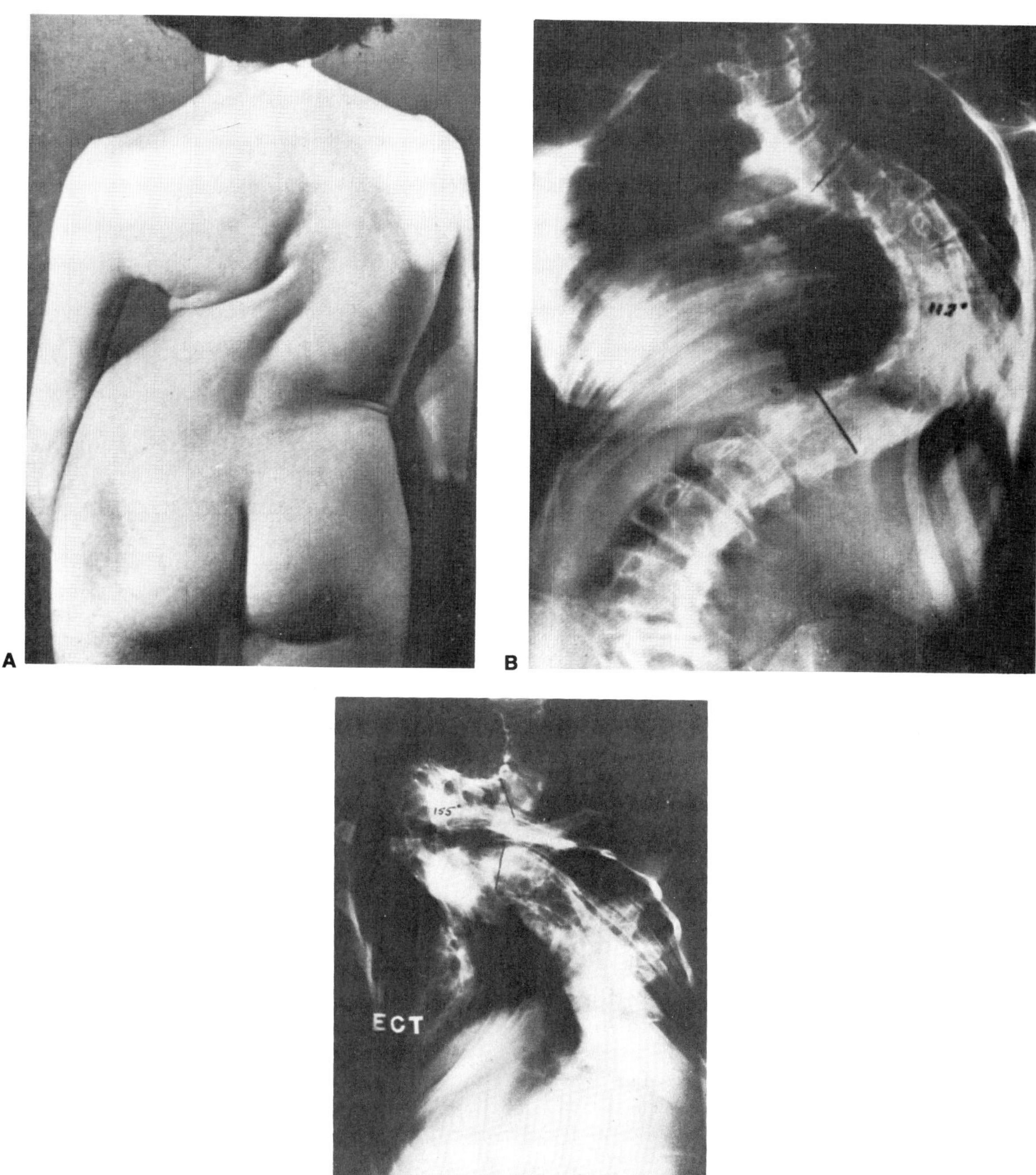

Figure 23-4. **(A)** External appearance of a patient with adolescent idiopathic thoracic scoliosis; **(B)** radiographic appearance. The spinal curvature places the ribs and ventilatory muscles in a disadvantageous mechanical situation, and such deformities are often associated with severe ventilatory restriction. **(C)** Chest radiograph of an adolescent boy with severe kyphoscoliosis following poliomyelitis at age 10. The lung volumes are severely reduced. Patients with such conditions frequently develop chronic ventilatory insufficiency and eventual frank ventilatory failure. (From James,[23] with permission.)

chest radiographs of two patients with this type of spinal disorder who would be expected to have severe restrictive impairment. The spinal deformity results in decreased chest wall compliance and diminished lung volumes, which may ultimately lead to respiratory failure. Although surgical correction is considered for adolescents with severe cases, there is a high (50 percent) complication rate in adults undergoing corrective surgery.[24]

Obesity

Obesity is a common disorder characterized by excess adipose tissue. The increased weight pressing on the thoracic cage and abdominal wall may result in diminished chest wall compliance[25] and sometimes in reduced compliance of the lung itself as well.[26] The restrictive defect is generally proportional to the degree of obesity and is reversible with weight loss.

Disorders of the Muscles and Nerves

Disorders of the muscles (the engine) and the nerves (the wiring) restrict ventilation by causing inadequate muscular force, which is due to muscular dysfunction or to insufficient neural function. Prognosis and severity vary as a function of the underlying cause, and in some cases respiratory failure may ultimately result. Some of the more common causes of muscle and nerve dysfunction are discussed in this section, and additional discussion can be found in Chapters 26 and 90.

Following upper abdominal surgery a mild and temporary diaphragmatic dysfunction occurs (see Ch. 41), which persists despite epidural narcotic pain control. A restrictive pattern is found, hypoxemia develops, and atelectasis appears radiographically in the basilar areas of the lung; however, recovery normally takes place over 2 to 7 days.[27]

Ventilatory Muscles

Disorders of the ventilatory muscles (Ch. 26) are usually associated with a systemic illness affecting other muscles as well. Polymyositis is a generalized muscle disease characterized by infiltration of the muscles with leukocytes. This disorder manifests as diffuse muscle weakness and tenderness, and patients may demonstrate pulmonary restriction on lung function testing, depending on the severity of involvement. Interstitial lung disease may be present as well. Pulmonary restriction may therefore derive from weakness of the respiratory muscles as well as from increased stiffness of the lung due to the presence of interstitial lung disease. Corticosteroid administration may result in clinical remission, but patients may eventually die of respiratory failure.[28] The muscular dystrophies also result in pulmonary restriction due to muscle weakness.[29] Treatment is supportive in nature, and death is usually due to respiratory failure if long-term mechanical ventilation (Ch. 101) is not undertaken.[30]

Shock due to cardiac insufficiency may result in impaired delivery of O_2 to the muscles of respiration as a result of reduced cardiac output.[31] Septic shock may be complicated by a reduced ability of the respiratory muscles to extract O_2 from the blood.[32] Respiratory muscle weakness ensues in either case, and respiratory failure may result. The hyperinflation in chronic obstructive pulmonary disease (COPD) contributes to fatigue (and thereby weakness) of the respiratory muscles by increasing the work of breathing and by decreasing the maximum pressure that the muscles can develop.[33]

Pancuronium and succinylcholine are two drugs used commonly in the intensive care and anesthesiology settings that result in acute, reversible paralysis of the ventilatory (and other) muscles. Pancuronium (Pavulon) is a nondepolarizing neuromuscular blocking agent, which competes for cholinergic receptors at the motor end-plate, and succinylcholine is a muscle relaxant, which combines with the cholinergic receptors at the motor end-plate to depolarize the muscle. The use of these agents represents the extreme of pulmonary restriction due to neuromuscular weakness.[34]

Ventilatory Nerves

Myasthenia gravis, toxic effects of certain antibiotics[35] (aminoglycosides and polymyxins), botulism,[36] and organophosphate toxicity[37] are all thought to cause weakness of the respiratory muscles through action on the neuromuscular junction. In myasthenia gravis the illness is antibody-mediated, prolonged, and often punctuated by bouts of respiratory muscle failure.[38] The other conditions that act on the neuromuscular junction are reversible providing that there is adequate ventilatory support of respiratory muscle failure during the recovery period.

The Guillain-Barré syndrome is an acute inflammatory polyneuropathy affecting the peripheral nerves. The maximum weakness occurs typically 10 to 30 days following onset and characteristically has an ascending pattern. Pulmonary restriction and respiratory failure (occurring in 10 to 20 percent of those afflicted) is caused by inflammatory nerve injury and the reduction of conducted nerve impulses to the respiratory muscles.[39]

Isolated neuropathy of the phrenic nerves may occur in the setting of trauma or cardiac surgery, for a wide variety of other reasons, and many times for unknown reasons (idiopathic neuropathy). The result is paralysis or paresis of the ipsilateral hemidiaphragm. The chest radiograph usually reveals ipsilateral hemidiaphragmatic elevation if the neuropathy is unilateral[40] or the appearance of reduced lung volumes (small lungs) if it is bilateral. Pulmonary restriction and dyspnea are more notable in bilateral involvement, and prognosis is generally worse.[41]

Lesions of the cervical and thoracic spinal cord damage the nerves that transmit respiratory signals. Generally, the higher the injury or lesion, the more profound the effect on respiratory muscle innervation (see Ch. 90). Injuries above the C4 level result in near complete paralysis of ventilatory muscles, while thoracic spinal cord injuries result primarily in impaired cough and expiratory muscle weakness.[42]

References

1. Von Euler C: On the role of proprioceptors in perception and execution of motor acts with special reference to breathing. pp. 139–149. In Penguelly D, Rebuck AS, Campbell EJM (eds): Loaded Breathing. Churchill-Livingstone, Edinburgh, 1974

2. Turner-Warwick M: Widespread pulmonary fibrosis. pp. 755–769. In Fishman AP (ed): Pulmonary Diseases and Disorders. 2nd Ed. McGraw-Hill, New York, 1988
3. Crystal RG, Bitterman PB, Rennard SI et al: Interstitial lung diseases of unknown cause. Disorders characterized by chronic inflammation of the lower respiratory tract. N Engl J Med 1984;310:154–166, 235–244
4. Livingstone JL, Lewis JG, Reid L, Jefferson KE: Diffuse interstitial pulmonary fibrosis. A clinical, radiological and pathological study based on 45 patients. Q J Med 1964;33:71–103
5. Cherniack RM, Crystal RG, Kalica AR: Current concepts in idiopathic pulmonary fibrosis: A road map for the future. Am Rev Respir Dis 1991;143:680–683
6. Crystal RG, Ferrans VJ: Reactions of the interstitial space to injury. pp. 711–737. In Fishman AP (ed): Pulmonary Diseases and Disorders. 2nd Ed. McGraw-Hill, New York, 1988
7. Carrington CB, Gaensler EA, Contu RE et al: Natural history and treated course of unusual and desquamative interstitial pneumonia. N Engl J Med 1978;298:1801–1809
8. Turner-Warwick M, Burrows B, Johnson A: Cryptogenic fibrosing alveolitis: Clinical features and their influence on survival. Thorax 1980;35:171–180
9. Fanburg BL, Pitt EA: Sarcoidosis. pp. 1486–1499. In Murray JF, Nadel JA (eds): Textbook of Respiratory Medicine. WB Saunders, Philadelphia, 1988
10. Sharma OP: Sarcoidosis. pp. 1742–1746. In Kelley WN (ed): Textbook of Internal Medicine. 2nd Ed. JB Lippincott, Philadelphia, 1992
11. Hunninghake GW, Crystal RG: Pulmonary sarcoidosis, a disorder mediated by excess helper T-lymphocyte activity at sites of disease activity. N Engl J Med 1981;305:429–434
12. American Thoracic Society: Treatment of sarcoidosis. A statement by the Committee on Therapy. Am Rev Respir Dis 1971;103:433–434
13. Armstrong D, Bernard EM: Pneumocystosis. pp. 1539–1543. In Kelley WN (ed): Textbook of Internal Medicine. JB Lippincott, Philadelphia, 1992
14. Murray JF, Mills J: Pulmonary infectious complications of human immunodeficiency virus infection. Am Rev Respir Dis 1990;141:1356–1372, 1582–1598
15. Leigh TR, Parsons P, Hume C et al: Sputum induction for diagnosis of *Pneumocystis carinii* pneumonia. Lancet 1989;2:205–206
16. Petersen C, Slutkin G, Mills J: Parasitic Infections. pp. 950–985. In Murray JF, Nadel JA (eds): Textbook of Respiratory Medicine. WB Saunders, Philadelphia, 1988
17. Johnson NT, Pierson DJ: The spectrum of pulmonary atelectasis: Pathophysiology, diagnosis, and therapy. Respir Care 1986;31:1107–1120
18. Carr DT, Holoye PY: Neoplasms of the lungs. pp. 1169–1270. In Murray JF, Nadel JA (eds): Textbook of Respiratory Medicine. WB Saunders, Philadelphia, 1988
19. Legha SS, Mugia FM: Pleural mesothelioma: Clinical features and therapeutic implications. Ann Intern Med 1977;87:613–621
20. Light RW: Tumors of the pleura. pp. 1770–1780. In Murray JF, Nadel JA (eds): Textbook of Respiratory Medicine. WB Saunders, Philadelphia, 1988
21. Okike N, Bernatz PE, Woolner LB: Localized mesothelioma of the pleura: Benign and malignant variants. J Thorac Cardiovasc Surg 1978;75:363–372
22. Light RW: Chylothorax, hemothorax, and fibrothorax. pp. 1760–1769. In Murray JF, Nadel JA (eds): Textbook of Respiratory Medicine. WB Saunders, Philadelphia, 1988
23. James J: Scoliosis. 2nd Ed. Churchill-Livingstone, Edinburgh, 1976
24. Swank S, Lonstein J, Moe J et al: Surgical treatment of adult scoliosis. J Bone Joint Surg 1981;63:268–287
25. Suratt P, Wilhoit S, Hsiao H et al: Compliance of the chest wall in obese subjects. J Appl Physiol 1984;57:403–407
26. Sharp J, Henry J, Sweany S et al: The total work of breathing in normal and obese men. J Clin Invest 1964;43:728–739
27. Ford GT, Whitelaw WA, Rosenal TW et al: Diaphragm function after upper abdominal surgery in humans. Am Rev Respir Dis 1983;127:431–436
28. Dickey BF, Myers AR: Pulmonary disease in polymyositis/dermatomyositis. Semin Arthritis Rheum 1984;14:60–76
29. Inkley SR, Oldenburg FC, Vignos PJ: Pulmonary function in Duchenne muscular dystrophy related to stage of disease. Am J Med 1974;56:279–306
30. Pierson DJ, Kacmarek RM: Home ventilator care. In Casaburi R, Petty TL (eds): Principles and Practice of Pulmonary Rehabilitation. WB Saunders, Philadelphia, 1992 (in press)
31. Aubier M, Trippenbach T, Roussos C: Respiratory muscle fatigue during cardiogenic shock. J Appl Physiol 1981;51:499–508
32. Hussain SNA, Simkus G, Roussos C: Respiratory muscle fatigue, a cause of ventilatory failure in septic shock. J Appl Physiol 1985;58:2027–2032
33. Roussos C, Fixley M, Gross D, Macklem PT: Fatigue of inspiratory muscles and their synergistic behavior. J Appl Physiol 1979;47:897–904
34. Kimball W, Loring SH, Basta SJ et al: Effects of paralysis with pancuronium on chest wall statics in awake humans. J Appl Physiol 1985;58:1638–1645
35. Lindesmith LA, Baines RD, Bigelow DB, Petty TL: Reversible respiratory paralysis associated with polymyxin therapy. Ann Intern Med 1968;68:318–327
36. Schmidt-Nowara WW, Samet JM, Rosario PA: Early and late pulmonary complications of botulism. Arch Intern Med 1983;143:451–456
37. Taylor P: Anticholinesterase agents. pp. 110–129. In Gilman AG, Gilman LS, Rall TW, Murad F (eds): The Pharmacological Basis of Therapeutics. 7th Ed. Macmillan, New York, 1985
38. Dau P: Respiratory failure in myasthenia gravis. Chest 1985;85:721–722
39. Gracey DR, McMichan JC, Divertie MB, Howard FM: Respiratory failure in Guillain-Barré syndrome. Mayo Clin Proc 1982;57:742–746
40. Riley EA: Idiopathic diaphragmatic paralysis. Am J Med 1962;32:404–416
41. McCredie M, Lovejoy FW, Kaltreider NL: Pulmonary function in diaphragmatic paralysis. Thorax 1962;17:213–217
42. Arora NS, Suratt PM, Rochester DF: Respiratory muscle and ventilatory function in spinal cord injury. Clin Res 1978;26:443a
43. Naidich DP, Zerhouni EA, Siegleman SS: Computed Tomography and Magnetic Resonance of the Thorax. 2nd Ed. Raven Press, New York, 1991
44. Katzenstein AA, Askin FB: Surgical Pathology of Non-Neoplastic Lung Disease. pp. 1–430. In Bennington JL (ed): Major Problems in Pathology. Vol. 13. WB Saunders, Philadelphia, 1982

Chapter 24

Disorders of the Pulmonary Circulation

Steven M. Weiss
David J. Pierson

CHAPTER OUTLINE

The pulmonary circulation serves as a vital link between the cardiovascular and respiratory systems, since it is in the pulmonary capillaries that O_2 is transferred to hemoglobin. No physiologic process is more fundamental to survival, and with its complexity comes many opportunities for disruption of normal function by disease. This chapter explores the basic pathophysiologic mechanisms that may impair pulmonary vascular function and describes the major disease processes associated with this impairment.

PATHOPHYSIOLOGY OF PULMONARY VASCULAR DISEASE

Table 24-1 lists the general categories of disorders that can cause pulmonary vascular impairment. Emphysema is an example of an obstructive disease, which can cause diffuse or global destruction of the pulmonary vascular bed by damaging large numbers of individual alveolar subunits.[1] Pulmonary fibrosis and asbestosis represent restrictive processes, which affect the pulmonary circulation, primarily causing damage to lung parenchyma and secondarily involving the vascular bed.[2] Systemic vasculitis involving the lung can also cause direct and widespread damage to the pulmonary circulation.[3] Primary pulmonary hypertension (PPH), a disease of unknown cause, also produces widespread changes in the pulmonary circulation.[3,4] The pulmonary vascular bed may also become obstructed by more localized disease processes such as pulmonary thromboembolism[5] or emboli composed of tumor cells.

All these processes can eventually lead to cor pulmonale and right heart failure. Cor pulmonale refers to right ventricular hypertrophy secondary to pathology in the lungs,[6–8] and right ventricular failure typically occurs as a late clinical manifestation. Figure 24-1 schematically depicts several types of pulmonary vascular injury that may lead to cor pulmonale in chronic obstructive pulmonary disease (COPD), the most common disorder in which it is encountered clinically.[9] As discussed in Chapter 10, hypoxic pulmonary

Table 24-1. Diseases and Disorders Producing Pulmonary Vascular Impairment

Generalized pulmonary vascular obstruction or destruction
Emphysema
Pulmonary fibrosis
Primary pulmonary hypertension
Pulmonary vasculitis
Fat embolism
Amniotic fluid embolism
Parasitic embolism
Air embolism
Localized pulmonary vascular obstruction or destruction
Pulmonary thromboembolism
Tumor embolism
Septic embolism
Cor pulmonale
Left ventricular failure
Pulmonary arteriovenous malformations
Intracardiac shunts

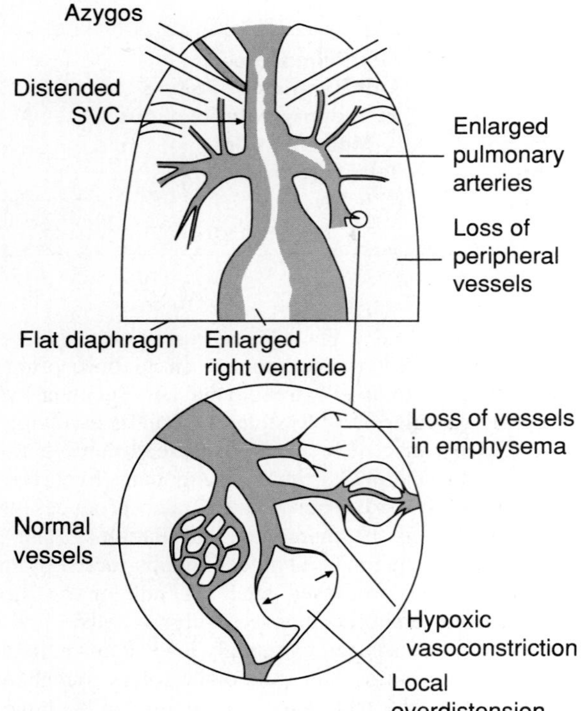

Figure 24-1. Schematic representation of (**A**) chest radiographic and (**B**) pulmonary vascular changes found in severe COPD with pulmonary hypertension and cor pulmonale. (Adapted from Butler,[9] with permission.)

vasoconstriction (HPV) is a normal physiologic response to alveolar hypoxia and plays an important role in the development of cor pulmonale in COPD.[10] Destruction of lung parenchyma, such as occurs in emphysema can also lead to loss of pulmonary capillary surface area and contribute to cor pulmonale. Cor pulmonale may also result when there is sustained alveolar hypoxia without extensive lung disease, as in chronic mountain sickness, alveolar hypoventilation syndromes associated with obesity, and obstructive sleep apnea.

Numerous congenital or developmental abnormalities, including arteriovenous (AV) malformations and atrial or ventricular septal defects, can also cause pulmonary hypertension and eventually lead to right heart failure.[3] These conditions must be distinguished from the situation in cor pulmonale, however, in which the cardiac disorder is due primarily to pulmonary disease. One of the most common causes of pulmonary vascular impairment is pulmonary edema secondary to left ventricular failure, as discussed in Chapter 10. In this case the lungs are initially normal but become congested because of inadequate left ventricular function. When the left ventricle fails, plasma backs up in the pulmonary veins and eventually seeps through capillaries and into the alveolar spaces. If unchecked, this process can lead to right heart failure, as the thin-walled right ventricle struggles to pump blood through the increased resistance in the pulmonary vasculature.[11,12]

Blood flow through the lungs should be thought of as a dynamic process, which changes with different conditions. For example, with increases in pulmonary artery pressures during exercise or in certain disease states, blood flow to the upper lobes increases, whereas under normal circumstances these zones receive less blood flow than do the lower portions of the lungs. Another important mechanism regulating pulmonary blood flow is HPV.[10,13] If an area of lung is underventilated, alveolar hypoxia triggers the vascular smooth muscle and endothelial lining cells to contract, shunting blood away from the area of underventilated lung. If HPV did not occur and blood were not shunted away from an area of atelectasis or consolidation, all the deoxygenated blood returning from that area would eventually join the systemic circulation and cause substantial lowering of arterial O_2 pressure (PaO_2). Instead, blood is shunted away from hypoventilated areas so that more blood flow is directed toward functioning alveoli.

GENERALIZED PULMONARY VASCULAR OBSTRUCTION OR DESTRUCTION

Emphysema

As discussed in Chapter 22, the clinical syndrome of COPD results from the cumulative effects of emphysema, chronic bronchitis, and asthma.[14–17] Both asthma and chronic bronchitis primarily involve the conducting airways, but emphysema damages alveolar walls and their adjacent pulmonary capillaries.[18] Emphysema, therefore, is both a disease that produces airway obstruction and a disorder of the pulmonary circulation. Alveolar damage can lead to ventilation/perfusion ($\dot{V}/\dot{Q}$) mismatching and alveolar hypoxia. Elastic fibers that are normally contained in the lung parenchyma are lost in emphysema (Fig. 24-2). Damage to the alveolar and interstitial tissue in emphysema also causes disruption of the adjacent capillary bed. However, actual destruction of the pulmonary vascular bed by emphysema plays a less important role than HPV in producing an increased pulmonary vascular resistance.

As much of the alveolar-capillary interface is destroyed by emphysema, the diffusing capacity for carbon monoxide (DLCO), which assesses alveolar-capillary surface area, is reduced.[19] As discussed further in Chapter 62, while patients whose COPD is predominantly chronic bronchitis and/or asthma may have normal or near normal values for DLCO, individuals with predominantly emphysema (as in alpha-1-antitrypsin deficiency) tend to have reductions in DLCO that are as severe as their airflow obstruction. As mentioned above, however, although alveolar surface area and hence DLCO may be profoundly reduced in patients with emphysema, this is not the main cause of the elevated pulmonary vascular resistance and pulmonary arterial pressures observed in such individuals, which are due primarily to HPV.[20] Even when capillary destruction reduces the DLCO to 40 percent or less of predicted values, HPV remains the main mechanism for increased pulmonary vascular resistance.[20,21] Secondary erythrocytosis in COPD also contributes to increased pulmonary arterial pressures, as discussed later in this chapter.

Pulmonary Fibrosis

Interstitial pulmonary fibrosis is a restrictive disorder, which often begins as an inflammatory infiltrate involving the alveolar walls and which can lead to scarring and destruction of lung parenchyma[22,23] (see Ch. 23). Most cases are labeled as idiopathic pulmonary fibrosis (IPF), since no etiologic agent can be identified. However, in other cases a causative agent is strongly suspected. Examples of such agents include certain drugs (e.g., amiodarone, methotrexate, bleomycin, and nitrofurantoin),[24] inert compounds such as silica and asbestos,[25] inhaled antigens such as organic dusts (farmer's lung)[26] or avian proteins (pigeon breeder's lung), and pulmonary infections with either viral or bacterial pathogens. Interstitial fibrosis may also occur in association with numerous collagen-vascular disorders, including progressive systemic sclerosis (scleroderma), rheumatoid arthritis, polymyositis, Sjögren's syndrome, and occasionally systemic lupus erythematosus.[27]

Although IPF may occur at any age, it most frequently affects patients in the fifth and sixth decades of life. Large series have shown an approximately 2:1 male predominance.[28] The most common presenting symptom is dyspnea, which is classically more pronounced with exertion. A nonproductive cough, atypical chest pain, and fatigue may also be present. Physical examination typically reveals distinctive, inspiratory crackles ("velcro rales") on auscultation over the lower lung fields. Clubbing is present in nearly half of all patients with IPF. Cyanosis and signs of right ventricular failure may become evident as the disease progresses.[29] The chest radiograph typically shows a diffuse interstitial infiltrate, although signs of pulmonary hypertension may also be seen later in the course. A distinguishing characteristic of pulmonary fibrosis secondary to asbestos exposure is the presence of calcified plaques on the parietal pleural surface.[30] These plaques can also occur in patients exposed to asbestos who do not develop pulmonary fibrosis. However, pleural involvement is rare in other forms of pulmonary fibrosis.

Although there are numerous causes of pulmonary fibrosis, the lung's inflammatory response is rather stereotypical regardless of the inciting agent.[22] Early in the course of IPF, inflammatory cells collect in the airspace and interstitium. Collagen and other fibrous tissue are then deposited in the interstitium, which further disrupts the normal architecture. Capillaries supplying the alveolar septae are obliterated as the fibrous tissue infiltrates into their structure as well. This is the primary mechanism of pulmonary vascular destruction in IPF and results in significant loss of capillary surface area.[22,31] As capillary surface area is reduced, pulmonary vascular resistance increases and pulmonary hypertension may develop.

As the disease progresses and interstitial fibrosis develops, the alveolar-capillary interface required for effective gas exchange is lost, as reflected in a lowering of the DLCO. Pulmonary function tests reveal a restrictive pattern and a reduction in lung compliance. Dead space ventilation is often increased as more of the pulmonary vascular bed is lost and effective ventilation is wasted on nonperfused regions of lung. As alveolar function declines, patients may develop hypoxemia, which typically worsens with exercise. Lung biopsy is often needed to demonstrate the characteristic pathology of IPF and to rule out other disorders.

Most treatment regimens for pulmonary fibrosis are aimed at arresting the inflammatory response before further fibrosis can occur. For this reason, corticosteroids and other anti-inflammatory drugs are often given in an attempt to prevent further inflammatory reaction and scar tissue formation.[31] Despite these interventions, however, prognosis for patients with IPF remains poor, and mean survival from the time of diagnosis is less than 5 years.[31,32] Nevertheless, the course of the disease in different individuals may be highly variable.[29,31] Some patients remain nearly asymptomatic for long periods despite a radiographic picture of extensive interstitial fibrosis.

Primary Pulmonary Hypertension

PPH is a disease characterized by progressive obliteration of the small pulmonary arteries.[4,33] It is a rare condition of

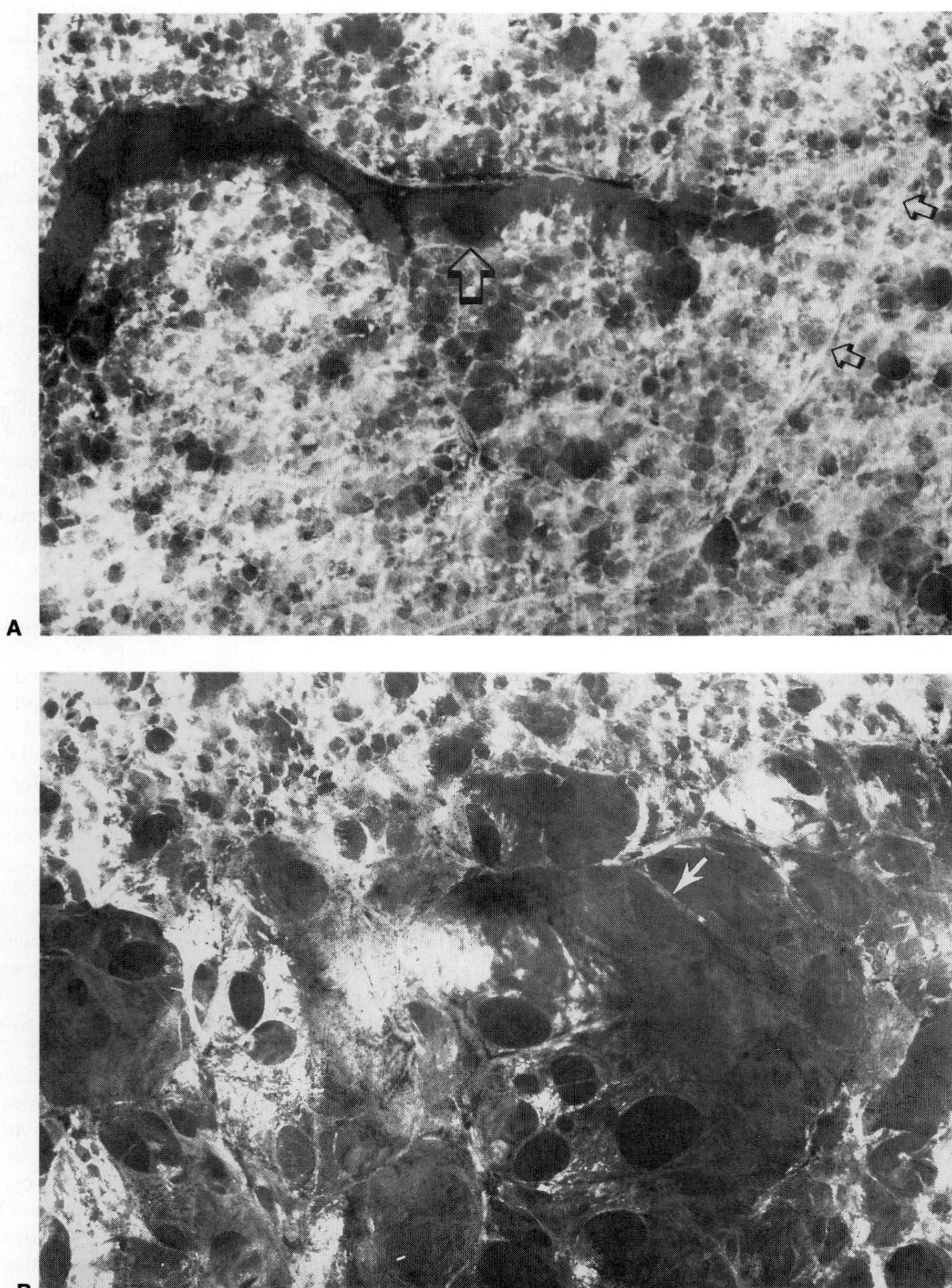

Figure 24-2. Microscopic sections of normal lung as compared with emphysematous lung, to illustrate loss of vascular area along with alveolar tissue. (**A**) Dissecting microscope view of normal lung tissue prepared by freeze drying after air inflation (× 15). Large arrow, branch bronchiole projecting into tissue; small arrows, secondary lobular septum. (**B**) Section of lung with centrilobular emphysema, with specimen preparation and magnification the same as in Figure A. In the lower portion of the section, architecture has been completely destroyed, leaving an empty space, a bleb, demarcated by membranes, sometimes with branching vessels (arrow). *(Figure continues.)*

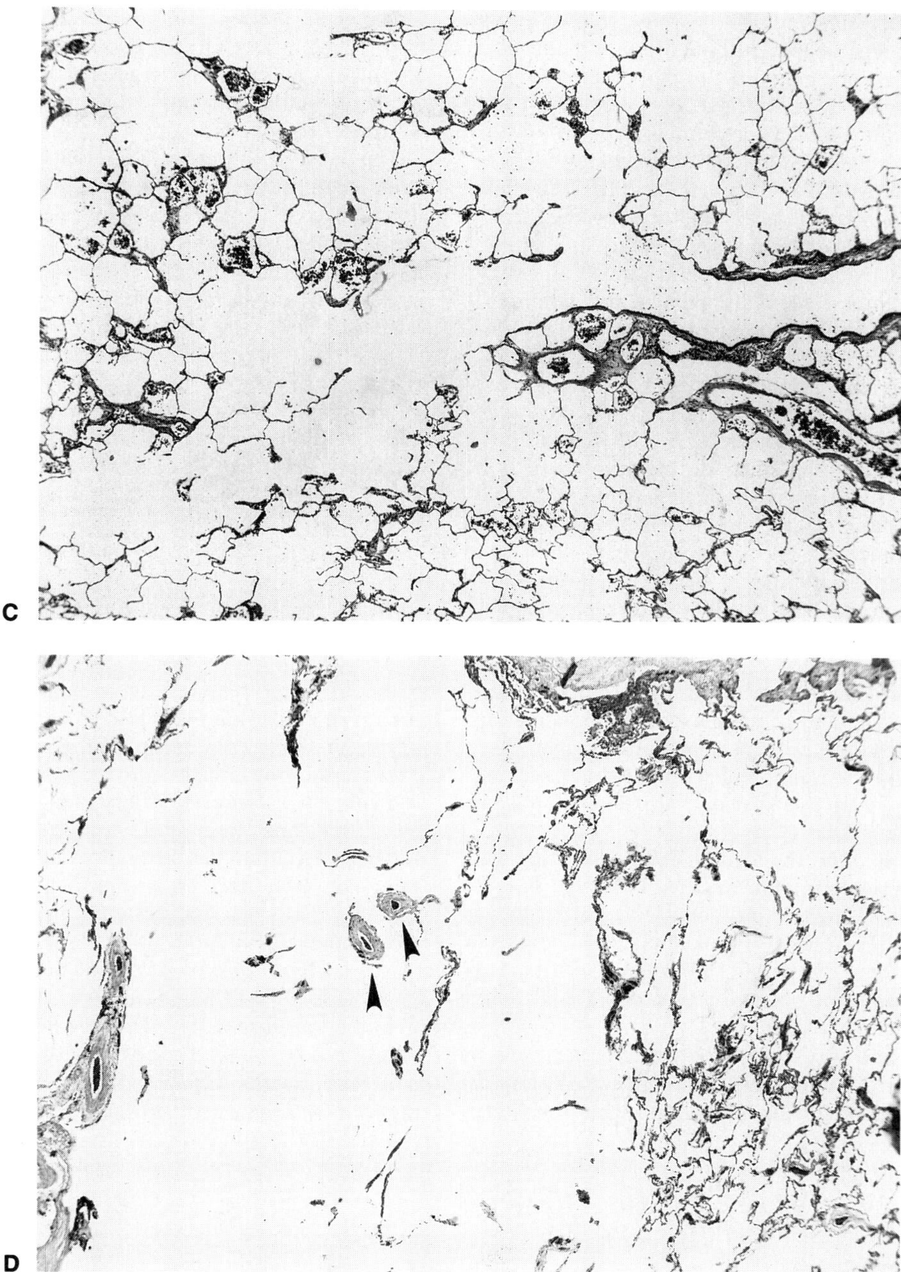

Figure 24-2 (*Continued*). (**C**) Normal alveolar histology (H&E, ×18). A respiratory bronchiole is seen at right, extending into the branching alveolar duct surrounded by alveoli. Every alveolar septum is continuous and attached to surrounding tissue. (**D**) Histopathology of centrilobular emphysema, with preparation and magnification the same as in Figure C. Large central space contains many isolated strands of alveolar septal tissue and several cross sections of small vessels (arrowheads) representing the strands of tissue seen in Figure B. (From Pratt,[98] with permission.)

uncertain etiology and primarily affects young women in the third and fourth decades of life. Although the pathogenesis of PPH remains uncertain, many of the pathologic changes found in the pulmonary vascular bed have been well described.[34] These include medial or intimal hypertrophy of pulmonary arterioles, which is typically followed by fibrosis and destruction of the vascular architecture. These changes occur diffusely throughout the lungs and account for the $\dot{V}/\dot{Q}$ mismatching and hypoxemia observed in the disease.

Patients with PPH usually present with fatigue and dyspnea on exertion.[35] Substernal chest pain is also common, although coronary artery disease is rarely present.[36] Elevated pulmonary artery pressures may cause rupturing of microvascular aneurysms, which may lead to hemoptysis. The physical examination of patients in the early course of PPH may be relatively unremarkable. As the disease progresses, however, the patient often develops signs of pulmonary hypertension and cor pulmonale, including an accentuated second (pulmonary) component to the second heart sound, hepatomegaly, and peripheral edema.[35,37] As right ventricular afterload increases, the systolic murmur of tricuspid regurgitation can frequently be heard. Cyanosis is often a late phenomenon in PPH and may be most notable following exercise. Clubbing is rarely encountered.

Laboratory abnormalities in PPH are nonspecific. Approximately 15 to 20 percent of patients have a positive antinuclear antibody test and positive rheumatoid factor, suggesting that a possible autoimmune component may contribute to the etiology of this disease.[4] Arterial blood gas analysis typically reveals a compensated respiratory alkalosis, and the PaO_2 is often reduced.[33] Exercise testing frequently reveals physiologic abnormalities that may not be apparent at rest. These include an increased alveolar-to-arterial PO_2 gradient [$P(A\text{-}a)O_2$], hypoxemia, and increased dead space ventilation.[33,35] Even in the presence of resting hypoxemia, only a minority of patients with PPH develop secondary polycythemia.

Several mechanisms may be responsible for the hypoxemia present in PPH. As with most other diffuse pulmonary diseases, $\dot{V}/\dot{Q}$ mismatching is the primary process involved. Destruction of the pulmonary vascular bed causes an abnormally low D_LCO and contributes to hypoxemia during exercise.[3,33] As right heart pressures rise, right-to-left intracardiac shunting through a patient foramen ovale can lead to further hypoxemia.

The chest radiograph in PPH may show prominence of the central pulmonary arteries, with peripheral oligemia (i.e., a lack of vascular markings in the peripheral lung zones).[4,37] Peripheral oligemia reflects partial destruction of the pulmonary vascular bed. In the later stages of PPH, the chest radiograph may reveal hypertrophy of the right ventricle as well. Similarly, the electrocardiogram (ECG) may disclose right atrial enlargement, right ventricular hypertrophy, or right axis deviation.[4,35] In addition to its role in evaluating ventricular function, the echocardiogram can be used to measure pulmonary artery pressures by employing Doppler techniques. Intracardiac shunting can often be identified by echocardiogram following injection of microbubbles into the venous circulation.

Right heart catheterization has traditionally been employed in patients with suspected pulmonary hypertension to measure pressures in the right ventricle and pulmonary outflow tract and to calculate cardiac output as well as systemic and pulmonary vascular resistances. During right heart catheterization, response to pulmonary vasodilators and O_2 therapy can also be measured to assess their potential therapeutic benefit. Pulmonary angiography is also necessary to exclude the presence of thromboembolic disease.

Typically, pulmonary artery pressure and pulmonary vascular resistance are markedly increased in patients with PPH, while pulmonary arterial wedge pressure and systemic vascular resistance remain normal.[35] Table 24-2 compares normal pulmonary and systemic pressures with those typically found in PPH and other forms of pulmonary vascular disease. Open lung biopsy is sometimes considered in patients suspected of having PPH to rule out other potentially treatable disorders.[34,38] Therapy for PPH remains disappointing, and most patients progress toward death over a period of months, although some survive 3 to 5 years from the time of diagnosis.[39] Vasodilating drugs such as nitrates,

Table 24-2. Representative Central Vascular Pressures in Different Forms of Pulmonary Vascular Disease

	Vascular Pressure (mmHg)			
Condition	Right Atrium	Pulmonary Artery (systolic/diastolic)	Pulmonary Artery (mean)	Pulmonary Capillary Wedge Pressure
Normal	4–6	15–20/4–8	14–16	8–12
Emphysema (without cor pulmonale)	4–6	25–30/8–10	16–18	8–12
Chronic cor pulmonale in COPD	8–12	35–40/10–20	26–30	8–12
Primary pulmonary hypertension	12–16	45–100/20–40	45–60	8–12
Acute pulmonary embolism (in patient without underlying pulmonary vascular disease)	6–10	40–45/10–20	26–30	4–6
Left ventricular failure	4–12	30–40/15–25	22–26	20–25 +

calcium channel blockers, angiotensin-converting enzyme inhibitors, and prostaglandins have been used, but unfortunately most of these agents lower systemic vascular resistance as well as pulmonary vascular resistance and do not appear to improve survival.[40–42] However, recent studies have suggested that anticoagulants may improve survival in PPH.[39,43] Lung or heart-lung transplantation has helped some patients, although this procedure is not widely available and remains an expensive and complicated form of therapy.

Pulmonary veno-occlusive disease, through unknown mechanisms, causes thrombosis and obstruction of pulmonary venules by intimal hypertrophy and fibrosis.[44] Like PPH, pulmonary veno-occlusive disease is a rare condition, and therapy is often ineffective. The disease tends to affect children and young adults, with a male predominance.

Pulmonary Vasculitis

Like PPH, other diseases can cause widespread destruction of the pulmonary vascular bed and eventually lead to pulmonary hypertension. The term *pulmonary vasculitis* refers to a diverse group of disorders, which have in common the inflammation and destruction of the pulmonary vasculature.[3,45,46] Pulmonary vasculitis may occur as part of a generalized collagen vascular disease,[47] such as progressive systemic sclerosis (scleroderma), rheumatoid arthritis, or systemic lupus erythematosus. These disorders may cause generalized inflammatory destruction of the lung parenchyma, which can extend to involve the adjacent pulmonary vasculature.

Many of the pulmonary vasculitides are classified according to the type of inflammatory lesion that they produce. For example, in *Wegener's granulomatosis*[48] the inflammatory response is characterized by necrotizing granulomas along the blood vessel walls. Wegener's granulomatosis usually afflicts patients in the fourth to sixth decades of life and has a slight male predominance. Necrotizing granulomatous lesions involve the upper and lower respiratory tracts, and patients may present with rhinorrhea, sinusitis, cough, or hemoptysis. In addition to respiratory disease, most patients with Wegener's granulomatosis have necrotizing glomerulonephritis, and many have disseminated vasculitis as well. Prior to the advent of modern cytotoxic therapy, most patients with this disease died within 6 months of presentation because of progressive renal failure, disseminated vasculitis, and respiratory insufficiency. Current therapy combines cyclophosphamide with prednisone and achieves long-term remission in over 90 percent of patients.

Allergic granulomatosis, or *Churg-Strauss syndrome*,[49] is another form of vasculitis that affects the pulmonary circulation. This disorder is characterized by asthma, blood eosinophilia, extravascular necrotizing granulomas, and an intense vasculitis involving the pulmonary circulation. The skin and central nervous system are frequently involved as well. Patients with Churg-Strauss syndrome often respond favorably to corticosteroid therapy.

Diffuse Embolization to the Pulmonary Circulation

Fat Embolism

Many so-called embolic diseases are noteworthy because their pathogenesis involves diffuse disruption of the pulmonary circulation rather than focal abnormalities as their names imply. The fat embolism syndrome, for example, occurs when liquid fat droplets from a fractured long bone embolize diffusely to the pulmonary capillaries. The major pathophysiologic consequences of this syndrome appear to derive more from the inflammatory reaction caused by the degradation of the triglycerides to free fatty acids by lipases than from the mechanical obstruction from the fat droplets themselves.[50] A diffuse vasculitis and capillary leak syndrome can occur following release of these free fatty acids. The clinical presentation of the fat embolism syndrome includes the triad of dyspnea, petechiae, and mental confusion, typically occurring in the first 24 to 48 hours after traumatic long bone fractures.[50,51] The diffuse, acute lung injury can lead to the adult respiratory distress syndrome (ARDS). There is no treatment other than supportive care, including supplemental O_2 mechanical ventilation, and positive end-expiratory pressure (PEEP) if required.[51]

Amniotic Fluid Embolism

Amniotic fluid embolism represents another unusual form of embolism, in which generalized disruption of the pulmonary vasculature accounts for the pathophysiology.[52] In this disorder amniotic fluid enters the venous circulation through the pelvic veins either during labor or early in the postpartum period. The clinical syndrome is characterized by sudden dyspnea, cyanosis, tachycardia, and hypotension. Some of the particulate matter within amniotic fluid may cause obstruction of the pulmonary vasculature, but this syndrome appears to be secondary mainly to a severe coagulopathy produced by the highly thromboplastic nature of amniotic fluid.[52] Treatment is supportive, with mechanical ventilation if required and repletion of fibrinogen and other coagulation factors.

Parasitic Embolism

Parasites can also embolize to the lung. The ova and flukes of schistosomiasis, for example, can lodge in the pulmonary circulation, where they can incite an intense inflammatory reaction, which can cause destruction of the pulmonary vascular bed.[53] This can lead to an elevation in pulmonary vascular resistance and eventually to pulmonary hypertension with cor pulmonale.[54] Although rare in the United States, schistosomiasis is a common cause of pulmonary hypertension and cor pulmonale in many parts of the world.

Air Embolism

Air embolism represents another form of nonthrombotic embolism, which is becoming more common with the use of large-bore central venous catheters as well as increasingly complex thoracic and neurosurgical procedures.[55,56] If a sufficient quantity of air enters the venous circulation, it can embolize to the pulmonary capillary bed and cause a diffuse capillary leak, resulting in an ARDS-like syndrome.[55] Some of the air bubbles may pass into the systemic circulation, either by diffusing through the lungs or by passing through a patent foramen ovale. Once air has entered the systemic circulation, it can embolize to the brain or other organs, interfering with organ perfusion and producing serious illness or death.

LOCALIZED PULMONARY VASCULAR OBSTRUCTION OR DESTRUCTION

Pulmonary Thromboembolism

Pulmonary thromboembolism (PTE) occurs when blood clots originating in peripheral veins travel through the venous system and become lodged in the pulmonary arterial bed, occluding a portion of the pulmonary circulation.[5,57–60] Acute PTE can produce a striking example of the effects of a sudden, localized disruption of a portion of the pulmonary vascular bed. The incidence of PTE in the United States probably exceeds 500,000 cases per year.[61] Approximately 50,000 of affected individuals die as a consequence of their embolism.[57,58] The incidence of deep venous thrombosis (DVT), which remains the major risk factor for pulmonary embolism, is approximately 5 million per year.[61] The overwhelming majority of pulmonary emboli arise from DVT in the lower extremities. Either the entire DVT or a portion of it then travels through the venous circulation and eventually lodges in the pulmonary vasculature, creating a pulmonary embolism. Less commonly, thrombi can arise in one of the deep pelvic veins or in the right ventricle.

A venous thrombosis occurs when fibrin, platelets, and other clotting factors aggregate within the lumen of the vessel and then adhere to its wall. Virchow described the three primary risk factors for venous thrombosis over a century ago; these factors, known as *Virchow's triad*, are venous stasis, injury to the vessel wall, and alterations in the normal coagulation or fibrinolytic systems.[5,57] Conditions that increase the risk of DVT and subsequent PTE, including pregnancy, obesity, pelvic or lower extremity trauma or surgery, administration of estrogen-containing compounds, and certain types of malignancy, probably act by producing one or more of these risk factors.[5,62]

After a thrombus has formed, the body's natural fibrinolytic system usually dissolves it over 7 to 10 days.[63] If part of the thrombus fails to dissolve, it becomes incorporated into the vessel wall in a process called organization. During the 7 to 10 days required for resolution of a thrombus, a portion of the clot can break off and embolize to the lungs. Once PTE has occurred, several physiologic changes may follow.[63] As a clot lodges in the pulmonary vascular bed, pulmonary vascular resistance increases, raising pulmonary artery pressure and right ventricular afterload.[64,65] If the embolus is sufficiently large, acute right ventricular failure (acute cor pulmonale) and hemodynamic collapse may occur.[5,57,58]

Hypoxemia is usually present in acute PTE and has several potential mechanisms.[57,66] When an embolus lodges in a pulmonary artery or arteriole, dead space increases, since a portion of the lung continues to be ventilated but is no longer perfused. The area of underperfused lung may then become hypoventilated as pneumoconstriction occurs, and altered $\dot{V}/\dot{Q}$ relationships may result. Hyperventilation frequently accompanies acute PTE, although the mechanisms for this phenomenon are unclear. A late consequence of PTE is loss of pulmonary surfactant in the alveolar regions supplied by the embolized vessels. This may occur 24 hours after the initial embolism and result in alveolar edema and atelectasis in the involved area. As pulmonary artery pressure rises, there may be enhanced perfusion to areas of hypoventilated lung that were relatively protected by HPV prior to the rise in pulmonary vascular resistance caused by the embolism.[66]

Unfortunately for the clinician, the signs and symptoms of PTE are nonspecific and unreliable.[59,60,67] Dyspnea is the most common symptom; pleuritic chest pain and hemoptysis are encountered less frequently. On physical examination, tachypnea is often present. Tachycardia, hypotension, and signs of acute right ventricular failure may be present with a large embolism. Examination of the lower extremities may reveal evidence of DVT, but a negative examination in no way excludes the presence of clot. Only 50 percent of patients with documented DVT will have physical signs of thrombophlebitis (e.g., swelling, warmth, redness, tenderness) to suggest the diagnosis.[57,60]

Laboratory findings are also nonspecific.[5,59,60] Arterial blood gas measurements usually reveal acute respiratory alkalosis with an increased $P(A\text{-}a)O_2$, generally accompanied by hypoxemia.[66] The chest radiograph with pulmonary embolism is typically normal, but it may suggest hypoperfusion of certain lung zones or show nonspecific abnormalities such as small areas of discoid atelectasis.[68] If pulmonary infarction occurs, which is an uncommon complication of PTE in otherwise healthy individuals, a pleural effusion or wedge-shaped peripheral infiltrate may be seen on the chest radiograph.[68] The ECG typically shows only sinus tachycardia but may reveal evidence of right ventricular strain. The main value in obtaining a chest radiograph and ECG in suspected PTE is to rule out other conditions, such as pneumonia, pneumothorax, or myocardial infarction, that can mimic its presentation.

When the diagnosis of pulmonary embolism is suspected, a $\dot{V}/\dot{Q}$ scan should be performed.[69,70] In this study, described in more detail in Chapter 57, the patient inhales a radioactive inert gas such as xenon 133 (Xe 133), and a gamma camera images the chest while the patient is breathing the labeled gas. A perfusion scan is then performed by injecting approximately 5×10^5 macroaggregates of technetium 99 (Tc 99m)-labeled human albumin into the patient's vein. These tiny particles are trapped by the pulmonary vasculature and stay in the lungs for about 6 to 8 hours until they are degraded. The chest is once again imaged with a gamma camera, and an outline of the pulmonary circulation is obtained.

Pulmonary embolism is suspected if the $\dot{V}/\dot{Q}$ scan reveals an area of ventilation-perfusion mismatch, such as a lung segment that is being ventilated but not perfused (see Fig. 57-19). A normal perfusion scan makes the diagnosis of pulmonary embolism very unlikely.[70] The study can be equivocal if an area with a matched ventilation and perfusion defect is identified. In this case, the perfusion defect might be secondary to HPV in an area of lung that is being hypoventilated.

If the $\dot{V}/\dot{Q}$ scan is equivocal and the clinical suspicion for PTE is high, the clinician may wish to proceed with a pulmonary angiogram.[71] This procedure poses some risk to the patient since it is an invasive technique and involves injection of contrast dye, which may be nephrotoxic. During a pulmonary angiogram, right heart catheterization is performed and dye is injected into the pulmonary circulation. If an embolus is present, it will be represented as a filling defect in one or more of the pulmonary arteries on the radiographic image (see Fig. 57-20).

Once the diagnosis of PTE is established, anticoagulation therapy should be started.[72,73] Intravenous heparin remains the treatment of choice during the acute stage of proximal DVT or PTE. Although heparin will not dissolve a thrombus that has already formed, it will prevent further clot formation, while allowing the patient's own fibrinolytic system to organize and degrade the thrombus. Heparin therapy is typically replaced by oral anticoagulation with warfarin (coumadin), which is continued for at least 3 to 6 months.[72,73] Some patients may require lifelong prophylaxis. If anticoagulation therapy is contraindicated because of a high risk of hemorrhage, a filter can be placed in the inferior vena cava.[74] This device can prevent further clots that may embolize from lower extremity or pelvic veins from reaching the pulmonary circulation.

Other Conditions

Occasionally, bodies other than venous thrombi can become lodged in a pulmonary artery and cause localized obstruction of the pulmonary vascular bed. *Tumor emboli*, for example, represent intravascular spread of solid tumors that enter the venous circulation and obstruct a portion of the pulmonary circulation. A *septic embolism* occurs when a venous thrombus becomes infected with bacteria and then embolizes to the lung. In the past most septic emboli occurred as complications of septic pelvic thrombophlebitis associated with septic abortions.[75] Today, however, most septic emboli occur as a consequence of intravenous drug abuse or of iatrogenic infections from indwelling venous catheters.[76]

Intravenous drug users are also at risk for causing damage to their pulmonary vasculature from impurities that may lace the drugs that they are injecting.[77,78] Talc is an example of a chemical substance that is often mixed with heroin and can cause a granulomatous vasculitis in the lungs, with ultimate development of pulmonary fibrosis.[79] When used intravenously, methylphenidate (Ritalin) can also lead to an inflammatory pulmonary vascular sclerosis, with subsequent development of severe airflow obstruction.[78,80] These diagnoses are important to recognize, since their clinical course and management differ from those of PTE secondary to DVT.

COR PULMONALE

Cor pulmonale is right ventricular hypertrophy or dilatation due to increased right ventricular afterload resulting from disease of the lung parenchyma or pulmonary circulation.[6–8] The clinical manifestations of cor pulmonale usually become evident only after the disease has progressed to the stage of right ventricular failure. It should be noted that the definition of cor pulmonale excludes right ventricular abnormalities that are secondary to left ventricular failure, mitral valve disease, or congenital heart disease. Any disorder that produces either sustained HPV or obliteration of the pulmonary vascular bed can lead to cor pulmonale[7] (Table 24-3).

The severity of pulmonary hypertension and cor pulmonale in patients with chronic respiratory disease strongly correlates with mortality. Bishop reported a significantly lower survival rate in patients with chronic bronchitis and pulmonary hypertension than in similar patients with normal pulmonary arterial pressures[81] in a study of 128 patients with chronic bronchitis who were followed for 5 years. Of patients with a normal pulmonary arterial pressure, 90 percent were alive at the end of the 5 years; by contrast, less than 10 percent of patients with mean pulmonary arterial pressures of 45 mmHg or higher survived for 5 years[81] (Fig. 24-3).

Occasionally cor pulmonale can develop acutely, as in acute PTE. More typically, however, cor pulmonale progresses over a period of months or years because of contin-

Table 24-3. Conditions Associated with Cor Pulmonale

Diseases associated with hypoxic pulmonary vasoconstriction
COPD
Bronchiectasis
Chronic mountain sickness
Cystic fibrosis
Idiopathic alveolar hypoventilation
Obesity hypoventilation syndrome
Neuromuscular disease
Kyphoscoliosis
Pleuropulmonary fibrosis
Upper airway obstruction
Diseases producing obstruction or obliteration of the pulmonary vasculature
Pulmonary embolism
Pulmonary fibrosis
Pulmonary lymphangitic carcinomatosis
Idiopathic pulmonary hypertension
Progressive systemic sclerosis (scleroderma)
Sarcoidosis
Intravenous drug use
Pulmonary vasculitis
Pulmonary veno-occlusive disease

(From Rubin,[7] with permission.)

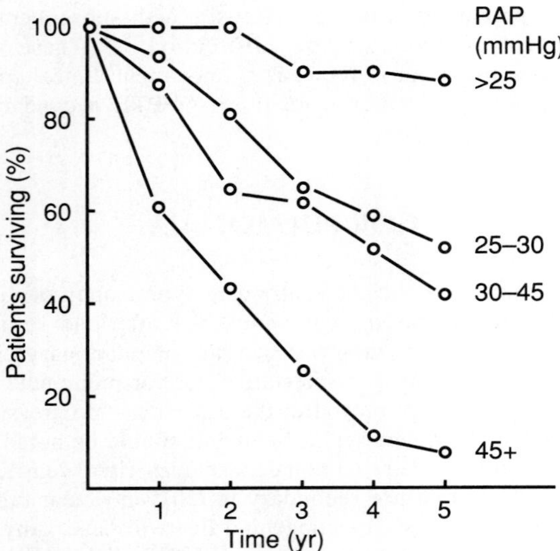

Figure 24-3. Adverse effect of pulmonary hypertension on patient survival in chronic bronchitis. Five-year survival decreases dramatically with increasing mean pulmonary arterial pressure (PAP). (From Rubin,[7] with permission.)

ued destruction of lung parenchyma and pulmonary vascular bed or sustained alveolar hypoxia.[64,65,82,83] The pathophysiologic sequence through which cor pulmonale develops is diagrammed in Figure 24-4.

The symptoms of cor pulmonale are nonspecific and often are dominated by symptoms from the underlying respiratory disease. Many patients experience dyspnea, cough, fatigue, poor exercise tolerance, and discomfort related to hepatic congestion and peripheral edema.[84,85] On physical examination there is evidence of right heart failure with distension of the jugular veins, hepatomegaly, and ankle edema. Auscultation of the heart reveals a prominent second heart sound (S_2) with accentuation of the pulmonic component. A right-sided fourth heart sound (S_4) may often be heard as the hypertrophied right ventricle becomes stiff and noncompliant. Murmurs of pulmonary and tricuspid insufficiency may be present as well.[86]

In patients with pulmonary hypertension and cor pulmonale the chest radiograph may show enlargement of the pulmonary arteries as well as hypertrophy of the right ventricle[8] (Fig. 24-5). The ECG may show evidence of right axis deviation, P pulmonale, right bundle branch block, or right ventricular strain.[8] Laboratory analysis may reveal evidence of secondary erythrocytosis precipitated by chronic hypoxemia. An elevated hemoglobin concentration may serve as an adaptation to chronic tissue hypoxia. Erythropoietin, a hormone produced by the kidney, increases in response to chronic tissue hypoxia. Elevated levels of erythropoietin increase the bone marrow's production of red blood cells, thereby increasing the hemoglobin concentration so that more O_2 can be delivered to hypoxic tissues. In the late stage of cor pulmonale arterial blood gas analysis may reveal a compensated respiratory acidosis with an increased $P(A\text{-}a)O_2$.

Right ventricular function and pulmonary pressures can often be measured noninvasively by an echocardiogram.[80] A radionuclide ventriculogram may be employed to estimate right ventricular function as well. Right heart catheterization remains the most accurate means of assessing pulmonary pressures and right heart function, but this is an invasive procedure and carries the risks associated with the use of contrast dyes.

Therapy for chronic cor pulmonale is primarily aimed at controlling or reversing the underlying pulmonary disorder and relieving the associated alveolar hypoxia and hypoxemia[8,83] (see Ch. 63). Patients with chronic hypoxemia and cor pulmonale complicating COPD should be treated with supplemental O_2.[8,10,83] In a select group of such patients, long-term O_2 therapy has been shown to reduce mortality by slowing the progression of pulmonary hypertension and right heart failure.[87,88] Diuretics are often employed to

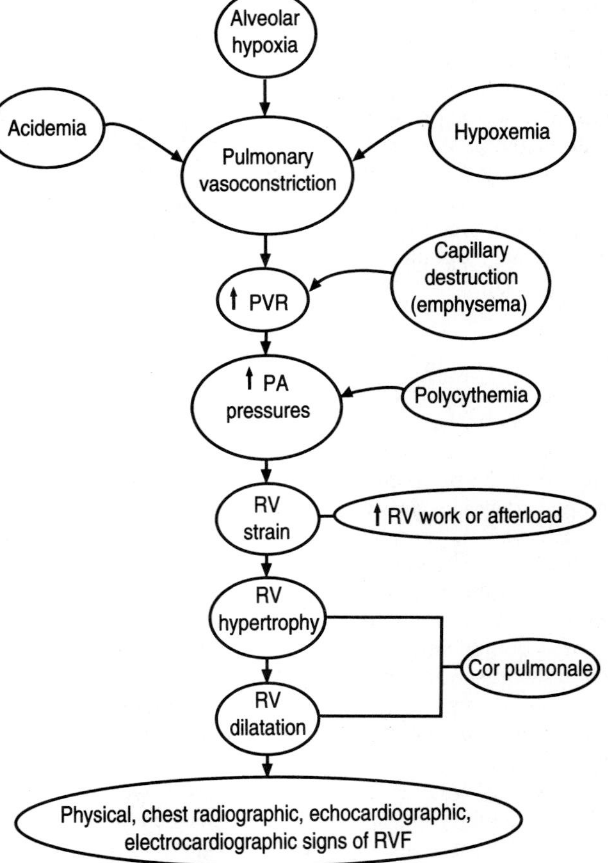

Figure 24-4. Pathogenesis of cor pulmonale in COPD. PVR, pulmonary vascular resistance; PA, pulmonary artery; RV, right ventricle; RVF, right ventricular failure.

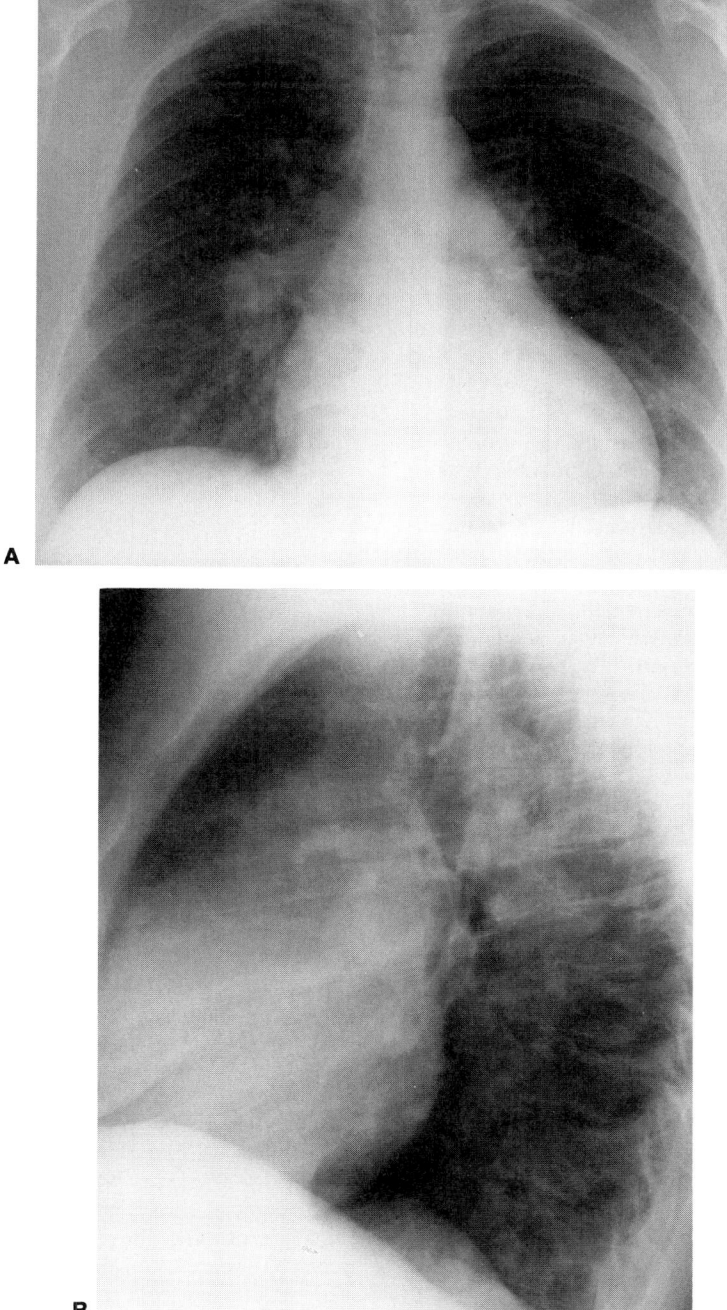

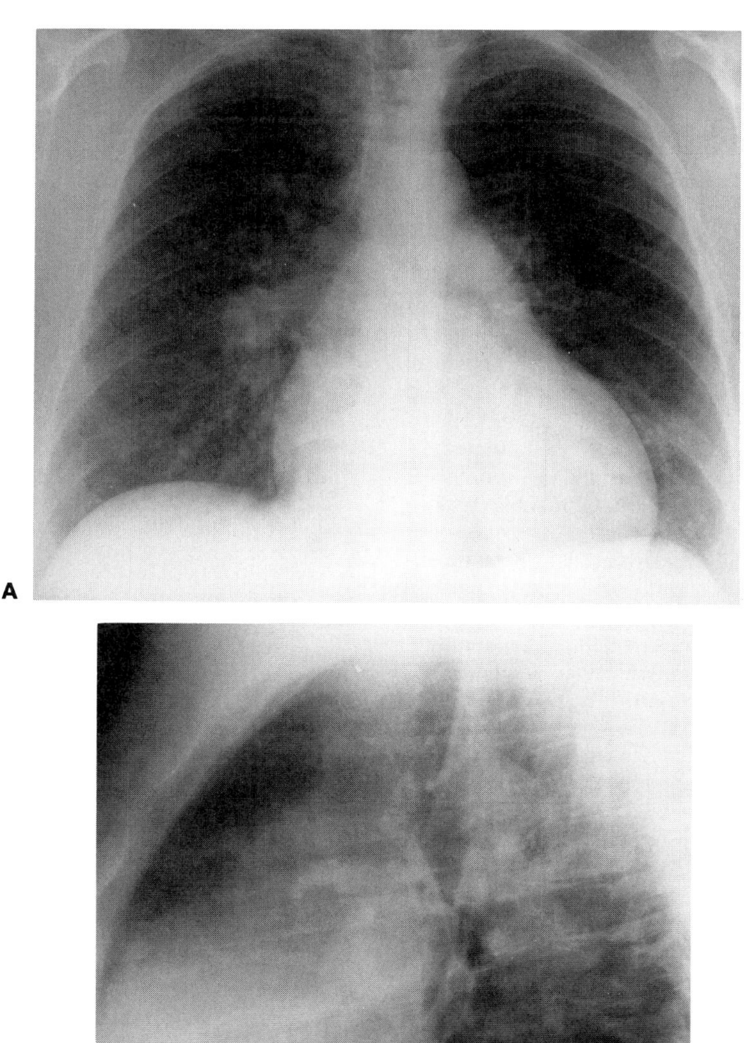

Figure 24-5. (**A**) Posteroanterior and (**B**) lateral chest radiographs of a 31-year-old woman with severe cor pulmonale secondary to primary pulmonary hypertension. The heart is markedly enlarged, which on lateral projection is seen to be due virtually entirely to right ventricular enlargement. The right and left pulmonary arteries are massively enlarged and appear almost as mass lesions.

reduce peripheral edema. Various pulmonary vasodilators have been tried in pulmonary hypertension, but their usefulness is often limited by concurrent effects on systemic vascular resistance, and they do not have a prominent role in management.[83]

LEFT VENTRICULAR FAILURE

Pulmonary vascular congestion leading to pulmonary edema often stems from left ventricular failure. Fluid can leak from the pulmonary capillaries and into the alveolar space as a consequence of elevated pressures created by the failing left heart.[12] As pulmonary edema worsens, right heart failure may occur as a consequence of increased pulmonary vascular resistance and rising right ventricular afterload. It should be emphasized, however, that cor pulmonale by definition represents disease of the right ventricle secondary to intrinsic pulmonary vascular abnormalities. This must be differentiated from the right heart failure that stems primarily from left ventricular failure or congenital heart disease.

The most common cause of left heart failure is acute myocardial infarction or ischemia[12]; other causes include pericardial tamponade, constrictive pericarditis, mitral stenosis, and mitral insufficiency. Certain toxins such as alcohol and some cancer chemotherapeutic agents, viral infections, and chronic systemic arterial hypertension are other potential causes of left ventricular failure. Treatment for pulmonary edema due to left ventricular failure consists of the administration of diuretics, nitrates, positive ionotropes, and vasodilators designed to reduce left ventricular afterload[77] (see Ch. 77).

PULMONARY ARTERIOVENOUS MALFORMATIONS

Various congenital and developmental abnormalities can cause clinical disease affecting the pulmonary circulation. In pulmonary arteriovenous fistulas, for example, blood travels from pulmonary arteries to pulmonary veins without passing through a capillary bed.[89,90] This results in the return of deoxygenated blood to the systemic circulation (right-to-left shunt). About half of patients with pulmonary arteriovenous fistulas have vascular malformations in other organs, including the skin and gastrointestinal tract. Approximately 15 percent of patients with hereditary hemorrhagic telangiectasia (Osler-Weber-Rendu syndrome) have pulmonary arteriovenous fistulas.[91]

Patients with pulmonary arteriovenous fistulas typically present either with hemoptysis or with dyspnea related to hypoxemia.[3,89] Physical examination may reveal telangiectasias on the skin or mucous membranes, and clubbing may be present.[89,90] Erythrocytosis is frequently encountered on laboratory examination.[3,90] On the chest radiograph the AV malformation may show up as an irregular peripheral density, often in the lower lobes; frequently, however, the plain radiograph is unremarkable. In some cases the diagnosis may be made by computed tomography (CT)[92] of the chest with injection of contrast, although pulmonary angiography is usually necessary to confirm the size and location of the malformation (Fig. 24-6).

Hypoxemia in patients with pulmonary arteriovenous fistulas may be profound and often fails to improve significantly even when the patient inspires 100 percent O_2,[3,90] since the shunted blood is not exposed to alveolar gas. Treatment should be considered if hemoptysis has occurred, if significant hypoxemia is present, or if the fistulas are noted to be increasing in size radiographically.[3,89,90] Definitive management includes either surgical resection of the malformation or obliterative therapy by angiographic embolization of inert material into the fistula.[93]

INTRACARDIAC SHUNTS

Left-to-right intracardiac shunts can produce multiple physiologic consequences and lead to right heart failure by causing an elevation of right ventricular preload and an increase in pulmonary blood flow.[3] *Atrial septal defects* (ASDs) most commonly occur as developmental anomalies, as in the case of an ostium secundum, which creates an abnormal communication between the two atrial chambers. Patients with a left-to-right shunt from an ASD may develop right ventricular overload, atrial dysrhythmias, and pulmonary hypertension from the increased pulmonary blood flow.[94,95] Eventually they may develop right-to-left shunting of blood as right ventricular end-diastolic volume and pressure increase.

The ECG in ASD typically reveals right axis deviation and right ventricular hypertrophy. The anatomic defect can often be visualized by an echocardiogram with color Doppler flow examination. The sensitivity of the echocardiogram is increased with a bubble study, in which tiny air bubbles injected into the venous circulation can be seen crossing the septal defect. Operative repair is required in most cases of ASD when a significant shunt is present.[94,95] Ideally, this procedure should be performed prior to development of clinical pulmonary hypertension.

Ventricular septal defects (VSDs) are another cause of left-to-right shunts. These defects most often occur in the presence of other developmental anomalies but can also occur as isolated congenital malformations. Occasionally a VSD may result from rupture of the intraventricular septum following myocardial infarction. Surgical correction is indicated when the shunt produces significant hemodynamic compromise or pulmonary hypertension.[94,95]

A *patent ductus arteriosus* can cause either left-to-right or right-to-left shunting of blood.[94] The ductus arteriosus is a blood vessel leading from the pulmonary artery to the aorta, which is open during fetal life and serves to shunt blood away from the fetal pulmonary circulation (see Ch. 3). Shortly after birth, the ductus arteriosus normally closes. If this does not occur, blood can be shunted from the high-pressure systemic circulation to the low-pressure pulmonary circulation. If not surgically corrected, this condition can lead to pulmonary

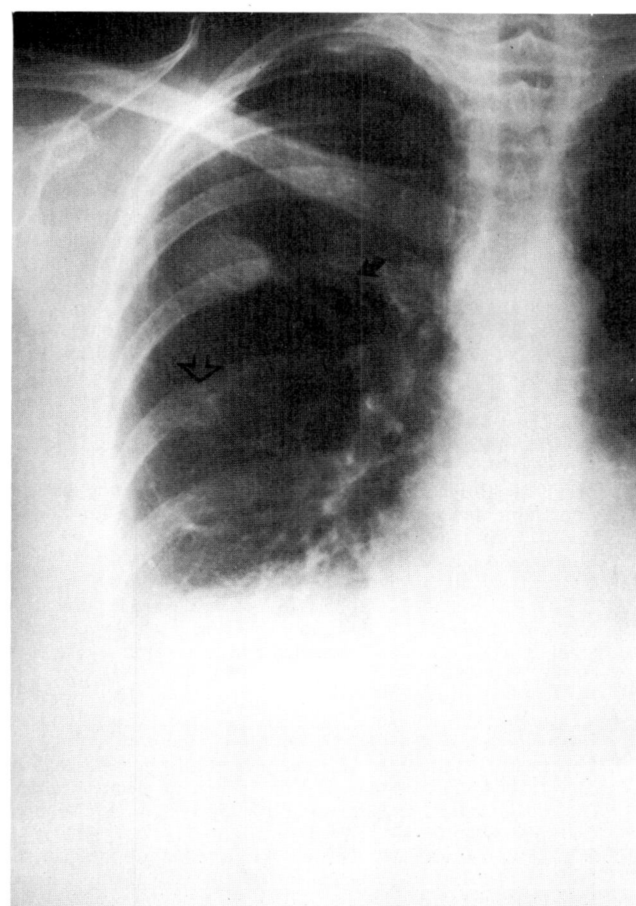

A

Figure 24-6. Chest radiograph and pulmonary angiogram in a patient with pulmonary arteriovenous malformations complicating the Osler-Weber-Rendu syndrome, who presented with hemoptysis. (A) The posteroanterior standard radiograph shows rounded, ill-defined densities at the levels of posterior ribs 6 and 7, the latter indicated by the open arrow; there is also a large feeding vessel (black arrow) and a pleural effusion (hemothorax). (B) The angiogram, taken during the pulmonary arterial phase following contrast injection, shows the two rounded densities to be large arteriovenous malformations (1 and 2); a third malformation (3) is seen medially overlying the spine. LPA, left pulmonary artery; RPA, right pulmonary artery. (From Blank,[99] with permission.)

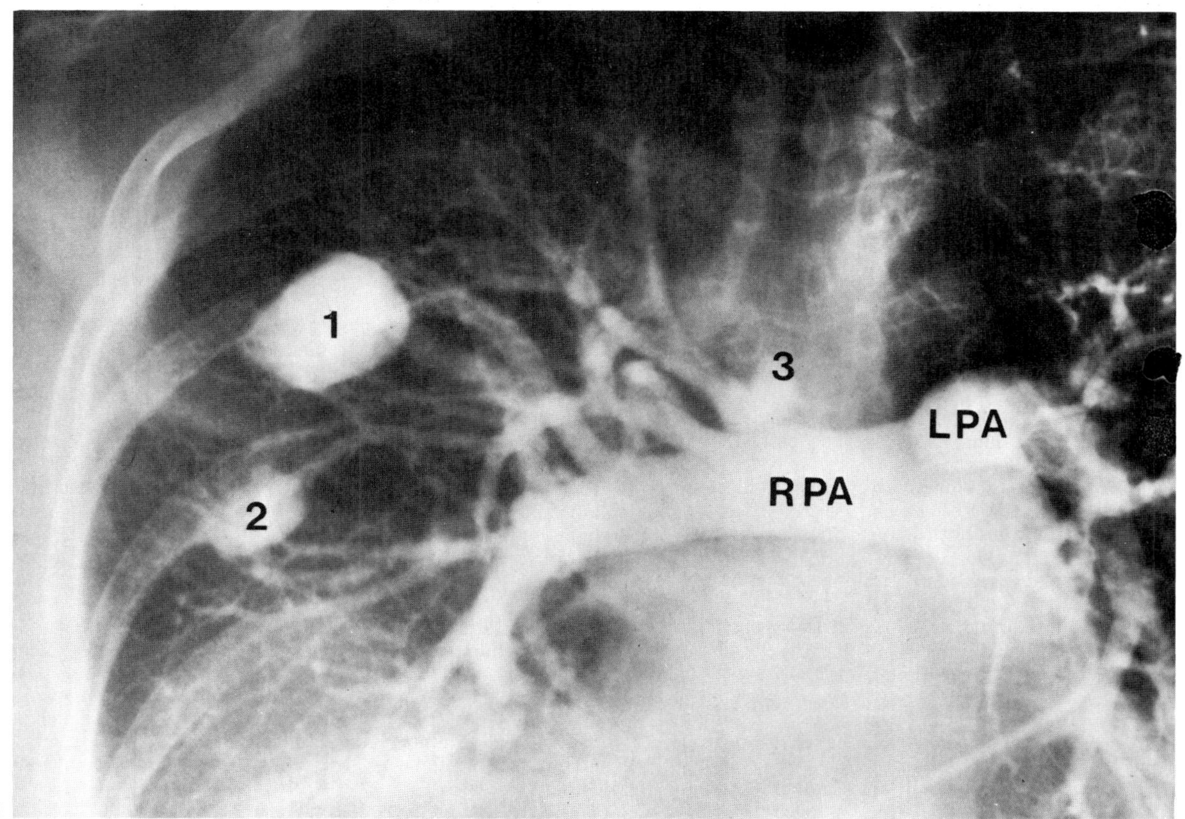

B

vascular congestion and pulmonary hypertension. The end result can be right-to-left shunting and cyanosis as right heart failure occurs. This represents an example of Eisenmenger syndrome, in which pulmonary vascular resistance is equal to or greater than systemic vascular resistance.[96] Eisenmenger syndrome can also occur in the setting of right-to-left shunting with an ASD or VSD.[96,97] As pulmonary vascular resistance and pulmonary artery pressures increase, medical hypertrophy and intimal fibroplasia may develop in the pulmonary arterioles. Patients may die from right heart failure, endocarditis, or aneurysmal dilatation and rupture of the patent ductus. Surgical ligation of a patent ductus arteriosus can result in dramatic clinical improvement and the return of normal physiology.[94,95] Ideally, surgical therapy should be employed prior to development of severe pulmonary vascular disease and pulmonary hypertension.[94,96,97]

References

1. Snider GL: Chronic bronchitis and emphysema. pp. 1069–1107. In Murray JF, Nadel JA (eds): Textbook of Respiratory Medicine. WB Saunders, Philadelphia, 1988
2. Hay JG, Turner-Warwick M: Interstitial pulmonary fibrosis. pp. 1445–1461. In Murray JF, Nadel JA (eds): Textbook of Respiratory Medicine. WB Saunders, Philadelphia, 1988
3. Luce JM: Vasculitis, primary pulmonary hypertension, and arteriovenous fistulas. pp. 1328–1358. In Murray JF, Nadel JA (eds): Textbook of Respiratory Medicine. WB Saunders, Philadelphia, 1988
4. Rich S, Brundage BH: Primary pulmonary hypertension: Current update. JAMA 1984;251:2252–2254
5. Moser KM: Venous thromboembolism. Am Rev Respir Dis 1990;141:235–249
6. World Health Organization: Chronic cor pulmonale. A report of the expert committee. Circulation 1963;27:594–615
7. Rubin LJ: Pulmonary hypertension secondary to lung disease. pp. 291–320. In Weir EK, Reeves JT (eds): Pulmonary Hypertension. Futura Publishing, Mt. Kisco, NY, 1984
8. Butler J: Cor pulmonale. pp. 1410–1433. In Murray JF, Nadel JA (eds): Textbook of Respiratory Medicine. WB Saunders, Philadelphia, 1988
9. Butler J: Introduction to clinical respiratory disease. pp 153–161. In Culver BH (ed): The Respiratory System. Syllabus for Human Biology. University of Washington Health Sciences Academic Services, Seattle, WA, 1990
10. Fishman AP: Hypoxia on the pulmonary circulation. How and where it acts. Circ Res 1976;38:221–231
11. Parmley WW: Pathophysiology of congestive heart failure. Am J Cardiol 1985;56:7A–11A
12. Schlant RC, Sonnenblick EH: Pathophysiology of heart failure. pp. 387–417. In Hurst JW, Schlant RC (eds): The Heart. 7th Ed. McGraw-Hill, New York, 1990
13. Herget J, McMurtry IF: Possible mechanisms of hypoxic pulmonary vasoconstriction. Prog Respir Res 1985;20:5–10
14. Petty TL: Definitions in chronic obstructive pulmonary disease. Clin Chest Med 1990;11:363–373
15. Matthys H: Definition and assessment of asthma. Lung, Suppl. 1990;168:51–56
16. Clausen JL: The diagnosis of emphysema, chronic bronchitis, and asthma. Clin Chest Med 1990;11:405–416
17. Burrows B: Differential diagnosis of COPD. Chest, suppl. 2, 1990;97:16S–18S
18. Senior RM, Kuhn C: The pathogenesis of emphysema. pp. 1209–1218. In Fishman AP (ed): Pulmonary Diseases and Disorders, Vol. 2. 2nd Ed. McGraw-Hill, New York, 1988
19. Symonds G, Renzetti AD Jr, Mitchell MM: The diffusing capacity in pulmonary emphysema. Am Rev Respir Dis 1974;109:391–394
20. Wiedemann HP, Matthay RA: Cor pulmonale in chronic obstructive pulmonary disease. Circulatory pathophysiology and management. Clin Chest Med 1990;11:523–545
21. Matthay RA, Niederman MS, Wiedemann HP: Cardiovascular-pulmonary interaction in chronic obstructive pulmonary disease with special reference to the pathogenesis and management of cor pulmonale. Med Clin North Am 1990;74:571–618
22. Dunnill MS: Pulmonary fibrosis. Histopathology 1990;16: 321–329
23. Crystal RG, Bitterman PB, Rennard SI et al: Interstitial lung diseases of unknown cause. N Engl J Med 1984;310:154–166, 235–244
24. Smith GJ: The histopathology of pulmonary reactions to drugs. Clin Chest Med 1990;11:95–117
25. Morgan WKC, Seaton A: Occupational Lung Diseases. 2nd Ed. WB Saunders, Philadelphia, 1984
26. Braun SR, doPico GA, Tsiatis A et al: Farmer's lung disease: Long term clinical and physiological outcome. Am Rev Respir Dis 1979;119:185–191
27. Wiedemann HP, Matthay RA: Pulmonary manifestations of the collagen vascular diseases. Clin Chest Med 1989;10:677–722
28. Crystal RG, Fulmer JD, Roberts WC et al: Idiopathic pulmonary fibrosis: Clinical, histologic, radiographic, physiologic, scintigraphic, cytologic, and biochemical aspects. Ann Intern Med 1976;85:769–788
29. Panos RJ, Mortenson RL, Niccoli SA et al: Clinical deterioration in patients with idiopathic pulmonary fibrosis; causes and assessment. Am J Med 1990;88:396–404
30. Craighead JE, Abraham JL, Churg A et al: The pathology of asbestos-associated diseases of the lungs and pleural cavities: Diagnostic criteria and proposed grading system. Arch Pathol Lab Med 1982;106:544–596
31. Crystal RG, Gadek JE, Ferrans VJ: Interstitial lung disease: Current concepts of pathogenesis, staging and therapy. Am J Med 1981;70:542–568
32. Fulmer JD: The interstitial lung diseases. Chest 1982;82:172–178
33. Weir EK: Diagnosis and management of primary pulmonary hypertension. pp. 115–168. In Weir EK, Reeves JT (eds): Pulmonary Hypertension. Futura Publishing, Mt. Kisco, NY, 1984
34. Bjornsson J, Edwards WD: Primary pulmonary hypertension: A histopathologic study of eighty cases. Mayo Clin Proc 1985;60:16–25
35. Hawkins JW, Dunn MI: Primary pulmonary hypertension in adults. Clin Cardiol 1990;13:382–387
36. Zimmerman D, Parker BM: The pain of pulmonary hypertension: Fact or fancy? JAMA 1981;246:2345–2346
37. Randall PA, Heitzman ER, Bull MJ et al: Pulmonary arterial hypertension: A contemporary review. Radiographics 1989; 9:905–927
38. Wagenvoort CA: Lung biopsy specimens in the evaluation of pulmonary vascular disease. Chest 1980;77:614–625
39. Fuster V, Steele PM, Edwards WD et al: Primary pulmonary hypertension: Natural history and the importance of thrombosis. Circulation 1984;70:580–587
40. Hjemdahl-Monsen CE, Fuster V: Pulmonary hypertension: New directions in therapy. Prim Cardiol 1986;12:115–129
41. Rich S, Brundage BH, Levy PS: The effect of vasodilator therapy on the clinical outcome of patients with primary pulmonary hypertension. Circulation 1985;71:1191–1196
42. Packer M: Vasodilator therapy for primary pulmonary hypertension: Limitations and hazards. Ann Intern Med 1985; 103:258–270
43. Frank H, Mlczock J, Lang I: Influence of warfarin therapy in primary pulmonary hypertension. Prog Respir Res 1990; 26:119–124
44. Wagenvoort CA, Wagenvoort N, Takahashi T: Pulmonary veno-occlusive disease: Involvement of pulmonary arteries and review of the literature. Hum Pathol 1985;16:1033–1041
45. Dreisin RB: Pulmonary vasculitis. Clin Chest Med 1982; 3:607–618

46. Fulmer JD, Kaltreider HB: The pulmonary vasculitides. Chest 1982;82:615–624
47. Hunninghake GW, Fauci AS: State of the art: Pulmonary involvement in the collagen vascular diseases. Am Rev Respir Dis 1979;119:471–503
48. Fauci AS, Haynes BF, Katz P et al: Wegener's granulomatosis: Prospective clinical and therapeutic experience with 85 patients for 21 years. Ann Intern Med 1983;98:76–85
49. Chumbley LC, Harrison EG Jr, DeRemee RA: Allergic granulomatosis and angiitis (Churg-Strauss syndrome): Report and analysis of thirty cases. Mayo Clin Proc 1977;52:477–484
50. Gossling HR, Donohue TA: The fat embolism syndrome. JAMA 1979;241:2740–2742
51. Vincent JM, Hudson LD: Fat embolism. pp. 1951–1953. In Kelley WN (ed). Textbook of Internal Medicine. JB Lippincott, Philadelphia, 1989
52. Sperry K: Amniotic fluid embolism: To understand an enigma. JAMA 1986;255:2183–2186
53. Mahmoud AAF: Schistosomiasis. pp. 443–457. In Warren KS, Mahmoud AAF (eds): Tropical and Geographic Medicine. McGraw-Hill, New York, 1984
54. Sadigursky M, Andrade ZA: Pulmonary changes in schistosomal cor pulmonale. Am J Trop Med Hyg 1982;31:779–784
55. O'Quin RJ, Lakshminarayan S: Venous air embolism. Arch Intern Med 1982;142:2173–2176
56. Peters JL, Armstrong R, Bradford R et al: Air embolism: A serious hazard of central venous catheter systems. Intensive Care Med 1984;10:261–262
57. Moser KM: Pulmonary embolism. pp. 1299–1327. In Murray JF, Nadel JA (eds): Textbook of Respiratory Medicine. WB Saunders, Philadelphia, 1988
58. Rosenow EC III, Osmundson PJ, Brown ML: Pulmonary embolism. Mayo Clin Proc 1981;56:161–178
59. Dehring DJ, Arens JF: Pulmonary thromboembolism: Disease recognition and patient management. Anesthesiology 1990; 73:146–164
60. Otoya J, Nemcek AA Jr, Green D: Venous thromboembolism (clinical conference). Chest 1989;96:1169–1174
61. Coon WW: Venous thromboembolism: Prevalence, risk factors and prevention. Clin Chest Med 1984;5:391–401
62. Coffman JD: Deep venous thrombosis and pulmonary emboli: Etiology, medical treatment, and prophylaxis. Thorac Imaging 1989;4:4–7
63. Benotti JR, Dalen JE: The natural history of pulmonary emboli. Clin Chest Med 1984;5:403–410
64. Palevsky HI, Weiss DW: Pulmonary hypertension secondary to chronic thromboembolism (clinical conference). J Nucl Med 1990;31:1–9
65. Moser KM, Auger WR, Fedullo PF: Chronic major vessel thrombo-embolic pulmonary hypertension. Circulation 1990; 81:1735–1743
66. Huet Y, Lemaire F, Brun-Buisson C et al: Hypoxemia in acute pulmonary emboli. Chest 1985;88:829–836
67. Hirsh J (ed): Venous thromboembolism: Prevention, diagnosis, and treatment. Chest suppl 5, 1986;89:369S–437S
68. Greenspan RH, Ravin CE, Polansky SM et al: Accuracy of the chest radiograph in diagnosis of pulmonary emboli. Invest Radiol 1982;17:539–543
69. Hull RD, Hirsh J, Carter CJ et al: Diagnostic value of ventilation perfusion lung scanning in patients with suspected pulmonary emboli. Chest 1985;88:819–828
70. Saltzman HA, Alavi A, Greenspan RH et al: Value of the ventilation perfusion scan in acute pulmonary emboli. (PIOPED study). JAMA 1990;263:2753–2759
71. Hull RD, Hirsh J, Carter CJ et al: Pulmonary angiography, ventilation lung scanning, and venography for clinically suspected pulmonary embolism with abnormal perfusion lung scan. Ann Intern Med 1983;98:891–899
72. Hyers TM, Hull RD, Weg JG: Antithrombotic therapy for venous thromboembolic disease. Chest 1989;95:37S–51S
73. Hyers TM: Venous thromboembolic disease: Diagnosis and use of antithrombotic therapy. Clin Cardiol, suppl. 4, 1990;13: V123–V128
74. Kanter B, Moser KM: The Greenfield vena cava filter. Chest 1988;93:170–175
75. Collins CG: Suppurative pelvic thrombophlebitis II: Symptomatology and diagnosis. Surgery 1951;30:311–327
76. Hershey CO, Tomford JW, McLaren CE et al: The natural history of intravenous catheter associated phlebitis. Arch Intern Med 1984;144:1373–1375
77. Heffner JE, Harley RA, Schabel SI: Pulmonary reactions from illicit substance abuse. Clin Chest Med 1990;11:151–162
78. Schmidt RA, Glenny RW, Godwin JD: Panlobular emphysema in young intravenous ritalin abusers. Am Rev Respir Dis 1991;143:649–656
79. Robertson CH Jr, Reynolds RC, Wilson JE: Pulmonary hypertension and foreign body granulomas in intravenous drug abusers. Am J Med 1976;61:657–664
80. Sherman CB, Hudson LD, Pierson DJ: Severe precocious emphysema in intravenous methylphenidate (ritalin) abusers. Chest 1987;92:1085–1107
81. Bishop JM: Hypoxia and pulmonary hypertension in chronic bronchitis. Prog Respir Res 1975;9:10–16
82. Peacock A: Pulmonary hypertension due to chronic hypoxia. Br Med J 1990;300:763
83. Palevsky HI, Fishman AP: Chronic cor pulmonale: Etiology and management. JAMA 1990;263:2347–2353
84. Murphy ML, Dinh H, Nicholson D: Chronic cor pulmonale. Dis Mon 1989;35:653–718
85. Fishman AP: State of the art: Chronic cor pulmonale. Am Rev Respir Dis 1976;114:775–794
86. Yock PG, Popp RL: Non-invasive estimation of right ventricular systolic pressure by Doppler ultrasound in patients with tricuspid regurgitation. Circulation 1984;70:657–662
87. Bishop JM: Effects of long term oxygen therapy on mortality and morbidity in chronic obstructive pulmonary disease. Prog Respir Res 1985;20:55–59
88. Howard P: Natural history of obstructive airways disease and hypoxia. Implications for therapy. Lung suppl. 168, 1990; 743–750
89. Prager RL, Laws KH, Bender HW Jr: Arteriovenous fistula of the lung. Ann Thorac Surg 1983;36:231–239
90. Dines DE, Arms RA, Bernatz PE et al: Pulmonary arteriovenous fistulas. Mayo Clin Proc 1974;49:460–465
91. Hodgson CH, Burchell HB, Good CA et al: Hereditary hemorrhagic telangiectasia and pulmonary arteriovenous fistula: Survey of a large family. N Engl J Med 1959;261:625–636
92. Rankin S, Faling LJ, Pugatch RD: CT diagnosis of pulmonary arteriovenous malformations. J Comput Assist Tomogr 1982;6:746–749
93. Terry PB, White RI Jr, Barth KH et al: Pulmonary arteriovenous malformations: Physiologic observations and results of therapeutic balloon embolization. N Engl J Med 1983;308:1197–1200
94. Rabinovitch M: Pulmonary hypertension. pp. 856–886. In Adams FH, Emmanouilides GC, Riemenschneider TA (eds): Moss' Heart Disease in Infants, Children and Adolescents, 4th Ed. Williams & Wilkins, Baltimore, 1989
95. Kirklin JW, Barratt-Boyes BG: Cardiac Surgery. Churchill Livingstone, New York, 1986
96. Graham TP Jr: The Eisenmenger syndrome. pp. 567–581. In Roberts WC (ed): Adult Congenital Heart Disease. FA Davis, Philadelphia, 1987
97. Rutledge JM, Boor PJ: Eisenmenger's: A case study and review of the syndrome and complex. Am J Cardiovasc Pathol 1989;2:285–294
98. Pratt PC: Emphysema and chronic airways disease. pp. 651–669. In Dail DH, Hammar SP (eds): Pulmonary Pathology. Springer-Verlag, New York, 1988
99. Blank N: Chest Radiographic Analysis. Churchill Livingstone, New York, 1989, pp. 329–330

Chapter 25

Disorders of the Regulation of Ventilation

Robert B. Schoene

CHAPTER OUTLINE

In any individual the control of ventilation can be defined by several parameters, such as resting ventilation, the level at which the subject maintains alveolar ventilation—that is, the set point for CO_2 partial pressure (PCO_2)—and the ventilatory responses to various stimuli such as hypoxia, increased CO_2, and exercise. These responses are usually consistent in any one subject, although there is a normal distribution between subjects. For instance, a person who at rest has a slightly higher than normal PCO_2 usually also has relatively blunted ventilatory responses to hypoxia (HVR), hypercapnia (HCVR), and exercise. So long as one's ventilatory drives are somewhere in the normal range, there is a margin of safety in terms of maintaining adequate oxygenation and normal pH. Healthy individuals can function quite adequately with high or low ventilatory drives, and therefore it is difficult to define "abnormal" drives.

Having a ventilatory drive at one or the other end of the bell-shaped curve may in fact convey certain advantages in some activities. For instance, there has been an association between blunted ventilatory drives and high levels of performance in certain athletic activities.[1–4] Highly fit, aerobic athletes who compete at low altitude have been shown to have blunted ventilatory drives and ventilatory responses to exercise. This characteristic may allow them to exercise with a lower work of breathing and less dyspnea, and if they have other characteristics that are advantageous to their particular sport, they may excel. On the other hand, certain individuals who climb to extreme altitude have been shown to have brisk ventilatory responses, which may be essential to maintaining a viable level of oxygenation.[5–7] These associations may in fact be just that—associations—and not evolutionary developments per se.

If one is healthy, one can tolerate most levels of ventilatory drive and survive quite well. On the other hand, if an individual has very high or very low drives and if certain pathophysiologic processes occur, drives at one or the other end of the spectrum may be accentuated by that process or may not allow the individual to respond adequately to maintain oxygenation and ventilation. Therefore, the purpose of this chapter is to review some of the disease entities that either are primary drive disorders or are accentuated by ventilatory drives at one or the other end of the range.

CLINICAL DISORDERS OF VENTILATORY DRIVE

One must differentiate between distinct disease entities caused primarily by abnormal ventilatory drives and other diseases whose characteristics are merely accentuated by or associated with blunted or vigorous drives. It is important to differentiate between those patients who "won't breathe" (e.g., have ventilatory capability but blunted drives) and those who "can't breathe" (e.g., have reduced ability to ventilate whatever the state of their ventilatory drives). Those who won't breathe are obviously most in danger of following an inexorable course to death. For instance, infants who succumb to sudden infant death syndrome (SIDS) probably have some primary dysfunction of their ventilatory control mechanism, which causes dysrhythmic or apneic periods during sleep, resulting in asphyxia.[8] Altered control of ventilation may also be a factor in adults who have various forms of sleep apnea and suffer sudden death (see Ch. 27).

Primary Alveolar Hypoventilation Syndrome

A rare but classic example of dysfunctional control of breathing is the primary alveolar hypoventilation syndrome.[9,10] Although it may be more common than has been documented, only about 30 cases have been reported in the medical literature. It usually occurs in men in the third or fourth decade of life and is associated with cyanosis, somnolence, cor pulmonale, and polycythemia, which are all ravages of chronic hypoxemia. Pulmonary function tests are normal, and the patients are not obese. They do not have an appropriate ventilatory response during exercise and tend to retain CO_2. If asked to do so, they can hyperventilate, but measured HVR and HCVR are absent or markedly blunted. There also seems to be some hereditary transmission of this disease, although there is no clear association with other neurologic disorders. Patients usually experience progressive respiratory failure, and since respiratory stimulants do not seem to work on their peripheral or central chemosensor, mechanical augmentation of ventilation, such as the use of diaphragmatic pacing or nocturnal mechanical ventilation, becomes necessary.

Ondine's Curse

Another entity, which is probably a primary dysfunction of respiratory control centers, has been termed *Ondine's curse*.[11] The eponym refers to the mythologic story and subsequent French play about a young man who jilted his lover, the sea nymph Ondine. Her father in revenge cursed him with a condition that would cause him to stop breathing and subsequently die when he fell asleep. He, therefore, was sentenced to constant wakefulness. Patients with classic Ondine's curse are not too dissimilar from those with primary alveolar hypoventilation syndrome except that the disorder of their central control mechanism is accentuated with sleep. Like central hypoventilation syndrome, Ondine's curse can be fatal.

Obesity Hypoventilation Syndrome

Another literary eponym, the pickwickian syndrome, is derived from the Charles Dickens novel *The Pickwick Papers*, in which one of the characters is an obese, plethoric, hypersomnolent boy. This disorder is probably more properly described by the term *obesity hypoventilation syndrome*.[12–15] By definition patients are obese, sometimes markedly so, which produces an increased work of breathing from their overloaded chest wall. There are decreases in functional residual capacity (FRC), expiratory reserve volume (ERV), and vital capacity (VC), probably secondary to the obese chest wall. The VC and inspiratory capacity (IC) of these patients also are lower than those of normal obese individuals. There is some evidence of muscle weakness; however, when asked to hyperventilate, they generally can.

Most studies show that these individuals have blunted ventilatory drives as measured by the ventilatory response alone[15]; however, other studies have shown a spectrum of mouth occlusion pressure ($P_{0.1}$) and diaphragmatic electromyogram (EMG_{di}) responses, which suggests that there may be some mechanical inefficiency and/or impairment of neuromuscular coupling, resulting in overt hypoventilation.[12] These individuals should not be confused with obese "type B" patients with chronic obstructive pulmonary disease (COPD), who are also hypoxemic and hypercapnic, for patients with obesity hypoventilation syndrome do for the most part respond to respiratory stimulants, as discussed in Chapter 66.

Hyperventilation Syndrome

It is difficult to state that hyperventilation syndrome is a primary disorder of the ventilatory control mechanisms. This common entity is episodic and is characterized by anxiety, breath hunger, and tingling of the hands and perioral area.[16] Affected individuals have a marked respiratory alkalosis, and when the episode abates, they usually have normal resting blood gases. There may be some definable event that triggers hyperventilation; however, for the most part it is difficult for the patient to recall anything specific. Reassurance and psychological counseling are often quite helpful. Immediate treatment by having the subject rebreathe into a paper bag or rebreathing circuit is usually successful in terminating the somatic symptoms, such as the tingling and dyspnea, and subsequently, the anxiety.

VENTILATORY DRIVES IN OTHER DISEASES AND SETTINGS

As already discussed, a wide range of ventilatory drives are considered normal; however, concomitant pathologic conditions may be aggravated in patients whose ventilatory drives fall at the high or low end of the spectrum. For instance, dyspnea can be accentuated in patients with high ventilatory drives, while hypoxemia and hypercapnia can be worsened in individuals with very blunted ventilatory drives. There is certainly considerable overlap, and the issues are not always clear. However, a discussion of some of the associations between drives and disease should be helpful.

Chronic Obstructive Pulmonary Disease

One of the few descriptions that medical students never forget is the terminology "pink puffers" and "blue bloaters," further discussed in Chapters 22 and 62. These terms provide poignant portraits of differences in ventilatory responses in patients with COPD. Although most patients with COPD cannot be categorized in this manner, certain types can be, and these differences are believed to be secondary to differences in ventilatory drive.

Classically the blue bloater (type B) is the severely hypoxemic and hypercapnic patient with markedly blunted respiratory drives to CO_2 and hypoxia, but whose remnant of an HVR is the sole stimulus that is adequate to maintain some alveolar ventilation and oxygenation. On the other hand, the pink puffer (type A) also has obstructive disease, but high inherent respiratory drives have imposed a tremendous work of breathing on the patient as the central nervous system over-responds to the lungs' mechanical dysfunction. Such patients tend to maintain quite viable levels of O_2 pressure (PO_2), usually in the 70 mmHg range at sea level, and many do so at least until their obstruction worsens irreversibly. These characteristics impose a high metabolic demand on these patients during rest and exercise, so that unlike the blue bloater who tends to be moderately obese, these patients are usually quite cachectic.

As discussed in Chapter 14, some patients with even mild restrictive disease end up with inordinately high levels of ventilation. The augmentation in their chemosensitivity is thought to be secondary to increased J receptor afferent input to the central nervous system, which results in a high ventilatory drive output. These individuals are usually quite dyspneic, and until their gas exchange or mechanical dysfunction approaches the terminal stage, they tend to hyperventilate with low tidal volume/high frequency patterns of breathing. Their resting ventilatory drives and $P_{0.1}$ values are quite high, and their exercise ventilation is characterized by a high ventilatory equivalent.

Hypoventilators

Most patients with COPD tend to retain CO_2 if their forced expiratory volume in 1 second (FEV_1) falls much below 1.0 L[17]; however, each patient is different, and this value is by no means absolute. There are many factors, particularly those related to mechanics and gas exchange, that dictate how much respiratory acidosis these patients are going to live with, but inherent and/or acquired chemosensitivity may play a role by accentuating their level of alveolar hypoventilation.

In patients who hypoventilate it is important to differentiate between ventilatory *result* and ventilatory *drive*. For instance, normocapnic COPD patients have mildly decreased HCVR, but when other measurements of "drive," such as $P_{0.1}$ and EMG_{di}, are used, results tend to be increased, suggesting that the brain is responding with a high output in order for the patient to overcome the mechanical inefficiency due to the lung disease.[18,19] Patients who retain CO_2 have blunted HCVR levels as well as $P_{0.1}/PCO_2$ responses, although their resting $P_{0.1}$ levels are higher than normal.[19] These findings suggest a high resting drive but very blunted chemoreceptor gain to CO_2. It is difficult to study HVR in these patients, because making them hyperoxic usually blunts any resting drive and causes them to hypoventilate, often to a dangerous level of respiratory acidosis. One study of HVR has shown blunted responses with respect to both ventilation and $P_{0.1}$ level.[19] These findings suggest that blunted respiratory drives may be a risk factor for CO_2 retention and may explain the variations seen among individuals between CO_2 retention and FEV_1.

It has been difficult to determine whether these characteristics are inherited or acquired. Several studies have shown that hypoventilators with COPD have a familial predisposition to blunted HVR and HCVR.[20,21] It has been difficult to discern accurately whether changes in drive can occur, since longitudinal studies are next to impossible. Some high altitude studies have shown that many years of exposure to hypoxia can lead to blunted HVR,[22] but most of these data do not necessarily pertain to COPD patients. Normal subjects exposed to 1.5 percent CO_2 for 40 days increased their resting ventilation by 35 percent while their PCO_2 increased by 4.5 mmHg with a decrease in HCVR.[23] Some of this alteration in chemosensitivity may be related to increased buffering capacity in the brain with chronic CO_2 exposure. The possibility of correcting for this alteration and buffering has not been studied in a systematic fashion.

From all these data it is clear that many factors contribute to CO_2 retention, including decreased responses to respiratory loading, chronic muscle fatigue, mechanical inability to respond to increased central drives, altered chest wall configuration and diaphragmatic flattening, and inherent or acquired blunted ventilatory drives; thus all these factors, to a greater or lesser degree, contribute to a patient's chronic respiratory failure.

Hyperventilators

Patients with COPD who over-respond to the mechanical inefficiency and resistive loading of their airways pay a high price for maintaining adequate oxygenation and ventilation. Even though many of these patients tend to be hypocapnic, they generally ventilate with small tidal volumes and high frequencies and a high work of breathing. Their resting central drives, as measured by $P_{0.1}$ and by HVR and HCVR, are also elevated.[24] Even though their mechanical dysfunction may be as impaired as that of patients who retain CO_2, their attempt to compensate is more than likely driven by their brain's perception of their inefficiency.

Respiratory Failure and Mechanical Ventilation

An understanding of respiratory drives in patients receiving mechanical ventilation in the intensive care unit is important as the clinician tries to decide when and how to wean them from ventilatory support. This is particularly difficult because of the wide spectrum of patients who need mechanical ventilation, which includes the young, previously healthy individual with a sedative overdose whose lung mechanics and gas exchange are normal but whose drives are exogenously blunted with medication, the patient with severe COPD and respiratory failure, and the patient with adult respiratory distress syndrome (ARDS) and very stiff lungs. Nutritional factors, respiratory muscle fatigue, numerous pharmacologic agents, dynamic mechanical dysfunction, and alterations in ventilatory drives all increase the difficulty of weaning from the ventilator.

Numerous *weaning parameters* are used to help the clinician judge whether the patient can be taken off ventilatory support (see Ch. 86), most of which examine gas exchange and pulmonary mechanical capabilities. Although it is often felt that some patients are ventilator-dependent because of insufficient ventilatory drive, the contrary is often the case. Two studies have used $P_{0.1}$ measurements to evaluate the possibility of assessing weanability by measurement of ventilatory drives. Sassoon et al.[25] showed that patients who failed to wean after a T-piece trial had much greater $P_{0.1}$ values (8.35 versus a normal value of about 2.5 cmH_2O). This information suggested that those who failed already had a very high central drive output and could not further increase central drive to sustain spontaneous ventilation requirements. Montgomery et al.[26] found similar results when $P_{0.1}$ measurements were made during exogenous CO_2 stimulation. Patients who could not wean from ventilator support had very high $P_{0.1}/PaCO_2$ responses, again suggesting that they could not call on greater drive to produce a higher ventilatory response. It must therefore be the clinician's role to judge patients' weanability on the basis of all the standard weaning parameters as well as to try to obtain insight into their underlying drive and reserve.

High Altitude

Millions of people live in an environment of global hypoxia. Habitation for years and generations in this environment usually results in decreased hypoxic chemosensitivity.[22] Fortunately, however, enough drive is present in most individuals so that viable levels of oxygenation and ventilation are maintained. Several studies give insight into characteristics of ventilatory drive that may contribute to acute altitude illnesses and chronic mountain sickness (CMS).[27–29] Whereas it seems quite obvious, and has been well documented, that most individuals who ascend to extreme altitude have intact HVRs, sojourners at moderate altitude, who have a wide spectrum of drives, are subject to acute mountain sickness (AMS) and to the more severe forms of altitude illness, such as high altitude pulmonary edema (HAPE) and cerebral edema (HACE). These entities are discussed more thoroughly in Chapter 16. Briefly, these studies show that individuals who develop AMS and HAPE have more blunted HVRs and lower resting ventilations than those who ascend to moderate altitudes without illness.[27–29]

The syndrome of CMS is basically one of hypoventilation relative to that of individuals who live successfully at the same altitude.[30,31] It is difficult to ascertain why some high altitude native populations have a high incidence of CMS while others do not. As is discussed in greater detail in Chapter 16, some studies suggest that blunted ventilatory drives in the high altitude population of South America predispose these individuals to a higher incidence of CMS, whereas natives of the Himalayas, where there is a very low incidence of CMS, may have somewhat higher drives.

References

1. Merchant JA: Occupational Respiratory Disorders. Dept. of Health and Human Services, Publication No. NIOSH 86-102. U.S. Government Printing Office, Washington, DC, 1986
2. Parkes WR: Occupational Lung Disorders. 2nd Ed. Butterworth, London, 1982
3. Saunders NA, Ledder SR, Rebuck AS: Ventilatory responses to carbon dioxide in young athletes: A family study. Am Rev Respir Dis 1976;113:497–502
4. Schoene RB, Robertson HT, Pierson DJ, Peterson AP: Respiratory drives and exercise in the menstrual cycle in athletic and non-athletic women. J Appl Physiol 1981;50:1300–1305
5. Schoene RB: The control of ventilation in climbers to extreme altitude. J Appl Physiol 1982;53:886–890
6. Schoene RB, Lahiri S, Hackett PH et al: The relationship of hypoxic ventilatory response to exercise performance on Mt. Everest. J Appl Physiol 1984;56:1478–1483
7. Masuyama S, Kimura H, Sugita T et al: Control of ventilation in extreme-altitude climbers. J Appl Physiol 1986;61:500–506
8. Phillipson EA: Sleep disorders. pp. 1841–1860. In Murray JF, Nadel JA (eds): Textbook of Respiratory Medicine. WB Saunders, Philadelphia, 1988
9. Wolkove N, Altose MD, Kelsen SG, Cherniack NS: Respiratory control abnormalities in alveolar hypoventilation. Am Rev Respir Dis 1980;122:163–167
10. Reichel J: Primary alveolar hypoventilation. Clin Chest Med 1980;1:119–125
11. Severinghaus JR, Mitchell RA: Ordine's curse: Failure of respiratory center automaticity while asleep. Clin Res 1962;10:122
12. Lopata M, Freilien RA, Onal E et al: Ventilatory control in the obesity hypoventilation syndrome. Am Rev Respir Dis 1977; 115:65–68
13. Lyons HA, Huang CT: Therapeutic use of progesterone in alveolar hypoventilation associated with obesity. Am J Med 1968; 44:881–888
14. Sutton FD, Zwillich CW, Creagh CE et al: Progesterone for outpatient treatment for pickwickian syndrome. Ann Intern Med 1975;83:476–479
15. Zwillich CW, Sutton FD, Pierson DJ et al: Decreased hypoxic ventilatory drive in the obesity-hypoventilation syndrome. Am J Med 1975;59:343–348
16. Cherniack NS: Hyperventilation syndromes. pp. 1861–1866. In Murray JF, Nadel JA (eds): Textbook of Respiratory Medicine. WB Saunders, Philadelphia, 1988

17. Cherniack NS: Clinical assessment of the chemical regulation of ventilation. Chest 1976;70:274–279
18. Lourenco RV, Miranda JM: Drive and performance of the ventilatory apparatus in COPD. N Engl J Med 1967;279:53–59
19. Park SS: Respiratory control in COPD. Clin Chest Med 1980; 1:73–79
20. Mountain R, Zwillich CW, Weil JV: Hypoventilation in obstructive lung disease: The role of familial factors. N Engl J Med 1978;298:251–255
21. Fleetham JA, Arnup ME, Anthonisen NR: Familial aspects of ventilatory control in patients with chronic obstructive pulmonary disease. Am Rev Respir Dis 1984;129:3–7
22. Weil JV, Byrne-Quinn E, Sodal IE et al: Acquired attenuation of chemoreceptor function in chronically hypoxic man at high altitude. J Clin Invest 1971;50:186–195
23. Schaefer KE, Hastings JB, Carey CR: Respiratory acclimatization to carbon dioxide. J Appl Physiol 1963;18:1071–1078
24. Aubier M, Murciano D, Fournier M et al: Central respiratory drive in acute respiratory failure in patients with COPD. Am Rev Respir Dis 1980;122:191–199
25. Sassoon CSH, Te T, Mahutte CK et al: Airway occlusion pressure ($P_{0.1}$) as a reliable predictor to weaning? Abstracted. Chest, suppl. 1, 1985;88:38S
26. Montgomery AB, Holle RHO, Neagley SR et al: Prediction of successful ventilator weaning using airway occlusion pressure and hypercapnic challenge. Chest 1987;91:496–499
27. King AB, Robinson SM: Ventilation response and hypoxia in acute mountain sickness. Aviat Space Environ Med 1972; 43:419–421
28. Hackett PH, Rennie D, Hofmeister SE et al: Fluid retention and relative hypoventilation in acute mountain sickness. Respiration 1982;45:321–329
29. Hackett PH, Roach RC, Schoene RB et al: Abnormal control of ventilation in high altitude pulmonary edema. J Appl Physiol 1988;64:1268–1272
30. Kryger M, McCullough R, Doekel R et al: Excessive polycythemia of high altitude. Role of ventilatory drive and lung disease. Am Rev Respir Dis 1978;118:659–666
31. Monge-M C: La enfermedad de los Andes. Sindromes eritremicos. Ann Fac Med Univ San Marcos (Lima) 1928;11:1–316

Chapter 26

Ventilatory Muscle Dysfunction

Robert M. Kacmarek

CONTENT OUTLINE

Ventilatory muscles, although having large reserves, are as susceptible to dysfunction as any other voluntary muscles. Dysfunction is commonly referred to as fatigue, although fatigue is the extreme of dysfunction. As noted below, fatigue is easily defined, the factors causing it are easily outlined, and its presence is easily identified in controlled laboratory settings. However, at the bedside numerous factors affect ventilatory function, making the diagnosis of fatigue difficult. In this chapter muscle dysfunction and fatigue are defined and factors causing dysfunction are discussed.

FATIGUE

Fatigue of any muscle is defined as "the inability of a muscle to maintain the required or expected force with continued or repeated contraction."[1] Acute ventilatory muscle fatigue may be defined as the inability of the ventilatory muscles to sustain a contractile force, while chronic respiratory muscle fatigue may be defined as the inability of the ventilatory muscles to generate a contractile force.[2] In general, dysfunction of the ventilatory muscles is the result of a mismatch between ventilatory muscle energy demands and energy availability. Table 26-1 outlines the primary factors affecting energy demand and energy availability.

Most of the effort required for breathing is performed by the inspiratory muscles, expiration is usually passive, and the energy required for expiration is mainly provided by the elastic recoil of the lung/thorax system.[3] Expiratory muscles are normally only recruited during marked ventilatory stress or chronic airflow limitation.

Ventilatory muscle fatigue may occur anywhere along the command chain of voluntary skeletal muscle contraction[4] (Fig. 26-1). Overall, fatigue is classified as *central* or *peripheral*,[1] although Rochester has defined a condition referred to as incipient fatigue.[5] Central fatigue is manifested by an exertion-induced decrease in neural drive, which is reversible.[6] During central fatigue, information from chemical or proprioceptive changes in the muscle via either the phrenic nerve or the vagus nerves are believed to inhibit motor activity of ventilatory muscles.[7] The exact central nervous system mechanisms responsible for this inhibition are unknown, although numerous centers in the brain have been implicated.[8,9] Elimination of inhibiting factors resolves this type of fatigue.

There are two types of peripheral fatigue, transmission and contractile fatigue.[1] Most of the data on transmission fatigue have been accumulated in vitro during high-frequency stimulation of muscle units. The data point to one of three locations as the site of fatigue: (1) failure of conduction through axonal fibers[10]; (2) inadequate neurotransmitter function[11]; and (3) altered sensitivity of the motor end place of the muscle.[12] Contractile fatigue is believed to be of two types.[7] Type 1, induced by high-frequency (50 to 100 Hz) stimulation of

Table 26-1. Factors Predisposing to Inspiratory Muscle Fatigue

Factors affecting inspiratory muscle demand
Work of breathing
Minute ventilation
Frequency
Tidal volume
Compliance
Resistance
Muscle strength
Lung volume
Prematurity
Neuromuscular disease
Nutritional state
Muscle efficiency
Ventilatory load
Fiber length
State of contraction
Factors affecting inspiratory muscle energy availability
Energy stores
Muscle blood flow
O_2 content of arterial blood
Blood substrate levels
Ability to extract sources of energy
Energy stores
Nutritional status
Metabolic disorders

(Modified from Roussos and Moxham,[1] with permission.)

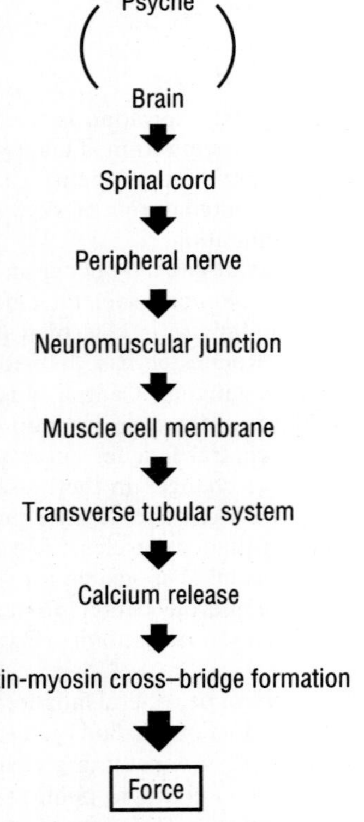

Figure 26-1. Command chain for voluntary contraction of skeletal muscle. The development of muscle dysfunction or fatigue can occur as a result of alterations at any point in this chain. (From Edwards,[4] with permission.)

the muscle, is manifested by a decreased response at these frequencies. Type 2, or low-frequency, fatigue is a reduced response to stimulation in the range in which respiratory muscles normally function (10 to 20 Hz). The terms *high-* and *low*-frequency refer to the frequency at which nerve impulses reach the diaphragm via the phrenic nerve. In general, high-frequency fatigue is resolved with rest for a few hours, while low-frequency fatigue requires at least 12 to 24 hours of rest to resolve.[7] Patients requiring mechanical ventilation because of ventilatory muscle dysfunction normally require 24 to 48 hours of ventilatory control to ensure that both transmission and contractile peripheral fatigue are resolved.

Rochester[5] has coined the term *incipient fatigue* to indicate the earliest physiologic response to severe muscle stress before actual fatigue occurs. During this period, relaxation rates of the muscle slow, but contractile strength at low frequencies may be enhanced.[13] It is believed that central output during this period is reduced without overall impairment of muscle function.[9] This adaptation is believed to prevent or forestall overt fatigue (Table 26-2).

ENERGY DEMAND VERSUS ENERGY AVAILABILITY

As stated earlier, ventilatory muscle dysfunction is a result of an imbalance between energy demands and energy availability, as summarized in Table 26-1. Three factors that determine energy demand are work of breathing, muscular strength, and muscle efficiency. Energy supply and the body's energy stores determine energy availability.

Work of Breathing

Work, as defined previously (see Ch. 5) and used in reference to the respiratory system, is equal to the product of pressure times volume; that is, the greater the pressure gradient required to move a given tidal volume (V_T), the greater the work of breathing. Thus, any factor that increases volume or pressure increases the load on the ventilatory muscles. Rapid respiratory rates, large V_T, or high minute ventilation all translate into increased work load. Respiratory rate and minute ventilation are the most sensitive indicators of increased work load.[14–16] It is generally believed that sustained respiratory rates higher than 35 per minute enhance muscle dysfunction.[14,15] As minute volume increases for sustained periods, we near thresholds that may result in fatigue.[15,16] Figure 26-2 illustrates the relationship between percentage of maximum voluntary ventilation and the time it can be sustained before high-frequency contractile fatigue sets in. The maximum sustainable volume is the maximum minute ventilation that can be maintained without fatigue. In the normal, healthy individual this is about 60 percent of maximum voluntary ventilation.[17]

At normal respiratory rates and V_T in the spontaneously breathing individual, lung and chest wall compliance (elastic

Table 26-2. Types of Fatigue

Type	Subdivision	Manifestation	Mechanism[a]	Recovery
Central	—	Exercise-induced decrease in neural drive	Chemical or proprioceptive changes inhibit drive via phrenic or vagus nerves	Rapid (hours)
Peripheral	Transmission	Inhibition of transfer of motor activity to the muscle	Conduction failure Neurotransmitter failure Membrane transfer failure	Rapid (hours)
Peripheral	Contractile, high frequency	Decreased response at 50–100 Hz stimulation	Accumulation of metabolic by-products	Rapid (hours)
Peripheral	Contractile, low frequency	Decreased response at 10–20 Hz stimulation	Muscle injury	Lengthy (>12 to 24 h)
Incipient fatigue	—	Decreased relaxation rate, enhanced contractile strength at low frequencies	Reduced neural output to spare muscle function	Rapid (hours)

[a] Mechanisms are all speculative; none have been definitively documented.

resistance) and airway resistance (flow resistance) are the factors that most affect work load. Figure 26-3 graphically depicts the relationships among elastic resistance, flow resistance, and ventilatory rate. In general, an unconscious attempt is made by an individual to assume a ventilatory pattern resulting in the least work, as indicated in Figure 26-3. With normal elastic and flow resistances, the respiratory rate resulting in the least work of breathing is about 15 breaths per minute.[18] If elastic resistance increases (Fig. 26-3B), work is minimized if rate is increased; that is, minimal but more frequent distortion of the lung and chest wall results in less overall work. On the other hand, an increase in flow resistance (Fig. 26-3C) requires a slower than normal respiratory rate to minimize work. Work becomes markedly elevated when the individual with increased flow resistance, such as a patient with chronic obstructive pulmonary disease (COPD), tries to breathe rapidly or the patient with restrictive lung disease (increased elastic resistance) attempts to breathe slowly and deeply.[18]

In intubated patients who require ventilatory assistance, numerous factors can affect work load, including endotracheal tubes,[19] demand valves,[20] peak flow settings,[21] or the presence of intrinsic positive end-expiratory pressure (auto-PEEP).[22] These factors are discussed in detail in Chapter 87.

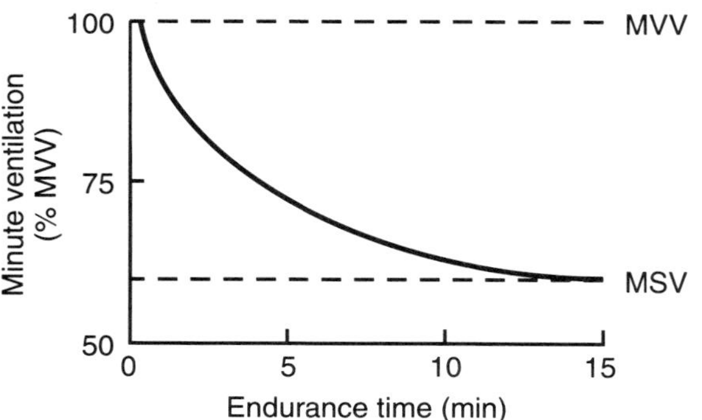

Figure 26-2. The relationship between minute ventilation, expressed as a percentage of maximum voluntary ventilation (%MVV), and endurance time is illustrated. MVV can only be maintained for about 15 to 30 seconds, whereas 75 percent of MVV may be sustained for 4 minutes. Maximal sustainable ventilation is referred to as 60 percent of MVV normally sustainable for 15 minutes in health. (From Rochester et al.,[17] with permission.)

Muscular Strength

The strength of the ventilatory muscles is affected by numerous factors, including lung volume, atrophy, prematurity, neuromuscular disease, and nutritional state.[1] The lung volume at which contraction of ventilatory muscles occurs greatly affects the strength of contraction. At the functional residual capacity (FRC) level or below, inspiratory muscles are capable of exerting their maximal force, while as lung volume increases above the FRC level, inspiratory muscle fibers shorten and the force they can generate diminishes.[3,23] Figure 26-4 illustrates the length-tension curve of inspiratory muscles.[24] The ventilatory muscle length producing maximum tension, and thus maximum strength, is at or below FRC level. As length decreases from this point, tension or strength diminishes. Hyperinflation, as noted in COPD, shortens inspiratory muscle length, especially that of the diaphragm. These disadvantaged muscles are incapable of exerting their normal force.

Muscles that have atrophied, as in the patient receiving controlled mechanical ventilation for several weeks, have diminished strength and may require retraining to return to normal strength. The duration of controlled ventilation required before atrophy of ventilatory muscles occurs is questionable. However, the greater the duration of controlled ventilation, the greater the likelihood of atrophy. It is un-

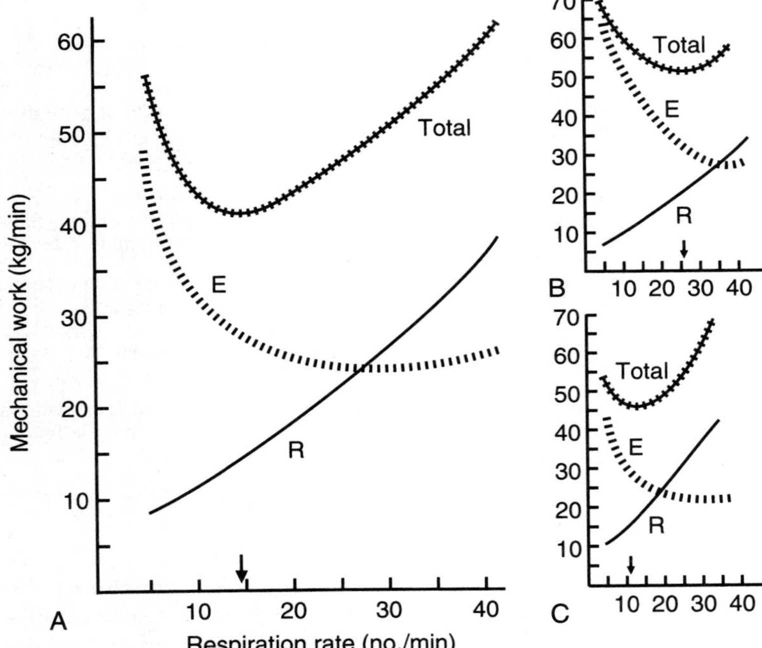

Figure 26-3. The relationship between respiratory rate and mechanical work of breathing at a given alveolar ventilation. **(A)** In the healthy individual an increase in respiratory rate is associated with a fall in V_T, so that elastic work (E) is reduced, but the increase in rate and therefore, in airflow resistance, results in a rise in the work required to overcome flow resistance (R). As a result of these divergent effects, there is a respiratory rate at which the total work of breathing is minimal. **(B)** In a patient with a restrictive disorder, the elastic work is greater at any respiratory rate, and as a result the total work of breathing is minimal at a higher respiratory rate than in the healthy individuals. **(C)** In a patient with an obstructive disorder, the flow resistive work is greater at any respiratory rate, so that the total work is least at a lower respiratory rate than in the healthy individual. (From Cherniack and Cherniack,[18] with permission.)

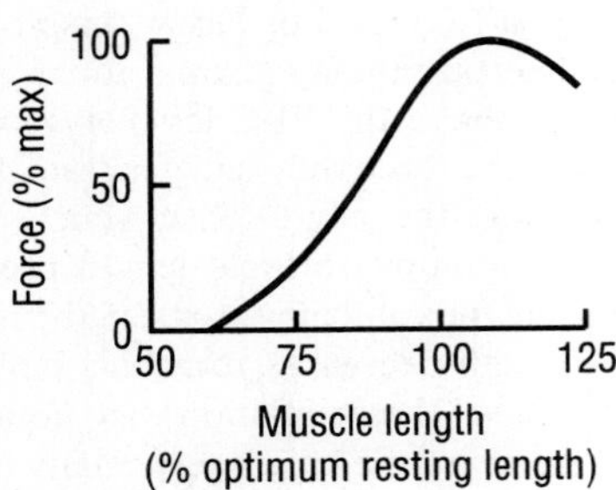

Figure 26-4. The length-tension (force) curve of a normal diaphragm is shown. Force is expressed as a percentage of maximum tension (%max) developed during isometric contraction. Length is expressed as a percentage of optimal resting length. Note that maximum force is generated at 100 percent of optimal length. As length increases beyond or decreases below this optimal value, the force generated during contraction diminishes. (From Rochester and Braun,[24] with permission.)

likely that up to 48 hours of controlled ventilation will adversely affect muscle function, while the effort required to trigger assisted ventilation or demand valves seems to be sufficient to prevent muscular atrophy.

Prematurity may result in gross ventilatory muscle strength alterations, as do neuromuscular diseases. Nutritional deficits diminish ventilatory muscle strength and efficiency and decrease diaphragmatic mass and thickness, as well as decreasing the ventilatory response to hypoxemia and increasing susceptibility to pulmonary infection.[25] (See Ch. 51 for a detailed discussion of nutritional effects on ventilation.)

Muscular Efficiency

As the efficiency of ventilatory muscle contraction diminishes, energy demands increase. Ventilatory muscles are normally relatively *inefficient*, functioning at a 10 to 20 percent efficiency level.[26] Ventilatory muscle efficiency is reduced by chronic lung disease, decreased fiber length (hyperinflation), and isometric, as opposed to isotonic, contraction.[26] In addition, any factor increasing ventilatory load, such as mucosal edema, secretions, or altered lung and chest wall compliance, decreases muscular efficiency.[2]

Energy Supply

In order for any cell to function normally, sufficient nutrients must be supplied to it per unit time to meet its energy demand.[25] These include O_2 and normal energy substrates (i.e., glucose, free fatty acids, and protein). In the short term, O_2 is the substance most important to muscle function. Without sufficient O_2 supply, normal aerobic metabolism stops and is replaced with anaerobic metabolism. However, production of adenosine triphosphate (ATP) is markedly decreased with this transition. In addition to adequate O_2 partial pressure (PO_2) and hemoglobin content, cardiac output must be sufficient and its distribution must be appropriate to ensure adequate energy supply. In severe ventilatory failure in the critically ill patient, up to 30 to 40 percent of cardiac output may be perfusing the diaphragm.[27] Energy supply may be disrupted by an inability to extract or properly carry nutrients as a result of sepsis or cyanide poisoning.

Energy Stores

During periods of prolonged stress, energy supply may be compromised. During these periods patients must rely on energy stores to provide sufficient energy to prevent fatigue. Metabolic disorders (hypermetabolic states) or severe trauma, sepsis, or postoperative states may inhibit the recruitment of energy stores and increase the likelihood of muscular fatigue.[26]

References

1. Roussos C, Moxham J: Respiratory muscle fatigue. In Roussos C, Macklen PT: The Thorax. Part B. Marcel Dekker, New York, 1985
2. Tobin MJ: Respiratory muscle involvement in chronic obstructive pulmonary disease and asthma. Prob Respir Care 1990; 3:375–395
3. Macklen PT, Macklem DM, DeTroyer A: A model of inspiratory muscle mechanics. J Appl Physiol 1983;55:547–557
4. Edwards RHT: Physiological analysis of skeletal muscle weakness and fatigue. Clin Sci M 1978;54:463–470
5. Rochester DF: Does respiratory muscle rest relieve fatigue or incipient fatigue? Am Rev Respir Dis 1988;138:516–517
6. Aldrich TK: Respiratory muscle fatigue. Prob Respir Care 1990;3:329–342
7. Edwards RHT: The diaphragm as a muscle: Mechanisms underlying fatigue. Am Rev Respir Dis, suppl. 1979;119:81–84
8. Road J, Vahi R, DelRio P, Grassino A: *In vivo* contractile properties of fatigued diaphragm. J Appl Physiol 1987;63:471–478
9. Bigland-Ritchie B, Dawson NJ, Johansson RS, Lippold OCJ: Reflex origin for the slowing of motoneurone firing rates in fatigue of human voluntary contractions. J Physiol (Lond) 1986;379:451–459
10. Krnjevic K, Miledi R: Failure of neuromuscular propagation in rats. J Physiol (Lond) 1958;140:440–461
11. Scardella AT, Parisi RA, Phair DK et al: The role of endogenous opioids in the ventilatory response to acute flow-restrictive loads. Am Rev Respir Dis 1986;133:26–31
12. Kurihara T, Brooks JE: The mechanism of neuromuscular fatigue. Arch Neurol 1975;32:168–174
13. Bigland-Ritchie B, Johansson R, Lippold OCJ, Woods JJ: Contractile speed and EMG changes during fatigue of sustained maximal voluntary contractions. J Neurophysiol 1983;50:313–324
14. Tobin MJ, Chadhats HC, Jenouri G et al: Breathing patterns. 1. Normal subjects. Chest 1983;84:202–210
15. Tobin MJ, Perez W, Guenther SM et al: The pattern of breathing during successful and unsuccessful trials of weaning from mechanical ventilation. Am Rev Respir Dis 1986;134:1111–1118
16. Cohen C, Zagelbaum G, Gross D et al: Clinical manifestations of inspiratory muscle fatigue. Am J Med 1982;73:308–316
17. Rochester DF, Arora NS, Brawn NMV et al: The respiratory muscles in chronic obstructive pulmonary disease (COPD). Bull Eur Physiopathol Respir 1979;15:951–960
18. Cherniack RM, Cherniack L: Respiration in Health and Disease. 3rd Ed. WB Saunders, Philadelphia, 1983
19. Wright PE, Marini JJ, Bernard GR: *In vitro* versus *in vivo* comparison of endotracheal tube airflow resistance. Am Rev Respir Dis 1989;140:10–16
20. Katz JA, Kraemer RW, Gjerde GE: Inspiratory work and airway pressure with continuous positive airway pressure delivery systems. Chest 1985;88:519–526
21. Marini JJ, Capps JS, Culver BH: The inspiratory work of breathing during assisted ventilation. Chest 1985;87:612–618
22. Smith TC, Marini JJ: Impact of PEEP on lung mechanics and work of breathing in severe airflow obstruction. J Appl Physiol 1988;65:1488–1499
23. Bradburne RM, McCool FD: The respiratory muscles: structural and functional consideration. Probl Respir Care 1990;3:257–276
24. Rochester DF, Brawn NMV: The respiratory muscles. Basics RD 1978;6:1–10
25. Lewis MI, Belman MJ: Nutrition and respiratory muscle function. Probl Respir Care 1990;3:343–359
26. Roussas C: Energetics. pp. 437–492. In Roussos C, Macklen PT (eds): The Thorax. Part A. Marcel Dekker, New York, 1985
27. Rochester DF: Respiratory muscle blood flow and metabolics. pp. 393–436. In Roussos C, Macklen PT: The Thorax. Part A. Marcel Dekker, New York, 1985

Chapter 27

The Physiology and Pathophysiology of Sleep and Sleep-Disordered Breathing

Eugene C. Fletcher

CHAPTER OUTLINE

NORMAL AND ABNORMAL SLEEP ARCHITECTURE

The scientific investigation of sleep is a relatively recent addition to the many facets of medicine in which we now concentrate research, teaching, and provision of clinical care. The earliest systematic research involving sleep appeared in the late 1800s and, in accordance with the tools of the time, used simple observation or "behavioral" appearance to assess sleep. Simple physiologic parameters of respiration, heart rate, and blood pressure were quantitated and correlated with waking body functions. While the electroencephalograph (EEG) was devised and used in animals in the late nineteenth century, it was not until 1929 that this most valuable tool was applied to the study of human brain waves.[1,2]

The age of modern sleep research can probably be best dated from the landmark 1935 article by Loomis et al., which described cerebral cortical rhythms unique to sleep.[3] No less important was the description by Aserinsky and Kleitman[4,5] of rapid eye movement (REM) sleep and its association with dreaming. For many years, however, there was considerable nonuniformity of terminology, leading to misunderstanding and difficulty in communication regarding sleep staging. In a monumental effort to resolve differences and provide a common language among polysomnographers (as scientists involved in sleep research came to be called), Rechtschaffen and Kales[6] published their now famous and widely used manual of terminology and techniques for staging human sleep.

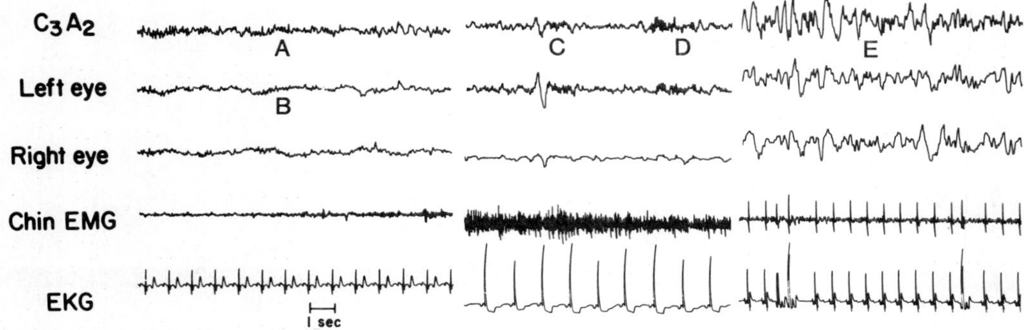

Figure 27-1. Stages of non-REM sleep. C_3A_2 is the EEG channel monitored, and the electro-occulograph channels are labeled left eye and right eye. The left panel shows stage 1 sleep, characterized by **(A)** low-amplitude, mixed-frequency EEG activity and **(B)** slow rolling eye movements. The middle panel shows a brief period of stage 2 sleep characterized by **(C)** K complex and **(D)** sleep spindles. **(E)** The right panel shows a segment of stage 3 or stage 4 sleep characterized by high-amplitude slow waves.

While it is beyond the scope of this text to describe sleep staging in detail, it is important for the student of this discipline to appreciate the basic stages of sleep and some of the differences in body physiology associated with the different stages.

Stages of Sleep

Sleep is classified as either REM or non-REM depending on the presence or absence of rapid eye movements, the amount of muscle tone present, and other characteristics of cortical EEG activity. Non-REM sleep is divided into stages 1 through 4. Stage 1, or light sleep, is a transitional stage often seen between the waking state and other stages of deeper sleep (Fig. 27-1). About 5 to 10 percent of the total night's sleep should be stage 1 (Table 27-1). It is usually the first stage experienced at sleep onset and is often seen preceding or following periods of REM sleep. Slow rolling eye movements may be seen on leads placed over the lateral canthus of the eyes. The respiratory pattern is frequently irregular in normal subjects; this may be related to oscillation between waking and sleeping breathing control mechanisms, including variations in the CO_2 set point. Apneas are frequently seen at sleep onset and are not usually considered pathologic. In addition, patients with severe sleep apnea will experience a high proportion of stage 1 sleep throughout the night since they arouse so frequently and do not progress through the usual stages of sleep.

About 40 to 60 percent of total sleep time should be spent in stage 2 sleep (Table 27-1), during which short bursts of 12 to 14 cycle/s wave activity (sleep spindles) and/or K complexes are superimposed on the underlying EEG pattern (Fig. 27-1). The respiratory pattern of stage 2 is usually quite

Table 27-1. Average Values for Sleep Stage Distribution for Men[a]

Report Indices	Age (yr) 20–29	30–39	40–49	50–59
Time in bed (min)	442 (12.2)	435 (20.5)	429 (39.2)	423 (44.9)
Sleep period time (min)	425 (14.4)	428 (23.2)	414 (36.9)	407 (45.9)
Total sleep time (min)	419 (14.5)	421 (21.9)	389 (46.5)	390 (49.5)
Sleep efficiency index	95% (0.04)	97% (0.02)	91% (0.06)	92% (0.04)
Stage 0 (% SPT)	1.3 (1.1)	1.5 (1.9)	6.2 (5.6)	4.3 (2.3)
Stage 1 (% SPT)	4.4 (1.6)	5.7 (3.4)	7.5 (3.0)	7.5 (3.9)
Stage 2 (% SPT)	45.5 (5.2)	56.9 (7.4)	54.7 (11.1)	61.7 (10.3)
Stage 3 (% SPT)	6.2 (1.4)	5.7 (1.46)	5.4 (3.3)	3.2 (4.8)
Stage 4 (% SPT)	14.5 (4.4)	6.8 (5.2)	3.2 (6.3)	1.6 (3.2)
Stage REM (% SPT)	28.0 (5.7)	23.5 (3.9)	22.8 (4.0)	21.4 (4.0)
Sleep latency onset	14.5 (4.4)	5.8 (3.9)	10.0 (7.9)	11.9 (10.5)

[a] Time in bed (TIB): Time from lights out at night until the subject gets out of bed in the morning. Sleep period time (SPT): Time from first sleep at bedtime until final awakening in the morning. Total sleep time (TST): SPT less any time that the subject spent awake during the night after falling asleep. Sleep efficiency index: TST divided by TIB. Sleep latency onset: Time from lights out until the appearance of the first sleep stage, either stage 1 or stage 2. Numbers in parenthesis are ±1 standard deviation.

(Adapted from Williams et al.,[9] with permission.)

regular but may show some of the same cyclic changes seen in stage 1 sleep. Pathologic apnea may be seen during stage 2 sleep.

Stages 3 and 4 sleep are usually discussed together and termed *slow-wave sleep* because of the characteristic high-amplitude, low-frequency activity on the EEG channel (Fig. 27-1). Indeed, the only difference between stage 3 and stage 4 sleep is in the quantity of these slow waves, stage 3 being 20 to 50 percent and stage 4 more than 50 percent composed of slow-wave activity. Respiration as a rule is very regular during stages 3 and 4 sleep, and apneas are almost never present. Conversely, patients with severe sleep apnea frequently never experience slow-wave sleep. Slow-wave sleep usually occupies 20 percent of sleep in younger people and may decrease to around 5 percent in late middle age (Table 27-1).

The EEG in REM sleep is characterized by high-frequency, low-voltage EEG activity, which appears much like that of stage 1 sleep. Virtually all electromyographic (EMG) leads are silent owing to the diffuse loss of skeletal muscle tone. Phasic bursts of eye movement are present, giving it the name rapid eye movement sleep (Fig. 27-2). Changes in cardiac rate, respiration, and blood pressure occur, which are related to fluctuations in autonomic tone. Bulbocavernosus engorgement causes penile erection in males and is the basis for the study of *nocturnal penile tumescense*.[7] The respiratory control mechanisms during REM sleep, believed to be similar to those active during the awake state, result in irregular rhythm, increased frequency, and decreased tidal volume (V_T).[8] There may be short periods of apnea during the bursts of REM but these are not generally considered pathologic. The dramatic decreases in muscle tone, irregular respiratory control, and autonomic instability make REM sleep more vulnerable to respiratory problems associated with apnea, hypopnea, and oxyhemoglobin desaturation. It is usually during REM sleep that the longest episodes of apnea and the deepest oxyhemoglobin desaturations are seen. REM sleep appears periodically throughout the night, usually starting 90 minutes after sleep onset and recurring at 90-minute intervals.

Disturbances of Normal Sleep Architecture

Sleep architecture refers to the normal distribution and frequency of the above-mentioned sleep stages. Although the patterns of appearance of these stages vary with age and sex, they are well defined in healthy individuals[9] (Table 27-1). Thus, we are able to recognize disturbances of sleep architectural patterns in disease states affecting sleep. Such nocturnal breathing disorders as sleep apnea and chronic lung disease will interfere with usual sleep patterns by creating frequent arousals from a given stage as well as frequent shifts from one stage to another. These arousals and stage shifts usually go unrecognized by the patient but may become manifest as feelings of "poor sleep" or of not feeling "rested" after a night's sleep. For example, termination of

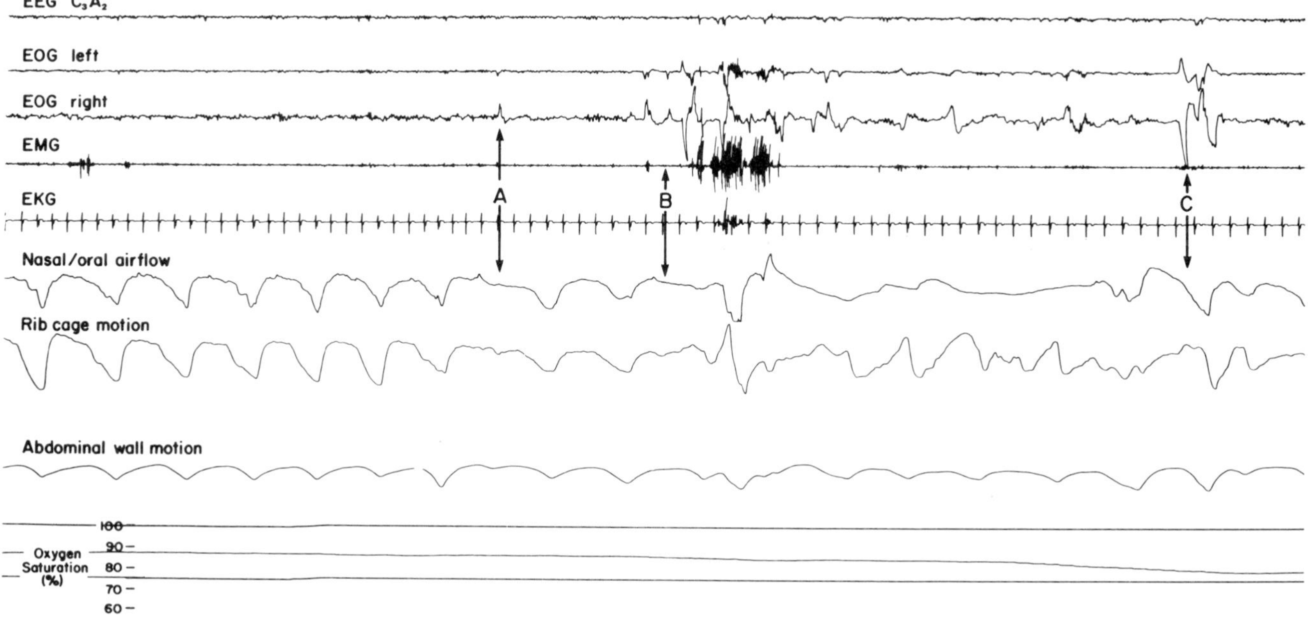

Figure 27-2. REM sleep, characterized by low-amplitude, mixed-frequency EEG waves (top channel) with absent EMG activity (fourth channel) and bursts of REM (second and third channels). Of note are the areas of **(A)** hypopnea and **(B & C)** apnea, coinciding with bursts of eye movement. The effect of these disordered breathing events is evidenced by the fall in SaO_2 on the bottom channel. (From Fletcher,[74] with permission.)

each apnea episode in patients with obstructive sleep apnea requires transient arousal from the sleep stage.

While the patient may not be aware that the EEG manifests an arousal pattern for several seconds after each apneic episode, 400 to 500 such episodes during the night accompanied by as many arousals certainly constitute a radical interruption of the usual sleep architecture. In addition, these frequent arousals in some way prevent progression through the usual sequence of sleep stages, and thus a patient with severe sleep apnea may never progress beyond stage 1 and 2 sleep, never experience or undergo only small amounts of slow-wave sleep, and have fragmentation of REM sleep periods.[10] While there is tacit acceptance of this disturbance of sleep architecture as the cause of daytime hypersomnolence so frequently seen in the more severe cases of obstructive sleep apnea, two recent studies[11] have challenged this concept. Orr and Martin,[11] examining the EEGs of patients with similar degrees of apnea and disturbance of sleep architecture, found the major difference between "sleepy" and "nonsleepy" patients to be the degree of nocturnal oxyhemoglobin desaturation, those with worse desaturation having the more marked symptoms. A similar study in the elderly supports this concept.[12] Likewise, the usual sleep architecture of patients with severe chronic obstructive pulmonary disease (COPD) may be interrupted by frequent arousals, stage shifts, maldistribution of stages, and decreased occurrence of slow-wave and REM sleep.

An interesting finding is the effect of hospitalization on normal sleep architecture. Williams[13] has reviewed recent publications on the effect of intensive care hospitalization on patients' sleep EEG. To summarize the findings of several studies, there is a generalized decrease in sleep efficiency (total sleep time in relation to total time in bed), marked fragmentation of sleep, a higher percentage of stage 1 and 2 sleep, a low percentage and fewer periods of REM sleep, and a conspicuous absence of stage 3 and 4 sleep. For example, Elwell et al. studied five open-heart surgery patients for 3 nights before surgery, while in the recovery room, and for 4 consecutive nights after transfer from the recovery room.[14] There was no slow-wave sleep before surgery or after surgery. In addition, REM sleep was markedly decreased and fragmented, and neither REM sleep nor slow-wave sleep had returned to anywhere near expected baseline levels during the period of the study. It has been postulated that "ICU [intensive care unit] psychosis" may result from this intense disturbance of sleep architecture and sleep deprivation.

The typical report from a sleep laboratory studying patients for sleep pathology will include information on the latency to sleep onset (which may be altered in patients with apnea and lung disease), percentage of total time spent in sleep, distribution of sleep stages, number, type, and duration of apneas, and the presence of cardiac arrhythmias. Minimal oxyhemoglobin desaturation associated with respiratory events should be included, and new on-line analysis of nocturnal oxyhemoglobin desaturation allows specific quantitation of the time spent at chosen level of saturation.[15] All the above information should be evaluated in the light of clinical symptoms, medical history, and condition of the patient in order to arrive at appropriate therapeutic decisions.

RESPIRATORY CONTROL AND THE PATHOPHYSIOLOGY OF APNEA DURING SLEEP

Regulation of Ventilation during Sleep

Since the early 1980s rapid progress has been made in the understanding of events leading to abnormalities of respiration during sleep in such disease states as obstructive and central sleep apnea and chronic lung disease. To appreciate the process leading to sleep respiratory abnormalities, one must have some basic understanding of the control of breathing during sleep and how it varies from awake control. The key to acute changes in breathing control during all stages of alertness and sleep is peripheral receptor chemosensitivity to CO_2 and, to a lesser extent, levels of oxygenation. An excellent review on the control of breathing and the effects of sleep on such control is available.[8]

Basically, the central respiratory controller located in the medullary center regulates breathing by a complicated system of feedback receptors and output effectors.[16] The feedback receptors include a variety of chemoreceptors (peripheral aortic and carotid), which are sensitive to acute blood gas changes and central chemoreceptors, which are more attuned to chronic breathing control. In addition, a variety of peripheral mechanoreceptors located in the lungs, in the proximal and distal airways, and probably in skeletal muscles send continuous signals to the central respiratory controller regarding the adequacy of respiration. One major difference in respiratory control in the waking versus sleeping states is that in the former cerebral cortical activity is continuously superimposed on the more basic, automatic control of breathing. Thus, the volitional acts of speaking, breath holding, hypoventilation, and hyperventilation may supersede the respiratory controller's drive to maintain chemical and mechanical homeostasis.

During sleep the level of respiration is predominantly dependent on peripheral chemoreceptor sensitivity, especially to the CO_2 set point. During non-REM sleep, there is an approximate 3 to 9 mmHg increase in basal CO_2 level due to alveolar hypoventilation. Such hypoventilation results from a reduction in the output of the central respiratory controller, coinciding with loss of the cortical drive of wakefulness.[17] A similar degree of hypoventilation occurs in patients with chronic CO_2 retention states such as chronic alveolar hypoventilation and COPD.[18] Controlling mechanisms during REM sleep are much harder to evaluate because of the inherent variation in respiration during this stage. Obvious differences in respiratory control within REM sleep are exhibited by the marked tendency to apnea and hypoventilation during the phasic bursts of rapid eye movement and more stable breathing of tonic REM sleep

(Fig. 27-2). In general, however, studies show that acute ventilatory responsiveness is even further depressed during REM sleep[19,20] (Fig. 27-3).

Periodic Breathing and the Apnea Threshold

To understand the mechanisms basic to both central and obstructive apnea, knowledge of the concepts of periodic

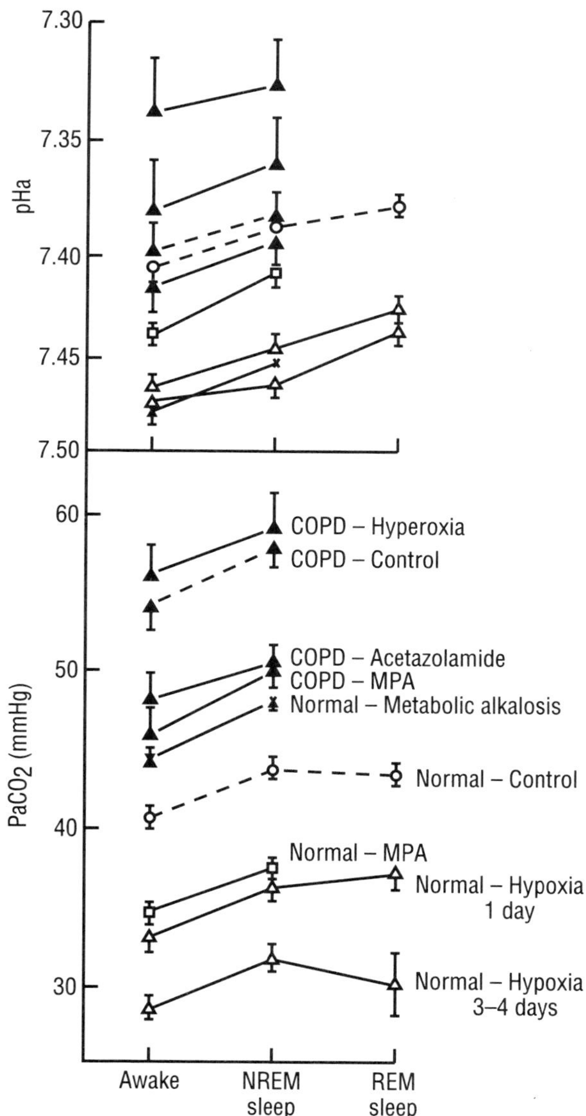

Figure 27-3. The effect of sleep state under various conditions on $PaCO_2$ and arterial pH (pHa). Under all conditions (normal, COPD, COPD with hyperoxia, acetazolamide, MPA), there is a fall in pH and an increase in $PaCO_2$ during non-REM (NREM) sleep. The change is more variable during REM sleep. MPA, medroxyprogesterone. (From Dempsey and Skatrud,[18] with permission.)

breathing and the apnea threshold is required. When a normal person is exposed to hypoxia, as at high altitude, a well known phenomenon known as *periodic breathing* results during sleep.[21,22] This consists of alternating short periods of hypopnea or apnea followed by short periods of hyperventilation. A somewhat similar phenomenon observed during both the awake and asleep states is Cheyne-Stokes breathing, the mechanism of which has been well described by Cherniak and colleagues.[23] Briefly, what happens is that the primary stimulus, hypoxia, induces a brief hyperventilation, which in turn elevates arterial O_2 tension (PaO_2) and lowers arterial CO_2 tension ($PaCO_2$). Since the peripheral and medullary chemoreceptors are highly sensitive to $PaCO_2$, respiratory drive is immediately reduced, which results in hypoventilation or apnea until $PaCO_2$ increases to its central set point and the stimulus to breathe again returns.

The level below which $PaCO_2$ must fall to result in decreased respiratory motor output (which in turn inhibits breathing) is termed the *apnea threshold*.[18] During this period of apnea or hypopnea, arterial oxyhemoglobin saturation (SaO_2) may fall, adding an additional stimulus to the tendency to postapneic hyperventilation (Fig. 27-4). This apnea threshold is present during both sleep and awake states but is not so obvious during awake breathing because of the masking effect of volitional cortical control of breathing. A classic description of the interaction of arterial hypoxia, hypocapnia, and hypercapnia in producing periodic breathing and central apnea was recently published by Dempsey and Skatrud[18] and is recommended for further understanding of this important concept.

The gap in our understanding of the relationship between central and obstructive apnea is rapidly narrowing. In order to understand this relationship, one should have knowledge of the relationship of upper airway anatomy and physiology to airway patency during sleep.

Mechanisms of Apnea during Sleep

The reason that some people obstruct their upper airways during inspiration while asleep yet others do not is not completely known. Observations of the anatomic and functional behavior of the airway have been made in both the physiologic and the pathologic state. From these we have come to understand the mechanism for obstruction to be a *balance* between negative inspiratory forces (pressures) within the airway, tending to collapse the pharynx, and forces tending to maintain airway patency (constriction of the pharyngeal muscles), resulting in airway dilatation. Inspiration is a complex action, involving contraction of the diaphragm with downward movement that creates negative intrathoracic pressure, which is transmitted to the pharynx (Fig. 27-5). At the same time, the pharyngeal muscles contract, "holding open" the pharynx and allowing inward airflow. If for any reason the negative pressure exceeds the constricting forces tending to keep the airway open, there is inspiratory collapse and airflow stops, resulting in obstructive apnea. Occlusion is felt to result from an *imbalance* of forces, which favor

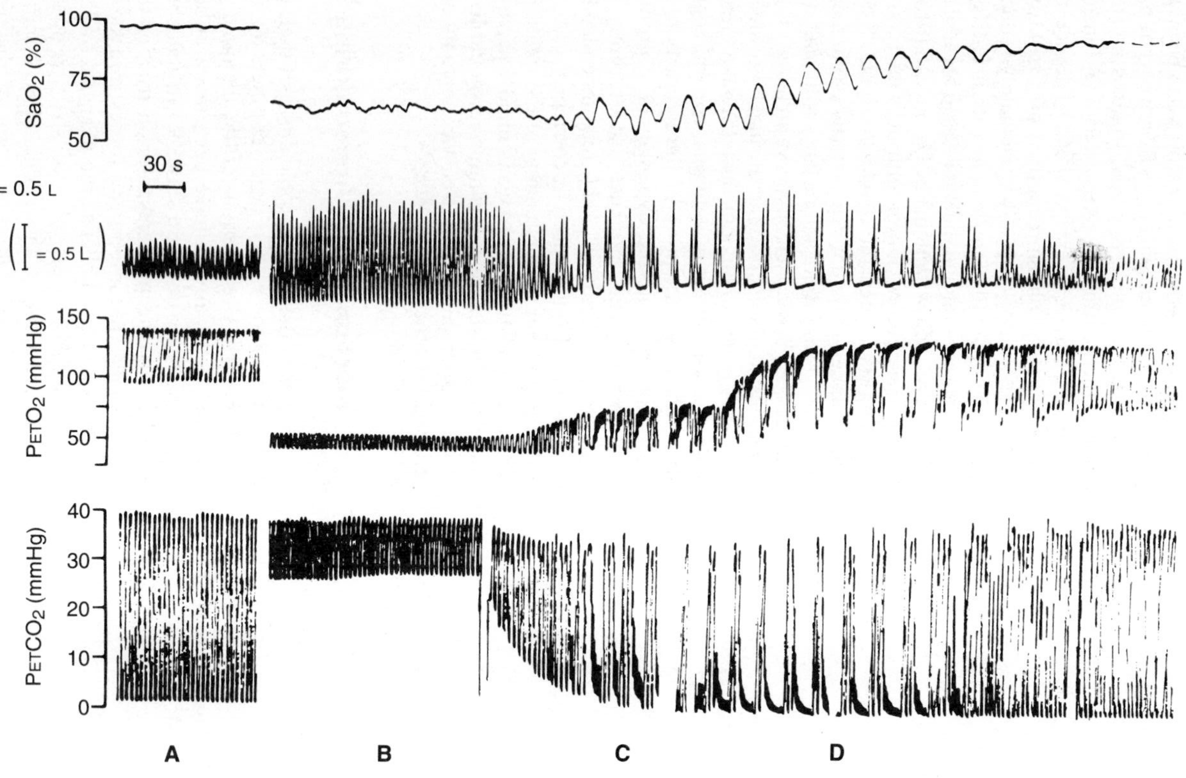

Figure 27-4. The development of periodic breathing (central apnea) in a normal (non-REM) sleeping subject in response to induced hypoxia. **(A)** normoxia showing the baseline SaO_2 (top channel), normal V_T (second channel), baseline end-tidal PO_2 ($P_{ET}O_2$) (third channel), and baseline $P_{ET}CO_2$ (bottom channel). **(B)** Isocapnic hypoxia (induced by lowering the inspired O_2 fraction (F_IO_2) and addition of CO_2 to breathing mixture). V_T and respiratory rate increase while SaO_2 and $P_{ET}O_2$ fall. Respiration remains regular. **(C)** Addition of CO_2 to the breathing mixture is stopped and the CO_2 is allowed to fall. This results first in a cyclic breathing pattern followed by 10-second central apneas as CO_2 oscillates above and below the apnea threshold. **(D)** Restoration of normoxia initially prolongs the apneic episodes, but as CO_2 rises above the apnea threshold, normal breathing rhythm is restored. (From Dempsey and Skatrud,[18] with permission.)

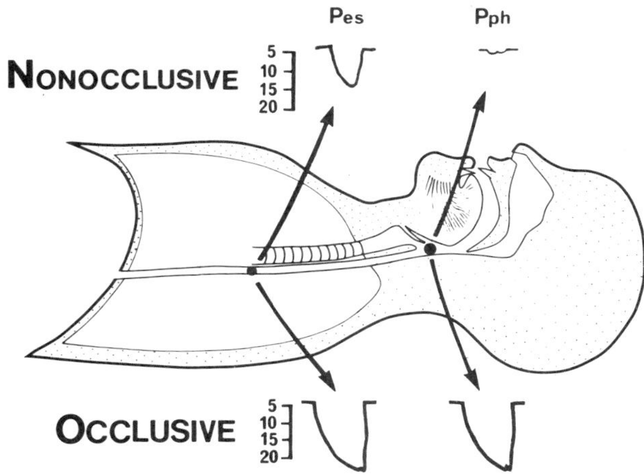

Figure 27-5. Diagram illustrating the transmission of negative pressure from the thoracic space through the trachea into the pharynx. With a patent airway (marked Pes and Pph), there are only small variations in hypopharyngeal pressure during inspiration. With a narrow airway or high resistance, thoracic pressure is transmitted to the pharynx. (From Block et al.,[26] with permission.)

those that promote airway closure and overcome those directed at maintaining patency. The occlusion is broken when the imbalance is overcome by changes in pharyngeal muscle tone brought about by arousal, as well as by increased inspiratory pressure.

Remmers and colleagues[24] have provided the classic description of this mechanism. Figure 27-6 shows peak genioglossal EMG activity plotted against simultaneous intrapharyngeal *negative* pressure during numerous inspiratory efforts. Those efforts resulting in occlusion (open circles) all fall to the left (representing a high pressure/EMG activity ratio) and those resulting in airflow (closed circles) fall to the right (representing a low pressure/EMG activity ratio) of a 45-degree line. Put simply, if the ratio of negative inspiratory pressure to pharyngeal muscle activity is high, obstruction will result. If the ratio is low, patency of the airway will be maintained throughout inspiration. Figure 27-7 shows hysteresis loops (recorded during continuous measurement of EMG activity and airway pressure throughout the entire inspiratory-expiratory cycle) of several breaths during periods of increased pharyngeal resistance. At a pharyngeal resistance of 49, the inspiratory pressure/EMG activity ratio remains low and to the right of the line of identity, and no obstruction results. As pharyngeal resistance increases, the inspiratory limb of the loop falls near the line describing occlusion. At high resistances the inspiratory portion of the loop crosses the line of identity, and occlusion results.

One can readily see that anything that increases negative intrapharyngeal pressure during inspiration (increased resistance upstream, such as may be due to nasal occlusion or to narrowing of the nasopharyngeal airway) or lowers EMG activity (alcohol, hypoxia, central factors) will tend to produce occlusion. It is easy to see from these studies how mechanical factors may predispose to occlusion, especially the subtle anatomic narrowing that has been theorized to occur in obese patients (Table 27-2). Anatomic narrowing leads to increased airway resistance. Overcoming this requires more negative inspiratory pressure. This results in a greater tendency toward collapse of this compliant airway if pharyngeal muscle tone does not increase to meet the demand. In addition, multiple functional factors have been shown to influence upper airway closure (Table 27-3).

Interaction of Central and Peripheral Mechanisms in Sleep Apnea

Can there be a relationship between the two distinct types of apnea—*central*, in which there is no central respiratory output and hence no respiratory effort (described above under periodic breathing), and *obstructive*, in which central respiratory output is at maximum but pharyngeal closure prevents airflow? This point is addressed in Dempsey and Skatrud's[18] discussion of the underlying chemical mechanisms that relate periodic breathing to obstructive sleep apnea. The initial event appears to be a slight fall in blood O_2 tension such as might result during the onset of the mild hypopnea that accompanies the beginning of stage 2 sleep. In normal subjects the onset of mild hypoxemia, while tend-

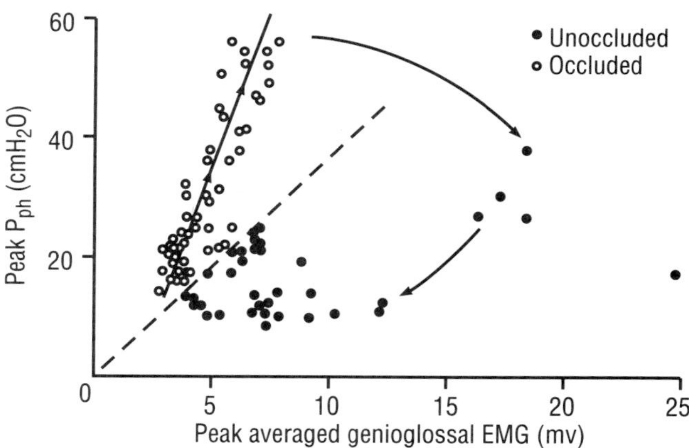

Figure 27-6. Linear regression analysis of peak negative intrapharyngeal pressure versus peak averaged genioglossal EMG activity during five obstructed respiratory cycles. The open circles represent occluded efforts and the closed circles represent unoccluded efforts. The line of identity separates occluded from unoccluded efforts and arrows indicate the time sequence (beginning at the far right). As the ratio of pressure/EMG activity increases (moves to the left), the tendency to collapse the airway becomes greater until the ratio passes the line of identity and all breaths are obstructed. As respiratory effort increases, EMG activity also increases (moves back to the right), and finally the obstructed breaths are broken as the pressure/EMG ratio decreases. (From Remmers et al.,[24] with permission.)

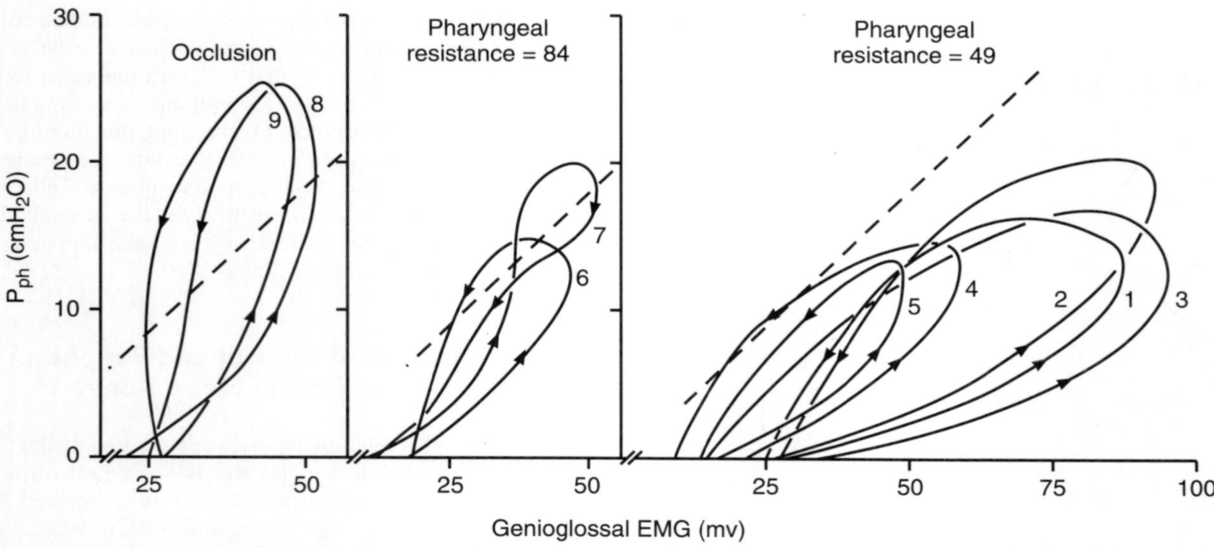

Figure 27-7. Hysteresis loops of pressure versus EMG activity of nine consecutive breaths in the same patient whose patterns are shown in Figure 27-6. Each loop represents a single complete breath, with inspiration moving up and to the right and expiration down and to the left. Breaths 1 through 5 are unobstructed (all are to the right of the obstruction line) and have a low pressure/EMG activity ratio. Breaths 6 and 7 move closer to the obstruction line (moderate pressure/EMG ratio), and pharyngeal resistance is noted to have increased over that of the right panel. The inspiratory limbs of breaths 8 and 9 cross the occlusion line, and no airflow occurs as these breaths are occluded (high pressure/EMG ratio). (From Remmers et al.,[24] with permission.)

Table 27-2. Mechanical Factors Influencing Pharyngeal Closure

Compliance: The tone of the pharyngeal muscles has the most direct effect on compliance of the upper airway. The oropharynx is the most compliant area and therefore has the greatest tendency to collapse when muscular tone decreases, as during REM sleep.[25]

Surface Adhesive Forces: Once opposing mucosal surfaces approximate, the force needed to overcome mechanical resistance to opening is greater. Thus, anatomically smaller airways may require higher muscular tone to maintain patency.[26]

Airway Configuration: Both change in body position from upright to supine and forward flexion of the neck reduce upper airway cross-sectional area.[27,28]

Anatomic Narrowing: Aside from obvious anatomic narrowing of the pharyngeal airway from strictures, retroplacement or shortening of the mandible (retroagnathia), and tumors, evidence of anatomic narrowing of the airway has been well demonstrated by computed tomography (CT).[29,30] This does not appear to be a simple matter of increased fat in the airway, but it may be a combination of fat and/or tissue edema and chronic inflammation resulting from the repeated vibrational trauma of snoring (Cohen M, personal communication).

Upper Airway Resistance: As resistance to airflow above the level of the pharynx increases, the negative pressure required to meet airflow requirements also increases. Thus, blockage of the nasal passage resulting from mucosal swelling (rhinitis) or nasal packs for bleeding may contribute to inspiratory obstruction.[31,32]

ing to induce periodic breathing as discussed above, stimulates the upper airway pharyngeal muscles to maintain airway patency.

Snoring patients, who have a reduced upper airway cross-sectional area because of either low upper airway muscle tone and/or actual anatomic airway narrowing, show a different response to hypoxia. In such patients the onset of non-REM sleep alone increases pharyngeal airway resistance about 10-fold, probably owing to sleep-related relaxation of pharyngeal muscles (Table 27-3). Both hypoxemia and elevation of systemic blood pressure have been described with snoring.[40,41] The hypoxemia stimulates ventilation, resulting in mild hypocapnia (which would tend to depress ventilation), but the net effect is increased ventilatory drive and upper airway tone. The subsequent hyperpnea allows a greater fall in PCO_2, causing decreased upper airway pharyngeal muscle stimulation with reduced diaphragmatic activity. This leads to a large increase in upper airway resistance with low respiratory drive, causing obstructive hypopnea. The subsequent hypoxia causes reflex hyperpnea, during which upper airway resistance falls (hypoxic stimulation of upper airway muscles) and ventilatory drive increases (increased diaphragmatic EMG). If these oscillations in PCO_2 following hyperpnea continue but the lowest PCO_2 remains above the central apnea threshold, obstructive hypopneas result. If PCO_2 falls below the central apnea thresh-

Table 27-3. Functional Factors Affecting Upper Airway Tone

Lung Volume: Increasing lung volume has a negative feedback inhibition on selected pharyngeal muscles. Thus, at inappropriately low lung volumes for a given respiratory effort, stimulation of the upper airway muscles to maintain patency (and avoid obstruction) will continue.[33]

Chemosensitivity: Pharyngeal muscle tone increases with hypercapnia, hypoxemia, or both (asphyxia). Conversely, hypocapnia lowers upper airway muscle tone. Thus, cyclical changes in $PaCO_2$ and lowering of $PaCO_2$ below the *central apnea threshold* (see text) could create an imbalance of forces, leading to airway closure.[33]

Upper Airway Receptors: Three types of pharyngeal receptors cause stimulation of upper airway tonic muscle activity: pressure receptors responding to negative intrapharyngeal pressure, flow receptors responding to temperature changes in the airway, and proprioceptors activated by laryngeal movements. With the exception of the flow receptors, obstruction to airflow would result in activation of these receptors and stimulation of pharyngeal dilator muscles.[34]

Pharmacologic Agents: General anesthetics, alcohol, and sedatives (diazepam) have been well demonstrated to decrease upper airway muscle activity, thus predisposing to the development of inspiratory obstruction.[35–38] Conversely, protriptyline increases upper airway muscle activity.[39]

State of Wakefulness: There is differential activation and suppression of respiratory muscle activity with sleep onset. For example, both tonic and phasic upper airway muscle activity decrease with the onset of non-REM sleep, while diaphragm activity remains constant. REM sleep is accompanied by a further decrease in upper airway muscle tone. Thus, the sleep state produces a tendency toward increased upper airway resistance while preserving forces tending to maintain negative inspiratory pressure.[33]

old, central apneas result. A graphic example of the relationship of central periodic breathing, hypoxia, hypocapnia, and obstructive hypopneas can be found in Dempsey and Skatrud's work.[18]

This theory of the relationship of central respiratory drive to neural control of pharyngeal airway patency finally allows abandonment of the simplistic view of pure anatomic airway narrowing as a cause of obstructive apnea. We can now combine mechanical *and* functional factors with the long suspected disturbances of central respiratory control. For example, a 1986 publication by Issa and Sullivan[42] shows that the use of nasal continuous positive airway pressure (CPAP), which in effect "splints" the airway open during obstructed inspiration, will also relieve apneas of *central* origin. Attempts are now being made to explain the origin of mixed apneas and their relationship to both central and obstructive apnea.[43] Other authors are now addressing the effects of hypercapnia and hyperoxia on differential stimulation of upper airway muscles versus diaphragmatic and chest wall muscle drive in altering obstructive apnea.[44]

SLEEP RESPIRATORY DYSFUNCTION ASSOCIATED WITH CHRONIC LUNG DISEASE

Obstructive sleep apnea is a popular topic and tends to receive the greatest amount of the attention given to sleep-disordered breathing. Nonapneic oxyhemoglobin desaturation during sleep in patients with chronic lung disease will become an increasingly popular topic, if not because of the rapid increase in knowledge about it, then because of the sheer numbers of patients with lung disease for whom nocturnal desaturation will become a clinical issue.

Patterns of Nocturnal Desaturation in Patients with Chronic Lung Disease

Patients with abnormal lungs or chest wall bellows (Table 27-4) have two types of oxyhemoglobin desaturation, frequent short episodes and long periods of nonapneic desaturation. The more common short desaturation episodes last from a few seconds to a few minutes and are related to either obstructive or central hypopnea.[57] These episodes tend to be frequent throughout both non-REM and REM sleep and usually cause only mild desaturation (Fig. 27-8), which is easily corrected by low-flow supplemental O_2 and probably places no major stress on the cardiovascular system.

The longer desaturation episodes occur mainly during REM sleep and are uniformly associated with decreased respiratory effort[45,58] (Fig. 27-9). They too are often corrected by low-flow O_2.[59] No specific waking pulmonary function test can predict which patients with COPD will show REM-related desaturation during sleep. However, patients who are "blue bloaters" and patients with daytime resting arterial hypoxemia are more likely to be affected than patients with a "pink puffer" appearance.[60–62] In patients with advanced

Table 27-4. Chronic Disease of the Lung and Thorax Associated with Nonapneic Oxyhemoglobin Desaturation

Diseases of the Lung Parenchyma
- COPD[44]
- Interstitial fibrosis[45,46]
- Cystic fibrosis[47,48]

Diseases of the Chest Wall Bellows
- Bilateral diaphragmatic paralysis[49,50]
- Kyphoscoliosis[51,52]
- Myasthenia gravis[53]
- Muscular dystrophy[49,54]
- Myotonic dystrophy[55]
- Postpoliomyelitis[56]

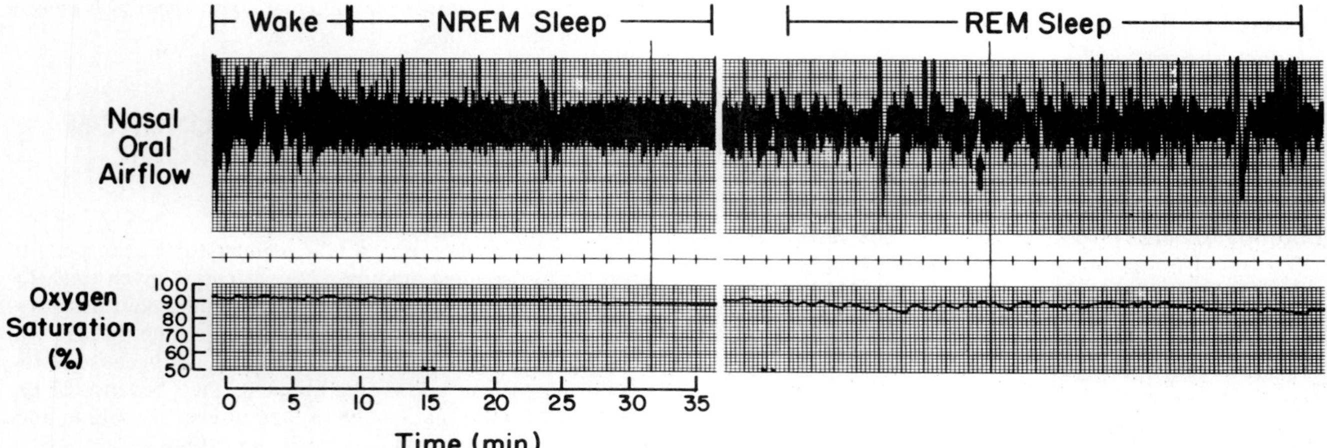

Figure 27-8. Slow speed (3 mm/min) strip chart recording of SaO_2 (bottom panel) measured by ear oximeter, and nasal airflow (top panel) measured by thermistor. While the patient, who has COPD, is awake, respiration is irregular (cortical modulation) and SaO_2 remains above 90 percent. During non-REM sleep, respiration is regular and SaO_2 is stable at around 90 percent. During REM sleep, respiration is again irregular, with frequent short hypopneas (arrow) and consequent 2 to 6 percent drops in SaO_2. These short hypopneas and mild desaturation are probably of little hemodynamic consequence. (From Fletcher,[74] with permission.)

COPD, altered respiratory drives, including blunted hypercarbic and hypoxic drives, have been shown to correlate with nocturnal desaturation.[63–65] A 1987 study examined the occurrence of REM-related oxyhemoglobin desaturation in patients with chronic lung disease and a PaO_2 above 60 mmHg.[66] This study identified a history of chronic bronchitis, lower daytime PO_2, and higher PCO_2 as factors predictive of desaturation.

Mechanisms of Desaturation during REM Sleep

There has been much debate over the cause of REM-related oxyhemoglobin desaturation. Since hypoxemia must result from either alveolar hypoventilation or abnormalities of gas exchange, one or both of these hypoxia-causing mechanisms must account for the desaturation. Alveolar hypoventilation can be recognized by the accompanying increase in $PaCO_2$ and decrease in airflow parameters. There is no doubt that some degree of alveolar hypoventilation occurs during REM sleep in patients with chronic lung disease. Direct measurements of minute ventilation during REM sleep by inductance plethysmography have shown at least a 25 percent decrease in minute ventilation in such patients.[45] Other authors claim that alveolar hypoventilation accounts for almost all the hypoxemia.[67] One piece of evidence against this is the lack of significant CO_2 retention, which should result from alveolar hypoventilation. Direct measurement of $PaCO_2$ during REM sleep desaturation in COPD patients showed only a 3.2 mmHg increase. A graphic representation of the minimal increase in PCO_2 as measured by a transcutaneous CO_2 electrode can be seen in an article by Goldstein and colleagues.[58] Another piece of evidence against pure alveolar hypoventilation during REM sleep is the relatively complete correction of desaturation by low-flow supplemental O_2.[45]

Koo et al.,[68] who were among the first authors to publish an accurate description of REM desaturation in COPD patients, proposed, on the basis of calculated decreases in the alveolar to arterial O_2 gradient [$P(A\text{-}a)O_2$], that deterioration in gas exchange occurs during REM sleep. Flick and Block[69] have reported similar findings. By using a slightly more sophisticated measure of gas exchange, simultaneous mixed venous and arterial blood gases were drawn before and during the REM sleep desaturations and used to calculate venous admixture. A clear increase in venous admixture demonstrated that worsening ventilation/perfusion ($\dot{V}/\dot{Q}$) mismatch accounts for a large portion of the desaturation seen in COPD patients.[45]

The actual mechanism of REM desaturation is not well understood but is probably closely related to lung volume during sleep. Generalized muscle paralysis or decreased tone is a physiologic occurrence during REM sleep and has been demonstrated in normal sleeping infants,[70] normal adults, patients with cystic fibrosis, and patients with COPD by a variety of methods.[48,71–73] Teleologically, this may represent the body's effort to protect itself against injury by not allowing sleepers to act out their dreams. In normal subjects this small drop in muscle tone probably causes a mild decrease in functional residual capacity (FRC), which is not noticed because the lungs stay well above closing volume (CV).

Below CV, the point at which some airways collapse owing to low alveolar volume and high surface tension, maldistribution of ventilation results in lowering of $\dot{V}/\dot{Q}$ relationships and perhaps outright shunting. In the chronic bron-

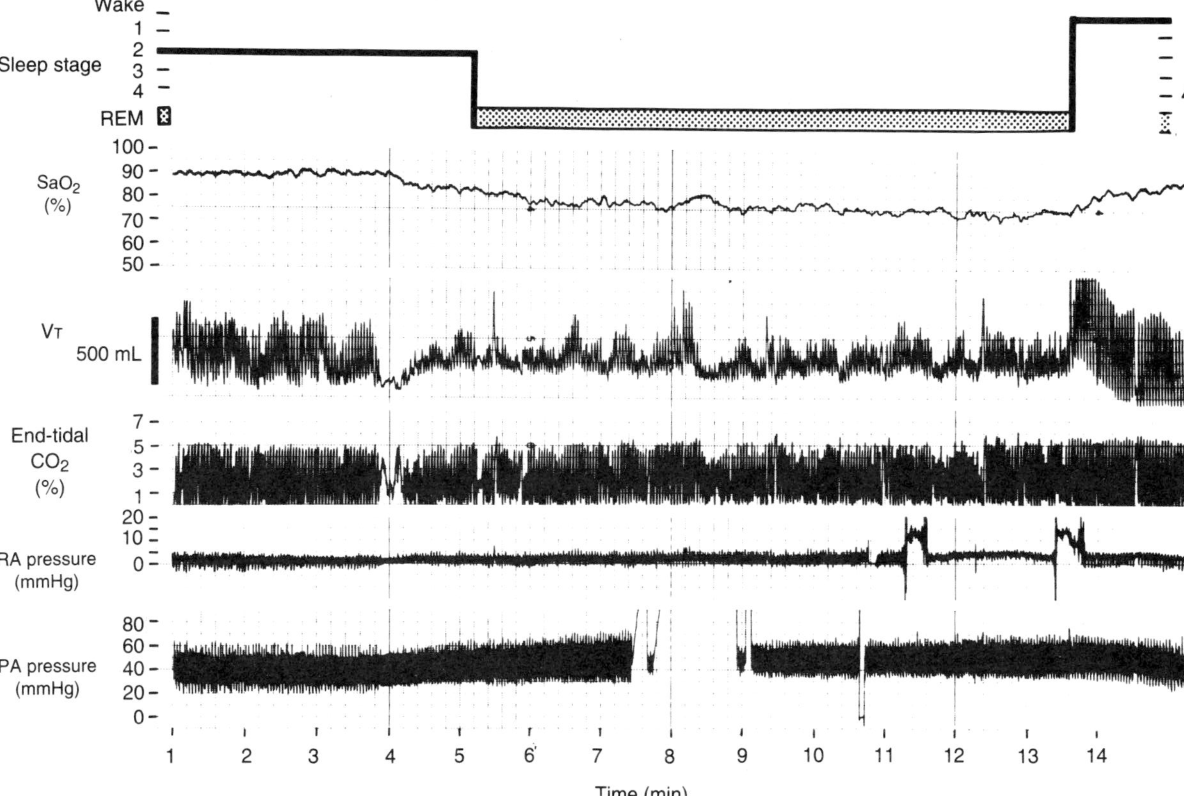

Figure 27-9. Transition in breathing pattern from non-REM to REM sleep in a patient with severe COPD and daytime hypoxemia. Coinciding approximately with EEG-scored REM sleep is a short apnea, followed by irregular breathing with alternating hypopnea and hyperpnea (see V_T). The SaO_2 falls progressively to just below 75 percent. Upon arousal, supranormal V_T levels result in resaturation. Note that end-tidal CO_2 barely increases. The fine negative deflections seen beneath the heavy solid line representing right atrial (RA) pressure (second channel from bottom) in non-REM sleep are a result of negative inspiratory efforts. These decrease or drop out during REM sleep, indicating a decrease in central breathing drive during that stage. The transient increase in pulmonary artery pressure (bottom channel) should also be noted. (From Fletcher et al.,[45] with permission.)

chitic form of COPD, gas exchange is already abnormal, and a high FRC compensates for loss of elastic recoil. This high FRC keeps many alveoli above CV, which is increased in COPD patients. CV also increases with age and with the supine position. Since the diaphragm is flattened in many COPD patients, loss in intercostal muscle tone also would predictably have a greater effect than in normal subjects. Added to this is the hypoventilation from the decreased V_T. When the subject emerges from REM sleep, muscle tone returns, FRC increases to pre-REM levels, ventilation distribution improves, and hypoventilated alveoli re-expand, correcting the $\dot{V}/\dot{Q}$ mismatch (Fig. 27-10). One can easily see how the abnormal bellows of chest wall disease would cause a similar REM-related desaturation.

Other factors may contribute to the development of nocturnal hypoxemia in COPD patients, and although extensive discussion of these is beyond the scope of this chapter, appropriate references provide additional sources of information. Entering sleep at a low position on the oxyhemoglobin dissociation curve by virtue of bad gas exchange or CO_2 retention from alveolar hypoventilation would tend to cause greater nocturnal desaturation. This is because a fall in PaO_2 starting on the steep portion of the curve causes a much greater decrease in SaO_2 than an equivalent fall in PaO_2 beginning on the flat portion of the curve.[74] Airway resistance both in the lower airways[75] and upper airways[76] may increase during REM sleep, adding to the work of breathing and contributing to hypoxemia. A depressed cough reflex[77] and decreased mucociliary clearance[78] may allow pooling of secretions, which adds to ventilation maldistribution. Chemoresponsiveness may be further depressed during REM sleep, which interferes with the patient's ability to compensate for progressive hypoxemia.[79]

EFFECTS OF SLEEP DISORDERS ON CARDIOVASCULAR FUNCTION

While the daytime symptoms of obstructive sleep apnea may be quite bothersome and embarrassing to the patient, the cardiac and hemodynamic sequelae may be of much

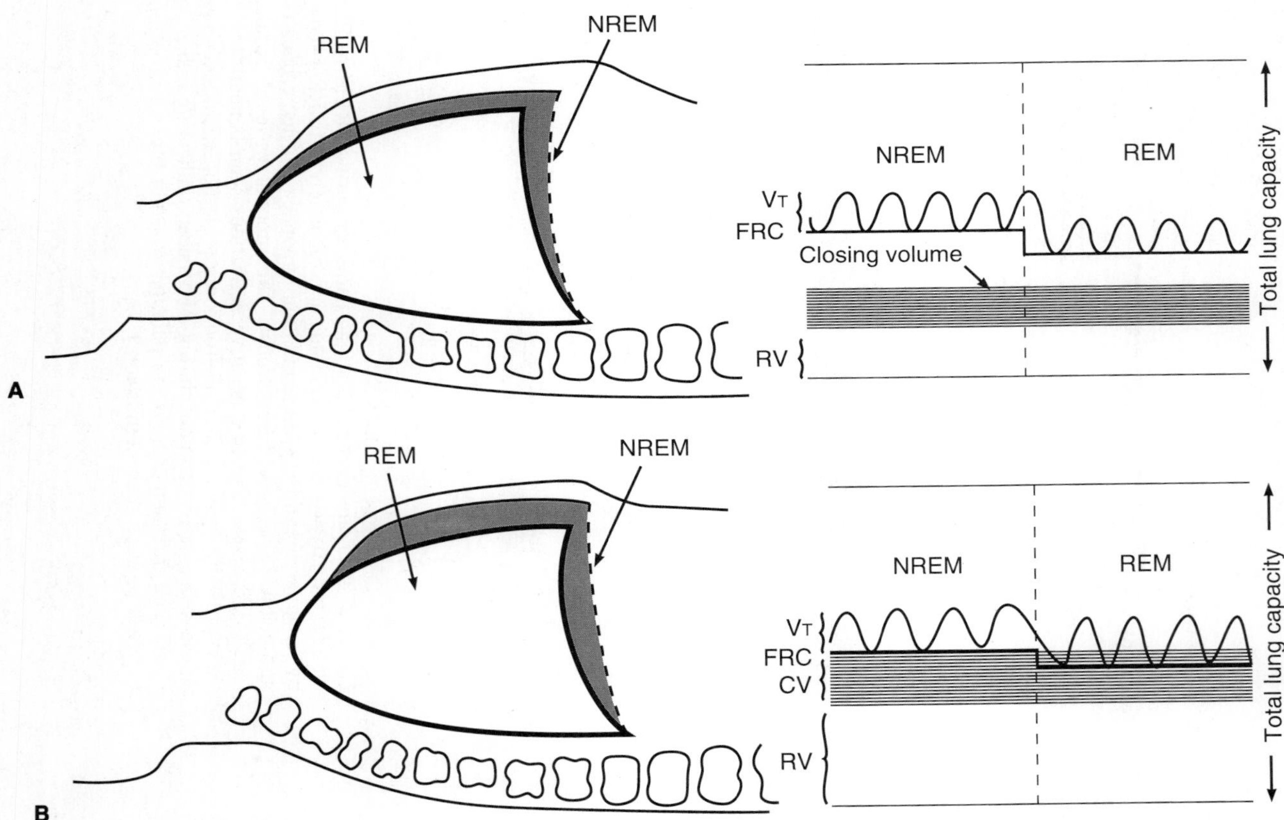

Figure 27-10. Diagrammatic representation of the thorax in transition from non-REM (NREM) to REM sleep in **(A)** normal patients and **(B)** patients with COPD. Although FRC falls during REM sleep in both situations, it remains above closing volume (CV) in normal subjects, and ventilation distribution remains adequate to maintain SaO_2. In the patient with COPD, the fall in FRC places many lung units below closing volume, and maldistribution of ventilation occurs, lowering the $\dot{V}/\dot{Q}$ ratio. This, in combination with hypoventilation, results in hypoxemia. (From Fletcher,[74] with permission.)

greater concern, since the ultimate expression of these may be death. These sequelae can be conveniently separated into three categories: (1) the effect on the systemic circulation (systemic hypertension); (2) the effect on the pulmonary circulation (pulmonary hypertension, cor pulmonale), and (3) the effect on the heart (ventricular irritability with arrhythmias and conduction abnormalities).

Effects on Systemic Arterial Pressures

The normal response of systemic pressure to sleep is a gradual fall in both systolic and diastolic pressure by about one-third until early morning, at which time the pressure gradually returns to baseline waking levels.[80] This is also true in hypertensive patients. However, acute elevation in systemic pressure immediately coincides with apneic hypoxemia and is presumed to result from generalized sympathetic discharge. Shepard[81] has shown the acute increase to be fairly uniform among apnea patients, both systolic and diastolic pressure increasing by about 25 percent. There is a high correlation with the degree of desaturation; however, owing to a great variability among subjects, it can only account for 30 percent of this increase. A subacute elevation in systemic pressure may occur over the course of the night in patients with frequent or repetitive apnea. That is, their pressure may not return to baseline following rapidly repetitive apnea and the usual diurnal fall in systemic pressure will be lost[82] (Fig. 27-11).

In addition to abnormalities of nocturnal systemic pressure, sustained daytime systemic hypertension is seen in up to 50 percent of patients with obstructive sleep apnea syndrome. Tracheostomy reverses this phenomenon and can cure the sustained systemic hypertension. Recent evidence indicates that both the nocturnal elevations and the sustained daytime systemic hypertension may result from increased sympathetic tone.[83] Three independent studies have investigated the incidence of sleep apnea among middle-aged men with essential hypertension to determine if occult sleep apnea could be a significant contributor to this problem[84–86] (Fig. 27-12). All three studies agree that in this population there is about a 30 percent incidence of obstructive sleep apnea. However, one cannot be certain of the contribution of apnea to hypertension for two reasons: the definition of "significant" apnea varies according to the author (more than 5 episodes per hour, more than 10 per hour, etc.) and although the hypertension was ameliorated in the majority of cases, it was not always cured by treatment of the apnea.

Effects on the Pulmonary Circulation

The acute pulmonary vascular response to the asphyxia created by apnea is pulmonary artery vasoconstriction mediated by local receptors in the lung. This, of course, increases pulmonary artery resistance, pulmonary artery pressure, and right ventricular afterload. Another contributing factor to right ventricular strain may be the greater preload from increased venous return as a result of the high negative intrathoracic pressure created by the Mueller maneuver (inspiration against a closed glottis). Cinefluoroscopic increase in heart size has been demonstrated.[87] The subacute rise in pressure that is seen in the systemic circulation over the course of the night has been described for the pulmonary circulation as well[82,88] (Fig. 27-11).

The contribution of nocturnal hypoxemia from pure obstructive sleep apnea to chronic pulmonary hypertension and cor pulmonale has recently been questioned by Bradley et al.,[89] who propose that cor pulmonale does not occur in sleep apnea unless associated with daytime hypoxemia and expiratory airflow abnormalities from underlying lung disease. Only 6 of 50 consecutively studied apnea patients had "clinical evidence" of right heart failure. The two features that separated these six from an age- and weight-equivalent group of eight apnea patients without cor pulmonale was the presence of daytime hypoxemia (PaO_2 52 versus 73 mmHg, respectively) and expiratory airflow limitation (57 versus 105 percent of predicted 1-second forced expiratory volume [FEV_1], respectively). These authors concluded that cor pulmonale occurs in obstructive apnea patients only in the presence of daytime hypoxemia caused by obstructive lung disease. To this however, must be added one of the major causes of daytime hypoxemia in apnea patients, namely, the obesity-hypoventilation syndrome. Indeed, the average body weight of the six cor pulmonale patients in their study was 186 percent of ideal and they may well have been hypercarbic and hypoxemic on the basis of obesity-hypoventilation.

In general, pulmonary hypertension and right heart dysfunction generated by obstructive apnea are milder, and the normalization of pulmonary hemodynamics following treatment is more rapid, in apnea patients without lung disease than in those with it[90] (Fig. 27-13). In five severely symptomatic apnea patients without lung disease, the highest mean pulmonary artery pressure was 30 mmHg, and all pressures returned to near normal (20 mmHg) by the end of 2 years following tracheotomy. Pulmonary artery pressure in nine symptomatic apnea patients with COPD ranged up to 60 mmHg and *did not* return to normal within 2 years of tracheotomy. In 10 subjects with apnea and COPD treated by "less than curative" measures (drugs, O_2, upper airway surgery) the pulmonary artery pressure remained at its baseline level at the end of 2 years. It is noteworthy that in the group with tracheostomies, daytime arterial blood gases improved significantly without any weight loss or improvement in pulmonary function, which indicates that elimination of nocturnal apnea and hypoxemia improved the daytime drive to breathe. This issue has been examined closely in an article examining the relationship of chronic hypercapnia to obstructive sleep apnea or the pickwickian syndrome.[91]

Effects on Cardiac Function

Reduction in heart rate during obstructive and central apneas has been well documented and studied.[92] A "rebound"

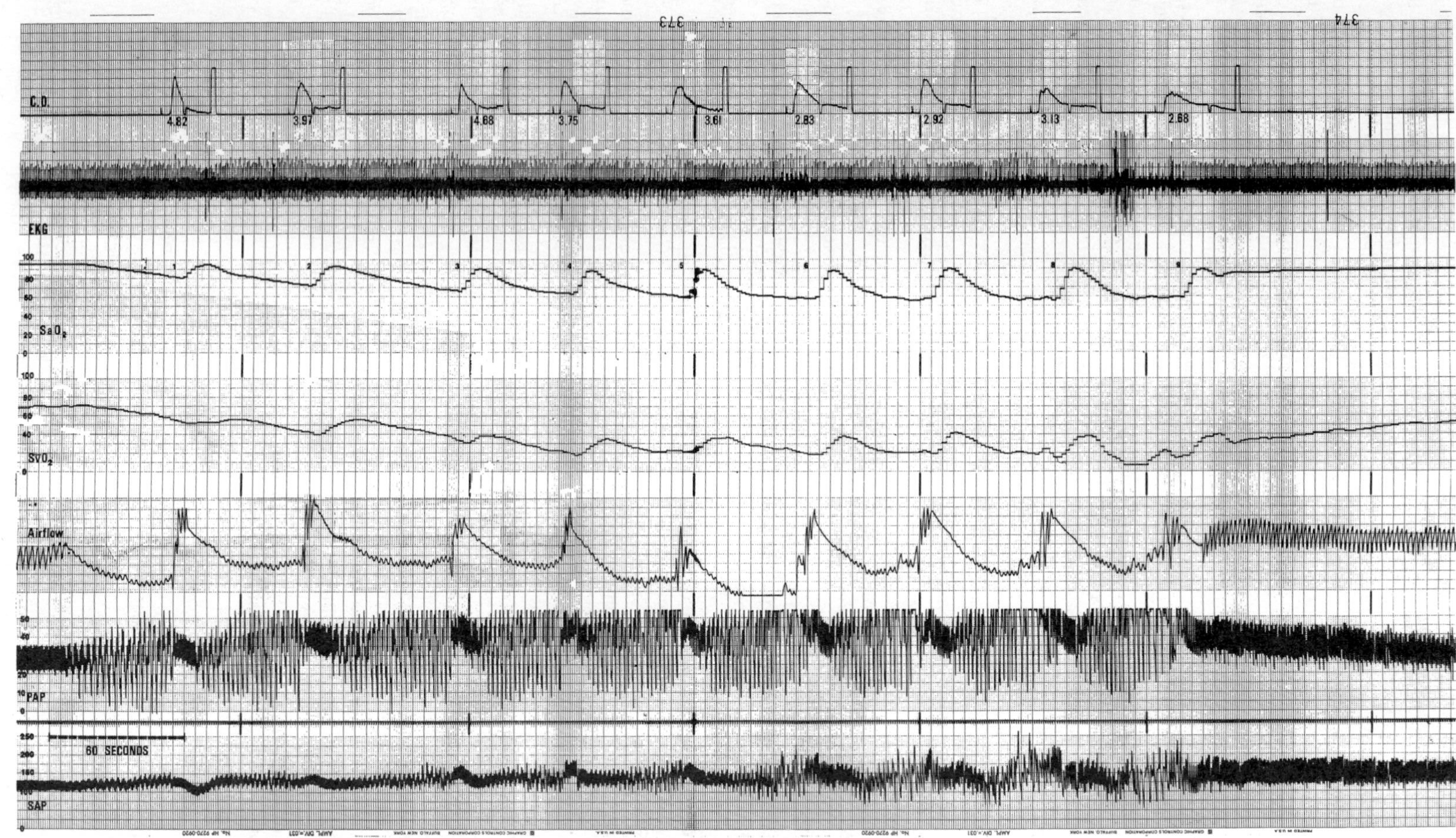

Figure 27-11. Series of repetitive apneic episodes artificially induced by endotracheal tube obstruction in an adult male baboon. Three breaths are allowed for recovery between apneas. Channel 1: cardiac output; channel 2: ECG; channel 3: SaO_2; channel 4: mixed venous oxyhemoglobin saturation ($S\bar{v}O_2$); channel 5: endotracheal tube airflow; channel 6: pulmonary artery pressure; channel 7: systemic arterial pressure. Note the steady, progressive ''stair step'' rise in systemic and pulmonary artery pressures with each successive apnea. While pulmonary artery pressure begins to fall after the last sequential apnea, systemic artery pulse and mean pressure remain elevated.

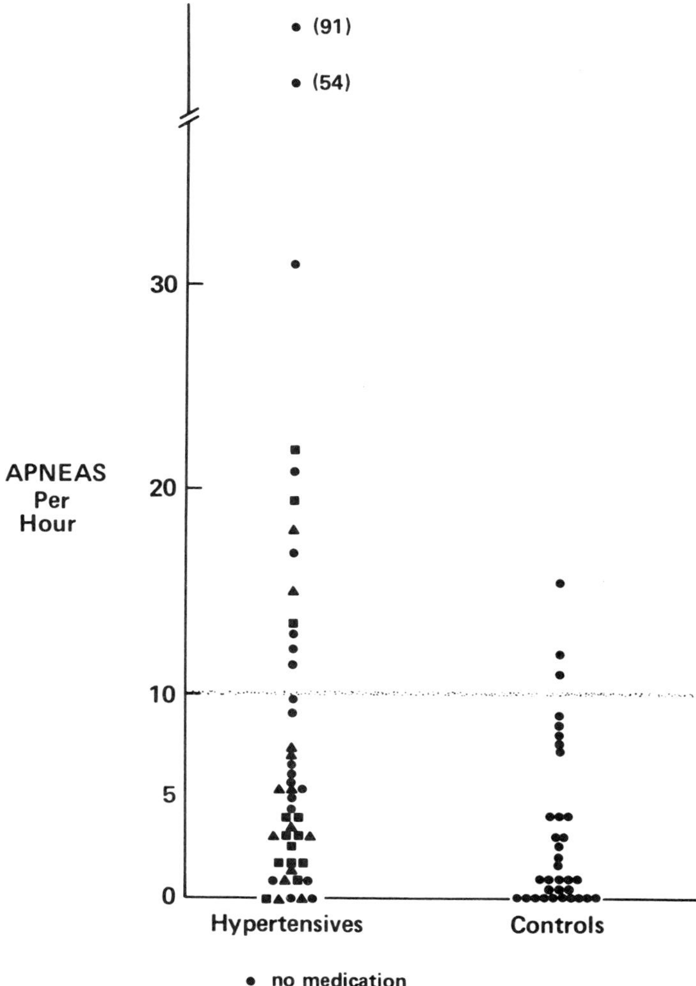

Figure 27-12. Comparison of the apnea index in a group of middle-aged men with essential hypertension versus an age-matched group of normotensive men. When an apnea index of 10/h is used as a cutoff, about 30 percent of the hypertensive men have "sleep apnea," while only 9 percent of the controls would receive this diagnosis. (From Fletcher et al.,[86] with permission.)

type of tachycardia is often seen in the terminal portion (3 to 10 seconds) of an obstructive apnea. The bradycardia associated with apnea is dependent on three things: (1) hypoxemia—the inhalation of pure O_2 before breath holding or apnea ameliorates the bradycardia; (2) absence of chest movement—rebreathing experiments that allow thoracic movement while achieving levels of asphyxia comparable with those achieved in apnea ameliorate the bradycardia; and (3) vagal tone—atropine blocks the reflex bradycardia due to apnea. The major clinical significance of this bradycardia or increased vagal tone may lie in its relationship to occasional episodes of complete heart block that develop during apnea and in the potential for reducing cardiac output.

It is quite difficult to examine changes in cardiac output by the thermal dilution technique. Many apneic episodes must be measured because only one injection at the beginning and one at the end of the episode are possible. By using impedance cardiography Lin et al.[93] observed a decrease in cardiac output during 90-second breath holds starting 30 seconds into the hold. This was related to a 30 percent fall in heart rate.

Marked sinus arrhythmia (a variation of more than 30 bpm) is observed in 78 to 100 percent of patients with obstructive sleep apnea. Miller[94] found no difference in ventricular ectopic frequency between wakefulness and sleep in apnea patients, and Guilleminault et al.[95] reported that ectopic activity increased during sleep in only 14 percent of 400 apnea patients studied. Episodes of unsustained ventricular tachycardia were observed in eight patients in association with apnea-induced oxyhemoglobin desaturation to less than 65

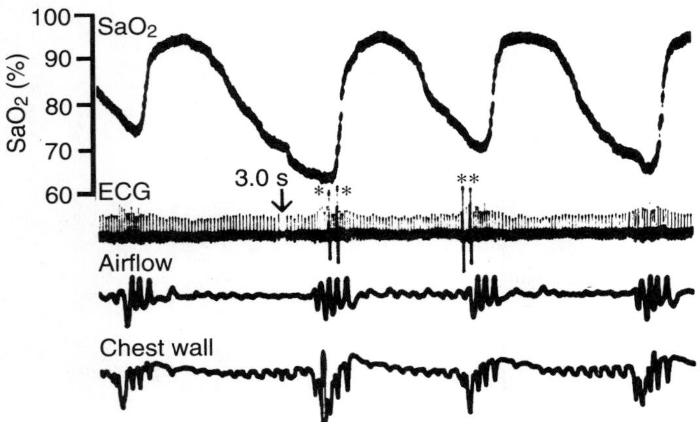

Figure 27-13. Segment of a sleep apnea patient's recording, demonstrating multiple premature ventricular contractions (PVCs) occurring in relation to apnea desaturation. Note that the PVCs (*) occur during the period of resumed airflow (cardioacceleration), not during the apnea itself. This could be due to a washing out of anaerobic metabolites from the anoxic myocardium and/or a shift from dominant parasympathetic control of the heart to sympathetic control. In this patient PVCs appeared only when the lowest SaO_2 due to apnea approached 60 percent. (From Shepard,[106] with permission.)

percent. Shepard et al.[96] have partially explained this discrepancy. Examining 31 apnea patients for nocturnal ectopic activity, he found no difference in daytime and sleeping activity as long as the SaO_2 remained above 60 percent. In patients in whom desaturation to below 60 percent occurred, the frequency of premature ventricular contractions (PVCs) increased nearly threefold as compared with when saturation was greater than 90 percent (Fig. 27-13). Ventricular ectopy usually occurred during the period of cardiac acceleration immediately following the resumption of ventilation. It may be that the shift from parasympathetic-dominant to sympathetic dominant neural activity following apnea termination acts to lower the ectopic threshold of the myocardium. Also, mechanical stresses or biochemical changes associated with reoxygenation of hypoxic myocardium may be involved in the generation of the ventricular ectopy. In a recent study examining the effect of supplemental O_2 on ventricular arrhythmias in apnea patients with concomitant lung disease, the only patients who had baseline complex arrhythmias were those with a history of previous acute myocardial infarction (AMI), angina, or evidence of left ventricular failure.[97]

MacGregor et al.[98] have reported respiratory death in 6 of 25 patients admitted to the hospital from 1959 to 1969 with what was probably sleep apnea. Five of these were sudden deaths, usually unobserved and occurring presumably during sleep. All five occurred before 1966, 3 years prior to the first reported treatment of obstructive sleep apnea by tracheotomy. Death most likely resulted from severe hypoxemia with induction of a malignant cardiac arrhythmia, but recent reports suggest that acute left ventricular failure may accompany severe apnea.[99] Observed, reported deaths in sleep apnea are so rare that it is difficult to form an opinion about the immediate mode of death. More important, it is difficult to establish which apnea patients are at risk for sudden death. In my experience (four known apnea deaths during sleep), all four patients had concomitant COPD and alveolar hypoventilation as well as severe cor pulmonale and had refused to undergo tracheotomy (prior to CPAP availability). It is very likely that patients with underlying coronary artery disease and sleep apnea may also be at high risk for death during sleep.

The incidence of obstructive apnea has been reported to be increased in patients with coronary artery disease. De Olazabal et al.[100] studied 17 middle-aged men with symptomatic coronary artery disease (documented by angiography) using nocturnal polysomnography. Of these patients, 13 had breathing abnormalities during sleep, which took the form of Cheyne-Stokes breathing in two cases and obstructive sleep apnea in the others. The apnea index among the 13 was 20 episodes per hour. O_2 desaturation occurred in 10 of the patients, with a mean fall in saturation of 11 percent. Along with Cheyne-Stokes respiration, central apnea is now a reported nocturnal breathing dysrhythmia among patients with left ventricular failure. A 1984 study reported two of nine patients with compensated left ventricular failure to have greater than 30 apneic episodes per night.[101] In two of four subjects studied, the frequency of central apnea episodes decreased from 230 and 50 per night to 42 and zero, respectively, following treatment of the congestive heart failure, and a 1987 study reported a significant decrease in sleep-disordered breathing following cardiac transplant in five of six patients.[102]

Hypopnea and gas exchange abnormalities during REM sleep have been proposed as components of a mechanism that can cause sustained pulmonary hypertension in COPD patients. It has been clearly demonstrated that the prolonged, profound (lower than 50 percent in some cases) oxyhemoglobin desaturation that accompanies REM sleep causes transient elevations in pulmonary artery pressure even in patients with only mild daytime hypoxemia.[21,69,103] It has therefore been proposed that prophylactic O_2 during sleep in patients with COPD and sleep desaturation might delay the onset of pulmonary hypertension and decrease the morbidity of the disease.[104,105] This hypothesis as well as the effect of nocturnal desaturation on longevity in COPD patients is being further investigated.[107–110]

References

1. Caton R: The electric currents of the brain. Br Med J 1875; 2:278
2. Berger H: Über das Elektroencephalogramm des Menschen. Arch Psychiatr Nervenkr 1929;87:527–570
3. Loomis AL, Harvey EN, Hobart GA: Potential rhythms of the cerebral cortex during sleep. Science 1935;81:597–598
4. Aserinsky E, Kleitman N: Regularly occurring periods of eye motility, and concomitant phenomena, during sleep. Science 1953;118:273–274
5. Aserinsky E, Kleitman N: Two types of ocular motility occurring in sleep. J Appl Physiol 1955;8:1–10
6. Rechtschaffen A, Kales A (eds): A Manual of Standardized Terminology, Techniques and Scoring System for Sleep Stages of Human Subjects. NIH Publication 204. National Institutes of Health, Washington, D.C., 1968
7. Fisher C, Gross J, Zuch J: Cycle of penile erections synchronous with dreaming (REM) sleep. Arch Gen Psychiatry 1965; 2:29
8. Phillipson EA: State of the art: Control of breathing during sleep. Am Rev Respir Dis 1978;118:909–939
9. Williams RL, Karacan I, Hursch CJ: Electroencephalography of Human Sleep: Clinical Applications. John Wiley & Sons, New York, 1974
10. Guilleminault C, van den Hoed J, Mitler MM: Clinical overview of the sleep apnea syndromes. pp. 1–12. In Guilleminault C, Dement WC (eds): Sleep Apnea Syndromes. Alan R Liss, New York, 1978
11. Orr WC, Martin RJ: Hypersomnolent and non-hypersomnolent patients with upper airway obstruction during sleep. Chest 1979;75:418–422
12. Sink J, Bliwise DL, Dement WC: Self-reported excessive daytime somnolence and impaired respiration in sleep. Chest 1986; 90:177–180
13. Williams RL: Sleep disturbances in various medical and surgical conditions. pp. 285–302. In Williams RL, Karacan I (eds): Sleep Disorders: Diagnosis and Treatment. John Wiley & Sons, New York, 1978
14. Elwell EL, Frankel BL, Snyder F: A polygraphic sleep study of five cardiotomy patients. Sleep Res 1974;3:133
15. Slutsky AS, Strohl KP: Quantification of oxygen saturation during episodic hypoxemia. Am Rev Respir Dis 1980;121:893–895
16. Berger AJ, Mitchell RA, Severinghaus JW: Regulation of respiration. N Engl J Med 1977;297:92–97, 138–143, 194–201
17. Remmers JE: Effects of sleep on control of breathing. pp. 111–147. In Widdicombe JG (ed): Respiratory physiology. Vol. 3. University Park Press, Baltimore, 1981
18. Dempsey JA, Skatrud JB: A sleep-induced apneic threshold and its consequences. Am Rev Respir Dis 1986;133:1163–1170
19. Berthon-Jones M, Sullivan CE: Ventilatory and arousal responses to hypoxia in sleeping humans. Am Rev Respir Dis 1982;125:632–629
20. Douglas NJ, White DP, Weil JV et al: Hypoxic ventilatory response decreases during sleep in normal men. Am Rev Respir Dis 1982;125:286–289
21. Berssenbrugge A, Dempsey JA, Iber C et al: Mechanisms of hypoxia-induced periodic breathing during sleep in humans. J Physiol (Lond) 1983;343:507–524
22. Berssenbrugge A, Dempsey JA, Skatrud J: Effects of sleep state on ventilatory acclimatization to chronic hypoxia. J Appl Physiol 1984;57:1089–1096
23. Cherniack NS, Longobardo GS: Cheyne-Stokes breathing and instability in physiologic control. N Engl J Med 1973;288:952–957
24. Remmers JE, deGroot WJ, Sauerland EK et al: Pathogenesis of upper airway occlusion during sleep. J Appl Physiol 1978; 44:931–938
25. Reed WR, Roberts JL, Thach BT: Factors influencing regional patency and configuration of the human infant upper airway. J Appl Physiol 1985;58:635–644
26. Block AJ, Faulkner JA, Hughes RL et al: Factors influencing upper airway closure. Chest 1984;86:114–122
27. Fouke JM, Galbraith FM, Strohl KP: Effect of subject position on upper airway geometry. FASEB J 1985;44:A2498
28. Safar P, Escarraga LA, Chang F: Upper airway obstruction in the unconscious patient. J Appl Physiol 1959;14:760–764
29. Haponik EF, Smith PL, Bohlman ME et al: Computerized tomography in obstructive sleep apnea. Am Rev Respir Dis 1983; 127:221–226
30. Bohlman ME, Haponik EF, Smith PL et al: CT demonstration of pharyngeal narrowing in adult obstructive sleep apnea. AJR 1983;140:543–548
31. Taasan VC, Wynne JW, Cassisi N, Block AJ: The effect of nasal packing on sleep disordered breathing and nocturnal oxygen desaturation. Laryngoscope 1981;19:116–172
32. Zwillich CW, Pickett C, Hanson RN, Weil JV: Disturbed sleep and prolonged apnea during nasal obstruction in normal men. Am Rev Respir Dis 1981;124:158–160
33. Kunna S, Remmers J: Pathophysiology and mechanisms of sleep apnea. pp. 63–94. In Fletcher EC (ed): Abnormalities of Respiration during Sleep: Diagnosis, Pathophysiology, and Treatment. Grune & Stratton, Orlando, FL, 1986
34. Van Lunteren E, Van de Graaf WB, Parker DM et al: Nasal and laryngeal reflex responses to negative upper airway pressure. J Appl Physiol 1984;56:746–752
35. Bonora M, Shields GI, Knuth SL et al: Selective depression by ethanol of upper airway respiratory motor activity in cats. Am Rev Respir Dis 1984;130:156–161
36. Hwang J, St. John WM, Bartlett D Jr: Respiratory-related hypoglossal nerve activity: Influence of anesthetics. J Appl Physiol 1983;55:785–792
37. Nishino T, Shirahata M, Yonezawa T, Honda Y: Comparison of changes in the hypoglossal and phrenic nerve activity in response to increasing depth of anesthesia in cats. Anesthesiology 1984;60:19–24
38. Dolly FR, Block AJ: Effect of flurazepam on sleep-disordered breathing and nocturnal oxygen desaturation in asymptomatic subjects. Am J Med 1982;73:239–243
39. Bonora M, St. John WM, Bledsoe TA: Differential elevation by protriptyline and depression by diazepam of upper airway respiratory motor activity. Am Rev Respir Dis 1985;131:41–45
40. Lugaresi E, Coccagna G, Cirignotta F: Snoring and its clinical implications. pp. 13–21. In Guilleminault C, Dement WC (eds): Sleep Apnea Syndromes. Alan R Liss, New York, 1978
41. Block AJ, Boysen PG, Wynne JW et al: Sleep apnea, hypopnea and oxygen desaturation in normal subjects—a strong male predominance. N Engl J Med 1979;300:513–517
42. Issa FG, Sullivan CE: Reversal of central sleep apnea using nasal CPAP. Chest 1986;90:165–171
43. Sanders MH: Nasal CPAP effect on patterns of sleep apnea. Chest 1984;86:839–844
44. Hudgel DW, Hendricks C, Dadley A: Alteration of apnea time in obstructive sleep apnea by O_2 and CO_2 inhalation, abstracted. Am Rev Respir Dis 1987;135:A185
45. Fletcher EC, Gray BA, Levin DC: Nonapneic mechanisms of arterial oxygen desaturation during rapid-eye-movement sleep. J Appl Physiol 1983;54:632–639
46. Bye PT, Issa F, Bethan-Jones M, Sullivan CE: Studies of oxygenation during sleep in patients with interstitial lung disease. Am Rev Respir Dis 1984;129:27–32
47. Francis PWJ, Muller NL, Gurwitz D et al: Hemoglobin desaturation. Its occurrence during sleep in patients with cystic fibrosis. Am J Dis Child 1980;134:734–740

45. Fletcher EC, Gray BA, Levin DC: Nonapneic mechanisms of arterial oxygen desaturation during rapid-eye-movement sleep. J Appl Physiol 1983;54:632–639
46. Bye PT, Issa F, Bethan-Jones M, Sullivan CE: Studies of oxygenation during sleep in patients with interstitial lung disease. Am Rev Respir Dis 1984;129:27–32
47. Francis PWJ, Muller NL, Gurwitz D et al: Hemoglobin desaturation. Its occurrence during sleep in patients with cystic fibrosis. Am J Dis Child 1980;134:734–740
48. Muller NL, Francis PWJ, Gurwitz D et al: Mechanism of hemoglobin desaturation during rapid-eye-movement sleep in normal subjects and in patients with cystic fibrosis. Am Rev Respir Dis 1980;121:463–469
49. Newsom-Davis J, Goldman DM, Loh L, Casson M: Diaphragm function and alveolar hypoventilation. Q J Med 1975;45:87–100
50. Amis TC, Ciofetta G, Hughes JMB, Loh L: Regional lung function in bilateral diaphragmatic paralysis. Clin Sci 1980;59:485–492
51. Mezon BL, West P, Israels J, Kryger M: Sleep breathing abnormalities in kyphoscoliosis. Am Rev Respir Dis 1980; 122:617–621
52. Guilleminault C, Kurland G, Winkle R, Miles LE: Severe kyphoscoliosis, breathing and sleep. Chest 1981;79:626–630
53. Skatrud J, Iber C, McHugh W et al: Determinants of hypoventilation during wakefulness and sleep in diaphragmatic paralysis. Am Rev Respir Dis 1980;121:587–593
54. Martin RJ: Neuromuscular and skeletal abnormalities with nocturnal respiratory disorders. pp. 251–282. In Martin RJ (ed): Cardiorespiratory Disorders During Sleep. Futura Publishing, Mount Kisco, NY, 1990
55. Coccagna G, Mantovani M, Parchi CL et al: Alveolar hypoventilation and hypersomnia in myotonic dystrophy. Neurol Neurosurg Psychiatry 1975;38:977–984
56. Guilleminault C, Motta J: Sleep apnea syndrome as a long term sequela of poliomyelitis. pp. 309–315. In Guilleminault C, Dement WC (eds): Sleep Apnea Syndromes. Alan R Liss, New York, 1978
57. Arand DL, McGinty DJ, Littner MR: Respiratory patterns associated with hemoglobin desaturation during sleep in chronic obstructive pulmonary disease. Chest 1981;80:183–190
58. Goldstein RS, Ramcharan V, Bowes G et al: Effect of supplemental nocturnal oxygen on gas exchange in patients with severe obstructive lung disease. N Engl J Med 1984;310:425–429
59. Fletcher EC, Levin DC: Cardiopulmonary hemodynamics during sleep in subjects with chronic obstructive pulmonary disease: The effect of short and long term oxygen. Chest 1984; 85:6–14
60. Douglas NJ, Calverley PM, Leggett RJ et al: Transient hypoxemia during sleep in chronic bronchitis and emphysema. Lancet 1979;1:1–4
61. Flenley DC, Calverly PM, Douglas NJ et al: Nocturnal hypoxemia and long-term domiciliary oxygen therapy in "blue and bloated" bronchitics. Physiopathologic correlations. Chest 1980;77:305–307
62. Demarco FJ, Wynne JW, Block AJ et al: Oxygen desaturation during sleep as a determinant of the blue and bloated syndrome. Chest 1981;79:621–625
63. Littner MR, McGinty DJ, Arand DL: Determinants of oxygen desaturation in the course of ventilation during sleep in chronic obstructive pulmonary disease. Am Rev Respir Dis 1980; 122:849–857
64. Fleetham JA, Bradley CA, Kryger MH, Anthonisen NR: The effect of low flow oxygen therapy on chemical control of ventilation in patients with hypoxemic COPD. Am Rev Respir Dis 1980;833–840
65. Goethe B: Effect of chemosensitivity on arterial oxygen saturation during sleep, abstracted. Am Rev Respir Dis 1979; 119:119
66. Fletcher EC, Miller J, Divine GW et al: Nocturnal oxyhemoglobin desaturation in COPD patients with arterial oxygen tensions above 60 torr. Chest 1987;92:604–608
67. Hudgel DW, Martin RJ, Capehart M, Johnson B: Contribution of hypoventilation to sleep oxygen desaturation in chronic obstructive pulmonary disease. J Appl Physiol 1983;55:669–677
68. Koo KW, Sax DS, Snider GL: Arterial blood gases and pH during sleep in chronic obstructive pulmonary disease. Am J Med 1985;58:663–670
69. Flick MR, Block AJ: Continuous in-vivo monitoring of arterial oxygenation in chronic obstructive lung disease. Ann Intern Med 1977;86:725–730
70. Henderson-Smart DJ, Read DJ: Reduced lung volume during behavioral active sleep in the newborn. J Appl Physiol 1979; 46:1081–1085
71. Tusiewicz K, Moldofsky H, Bryan AC, Bryan MH: Mechanics of the rib cage and diaphragm during sleep. J Appl Physiol 1977; 43:600–602
72. Hudgel DW, Devadatta P: Decrease in functional residual capacity during sleep in normal humans. J Appl Physiol 1984; 57:1319–1322
73. Tabachnik E, Muller NL, Bryan AC, Levison H: Changes in ventilation and chest wall mechanics during sleep in normal adolescents. J Appl Physiol 1981;51:557–566
74. Fletcher EC: Sleep, breathing, and oxyhemoglobin saturation in chronic lung diseases. pp. 158–180. In Fletcher EC (ed): Abnormalities of Respiration during Sleep: Diagnosis, Pathophysiology, and Treatment. Grune & Stratton, Orlando, FL, 1986
75. Hetzel MR, Clark TJH: Does sleep cause nocturnal asthma? Thorax 1979;34:749–754
76. Hudgel DW, Martin RJ, Johnson B, Hill P: Mechanics of the respiratory system and breathing pattern during sleep in normal humans. J Appl Physiol 1984;56:133–137
77. Phillipson EA, Goldstein RS: Breathing during sleep in chronic obstructive pulmonary disease. Chest 1984;85:24S–30S
78. Bateman JRM, Pavia D, Clarke SW: The retention of lung secretions during the night in normals. Clin Sci 1978;55:523–527
79. Berthan-Jones M, Sullivan CE: Ventilatory and arousal responses to hypoxia in sleeping humans. Am Rev Respir Dis 1982;125:632–639
80. Richardson DW, Honour AJ, Fenton GW et al: Variation in arterial pressure throughout the day and night. Clin Sci 1964; 26:445–460
81. Shepard JW Jr: Gas exchange and hemodynamics during sleep. Med Clin North Am 1985;69:1234–1263
82. Schroeder JS, Motta J, Guilleminault C: Hemodynamic studies in sleep apnea. pp. 177–196. In Guilleminault C, Dement WC (eds): Sleep Apnea Syndromes. Alan R Liss, New York, 1978
83. Fletcher E, Miller J, Schaaf J et al: Urinary catecholamines before and after tracheostomy in obstructive sleep apnea. Sleep 1987;10:35–44
84. Kales A, Bixler EO, Cadieux RJ et al: Sleep apnoea in a hypertensive population. Lancet 1984;2:1005–1008
85. Lavie P, Ben-Yosef R, Rubin AE: Prevalence of sleep apnea syndrome among patients with essential hypertension. Am Heart J 1984;108:373–376
86. Fletcher EC, DeBehnke RD, Lovoi MS et al: Undiagnosed sleep apnea among patients with essential hypertension. Ann Intern Med 1985;103:190–194
87. Lugaresi E, Cirignotta F, Coccagna G et al: Clinical significance of snoring. pp. 283–298. In Saunders NA, Sullivan CE (eds): Sleep and Breathing. Marcel Dekker, New York, 1984
88. Tilkian AG, Guilleminault C, Schroeder JS et al: Hemodynamics in sleep-induced apnea: Studies during wakefulness and sleep. Ann Intern Med 1976;85:714–719
89. Bradley TD, Rutherford R, Grossman RF et al: Role of daytime hypoxemia in the pathogenesis of right heart failure in the obstructive sleep apnea syndrome. Am Rev Respir Dis 1985; 131:835–839
90. Fletcher EC, Schaaf JW, Miller J, Fletcher JG: Long-term cardiopulmonary sequelae in patients with sleep apnea and chronic lung disease. Am Rev Respir Dis 1987;135:525–533
91. Rapoport DM, Garay SM, Epstein H, Goldring RM: Hypercapnia in the obstructive sleep apnea syndrome: A reevaluation of the "pickwickian syndrome." Chest 1986;89:627–635

92. Zwillich C, Devlin T, White D et al: Bradycardia during sleep apnea: Characteristics and mechanism. J Clin Invest 1982; 69:1286–1292
93. Lin YC, Shida KK, Hong SK: Effects of hypercapnia, hypoxia, and rebreathing on circulatory response to apnea. J Appl Physiol 1983;54:172–177
94. Miller WP: Cardiac arrhythmias and conduction disturbances in the sleep apnea syndrome. Am J Med 1982;73:317–321
95. Guilleminault C, Connolly SJ, Winkle RA: Cardiac arrhythmia and conduction disturbances during sleep in 400 patients with sleep apnea syndrome. Am J Cardiol 1983;52:490–494
96. Shepard JW Jr, Garrison MW, Grither DA et al: Relationship of ventricular ectopy to nocturnal O_2 desaturation in patients with obstructive sleep apnea. Chest 1983;88:335–340
97. Alford NJ, Fletcher EC, Nickeson D: Effects of acute oxygen in patients with sleep apnea and chronic obstructive lung disease. Chest 1986;89:30–38
98. MacGregor MI, Block AJ, Ball WC Jr: Serious complications and sudden death in the pickwickian syndrome. Johns Hopkins Med J 1970;126:279–295
99. Chaudhary BA, Ferguson DS, Speir WA Jr: Pulmonary edema as a presenting feature of sleep apnea syndrome. Chest 1982; 82:122–124
100. De Olazabal JR, Miller MJ, Cook WR, Mithoefer JC: Disordered breathing and hypoxia during sleep in coronary artery disease. Chest 1982;82:548–552
101. Dark DS, Pingleton SK, Drieling R et al: Sleep disordered breathing and desaturation in stable severe congestive heart failure. Am Rev Respir Dis 1984;129:A58
102. Loggan M, Gollub S, Pingleton SK, Kerby GR: The effect of cardiac transplantation upon sleep disordered breathing. Am Rev Respir Dis 1987;135:A232
103. Fletcher EC, Levin DC: Cardiopulmonary hemodynamics during sleep in subjects with chronic obstructive pulmonary disease: The effect of short and long term oxygen. Chest 1984; 85:6–14
104. Flenley DC: Clinical hypoxia: Causes, consequences, and correction. Lancet 1978;1:542–546
105. Block AJ, Boysen PG, Wynne JW: The origins of cor pulmonale, a hypothesis. Chest 1979;75:109–110
106. Shepard JW Jr: Hemodynamics in obstructive sleep apnea. pp. 39–62. In Fletcher EC (ed): Abnormalities of Respiration during Sleep: Diagnosis, Pathophysiology, and Treatment. Grune & Stratton, Orlando, FL, 1986
107. Fletcher EC, Luckett RA, Miller T et al: Pulmonary vascular hemodynamics in chronic lung disease patients with and without nocturnal oxyhemoglobin desaturation during sleep. Chest 1989;95:757–764
108. Fletcher EC, Luckett RA, Miller T, Fletcher JG: Exercise hemodynamics and gas exchange in patients with chronic obstructive pulmonary disease, sleep desaturation, and a daytime PaO_2 above 60 mmHg. Am Rev Respir Dis 1989;140:1237–1245
109. Fletcher EC, Scott D, Qian RA et al: Evolution of nocturnal oxyhemoglobin desaturation in patients with chronic obstructive pulmonary disease and a daytime PaO_2 above 60 torr. Am Rev Respir Dis 1991;144:401–405
110. Fletcher EC, Donner CF, Midgren B et al: Survival in COPD patients with a daytime $PaO_2 > 60$ torr with and without nocturnal oxyhemoglobin desaturation (NOD). Chest (in press)

Chapter 28

Disorders of Water, Solute, and Acid-Base Balance

John M. Luce

CHAPTER OUTLINE

DISORDERS OF EXTRACELLULAR FLUID VOLUME REGULATION

General Principles

As noted in Chapter 13, the effects of intravascular volume loss and hypoperfusion are so potentially deleterious that extracellular fluid (ECF) volume is defended even to the detriment of ECF osmolality in certain circumstances.[1,2] The stimulus for this defense is the perception by the body of an inadequate volume in the arterial tree and, to some extent, the venous side of the circulation. The inadequate volume results either from a fall in cardiac output or from peripheral arterial vasodilation. The body's defense is called the *integrated volume response*.[2] It has three aspects: (1) an increase in autonomic nervous system output and the release of catecholamines, which increase blood pressure by increasing arteriolar resistance and heart rate and decreasing venous capacitance; (2) the release of antidiuretic hormone (ADH; vasopressin) by the pituitary gland, which induces the kidney to retain water; and (3) the renal release of renin, a hormone that causes the creation of angiotension II, which enhances peripheral vasoconstriction, induces aldosterone secretion by the kidneys, and stimulates thirst. Aldosterone in turn prompts the kidneys to conserve Na^+ in exchange for K^+ and H^+, whereas thirst prompts patients to increase their water intake even to the point of ECF hypotonicity.[2–5]

Hypovolemia

Volume depletion, or hypovolemia, is a state in which ECF volume is decreased either acutely or on a chronic basis. Hypovolemia occurs when the rate of Na^+ and water intake by the body is less than the loss of these substances, although input and output may be equal in chronically volume-depleted states.[3] Total body water always is decreased during volume depletion. Total body Na^+ usually is decreased as well, but hypovolemia can occur with any Na^+ concentration because the Na^+ concentration represents only the relative amounts of Na^+ and water in serum or plasma and not the total amounts of these substances in the body.

Causes and Clinical Settings

The major causes of hypovolemia can be divided into those that involve renal or extrarenal Na^+ and those that involve water loss.[3–5] Clinically, disorders in the latter category are most common, perhaps the most dramatic being hemorrhage, in which whole blood may be lost rapidly. Whole blood is made up of plasma, of which 95 percent is water and 5 percent is solute, and formed elements, mainly red blood cells. In a 70-kg individual whose intravascular volume is 5 L and whose hematocrit is 40 to 45 percent, plasma volume is approximately 3 L and the total volume of formed blood elements is 2 L. A bleeding patient whose plasma may be assumed to have a normal Na^+ concentration of 140 mEq/L and a normal osmolality will lose formed blood elements and fluid that is isotonic with plasma (i.e., has the same osmolality).

Although hemorrhage is perhaps the most dramatic manifestation of isotonic fluid loss, the same loss can occur in patients with extensive burns when plasma weeps from the burned surface. By contrast, hypotonic fluid loss is the rule during extensive sweating inasmuch as sweat contains as few as 50 mEq/L of Na^+. Gastrointestinal fluid losses due to vomiting, diarrhea, or tube drainage may be hypotonic or isotonic depending on the site of loss. For example, gastric juice lost by vomiting contains approximately 50 mEq/L of Na^+, 10 mEq/L of K^+, and 90 mEq/L of H^+, whereas diarrheal fluid contains 130 mEq/L of Na^+ and 10 mEq/L of K^+. The concentrations of major solutes in body fluids are outlined in Table 13-1.

Nonrenal causes of hypovolemia include hormonal deficiency states and kidney disease. Of the hormonal deficiencies perhaps the most common is central diabetes insipidus (DI), which results from a diminution in the secretion of ADH by the pituitary gland. Seen for the most part in patients with intracranial processes such as head trauma or following brain surgery, central DI may lead to the loss of up to 18 L/d of water that normally would be conserved by the kidneys. Aldosterone deficiency also may produce hypovolemia through renal Na^+ wasting, such as is seen in states of adrenal insufficiency related to primary failure of the adrenals (Addison's disease). This condition usually leads to chronic Na^+ loss and is associated with hypokalemia and metabolic acidosis because of interference with the exchange of Na^+ for K^+ and H^+ by the distal tubules in the kidneys.[2]

Renal disorders of Na^+ and water conservation include those in which the kidneys themselves are damaged and those in which they passively allow a loss of fluid from the body. Examples of the first category include nephrogenic DI, in which ADH is released by the pituitary gland but the diseased kidneys cannot concentrate urine in response to the hormone; renal tubular acidosis (discussed later in this chapter), in which Na^+ is lost owing to a defect in the collecting tubules; and chronic renal failure due to any cause, in which there is an obligatory loss of Na^+. Examples of situations in which the kidneys merely allow Na^+ and water loss are (1) excessive diuretic administration, in which agents such as furosemide that inhibit Na^+ uptake in the ascending limb of the loop Henle prompt the excretion of hypotonic fluid containing approximately 70 mEq/L of Na^+; and (2) the accumulation or administration of solutes such as glucose and mannitol that cause an osmotic diuresis of water, Na^+, and K^+.

Clinical Manifestations

The clinical manifestations of volume deficiency depend largely on the type of fluid lost from the body, the extent of the integrated volume response, and the net effect of the Starling forces,[1,2] discussed in Chapter 13. To reiterate briefly, the Starling forces represent the sum of the Starling equation for fluid flux across capillary membranes. The flux (F) is equal to $k(P_{cap} - P_{is}) - \sigma(\pi_{cap} - \pi_{is})$, where k is a permeability factor describing how readily water traverses the capillary membranes; P_{cap} is capillary hydrostatic pressure, the pressure of the volume of water (plasma) in the capillary; P_{is} is the hydrostatic pressure in the interstitium, a part of the ECF that surrounds the capillary; σ is a reflection coefficient describing how well the capillary membrane keeps proteins on one side; π_{cap} is capillary oncotic pressure; and π_{is} is interstitial oncotic pressure. Assuming that capillary membrane integrity is intact and that k and σ stay constant, water normally passes out of the capillary at its arterial end, where P_{cap} is higher than π_{cap}, and re-enters the capillary at its venular end, where the situation is reversed (see Fig. 13-3). The net effect of the Starling forces, then, is to keep water within the intravascular space and thereby maintain blood volume.

Compensated Hemorrhagic Shock

During acute hemorrhage as much as one-tenth of the total blood volume of 5 L may be lost with little obvious physiologic effect. However, loss of more than 500 mL of blood usually is manifested by a drop in diastolic blood pressure when patients assume an upright posture. This postural blood pressure change is paralleled by postural tachycardia mediated by catecholamines. The catecholamines and circulating angiotension tend to restore blood pressure and to divert the cardiac output to vital organs such as the brain and the heart. At a microcirculatory level, the catecholamines cause arteriolar vasoconstriction, which in turn lowers capillary hydrostatic pressure, favoring fluid flow into the vessels from the surrounding interstitium. Thirst becomes intense, prompting patients to drink water if it is available; and renal excretion of Na^+ begins to fall off, resulting in reduction of the urinary Na^+ concentration. Intravascular volume is at least partially restored, and patients are said to be in compensated hemorrhagic shock.[2]

Decompensated Hemorrhagic Shock

As bleeding continues and much more than 1 L of blood is lost, the compensatory mechanisms to restore vital organ perfusion may become inadequate. Now hypotension and tachycardia may persist in any position. Mental status becomes depressed as cerebral perfusion diminishes; urine output falls below 20 mL/h due to inadequate renal blood flow; and patients with coronary artery disease may experience chest pain because of myocardial ischemia. Patients now appear pale and cold owing to poor skin perfusion, and they develop metabolic acidosis (discussed later in this chapter) because of tissue ischemia and hypoxia. The hypoxia is caused in part by poor perfusion and in part because the O_2-conveying capacity of the blood is reduced owing to the decrease in red blood cells.

Patients with this clinical profile are said to be in decompensated shock. Without prompt treatment their shock will become irreversible. Such irreversibility stems from cellular damage caused by ischemia and hypoxia and is aggravated by the intense vasoconstriction mediated by the release of catecholamines and angiotension II that is part of the body's defense against hypovolemia. Because of the vasoconstriction and the decrease in blood volume, formed blood elements tend to agglutinate in the bloodstream, again compromising tissue perfusion. Also, because of the ongoing cellular damage, capillary permeability increases, leading to loss of water and protein from the intravascular to the interstitial space and a further collapse of the circulation.

Other Clinical Settings

Massive isotonic fluid loss also may occur with diarrhea, and although red blood cells and other formed elements usually are not lost in this condition, severe shock nevertheless may ensue. The loss of hypotonic fluids through sweating or processes such as DI causes much less circulatory compromise, however, because water, but little or no Na^+, is lost. For example, in a 70-kg patient whose total body water is 40 L and whose hematocrit is 45 percent, the rapid loss of 1 L of hypotonic fluid would reduce intravascular volume by only 7 percent. Blood pressure and pulse would remain normal as a result, and thirst would be minimal. The patient might manifest only slightly sunken eyeballs, poor skin turgor, and other signs of volume deficiency—the same signs seen in patients with more chronic forms of volume loss.

Monitoring

Because such signs may be difficult to detect and because volume status may change frequently and rapidly, clinicians may employ a variety of monitoring techniques, especially in critically ill patients. Such monitoring may be as noninvasive as the daily recording of weight gain or loss or Na^+ and water intake and output, as discussed in Chapter 13. Ongoing measurement of blood pressure and pulse by means of intra-arterial catheters may be called for in certain situations, as may measurement of urine output via bladder catheterization. Measurements of urinary Na^+ concentration and other indices of renal Na^+ excretion also may contribute to the assessment of volume status.

When these measures are not sufficient, clinicians may use invasive forms of hemodynamic monitoring. These include measurement of pressure in the right atrium through an indwelling catheter in the superior or inferior vena cava. Unfortunately, the central venous pressure (CVP) measured in this fashion may be elevated owing to decreased compliance of the right ventricle or increases in pulmonary artery pressure and therefore may not indicate pressure in the left side of the heart, which is a more accurate reflection of intravascular volume. As a result, clinicians may prefer to place a flow-directed (Swan-Ganz) catheter into the pulmonary circulation to measure the pulmonary artery wedge or occlusion pressure, as discussed in Chapters 13 and 50.

Treatment

Even when the pulmonary artery wedge pressure is available, management of hypovolemic patients frequently requires empirical or individually adjusted administration of fluids containing Na^+, water, and formed blood elements in proportions and amounts dictated by the substances that have been lost from the body and the rate at which they were depleted. Generally speaking, clinicians should restore the intravascular volume with little regard for the disturbances of osmolality that may result, just as the body does. The most appropriate replacement fluid for massive hemorrhage is either whole blood or its major constituents, red blood cells and plasma.

Until these fluids are available, isotonic or "normal" saline or Ringer's lactate should be given by the intravenous route. Because Na^+ will distribute throughout the ECF space, only one-third of which is blood, 1 L of isotonic saline will restore the intravascular volume by approximately 300 mL. Nevertheless, because interstitial fluid has shifted into the bloodstream during the body's compensation for shock, the 700 mL of saline that is not intravascular is helpful in repleting the interstitial fluid space; this is a cornerstone of what is called *crystalloid therapy*.[6–8]

Another approach to treating hypovolemia due to hemorrhage and certain other conditions is either to give increased concentrations of Na^+ contained in fluids such as hypertonic saline or to administer other osmotically active substances such as synthetic starches or human albumin. The theory behind this is that such substances remain in the bloodstream and tend to draw water from the interstitium into the intravascular space. Intravenous albumin administration, which also is called *colloid therapy*, will indeed support the circulation. At the same time, however, albumin does not help to rehydrate the interstitium. Furthermore, albumin has a limited half-life in the bloodstream and is quite expensive. Finally, during the later stages of shock and in other conditions of increased capillary permeability (see under Apparent Hypovolemia) the albumin may leak into the interstitium and draw water with it. For these reasons, colloid therapy is preferred to crystalloid therapy primarily when, following initial saline replacement, the intravascular albumin concentration is low.

Volume replacement for profuse diarrhea or other causes of isotonic fluid loss usually involves intravenous administration of normal saline or Ringer's lactate. Hypotonic fluid losses due to sweating, DI, or other conditions should be treated with substances such as 5 percent dextrose in water (D_5W) that contain little or no Na^+. Because D_5W lacks Na^+, it is distributed equally within the ECF and intracellular fluid (ICF) compartments. In addition, because two-thirds of total body water is intracellular and one-third is extracellular and because one-third of extracellular water is intravascular, a 1-L infusion of D_5W will expand the bloodstream by only 100 mL. For this reason D_5W would be inappropriate in hemorrhaging patients, although it might be satisfactory in patients with DI. The intravenous solutions and the additions used to maintain water and solute balance are outlined in Table 13-2.

Apparent Hypovolemia

As discussed earlier, hypovolemia requires a decrease in ECF volume. Apparent hypovolemia is said to exist when overall ECF volume is normal or even increased but volume has shifted within the ECF compartment from the intravascular to the interstitial space. Such shifts occur in conditions of increased capillary permeability, such as bacterial sepsis, extensive burns, pancreatitis, and the adult respiratory distress syndrome (ARDS), in which the pulmonary capillaries are involved. The general or local increase in capillary permeability associated with these conditions causes an unbalancing of the Starling equation (discussed earlier) and leads to a displacement of both water and small proteins, including albumin, thereby further dehydrating the bloodstream. The end result is a collection of interstitial ECF that is called edema. This edema may collect in the subcutaneous tissue of patients with sepsis or burns and in the lungs of patients with ARDS. Patients with these diseases may appear severely volume-depleted even though their overall ECF volume is intact.[2]

The differentiation of apparent from real hypovolemia may be difficult, and determination of pulmonary artery wedge pressure may be required. Treatment of apparent hypovolemia also is difficult because administration of additional fluid may overly expand the ECF space, causing hypervolemia and augmenting edema formation. Some clinicians give vasoactive agents to patients with sepsis or ARDS to support blood pressure, improve cardiac output, and constrict arterioles and thereby reduce capillary hydrostatic pressure. Others administer albumin to increase intravascular osmotic pressure and draw water from the interstitium, all the while risking albumin leakage into the interstitial space. The most logical approach is to restore capillary integrity by treating the underlying processes, for example, by giving antibiotics in sepsis, but this approach also may not work.

Hypervolemia

Volume expansion, or hypervolemia, is a state in which ECF volume is increased either acutely or on chronic basis. Hypervolemia occurs when the rate of Na^+ and water intake by the body is greater than the loss of these substances, although input and output may be equal in chronically volume-expanded states. Total body water always is increased during volume expansion. Total body Na^+ usually is increased as well, but hypervolemia can occur with any Na^+ concentration because the Na^+ concentration represents only the relative amounts of Na^+ in serum or plasma and not the total amount in the body.

Causes

When water and Na^+ intake increases, the body normally excretes these substances because the integrated volume response is no longer operative. Hypervolemia happens either because the response is not damped as a result of the body's perception that intravascular volume is not adequate, because hormonal secretion cannot be regulated, or because the kidneys cannot excrete a Na^+ and water load.

Edematous Conditions

The first situation, in which intravascular volume appears inadequate, is characterized by unbalancing of the Starling forces and edema formation. Foremost among the edematous conditions is congestive heart failure, in which despite a normal or even increased intravascular volume, low cardiac output stimulates adrenergic nervous system activity, ADH secretion by the pituitary gland, and renin release by the kidneys, so that Na^+ and water are retained. The increased capillary hydrostatic pressure that results from Na^+ and water retention in patients with congestive heart failure leads to a flux of intravascular fluid into the interstitial space.[1–5]

A second edematous condition is hepatic cirrhosis, in which peripheral arterial vasodilation diminishes vascular filling and stimulates Na^+ and water retention; these substances in turn translocate into the interstitium owing to increased hydrostatic pressure in the portal circulation and decreased oncotic pressure in the bloodstream secondary to a diminution in albumin synthesis by the liver. A third edematous condition is the nephrotic syndrome, in which decreased oncotic pressure due to albumin wasting by the kidneys in combination with intrarenal mechanisms, leads to Na^+ and water retention. In all three conditions water retention may exceed the Na^+ retention, so that hyponatremia and hypotonicity develop.[4,5]

Excess Hormone Secretion

The hormones that in excess may cause hypervolemia are ADH and aldosterone. The former substance may be released by the pituitary not only in response to volume depletion (or hypotonicity, see p. 283) but also in response to drugs such as narcotics and barbiturates and because of severe pain. Excess vasopressin or vasopressin-like material also may be present in the syndrome of inappropriate ADH production (SIADH), which occurs with intracranial processes such as head trauma that activate the pituitary and also with certain neoplasms that independently secrete an ADH-like substance. Solitary water retention is the rule in these conditions of ADH excess, and therefore edema is not present because the excess water distributes between the ECF and ICF, but dilutional hyponatremia does occur. This is not the case with disorders of aldosterone excess, including hyperaldosteronism due to various tumors, in which volume expansion is due primarily to Na^+ retention by the kidneys.[2–5]

Impaired Renal Excretion

The third cause of hypervolemia is impaired renal excretion of Na^+ and water. As noted earlier, chronic renal failure usually is associated with Na^+ and water depletion and hypovolemia. However, acute diseases of the renal glomeruli may limit the kidney's ability to handle Na^+ and water and lead to the retention of these substances. The increased capillary hydrostatic pressure that results from this retention may be responsible for edema formation. Indeed, volume excess may become so pronounced during acute glomerulonephritis that congestive heart failure develops.

Assessment and Treatment

Volume expansion usually can be readily identified by the presence of generalized edema. The blood pressure may be elevated, especially in congestive heart failure, or it may be normal or low, as is often the case in cirrhosis. Neck vein distension is a clue to the presence of elevated right atrial pressure, which again, is most commonly seen in congestive heart failure. A more accurate reading of the CVP may be obtained by a catheter in the superior vena cava; alternatively, the left ventricular end-diastolic pressure may be approximated by measurement of the pulmonary artery wedge or occlusion pressure. Further evaluation of the exact etiology of volume excess may require tests of heart, liver, kidney, and hormonal function.[1,2]

The treatment of hypervolemia naturally depends on its acuteness, severity, and underlying cause. In addition, therapy should be individualized depending on whether patients have primary Na^+ or water retention. For example, patients with mild primary water excess due, for example, to SIADH, usually respond to water restriction; this also helps manage their hyponatremia (see under Hypotonicity). On the other hand, Na^+ restriction, removal, or both may be appropriate in edematous patients. Removal of Na^+ may be accomplished by the administration of loop diuretics such as furosemide that inhibit Na^+ uptake in the ascending loop of Henle or by spironolactone and other agents that inhibit Na^+ reabsorption in the distal tubule. These latter drugs also suppress K^+ excretion and may cause hyperkalemia.

DISORDERS OF EXTRACELLULAR FLUID OSMOLALITY REGULATION

General Principles

Although preservation of ECF volume is paramount, the body also strives to maintain ECF osmolality within the range of 280 to 295 mOsm/kg H_2O through a process of osmoregulation that requires the activation or inhibition of ADH release by the pituitary gland. The process also serves to keep the ECF Na^+ concentration within the range of 135 to 145 mEq/L because Na^+ is the most abundant and osmotically active solute in the ECF. Because all membranes are permeable to water and because ECF osmolality and Na^+ concentration are kept constant, the ratio of solute to water is kept constant in all body compartments. At the same time, as body water balance is maintained by osmoregulation, the volume of body cells is kept constant. This is particularly important in the central nervous system, where cell shrinkage or swelling may have disastrous consequences.[1,2,9]

Although Na^+ is the most osmotically active ECF solute, other solutes also exert an osmotic effect. These include glucose, blood urea nitrogen (BUN), and substances (e.g., ethanol and mannitol) that may be introduced into the body. Serum osmolality is determined by the following equation:

$$(2)\,(Na^+) + \left(\frac{\text{glucose}}{18}\right) + \left(\frac{\text{BUN}}{2.8}\right) \qquad (1)$$

The normal serum Na^+ concentration is 140 mEq/L, the glucose concentration is approximately 100 mg/dL, and the BUN concentration is 10 mg/dL; as a result, serum osmolality is about 285 mOsm/kg H_2O. The osmolar contributions of ethanol and mannitol may be obtained by dividing their serum or plasma concentrations in milligrams per deciliter by 4.6 and 9, respectively, as discussed in Chapter 13.

Although all solutes affect ECF osmolality, only those such as Na^+ and mannitol that preferentially remain in that compartment exert an osmotic effect that can draw water from the ICF into the ECF. The same is true of circulating glucose, whose entry into cells is regulated by hormones and other factors. Because of their normally fixed location in one body compartment, these solutes are called *impermeant.* The term *tonicity* is used to describe the osmotic equivalence of fluids that contain impermeant solutes; these fluids necessarily have the same osmolality as they do tonicity. Thus, isotonic saline is also iso-osmolar, whereas hypotonic saline is hypo-osmolar. Hypotonicity results when the concentration of ECF solutes, in most cases Na^+, decreases and causes net ICF volume excess due to an imbalance of the Starling forces. On the other hand, hypertonicity occurs when ECF solutes increase and cause net ICF volume depletion.[1,2,9]

Hypotonicity

As noted earlier, hypotonicity occurs when ECF solutes are decreased relative to water so that serum osmolality falls and water shifts to the ECF. For practical purposes this is reflected in a decrease in the serum Na^+ concentration to 135 mEq/L or less. The water excess that exists in this situation can be calculated from the formula:

Water excess,

$$L = \left(\frac{140 - \text{serum } Na^+ \text{ concentration}}{140}\right) \times [(0.6)\,(\text{body weight, kg})] \qquad (2)$$

Although the low Na^+ concentration is referred to as a *hy-*

ponatremia, this term does not necessarily indicate the body's Na^+ content. In fact, hypotonicity may exist when the Na^+ content is normal, decreased, or increased. The major clinical manifestation of hypotonicity is water intoxication, which is characterized by apathy and a decline in mental function, which may progress to generalized seizures. Water intoxication is caused by swelling of cells in the central nervous system, a condition called cerebral edema. Other symptoms associated with hypotonicity reflect concomitant abnormalities of Na^+ content and ECF volume.

Hypotonicity with a Normal Na^+ Content

Hypotonicity with a normal Na^+ content and ECF volume is seen in patients with SIADH. The diagnosis of this condition is suggested by the combination of serum hypo-osmolality, urine hyperosmolality, a urine Na^+ concentration greater than 50 mEq/L, and a normal or increased intravascular volume, as discussed earlier. Usually the hypotonicity is not severe; patients may be asymptomatic and require mild water restriction. If the hypotonicity is severe (serum Na^+ concentration, 110 mEq/L or less), if the patient is having convulsions, or if both circumstances exist, a combination of hypertonic fluids rich in Na^+ should be given, along with furosemide or other diuretics that cause the kidneys to excrete hypotonic urine with a lower Na^+ content.[3,8]

Hypotonicity with a Decreased Na^+ Content

Hypotonicity with decreased Na^+ content and ECF volume is seen for the most part in patients who lose large amounts of Na^+ and water from their kidneys, gastrointestinal tract, or bloodstream and replace only the water they have lost. The water is retained because the body releases ADH to maintain ECF volume, but the water equilibrates in the intracellular and extracellular compartments, and ECF volume is not restored. The inadequate intravascular volume in such patients may cause postural changes and symptoms of poor organ perfusion. The urine Na^+ will be less than 20 mEq/L, and urine osmolality will be greater than serum osmolality. Very severe volume depletion should be treated with hypertonic fluids, but isotonic NaCl is sufficient when volume depletion is not so severe.

Hypotonicity with an Increased Na^+ Content

Hypotonicity with an increased Na^+ content and ECF volume occurs primarily in patients with congestive heart failure, cirrhosis, or nephrosis. Although intravascular volume is increased in all three conditions, the body preserves volume and the kidneys retain water because the pituitary liberates ADH. Osmolality may be normalized in some patients with hypotonicity and Na^+ excess if they are given diuretics followed by hypertonic fluids. However, Na^+ repletion of this sort usually worsens edema and other manifestations of Na^+ excess without improving the serum Na^+ concentration because the body retains more water to restore osmolality and perhaps also because it still senses that the ECF volume is low. Therefore most patients do best with a combination of Na^+ and water restriction.

Hypertonicity

Hypertonicity occurs when ECF solutes increase relative to water so that serum osmolality rises and water shifts from the ICF. In most but not all situations, Na^+ is the solute in excess, and the serum Na^+ is 145 mEq/L or more. The water deficit that exists in this situation can be calculated from the formula:

Water deficit,

$$\text{L} = \left(\frac{\text{serum Na}^+ \text{ concentration} - 140}{140}\right) \times [(0.6)\,(\text{body weight, kg})] \quad (3)$$

Although the high Na^+ concentration is referred to as *hypernatremia*, total body Na^+ content may be normal, low, or high.

The major clinical sign of hypertonicity is thirst (assuming patients can communicate). The major clinical symptoms are lethargy and obtundation caused by the depleted water content of cells in the central nervous system, a condition called cerebral dehydration. Presumably because of their vulnerability to dehydration, brain cells can protect themselves by gradually generating intracellular solutes, called idiogenic osmoles, which attract extra water in the face of overall ICF water depletion. Thus, too rapid a return of serum osmolality to normal in hypertonic patients may cause rebound cerebral edema and water intoxication. Other symptoms of hypertonicity relate to associated abnormalities in Na^+ content and ECF volume or to the effects of solutes other than Na^+.[1,9]

Hypertonicity with a Normal Na^+ Content

Hypertonicity with a normal Na^+ content and ECF volume, or pure water depletion, is seen in patients who either lack access to water or who lose it from the respiratory tract because of greatly increased minute ventilation or because they are breathing unhumidified gases. This condition can be corrected by water administration.[1]

Hypertonicity with a Decreased Na^+ Content

Hypertonicity with a decreased Na^+ content and ECF volume is seen in patients who lose water and Na^+ and cannot replace their losses. Such losses may occur through the skin in patients who sweat profusely since sweat is hypotonic. They also may originate from the gastrointestinal tract in patients with severe vomiting or diarrhea, or they may originate from the kidneys, either when osmotically active substances such as glucose or mannitol draw water and Na^+ from the body or when central or nephrogenic DI exists. The urine Na^+ should be greater than 50 mEq/L in both forms of DI unless volume depletion is severe, and the osmolality of the urine should be less than that of serum. Patients with central DI usually increase urine osmolality and correct hypertonicity when given exogenous vasopressin, whereas patients with nephrogenic DI do not. Acute hypertonicity with symptoms of intravascular volume inadequacy should be treated with isotonic fluids. Once ECF volume has been restored, the abnormality in osmolality can be treated by water administration. Water should be given orally or intravenously as D_5W at a rate of less than 500 mL/h if possible to avoid rebound water intoxication.

Hypertonicity with an Increased Na^+ Content

Hypertonicity with an increased Na^+ content and ECF volume is seen in patients given large amounts of Na^+ in the form of salt (NaCl) tablets, sodium bicarbonate ($NaHCO_3$), or hypertonic fluids. Total ECF solute content is approximately 4000 mOsm in 70-kg adults. ECF solute content in a patient given 20 ampules of $NaHCO_3$, each containing 44 mEq Na^+, during cardiopulmonary resuscitation will increase by 1760 mOsm. The serum Na^+ concentration will rise from 140 to 160 mEq/L, and 4000 mL of water will shift from the ICF to the ECF. This ECF overload in turn might cause sudden pulmonary edema and severe cerebral dehydration, as the brain cells will not have enough time to generate idiogenic osmoles. Insults of this sort require rapid treatment with furosemide to induce renal Na^+ and water loss and with water, usually given intravenously, to correct osmolality. Patients whose serum Na^+ exceeds 180 mEq/L may require hemodialysis to restore water and solute balance.[1,9]

Hypertonicity Due to Hyperglycemia

Hyperglycemia, an increase in serum glucose concentration, may occur inadvertently in patients receiving hyperalimentation fluids rich in carbohydrates. Although hypertonicity will occur in this situation, total body Na^+ and water will not be affected. Alternatively, hyperglycemia may occur gradually in patients with diabetic ketoacidosis or hyperosmolar nonketotic coma, conditions characterized by lack of insulin or by a decreased tissue responsiveness to the hormone. These patients may experience profound renal Na^+ and water losses and may not replace their losses adequately. Hyperglycemia attracts water from the ICF to the ECF and artifactually lowers the serum Na^+ concentration in all circumstances, so that the rise in Na^+ concentration seen in hypertonicity due to Na^+ alone may or may not be present, depending on whether more Na^+ or more water has been lost.[1,9]

The serum Na^+ concentration can be expected to fall by 1.6 mEq/L for every 100 mg/dL rise in the glucose concentration over its normal level of approximately 100 mg/dL. Calculation of the true Na^+ concentration by this method should tell the clinician what the patient's Na^+ concentration will be after hyperglycemia is corrected by insulin. Since total body Na^+ is likely to be low unless hyperglycemia is acute, regardless of the true serum Na^+ concentration, water should not be given initially to correct the hyperosmolality caused by glucose. Instead, the patient should receive isotonic fluids to ensure intravascular volume adequacy.

Once intravascular volume has been restored, the patient may be given water to correct hypertonicity due to an increased Na^+ concentration, if it exists. The rapidity of water administration should reflect its rate of loss when hyperglycemia was present. Overly aggressive rehydration during correction of hyperglycemia is particularly hazardous in patients with hyperosmolar nonketotic coma. In such patients, water once held in the ECF by its high glucose concentration, which may approach 2000 mg/dL, shifts rapidly into the ICF and may cause water intoxication as it enters cerebral cells.

Hypertonicity Due to Solutes Other Than Na^+ and Glucose

Hypertonicity also may result from the presence of mannitol and other impermeant solutes, such as glycerol or sorbitol, in the ECF. These substances may cause a Na^+ and water diuresis and may also artifactually lower the serum Na^+ concentration by diluting the ECF, as does glucose. Treatment of hypertonicity due to these solutes is similar to that for hyperglycemia in that attention is focused first on ECF volume protection and then on correction of hyperosmolality.[9]

DISORDERS OF POTASSIUM BALANCE

General Principles

In Chapter 13 the point was made that K^+ is the major intracellular anion in the body. Approximately 98 percent of total body K^+, which amounts to some 3400 mEq in a 70-kg individual, is found in the ICF, primarily in skeletal muscle; only 2 percent of total body K^+, amounting to between 50 and 75 mEq, is found in the ECF. The ICF therefore serves as the body's major reservoir of K^+, and as such it helps protect the constancy of the ECF K^+ concentration. This concentration normally ranges between 3.5 and 5.5 mEq/L because the 50 to 75 mEq is distributed throughout the 14-L ECF volume of a 70-kg individual. In a chronic, steady-state condition, then, a 1 mEq/L rise or fall in the serum or plasma K^+ concentration usually reflects an increase or decrease in intracellular K^+ of between 100 and 200 mEq/L. The clinical consequences of these changes are due less to gains or losses in total body K^+ than to alterations in the K^+ concentration, which in turn affect the ratio of K^+ in the ICF and ECF.[1,10]

K^+ balance in the body is maintained by three processes, any or all of which may become disturbed and produce imbalance. The first process is K^+ intake, which involves dietary K^+ consumption and the release of K^+ from the breakdown of muscle and other cells. Daily K^+ intake usually amounts to 100 mEq in a 70-kg individual and is balanced by the second process, K^+ excretion. Normally only small amounts of the solute are excreted by the skin and gastrointestinal tract, so K^+ excretion for the most part involves secretion by the renal tissues. Such secretion is governed by factors such as Na^+ delivery to the tubules, changes in ECF acidity and alkalinity, the presence of unabsorbable anions such as phosphate and sulfate, and the effects of the hormone aldosterone, which causes an exchange of Na^+ for K^+ in defense of ECF volume, as previously discussed. From the discussion it seems that K^+ imbalance will occur if intake or output rises or falls excessively without a commensurate change in the other process.

The third process that affects K^+ balance is the shift of the solute between the ICF and ECF. This shift may involve the active transport of K^+ into cells by beta-adrenergic stimulation, by the hormones insulin and aldosterone, or the passive transport that occurs in the presence of increased ECF alkalinity. Alternatively, K^+ may enter cells in the presence of increased ECF acidity or hypertonic fluids or as a result of alpha-adrenergic stimulation. When these conditions are acute, total body K^+ need not change because K^+ is never added to or lost from the body. Nevertheless, serious problems may result from alterations in the ECF K^+ concentration and the distribution of K^+ between the ICF and the ECF.[11]

Hypokalemia

As suggested by the previous discussion, hypokalemia may be due to inadequate K^+ intake, excess K^+ loss, or a shift of K^+ into cells from the ECF. Inadequate intake is seen for the most part in patients who are malnourished either because of alcoholism or because of eating "tea and toast" diets, or in hospitalized patients who receive too little K^+ in intravenous fluids. Excess K^+ losses can be divided into those due to renal or to extrarenal causes. Renal K^+ loss may be due to conditions that increase mineralocorticoid levels, including primary aldosteronism, secondary aldosteronism related to congestive heart failure, and Cushing's syndrome and other causes of glucocorticoid excess. An increased delivery of Na^+ and water to the distal renal tissues also enhances K^+ secretion, so diabetes and the osmotic diuresis caused by mannitol administration produce K^+ loss. Renal tubular acidosis, especially the proximal type treated with HCO_3^-, is associated with renal K^+ wasting. Finally, furosemide and other diuretics may cause hypokalemia on a renal basis. Extrarenal K^+ loss may involve the skin, especially in athletes and other persons who sweat profusely, and the gastrointestinal tract, especially in patients with protracted vomiting or diarrhea.[12]

Intracellular shifts of K^+ that result in hypokalemia are seen most commonly in alkalosis, an acid-base disturbance discussed later in this chapter. Insulin also causes a shift of K^+ from the ECF into the ICF, but it rarely reduces the K^+ concentration enough to produce symptoms. The same is true following endogenous or exogenous beta-adrenergic stimulation, including that caused by parenteral or aerosolized bronchodilators.[13,14] Thyrotoxicosis, a state of advanced hyperthyroidism, may be associated with severe hypokalemia, as may a rare familial condition called periodic hypokalemic paralysis.

Many patients with mild hypokalemia whose K^+ levels remain above 3 mEq/L have no symptoms at all. However, when the K^+ concentration falls much lower than this, muscle weakness is likely to occur because the aggravated increase in ICF/ECF K^+ ratio hyperpolarizes the muscle cells and then prolongs repolarization.[15,16] Lower K^+ levels may lead to areflexic paralysis and can cause respiratory failure due to weakness of the diaphragm and other respiratory muscles. At the same time, large K^+ losses from skeletal muscle may be associated with rhabdomyolysis, the appearance of myoglobin in urine, and subsequent renal failure. Rhabdomyolysis may be seen in trauma patients with crush injuries and in athletes or military recruits following extreme exercise.[17]

In parallel with its effects in skeletal muscle, hypokalemia alters the polarization of cardiac muscle. This leads to characteristic electrocardiographic (ECG) manifestations, including depression of the ST segment and T wave and elevation of the U waves (Fig. 28-1). These changes usually are without clinical consequence and are significant only in gauging the severity of hypokalemia. However, especially in patients treated with digitalis, profound falls in the K^+ level may be associated with life-threatening dysrhythmias.[12]

The treatment of hypokalemia involves correction of its underlying cause and restoration of the K^+ concentration. This restoration usually should be gradual because the ICF/ECF K^+ ratio is more important than the absolute K^+ level. Thus, approximately 60 mEq/d of K^+ should be given to patients when K^+ concentration is 3 mEq/L or higher; oral administration is preferable. If the K^+ concentration is between 2 and 3 mEq/L, 100 mEq/d of K^+ may be given in addition to that needed to replace ongoing losses. Patients with severe symptoms or ECG changes and asymptomatic patients whose K^+ concentration is less than 2.0 mEq/L usually should receive intravenous K^+ at the rate of 20 to 40 mEq/h. Such patients should receive ECG monitoring and should have their K^+ levels checked to avoid unintentional hyperkalemia.[10]

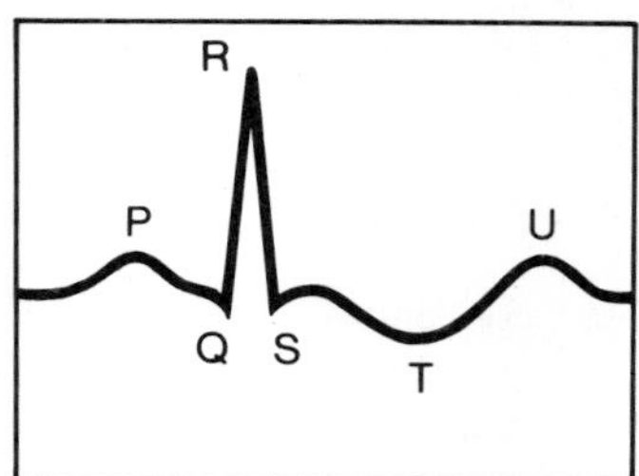

Figure 28-1. ECG changes in hypokalemia. Note ST depression and prominent U wave. (From Ott,[12] with permission.)

Hyperkalemia

Hyperkalemia may be caused by increased K^+ intake, decreased K^+ excretion, or a shift of K^+ from cells to the ECF. Acute or chronic increases in the K^+ concentration due to exogenous K^+ administration are uncommon in normal persons because the ICF acts as a reservoir for excess K^+ and because renal excretion should increase in this circumstance. However, some patients with abnormal renal function who consume large amounts of K^+ in foods such as bananas may become hyperkalemic, as may patients who receive K^+ in intravenous antibiotics or fluids. Diminished excretion of K^+ from the kidneys is seen for the most part in patients with renal failure due to decreased delivery of K^+ to the tubules. In the absence of renal failure, tubular secretion of K^+ may be decreased by hypoaldosteronism, Addison's disease, or diuretics such as spironolactone.[18,19]

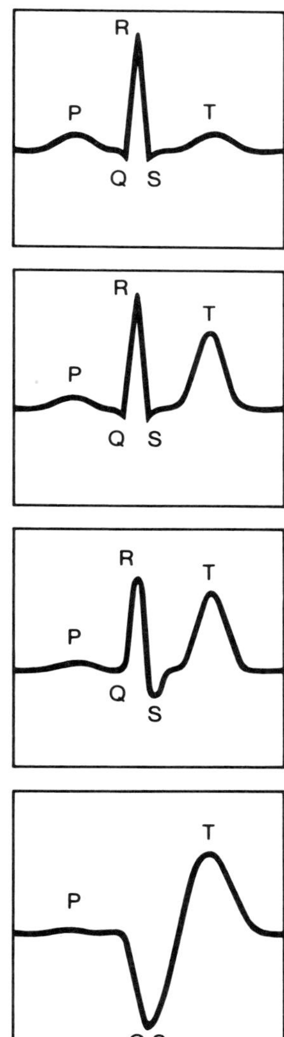

Figure 28-2. Progression of ECG changes in hyperkalemia. The T wave becomes symmetrically peaked, the P wave disappears, and the QRS evolves into a sine wave. (From Ott,[12] with permission.)

Perhaps the most common cause of hyperkalemia due to transcellular shifts of the solute is acidosis (discussed later in this chapter). Cell destruction associated with trauma, the lysis of certain tumors, hemolysis of red blood cells, and rhabdomyolysis all may increase the K^+ concentration. Hyperkalemia also may be caused by the administration of succinylcholine, which depolarizes muscle; by beta-adrenergic blockade due to drugs such as propranolol; and by familial hyperkalemic periodic paralysis.

Although hyperkalemia may cause muscle paralysis, its major toxic effect is cardiac dysrhythmias related to depolarization of heart muscle cells as a result of the decreased ICF/ECF K^+ ratio. The earliest ECG manifestation of hyperkalemia is peaking of the T wave, which occurs at a K^+ concentration of around 6.5 mEq/L. This is followed by a loss of P waves and a widening of the QRS complex, which eventually evolves into a sine wave (Fig. 28-2). At this point if not earlier, ventricular fibrillation, a potentially fatal dysrhythmia, is common.[18]

The treatment of hyperkalemia involves attention to its underlying cause, rapid reversal of ECG abnormalities, and removal of K^+ from the body. Ca, which does nothing to the K^+ level, but counteracts the effects of hyperkalemia on heart muscle excitability, should be given as Ca gluconate intravenously when P waves are absent and the QRS complex on the ECG is widened. Thereafter, or as a first step if the ECG is less abnormal, the intravenous combination of glucose, insulin, and $NaHCO_3$ will promote K^+ shift into cells. The $NaHCO_3$ must be given in a separate intravenous line from that of Ca to avoid precipitation of the latter. Finally, exchange resins such as kayexelate can be given orally or by enema to exchange Na^+ for K^+ in the gut. If renal failure has contributed to the hyperkalemia, dialysis may be required.[18]

DISORDERS OF ACID-BASE BALANCE

General Principles

As noted in Chapter 13, the body's acid-base status may be quantified in terms of either the serum or the plasma concentration of H^+ or the negative logarithm of that concentration, the pH. H^+ is generated by the regular production of nonvolatile acids through cellular metabolism and normally is excreted by the kidneys in a process that regenerates HCO_3^-, the normal concentration of which is 24 mEq/L, with a range of 22 to 26 mEq/L. At the same time, cellular respiration accounts for the production of the volatile acid CO_2, which is excreted by the lungs. The partial pressure of CO_2 in systemic arterial blood ($PaCO_2$) represents a balance between CO_2 production ($\dot{V}CO_2$) and alveolar ventilation ($\dot{V}_A$) in the body. It normally is 40 mmHg at sea level, with a range of 35 to 45 mmHg.

The systemic arterial pH (pHa) normally is 7.40, with a range of 7.35 to 7.45. It is maintained at that level by the kidneys and lungs on a regular basis. However, acute perturbations in acid production and elimination are compensated primarily by the H_2CO_3/HCO_3^- buffering system, in which H_2CO_3 is formed by hydration of CO_2 in the presence of the enzyme carbonic anhydrase (CA) by the reaction:

$$CO_2 + H_2O \overset{CA}{\rightleftharpoons} H_2CO_3 \rightleftharpoons H^+ + HCO_3^- \quad (4)$$

The Henderson-Hasselbalch equation describing the dissociation of H_2CO_3 (see Ch. 1) may be written as

$$pH = 6.1 + \log \frac{HCO_3^- \text{ concentration}}{(0.3)\,(PaCO_2)} \quad (5)$$

Implicit in this equation is the concept that changes in the body's HCO_3^- concentration reflect metabolic acid-base balance, whereas change in the $PaCO_2$ reflects respiratory acid-base balance. At the same time, since changes in HCO_3^- are controlled by the kidneys and $PaCO_2$ is controlled by the lungs, the Henderson-Hasselbalch equation can be rewritten as

$$pH = pK + \log \frac{\text{kidneys}}{\text{lungs}} \quad (6)$$

to conceptualize how metabolic acid-base changes are compensated by respiratory acid-base changes and vice versa.

The relative acidity of blood with a pH of 7.35 or less is called *acidemia*, whereas the relative alkalinity of blood with a pH of 7.45 or more is called *alkalemia*. These terms are preferable to the words acidosis and alkalosis, which are used to describe the processes through which acidemia and alkalemia occur. Respiratory acidosis and alkalosis are disturbances in the production or elimination of volatile acid. Respiratory acidosis results from an increase in $PaCO_2$ that is due to an increase in the ratio $\dot{V}CO_2/\dot{V}A$; this increase in $PaCO_2$ is called hypoventilation because $\dot{V}A$ is decreased relative to $\dot{V}CO_2$. On the other hand, respiratory alkalosis results from a decrease in $PaCO_2$ that occurs because the ratio $\dot{V}CO_2/\dot{V}A$ decreases; this decrease in $PaCO_2$ is called hyperventilation because $\dot{V}A$ is increased relative to $\dot{V}CO_2$.

Metabolic acidosis and alkalosis are disturbances in the production or elimination of nonvolatile acid. Metabolic acidosis results from a decrease in HCO_3^- that occurs because HCO_3^- is lost from or H^+ is added to the body. The HCO_3^- may be lost in diarrheal fluid or because the kidney malfunctions and either wastes HCO_3^- or fails to regenerate it; alternatively, H^+ may enter the body in the form of HCl. On the other hand, metabolic alkalosis results from an increase in HCO_3^- that occurs because H^+ is lost from or HCO_3^- is added to the body. In this case, H^+ may be lost through protracted vomiting; HCO_3^- retention usually occurs because of ECF volume concentration, increased delivery of Na^+ to the kidney, or an excess of aldosterone.[20]

Respiratory Acidosis

Respiratory acidosis, as noted previously, is caused by alveolar hypoventilation and by definition can be present only when the $PaCO_2$ exceeds approximately 45 mmHg. This elevation in $PaCO_2$ is also called hypercapnia. Acute respiratory acidosis usually is a primary disorder seen in sedative drug overdosage, respiratory arrest, or exacerbations of obstructive and restrictive lung disease. Respiratory acidosis also may serve as compensation for metabolic alkalosis, although a $PaCO_2$ over 50 mmHg for purely compensatory reasons is unusual. Although the acidemia of uncompensated respiratory acidosis generally depresses cardiovascular and cerebral function, hypercapnia may increase cardiac irritability through activation of the sympathetic nervous system. It also increases cerebral blood flow. Since CO_2 crosses the blood-brain barrier, acute hypercapnia is a potent stimulus of ventilation in persons who are physically able to breathe.[21]

Systemic arterial blood gas analysis of a patient with acute respiratory acidosis might reveal a pH of 7.30, a $PaCO_2$ of 50 mmHg, and a HCO_3^- of 25 mEq/L. It should be noted that the patient is acidemic (pH, 7.30), has respiratory acidosis ($PaCO_2$, 50 mmHg), and has no metabolic change (HCO_3^-, 25 mEq/L). The normal HCO_3^- concentration in this case, coupled with a decrease in pH that is proportional to the increase in $PaCO_2$, indicates the acuteness of the acid-base disorder.

Acute respiratory acidosis is defended against by buffering and eventually by renal retention of HCO_3^-, that is, by metabolic alkalosis. Although acute respiratory acidosis can be treated by administration of alkali, this is neither indicated nor necessary if the $PaCO_2$ can be lowered by increasing $\dot{V}A$. If the patient cannot achieve this increase spontaneously, mechanical ventilation may be required. If uncorrected, acute respiratory acidosis may progress to the chronic respiratory acidosis seen in patients with severe obstructive or restrictive lung disease. Such patients become adjusted to the high $PaCO_2$ associated with this condition, and because the pH is near normal, aggressive therapy of the acid-base disorder is not required. However, intervention often is mandated by the superimposition of acute respiratory acidosis on chronic respiratory acidosis, as frequently occurs when pulmonary patients develop bronchitis or pneumonia and experience acute hypercapnic respiratory failure.[21]

Respiratory Alkalosis

Respiratory alkalosis results from alveolar hyperventilation and is characterized by a decrease in the $PaCO_2$ to below 35 mmHg. This decrease is also called hypocapnia. Acute respiratory alkalosis may result from anxiety in patients with the acute hyperventilation syndrome. Nonetheless, because a decreased $PaCO_2$ also may accompany shock, sepsis, salicylate intoxication, or overvigorous mechanical ventilation, the diagnosis of hyperventilation syndrome should be one of exclusion. Respiratory alkalosis also may serve as compensation for metabolic acidosis and in such circumstances may be quite profound. The alkalemia associated with uncompensated respiratory alkalosis increases cardiac and cerebral irritability. In addition, hypocapnia decreases cerebral blood flow, and the exchange of extracellular K^+ and Ca for intracellular H^+ increases neuromuscular irritability. As a result, cardiac dysrhythmias and seizures may occur in patients with this disorder.[21]

Systemic arterial blood gas analysis of a patient with acute respiratory alkalosis might reveal a pH of 7.48, a $PaCO_2$ of 30 mmHg, and a HCO_3^- of 22 mEq/L. It should be noted that the patient is alkalemic (pH, 7.48), has respiratory alkalosis ($PaCO_2$, 30 mmHg), and has no metabolic change (HCO_3^-, 22 mEq/L). Here again, the normal HCO_3^- concentration, coupled with an increase in pH that is proportional to the decrease in $PaCO_2$, indicates the acute nature of the acid-base disorder.

The treatment of acute respiratory alkalosis usually is aimed at its underlying cause. This includes reduction of the minute ventilation of alkalemic patients on mechanical ventilators; correction with metabolic acids such as dilute HCl is rarely required. Chronic respiratory alkalosis is seen in individuals living at high altitudes, who are stimulated to hyperventilate by the low ambient inspired O_2 pressure, in patients with restrictive lung disease, and in persons undergoing long-term mechanical ventilation. Since the pH is near normal in such situations, treatment of the acid-base disorder is not required.[21]

Metabolic Acidosis

Metabolic acidosis results from either the loss of HCO_3^- or the addition of H^+ to the body. It is characterized by a reduced HCO_3^- concentration. Metabolic acidosis may be divided into two types depending on whether an anion gap is present. As discussed in Chapter 13, the total number of cations—Na^+ and K^+—and anions—Cl^-, HCO_3^- and small amounts of phosphate, sulfate, and other metabolic salts—must be equal for serum or plasma to maintain electrical neutrality. A 10 mEq/L difference between the Na^+ concentration and the sum of the Cl^- and HCO_3^- concentrations is usually reported in serum samples sent to the laboratory, however, because phosphates, sulfates, and other anions are not measured.[1]

Although HCO_3^- is generally reduced in all forms of metabolic acidosis, the concentration of Cl^- increases when exogenous acids such as HCl are ingested, when metabolic acidosis is a compensation for respiratory alkalosis, or in renal tubular acidosis. In these instances the anion difference or gap does not increase. However, in other disorders the fall in HCO_3^- is not balanced by a rise in Cl^- but instead by other unmeasured anions, and an anion gap greater than 10 mEq/L occurs (see Fig. 13-5). In addition to phosphate and sulfate, which may accumulate in renal failure, these unmeasured anions include lactate, the result of anaerobic metabolism; acetate and other products of the breakdown of ketones that occurs during starvation and in diabetes, in which glucose is not metabolized; and certain acidic compounds such as salicylates,[22–25] (Table 28-1). Acute metabolic acidosis with an anion gap due to lactate accumulation is particularly common in patients with poor tissue perfusion, respiratory failure, or both.[26,27]

Systemic arterial blood gas analysis of a patient with acute

Table 28-1. Causes of Metabolic Acidosis

With an increased anion gap
Uncontrolled diabetes mellitus
Renal failure
Lactic acidosis
Ingestion of
Ethyl alcohol, with starvation and production of keto acids
Salicylate
Methyl alcohol
Paraldehyde
Ethylene glycol
With a normal anion gap
Diarrhea or loss of other gastrointestinal fluids with high HCO_3^- concentrations
Renal tubular acidosis
Ureterosigmoidostomy
Administration of
HCl
NH_4Cl
Carbonic anhydrase inhibitors

NH_4Cl, ammonium chloride
(From Luce et al.,[1] with permission.)

metabolic acidosis might reveal a pH of 7.22, a $PaCO_2$ of 20 mmHg, and a HCO_3^- of 10 mEq/L, with simultaneous serum electrolytes of Na^+, 140 mEq/L; K^+, 4 mEq/L; Cl^-, 100 mEq/L; and HCO_3^-, 10 mEq/L. It should be noted that the patient is acidemic (pH, 7.22), has a compensatory respiratory alkalosis ($PaCO_2$, 20 mmHg), has a metabolic acidosis (HCO_3^-, 10 mEq/L), and has an anion gap [$Na^+ - (Cl^- + HCO_3^-) = 30$ mEq/L]. Even though two acid-base disorders are present, the acidemic pH suggests that metabolic acidosis is the primary disturbance and that respiratory alkalosis is compensatory. The acuteness of the disorders cannot be determined.

Whatever its cause, metabolic acidosis is a severe acid-base disturbance because pH falls precipitously and body stores of HCO_3^- are depleted. Respiratory alkalosis may provide some compensation, but many patients with lung disease cannot hyperventilate for prolonged periods. Therapy for acute metabolic acidosis is aimed at the underlying disorder, for example at the prevention of anaerobic metabolism and excess lactic acid production by increasing blood supply to a patient's tissues or at the prevention of ketone metabolism by supplying a diabetic patient with insulin. When this will not suffice or when the pH is below 7.0 or the HCO_3^- concentration below 5 mEq/L, HCO_3^- (in the form of $NaHCO_3$) often is given despite controversy about the possible toxicity of the treatment.[28,29]

The dose of HCO_3^- in milliequivalents per liter may be calculated as follows: HCO_3^- mEq needed = (normal HCO_3^- concentration − measured HCO_3^- concentration) (0.4 × body weight in kg). $NaHCO_3$ usually is given in one-ampule (44 mEq) boluses, and the pH and serum HCO_3^- concentration are followed closely to avoid overcompensation and the creation of metabolic alkalosis. The patient's intravascular volume status also must be monitored, for the Na^+ administered in $NaHCO_3$ remains in the ECF and attracts water from the ICF; this latter action may cause coma, owing to hypertonicity of cells in the central nervous system. Chronic metabolic acidosis, such as may occur in patients with chronic diarrhea or renal failure, may also require supplemental HCO_3^- to replenish body HCO_3^- stores and to prevent the dissolution of bone, which serves as a buffer when HCO_3^- is low. Clinicians should bear in mind that HCO_3^- ultimately will be converted into CO_2 and cause respiratory acidosis unless the CO_2 can be eliminated by the lungs. For this and other reasons, dichloroacetate may provide better therapy.[30]

Metabolic Alkalosis

Metabolic alkalosis results from the loss of H^+ or the addition of HCO_3^- to the body. It is usually generated by the loss of H^+, Na^+, and K^+, either from the gastrointestinal tract during vomiting or nasogastric suctioning or from the kidneys in patients taking diuretics, such as thiazides, that block the renal reabsorption of Cl^-. ECF volume is decreased in all these situations, so that the metabolic alkalosis is maintained by enhanced renal reabsorption of $NaHCO_3$ in an effort to support ECF volume.[31,32] Total body Cl^- stores also are reduced, since Cl^- is the major anion for the cations lost from the body, and the urinary Cl^- concentration should be less than 10 mEq/L[33] (Table 28-2). This indicates that the alkalosis should be Cl^- responsive, that is, it should be correctable with Cl^-. Metabolic alkalosis can also occur with a normal or high ECF volume in patients with severe K^+ depletion and hyperaldosteronism, in which case the urinary Cl^- concentration should be greater than 10 mEq/L. This indicates that the alkalosis may not respond to Cl^- alone.

Systemic arterial blood gas analysis in a patient with metabolic alkalosis might reveal a pH of 7.50, a $PaCO_2$ of 45 mmHg, and a HCO_3^- of 35 mEq/L, with simultaneous serum electrolytes of Na^+, 140 mEq/L; K^+, 4 mEq/L; Cl^-, 100 mEq/L; HCO_3^-, 35 mEq/L; and a urine Cl^- of 5 mEq/L. It should be noted that the patient is alkalemic (pH, 7.50) and has respiratory acidosis ($PaCO_2$, 45 mmHg), metabolic alkalosis (HCO_3^-, 35 mEq/L), and a low urine Cl^- concentration (5 mEq/L). Even though two acid-base disturbances are present, the alkalemic pH suggests that metabolic alkalosis is the primary disturbance and that respiratory acidosis is compensatory. The acuteness of the disturbance cannot be determined.

Table 28-2. Causes of Metabolic Alkalosis

With low urine chloride
Vomiting, nasogastric suction
Diuretic therapy
With normal or high urine chloride
Increased mineralocorticoid activity
Hyperaldosteronism
Cushing's syndrome
Exogenous glucocorticosteroid administration
Exogenous alkali administration

The formula used earlier to determine HCO_3^- depletion may be used to estimate Cl^- depletion by substituting Cl^- for the final calculated HCO_3^-, since a reciprocal relationship exists between HCO_3^- and Cl^-. For practical purposes Cl^- is usually given as NaCl while serum electrolytes are monitored. Supplemental K^+ is needed for patients who are not Cl^- responsive; it can usually be given as KCl. In fact, some clinicians give KCl to all patients with metabolic alkalosis without worrying about why it has occurred. Patients whose ECF volume is normal or increased or in whom metabolic and respiratory alkalosis coexist may be treated with dilute HCl, although this is seldom necessary.

Combined Acid-Base Disorders

Combinations of the aforementioned disorders occur commonly and are particularly severe if the respiratory and metabolic processes are in the same direction, as in the case of combined respiratory and metabolic alkalosis just cited. When this occurs, the blood pH is so alkalemic (or acidemic, in the case of combined respiratory and metabolic acidosis) that the question of whether one process is compensatory for the other is rarely raised. This question does arise, however, when the processes oppose each other and the possibility exists that one is primary. One approach to this problem is to use empirically developed nomograms that plot changes in pH, $PaCO_2$, and HCO_3^- concentrations in various states (Fig. 28-3). Another approach is to remember that because secondary compensation rarely returns the pH to normal and never overshoots in the opposite direction, the primary process is likely to be reflected in the pH.[34]

Unfortunately, the situation becomes more complex when three acid-base disturbances are present. When this occurs, the anion gap should be calculated; if the gap is greater than 10 mEq/L, a primary metabolic acidosis must exist because compensatory metabolic acidosis is of the non-anion gap variety. Next, the excess anion gap, which is the difference between the measured anion gap and the normal gap of 10 mEq/L, should be calculated and added to the measured HCO_3^- concentration. This will yield the HCO_3^- concentration before the most recent acid-base disorder occurred. If the sum is greater than 26 mEq/L, an underlying metabolic alkalosis must be present; if the sum is less than 22 mEq/L, an underlying non-anion gap metabolic acidosis must be present.[35]

Systemic arterial blood gas analysis of a patient with a triple acid-base disorder might reveal a pH of 7.48, a $PaCO_2$ of 20 mmHg, and a HCO_3^- of 15 mEq/L, with simultaneous serum electrolytes of Na^+, 140 mEq/L; K^+, 4 mEq/L; Cl^-, 100 mEq/L; and HCO_3^-, 15 mEq/L. It should be noted that the patient is alkalemic (pH, 7.48) and has respiratory alkalosis ($PaCO_2$, 20 mmHg), metabolic acidosis (HCO_3^-, 15 mEq/L, and has an anion gap [$Na^+ - (Cl^- + HCO_3^-) =$ 25 mEq/L]. The excess anion gap is 15 mEq/L (25 mEq/L − 10 mEq/L). When this is added to the measured HCO_3^- (15 mEq/L), the "original" HCO_3^- amounts to 30 mEq/L, so the patient has metabolic alkalosis as well.

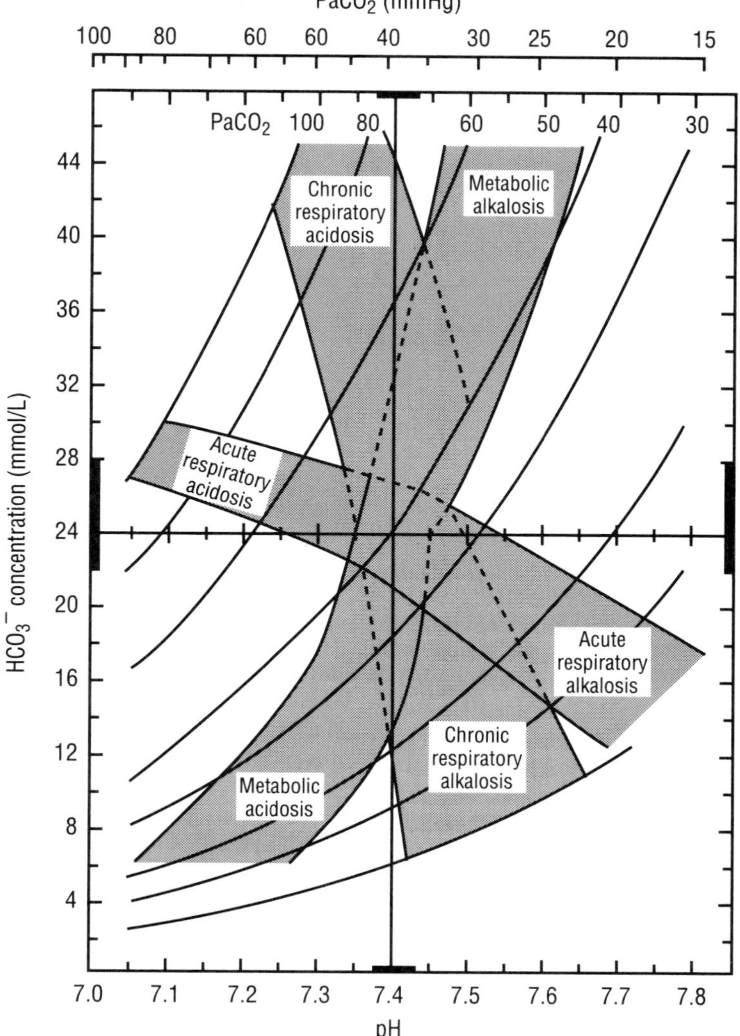

Figure 28-3. Acid-base nomogram of changes in blood pH, $PaCO_2$ and HCO_3^- concentration, the acid-base disorder can be named by finding the point at which variables intersect on the nomogram. (From Luce et al.,[1] with permission.)

References

1. Luce JM, Tyler ML, Pierson DJ: Intensive Respiratory Care. 2nd Ed. WB Saunders, Philadelphia, 1992 (in press)
2. Andreoli TE: Disorders of fluid volume, electrolyte, and acid-base balance. pp. 528–557. In Wyngaarden JB, Smith LH (eds): Cecil's Textbook of Medicine. 18th Ed. WB Saunders, Philadelphia, 1988
3. Schrier RW, Berl T: Disorders of water metabolism. pp. 1–44. In Schrier RW (ed): Renal and Electrolyte Disorders. Little Brown, Boston, 1976
4. Schrier RW: Pathogenesis of sodium and water retention in high-output and low-output cardiac failure, nephrotic syndrome, cirrhosis, and pregnancy, part one. N Engl J Med 1988;319:1065–1072
5. Schrier RW: Pathogenesis of sodium and water retention in high-output and low-output cardiac failure, nephrotic syndrome, cirrhosis, and pregnancy, part two. N Engl J Med 1988;319:1127–1134
6. Ayus JC, Krothapalli RK, Arieff AI: Treatment of symptomatic hyponatremia and its relation to brain damage. N Engl J Med 1987;317:1190–1195
7. Arieff AI: Hyponatremia, convulsions, respiratory arrest, and permanent brain damage after elective surgery in healthy women. N Engl J Med 1986;314:1529–1535
8. Sterns RH: Severe symptomatic hyponatremia: Treatment and outcome. Ann Intern Med 1987;107:656–664
9. Feig PU, McCurdy DK: The hypertonic state. N Engl J Med 1977;297:1444–1454
10. Gabow P: Disorders of potassium metabolism. pp. 143–165. In Schrier RW (ed): Renal and Electrolyte Disorders. Little Brown, Boston, 1976
11. Adrogue HJ, Madias NE: Changes in plasma potassium concentration during acute acid-base disturbances. Am J Med 1981;71:456–467

12. Ott SM: Hypokalemia. pp. 307–310. In Luce JM, Pierson DJ (eds): Critical Care Medicine. WB Saunders, Philadelphia, 1988
13. Gelmont DM, Balmes JR, Yee A: Hypokalemia induced by inhaled bronchodilators. Chest 1988;94:763–766
14. Brown MJ, Brown DC, Murphy MB: Hypokalemia from beta$_2$-receptor stimulation by circulating epinephrine. N Engl J Med 1979;309:1414–1419
15. Nardone DA, McDonald WJ, Girard DE: Mechanisms in hypokalemia: Clinical correlation. Medicine (Baltimore) 1978;57:435–446
16. Knochel JP: Neuromuscular manifestations of electrolyte disorders. Am J Med 1982;72:521–535
17. Gabow PA, Kaehny WD, Kelleher SP: The spectrum of rhabdomyolysis. Medicine (Baltimore) 1982;61:141–152
18. Ott SM: Hyperkalemia. pp. 302–306. In Luce JM, Pierson DJ (eds): Critical Care Medicine. WB Saunders, Philadelphia, 1988
19. Cox M, Sterns RH, Singer I: The defense against hyperkalemia: The roles of insulin and aldosterone. N Engl J Med 1978;299:525–532
20. Ott SM, Luce JM: Acid-base disturbances. pp. 271–283. In Luce JM, Pierson DJ (eds): Critical Care Medicine. WB Saunders, Philadelphia, 1988
21. Narins RG, Jones ER, Stom MC et al: Diagnostic strategies in disorders of fluid, electrolyte and acid-base homeostasis. Am J Med 1982;72:496–520
22. Emmett M, Narins RG: Clinical use of the anion gap. Medicine (Baltimore) 1977;56:38–54
23. Gabow PA, Kaehny WD, Fennessey PV et al: Diagnostic importance of an increased serum anion gap. N Engl J Med 1980;303:854–858
24. Foster DW, McGarry JD: The metabolic derangements and treatment of diabetic ketoacidosis. N Engl J Med 1983;309:159–169
25. Gabow PA, Anderson RJ, Potts DE, Schrier RW: Acid-base disturbances in the salicylate-intoxicated adult. Arch Intern Med 1978;138:1481–1484
26. Oliva PB: Lactic acidosis. Am J Med 1970;48:209–225
27. Kreisberg RA: Lactate homeostasis and lactic acidosis. Ann Intern Med 1980;92:227–237
28. Morris LR, Murphy MB, Kitabchi AE: Bicarbonate therapy in severe diabetic ketoacidosis. Ann Intern Med 1986;105:836–840
29. Stacpoole PW: Lactic acidosis: The case against bicarbonate therapy. Ann Intern Med 1986;105:276–279
30. Stacpoole PW, Harman EM, Curry SH et al: Treatment of lactic acidosis with dichloroacetate. N Engl J Med 1983;309:390–396
31. Cogan MG, Liu FY, Berger BE et al: Metabolic Alkalosis. Med Clin North Am 1983;67:903–914
32. Seldin DW, Rector FC: The generation and maintenance of metabolic alkalosis. Kidney Int 1972;1:306–321
33. Sherman RA, Eisinger RP: The use (and misuse) of urinary sodium and chloride measurements. JAMA 1982;247:3121–3124
34. Narins RG, Emmett M: Simple and mixed acid-base disorders: A practical approach. Medicine (Baltimore) 1980;59:161–187
35. Haber RJ: A practical approach to acid-base disorders. West J Med 1991;155:146–151

Chapter 29

Respiratory Failure: Introduction and Overview

David J. Pierson

CHAPTER OUTLINE

COMPONENTS OF NORMAL RESPIRATION: WHAT CAN GO WRONG

Only with a thorough understanding of normal respiration and the ways in which its components may become disturbed can the clinician take a physiologic approach to therapy for respiratory failure. As discussed more thoroughly in Chapter 2 and summarized in Table 29-1, the three basic respiratory functions are ventilation of the alveoli, oxygenation of the blood, and oxygenation of the tissues. Each in turn has two components: alveolar ventilation both supplies O_2 to the lung's gas exchange surface and removes CO_2; blood oxygenation involves attaining both a certain partial pressure (PaO_2) and content (CaO_2) of O_2 in arterial blood; and tissue oxygenation requires both the appropriate delivery of O_2 to, and its normal utilization by, the organs and tissues of the body. As Table 29-1 shows, the six components can be evaluated clinically by arterial blood gas measurements and other common laboratory assessments.

DEFINITIONS OF RESPIRATORY FAILURE

Interference with any of the three functions, with their respective components, or with the physiologic determinants listed in Table 29-1, produces a respiratory abnormality. Whether this abnormality leads to clinical impairment, to respiratory insufficiency, or to frank respiratory failure depends on its severity and on the rapidity with which it occurs. Unfortunately, there are no standardized terms or expressions for describing different degrees of respiratory dysfunction, and therefore, respiratory failure has no universally accepted definition, and the same terms are often used differently by different clinicians. In this chapter the following definitions, which are admittedly arbitrary, are used:

Physiologic abnormality: A measurement of any respiratory function that lies outside the predicted or accepted normal range and may or may not cause symptoms or clinical impairment

Table 29-1. Determinants and Assessment of the Basic Components of Respiration

Main Function	Physiologic Components	Physiologic Determinants	Clinical Assessment
Alveolar ventilation	CO_2 removal	Load (how much CO_2 is produced: $\dot{V}CO_2$) Efficiency (dead space ventilation; V_D/V_T)	$PaCO_2$
	Alveolar oxygenation	Alveolar gas equation	$PaCO_2$; $P(A\text{-}a)O_2$
Blood oxygenation	Arterial O_2 tension	P_IO_2; $\dot{V}_A$; matching of $\dot{V}_A$ and $\dot{Q}$; R → L shunt (diffusion limitation)	PaO_2
	CaO_2	SaO_2; quantity and function of available hemoglobin; PaO_2	SaO_2; Hb; (PaO_2)
Tissue oxygenation	O_2 transport	CaO_2; cardiac output	CaO_2; $\dot{Q}_T$
	Tissue O_2 utilization	Delivery of O_2 to tissues; ability of tissues to utilize available O_2	$\dot{V}O_2$

Respiratory impairment: A clinically significant respiratory dysfunction, resulting in an abnormality of sufficient degree to be noticeable by the patient

Respiratory insufficiency: Impairment in respiratory function severe enough to prohibit certain activities that the patient might normally pursue, and to interfere with daily living; occurring in association with measurements of respiratory mechanics and/or gas exchange that are markedly abnormal

Respiratory failure: Abnormality of one or more aspects of respiratory function of sufficient degree to threaten the life of the individual

Table 29-2 illustrates the intended use of these terms, using as examples the range of clinical findings observed in a patient with chronic obstructive pulmonary disease (COPD).

Acute respiratory failure may be defined more specifically as any abnormality in alveolar ventilation, oxygenation of the arterial blood, or tissue oxygenation that is severe enough and occurs rapidly enough to create an emergent threat to the life of the patient. In certain circumstances abnormalities of similar degree may develop gradually and be tolerated for weeks or longer by a patient with chronic respiratory insufficiency. Such a state of *chronic respiratory failure* threatens the patient's life but without the emergent connotation of its acute counterpart. The hypothetical patient whose arterial blood gas values are shown at the bottom of Table 29-2 is in acute, not chronic, respiratory failure, as indicated by the severe reduction in arterial pH.

As discussed later, it is not possible to assess the adequacy of oxygenation and ventilation by physical signs alone. With a few exceptions (see Chs. 32 to 34), acute respiratory failure produces readily detectable changes in PaO_2 and/or arterial CO_2 partial pressure ($PaCO_2$) and pH, so that its diagnosis relies primarily on arterial blood gas measurements. Unfortunately, the criteria used by different authorities vary. Most commonly used are a PaO_2 of less than 60 mmHg and/or a $PaCO_2$ exceeding 45 or 50 mmHg.[1,2]

Table 29-2. Terms Used in Describing the Severity of Respiratory Dysfunction: Examples as Applied to Patients with COPD

Term	Physiologic Correlates: Mechanics	Physiologic Correlates: Gas Exchange	Clinical Status
Normal	FEV_1 3.6 L (100% pred) FEV_1/FVC 0.80	—	No limitation
Physiologic abnormality	FEV_1 2.6 L (72% pred) FEV_1/FVC 0.62	—	No limitation
Respiratory impairment	FEV_1 1.8 L (50% pred) FEV_1/FVC 0.50	$PaCO_2$ 40 mmHg, pH 7.40,[a] PaO_2 80 mm Hg[b]	Interference with activities requiring more than moderate exertion
Chronic respiratory insufficiency	FEV_1 0.8 L (25% pred) FEV_1/FVC 0.38	$PaCO_2$ 55 mmHg, pH 7.38,[c] PaO_2 64 mm Hg[d]	Severe interference with activities of daily living
Acute respiratory failure	—	$PaCO_2$ 75 mmHg, pH 7.24,[e] PaO_2 44 mm Hg[f]	Acute threat to patient's life (possibility of severe complication or death within hours)

[a] Normal.
[b] Normoxemia for age.
[c] Compensated respiratory acidosis.
[d] Mild hypoxemia.
[e] Uncompensated respiratory acidosis.
[f] Severe hypoxemia.

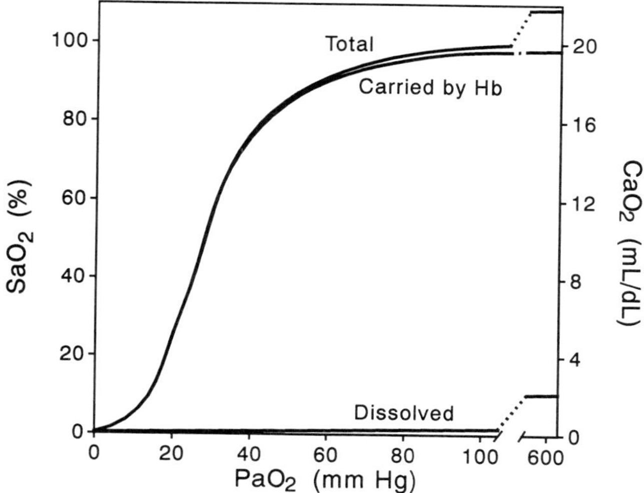

Figure 29-1. Relationships among PaO_2 (horizontal axis), SaO_2 (left vertical axis), and CaO_2 (right vertical axis). CaO_2 is primarily determined by the quantity of functional hemoglobin present (graph assumes normal hemoglobin of 15 g/dL). Almost no O_2 in addition to that bound to hemoglobin is carried in the blood at PaO_2 values usually encountered in clinical respiratory care. As PaO_2 falls, both SaO_2 and CaO_2 diminish rapidly once the "hump" of the curve is reached (PaO_2 values below 50 to 60 mmHg).

Although healthy individuals can journey to high altitude and experience PaO_2 values in the 40 to 50 mmHg range without immediate harm and although chronic hypoxemia may be tolerated for months by some patients, an *acute* impairment in blood oxygenation such that CaO_2 (i.e., hemoglobin saturation) drops substantially is a potential threat to life. This happens when PaO_2 falls far enough for the oxyhemoglobin saturation (SaO_2) curve to curve more sharply downward (Fig. 29-1), causing more substantial decreases in SaO_2. Hypoxemia thus becomes progressively more threatening at PaO_2 values below about 50 mmHg.[3]

Acute hypercapnia causes a threat to life in proportion to the degree of *acidemia* produced, as shown in Table 29-3. Patient A has life-threatening acute respiratory acidosis, while patient B has respiratory acidosis and metabolic alkalosis that offset each other, as occurs in chronic hypercapnia, producing a normal pH. This example shows that it is the pH, not the $PaCO_2$ per se, that defines a state of acute respiratory failure in cases of hypercapnia. A clinically useful definition of acute respiratory failure of this type is any acute rise in $PaCO_2$ (from normal or from the patient's baseline value) that causes arterial pH to fall below 7.30.[3]

Table 29-3. Comparison Showing Degree of Acidemia in Acute Respiratory Failure

	Patient A	Patient B
$PaCO_2$ (mmHg)	55	55
HCO_3^- (mEq/L)	24	34
Arterial pH (units)	7.25	7.40

Table 29-4. Clinical Categories of Acute Respiratory Failure

General Category	Clinical Determinants
Failure of alveolar ventilation	↑ $PaCO_2$; ↓ arterial pH; (↓ PaO_2)
Failure to oxygenate the arterial blood	
Hypoxemia	↓ PaO_2
Inadequate CaO_2	↓ SaO_2 and/or ↓ functional hemoglobin
Failure of tissue oxygenation	
Inadequate systemic O_2 transport	↓ CaO_2, and/or ↓ cardiac output
Inadequate tissue O_2 extraction	↓ $\dot{V}O_2$

From the foregoing, acute respiratory failure may be divided conceptually into *ventilation failure* (impaired CO_2 excretion) and *oxygenation failure*,[1,3–5] and further subdivided into the five categories shown in Table 29-4. In the remaining sections of this chapter each of these categories is characterized pathophysiologically; corresponding clinical descriptions and examples are provided in Chapters 30 through 35.

FAILURE OF ALVEOLAR VENTILATION

$PaCO_2$ is essentially equivalent to alveolar PCO_2 (P_ACO_2), which according to the alveolar ventilation equation (see Ch. 10) is determined by the ratio of CO_2 production ($\dot{V}CO_2$) to alveolar ventilation ($\dot{V}_A$, the ventilation of alveoli exposed to pulmonary perfusion).[6] If $\dot{V}CO_2$ increases without a com-

Table 29-5. Mechanisms of Hypercapnic Respiratory Failure (Ventilatory Failure)

- Decreased overall ventilation
  - Failure of ventilatory drive (insufficient output from medullary respiratory centers to maintain adequate alveolar ventilation)
  - Failure of transmission of the drive impulse to the respiratory pump (failure of nerve conduction from central nervous system to respiratory muscles)
  - Failure of the respiratory pump
    - Insufficient response from the respiratory muscles
    - Insufficient movement of the thorax
  - Failure of the conducting airways
    - Localized upper airway obstruction
    - Generalized lower airway obstruction
  - Failure of gas exchange (impairment of $\dot{V}/\dot{Q}$ relationships severe enough to impair CO_2 elimination)
- Increased CO_2 production (even in presence of normal overall ventilation)
- Increased dead space ventilation (even in presence of normal overall ventilation)
- Exogenous CO_2 inhalation

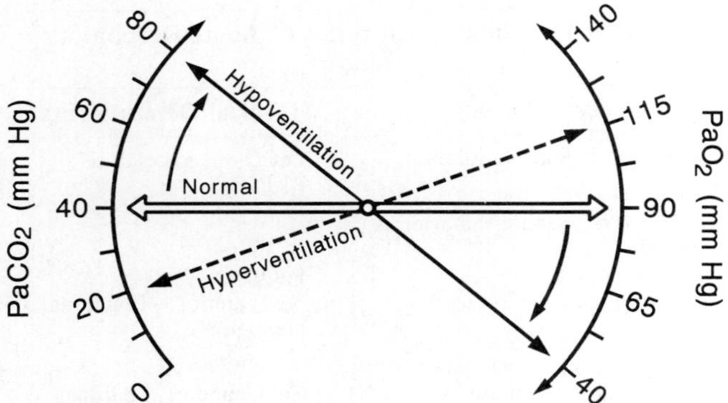

Figure 29-2. Schematic depiction of how PaO_2 and $PaCO_2$ change in opposite directions, assuming an unchanging $P(A\text{-}a)O_2$ and a respiratory exchange ratio of 0.8. Alveolar hypoventilation raises $PaCO_2$ above the normal value of 40 mmHg and decreases PaO_2 proportionally. Hyperventilation produces the opposite effect (dashed line).

pensatory increase in $\dot{V}_A$ or if $\dot{V}_A$ falls (either because overall ventilation falls or dead space ventilation increases), then $PaCO_2$ will increase proportionally. These possible mechanisms for failure of alveolar ventilation (hypercapnic respiratory failure or ventilatory failure) are outlined in more detail in Table 29-5.

The effectiveness of CO_2 excretion affects oxygenation as well as acid-base status, as described by the alveolar gas equation:

$$P_AO_2 = P_IO_2 - \frac{PaCO_2}{R}$$

This equation states that, if inspired PO_2 (P_IO_2) does not change, an increase in $PaCO_2$ will decrease P_AO_2 by an amount equal to the increase in $PaCO_2$ (divided by the respiratory exchange ratio [R], which corrects for a ratio of CO_2 production to O_2 consumption different from unity). If the alveolar to arterial PO_2 difference [$P(A\text{-}a)O_2$] does not change and a large right-to-left shunt is not present, this fall in P_AO_2 will cause an equal fall in PaO_2. PaO_2 and $PaCO_2$ are thus linked like the pans on a balance scale or the ends of the needle in a compass (Fig. 29-2). In the presence of a normal R value of 0.8, every 8 mmHg increase in $PaCO_2$ will produce a 10 mmHg fall in PaO_2.

FAILURE OF BLOOD OXYGENATION

Hypoxemia

There are five possible physiologic mechanisms for hypoxemia (PaO_2 less than normal): (1) alveolar hypoventilation; (2) ventilation-perfusion ($\dot{V}/\dot{Q}$) mismatch; (3) right-to-left shunt; (4) decreased ambient O_2 tension; and (5) diffusion limitation. The clinical settings in which each characteristically occurs are described in Chapter 31. Most important clinically are alveolar hypoventilation, $\dot{V}/\dot{Q}$ mismatch, and right-to-left intrapulmonary shunt. The effects of each of these on PaO_2 can be understood more readily through the series of diagrams shown in Figures 29-3 to 29-6.

Hypoxemia Due to Alveolar Hypoventilation

Figure 29-3A shows normal alveolar oxygenation and ventilation, while Figure 29-3B depicts what would happen if $\dot{V}_A$ were reduced by 50 percent while the patient's metabolism (i.e., $\dot{V}O_2$ and $\dot{V}CO_2$) remained the same. On the oxygenation side (left portions of Fig. 29-3A and B), if O_2 removal from the lung remained the same while O_2 supply (ventilation) diminished by half, P_AO_2 (and hence PaO_2) would also diminish by half. On the ventilation side the reverse would occur: the same CO_2 load would be presented to the

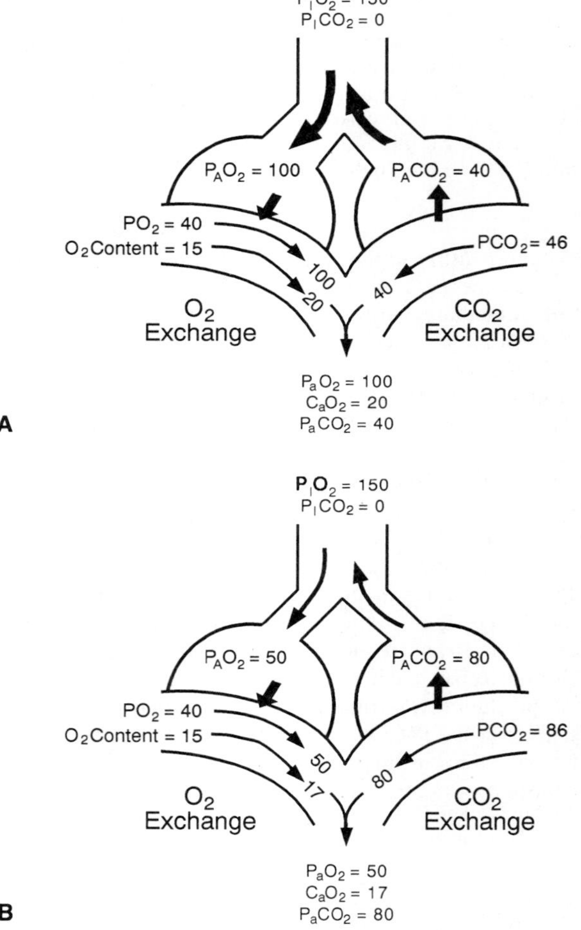

Figure 29-3. Conceptual diagram of hypoxemia due to alveolar hypoventilation. Both idealized lung units depict oxygenation on the left and ventilation on the right; $P(A\text{-}a)O_2$ is zero in this example. **(A)** Normal alveolar gas exchange. **(B)** Alveolar hypoventilation, with $\dot{V}_A$ half of normal. For further explanation see text.

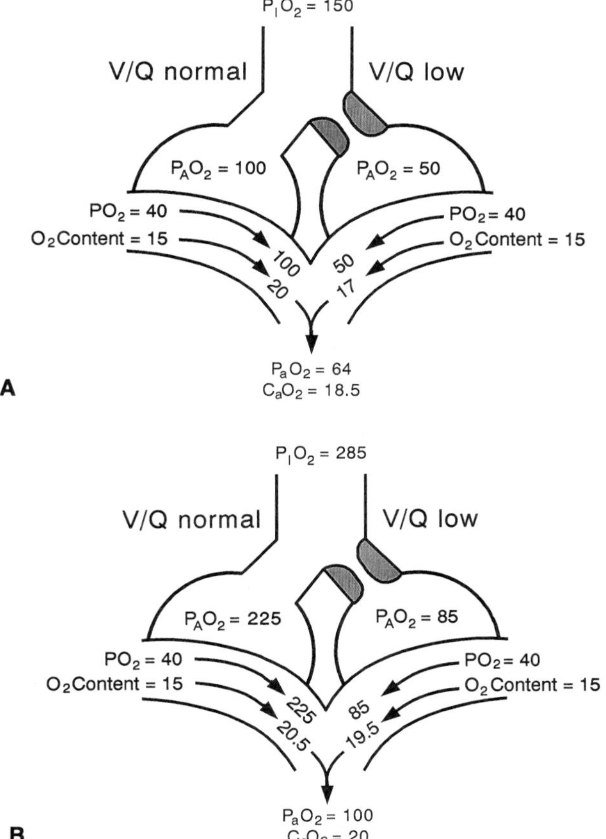

Figure 29-4. Hypoxemia due to $\dot{V}/\dot{Q}$ mismatch, showing the effect of supplemental O_2. $\dot{V}/\dot{Q}$ is normal on the left side of each idealized lung unit and low on the right. Only O_2 exchange is shown, and P(A-a)O_2 is assumed to be zero. **(A)** With room air, not enough O_2 reaches the poorly ventilated alveolus to fully saturate its capillary blood; **(B)** with 40 percent O_2, PAO_2 in this alveolus is raised enough to make its capillary PO_2 nearly normal. Note that the PaO_2 in the mixed effluent from the two capillaries is determined by the average of the O_2 *contents* of the two streams, not by their PaO_2 values.

lung, but only half as much of it would be removed, so that PaCO_2 would double.

When hypoxemia is due solely to alveolar hypoventilation [i.e., elevated PaCO_2 with normal P(A-a)O_2], its correction does not require supplemental O_2; simply restoring $\dot{V}$A to normal will also return PaO_2 to normal.

Hypoxemia Due to Low $\dot{V}/\dot{Q}$

Although the matching of $\dot{V}$A to capillary perfusion normally varies somewhat in different regions of the lung, the overall effect is one of approximately equal matching ($\dot{V}/\dot{Q}$ = 1). When overall ventilation is decreased in relation to overall perfusion, hypoxemia results, as shown schematically in Figure 29-4A. Some ventilation is present in the affected low $\dot{V}/\dot{Q}$ areas but not enough to fully oxygenate the blood perfusing those areas. Hypoxemia caused by this mechanism is readily corrected, however, by simply increasing the "driving pressure" of O_2 into the low $\dot{V}/\dot{Q}$ alveoli by administration of supplemental O_2 (Fig. 29-4B).

Hypoxemia Due to Right-to-Left Shunt

If deoxygenated blood passes through the lung without being exposed to *any* $\dot{V}$A as occurs when there is an anatomic right-to-left shunt or when alveoli are collapsed or filled with

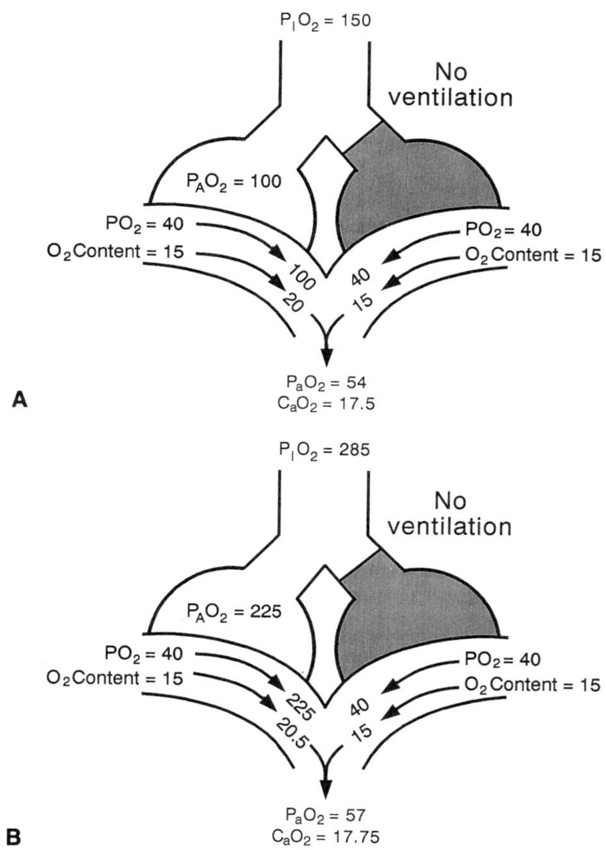

Figure 29-5. Alveolar-capillary diagram of intrapulmonary right-to-left shunt, showing why supplemental O_2 fails to correct the hypoxemia. Only O_2 exchange is shown, and P(A-a)O_2 is assumed to be zero. **(A)** With room air, although blood leaving the normal alveolar-capillary unit is normally saturated, blood passing the capillary on the right "sees" no O_2, since its alveolus is unventilated, and it leaves the unit unsaturated. When the two effluent streams mix, the resulting PaO_2 is determined by the average of their O_2 contents, not by their PO_2 values. **(B)** Addition of 40 percent O_2 fails to correct the hypoxemia, since O_2 content is not significantly raised in the normal unit and capillary blood in the unventilated unit still "sees" no O_2. Even 100 percent O_2 would not completely reverse the oxygenation defect in this example. Compare with Figure 29-4.

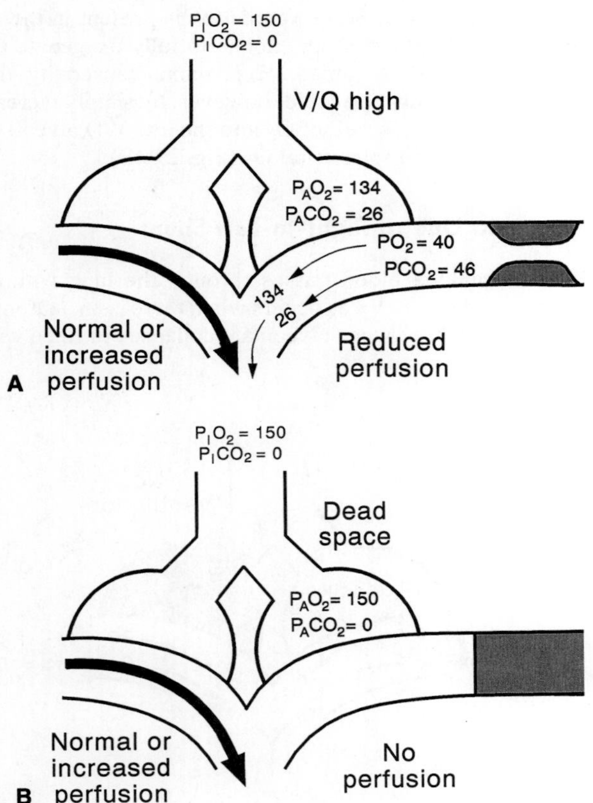

Figure 29-6. Alveolar diagrams depicting lung units with **(A)** high $\dot{V}/\dot{Q}$ and **(B)** dead space. Areas of high $\dot{V}/\dot{Q}$ experience alveolar hyperventilation, and capillary blood leaves them with higher PaO_2 and lower $PaCO_2$ than in the normal units. Because these areas are poorly perfused, they impair the efficiency of overall gas exchange. When some alveoli are not perfused at all (dead space—infinitely high $\dot{V}/\dot{Q}$ units), their ventilation is wasted, and overall ventilation must be increased in order to maintain normal CO_2 excretion.

fluid, it leaves the lung still deoxygenated. As shown in Figure 29-5A, this results in hypoxemia. A shunt is thus the ultimate low $\dot{V}/\dot{Q}$ unit. However, in contrast to what happens when PIO_2 is raised in the presence of low $\dot{V}/\dot{Q}$ units, supplemental O_2 fails to normalize PaO_2 when hypoxemia is due to shunt (Fig. 29-5B). This essential difference between the two main physiologic mechanisms of oxygenation failure has important therapeutic implications, since measures other than adding supplemental O_2 must be employed if hypoxemia due to shunt is to be corrected.

Removal of CO_2 is usually not affected when hypoxemia is due to $\dot{V}/\dot{Q}$ mismatch. This is because the shape of the CO_2 dissociation curve favors excretion in its physiologic range, making it easier for CO_2 to leave than for O_2 to enter the capillary blood, and also because patients can usually augment ventilation sufficiently in response to the hypercapnic stimulus to maintain normocapnia.[7,8]

Figure 29-6 shows schematically why $\dot{V}/\dot{Q}$ mismatching dominated by *high* rather than low $\dot{V}/\dot{Q}$ areas is not an important cause of hypoxemia. Instead, abnormally high $\dot{V}/\dot{Q}$ (the extreme of which is alveolar dead space) may cause ventilatory failure if overall ventilation cannot increase appropriately. If dead space doubled while minute ventilation remained the same, $\dot{V}A$ would decrease by half and $PaCO_2$ would double, just as occurs with overall hypoventilation (Fig. 29-2).

Decreased Ambient Oxygen Tension

Normal individuals who travel to high altitude may experience hypoxemia due to low ambient PO_2 and thus low PIO_2 (see Ch. 16). Patients with cardiorespiratory disease who live at moderate elevation (e.g., Denver's 1600 m) develop hypoxemia earlier, and may require supplemental O_2 in the presence of less severe disease, than if they lived at sea level. The possibility of altitude-related hypoxemia must be considered when individuals with chronic cardiorespiratory disease travel or are transferred between institutions, as discussed in Chapters 100 and 96, respectively. Consumption of O_2 through combustion during a fire can produce a life-threatening fall in PIO_2. Patients receiving supplemental O_2 may experience severe hypoxemia if this therapy is unwisely or inadvertently interrupted.

Decreased PIO_2 is the only physiologic mechanism aside from alveolar hypoventilation by which hypoxemia occurs in the presence of normal $P(A\text{-}a)O_2$.

Hypoxemia Due to Diffusion Limitation

Hypoxemia due to diffusion limitation may occur during strenuous exercise at high altitude[9] but is not clinically important in most patients with cardiorespiratory disease.[3,4,6,10] Individuals with lung disease often have thickened alveolar-capillary membranes when their lungs are examined at autopsy, and this gave rise to the concept of "alveolar-capillary block" as the cause of their hypoxemia during life. However, only in exceptional circumstances (e.g., high cardiac output states at altitudes substantially above sea level) could this be considered a possible contributory factor in clinical hypoxemia; such hypoxemia would be readily corrected by administration of small amounts of supplemental O_2.[11]

Decreased Arterial Oxygen Content

Life-threatening oxygenation failure can occur in the presence of a normal PaO_2 if the amount of functional hemoglobin is inadequate. Figure 27-1 shows that only a small quantity of O_2 is present in blood apart from that bound to hemoglobin, even when PaO_2 is raised to very high levels. The importance of hemoglobin in acute respiratory failure is illustrated by Figure 29-7, which depicts CaO_2 in relation to PaO_2 at four different hemoglobin levels. CO poisoning and other disorders can produce a similar effect despite normal quantities of hemoglobin by rendering the hemoglobin dysfunctional.

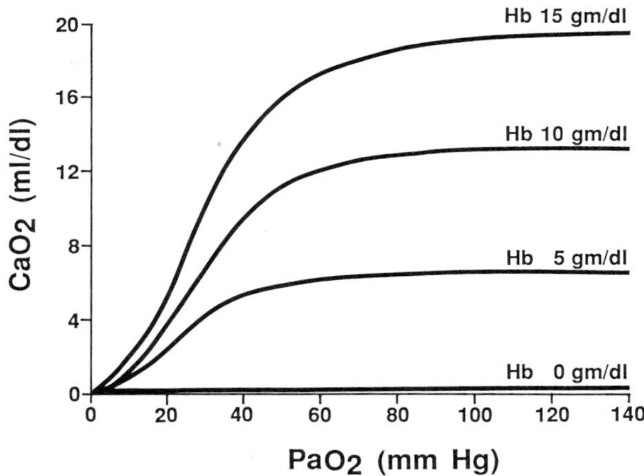

Figure 29-7. Relationship of CaO_2 to PaO_2 in the presence of different hemoglobin concentrations. Blood with 15 g/dL of hemoglobin (the normal amount), when fully saturated, contains 20 mL O_2 per 100 mL blood. Despite normal or even elevated PaO_2, however, the blood of a patient with anemia contains a markedly reduced amount of O_2.

FAILURE OF TISSUE OXYGENATION

Inadequate Systemic Oxygen Transport

Normal oxygenation of the arterial blood does not in and of itself ensure normal respiration. Sufficient O_2 must be transported to respiring tissues to meet their metabolic needs.[4,5] Systemic O_2 transport (DO_2) comprises both CaO_2 and cardiac output ($\dot{Q}_T$):

$$DO_2 = (CaO_2)(\dot{Q}_T)$$

Normal CaO_2 is about 20 mL/dL, and $\dot{Q}_T$ is roughly 5 L/min in an average-sized adult at rest, so that DO_2 is normally approximately 1 L/min. Any process that reduces DO_2 sufficiently to threaten the life of the individual, whether it is primarily "respiratory" (affecting blood oxygenation) or "cardiac" (affecting $\dot{Q}_T$), will result in acute respiratory failure due to inadequate systemic O_2 transport.

Inadequate Tissue Oxygen Extraction

The final step in respiration, and thus the "bottom line" with respect to its adequacy, is the uptake and intracellular utilization of O_2 by the tissues themselves. O_2 consumption ($\dot{V}O_2$) is defined by the Fick equation as the quantity of O_2 transported to the tissues minus the amount that returns to the heart unused: $\dot{V}O_2$ is systemic (outbound) O_2 transport ($CaO_2 \times \dot{Q}_T$) minus mixed venous (inbound) O_2 transport ($C\bar{v}O_2 \times \dot{Q}_T$), or

$$\dot{V}O_2 = [\dot{Q}_T][C(a\text{-}\bar{v})O_2]$$

where $C(a\text{-}\bar{v})O_2$ is the difference between arterial and mixed venous O_2 contents.

The relationship described by the Fick equation assumes that oxygen extraction by the tissues will proceed normally once sufficient O_2 is delivered to them.[4,5] Individual tissue beds normally adjust regional perfusion to meet their O_2 needs, presumably through hormonal mechanisms. However, there are circumstances in which the process of tissue O_2 extraction itself is impaired, independently of DO_2; this causes acute respiratory failure, either because the cells' internal mechanisms for using O_2 are disrupted (as in cyanide poisoning) or because blood reaching tissue beds is diffusely shunted past them (as may occur in septic shock). With decreased tissue uptake, $C\bar{v}O_2$ rises and $C(a\text{-}\bar{v})O_2$ is reduced; in extreme situations blood returns to the right side of the heart still fully oxygenated. Chapter 34 further describes the clinical settings in which this phenomenon can occur.

CLINICAL MANIFESTATIONS OF ACUTE RESPIRATORY FAILURE

Acute respiratory failure cannot be diagnosed accurately by history or physical examination regardless of the physiologic mechanism by which it occurs. This is because its clinical manifestations are notoriously nonspecific—they may be absent in profound hypoxia or respiratory acidosis, and they are observed in many other conditions besides respiratory failure.

Symptoms and signs of acute respiratory failure (Table 29-6) are caused by tissue hypoxia and acidosis, the manifestations of which are primarily cardiovascular and neurologic rather than respiratory.[3] Dyspnea, tachypnea, and other signs of respiratory distress are often absent. Restlessness, confusion, and other disturbances of consciousness are common, as are headache, tremor, and asterixis. However, these do not distinguish between oxygenation failure and ventilation failure and do not correlate with the severity of the abnormality.

It was demonstrated long ago that bedside assessments of oxygenation and ventilation are notoriously unreliable even in the hands of experienced observers.[12,13] Although in some patients cyanosis reflects the expected presence of 5 g/dL of deoxygenated hemoglobin in arterial blood, it is absent in

Table 29-6. Clinical Manifestations of Acute Respiratory Failure

Symptoms	Signs
(Dyspnea)	(Respiratory distress)
Restlessness	(Cyanosis)
Confusion	Tachycardia
Agitation	Cardiac arrhythmias
Headache	Hypertension
Tremor	Hypotension
Asterixis	Lethargy
Diaphoresis	Coma

others who are profoundly hypoxemic, and still others have this sign despite normal PaO_2 and CaO_2.[12] Likewise, the bedside prediction of effective $\dot{V}_A$ and $PaCO_2$, even by skilled clinicians, has been shown to be haphazard.[13] These points emphasize that acute respiratory failure, even when appropriately suspected on clinical grounds, requires arterial blood gas measurement or other laboratory tests for accurate diagnosis.

References

1. Johanson WG Jr, Peters JI: Respiratory failure. General principles and diagnostic approach. pp. 1973–1975. In Murray JF, Nadel JA (eds): Textbook of Respiratory Medicine. WB Saunders, Philadelphia, 1988
2. Pontoppidan H, Geffen B, Lowenstein E: Acute respiratory failure in the adult. N Engl J Med 1972;287:690–698, 743–752, 799–806
3. Pierson DJ: Acute respiratory failure. pp. 75–126. In Sahn SA (ed): Pulmonary Emergencies. Churchill Livingstone, New York, 1982
4. Pierson DJ, Luce JM: Cardiopulmonary components of respiratory failure. pp. 1–9. In Fallat RJ, Luce JM (eds): Cardiopulmonary Critical Care Management. Churchill Livingstone, New York, 1988
5. Luce JM, Pierson DJ: Critical Care Medicine. WB Saunders, Philadelphia, 1988
6. Culver BH (ed): Syllabus: Human Biology 541—The Respiratory System. University of Washington School of Medicine, Health Sciences Academic Services, Seattle, 1988, pp. 27–68
7. West JB: State of the art: Ventilation-perfusion relationships. Am Rev Respir Dis 1977;116:919–943
8. West JB: Ventilation, blood flow, and gas exchange. pp. 47–84. In Murray JF, Nadel JA (eds): Textbook of Respiratory Medicine. WB Saunders, Philadelphia, 1988
9. Torre-Bueno JR, Wagner PD, Saltzman HA et al: Diffusion limitation in normal humans during exercise at sea level and simulated altitude. J Appl Physiol 1985;58:989–995
10. Murray JF: Pathophysiology of acute respiratory failure. Respir Care 1983;28:531–541
11. Murray JF: Update: Pathophysiology of acute respiratory failure. p. 15. In Pierson DJ (ed): Respiratory Intensive Care. Daedalus Press, Dallas, 1986
12. Comroe JH Jr, Botelho S: The unreliability of cyanosis in the recognition of arterial anoxemia. Am J Med Sci 1947;214:1–6.
13. Mithoefer JD, Bossman OG, Thibeault DW, Mead GD: The clinical estimation of alveolar ventilation. Am Rev Respir Dis 1968; 98:868–871

Chapter 30

Ventilatory Failure

Leonard D. Hudson
David J. Pierson

CHAPTER OUTLINE

Ventilatory failure represents one of the categories of respiratory failure, as described in Chapter 29. Ventilatory failure is present when ventilation is inadequate to keep up with the metabolic demands of the body, which results in an increase in the partial pressure of CO_2 in the arterial blood ($PaCO_2$), or respiratory acidosis. Thus, ventilatory failure is defined by an elevation in $PaCO_2$. When this increase occurs acutely (without time to allow a concomitant rise in serum HCO_3^-), respiratory acidosis produces a fall in arterial pH (acidemia).

Ventilatory failure also may produce hypoxemia by a mechanism described in detail in Chapter 10 on pulmonary perfusion, ventilation, and gas exchange. To summarize briefly, if ventilation is not adequate to remove CO_2, so that the alveolar partial pressure of CO_2 (P_ACO_2) rises, then ventilation is also insufficient to bring in enough O_2, which results in a decrease in the alveolar partial pressure of O_2 (P_AO_2). Since at any given barometric pressure the total pressure available for all gases in the alveolar space is fixed and since other gases are present in relatively fixed amounts (e.g., N_2 is neither produced nor absorbed in the body to any clinically significant extent), the alveolar values for the partial pressures of CO_2 and O_2 are interrelated. If hypoventilation occurs and the P_ACO_2 rises, the P_AO_2 must decrease in a reciprocal fashion (see Fig. 29-2). The changes in these values are related to each other by the alveolar gas equation

$$P_AO_2 = P_IO_2 - \frac{P_ACO_2}{R} \quad (1)$$

The respiratory exchange ratio (R) represents the rate at which O_2 is absorbed relative to the rate at which CO_2 is produced. In this equation it is assumed that the $PaCO_2$ reflects the P_ACO_2. Therefore, if the inspired O_2 pressure (P_IO_2) is known, the equation can be solved for P_AO_2. (P_IO_2 can be calculated from the barometric pressure and the inspired O_2 fraction [F_IO_2].) The difference between the P_AO_2 and PaO_2 [$P(A\text{-}a)O_2$] can then be assessed. Whenever hypercapnia is present during hypoxemia, alveolar hypoventilation is making some contribution to that hypoxemia: if $P(A\text{-}a)O_2$ is normal, hypoventilation alone is causing the hypoxemia; if $(P_A\text{-}a)O_2$ is increased, another mechanism(s) (e.g., ventilation/perfusion [$\dot{V}/\dot{Q}$] mismatch or shunt) contributes to the hypoxemia.[1]

There are three mechanisms by which hypoventilation can occur: (1) a decrease in minute ventilation ($\dot{V}_E$) resulting in a decrease in alveolar ventilation ($\dot{V}_A$); (2) a normal or even increased $\dot{V}_E$ but an increase in the dead space ($\dot{V}_D$) or wasted ventilation component, resulting in relative reduction in $\dot{V}_A$; and/or (3) an increase in CO_2 production ($\dot{V}CO_2$). The causes of ventilatory failure under these categories are shown in Table 30-1, and the clinical situations related to each of these physiologic abnormalities are discussed below.

DECREASED ALVEOLAR VENTILATION

A decrease in $\dot{V}_A$ can result from dysfunction of any of the components of the respiratory system including (1) the central drive to ventilation; (2) the nerve transmission of the central message to breathe; (3) the muscles of ventilation; (4) the bony and fibrous tissue components of the thorax; and (5) the lungs and airways. Each of these sites or types of defects must be considered in seeking the possible etiology of the hypoventilation.

In approaching the etiology of hypoventilation, first, one can divide patients with hypoventilation into those who "*won't* breathe" versus those who "*can't* breathe" (as also discussed in Chs. 25 and 66). Patients who *won't breathe* have an abnormality in their central ventilatory drive without severe impairment of the mechanics of ventilation. This can be due either to a structural brain stem lesion, to suppression of the ventilatory drive center by drugs, or to failure to appreciate stimuli that ordinarily trigger the respiratory center to increase drive (such as abnormalities of the carotid body chemoreceptors or of the afferent limb of cranial nerve IX). Those patients who *can't breathe* are mechanically incapable of ventilating more, and there may be several etiologies for this condition, including defects in neuromuscular transmission, respiratory muscle weakness or fatigue, restriction of the bony thorax, or diseases of the airways. As a general clinical point, patients with reduced central drive to breathe usually are not dyspneic, even in the face of significant hypercapnia, whereas patients with abnormalities of other respiratory system components but with intact ventilatory drive usually have a sensation of shortness of breath.

Decreased Central Drive

A decreased central ventilatory drive can result from structural abnormalities of the brain. In this situation the brain stem is involved, and usually other central neurologic deficits are obvious. By far the most common cause of central ventilatory drive loss is pharmacologic depression of the respiratory control center of the brain, either iatrogenic or resulting from a deliberate or accidental drug overdose.[2–6]

Patient Example 30-1

Decreased Central Ventilatory Drive—Acute (Drug Overdose)

A 26-year-old man with a past history of depression and several previous suicide gestures is found unresponsive with several empty medication bottles nearby. His pulse and blood pressure are normal, but his respiratory rate is 8 breaths per minute and he is cyanotic. Determinations of arterial blood gas (ABG) levels when breathing air show pH 7.22, $PaCO_2$ 72 mmHg, and PaO_2 46 mmHg. His calculated $P(A\text{-}a)O_2$ is 14 mmHg, indicating that alveolar hypoventilation is the sole cause of his hypoxemia and also suggesting that significant aspiration or other pulmonary complication of his polydrug overdose has not occurred.

Sleep-disordered breathing syndromes (sleep apnea) are associated with periodic hypoventilation during sleep.[7] However, occasionally they can be associated with persistent hypoventilation even in the waking state. Patients with this abnormality probably have an abnormal central drive to breathe while awake, and those with the obesity-hypoventilation (pickwickian) syndrome probably require an abnormal central drive to breathe in addition to the added stress of obesity, which restricts chest movement and increases the work of breathing.[5,8] In addition, hypoventilation can be idiopathic central hypoventilation.[5] These abnormalities are most frequently associated with chronic hypoventilation with a compensated respiratory acidosis and are rarely the cause of acute ventilatory failure. However, these patients may not respond with normal compensatory hyperventilation when other acute disease processes (e.g., pneumonia) affect the respiratory system. Thus, their level of hypoxemia may be disproportionate to that seen in patients with similar acute lung abnormalities but with normal ventilatory drives.

Patient Example 30-2

Decreased Central Ventilatory Drive—Chronic (Pickwickian Syndrome)

A 62-year-old man with a lifetime history of morbid obesity and heavy snoring reports that he has gained 40 pounds in the last 4 months (to 280 pounds) and is having increasing trouble staying awake while driving his delivery van; last week he was involved in a minor traffic accident after dozing off at the wheel and running a red light. He denies dyspnea or other respiratory symptoms. On physical examination he is somnolent, plethoric, and cyanotic, with moderately elevated blood pressure. He has cardiomegaly and signs of right-sided heart failure, including pitting pedal edema and distended neck veins. Basilar crackles heard on initial auscultation clear after several deep breaths. His hematocrit is 58 percent, and his ABG levels while breathing air show pH 7.38, $PaCO_2$ 55 mmHg, and PaO_2 52 mmHg. After several deep breaths his ABG levels are pH 7.56, $PaCO_2$ 35 mmHg, and PaO_2 90 mmHg.

Table 30-1. Clinical Classification of Ventilatory Failure

Site or Type of Defect	Mechanism or Category	Clinical Examples
Ventilatory drive	Pharmacologic	Drug overdose (opiates, sedatives, alcohol); general anesthesia
	Congenital	Sudden infant death syndrome (SIDS); Ondine's curse
	Acquired	Cerebrovascular accident; tumor; trauma; carotid body resection
	Combination	Obesity hypoventilation (pickwickian) syndrome; idiopathic alveolar hypoventilation syndromes; type B ("blue bloater") COPD
Neural transmission to the respiratory muscles	Cervical spinal cord injury	Trauma; tumor; vascular accident
	Demyelinating peripheral neuropathy	Guillain-Barré syndrome
	Anterior horn cell disease	Poliomyelitis; amyotrophic lateral sclerosis
	Phrenic nerve lesion	Trauma; cardiac surgery (cold cardioplegia); infiltration by tumor; idiopathic
Respiratory muscles	Pharmacologic	Paralytic agents (pancuronium, atracurium, curare); aminoglycoside toxicity
	Primary disease of muscle	Muscular dystrophy; polymyositis; dermatomyositis
	Disorders of the neuromuscular junction	Myasthenia gravis; botulism; tetanus; tick paralysis
	Electrolyte and metabolic disturbances	Hypophosphatemia; hypokalemia; hypomagnesemia; myxedema
	Excessive work of breathing in absence of primary neuromuscular disease	Acute exacerbation of COPD; status asthmaticus; intubation with small endotracheal tube
Bony thorax	Decreased mobility	Kyphoscoliosis; traumatic asphyxia; postoperative splinting; tight casts or bandages; massive pneumo- or hydrothorax; diffuse pleural thickening or malignancy; massive obesity
	Loss of rigidity	Severe flail chest
Conducting airways	Localized upper airway obstruction	Foreign body; tumor; croup; laryngeal spasm or edema; epiglottitis; obstructive sleep apnea; obstructed endotracheal tube
	Diffuse lower airway obstruction	Acute exacerbation of COPD; status asthmaticus
Increased dead space ventilation	Very high $\dot{V}/\dot{Q}$	ARDS; severe COPD
	External dead space	Ventilator tubing; other apparatus
	Generalized pulmonary hypoperfusion	Hypovolemic or cardiogenic shock; during CPR; excessive pulmonary hyperinflation (applied or auto-PEEP)
	Localized pulmonary hypoperfusion	Pulmonary thromboembolism[a]; venous air embolism
Increased CO_2 production	Inflammation; hypermetabolism	Fever; sepsis; burns; severe trauma
	Muscle activity	Shivering; fasciculations; tetany; agitation; seizures
	Excessive caloric intake	Increased overall caloric intake
	Increased respiratory quotient	Increased proportion of total intake by carbohydrate
Exogenous CO_2 inhalation	Increased $P_{I}CO_2$	Laboratory or industrial accident; therapeutic use

COPD, chronic obstructive pulmonary disease; ARDS, adult respiratory distress syndrome.
[a] In absence of ability to compensate with increased overall ventilation.

Comment

This patient has the pickwickian (obesity-hypoventilation) syndrome, with chronic hypoventilation related to a combination of decreased central ventilatory drive and increased work of breathing. His initially increased $P(A\text{-}a)O_2$ is consistent with $\dot{V}/\dot{Q}$ abnormalities from poor lung expansion, which are corrected by voluntary deep breathing; most of his hypoxemia is due to hypoventilation.

The following topics are discussed in more detail elsewhere in the text: the pickwickian syndrome, Chapter 25; the sleep apnea syndrome, Chapter 27; the approach to drive disorders including use of progesterone, Chapter 66; and the approach to patients with cor pulmonale, Chapter 63.

Abnormalities of Neural Transmission

Diseases of the peripheral nerves rarely involve the nerves supplying the muscles of ventilation to such an extent that hypoventilation develops.[6] Of the peripheral polyneuropathies that do result in hypoventilation, the Guillain-Barré syndrome is most common.[9] This syndrome is a rapidly evolving neuropathy, with weakness ranging from minimal leg weakness to total paralysis of all extremities and trunk, bulbar, and facial paresis. Pathologic examination has shown demyelination of the involved nerves. Approximately three-fourths of patients with Guillain-Barré syndrome recall a previous infection, which has prompted the unproven suggestion that this disorder is a reaction to a viral or bacterial infection. The cerebrospinal fluid changes are characteristic, involving an elevated protein level but few cells. Weakness usually begins in the legs and progresses over several days, although major weakness can develop within 24 hours or less. Evolution is complete after 2 weeks in more than 50 percent of patients and after 4 weeks in more than 90 percent. Measurement of vital capacity (VC) and maximal inspiratory force (MIF) on a daily or even more frequent basis is recommended during evolution of the weakness in order to monitor the threat of acute ventilatory failure.

Patient Example 30-3

Abnormal Neural Transmission of Drive Impulse to Bellows—Acute (Guillain-Barré Syndrome)

A 35-year-old woman develops weakness and mild tingling in her legs about 2 weeks after an apparent viral upper respiratory infection. The weakness ascends and progresses over the next several days, and she begins to experience dyspnea and is admitted to the intensive care unit. Physical examination shows a reflexic, flaccid paralysis of the extremities. Cerebrospinal fluid protein is elevated, but all other laboratory tests are normal. Her VC is initially 20 mL/kg but falls over the next 72 hours to 10 mL/kg; MIF declines from 30 to 20 cmH_2O during this time. Her ABG levels on admission show acute respiratory alkalosis and a mildly increased $P(A\text{-}a)O_2$; on the third day ABG determinations while breathing room air show pH 7.33, $PaCO_2$ 52 mmHg, and PaO_2 58 mmHg.

Comment

This patient has Guillain-Barré syndrome. Her calculated initial $P(A\text{-}a)O_2$ is 27 mmHg, which suggests that $\dot{V}/\dot{Q}$ abnormalities from poor lung expansion in addition to hypoventilation are contributing to the hypoxemia. Elective intubation and initiation of mechanical ventilation would be prudent at this time in view of the progressive nature of her muscle weakness and current VC and MIF values.

See Chapters 52, 72, 81, and 90, respectively, for further discussion of assessment of ventilatory muscle function, airway management, indications for mechanical ventilation, and respiratory care of the paralyzed patient.

Prior to the development of the polio vaccine, acute poliomyelitis was a common cause of ventilatory failure. In fact, mechanical ventilation was first developed on a practical large-scale basis to manage patients with ventilatory failure secondary to poliomyelitis. Fortunately, acute poliomyelitis with ventilatory insufficiency is now extremely rare, at least in developed countries. Another disease involving the anterior horn cells with ventilatory nerve paralysis is amyotrophic lateral sclerosis (ALS), also known as Lou Gehrig's disease. Ventilatory failure is a frequent cause of death in patients with ALS.[6]

Bilateral abnormalities of the phrenic nerves can result in hypoventilation. This occasionally occurs postoperatively and has been described with the prolonged use of iced cardioplegic solution during open heart surgery. Fortunately, this is rare.

Abnormal Bellows Function

The central signal to breathe and its transmission to the chest may be normal but the chest bellows (i.e., the usually flexible bony thorax and the ventilatory muscles that move the thoracic cage and abdomen) may not be able to respond so as to allow the lungs to ventilate in a normal fashion. This inability to respond may be due either to abnormalities of the thorax itself or to dysfunction of the ventilatory muscles.

Abnormalities of Ventilatory Muscle Function

Several disorders involve abnormalities of neurotransmission at the neuromuscular junction.[6] Probably the most frequent of these is the use of muscle-paralyzing agents such as pancuronium bromide (Pavulon). Myasthenia gravis involves the respiratory muscles in most cases but usually not until months or years after the onset of symptoms. Botulism can result in severe paralysis with respiratory failure and usually also involves the cranial nerves. Tetanus can also be associated with muscle failure with hypoventilation.

Patient Example 30-4

Decreased Chest Bellows Function—Acute (Muscle Relaxant Drug)

A 58-year-old woman without prior history of cardiopulmonary disease undergoes an uneventful cholecystectomy. During the 45-minute surgery she receives a total of 9 mg pancuronium bromide as a muscle relaxant. At the conclusion of the surgery she is given 1 mg neostigmine and 0.4 mg atropine intravenously to reverse the paralysis. She is extubated in the recovery room and a few minutes later is noted to be tachypneic, tachycardic, and diaphoretic and her ABG levels while breathing nasal O_2 at 2 L/min indicate pH 7.26, $PaCO_2$ 64 mmHg, and PaO_2 86 mmHg. She is awake and alert. Her VC is 8 mL/kg and her MIF 18 cmH_2O.

Comment

The problem here is incomplete reversal of a depolarizing muscle relaxant drug. Upon administration of an additional 4 mg neostigmine and 1.5 mg atropine this patient's full strength promptly returned and her ventilation normalized.

For further discussion of assessment for extubation and assessment for weaning see Chapters 53 and 86, respectively.

Several abnormalities involving skeletal muscle can result in ventilatory failure.[10–13] The ventilatory muscles are involved in almost all generalized myopathies, and ventilatory failure is particularly common in Duchenne type muscular dystrophy. The inflammatory myopathies, including polymyositis and dermatomyositis, also affect the respiratory muscles in a high percentage of cases.

Patient Example 30-5

Decreased Chest Bellows Function—Chronic (Duchenne Type Muscular Dystrophy)

A 19-year-old man with Duchenne type muscular dystrophy has been wheelchair-bound for 6 years, and during the last year he has been hospitalized twice with pneumonia. In the last month he has complained of dyspnea and has developed an intermittent cough. He has had periods of confusion and complains of severe headaches on awakening in the morning. Physical examination shows cyanosis, tachypnea, reduced chest and abdominal movement, and coarse rhonchi on inspiration. ABG levels while breathing air show pH 7.34, $PaCO_2$ 76 mmHg, and PaO_2 44 mmHg. His calculated $P(A\text{-}a)O_2$ is 11 mmHg, which indicates pure hypoventilation as the etiology for his hypoxemia.

For further discussion of respiratory muscle dysfunction and of elective long-term nocturnal mechanical ventilation see Chapters 26 and 101, respectively.

Electrolyte abnormalities, including hypophosphatemia, hypomagnesemia, and hypokalemia, can depress muscle function and result in ventilatory failure.[14] Hypophosphatemia and hypomagnesemia may be unrecognized in patients with chronic nutritional deficiencies, especially chronic alcoholics, and their contribution to ventilatory failure may elude recognition and diagnosis.

The ventilatory failure associated with severe myxedema is probably multifactorial, including a component of decreased central drive to ventilation. However, ventilatory failure in these patients is in part attributed to abnormal muscle function.

Finally, ventilatory muscle fatigue (also frequently referred to as *respiratory* muscle fatigue) has been well documented as a contributing factor to acute ventilatory failure, particularly in patients with chronic obstructive pulmonary disease (COPD) and elevated work of breathing on a chronic basis.[10,12,13]

Patient Example 30-6

Decreased Chest Bellows Function—Acute Ventilatory Muscle Fatigue (Weaning Failure)

A 66-year-old woman with severe COPD develops fever and abdominal pain and undergoes an emergency cholecystectomy for acute cholecystitis. Her postoperative course is complicated by persistent fever and severe bronchospasm. After 1 week an attempt to wean her from the ventilator is made, and she is switched from full ventilatory support to a T-piece. Her ABG levels prior to the weaning attempt show good oxygenation and normal acid-base balance. As the trial of spontaneous ventilation begins, her heart rate is 100 bpm and her respiratory rate 20 breaths per minute, and she appears comfortable. After 5 minutes, however, her respiratory rate begins to increase, and dyssynchronous movements of her chest and abdomen are noted. During the next 15 minutes she becomes tachycardic and more and more tachypneic; paradoxical respirations continue, and she becomes diaphoretic and increasingly agitated. An arterial blood specimen shows acute respiratory acidosis, and she is returned to the ventilator.

The monitoring of respiratory muscle function during a weaning attempt is discussed in Chapter 52, and the sequence of this patient's ventilatory muscle fatigue and the development of acute ventilatory failure are illustrated graphically in Figure 52-4.

Signs of ventilatory muscle fatigue, such as rapid shallow breathing, are frequently nonspecific. However, paradoxical abdominal breathing (in which the abdomen moves inward when the chest is moving outward) and respiratory alternans (breathing for short periods with the chest wall ventilatory muscles, then changing to breathing primarily with the diaphragm and alternating between these patterns) have been described as more specific signs of respiratory muscle fatigue. However, it has been suggested that these may simply reflect an increased load rather than true muscle fatigue. Nonetheless, they appear to be useful physical diagnostic signs of a situation in which ventilatory failure may be either present or impending, with ventilatory muscle fatigue contributing to the hypoventilation.

Disorders of the Thorax

Disorders of the bony thoracic cage or other components of the thorax besides the lungs themselves may contribute to ventilatory failure.[15,16] Severe kyphoscoliosis is frequently associated with ventilatory failure.[17] However, significant $\dot{V}/\dot{Q}$ mismatching is usually also present, which contributes to the hypoxemia. Trauma resulting in a severe flail chest can lead to ventilatory failure; this must be assessed in each patient because the physiologic consequences of a flail chest vary markedly. Most patients with flail chest maintain relatively normal gas exchange despite multiple rib fractures and paradoxical movement of the chest wall with inspiratory effort (see Ch. 91). Abnormalities of the pleural space, such as pneumothorax, hydrothorax, hemothorax, or diffuse pleural involvement, may rarely be associated with hypoventilation. Usually these abnormalities must be striking in their extent in order to contribute to hypoventilation. Finally, severe obesity can contribute to both a restrictive ventilatory defect and increased work of breathing and result in hypoventilation. However, such patients usually also have a reduction in their central ventilatory drives. Thus, restriction of the thorax due to a variety of causes rarely results in pure ventilatory failure. If hypoventilation is present, usually there is a combined disorder.

Patient Example 30-7

Decreased Chest Bellows Function—Chronic (Kyphoscoliosis)

A 47-year-old woman developed severe kyphoscoliosis during her early adolescence, resulting in short stature and external deformity but not preventing her from completing her education and working for 25 years as a bookkeeper. Her work attendance was excellent until the last 3 years; in that time she has had several chest infections each year and has been hospitalized twice. Over the last 6 months her previously intermittent cough has been persistent and productive of large amounts of yellow sputum, and she has developed pedal edema. On examination she has tachypnea, clubbed fingers, cyanosis, pitting edema to midcalf, little discernible chest motion on respiration, distended neck veins, and coarse rhonchi throughout both lung fields on auscultation. Her chest radiograph shows cardiomegaly and enlarged main pulmonary arteries in addition to severe kyphoscoliosis. Her hematocrit is 58 percent. ABG levels while breathing air show pH 7.38, $PaCO_2$ 58 mmHg, and PaO_2 48 mmHg.

Comment

The problem here is failure of the pump; hypoxemia is due both to hypoventilation and to $\dot{V}/\dot{Q}$ mismatching (the calculated $P(A\text{-}a)O_2$ is 30 mmHg), and the patient has developed cor pulmonale. Like many patients with chronic respiratory insufficiency due to kyphoscoliosis, she has features of bronchiectasis as well.

More detailed discussions of the approach to chronic hypoxemia/cor pulmonale, long-term O_2 therapy, and long-term home ventilation are provided in Chapters 63, 99, and 101, respectively.

Airways Obstruction

Severe diffuse abnormalities of the lungs can result in ventilatory failure,[14,18–20] although pure alveolar hypoventilation is unusual. Airflow obstruction is the most frequent pulmonary cause of hypoventilation. Conditions producing upper airway obstruction, such as laryngeal edema, epiglottitis, or croup, can cause hypoventilation but only when these conditions are extreme and the airway is near total obstruction. Until that point patients frequently have had hyperventilation in response to the compromised airway. Generalized lower airway obstruction as in severe COPD or asthma can be associated with hypoventilation, but frequently abnormalities in central ventilatory drive, muscle fatigue, or dead space also contribute.

Patient Example 30-8

Airway Obstruction—Chronic (COPD)

A 68-year-old man has smoked between one and two packs of cigarettes daily for 45 years. He has had a long-standing daily productive cough and progressive exertional dyspnea over the last 15 years. For the last 7 years he has been under a physician's care for COPD; after documentation of chronic hypoxemia while clinically stable despite maximal medical therapy he was placed on continuous home O_2 therapy 3 years ago. He can currently walk one-half block slowly. His forced expiratory volume in 1 second (FEV_1) is 0.6 L. A chest radiograph shows hyperinflation, flattened hemidiaphragms, and diminished vascular markings in the peripheral lung fields. With the patient in a clinically stable state, ABG levels while breathing O_2 at 2 L/min show pH 7.38, $PaCO_2$ 55 mmHg, PaO_2 65 mmHg, and HCO_3^- 33 mEq/L.

Comment

This patient has chronic hypoventilation with complete metabolic compensation of the respiratory acidosis. The hypoxemia is due to a combination of hypoventilation and $\dot{V}/\dot{Q}$ mismatching related to his COPD.

See Chapters 22, 62, 63, and 99, respectively, for further discussion of the clinical description of COPD, the approach to COPD management, indications for long-term O_2 therapy, and long-term O_2 therapy.

Patient Example 30-9

Airway Obstruction—Acute-on-Chronic (COPD) plus Ventilatory Muscle Fatigue

The patient described in Example 30-8 develops an acute exacerbation of his COPD, with increased dyspnea, change in sputum color to yellow, weakness, and anorexia. On examination he is diaphoretic, sitting bolt upright, and so dyspneic that he cannot complete a sentence in a single breath. His respiratory rate is 25 breaths per minute, his heart rate 120 bpm, and his blood pressure normal. He is cyanotic while receiving nasal O_2 at 2 L/min. Paradoxical thoracoabdominal breathing is present, and wheezes, crackles, and rhonchi are heard scattered throughout all lung fields. His blood leukocyte count is normal, his sputum Gram stain shows many leukocytes and mixed bacteria, and his chest radiograph is unchanged. While he is breathing O_2 at 2 L/min, his ABG levels show pH 7.24, $PaCO_2$ 86 mmHg, PaO_2 45 mmHg, and HCO_3^- 36 mEq/L.

The worsening hypoventilation and subsequent acidosis are likely related both to increased airflow obstruction from the bronchitic exacerbation and to ventilatory muscle fatigue.

For a discussion of the approach to acute exacerbation of COPD see Chapter 64 and for discussions of paradoxical respiration see Chapters 26 and 52.

INCREASED DEAD SPACE

What accounts for an elevated $PaCO_2$ when minute ventilation is actually increased? Although there are a variety of clinical etiologies for this situation, there are only two possible physiologic explanations: either dead space (wasted ventilation) is increased or CO_2 production is increased.[1] A combination of these two mechanisms is often present.

Many pulmonary diseases can result in increased V_D, which is that volume of each breath that is inhaled but does not reach functioning terminal respiratory units and is therefore wasted with respect to gas exchange. Dead space can be divided into *anatomic dead space,* the volume of the upper respiratory tract and conducting airways from which alveoli do not arise and thus in which gas exchange cannot take place, and alveolar or *physiologic dead space,* to which all terminal respiratory units that are overventilated relative to their perfusion contribute. The combination of the anatomic and physiologic dead spaces represents the total wasted ventilation or $\dot{V}_D$. An estimate of $\dot{V}_D$ is easily determined from measurements of CO_2 tension on simultaneously collected samples of expired air and arterial blood by using a modification of the Bohr equation that assumes that $PaCO_2$ equals P_ACO_2:

$$\dot{V}_D = \left(\frac{PaCO_2 - P_ECO_2}{PaCO_2}\right)(\dot{V}_E) \qquad (2)$$

where P_ECO_2 is expired CO_2 pressure.

$\dot{V}_E$ equals $\dot{V}_A$ plus $\dot{V}_D$. When an increase in dead space is present and the patient has a normal $\dot{V}_E$, the $\dot{V}_A$ component must be reduced. Patients with intact ventilatory drive respond to this situation with an increase in $\dot{V}_E$; however, when very high $\dot{V}_D$ is present, the patient may not be able to adequately compensate by increasing $\dot{V}_E$ over long periods. Relative alveolar hypoventilation in relation to the metabolic demands then ensues, and $PaCO_2$ rises.

The classic example of an area of increased physiologic dead space is that associated with acute pulmonary embolism. The ventilation to the affected lung area may remain intact, but the blood flow is markedly reduced, resulting in wasted ventilation. In fact, even patients with large pulmonary emboli usually can compensate for the increased dead space in the affected area by increasing ventilation to other areas of lung with relatively normal blood flow, and so ventilatory failure is unusual, although hypoxemia related to other mechanisms is the rule (see Ch. 31).

Increase in $\dot{V}_D$ is common in the adult respiratory distress syndrome (ARDS).[21] This effect occurs early in the lung injury process but frequently worsens as lung remodeling and scarring develop in the first and second weeks in those patients who do not rapidly resolve their lung injury. Mechanical ventilation and positive end-expiratory pressure (PEEP) contribute to development of dead space in these patients. Generally patients with ARDS, including those with greatly increased dead space, do not develop ventilatory failure with hypercapnia despite the presence of severe hypoxemia. Patients are able to compensate for both the wasted ventilation related to areas of dead space and the lack of CO_2 removal from the blood in airless lung areas by increasing ventilation in lung areas that have relatively good $\dot{V}/\dot{Q}$ matching. This is possible because lung injury in the ARDS patient, although appearing to be diffuse and homogeneous on the chest x-ray, is in fact widespread but patchy. As described in Chapter 35, some areas of the lung are severely involved, but often adjacent areas are relatively preserved.

The reason that increasing ventilation to these areas is able to compensate for the abnormality in CO_2 removal but not for the abnormality in oxygenation relates to differences in the hemoglobin-CO_2 and oxyhemoglobin dissociation curves and to a lesser extent to differences in the diffusivity of CO_2 as compared with O_2. The hemoglobin-CO_2 dissociation curve is a flat line such that increases in ventilation have tremendous effects on lowering CO_2 content. The oxyhemoglobin dissociation curve has a sigmoid shape, and the relatively normal areas of the lung result in a local PaO_2 that falls on the relatively flat portion of the curve; thus, large increases in ventilation have relatively little effect on increasing overall arterial O_2 content. However, some patients with ARDS have such severe abnormalities in dead space ventilation that they indeed do retain CO_2. These patients usually also have increased CO_2 production (see below). In fact, in the initial description of ARDS by Ashbaugh et al.[22] in 1967, 2 of the 12 patients described had significant hypercapnia.

INCREASED CARBON DIOXIDE PRODUCTION

An elevation in CO_2 production ($\dot{V}CO_2$) can contribute to ventilatory failure; however, if the respiratory system is entirely normal, a rise in $\dot{V}CO_2$ does not result in hypercapnia. Ventilatory failure, therefore, requires not only an increase in $\dot{V}CO_2$ but also either a failure to respond to the stimulus of a rising $PaCO_2$ because of abnormal ventilatory drive or a disease of the respiratory nerves, bellows, or lungs such that the patient is not able to respond with an adequate rise in $\dot{V}_E$ to compensate for the elevation in $\dot{V}CO_2$. An increase in $\dot{V}CO_2$ reflects an increase in metabolic rate, which can be related to increased muscular activity (e.g., seizures or severe shivering with accompanying increased O_2 utilization and CO_2 production) or to fever.

The $\dot{V}CO_2$ is also affected by the respiratory quotient (RQ). Oxidation of carbohydrates, protein, and fats in the body is necessary to produce the energy required for maintenance of life and bodily functions. The principal breakdown products of this oxidation are CO_2 and H_2O. The RQ is the ratio of metabolic CO_2 production to the O_2 consumption of the tissues ($\dot{V}CO_2/\dot{V}O_2$). As discussed in Chapter 51, the RQ varies for each of the substrates being metabolized: for carbohydrate it equals 1.0, for fat 0.7, and for protein 0.8. When a critically ill patient is being nourished primarily with carbohydrates, relatively more CO_2 is produced for the amount of O_2 consumed than when fats are being administered. Thus, how the patient is being fed can have some effect on the amount of CO_2 produced.

References

1. Dantzker DR: Pulmonary gas exchange. pp. 1684–1688. In Kelley WN (ed): Textbook of Internal Medicine. 2nd Ed. JB Lippincott, Philadelphia, 1992
2. Mellins RB, Balfour HH Jr, Turino GM, Winters RW: Failure of automatic control of ventilation (Ondine's curse). Medicine (Baltimore) 1970;49:487–504
3. Plum F, Leigh RJ: Abnormalities in central mechanisms. pp. 989–1067. In Hornbein TF (ed): Regulation of Breathing. Vol. 2. Marcel Dekker, New York, 1981
4. Zwillich CW: Control of ventilation. pp. 1689–1691. In Kelley WN (ed): Textbook of Internal Medicine, 2nd Ed. JB Lippincott, Philadelphia, 1992
5. Zwillich CW: Diseases of ventilatory control. pp. 1790–1794. In Kelley WN (ed): Textbook of Internal Medicine, 2nd Ed. JB Lippincott, Philadelphia, 1992
6. Bennett DA, Bleck TP: Diagnosis and treatment of neuromuscular causes of acute respiratory failure. Clin Neuropharmacol 1988;11:303–347
7. White DP: Sleep apnea syndrome. pp. 1794–1798. In Kelley WN (ed): Textbook of Internal Medicine. 2nd Ed. JB Lippincott, Philadelphia, 1992
8. Zwillich CW, Sutton FD, Pierson DJ et al: Decreased hypoxic ventilatory drive in the obesity-hypoventilation syndrome. Am J Med 1975;59:343–348
9. Moore P, James O: Guillain-Barré syndrome: Incidence, management and outcome of major complications. Crit Care Med 1981;9:549–555
10. Grassino A, Macklem PT: Respiratory muscle fatigue and ventilatory failure. Annu Rev Med 1984;35:625–647
11. Tobin MJ (ed): The respiratory muscles. In Branson RD, MacIntyre NR (eds): Problems in Respiratory Care. JB Lippincott, Philadelphia, 1990
12. Belman MJ (ed): Respiratory muscles: Function in health and disease. Clin Chest Med 1988;9:175–361
13. Roussos C, Macklem RP: The respiratory muscles. N Engl J Med 1982;307:786–797
14. Sherman CB, Osmanski JP, Hudson LD: Acute exacerbations in COPD patients. pp. 443–456. In Cherniak NS (ed): Chronic Obstructive Pulmonary Disease. WB Saunders, Philadelphia, 1991
15. Bergofsky EH: Respiratory failure in disorders of the thoracic cage. Am Rev Respir Dis 1979;119:643–669
16. Rochester DF, Findley LJ: The lungs and neuromuscular and chest wall diseases. pp. 1942–1971. In Murray JF, Nadel JA (eds): Textbook of Respiratory Medicine. WB Saunders, Philadelphia, 1988
17. Bergofsky E, Turino G, Fishman A: Cardiorespiratory failure in kyphoscoliosis. Medicine (Baltimore) 1959;38:263–317
18. Lane DJ, Howell JBL, Giblin B: Relation between airways obstruction and CO_2 tension in chronic obstructive airways disease. Br Med J 1968;3:707–709
19. Hudson LD: Acute respiratory failure in patients with chronic obstructive pulmonary disease. pp. 155–172. In George RB, Bone RC, Hudson LD (eds): Acute Respiratory Failure. Churchill Livingstone, New York, 1987
20. Schmidt GA, Hall JB: Acute on chronic respiratory failure: Assessment and management of patients with COPD in the emergent setting. JAMA 1989;261:3444–3453
21. Pepe PE, Hudson LD: Acute respiratory failure. pp. 47–55. In Callaham ML (ed): Current Practice of Emergency Medicine. 2nd Ed. BC Decker, Philadelphia, 1991
22. Ashbaugh DJ, Bigelow DB, Petty PL, Levine BE: Acute respiratory distress in adults. Lancet 1967;2:319–323

Chapter 31

Hypoxemia

Leonard D. Hudson
David J. Pierson

CHAPTER OUTLINE

This chapter deals with clinical examples of the physiologic mechanisms by which hypoxemia occurs, as described in Chapter 29. The rational practice of respiratory care depends on continuously relating a given clinical situation involving hypoxemia to the pathophysiologic mechanisms causing the hypoxemia. In approaching this relationship there are four clinical aspects to be dealt with: (1) the clinical setting (including diagnosis or differential diagnosis); (2) arterial blood gas (ABG) results; (3) chest radiographic findings; and (4) response in the arterial O_2 partial pressure (PaO_2) to the administration of O_2. In some cases the diagnosis and chest radiographic findings will dictate a particular approach to administration of O_2; in other cases, the response in the PaO_2 to O_2 administration will provide information about the mechanism of hypoxemia and thus will help to define the differential diagnostic possibilities. Table 31-1 presents a practical diagnostic approach to the patient with hypoxemia that involves these four factors. Examples of the interplay between these factors and their clinical usefulness are given in the following discussion, which provides a clinical perspective on each of the five physiologic mechanisms for hypoxemia: low inspired O_2 tension (P_IO_2), alveolar hypoventilation, ventilation/perfusion ($\dot{V}/\dot{Q}$) mismatch, right-to-left shunt, and diffusion limitation.[1,2]

LOW INSPIRED OXYGEN PRESSURE

Decreased Inspired Oxygen Fraction at Normal Barometric Pressure

Clinical examples of hypoxemia caused by a low P_IO_2 are of two types: (1) those due to an inspired O_2 fraction (F_IO_2) lower than that usually found in air (i.e., less than 0.21); and (2) those due to breathing a mixture with an F_IO_2 of 0.21 at a low atmospheric pressure, which results in a P_IO_2 substantially lower than that found at sea level. In turn, there are two types of clinical situations resulting in inhalation of a low F_IO_2 mixture. The first is the accidental inhalation of a mixture with a low F_IO_2, which is encountered when victims find themselves in a hostile environment. Examples include being in the immediate area of a fire, which is consuming the O_2, leaving a gas mixture that has an O_2 content significantly less than 21 percent. This could also result from the escape of non-oxygen-containing gases in large quantities in a closed space, with dilution of the available O_2 resulting in a low F_IO_2 mixture. An example is a faulty fire extinguishing system in the hold of a ship in which CO_2 is released acutely in large quantities and dilutes the available O_2. A

Table 31-1. Diagnostic Approach to the Patient with Hypoxemia

1. Establish a working diagnosis or differential diagnosis based on the available clinical history and physical examination
2. Examine the arterial blood gases for the following:
   a. Whether hypoxemia is present
   b. The degree of hypoxemia
   c. Whether alveolar hypoventilation is present
   d. From the alveolar gas equation
   $$\left(P_{AO_2} = P_{IO_2} - \frac{PaCO_2}{R}\right)$$
   calculate whether alveolar hypoventilation accounts for all the hypoxemia [i.e., $P(A\text{-}a)O_2$ normal] or whether some other mechanism is present [i.e., $P(A\text{-}a)O_2$ increased]
3. Examine the chest radiograph:
   a. Clear lung fields or mild abnormalities suggest hypoxemia due to hypoventilation or low $\dot{V}/\dot{Q}$
   b. Significant airspace filling and consolidation suggest hypoxemia secondary to intrapulmonary shunt
4. On the basis of the first three steps, determine the likely mechanism of oxygenation abnormality (hypoventilation, low $\dot{V}/\dot{Q}$, or shunt) and initiate O_2 therapy accordingly:
   a. Small O_2 supplements for hypoventilation and/or low $\dot{V}/\dot{Q}$
   b. Large O_2 supplements for shunt
5. Assess the response of the PaO_2 to the amount of O_2 administered in step 4; revise the suspected mechanism(s) and broaden the differential diagnosis accordingly

reduction in FIO_2 will result in a low PIO_2 and eventually a low PaO_2. In these situations no lung impairment or lung disease need be present to result in a low PaO_2, and in such cases the chest radiograph is normal. However, this mechanism obviously could further impair any individual with preexisting lung disease and add to other mechanisms causing hypoxemia.

Patient Example 31-1

Decreased FIO_2 in the Workplace

Two repairmen are working on the roof of a nearly empty silo containing silage from the previous season. One of them accidentally drops a wrench and climbs down into the silo to retrieve it. When he does not return his companion looks into the silo and sees him lying motionless and unresponsive on the floor below.

Comment

This victim suffers asphyxia from breathing stale air in an enclosed, unventilated space in which methane and other gases have built up as a result of fermentation, lowering the FIO_2. Fatal hypoxia can be the result despite normal lung and cardiac function. Rescue in such situations can be both difficult and dangerous.

The second example of inhalation of a low FIO_2 mixture occurs when such a mixture is inadvertently administered in a medical situation. Several examples of this have been reported. A gas other than O_2 has been delivered from a hospital gas administration system, resulting in an FIO_2 lower instead of higher than that of room air. Other mistakes in administration of gas mixtures from tank systems to individual patients can occur, with the same result. Again, a patient does not have to have lung disease in order for a low PaO_2 to result from this clinical situation.

Therapy in these two situations is obvious. First, the patient must be removed from the hostile environment that resulted in the low FIO_2. Following that, whether administration of supplemental O_2 is required depends on any other injuries or insults that the patient might have received. For example, if CO also is suspected to be present in a fire environment, administration of a high FIO_2 mixture is warranted to hasten the removal of CO from hemoglobin. If the patient has an impaired level of consciousness, administration of supplemental O_2 is prudent. In the case of inadvertent medical administration of a low FIO_2 mixture, the major problem is identifying the mistake in gas administration; once the technical error is discovered, the corrective measures are obvious.

A more common occurrence in the hospital setting is the inadvertent administration of less supplemental O_2 than intended to a patient with hypoxemia due to other mechanisms. O_2 masks or nasal cannulas may become dislodged or be removed by confused patients, or the O_2 flow may be set incorrectly or accidentally decreased. A similar mishap may occur during mechanical ventilation in the intensive care unit (ICU), as shown by the example below. It is important that the clinician consider an interruption or decrease in the ordered O_2 therapy as a possible cause whenever a patient receiving supplemental O_2 develops new or worsened hypoxemia.

Patient Example 31-2

Decreased FIO_2 during Mechanical Ventilation

A patient is receiving postoperative mechanical ventilation after open heart surgery. With full ventilatory support and FIO_2 0.40 following reversal of anesthesia in the recovery room, ABG values were pH 7.40, $PaCO_2$ 40 mmHg, and PaO_2 110 mmHg. Shortly after transfer to the ICU the patient is noted to be tachycardic, restless, and "overbreathing" the ventilator, and the bedside pulse oximeter reads 80 percent saturation. ABG values at this time show pH 7.46, $PaCO_2$ 33 mmHg, and PaO_2 50 mmHg. The patient is removed from the ventilator and given manual ventilation with 100 percent O_2, which results in prompt disappearance of distress and desaturation. Inspection of the ventilator reveals that the FIO_2 knob had inadvertently been set at 0.21 instead of 0.40.

Comment

Although this patient's oxygenation is impaired by one or more of the other mechanisms discussed in the following sections, the acute hypoxemia in this instance was due to unintentional administration of a lower F_{IO_2} than that required to correct the hypoxemia.

The approach to the agitation and dyspnea that develop during mechanical ventilation is discussed in Chapter 84.

Decreased Barometric Pressure at High Altitude

Inhalation at a low P_{IO_2} and a normal F_{IO_2} (0.21) occurs at high altitude.[3] Examining the differences in the P_{IO_2} at sea level versus that at 1 mile (5280 ft) altitude serves to exemplify this. Assuming an average barometric pressure at sea level of 760 mmHg, the P_{IO_2} is approximately 150 mmHg (760 − 47 mmHg water vapor pressure = 713 × 0.21 F_{IO_2} = 150 mmHg). Assuming an average $PaCO_2$ of 40 mmHg and a respiratory exchange ratio (R) of 0.8 and calculating from the alveolar gas equation, this would result in an alveolar O_2 pressure (P_{AO_2}) of approximately 100 ($P_{AO_2} = P_{IO_2} - \frac{P_{ACO_2}}{R}$ or $P_{AO_2} = 150 - \frac{40}{0.8} = 100$). At an altitude of 1 mile the average barometric pressure is 630 mmHg, resulting in an average P_{IO_2} of 122 [(630 − 47) × 0.21]. Using an average $PaCO_2$ of 36 at this altitude (reflecting a slight increase in ventilation due to the relative hypoxemia and the increase in hypoxic ventilatory drive that occur at this altitude) and again calculating from the alveolar air equation, the average P_{AO_2} is approximately 77 mmHg. Thus a normal PaO_2 at sea level ranges from approximately 80 to 95 mmHg whereas the normal value at 1 mile altitude is 65 to 75 mmHg.

Obviously, altitudes higher than 1 mile have more striking effects on the P_{IO_2} and resultant P_{AO_2} and PaO_2. The extreme example of these altitude effects on earth is provided by the measurements of the barometric pressure and subsequent calculations of alveolar gases that were made on a scientific expedition to Mount Everest (altitude 29,028 ft). The measured barometric pressure at the top of Mount Everest is 253 mmHg (measured October 24, 1981), and thus the P_{IO_2} is 43 mmHg. Individuals breathing air at this altitude markedly hyperventilate owing to stimulation of their hypoxic ventilatory drive. Assuming a P_{ACO_2} of 10 mmHg would result in a calculated P_{AO_2} of 31 to 32 mmHg.

Inhalation of a low P_{IO_2} mixture is of practical importance in the patient with lung disease who is flying on a commercial airline[4] (see Ch. 100). The cabin pressure in a commercial airliner is generally planned to be similar to the barometric pressure at approximately 8000 ft although recent actual measurements of several flights involving multiple airlines showed a range in cabin altitude from sea level to 8915 ft, with a mean of 5673 ft and a median of 6214 ft.[5] This could obviously have a major effect on a patient with pre-existing lung disease who flies on a commercial airliner and is subjected to barometric pressure similar to that found at 8000 to 9000 feet.

Patient Example 31-3

Decreased P_{IO_2} (Air Travel)

A 68-year-old woman with severe chronic obstructive pulmonary disease (COPD) develops acute respiratory distress during a commercial airline flight to visit her daughter in another state. The flight attendants administer supplemental O_2 by mask, the woman's distress abates, and she falls asleep. After the plane lands at its sea-level destination, the patient is examined and found to be in no acute distress, and the following ABG values are obtained: pH 7.38, $PaCO_2$ 52 mmHg, and PaO_2 60 mmHg.

Comment

Although she does not have resting hypoxemia severe enough to warrant long-term O_2 therapy (see Ch. 63), this patient's PaO_2 fell significantly during the flight, probably to 50 mmHg or lower. Because of her airflow obstruction she was unable to relieve the hypoxemia by hyperventilating, and both the low PaO_2 and her increased efforts to breathe contributed to her dyspnea. Administration of mask O_2 (perhaps enough to effectively eliminate her hypoxic ventilatory drive) relieved her distress but may have led to acute respiratory acidosis because of her underlying CO_2 retention. Such patients should undergo a preflight assessment of O_2 need, as described in Chapter 100.

ALVEOLAR HYPOVENTILATION

Clinical examples of ventilatory failure and the effect of alveolar hypoventilation on hypoxemia have been covered in Chapter 30. In brief summary, there are many causes of alveolar hypoventilation, including (1) decreased ventilatory drive; (2) abnormal neural transmission of the respiratory signal; (3) failure of the ventilatory pump (either muscular failure or abnormalities of the bony thorax); (4) severe airway obstruction; (5) the existence of a very high dead space; or (6) markedly increased CO_2 production. Any of these can result in alveolar hypoventilation (by definition an increase in $PaCO_2$). Calculations from the alveolar gas equation allow determination of whether alveolar hypoventilation is the sole cause of the hypoxemia; this is necessary since a patient with alveolar hypoventilation also can simultaneously have any of the other mechanisms of hypoxemia.

Patient Example 31-4

Hypoxemia Only Partly Due to Hypoventilation (Drug Overdose)

A 20-year-old woman with a past history of depression and several previous suicidal gestures is found unresponsive with several empty medication bottles nearby. Vomitus is present on the bed and around her mouth. ABG levels when breathing room air show pH 7.22, $PaCO_2$ 72 mmHg, and PaO_2 34 mmHg. Her calculated alveolar-arterial O_2 pressure difference [$P(A\text{-}a)O_2$] is 26 mmHg, which suggests that alveolar hypoventilation accounts for only part of the observed hypoxemia. On the basis of the circumstances, aspiration of gastric contents is a likely explanation for the additional $\dot{V}/\dot{Q}$ mismatch and/or right-to-left shunt. These findings should be compared with those in Patient Example 30-1.

In approaching the patient with hypoxemia one of the first steps is to examine the ABG levels and see whether alveolar hypoventilation is present. If it is, the next step is to calculate P_AO_2 from the alveolar gas equation (see Table 31-1 and Ch. 29) and then to calculate the $P(A\text{-}a)O_2$. If the $P(A\text{-}a)O_2$ is normal, alveolar hypoventilation alone accounts for the hypoxemia present. However, if the $P(A\text{-}a)O_2$ is increased or widened, another mechanism, either $\dot{V}/\dot{Q}$ mismatch or shunt, is present. Subsequently steps must be taken as described below to determine which of these mechanisms is responsible for the hypoxemia not accounted for by alveolar hypoventilation.

VENTILATION/PERFUSION MISMATCH (LOW $\dot{V}/\dot{Q}$ RATIO)

Mismatching of ventilation and perfusion can occur either with a reduction in ventilation out of proportion to perfusion or with an increase in ventilation relative to perfusion.[2] The latter situation, increased $\dot{V}/\dot{Q}$, results in dead space or wasted ventilation, as described in Chapter 30. The term *$\dot{V}/\dot{Q}$ mismatch* is usually used to describe a *reduction* in ventilation in relation to perfusion. Hypoxemia results only when ventilation is reduced out of proportion to perfusion. This is because a continuing blood supply is necessary for the reduction in ventilation to be reflected in a reduced arterial blood O_2 content.

When no ventilation exists to an area of lung but perfusion continues, this extreme form of $\dot{V}/\dot{Q}$ mismatch is called a *shunt*. (The mechanism of shunt is discussed in the next section.) However, it is important to note that differentiation between low $\dot{V}/\dot{Q}$ ($\dot{V}/\dot{Q}$ mismatch) and shunt has important physiologic and clinical implications. This important difference is reflected in the response to O_2 administration of an area of low $\dot{V}/\dot{Q}$ as compared with the response of an area of shunt. With a low $\dot{V}/\dot{Q}$ area, the airway is still open to the alveoli even though the alveoli are grossly underventilated. Therefore, when O_2 is given, in time it diffuses down to the alveolar level, displacing the N_2 and resulting in a high P_AO_2; this results in improved oxygenation of the blood flowing by the underventilated alveoli. In an area of shunt the alveoli either are full of fluid, pus, or other material or are collapsed. When O_2 is administered, the area of shunt receives no increase in O_2 because no ventilation is present, and therefore the blood flowing by that region of lung has *no* change in its O_2 content. The only improvement in oxygenation in a lung that has an area or areas of shunt occurs in the nonshunt regions. The important practical difference is that the hypoxemia resulting from low $\dot{V}/\dot{Q}$ areas can be corrected by a small supplementation in O_2 because this O_2 will reach the alveolar level and be absorbed into the blood. However, hypoxemia due to shunt will show only slight improvement with high amounts of supplemental O_2.

The response to O_2 administration either confirms the suspected mechanism and helps to substantiate the working diagnosis or causes the clinician to question the presumed hypoxemia mechanism and diagnosis. As an example, let us consider a patient who is thought to have low $\dot{V}/\dot{Q}$ as the mechanism for hypoxemia but shows no change in PaO_2 with administration of 3 L/min of O_2 by nasal prongs and only a slight increase in PaO_2 with administration of high-flow O_2 by face mask. This information would suggest that a shunt is present, leading to consideration of pathologic processes that cause shunts, and would raise new possibilities in the differential diagnosis.

Low $\dot{V}/\dot{Q}$ usually results when the alveoli are open but airflow to the alveoli is diminished, which classically occurs with partial obstruction of the airways. Examples include COPD, often with superimposed acute further diminution in airflow (e.g., due to increased secretions related to an acute bronchitis).[6–8] Another classic example is that of an acute asthmatic attack with significant bronchospasm, resulting in poor airflow but with the alveoli open and continuing blood flow to those alveoli.

Frequently the blood flow in an area of low $\dot{V}/\dot{Q}$ is also somewhat reduced from normal owing to so-called hypoxic vasoconstriction, a phenomenon in which the blood flow to alveoli is self-regulated and diminishes in response to low P_AO_2. However, the reduction in blood flow often is inadequate to match the reduction in ventilation, and a low $\dot{V}/\dot{Q}$ ratio still exists. Certain vasoactive drugs can reduce hypoxic vasoconstriction and cause significant worsening of arterial oxygenation. This is particularly true of vasodilators such as hydralazine and nitroprusside, which cause dilation of the pulmonary as well as the systemic vasculature.

Patient Example 31-5

Hypoxemia Due to $\dot{V}/\dot{Q}$ Mismatch (Acute Asthma)

A 30-year-old man with long-standing asthma presents to a hospital emergency department with wheezing and dyspnea, which have worsened over several hours despite frequent use of aerosol bronchodilator. He is in moderate respiratory distress, is using his accessory ventilatory muscles, and has widespread wheezes on chest auscultation. His peak expiratory flow rate is 100 L/min (35 percent of the predicted value). ABG values with the patient breathing room air are pH 7.48, $PaCO_2$ 32 mmHg, and PaO_2 59 mmHg. The $P(A\text{-}a)O_2$ is 50 mmHg. Administration of O_2 by nasal cannula at 2 L/min results in ABG values of pH 7.42, $PaCO_2$ 38 mmHg, and PaO_2 125 mmHg.

Comment

The exact FIO_2 cannot be known when using nasal prongs (see Ch. 75), so that $P(A\text{-}a)O_2$ cannot be calculated. From the large increase in PaO_2, however, it is clear that $\dot{V}/\dot{Q}$ mismatching was the primary mechanism of this patient's initial hypoxemia.

The approach to patient assessment and management in acute asthma is discussed in Chapter 62.

In using the approach presented in Table 31-1, if a patient with known asthma has symptoms and signs typical of an acute asthmatic attack, a $\dot{V}/\dot{Q}$ mismatch should be suspected. Low $\dot{V}/\dot{Q}$ should also be suspected if a patient with known COPD reports increasing sputum production, a change in sputum color, and increasing dyspnea. One of the next steps in the process is to examine the patient's chest radiograph. In general, if a low $\dot{V}/\dot{Q}$ area is present, this will not be apparent on the chest radiograph, and the chest film either will be the same as in the patient's usual chronic state or will show increased air trapping. However, no airless lung will be present (Fig. 31-1). On the other hand, if a shunt is present, this is caused by alveoli being filled or by collapse of alveoli. In either case, airspace filling or airless lung should be apparent on the chest radiograph, appearing as opacities in the usual air-filled lung (Fig. 31-2). In a patient whose clinical situation suggests low $\dot{V}/\dot{Q}$ as the cause of hypoxemia, a "clear" chest radiograph supports this impression; if airless lung or areas of consolidated lung are present, shunt should be suspected as a mechanism of hypoxemia in addition to low $\dot{V}/\dot{Q}$.

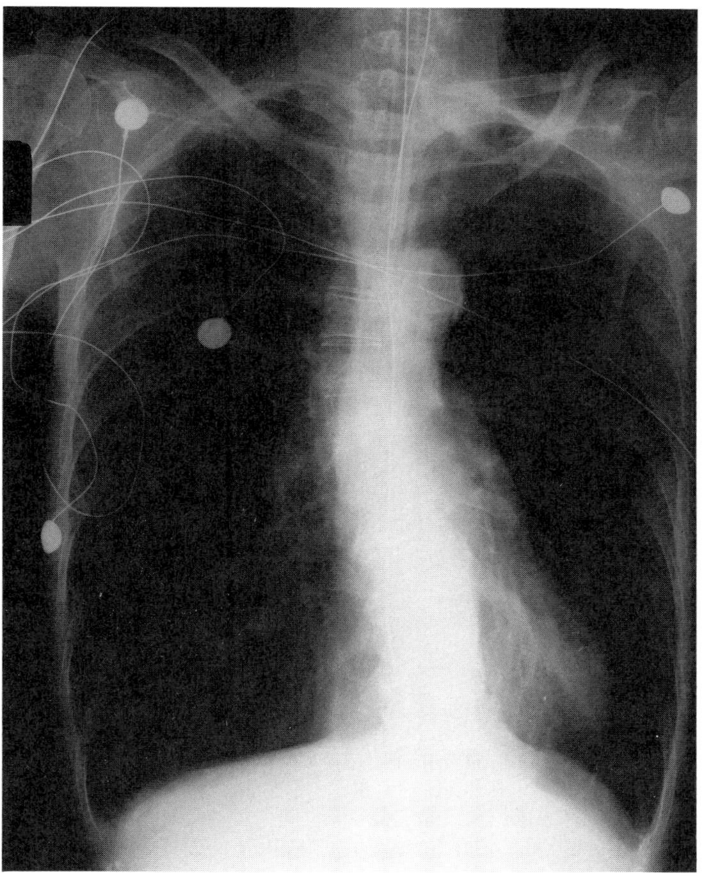

Figure 31-1. Chest radiograph of a patient with severe COPD, taken during an acute exacerbation. The lung fields are hyperlucent with no evidence for consolidation or airspace filling. Hypoxemia present in such a patient would be expected to be due primarily to $\dot{V}/\dot{Q}$ mismatching (with or without alveolar hypoventilation) rather than to shunt and should respond satisfactorily to the administration of low-flow supplemental O_2. (From Pierson,[9] with permission.)

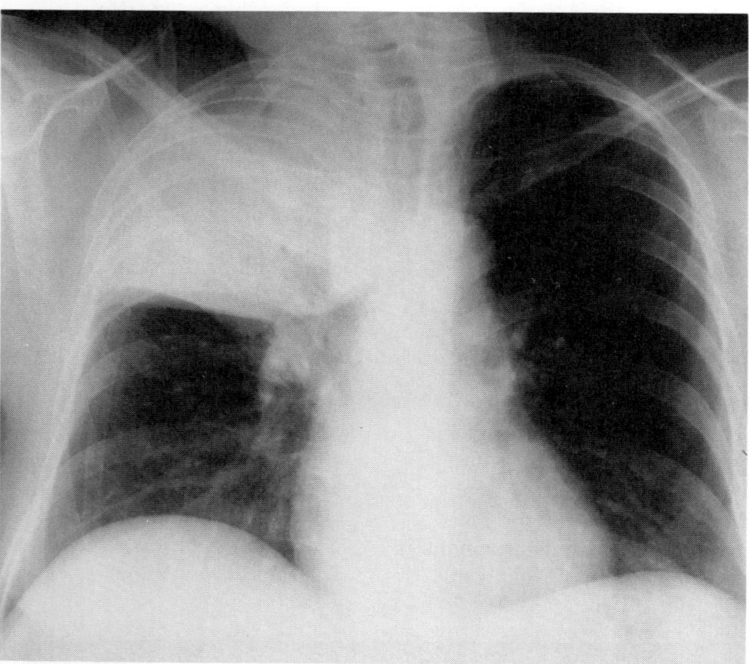

Figure 31-2. Chest radiograph of a 40-year-old woman with pneumococcal pneumonia, showing dense consolidation of the right upper lobe. The lung fields are otherwise clear. Hypoxemia in such a patient typically is due primarily to shunt, and it may be difficult or impossible to raise the PaO_2 into the normal range by using supplemental O_2. (From Pierson,[9] with permission.)

If low $\dot{V}/\dot{Q}$ is suspected as the mechanism of hypoxemia, appropriate O_2 therapy consists of administration of a small amount of O_2 above that in air (e.g., 1 to 2 L/min O_2 delivered by nasal cannula). If, in fact, low $\dot{V}/\dot{Q}$ is the only cause of the hypoxemia, one expects a substantial improvement in the arterial O_2 level related to this therapy. For example, if the initial PaO_2 is 45 mmHg in a patient with COPD and an acute exacerbation, one might expect administration of 2 L/min of O_2 by nasal prongs to result in a PaO_2 of 55 to 60 mmHg. If there is no improvement in the arterial oxygenation with administration of supplemental O_2, shunt should be suspected and evidence for this sought by obtaining a chest radiograph if one was not already taken.

RIGHT-TO-LEFT SHUNT

The concept of a shunt has been described above in the section dealing with low $\dot{V}/\dot{Q}$. An intrapulmonary shunt is called a right-to-left shunt because essentially blood from the right side of the heart bypasses any chance of receiving O_2, since it does not flow by alveoli that are open and capable of gas exchange but goes directly to the left side of the heart, where it is pumped in a deoxygenated state to the body tissue beds.[2] It is also possible to have an intracardiac shunt in which blood passes through a defect directly from the right side of the heart to the left side of the heart. Normal pressures within the heart cause a pressure gradient such that blood usually flows from the left side to the right side if a defect is present, although it is possible for a small amount of blood to flow from right to left, which also may occur if the pressures in the right side of the heart gradually increase to the level of systemic pressures. Occasionally shunts can occur in the lung through small direct arteriovenous (A-V) connections, which may be either congenital defects (so-called A-V malformations) or connections that develop in patients with severe chronic liver disease. Neither of these types of vascular abnormalities are readily visible on a standard chest radiograph, although large A-V malformations can sometimes be detected.

Two clues to the presence of a shunt are found in the laboratory workup. First, the degree of hypoxemia due to a shunt is usually severe. Second, as described above, the chest radiograph usually shows significant opacities representing either fluid-filled lung or collapsed lung (Fig. 31-2). If the chest radiographic findings are thought to be acute and if they correlate with the acute clinical history, a shunt should be anticipated. Its presence is confirmed by the response to O_2 administration, again as discussed under the section dealing with $\dot{V}/\dot{Q}$ mismatch.

Patient Example 31-6

Hypoxemia Due to Shunt (Lobar Pneumonia)

A 40-year-old woman with a history of chronic alcoholism and heavy cigarette smoking is brought to the hospital with a 2-day history of shaking chills, high fever, pleuritic chest pain, and cough productive of rusty sputum. Physical examination reveals dullness to percussion and accentuated tactile fremitus over the right upper thorax posteriorly, with bronchial breath sounds and inspiratory crackles in this area. The patient's chest radiograph (Fig. 31-2) confirms the presence of right upper lobe consolidation. Initial ABG determinations with the patient breathing room air show pH 7.32, $PaCO_2$ 33 mmHg, and PaO_2 36 mmHg. High-flow O_2 (F_IO_2 1.00) is administered by mask, and the patient's PaO_2 rises only to 56 mmHg. Cultures of sputum and blood are subsequently positive for *Streptococcus pneumoniae*.

Comment

The relative lack of response of this patient's hypoxemia to administration of high-F_IO_2 supplemental O_2 confirms that it is due to right-to-left intrapulmonary shunt.

The approach to acute hypoxic respiratory failure is discussed in Chapter 65, the approach to lobar pneumonia and other infections in Chapter 68, and techniques for administering high-F_IO_2 supplemental O_2 to nonintubated patients in Chapter 75.

If an intrapulmonary shunt is present, the alveoli are either totally full or collapsed. Therefore when considering possible etiologies, one should think of pathologic processes that fulfill these requirements. Although the number of disease processes that can lead to shunting are multiple, the actual pathologic processes are relatively limited. The alveolar spaces can either be filled with fluid as in cardiogenic pulmonary edema or early adult respiratory distress syndrome (ARDS) or they can be filled with other material, particularly a cellular exudate as in pneumonia.[8,10,22] Collapse can either be diffuse patchy microatelectasis such as occurs in ARDS and is presumably related to the effect of protein-rich edema fluid on inactivating surfactant (see Ch. 35), or can be focal, as with lobar or whole-lung atelectasis. This in turn can be either obstructive atelectasis, in which the airway is blocked with collapse distal to the area of blockage (if collateral ventilation is not adequate to maintain the patency of the alveolar spaces) or absorptive atelectasis, in which the airway remains open. Many variations on these processes exist, but the basic types of abnormalities are relatively limited.

Changes in cardiac output can have marked effects on arterial oxygenation when an intrapulmonary shunt is present.[12] A change in cardiac output results in a change in the oxygenation of the mixed venous blood returning to the heart. This is reflected by changes in the mixed venous oxygenation as measured by (1) O_2 partial pressure ($P\bar{v}O_2$), (2) O_2 saturation ($S\bar{v}O_2$), and (3) O_2 content ($C\bar{v}O_2$) in the mixed venous blood. Teleologically, this represents a mechanism protecting tissue oxygenation. When cardiac output is low, with a reduction in blood flow to tissue beds, those tissues extract more O_2 from the blood perfusing them in order to maintain their oxygenation. This, however, results in a lower $C\bar{v}O_2$. When this mixed venous blood passes through the lungs, that portion that flows through an area of shunt receives no increase in oxygenation. Thus, this shunted blood will be mixed with the blood from areas of the lung in which shunt is not present. The final arterial O_2 content is determined by the relative contributions of blood from shunt and nonshunt lung regions. Because the mixed venous blood has a lower O_2 content, the blood returning to the left side of the heart after passing through the shunt will also have a lower O_2 content; this will have a significant effect in reducing the arterial oxygenation. If an intrapulmonary shunt were not present, the blood would flow through areas of the lung where it would receive at least some increase in O_2, and the effect of cardiac output on arterial oxygenation would not be clinically important. Therefore, the effect of cardiac output is clinically important only when significant shunt is present. There are situations in which a reduction in cardiac output does not result in increased tissue extraction of O_2 (considered further in Chs. 33 and 34).

DIFFUSION ABNORMALITY

Although an abnormality in the diffusion of O_2 across the alveolar-capillary membrane is a possible mechanism of hypoxemia, it usually is not a clinically significant factor and therefore can be ignored for purposes of simplicity. The reason that diffusion abnormalities do not usually affect oxygenation is related to the time available for a red blood cell to receive O_2 as it passes through a capillary bed. Given a relatively normal cardiac output, the hemoglobin is fully saturated with O_2 in about one-third of the time that the red blood cell is exposed to available O_2 in the capillary. Even with severe diffusion problems there usually is enough time for the hemoglobin to become saturated with O_2 and to compensate for the diffusion abnormality. Exceptions to this are possible (e.g., in an exercising individual in whom cardiac output is markedly increased and thus transit time through the capillary is decreased). It also can be the case in any other condition in which the cardiac output is increased and the transit time of the red blood cell through the capillary is decreased. Because critically ill patients, especially those with multiple trauma or sepsis, frequently have an elevated cardiac output, this condition could hold true in patients in an ICU. However, even if this mechanism does affect oxygenation, the other mechanisms causing hypoxemia, particularly low $\dot{V}/\dot{Q}$ and shunt, outweigh any contribution from a diffusion abnormality.

References

1. Weibel ER: The Pathway for Oxygen. Harvard University Press, Cambridge, MA, 1984
2. West JB: Ventilation/Blood Flow and Gas Exchange. 4th Ed. Blackwell Scientific Publications, Oxford, 1985
3. Schoene RB: Diseases of high altitude. pp. 1805–1807. In Kelley WN (ed): Textbook of Internal Medicine. 2nd Ed. JB Lippincott, Philadelphia, 1992
4. Dillard TA, Berg BW, Rajagopal KR et al: Hypoxemia during

air travel in patients with chronic obstructive pulmonary disease. Ann Intern Med 1989;111:362–367

5. Cottrell JJ: Altitude exposures during aircraft flight. Chest 1988;92:81–84
6. Sherman CB, Osmanski JP, Hudson LD: Acute exacerbations in COPD patients. pp. 443–456. In Cherniack NS (ed): Chronic Obstructive Pulmonary Disease. WB Saunders, Philadelphia, 1991
7. Hudson LD: Acute respiratory failure in patients with chronic obstructive pulmonary disease. pp. 155–172. In George RB, Bone RC, Hudson LD (eds): Acute Respiratory Failure. Churchill Livingstone, New York, 1987
8. Pepe PE, Hudson LD: Acute respiratory failure. pp. 47–55. In Callaham ML (ed): Current Practice of Emergency Medicine. 2nd Ed. BC Decker, Philadelphia, 1991
9. Pierson DJ: Acute respiratory failure. pp. 75–126. In Sahn SA (ed): Pulmonary Emergencies. Churchill Livingstone, New York, 1982
10. Maunder RJ, Hudson LD: Management of the adult respiratory distress syndrome. pp. 1861–1865. In Kelley WN (ed): Textbook of Internal Medicine. 2nd Ed. JB Lippincott, Philadelphia, 1992
11. Wiedemann HP, Matthay MA, Matthay RA (eds): Acute lung injury (symposium). Crit Care Clin 1986;2:377
12. Dantzker DR: The influence of cardiovascular function on gas exchange. Clin Chest Med 1983;4:149–159

Chapter 32

Inadequate Blood Oxygen Content

Leonard D. Hudson
David J. Pierson

CHAPTER OUTLINE

MECHANISMS

In considering the clinical problems of getting O_2 from inhaled air to the tissues of the body in which metabolism takes place, one must consider all the variables that can affect this, including variables other than simply the function of the lungs and their role in delivering O_2 into the arterial blood.[1,2] One of these major variables is arterial O_2 content (CaO_2), which represents the total amount of O_2 carried in the blood. The variables affecting CaO_2 are arterial O_2 saturation (SaO_2), hemoglobin concentration, and to a lesser extent arterial O_2 tension (PaO_2).

CaO_2 is equal to the amount of O_2 carried by the hemoglobin in the blood plus the normally smaller amount of O_2 dissolved in the blood. These relationships, discussed more fully in Chapter 11, are expressed by the formula for CaO_2:

$$CaO_2 = [(1.34 \text{ mL } O_2/\text{g Hb})(\text{g Hb}/100 \text{ mL blood})(SaO_2)] + [(0.003 \text{ mL } O_2/100 \text{ mL blood})(PaO_2)] \quad (1)$$

This formula reveals that the greatest amount of O_2 is carried on the hemoglobin, with 1.34 mL of O_2 available for each gram of hemoglobin that is fully saturated with O_2, whereas only 0.003 mL of O_2 is the maximum amount in each 100 mL of blood for each millimeter of Hg of PaO_2.

Abnormalities of PaO_2 are dealt with in Chapter 31 on hypoxemia. This leaves two additional variables that could be abnormal in clinical situations and thereby lower the CaO_2. The first is the quantity of hemoglobin (i.e., the hemoglobin concentration) in the blood; because most of the O_2 is carried on the hemoglobin, the hemoglobin concentration becomes a critical variable. The other variable, the SaO_2, usually is directly related to the PaO_2 by the oxyhemoglobin dissociation curve (see Ch. 11). However, there are certain clinical situations in which PaO_2 is normal but SaO_2 is quite abnormal; the main example encountered clinically is CO intoxication.

CHANGES IN HEMOGLOBIN CONCENTRATION

When anemia is present, as measured by a reduction in hemoglobin concentration (and usually reflected by a reduction in the hematocrit), the CaO_2 is decreased in direct proportion to the reduction in hemoglobin concentration. For example, if the hemoglobin concentration were decreased to half the normal value, the CaO_2 would be decreased by approximately half (see Fig. 29-7).

Patient Example 32-1

Acute Anemia (Massive Hemorrhage from Duodenal Ulcer)

A 50-year-old man with a history of peptic ulcer disease has been taking aspirin for 2 days because of back pain and has been experiencing intermittent upper abdominal discomfort. He is brought to the emergency department by ambulance after suddenly vomiting a large amount of blood. On arrival he is tachycardic and hypotensive. His initial hematocrit is 44 percent with a hemoglobin of 16 g/dL. Arterial blood gas (ABG) evaluation with the patient breathing room air shows pH 7.40, $PaCO_2$ 40 mmHg, PaO_2 90 mmHg, and SaO_2 98 percent. One hour later, after several liters of rapid intravenous volume replacement with saline, his hematocrit is 22 percent (hemoglobin 8) and his ABG values: pH 7.36, $PaCO_2$ 32 mmHg, PaO_2 98 mmHg, and SaO_2 99 percent. Serum electrolytes indicate that his metabolic acidosis is accompanied by an increased anion gap.

Comment

This patient's bleeding ulcer (exacerbated by the use of aspirin) causes acute depletion of central circulating blood volume, with markedly decreased cardiac preload and an element of acute hemoconcentration, which initially maintains a normal hemoglobin concentration. His CaO_2 on admission, however, is normal:

$$CaO_2 = (1.34)\ (16)\ (.98) + (0.003)\ (90)$$
$$= 21.28 \text{ mL/dL}$$

After vigorous fluid resuscitation (producing hemodilution) and perhaps some additional bleeding the patient's hemoglobin has fallen to half its initial value. Although his PaO_2 has risen because of hyperventilation and his SaO_2 remains normal, his CaO_2 is now only about half its initial value:

$$CaO_2 = (1.34)\ (8)\ (99) + (0.003)\ (98)$$
$$= 10.78 \text{ mL/dL}$$

The metabolic acidosis reflects anaerobic metabolism at the tissue level in the face of decreased O_2 delivery in this middle-aged man, whose cardiac output does not increase sufficiently to make up the deficit in O_2 delivery.

Patient Example 32-2

Chronic Anemia (Menorrhagia)

A 23-year-old woman visits her physician because of fatigue and dyspnea on exertion. She has been having exceptionally heavy menstrual periods for the last 6 months. She is pale, with a bounding pulse, a heart rate of 116, and a normal blood pressure. Her hematocrit is 15 percent with a hemoglobin of 5.6 g/dL. ABG analysis shows pH 7.40, $PaCO_2$ 40 mmHg, PaO_2 90 mmHg, and SaO_2 98 percent.

Comment

This patient's CaO_2 is

$$(1.34)\ (5.6)\ (.98) + (0.003)\ (90) = 7.62 \text{ mL/dL}$$

This young, otherwise healthy patient is able to compensate fully for a decreased CaO_2 (at least at rest) by increasing cardiac output, as confirmed by her bounding pulse and tachycardia. The adequacy of her cardiac compensation is further shown by her lack of metabolic acidosis. ABG analysis might not ordinarily be included in this patient's initial evaluation, but it illustrates how patients can have markedly reduced CaO_2 (despite normal PaO_2 and SaO_2 values) but still maintain adequate O_2 transport if they are otherwise healthy and the peripheral O_2 need is not excessive.

ABNORMALITIES OF ARTERIAL OXYGEN SATURATION INDEPENDENT OF PaO_2

The SaO_2 can be reduced in the face of a normal PaO_2 when the hemoglobin is bound by a substance other than O_2.[3–5] The major clinical example of this occurs in CO intoxication.[6] In these cases the PaO_2 is frequently normal or can even be high if O_2 is being administered, but the hemoglobin is bound by CO and the SaO_2 is reduced. For example, if 40 percent of the hemoglobin is bound by CO, only 60 percent of the hemoglobin is available for binding with O_2; thus, although the hemoglobin available for binding with O_2 may be completely saturated, the maximal possible SaO_2 value is 60 percent. In addition to this anemia-like effect, CO binding of hemoglobin causes a severe shift to the left in the oxyhemoglobin dissociation curve, so that O_2 is bound more tightly to the hemoglobin and thus O_2 is not as easily unloaded at the tissue level, as described further in Chapter 34.

Patient Example 32-3

Decreased CaO_2 Because of Abnormal Hemoglobin (CO Poisoning)

A 68-year-old woman is pulled unresponsive from the bedroom of her burning home. The fire was concentrated in the kitchen, but the bedroom was densely filled with smoke. On arrival in the emergency department the patient is lethargic and confused but has no evidence of cutaneous burns. She appears in no respiratory distress and is not cyanotic but is tachycardiac and tachypneic. Her hematocrit is 36 percent and her hemoglobin concentration 13.5 g/dL. ABG analysis with the patient breathing room air shows pH 7.28, $PaCO_2$ 32 mmHg, and PaO_2 90 mmHg; the ABG report gives the SaO_2 as 96 percent. The patient is placed on 100 percent O_2 by mask, and her PaO_2 rises to 570 mmHg (SaO_2 100 percent). A carboxyhemoglobin (COHb) level on the initial ABG specimen, measured by co-oximetry, is 45 percent.

Comment

The COHb of 45 percent means that this patient's effective hemoglobin concentration (that available for binding with O_2) is 13.6 × (100 percent − 45 percent) or 7.4 g/dL. Thus, her initial CaO_2 is

$$(1.34)\ (7.4)\ (.96) + (0.003)\ (90) = 9.78\ \text{mL/dL}$$

When receiving supplemental O_2 ($F_{IO_2} = 1.0$) her CaO_2 is

$$(1.34)\ (7.4)\ (1.00) + (0.003)\ (570) = 11.63\ \text{mL/dL}$$

Thus, although the contribution of dissolved O_2 to CaO_2 is usually very small, placing a patient on 100 percent O_2 can produce a modest increase in CaO_2 [providing the $P(A\text{-}a)O_2$ is normal]. Hyperbaric O_2, if immediately available, can augment dissolved O_2 to the extent that CaO_2 is normal; however, the decay curve of COHb at an F_{IO_2} of 1.0 is such that a chamber must be close at hand if this is to be efficacious, at least from the standpoint of displacing CO from the patient's hemoglobin (see Ch. 80 for further discussion).

As discussed in Chapters 80 and 94, the half-life of carboxyhemoglobin (the time it takes for the carboxyhemoglobin level to fall to 50 percent of its initial value) when breathing room air is approximately 4 hours. This can be enhanced by breathing a high F_{IO_2} mixture and increasing the competition for hemoglobin binding sites between O_2 and CO. The half-life of carboxyhemoglobin when the F_{IO_2} is 1.0 is approximately 40 minutes.

It is important to be aware that many hospital laboratories *calculate* the SaO_2 rather than measuring it directly. The SaO_2 is calculated from the PaO_2 and pH from a table of normal interrelationships among these three variables. If a patient has a normal PaO_2, the *calculated* SaO_2 also would be normal (nearly 100 percent) even in the face of significant CO intoxication. A directly measured SaO_2 would more closely reflect the actual SaO_2 (even though the presence of carboxyhemoglobin may affect this measurement to some degree). Therefore, if CO intoxication is clinically suspected, the clinician should request that the laboratory directly measure both the carboxyhemoglobin level and the SaO_2.

References

1. Bryan-Brown CW, Gutierrez G: Gas transport and delivery. pp. 491–499. In Shoemaker WC, Ayres S, Grenvik A et al (eds): Textbook of Critical Care. 2nd Ed. WB Saunders, Philadelphia, 1989
2. Gutierrez G, Bismar H: Oxygen transport and utilization. pp. 199–230. In Dantzker DR (ed): Cardiopulmonary Critical Care. 2nd Ed. WB Saunders, Philadelphia, 1991
3. Sharrar SR, Heimbach DM, Hudson LD: Management of inhalation injury in patients with and without burns. pp. 195–214. In Haponik E, Munster AM (eds): Respiratory Injury: Smoke Inhalation and Burns. McGraw-Hill, New York, 1990
4. Jederlinic PJ, Irwin RS: Acute inhalation injury. pp. 624–645. In Rippe JM, Irwin RS, Alpert JS, Fink MP (eds): Intensive Care Medicine. 2nd Ed. Little Brown, Boston, 1991
5. Dolan MC: Carbon monoxide poisoning. Can Med Assoc J 1985;133:392–399
6. Wald PH, Balmes JR: Respiratory effects of short-term, high-intensity toxic inhalations: Smoke, gases, and fumes. Intensive Care Med 1987;2:260–266

Chapter 33

Inadequate Oxygen Transport

Leonard D. Hudson
David J. Pierson

CHAPTER OUTLINE

MECHANISMS

As discussed in Chapter 32, failure of the process of respiration occurs when O_2 is not delivered in an adequate amount for the tissues to continue with normal metabolism. This can occur when the arterial O_2 tension (PaO_2) is normal and even when arterial O_2 content (CaO_2) is normal but the delivery of blood containing a normal CaO_2 is abnormally low.[1,2] Tissue O_2 delivery (DO_2) is equally dependent on cardiac output ($\dot{Q}T$) and CaO_2:

$$DO_2 = (\dot{Q}T)\ (CaO_2) \quad (1)$$

Thus, cardiac function has a major effect on DO_2.[3,4] In addition to total tissue DO_2 the clinician is interested in individual organ function, which in turn is dependent on adequate delivery of O_2 to the involved organ. Thus, *distribution* of $\dot{Q}T$ also becomes a factor in assessing the tissue DO_2 to specific organs.

In the critically ill patient cardiopulmonary interactions are possible that can affect ultimate transport of O_2 to the tissues. In addition, hematologic changes in either blood composition (increased or decreased hemoglobin concentration) or blood volume can affect the function of both the lungs and the heart.[5] The clinician must be aware of these interactions and must attempt to assess each of the independent effects. Examples include the effect of hypoxemia on cardiac function in a patient with coronary artery disease and already compromised blood flow to cardiac muscle; primary cardiac disease with heart failure resulting in congestion of the lungs, which affects pulmonary gas exchange; the effect of hypovolemia in reducing cardiac contractility; hypervolemia contributing to congestive heart failure in the patient with an already compromised cardiac pump; and the effect of mechanical ventilation and other ventilatory modalities such as positive end-expiratory pressure (PEEP) on decreasing venous return and thus decreasing $\dot{Q}T$.[6] The clinician must isolate all these individual effects and determine how they might independently change lung function and arterial oxygenation, CaO_2, and cardiac function as manifested by cardiac output.

Cardiac dysfunction affecting O_2 transport in critically ill patients can be divided into four mechanisms: (1) primary cardiac disease; (2) effects of changes in circulating blood volume on cardiac function; (3) pulmonary effects on cardiac function; and (4) exogenous circulating depressants, including cardiodepressant drugs or toxins.

PRIMARY CARDIAC DISEASE

Probably the most prevalent cause of reduced $\dot{Q}T$ in a critically ill patient is, at least in part, primary cardiac disease.[7,8]

Coronary artery disease (CAD) or ischemic heart disease is the most common form of cardiac disease encountered in critically ill patients. Cardiac ischemia may be the primary event bringing the patient to the intensive care unit (ICU), or ischemia may be exacerbated by other conditions or therapies in a critically ill patient with previously stable CAD. For example, addition of acute arterial hypoxemia in the patient with compromised coronary artery blood flow from CAD could induce or exaggerate cardiac ischemia.

Patient Example 33-1

Effect of Primary Cardiac Disease on Tissue Oxygenation (Acute Myocardial Infarction with Pulmonary Edema)

A 58-year-old man is admitted to the coronary care unit with an acute anterior myocardial infarction and cardiogenic pulmonary edema. His cardiac function stabilizes with aggressive drug therapy, and his hypoxemia improves when he is given supplemental O_2 by mask. On the second hospital day he develops chest pain and hypotension, and the pulse oximeter signals acute desaturation. Gas exchange and hemodynamic data are as follows:

	PaO_2 (mmHg)	$\dot{Q}_T$ (L/min)
Baseline	90	5.0
Hypotension	52	2.5

An electrocardiogram indicates extension of his myocardial infarction, and his $\dot{Q}_T$ is restored to its baseline value during infusion of dobutamine; at this time his PaO_2 returns to its previous value without other changes in therapy.

Comment

Some right-to-left intrapulmonary shunt remained from the resolving pulmonary edema, and when $\dot{Q}_T$ dropped by 50 percent (in the face of constant peripheral O_2 demand) the patient's hypoxemia worsened because of a fall in mixed venous O_2 content. Restoring $\dot{Q}_T$ allowed the same peripheral O_2 extraction to use a smaller proportion of the CaO_2, so that the mixed venous saturation was higher and the blood passing through the intrapulmonary shunt exerted less effect on the mixed arterial blood.

For further discussion of the above effect see Chapter 10. Dobutamine and other sympathomimetic amines used in congestive heart failure are discussed in Chapter 77.

Cardiomyopathies are also associated with poor pumping action of the heart. Although ischemic cardiomyopathy is the most common etiology in North America, other causes exist; these include alcoholic cardiomyopathy, viral cardiomyopathy, and infiltrative diseases affecting the heart, including sarcoidosis, amyloidosis, and certain tumors.[7] The heart is frequently dilated when a cardiomyopathy is present.

VOLUME CHANGES AFFECTING CARDIAC FUNCTION

The primary volume change affecting cardiac function is relative hypovolemia, a decrease in circulating central blood volume. The force generated by the contraction of any muscle is dependent in part on the resting length of that muscle. When the normal muscle is in a stretched or lengthened position, contraction of the muscle will generate a greater force. Therefore, in order for the normal heart to achieve maximal contraction and thus stroke volume and $\dot{Q}_T$, adequate filling volumes of the cardiac chambers, particularly the left ventricle, are required. When hypovolemia exists, the cardiac muscle fibers are relatively short and have submaximal contractile force. This relationship is known as the Frank-Starling curve and is described in greater detail in Chapter 77.[7,8]

Patient Example 33-2

Effect of Changes in Circulating Blood Volume on DO_2 (Large-Volume Paracentesis in Hepatic Failure)

A 62-year-old man with alcoholic cirrhosis of the liver and severe portal hypertension is admitted to the hospital with massive ascites. On the second hospital day paracentesis is performed to decrease his ascites, and 4.5 L of peritoneal fluid is removed over a 20-minute period. One hour later the patient is noted to be obtunded and hypotensive, and assessment by arterial blood gas (ABG) and blood chemistry analyses shows normoxemia with an incompletely compensated, anion-gap metabolic acidosis. Vigorous administration of intravenous fluids initially raises the patient's blood pressure, but over the next 4 hours he is found to have acute pulmonary edema and is transferred emergently to the ICU.

Comment

Patients with portal hypertension may accumulate massive amounts of peritoneal fluid, which collects because of hydrostatic forces favoring fluid movement from the vascular space into the peritoneum. If a large amount of this ascitic fluid is suddenly removed, the hydrostatic pressure gradient into the abdominal cavity may cause acute intravascular hypovolemia as fluid moves from the blood into the peritoneum. In such cases cardiovascular collapse due to decreased preload may occur. Then, in the face of the decrease in serum oncotic forces often occurring in such patients as a result of hypoalbuminemia, vigorous crystalloid administration may precipitate acute pulmonary edema. The development of an anion-gap metabolic acidosis soon after paracentesis suggests that intravascular volume depletion resulted in decreased DO_2 (in this case all from a fall in $\dot{Q}_T$, since there was no hypoxemia) to a degree that led to anaerobic metabolism in some tissue beds.

Chapters 13 and 28 discuss body fluid regulation and the effects of disease on intravascular and extravascular fluid compartments.

In the abnormal heart it is possible that the cardiac muscle can be "overstretched," with a resulting decrease in contractility. There is some controversy about whether this so-called descending limb of the Frank-Starling curve actually exists, but clinically there are situations in which this phenomenon seems to occur. Obviously, if congestive heart failure is present with exudation of fluid into the lungs due to high pulmonary microvascular pressures, a further increase in blood volume will exacerbate this exudation of fluid, thus worsening pulmonary function and gas exchange.

PULMONARY EFFECTS ON CARDIAC FUNCTION

Significant cardiopulmonary interactions exist that can result in adverse effects on cardiac function. The primary pulmonary effect on the heart results from any change in the lungs that leads to an increase in intrathoracic pressure. This effect can be seen with mechanical ventilation alone but is especially a factor when PEEP is employed.[4,6,9] With these respiratory modalities, alveolar volume is increased by the application of a positive pressure (regardless of whether the ventilator is pressure- or volume-limited). The increased alveolar volume is thus associated with an increase in alveolar pressure, some of which is transmitted to the pleural space, resulting in an increased intrapleural pressure. The venae cavae, the great veins returning blood from the tissues of the body to the right side of the heart, are exposed to the effect of pleural pressure as they course through the thorax. Thus, an elevated intrapleural pressure will exert pressure on the compressible venae cavae and can result in compression of these vessels, with a consequent reduction in venous return to the right side of the heart. Because of the decrease in venous return less blood will be pumped from the left side of the heart and $\dot{Q}_T$ will fall. In addition to the effect of pleural pressure on the great veins, the lungs themselves, which are distended, will press directly on the heart and can further restrict blood return to the heart. Another possible mechanism by which PEEP can result in reduced cardiac output is its distending effect on alveolar volume.[4] As alveolar volume increases, the capillaries running through the alveolar wall are stretched, their lumen size is reduced, and the resistance to blood flow through these capillaries is increased. If this results in an overall increase in pulmonary vascular resistance, $\dot{Q}_T$ can be adversely affected. Within the usual range of alveolar volumes and pressures exerted by normal use of mechanical ventilation and PEEP, the predominant effect on $\dot{Q}_T$ results from a reduction in venous return. These phenomena are discussed in further detail in Chapter 65.

Patient Example 33-3

Adverse Pulmonary Effects on Cardiac Function (PEEP)

A patient with the adult respiratory distress syndrome (ARDS) has persistent hypoxemia (PaO_2, 55 mmHg) despite an inspired O_2 fraction (FIO_2) of 0.7, and PEEP at 10 cmH_2O is added. The patient's PaO_2 promptly rises to 110 mmHg. Has the patient's overall oxygenation been improved, and should the PEEP be continued at this level? Gas exchange and cardiac function data before and after the PEEP was added are as follows (FIO_2 and all other management variables remained the same):

PEEP (cmH_2O)	PaO_2 (mmHg)	SaO_2 (%)	CaO_2 (mL/dL)	$\dot{Q}T$ (L/min)
0	55	86	17.5	6.0
10	110	99	20.2	4.0

Comment

While it might initially appear that the improvement in blood oxygenation means that the patient has been helped, examining $\dot{Q}_T$ and DO_2 in addition to the oxygenation parameters is necessary to adequately assess the response to PEEP. Increasing mean intrathoracic pressure diminished cardiac preload and resulted in a 33 percent fall in $\dot{Q}_T$. The effects of PEEP on DO_2 in this example were therefore

$$DO_2 = (17.5)(6.0) = 1050 \text{ mL/min}$$

on 0 PEEP, and

$$DO_2 = (20.2)(4.0) = 808 \text{ mL/min}$$

on 10 cmH_2O PEEP. Thus, the application of 10 cmH_2O PEEP in this patient resulted in a decrease in DO_2 despite "improved oxygenation."

Further discussion of the hemodynamic effects of PEEP can be found in Chapters 76 and 84, while the clinical approach to application of PEEP in this and other circumstances is discussed in Chapter 65.

EXOGENOUS CARDIAC DEPRESSANTS

Certain drugs can act as myocardial depressants. The category of drugs that most commonly have this effect consists of the beta-adrenergic blocking agents. In fact, beta blockers are frequently employed for this specific use. For example, in a patient with a dissecting aortic aneurysm, beta blockers are administered in order to decrease the force of the contraction and thus to lower high peak pressure in the aortic jet of blood resulting from left ventricular contraction so as to lessen the risk of propagation of the dissection. Occasionally, beta-blocking agents are given to a patient with unsuspected cardiac disease that was not previously manifested; this can precipitate congestive heart failure accompanied by a reduction in $\dot{Q}_T$ and thus decreased O_2 transport. Endotoxemia seen with sepsis syndrome and septic shock due to bacterial infection has been shown to be associated with a cardiac depressant factor that reduces contractility. However, in this situation the cardiac output is usually elevated, and this depressed contractility is shown only by a reduction in ejection fraction. Therefore, the $\dot{Q}_T$ may not be a factor in terms of decreasing DO_2 in sepsis syndrome. On the other hand, changes in distribution of blood flow to certain tissue beds of the body may occur, and local O_2 transport may be reduced. Also, some patients with sepsis syndrome may have a reduced $\dot{Q}_T$.

Cardiac function, as measured by $\dot{Q}_T$, has a tremendous effect on the transport of O_2 to the tissues of the body. The clinician must remember that $\dot{Q}_T$ and CaO_2 are equal partners in the equation of tissue DO_2, and every attempt must be made to maintain adequate $\dot{Q}_T$ in the critically ill patient. This is particularly important since many of the interventions used in critically ill patients, particularly those with severe pulmonary disease, carry the undesired potential side effect of reduction in $\dot{Q}_T$, an adverse effect that can often be avoided either by careful titration of the intervention (e.g., PEEP) or by use of some compensating therapeutic measure (such as increasing blood volume). However, all the interactions must be weighed, so that the end result is beneficial to the patient.

References

1. Gutierrez G, Bismar H: Oxygen transport and utilization. pp. 199–230. In Dantzker DR (ed): Cardiopulmonary Critical Care. 2nd Ed. WB Saunders, Philadelphia, 1991
2. Bryan-Brown CW, Gutierrez G: Gas transport and delivery. pp. 491–499. In Shoemaker WC, Ayres S, Grenvik A et al (eds): Textbook of Critical Care. 2nd Ed. WB Saunders, Philadelphia, 1989
3. Dantzker DR: The influence of cardiovascular function on gas exchange. Clin Chest Med 1983;4:149–159
4. Craig KC, Pierson DJ, Carrico CJ: The clinical application of positive end-expiratory pressure (PEEP) in the adult respiratory distress syndrome (ARDS). Respir Care 1985;30:184–201
5. Gilbert EM, Haupt MT, Mandanas RY et al: The effect of fluid loading, blood transfusion and catecholamine infusion on oxygen delivery and consumption in patients with sepsis. Am Rev Respir Dis 1986;134:873–878
6. Potkin RT, Hudson LD, Weaver LJ, Trobaugh G: Effect of positive end-expiratory pressure on right and left ventricular function in patients with the adult respiratory distress syndrome. Am Rev Respir Dis 1987;135:307–311
7. Zelis R, Sinoway LI: Pathophysiology of congestive heart failure. pp. 104–112. In Kelley WN (ed): Textbook of Internal Medicine. 2nd Ed. JB Lippincott, Philadelphia, 1992
8. Vatner SF, Cox DA: Circulatory function and control. pp. 96–104. In Kelley WN (ed): Textbook of Internal Medicine. 2nd Ed. JB Lippincott, Philadelphia, 1992
9. Broaddus VC, Berthiaume Y, Biondi JW et al: Hemodynamic management of the adult respiratory distress syndrome. J Crit Care 1987;2:190

Chapter 34

Failure of Peripheral Oxygen Extraction

Leonard D. Hudson
David J. Pierson

CHAPTER OUTLINE

The pathway of O_2 from inhaled air to tissue metabolism involves extraction of the O_2 available in the blood and delivered to the tissues. The O_2 must be extracted in a form that allows it to be used by the cells, and the cells must have the capacity to use the O_2 in their metabolism. Two categories of abnormalities can adversely affect this final step: (1) conditions that cause the O_2 to be more tightly bound to the hemoglobin so that the O_2 cannot be readily extracted by the tissues; and (2) conditions that poison the intracellular machinery by which O_2 is metabolized.

OXYGEN-HEMOGLOBIN BINDING AFFINITY

The affinity of O_2 binding to hemoglobin is described by the shape and position of the oxyhemoglobin dissociation curve (Fig. 34-1). When the curve is shifted to the right (and downward), the affinity is lower and less O_2 is taken up per gram of hemoglobin as the blood travels through the lung; however, at the tissue level at which the O_2 tension (PO_2) is lower, the O_2 is also bound less tightly, and therefore, the hemoglobin gives up O_2 to the tissues more readily. In other words, it is easier for the tissues to extract the O_2 that is present on the hemoglobin. The net result of a rightward shift of the curve, therefore, is usually an increase in total O_2 delivery to the tissues. On the other hand, if the curve is shifted to the left and upward, slightly more O_2 is added to the hemoglobin in the lungs, where the PO_2 is high. At the tissue level, where the PO_2 is low, however, the O_2 is bound more tightly to the hemoglobin and is not as easily extracted by the tissues. Thus, the amount of O_2 available for tissue utilization is decreased. There are a variety of variables that affect the position of the oxyhemoglobin dissociation curve (Table 34-1), among the most important of which is the acid-base status. Acidosis shifts the curve to the right, thus causing O_2 to be unloaded more readily, whereas alkalosis shifts the curve to the left, resulting in poorer tissue O_2 extraction.

The shift of the curve is mediated in part by the presence of 2,3-diphosphoglycerate (2,3-DPG). When donated blood used for transfusions is stored, the 2,3-DPG levels decrease. Thus, when a large amount of blood is transfused, the O_2 will be relatively tightly bound to the hemoglobin. Once the blood has been transfused, the 2,3-DPG level is usually regenerated within hours, so that this effect is a relatively transient one.

The clinical situation in which the affinity of O_2 for hemoglobin is extraordinarily high, with a resulting very im-

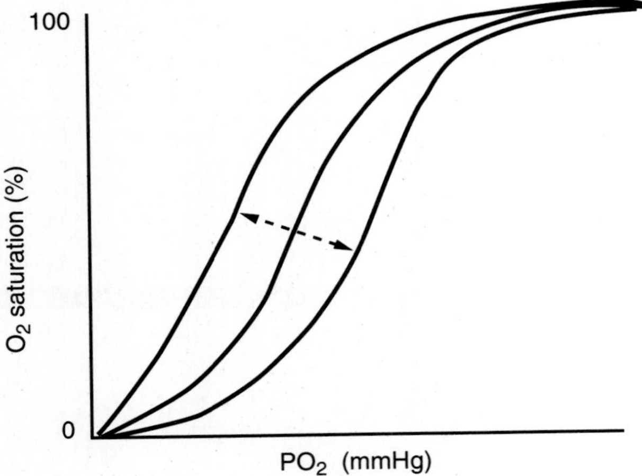

Figure 34-1. Oxyhemoglobin dissociation curve, showing effects of left and right shift (see text).

portant clinical effect, is CO intoxication.[1–5] The presence of a substantial amount of carboxyhemoglobin markedly affects the O_2 binding affinity in the remaining hemoglobin; thus, O_2 that *is* present on hemoglobin is very poorly released at the tissue level. This, in large measure, accounts for the striking neurologic effects of CO intoxication. For example, most patients with a carboxyhemoglobin level of 50 percent are comatose, and frequently they develop anoxic encephalopathy. If the only effect of a carboxyhemoglobin level of 50 percent were to bind half the hemoglobin so that it would not be available for O_2, one would expect an effect identical to that of a relatively severe anemia in which the hemoglobin or hematocrit is reduced to half the baseline value. However, patients with gastrointestinal bleeding (or other causes of acute anemia) are frequently seen with reductions in hematocrit to approximately half of the baseline value with no evidence of cerebral hypoxia and certainly no devastating effects of anoxic cephalopathy. Presumably the major difference between the two situations is the tenacity with which the O_2 and hemoglobin are bound. There is probably an additional effect due to CO poisoning of the oxidative enzyme system, which could also contribute to the dramatic neurologic effects.

Table 34-1. Causes of Shifts in the Oxyhemoglobin Dissociation Curve

	Left Shift	Right Shift
Effect on tissue O_2 availability	↓	↑
Causes	Alkalosis	Acidosis
	↓ PCO_2	↑ PCO_2
	↓ Temperature	↑ Temperature
	↓ 2,3-DPG	↑ 2,3-DPG
	CO	

POISONING OF THE INTRACELLULAR OXIDATIVE ENZYME SYSTEM

The primary enzyme system present at the cellular level that promotes the role of O_2 in cell metabolism is the cytochrome oxidase system. If this system is poisoned or otherwise affected so that it does not function normally, O_2 is not extracted and used in normal fashion. The primary clinical situation in which this occurs is probably cyanide intoxication or poisoning,[6,7] which can occur in several ways, including (1) ingestion of cyanide, which can either be a deliberate suicide attempt or accidental (including highly publicized cases of drug tampering[8,9]); (2) accidental inhalation of cyanide gas, particularly in a fire environment with smoke inhalation[10,11]; and (3) formation of cyanide as a breakdown product of nitroprusside, a drug used in the critical care unit to reduce cardiac afterload.[12,13]

Patient Example 34-1

Cyanide Ingestion

A 30-year-old man attempted suicide by ingesting potassium cyanide. Immediately after swallowing it, he had second thoughts and called 911. Paramedics arrived within 5 minutes to find the patient markedly anxious, tachycardic, hypotensive, vomiting, and complaining of headache, dizziness, and palpitations. While intravenous access was being established and a commercial cyanide antidote kit readied for administration, the patient became unresponsive and apneic and suffered a generalized seizure. His skin was noted to have an unusual pinkish hue, and one observer detected an odor of bitter almonds in exhaled air following intubation.

Cyanide binds to the enzyme cytochrome oxidase found in mitochondria. This enzyme is inhibited and the electron transport chain involved in O_2 metabolism is disrupted, either decreasing or prohibiting oxidative phosphorylation. The end result is a change from aerobic to anaerobic metabolism, with decreased adenosine triphosphate (ATP) production (important as a cell energy source), depletion of cell energy stores, generation of lactic acid with development of a metabolic acidosis, and tissue hypoxia.

Acute cyanide poisoning usually progresses rapidly to coma, convulsions, shock, respiratory failure, and death.[6,7,14] Early signs are nonspecific and can include anxiety, headache, tachypnea, and rapid respirations followed by nausea and vomiting. The odor of bitter almonds has been reported and is characteristic of cyanide. However, the ability to detect this odor is genetically determined and is often lacking, so that this is an unreliable clinical sign.

The binding of cyanide to cytochrome oxidase is reversible. The natural defense mechanism in the body is mediated by the presence of an enzyme known as rhodanase, which causes cyanide to be complexed with sulfur to form thiocyanate (SCN), which is much less toxic than cyanide itself.

However, the sulfur pool in the body is quite limited, and this limits the rate at which cyanide detoxification can occur. In clinical cyanide poisoning, treatment involves administration of nitrites.[6,14] These should be administered initially as an amyl nitrite pearl broken in gauze and held to the nose and mouth of a spontaneously breathing patient. Once intravenous access has been established, an infusion of sodium nitrite should be started. This should be followed with an intravenous bolus of sodium thiosulfate.

Patient Example 32-3 involving CO intoxication could also serve as an example of a patient who might have cyanide poisoning. In a forensic medical study of fire fatalities, all the victims had substantial levels of CO but half of those victims also had clinically significant cyanide levels at postmortem examination.[15] Cyanide gas is frequently formed in fires.[1,2] CO intoxication and cyanide intoxication are additive, if not synergistic, in effect, the end result being ineffective aerobic tissue metabolism and ultimately tissue hypoxia or anoxia.[10] This is especially manifest in the central nervous system. As discussed above, one of the minor effects of CO is the same as or similar to the major effect of cyanide, but CO has other effects, as already described.

Patient Example 34-2

Cyanide Poisoning due to Administration of Sodium Nitroprusside

A 58-year-old woman with chronic renal insufficiency and long-standing, poorly controlled hypertension developed severe congestive heart failure in the setting of a hypertensive crisis. Sodium nitroprusside was administered by continuous infusion at 0.5 μg/kg/min, but her condition proved difficult to control and progressively higher doses were required over the next 24 hours. With the infusion at 6 μg/kg/min the patient developed restlessness, muscle spasms, and new ventricular dysrhythmias and was noted to be confused. Analysis of arterial and mixed venous blood specimens (with the patient breathing nasal O_2 at 4 L/min) revealed the following:

	Arterial Blood	Mixed Venous Blood
pH (units)	7.22	7.15
PCO_2 (mmHg)	26	32
PO_2 (mmHg)	140	65

Comment

This patient's mental status changes, cardiac dysrhythmias, muscle spasms, and (anion-gap) metabolic acidosis are all explainable by cyanide toxicity related to nitroprusside administration. Her hyperventilation is in response to the metabolic acidosis; arterial oxygenation is excellent, but the abnormally high mixed venous PO_2 reflects decreased peripheral O_2 extraction.

Nitroprusside is metabolized to thiocyanate, which is subsequently eliminated over a half-life of 2 to 3 days. Thus the metabolites are most likely to accumulate in patients with renal insufficiency, in whom elimination is very slow. The adverse effects of nitroprusside, other than the predictable one of progressive hypotension, are related to thiocyanate and primarily are central nervous system effects, including agitation and toxic psychoses. Cyanide is the intermediate formed in metabolism of nitroprusside to thiocyanate. Rarely, cyanide toxicity can occur if nitroprusside is administered in such large doses that the reaction of cyanide with thiosulfate to form thiocyanate is overwhelmed.

The U.S. Food and Drug Administration (FDA) has recently advised that infusion of sodium nitroprusside at rates exceeding 2 μg/kg/min can result in potentially lethal cyanide levels.[13] The FDA further states that infusion rates exceeding 10 μg/kg/min should never be sustained for more than 10 minutes.[13] If required, however, high rates of infusion can safely be administered if sodium thiosulfate or hydroxocobalamin is given concomitantly.[12,16,17] Even when precautions are used, however, the clinician should not overlook cyanide poisoning as a possible cause for unexplained central nervous system dysfunction, metabolic acidosis, or cardiovascular instability when sodium nitroprusside is administered. Treatment involves immediate discontinuation of the infusion, administration of 100 percent O_2, and prompt use of a commercially available cyanide antidote kit (e.g., Lilly Cyanide Antidote Kit, Eli Lilly, Indianapolis, IN).[12]

RELATIONSHIP BETWEEN OXYGEN UPTAKE AND OXYGEN DELIVERY

This chapter would not be complete without a brief discussion of the issue of the interrelationship between O_2 utilization or uptake ($\dot{V}O_2$) and O_2 delivery or supply (DO_2).[18,19] In the normal individual $\dot{V}O_2$ is independent of DO_2 over a wide DO_2 range. When DO_2 reaches a very low critical level, $\dot{V}O_2$ becomes dependent on O_2 supply and therefore falls with any further decrease in DO_2 (Fig. 34-2). Investigators have described an abnormal relationship between $\dot{V}O_2$ and O_2 supply in several abnormal states, particularly critical illnesses, and most especially sepsis syndrome, septic shock, and the adult respiratory distress syndrome (ARDS), in which O_2 utilization is dependent on O_2 delivery at a much higher DO_2 level than in the normal individual.[20–22] Thus, as DO_2 is reduced, O_2 uptake is also reduced over a wide range of DO_2 (Fig. 34-2). Although one can argue that this could be some sort of compensatory mechanism, ultimately tissues undergo reduction in aerobic metabolism because of a lack of available O_2. This is a controversial area[18,19,23]; the data suggesting that $\dot{V}O_2$ is supply-dependent in critically ill patients have been questioned on a methodologic basis. Most of the data suggesting this relationship have relied on variables in measuring or calculating $\dot{V}O_2$ that are also involved

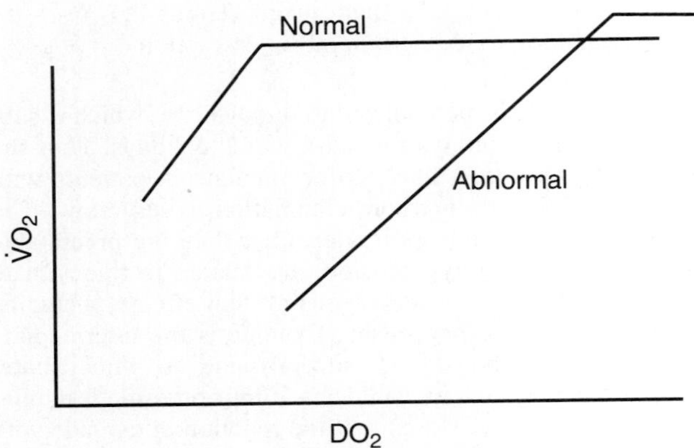

Figure 34-2. O_2 utilization and supply relationship.

in determining DO_2. When $\dot{V}O_2$ and DO_2 delivery have been measured by totally independent means, some investigators have not been able to find this relationship. Therefore, the clinical importance of this issue is unsettled at present.

References

1. Sharrar SR, Heimbach DM, Hudson LD: Management of inhalation injury in patients with and without burns. pp. 195–214. In Haponik E, Munster AM (eds): Respiratory Injury: Smoke Inhalation and Burns. McGraw-Hill, New York, 1990
2. Wald PH, Balmes JR: Respiratory effects of short-term, high-intensity toxic inhalations: Smoke, gases, and fumes. J Crit Care 1987;2:260
3. Kizer KW: Toxic inhalations. Emerg Med Clin North Am 1984;2:649–666
4. Jederlinic PJ, Irwin RS: Acute inhalation injury. pp. 624–645. In Rippe JM, Irwin RS, Alpert JS, Fink MP (eds): Intensive Care Medicine. 2nd Ed. Little Brown, Boston, 1991
5. Dolan MC: Carbon monoxide poisoning. Can Med Assoc J 1985;133:392–399
6. Hall AH: Systemic asphyxiants: Cyanide and cyanogens, hydrogen sulfide, methemoglobin inducers. pp. 1248–1258. In Rippe JM, Irwin RS, Alpert JS, Fink MP (eds): Intensive Care Medicine. 2nd Ed. Little Brown, Boston, 1991
7. Hall AH, Rumack BH: Clinical toxicology of cyanide. Ann Emerg Med 1986;15:1067–1074.
8. Wolnik KA, Fricke FL, Bonnin E et al: The Tylenol tampering incident—tracing the source. Anal Chem 1984;56:466A–470A, 474A
9. Hall AH, Linden CH, Kulig KW, Rumack BH: Cyanide poisoning from laetrile: Role of nitrate therapy. Pediatrics 1986;78:269–272
10. Clark CJ, Campbell D, Reid WH: Blood carboxyhemoglobin and cyanide levels in fire survivors. Lancet 1981;1:1332–1333
11. Jones J, McMullen MJ, Dougherty J: Toxic smoke inhalation: Cyanide poisoning in fire victims. Am J Emerg Med 1987;5:317–321
12. Curry SC, Arnold-Capell P: Nitroprusside, nitroglycerin, and angiotensin-converting enzyme inhibitors. Crit Care Clin 1991;7:555–582
13. Holland MA, Kozlowski LM: Clinical features and management of cyanide poisoning. Clin Pharm 1986;5:737–741
14. Symington IS, Anderson RA, Thomson I et al: Cyanide exposure in fires. Lancet 1978;2:91–93
15. Cottrell JE, Casthely P, Brodie JD et al: Prevention of nitroprusside-induced cyanide toxicity with hydroxocobalamin. N Engl J Med 1978;298:809–811, 813
16. Hall AH, Kulig KW, Rumack BH: Drug- and chemical-induced methemoglobinemia: Clinical features and management. Med Toxicol 1986;1:253–260
17. Bryan-Brown CW, Gutierrez G: Gas transport and delivery. pp. 491–499. In Shoemaker WC, Ayres S, Grenvik A et al (eds): Textbook of Critical Care. WB Saunders, Philadelphia, 1989
18. Gutierrez G, Bismar H: Oxygen transport and utilization. pp. 199–230. In Dantzker DR (ed): Cardiopulmonary Critical Care. 2nd Ed. WB Saunders, Philadelphia, 1991
19. Danek SJ, Lynch JP, Weg JG, Dantzker DR: The dependence of oxygen uptake on oxygen delivery in the adult respiratory distress syndrome. Am Rev Respir Dis 1980;122:387–395
20. Mohsenifar Z, Goldbach P, Tashkin DP, Campisi DJ: Relationship between O_2 delivery and O_2 consumption in the adult respiratory distress syndrome. Chest 1983;84:267–271
21. Fenwick JC, Dodek PM, Ronco JJ et al: Increased concentrations of plasma lactate predict pathologic dependence of oxygen consumption on oxygen delivery in patients with adult respiratory distress syndrome. J Crit Care 1990;5:81–86
22. Ronco JJ, Phang PT, Walley KR et al: Oxygen consumption is independent of changes in oxygen delivery in severe adult respiratory distress syndrome. Am Rev Respir Dis 1991;143:1267–1273
23. Annat G, Viale JP, Percival C et al: Oxygen delivery and oxygen uptake in the adult respiratory distress syndrome: Lack of relationship when measured independently in patients with normal blood lactate concentrations. Am Rev Respir Dis 1986;133:999–1001

Chapter 35

The Adult Respiratory Distress Syndrome

Richard J. Maunder
David J. Pierson

CHAPTER OUTLINE

HISTORY AND DEMOGRAPHICS

Although clinical recognition of the adult respiratory distress syndrome (ARDS) probably dates to biblical times, the syndrome was first described in the modern medical literature by Ashbaugh et al.[1] in 1967. ARDS is characterized by acute respiratory insufficiency, often in the setting of trauma, sepsis, or another precipitating clinical event, with severe hypoxemia, generalized pulmonary infiltrates, and a decline in pulmonary compliance. For research purposes specific criteria have been developed to determine whether a patient has ARDS. From the clinical perspective the syndrome is more properly viewed as a spectrum of illness, ranging from mild lung injury to the severe, fulminant respiratory failure commonly associated with the term ARDS.

Typically, ARDS is triggered by an illness or injury that may not involve the lung initially. Systemic infection and sepsis syndrome account for the largest number of cases in most centers, and if viral and bacterial pneumonias are included as risk factors, an infectious etiology accounts for most cases.[2] Major traumatic injury is probably the second leading cause of ARDS, followed by aspiration of gastric contents, drug overdose, pancreatitis, near drowning, toxic gas inhalation, and a variety of less common precipitating illnesses.[2,3] Often, the etiology of ARDS is classified according to whether the inciting event represents a systemic insult (e.g., sepsis, soft tissue trauma, pancreatitis) or a direct injury to the lung (chest trauma, toxic gases, near drowning).[3] Regardless of etiology, it appears that the lung responds in a fairly predictable fashion and that prognosis is not directly related to etiology.

The incidence of ARDS in the United States has been estimated at 150,000 cases per year on the basis of a 1972 workshop sponsored by the National Institutes of Health. Mortality in several recently published series is approximately 60 percent, which is comparable with the mortality originally reported by Ashbaugh et al.[1,4]

PATHOGENESIS

Despite intensive clinical and laboratory investigations, the pathogenesis of ARDS has not been fully elucidated. Lung inflammation is a prominent feature of the syndrome. Data obtained through lung histology and bronchoalveolar lavage indicate that neutrophil accumulation is a consistent finding in ARDS and have led most workers to the hypothesis that the lung injury process is mediated by activated neutrophils and by the toxic inflammatory products that they release.[5] Nonetheless, ARDS has been observed in bone marrow transplant recipients and other patients with profound depletion of circulating neutrophils.[6] Even if neutrophils are not required for lung injury, it certainly appears that they are capable of amplifying the response to other stimuli.

Cellular Inflammation

Bronchoalveolar lavage studies have shown that in the first 24 hours following onset of ARDS there is a profound increase in alveolar inflammatory cells, with a predominance of neutrophils in virtually all cases.[7] Over the next several days, the inflammatory response evolves into a picture in which alveolar macrophages begin to predominate.[8] Although some investigators have suggested that the macrophage may participate in the lung injury process, this cell certainly plays a role in the resolution of acute inflammation as well. Not only does the macrophage produce a number of anti-inflammatory and regulatory factors, but it also is capable of removing alveolar debris, pro-inflammatory mediators, bacteria, and even neutrophils that have accumulated in the alveolar space.[8] As Metchnikoff observed in the nineteenth century, "the macrophages eat the microphages." If the inflammatory process fails to shift in the direction of macrophage predominance, there is perpetuation of acute inflammation and ongoing lung injury rather than resolution and repair. This may occur because of ongoing activation of inflammatory pathways from localized or systemic infection, or it may represent a failure of the normal orchestration of inflammation due to host factors.

Biochemical Mediators of Inflammation

Investigators have sought for years to discover the pivotal inflammatory mediator responsible for acute lung injury, anticipating that prevention or cure of ARDS might be possible by using pharmacologic blockade. While dozens of mediators have been implicated, none has been demonstrated to be primarily responsible for initiating the tissue damage associated with ARDS. From a biochemical standpoint it appears that the inflammatory process is complex and multifaceted—it is characterized by cytokines, which attract and activate inflammatory cells (endotoxin, tumor necrosis factor, interleukins, platelet-activating factor); by release of toxic inflammatory products (oxygen radicals, elastase); and by the activation of multiple "cascades" of inflammation, such as the complement pathway, prostaglandins, kinins, and the coagulation system.[9] Each of these factors has been shown in some way to participate in the sequence of events linking the initial clinical insult, such as trauma or sepsis, to the pulmonary tissue injury associated with full-blown ARDS. Blocking agents have been tested in numerous clinical trials, and although some have shown promise, none has emerged as an approved standard therapy for ARDS.[10]

STRUCTURAL CHANGES

Epithelial Damage and Edema

The earliest changes in the lung during development of ARDS involve type I alveolar epithelial cells—the "pancake-like" squamous cells covering approximately 95 percent of the alveolar surface area in the normal lung, which form a protective lining that at the same time is thin enough to facilitate the exchange of gas between the airspace and the lung capillaries.[11] These cells are extremely susceptible to injury. Within a few hours after the onset of alveolar inflammation, they swell and become detached from the underlying basement membrane, leaving the gas exchange barrier denuded and prone to the leakage of edema fluid. The endothelial cells lining alveolar capillaries also undergo significant changes, with cell swelling and loss of the normal barrier function. The combination leads to accumulation of protein-rich edema fluid within the alveolar walls (interstitial space) and the alveolar space.[11]

Among the high molecular weight proteins leaking into the interstitium and alveoli are coagulation factors such as fibrinogen, which not only contribute to the inflammatory process but also cause gelling of the accumulated edema fluid; this, in part explains the markedly delayed alveolar liquid clearance in ARDS. Clearance of alveolar fluid involves cellular transport of sodium with secondary movement of water across the healthy epithelial surface. While this is effective in clearing the transudative fluid of congestive heart failure, in patients with ARDS it leads to the concentration of protein, which acts as an osmotic force, pulling fluid into the alveoli. Another reason that the clearance of ARDS edema fluid is often slower is that the epithelial cells responsible for fluid absorption are often functionally impaired and unable to transport fluid and electrolytes. Surfactant, normally present on the surface of alveolar lining cells, is reduced in quantity and rendered less active by the presence of plasma proteins in the alveolar space.

Lung Repair

Over the next 24 to 48 hours, the denuded basement membrane surface becomes covered by a layer composed of fibrin and other proteins known as a *hyaline membrane*, familiar to many as the descriptor from which infant respiratory dis-

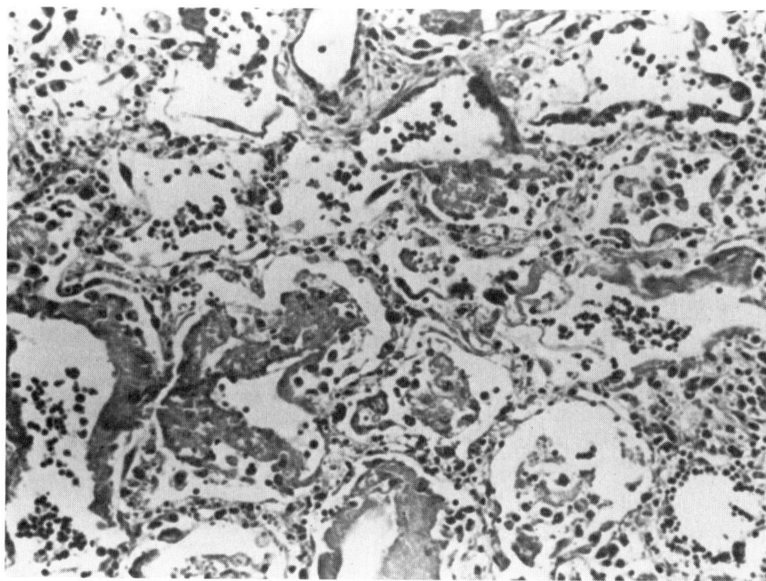

Figure 35-1. Histologic appearance in ARDS about 1 week following injury. There is prominent interstitial inflammation, and hyaline membranes are resolving but still seen in several areas. The cuboidal type II pneumocytes are proliferating, as is typical for this phase of the injury repair process. (H&E, × 180.) (From Katzenstein and Askin,[32] with permission.)

tress syndrome took its original name, *hyaline membrane disease*. At this point there has also been early proliferation of type II alveolar epithelial cells, the relatively hardy cuboidal cells that normally make up about 5 percent of the alveolar surface and are responsible for surfactant synthesis and other metabolic functions of the lung[11] (Fig. 35-1). As with other forms of lung injury, the repair process in ARDS is believed to involve proliferation of these cells followed by spreading along the alveolar surface, often on top of hyaline membranes, and eventually by differentiation into type I cells, which are better suited to the gas exchange and barrier function of the lung.

Pulmonary Fibrosis

Although pulmonary fibrosis (scarring) is often thought of as a chronic process, which may take months or even years to develop, the cells responsible for scar formation appear to be activated and increased in number by as early as 3 to 5 days in patients with ARDS.[12] These cells, known as *fibroblasts*, migrate from their normal location in the interstitial space into the alveolar space, where the fibrin matrix, referred to earlier, serves as a scaffolding for the deposition of collagen. Although inflammatory lung diseases are commonly characterized by fibrosis, intra-alveolar fibrosis is unique to ARDS. Lung scarring appears to be a dynamic process, representing a balance between collagen synthesis by the fibroblasts and collagen degradation by the collagenase enzymes produced by macrophages and other inflammatory cells. Thus, although relentless progression of fibrosis is the rule in patients who die with ARDS, those who survive the lung injury process usually demonstrate reversal of fibrosis, as indicated by improvements in lung compliance, total lung capacity, and the characteristic honeycomb pattern on chest radiograph.

Pulmonary Vascular Changes

The pulmonary vasculature undergoes dramatic changes over the course of ARDS, particularly in those patients who have ARDS lasting more than 1 or 2 weeks. Morphometric studies have shown a progressive increase in the distance between the gas exchange surface and the pulmonary capillaries over time, which is primarily due to the accumulation of edema fluid within the interstitial space. At the same time there is a progressive decrease in capillary cross-sectional area.[11] In the earliest stages of lung injury, this may be due to pulmonary artery constriction under the influence of vasoactive mediators such as thromboxane A2, platelet-activating factor, and leukotrienes. Thereafter, capillary occlusion occurs as a result of microemboli and in situ thrombosis. In the later stages of ARDS vessels become distorted by pulmonary fibrosis, further compromising blood flow to the alveolar surface. Over time, there is permanent destruction of pulmonary vasculature, even in patients who eventually recover.

PHYSIOLOGIC CHANGES

Gas Exchange Abnormalities

The earliest and most common physiologic abnormality seen in patients with ARDS is hypoxemia, which is largely due to regional atelectasis and alveolar flooding, with resultant venoarterial shunting of blood.[13] There also appears to be a disturbance in hypoxic pulmonary vasoconstriction, the regulatory mechanism that would normally minimize blood flow to hypoxic lung regions, thereby minimizing the impact on overall gas exchange. In the early stages of ARDS, if the patient is breathing spontaneously, it is common for the arterial CO_2 pressure ($PaCO_2$) to be reduced as a result of hyperventilation.[13] This response may be due in part to hypoxemia, but it is primarily caused by stimulation of respiratory drive mediated by the pulmonary stretch receptors in response to low compliance and reduced lung volumes. After several days there is often an improvement in oxygenation as effective hypoxic pulmonary vasoconstriction returns. There also appears to be a shift from venoarterial shunting as the primary mechanism of hypoxemia to ventilation/perfusion ($\dot{V}/\dot{Q}$) heterogeneity. Although hyperventilation persists for the reasons outlined above, there is usually a progressive rise in the $PaCO_2$ level after 3 to 7 days of ARDS; this is due to the destruction of pulmonary capillaries with a resultant increase in dead space ventilation.[12] It is not uncommon to see dead space/tidal volume (V_D/V_T) ratios in excess of 75 percent in patients with ARDS.

Many believe that ARDS and some of the diseases commonly associated with the syndrome lead to a disturbance in the relationship between O_2 delivery (DO_2) and O_2 consumption ($\dot{V}O_2$) (see Ch. 34). Normally, $\dot{V}O_2$ is approximately 250 mL/min for an average-sized adult at rest and is relatively independent of DO_2, which is normally about 1000 mL/min, but it may vary in the critically ill patient as a result of changes in cardiac output and hemoglobin level. Several clinical studies have been published suggesting that in ARDS patients there is O_2 "hunger" at the tissue level, creating a pathologic dependency of $\dot{V}O_2$ on DO_2.[14,15] In these studies measured $\dot{V}O_2$ has increased when DO_2 is increased by blood transfusion or agents that increase cardiac output. It has been argued that O_2 transport variables should be carefully monitored in ARDS patients and that hemoglobin levels and cardiac output should be maximized.[16] However, some more recent carefully performed studies have not supported the earlier findings, and the value of aggressively manipulating DO_2 in ARDS patients remains speculative.[17]

Lung Mechanics

Most patients with ARDS show a reduction in lung compliance. In the early stages this is due to alveolar and interstitial edema as well as to regional microatelectasis from the loss of surfactant function. In the later stages atelectasis may persist, but pulmonary fibrosis becomes the major determinant of compliance. This increase in elastic recoil of the lung causes a reduction in functional residual capacity, which among other things further impairs oxygenation, since there is necessarily a reduction in the volume of fresh O_2 within the alveolar reservoir. Although the pulmonary function abnormalities in ARDS have been categorized as restrictive and are treated as such throughout this text, recent work both in experimental animals and in humans has suggested that there is also a component of airflow limitation that is reversible with the administration of bronchodilator agents.[18]

Pulmonary Hypertension

Pulmonary hypertension is common in patients with ARDS, particularly in the later stages. In the early stages pulmonary hypertension may be due to the vasoactive mediators mentioned above, particularly in patients with septic lung injury. The occlusion and eventual destruction of capillaries causes a progressive rise in pulmonary artery pressures beginning as early as 5 to 10 days after the onset of ARDS.[11] If this process proceeds rapidly, there may be right ventricular dysfunction with a drop in cardiac output. Usually, however, the process is gradual enough that adaptation of the right ventricle, compensating for the increased load, takes place. As mentioned above, capillary destruction also causes an increase in dead space ventilation and minute ventilation requirement.[11,12] This loss of capillary surface area for gas exchange manifests itself in pulmonary function testing as a reduction in the diffusing capacity for carbon monoxide (D_LCO), the most common and longest-lasting physiologic abnormality seen in survivors of ARDS.

CHEST RADIOGRAPHIC FINDINGS

The chest x-ray in ARDS characteristically shows generalized pulmonary infiltrates involving all lung fields[19] (Fig. 35-2 and also Fig. 57-13A). In most cases radiographic abnormalities appear simultaneously or after the development of gas exchange impairment, but occasionally diffuse pulmonary infiltrates are present for a day or more prior to the onset of clinical hypoxemia. Just as the syndrome itself represents a spectrum from mild to severe respiratory failure, the radiographic abnormalities also represent a spectrum from mild interstitial edema to virtual "white-out" of the lung fields. In contrast to cardiogenic pulmonary edema, the opacities seen in acute lung injury (ARDS) usually extend into the peripheral lung regions and upper lung fields. The pattern is often patchy and may be asymmetric. This is most evident with computed tomography (CT) of the chest (Fig. 35-3), which typically demonstrates heterogeneous lung involvement with preservation of normal lung regions in certain areas, similar to what is seen with careful pathologic evaluation.[20] Early in the course of ARDS the infiltrates are caused by alveolar and interstitial edema, along with regions of atelectasis. In the later stages (Fig. 35-4) pulmonary opac-

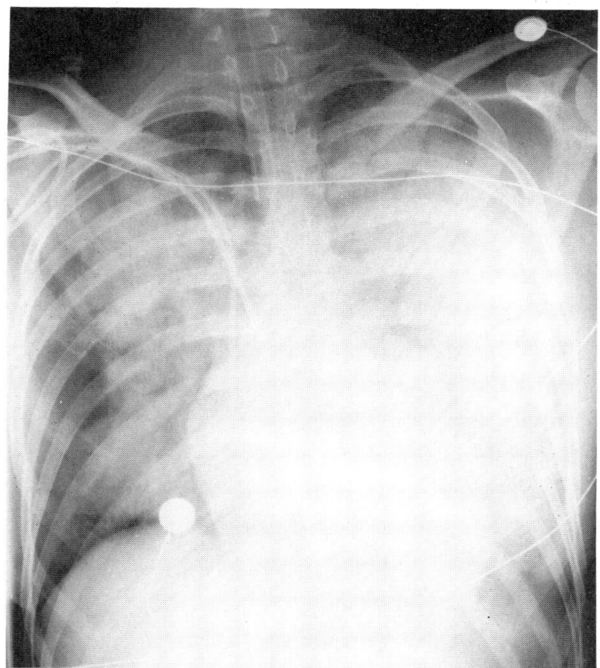

Figure 35-2. Chest radiographic appearance on admission in a case of heroin-induced noncardiogenic pulmonary edema, which progressed to ARDS. There is diffuse infiltration in all lung areas, at this stage relatively sparing the peripheral lung zones on the right. (From Pierson,[33] with permission.)

ities may represent infection or fibrosis complicating the basic process.

NATURAL HISTORY

Time Course

About one-third of patients who develop ARDS die within the first 72 hours, usually as a result of the underlying illness or injury that caused the ARDS in the first place.[4] Death in such cases is often due to irreversible septic shock, uncontrolled bleeding, or massive injuries to the brain or other vital organs. In another one-third of patients with ARDS, the underlying disease is controlled and there is fairly rapid resolution of the lung injury process and associated physiologic abnormalities. Such patients recover adequate lung function to permit weaning from the ventilator within the first week after onset of ARDS, and the recovery of lung function after leaving the hospital is usually rapid and complete. The remaining one-third of patients progress to what might be termed *chronic ARDS*, with ongoing acute alveolar inflammation, persistent hypoxemia, and poor lung compliance, necessitating continued ventilatory assistance. In these patients, the outcome is related to the severity of lung injury as well as to the development of complications.

Infectious Complications

The principal complications of ARDS are infectious complications, especially sepsis syndrome, and multiple organ failure.[4,21–23] Infections are extremely common in ARDS patients and have been clearly shown to be related to mortality. Among patients with ARDS due to noninfectious causes, the lungs are the most common site of secondary infections. There are a number of reasons for the increased susceptibility of ARDS patients to infection. Prolonged endotracheal intubation is a known risk factor for nosocomial pneumonia, the endotracheal tube itself serving as a direct conduit to the lungs for pathogens from the intensive care unit (ICU) environment. Prolonged endotracheal intubation has also been shown to impair the function of the mucociliary escalator and to enhance the adhesion of gram-negative bacteria to airway epithelial cells. Not only are the diseases that predispose patients to ARDS commonly associated with impaired immunity, but ARDS itself appears to produce defects in the function of alveolar inflammatory cells, impairing the ability to clear and kill microbial pathogens. Furthermore, the proteinaceous edema fluid found in the lungs of ARDS patients provides an excellent culture medium for bacteria. Patients who develop ARDS are six times as likely to develop sepsis syndrome than patients with similar illnesses or injuries who do not develop ARDS. Not only is the presence of infection associated with increased mortality, but sepsis syndrome is a direct or contributing cause of death in 72 percent of ARDS deaths.[4] One report came to the discouraging conclusion that among ARDS patients with infection, those receiving adequate antibiotic coverage fared no better than those judged to have received inadequate coverage.[22]

Multiple Organ Failure

When there is simultaneous dysfunction of several organ systems, the phenomenon is termed *multiple organ failure syndrome*. This complication, recognized only in recent years, is extremely common in patients with ARDS.[23,24] Through the early and middle 1970s, the failure of a single organ system was sufficient to cause death. However, with the advent of renal dialysis, devices to support ventilation, advances in hemodynamic support, and organ transplantation, we are able to avert or at least to postpone deaths that might be caused by the failure of a single organ, thus permitting the subsequent development of other organ failures. Despite these advances in technology, the mortality associated with multiple organ failure is extremely high, which suggests that the picture is more complex than some simple alterations in physiology.[25] Pinsky and Matuschak[26] have defined multiple organ failure as generalized malignant inflammation. It is virtually synonymous with the clinical entity that many have termed *sepsis syndrome*, in which the cardinal features of localized inflammation become manifest systemically, including *rubor* (generalized vasodilation with hypotension and low systemic vascular resistance), *tumor* (capillary leak with soft tissue edema), *calor* (fever), and

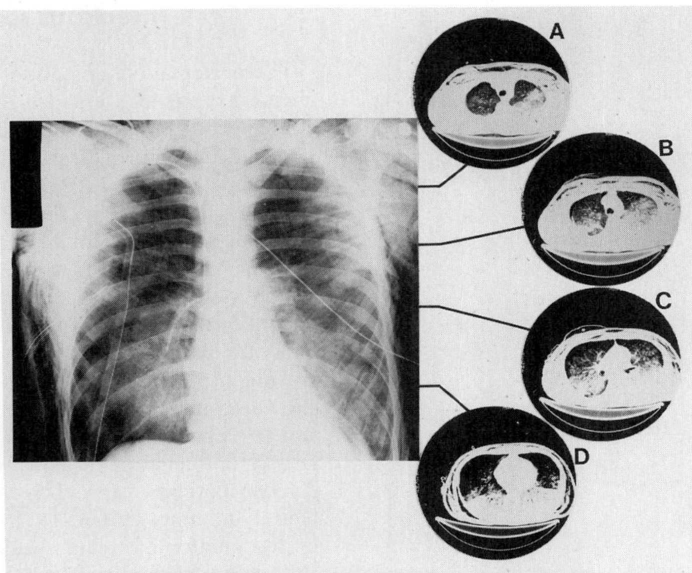

Figure 35-3. Portable anteroposterior chest radiograph and corresponding CT images taken from the indicated levels **(A–D)** in a patient with ARDS a few days after onset of illness. Pulmonary involvement is inhomogeneous and tends to be more prominent posteriorly, in the more dependent portions of lung. (Modified from Maunder et al.,[20] with permission.)

functio laesa (loss of organ function).[27] Consensus has not been reached as to a clinical definition of multiple organ failure syndrome, but most would agree that there must be measurable dysfunction of at least three organ systems. Some workers have applied organ failure scoring systems that take into account the severity of the functional abnormalities as well as the number of failing organs.

The incidence of multiple organ failure syndrome in patients with ARDS has been estimated at approximately 70 percent.[23] Organ failure is known to be associated with most of the systemic conditions that predispose patients to ARDS, most notably major traumatic injury and sepsis. Among trauma victims, the likelihood of developing multiple organ failure is increased in those of advanced age, female patients, those with hypothermia, and those who are hypertransfused.[28] The time to onset of multiple organ failure syndrome is variable but is somewhat earlier for patients with sepsis, and it appears that those with earlier onset have a greater risk of dying. Mortality is also determined by the number of organs failing, by the overall severity of organ dysfunction, by the duration of multiple organ failure, and by the age of the patient.[23,25,28] There are conflicting reports about whether certain organ failure combinations are uniformly fatal, with one group having reported no survivors among patients with simultaneous hepatic and respiratory failure and others having reported the primary importance of renal and central nervous system failure.[29] Our experience suggests that there are no uniformly fatal combinations.[28] Although respiratory failure is often the earliest, there is no predictable sequence of subsequent organ failures. In fact, many have argued that there is nothing unique about the respiratory system and that ARDS simply represents the failure of one among many organs in response to a systemic insult such as trauma or sepsis.[23,27]

The mechanism of multiple organ failure syndrome is incompletely understood. Theories of pathogenesis have centered on inflammatory pathways and regional organ ischemia, and many of the biochemical and cellular mediators implicated in ARDS are believed to be important in the development of the syndrome. Neutrophils and their products, endotoxin, tumor necrosis factor, and interleukin-1 have all been suggested as factors responsible for the initiation of organ dysfunction, which is presumably followed by secondary activation of other inflammatory cascades such as the coagulation system, complement, and the kinin pathway.[24,26,29] Regional organ ischemia may result from activation of the coagulation cascade with intravascular clot formation or from plugging of the microvasculature with aggregated and nondeformable neutrophils.

FUNCTIONAL RECOVERY IN SURVIVORS

Recovery of lung function in survivors of ARDS has been difficult to study systematically, and most reports are anecdotal. It is clear that some ARDS patients, probably those with relatively minor respiratory failure and a shorter course, progress to complete recovery of lung function within several months. Most patients have some degree of impairment in lung function when they leave the hospital, and most show

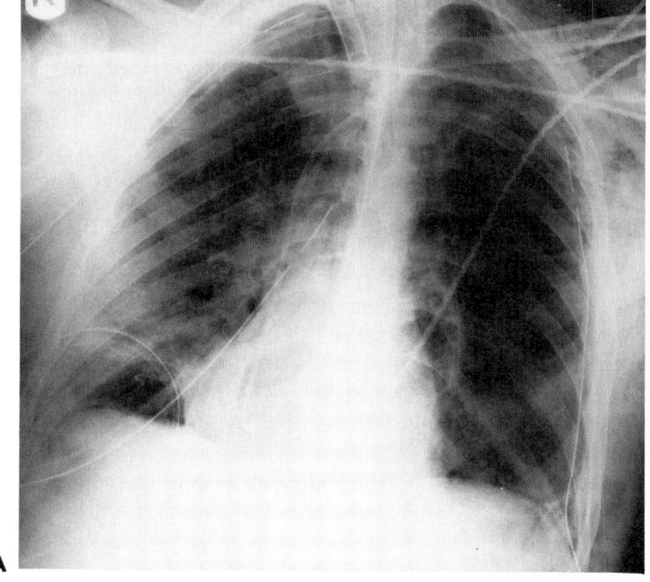

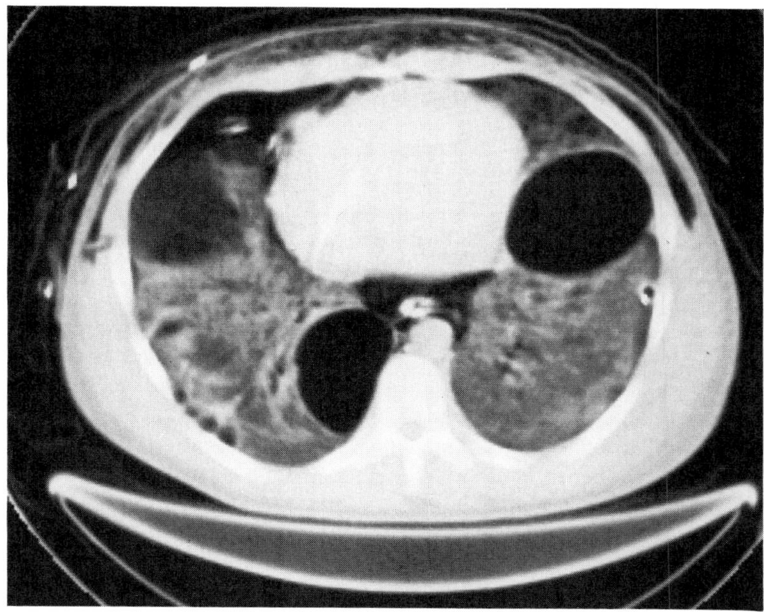

Figure 35-4. Typical radiographic and CT appearances in chronic ARDS 2 or 3 weeks after onset of illness. **(A)** Portable chest radiograph showing inhomogeneous distribution of airspace filling process. The patient had had multiple pneumothoraces and bronchopleural fistulae, and there are four chest tubes (three on the right, one on the left) visible on the film. **(B)** CT slice through the midchest region taken at the same time, demonstrating the marked inhomogeneity of parenchymal involvement. There are two large, cyst-like gas collections and a right-sided anterior pneumothorax. Subcutaneous emphysema is also noted, and chest tubes are present bilaterally. (From Pierson[34] with permission.)

improvement in the first 6 months even if they do not return to normal.[30,31] After that there appears to be a plateau in the recovery of pulmonary function, although some patients do continue to improve in their ability to perform work-related and everyday activities.

The most common and persistent abnormality in pulmonary function is a reduction in DLCO. This corresponds to the destruction of pulmonary vasculature described above and explains why many patients who are comfortable at rest have significant exercise limitation. Reduced lung volumes are seen in nearly all patients at the time of leaving the hospital, but most show improvement in the next several months, and the majority actually return to normal predicted values within 6 months to 1 year. This restrictive defect is probably related to lung scarring, and the improvement over time suggests that the process is somewhat dynamic, as described above.

A smaller proportion of patients show airflow limitation on pulmonary function testing, often developing this abnormality after leaving the hospital. The airflow obstruction is frequently, but not always, reversible with bronchodilator administration. Gas exchange abnormalities appear to be somewhat less common after ARDS, although many patients are hypoxemic at the time they leave the hospital, some requiring supplemental O_2 therapy. By 6 months the hypoxemia is infrequent, but some patients still demonstrate O_2 desaturation with exercise.

References

1. Ashbaugh DG, Bigelow DB, Petty TL, Levine BE: Acute respiratory distress in adults. Lancet 1967;2:319–323
2. Maunder RJ, Hudson LD: Clinical risks associated with the adult respiratory distress syndrome. pp. 1–21. In Zapol WM, Lemaire F (eds): Adult Respiratory Distress Syndrome. Marcel Dekker, New York, 1991
3. Hudson LD: Causes of the adult respiratory distress syndrome: Clinical recognition. Clin Chest Med 1983;3:195–212
4. Montgomery AB, Stager MA, Carrico CJ, Hudson LD: Causes of mortality in patients with the adult respiratory distress syndrome. Am Rev Respir Dis 1985;132:485–489
5. Swank DW, Moore SB: Roles of the neutrophil and other mediators in adult respiratory distress syndrome. Mayo Clin Proc 1989;64:1118–1132
6. Maunder RJ, Hackman R, Riff E et al: Occurrence of the adult respiratory distress syndrome in neutropenic patients. Am Rev Respir Dis 1986;133:313–316
7. McGuire WW, Spragg RG, Cohen AB et al: Studies on the pathogenesis of the adult respiratory distress syndrome. J Clin Invest 1982;69:543–553
8. Henson PM, Larsen GL, Henson JE et al: Resolution of pulmonary inflammation. FASEB J 1984;43:2799–2806
9. Brigham KL: Lung injury and repair in the adult. pp. 12–29. In Brigham KL, Stahlman MT (eds): Respiratory Distress Syndromes: Molecules to Man. Vanderbilt University Press, Nashville, 1990
10. Maunder RJ, Hudson LD: Pharmacologic strategies for treating the adult respiratory distress syndrome. Respir Care 1990;35:241–246
11. Bachofen M, Weibel ER: Structural alterations of lung parenchyma in the adult respiratory distress syndrome. Clin Chest Med 1982;3:35–56
12. Lamy M, Fallat RJ, Koeniger E et al: Pathologic features and mechanisms of hypoxemia in adult respiratory distress syndrome. Am Rev Respir Dis 1976;114:267–284
13. Ralph D, Robertson HT: Respiratory gas exchange in adult respiratory distress syndrome. Semin Respir Med 1981;2:114–122
14. Danek SJ, Lynch JP, Weg JG, Dantzker DR: The dependence of oxygen uptake on oxygen delivery in the adult respiratory distress syndrome. Am Rev Respir Dis 1980;122:387–395
15. Weg JG: Oxygen transport in adult respiratory distress syndrome and other acute circulatory problems: Relationship of oxygen delivery and oxygen consumption. Crit Care Med 1991;19:650–657
16. Shoemaker WC, Appel PL, Kram HB et al: Prospective trial of supranormal values of survivors as therapeutic goals in high-risk surgical patients. Chest 1988;94:1176–1186
17. Ronco J, Phang PT, Walley KR et al: Oxygen consumption is independent of changes in oxygen delivery in severe adult respiratory distress syndrome. Am Rev Respir Dis 1991;143:1267–1273
18. Wright PE, Bernard GR: The role of airflow resistance in patients with the adult respiratory distress syndrome. Am Rev Respir Dis 1989;139:1169–1174
19. Pistolesi M, Massimo M, Milne ENC, Giunti G: The chest roentgenogram in pulmonary edema. Clin Chest Med 1985;6:315–344
20. Maunder RJ, Shuman WP, McHugh JW et al: Preservation of normal lung regions in the adult respiratory distress syndrome: Analysis by computed tomography. JAMA 1986;255:2463–2465
21. Pingleton SK: Complications of acute respiratory failure. Am Rev Respir Dis 1988;137:1463–1493
22. Seidenfeld JJ, Pohl DF, Bell RC et al: Incidence, site, and outcome of infections in patients with the adult respiratory distress syndrome. Am Rev Respir Dis 1986;134:12–16
23. Villar J, Manzano JJ, Blazquez MA et al: Multiple organ failure in acute respiratory failure. J Crit Care 1991;6:75–80
24. Heyman SJ, Rinaldo JE: Multiple system organ failure in the adult respiratory distress syndrome. J Intensive Care Med 1989;4:192–200
25. Knaus WA, Draper EA, Wagner DP, Zimmerman JE: Prognosis in acute organ-system failure. Ann Surg 1985;202:685–693
26. Pinsky MR, Matuschak GM: Multiple systems organ failure: Failure of host defense homeostasis. Crit Care Clin 1989;5:199–220
27. Hudson LD: Multiple systems organ failure (MSOF): Lessons learned from the adult respiratory distress syndrome (ARDS). Crit Care Clin 1989;5:697–705
28. Cockrill BA, Kubilis PS, Anardi DM et al: Pulmonary and extrapulmonary organ system failure in patients with trauma or sepsis. Am Rev Respir Dis 1990;141:A515
29. Matuschak GM, Rinaldo JE: Organ interactions in the adult respiratory distress syndrome during sepsis: Role of the liver in host defense. Chest 1988;94:400–406
30. Ghio AJ, Elliott CG, Crapo RO et al: Impairment after adult respiratory distress syndrome. An evaluation based on American Thoracic Society recommendations. Am Rev Respir Dis 1989;139:1158–1162
31. Peters JI, Bell RC, Prihoda TJ et al: Clinical determinants of abnormalities in pulmonary functions in survivors of the adult respiratory distress syndrome. Am Rev Respir Dis 1989;139:1163–1168
32. Katzenstein AA, Askin FB: Surgical Pathology of Non-Neoplastic Lung Disease. In Bennington JL (ed): Major Problems in Pathology. Vol. 13. WB Saunders, Philadelphia, 1982
33. Pierson DJ: Acute respiratory failure. pp. 75–126. In Sahn SA (ed): Pulmonary Emergencies. Churchill Livingstone, New York, 1982
34. Pierson DJ: Alveolar rupture during mechanical ventilation: Role of PEEP, peak airway pressure, and distending volume. Respir Care 1988;33:472–486

Chapter 36

Infectious Disease Concepts

Jan V. Hirschmann

CHAPTER OUTLINE

Pneumonia and other respiratory tract infections are important in respiratory care and account for a substantial proportion of the clinician's interactions with patients. An understanding of basic infectious disease principles and familiarity with the clinical characteristics of the commonly encountered respiratory infections are important in all practice settings. To provide this background, this chapter first summarizes the normal respiratory tract flora, then reviews the ways in which respiratory infections are diagnosed, and finally provides concise descriptions of the most important individual infectious diseases affecting the respiratory system.

In this chapter the principles and specific infectious diseases mentioned above are discussed, but principles of therapy are deferred to Chapter 68. Infections in the immunocompromised host, including those affecting patients with the acquired immunodeficiency syndrome (AIDS) and other forms of human immunodeficiency virus (HIV) infection, are discussed in Chapter 69. Other infectious disease topics considered elsewhere in the book include sepsis syndrome (Ch. 35) and infection control in respiratory care (Ch. 97).

NORMAL RESPIRATORY FLORA

Understanding respiratory infections requires a knowledge of the microbiology of the upper airway. Although the lung defense mechanisms delineated in Chapter 17 normally keep the tracheobronchial tree and lung tissue sterile, most of the respiratory tract above the larynx harbors an abundant flora consisting primarily of numerous bacterial species.[1] Bacteria in this location, as elsewhere, possess certain distinguishing characteristics, the most important being morphology (shape), color on Gram stain, and growth capacity according to O_2 content. Bacteria are called *cocci* when spherical, *bacilli* when rod-like, and *spirochetes* when spiral. On Gram stain organisms are either blue (gram-positive) or red (gram-negative), depending on the nature of their cell walls. The O_2 tolerance of bacteria ranges widely: obligate anaerobes grow only in the complete absence of O_2, whereas obligate aerobes grow only in its presence. *Microaerophilic* organisms prefer a reduced but not absent O_2 content, while *facultative* bacteria can grow under all these conditions. Table 36-1 lists some common bacteria, described by their Gram staining characteristics, morphology, and O_2 tolerance.

The flora of the upper airway contains a remarkably diverse population of bacteria, both gram-positive and gram-negative, of all morphologic types and O_2 tolerance. For the remainder of this chapter the term *aerobe* will apply to obligate aerobes and microaerophilic and facultative bacteria. In the nose and nasopharynx the concentrations of aerobes and anaerobes per milliliter of nasal secretions are each about 10^3 organisms. In the oropharynx saliva contains about 10^7 aerobes and 10^8 anaerobes per milliliter, the tooth surfaces contain 10^6 of each per milliliter, and the gingival scrapings contain about 10^7 of each per milliliter. It may seem surprising that anaerobes are so abundant in the respiratory tract since ambient air is constantly being inhaled, but these organisms can survive in the crevices of the mucosa, particularly in the area between the teeth and the gingiva, where O_2 is absent. These anaerobic organisms are weak pathogens and ordinarily cause disease only when they enter normally sterile sites in large numbers.

Many of the aerobic organisms that colonize the upper airway, however, are more potent pathogens, which readily cause disease under certain circumstances. These include *Staphylococcus aureus*, found in the anterior nares of about 20 percent of normal people; *Streptococcus pneumoniae* (pneumococcus), present in the oropharynx in up to 70 percent of normal persons; *Haemophilus influenzae*, part of the normal flora in as many as 80 percent of the population; and *Moraxella catarrhalis*, also present in a high proportion of normal individuals. Each of these organisms can cause serious respiratory infections involving the sinuses, middle ear, and lung.

Table 36-1. Morphologic and Staining Properties of Bacterial Species

Gram-positive cocci
- Aerobic: *Micrococcus*
- Facultative: *Staphylococcus, Streptococcus*
- Anaerobic: *Peptococcus, Peptostreptococcus*

Gram-negative cocci
- Aerobic: *Moraxella, Neisseria*
- Facultative: None
- Anaerobic: *Veillonella*

Gram-positive bacilli
- Aerobic: *Bacillus, Nocardia*
- Facultative: *Corynebacterium, Lactobacillus*
- Anaerobic: *Actinomyces, Clostridium, Eubacterium, Proprionibacterium*

Gram-negative bacilli
- Aerobic: *Acinetobacter, Haemophilus, Legionella, Pseudomonas*
- Facultative: *Citrobacter, Enterobacter, Escherichia, Klebsiella, Morganella, Proteus, Providencia, Serratia*
- Anaerobic: *Bacteroides, Fusobacterium*

The ability to colonize these mucosal surfaces depends in part on the adhesion of organisms to epithelial cells. Gram-negative bacilli adhere considerably less readily to the epithelial cells of the upper respiratory tract than do the predominant gram-positive bacteria that constitute its normal flora. Another factor regulating the nature of the colonizing organisms is the state of dentition. Periodontal disease increases the number of anaerobic bacteria present in the oral cavity, while the absence of teeth reduces their density. Some of the organisms normally growing in the upper airway inhibit the growth of respiratory pathogens, perhaps through competition for nutrients or the production of antibacterial substances. Secretory IgA, an immunoglobulin present in the saliva, also probably helps to regulate the oral flora.

Alteration of this microbial milieu may allow gram-negative bacilli, such as *Escherichia coli* and *Pseudomonas aeruginosa*, to inhabit the upper airway.[2] Various illnesses increase the adhesion of these organisms to the respiratory epithelium. Antimicrobial therapy can eradicate the normal flora, allowing gram-negative organisms to fill the microbial void created. Hospitalization, by exposing the patient to a large number of gram-negative bacilli present in the hospital environment, also promotes colonization with these organisms, especially in intensive care units, where the combination of very ill patients, widespread antimicrobial use, and a profuse flora exists. A similar but less intense propensity for acquiring gram-negative bacilli in the oropharynx exists in nursing homes, especially among the very ill or debilitated. To a lesser extent alcoholism and diabetes mellitus also seem to encourage this colonization.[3]

The importance of this upper respiratory flora is that the organisms present are responsible for many respiratory infections. Disease can occur when the bacteria present in the upper respiratory tract, through various mechanisms including trauma or the presence of another infection, enter normally sterile tissue, such as lung parenchyma and paranasal sinuses. In general, the normal flora are less virulent in these circumstances than gram-negative bacilli and are usually more easily treated with antimicrobial therapy. Disease can also occur when organisms that are never part of the normal flora anywhere in the body, such as viruses, are inhaled or ingested. These microbes, unlike normal flora, are usually strongly pathogenic, capable of causing disease even when acquired in small numbers.

MICROBIAL DIAGNOSIS OF RESPIRATORY INFECTIONS

Methods used for the microbial diagnosis of respiratory infections include cultures, stains, and serology.[4]

Cultures

Culturing an organism from a normally sterile site provides definitive evidence of the etiology of an infection. Normally sterile sites that might grow organisms in respiratory infections are blood, when a severe infection such as pneumonia occurs; pleural fluid, when infection of the pleural cavity (empyema) develops; and lung tissue obtained by percutaneous biopsy or surgical excision. Very strong evidence for an infection's etiology also comes with culturing from respiratory secretions an organism that is rarely present in the airway flora without being pathogenic. Examples of such pathogens include viruses, most fungi except *Candida* spp., *Mycobacterium tuberculosis*, and a few other microbes.

Bacterial Cultures

Since expectorated sputum travels through the oropharynx, it is always contaminated by the resident flora there. The diagnosis of a pneumonia's etiology by culture of bacteria from sputum, therefore, is always an inference that the organisms cultured represent microbes present in the lung tissue rather than oropharyngeal bacteria contaminating the sputum. This inference is supported by an evaluation of the Gram stain of the sputum. If the slide shows numerous neutrophils and alveolar macrophages but few or no squamous epithelial cells, the specimen probably accurately reflects the bacteriology of the lung. If many squamous epithelial cells are present, significant contamination by upper airway secretions has occurred, since these cells are present in the upper airway but not in the lung. These issues receive more complete discussions in Chapter 58, but bacterial cultures of sputum without concomitant evaluation of a Gram stain of the specimen are very difficult to interpret, since the organisms commonly causing pneumonia may be present as normal or innocent colonizing flora in the upper respiratory tract. These bacteria can therefore be isolated from sputum samples that are heavily contaminated by upper airway flora, and their presence in the culture will mislead the clinician about the actual cause of the infection.

Bacterial cultures of sputum usually grow the responsible organism within 24 hours, allowing a presumptive identification at that point. Definitive speciation by biochemical or other tests may require an additional 24 hours or more in some cases. Susceptibility testing to various antimicrobial agents is usually completed by 48 hours after the specimen is submitted. Certain techniques, such as DNA probes and monoclonal antibody tests, may allow more rapid identification of organisms in the future, but currently these methods are neither perfected nor widely available.

Viral Cultures

Although viruses cause a preponderance of upper respiratory infections, viral cultures are not commonly warranted since most of these disorders are short-lived, self-limited processes for which no specific therapy exists. Viral cultures are useful for epidemiologic reasons during outbreaks of severe respiratory infections such as influenza, for which prevention by vaccination or prophylactic amantidine is available. In addition, viral cultures are helpful in certain kinds of respiratory infections in immunocompromised patients, in whom the identification of a viral etiology has important implications for prognosis and therapy, such as the ability to discontinue antimicrobial agents begun presumptively to treat another cause.

Since viruses are obligate intracellular parasites, they require living cells on which to propagate. Viral culture media, therefore, include live human or animal cells on which the specimen is inoculated. Viral cultures generally require several days to weeks to become positive, depending on the number and kind of viruses present in the specimen.

Mycobacterial Cultures

Most mycobacteria causing respiratory infections are slow-growing organisms that require special media. Sputum must undergo special decontaminating treatment to eliminate other bacteria before being inoculated onto the culture media. Growth generally occurs in 2 to 6 weeks although certain techniques allow more rapid presumptive identification.

Fungal Cultures

The isolation of pathogenic fungi other than *Candida* spp. usually requires inoculation onto special media. Growth of the organisms generally takes several days to weeks, depending on the particular species involved.

Stains

The Gram stain is the most important aid in the presumptive diagnosis of bacterial disease. Although precise identification of a species by Gram stain is impossible, the organism's color, shape, and grouping (e.g., pairs, clusters, chains) strongly suggest the likely bacterium involved, given the clinical information and the source of the specimen (see Ch. 68 and Table 68-1). For example, the presence of numerous lancet-shaped (oval) gram-positive cocci in pairs on the sputum Gram stain of a patient with pneumonia should strongly suggest *S. pneumoniae* (pneumococcus) as the cause. Although some other streptococcal species can have a similar appearance, they rarely cause pneumonia.

Immunofluorescent stains can detect the antigens of certain organisms in either respiratory secretions or tissue samples. The primary use of immunofluorescent staining of sputum is for rapid identification of *Legionella* as a cause of pneumonia. With tissue specimens, immunofluorescent techniques can accurately identify *Legionella*, certain viruses, and the bacillus causing plague.

For identification of mycobacteria, the acid-fast (Ziehl-Neelsen) stain of sputum and other samples is a time-honored method still widely employed. Fluorescent staining of the organism with the fluorochrome dyes rhodamine and auramine is, however, more rapid.

For identification of fungi, a potassium hydroxide (KOH) preparation of sputum or other purulent material sometimes allows visualization of the organism, particularly *Coccidioides immitis* or *Blastomyces dermatitidis*. For identification of fungi in tissue specimens, Gomori's methenamine silver (GMS), periodic acid-Schiff (PAS), or other staining techniques permit identification of the fungi. Occasionally, fungi may be seen on sputum submitted for cytologic evaluation.

Viruses are too small to be visible with light microscopy. Because they may cause certain changes in the nucleus or cytoplasm of infected cells, however, the presence of some viral infections, such as herpes simplex or cytomegalovirus, may be inferred on routine (hematoxylin & eosin) stains of tissue. Visualization of the organism itself requires electron microscopy, but since a high density of the virus must be present for it to be visible, this technique is rarely practiced in diagnosing respiratory infections. Immunofluorescent stains of tissue, however, are useful in detecting some viruses.

Serology

The detection of antibodies to an organism may help implicate it as a cause of an infection. The test result is usually expressed as the highest dilution of the serum in which a reaction with the antigen is still detectable (e.g., 1:8 or 1:32). A single specimen is usually not helpful since a low titer may mean that the serologic response to infection has not yet occurred, whereas a high titer may be present with an infection from the recent or even remote past that is unrelated to the current illness. Testing two specimens simultaneously—one obtained during the illness ("acute") and a second obtained 2 to 6 weeks later ("convalescent")—should yield at least a fourfold change in titer for a definitive diagnosis. Serology is most useful in diagnosing infections due to viruses, chlamydia, or mycoplasma but may be helpful with certain other bacteria (e.g., the cause of tularemia) and fungi (e.g., *C. immitis*).

UPPER RESPIRATORY TRACT INFECTIONS

The most important upper respiratory tract infections[5] are acute pharyngitis, the common cold, and the acute forms of sinusitis, epiglottitis, laryngotracheobronchitis (croup), and otitis media, as well as soft tissue infections of the neck.

Acute Pharyngitis

Acute pharyngitis is an inflammation of the pharynx most commonly caused by viruses. *Streptococcus pyogenes* (group A streptococcus) is responsible for about 15 percent of cases; other bacterial etiologies, which include *Corynebacterium diphtheriae, Corynebacterium hemolyticum*, and *Neisseria gonorrhoeae* (gonococcus), are uncommon or rare. The most prominent symptom is soreness, irritation, or scratchiness of the throat. With some viruses other symptoms are common, including rhinorrhea, nasal congestion, fever, myalgias, headache, and cough. On physical examination the pharynx may demonstrate edema and erythema, the tonsils may be enlarged and covered with an exudate, and cervical lymph nodes may be swollen and painful. Accurately differentiating streptococcal from viral causes of pharyngitis is difficult on clinical evaluation, although certain findings such as a pharyngeal exudate and tender, enlarged cervical lymph nodes make a streptococcal etiology more likely. Accordingly, a throat culture is the only reasonably precise way to diagnose streptococcal pharyngitis, although in only about 50 percent of those in whom the organism is isolated is it the cause as defined by serologic changes. The importance of diagnosing streptococcal pharyngitis is not in shortening the course by prompt antibiotic therapy, which has little effect in the duration of symptoms, but in preventing the complication of acute rheumatic fever, a rare but potentially serious disorder. Patients with pharyngitis in whom group A streptococci are isolated on culture should receive penicillin or erythromycin. The isolation of *C. diphtheriae, C. hemolyticum*, or gonococci also warrants antibiotic therapy, but there is no effective treatment of viral pharyngitis.

Rare complications of pharyngitis include upper airway obstruction because of enormous tonsillar enlargement; peritonsillar abscesses, which may require drainage; and retropharyngeal abscesses, which occur from suppurative infection in retropharyngeal lymph nodes. In these cases tracheal intubation or tracheotomy may be necessary.

Common Cold

The common cold[6] is caused by viruses of several species, most of which have several antigenically different types. These organisms may be transmitted by coughing or sneezing, but infected subjects may contaminate their own hands by nasal secretions and pass the virus to the hands of susceptible subjects by brief or extended hand contact. This mechanism of contagion emphasizes the importance of hand washing when infected health professionals care for patients.

The incubation period for colds is usually 2 to 3 days, the main symptoms being rhinorrhea, nasal obstruction, cough, sneezing, and sometimes a sore throat. The symptoms ordinarily persist for 1 to 2 weeks.

The common cold seems to predispose some patients to infections in which the normal resident flora of the upper airway enters the normally sterile sites of the paranasal sinuses, the middle ear, and sometimes the lungs to cause sinusitis, otitis media, and pneumonia, respectively. The responsible mechanism is unknown but probably involves damage to the mucociliary mechanisms involved in cleansing the upper and lower airway.

Viruses causing the common cold may also affect pulmonary function. In normal hosts minor changes in respiratory function are common; in patients with underlying obstructive lung disease these viruses can cause substantial worsening of airflow obstruction and may be responsible for many acute exacerbations of asthma and chronic bronchitis, including those in which purulent sputum is produced.

Acute Sinusitis

Acute sinusitis is an infection of one or more of the paranasal sinuses, which the cleansing action of the mucociliary system ordinarily keeps sterile. The most common predisposing factor to acute sinusitis is a preceding viral respiratory infection, but others include allergic rhinitis or anatomic abnormalities causing obstruction at the ostia draining the sinuses. These may be tumors, polyps, or foreign bodies, including nasal tubes in hospitalized patients.

Acute sinusitis usually causes facial pain and purulent nasal discharge. Other features present in many patients include fever, headache, and nasal congestion. Tenderness may be present over the sinus but its absence is common. Transillumination of the maxillary and frontal sinuses is useful in excluding infection in these areas if they are completely normal and in confirming infection if they are completely opaque. Equivocal findings are not diagnostically useful. The best simple diagnostic technique is to demonstrate opacity, air-fluid levels, or mucosal thickness on radiography or limited computed tomography (CT) of the sinuses (Fig. 36-1). In both children and adults the most common infecting organisms are *S. pneumoniae* and *H. influenzae*. *M. catarrhalis* is common in children but uncommon in adults. *S. aureus* is quite unusual in both age groups. In nosocomial sinusitis associated with nasal tubes, gram-negative bacilli are the most common cause.[7]

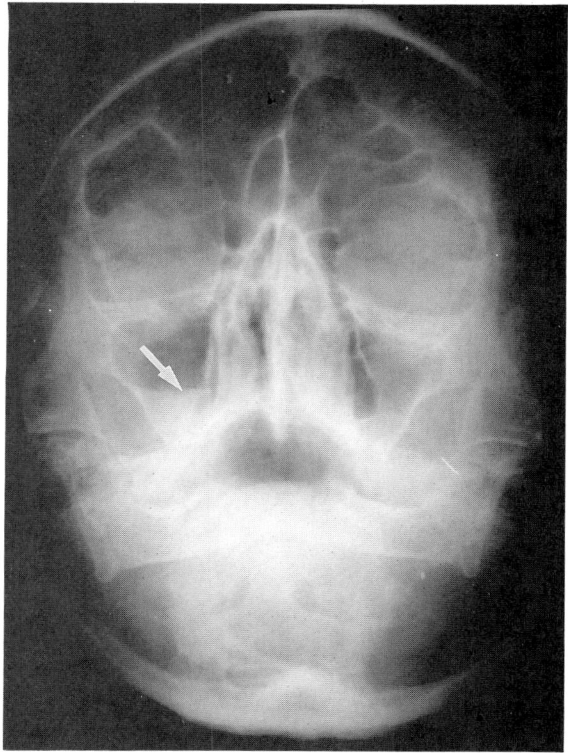

Figure 36-1. Upright sinus film of a patient complaining of right facial pain and purulent nasal drainage. The arrow indicates an air-fluid level in the right maxillary sinus, which taken together with the clinical presentation confirms the diagnosis of acute sinusitis.

Treatment includes nasal decongestants and antimicrobial agents effective against the likely organisms. In outpatients ampicillin (or amoxicillin) or sulfamethoxazole-trimethoprim should be effective. In nosocomial sinusitis aspiration of the infected sinus is probably wise to delineate the precise etiology.

Acute Epiglottitis

Acute epiglottitis,[8] more accurately termed *supraglottitis*, is a bacterial infection of the supraglottic structures, including the epiglottis, aryepiglottic folds, and ventricular bands. It occurs in both children and adults and may cause life-threatening upper airway obstruction. The most commonly responsible organism in both age groups is *H. influenzae*. The most common symptom is a sore throat, which is usually distinguishable on history from uncomplicated pharyngitis by its severity and by the complaint of marked pain on swallowing. When upper airway obstruction develops, dyspnea and stridor occur. Most patients are febrile and many have a hoarse or muffled voice, tender and enlarged cervical lymph nodes, and pooling of saliva. There is usually an increase in the white blood cell count in the blood.

The most helpful examination is indirect laryngoscopy to visualize the swollen epiglottis. Often considered dangerous in children because it can provoke airway obstruction, this procedure appears safe in adults and provides a definitive diagnosis. An alternative is lateral neck radiography, which will show a swollen epiglottis and edema of the arytenoid, aryepiglottic folds, and prevertebral soft tissues (Fig. 36-2). A definitive etiologic diagnosis is usually possible only if blood cultures are positive, which occurs in only about 40 percent of cases. Cultures of the naso- or oropharynx are not helpful since the causative organisms are part of the normal upper respiratory flora. Treatment includes antimicrobial therapy effective against *H. influenzae* and *S. pneumoniae*, the second most frequent cause. Choices include sulfamethoxazole-trimethoprim or a second-generation cephalosporin such as cefuroxime. Maintaining an adequate airway is critical, and most children undergo nasotracheal intubation. Adults without respiratory distress do not require intubation, but those with airway obstruction (about 20 percent of cases) should receive it, with tracheotomy indicated when intubation fails.

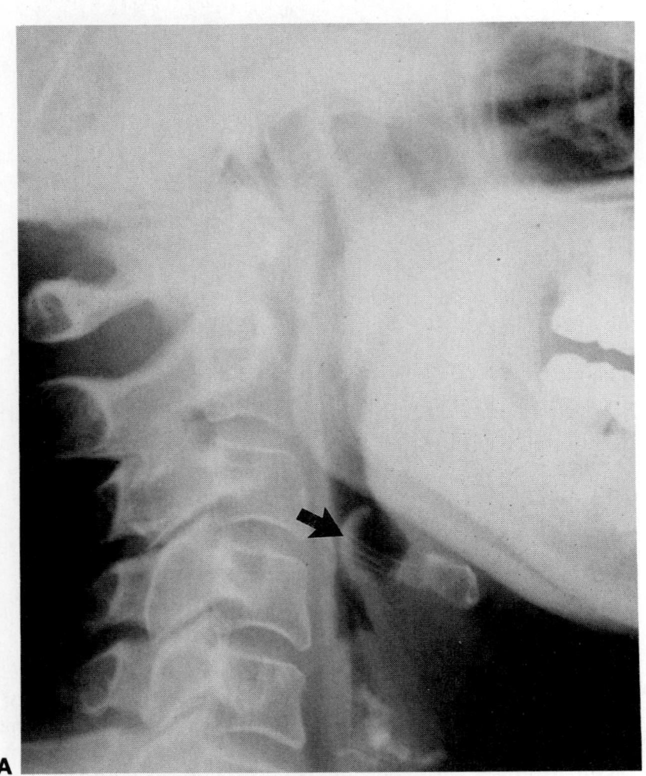

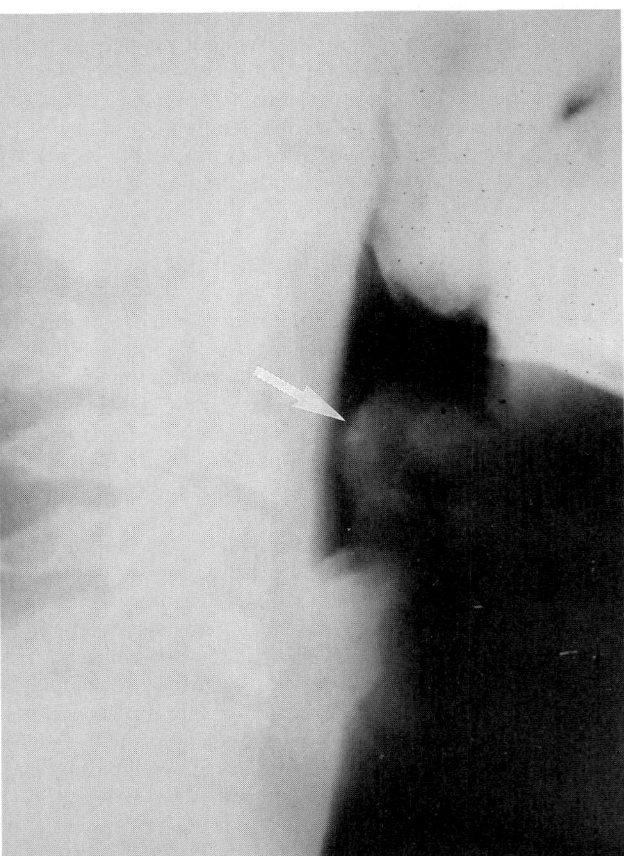

Figure 36-2. (**A**) Normal lateral soft-tissue neck radiograph. (**B**) Acute epiglottitis. This degree of swelling may critically compromise the airway and constitute an immediate threat to life. Arrows indicate the epiglottis.

Acute Laryngotracheobronchitis

Acute laryngotracheobronchitis (croup) is a viral respiratory infection of children, usually occurring between 3 months and 3 years of age. Several viruses may cause it, but parainfluenza is the most common. Both the upper airway and the lower respiratory tract are involved, with inflammation and obstruction being greatest at the subglottic area. Usually rhinorrhea, sore throat, fever, and a mild cough are present for 1 or more days before hoarseness, deepening cough, tachypnea, and inspiratory stridor develop, usually accompanied by chest wall retractions. The cough has a distinctive brassy sound resembling a seal's bark. The diagnosis is usually evident from the history and physical examination; possible confusion with inhalation of a foreign body or acute epiglottitis is resolved by a radiograph of the neck. In croup the films show *subglottic* swelling, whereas in acute epiglottitis the edema is in the *supraglottic* area. Treatment is supportive. Humidification of the inspired air may be beneficial but remains unproved. Seriously ill patients requiring hospitalization are often hypoxemic and need supplemental oxygen. A few become fatigued and develop acute respiratory failure, necessitating nasotracheal intubation, usually for about 3 to 4 days. The mortality rate of croup is about 1 to 2 percent.

Acute Otitis Media

Although predominantly a disorder of children, especially those between 6 months and 2 years of age, infection of the middle ear occurs in all ages. The basic pathogenic mechanism is impaired function of the eustachian tube, which impedes drainage and permits the secretions formed by the mucosa of the eustachian tube to collect behind the obstruction. There is a strong association with preceding upper respiratory viral infections, suggesting that inflammation caused by these organisms may produce the initial obstruction. Later, bacteria present in the normal respiratory flora cause suppuration. In both children and adults the most common organisms cultured from acute otitis media are *S. pneumoniae* and *H. influenzae*. Other frequent isolates include group A streptococci and *M. catarrhalis*.

The usual symptoms are ear pain, hearing loss, or drainage, sometimes accompanied by fever. In very young children irritability, poor eating, and lethargy may be the predominant signs. The diagnosis is confirmed by detection of fluid in the middle ear by otoscopy or tympanometry. This infection is usually managed with ampicillin or amoxicillin, sulfamethoxazole-trimethoprim, or a combination of erythromycin and a sulfonamide. Occasionally, otitis media occurs from eustachian tube obstruction associated with nasotracheal or endotracheal intubation and may cause fever that is unexplained until the ears are carefully examined.

Soft Tissue Infections of the Neck

Infections of certain areas of the neck are important in respiratory care because they can lead to upper airway obstruction.[9,10] These include infections in the submandibular and sublingual spaces, the lateral pharyngeal space, and the retropharyngeal and pretracheal spaces. The anatomy of these areas is complex, but the basic point is that inflammation, suppuration, and edema may compress the oropharynx or trachea, causing respiratory distress. One of the most important of these infections is Ludwig's angina, a bilateral infection of both the submandibular and sublingual spaces usually arising from periapical infection of the second and third mandibular molars. It begins in the floor of the mouth as a rapidly spreading, firm swelling, which causes elevation of the tongue, difficulty in eating and swallowing, and respiratory distress from neck and glottic edema. Patients with this disorder often require tracheal intubation or tracheotomy as well as parenteral antimicrobial therapy, usually penicillin or clindamycin.

Infection of the lateral pharyngeal space (pharyngomaxillary space), which lies in the lateral neck, may occur from dental infections, pharyngitis, or mastoiditis. It may cause upper airway obstruction by creating edema in the larynx. Retropharyngeal space infection, usually caused by the spread of pharyngitis to retropharyngeal lymph nodes in young children, can cause bulging of the posterior pharyngeal wall, narrowing the air column and occasionally rupturing into it to cause asphyxiation or laryngeal spasm. Infection of the pretracheal space usually develops from anterior esophageal perforation and readily compresses the trachea to cause dyspnea. Each of these infections requires surgical drainage and parenteral antibiotics effective against oropharyngeal flora, the bacteria commonly isolated from the infected material. Penicillin or clindamycin is the drug of choice.

LOWER RESPIRATORY TRACT INFECTIONS

The most important lower respiratory infections[11] are acute bronchitis and acute pneumonia.

Acute Bronchitis

Acute bronchitis is an inflammation of the tracheobronchial tree without involvement of the lung parenchyma. It is caused predominantly by viruses and sometimes by *Mycoplasma pneumoniae*, but bacteria are probably not responsible either as a primary etiology or as a complicating superinfection in the absence of pneumonia (lung tissue infection). A large number of viruses can cause acute bronchitis, including rhinovirus, influenza virus, adenovirus, coronavirus, and parainfluenza virus. In many of these infections rhinorrhea, nasal congestion, sore throat, and hoarseness are present in addition to the telltale cough, indicating tracheobronchial inflammation. The cough is usually nonproductive initially unless the patient has underlying lung disease, but sputum production, initially mucoid and then often purulent, commonly occurs later. In normal patients mild changes in pulmonary function develop, uncommonly causing symptoms, but in patients with underlying lung disease, especially chronic obstructive lung disease (COPD), marked bronchoconstriction may occur. Such episodes of acute viral bronchitis often initiate the symptoms of asthma, and they also probably explain a substantial number of acute exacerbations of chronic bronchitis, with increased cough, sputum production, and dyspnea. In normal hosts antimicrobial therapy, even for patients with purulent sputum, is ineffective in altering the course of acute bronchitis uncomplicated by pneumonia. In patients with chronic bronchitis during exacerbations, defined as increased cough and purulent sputum production, the value of antibiotics remains unconfirmed, and viruses or other factors may often be responsible.

Acute Pneumonia

Acute pneumonia is inflammation in the lung parenchyma, the portion of the lower respiratory system distal to the terminal bronchioles. Although the term *pneumonia* can apply to any inflammation, the most common cause is infection, usually bacterial. Organisms can reach the lung parenchyma by four routes: (1) inhalation of an airborne pathogen; (2) aspiration of microbes present in the upper respiratory tract; (3) hematogenous spread to the lungs of organisms present in a distant site; or (4) direct spread to the lung from a contiguous infection or from a penetrating wound. The first two mechanisms account for most pneumonias.

Inhalation

An airborne pathogen may originate from several sites. An infected patient may cough the organism into the air, a mechanism that accounts for the spread of disease due to *M. pneumoniae*, viruses, *M. tuberculosis*, and a few rare bacteria such as *Yersinia pestis*, the organism causing plague. The airborne pathogen may also originate from soil or water and be aerosolized by wind, equipment used in construction or other work in the environment, or machines that involve the spraying of water. Pneumonias resulting from this kind of pathogen spread include those due to *Legionella* spp. (Legionnaires' disease), *Nocardia asteroides*, and various fungi such as *Histoplasma capsulatum, C. immitis*, and *Cryptococcus neoformans*. A third source of airborne organisms causing pneumonia in humans is other animals. Examples include psittacosis, caused by *Chlamydia psittaci* found in birds, and Q fever, caused by *Coxiella burnetii* found in various animals, including cattle and sheep.

The pneumonias caused by airborne pathogens share several features that make accurate and prompt diagnosis difficult. These organisms are very pathogenic, capable of causing disease even if inhaled in small numbers. The density of the organisms in the lung tissue may therefore be small, and they may not grow readily on culture. Most of these pneumonias are not associated with much sputum production, which deprives the clinician of a valuable specimen to inoculate on appropriate media. Most of these organisms are not visible on Gram stain, which prevents the accurate inference about etiology that a revealing sputum specimen can provide in many types of pneumonias. These pathogens typically do not grow on the conventional media used to isolate bacteria. Even with appropriate cultures, growth is often slow and may represent a hazard to laboratory personnel since the organisms are capable of causing disease even when present in such low numbers. Strong evidence of the pneumonia's etiology often rests on serologic testing, which usually requires two blood specimens obtained several weeks apart, allowing only a retrospective diagnosis. All these points emphasize the great importance of inquiring about similar sickness in family or friends, recent travel, occupational or recreational exposure to certain environments, and animal contact in patients with pneumonia. For respiratory disease caused by airborne pathogens, this historical information may provide the only clue to the pneumonia's etiology.

Aspiration

The second pathogenic mechanism causing pneumonia is aspiration of organisms present in the oral cavity or pharynx into the lung. Such aspiration probably occurs frequently, even in normal hosts in small amounts, but pneumonia usually develops only in those with impaired lung defenses. The impairment may involve abnormal swallowing due to esophageal obstruction or motility disturbances; a diminished gag reflex from disorders such as neuromuscular disease or from alcoholism; or anatomic disruption from the presence of a tracheal tube. A main difference between the aspiration that occurs in normal persons and in these patients is probably the *volume* of upper respiratory tract contents that reaches the lung. Impaired mucociliary transport, predisposing the patient to pneumonia, may occur following certain viral infections, especially influenza, which causes necrosis of the bronchial mucosa. It also occurs with cigarette smoking, with tenacious sputum such as exists in cystic fibrosis, and with congenital abnormalities in ciliary function. Immunoglobulin disorders, whether congenital or acquired (such as multiple myeloma) predispose to pneumonias. Impaired white blood cell function, because of inadequate numbers, such as occurs in granulocytopenia due to cytotoxic drug therapy, or because of impaired neutrophil activity, also increases the risk of pneumonia.

In each of these cases the etiology of the pneumonia depends heavily on the flora present in the upper respiratory tract. If an organism capable of producing pneumonia by itself, such as pneumococcus or *H. influenzae*, is present in abundant numbers, this organism will usually be the sole cause. If pathogenic organisms are not present in adequate number and the volume of aspiration is great, a mixed aerobic-anaerobic infection caused by the normal mouth flora may occur, with anaerobes being most important. These organisms are weak pathogens individually but when present together in large numbers, can cause disease.

If the normal respiratory flora has been replaced by enteric gram-negative bacilli because of hospitalization, antimicrobial therapy, or other reasons, the risk of gram-negative bacillary pneumonia understandably increases. Consequently, pneumonias in hospitalized patients are much more likely to be from these organisms than are community-acquired pneumonias.

Certain abnormalities in lung defenses predispose to infections with specific bacteria. For example, pneumococci usually cause pneumonia in patients with hypogammaglobulinemia, and *P. aeruginosa* is the most frequent respiratory pathogen in cystic fibrosis. These factors—the volume of material aspirated, the acquisition in a community or a hospital setting, and the nature of the specific host defense impairment—help to predict the likely pathogen involved.

Hematogenous Spread

A third, uncommon, mechanism in the pathogenesis of pneumonias is hematogenous spread from a distant site, which may occur with certain unusual infections such as tularemia, in which the organism usually causes a cutaneous infection initially. A more frequent source of hemotogenous spread is a site of intravascular infection, especially in patients who use illicit intravenous drugs. The infection may be in a peripheral vein into which the drug was injected or on the tricuspid or pulmonic valve of the heart (endocarditis). Infected clots (septic emboli) from these sites travel by the bloodstream to lodge in the distal portions of the pulmonary arterial system, where they cause vascular occlusion. The infection spreads from the pulmonary vessels into the lung to cause pneumonia, often in several locations because numerous clots can dislodge from the original site of infection.

Direct Extension

A fourth, but very rare, mechanism of pneumonia is infection from penetrating trauma or spread from a contiguous site of infection. Penetrating trauma, if it causes an infection at all, is likely to produce one in the pleural cavity rather than the lung, and primary infections of the chest wall or pleural cavity rarely spread into the underlying lung. Occasionally, however, a malignant or infectious process in the esophagus or mediastinum will erode into the tracheobronchial tree or lung parenchyma to cause pneumonia. Alternatively, an intra-abdominal infection may transgress the diaphragm to infect the lung tissue. An example is an amebic liver abscess penetrating into the lung to cause a right lower lobe pneumonia.

Clinical Features

The clinical features of pneumonia are generally similar whatever the etiologic agent. Fever is common, but no particular pattern accurately identifies the responsible organism. Shaking chills (rigors), either single or multiple, suggest a bacterial rather than a viral or mycoplasmal etiology, but exceptions occur. Cough is present in most patients with pneumonia and may range from an unproductive one to one yielding abundant sputum. Hemoptysis may develop as a small amount of blood streaking the sputum or as a more profuse hemorrhage. Purulent sputum suggests a bacterial process but may be seen in pneumonia from any cause. The only really diagnostic characteristic of sputum is a putrid odor, which denotes an anaerobic infection.

Pleuritic chest pain—characterized as sharp, well localized, and exacerbated by cough, respiration, and movement of the chest—indicates inflammation of the parietal pleura. This symptom, common in bacterial pneumonias, is unusual in those due to viruses, mycoplasmas, or other nonbacterial causes such as psittacosis. Dyspnea is frequent with pneumonias but indicates the extensiveness of pulmonary involvement or the underlying lung disease rather than a specific etiology.

Often, especially in the elderly or debilitated patient, nonspecific extrathoracic symptoms predominate, such as confusion, unexplained fever, decreased appetite, or a general, poorly defined feeling of ill health. With bacteremia or with pneumonias due to certain organisms, myalgias, arthralgias, and headache may be severe, and in some patients a complication of the pulmonary infection, such as meningitis, may dominate the clinical picture.

In most patients the physical examination is abnormal. Tachycardia (heart rate higher than 100 bpm) usually accompanies fever, but a relative bradycardia may be present with certain infections such as psittacosis and Legionnaires' disease. Tachypnea (respiratory rate greater than 16 per minute) is common. With severe infections and especially with bacteremia, blood pressure may be reduced. Dullness to percussion over the area of the pneumonia is common. A frequent abnormality on auscultation is the presence of high-pitched crackles, heard best at the end of inspiration, sometimes only after coughing ("post-tussive rales"). These probably originate from air passing by purulent material in the airways. They may also represent the inspiratory opening of alveoli that had closed during exhalation from compression of the air sacs by inflammatory material. When the bronchi are patent and surrounded by consolidated lung, "bronchial" breath sounds occur. These are lower-pitched and better heard during exhalation than the normal breath sounds. With bronchial obstruction or the presence of pleural fluid, breath sounds may be absent or diminished in intensity. While several other abnormal sounds may occur (e.g., whispered pectoriloquy, etc) these generally provide no additional information of importance. The remainder of the physical examination may provide important clues about the cause of a pneumonia by revealing telltale skin lesions, metastatic foci of infection (such as meningitis or septic arthritis), the site of origin of a pneumonia resulting from hematogenous spread (e.g., a vein infected from the injection of illicit drugs), or a defect in host defenses (e.g., poor gag reflex).

Laboratory Data

The basic laboratory studies to obtain on a patient with pneumonia include a total and differential white blood cell count, blood cultures in seriously ill patients requiring hospitalization, a sputum specimen for Gram stain and culture, and a measurement of arterial blood gases if the patient has significant respiratory distress.

The white blood cell count is somewhat helpful in suggesting whether the process is bacterial. In general, a bacterial pneumonia will cause an increase in white blood cells (leukocytosis), in granulocytes (granulocytosis or neutrophilia), and in the percentage of immature forms ("a shift to the left"). In many nonbacterial pneumonias such as psittacosis, viral infections, or mycoplasma pneumonia, the white blood cells are usually normal in number and distribution. The neutrophils may demonstrate toxic granulation (prominent cytoplasmic granules), cytoplasmic vacuolization, and Dohle bodies (cytoplasmic inclusions); each of these changes is more common in bacterial than in nonbacterial infections. Blood cultures are frequently positive when the pneumonia arises from hematogenous spread, less commonly when it originates from aspiration of oropharyngeal contents. Sputum Gram stains and cultures, the most important diagnostic procedures in most pneumonias, are discussed thoroughly in Chapter 58.

Chest Radiographs

Abnormalities on chest radiographs are necessary to make a valid clinical diagnosis of pneumonia.[12] Only rarely, predominantly in patients with severe neutropenia or the acquired immunodeficiency syndrome (AIDS), will the initial chest radiograph be entirely normal when a parenchymal lung infection is present. Frequently, however, the radiographic abnormalities, which may be minor on initial films, become more extensive during the course of the infection. This can occur even with appropriate therapy because inflammation may continue despite effective eradication of the organisms that initiated it and because certain areas already infected were not radiographically visible because the inflammation had not elicited enough exudation of fluid.

The radiographic pattern cannot accurately predict a pneumonia's cause, but some configurations are more common with certain organisms than with others. Most pneumonias, whether bacterial or not, appear as *bronchopneumonias*, a term usually employed to describe an inhomogenous, patchy, nonlobar opacity that may be in a segmental distribution (Fig. 36-3). A *lobar pneumonia*, however, indicates a homogenous density that extends to involve the entire lobe (Fig. 36-4). This pattern is more common in bacterial than in nonbacterial pneumonia. A cavitary pneumonia indicates the presence of an air-fluid level within the area of opacity, which results from extensive tissue necrosis and nearly always indicates a bacterial, mycobacterial, or fungal etiology. It is, however, rare with *S. pneumoniae* or *H. influenzae* but common with *S. aureus*, enteric gram-negative bacilli, and anaerobes. A diffuse bilateral pneumonia often suggests a nonbacterial cause, especially a virus.

SPECIFIC PNEUMONIAS

Streptococcus pneumoniae Pneumonia

S. pneumoniae (pneumococcus), a resident in the upper airway of a large number of normal hosts, is the most common cause of bacterial pneumonia, which occurs when sufficient numbers of the organism are aspirated into the alveoli.[13–15] The classic description is the abrupt onset of fever, a single shaking chill, pleuritic chest pain, cough, and production of rust-colored sputum in a patient with a preceding viral upper respiratory tract infection. While that pattern may still occur, it was more common years ago, when younger, healthier patients were more frequently infected. Most patients with pneumococcal pneumonia currently are elderly, alcoholic, immunocompromised, or afflicted with chronic lung disease. In this group the clinical findings are usually less dramatic. Patients may have prominent respiratory complaints such as cough and sputum production but the onset may be insidious, with symptoms present for days before seeking medical attention. Many, especially alcoholic or elderly patients, have few or no respiratory complaints and have prominent symptoms of confusion, ill-defined malaise, or unexplained fever. Patients often expectorate no sputum, perhaps because pneumococcal pneumonia causes inflammation not in the bronchi and bronchioles but in the alveoli. The purulent material, therefore, is very distal in the respiratory system and may not be easily expectorated, especially in patients with a poor cough or muscle weakness.

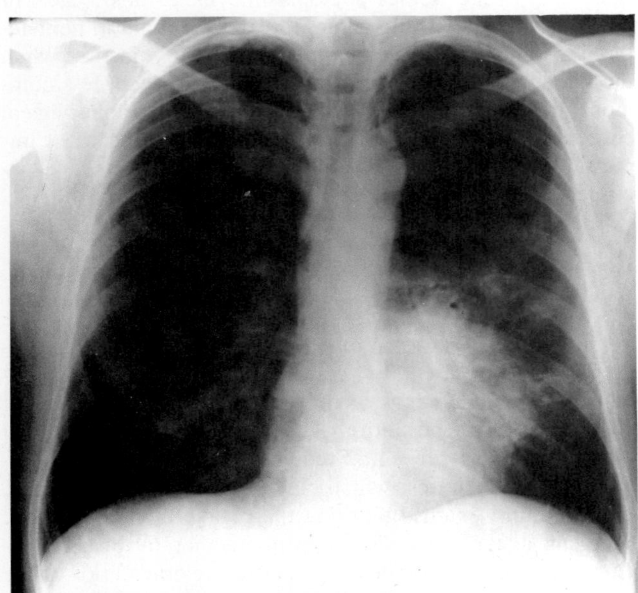

Figure 36-3. Patchy bronchopneumonia due to *S. pneumoniae*, involving the left lower lobe, as seen on the posteroanterior chest radiograph. (From Mandell et al.,[5] with permission.)

Most patients with pneumococcal pneumonia will have an elevated number of white blood cells with an increase in immature forms. Sometimes the white blood cell count is normal, but usually there is still a "shift to the left" (increased immature forms). A decreased white blood cell count (leukopenia) is frequent and is an unfavorable prognostic indicator. Blood cultures are positive for the organism in about 20 to 25 percent of patients. Occasionally, the serum bilirubin is modestly elevated because mild hemolysis (destruction of red blood cells) has released bilirubin into the bloodstream or because of slight inflammation of the liver itself. The chest radiograph typically demonstrates a pneumonia that involves one or more lobes. Because pneumococcal pneumonia is an alveolar-filling process, the radiographic pattern usually shows a fluffy homogeneous opacity surrounding visible, patent airways, producing an *air bronchogram*. Consolidation of much of an individual lobe is common as exudate spreads from alveolus to alveolus via the communicating channels (the alveolar pores of Kohn). Pleural effusions are common if diligently sought with decubitus views, but infected pleural fluid (empyema) occurs in less than 5 percent of cases.

Haemophilus influenzae Pneumonia

H. influenzae[16,17] is a gram-negative bacillus whose morphology on Gram stain ranges from nearly round organisms to long but slender bacilli. The organisms are therefore described as pleomorphic (many-shaped) gram-negative coccobacilli. *H. influenzae* is part of the normal upper respiratory flora and can exist as encapsulated or unencapsulated organisms. Most of those in the upper airway and those causing pneumonia in adults are unencapsulated. Those with capsules belong to one of six types, A to F, of which type B is most common and most virulent. *H. influenzae* pneumonias in children are usually due to type B.

Adult patients with *H. influenzae* pneumonia typically have COPD and/or alcoholism. Patients with chronic bronchitis are particularly at risk since their tracheobronchial tree is often colonized with this organism because of impaired mucociliary transport mechanisms. Healthy people, how-

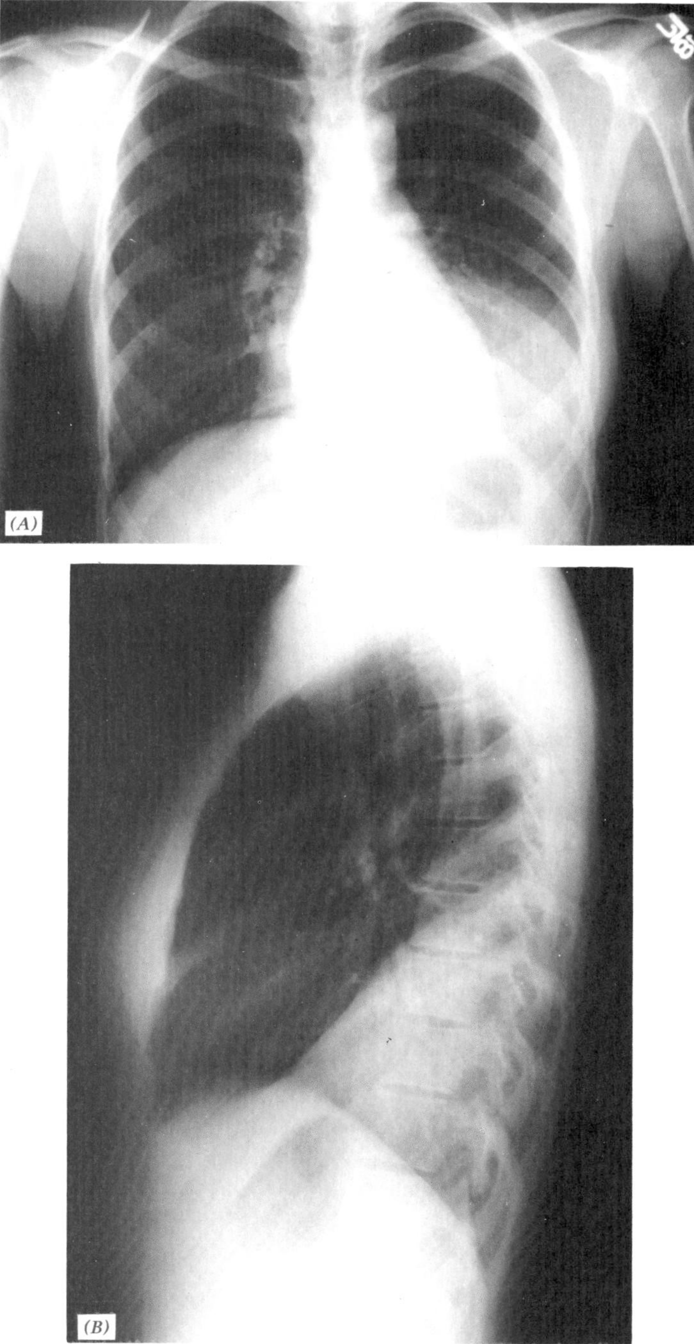

Figure 36-4. Lobar pneumonia due to *S. pneumoniae*, involving the left lower lobe: (**A**) frontal (posteroanterior) view; (**B**) lateral view. (From Mandell et al.,[5] with permission.)

ever, may also be affected, and in one study *H. influenzae* was the most common cause of bacterial pneumonia in military recruits. In some series it is the second most common cause of community-acquired bacterial pneumonia. It has no characteristic clinical features, ranging from a pneumonia with a dramatic onset of fever, chills, and sputum production to an insidious process with mild fever, increased sputum purulence, and worsening dyspnea.

Most patients have leukocytosis and an increased number of immature forms in the white blood cell count. *H. influen-*

zae pneumonia is pathologically a bronchopneumonia, with inflammation in the bronchi and surrounding parenchyma. The organism appears to be very irritating to the bronchi since sputum production is virtually uniform and profuse in infected patients. The chest radiograph usually demonstrates a patchy inhomogeneous pneumonia (bronchopneumonia) or, less commonly, a homogeneous alveolar (airspace) consolidation. Cavitation is very rare. Pleural effusions are common, and *H. influenzae* can cause a rapid pleural space infection.

Moraxella catarrhalis Pneumonia

M. catarrhalis (formerly *Branhamella catarrhalis*), a gram-negative coccus occurring in pairs (diplococci), is part of the normal respiratory flora. It can cause acute otitis media and acute sinusitis. It can also cause pneumonia, almost exclusively in patients with serious underlying disorders, especially COPD.[18] There are no distinctive clinical features, but the onset is not usually dramatic, and fever is generally mild.

Most patients have a leukocytosis, and there is often a striking increase in band forms. As with most pneumonias the lower lobes are predominantly involved on the chest radiograph. About equal numbers of cases have single and multiple lobe involvement, predominantly as patchy bronchopneumonia, but a few have an airspace infiltrate. Large pleural effusions are uncommon, cavitation rare.

Meningococcal Pneumonia

Neisseria meningitidis is a gram-negative diplococcus, which may be present in the upper respiratory tract transiently, intermittently, or chronically. The carriage rate in the general population varies considerably in different studies, with a prevalence rate of 2 to 15 percent in nonepidemic circumstances. It is an unusual cause of pneumonia, being especially likely to occur in military recruits or alcoholics.[19] Most cases have no distinctive clinical features, and the dramatic complications of meningococcemia (fever, hypotension, and purpuric skin lesions) or meningococcal meningitis rarely occur. Leukocytosis is usually present. The chest radiograph typically demonstrates unilateral airspace pneumonia. Cavitation rarely, if ever, occurs, but bilateral involvement and pleural effusions are occasional.

Staphylococcus aureus Pneumonia

S. aureus is present in the anterior nares of about 20 percent of the general population but is an unusual cause of pneumonia except in special circumstances.[20] Classically, *S. aureus* pneumonia follows an attack of influenza, although it is a less frequent cause than *S. pneumoniae* in that situation. Ordinarily, the patient, who usually has a serious underlying disease, has a typical attack of influenza and appears to be improving for a few days when fever recurs. Cough and sputum production develop, with evidence of pneumonia on physical examination and chest radiograph. Staphylococcal pneumonia may also be seen as septic pulmonary emboli complicating illicit intravenous drug use, the source of emboli being an infected vein or endocarditis on the tricuspid or pulmonic valves. In these patients or others with septic pulmonary emboli from intravascular infection, the onset is often associated with pleuritic chest pain, hemoptysis, and dyspnea. A third, very common, setting is in hospitalized patients who develop pneumonia.

A brisk leukocytosis is usual. The chest radiograph in patients without septic pulmonary emboli shows a bronchopneumonia, usually multilobar and often bilateral, with a marked tendency to cavitate. In children the abscess cavities may enlarge because of a check valve mechanism to form thin-walled pneumatoceles. This complication is unusual in adults. Pleural effusions are common and are often infected. When septic emboli occur, the chest film typically shows several nodules throughout the lung, especially at the periphery. Cavitation is common, as are pleural effusions. Cavities in all forms of staphylococcal pneumonia may erode into the pleural cavity to cause a pneumothorax, a pyopneumothorax, or an empyema.

Streptococcal Pneumonia

Group A streptococci (*S. pyogenes*) and group B streptococci (*S. agalactiae*) are gram-positive cocci, which form chains on Gram stain and occasionally cause pneumonia.[21,22] Group A streptococci colonize the throats of a small minority of adults. Group B streptococci are common in the oropharynx and seem to cause pneumonia in debilitated patients who are elderly, diabetic, receiving corticosteroid therapy, or afflicted with chronic renal failure or malignancies. The onset of group A streptococcal pneumonia is usually abrupt, with fever, shaking chills, and a cough productive of purulent, often bloody, sputum. The chest radiograph typically demonstrates a patchy pneumonia, which may cavitate. One striking feature is the remarkable tendency to cause rapid infection of the pleural space. Group B streptococcal pneumonia has no distinctive clinical features; cavitation or pleural effusions seem unusual, however.

Anaerobic Lung Infections

Anaerobic bacteria can cause three types of lung infections: anaerobic pneumonia, anaerobic necrotizing pneumonia, and lung abscess.[23] Empyemas (see subsequent section) can often complicate these infections. Since most anaerobes are weak pathogens individually, anaerobic lung infections generally involve several organisms rather than just a single species. Because infection usually develops only with aspiration of large volumes of upper airway contents, most infected patients have some predisposition to aspiration, such as impaired consciousness (from alcoholism, cerebrovascular disease, drug overdose, etc) or altered swallowing because of neuromuscular disease, esophageal obstruction, or other reasons. The distinction among the types of infection is based on radiographic appearance. A lung abscess has a cavity at least 2 cm in diameter, necrotizing pneumonia has several small areas of cavitation, and anaerobic pneumonia consists of an infiltrate without cavitation.

Patients with anaerobic pneumonia without cavitation generally have a history of a few days of fever, cough, and sputum production. The sputum is rarely putrid. The white blood cell count is ordinarily increased, with an average of about 14,000/mm^3. The sputum Gram stain in this as in other anaerobic pulmonary infections demonstrates a wide variety of organisms, including gram-positive cocci, gram-positive bacilli, gram-negative cocci, and gram-negative bacilli. Since anaerobes are normally present in expectorated sputum, samples to delineate the cause must come from transtracheal aspirates, percutaneous needle aspiration, surgical resection, or perhaps through bronchoscopy with a specialized sampling catheter. These procedures are not usually warranted, but such specimens have typically yielded a mixed flora of aerobic and anaerobic organisms. In about 35 percent of cases anaerobes alone are isolated. The anaerobes most frequently cultured are *Fusobacterium nucleatum* (a spindle-shaped gram-negative rod), *Bacteroides melaninogenicus* (a pleomorphic gram-negative bacillus), peptococci and peptostreptococci (gram-positive cocci in clusters and chains), and *Clostridium* spp. (gram-positive bacilli). Aerobic isolates include *S. pneumoniae*, *S. aureus*, and enteric gram-negative bacilli, but these organisms do not appear pathogenic in this circumstance, since treatment directed against anaerobes alone appears effective. The radiographs typically show an infiltrate in the dependent portion of the lung, especially in the basilar segments of the lower lobes.

Necrotizing pneumonia (Fig. 36-5) differs from anaerobic pneumonia not only in its radiographic appearance but also in its clinical presentation. The patients have been ill for a longer time before they seek medical attention, with most patients having been sick for more than 1 week. Putrid sputum is present in over half of cases. Leukocytosis is virtually universal, with white blood cell counts averaging 24,000/mm^3 compared with 14,000 in patients with anaerobic pneumonia without cavitation. The dependent portions of the lung are again involved, but the posterior segments of the upper lobes and superior segments of the lower lobes are more frequent sites than in anaerobic pneumonia. Anaerobes as the sole isolates are more common (70 percent), but the identity of the organisms is similar.

Although a lung abscess can occur with several different kinds of pulmonary infections, including those due to *S. aureus*, enteric gram-negative rods, and other organisms, a frequent form is due to a mixture of aerobic and anaerobic organisms. These patients typically have one to several weeks of symptoms, including fever, anorexia, weight loss, and sputum production, which is putrid in about half of cases. The white blood cell count is usually elevated, averaging about 14,000/mm^3. On chest radiography, the major finding is a fluid-containing cavity greater than 2 cm in diameter, usually located in a dependent portion—the posterior segments of the upper lobes or basilar segments of the lower lobes (Fig. 36-6).

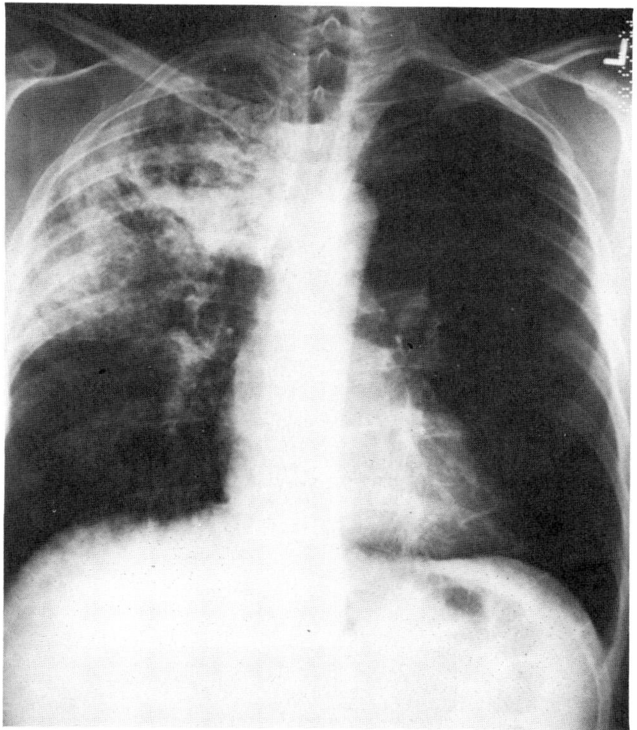

Figure 36-5. Necrotizing pneumonia. The patient was a middle-aged alcoholic man, who presented with a 3-week history of malaise, nausea, fever, chills, and a cough productive of copious foul-smelling sputum. There are multiple small cavitations throughout the right upper lobe. (From Mandell et al.,[5] with permission.)

Enteric Gram-negative Bacillary Pneumonia

Because enteric gram-negative bacilli are not part of the normal upper respiratory flora, they are rare causes of community-acquired pneumonia, even in patients known to have a higher carriage rate of these organisms, such as alcoholics, diabetics, and nursing home residents.[24] An exception is cystic fibrosis, in which colonization is common with *P. aeruginosa*, an organism that appears important in causing pneumonia and febrile exacerbations.

In hospitalized patients, especially those who are very ill, are in intensive care units, and have received antimicrobial therapy, enteric gram-negative rods colonize the oropharynx and become the most common cause of nosocomial pneumonia. The major organisms implicated are *Klebsiella* spp., *E. coli*, and *P. aeruginosa*.

The genus *Klebsiella* includes four species, two of which

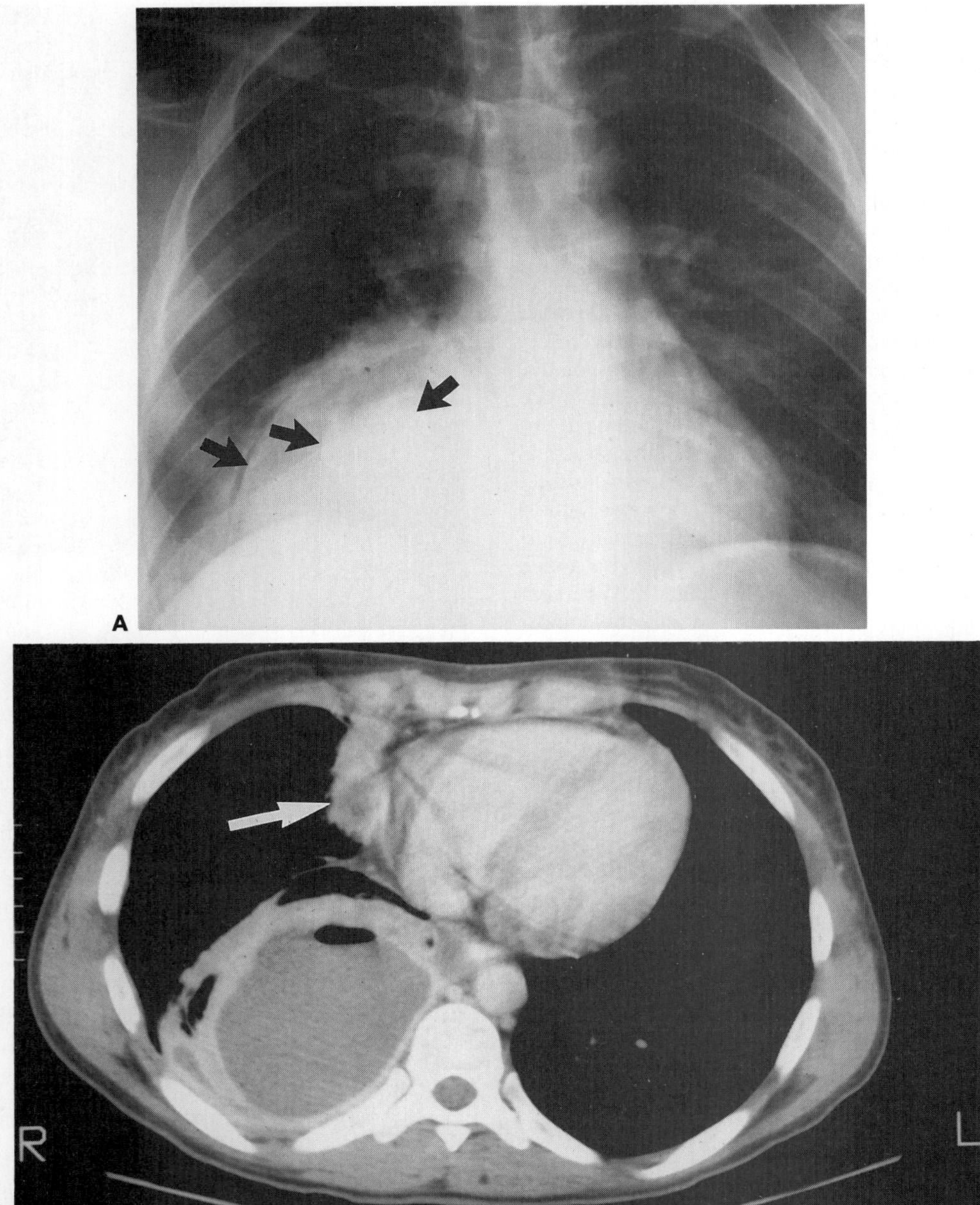

Figure 36-6. A multiloculated lung abscess affecting the right lung, seen on (**A**) posteroanterior chest radiograph and (**B**) computed tomography (CT) of the chest. The conventional chest film (Fig. A) suggests both anterior and posterior fluid collections, each containing air (small arrows). The larger, posterior mass does not obscure the superior heart border or the diaphragm, which are both anterior to it, whereas the smaller, anterior mass (large arrow) effaces the right heart border (silhouette sign). On CT scan (Fig. B), both anterior (arrow) and posterior abscess masses can be distinguished, each consisting of a thick, dense, outer rind encasing a less-dense fluid core. Several air collections are visible in the posterior abscess.

can cause pulmonary infections; these infections are predominantly due to *K. pneumoniae* and much less commonly to *K. oxytoca*. This organism is occasionally found in the oral flora of healthy persons and is part of the normal bowel flora. *E. coli* is also part of the normal bowel flora and can cause pneumonia when aspirated from the oropharynx or as a complication of bacteremia from another site such as an intra-abdominal infection or a urinary tract infection. *P. aeruginosa* is an obligate aerobe found widely in water, soil, and vegetation. It is rarely present in the oropharynx of healthy adults but may occasionally be part of the colonic flora or the skin flora. It is ubiquitous in hospitals, especially in moist environments, and is spread from patient to patient primarily via the hands of hospital personnel. Uncommon causes of gram-negative bacillary pneumonia, even in hospitalized patients, are *Enterobacter, Proteus, Morganella, Providencia*, and *Acinetobacter* spp.

Most commonly, enteric gram-negative bacilli cause pneumonia when they are aspirated into the lung from an oral site. Sometimes, especially with *E. coli* or *P. aeruginosa*, they may spread to the lung via the bloodstream from another site. Occasionally they cause pneumonia when inhaled from contaminated respiratory equipment, especially nebulizers.

The clinical features of gram-negative bacillary pneumonia are not different from those of other bacterial pneumonias. Patients with gram-negative bacillary pneumonia are usually quite ill, however, with high fever, dyspnea, and hypoxemia. Rarely, skin lesions known as *ecthyma gangrenosum* occur in patients with bacteremia. These are erythematous papules or plaques, which rapidly spread and develop bullae, purpura, and necrosis in the center. Common sites are the axilla and the anogenital area. The lesions usually occur with *P. aeruginosa* bacteremia but occasionally with other enteric gram-negative bacilli. Leukocytosis with increased band forms is usual with gram-negative bacillary pneumonia, but leukopenia may also occur. The sputum Gram stain shows gram-negative bacilli, which may be plump or slender, are usually uniform in size, and often show bipolar staining (increased areas of redness at the ends of the rods).

The radiographic patterns of gram-negative bacillary pneumonia are not distinctive. *Klebsiella* pneumonia may cause an airspace pneumonia with bulging fissures because of voluminous secretion, but such a pattern can also be seen with other organisms, including *S. pneumoniae*. *Klebsiella* pneumonia, like other gram-negative bacillary pneumonias, often causes cavitation and pleural effusions. *E. coli* pneumonia is also primarily an airspace pneumonia. With *P. aeruginosa* pneumonia three patterns may occur: extensive bilateral parenchymal consolidation, patchy areas of consolidation with cavitation, or bilateral widespread patchy or nodular shadows. Other organisms cause no distinctive patterns on chest radiographs, but they all have a tendency to cause cavitation and pleural effusions.

Legionella Pneumonia

More than 30 species of *Legionella* exist, although most cases of pneumonia are caused by *L. pneumophila*.[25] They are strictly aerobic pleomorphic gram-negative bacilli, rarely visible on routine Gram stain. They are widespread in the environment, mainly in moist conditions, such as stagnant lakes, soil, and mud. They also thrive in artificial aquatic environments such as plumbing systems, heat exchange units in cooling towers, air conditioners, and evaporative condensers. They prefer warm rather than cold water, especially at temperatures between about 40°C and 60°C. Disease occurs when the organism is inhaled from some aerosol source such as air conditioners, shower heads, or respiratory therapy devices. Person-to-person transmission of disease does not occur.

Legionella pneumonia accounts for about 1 percent of community-acquired pneumonia but has also been associated with hospital epidemics arising from contaminated air conditioning systems or plumbing. Although normal hosts can become infected, risk factors predisposing to pneumonia include cigarette smoking, diabetes mellitus, use of immunosuppressive medication (especially corticosteroids), cancer, and chronic lung, heart, or kidney disease.

The incubation period is about 2 to 10 days. Often a prodrome of weakness, malaise, myalgias, and headache occurs, but symptoms of an upper respiratory infection such as rhinorrhea or stuffy nose are rare. High fever and shaking chills are common and may precede any respiratory symptoms by several hours. Cough is usually moderate and unproductive or initially yields nonpurulent sputum. Pleuritic chest pain is common. Watery diarrhea, abdominal pain, nausea, and vomiting may all occur in the first few days of illness, and confusion or obtundation can be prominent. The fever is generally high (above 39°C), and there may be a relative bradycardia.

The white blood cell count usually reveals a leukocytosis with increased numbers of immature forms. Decreases in serum Na^+ and phosphate may occur, and proteinuria and elevated liver enzymes are frequent. The sputum Gram stain may demonstrate white blood cells, but the organisms are rarely visible. These bacteria do not grow in routine bacterial cultures but will grow in several days when inoculated onto special media. A direct fluorescent antibody test performed on a sputum sample is positive in about 70 percent of patients with the disease, with few false positive results. A serologic test (an indirect fluorescent antibody test) on specimens obtained 6 weeks apart in the acute and convalescent stages of the disease is diagnostic when a fourfold rise to at least 1:128 occurs; a single specimen showing a titer of at least 1:256 is strongly suggestive. Unfortunately, cross-reactions occur with other organisms, and this test usually allows only a retrospective diagnosis.

The chest radiographic appearance varies from rounded nodular infiltrates to patchy opacities to airspace pneumonia. The disease is bilateral in about half of patients, and many have pleural effusions, usually small. Cavitation is rare.

Mycoplasma pneumoniae Pneumonia

The mycoplasmas are the smallest free-living organisms, neither bacteria (because they lack a cell wall) nor viruses (because they grow on cell-free media). *M. pneumoniae* is a pathogen confined to humans and spread by inhalation of organisms coughed or sneezed into the air by an infected subject.[26] Close contact is usually required for disease transmission, which tends to occur in families, schools, and institutionalized populations. It is the most common cause of pneumonia in patients 5 to 20 years of age but may infect people of all ages. It is unusual, however, in patients over 40 years of age, and in them a history of contact with children is almost always present.

The incubation period is about 3 weeks, and the disease usually occurs as one of three syndromes: pharyngitis, tracheobronchitis, or pneumonia. Pneumonia probably occurs in about 5 percent of infected patients. The onset of pneumonia is usually insidious with headache, fever, and malaise, followed in 2 to 4 days by a cough, which is usually prominent and nonproductive but may yield small quantities of purulent or mucoid sputum. Sore throat, earache, hoarseness, and a sense of chilliness are common. The fever is often sustained and frequently exceeds 102°F (39°C). Chest discomfort is common, but genuine pleuritic pain is rare.

The white blood cell count is usually normal or mildly elevated. Levels of 15,000/mm^3 or more occur in 5 percent of cases. The sputum Gram stain shows white blood cells with a few oral bacteria, but mycoplasmas are too small to be visible. The diagnosis rests on isolating the organism on special media, a technique not widely used, or on various blood tests. About 50 percent of patients have elevated levels of cold hemagglutinins (above 1:128). These may also be elevated in other diseases, but the finding allows a presumptive diagnosis of mycoplasma pneumonia. A definitive serologic diagnosis requires a fourfold rise in complement fixation titer between acute and convalescent stage sera.

Psittacosis

Psittacosis[27] is caused by *C. psittaci*, an obligate intracellular organism, transmitted from birds to humans. Most cases are acquired from exotic birds, especially those of the psittacine order, including parrots, parakeets, budgerigars, macaws, cockatiels, and cockatoos. Other avian species are commonly infected, however, including domesticated turkeys and the common pigeon. It is reasonable to assume that any bird species is capable of transmitting the disease. The birds themselves may appear normal or may have such nonspecific features as ruffled feathers, drowsiness, diarrhea, weakness, and drainage from the eyes or nostrils. Since the organism is very infectious, contact with an infected bird need not be protracted or intimate. Mere exposure to an environment in which an infected bird has been present is enough to acquire the organism by inhalation. It is also an occupational disease of those processing poultry, especially those who pluck or eviscerate turkeys. Human-to-human transmission rarely occurs.

The incubation period is usually 1 to 2 weeks (up to 6 weeks) and is followed by an abrupt onset of fever, chills, sweating, myalgias, and headache. The muscle pains and headache are usually severe. Cough typically occurs a few days later and is often mild and usually unproductive. The temperature is usually high, often over 40°C, and, as in *Legionella* pneumonia, the heart rate occasionally may be lower than expected for the degree of fever. Palpable splenomegaly occurs in a small number of patients.

The white blood cell count is usually normal. Because the organisms are not visible, the sputum Gram stain usually reveals white blood cells and a few oral bacteria. The chest radiograph typically shows a patchy, unilateral lower lobe infiltrate but bilateral involvement is common, and occasionally an airspace pneumonia develops. Small pleural effusions can occur, but large ones are rare. Cavitation is virtually unknown. The diagnosis can be established by isolating the organism on cell culture lines (e.g., McCoy or HeLa), but the infectiousness of the organism makes this approach potentially hazardous to laboratory workers. Generally the diagnosis is established by demonstrating a fourfold rise in titer on complement fixation testing of acute and convalescent stage sera.

Chlamydia pneumoniae Pneumonia

Chlamydia pneumoniae, strain TWAR, apparently infects humans only, is transmitted from person to person, and can cause respiratory diseases, including pharyngitis, bronchitis, and pneumonia.[28] Serologic studies suggest that infection occurs sometime during the life of nearly everyone and that reinfection is common in adult life. The incubation period is uncertain but appears long (several weeks). Many infected patients have no symptoms; in those with pneumonia the onset is usually gradual, with sore throat and hoarseness common initially. A cough appears several days to 1 week or more later; fever is uncommon, but headache is frequent.

The white blood cell count is usually normal, and the chest radiograph typically reveals a subsegmental patchy opacity. Most reported cases have occurred in young adults; in older patients the disease may be more severe. This microorganism has been implicated in about 5 to 10 percent of adult community-acquired pneumonias. The definitive diagnosis depends on isolating the organism, which is usually difficult and requires special media, or demonstrating serologic changes with a microimmunofluorescent test, which is not widely available. Often, the diagnosis is suggested by clinical or epidemiologic features.

Q Fever

Q Fever[29] is caused by a rickettsia, *Coxiella burnetii*, a highly pleomorphic, obligate intracellular organism found in wild animals, in domestic livestock such as cattle, sheep, and goats, and occasionally in cats. Humans acquire the infection by inhaling organisms that contaminate the environment from placental and birth fluids of infected animals. Although it may cause abortion in animals, most infected animals are not ill. Human-to-human transmission of disease does not occur.

After an incubation period of 1 to 6 weeks, the disease begins abruptly with severe headaches, myalgias, chills, and fever frequently higher than 104°F (40°C). In many patients pneumonia does not develop; when it does, cough is often a late and mild symptom. Evidence of hepatitis (abdominal pain, hepatomegaly, elevated liver enzymes), can occur with or without pneumonia.

The white blood cell count is usually normal. Sputum, if produced, is unrevealing since the organism is not visible on Gram stain. As with *C. psittaci*, this agent is very infectious, and most laboratories do not attempt its isolation. Instead, the diagnosis requires at least a fourfold rise in titer between acute and convalescent stage sera obtained 2 to 4 weeks apart. The chest radiograph typically reveals a unilateral bronchopneumonia, sometimes with a small pleural effusion.

Viral Pneumonia

While viruses are a common cause of pneumonia in young children, they are a rare cause in immunocompetent adults.[30] In the absence of severely impaired cell-mediated immunity, virtually the only viruses that cause pneumonia with any frequency in adults are varicella and influenza. About 20 percent of young adults have not had varicella (chickenpox) during childhood and are therefore at risk for acquiring it from someone with either varicella or *herpes zoster*, the latter caused by the same virus reactivated from dormancy years after the initial varicella infection. The incubation period of varicella is about 2 weeks. After a short prodrome, which may include fever, myalgia, and arthralgia, skin lesions appear on the scalp or trunk as erythematous papules, which form small blisters (vesicles) that burst and develop a crust. The formation of new lesions usually ends by 4 days. Pneumonia, much more common in adults than in children, usually begins during the first few days after the rash appears. Tachypnea, cough, and dyspnea are the major clinical findings. The cause of the pneumonia is usually obvious because of the presence of the skin lesions, from which the virus can be isolated. With a typical clinical appearance, however, cultures are unnecessary. The chest radiograph typically demonstrates diffuse nodular or mixed interstitial-alveolar infiltrates (Fig. 36-7). Pleural effusion or pneumothorax can occur. Many years later calcification may appear in the areas of the nodules.

Influenza tends to occur in epidemics during the winter months. After an incubation period of 1 to 2 days, fever, chills, headache, myalgias, and arthralgias develop. The muscle aches may involve the back and extremities but may sometimes be prominent in the retro-orbital area, making movement of the eyes painful. Cough, rhinorrhea, sore throat, and hoarseness are also common. The fever is typically high and lasts 1 to 5 days. Because this virus causes destruction of the respiratory epithelium, influenza predisposes to bacterial pneumonia, especially from *S. pneumoniae, H. influenzae*, and *S. aureus*. A primary viral pneumonia or mixed viral-bacterial pneumonia may also occur. Those with primary viral pneumonia often have cardiovascular disease, but it may occur in healthy young people as well. Typically, there is the usual onset of influenza, but instead of improvement over several days, a rapid progression of fever, cough, dyspnea, and cyanosis follows. Leukocytosis is also

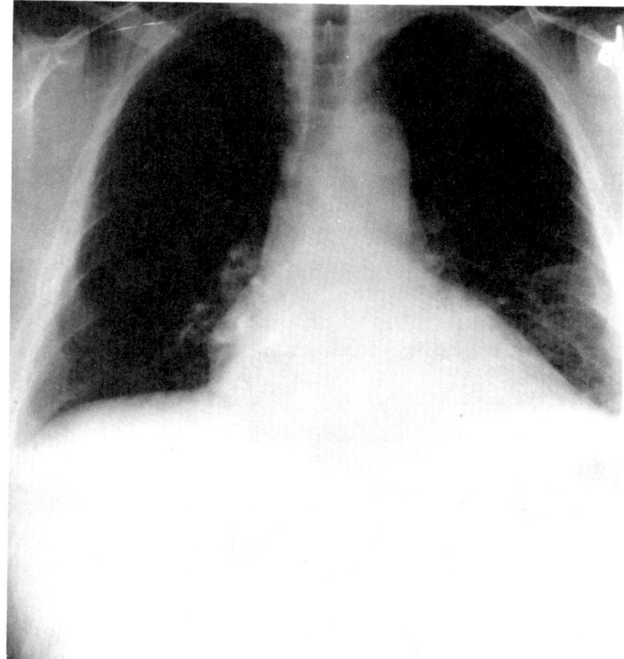

Figure 36-7. Viral pneumonia, showing a bilateral mixed interstitial-alveolar pattern. (From Mandell et al.,[5] with permission.)

typical, but the sputum Gram stain reveals only normal oral flora. The sputum viral culture is positive for influenza. The chest radiograph reveals diffuse bilateral patchy infiltrates resembling pulmonary edema. Sometimes a unilateral infiltrate occurs, usually with a considerably milder clinical picture.

Fungal Pneumonia

In the healthy host, certain fungi, especially *Histoplasma capsulatum* and *Coccidioides immitis*, can cause acute pneumonias.[31,32] Both fungi reside in the soil in certain geographically confined areas and can cause disease when inhaled.

C. immitis grows only in semiarid climates of the Western Hemisphere, mostly in the southwestern United States but also in Mexico and a few other countries of Central and South America. In the United States it is found in six states, mainly in California, Arizona, and western Texas but also in New Mexico, Utah, and Nevada. Most patients with infections have no symptoms, but about 2 weeks after inhalation of the organisms, some develop cough, fever, chest pain, and arthralgias. The diagnosis occasionally is made by growing the organisms from sputum, but it is highly infectious and such cultures should only be handled by experienced laboratories. Person-to-person transmission of disease, however, does not occur. Usually the diagnosis rests on serologic studies, especially the tube precipitins for acute disease. These tests usually become positive 1 to 3 weeks after symptoms begin. The chest radiograph typically reveals a unilateral homogeneous or patchy pneumonia, which may be associated with a pleural effusion and hilar or mediastinal lymph node enlargement. Cavitation may occur.

H. capsulatum grows in soil throughout the world, especially in areas contaminated by bird droppings. In the United States the organism is found mainly in the midwestern states. Most infected patients have no symptoms, but fever, headache, cough, and chest pain may occur. With the inhalation of large quantities of fungi, especially by persons with previous exposure to the organisms, dyspnea may develop. The white blood cell count is typically normal. The diagnosis is usually established by serologic testing with the complement fixation or the agar gel diffusion test. The chest radiograph ordinarily shows patchy infiltrates with or without ipsilateral hilar lymph node enlargement. Following inhalation of large numbers of organisms, the chest radiograph reveals diffuse small nodular infiltrates throughout both lungs. Person-to-person transmission of disease does not occur.

EMPYEMA

Thoracic empyema[33] has many differing definitions, but the simplest is an infection in the pleural cavity. Organisms can arrive there by extension from an underlying pneumonia; from a contiguous mediastinal, vertebral, or intra-abdominal infection; from penetrating trauma, including surgery or the insertion of chest tubes; or rarely, by hematogenous spread from an infection at a distant site. Most cases originate from a contiguous pneumonia or from thoracic surgery.

The usual symptoms are chest pain and fever. Dyspnea often occurs when the infection is extensive or when significant underlying cardiorespiratory disease is present. The onset may be dramatic but often is insidious; in patients with an underlying pneumonia signs of infection (e.g., fever or leukocytosis) may fail to improve as anticipated. With post-surgical or post-traumatic empyema, drainage of purulent material from the chest wound may occur. Other physical findings include diminished breath sounds and dullness to percussion over the involved area. Sometimes the overlying skin is warm, erythematous, and tender on palpation. The white blood cell count is usually elevated. The major clue comes from chest radiography, which reveals the presence of a pleural effusion. When the chest radiographs are confusing, diagnostic ultrasound or CT scans help to delineate the pleural fluid.

Definitive diagnosis of thoracic empyema requires thoracentesis, which usually yields purulent fluid with a high white blood cell count (usually more than 25,000/mm^3), a predominance of neutrophils, and, frequently, organisms visible on Gram stain. The identity of the infecting organisms varies according to the underlying cause. Extension from an underlying pneumonia may be due to a single pathogen such as *S. pneumoniae, S. aureus*, or enteric gram-negative rods, but many cases occur from an extension of a mixed aerobic-anaerobic pulmonary infection or one in which anaerobes alone are present. With purely anaerobic infections in the pleural cavity, as in the lung, several species rather than a single one are usually present. Post-traumatic or postoperative empyemas are typically due to a single organism, either *S. aureus, Streptococcus* spp., or an aerobic or facultative gram-negative bacillus.

TUBERCULOSIS

Tuberculosis[34,35] is caused by the bacterium *M. tuberculosis*, an obligate aerobic bacillus spread from person to person by "droplet nuclei." Patients with pulmonary tuberculosis can cough or sneeze the bacilli into the air. The surrounding moisture dries, and the organism remains suspended in the air, to be inhaled by others minutes to hours later. Because the upper airway and tracheobronchial tree are resistant to this bacillus, infection usually occurs only when it reaches the alveoli. If the person has not had previous infection, the organism replicates there and then spreads via lymphatics to the regional lymph nodes and subsequently into the bloodstream. This hematogenous dissemination probably occurs in all primary infections of tuberculosis but is asymptomatic or associated only with mild systemic complaints. These organisms may lodge in many different organs but prefer sites of high O_2 content, such as the upper lobes of the lung and the renal cortex. Several weeks after the initial infection, cell-mediated immunity against the organism develops; if adequate, the infection halts, and many organisms are destroyed. Live bacilli, however, remain in the body, dormant but capable of causing disease in the future if cell-mediated immunity wanes. In some patients the initial response to infection is inadequate, and progressive pulmonary and/or extrapulmonary disease occurs.

In developed countries the prevalence of active tuberculosis is low and few have been infected. Previous infection is indicated by a positive test to intracutaneous injection of tuberculin (purified protein derivative [PPD]), demonstrated by an area of induration of more than 10 mm in diameter 48 to 72 hours later. Even the elderly in many developed countries have not had previous exposure to tuberculosis. Consequently, primary tuberculosis, as described above, can occur in this age group as well as in the younger patient. Most cases of primary tuberculosis are asymptomatic, and the diagnosis is established, often in retrospect, by demonstrating a positive tuberculin test, sometimes in association with mild radiographic changes indicating previous infection. These include areas of linear opacity representing scars in either the upper or lower lobes, sometimes accompanied by enlarged or calcified hilar lymph nodes on the same side as the lung opacities. When symptoms occur, fever, cough, sputum production, sometimes with weight loss and hemoptysis, typically develop insidiously. In primary symptomatic tuberculosis, the chest radiograph often demonstrates a lower lobe unilateral infiltrate, which may be accompanied by ipsilateral hilar lymph node enlargement. Pleural effusions sometimes occur, and cavitation may develop.

Postprimary or reactivation tuberculosis occurs when a quiescent infection recrudesces, often many years after the initial event. This recurrence usually develops because of diminished cell-mediated immunity caused by old age, concomitant disease, or immunosuppressive therapy. Typically, the patient has a cough, sputum production, and fever, often with weight loss. The usual radiographic appearance is a unilateral or sometimes bilateral upper lobe opacification, characteristically in the apical or posterior segments. Cavitation, either in single or multiple areas, is common (Fig. 36-8).

The diagnosis rests on demonstrating the organism on cultures of sputum, other body fluids, or tissue. The organism requires 2 to 6 weeks to grow on the special media employed to isolate the tubercle bacillus, although new microbiologic techniques may allow presumptive identification of cultures in 1 to 2 weeks. An immediate presumptive diagnosis can be made when the expectorated sputum demonstrates the organism on special stains, either the Ziehl-Neelsen stain or one using fluorochrome dyes, auramine or rhodamine.

Miliary tuberculosis is a form of disseminated tuberculosis in which foci of infection, hematogenously spread throughout the body following either primary infection or reactivation, grow and proliferate, causing death in days to weeks if appropriate chemotherapy is not instituted. A characteristic picture on chest radiography is one in which all lung areas demonstrate fine, millet seed-sized nodules (Fig. 36-9). Because active pulmonary tuberculosis may not be present and the widespread pulmonary nodules originate in the circulation rather than the airways, sputum smears and even cultures are often negative for tubercle bacilli. Diagnosis

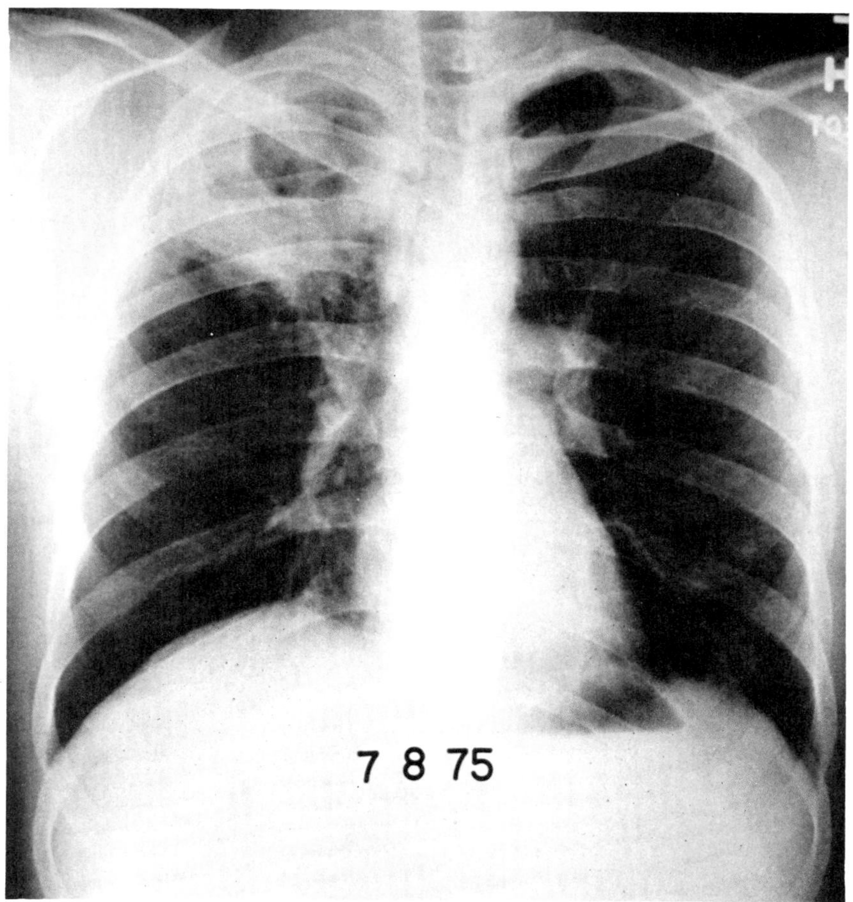

Figure 36-8. Cavitary tuberculosis involving mainly the right upper lobe. There is a large, thick-walled cavity surrounded by parenchymal infiltrate, and there has been loss of volume in the lobe as shown by the elevation of the transverse fissure. (From Mandell et al.,[5] with permission.)

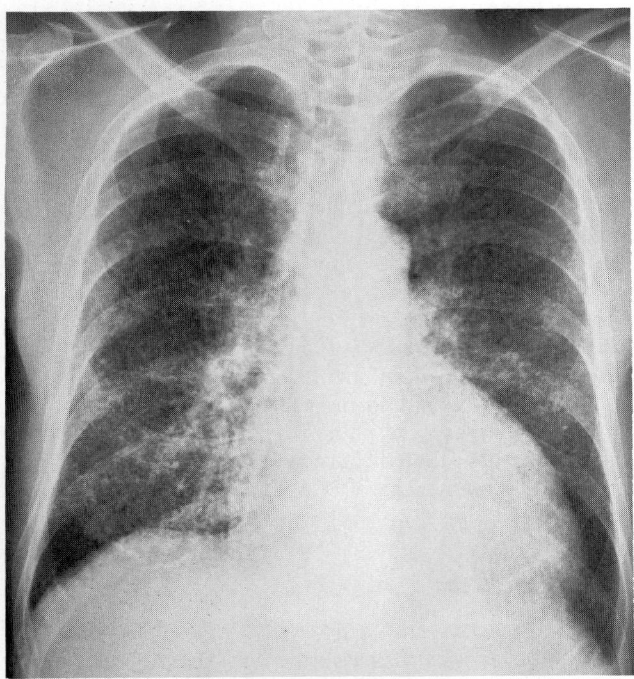

Figure 36-9. Miliary tuberculosis. There are fine, fairly discrete, nodular opacities distributed throughout all portions of both lungs. (From Blank,[36] with permission.)

usually requires transbronchial lung biopsy or examination of tissue from bone marrow, liver, or other sites.

References

1. Mackowiak PA: The normal microbial flora. N Engl J Med 1982;307:83–93
2. Toews GB: Nosocomial pneumonia. Am J Med Sci 1986;291:355–367
3. Mackowiak PA, Martin RM, Jones SR, Smith JW: Pharyngeal colonization by gram-negative bacilli in aspiration-prone persons. Arch Intern Med 1978;138:1224–1227
4. Lennette EH, Balows A, Hausler WT, Shadomy HJ et al (eds): Manual of Clinical Microbiology. 4th Ed. American Society for Microbiology, Washington, 1985
5. Mandell GL, Douglas RG, Bennett JE (eds): Principles and Practice of Infectious Diseases. 3rd Ed. Churchill Livingstone, New York, 1990; pp. 489–584
6. Lowenstein SR, Parrino TA: Management of the common cold. Adv Intern Med 1987;32:207–233
7. Caplan ES, Hoyt NJ: Nosocomial sinusitis. JAMA 1982; 247:639–641
8. Sheikh KH, Mostow SR: Epiglottitis—an increasing problem for adults. West J Med 1989;151:520–524
9. Blomquist IK, Bayer AS: Life-threatening deep fascial space infections of the head and neck. Infect Dis Clin North Am 1988;2:237–264
10. Bartlett JG, Gorbach SL: Anaerobic infections of the head and neck. Otolaryngol Clin North Am 1976;9:655–678
11. Mandell GL, Douglas RG, Bennett JE (eds): Principle and Practice of Infectious Diseases. 3rd Ed. Churchill Livingstone, New York, 1990, pp. 529–564
12. Fraser RG, Pare JAP, Pare PD et al: Diagnosis of Diseases of the Chest. 3rd Ed. WB Saunders, Philadelphia, 1988, pp. 774–1081
13. Kantor HG: The many radiologic facies of pneumococcal pneumonia. AJR 1981;137:1213–1220
14. Jay SH, Johanson WG, Pierce AK: The radiographic resolution of *Streptococcus pneumoniae* pneumonia. N Engl J Med 1975;293:798–801
15. Murphy TF, Fine BC: Bacteremic pneumococcal pneumonia in the elderly. Am J Med Sci 1984;288:114–118
16. Hirschmann JV, Everett ED: *Haemophilus influenzae* infections in adults: Report of nine cases and a review of the literature. Medicine (Baltimore) 1979;58:80–94
17. Pearlberg J, Haggar AM, Saravolatz L et al: *Hemophilus influenzae* pneumonia in the adult. Radiology 1984;151:23–26
18. Wright PW, Wallace RJ, Shepherd JR: A descriptive study of 42 cases of *Branhamella catarrhalis* pneumonia. Am J Med, suppl. 5s, 1990;88:5A-2S–5A-8S
19. Irwin RS, Woelk WK, Coudin WL: Primary meningococcal pneumonia. Ann Intern Med 1975;82:493–498
20. Kaye MG, Fox MJ, Bartlett JG et al: The clinical spectrum of *Staphylococcus aureus* pulmonary infection. Chest 1990;97:788–792
21. Braman SS, Donat WE: Explosive pleuritis: Manifestation of group A beta-hemolytic streptococcal infection. Am J Med 1986;81:723–726
22. Verghese A, Berk SL, Boelen LJ, Smith JK: Group B streptococcal pneumonia in the elderly. Arch Intern Med 1982;142:1642–1645
23. Bartlett JG, Finegold SM: Anaerobic infections of the lung and pleural space. Am Rev Respir Dis 1974;110:56–77
24. Levison ME, Kaye D: Pneumonia caused by gram-negative bacilli: An overview. Rev Infect Dis suppl. 4, 1985;7:S656–S665
25. Nguyen MLT, Yu VL: *Legionella* infection. Clin Chest Med 1991;12:257–268
26. Mansel JK, Rosenow EC, Smith TF, Martin JW: *Mycoplasma pneumoniae* pneumonia. Chest 1989;95:639–646
27. Hirschmann JV: Psittacosis. Med Grand Rounds 1982;1:57–66
28. Thom DH, Grayston JT: Infection with *Chlamydia pneumoniae* strain TWAR. Clin Chest Med 1991;12:245–256
29. Marrie TJ: Q fever pneumonia. Semin Respir Infect 1989;4:47–55
30. Ruben FL, Nguyen MLT: Viral pneumonitis. Clin Chest Med 1991;12:223–235
31. Bayer AS: Fungal pneumonias. Pulmonary coccidioidal syndrome. Chest 1981;79:575–582; 686–691
32. Goodwin RA, Loyd JE, Des Prez RM: Histoplasmosis in normal hosts. Medicine (Baltimore) 1981;60:231–266
33. Lemmer JH, Botham MJ, Orringer MB: Modern management of adult thoracic empyema. J Thorac Cardiovasc Surg 1985;90:849–855
34. Mangura BT, Mangura CT, Reichman LB: Tuberculosis and the atypical pneumonia syndrome. Clin Chest Med 1991;12:349–362
35. Bass JB, Farer LS, Hopewell PC, Jacobs RF: Treatment of tuberculosis and tuberculous infection in adults and children. Am Rev Respir Dis 1986;134:355–363
36. Blank N: Chest Radiographic Analysis. Churchill Livingstone, New York, 1989

Chapter 37

Effects of Smoking on the Cardiorespiratory System

David A. Schwartz

CHAPTER OUTLINE

> Tobacco is a filthy weed, and the custom is loathsome to the eye, hateful to the nose, harmful to the brain, dangerous to the lungs, and the black stinking fume thereof nearest resembling the horrible Stygian smoke of the pit that is bottomless.[1]

This somewhat dramatic but accurate condemnation of tobacco smoke was espoused by King James I in 1604. Unfortunately, many individuals have not heeded these remarks. Currently, more than one of every six deaths in the United States is directly related to cigarette smoking.[2,3] Smoking accounts for 30 percent of all cancer deaths (87 percent of all lung cancer is caused by cigarette smoking), 21 percent of deaths due to coronary artery disease, 18 percent of those caused by strokes, and 82 percent of deaths from chronic obstructive pulmonary disease (COPD).[2] In fact, it has recently been estimated that 390,000 Americans died in 1985 alone as a direct result of cigarette smoking.

This chapter reviews the basic epidemiology of cigarette-related morbidity and mortality in the context of injury and neoplasia to the heart and lungs. Although the vast majority of persons in the United States who develop COPD and/or lung cancer are or have been cigarette smokers, not all smokers develop these problems. This indicates that other etiologies (see Ch. 38) and/or factors specific to the host may contribute to the development of these diseases.

COMPOSITION OF CIGARETTE SMOKE

Tobacco is obtained from a variety of different plants of the nightshade family. Various species have been developed that have vastly different physical and chemical properties. The constituents of cigarettes are influenced further by soil, climate, and post-harvest processing. In fact, several techniques, including crop selection, reduced use of pesticides, improved curing methods, and use of filters, have substantially reduced the tar, nicotine, and other toxic components of cigarette smoke.

Cigarette smoke represents a complex mixture of respirable particles (over 2000 separate chemicals) and gaseous agents.[4,5] One cigarette produces approximately 500 mg of smoke with 5 to 10 percent particulate matter, 12 to 15 percent CO_2, and 3 to 6 percent CO. The major toxic components of cigarette smoke are listed in Table 37-1.

The toxicity of tobacco smoke is dependent on the toxicity of the smoke itself, the amount and depth of inhalation, and the duration of smoking. Although low-yield cigarettes ap-

Table 37-1. Major Toxic Components of Cigarette Smoke

Particulate chemicals
Cresols
Hydroquinone
Nicotine
Pesticides
Phenol
"Tar"
Gaseous components
Acetaldehyde
Acrolein
Acrylonitrile
Ammonia
Benzopyrene
Carbon monoxide
Formaldehyde
Hydrazine
Hydrogen cyanide
Nitrosamines
Oxides of nitrogen
Urethane
Vinyl chloride

pear to decrease the risks associated with lung cancer,[6,7] smokers tend to compensate,[8,9] and the use of low-yield cigarettes has not been shown to diminish the risk of developing COPD.[10,11] In fact, several studies[10–12] indicate that the primary health effect of low-yield cigarettes is to decrease the prevalence of cough and phlegm production. However, these modifications appear to have very little effect on the level or rate of decline of lung function. The cumulative exposure to cigarette smoke (cigarettes per day, years smoked, or pack-years) remains the most potent predictor of decline in lung function.[13,14] This relationship is illustrated in Figure 37-1, in which pack-years of smoking is shown to directly influence the forced expiratory volume in 1 second (FEV_1).

CARDIOVASCULAR DISEASE

Cigarette smoking has a direct impact on cardiovascular morbidity and mortality. Overall, it is associated with 30 percent of deaths due to chronic heart disease and has been

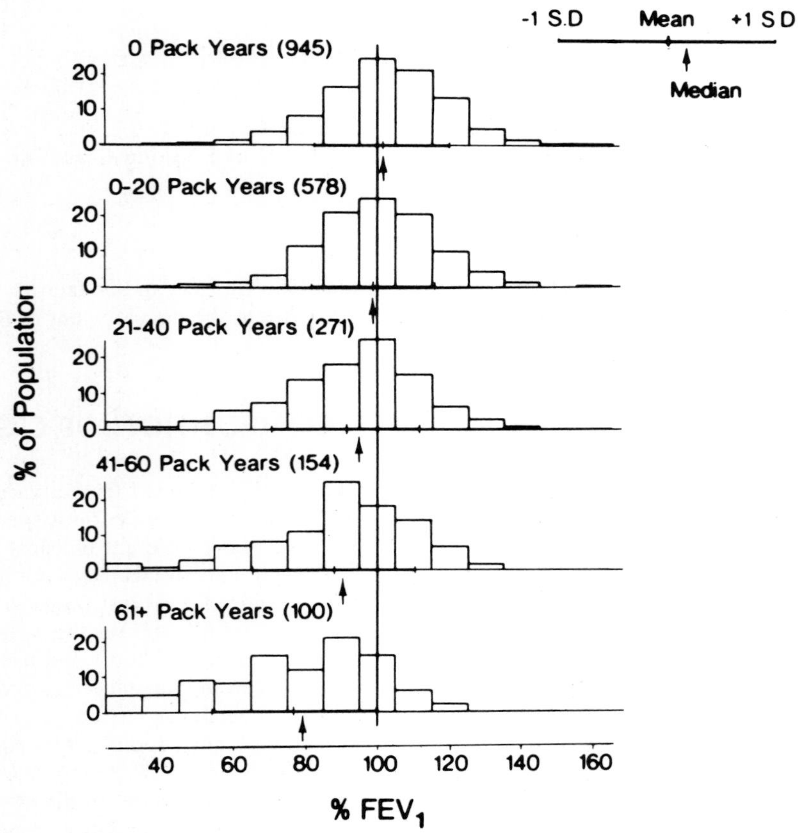

Figure 37-1. Distribution of percent predicted FEV_1 in subjects with different smoking histories. Means, medians, and ±1 SD of the data for each group are displayed on the x axis. Numbers in parentheses indicate the number of subjects in each smoking category. (From Burrows et al.,[13] with permission.)

reported to be a major contributor to morbidity and mortality from coronary artery disease, cerebrovascular disease, and peripheral vascular disease.[2] In fact, the most prevalent and potentially lethal consequence of cigarette smoking is premature coronary artery disease.

Cigarette smoking enhances the prevalence of clinical heart disease; however, it also results in a greater extent of clinically silent lesions.[15–17] An autopsy study demonstrated that heavy smokers had 50 percent more coronary atherosclerosis and 100 percent more abdominal aortic disease than nonsmokers.[17]

However, the mechanisms linking cigarette smoke and cardiac disease are not well understood. Components of cigarette smoke, such as nicotine and CO, may have direct physiologic effects on the cardiovascular system. In fact, the level of carboxyhemoglobin in smokers is directly related to the prevalence of atherosclerotic heart disease.[18] Of more interest is the potential ability of cigarette smoke to promote atherosclerosis by altering plasma lipoprotein levels,[19,20] directly damaging vascular endothelial cells, promoting platelet activation, and enhancing the mitogenic activity of smooth muscle cells and fibroblasts.[21] Although these cellular events are well substantiated in the laboratory, their importance in the pathogenic relation between cigarette smoke and heart disease is not well understood.

Cessation of smoking results in a dramatic and substantial reduction in death rates associated with cardiovascular heart disease.[22] Ten years following cessation, the cardiovascular heart disease death rate for former smokers is similar to that of lifetime nonsmokers. Moreover, smoking cessation decreases the mortality associated with coronary artery bypass surgery, reduces the morbidity and mortality associated with peripheral vascular disease, and decreases the mortality for postmyocardial infarction patients.

DISEASE OF THE AIRWAYS

The association between cigarette smoking and both chronic bronchitis and COPD has been well established through carefully designed epidemiologic studies that were completed by the mid-1960s.[23–32] These studies conclusively demonstrate that cough and phlegm production are more prevalent among cigarette smokers and that cigarette smokers are at risk for developing impaired lung function characterized by airflow obstruction. These findings are further supported by pathologic studies,[33,34] which demonstrated the focal inflammatory changes in the small airways and the centrilobular emphysema that are characteristically found in individuals with a history of prolonged cigarette use. In aggregate, these studies led to the 1964 landmark report by the U.S. Surgeon General, which authoritatively linked cigarette smoking and chronic airflow obstruction.[35]

Although there is clear and consistent evidence to support the causal relationship between cigarette smoking and chronic airflow obstruction, a number of important issues remain unresolved. In 1977, Burrows et al. showed that cumulative exposure to cigarettes is inversely related to the FEV_1[13] (Fig. 37-1). However, Fletcher and Peto[36] have shown that many cigarette smokers never develop airflow obstruction from smoking (Fig. 37-2). Thus, factors that are specific to the host, such as childhood infections, atopic status, occupational exposures, and protease phenotypes may influence the effect of cigarette smoke on the lungs. The relative importance of these factors in the development of COPD remains an area of intense investigation and controversy. Moreover, Figure 37-2 indicates that within 2 to 3 years of stopping smoking, the decline in lung function in former smokers is similar to that in nonsmokers. However, it appears that lost lung function is not regained after quitting

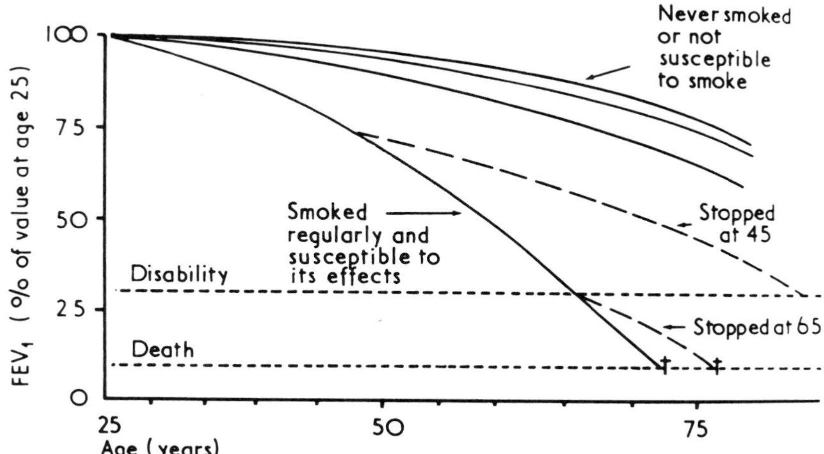

Figure 37-2. Decline in FEV_1 as a function of cigarette smoking and age in men. † denotes death due to COPD. (From Fletcher and Peto,[36] with permission.)

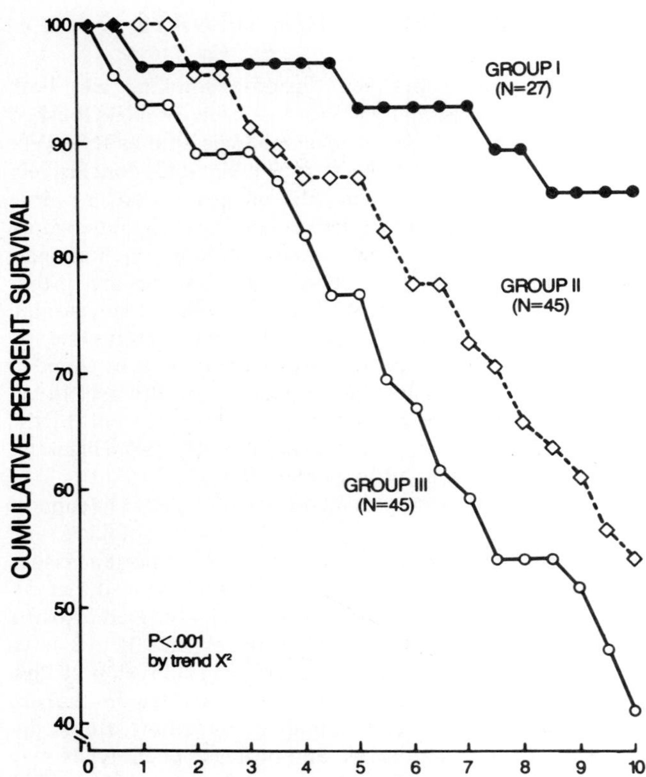

Figure 37-3. Comparison of 10-year survival rates between nonsmoking, nonatopic asthmatics (group I), nonatopic smokers with COPD (group III), and subjects with airflow obstruction who did not clearly fit into either group I or group III (group II). (From Burrows et al.,[38] with permission.)

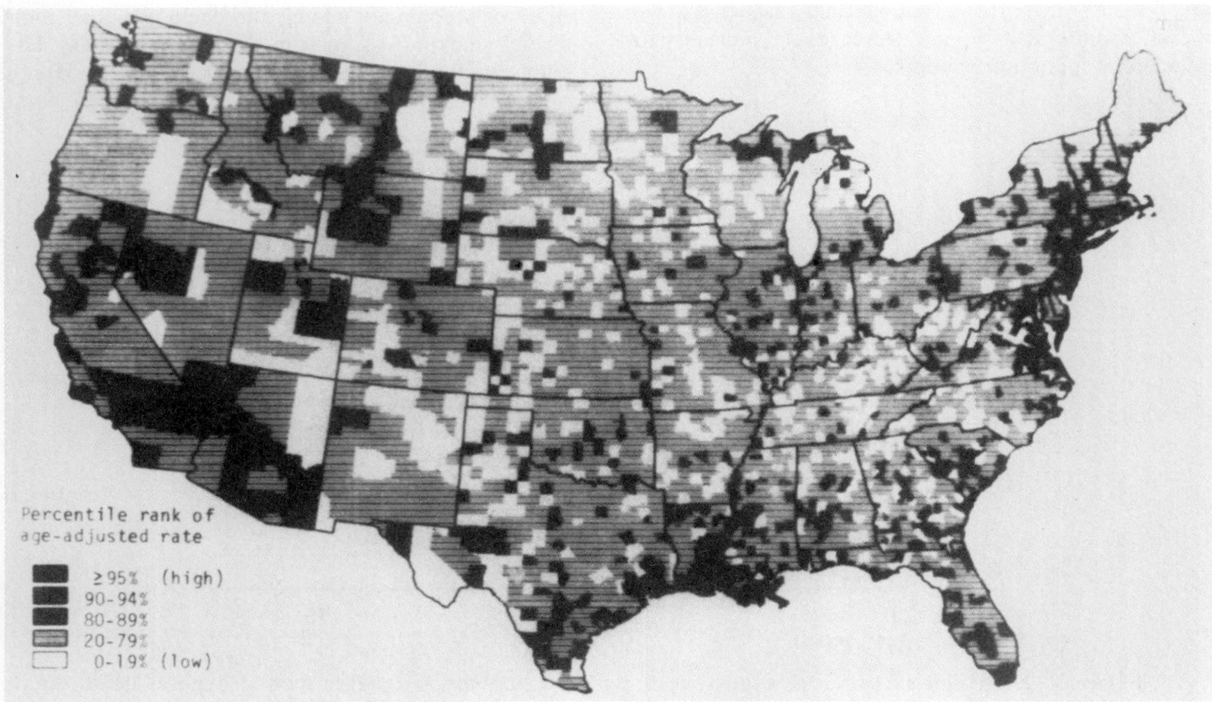

Figure 37-4. Age-adjusted lung cancer mortality for white men by county. (From Blot and Fraumeni,[47] with permission.)

cigarette smoking.[36,37] In 1987 Burrows et al.[38] showed that patients with asthmatic bronchitis have a different prognosis than those with typical COPD associated with smoking; the latter patients tend to lose lung function at a faster rate and to have a diminished 10-year survival (Fig. 37-3). Moreover, among persons with COPD, the postbronchodilator FEV_1 has been shown to be a better predictor of survival than the FEV_1 measured before use of bronchodilators.[38,39] These findings indicate that different pathogenic mechanisms are probably involved in asthmatic bronchitis and typical COPD, and that therapy directed at the asthmatic component of chronic airflow obstruction may improve survival. Although controversy still exists regarding the effect of passive smoking on chronic respiratory symptoms in adult nonsmokers,[40] several studies have shown an increased frequency of respiratory problems among children of smoking parents as compared with children of nonsmoking parents.[41,42]

LUNG CANCER

Lung cancer is the leading cause of cancer-related deaths among men and women in the United States.[43] Overall, lung cancer accounts for 16 percent of all new cases of cancer and 28 percent of all cancer deaths.[43] In 1987, according to the American Cancer Society estimates, 150,000 persons were newly diagnosed with lung cancer and 136,000 deaths were attributable to this disease. Although most investigators agree that over 85 percent of lung cancer cases are attributable to cigarette smoke, several studies indicate that work place and environmental exposures contribute to the development of between 5 and 30 percent of all cases of lung cancer.[44–46] This is further supported by the uneven distribution of lung cancer throughout the United States.[47] As indicated in Figure 37-4, the excess lung cancer-associated mortality may, in part, be caused by a variety of carcinogens that are present in our larger cities and seaports.

The risk of developing lung cancer is clearly dependent on the cumulative exposure to tobacco smoke. The intensity (number of cigarettes per day) and duration of smoking and the depth of inhalation factor into the probability of developing this neoplasm.[48,49] Thus, although heavy cigarette smokers continue to be at highest risk of developing lung cancer, people who smoke cigars or pipes[48] and persons passively exposed to cigarette smoke[50,51] are at greater risk than nonsmokers who have not been exposed.

Fortunately, the risk of developing lung cancer can be substantially reduced by avoiding exposure to cigarette smoke. In fact, even among heavy smokers, 10 to 15 years after quitting cigarettes the risk of developing lung cancer is similar to that of nonsmokers.[49,52]

EFFECTS OF SMOKING CESSATION

Although methods for smoking cessation are reviewed in Chapter 102, the salutary health effects of stopping smoking deserve further mention here. Cigarette smoking has been clearly shown to cause excess mortality by substantially increasing the incidence of atherosclerosis, strokes, chronic airflow obstruction, and lung cancer. In all cases cessation of smoking tends to diminish the risk of developing these diseases, and within 10 to 15 years after stopping, the risk of these tobacco-related diseases is similar to that of persons who never smoked.

References

1. Dunhill AH: The Gentle Art of Smoking. Stellar Press, Hatfield, U.K., 1976, p. 142
2. U.S. Department of Health and Human Services: Reducing the Health Consequences of Smoking: 25 Years of Progress. Department of Health and Human Services, Office on Smoking and Health. Government Printing Office, Washington, D.C., 1989
3. Smoking—attributable mortality and years of potential life lost—United States, 1984. MMWR 1987;36:693–697
4. Wynder EL, Hoffman D: Tobacco and health. N Engl J Med 1979;300:894–900
5. Smoking and Health: A report of the Surgeon General. Chapter 14: Constituents of Tobacco Smoke, No. 79-50066. U.S. Department of Health, Education, and Welfare, 1979
6. Lee PN, Garfinkel L: Mortality and type of cigarette smoked. J Epidemiol Community Health 1981;35:16–22
7. Remington J: The effect of filters on the incidence of lung cancer in cigarette smokers. Environ Res 1981;24:162–166
8. Kozlawski LT, Frecker RC, Khauw V, Pope MA: The misuse of "less-hazardous" cigarettes and its detection: Hole-blocking of ventilated filters. Am J Public Health 1980;70:1202–1203
9. Stepnez R: Would a medium-nicotine, low-tar cigarette be less hazardous to health? Br Med J 1981;283:1292–1296
10. Higenbottam T, Shipley MJ, Clark TJH, Rose G: Lung function and symptoms of cigarette smokers related to tar yield and number of cigarettes smoked. Lancet 1980;1:409–412
11. Schenker MB, Samet JM, Speizer FE: Effect of cigarette tar content and smoking habits on respiratory symptoms in women. Am Rev Respir Dis 1982;125:684–690
12. Sparrow D, Stefos T, Bosse R, Weiss ST: The relationship of tar content to decline in pulmonary function in cigarette smokers. Am Rev Respir Dis 1983;127:56–58
13. Burrows B, Knudson RJ, Clive MG, Lebowitz MD: Quantitative relationships between cigarette smoking and ventilatory function. Am Rev Respir Dis 1977;115:201–205
14. Beck GJ, Doyle CA, Schachter EN: Smoking and lung function. Am Rev Respir Dis 1981;123:149–155
15. Wilens SL, Plair CM: Cigarette smoking and arteriosclerosis. Science 1962;138:975–979
16. Sackett DL, Epid MS, Gibson RW: Relation between aortic atherosclerosis and the use of cigarettes and alcohol. N Engl J Med 1968;279:1413–1417
17. Strong JP, Richards ML: Cigarette smoking and atherosclerosis in autopsied men. Atherosclerosis 1976;23:451–457
18. Wald N, Howard S, Smith PG: Association between atherosclerotic disease and carboxyhaemglobin levels in tobacco smokers. Br Med J 1973;31:761–765
19. Hulley SB, Cohen R, Widdowson G: Plasma high-density lipoprotein cholesterol level: Influence of risk factor intervention. JAMA 1977;238:2269–2274
20. Phillips NR, Havel RJ, Kane JP: Levels and interrelationships of serum and lipoprotein cholesterol and triglycerides: Association with adiposity and the consumption of ethanol, tobacco, and beverages containing caffeine. Atherosclerosis 1981;1:13–18
21. Grundy SM: Atherosclerosis: Pathology, pathogenesis, and role of risk factors. Dis Mon 1983;29:1–58
22. Rogot E, Murray JL: Smoking and causes of death among US veterans: 16 years of observation. Public Health Rep 1980; 95:213–222

23. Brown RG, McKeown T, Whitfield AGW: A note on the association between smoking and disease in men in the seventh decade. Br J Prev Soc Med 1957;11:162–164
24. Greene BA, Berkowitz S: Tobacco bronchitis: An anesthesiologic study. Ann Intern Med 1954;40:729–742
25. Higgins ITT, Oldham PD, Cochrane AL, Gilson JC: Respiratory symptoms and pulmonary disability in an industrial town: Survey of a random sample of the population. Br Med J 1956;2:904–910
26. Lowell FC, Franklin W, Michelson AL, Schiller IW: Chronic obstructive pulmonary emphysema: A disease of smokers. Ann Intern Med 1956;45:268–275
27. Palmer KNV: The role of smoking in bronchitis. Br Med J 1954;1:1473–1474
28. Payne M, Kielsberg M: Respiratory symptoms, lung function and smoking habits in an adult population. Am J Public Health 1964;54:261–277
29. Franklin W: The effect of smoking on pulmonary function in a working adult population. J Clin Invest 1958;37:895–899
30. Edelman NH, Mittman C, Norris AH et al: The effects of cigarette smoking upon spirometric performance of community dwelling men. Am Rev Respir Dis 1966;94:421–429
31. Anderson DO, Ferris BG, Zickmantel R: The effect of tobacco smoking on the prevalence of respiratory disease. Can Med Assoc J 1965;92:26–31
32. Reid DD, Anderson DO, Ferris BG, Fletcher CM: An Anglo-American comparison of the prevalence of bronchitis. Br Med J 1964;1:1487–1491
33. Reid LM: Pathology of chronic bronchitis. Lancet 1954;1:275–278
34. Leopold JG, Gough J: The centrilobular form of hypertrophic emphysema and its relation to chronic bronchitis. Thorax 1957;12:219–235
35. U.S. Department of Health, Education, and Welfare: Smoking and Health: A Report of the Advisory Committee to the Surgeon General of the Public Health Service. U.S. Public Health Service Publication No. 1103. Washington, D.C., 1964
36. Fletcher C, Peto R: The natural history of chronic airflow obstruction. Br Med J 1977;1:1645–1648
37. U.S. Department of Health, Education, and Welfare: Smoking and Health: A Report of the Surgeon General. U.S. Public Health Service Publication PHS 79-50066. Washington, D.C., 1979
38. Burrows B, Bloom JW, Traver GA, Cline MG: The course and prognosis of different forms of chronic airways obstruction in a sample from the general population. N Engl J Med 1987;317:1309–1314
39. Anthonisen NR, Wright EC, Hodgkin JE, and the IPPB Trial Group: Prognosis in chronic obstructive pulmonary disease. Am Rev Respir Dis 1986;133:14–20
40. Fielding JE, Phenow KJ: Health effects of involuntary smoking. N Engl J Med 1988;319:1452–1460
41. Harlap S, Davies AM: Infant admissions to hospital and maternal smoking. Lancet 1974;1:529–532
42. Tager IB, Weiss ST, Munoz A et al: Longitudinal study of the effects of maternal smoking on pulmonary function in children. N Engl J Med 1983;309:699–703
43. Silverberg E: Cancer statistics. CA 1987;37:2–19
44. Doll R, Peto R: The causes of cancer: Quantitative estimates of available risks of cancer in the United States today. J Natl Cancer Inst 1981;66:1191–1308
45. Kjuus H, Langard S, Skjaerven R: A case-referent study of lung cancer, occupational exposures, and smoking. Scand J Work Environ Health 1986;12:210–215
46. Speizer FE: Overview of the risk of respiratory cancer from airborne contaminants. Environ Health Persp 1986;70:9–15
47. Blot WJ, Fraumeni JF: Changing patterns of lung cancer in the United States. Am J Epidemiol 1982;115:664–673
48. Hammond EC, Horn D: Smoking and death rates—Report on forty-four months of follow-up of 187,783 men. II. Death rates by cause. JAMA 1958;166:1294–1308
49. Doll R, Hill AB: Mortality in relation to smoking: Ten years observation of British doctors. Br Med J 1964;1:1399–1410
50. Sandler DP, Everson RB, Wilcox AJ: Passive smoking in adulthood and cancer risk. Am J Epidemiol 1985;121:37–48
51. Humble CG, Samet JM, Pathak DR: Marriage to a smoker and lung cancer risk. Am J Public Health 1987;77:598–602
52. Wynder EL: The etiology, epidemiology, and prevention of lung cancer. Semin Respir Med 1982;3:135–139

Chapter 38

Effects of Dusts, Fumes, and Other Inhaled Substances on the Respiratory System

David A. Schwartz

CHAPTER OUTLINE

Occupational and environmental agents are common causes of a variety of different lung disorders. Asthma, bronchitis, chronic obstructive pulmonary disease (COPD), bronchiolitis obliterans, interstitial fibrosis, hypersensitivity pneumonitis, and granulomatous lung disease can be caused by specific occupational exposures. Since the clinical manifestations of these diseases are similar regardless of the etiology, recognition of occupational and environmental lung diseases is primarily based on the information obtained from an exposure history.

The goal of the exposure history is to determine whether the disease process is specifically associated with previous occupational or environmental exposures. The essential items in an exposure history are outlined in Table 38-1. Given knowledge of the disease process, one should focus on the exposure history to solicit specific information regarding exposures that are pertinent to the type of lung disease (Table 38-2). For example, all patients with interstitial fibrosis should be asked whether they have been exposed to fibrogenic agents, such as asbestos, silica, coal dust, beryllium, or tungsten carbide. Once a positive exposure history has been identified, further information regarding the intensity, duration, and timing of the exposure is needed to clarify the exposure–disease relationship. Because many types of occupational lung disease are manifested following a latency of 20 to 40 years, it is important to identify jobs and exposures dating back to high school and the military service.

This chapter provides a conceptual framework with which to approach occupational and environmental lung diseases. Rather than focusing on specific diseases, such as asbestosis or metal fume fever, we will examine disease patterns to define etiologies and interventions that are appropriate to a specific disease process. This approach should provide the clinician with the information needed to readily address specific clinical problems. More comprehensive reviews of occupational and environmental lung diseases have recently been published[1–4] and should be consulted for further information.

AIRWAY DISORDERS

Diseases involving the airways include those that result in excess mucus production (bronchitis), increased airway

Table 38-1. Essential Items in an Exposure History

Identify and quantify exposures
Prioritize exposures
Quantity
Toxicity
Establish temporal relation
Exposures vs onset of disease
Exposures vs exacerbation of disease
Consider other workers
Similar symptoms in co-workers
Known occupational illnesses

reactivity (asthma), and collapse or fibrosis of small and large airways (bronchiectasis, peribronchial fibrosis, bronchiolitis obliterans, and COPD). In aggregate, these airway disorders constitute the overwhelming majority of lung diseases that are attributed to either occupational or environmental agents, which very likely reflects the relatively short latency between exposure and disease onset in these disorders, in contrast to the long latency that is characteristic of the parenchymal and neoplastic lung diseases.

Occupational Asthma

Occupational asthma is clinically and pathogenically identical to other forms of asthma, but is caused or exacerbated by specific occupational and/or environmental exposures.[5,6] Fortunately, the time interval between exposure and onset of symptoms is less than 12 hours and may be as short as a few minutes. Agents listed in Table 38-2 may cause or exacerbate asthma in as much as 10 to 20 percent of the exposed population. Overall, occupational asthma is thought to account for 1 to 5 percent of all asthma cases.[5,6]

Table 38-2. Occupational and Environmental Causes for Common Lung Diseases

Lung Disease	Occupational/Environmental Etiologies
Asthma	Animal proteins, wood dusts, toluene diisocyanate, noxious gases, metal fumes, and grain dusts
COPD	Mineral dusts, organic dusts, and noxious gases
Interstitial fibrosis	Asbestos, silica, coal dust, and tungsten carbide
Granulomatous lung disease	Beryllium
Hypersensitivity pneumonitis	Organic dusts, thermophilic bacteria, a variety of fungi, toluene diisocyanate, trimellitic anhydride, and animal proteins
Lung cancer	Asbestos, arsenic, bischloromethyl ether, chromium, soots/tar, nickel, and radiation

Direct damage to the airway mucosa can be caused by exposure to unusually high levels of an irritant vapor, fume, or smoke.[7,8] The symptoms of cough, dyspnea, and wheezing usually develop within minutes to hours following exposure and may be associated with extensive alveolar injury. Actually, the location of the lung injury and the onset of clinical symptoms are dependent on the water solubility of the gas and the extent of the exposure (Table 38-3). Airway symptoms with objective documentation of airway hyperreactivity may persist for several years after the incident; however, most patients return to their baseline function 3 to 6 months after the exposure. Following extensive exposure to these irritating gases a few individuals have been reported to develop chronic bronchitis, bronchiolitis obliterans, or COPD[9,10] (Table 38-3).

Chronic Obstructive Pulmonary Disease

As reviewed in Chapter 37, COPD affects over 20 million Americans and is the sixth most common cause of death in the United States.[11] Cigarette smoking is the single most important factor responsible for the development and progression of COPD, directly contributing to 82 percent of COPD mortality.[12] However, along with sex, age, and baseline pulmonary function, cigarette smoking accounts for only 50 to 70 percent of those who actually develop COPD.[13,14] Thus, other exposures and/or host factors may contribute to 30 to 50 percent of COPD cases. In fact, community-based longitudinal studies indicate that occupational dusts, fumes, and chemicals are associated with decreased lung function[15,16] and greater declines in FEV_1 over time.[14,17] Similarly, workers exposed to mineral dusts,[18–24] fumes,[25,26] and either sulfur dioxide (SO_2)[27] or oxides of nitrogen[28] have excess decline in lung function that appear to be directly related to these exposures. Furthermore, after controlling for age and smoking, employment in underground mining was found to be significantly related to histologic emphysema identified at autopsy.[29] In aggregate, these studies provide considerable evidence identifying occupational dusts, fumes, and chemicals as factors that are potentially important in the pathogenesis of COPD.

The identification of individuals who are at risk for developing asthma or COPD from occupational exposure involves use of a focused history to supplement specific tests of airway function. Adult-onset asthmatics and patients with COPD who do not have other established risk factors, such as cigarette smoking, atopy, and alpha-1-antitrypsin deficiency, are likely to have occupational or environmental determinants for their airflow obstruction. In asthma, one would expect to see a strong temporal relationship between exposures and exacerbations of airway symptoms. This can be documented further by observing whether these symptoms improve on weekends and vacations and if the exposures are associated with decrements in peak expiratory flow.[5,30,31] COPD is a chronic disorder, which takes many years to develop, and therefore a more extensive exposure

Table 38-3. Clinical Manifestations Associated with Exposure to Gaseous Respiratory Irritants[a]

			Acute Respiratory Manifestations		Chronic Respiratory Sequelae		
Irritant Gas	Water Solubility	Onset	Upper Airway Irritation	Parenchymal Injury	Bronchitis	Bronchiolitis Obliterans	Obstructive Lung Disease
Ammonia	High	Minutes	Severe	+	+	−	+
Sulfur dioxide	High	Minutes	Severe	+	−	+	+
Hydrogen chloride	High	Minutes	Severe	−	−	−	−
Chlorine	Intermediate	Minutes to hours	Moderate	+	+	−	+
Oxides of nitrogen	Low	Hours	Mild	+	−	+	−
Ozone	Low	Hours	Mild	−	−	−	−
Phosgene	Low	Hours	Mild	+	−	−	−

[a] −, exposure (as yet) not reported to be associated with clinical entity; +, exposure reported to be associated with clinical entity.

history, focusing on chronic exposure to mineral dusts, noxious gases, and organic dusts, is required.

PARENCHYMAL DISORDERS

The parenchymal lung diseases associated with occupational exposures may arise from a vast array of occupational exposures and can present as focal infiltrates or diffuse interstitial fibrosis. These diseases include hypersensitivity pneumonitis, granulomatous lung disease, and the pneumoconioses (interstitial fibrosis) and are caused by inhalation either of bioaerosols containing fungi or bacteria or of mineral dusts or metals (Table 38-2). Although the exposure history remains important, there is often a long time period between exposure and onset of lung disease. Therefore it is important to inquire about part-time jobs, military service, and hobbies that may involve specific respiratory exposures.

Hypersensitivity Pneumonitis

Hypersensitivity pneumonitis represents an immunologic reaction following the inhalation of a foreign substance.[32,33] Initially, persons may present with recurrent flu-like symptoms, which occur 4 to 12 hours following the exposure and are associated with patchy, fleeting infiltrates. Continued exposure may result in progressive constitutional symptoms, including weight loss and night sweats, and the development of diffuse interstitial fibrosis. Traditionally, serum-precipitating antibodies have been included in the diagnostic evaluation. However, since only the common antigens are included in the screening panels, 20 to 30 percent of those with hypersensitivity pneumonitis may have a negative test result. In most cases a lymphocytic alveolitis can be demonstrated by bronchoalveolar lavage[34,35] and in contrast to sarcoidosis, T-suppressor lymphocytes predominate in the lavage fluid.[34] In addition, loose granulomata with eosinophils are detected in up to 70 percent of the open lung biopsies. Since none of these tests are diagnostic of hypersensitivity pneumonitis, the diagnosis is usually made by excluding other similar disease processes and eliciting a constellation of clinical symptoms and signs that are consistent with this lung disease. Treatment should focus on identifying and eliminating the exposure and temporarily treating the constitutional symptoms with corticosteroids.

Berylliosis

Berylliosis is a granulomatous lung disease with many systemic manifestations.[36] Chronic beryllium disease may present as a radiographic finding without respiratory symptoms or may be associated with profound dyspnea and a restrictive pattern of lung dysfunction. Recently, bronchoalveolar lavage has been used to identify T lymphocytes that specifically proliferate, in vitro, in response to beryllium and are characteristic of berylliosis.[37] In addition to this specific proliferative response, berylliosis can be differentiated from sarcoidosis by exposure history and the distinct absence of either central nervous system disease or altered calcium metabolism in berylliosis. The disease course is highly variable even with cessation of exposure. Although no controlled trials have been performed, corticosteroids are thought to promote the resolution of chronic beryllium disease.

Pneumoconioses

Pneumoconioses are caused by inhalation of specific mineral dusts (Table 38-2) and are virtually indistinguishable from other forms of interstitial fibrosis. *Silicosis* and *coal workers' pneumoconiosis* (CWP) will tend to present as upper lobe nodular disease,[38] while *asbestosis* will usually present as lower lobe linear and irregular fibrosis, often associated with bilateral pleural fibrosis.[39] These diseases tend to be slowly progressive; however, acute, rapidly progressive silicosis has been reported following exposure to very high concentrations of silica. In addition, progressive massive fibrosis (PMF), usually in association with tuberculosis, is seen in patients with silicosis and CWP and can result in conglomerate fibrosis involving the upper lobes. Persons with asbestosis are likely to die from an asbestos-related lung disease—20 percent from progressive asbestosis, 39 percent from lung cancer, and 9 percent from mesothelioma.[40] Unfortunately, no treatment is currently available for any of the pneumoconioses. However, given the associations both of asbestosis with cancers of the lung and pleura and of silicosis with tuberculosis, close medical surveillance is recommended and appears warranted.

CANCERS OF THE LUNG AND PLEURA

Lung Cancer

Lung cancer is the leading cause of cancer-related deaths among men and women in the United States[41] and accounts for 75 percent of all occupational cancers.[42] Although most investigators agree that over 85 percent of the cases of lung cancer are attributable to cigarette smoke, several studies estimate that workplace and environmental exposures contribute to the development of 5 to 30 percent of all cases of lung cancer.[43–45] Because of the overwhelming effect of cigarette smoke, other putative environmental agents must be evaluated in the context of their interaction with this potent lung carcinogen. The best example of this is asbestos, which alone results in a five-fold excess risk of lung cancer. However, when a person is exposed to both asbestos and cigarette smoke, there is a 60- to 90-fold excess risk of lung cancer.[46] Because of this synergistic interaction, asbestos is as likely as is cigarette smoke to contribute to the development of lung cancer in a person exposed to both agents. With the exception of bischloromethyl ether, which is only associated with small cell carcinoma, the carcinogens listed in Table 38-2 are associated with all cell types of lung cancer.[47]

Mesothelioma

Mesothelioma has the longest latency of all types of asbestos-related lung diseases; because of exposures that occurred up to 1980, it is expected to increase in incidence through the first 5 or 10 years of the twenty-first century.[48,49] These tumors, which are unrelated to cigarette smoke and other forms of asbestos-related pleural disease, tend to be large, bulky pleura-based lesions and to present with marked chest pain due to chest wall invasion. The prognosis remains very poor, and neither surgery, chemotherapy, nor radiation therapy has any significant impact on the mean survival of 12 months.[50]

References

1. Merchant JA: Occupational Respiratory Disorders. Dept. of Health and Human Services, Publication No. NIOSH 86-102. U.S. Government Printing Office, Washington, DC, 1986
2. Parkes WR: Occupational Lung Disorders. 2nd Ed. Butterworth, London, 1982
3. Rom WN (ed): Environmental and Occupational Medicine. Little Brown, Boston, 1983
4. Weill H, Turner-Warwick M: Occupational Lung Diseases: Research Approaches and Methods. Marcel Dekker, New York, 1981
5. Chan-Yeung M, Lam S: Occupational asthma. Am Rev Respir Dis 1986;137:686–703
6. Brooks SM: Occupational asthma. Chest 1985;87:218s–222s
7. Brooks SM, Weiss MA, Bernstein IL: Reactive airways dysfunction syndrome (RADS). Chest 1985;88:376–384
8. Schwartz DA: Acute inhalational injury. Occup Med State Art Rev 1987;2:297–318
9. Epler GR, Colby TV: The spectrum of bronchiolitis obliterans. Chest 1983;83:161–162
10. Epler GR, Colby TV, McLoud TC et al: Bronchitis obliterans organizing pneumonia. N Engl J Med 1985;312:152–158
11. Weiss ST: Epidemiology of chronic lung disease: Risk factors and natural history. Compr Ther 1986;12:10–13
12. Chronic Disease Reports: Chronic obstructive pulmonary disease mortality—United States, 1980. MMWR 1989;38:549–561
13. Higgins MW, Keller JB, Landis JR et al: Risk of chronic obstructive pulmonary disease. Am Rev Respir Dis 1984;130:380–385
14. Krzyzanowski M, Jedrychowski W, Wysocki M: Factors associated with the change in ventilatory function and the development of chronic obstructive pulmonary disease in a 13 year follow-up of the Cracow study. Am Rev Respir Dis 1986; 134:1011–1019
15. Lebowitz M: Occupational exposures in relation to symptomatology and lung function in a community population. Environ Res 1977;44:59–67
16. Prediletto R, Viegi G, Paoletti P: Effects of occupational exposure on respiratory symptoms and lung function in a general population sample. Am Rev Respir Dis, suppl. 1987;135:A342
17. Korn RJ, Dockery DW, Speizer FE et al: Occupational exposures and chronic respiratory symptoms: A population based study. Am Rev Respir Dis 1987;136:298–304
18. Love RG, Miller BG: Longitudinal study of lung function in coal miners. Thorax 1982;37:193–197
19. Attfield MD: Longitudinal decline in FEV in United States coal miners. Thorax 1985;40:132–137
20. Siracusa A, Cicioni C, Volpi R et al: Lung function among asbestos cement factory workers: Cross-sectional and longitudinal study. Am J Ind Med 1984;5:315–325
21. Ohlson CG, Bodin L, Rydman T, Hogstedt C: Ventilatory decrements in former asbestos workers: A four year follow up. Br J Ind Med 1985;42:612–616
22. Pham QT, Mur JM, Tecelescu D et al: A longitudinal study of symptoms and respiratory function tests in iron miners. Eur J Respir Dis 1986;69:346–354
23. Pham QT, Mastrangelo G, Chau N, Haluszka J: Five year longitudinal comparison of respiratory symptoms and function in steel workers and unexposed workers. Bull Eur Physiopathol Respir 1979;15:469–480
24. Manfreda J, Johnson B, Cherniack RM: Longitudinal change of lung function: Comparison of employees of hardrock mining industry and general population, abstracted. Am Rev Respir Dis 1984;129:A142
25. Kauffmann F, Drouet D, Lellouch J, Brille D: Occupational ex-

posure and 12 year spirometric changes among Paris area workers. Br J Ind Med 1982;39:221–232
26. Kauffmann F, Drouet D, Lellouch J, Brille D: Twelve year spirometric changes among Paris area workers. Int J Epidemiol 1979;8:201–212
27. Manfreda J, Sidwall G, Maini K et al: Respiratory anomalies in employees of the hardrock mining industry. Am Rev Respir Dis 1982;126:629–634
28. Manfreda J, Johnston B: Occupational factors in the etiology of airflow obstruction, abstracted. Am Rev Respir Dis 1987;135:A341
29. Becklake MR, Irwig L, Kielkowski D et al: The predictors of emphysema in South African gold miners. Am Rev Respir Dis 1987;135:1234–41
30. Burge PS: Single and serial measurements of lung function in the diagnosis of occupational asthma. Eur J Respir Dis, suppl. 123, 1982;63:47–59
31. Cartier A, Pineau L, Malo JL: Monitoring of maximum expiratory peak flow rates and histamine inhalation tests in the investigation of occupational asthma. Clin Allergy 1984;14:193–196
32. Stankus RP, Salvaggio JE: Hypersensitivity pneumonitis. Clin Chest Med 1983;4:55–62
33. Fink JN: Hypersensitivity pneumonitis. J Allergy Clin Immunol 1984;74:1–15
34. Leatherman JW, Michael AF, Schwartz BA, Hoidal R: Lung T cells in hypersensitivity pneumonitis. Ann Intern Med 1984; 100:390–392
35. Cormier Y, Belanger J, Le Blanc P, Laviolette M: Bronchoalveolar lavage in farmer's lung disease: Diagnostic and physiological significance. Br J Ind Med 1986;43:401–405
36. Kriebel D, Brain JD, Sprince NL, Kazemi H: The pulmonary toxicity of beryllium. Am Rev Respir Dis 1988;137:464–473
37. Rossman MD, Kern JA, Elias JA et al: Proliferative response of bronchoalveolar lymphocytes to beryllium. Ann Intern Med 1988;108:687–693
38. Ziskind M, Jones RN, Weill H: Silicosis: State of the art. Am Rev Respir Dis 1976;113:643–657
39. Mossman BT, Gee JB: Asbestos-related diseases. N Engl J Med 1989;320:1721–1730
40. Berry G: Mortality of workers certified by pneumoconiosis medical panels as having asbestosis. Br J Ind Med 1981;38:130–137
41. Silverberg E: Cancer statistics. CA 1987;37:2–19
42. Doll R, Peto R: The causes of cancer: Quantitative estimates of avoidable risks of cancer in the United States today. J Natl Cancer Inst 1981;66:1193–1308
43. Bridbord K, Decoufle P, Fraumeni JF et al: Estimates of the fraction of cancer in the United States related to occupational factors. National Cancer Institute, National Institute of Environmental Health Sciences, National Institute of Occupational Safety and Health, 1978
44. Kvale G, Bjelke E, Heuch I: Occupational exposure and lung cancer risks. Int J Cancer 1986;37:185–190
45. Kjuus H, Langard S, Skjaerven R: A case-referent study of lung cancer, occupational exposure and smoking. III. Etiologic fraction of occupational exposures. Scand J Work Environ Health 1986;12:210–215
46. Hammond EC, Selikoff IJ, Seidman H: Asbestos exposure, cigarette smoking and death rates. Ann NY Acad Sci 1979;330:473–490
47. Ives JC, Buffler PA, Greenberg SD: Environmental associations and histopathologic patterns of carcinoma of the lung: The challenge and dilemma in epidemiologic studies. Am Rev Respir Dis 1983;128:195–209
48. Hillerdal G: Malignant mesothelioma 1982: Review of 4710 published cases. Br J Dis Chest 1983;77:321–343
49. Nicholson WJ, Perkel G, Selikoff IJ: Occupational exposure to asbestos: Population at risk and projected mortality—1980–2030. Am J Ind Med 1982;3:259–311
50. Chahinian AP, Pajak TF, Holland JF et al: Diffuse malignant mesothelioma. Ann Intern Med 1982;96:746–755.

Chapter 39

Drug-Induced Lung Disease

Pope L. Moseley

CHAPTER OUTLINE

Drug-induced lung diseases comprise a heterogenous group of clinical syndromes, including interstitial fibrosis, pulmonary edema, and asthma. In many instances one drug may cause several types of lung injury. For example, the antibiotic nitrofurantoin may cause chronic interstitial fibrosis, acute pulmonary infiltrates with eosinophilia, and pleural effusion.

The purpose of this chapter is to acquaint the clinician with the various drugs that injure the lung and to relate symptoms of lung injury to various drug exposures. In order to facilitate the recognition of clinical lung injury syndromes, this chapter is organized by clinical syndrome rather than by drug (Table 39-1). Thus, each drug may appear more than once. Associations between drugs and characteristic or particularly common presentations are listed in Table 39-2.

DRUGS THAT CAUSE CHRONIC INTERSTITIAL PULMONARY DISEASE

In general, drug-induced lung disease that results in interstitial infiltrates (Table 39-3) presents in a subacute, insidious fashion. The usual complaints are dyspnea on exertion and a dry, nonproductive cough. Physical examination will often reveal bibasilar or diffuse crackles. The chest x-ray will usually show a reticular pattern, although a nodular pattern has been reported with some drug exposures. Pulmonary function studies are variable, with a restrictive or mixed defect. In most drug-induced lung injury causing interstitial lung disease, diffusing capacity will be abnormal.

Bibasilar or Diffuse Infiltrates

Bleomycin

Bleomycin is an antitumor antibiotic useful in the treatment of testicular carcinoma, squamous cell carcinoma, and lymphoma. The overall incidence of bleomycin-induced interstitial disease is 5 to 10 percent of patients receiving the drug.[1]

Risk factors that increase the incidence of bleomycin toxicity are exposure to supplemental O_2 and radiation expo-

Table 39-1. Syndromes of Drug-Induced Lung Disease

Chronic interstitial disease
Diffuse/bibasilar
Upper lobe predominance
Pulmonary infiltrates with eosinophilia
Pulmonary edema
Unique syndromes
Pleural effusions
Bronchiolitis obliterans
Muscle paralysis
Pulmonary hemorrhage
Asthma

sure.[2,3] In this regard bleomycin participates in a radiation recall phenomenon, in which patients who have previously received radiation develop pulmonary toxicity during subsequent bleomycin therapy. Prior exposure to bleomycin also sensitizes patients to radiation injury. Unlike other types of radiation recall injury, the lung injury is not limited to the radiation port. Bleomycin toxicity is also increased by exposure to cyclophosphamide.[2]

The time course of bleomycin injury is variable and is also dependent on cumulative dose. The threshold dose for bleomycin toxicity is generally felt to be 400 U total dose[1]; however, patients have suffered lethal lung injury after 100 U of bleomycin.[4] Patients present with a dry cough, exertional dyspnea, and malaise. The diffusing capacity is used as a marker of bleomycin lung injury, a fall of 20 percent or more from baseline being indicative of pulmonary toxicity.

The outcome of bleomycin-induced lung disease is variable, with a mortality of 20 percent.[2] Unlike the acute eosinophilic syndrome of bleomycin lung disease (see below), steroids have not been shown to be beneficial in chronic bleomycin toxicity.

Busulfan

Busulfan is an alkylating agent used in the therapy of a number of myeloproliferative disorders and was the first cytotoxic agent to be associated with pulmonary toxicity.[5] The incidence of significant pulmonary toxicity is 5 percent. Autopsy studies, however, have noted significant histopathologic changes in half of patients who had received busulfan therapy.[6] While no increase in busulfan lung toxicity has been shown to occur with exposure to radiation or other cytotoxic drugs, there appears to be a threshold dose, busulfan toxicity having been reported only in patients who have received a 500-mg or higher total dose.[2] Other than this threshold dose, there is no dose dependence for busulfan toxicity.

Table 39-2. Common Associations between Drugs and Clinical Findings[a]

Pleural effusion	Nitrofurantoin
Pleuritic chest pain	Nitrofurantoin, methotrexate, amiodarone
Bronchoalveolar lavage useful in diagnosis	Nitrofurantoin (altered T-cell subsets), busulfan (bizarre cells)
Long latency	Cyclophosphamide, busulfan
Radiation recall	Bleomycin
Threshold dose for pulmonary toxicity	Bleomycin (400 U total dose), busulfan (500 mg total dose), amiodarone (400 mg/d)
Patient age	Bleomycin (older patients), nitrosoureas (younger patients)

[a] The drugs listed have the best established associations in each category.

Table 39-3. Drugs Associated with Chronic Interstitial Disease

Diffuse/bibasilar infiltrates
Bleomycin
Busulfan
Chlorambucil
Cyclophosphamide
Melphalan
Methotrexate
Mitomycin
Nitrofurantoin
Nitrosoureas
Penicillamine
Upper lobe predominance
Amiodarone
Gold

The chest x-ray is abnormal in nearly all cases of busulfan toxicity and shows a bibasilar infiltrate. Because busulfan lung injury causes a desquamative reaction, the chest x-ray may also reveal an alveolar infiltrative process, as is seen with desquamative interstitial pneumonitis.[6]

Unlike most other drug-induced lung injuries, in which abnormal cells merely serve as a marker of drug exposure, cytopathology is useful in the diagnosis of busulfan lung disease. Bizarre, atypical pneumocytes with inclusions may be seen in the sputum or in the bronchoalveolar lavage of patients with busulfan lung toxicity. These atypical cells correlate with the extent of pulmonary injury and not merely with drug exposure.

Therapy is supportive, with immediate withdrawal of the drug. Corticosteroids have not been shown to be effective. Busulfan lung disease carries a grave prognosis and may be progressive despite discontinuation of therapy. The mean survival after diagnosis has been reported as 5 months.[2]

Chlorambucil

Chlorambucil is an alkylating agent used in the treatment of hematologic malignancies. The onset of symptoms occurs 6 months to 3 years after the institution of therapy. Clinically, the syndrome of chlorambucil interstitial lung disease parallels that of other drug-induced interstitial diseases except that fever is a predominant finding. The overall mortality for chlorambucil-induced pulmonary toxicity is 50 percent. Case reports have demonstrated benefits from corticosteroid therapy; however, discontinuation of chlorambucil is the mainstay of therapy.

Cyclophosphamide

Cyclophosphamide is a nitrogen mustard, which is used in the treatment of numerous tumors as well as inflammatory conditions. The incidence of pulmonary toxicity from cyclophosphamide is low; however, its widespread use makes it an important cause of drug-induced interstitial disease.

Interstitial disease may occur immediately after as little as 2 weeks of cyclophosphamide exposure. There are also reports of lung injury 10 years after exposure.[2] In general, the interstitial disease follows exposures longer than 1 month. The incidence of lung toxicity is increased following use of cyclophosphamide in combination with bleomycin or mitomycin. Mortality is high (40 percent), and is not reduced by steroid therapy.[2]

Methotrexate

Methotrexate is a folic acid analogue used in the therapy of a number of malignancies as well as inflammatory conditions. As with cyclophosphamide therapy, the onset of toxicity may occur after a few weeks of therapy or after prolonged exposure (more than 10 years).[7] Toxicity is increased when patients receive methotrexate at daily or weekly rather than less frequent intervals.[8]

Patients with methotrexate interstitial disease present with cough and dyspnea on exertion. Fever is common. The mortality following methotrexate exposure is low (less than 1 percent). Corticosteroids may be helpful, since patients have developed methotrexate-induced pulmonary toxicity when steroids were tapered. Interestingly, some patients have improved even when maintained on methotrexate, and others have recovered from pulmonary toxicity and then received subsequent courses of methotrexate without further pulmonary injury. Given that methotrexate does cause interstitial fibrosis, these rechallenges with the drug are not without risk.

Mitomycin

Mitomycin is an antitumor antibiotic used in treatment of solid tumors. Pulmonary toxicity is a major limiting side effect of the drug. As with bleomycin, interstitial lung disease caused by mitomycin is increased by prior exposure to cyclophosphamide and concurrent exposure to supplemental O_2. Unlike bleomycin-induced damage, lung injury from mitomycin does not appear to be exacerbated by radiation therapy.

While the mortality for mitomycin-induced interstitial disease has been reported to be as high as 50 percent, the response to corticosteroids is dramatic. In this regard mitomycin-induced lung injury has been seen following the tapering of corticosteroids in various therapy protocols.[2]

Nitrofurantoin

Nitrofurantoin is an antibiotic used in the treatment of urinary tract infections. Since it is also used in chronic suppressive therapy of these infections, patients are often exposed to the drug for months to years. While nitrofurantoin is the most common cause of drug-induced lung injury, the chronic interstitial form of the disease is its least common manifestations of pulmonary toxicity. Chronic lung injury occurs after at least 4 to 6 months, and can be seen after years of continuous therapy.[9] Laboratory abnormalities may include elevated liver enzymes, elevated serum creatinine, and elevated antinuclear antibodies. Eosinophilia is not a feature of chronic nitrofurantoin toxicity. Bronchoalveolar lavage reveals a lymphocytic predominance with an inverted helper/suppressor ratio.[10] The prognosis of chronic nitrofurantoin toxicity is variable, with a 10 percent mortality rate. The majority of patients have persistent radiographic and functional abnormalities.

Nitrosoureas

The nitrosoureas, such as carmustine (BCNU), lomustine (CCNU), and semustine (methyl CCNU), are used in the treatment of central nervous system malignancies. The incidence of interstitial pulmonary toxicity may be as high as 30 percent with these agents. Age is a risk factor for the development of pulmonary toxicity; younger patients are at greater risk, but it is not clear whether this risk is due to more intensive chemotherapy. Overall mortality is 20 percent. Corticosteroids have not been shown to be effective therapeutically, and withdrawal of the nitrosourea is the main therapeutic intervention.

Prominent Upper Lobe Involvement

Amiodarone

Amiodarone is an antiarrhythmic agent, which has a 5 to 10 percent incidence of pulmonary toxicity. There appears to be a threshold dose, and in fact, pulmonary toxicity was unrecognized when the drug was initially used at lower doses (less than 400 mg/d).

Patients usually present 6 months to 1 year after onset of therapy with dyspnea on exertion, a nonproductive cough, and fever. Pleuritic chest pain may also be noted. Laboratory data commonly reveal an elevated erythrocyte sedimentation rate. Biopsy reveals lamellar inclusions in macrophages and lung parenchymal cells; however, these abnormalities reflect exposure to the drug and do not rule out other causes of interstitial lung disease. Thus, the biopsy is helpful only if it does *not* show these abnormal cells, since no cases of amiodarone pulmonary toxicity have been reported in the absence of these findings.

Treatment is discontinuation of the agent; however some patients have had resolution of pulmonary symptoms when the dose was lowered below 400 mg/d. As with lung toxicity induced by other drugs, however, continuation of the drug in the setting of toxicity may be dangerous. Case reports of corticosteroid use have yielded mixed results. Since several patients have developed amiodarone lung toxicity while on corticosteroids, these agents may not be effective therapy.

Gold

While gold-induced pulmonary toxicity has a low incidence, it often appears together with gold dermatitis. Symptoms other than dermatitis are cough, dyspnea on exertion, and fever. While the vast majority of patients survive, roughly half of them have residual pulmonary impairment. Patients with gold-induced pulmonary toxicity should have the gold shots discontinued. It is unclear whether corticosteroids or gold chelation with dimercaprol (British antilewisite) is helpful.[11]

DRUGS THAT CAUSE PULMONARY INFILTRATES WITH EOSINOPHILIA

A large number of drugs have been described as causing a hypersensitivity syndrome of pulmonary infiltrates with peripheral blood eosinophilia (Table 39-4), which is a form of hypersensitivity disease. Symptoms include fever, cough, and dyspnea. The infiltrates may be interstitial or alveolar.

The association of most drugs with this syndrome is based on sporadic case reports. Several drugs (described in greater detail below) have been found to cause a reproducible syndrome of infiltrates with eosinophilia. In general, this syndrome is acute and responds well to removal of the agent and/or steroid therapy. Since the syndrome can be progressive, it is important to recognize that it may be drug-related and to institute therapy.

Table 39-4. Drugs Associated with Pulmonary Infiltrates with Eosinophilia

Aspirin and NSAIDs
Bleomycin
Carbamazepine
Chlorpromazine[a]
Chlorpropamide
Cromolyn sodium[a]
Diphenylhydantoin (phenytoin)
Gold salts[a]
Imipramine
Methotrexate
Methylphenidate[a]
Nitrofurantoin
Para-aminosalicylic acid
Penicillamine[a]
Penicillin
Procarbazine
Propranolol[a]
Streptomycin
Sulfonamides
Tetracycline
Thiazides
Tolazamide[a]

[a] Only isolated case reports.

Aspirin and Other Nonsteroidal Anti-inflammatory Drugs

Aspirin and other nonsteroidal anti-inflammatory drugs (NSAIDs) have rarely been shown to cause an interstitial-acinar infiltrate with peripheral eosinophilia. More commonly, these agents have been associated with the development of bronchospasm or noncardiogenic pulmonary edema (see below). Patients with aspirin-induced hypersensitivity generally complained of dyspnea, a nonproductive cough, and wheezing. Blood chemistries reveal an elevated eosinophil count. Therapy is withdrawal of the agent, and prognosis once the agent is removed is excellent. The patient should not be rechallenged with this family of agents because of the risk of recurrence.

Bleomycin

The hypersensitivity reaction to bleomycin is the acute form of bleomycin lung toxicity. It appears to be an idiosyncratic reaction, and there are no established risk factors for it. The bleomycin-induced hypersensitivity reaction usually occurs after an initial dose of bleomycin or within the first 4 to 6 weeks of therapy. Patients present with dyspnea and a nonproductive cough. Pulmonary function studies reveal a restrictive defect with a low diffusing capacity. The chest radiograph is similar to that seen with chronic interstitial disease and reveals a diffuse reticular pattern greatest at the bases. Patients with acute bleomycin toxicity respond well to discontinuation of the drug and corticosteroid therapy. There appears to be no association between acute bleomycin hypersensitivity and the more insidious chronic interstitial disease.

Carbamazepine and Diphenylhydantoin

A few cases have been reported of pulmonary infiltrates with eosinophilia associated with the anticonvulsant agents carbamazepine and diphenylhydantoin. These patients presented with nonproductive cough, dyspnea, and myalgias within 6 weeks of initiation of therapy. Of interest, nearly all patients presented with significant temperature elevations to 41°C. In diphenylhydantoin-induced toxicity, several patients presented with lymphadenopathy and chest radiographic evidence of hilar adenopathy. The prognosis of anticonvulsant hypersensitivity lung disease is quite good once the drugs are stopped. Steroids have been used and may hasten resolution of symptoms. Since the numbers of patients affected are quite small, it is unknown whether the hypersensitivity reaction to one drug predisposes to hypersensitivity to the other.

Methotrexate

The hypersensitivity reaction to methotrexate is similar to that seen with bleomycin. It is an acute illness, which occurs within weeks of onset of therapy. Patients complain of constitutional symptoms such as fevers, chills, and myalgias in addition to dyspnea and cough. Methotrexate hypersensitivity lung disease is unique in that biopsies have shown the presence of noncaseating granuloma.[9] Thus, a lung biopsy may be helpful in the diagnosis of acute methotrexate pulmonary toxicity. Therapy is discontinuation of the drug and possibly corticosteroid therapy.

Nitrofurantoin

Possibly the most common manifestation of drug-induced pulmonary disease is the acute form of nitrofurantoin lung toxicity. Patients present with cough, arthralgia, fever, and dyspnea within 2 weeks of onset of therapy.[9] Of interest, in one large series 20 percent of patients had had a previous exposure to the drug, and of these patients, more than half of them had experienced a nonpulmonary side effect.[11] On physical examination, patients present with dry rales and occasionally wheezing. Laboratory examination reveals eosinophilia in more than three-fourths of patients and an elevated erythrocyte sedimentation rate in approximately 90 percent.[11] Pulmonary function studies show a restrictive defect with a low diffusing capacity. The chest x-ray reveals bibasilar interstitial infiltrates in most cases; however, there is usually an acinar component. Patchy infiltrates may also be seen. Pleural effusions are seen in approximately 25 percent of patients with acute nitrofurantoin toxicity,[9] and are generally unilateral (see below).

Therapy for this form of nitrofurantoin toxicity is withdrawal of the drug. Steroid therapy may be beneficial in patients who are severely ill. The prognosis of acute nitrofurantoin hypersensitivity is good. Unlike the chronic form of nitrofurantoin toxicity, the hypersensitivity reaction to nitrofurantoin is associated with resolution of symptoms. Since there are case reports of patients developing recurrent pulmonary toxicity on rechallenge with nitrofurantoin, it is wise to avoid re-exposure of patients to this agent.

Other Antibiotics

There are reports of interstitial infiltrates accompanied by fever, arthralgia, rash, and peripheral eosinophilia following an exposure to antibiotics such as penicillin, streptomycin, sulfonamides, and tetracycline. These patients improved rapidly after withdrawal of the agent. Most of them had had no prior history of allergy to the drug. Pulmonary toxicity may follow topical exposures to the agents. In the case of sulfonamides, pulmonary infiltrates and eosinophilia recurred with rechallenge. Thus, this reaction should be considered a significant drug reaction and rechallenge should be avoided.

Procarbazine

Procarbazine produces a syndrome of pulmonary injury associated with fever, constitutional symptoms, and skin rash. Patients have responded to discontinuation of the drug alone. The prognosis is good.

DRUGS ASSOCIATED WITH PULMONARY EDEMA

Pulmonary edema occurs as the result of exposure to a number of drugs (Table 39-5). Patients present with dyspnea, respiratory distress, and cough. In most cases drug-induced pulmonary edema is the result of a drug overdose. The mechanism for its development is believed to be the effect of the drugs on the central nervous system, which produces a combination of permeability and nonpermeability edema. Recent studies have suggested that constriction of the postcapillary venules may play a major role in development of this type of pulmonary edema.

Amphotericin B

Amphotericin B in combination with leukocyte transfusion has been reported as the cause of noncardiogenic pulmonary edema.[13] In these studies the patients presented with tachypnea, dyspnea, and cough. Most patients were hypoxemic and had evidence of alveolar hemorrhage, more than half of the patients required mechanical ventilation, and the mortality was over 30 percent.

While these studies have implicated amphotericin and leukocyte transfusion, follow-up studies have not been able to confirm these findings. Given the initial findings and the severity of the reaction, it is probably wise to avoid the use of amphotericin B and leukocyte transfusion within a short time.

Aspirin and Other Nonsteroidal Anti-inflammatory Drugs

In large overdoses aspirin, as well as other NSAIDs, may cause noncardiogenic pulmonary edema. In the majority of

Table 39-5. Drugs Associated with Pulmonary Edema

Aspirin
Amphotericin B
Colchicine[a]
Cytosine arabinoside[a]
Hydrochlorthiazide
Opiates
Tocolytic agents
Tranquilizers (neuroleptic malignant syndrome)

[a] Only isolated case reports.

cases, this pulmonary edema is also associated with the mental status changes of overdose. Patients generally present with confusion, various degrees of unresponsiveness, tachypnea, and dyspnea. Physical examination reveals diffuse rales. In patients in whom cardiopulmonary hemodynamics have been measured, the pulmonary capillary wedge pressure is normal. The chest x-ray reveals diffuse alveolar infiltrates consistent with pulmonary edema. In general, the outcome for patients with analgesic-induced pulmonary edema is good. Very few patients have required mechanical ventilation; most can be treated with supplemental O_2 and alkaline diuresis.

Hydrochlorothiazide

There have been several reports of noncardiogenic pulmonary edema following therapy with the diuretic hydrochlorothiazide. In the patients reported, there was no clear association with other toxicity from the drug, such as a hypersensitivity reaction, and the patients developed pulmonary edema after both initial and chronic exposures. In all cases patients reported the onset of tachypnea, tachycardia, dyspnea, cough, and chest pain within 1 hour of ingestion of a normal therapeutic dose. Clinically, most patients were in acute respiratory distress, with diffuse bibasilar rales and cyanosis. Therapy is supportive, and mechanical ventilation may be needed. The hydrochlorothiazide-induced pulmonary toxicity resolves quickly, and most patients recover within 24 hours. Rechallenge with hydrochlorothiazide is not recommended.

Opiates

Opiates are associated with pulmonary edema in the setting of overdose. Patients generally present with stupor and hypoventilation. The chest x-ray reveals diffuse alveolar infiltrates without cardiomegaly. Therapy is supportive, with mechanical ventilation if necessary. The use of naloxone has not been shown to alter the course of pulmonary edema, but the improvement in mental status and reversal of hypoventilation make it beneficial.

Tocolytic Agents

There has been an increasing recognition of the development of pulmonary edema in pregnant patients who receive the tocolytic agents ritodrine and terbutaline for treatment of premature labor. While these patients often receive significant intravenous fluids, it is clear that the development of pulmonary edema is related to the tocolytic agents themselves. The patients develop dyspnea, cough, and frothy sputum within 72 hours of therapy with the agent. Physical examination reveals diffuse rales, and the patients are often hypoxemic. The chest x-ray reveals diffuse alveolar infiltrates with no evidence of cardiomegaly. Therapy is immediate cessation of the tocolytic agent, supplemental O_2, and in severe cases mechanical ventilation. Response to therapy is rapid (24 to 48 hours). Mortality is low, and there is no evidence of increased fetal wastage.

Tranquilizers

The major tranquilizers are associated with pulmonary edema as part of the neuroleptic malignant syndrome. This syndrome is the acute onset of severe hyperpyrexia, muscle rigidity, autonomic dysfunction, and pulmonary edema. The chest x-ray reveals diffuse alveolar infiltrates consistent with pulmonary edema. Therapy is supportive, and recent case reports have suggested that bromocriptine and dantrolene may be helpful.[14] Although the syndrome is rare, mortality is approximately 20 percent.

UNIQUE DRUG-RELATED SYNDROMES

Several distinct, unique syndromes involving the respiratory system occur in association with the administration of various drugs (Table 39-6).

Pleural Effusions

Methotrexate

While the majority of patients with methotrexate pulmonary toxicity present with acute pulmonary infiltrates or chronic interstitial disease, some patients show an effusion on chest x-ray. The pleural effusion is often associated with pleuritic chest pain and fever and may be seen in association with pulmonary abnormalities such as interstitial infiltrates or atelectasis.[15] As with pulmonary toxicity from methotrexate, the pleural effusion associated with this drug may be self-limited, resolving spontaneously with or without withdrawal of the drug.

Methysergide

Methysergide is a rare cause of pleural effusion. The incidence of pleural effusion is unknown but is certainly lower

Table 39-6. Unique Syndromes Related to Drugs

Pleural effusions
Methotrexate
Methylsergide
Nitrofurantoin
Bronchiolitis obliterans
Gold
Penicillamine
Muscle paralysis
Aminoglycosides
Polymixins
Pulmonary hemorrhage
Penicillamine

than the incidence of methysergide-induced retroperitoneal fibrosis. Therapy is withdrawal of the drug; however, many individuals will develop diffuse pleural thickening.

Nitrofurantoin

The pleural disease caused by nitrofurantoin is related to acute pulmonary toxicity and begins within 2 weeks of the onset of therapy. Patients present with dyspnea, and fever occurs in 90 percent of patients.[16] Pleuritic chest pain occurs in more than 30 percent of patients, as does peripheral eosinophilia. The effusion is most often unilateral.

Bronchiolitis Obliterans

Gold

As stated above, the incidence of pulmonary reaction to gold salts is low. Bronchiolitis obliterans associated with gold is more acute in onset than the chronic interstitial disease described above. In this instance patients develop respiratory symptoms hours to weeks after receiving gold shots, presenting with fever, cough, and wheezing. The chest radiograph shows a diffuse nodular infiltrate, and pulmonary function studies reveal a restrictive defect. Biopsy confirms the diagnosis of bronchiolitis obliterans. Therapy of this syndrome includes withdrawal of gold therapy and administration of corticosteroids; some patients require a long course of corticosteroid therapy.

Penicillamine

Patients receiving penicillamine may develop bronchiolitis obliterans over months of therapy. The usual presentation is dyspnea and a mild productive cough. Eosinophilia is variably present. The chest x-ray may reveal a diffuse reticulonodular infiltrate or may be normal but pulmonary function studies are abnormal revealing a combined restrictive and obstructive defect. The development of obstructive disease in patients on penicillamine suggests bronchiolitis.[11] Therapy is removal of the drug and administration of corticosteroids. As with gold-induced bronchiolitis obliterans, a long course of steroid therapy may be necessary.

Muscle Paralysis

Although not a true pulmonary toxicity, the aminoglycosides and polymixins may produce respiratory compromise through neuromuscular paralysis. This response may be idiosyncratic or dose-dependent. Because these agents act synergistically with muscle relaxants to cause muscle weakness, extreme care should be taken when these antibiotics are administered in patients who receive muscle relaxants. Therapy is supportive, with mechanical ventilation if necessary. Therapy with neostigmine, 0.125 mg every 30 minutes, may be useful.[12]

Pulmonary Hemorrhage

Penicillamine

Penicillamine is a rare cause of a pulmonary-renal syndrome clinically indistinguishable from Goodpasture syndrome.[17] Patients present with a severe acute illness characterized by hemoptysis, tachypnea, hematuria, fever, and renal failure. The chest x-ray shows a diffuse alveolar "ground grass" infiltrate consistent with hemorrhage. Because of the large amount of blood in the lungs, the diffusing capacity is often elevated. Laboratory values show an elevated sedimentation rate and evidence of renal failure. The anti-glomerular basement membrane antibody is negative. The syndrome develops soon after therapy with penicillamine has begun; in almost all cases, the onset of symptoms has occurred within 1 week. Therapy is removal of the drug, corticosteroids, and cytotoxic therapy as in Goodpasture syndrome.[18]

DRUGS THAT CAUSE OR EXACERBATE ASTHMA

Drugs associated with asthma are aspirin, beta-blockers, tartrazine dyes, and vinca alkaloids.

Aspirin, NSAIDs, and Tartrazine Dyes

Aspirin, NSAIDs, and tartrazine dyes are grouped together because there is cross-reactivity between them. Approximately 1 percent of the population responds to these agents with urticaria, rhinitis, and mild wheezing.[12] However, as many as 20 percent of patients with the diagnosis of asthma may develop life-threatening bronchospasm following exposure to one of these agents. Patients who have aspirin sensitivity and asthma often also have nasal polyposis (triad syndrome). Owing to the life-threatening nature of the bronchospasm, patients with a history of sensitivity to one of these agents should avoid all of them.

Beta-Blockers

Beta-blockers cause bronchospasm by virtue of their beta-adrenergic blockade. The degree of respiratory impairment from exposure is dose-dependent; however, reactions have occurred following small doses of beta-blockers in ophthalmic preparations. In patients with a history of asthma, beta-blockers may worsen the overall respiratory condition without producing acute bronchospastic events. Even the selective beta-blockers have been reported to cause pulmonary symptoms. Thus, in patients with a history of reactive airway disease it is wise to avoid all beta-blocker preparations.

Vinca Alkaloids

Vinca alkaloids, used as antitumor agents, have rarely been associated with wheezing and bronchospasm within minutes to hours after exposure. Pulmonary infiltrates may be present, and several patients with this syndrome have required mechanical ventilation. Unlike most bronchospastic disease, the bronchospasm associated with vinca alkaloids carries with it a high mortality. Patients have developed acute shortness of breath, wheezing, and dyspnea, followed by pulmonary infiltrates and progressive respiratory failure. Corticosteroids may be of value and should be instituted immediately if this syndrome develops.

References

1. Bennett JM, Reich SD: Bleomycin. Ann Intern Med 1979; 90:945–948
2. Cooper JAD, White DA, Matthay RA: Drug-induced pulmonary disease. Part 1: Cytotoxic drugs. Am Rev Respir Dis 1986; 133:321–340
3. Goldiner PL, Carlon GC, Cvitovic E et al: Factors influencing postoperative morbidity and mortality in patients treated with bleomycin. Br Med J 1978;1:1664–1667
4. Iacovino JR, Leitner J, Abbas AK et al: Fatal pulmonary reaction from low doses of bleomycin. An idiosyncratic tissue response. JAMA 1976;235:1253–1255
5. Oliner H, Schwartz R, Rubio F et al: Interstitial pulmonary fibrosis following busulfan therapy. Am J Med 1961;31:134–139
6. Heard BE, Cooke RA: Busulfan lung. Thorax 1968;23:187–193
7. Kaplan RL, Waite DH: Progressive interstitial lung disease from prolonged methotrexate therapy. Arch Dermatol 1978;114:1800–1802
8. Ginsberg SJ, Comis RL: The pulmonary toxicity of antineoplastic agents. Semin Oncol 1982;9:34–51
9. Rosenow EC, Martin WJ: Drug-induced interstitial lung disease. pp. 123–137. In Schwartz MI, King TE (eds): Interstitial Lung Disease. BC Decker, Philadelphia, 1988
10. Brutinel W, Martin W: Chronic nitrofurantoin reaction associated with T-lymphocyte alveolitis. Chest 1986;89:150–152
11. Cooper JAD, White DA, Matthay RA: Drug-induced pulmonary disease. Part 2: Noncytotoxic drugs. Am Rev Respir Dis 1986; 133:488–505
12. Taraska VA: Drug-induced lung disease. pp. 178–183. In Cherniack RM (ed): Current Therapy of Respiratory Disease. Vol. 2. BC Decker, Toronto, 1986
13. Wright DG, Robichaud KJ, Pizzo PA et al: Lethal pulmonary reactions associated with the combined use of amphotericin B and leukocyte transfusions. N Engl J Med 1981;304:1185–1189
14. Granato JE, Stern BJ, Fingel A et al: Neuroleptic malignant syndrome: Successful treatment with dantrolene and bromocriptine. Ann Neurol 1983;14:89–90
15. Sostman HD, Matthay RA, Putman CE: Methotrexate-induced pneumonitis. Medicine (Baltimore) 1976;55:371–388
16. Hailey FJ, Glascock HW, Hewitt WF: Pleuropneumonic reactions to nitrofurantoin. N Engl J Med 1969;281:1087–1090
17. Sternlieb I, Bennett B, Scheinberg IH: D-Penicillamine induced Goodpasture's syndrome in Wilson's disease. Ann Intern Med 1975;82:673–676
18. Matloff DS, Kaplan MM: D-Penicillamine-induced Goodpasture's-like syndrome in primary biliary cirrhosis. Successful treatment with plasmapheresis and immunosuppressives. Gastroenterology 1980;78:1046–1049

Chapter 40

Disorders of Body Temperature

David J. Pierson

CHAPTER OUTLINE

Homeostasis, the constancy of the body's internal milieu that permits its many chemical and physical systems to function optimally, depends strongly on maintenance of a constant, normal body temperature. Unlike some animals (poikilotherms), which have adapted to an inconstant environment by evolving the ability to tolerate a range of body temperatures, humans and other homeotherms have a tightly controlled system for maintaining the same body temperature despite widely varying external temperatures and physical activities.

Under normal conditions heat production and dissipation are regulated to keep the body's core temperature at 37°C (98.6°F), with a normal range of about ±1°C (±1.4°F). An average-sized resting adult produces heat at the rate of 60 to 70 kcal/h.[1] Heat production rises with exertion or excitement and in the presence of increased catecholamines, thyroid hormone, and other endogenous factors; it can be increased manyfold, transiently to as much as 1000 kcal/h during extreme exertion.[1]

The central controller of body temperature is the hypothalamus, which senses temperature, establishes the normal "set point," and mediates increases in heat production or heat dissipation in order to achieve and maintain this set point. Beyond the heat generated normally by the body's "respiratory engine" (see Ch. 2), heat production can be increased by shivering (which can raise the basal rate as much as fivefold) and by various behavioral modifications. Heat conservation, as in a cold room, is accomplished by constriction of cutaneous blood vessels (diverting blood from the body's "shell" to its "core") and to a small extent by piloerection.

To increase heat loss, as with strenuous exercise or high environmental temperatures, the cutaneous vessels dilate, blood is diverted from the splanchnic bed to the periphery, and eccrine glands in the skin are activated, causing sweating. These changes increase heat loss through conduction, convection, and evaporation.

Normal functioning of the body's temperature-regulating system requires an intact hypothalamus, autonomic nervous system (to mediate vasomotor changes and sweating), and peripheral somatic nervous system (the sensory branch to correctly perceive temperature and the motor branch to mediate shivering and piloerection). When this system becomes deranged or is unable to keep up with heat gain or loss, life-threatening hyper- or hypothermia can result.

HYPERTHERMIA

An elevated body temperature is seen in four types of disorders[2] (Table 40-1). *Fever* is a disorder of thermoregulation, in which there is an upward displacement of the set point of the hypothalamic thermostat; the body responds by

Table 40-1. Classification of Disorders Characterized by Elevated Body Temperature

Fever
Environmental heat illness
Minor illness associated with heat exposure
Heat syncope
Heat edema
Heat tetany
Heat cramps
Heat exhaustion
Heat stroke
Classical heat stroke
Exertional heat stroke
Malignant hyperthermia
Neuroleptic malignant syndrome

actively raising body temperature to this new, higher set point. In the other three types of disorder hyperthermia occurs because heat gain or heat production exceeds the body's ability to dissipate it.

Fever

Although fever may occasionally be caused by a primary disorder of the hypothalamus, causing the body's thermostat to be set inappropriately high, in most instances it results from the normal response of the hypothalamus to temperature-increasing (pyrogenic) stimulation.[3,4] The most familiar such stimulus is infection. Infectious agents such as viruses, gram-positive and gram-negative bacteria, and fungi produce or act as exogenous pyrogens, substances that stimulate bone marrow-derived phagocytes (e.g., neutrophils or macrophages) to release a substance called *endogenous pyrogen*. This agent has been isolated and purified and can induce fever in experimental animals at doses as small as 35 ng.[3] In response to endogenous pyrogen (which can also be released by noninfectious stimuli), the body's thermogenic mechanisms are brought into action in order to achieve and maintain a new, higher hypothalamic temperature set point. This is the cause of the piloerection ("goose-bumps") and shivering that occur commonly in the early stages of infectious illnesses.

With true fever, body temperature seldom exceeds 41°C (105.8°F). Higher temperatures than this are usually the result of additional thermogenesis, as with seizures.

Because fever is a normal adaptive response to infection and other stress, automatically attempting to decrease it with antipyretics or other measures would seem illogical and perhaps counterproductive. In certain circumstances, however, the high temperature itself should be treated. An example is sometimes encountered in febrile patients with severe adult respiratory distress syndrome (ARDS), whose elevated temperatures increase O_2 consumption sufficiently to prevent satisfactory arterial and tissue oxygenation: because O_2 consumption increases 7 to 8 percent for each degree Celsius above 37, reducing core temperature by 2 to 4°C can significantly decrease O_2 demands.

The scientific basis for treating fever in other familiar settings is less clear. Examples of such settings include the attempted prevention of febrile seizures in small children and the treatment of high fever in pregnancy in attempt to prevent fetal developmental defects. Fever is sometimes treated for reasons of comfort although cooling blankets and other techniques used in the intensive care unit (ICU) can sometimes make patients more uncomfortable than their fever.

Environmental Heat Illness

Healthy individuals become acclimated to high environmental temperatures on repeated or prolonged exposure. Their skeletal muscles work more efficiently and generate less heat, their cardiac outputs and circulating blood volumes increase, and they produce increased quantities of sweat while losing less salt.[1] Several non-life-threatening but bothersome manifestations of heat stress occur mainly in nonacclimatized individuals. These include the following:

Heat syncope: Orthostatic dizziness or fainting following exposure to high environmental temperatures

Heat edema: Transient peripheral or generalized edema, seen mainly in women and during heat acclimatization, secondary to salt retention brought on by increased aldosterone secretion

Heat tetany: Focal muscle contractions related to acute respiratory alkalosis, which sometimes develops an initial exposure to high environmental temperatures.

Heat cramps: Painful muscle contractions occurring during or after work in the heat, usually seen in athletes or highly acclimatized workers and due to consumption of large quantities of water without salt supplementation

The more severe, potentially life-threatening environmental heat illnesses include heat exhaustion and two forms of heat stroke. *Heat exhaustion* is caused by excessive loss of body water and/or electrolyte depletion due to high environmental temperature. Free water depletion is seen typically in infants, very old people, or others who are unable to communicate their need for water; it can also result from excessive salt intake. The salt depletion form of heat exhaustion develops in the setting of profuse sweating or when continued water intake is not accompanied by ingestion of salt. Its symptoms include weakness, fatigue, severe headache, nausea, vomiting, diarrhea, and diffuse myalgias; these usually respond promptly to salt repletion.[1]

Heat stroke is a medical emergency characterized by extreme hyperthermia, usually above 40.6°C (105°F), plus central nervous system dysfunction and (usually) cessation of sweating. In most instances a person with true heat stroke will die if the condition is not recognized promptly and measures to lower body temperature are not taken immediately.[1] Full recovery can usually be anticipated if such cooling can be accomplished quickly and if the numerous recognized complications (see below) are anticipated and managed appropriately.

There are two distinct forms.[1,2] *Classic heat stroke* occurs in sedentary or confined persons who are exposed to high surrounding temperatures for several days, as can occur during summer heat waves. Conditions that increase a person's susceptibility to classic heat stroke include diabetes mellitus, hyperthyroidism, alcoholism, malnutrition, and anything that impairs sweat production, such as old healed burns or scleroderma. Patients with classic heat stroke present with marked hyperthermia, lethargy or coma, and hot, dry, flushed skin. The usual acid-base abnormality encountered in such patients is acute respiratory alkalosis.

Exertional heat stroke occurs in the setting of heavy muscular exertion in a hot, typically humid environment.[1] Athletes competing in outdoor endurance events in hot surroundings and laborers working in conditions of very high temperature and humidity are typical victims of this form of heat injury. Severe central nervous system dysfunction (including bizarre behavior) and profound volume depletion are characteristic. Sweating often persists, resulting in paradoxically cool, clammy skin. Body core temperature can be extreme, higher than 44.5°C (112°F).

Rhabdomyolysis is common in exertional heat stroke. Other common manifestations include disseminated intravascular coagulation, severe lactic acidosis, hyperuricemia, hypocalcemia, and hyperkalemia. Severe metabolic acidosis is frequent, and serum HCO_3^- levels may be unmeasurable.[1] Creatine kinase in serum often reaches very high levels because of the rhabdomyolysis. Acute renal failure occurs in perhaps one-third of patients. If the disorder is untreated, mortality is virtually 100 percent; with appropriate treatment it should be 10 percent or less.

Successful management of heat stroke hinges on rapidly decreasing core body temperature; the goal should be to lower it to 38°C within 1 hour.[1] The traditional cooling technique consists either of (1) immersing the patient in a tub of ice water and briskly rubbing the extremities or (2) rubbing the patient's wetted skin with plastic bags filled with ice while directing the flow from a large fan over the patient. A newer, less uncomfortable but incompletely proven technique involves supporting the patient on a mesh sling in the path of a warmed airstream containing atomized water.[5] Cooling is achieved by vaporization of the spray from the patient's warm skin. This technique has been reported to decrease core temperature at a rate of 0.06°C/min.[1]

Malignant Hyperthermia

Malignant hyperthermia is a pharmacogenetic disorder in which acute hypermetabolic reactions in skeletal muscle are triggered by exposure to inhalational anesthetics, skeletal muscle relaxants, or occasionally other factors.[2,6,7] It is most common in children undergoing anesthesia, among whom the potential incidence may be as high as 1 in 15,000 cases.[8] In adults the susceptibility to this disorder is much less, and it has recently been estimated that the fulminating syndrome presently occurs in perhaps 1 in 250,000 anesthesias.[6]

Malignant hyperthermia is believed to be due to sudden massive release of calcium from muscle sarcoplasmic reticulum in genetically susceptible individuals on exposure to the triggering agent. It is characterized by the acute development of muscle rigidity, cardiovascular instability, signs of hypermetabolism, and rapidly rising body temperature—as much as 1°C/5 min (Table 40-2). A dramatic increase in CO_2 production can cause end-tidal CO_2 tension ($P_{ET}CO_2$) to double in 10 to 15 minutes.[9] This condition has been described as an anesthesiologist's nightmare in that the fulminating syndrome can emerge rapidly and be fatal if not managed quickly and correctly.

Management consists of immediately discontinuing administration of any potential triggering agent and quickly giving the drug dantrolene (a direct-acting muscle relaxant) intravenously. An initial dose of 2.5 mg/kg is followed by additional doses as needed up to 10 mg/kg. Early management also includes vigorous hyperventilation and volume resuscitation, plus careful monitoring for cardiac arrhythmias and other complications.

Confirmation of the diagnosis and detection of susceptible individuals require muscle biopsy. A fresh, intact strip of skeletal muscle is tested for response to small amounts of caffeine and halothane, which cause vigorous contraction when the genetic defect is present but have no effect on muscle tissue from normal individuals.

Neuroleptic Malignant Syndrome

The neuroleptic malignant syndrome (NMS) has similar manifestations to malignant hyperthermia (Table 40-2), although these are usually less dramatic and both the clinical setting and the pathophysiology are different.[2,10,11] NMS is an idiosyncratic reaction to neuroleptic (antipsychotic) drugs and hence is usually seen in patients with major psychiatric disorders. The drugs most commonly associated with NMS are members of the phenothiazine and butyrophenone families, of which haloperidol, chlorpromazine, and fluphenazine have accounted for the greatest number.[11] Although the pathogenesis is incompletely understood, NMS appears to involve blockade of dopaminergic receptors in the hypothalamus, spinal cord, and corpus striatum. It is not a primary disorder of skeletal muscle, and there is no known genetic predisposition.

Patients who develop NMS have usually been taking neuroleptic agents for a period of days or months, sometimes years, at usual recommended doses. Typically, over a period of 1 to 3 days patients develop hyperthermia (which can reach 41°C or higher), characteristic "lead pipe" skeletal muscle rigidity, fluctuating consciousness, and signs of autonomic dysfunction such as diaphoresis, tachycardia, cardiac arrhythmias, and blood pressure instability. Rigidity and akinesia develop concomitantly with or shortly before

Table 40-2. Clinical Features of Malignant Hyperthermia and Neuroleptic Malignant Syndrome

	Malignant Hyperthermia	Neuroleptic Malignant Syndrome
Precipitating factors	Inhalational anesthetics (e.g., halothane, cyclopropane, enflurane, isoflurane) Depolarizing muscle relaxants (e.g., succinylcholine, decamethonium) Stress of surgery	Neuroleptic drugs (e.g., haloperidol, chlorpromazine, fluphenazine)
Genetic predisposition	Yes	None known
Localization of thermoregulatory defect	Sarcoplasmic reticulum of skeletal muscle	Central nervous system
Onset	Minutes (usually) to hours after contact with agent	Days (usually) to years after starting drug
Presenting physical signs	Masseter muscle spasm Increased $P_{ET}CO_2$; tachypnea Tachycardia; arrhythmias; rigidity; sweating Rapidly rising core temperature	Muscular rigidity; dystonia Tachycardia; diaphoresis; tachypnea Temperature elevation
Laboratory findings	Respiratory and metabolic acidosis Hyperkalemia; hypercalcemia; hypernatremia Elevated creatine kinase Elevated liver enzymes	Nonspecific electrolyte disturbances; possible leukocytosis and enzyme elevations
Diagnosis	Muscle biopsy (caffeine-halothane contraction test)	Clinical setting; must be differentiated from heat stroke and lethal catatonia
Treatment	Dantrolene Immediate discontinuation of offending agent Hyperventilation; ICU monitoring and support	Discontinuation of offending drug Dantrolene; bromocriptine
Mortality	Unrecognized & untreated: 75–100% With appropriate treatment: 5–10%	Untreated: 20–30% With appropriate treatment: <5%

the onset of hyperthermia. Masseter muscle spasm may occur but is neither as uniform nor as marked as in malignant hyperthermia. Laboratory changes are nonspecific and less dramatic than in malignant hyperthermia. Rhabdomyolysis, elevated muscle and liver enzymes, and leukocytosis may occur. Untreated, NMS has a mortality rate as high as 20 to 30 percent.

The incidence is variously reported as 0.15 to 0.5 percent of patients receiving the offending drugs.[10,11] Certain patient groups appear to be relatively predisposed to the development of NMS; examples are individuals with organic brain syndrome, dehydration, physical exhaustion, and exposure to high environmental temperatures.[11]

The diagnosis is made clinically, primarily on the basis of the setting and manifestations. Other conditions with which NMS can be confused are classic heat stroke and lethal catatonia, a rare primary psychiatric disorder characterized by progressive mental excitement, with fever, continuous motor activity, and in some cases muscle rigidity.[10,11]

Therapy is not as firmly established for NMS as for malignant hyperthermia but in most respects is similar. Although less acute than malignant hyperthermia, NMS should nonetheless be approached as a life-threatening illness. Prompt diagnosis is important (and often difficult in patients with complicating major behavioral disturbances) so that the offending drug can be discontinued. Although there are no controlled studies, the existing literature supports the use of dantrolene.[10,12] Bromocriptine, a dopamine agonist, also appears to be helpful and can be administered concomitantly with dantrolene.

HYPOTHERMIA

Hypothermia is present when the core body temperature is less than 35°C (95°F). Its severity, clinical manifestations, and prognosis depend substantially on the lowest temperature reached, and hypothermia is classified accordingly as mild (32 to 35°C or 90 to 95°F), moderate (30 to 32°C or 86 to 89°F), and severe (under 30°C or 86°F).[2,13–17] The severity of hypothermia is often underestimated on initial evaluation because standard clinical thermometers read only down to 34°C (94°F). An electronic or special low-reading mercury thermometer should be used whenever a reading near 34°C is obtained. It is also important to measure core (e.g., rectal) rather than mouth or axillary temperature.

Physiologic Effects and Clinical Manifestations

O_2 consumption and CO_2 production fall relatively linearly at 7 to 9 percent per degree Celsius down to roughly 20°C, so that both are about 50 percent of normal at 28 to 30°C and 20 percent at 18 to 20°C.[14,17]

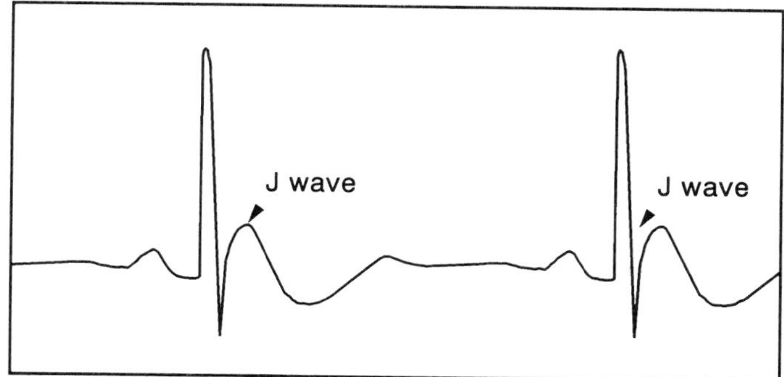

Figure 40-1. Characteristic electrocardiographic J wave of hypothermia.

Cardiovascular alterations with increasing hypothermia relate primarily to cardiac conduction and susceptibility to arrhythmias. Electrocardiographic changes include increased P-R interval, widening QRS complexes, S-T depression, and T-wave inversion, along with the characteristic J wave first described by Osborn[18] (Fig. 40-1), which is considered pathognomonic for hypothermia. Arrhythmias occur with increasing frequency and clinical severity below about 29°C. Most serious of these is ventricular fibrillation, which may be unresponsive to electrical defibrillation until the patient is rewarmed to at least 30°C. In the past some authorities have cautioned against instrumentation of the heart in hypothermia lest ventricular fibrillation be induced. However, most clinicians now agree that if Swan-Ganz catheterization is clearly indicated for hemodynamic assessment and management, this should be done regardless of the patient's temperature.

Respiratory effects include bradypnea, down to rates of 7 to 12 breaths per minute at 30°C and 4 to 7 breaths per minute in the mid-20°C range.[14] Decreases in mentation and in the

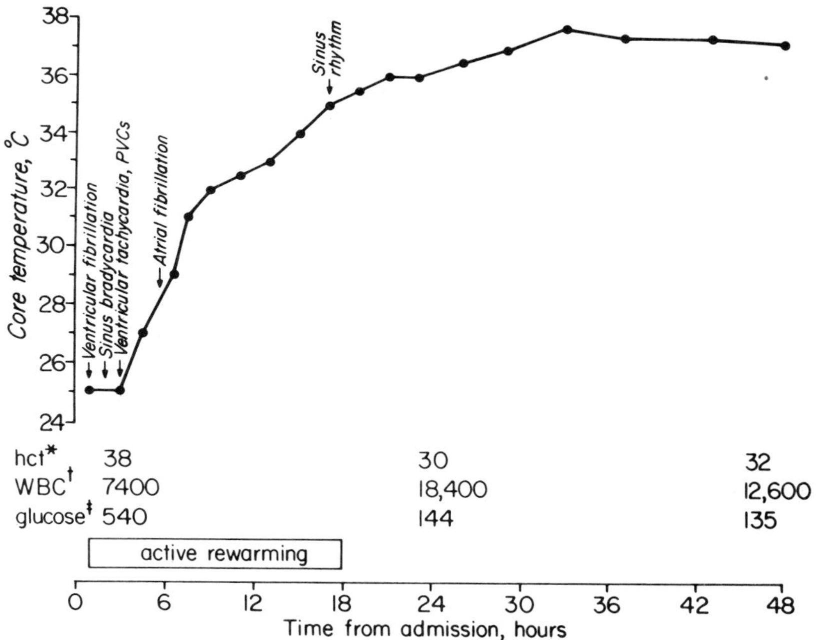

Figure 40-2. Clinical course of severe accidental hypothermia in a 75-year-old woman, illustrating several typical physiologic changes. Active rewarming consisted of warm water enemas and gastric lavage plus administration of warmed intravenous fluids. Initial ventricular arrhythmias gave way to atrial fibrillation as warming occurred, and the latter resolved spontaneously. PVCs, premature ventricular contractions; hct, hematocrit (percent); WBC, blood leukocyte count, cells per milliliter. (From Stanton and Pierson,[19] with permission.)

cough reflex, combined with cold-induced bronchorrhea, may lead to aspiration and difficulty in clearing respiratory secretions.[13] Both anatomic and physiologic dead space increase progressively with hypothermia.

Changes in central nervous system function are highly variable. As core temperature falls below 35°C, most patients become disoriented, forgetful, and unable to engage in rational conversation. Hallucinations and argumentativeness are common. Consciousness decreases progressively, and most individuals are semiconscious at 30°C. Seizures may occur. Discoordination is due in part to decreased nerve conduction velocity, from 30 m/s at 35°C to 26 m/s at 23°C, to 12 m/s at 21°C.[14] Peripheral reflexes (including pupillary reflexes) are generally lost at 26 to 27°C. Central nervous system electrical activity ceases by 18°C.

Decreased renal tubular reabsorption produces diuresis of both water and nitrogen with hypothermia. Acute tubular necrosis may occur. Hematologic changes include hemoconcentration, with associated increases in blood viscosity and hematocrit, and leukocytosis, due primarily to demargination. Coagulation is slowed but returns to normal on rewarming.

One of the most important endocrine changes in hypothermia is a loss of peripheral effect of insulin below about 31°C, resulting in hyperglycemia. Administration of insulin to a hypothermic patient is thus ineffective while core temperature remains low but may lead to serious hypoglycemia on rewarming. Hypoglycemia may also occur spontaneously in hypothermic patients. Endogenous corticosteroid levels are increased and changes in thyroid hormones are variable during hypothermia. Pancreatitis is a not uncommon finding.

Figure 40-2 graphically depicts the course of one patient's physiologic complications during rewarming from profound hypothermia and illustrates several of the changes described above.[19]

Table 40-3. Clinical Settings Associated with Hypothermia

Description	Settings
Accidental	
Anyone (including fit, healthy host)	Recreational environmental exposure Cold water immersion Following trauma
Vulnerable host (neonate, elderly, immobile)	Any of above plus cool surroundings
Deliberate	Cardiopulmonary bypass Treatment of Reye syndrome
Drug-induced	Alcohol, opiates, barbiturates, phenothiazines, anesthetics, possibly others
Generalized central nervous system dysfunction	Spinal cord injury Cerebrovascular accident Hypopituitarism
Hypothalamic dysfunction	Head trauma Wernicke's encephalopathy Anorexia nervosa Pinealoma (other tumors)
Associated with serious systemic illness	Sepsis Disseminated malignancy Malnutrition Cardiovascular collapse
Endocrine and metabolic disorders	Hypothyroidism Hypoadrenalism Hypoglycemia Malnutrition
Loss of protective effect of skin	Burns Severe exfoliation (e.g., drug-induced or Stevens-Johnson syndrome) Erythrodermas

Clinical Settings

Although most of the physiologic effects just discussed are primarily features of the level to which core temperature falls, the clinical implications and prognosis of hypothermia depend largely on who the patient is and on the cause of the hypothermia.[13–15,20–22] Table 40-3 lists several general categories into which hypothermic patients can be placed, each with characteristic clinical implications.

Accidental hypothermia may be defined as a spontaneous decrease in core temperature, usually in a cold environment and usually without specific hypothalamic dysfunction. The body size, fitness, and general health of the affected individual determine the severity of cold exposure required to produce clinical hypothermia. Newborns, the elderly, quadriplegics, and other individuals who are immobile are particularly susceptible to hypothermia, even in only modest cold. Surveys in England during the winter have found as many as 15 percent of otherwise healthy old people living alone to have body temperatures below 35°C[23]; such "subclinical" hypothermia can also occur in the warmer seasons of the year, although this is less frequent.

Overall mortality among 401 hypothermic patients in one large multicenter study was 17 percent.[24] The prognosis was less favorable in those with the most severe hypothermia. Among the various categories listed in Table 40-3, patients who present with low body temperature in the setting of severe underlying systemic disease such as sepsis or disseminated malignancy have a less favorable prognosis than most of those in the other groups.[13,21] In one study of a series of patients who were hypothermic on admission to the ICU, those with bacteremia had lower systemic vascular resistances and higher cardiac indices than those with negative blood cultures, although most cardiovascular and laboratory indices were not different in the two groups.[20] Thus, distinguishing clinically between different patient groups may not always be possible initially.

Management

Management consists of removing the patient from the cold, treating concomitant conditions, careful monitoring, good general ICU care, and specific rewarming measures.

Although there is a tendency to focus on the last of these, the other aspects of management are at least as important as the rewarming method used[2,13,15,16] (Table 40-4). Because of the risk of ventricular fibrillation, care should be taken with endotracheal intubation, passage of catheters into the central circulation, and other manipulations that might trigger arrhythmias. However, necessary procedures should not be deferred or delayed for this reason. Despite higher mortality in the presence of serious infection, there is no evidence that routinely administering antibiotics to hypothermic patients is efficacious.

Passive rewarming should be adequate in mild hypothermia, particularly that which has developed gradually, as in the elderly. Such patients should be wrapped warmly in blankets and cared for in a warm room. *Active rewarming* is advisable when core temperature is below 32°C (89.6°F), although controversy persists over which of the various techniques is best. It was formerly believed that aggressive surface rewarming resulted in sudden cutaneous vasodilation, with return of large volumes of cold, acidotic, toxin-laden blood to a central circulation that was unable to respond normally. For this reason, until recently, active core rewarming was the treatment of choice. However, in the presence of vigorous fluid resuscitation and appropriate hemodynamic monitoring, either core or surface techniques can probably be used, the choice depending in part on local availability and the clinician's experience with the different methods.

The most efficient method of altering body temperature is extracorporeal circulation. This technique is used extensively during cardiac surgery. Warming or cooling via transfer of heat from liquids is highly efficient because 1 g of water either gives up or takes on 1 cal of heat (1000 cal = 1 kcal, as used in assessment of nutritional needs) per degree Celsius temperature change. Thus, massive heat transfer occurs as the total cardiac output is warmed externally and then recirculated.

On the other hand, the least efficient method of adding or removing heat is via the respiratory tract. The potential for heat transfer is minimal because of the small amount of water carried even in the densest aerosol. If 5 g of water is *nebulized*, only about 1 g is actually inhaled; thus, even if gas is heated to 44°C, the quantity of heat transfer is insignificant in relation to the amount needed to effect a total-body temperature change. Heated *humidified* gas is even less effective, since at 37°C and 100 percent humidity only 43.8 mg of water is present in 1 L of gas. Heating to 44°C increases the water content to approximately 52 mg/L of completely water-saturated gas. Gas delivered to the respiratory tract should be maintained at normal body temperature, as the minor quantity of heat transferred at elevated inhaled gas temperature does not outweigh the risk of local tissue damage by the elevated temperatures. The heat capacity of air is so small that this type of "rewarming" plays no significant part in the therapy of hypothermia.

The optimum rate of rewarming has also been controversial. Most authorities still recommend relatively slow rewarming—for example, not faster than 1°C/h.[2,15,16] However, recent studies suggest that with aggressive support and monitoring it may be possible to rewarm severely hypothermic patients to 37°C within 2 to 3 hours of admission without serious complications.[25,26] Such an approach would seem particularly appropriate for patients with refractory ventricular arrhythmias. However, further experience with more rapid rewarming, whether by surface[25] or core[26] approaches, will be required before this can be routinely recommended.

Table 40-4. Available Methods of Rewarming in Hypothermia

Passive rewarming
Insulation from further heat loss
Administration of fluids and metabolic substrates for endogenous heat generation
Active surface rewarming
Immersion in warm water
Heating blankets
Radiant warmers
"Tropical rooms"
Active core rewarming
Heated intravenous fluids
Gastric lavage with warm water
Warm water enemas
Peritoneal lavage with warmed fluids
Pleural or mediastinal irrigation
Extracorporeal circulation

The prognosis of severe hypothermia is dependent in large part on the patient's previous state of health and on whether the hypothermia is due to overwhelming environmental exposure or to serious underlying illness. Because of the loss of such indices as pupillary reflexes, peripheral pulses, or even cardiac electrical activity at very low temperatures, hypothermic patients should not be considered "dead" until they are "warm and dead." A 1988 report of full recovery in a child with an initial core temperature of 19°C after 66 minutes' submersion in cold water[27] illustrates this principle.

EFFECTS OF TEMPERATURE ON BLOOD GASES

In accordance with Charles's law (see Ch. 1), the partial pressures of gases in a given sample of blood decrease with decreasing temperature and increase with increasing temperature. The pH and plasma HCO_3^- concentration also change, the pH slightly rising as temperature falls. Table 40-5 illustrates these points in relation to a specimen of blood with normal arterial blood gas values at 37°C. If this specimen is heated or cooled anaerobically, the measured gas tensions, pH, and HCO_3^- level will vary as shown. The arterial blood in a hypothermic or hyperthermic patient will undergo the same changes provided that ventilation and metabolism remain the same. Table 40-6 provides correction factors for calculating actual PO_2, PCO_2, and pH values in patients when their core temperatures are different from the 37°C at which the blood gas electrode is maintained.

Whether to report blood gas values as they are measured (i.e., at 37°C) or "corrected" to the actual values present in

Table 40-5. Changes in Blood Gas Values with Temperature[a]

Variable	Temperature				
	25°C	29°C	33°C	37°C	41°C
pH (U)	7.58	7.52	7.46	7.40	7.34
PCO_2 (mmHg)	18	26	33	40	47
PO_2 (mmHg)	44	58	76	100	124
HCO_3^- (mEq/L)	17	21	23	24	25

[a] Values at 41°C, 33°C, 29°C, and 25°C, that would correspond to the normal values shown at 37°C, if only the temperature changed.

the patient's blood is a matter of long-standing controversy.[28–31] Likewise, whether to manage patients by attempting to maintain normal values at 37°C or at their actual body temperatures is an unresolved and hotly debated question.

This issue is most often dealt with in the operating room in connection with deliberate hypothermia for cardiac surgery. There are two separate schools adhering to the "pH-stat" and "alpha-stat" concepts, and they manage the patient's acid-base status differently. The pH-stat approach seeks to keep arterial pH at 7.40 at the patient's actual body temperature. This means that for a hypothermic patient, a pH that is "normal" in the patient will be acidotic when measured at 37°C. The alpha-stat approach[28] seeks to keep the total CO_2 content of the blood constant with respect to normal body temperature; with this approach, a pH of 7.40 and PCO_2 of 40 mmHg when measured at 37°C are the desired values, even though the pH is actually higher and the PCO_2 lower than those at the patient's current temperature.

A good study published in 1990 randomly allocated 86 patients to be managed during hypothermic cardiac surgery by either the pH-stat or the alpha-stat technique and carefully examined a number of physiologic and neuropsychological variables both immediately after the procedure and months later.[32] No differences were found in any variable. This supports the notion that for anesthetic management it probably does not matter which approach the clinician uses to regulate acid-base status.

For patients with hypothermia or hyperthermia being assessed in the emergency room or managed in the ICU, whether the reporting of blood gas values should be as measured at 37°C or as "corrected" for the patient's actual temperature will likely continue to be the focus of debate. The issue is handled differently in different institutions, and either way is probably satisfactory as long as the clinician knows which method is being used and understands the implications of the results for the patient.

Table 40-6. Temperature Correction Factors for Arterial Blood Gas Values

Temperature		Correction Factor[a]		
°C	°F	PO_2[b]	PCO_2[c]	pH[d]
43.4	110	1.43	1.28	−0.09
42.2	108	1.35	1.25	−0.08
41.1	106	1.26	1.19	−0.06
40.0	104	1.19	1.14	−0.04
38.9	102	1.11	1.08	−0.03
37.0	98.6	1.00	1.00	0
35.0	95	0.89	0.92	+0.03
32.2	90	0.76	0.82	+0.07
31.1	88	0.72	0.78	+0.09
30.0	86	0.67	0.74	+0.10
28.9	84	0.63	0.71	+0.12
27.8	82	0.59	0.68	+0.14
26.7	80	0.56	0.64	+0.15
25.6	78	0.52	0.61	+0.17
24.4	76	0.49	0.59	+0.18
23.3	74	0.46	0.56	+0.20
22.2	72	0.43	0.53	+0.22
21.1	70	0.40	0.50	+0.24
20.0	68	0.37	0.47	+0.25

[a] To correct for temperature, *multiply* for PO_2 and PCO_2 and *add* for pH.

[b] The corrections shown for PO_2 are approximations. Change in PO_2 with temperature is nonlinear and depends on O_2 saturation: it is 1.3%/°C (0.72%/°F) when PO_2 is >500 mmHg and increases to 7.2%/°C (4.0%/°F) when saturation is <90%.

[c] PCO_2 decreases 4.5%/°C (2.4%/°F) fall in temperature.

[d] pH increases 0.015 U/°C (0.008 U/°F) fall in temperature.

References

1. Knochel JP: Heat stroke and related heat stress disorders. Dis Mon 1989;35:301–378
2. Farmer JC: Temperature-related injuries. pp. 693–700. In Civetta JM, Taylor RW, Kirby RR (eds): Critical Care. JB Lippincott, Philadelphia, 1988
3. Bernheim HA, Block LH, Atkins E: Fever: Pathogenesis, pathophysiology, and purpose. Ann Intern Med 1979;91:261–270
4. Styrt B, Sugarman B: Antipyresis and fever. Arch Intern Med 1990;150:1589–1597
5. Costrini A: Emergency treatment of exertional heatstroke and comparison of whole-body cooling techniques. Med Sci Sports Exerc 1990;22:15–18
6. Symposium on Malignant Hyperthermia. Acta Anaesthesiol Belg 1990;41:61–132
7. Muldoon SM, Boggs SD, Freas W: Malignant hyperthermia. pp. 109–114. In Shoemaker WC, Ayres S, Grenvik A et al. (eds): Textbook of Critical Care. 2nd Ed. WB Saunders, Philadelphia, 1989
8. Vakharia N, Hall R: Malignant hyperthermia: A review of current concepts. Respir Care 1990;35:977–986
9. Baudendistel L, Goudsouzian N, Cote C, Strafford M: End-tidal CO_2 monitoring. Its use in the diagnosis and management of malignant hyperthermia. Anaesthesia 1984;39:1000–1003
10. Guze BH, Baxter LR Jr: Neuroleptic malignant syndrome. N Engl J Med 1985;313:163–166
11. Ebadi M, Pfeiffer RF, Murrin LC: Pathogenesis and treatment of neuroleptic malignant syndrome. Gen Pharmacol 1990;21:367–386
12. Rosenberg MR, Green M: Neuroleptic malignant syndrome. Review of response to therapy. Arch Intern Med 1989;149:1927–1931
13. Reuler JB: Hypothermia: Pathophysiology, clinical settings, and management. Ann Intern Med 1978;89:519–527
14. Paton BC: Accidental hypothermia. Pharmacol Ther 1983;22:331–377
15. Elder PT: Accidental hypothermia. pp. 101–109. In Shoemaker WC, Ayres S, Grenvik A et al (eds): Textbook of Critical Care. 2nd Ed. WB Saunders, Philadelphia, 1989
16. Miller JW Jr: Hypothermia. pp. 639–656. In Kravis TC, Warner

CG (eds): Emergency Medicine. 2nd Ed. Aspen Publishers, Rockville MD, 1987

17. Rupp SM, Severinghaus JW: Hypothermia. pp. 1995–2022. In Miller RD (ed): Anesthesia. 2nd Ed. Churchill Livingstone, New York, 1986
18. Osborn JJ: Experimental hypothermia: Respiratory and blood pH changes in relation to cardiac function. Am J Physiol 1953;175:389–398
19. Stanton BL, Pierson DJ: Accidental hypothermia: A case report. Respir Care 1981;26:56–59
20. Morris DL, Chambers HF, Morris MG, Sande MA: Hemodynamic characteristics of patients with hypothermia due to occult infection and other causes. Ann Intern Med 1985;102:153–157
21. Hudson LD, Conn RD: Accidental hypothermia: Associated diagnoses and prognosis in a common problem. JAMA 1974; 227:37–40
22. Luna GK, Maier RV, Pavlin EG et al: Incidence and effect of hypothermia in seriously injured patients. J Trauma 1987;27:1014–1018
23. Salvosa CB, Payne PR, Wheeler EF: Environmental conditions and body temperatures of elderly women living alone or in local authority homes. Br Med J 1971;4:656–659
24. Danzl DF, Pozos RS, Auerbach PS et al: Multicenter hypothermia survey. Ann Emerg Med 1987;16:1042–1055
25. Zachary L, Kucan JO, Robson MC, Frank DH: Accidental hypothermia treated with rapid rewarming by immersion. Ann Plast Surg 1982;9:238–241
26. Gentilello LM, Cortes V, Moujaes S et al: Continuous arteriovenous rewarming: Experimental results and thermodynamic model simulation of treatment for hypothermia. J Trauma 1990; 30:1436–1449
27. Bolte RG, Black PG, Bowers RS et al: The use of extracorporeal rewarming in a child submerged for 66 minutes. JAMA 1988; 260:377–379
28. Rahn H, Reeves RB, Howell BJ: Hydrogen ion regulation, temperature, and evolution. Am Rev Respir Dis 1975;112:165–172
29. Prough DS, Stump DA, Troost BJ: $PaCO_2$ management during cardiopulmonary bypass: Intriguing physiologic rationale, convincing clinical data, evolving hypothesis? Anesthesiology 1990;72:3–6
30. Swain JA: Hypothermia and blood pH. A review. Arch Intern Med 1988;148:1643–1646
31. Kelman GR, Nunn JF: Nomograms for correction of blood PO_2, PCO_2, pH, and base excess for time and temperature. J Appl Physiol 1966;21:1484–1490
32. Bashein G, Townes BD, Nessly ML et al: A randomized study of carbon dioxide management during hypothermic cardiopulmonary bypass. Anesthesiology 1990;72:7–15

Chapter 41

Effects of Anesthesia and Surgery on the Respiratory System

Kenneth Davis, Jr.
Daniel J. Johnson

CHAPTER OUTLINE

The care of the surgical patient requires close monitoring of perioperative pulmonary function. Pulmonary complications, resulting from intraoperative and postoperative changes in respiratory physiology, can occur in 2 to 70 percent of surgical patients. These alterations in pulmonary function are multifactorial and depend on anesthetic techniques, intraoperative positioning, and surgical procedure. Abnormalities in gas exchange such as hypoxia and hypercarbia result from this combination of factors. This chapter discusses the various effects that anesthesia and surgery have on the respiratory system, including postoperative changes, complications, and their management.

EFFECTS OF ANESTHESIA

The induction of general anesthesia can cause changes in pulmonary physiology based on a variety of effects. Airway control, pharmacologic therapy, and changes in intravascular volume and its distribution are essential components of general anesthesia. The anesthesiologist can control certain respiratory parameters such as inspired O_2, tidal volume (V_T), minute ventilation, the airway, and dead space. On the other hand, there is little or no control over patient position, surgical procedure, drug effects, pre-existing disease, and patient age. All these factors can affect the respiratory system in various ways, but the end result is alteration in gas exchange.

Hypoxemia

The primary change in respiratory function brought about by the induction of general anesthesia is a reduction in functional residual capacity (FRC) (Table 41-1). This reduction has several proposed explanations, but the effect on alveolar-arterial O_2 gradient is well established.[1] The diminished FRC increases the number of poorly ventilated but well perfused lung units, and ventilation/perfusion ($\dot{V}/\dot{Q}$) mismatching results. This corresponds to an increase in "zone 3" lung

Table 41-1. Factors That Alter Functional Residual Capacity during Anesthesia

Hypoventilation
Tracheal intubation
Altered ventilatory muscle mechanics
Chest wall paralysis
Diaphragmatic paralysis
Supine position

units and an increased intrapulmonary shunt with consequent hypoxemia. General anesthesia may increase shunt by as much as 10 percent,[2] and this increase is primarily due to atelectasis and decreased FRC.

This change in lung volume has been explained in a variety of ways. Hypoventilation can, in part, be responsible, so that careful attention should be paid to V_T during general anesthesia. Inadequate V_T can cause progressive decreases in arterial O_2 pressure (PaO_2) and compliance during anesthesia.[3] Once again, atelectasis or microatelectasis appears to be responsible.[4] Conventional radiography has failed to demonstrate the presence of atelectasis during anesthesia, but computed tomography (CT) has demonstrated densities in dependent lung regions when performed on anesthetized patients.[5,6] These densities constituted up to 7 percent of the intrathoracic area, occurred within 10 minutes of induction, and were located in the caudal rather than the cephalic regions. The area of atelectasis corresponded with the increase in intrapulmonary shunt in these patients. Densities persisted for at least 1 hour postoperatively and for 24 hours in over half the patients.

Tracheal intubation and altered ventilatory muscle mechanics can also contribute to lower FRC. Tracheal intubation can lead to small airway closure, thought to be related to airway reflex mechanisms.[7] These changes occur whether the patient is paralyzed or breathing spontaneously. Anesthetic agents and paralysis decrease chest wall and diaphragm tone. In a spontaneously breathing patient, anesthesia alters rib cage motion, decreasing the anteroposterior chest wall diameter and correspondingly increasing the lateral diameter.[8,9] This results in a loss of FRC and increases the distribution of low $\dot{V}/\dot{Q}$ lung units.

Relaxation of chest wall muscles under anesthesia further reduces FRC by decreasing the elastic recoil of the respiratory muscles and increasing the elastic recoil of the lung.[10] Studies in healthy volunteers have shown that a 20 percent reduction in FRC by chest wall restriction had no effect on $\dot{V}/\dot{Q}$ matching or shunt.[11] Under anesthesia, however, compensatory mechanisms such as increased diaphragmatic movements are not possible when decreased chest wall tone and airway closure contribute to the adverse physiologic effects brought on by a decrease in FRC.

Chemical paralysis prevents chest wall and diaphragmatic movement. The diaphragmatic motion can be affected by anesthesia independently of paralysis,[12] and the supine position exacerbates these alterations. In spontaneously breathing patients, the greatest displacement of the diaphragm occurs in the most dependent region regardless of position. With muscle paralysis, the opposite occurs, and the greatest displacement of the diaphragm is in the nondependent region. This effect may worsen $\dot{V}/\dot{Q}$ mismatching, which occurs with mechanical ventilation. In addition, paralysis presumably allows for the intrusion of intra-abdominal contents into the chest cavity caused by the weight of the intra-abdominal organs. Curiously, however, Jones et al.,[13] found no change in either abdominal or rib cage circumference following induction of anesthesia and suggested that a reduction of FRC could be explained by a central redistribution of blood volume. This finding has been confirmed by CT scanning, which has shown a cranial shift of the diaphragm, reduction of FRC, and a shift of blood to the abdomen after the induction of anesthesia.[14]

Inhalation agents can potentially aggravate the hypoxia caused by atelectasis through the inhibition of hypoxic pulmonary vasoconstriction (HPV). This phenomenon has been observed in vitro[15,16] but may be of little clinical significance in human subjects.[17,18] As discussed in Chapter 10, HPV is an autoregulatory mechanism that enables pulmonary vessels to constrict in response to alveolar hypoxia. Perfusion to nonventilated lung segments is therefore decreased and blood flow to better oxygenated regions thereby promoted. Venous admixture and hypoxemia are consequently diminished. HPV results from either the direct effects of alveolar hypoxia on adjacent vessels or the indirect effects of vasoactive substances released in response to alveolar hypoxia.

With inhibition of HPV, unventilated lung units continue to receive blood flow, which results in an increased intrapulmonary shunt, a widened alveolar-arterial O_2 tension difference [$P(A\text{-}a)O_2$], and relative hypoxemia. This does not appear to have clinical significance, and the inhibition of HPV appears to be related to pre-existing vascular distension.[18] PaO_2 appears to be maintained in spite of impaired HPV. Whether the use of other direct arteriolar vasodilators, such as nitroprusside or dobutamine, during anesthesia, can further inhibit HPV and produce clinically significant hypoxemia is not known.

One aspect of anesthesia that is controlled by the anesthetist and may affect oxygenation is intravenous fluid administration. Augmentation of intravascular volume is essential to counter the effects of vasodilating agents during general or regional anesthesia. Subsequent redistribution of this volume into the central circulation can raise hydrostatic pressure in the pulmonary circulation, potentially aggravating pre-existing hypoxemia because of decreased FRC and increased shunt. These shifts in intravascular volume can occur up to several days postoperatively when the sequestered fluid undergoes postinjury mobilization.

If gas exchange abnormalities during anesthesia are due to decreased FRC, positive end-expiratory pressure (PEEP) would presumably reverse this situation. CT has demonstrated the development of dependent lung densities during the first 5 to 15 minutes after induction of anesthesia.[5] PEEP was shown to decrease the area of atelectasis without decreasing the shunt.[19] Additionally, PEEP and large V_T do not fully overcome the changes in diaphragmatic function caused by anesthesia. PEEP is not routinely used during general anesthesia as it can adversely affect cardiac output, especially in a hypovolemic patient.

Hypercapnia

Certain manipulations during general anesthesia serve to increase dead space ventilation, which can result in hypercapnia. These primarily relate to airway manipulation and patterns of mechanical ventilation. Anatomic dead space can be increased by as much as 46 percent by the anesthesia apparatus and tracheal intubation.[20,21] *Dead space ventilation* is defined as the volume of gas not involved in gas exchange. Physiologic dead space is divided into *anatomic*, which is the volume of gas occupying the larger airways (1 mL/lb [2.2 mL/kg] body weight), and *alveolar*, which is gas contained in unperfused or poorly perfused alveoli. Alveolar dead space corresponds to "zone 1" (high $\dot{V}/\dot{Q}$ ratio) lung units.

In addition, anesthetic agents can aggravate the changes caused by intubation as described above. Halothane, cyclopropane, and nitrous oxide (N_2O) increase both anatomic and alveolar dead space. The increase in dead space/tidal volume ratio (V_D/V_T) progresses with time, and the exact mechanism of action remains unclear.[22]

Inhalation agents also diminish the ventilatory response to hypoxemia,[23] which appears to be mediated by direct action on the carotid body chemoreceptors.[24] Additionally, these agents depress the ventilatory response to changes in $PaCO_2$. These factors are more pertinent in spontaneously breathing patients and in the immediate postoperative period. Inhalation agents can also decrease V_T in spontaneously breathing patients. This decrease is dose-dependent and unaffected by $PaCO_2$.

EFFECTS OF SURGERY

The effects of the surgical procedure on respiratory physiology depend primarily on patient position, the operation performed, and the operative techniques that may be employed. The supine position is the one most commonly used for a wide range of surgical procedures; in this position the orientation of the zone 1, 2, and 3 lung units is from anterior to posterior rather than superior to inferior. A decrease in FRC of approximately 0.5 to 1.0 L occurs. As FRC decreases, it approaches and may even fall below the closing volume (CV), that is, the volume above residual volume (RV) at which small airways close. Smoking, obesity, and aging also decrease FRC,[25,26] and with advancing age FRC approaches the closing capacity (CV plus RV). This would, therefore, lead to $\dot{V}/\dot{Q}$ mismatch with an increase in shunt. Supine positioning also affects diaphragm function by altering diaphragm displacement, leading to the effects described previously. Prone and decubitus positioning have analogous effects.

The operation performed and the body cavity entered have dramatic effects on pulmonary function. Upper abdominal and thoracic surgery are associated with large decreases in lung volume (Fig. 41-1). Surgery not involving the thorax or abdomen does not substantially alter vital capacity (VC) or lung volume.[27,28] Pulmonary resection performed in the decubitus position can potentially divert blood from the right heart circulation into poorly ventilated lung, thus increasing shunt.

Surgical procedures involving the airways have a more direct effect on pulmonary physiology. This effect relates to the types of airway control and ventilation employed. Special circumstances include single lung ventilation using a double-lumen endotracheal tube and high-frequency jet ven-

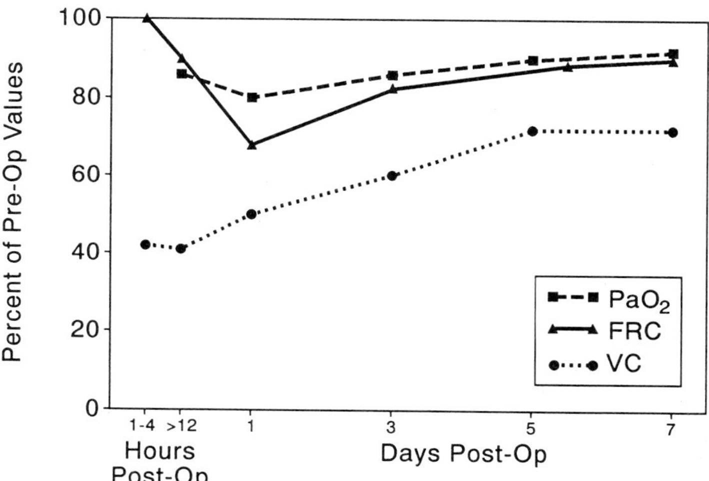

Figure 41-1. Postoperative VC, FRC, and PaO_2 (F_IO_2 = 0.21) following upper abdominal surgery. F_IO_2, fraction of inspired O_2. (Adapted from Craig,[34] with permission.)

tilation used during bronchoscopic procedures. Operations performed on the tracheobronchial tree at times require periods of hypoventilation or apnea, resulting in closure of small airways.

POSTOPERATIVE CONSIDERATIONS

Pulmonary problems (atelectasis, pneumonia, pulmonary edema, and bronchitis) are among the most common causes of postoperative morbidity. Their incidence is highest following upper abdominal or thoracic surgery. Risk factors for the development of postoperative pulmonary complications include chronic obstructive pulmonary disease, smoking, obesity, advanced age, site of incision, cardiovascular disease, and prolonged anesthesia.[29] A decrease in VC by as much as 50 to 60 percent is one of the most dramatic early changes in postoperative pulmonary function.[29] The degree of postoperative morbidity is closely related to the type of surgery performed. Vertical laparotomy incisions are associated with a higher morbidity than transverse incisions.[30–32] Lower abdominal surgery is associated with a 25 to 30 percent lower rate of morbidity,[33] while surgery outside the thorax or abdomen does not alter VC or lung volume.[27,28]

Postoperative Hypoxemia

Postoperative hypoxemia has been divided into early and late phases[34] (Table 41-2). The early phase, due to anesthetic drugs and techniques, is most likely an extension of the abnormalities in gas exchange that occur during anesthesia and may last up to 2 hours postoperatively. The normal hypoxic ventilatory drive is abolished by concentrations of halothane or enflurane as low as one-tenth of the maximum allowable concentration,[23] which may be present during the immediate postoperative period.

Alterations in the relationship between FRC and CV also continue into the postoperative period.[35] Additionally, respiratory reserve is decreased by pre-existing disease. Anesthetic agents depress ciliary activity, increase mucus secretion, and decrease mucus clearance.[36] Intubation also contributes to these abnormalities. The maximum decrease in FRC occurs in the first 48 hours, and in uncomplicated situations FRC returns to baseline by the fifth postoperative day.

The late phase of postoperative hypoxemia is believed to be due to the administration of opioid drugs. Pain, abdominal distension, and immobilization can also contribute during this phase, which is characterized by a decrease in FRC to less than 60 percent of preoperative values.[33] Narcotics tend to depress respiratory rate and minute ventilation without affecting V_T. Hypoxemia results from these changes, although hypercapnia can be observed. The hypoxemia is due to unpredictable and short-lived disturbances in ventilatory patterns.[37] In a study of cholecystectomy and hip replacement patients randomly assigned to either regional bupivicaine or intravenous morphine for pain control, the morphine group demonstrated numerous episodes of arterial desaturation (to less than 80 percent oxyhemoglobin saturation) during disturbances in ventilatory patterns.[38] No patient in the regional analgesia group fell below 87 percent oxyhemoglobin saturation during the 24-hour postoperative period.

Table 41-2. Mechanisms of Postoperative Hypoxemia

Early	
	Decreased FRC (effects of general anesthesia)
	Residual loss of hypoxic drive (inhalation agents)
Late	
	Hypoventilation (narcotic analgesics)
	Atelectasis (splinting from pain)

Atelectasis is the most common postoperative pulmonary complication and generally occurs within the first 3 days. This condition is characterized by decreased FRC and may be an extension of changes that occur during general anesthesia. In most cases it is not clinically significant and does not require specific therapy. Atelectasis can be plate-like or discoid involving the bases, segmental, lobar, or miliary (diffuse). Clinical signs include fever, tachypnea, tachycardia, diminished breath sounds, tubular breathing, and rales (crackles) on auscultation.

This clinical problem has been studied experimentally in postoperative patients by using radiopaque tantalum powder. Mucus, which collects this powder, was cleared from the lungs of postoperative orthopaedic patients sooner than from patients who underwent abdominal vascular surgery.[39] The latter group showed pooling of tantalum-labeled mucus in dependent regions followed by segmental or lobar atelectasis. In this group clearance was delayed until lung re-expansion occurred.

Prevention and Treatment of Postoperative Complications

Prevention of postoperative pulmonary complications (see Ch. 89) can begin in the preoperative period. Cessation of smoking at least 8 weeks before surgery,[39] bronchodilator therapy, and antibiotics when purulent sputum is present are useful measures in high-risk patients.[40] Preoperative teaching of coughing, deep breathing techniques, and the use of incentive spirometry (discussed below), with reinforcement in the postoperative period, is more beneficial than postoperative teaching alone because of the influences of pain and analgesics.

The treatment of atelectasis should be directed toward prevention. Intraoperative factors cannot always be controlled, but early postoperative intervention is mandatory. Prevention of atelectasis should start, where appropriate, with adequate preoperative teaching. This is not always possible, especially in emergency situations. Therefore, postoperative care should be aimed at increasing lung volume and FRC to near preoperative levels (see Ch. 73). Early ambulation postoperatively may increase FRC by as much as 10 to 20 percent.[27,32] Intermittent positive pressure breathing (IPPB) was traditionally used as a routine postoperative treatment; however, little or no real benefit has been shown with this modality because it tends to increase end-inspiratory pressure instead of volume.[41,42] Additionally, the need for trained personnel and specialized equipment makes this treatment not very cost-effective.

Other methods that have been used include blow bottles and chest physiotherapy (CPT). Blow bottles increase expiratory resistance, thus increasing airway pressure.[43] No studies have shown any direct benefit, and the indirect benefit comes from the deep inspiration taken prior to blowing into the bottle. CPT is a generalized term referring to supervised activities such as deep breathing, coughing, nasotracheal suctioning, patient turning, postural drainage, and percussion (with vibratory devices or cupped hands on the chest wall and the patient so positioned as to drain the affected bronchus). CPT is probably more effective in treating established atelectasis or lobar collapse and is not a good preventive measure since it does not directly alter lung volume. It appears to be beneficial for improving mucociliary clearance, especially in patients with large volumes of secretions.[44]

Incentive spirometry, when used routinely, may be the most efficient and cost-effective method for preventing postoperative atelectasis. It relies on a sustained, voluntary inspiration, which can open closed airways and increase FRC. This method does, however, require a certain amount of patient compliance and encouragement from staff.

The treatment of established atelectasis or lobar collapse may involve any of the effective treatment methods discussed above (see Ch. 74). Continuous positive airway pressure (CPAP), via either a mask or endotracheal tube, mechanical ventilation, and bronchoscopy may also be necessary depending on the extent of lung collapse. Mask CPAP has been shown to improve oxygenation in patients with postoperative hypoxemia by opening alveoli and increasing FRC.[45,46] Up to 15 cmH_2O pressure can be applied with low resistance end-expiratory valves. Mask CPAP should be used with caution in patients with basilar skull fractures or anastomoses of the upper gastrointestinal tract. Potential complications include skin erosion due to the tight-fitting mask, aerophagia, gastric distension, and vomiting with tracheal aspiration.

References

1. Hickey RF, Visick W, Fairley HB et al: Effects of halothane anesthesia on functional residual capacity and alveolar-arterial oxygen tension difference. Anesthesiology 1973;38:20–24
2. Nunn JF: Factors influencing the arterial oxygen tension during halothane anesthesia with spontaneous respiration. Br J Anaesth 1964;36:326–341
3. Bendixen HH, Hedley-Whyte J, Laver MB: Impaired oxygenation in surgical patients during general anesthesia with controlled ventilation. N Engl J Med 1963;269:991–996
4. Bendixen HH, Bullwinkel B, Hedley-Whyte J et al: Atelectasis and shunting during spontaneous ventilation in anesthetized patients. Anesthesiology 1964;25:297–301
5. Brismar B, Hedenstierna G, Lundquist H et al: Pulmonary densities during anesthesia with muscular relaxation—a proposal of atelectasis. Anesthesiology 1985;62:422–428
6. Tokics L, Hedenstierna G, Strandberg A et al: Lung collapse and gas exchange during general anesthesia: Effects of spontaneous breathing, muscle paralysis and positive end-expiratory pressure. Anesthesiology 1987;66:157–167
7. Jones JG, Sapsford DJ, Wheatley RG: Post-operative hypoxaemia: Mechanism and time course. Anesthesia 1990;45:566–573
8. Vellody VPS, Nassery M, Balusaraswuthe K et al: Compliances of human rib cage and diaphragm-abdomen pathways in relaxed versus paralyzed states. Am Rev Respir Dis 1978;118:479
9. Vellody VPS, Nassery M, Druz WS et al: Effects of body position change on a thoracoabdominal motion. J Appl Physiol 1978;45:581–589
10. Westbrook PR, Stubbs SE, Sessler AD et al: Effects of anesthesia and muscle paralysis on respiratory mechanics in normal man. J Appl Physiol 1973;34:81–86
11. Tokics L, Hedenstierna G, Brismar B et al: Thoracoabdominal restriction in supine men: CT and lung function measurements. J Appl Physiol 1988;64:599–604
12. Froese AB, Bryan AC: Effects of anesthesia and paralysis on diaphragmatic mechanics in man. Anesthesiology 1974;41:242–255
13. Jones JG, Faithfull D, Jordan C et al: Rib cage movement during halothane anesthesia in man. Br J Anaesth 1979;51:399–407
14. Hedenstierna G, Tokics L, Strandberg AA et al: Correlation of gas impairment to development of atelectasis during anesthesia and muscle paralysis. Acta Anaesthiol Scand 1986;30:183–191
15. Bredesen J, Bjertnaes L, Lange A: Effects of anesthetics on the pulmonary vasoconstriction response to acute alveolar hypoxia. Microvasc Res 1975;10:236
16. Sykes MK, Davies DM, Chakrebarti MK: The effects of halothane, trichlorethylene and ether on the hypoxic pressor response and pulmonary vascular resistance in the isolated perfused lung. Br J Anaesth 1973;45:655–663
17. Benumof JL: One-lung ventilation and hypoxic pulmonary vasoconstriction: Implications for anesthetic management. Anesth Analg 1985;64:821–833
18. Eisenkraft JB: Hypoxic pulmonary vasoconstriction and anesthetic drugs. Mt Saini J Med (NY) 1987;54:290–296
19. Strandberg AA, Tokics L, Brismar B et al: Atelectasis during anesthesia and in the post-operative period. Acta Anesthesiol Scand 1986;30:154–158
20. Kain ML, Panday S, Nunn JF: The effect of intubation on the dead space during halothane anesthesia. Br J Anaesth 1969;41:94
21. Nunn JF, Campbell EJM, Peckett BW: Anatomical subdivision of the volume of respiratory dead space and effects of position of the jaw. J Appl Physiol 1959;14:174–176
22. Askrog VF, Pender JW, Smith TC et al: Changes in respiratory dead space during halothane, cyclopropane and nitrous oxide anesthesia. Anesthesiology 1964;25:342–352
23. Knill RL, Gelb AW: Ventilatory response to hypoxia and hypercapnia during halothane sedation and anesthesia in man. Anesthesiology 1978;49:244–251
24. Ward DS: Stimulation of hypoxic ventilatory drive by droperidol. Anesth Analg 1984;3:106–110
25. Craig DB, Wahba WM, Don HF et al: Closing volume and its relationship to gas exchange in seated and supine positions. J Appl Physiol 1971;31:717–721
26. Leblac P, Ruff F, Melic-Emili J: Effects of age and body position on airway closure in man. J Appl Physiol 1970;28:448–451
27. Tisi GM: Preoperative evaluation of pulmonary function. Am Rev Respir Dis 1979;119:293–318
28. Anscomb AR, Buxton RS: Effect of abdominal operations on total lung capacity and its subdivisions. Br Med J 1958;2:84–87
29. Jackson CV: Preoperative pulmonary evaluation. Arch Intern Med 1988;148:2120–2127
30. Elman A, Lagonnet F, Dixsant G et al: Respiratory function is impaired less by transverse than by median vertical supraumbilical incisions. Intensive Care Med 1981;7:235–239

31. Ali J, Khan TA: The comparative effects of muscle transection and median upper abdominal incisions of postoperative pulmonary function. Surg Gynecol Obstet 1979;148:863–866
32. Halasz NA: Vertical versus horizontal laparotomies. Arch Surg 1964;88:911–914
33. Meyers JR, Lembeck L, O'Kane H et al: Changes in functional residual capacity of the lung after operation. Arch Surg 1975;110:526–583
34. Craig DB: Postoperative recovery of pulmonary function. Anesth Analg 1981;60:46–52
35. Schweiger I, Gamulin Z, Suter PM: Lung function during anesthesia and respiratory insufficiency in the postoperative period: Physiological and clinical implications. Acta Anesthesiol Scand 1989;33:527–534
36. Gamsu G, Singer MM, Vincent HH et al: Post-operative impairment of mucous transport in the lung. Am Rev Respir Dis 1976;114:673–679
37. Catling JA, Pinto DM, Jordan C et al: Respiratory effects of analgesia after cholecystectomy: Comparison of continuous and intermittent papaveritum. Br Med J 1980;281:478–480
38. Catley DM, Thornton C, Jordan C et al: Pronounced, episodic oxygen desaturation in the post-operative period: Its association with ventilatory pattern and analgesic regimen. Anesthesiology 1985;63:20–28
39. Werner MA, Divertie MB, Tinker JH: Pre-operative cessation of smoking and pulmonary complications in coronary artery bypass patients. Anesthesiology 1984;60:380–383
40. Tarkan S, Moffitt EA, Sessler AD et al: Risk of anesthesia and surgery in patients with chronic bronchitis and chronic obstructive pulmonary disease. Surgery 1973;74:720–726
41. Pontoppidan H: Mechanical aids to lung expansion in non-intubated surgical patients. Am Rev Respir Dis 1980;122:109–119
42. O'Donohue WJ: National survey of the usage of lung expansion modalities for the prevention and treatment of post-operative atelectasis following abdominal and thoracic surgery. Chest 1985;87:76–80
43. Colgan FJ, Mahoney PD, Fanneng GL: Resistance breathing (blow bottles) and sustained hyperinflations in the treatment of atelectasis. Anesthesiology 1970;32:543–550
44. Kirilloff LH, Owens GR, Rogers RM et al: Does chest physical therapy work? Chest 1985;88:436–444
45. DeHaven CB, Hurst JM, Branson RD: Post-extubation hypoxemia treated with a continuous positive airway pressure mask. Crit Care Med 1985;13:46–48
46. Hurst JM, DeHaven CB, Branson RD: Use of CPAP mask is the sole mode of ventilatory support in trauma patients with mild to moderate respiratory insufficiency. J Trauma 1985;25:1065–1068

Chapter 42

Respiratory Disease in Children

Patricia B. Koff
Steven H. Abman

CHAPTER OUTLINE

The airway of the child is much smaller than that of the adult and as a result is prone to obstruction that may significantly affect gas exchange, such that disease that frequently goes untreated in the adult may be life-threatening in the small child. Childhood diseases associated with significant morbidity and mortality affect both the upper and the lower airway. This chapter presents an overview of the pathophysiology and the management of potentially life-threatening childhood diseases. Disorders such as respiratory distress syndrome (hyaline membrane disease) that are unique to the newborn period are beyond the scope of this book and are accordingly omitted from this discussion.

UPPER AIRWAY DISEASES

Several infectious agents cause the acute onset of upper airway obstruction in the pediatric patient. Although many causes have distinctive clinical presentations, the overlap of clinical findings should be appreciated. Table 42-1 provides a comparison of the most common upper airway pediatric infections.

Differential diagnosis between croup, epiglottitis, tracheitis, and foreign body aspiration often hinges on the patient's history. An abrupt onset is most often seen with epiglottitis or foreign body aspiration. Airway obstruction that occurs after an upper respiratory infection is more commonly associated with croup or tracheitis. Age is another factor in considering the likelihood of one particular problem versus another. Rarely does a child under 2 years of age develop epiglottitis, while croup is commonly seen between the ages of 6 months and 3 years. Lateral neck radiographs may supply information for differential diagnosis, but the time involved in obtaining them and the positioning required may outweigh their usefulness, especially in the unstable patient suspected of having epiglottitis.

Epiglottitis

Perhaps the most dramatic respiratory illness that affects children is epiglottitis (Table 42-2). A previously healthy child can develop what appears to be a routine sore throat with cough and fever and within 6 to 8 hours be afflicted

Table 42-1. Infectious Causes of Upper Airway Obstruction in Children

Disease	Age	Season	History	Clinical Signs
Epiglottitis	3–7 yr	None	Abrupt onset	Anxiety, high fever, drooling, rare cough
Croup	6 mo–3 yr	Late fall/winter	URI	Stridor, barking cough, mild fever, hoarseness
Bacterial tracheitis	Varies	None	Croup	Croup-like illness, high fever, toxicity
Retropharyngeal abscess	<3 yr	None	URI	Acute pharyngitis, high fever, drooling, hyperextension of head

URI, upper respiratory infection.

with severe airway obstruction requiring immediate intervention.

The infection is usually caused by *Haemophilus influenzae* type b, a bacterium that requires treatment with antibiotics. While allowing time for effective antibiotic treatment, airway obstruction must be relieved. This is accomplished most commonly now by intubation in the operating room shortly after arrival in the emergency department. Treatment with inhaled sympathomimetic drugs has little effect on these children and may waste valuable time.

Once epiglottitis has been confirmed in the operating room and intubation has been performed (or tracheotomy in the difficult-to-intubate patient), the child is transferred to the pediatric intensive care unit (ICU), where antibiotic therapy is started. Children with epiglottitis are usually kept sedated and restrained. O_2 therapy is typically required, and mechanical ventilation may also be necessary.

After 24 to 72 hours extubation is considered. A decision to extubate is generally based on resolution of fever, breathing around the artificial airway, and direct visualization of the epiglottis.[1] The 10-day course of antibiotics is then completed on the ward and at home.

While the incidence of epiglottitis is relatively small in comparison with other childhood respiratory illnesses (approximately 3 to 11 children per 20,000 admissions),[2–4] its severity is dramatic. With appropriate intervention the outcome is good, however, and nearly all children recover without long-term effects of the disease.

Croup

Croup, or acute laryngotracheitis (Table 42-3), is a common cause of airway obstruction in children. Generally it is not severe, so relatively few patients will require hospital admission. Croup is a viral illness. Parainfluenza virus is the most common agent, but other viruses may also be responsible including adenoviruses, influenza A and B viruses, and respiratory syncytial virus (RSV). *Mycoplasma pneumoniae* may also cause some cases of croup. Patients with croup typically present with a history of upper respiratory infections, a characteristic "brassy" cough, stridor, and retractions. A fever may also be present.

Depending on the severity of the signs and symptoms, a child may be treated at home with a cool mist nebulizer or may require admission to the hospital ward or ICU. The degree of stridor at rest is a key determinant, as is the level of oxygenation. Pulse oximetry is commonly used to assess these children because arterial blood gas sampling causes agitation, which may further aggravate the respiratory distress.

Treatment in the hospital focuses on "croup tent" therapy with O_2 if needed and racemic epinephrine treatments. Some patients may require mechanical ventilation if respiratory distress is severe and fatigue occurs; an arterial line is usually placed in these patients for ongoing monitoring of arterial CO_2 tension ($PaCO_2$) and acid-base balance. Of the 10 percent of children who are afflicted with croup, only 2 percent require hospitalization.[5] The disease usually resolves within 2 to 4 days.

Bacterial Tracheitis

Children who develop bacterial tracheitis often have croup early in their course. Symptoms are similar, but the causative agent for bacterial tracheitis is usually *Staphylococcus aureus* or occasionally *H. influenzae*. Inspiratory stridor rapidly becomes more marked, fever rises, and the patient begins to appear toxic.[6] The disease state is also referred to as *pseudomembranous croup* because sloughing of the respiratory epithelium occurs and large amounts of secretions and

Table 42-2. Epiglottitis

Etiology	Pathophysiology	Treatment
H. influenzae b	Inflammation of the epiglottis, aryepiglottis folds, and arytenoid cartilages	Establish airway, antibiotics

Table 42-3. Croup

Etiology	Pathophysiology	Treatment
Parainfluenza and other viruses	Inflammation of larynx and subglottic tracheal wall	Croup tent, racemic epinephrine, fluids, O_2

debris begin to fill the airway. Intubation may be necessary. Lateral soft tissue radiographs of the neck reveal subglottic narrowing and the presence of foreign material.

Antibiotics are required for treatment, as are fluids, O_2, and ongoing monitoring via pulse oximetry or transcutaneous electrodes. Mechanical ventilation may be required in some cases.

Retropharyngeal Abscess

Another upper airway disease caused by infectious agents is retropharyngeal abscess (i.e., abscess of the lymph nodes in the walls of the pharynx). It is usually caused by *Staphylococcus* or *Streptococcus spp.* and produces a clinical picture similar to those of the diseases discussed above. Acute pharyngitis and high fever are usually present. Antibiotics are required for treatment.

FOREIGN BODY ASPIRATION

Foreign body aspiration (Table 42-4) contributes significantly to the morbidity and mortality of early childhood; children between 6 months and 4 years are at greatest risk. Clinically, upper airway obstruction presents with the acute onset of choking, drooling, cough and stridor (if partial) or the inability to vocalize or cough (if complete). It is possible for several hours or days to pass before symptoms appear if the foreign body has been aspirated into the lower airways and did not occlude a large airway.

In the presence of acute untreated obstruction, progressive cyanosis, loss of consciousness, seizures, and cardiopulmonary arrest may follow. Although foreign bodies within the esophagus may compress the airway and cause respiratory distress, the site of obstruction is more commonly the supraglottic airway, leading to laryngospasm. A history of a young child running with food, small toy, or other object in the mouth is common, as is one of an older sibling feeding the younger child age-inappropriate food.

Lower respiratory tract obstruction generally presents with the onset of cough, wheezing, or respiratory distress. Physical examination may reveal asymmetric breath sounds or localized wheezing or rales. These signs may decrease or disappear over time; however, if the signs are untreated, bronchiectasis or recurrent "pneumonias" may develop.

Table 42-4. Foreign Body Aspiration

Signs of obstruction
Acute onset of choking, drooling, cough and/or stridor
Asymmetric breath sounds
Forced expiratory radiograph shows mediastinal shift away from affected side
Treatments (depending on degree of obstruction)
Spontaneous cough
Back blows or Heimlich maneuver
Rigid bronchoscopy

Any child with chronic cough or recurrent respiratory infections should be evaluated for possible previous foreign body aspiration.

If aspiration is suspected, inspiratory and forced expiratory (using manual abdominal compression if necessary) chest x-rays should be obtained. A forced expiratory radiograph shows mediastinal shift away from the affected side. If a bronchus is obstructed, volume loss and consequently atelectasis may occur.

The emergency treatment of upper airway obstruction due to an aspirated foreign body includes allowing children to use their own cough reflex to remove the object if only partial obstruction is present. Acute intervention in infants less than 1 year old includes placing the child in a face-down position over the rescuer's arm with the head positioned below the trunk. Four back blows are delivered rapidly between the scapulae (Fig. 42-1). If still obstructed the infant should be rolled over, and four chest compressions, as performed in cardiopulmonary resuscitation (CPR) should be delivered. This sequence should be repeated until the obstruction is relieved. Blind probing of the airway in an attempt to dislodge the foreign body is discouraged. If the foreign body can be visualized, careful removal with the fingers or available instruments (Magill forceps) can be attempted. The abdominal thrust technique (Heimlich maneuver) is recommended in older children.

Lower respiratory tract foreign body aspiration usually requires rigid bronchoscopy for removal of the object.[7] Simultaneous fluoroscopy or bronchography may also be useful.[6]

LOWER AIRWAY DISEASES

Childhood Asthma

The definition of asthma, diffuse obstructive disease characterized by hyperreactivity of the trachea and bronchi, is the same for adults and children. The mechanism precipitating bronchoconstriction in children is often linked to an allergic mechanism, although infections and exercise may also induce bronchoconstriction. The significant fact about childhood asthma is that it is the most common chronic disease of childhood; it is also the leading cause of school absence. In recent years there have also been alarming reports of the increasing frequency of hospital admissions and deaths from childhood asthma.[8–15]

In diagnosing asthma in infants and young children, several other possible diseases must be considered (Table 42-5). Given that wheezing is present with most of these other problems, there at first may be a hesitancy to diagnose asthma. Clearly though, it can be identified in infants by 6 to 7 months of age and in most children onset occurs before 2 years of age.[15,16] The presence of chronic cough and dyspnea may also be indicative of asthma; not all children with asthma may wheeze.

Severity of asthma is assessed by evaluating color, mental state, inspiratory breath sounds, accessory muscle use, ex-

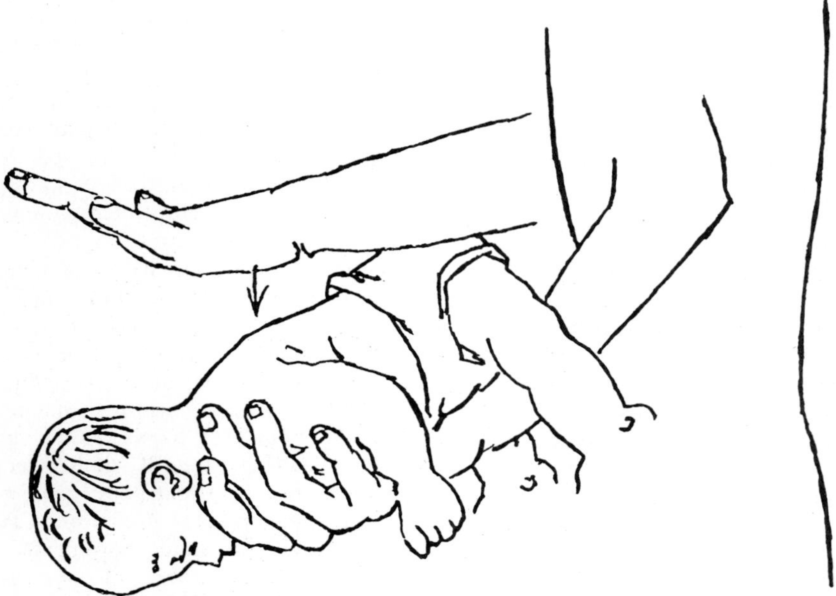

Figure 42-1. Positioning of child and application of back blows during suspected foreign body airway obstruction.

piratory wheezing, and oxygenation.[17] Arterial blood gases are relied on to confirm clinical scoring objectively. Initially $PaCO_2$ is reduced; a rising $PaCO_2$ above 40 mmHg indicates impending respiratory failure and the potential need for mechanical ventilation.

Management of childhood asthma is similar to that in adults, with inhaled adrenergic agents serving as the cornerstone. The use of metered dose inhalers for maintenance therapy poses a problem with the younger pediatric patient, but spacer devices have been shown to be helpful in effectively delivering medications without the need for coordinating deep breaths and spray activating.[18,19] Other chronic therapies may include oral theophylline and cromolyn sodium.

During an acute attack, O_2 is often necessary, and high-dose nebulized albuterol (0.15 mg/kg) delivered every 20 minutes for six doses has proved beneficial.[20] If a child requires hospitalization, an intravenous infusion of theophylline is often used. Subcutaneous epinephrine is another frequently used emergency department treatment. In extreme cases, before instituting mechanical ventilation a continuous infusion of isoproterenol or terbutaline has been used, usually with discontinuation of other beta-adrenergic drugs in an effort to avoid cardiac arrhythmias. The patient must be closely monitored for all side effects, which can include tremor, arrhythmias, myocardial ischemia or infarction, and worsening hypoxemia due to ventilation-perfusion mismatching.

If mechanical ventilation is required, a volume-cycled ventilator as opposed to a pressure-limited, time-cycled ventilator is desirable. Use of the volume ventilator allows consistent delivery of ventilation in the face of changing airway resistance.

Table 42-5. Differential Diagnosis of "Asthma" in Childhood

Consideration	Review Factors
Congenital malformations	History, age of onset, physical findings, and laboratory tests
Foreign bodies	Sudden onset in previously healthy children, inspiratory and expiratory chest radiographs
Infections	Viral most common, presence of stridor, barking cough
Acute bronchiolitis	Viral syndrome, age: occurs during first 2 years of life

Bronchiolitis

Bronchiolitis (Table 42-6) is one of the most common acute causes of hospitalizations of young infants, especially during winter months. Although RSV accounts for the majority of bronchiolitis infections, other pathogens, especially parainfluenza virus, may be the source of the infection. Children who require hospitalization for bronchiolitis often have an underlying cardiopulmonary disorder.

The usual course of RSV bronchiolitis is 1 to 2 days of fever, rhinorrhea, and cough, followed by tachypnea, wheezing, and retractions. Preterm newborns and young in-

Table 42-6. Bronchiolitis

Etiologies
Respiratory syncytial virus (RSV)
Parainfluenza
Clinical signs
Rhinorrhea
Fever
Cough
Tachypnea
Wheezing, rales, rhonchi
Apnea
Treatment
Humidification
Saline nose drops and suctioning
O_2, ventilation
Ribavirin[a]
ECMO[b]

[a] Use of ribavirin remains controversial.
[b] ECMO has been evaluated in limited cases.[25]

fants may present with apnea. Rales, rhonchi, and wheezes may be apparent on auscultation. Chest radiographs reveal hyperinflation, peribronchiolar thickening, and subsegmental and lobar consolidation. Nasal washings tested with immunofluorescent antibody staining can positively identify the RSV.[21] The peripheral white blood cell count may be normal or show a mild lymphocytosis. Severe airway obstruction typically lasts 3 days and usually resolves during the next 3 days. Otitis media and superimposed bacterial (especially pneumococcal) pneumonia may develop.

Treatment of bronchiolitis in the home includes providing adequate humidification for the copious secretions that are usually present and parental instruction in nasal suctioning. Saline nose drops are also recommended. Hospitalization is frequently required for children less than 2 years of age and in patients with hypoxemia in room air, apnea, moderate tachypnea with feeding difficulties, or marked respiratory distress. If an underlying chronic cardiopulmonary disorder such as congenital heart disease, bronchopulmonary dysplasia, or cystic fibrosis (CF) is present, hospitalization and aggressive treatment are usually required.

Supportive therapy includes supplemental O_2, intravenous hydration, beta-adrenergic bronchodilators administered via nebulization, theophylline, or corticosteroids. Arterial blood gas determinations or noninvasive measurements of oxygenation as well as pulse oximetry or transcutaneous monitors should be used to assess O_2 requirements and response to therapy.

Ribavirin, an antiviral drug with specific activity against RSV, is being used in some centers for children with coexistent cardiopulmonary disease or immunodeficiency, recent transplant recipients, and patients undergoing chemotherapy for malignancy. Its delivery requires use of a specific nebulizer, the small particle aerosol generator (SPAG). Currently, nebulizer therapy runs continuously for 12 to 18 hours each day for a 3- to 5-day course. Ribavirin may be delivered by hood, tent, or in-line with mechanical ventilation, provided certain safety precautions are taken.[22] The efficacy of ribavirin continues to be questioned, and its possible effects on staff members require additional investigation. Many centers have restricted its use to only those patients who have underlying cardiopulmonary disorders and who are in severe distress.[23] Some facilities use ribavirin during a relatively quiet period, usually at night, in order to limit exposure of staff and family members. Special equipment (ribavirin hood), such as that shown in Figure 42-2, is available from the drug's manufacturer to reduce the circulating levels of the drug.[24] However, the ribavirin hood by itself does not reduce environmental levels of ribavirin below recommended safe levels.[25] We (DJP and RMK) therefore recommend that a double-tent drug scavenging system (Fig. 42-3) be used whenever ribavirin is administered to spontaneously breathing individuals.[26,27] Proper use of these systems virtually eliminates environmental levels of ribavirin.

The use of extracorporeal membrane oxygenation (ECMO) is being investigated for the treatment of severe bronchiolitis. Twelve compassionate use cases were reported between 1983 and 1988 in nine centers.[28] However, ECMO cannot be considered to be part of the standard therapeutic armamentarium for patients with bronchiolitis.

The prognosis of patients with bronchiolitis is generally excellent, although children with pulmonary hypertension, bronchopulmonary dysplasia, or CF have high morbidity and mortality. Frequently, hospitalized bronchiolitic patients re-

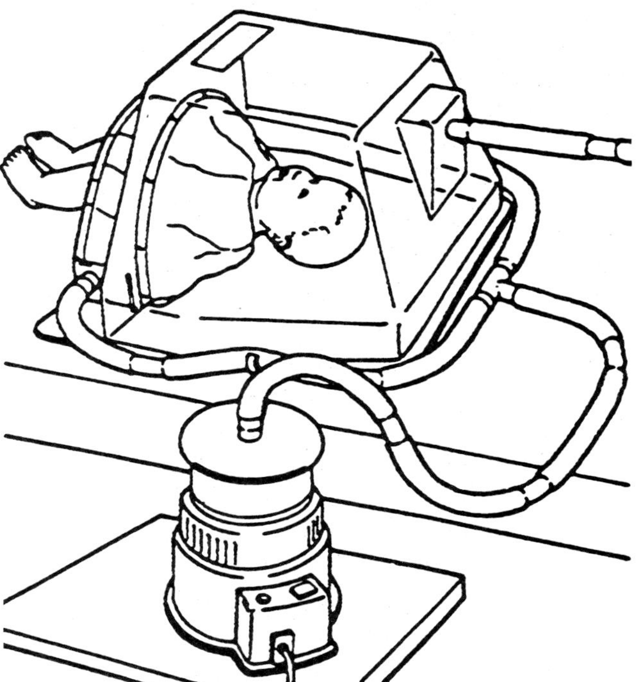

Figure 42-2. Ribavirin aerosol delivery hood with single vacuum scavenging device. (Courtesy of ICN Pharmaceuticals Inc., Costa Mesa, CA.)

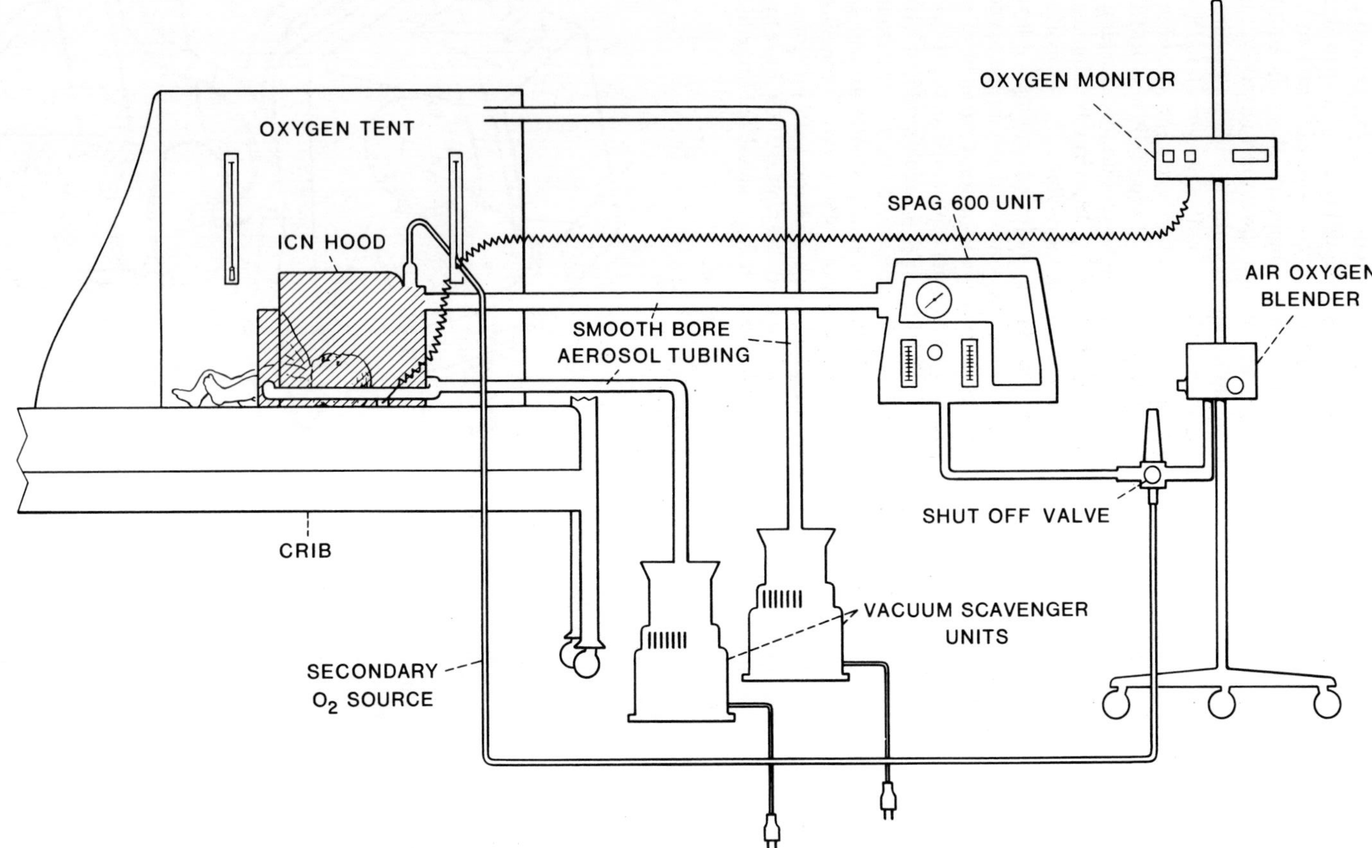

Figure 42-3. Double tent-hood ribavirin delivery system with two vacuum scavenging devices. A secondary O_2 source is necessary to ensure $F_{I}O_2$ when the SPAG unit is turned off and aerosolized ribavirin is being cleared before tent is entered. Smooth-bore aerosol tubing is used to reduce noise and increase flow to filtering devices. (From Kacmarek and Kratohvil,[27] with permission.)

quire home O_2 for a relatively brief time upon discharge. Recurrent episodes of wheezing may follow acute infection in almost half of hospitalized patients.

Cystic Fibrosis

CF is the most common fatal genetic disease in whites; its incidence is estimated at 1 in 2000 births. Although much less common, it is also found in blacks (1 in 17,000) and orientals (1 in 100,000). It can now be identified through a newborn screen. Life expectancy for CF patients has increased since the early 1970s, with many patients reaching adulthood. The current median age of survival is 26 years.

Recent genetic studies of CF have identified a mutation on human chromosome 7. This mutation accounts for a large majority of but not all CF cases. Although the basic defect remains unknown, it appears to involve an abnormality in the regulation of the chloride channel in secretory epithelial cells. This defect is believed to cause the characteristic abnormalities in sweat electrolytes and secretions of the lung, pancreas, intestine, liver, and other sites, which subsequently cause multiple organ dysfunction.

The clinical manifestations of CF are diverse. The leading cause of morbidity and mortality is progressive respiratory failure due to chronic endobronchial infection and inflammation. *Pseudomonas aeruginosa* is the major bacterial pathogen of CF; *S. aureus* and a newly designated strain of *Pseudomonas*, *P. cepacia*, are other frequent pathogens. The signs and symptoms of CF vary depending on disease severity and the degree of bacterial infection. A chronic productive cough is almost always present, and patients frequently develop a barrel-chested appearance. Although clinical courses are variable, recurrent hospitalizations for respiratory exacerbations and gastrointestinal and nutritional problems are common.

Ongoing respiratory treatment for these patients focuses on use of inhaled beta-adrenergic bronchodilators to relieve reversible obstruction and improve ciliary activity. Nebulizer treatments are usually followed by aggressive bronchial drainage. During acute infections and hospitalizations, these treatments are generally continued, along with the use in some cases of inhaled antibiotics. Long-term use of inhaled tobramycin is being investigated and may prove helpful in delaying and stopping the typical decline in pulmonary function.[39]

Lung transplantation has received increasing interest for CF patients. British surgeons have currently performed the largest number of such operations; their techniques favor heart-lung transplants. The 1-year survival rate from their group is 74 percent. Centers in Toronto and Pittsburgh use the double-lung transplantation procedure.[30]

As mentioned earlier, life expectancy is increasing for CF patients. With the identification of the first gene disorder, increasing transplantation experience, improving antibiotic therapy, and investigational use of inhaled amiloride[31] along with other inhaled therapeutic agents, hope remains high for improving the life expectancy even more for patients with this disease.

Bronchopulmonary Dysplasia

Bronchopulmonary dysplasia (BPD), a secondary chronic lung disease in pediatric patients, is defined according to the clinical course of the newborn infant (Table 42-7). The following criteria are used in making the diagnosis of BPD: (1) acute respiratory distress in the first week of life (mostly in preterm infants with hyaline membrane disease); (2) treatment with mechanical ventilation and O_2; and (3) persistent signs of chronic respiratory distress, including physical signs, chest radiographic findings, and O_2 requirements after the first month of life. Immaturity, O_2 toxicity, barotrauma, and inflammation are considered the major risk factors. The exact definition and cause of BPD remain controversial.

The clinical picture of BPD typically includes tachypnea, mild retractions, rales, and wheezing. Signs of right-sided heart failure such as peripheral edema, hepatomegaly, and jugular venous distension are also often present. The clinical course is widely variable, ranging from mild O_2 requirements, which resolve steadily over a few months, to more severe effects requiring tracheotomy and home mechanical ventilation.

Given that the development of BPD is linked to management of the patient during the neonatal period, some centers are exploring the use of less stringent criteria for weaning patients with respiratory distress syndrome from mechanical ventilation.[31] Ideally, prevention through improved neonatal management is preferable to treatment for this disease, which seems to be largely iatrogenic in etiology.

Management of BPD patients typically includes bronchodilators, O_2, and chest physiotherapy. Cromolyn sodium and steroids are also sometimes used. Recurrent pulmonary edema leads to the frequent use of chronic diuretic therapy. Volume contraction, hypokalemia, hyponatremia, and alkalosis are common side effects of the diuretics.

Serial monitoring of oxygenation through the use of blood gases, pulse oximeters, or transcutaneous monitors is important. Increasing interest is being placed on the rate at which low flow O_2 can be decreased[32]; monitoring is essen-

Table 42-7. Bronchopulmonary Dysplasia

History
Acute respiratory distress in first week of life
Treatment with mechanical ventilation and O_2
Persistent signs of chronic respiratory distress
Physical examination
Tachypnea, retractions, wheezing, rales
Arterial blood gases
Hypercapnia, hypoxemia
Chest radiograph
Cystic & atelectatic areas
Treatment
Varies with severity
Bronchodilators, O_2, ventilation, chest physiotherapy
Cromolyn sodium
Diuretics
Steroids

tial for safe reduction in O_2 therapy. Serial monitoring for the development of cor pulmonale is also important. Clinical management should include attention to nutrition and growth, development, metabolic status, and neurologic status.

While the mortality rate is high for patients with the most severe advanced BPD, prognosis is favorable for most patients. Long-term care, often in the form of chronic O_2 therapy, is commonly needed.

APPARENT LIFE-THREATENING EPISODES AND SUDDEN INFANT DEATH SYNDROME

An apparent life-threatening episode (ALTE) is defined as an episode that is frightening to the observer and is characterized by some combination of apnea, cyanosis or pallor, and a marked change in muscle tone (usually extreme limpness). Infants who have had an ALTE are at an increased risk of subsequently dying from sudden infant death syndrome (SIDS); consequently, *near-miss SIDS* is another term used.[33]

Clinical evaluation of these patients includes obtaining a clear description of the event to determine if any association can be made with the infant being awake or asleep or with feedings, crying, or signs of acute infection. Knowledge of the duration of the episode, the resuscitative efforts needed, and the infant's responses are all critical to investigating the source of the problem. A history of developmental delays, neurologic abnormalities, signs of chronic disease, or child abuse or neglect is also helpful.

Physical examination may help to direct the laboratory evaluations needed. Sleep studies to assess respiratory pattern and oxygenation are often diagnostic. Chest radiographs, electrocardiograms, barium swallows, esophageal pH studies, air laryngotracheograms, electroencephalograms, and serum electrolyte and hematocrit determinations may all be helpful. A thorough psychosocial assessment is also an important part of the evaluation.

Therapy is directed toward the identified cause. Indications for the use and duration of home apnea monitoring and respiratory stimulants remain controversial. The National Institutes of Health have developed a consensus statement on home monitoring.[34]

Sudden infant death syndrome (SIDS) or "crib death" occurs at an estimated frequency of 1 to 2 infants per 1000. It generally occurs between the ages of 1 and 6 months, with a peak incidence at about 2 months. Most deaths occur between midnight and 8 AM. Mild symptoms of upper respiratory infection may be present, but whether infection plays an important role is not known. Risk factors include low birth weight; adolescent, drug-addicted, or smoking mothers; and a family history of previous SIDS deaths (Table 42-8).

The diagnosis of SIDS is based on the clinical setting and a postmortem examination that rules out other causes of death. Therapy is directed toward providing family support during the immediate crisis as well as follow-up counseling by local resources. The National SIDS Foundation is an excellent resource for providing this support.

Table 42-8. Risk Factors for Sudden Infant Death Syndrome

Low birth weight
Adolescent mother
Drug-addicted mother
Smoking mother
Previous family history of SIDS

CONGENITAL RESPIRATORY LESIONS

Upper Respiratory Tract Lesions

There are several congenital upper respiratory abnormalities, generally presenting with inspiratory stridor at birth or within the first months of life (Table 42-9).

Laryngomalacia is one of the most common causes. The epiglottis and arytenoid cartilages collapse into the airway during inspiration, causing stridor. Diagnosis is readily made by flexible bronchoscopy. Although tracheotomy may be required, most children resolve their stridor with the first 2 years of life.

Other common congenital upper respiratory problems include choanal atresia (bilateral or unilateral) micrognathia (as in Pierre-Robin syndrome), laryngeal web, vocal cord paralysis, and subglottic hemangioma.

Table 42-9. Congenital Upper Respiratory Problems

Type	Description	Problems
Laryngomalacia	Epiglottis and arytenoid cartilages collapse into airway	Stridor
Choanal atresia	Obstruction of one or both nasal passages	Airway obstruction
Micrognathia	Hypoplastic mandible	Pharyngeal airway obstruction
Laryngeal web	Glottis is covered by web	Airway obstruction and weak or absent cry
Vocal cord paralysis	Nonfunctional vocal cord (may be unilateral)	Weak cry or occasional stridor
Subglottic hemangioma	Reddish blue soft subglottic lesion	Stridor, hoarse cry

Table 42-10. Congenital Intrathoracic Lesions

Lesion	Features
Tracheomalacia	Air laryngotracheogram or flexible bronchoscopy for diagnosis
Vascular rings	Variable clinical presentation: stridor, wheezing, or obstructive apnea may be present; esophageal and tracheal compression are most common
Tracheoesophageal fistula	Cough, choking, respiratory distress, & abdominal distension shortly after birth; attempt at passing nasogastric tube is suggested; chest x-ray will show tube usually coiled in blind pouch
Pulmonary hypoplasia	Incomplete lung growth often associated with space-taking lesions: diaphragmatic hernia, fetal hydrops, extralobar sequestration
Pulmonary sequestrations	Localized masses of pulmonary parenchyma—may be anatomically separate from lung
Congenital lobar emphysema	Presents in newborn period with respiratory distress; chest x-ray shows overdistension of affected lobe
Cystic adenomatoid malformations	Presents with marked respiratory distress within the first days of life; gland-like space-occupying cysts; surgical resection required

Intrathoracic Lesions

Congenital intrathoracic lesions are diverse and have variable clinical presentations, ranging from severe neonatal respiratory distress to mild chronic cough in older adolescents.[35] Table 42-10 provides a summary list of these lesions and their diagnostic features. Any child with a history of respiratory problems not directly attributable to other disease states discussed earlier may require evaluation for congenital structural lesions.

ACUTE RESPIRATORY FAILURE

Several anatomic and physiologic factors make young children more vulnerable than adults to acute respiratory failure (ARF), including:

- Smaller airway diameters
- Easy fatiguability of diaphragm and other respiratory muscles
- Decreased intra-alveolar connections (pores of Kohn)

In addition, most pediatric cardiopulmonary arrests are related to respiratory problems as opposed to cardiac abnormalities.

ARF is the inability of the respiratory system to effectively provide sufficient O_2 delivery or CO_2 removal. It occurs in a variety of clinical settings (including most of those discussed earlier in this chapter) and presents with variable physical findings depending on the exact etiology and physiologic response.

The clinical severity of respiratory insufficiency may not be appreciated without arterial blood gas measurements. Some situations in which severity cannot be assessed include hypoxemia as indicated by clinical cyanosis (unreliable except with extreme hypoxemia) and depression of the ventilatory center leading to marked hypercarbia without associated respiratory distress. Although pulse oximetry and transcutaneous PO_2 monitoring are helpful to noninvasively demonstrate serial changes in oxygenation, measurements of arterial blood gas tensions are necessary for a full assessment of acid-base balance.

Early recognition of the high-risk patient for ARF in various clinical settings is important so that caregivers can anticipate the clinical course and provide intervention prior to cardiopulmonary arrest. Table 42-11 provides a systematic approach for treating the child who is at risk for ARF, and Table 42-12 lists specific information on endotracheal tubes and chest tube sizes.

ADULT RESPIRATORY DISTRESS SYNDROME IN CHILDREN

Children can be just as susceptible to the adult respiratory distress syndrome (ARDS) as are adults. While the exact incidence of ARDS in children is not known, it has been reported in patients as young as 2 weeks.[36]

The pathophysiologic hallmark of this disease is the presence of nonhydrostatic (permeability) pulmonary edema due to injury to the alveolar-capillary membrane.

The causes of ARDS in children range from near drown-

Table 42-11. Systematic Approach to Acute Respiratory Failure in Children

Anticipate high risk	Provide clinical setting for early monitoring and intervention prior to arrest
Assess respiratory distress	Physical examination: mentation, cyanosis, apnea, rate, severity of distress (accessory muscle use, grunting, retractions, paradoxical effort, breath sounds, O_2 response via pulse oximetry) Laboratory: arterial blood gas levels, chest x-ray
Initiate basic CPR if in arrest	Follow American Heart Association standards
Provide other therapy	Dependent on severity of clinical findings

Table 42-12. Age-Dependent Changes in Pediatric Sizes of Endotracheal Tubes and Chest Tubes

Age	Endotracheal Tube Size (mm)	Chest Tube Size (French)
Premature		
<1000 g	2.5–3.0	10
1000–2500 g	3.0–3.5	10–14
Newborns–6 mo	3.0–3.5	12–18
6 mo–1 yr	3.5–4.0	14–20
1–2 yr	4.0–5.0	14–24
2–6 yr	(age + 16)/4	20–32
6–12 yr	(age + 16)/4	28–38

ing, trauma, and lung infections to those often associated with adult ARDS, such as sepsis and burns (see Ch. 35).

Treatment is primarily supportive, along with treatment of the underlying disorder. The goal of therapy in ARDS focuses on maximizing tissue O_2 delivery. Volume ventilation, as opposed to pressure-limited ventilation, is desired in order to ensure delivery of tidal volume in the face of varying lung compliance. Increased mean airway pressure is often needed and is usually provided by use of high levels of PEEP. The use of pulmonary artery catheters in monitoring and the subsequent administration of fluids are less common in children than in adults.[36–38] Monitoring of the pathophysiologic changes in ARDS is essential, however, and if a pulmonary artery catheter is not in place, often a central venous catheter will be used. Intake and output as well as daily weights are determined. Hourly monitoring of vital signs, pulse oximetry, end-tidal CO_2 monitoring, and arterial blood gas measurements are also commonly performed in the management of these patients.

Prognostic information for pediatric ARDS patients is limited, but mortality of 28.5 to 95 percent has been reported.[36–39] Follow-up studies show that children frequently have cough and exertional dyspnea, as well as abnormal chest radiographs and decreased lung volumes in some cases.[40]

References

1. Backofen JE, Rogers MC: Upper airway disease. pp. 189. In Rogers MC (ed): Textbook of Pediatric Intensive Care. Vol. 1. Williams & Wilkins, Baltimore, 1987
2. Faden HS: Treatment of Haemophilus influenza Type b, epiglottitis. Pediatrics 1979;63:402–408
3. Vernon DD, Sarnaik AP: Acute epiglottitis in children: A conservative approach to diagnosis and management. Crit Care Med 1986;14:23–29
4. Barker F: Current management of croup and epiglottitis. Pediatr Clin North Am 1979;36:565–582
5. Denny FW, Murphy TF, Wallace WA et al: Croup: An 11-year study in a pediatric practice. Pediatrics 1983;71:871–880
6. Tooley WH, Lipow HW: Inspiratory obstruction. pp. 410–412. In Rudolph AM (ed): Pediatrics. 18th Ed. Appleton & Lange, East Norwalk, CT, 1987
7. Green CG: Assessment of the pediatric airway by flexible bronchoscopy. Respir Care 1991;36:555–565
8. Halfon N, Newacheck EW: Trends in the hospitalization for acute childhood asthma, 1970 to 1984. Am J Public Health 1986;76:1308–1319
9. Mullally DI, Howard WA, Hubbard TJ et al: Increased hospitalizations for asthma among children in the Washington DC area during 1961–1981. Ann Allergy 1984;53:15–23
10. Dawson KP, Allan J, Horwood TJ: Trends in hospital admission for children with acute asthma in Christchurch, New Zealand 1974–1983. Aust Paediatr J 1986;22:71–79
11. Mitchell EA: International trends in hospital admission rates for asthma. Arch Dis Child 1985;60:376–384
12. Anderson HR: Increase in hospitalization for childhood asthma. Arch Dis Child 1987;53:295–308
13. Infante-Rivard C, Sukia SE, Roberge D et al: The changing frequency of childhood asthma. J Asthma 1987;24:283–294
14. Gergen PJ, Mullally DI, Evans R III: National survey of prevalence of asthma among children in the United States, 1976–1980. Pediatrics 1988;81:1–12
15. Richards W: Hospitalization of children with status asthmaticus: A review. Pediatrics 1989;111:84–101
16. Easton J, Hillman B, Shapiro F: Management of asthma. Pediatrics 1981;68:874–882
17. Downes JJ, Heiser MS: Status asthmaticus in children. In Gregory GA (ed): Respiratory Failure in the Child. Churchill Livingstone, New York, 1981
18. Levison H, Reilly PA, Worsly GH: Spacing devices and metered-dose inhalers in childhood asthma. J Pediatr 1985;107:662–673
19. Consensus conference on clinical aerosol administration. Respir Care 1991;36:916–921
20. Schuh S, Parkin P, Pajan K et al: High, versus low-dose, frequently administered, nebulized albuterol in children with severe, acute asthma. Pediatrics 1989;83:513–521
21. Kurth CD, Goodwin SR: Obstructive airway diseases in infants and children. pp. 93–114. In Koff PB, Eitzman DV, New J (eds): Neonatal and Pediatric Respiratory Care. CV Mosby, St. Louis, 1988
22. Demers R, Parker J, Frankel LR, Smith DW: Administration of ribavirin to neonatal and pediatric patients during mechanical ventilation. Respir Care 1986;31:1188–1197
23. Division of Occupational Hygiene, Department of Labor and Industries, The Commonwealth of Massachusetts: Ribavirin Alert. DOH #1558, July 1989
24. Aerosol delivery hood with vacuum unit. Instruction insert. Part No. 9035. ICN Pharmaceuticals, Inc. Costa Mesa, CA, 1988
25. Kacmarek RM: Ribavirin and pentamidine aerosols: Caregiver beware! (Editorial) Respir Care 1990;35:1034–1036
26. Charney W, Corkery KJ, Kramer R: Engineering administration controls to contain the delivery of aerosolized ribavirin: Results of simulation and application to one patient. Respir Care 1990;35:1042–1048
27. Kacmarek RM, Kratohvil J: The use of scavenging systems to reduce the environment concentration of ribavirin. Respir Care 1992;37:37–45
28. Steinhorn RH, Green TP: Use of extracorporeal membrane oxygenation in the treatment of respiratory syncytial virus bronchiolitis: The national experience, 1983 to 1988. J Pediatr 1990;116:338–346
29. MacLusky IB, Gold R, Corey M, Levison H: Long-term effects of inhaled tobramycin in patients with cystic fibrosis colonized with *Pseudomonas aeruginosa*. Pediatr Pulmonol 1989;7:42–53
30. Rodman DM: Cystic Fibrosis; Medical Grand Rounds, University of Colorado Health Sciences Center, Denver, 1989
31. Kraybill EN, Runyan DK, Bose CL, Khan JH: Risk factors for chronic lung disease in infants with birth weights of 751 to 1000 grams. J Pediatr 1989;115:1–12
32. Vain NE, Prudent LM, Stevens DP et al: Regulation of oxygen concentration delivered to infants via nasal cannulas. Am J Dis Child 1989;143:1458–1463
33. Chesrown SE: Sudden infant death syndrome and apnea dis-

orders. pp. 158–168. In Koff PB, Eitzman DV, New J (eds): Neonatal and Pediatric Respiratory Care. CV Mosby, St. Louis, 1988

34. Consensus statement: NIH consensus development conference on infantile apnea and home monitoring. Pediatrics 1987;79:292–301
35. Larsen GL, Abman SH, Fan LL et al: The respiratory system and mediastinum. pp. 364–411. In Hathaway WE, Hay WW, Groothuis JR, Paisley JW (eds): Current Pediatric Diagnosis and Treatment. 10th Ed. Lange, San Mateo, CA, 1991
36. Pfenninger J, Gerber A, Tschappeler H: Adult respiratory distress syndrome in children. J Pediatr 1982;101:3–12
37. Lyrene RK, Truog WE: Adult respiratory distress syndrome in a pediatric intensive care unit: Predisposing condition, clinical course, and outcome. Pediatrics 1981;67:790–797
38. Holbrook PR, Taylor G, Pollack MM, Fields AI: Adult respiratory distress syndrome in children. Pediatr Clin North Am 1980;27:3–13
39. Nussbaum E: Adult-type respiratory distress syndrome in children. Clin Pediatr 1983;22:401–409
40. Fanconi S, Kraimer R, Weber J et al: Long-term sequelae in children surviving adult respiratory distress syndrome. J Pediatr 1985;106:218–227

Chapter 43

Respiratory Effects of Diseases and Conditions Primarily Affecting Other Organs and Systems

Charles B. Sherman
Elizabeth Tarnell

CHAPTER OUTLINE

The lungs are often involved in diseases that primarily affect other organs of the body (Table 43-1). Pulmonary involvement associated with nonthoracic diseases may be relatively benign (e.g., pleural effusions) or can be severe enough to lead to the ultimate demise of the patient (e.g., aspiration pneumonia). This chapter reviews the pulmonary manifestations of certain gastrointestinal, renal, collagen vascular, and hematologic diseases and discusses the effects of pregnancy and several miscellaneous diseases on pulmonary function. It is hoped that the information given in this chapter will help the clinician to understand and anticipate pulmonary abnormalities that may develop in patients with mainly nonthoracic diseases.

THE LUNG AND GASTROINTESTINAL DISEASE

Liver Disease

Cirrhosis is an irreversible scarring of the liver resulting from infectious, inflammatory, metabolic, and toxic injuries.[1] As the architecture of the liver becomes more distorted, an increase in portal vein pressure may occur and lead to the development of portal-systemic collaterals, bleeding esophageal and gastric varices, splenomegaly, ascites, and/or encephalopathy.[2]

Table 43-1. The Common Pulmonary Manifestations of Nonthoracic Diseases and Treatments

Condition	Pulmonary Manifestations
Gastrointestinal	
Cirrhosis	Hypoxemia Pleural effusions Pulmonary hypertension
Gastroesophageal reflux and aspiration	Asthma/bronchospasm Recurrent pneumonias Interstitial fibrosis
Renal	
Chronic renal failure	Pleurisy and pleural effusions Interstitial fibrosis Pulmonary edema
Nephrotic syndrome	Pleural effusions Pulmonary emboli
Goodpasture's syndrome	Alveolar hemorrhage
Hemodialysis	Hypoxemia
Peritoneal dialysis	Basilar atelectasis Hypoxemia
Hematologic	
Leukemia	Pulmonary infiltrates Hilar/mediastinal adenopathy Pleural effusions "Factitious" hypoxemia
Lymphoma	Pulmonary nodules Pulmonary infiltrates Hilar/mediastinal adenopathy
Multiple myeloma	Parenchymal mass Paratracheal (parahilar) masses Pulmonary infiltrates
Sickle cell disease	Pulmonary infiltrates Hypoxemia Microvascular thrombosis
Collagen vascular	
Rheumatoid arthritis	Pleural effusion/pleurisy Rheumatoid nodules Interstitial fibrosis
Systemic lupus erythematosus	Pleurisy with or without effusions Lupus pneumonitis Hemorrhagic alveolitis Interstitial fibrosis Respiratory muscle dysfunction
Progressive systemic sclerosis (scleroderma)	Interstitial fibrosis Pulmonary hypertension
Miscellaneous	
Neurogenic pulmonary edema	Pulmonary edema
Hypothyroidism	Blunting of respiratory drives Obstructive sleep apnea Diaphragmatic dysfunction Respiratory muscle weakness Pleural effusions
Hyperthyroidism	Heightened respiratory drives
Wegener's granulomatosis	Parenchymal cavitary lesions Nasopharyngeal ulcerative lesions

A variety of pulmonary manifestations may complicate cirrhosis and its sequelae. *Hypoxemia* is the most common respiratory abnormality detected.[3] Although the hypoxemia is generally mild and not associated with any symptoms, in a minority of patients with more severe liver disease significant arterial hypoxemia may be found.[3] These patients often present with dyspnea, exercise intolerance, jaundice, ascites, clubbing, cyanosis, and cutaneous spider angiomas.[3,4]

Several pathogenic mechanisms have been proposed to explain the observed hypoxemia. Regional areas of low ventilation/perfusion ($\dot{V}/\dot{Q}$) ratio may cause the low O_2 partial pressure (PO_2).[5–7] Peribronchiolar edema from low plasma oncotic pressure can cause compression of smaller airways, leading to early alveolar closure at low lung volumes.[5] Similarly, pleural effusions, massive ascites, and/or splenomegaly may cause basilar atelectasis and impair regional ventilation. Some researchers have suggested that failure of hypoxic pulmonary vasoconstriction (HPV), the normal response by which blood flow is directed away from areas of low ventilation, permits these areas of low $\dot{V}/\dot{Q}$ to persist.[8] However, a 1981 study showed that most mildly to moderately decompensated cirrhotic patients had a degree of HPV similar to that of normal patients.[9]

Anatomic shunting may also explain the hypoxemia. Pathologic specimens from cirrhotic patients have demonstrated pleural and parenchymal arteriovenous connections, predominantly in the lower lobes.[3,4,10,11] Although right-to-left shunting was originally thought to result from communications between portal and systemic veins, it is most likely secondary to blood flow through these pulmonary vascular abnormalities. Two unusual findings in patients with cirrhosis, platypnea (dyspnea in the upright position) and orthodeoxia (arterial desaturation in the upright position), may be explained by increased blood flow through these anatomic shunts in the upright position.[10] It is difficult to determine how much of the observed hypoxemia in patients with liver disease is caused by areas of low $\dot{V}/\dot{Q}$ ratio and how much by anatomic shunting.

Pleural effusions are often found in patients with cirrhosis. They are believed to result from transdiaphragmatic transport of ascitic fluid, either via lymphatics or through defects in the diaphragm.[12] Hypoproteinemia and azygos hypertension secondary to portal hypertension may also be responsible for pleural fluid accumulation.[2] The effusions may accumulate rapidly, are usually bilateral, and are transudative in character. Therapy focuses on lessening the rate of ascites formation by improving intravascular osmotic pressure and reducing portal hypertension rather than on removing pleural fluid by repeated thoracentesis. Some patients with refractory ascites and significant pleural effusions may benefit from pleurodesis.[13]

Pulmonary hypertension, unrelated to left-sided heart failure, has been observed in some patients with cirrhosis regardless of the etiology of their underlying liver disease.[14,15] Demographically, these patients are young, usually female, and resemble those at risk for the development of primary pulmonary hypertension (PPH).[15] Pathologically, the lesions seen in most cases are indistinguishable from the plexogenic arteriopathy found in PPH.[16] The cause of the pulmonary hypertension remains unknown. One hypothesis is that recurrent pulmonary emboli from the portal circulation are responsible, but pathologic studies have not consistently confirmed this association.[14] Alternatively, mediators that are usually detoxified by normal hepatic function might bypass the liver in cirrhotics to produce pulmonary vasoconstriction and vascular injury.[14] Few data currently exist to support this mechanism.

A clinicopathologic syndrome similar to PPH also occurs in patients with chronic active hepatitis (CAH), an inflammatory process of the liver that fails to resolve within 6 months.[17] In contrast to the pulmonary hypertension described above, this entity appears to be part of an immunologically or humorally mediated multisystem disorder.[18,19]

Finally, *interstitial pneumonitis* has been associated with chronic active hepatitis and primary biliary cirrhosis (PBC), a disease characterized by destruction of small bile ductules in the liver.[1,20–24] The pulmonary fibrosis is thought to result from the underlying systemic autoimmune disorder. In several case reports, corticosteroid therapy has been shown to help modulate the course of lung involvement.[20]

Chronic Aspiration Syndromes

Several risk factors predispose patients to chronic aspiration; these include esophageal disorders, neurologic impairment (e.g., depressed consciousness, cerebrovascular accidents), neuromuscular diseases (e.g., myasthenia gravis, amyotrophic lateral sclerosis, multiple sclerosis), and mechanical abnormalities of the pharynx and larynx.[25]

Of all the esophageal disorders, *gastroesophageal reflux* (GER) is the most commonly associated with chronic aspiration. Failure of the lower esophageal sphincter allows gastric acid and particulate matter to regurgitate into the esophagus and subsequently into the lungs. Refluxed acid passing into the bronchial tree can cause asthma, chronic bronchitis, recurrent pneumonias, and if long term, bronchiectasis and pulmonary fibrosis.[26–30] Clinically, patients often present with symptoms of nonproductive cough, nocturnal wheezing, and/or hoarseness.[25,26] Two mechanisms have been proposed to explain the observed bronchospasm found in certain patients with GER. Microaspiration of gastric contents into the tracheobronchial tree may act as a direct irritant stimulus for bronchospasm.[31] Alternatively, vagal stimulation associated with GER may trigger bronchospasm apart from any direct airway damage.[32] Esophageal monitoring with demonstration of very low pH measurements in the more proximal esophagus is required for diagnosis of GER.[33] Therapy consists of standard antireflux measures, elevation of the head of the bed, avoidance of food or liquids right before bedtime, use of antacids or H_2 blockers (e.g., ranitidine), avoidance of cigarettes and alcohol, and weight loss.[33] Antireflux surgery is reserved for those patients failing conservative medical treatment.[34]

Other esophageal disorders associated with aspiration include achalasia, scleroderma, Zenker's diverticulum, lower esophageal diverticula, esophageal tumors, tracheoesophageal fistulas secondary to tumor, trauma, or tracheostomy.[25] These entities may produce any of the pulmonary disorders previously described.

Aspiration of medicinal compounds, especially mineral oil, can produce a distinct clinical entity called *lipoid pneumonia*.[35,36] This disease is often misdiagnosed as bacterial pneumonia until a more careful history is obtained. Chronic aspiration of mineral oil, taken as a laxative by the elderly, may produce few symptoms due to the benign chemical nature of the substance.[35] However, considerable basilar infiltrates may be detected on chest radiography. Histologically, the lung tissue contains numerous lipid-laden macrophages, with areas of fibrosis and foreign-body granuloma formation.[35] The natural course of lipoid pneumonia is variable; the infiltrates may resolve on discontinuing the mineral oil, or the patient may die from cor pulmonale secondary to considerable fibrosis.[36] Prednisone may be of value in the treatment of lipoid pneumonia.[37]

THE LUNG AND RENAL DISEASE

Chronic Renal Failure

Stable, chronic renal failure (CRF) is usually associated with few thoracic manifestations. Spirometry and ventilatory control are typically normal.[38] In some patients, however, a mild restrictive ventilatory defect with a low diffusing capacity associated with interstitial fibrosis secondary to uremia may be found.[39] Clinically significant pleural disease is uncommon.[40] Pleural disease is usually the result of uremia and can manifest as pleural friction rubs, pleural thickening, or effusions. Patients with pleurisy usually present with fever and pleuritic pain. Analysis of the pleural fluid commonly reveals an exudative, serosanguinous fluid with few inflammatory cells.[41] Other causes of pleural effusions in patients with CRF include tuberculosis, pulmonary infarction, and congestive heart failure. Pulmonary edema can result from fluid overload (cardiogenic pulmonary edema) or uremia-induced capillary leak in patients with severe renal dysfunction.[42]

Nephrotic Syndrome

The nephrotic syndrome is commonly seen in patients with glomerular disease and is defined by proteinuria, peripheral edema, hyperlipidemia, and renal failure.[43] As part of the syndrome, large amounts of protein are excreted in the urine (more than 3.5 g/d). This loss of intravascular protein leads to a low osmotic pressure and allows edema formation throughout the body. The two most common thoracic manifestations of the nephrotic syndrome are pleural effusions and pulmonary emboli.[40] Effusions, caused by low osmotic pressure, are usually bilateral and transudative in character. Clotting factor abnormalities associated with the nephrotic syndrome may predispose patients to renal vein thrombosis and recurrent pulmonary emboli.[44,45]

Goodpasture's Syndrome

Goodpasture's syndrome is an uncommon immune disease that causes both alveolar hemorrhage and glomerulonephritis. It results from linear deposition of antibodies directed at basement membranes in both the lungs and the kidneys.[43] Males are more frequently affected than females; the median age for the disease is approximately 21 years.[46] Hemoptysis is often the presenting complaint, followed in weeks or months by hematuria. Rales and rhonchi can be heard over the lower lung fields, and the chest radiograph may show alveolar-filling infiltrates at the bases. Mild restriction may be detected on pulmonary function testing; the diffusing capacity is usually supernormal owing to extravascular deposition of hemoglobin.[47]

Diagnosis is made by detecting anti-glomerular basement membrane antibodies in the serum or in tissue from the lung or kidney.[48] The cause of the spontaneous induction of these antibodies is unknown. Smoking may act as a trigger for their development, but infection is not thought to play any pathogenic role. Spontaneous remissions have been reported, but usually steroids, azathioprine, and/or plasmapheresis is required to treat the disease.[49–55]

Hemodialysis

Patients with end-stage renal disease require alternative methods to maintain excretory function. One common technique, *hemodialysis,* is a process by which urea and other low molecular weight solutes are removed from the blood by diffusion across a semipermeable membrane, the artificial kidney. A chemical gradient from blood to dialysis fluid (dialysate) allows this process to occur, and by increasing the hydrostatic pressure difference across the membrane, ultrafiltration, or the removal of fluid, may also be achieved.[55] The patient is attached to the dialysis machine via tubing that sends arterial blood for dialysis and returns venous blood after the process. Patients who require chronic hemodialysis often undergo surgical creation of an arteriovenous fistula or placement of a prosthetic arteriovenous graft in the forearm to facilitate connection to the dialysis machine. Hepatitis B and the dysequilibrium syndrome are two common untoward affects of hemodialysis.[55] The dysequilibrium syndrome results from more rapid removal of solutes from the plasma than from the intracellular space, which creates an osmotic gradient that promotes cerebral edema and causes headache, confusion, and other neurologic signs.

Hemodialysis can be associated with important gas exchange impairment. During dialysis arterial CO_2 partial pressure ($PaCO_2$) is maintained, but arterial O_2 partial pressure (PaO_2) may drop by as much as 20 percent from baseline.[56] Two possible explanations for these observations have been advanced: white blood cells may accumulate in the lungs during dialysis, causing a $\dot{V}/\dot{Q}$ mismatch and consequently a decrease in PaO_2[57]; alternatively, CO_2 may be partially removed in the dialysis bath, which lowers the respiratory exchange ratio ($PaCO_2/PaO_2$). This reduction in the ratio is associated with a decrease in minute ventilation, which maintains alveolar CO_2 partial pressure (P_ACO_2) but lowers alveolar O_2 partial pressure (P_AO_2),[58] and the reduction in P_AO_2 is quickly followed by a drop in PaO_2 (Fig. 43-1). Support for this mechanism comes from the observation that use of a bicarbonate bath, which decreases removal of CO_2, rather than an acetate bath can minimize the reduction in minute ventilation and consequently in PaO_2.[59] Most researchers believe this latter explanation to be the more appropriate one. Clinically, patients with significant lung disease may require supplemental O_2 to counter their hypoxemia. Most patients undergoing hemodialysis, however, need no intervention.

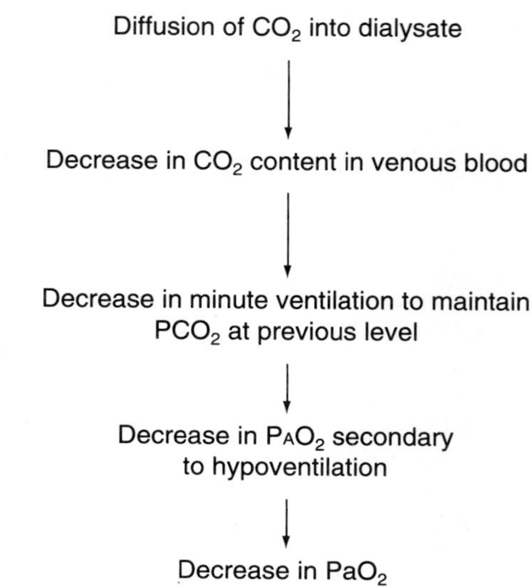

Figure 43-1. Proposed mechanism by which hemodialysis can cause hypoxemia.

Continuous Ambulatory Peritoneal Dialysis

Peritoneal dialysis is another method for maintaining excretory function in patients with either acute or chronic renal disease. This technique is similar in principle to hemodialysis, except that the peritoneal membrane serves as the semipermeable membrane for solute removal. A special catheter, the Tenckhoff peritoneal dialysis catheter, is placed in the abdominal cavity, and continuous exchange of 2 to 3 L of dialysate allows for removal of fluid and naturally occurring waste products. Peritonitis is the most serious complication of continuous ambulatory peritoneal dialysis (CAPD).[55]

In patients without underlying lung disease, the abdominal distension and elevation of the diaphragm that result from the instillation of dialysate may cause physiologically benign basilar atelectasis.[60] However, in patients with limited pulmonary reserve and/or ventilatory function, shortness of breath and hypoxemia may result during CAPD, especially if 3 L or more of dialysate is used.[61]

THE LUNG AND HEMATOLOGIC DISEASE

Leukemia

Leukemia is a disease in which the bone marrow is replaced by abnormally proliferating precursors of white blood cells. Leukemic involvement of the lungs may result in pulmonary infiltrates, hilar or mediastinal adenopathy, or pleural effusions.[62,63] Patients may complain of a nonproductive cough or dyspnea on exertion; cyanosis may be found on examination. Significant hypoxemia can result from microvascular plugging by white blood cells (leukostasis), especially when cell counts exceed 50,000/mL.[64,65] Alternatively, in the presence of extreme leukocytosis, the low PaO_2 may represent increased O_2 consumption by the white blood cells in the blood sample rather than true hypoxemia.[66] Acute and chronic myelocytic leukemia are most often associated with gas-exchange abnormalities.[67] Biopsy specimens are often required to confirm that the findings on chest radiography are the result of leukemia and not of an infectious process such as tuberculosis or another bacterial pathogen.[68] Chemotherapeutic agents are required for resolution of thoracic manifestations of the leukemias.

Lymphoma

Lymphoma is a malignant condition in which lymph tissue is replaced by abnormal lymphocytes. Two major types of lymphomas have been identified: Hodgkin's lymphomas are characterized by Reed-Sternberg cells and classified as nodular sclerosis, lymphocyte predominance, mixed cellularity, and lymphocyte depletion types[69]; non-Hodgkin's lymphomas are a heterogeneous group and account for the greatest number of lymphomas. The cause of both types is still unknown, although viruses, radiation, and immunodeficiency have been suspected.[70]

Non-Hodgkin's lymphoma has been reported in 5 to 10 percent of patients with the acquired immunodeficiency syndrome (AIDS).[71,72] These tumors tend to be very aggressive, with rapid doubling times. Most patients present with fever, weight loss, malaise, and/or neurologic symptoms. Rapid growth of lymph nodes and/or dementia is commonly seen. Chemotherapeutic treatment is limited because of the underlying immunodeficiency state.

Lymphomatous involvement of the lungs usually occurs as part of a systemic disease process. Nodules, infiltrates, and hilar or mediastinal adenopathy are common pulmonary manifestations.[73–75] Of all the lymphomas, nodular sclerosis Hodgkin's disease is most often associated with these findings.[73] Rarely, a lobar infiltrate will be the only manifestation of disease.[74] Patients with thoracic involvement may present with cough, chest pain, or fever, but some may be asymptomatic. Radiation therapy or, when advanced disease is found, combination chemotherapy is required to treat pulmonary involvement with lymphomas.[69,70]

As discussed in Chapter 39, many of the chemotherapeutic agents used to treat leukemia, lymphoma, and other malignancies can in themselves produce a variety of pulmonary disorders.

Multiple Myeloma

Multiple myeloma is a malignancy characterized by an abnormally large number of malfunctioning plasma cells. Bony invasion by these cells may cause hypercalcemia and hypercalciuria and lead to impaired renal function. In addition, the malignant plasma cells secrete antibodies, most commonly IgG or IgA, and parts of antibodies called light chains.[76] These so-called M-proteins, detected in serum and urine, have been associated with Raynaud's phenomenon, coagulation disorders, and hyperviscosity of the blood.[76]

Thoracic involvement with multiple myeloma is varied. "Punched out" lesions in the ribs and thoracic vertebrae may be seen on chest radiography.[77] Further, soft tissue masses (plasmacytomas) may extend from the bone marrow into the thorax, where they appear as lung masses.[78] Occasionally, paratracheal and parahilar masses are found, which when biopsied reveal multiple myeloma.[77] Parenchymal infiltrates may occasionally result from myeloma but more often represent an infectious process.[77] Treatment of multiple myeloma and its pulmonary manifestations consists of corticosteroids and chemotherapeutic agents; cure is not attainable but remission is common in most patients.[76]

Sickle Cell Disease

Sickle cell disease affects approximately 50,000 people in the United States, most of whom are of African ancestry.[79] The disease results from change of a single base in the DNA coding of the globin chain of the hemoglobin molecule, allowing the formation of hemoglobin S. This genetic abnormality causes the membrane of the red blood cell to become grossly deformed under conditions of low O_2 level.[80] The major manifestations of the disease, hemolytic anemia, high-output cardiac failure, pulmonary and splenic infarction, and bone pain, all result from plugging of misshapen red blood cells in the vascular bed.[80] Conditions that cause hypoxemia, such as pneumonia, travel to high altitude, or flying in unpressurized aircraft can predispose sickle cell patients to exacerbation of their disease, often called a "crisis."

Recurrent episodes of pleuritic chest pain, tachypnea, dyspnea, fever, elevated white blood cell count, and pulmonary infiltrates are common in patients with sickle cell disease.[81,82] It is often difficult to distinguish whether an underlying bacterial infection (usually caused by *Streptococcus pneumoniae* or *Mycoplasma pneumoniae*) or microvascular thrombosis is responsible for these symptoms. Antibiotics, O_2, fluids, and pain medications are usually given concurrently.[83,84] Patients with more severe recurrence of the chest "crisis" may develop pulmonary hypertension and cor pulmonale.[85–88]

Patients with other hemoglobulinopathies may have a combination of hemoglobin S with another type of hemoglobin molecule. Individuals with sickle cell trait have both hemoglobin A and S, and as a result are usually asymptomatic without an associated anemia.[80] In patients with hemoglobin SC or SD disease, a chronic anemia may be present but is usually less severe than in SS disease. Furthermore, these patients may have splenomegaly rather than the virtual absence of the spleen. Patients with SC disease, however, may have more significant ocular complications than patients with SS disease.[80] In all these hemoglobinopathies, pulmonary involvement is rare.

THE LUNG AND COLLAGEN VASCULAR DISEASE

Rheumatoid Arthritis

Rheumatoid arthritis is a systemic disease characterized primarily by inflammation of the joint lining, the synovium, but also associated with extra-articular involvement of the skin, eye, cardiovascular system, and nervous system.[89] Women are more often affected by the joint disease than men.

There are three common pulmonary findings with rheumatoid arthritis: (1) pleurisy with or without effusions, (2) rheumatoid nodules, and (3) interstitial fibrosis[90] (Table 43-2). These changes may be seen by themselves or in various combinations.

Pleural Disease

Pleural disease is the most common pulmonary manifestation of rheumatoid arthritis. Middle-aged men are more often affected than women, and unilateral disease is more common than bilateral involvement.[91] Patients with pleural involvement are usually asymptomatic but may present with pleurisy or dyspnea if a large effusion is present.

Pleural fluid is characteristically an exudate with a very low glucose value (less than 25 mg/dL).[92] Furthermore, rheumatoid factor, an immune marker, may be higher in the fluid than in the serum.[93] This finding is, however, nonspecific, being also present in other collagen vascular diseases.[94] Pleural effusions may spontaneously resolve over 6 months, leaving only minor residual pleural thickening, or may be present for several years.[95] Corticosteroids may shorten the time required for resolution but are generally not indicated.[95–97]

Table 43-2. Pulmonary Manifestations of Rheumatoid Arthritis, Systemic Lupus Erythematosus, and Scleroderma

Pulmonary Manifestation	Rheumatoid Arthritis	Systemic Lupus Erythematosus	Scleroderma
Pleural effusion	++	+++	+
Acute pneumonia	0	+	0
Interstitial fibrosis	++	+	+++
Pulmonary nodules	++	0	0
Pulmonary hypertension	+	0	++
Diaphragm dysfunction	0	+	0

(Modified from Myers,[195] with permission.)

Rheumatoid Nodules

Rheumatoid nodules are rounded, homogeneous masses of 0.3 to 0.7 cm diameter, which are found in the peripheral lung fields of patients with rheumatoid arthritis.[98] They are more often found in men than women and may be single or multiple. Histologically, they are identical to the subcutaneous nodules found in the upper extremities during flares of the disease.[99] Rheumatoid nodules usually do not result in symptoms; however, large space-occupying nodules may cause dyspnea and gas-exchange alterations.[100] Radiographically the nodules may cavitate, enlarge, or spontaneously resolve.[99] No specific therapy had been shown to be effective; treatment of the underlying rheumatoid disease is all that is required in most cases. A single nodule in a patient with rheumatoid disease must be further evaluated for malignancy, as guided by clinical presentation.

Interstitial Fibrosis

Interstitial fibrosis may develop during the course of rheumatoid arthritis and is indistinguishable from other forms of idiopathic pulmonary fibrosis.[101–103] Patients complain of dyspnea on exertion and a nonproductive cough. Crackles and clubbing are found on physical examination. Crackles are soft, high-pitched lung sounds that result from the sudden opening of small airways.[104] Significant hypoxemia may be found on arterial blood gas analysis. The role of steroids in preserving pulmonary function in patients with fibrosis related to rheumatoid arthritis is controversial.[102,103]

Systemic Lupus Erythematosus

Systemic lupus erythematosus (SLE) is an inflammatory multiorgan disease, which causes fever, fatigue, arthritis, a butterfly-shaped facial rash, lymphadenopathy, personality changes, and anemia.[105] There are five main pulmonary manifestations of SLE: (1) pleurisy with or without effusions, (2) lupus pneumonitis, (3) hemorrhagic alveolitis, (4) interstitial fibrosis, and (5) respiratory muscle dysfunction[106] (Table 43-2). These disorders may precede or follow other nonpulmonary organ involvement with SLE.[107]

Pleural Involvement

As in rheumatoid arthritis, pleural involvement is the most common thoracic manifestation in patients with SLE.[108] Effusions, if present, are usually small and unilateral. Analysis of the fluid reveals an exudate of high or low glucose content.[93] The most specific findings are an elevated antinuclear antibody (ANA) titer greater than 1:160 and a fluid to serum ANA ratio greater than unity.[109] Further, finding LE cells on Wright's stain of the pleural fluid is virtually pathognomonic for lupus-associated pleural disease.[110]

Lupus Pneumonitis

Patients with lupus pneumonitis present with fever, nonproductive cough, and patchy alveolar infiltrates on chest radiography.[111] Deposition of immune complexes and complement within alveolar membranes and capillary vessels is thought to be responsible for the observed clinical manifestations.[112] A vigorous search for an infectious etiology is necessary before the diagnosis of lupus pneumonitis can be made. Treatment consists of administration of steroids and/or azathioprine, along with supplemental O_2 as needed.[113]

Hemorrhagic Alveolitis

Hemorrhagic alveolitis is a rare but potentially lethal complication of SLE.[114,115] Dyspnea, hemoptysis, diffuse alveolar or interstitial infiltrates, and a reduction in hemoglobin are the main clinical findings.[114] Immune complex-mediated alveolar damage has been suggested as responsible for the alveolar hemorrhage.[116] High doses of steroids and/or azathioprine constitute the most effective treatment for this disease process.[115]

Interstitial Fibrosis

The interstitial fibrosis associated with SLE is similar to other forms of diffuse interstitial diseases. Symptoms of dyspnea on exertion and a nonproductive cough in conjunction with basilar fibrosis on chest radiography and a restrictive ventilatory defect on pulmonary function testing strongly suggest the diagnosis.[117,118] Histologically, fibrosis of the alveoli with or without demonstration of immune complexes is seen.[119] Treatment with steroids and cytotoxic agents (cyclophosphamide and azathioprine) has been tried, with varying results.[120]

Respiratory Muscle Weakness

Respiratory muscle weakness may develop in patients with SLE and can result in dyspnea on exertion.[121–123] Severe inflammation of muscle fibers in the diaphragm can cause diaphragmatic elevation with lower lobe atelectasis.[122,123] Over time, continued elevation of the diaphragm can lead to significant decreases in lung volumes or to the "shrinking lung" syndrome.[121]

Progressive Systemic Sclerosis (Scleroderma)

Progressive systemic sclerosis (PSS) is a systemic disease characterized by inflammation and fibrosis of the skin, esophagus, liver, and heart, with vascular lesions in the kidneys.[124] Pulmonary involvement with PSS often follows other manifestations of the disease. Interstitial fibrosis is the most common pulmonary finding.[125,126] Patients with PSS may develop dyspnea on exertion and have crackles in the lower lung fields on chest auscultation. Chest radiography often shows bibasilar interstitial fibrosis. Treatment for the interstitial fibrosis remains supportive; steroids and immunosuppressive drugs have not been shown to be effective.

A small number of patients with PSS may develop pulmonary hypertension out of proportion to the amount of pulmonary fibrosis present.[127,128] Pathologic changes within the vessel walls include proliferation of the endothelium and medial hyperplasia.[128] Right-sided heart failure usually follows the development of significant pulmonary hypertension. Administration of supplemental O_2 remains the most effective treatment. Pleuritis, pleural effusions, or lobar lung involvement is rare in patients with PSS.[129]

THE LUNG AND PREGNANCY

Pregnancy is associated with several mechanical and biochemical changes that may significantly alter pulmonary function and gas exchange. Most pregnant women experience mild dyspnea but are not significantly impaired. However, pregnant women with asthma or sarcoidosis may experience worsening of their respiratory symptoms and function. This section outlines pregnancy-associated modifications in anatomy and pulmonary function and discusses the effect of pregnancy on respiratory infections, including tuberculosis, asthma, sarcoidosis, and thromboembolic disease (Table 43-3).

Table 43-3. The Pulmonary Manifestations of Pregnancy

Anatomic alterations
Elevation of the diaphragm
Increase in transverse diameter of the chest
Pulmonary function changes
10–25% decrease in FRC
10% increase in inspiratory capacity
28% increase in V_T
No significant change in TLC
Gas exchange alterations
Hyperventilation (PCO_2 27–32 mmHg)
Increase in $P(A\text{-}a)O_2$ secondary to early closure of basilar alveoli
Respiratory infections
Increased risk of varicella and influenza pneumonia
Effect of pregnancy on course of tuberculosis is minimal
Respiratory diseases
Asthma: those with severe disease prior to conception may have worsening of their disease
Sarcoidosis: those with active alveolitis prior to conception may have worsening of their disease
Pulmonary embolism: risk greatest right after delivery

Anatomic Alterations

Anatomic changes with pregnancy include elevation of the diaphragm and increase in the transverse diameter of the chest.[130,131] These changes occur early, before the uterus has greatly expanded, and may be the result of increased levels of progesterone, estrogen, prostaglandins, or corticosteroids.[132] In the later stages of pregnancy, uterine expansion contributes to these anatomic alterations.

Pulmonary Function Changes

Pulmonary function testing is greatly modified as a result of the anatomic changes. Diaphragmatic elevation causes a 10 to 25 percent decrease in functional residual capacity (FRC).[133–135] Normal contraction of the diaphragm and the inspiratory muscles allows a 10 percent increase in inspiratory capacity and a 28 percent increase in tidal volume (V_T). Total lung capacity (TLC), therefore, is maintained until just prior to delivery, when it may fall slightly owing to further expansion of the uterus.[136,137]

Gas Exchange Alterations

Hyperventilation occurs during pregnancy. Progesterone stimulates an increase in both respiratory rate and V_T, resulting in augmentation of minute ventilation. This increase in minute ventilation is associated with dyspnea in approximately 60 to 70 percent of women.[138–141] Resting $PaCO_2$ drops to 27 to 32 mmHg; pH is maintained as renal wasting of bicarbonate follows.[142] Although the decline in $PaCO_2$ is associated with an increase in P_AO_2, the alveolar-arterial O_2 difference $[P(A\text{-}a)O_2]$ increases because of early closure of basilar alveoli at FRC.[143,144]

Respiratory Infections

Pregnant women are at increased risk of developing varicella and influenza pneumonia.[145,146] No similar risk for bacterial pneumonias has been reported. The effect of pregnancy on the course of tuberculosis is minimal[147,148]; the usual recommendations for treatment and prophylaxis remain unchanged. Isoniazid, rifampin, and ethambutal have not been shown to have a significant teratogenic effect on the fetus, although they all cross the placental membrane.[149] By contrast, streptomycin and ethionamide have been associated with an increased risk of congenital abnormalities and are contraindicated during pregnancy.[150,151]

Asthma

The course of asthma during pregnancy is variable and related to the severity of disease prior to conception.[152,153] Asthmatic women with severe disease may worsen during pregnancy, but usually those with mild or moderate asthma experience no change or slight improvement in their airway disease.[154] Increase in endogenous corticosteroids may explain improvement during pregnancy.[154] Fortunately, methylxanthines, beta-agonists, and anticholinergic bronchodilators are safe to use during pregnancy.[155] Exogenous corticosteroids have been associated with cleft palate in the fetus but are considered by most pulmonologists to be indicated when severe exacerbations develop.[156,157]

Sarcoidosis

As with asthma, the natural history of sarcoidosis is variable during pregnancy. Those women with inactive disease usually continue to demonstrate stable pulmonary function throughout their pregnancy.[158,159] However, women with active alveolitis prior to conception may have worsening of their disease and require corticosteroid therapy.[160] A subset of women with active disease prior to conception may actually improve during pregnancy, only to have their symptoms recur 3 to 6 months after delivery.[161]

Thromboembolic Disease

Several large series have estimated the incidence of *deep venous thrombosis* (DVT) to be 1.2 percent and that of *pulmonary embolism* to be 0.2 to 0.4 percent during pregnancy.[162–164] These values are probably underestimates since the diagnosis of DVT or pulmonary embolism during pregnancy is difficult, as venography, radiolabeled fibrinogen studies, and pulmonary angiography are associated with considerable risk to the fetus.[165] The risks of DVT and pulmonary embolism after delivery are significantly greater than during pregnancy; this is probably related to coagulation abnormalities found at the time of delivery.[162] Heparin is the drug of choice for treatment of thromboembolic disease during pregnancy since it does not cross the placental barrier.[166] Heparin therapy can be used up until the time of delivery and in the immediate postpartum period. Coumadin is contraindicated, especially in the first trimester, since it may cause fetal cerebral hemorrhage and congenital defects.[167]

Amniotic fluid embolism is a rare event that is associated with high maternal mortality. Amniotic fluid enters the venous circulation via uterine veins during delivery and may result in the adult respiratory distress syndrome (ARDS).[168,169] Additionally, hypotension with cardiovascular collapse and disseminated intravascular coagulation with hemorrhaging may develop.[168,169] Associated risk factors include traumatic vaginal delivery, advanced maternal age, multiparity, and intrauterine fetal demise.[169] Treatment is limited to supportive measures.[170]

THE LUNG AND MISCELLANEOUS DISEASES

Neurogenic Pulmonary Edema

Central nervous system injuries can result in a form of pulmonary edema called neurogenic pulmonary edema

(NPE).[171–174] The two most common insults associated with NPE are seizures and head trauma.[174] Increased intracranial pressure is most likely responsible for the edema formation; both a hydrostatic and a capillary leak mechanism have been postulated.[175–178] Typically, NPE develops minutes to hours after injury and presents with hypoxemia and bilateral perihilar infiltrates on the chest radiograph. Most episodes are well tolerated, but in some patients NPE may proceed to an entity indistinguishable from ARDS. Successful management depends on early recognition and institution of supportive measures, especially supplemental O_2. In patients who develop overt ARDS, implementation of positive end-expiratory pressure (PEEP) therapy must be undertaken cautiously as increased intracranial pressure may result.[179,180]

Thyroid Disease

Hypothyroidism

Hypothyroidism is associated with several pulmonary function abnormalities. Blunting of both hypoxic and hypercapnic respiratory drives has been documented in patients with varying degrees of hypothyroidism.[181,182] The mechanisms responsible for these disturbances are unknown, but replacement therapy with thyroid hormone usually results in restoration of drive function.[182] Additionally, patients with hypothyroidism may have obstructive sleep apnea, which is partially related to their obesity and the myxedematous changes often found in the tissue of the posterior pharynx.[183] Again, hormone replacement therapy with or without weight loss may significantly lessen the number of obstructive apnea episodes experienced.[184] Other manifestations of hypothyroidism include diaphragmatic dysfunction,[185,186] respiratory muscle weakness,[187] and pleural effusions.[188]

Hyperthyroidism

Patients with hyperthyroidism may have heightened respiratory drives, causing dyspnea in some individuals.[189] These abnormalities are reversed with thyroid ablation.[189] Case reports have demonstrated that when asthma and hyperthyroidism occur together, treatment of the thyroid condition may markedly improve the clinical course of the asthma.[190]

Wegener's Granulomatosis

Wegener's granulomatosis is a systemic disease resulting in extensive damage to small blood vessels. The lung is involved in over 90 percent of cases.[191] Most patients present with ulcerative lesions of the nasopharynx, cavitary lesions in the lungs, and glomerular involvement of the kidneys.[192] Diagnosis often requires tissue confirmation.[193] Treatment consists of immunosuppressive therapy with agents such as corticosteroids and cyclophosphamide, which can produce a 90 percent remission rate.[191] A 1985 report of successful treatment with trimethaprim-sulfamethoxazole suggests the possibility of an infectious trigger or etiology for this disorder.[194]

References

1. Bass NM, Van Dyke RW: Cirrhosis of the liver and its complications. pp. 327–333. In Andreoli TE, Carpenter CCJ, Plum F, Smith LH (eds): Cecil Essentials of Medicine. WB Saunders, Philadelphia, 1990
2. Boyer TD: Major sequelae of cirrhosis. pp. 847–852. In Wyngaarden JB, Smith LH (eds): Cecil Textbook of Medicine. WB Saunders, Philadelphia, 1988
3. Davis HH, Schwartz DJ, Lefrak SS et al: Alveolar capillary oxygen disequilibrium in hepatic cirrhosis. Chest 1978;73:507–511
4. Wolfe JD, Tashkin DP, Holly FE et al: Hypoxemia of cirrhosis, detection of abnormal small pulmonary vascular channels by a quantitative radionuclide method. Am J Med 1977;63:746–754
5. Furukawa T, Hara N, Yasumoto K et al: Arterial hypoxemia in patients with hepatic cirrhosis. Am J Med Sci 1984;287:10–13
6. Kennedy TC, Knudson RJ: Exercise-aggravated hypoxemia and orthodeoxia in cirrhosis. Chest 1977;72:305–309
7. Castaing Y, Manier G: Hemodynamic disturbances and $\dot{V}_A/\dot{Q}$ matching in hypoxemic cirrhotic patients. Chest 1989;96:1064–1069
8. Daoud FS, Reeves JT, Schaefer JW: Failure of hypoxic pulmonary vasoconstriction in patients with liver cirrhosis. J Clin Invest 1972;51:1076–1080
9. Naeije R, Hallemans R, Mols P et al: Hypoxic pulmonary vasoconstriction in liver cirrhosis. Chest 1981;80:570–574
10. Robin ED, Laman D, Horn BR et al: Platypnea related to orthodeoxia caused by true vascular lung shunts. N Engl J Med 1976;294:941–943
11. Bank ER, Thrau JH, Dantzker DR: Radionuclide demonstration of intrapulmonary shunting in cirrhosis. AJR 1983; 140:967–969
12. Lieberman FL, Peters RL: Cirrhotic hydrothorax. Arch Intern Med 1970;125:114–117
13. Falchuck KR, Jacoby I, Colucci WS et al: Tetracycline-induced pleural symphysis for recurrent hydrothorax complicating cirrhosis. Gastroenterology 1977;72:319–321
14. Lebrec D, Capron JP, Dhumeaux D et al: Pulmonary hypertension complicating portal hypertension. Am Rev Respir Dis 1979;120:849–856
15. McDonnell PJ, Toye PA, Hutchins GM: Primary pulmonary hypertension and cirrhosis: Are they related? Am Rev Respir Dis 1983;127:437–441
16. Matsubara O, Nakamura T, Uehara T et al: Histometrical investigation of the pulmonary artery in severe hepatic disease. J Pathol 1984;143:31–37
17. Bass NM, Van Dyke RW: Acute and chronic hepatitis. pp. 319–325. In Andreoli TE, Carpenter CCJ, Plum F, Smith LH (eds): Cecil Essentials of Medicine. WB Saunders, Philadelphia, 1990
18. Morrison EB, Gaffney FA, Eigenbrodt EH et al: Severe pulmonary hypertension associated with macronodular (postnecrotic) cirrhosis and autoimmune phenomena. Am J Med 1980; 69:513–519
19. Cryer PE, Kissane JM: Chronic active hepatitis and pulmonary hypertension. Am J Med 1977;63:604–613
20. Williams AJ, Marsh J, Stableforth DE: Cryptogenic fibrosing alveolitis, chronic active hepatitis and autoimmune hemolytic anemia in the same patient. Br J Dis Chest 1985;79:200–203
21. Kleiner-Baumgarten A, Schlaeffer R, Keynan A: Multiple autoimmune manifestations in a splenectomized subject with HLA-B8. Arch Intern Med 1983;143:1987–1989
22. Golding PL, Smith M, Williams R: Multisystem involvement in chronic liver disease. Am J Med 1973;55:772–782

23. Rodriguez-Roisin R, Pares A, Bruguera M et al: Pulmonary involvement in primary biliary cirrhosis. Thorax 1981;36:208–212
24. Weissman E, Becker NH: Interstitial lung disease in primary biliary cirrhosis. Am J Med Sci 1983;285:21–27
25. Hughes RL, Craig RM, Freilich RA et al: Aspiration and occult esophageal disorders. Chest 1981;80:489–495
26. Goodall RJR, Eans JE, Coopner DN et al: Relationship between asthma and gastroesophageal reflux. Thorax 1981; 36:116–121
27. Ducolone R, Vandvenne A, Jouin H et al: Gastroesophageal reflux in patients with asthma and chronic bronchitis. Am Rev Respir Dis 1987;135:327–332
28. Sladen A, Zanca P, Hadnott WH: Aspiration pneumonitis—the sequelae. Chest 1951;59:448–450
29. Mays EE, Dubois JJ, Hamilton GB: Pulmonary fibrosis associated with tracheobronchial aspiration. Chest 1976;69:512–515
30. Boyle JT, Tuchman DN, Altschuler SM et al: Mechanisms for the association of gastroesophageal reflux and bronchospasm. Am Rev Respir Dis 1985;131:S16–S20
31. Mansfield LE, Stein MR: The role of the vagus nerve in airway narrowing caused by intraesophageal hydrochloric acid provocation and distention. Ann Allergy 1981;47:431–434
32. Pellegrini CA, DeMeester TR, Johnson LF et al: Gastroesophageal reflux and pulmonary aspiration: Incidence, functional abnormality, and results of surgical therapy. Surgery 1979;86:110–119
33. Altorki NK, Skinner DB: Pathophysiology of gastroesophageal reflux. Am J Med 1989;86:685–689
34. Barish CF, Wu WC, Castell DO: Respiratory complications of gastroesophageal reflux. Arch Intern Med 1985;145:1882–1888
35. Scully RE, Galdabini JJ, McNeely BU: Case records of the Massachusetts General Hospital, Case 19-1977. N Engl J Med 1977;296:1105–1111
36. Kennedy JD, Costello P, Balikian JP et al: Exogenous lipoid pneumonia. AJR 1981;136:1145–1149
37. Ayvazian LF, Steward DS, Merkel CG et al: Diffuse lipoid pneumonitis successfully treated with prednisone. Am J Med 1967;43:930–934
38. Lee HY, Stretton TB, Barnes AM: The lungs in renal failure. Thorax 1975;30:46–53
39. Forman JW, Ayers LN, Miller WC: Pulmonary diffusing capacity in chronic renal failure. Br J Dis Chest 1981;75:81–87
40. Senior RM, Lefrak SS: The lungs and abdominal disease. pp. 1894–1905. In Murray JF, Nadel JA (eds): Textbook of Respiratory Medicine. WB Saunders, Philadelphia, 1988
41. Nidus BD, Matalon R, Cantacuzino D et al: Uremic pleuritis—a clinicopathologic entity. N Engl J Med 1969;281:255–256
42. Crosbie WA, Snowden S, Parsons V: Changes in lung capillary permeability in renal failure. Br Med J 1972;4:388–390
43. Couser WG: Glomerular disorders. pp. 582–602. In Wyngaarden JB, Smith LH (eds): Cecil Textbook of Medicine. WB Saunders, Philadelphia, 1988
44. Vigano-D'Angelo S, D'Angelo A, Kaufman CE et al: Protein S deficiency occurs in the nephrotic syndrome. Ann Intern Med 1987;107:42–47
45. Llach F: Nephrotic syndrome: Hypercoagulability, renal vein thrombosis, and other thromboembolic complications. pp. 121–144. In Brenner BM, Stein JH (eds): Nephrotic Syndrome. Churchill Livingstone, New York, 1982
46. Hay JG, Turner-Warwick M: Pulmonary hemosiderosis, hemorrhagic syndromes, and other rare infiltrative disorders. pp. 1501–1514. In Murray JF, Nadel JA (eds): Textbook of Respiratory Medicine. WB Saunders, Philadelphia, 1988
47. Ewan PW, Jones HA, Rhodes DG et al: Detection of intrapulmonary hemorrhage with carbon monoxide uptake: Application in Goodpasture's syndrome. N Engl J Med 1976; 295:1391–1396
48. Beechler CR, Enquist RW, Hunt KK et al: Immunofluorescence of transbronchial biopsies in Goodpasture's syndrome. Am Rev Respir Dis 1980;121:869–872
49. Teichmann S, Briggs WA, Kneiser MR et al: Goodpasture's syndrome: Two cases with contrasting early course and management. Am Rev Respir Dis 1976;113:223–232
50. Proskwy AJ, Weatherbee L, Easterling RE et al: Goodpasture's syndrome. Am J Med 1970;48:162–173
51. Hayslett JP, Berte JB, Kashgarian M: Successful treatment of renal failure in Goodpasture's syndrome. Arch Intern Med 1971;127:953–957
52. Lang CH, Brown DC, Staley N et al: Goodpasture's syndrome treated with immunosuppression and plasma exchange. Arch Intern Med 1977;137:1076–1078
53. Johnson JP, Whitman W, Briggs WA et al: Plasmapheresis and immunosuppressive agents in anti-basement membrane antibody induced Goodpasture's syndrome. Am J Med 1978; 64:354–358
54. Swainson CP, Robson JS, Urbaniak SJ et al: Treatment of Goodpasture's disease by plasma exchange and immunosuppressives. Clin Exp Immunol 1978;32:233–241
55. Luke RG: Treatment of irreversible renal failure. pp. 573–577. In Wyngaarden JB, Smith LH (eds): Cecil Textbook of Medicine. WB Saunders, Philadelphia, 1988
56. Burns CB, Scheinhorn DJ: Hypoxemia during hemodialysis. Arch Intern Med 1982;142:1350–1353
57. Eknoyan G: Side effects of hemodialysis. N Engl J Med 1984; 311:915–917
58. Quebbeman EJ, Maierhofer WJ, Piering WF: Mechanisms producing hypoxemia during hemodialysis. Crit Care Med 1984; 12:359–363
59. Hunt JM, Chappell TR, Henrich WL et al: Gas exchange during dialysis: Contrasting mechanisms contributing to comparable alterations with acetate and bicarbonate buffers. Am J Med 1984;77:255–260
60. Singh S, Dale A, Morgan B et al: Serial studies of pulmonary function in continuous ambulatory peritoneal dialysis: A prospective study. Chest 1984;86:874–877
61. Twardowski ZT, Prowant BF, Nolph KD et al: High volume, low frequency continuous ambulatory peritoneal dialysis. Arch Intern Med 1954;93:528–540
62. Bodey GP, Powell RD Jr, Hersh EM et al: Pulmonary complications of acute leukemia. Cancer 1966;19:781–793
63. Tenholder MF, Hooper RC: Pulmonary infiltrates in leukemia. Chest 1980;78:468–473
64. Bloom R, Taveira D, Silva AM: Reversible respiratory failure due to intravascular leukostasis in chronic myelogenous leukemia, relationship of O_2 transfer to leukocyte count. Am J Med 1979;67:679–683
65. Frost T, Isbister JP, Ravich RB: Respiratory failure due to leukostasis in leukemia. Med J Aust 1981;2:94–95
66. Chillar RK, Belman MJ, Farbstein M: Explanation for apparent hypoxemia associated with extreme leukocytosis: Leukocytic oxygen consumption. Blood 1980;5:922–924
67. Klatte EC, Yardley J, Smith EB et al: The pulmonary manifestations and complications of leukemia. AJR 1963;89:598–609
68. Rosenow EC, Wilson WR, Cockerill FR: Pulmonary disease in the immunocompromised host. Mayo Clin Proc 1985;60:473–487
69. Glick JH: Hodgkin's lymphoma. pp. 1014–1022. In Wyngaarden JB, Smith LH (eds): Cecil Textbook of Medicine. WB Saunders, Philadelphia, 1988
70. Portlock CS: The non-Hodgkin's lymphomas. pp. 1009–1013. In Wyngaarden JB, Smith LH (eds): Cecil Textbook of Medicine. WB Saunders, Philadelphia, 1988
71. Ziegler JL, Beckstead JA, Volberding PA et al: Non-Hodgkin's lymphoma in 90 homosexual men. N Engl J Med 1984;311:565–570
72. Levine AM, Meyer PR, Begandy MK et al: Development of B-cell lymphoma in homosexual men. Ann Intern Med 1984; 100:7–13
73. Ellman P, Bowdler AJ: Pulmonary manifestations of Hodgkin's disease. Br J Dis Chest 1960;54:59–71
74. Filly B, Blank N, Castellino RA: Radiographic distribution of intrathoracic disease in previously untreated patients with

Hodgkin's disease and non-Hodgkin's lymphoma. Radiology 1976;120:277–281
75. Robbins LL: The roentgenological appearance of parenchymal involvement of the lung by malignant lymphoma. Cancer 1953; 6:80–88
76. Salmon SE: Plasma cell disorders. pp. 1026–1036. In Wyngaarden JB, Smith LH (eds): Cecil Textbook of Medicine. WB Saunders, Philadelphia, 1988
77. Kintzer JS, Rosenow EC, Kyle RA: Thoracic and pulmonary abnormalities in multiple myeloma: A review of 958 cases. Arch Intern Med 1978;138:727–730
78. Kilburn KH, Schmidt AM: Intrathoracic plasmacytoma. Arch Intern Med 1960;106:802–809
79. Konotey-Ahula FID: The sickle cell diseases. Clinical manifestations including the "sickle crisis." Arch Intern Med 1974; 133:611–619
80. Forget BG: Sickle cell anemia and associated hemoglobulinemias. pp. 936–943. In Wyngaarden JB, Smith LH (eds): Cecil Textbook of Medicine. WB Saunders, Philadelphia, 1988
81. Bromberg PA: Pulmonary aspects of sickle cell disease. Arch Intern Med 1974;133:652–657
82. Charache S, Scott JC, Charache P: Acute chest syndrome in adults with sickle cell anemia: Microbiology, treatment and prevention. Arch Intern Med 1979;139:67–69
83. Charache S: Treatment of sickle cell anemia. Annu Rev Med 1981;32:195–206
84. Alavi JB: Sickle cell anemia: Pathophysiology and treatment. Med Clin North Am 1984;68:545–556
85. Collins FS, Orringer EP: Pulmonary hypertension and cor pulmonale in the sickle hemoglobinopathies. Am J Med 1982; 73:814–821
86. Sproule BJ, Halden ER, Miller WF: A study of cardiopulmonary alterations in patients with sickle cell disease and its variants. J Clin Invest 1958;39:486–495
87. Moser KM, Shea JG: The relationship between pulmonary infarction, cor pulmonale, and the sickle states. Am J Med 1957; 22:561–579
88. Yater WN, Hansmann GH: Sickle cell anemia: A new cause of cor pulmonale. Am J Med Sci 1936;191:474–484
89. Ho G, Kammer GM: Rheumatoid arthritis. pp. 640–643. In Andreoli TE, Carpenter CCJ, Plum F, Smith LH (eds): Cecil Essentials of Medicine. WB Saunders, Philadelphia, 1990
90. Walker WC, Wright V: Pulmonary lesions and rheumatoid arthritis. Medicine (Baltimore) 1968;47:501–520
91. Scadding JG: The lungs in rheumatoid arthritis. Proc R Soc Med 1969;62:227–238
92. Carr DT, Mayne TG: Pleurisy with effusion in rheumatoid arthritis with reference to the low concentration of glucose in pleural fluid. Am Rev Respir Dis 1962;85:345–350
93. Halla JT, Schrohenloher RE, Volanakis JE: Immune complexes and other laboratory features of pleural effusions. Ann Intern Med 1980;69:507–511
94. Levine H, Szanto M, Griekle HG et al: Rheumatoid factor in non-rheumatoid pleural effusions. Ann Intern Med 1968; 69:487–492
95. Walker WC, Wright V: Rheumatoid pleuritis. Ann Rheum Dis 1967;26:467–474
96. Hunninghake GW, Fauci AS: Pulmonary involvement in the collagen vascular diseases. Am Rev Respir Dis 1979;119:471–503
97. Mays EE: Rheumatoid pleuritis: Observations in eight cases and suggestions for making the diagnosis in patients without the "typical findings." Chest 1968;53:202–214
98. Horler AR, Thompson M: The pleural and pulmonary complications of rheumatoid arthritis. Ann Intern Med 1959; 51:1179–1203
99. Sienewicz DJ, Martine JR, Moore S et al: Rheumatoid nodules in the lung. J Can Assoc Radiol 1962;13:73–80
100. Gordon DA, Stein JL, Broden I: The extra-articular features of rheumatoid arthritis. Am J Med 1973;54:445–452
101. Cervantes-Perez P, Toro-Perez AH, Rodriguez-Jurado P: Pulmonary involvement in rheumatoid arthritis. JAMA 1980; 243:1715–1719
102. Popper MS, Bogdonoff ML, Hughes RL: Interstitial rheumatoid lung disease: A reassessment and review of the literature. Chest 1973;62:243–250
103. Stack BHR, Grant IWB: Rheumatoid interstitial lung disease. Br J Dis Chest 1965;59:202–211
104. Loudon R, Murphy RLH: State of the art. Lung sounds. Am Rev Respir Dis 1984;130:663–673
105. Ho G, Kammer GM: Systemic lupus erythematosus. pp. 643–646. In Andreoli TE, Carpenter CCJ, Plum F, Smith LH (eds): Cecil Essentials of Medicine. WB Saunders, Philadelphia, 1990
106. Gross M, Esterly JR, Earle RH: Pulmonary alterations in systemic lupus erythematosus. Am Rev Respir Dis 1972;105:572–577
107. Haupt HM, Moore GW, Hutchins GM: The lung in systemic lupus erythematosus: Analysis of the pathologic changes in 120 patients. Am J Med 1981;71:791–798
108. Harvey AM: Systemic lupus erythematosus: Review of the literature and clinical analysis of 138 cases. Medicine (Baltimore) 1954;33:291–337
109. Leechawengwong M, Berger HW, Sukumaran M: Diagnostic significance of antinuclear antibodies in pleural effusion. Mt Sinai J Med (NY) 1979;46:137–139
110. Carel RS, Shapiro MS, Shoham D et al: Lupus erythematosus cells in pleural effusion. Chest 1977;72:670–672
111. Matthay RA, Schwarz MI, Petty TL: Pulmonary manifestations of systemic erythematosus: Review of twelve cases of acute lupus pneumonitis. Medicine (Baltimore) 1974;54:397–409
112. Inoue T, Kanayana Y, Ohe A et al: Immunopathologic studies of pneumonitis in systemic lupus erythematosus. Ann Intern Med 1979;91:30–34
113. Smith CM: The lungs in systemic lupus erythematosus, progressive systemic sclerosis and its variants, polymyositis, dermatomyositis, and mixed connective tissue disease. pp. 381–386. In Bordow RA, Moser KM (eds): Manual of Clinical Problems in Pulmonary Medicine. Little Brown, Boston, 1985
114. Eagan JW, Memoli VA, Roberts JL et al: Pulmonary hemorrhage in systemic lupus erythematosus. Medicine (Baltimore) 1978;57:545–560
115. Gamsu G, Webb WR: Pulmonary haemorrhage in systemic lupus erythematosus. J Can Assoc Radiol 1978;29:66–68
116. Churg A, Franklin W, Chan KL et al: Pulmonary hemorrhage and immune complex deposition in the lung: Complications in a patient with systemic lupus erythematosus. Arch Pathol Lab Med 1980;104:388–391
117. Eisenberg H: The interstitial lung diseases associated with the collagen-vascular disorders. Clin Chest Med 1982;3:565–578
118. Eisenberg H, Dubois EL, Sherwin RP et al: Diffuse interstitial lung disease in systemic lupus erythematosus. Ann Intern Med 1973;79:37–45
119. Olsen EG, Lever JV: Pulmonary changes is systemic lupus erythematosus: Br J Dis Chest 1972;66:71–77
120. Azathioprine in systemic lupus erythematosus. (Editorial.) Lancet 1973;1:704–705
121. Hoffbrand BI, Beck ER: Unexplained dyspnoea and shrinking lungs in systemic lupus erythematosus. Br Med J 1965;1:1273–1277
122. Gibson GJ, Edmonds JP, Hughes GRV: Diaphragmatic function and lung involvement in SLE. Am J Med 1977;63:926–932
123. Martens J, Demedts M, VanMeenen MI et al: Respiratory muscle dysfunction in systemic lupus erythematosus. Chest 1983; 84:170–175
124. Ho G, Kammer GM: Scleroderma. pp. 650–651. In Andreoli TE, Carpenter CCJ, Plum F, Smith LH (eds): Cecil Essentials of Medicine. WB Saunders, Philadelphia, 1990
125. Hayman LO, Hunt RE: Pulmonary fibrosis and generalized scleroderma: Report of a case and review of the literature. Chest 1952;21:691–704
126. Taormina VJ, Miller WT, Gefter WB et al: Progressive sys-

temic sclerosis: Variable pulmonary features. AJR 1981;137: 277–285
127. Young RH, Mark GJ: Pulmonary vascular changes in scleroderma. Am J Med 1978;64:998–1004
128. Naeye RL: Pulmonary vascular lesions in systemic scleroderma. Chest 1963;44:374–380
129. Opie LH: The pulmonary manifestations of generalized scleroderma: Progressive systemic sclerosis. Chest 1955;28:665–680
130. Prowse CM, Gaensler EA: Respiratory and acid-base changes during pregnancy. Anesthesiology 1965;26:381–392
131. Gee JBL, Packer BS, Millne JE et al: Pulmonary mechanics during pregnancy. J Clin Invest 1967;46:945–952
132. Krumholz RA, Echt CR, Ross JC: Pulmonary diffusing capacity, capillary blood volume, lung volumes, and mechanics of ventilation in early and late pregnancy. J Lab Clin Med 1964; 63:648–655
133. Gazioglue K, Kaltreider NL, Rosen M et al: Pulmonary function during pregnancy in normal women and in patients with cardiopulmonary disease. Thorax 1970;25:445–450
134. Rubin A, Russo N, Goucher D: The effect of pregnancy upon pulmonary function in normal women. Am J Obstet Gynecol 1956;72:963–969
135. Alaily AB, Carroll KB: Pulmonary ventilation in pregnancy. Br J Obstet Gynaecol 1978;85:518–524
136. Cugell DW, Frank NR, Gaensler EA et al: Pulmonary function in pregnancy: Serial observations in normal women. Am Rev Respir Dis 1953;67:568–597
137. Gaensler EA, Patton WE, Verstraeten JM et al: Pulmonary function in pregnancy: Serial observations in patients with pulmonary insufficiency. Am Rev Respir Dis 1953;67:779–797
138. Milne JA, Howie AD, Pack AI: Dyspnoea during normal pregnancy. Br J Obstet Gynaecol 1978;85:260–263
139. Gilbert R, Epifano L, Auchincloss JH: Dyspnea of pregnancy: A syndrome of altered respiratory control. JAMA 1962; 182:1073–1077
140. Gilbert R, Auchincloss JH: Dyspnea of pregnancy: Clinical and physiological observations. Am J Med Sci 1966;252:270–276
141. Lehmann V: Dyspnea in pregnancy. J Perinat Med 1975;3:154–160
142. Dayal P, Murata Y, Takamura H: Antepartum and postpartum acid-base changes in maternal blood in normal and complicated pregnancies. Br J Obstet Gynaecol 1979;79:612–624
143. Bevan DR, Holdcroft A, Loh L et al: Closing volume and pregnancy. Br Med J 1974;1:13–15
144. Holdcroft A, Bevan DR, O'Sullivan JC et al: Airway closure and pregnancy. Anaesthesia 1977;32:517–523
145. Oxorne H: The changing aspects of pneumonia complicating pregnancy. Am J Obstet Gynecol 1955;70:1057–1063
146. Hopwood HG: Pneumonia in pregnancy. Obstet Gynecol 1965; 25:875–879
147. De March AP: Tuberculosis and pregnancy: Five- to ten-year review of 215 patients in their fertile age. Chest 1975;68:800–804
148. Schaefer G, Zervoudakis IA, Fuchs FF et al: Pregnancy and pulmonary tuberculosis. Obstet Gynecol 1975;46:706–715
149. Scheinhorn DJ, Angelillo VA: Antituberculous therapy in pregnancy: Risks to the fetus. West J Med 1977;127:195–198
150. Robinson GC, Cambon KG: Hearing loss in infants of tuberculous mothers treated with streptomycin during pregnancy. N Engl J Med 1964;271:949–951
151. Potworowska M, Sianozecka E, Szufladowicz R: Ethionamide treatment and pregnancy. Pol Med J 1966;5:1152–1158
152. Weinstein AM, Dubin BD, Podleski WK et al: Asthma and pregnancy. JAMA 1979;241:1161–1165
153. Gluck JC, Gluck PA: The effects of pregnancy on asthma: A prospective study. Ann Allergy 1976;37:164–168
154. Bahna SL, Bjerkedal T: The course and outcome of pregnancy in women with bronchial asthma. Acta Allergol 1972;27:397–406
155. Weinberger SE, Weiss ST, Cohen WR et al: Pregnancy and the lung. Am Rev Respir Dis 1980;121:559–581
156. Snyder RD, Synder D: Corticosteroids for asthma during pregnancy. Ann Allergy 1978;41:340–341
157. Fainstat T: Cortisone-induced congenital cleft palate in rabbits. Endocrinology 1954;55:502–508
158. O'Leary JA: Ten-year study of sarcoidosis and pregnancy. Am J Obstet Gynecol 1962;84:462–466
159. Dines DE, Banner EA: Sarcoidosis during pregnancy: Improvement in pulmonary function. JAMA 1967;200:726–727
160. Grossman JH, Littner MR: Severe sarcoidosis in pregnancy. Obstet Gynecol, suppl. 1977;50:81s–84s
161. Fried KH: Sarcoidosis and pregnancy. Acta Med Scand, suppl. 1964;176:218–221
162. Henderson SR, Lund CJ, Creasoman WT: Antepartum pulmonary embolism. Am J Obstet Gynecol 1972;112:476–486
163. Handin RI: Thromboembolic complications of pregnancy and oral contraceptives. Prog Cardiovasc Dis 1974;16:395–405
164. Aaro LA, Juergens JL: Thrombophlebitis associated with pregnancy. Am J Obstet Gynecol 1971;109:1128–1136
165. Howie PW: Thromboembolism. Clin Obstet Gynaecol 1977; 4:397–417
166. Flessa HC, Kapstrom AB, Glueck HI et al: Placental transport of heparin. Am J Obstet Gynecol 1965;93:570–573
167. Pettifor JM, Benson R: Congenital malformations associated with the administration of oral anticoagulants during pregnancy. J Pediatr 1975;86:459–462
168. Courtney LD: Amniotic fluid embolism. Obstet Gynecol Surv 1974;29:169–177
169. Peterson EP, Taylor HB: Amniotic fluid embolism: An analysis of 40 cases. Obstet Gynecol 1970;35:787–793
170. Chung AF, Merkatz IR: Survival following amniotic fluid embolism with early heparinization. Obstet Gynecol 1973;42:809–814
171. Archibault RB, Armstrong JD: Recurrent postictal pulmonary edema. Postgrad Med 1978;63:210–213
172. Carlson RW, Schaeffer RC, Michaels SG et al: Pulmonary edema following intracranial hemorrhage. Chest 1979;76:731–734
173. Neurogenic pulmonary edema, clinical commentary. Clin Chest Med 1985;6:473–489
174. Malik AB: Mechanisms of neurogenic pulmonary edema. Circ Res 1985;57:1–18
175. van der Zee H, Malik AB, Lee BC: Lung fluid and protein exchange during intracranial hypertension and role of sympathetic mechanism. J Appl Physiol 1980;48:273–280
176. Theodore J, Robin E: Speculations on neurogenic pulmonary edema. Am Rev Respir Dis 1976;113:405–411
177. Bowers RE, McKeen CR, Park KE et al: Increased pulmonary vascular permeability follows intracranial hypertension in sheep. Am Rev Respir Dis 1979;119:637–641
178. Melon E, Bonnet F, Lepresle E et al: Altered capillary permeability in neurogenic pulmonary edema. Intensive Care Med 1985;11:323–325
179. Huseby JS, Pavlin EG, Butler J: Effect of positive end-expiratory pressure on intracranial pressure in dogs. J Appl Physiol 1978;44:25–27
180. Grasberger RC, Spatz EL, Mortara RW et al: Effect of high-frequency ventilation vs conventional mechanical ventilation on intracranial pressure in head-injured dogs. J Neurosurg 1984;60:1214–1218
181. Zwillich CW, Pierson DJ, Hofeldt FD et al: Ventilatory control in myxedema and hypothyroidism. N Engl J Med 1975; 292:662–665
182. Ladenson PW, Goldenheim PD, Ridgeway EC: Prediction and reversal of blunted ventilatory responsiveness in patients with hypothyroidism. Am J Med 1988;84:877–883
183. Skatrud J, Iber C, Ewart R et al: Disordered breathing during sleep in hypothyroidism. Am Rev Respir Dis 1981;124:325–329
184. Orr WC, Males JL, Imes NK: Myxedema and obstructive sleep apnea. Am J Med 1981;70:1061–1066
185. Hamly FH, Timma RM, Mihn VD et al: Bilateral phrenic paralysis in myxedema. Am Rev Respir Dis 1975;111:A911–A912

186. Martinez FJ: Hypothyroidism; a reversible cause of diaphragmatic dysfunction. Chest 1989;96:1059–1063
187. Laroche CM, Cairns T, Moxham J et al: Hypothyroidism presenting with respiratory muscle weakness. Am Rev Respir Dis 1988;138:472–474
188. Sachder Y, Hall R: Effusions into body cavities in hypothyroidism. Lancet 1975;1:564–565
189. Zwillich CW, Matthay M, Potts DE et al: Thyrotoxicosis: Comparison of effects of thyroid ablation and beta-adrenergic blockade on metabolic rate and ventilatory control. J Clin Endocrinol Metab 1978;46:491–499
190. Settipane G, Schoenfeld E, Hamolsky MW: Asthma and hyperthyroidism. J Allergy Clin Immunol 1972;49:348–355
191. Fauci AS, Haynes BF, Katz P et al: Wegener's granulomatosis: Prospective clinical and therapeutic experience with 85 patients for 21 years. Ann Intern Med 1983;98:76–85
192. Israel HL, Patchefsky AS: Wegener's granulomatosis of lung: Diagnosis and treatment. Ann Intern Med 1971;74:881–891
193. DeRemee RA, McDonald TJ, Harrison EG Jr et al: Wegener's granulomatosis, anatomic correlates, a proposed classification. Mayo Clin Proc 1976;51:777–781
194. DeRemee RA, McDonald TJ, Weiland LH: Wegener's granulomatosis: Observations on treatment with antimicrobial agents. Mayo Clin Proc 1985;60:27–32
195. Myers AR: Pulmonary manifestations of collagen vascular diseases. p. 909–921. In Fishman AP (ed): Pulmonary Diseases and Disorders. McGraw-Hill, New York, 1980

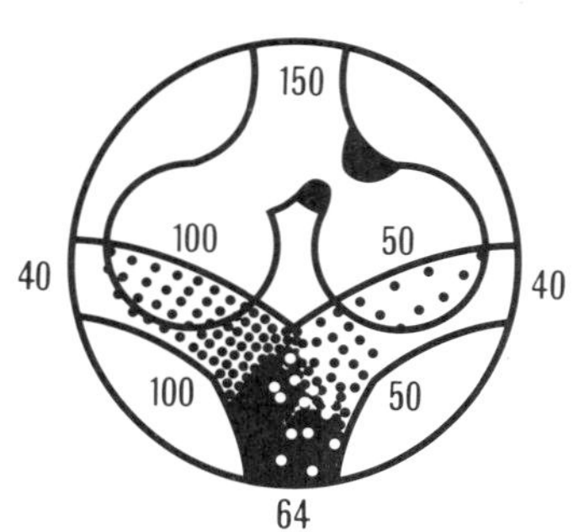

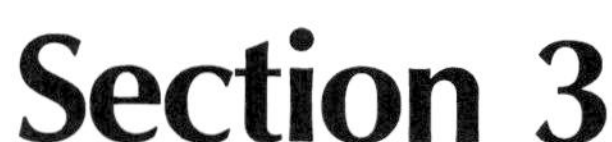
Section 3

Assessment of Respiratory Function and Diagnostic Techniques

Chapter 44

Clinical Skills in Respiratory Care

David J. Pierson
Robert L. Wilkins

CHAPTER OUTLINE

The first two sections of this book deal with the biomedical side of respiratory care—the structure and function of the cardiorespiratory system and the pathology and pathophysiology of respiratory disease. Clinical practice that is rational, effective, and safe requires a thorough understanding of these areas. However, biomedical knowledge and technical skills are not enough. Disease happens to people, not to organs or physiologic systems in isolation. Respiratory care as described in this book requires expertise in interacting with patients and other health care professionals as well as in biomedical science.

This is the first of several chapters to focus on this second side of respiratory care. Later chapters also dealing primarily with the human rather than the biomedical aspects include discussions of psychosocial assessment (Ch. 60), ethical issues (Ch. 103), the psychosocial impact of critical care (Ch. 104), and issues of sexuality, intimacy, and communication encountered in clinical practice (Ch. 105). However, effective application of the pathophysiologic approach to practice, as described in the 61 chapters that follow this one, also relies on elements of this human, interpersonal, essentially noncognitive side of respiratory care. The clinical evaluation skills described in this chapter are necessary components of all the assessments, approaches, and therapies discussed in this book.

Clinical assessment skills may be defined as that collection of intellectual and manual capabilities that enable a health care professional to interact effectively with patients and others in the professional arena. These capabilities include interviewing, history taking, physical examination, and medical record keeping. In addition, to function effectively in patient care clinicians need to master certain behaviors and communication skills, not only with respect to patients and their families but also in interactions with other health care professionals. This chapter reviews each of these attributes of the skillful clinician. For additional discussion of the material covered in this chapter the reader is referred to several authoritative texts,[1–4] as well as to chapters in other books dealing with the medical history and physical examination.[5–8]

ISSUES OF PROFESSIONALISM

Several attributes of a profession distinguish it from a trade or other type of occupation.[9,10] A profession relies heavily on a systematic body of theory (e.g., the scientific foundations of respiratory care) in addition to whatever technical skills are required. Members of a profession are permitted to behave in certain ways and to do things to other people that other members of society cannot. A profession has its own regulative code of ethics, which determines how access is gained to the profession's services and also establishes mechanisms of internal standards for such activities as ongoing quality assurance. This code of ethics also establishes working relationships and codes of conduct for interaction with members of other professions. Finally, a profession has its own culture, which in turn determines the environment in which that profession's practice occurs, establishes the mechanism by which new practitioners are added, and sets standards for continuing education and inquiry for all the profession's members.

These attributes pertain to all professionals involved in the assessment and management of patients with respiratory illness—physicians, respiratory care practitioners, nurses, and trainees in these fields—and they also carry distinct responsibilities. Other professionals and the public expect certain attitudes and behaviors from the members of these professions that are different from those that apply to other workers or to individuals outside the health care setting. Patients are not customers, clients, or business associates. Clinicians have powers and privileges in their interactions with patients that others do not. It is important that they be aware of these powers and privileges and know the expectations and responsibilities that come with them.

Table 44-1 gives 10 illustrations of professionalism in patient interactions in the form of guidelines of professional etiquette. As the "consumers" of health care, patients are often influenced more by "quality of service" than by "quality of care." The most up-to-date, scientifically enlightened tests and treatments may leave patients distrustful and dissatisfied if the people who carry them out do not behave professionally and do not treat their patients with courtesy and respect.

Clinicians must not forget that the patient is the reason all health care personnel are here. The health care professions exist to serve patients, not the other way around. All members of the health care team should remember this point, especially in times of heavy work load and disagreement.

The hospital can be a stressful workplace, and clinicians are often called on to perform intense, sometimes life-saving work when they are physically and emotionally fatigued. In such circumstances the use of "gallows humor" and the hospital's unique vocabulary of colorful expressions and

Table 44-1. Ten Golden Rules of Clinical Etiquette

1. **Maintain a professional appearance whenever you come into contact with patients or their families**
   Dress codes vary among hospitals, clinics, and home care services and also according to the clinician's role. However, whether appropriate dress includes a white laboratory coat, conventional business wear, or a scrub suit, it (and the person in it) should be clean and reasonably neat.
2. **Identify yourself—not only by name but also by role**
   Always wear a name tag when dealing with patients and explain why you are there. Attending physicians, residents, students, respiratory care practitioners, nurses, and others use the same medical terms and may dress similarly. Patients may assume that anyone in hospital dress is a doctor, and there can be serious medical, psychological, and even legal consequences if misconceptions are not corrected.
3. **Do not call adult patients by their first names**
   What may be intended as a means of "breaking the ice" and establishing rapport is perceived by many patients as condescending and insulting. In general, patients older than high school age should be called "Ms," "Miss," "Mrs," or "Mr." Use of a patient's first name requires that person's permission, would generally be considered only after numerous contacts, and would seldom be appropriate on a first encounter.
4. **Respect and preserve the patient's modesty**
   Draw the curtains. Do not uncover the patient in view of visitors or other patients. Remember that boys and men are often as modest as girls and women.
5. **Do not rest your foot on the bed frame or sit on the patient's bed without permission**
   Hospitalization renders patients vulnerable in many ways, and such uninvited invasions of their "territory" may cause unnecessary distress.
6. **Do not talk about patients in the elevator** (or in the hallways, in the cafeteria, or on a bus, or in other public places)
   Being a health professional allows one access to privileged, personal information that should not be shared, intentionally or unintentionally, with anyone not directly caring for the patient. Offhand remarks heard by family members in the elevator can cause great distress and interfere with clinician-patient relationships. Inappropriate use of such information is not only unethical but also against the law.
7. **Do not discuss prognosis or other sensitive issues with others in front of the patient**
   Patients may misinterpret snatches of conversation, or think remarks about another patient apply to them. Such terms as "death," "terminal," and "cancer" are especially upsetting and should be avoided around patients.
8. **Do not argue in front of the patient**
   Differences of opinion and disciplinary actions should take place well out of patients' earshot. Displays of anger have no place in patient care areas.
9. **Do not criticize the actions of other members of the health care team to or within earshot of the patient**
   You may not agree with Dr. so-and-so's diagnosis or treatment plan, but to voice this disagreement in front of the patient or family members is harmful to clinician-patient relationships and, indirectly, to the team's effectiveness.
10. **Keep disagreements and criticism out of the patient's chart**
    Such things should be dealt with one-on-one, in person, and not in the permanent (legal) record.

slang[11,12] can provide a welcome relief from stress and fatigue. However, while terms such as "gomer,"[11] "dirtball,"[13] and others may be permanent fixtures of hospital folk speech,[11] they can cause great hurt and erode the trust of patients and families in their caregivers when used at the wrong time or in the wrong place. Such expressions must never be used around patients and should be avoided whenever strangers or lay persons are present.

IMPROVING CLINICIAN-PATIENT COMMUNICATION

> What the scalpel is to the surgeon, words are to the clinician. When he uses them effectively, his patients do well. If not, the results can be disastrous.[14]

This quote from Philip Tumulty, a master bedside teacher,[14,15] emphasizes the importance of effective communication between patient and clinician, whether the latter is a physician, a respiratory care practitioner, or another member of the health care team whose work requires direct interaction with patients. Some people are naturally better communicators and more comfortable in talking with patients than others. However, there are several principles of effective communication that can be learned and practiced by anyone, which if followed will increase patients' comprehension and compliance with their care[14] (Table 44-2).

Table 44-2. Guidelines for Talking with Patients

1. Almost all patients, regardless of intellectual capacity, are naive and simplistic when dealing with their own health problems. One should assume nothing, start from basic facts, and build upward. A brilliant person is often a dull patient. A less endowed patient is often like a child.
2. Patients quickly forget what they are told and are easily confused if told too much at once. Therapeutic conversation should be administered in small but continued dosages in a preplanned fashion.
3. Very often, patients will retain only the part of the conversation that agrees with their own ideas or is pleasant to them. Gentle, firm, persistent reiteration is essential if important concepts are to be acted upon. One must emphasize and re-emphasize, again and again.
4. Because of anxiety and tension, patients are easily confused and poorly retentive. Therefore, dissipation of anxiety and tension is always the first order of business. Frequently, one accomplishes more with subsequent conversations than with the initial one as rapport develops and first fears fall away. First conferences often merely set the stage for subsequent effective ones. One proceeds in a stepwise manner. If the first consultation is not well handled, not much can be expected later.
5. Effective conversation with patients must be planned ahead and cannot be merely "off the cuff."
6. Careless or ill planned conversations can be disastrous to patients. Phrases or words having so little meaning to clinicians that they may not even recall saying them may be seized upon by patients and may have a profound effect upon them.
7. Needless details and technicalities should be avoided. They probably will not be understood and may prompt a host of new anxieties.
8. Above all else, clinicians should be protective of the patient's position and not of their own. They must be wise censors, filtering out matters that will either cause needless anxieties or fail to produce positive motivation. Clinicians who are impelled to tell the patient or the family (or both) *all* the facts are frequently protecting their own insecurity.

(From Tumulty,[14] with permission.)

THE MEDICAL INTERVIEW

The primary purpose of the medical interview is to obtain an accurate and pertinent assessment of the patient's state of health.[16] The interview may be broad and general or more focused, depending on the circumstances under which it takes place, but in all cases it has distinguishing characteristics that the clinician must appreciate. A medical interview is not just conversation but rather a complex process involving specialized interviewing skills and the acquisition of specific information.

The roles of both interviewers and interviewees are different from those of participants in an ordinary conversation. Interviewers have a specific job to do, subject to the previously mentioned privileges and responsibilities of a professional, and as a result of the professional setting (as opposed to the context for conversation) interviewees respond with information that they might not otherwise divulge.

Three aspects of the medical interview may influence the quantity and quality of information that it yields and also whether the interaction is smooth and pleasant or awkward and distressful for both participants. These are the physical setting in which the interview occurs, the clinician's skills at professional interviewing in general, and the clinician's proficiency in asking and responding to questions.

Physical Setting and Privacy Issues

Patients are more comfortable and more likely to provide complete, accurate information if the interview takes place in a quiet environment without extraneous noise or other distraction. While this is not always possible in a busy hospital or clinic, the interview environment can be improved by drawing the curtains around the patient's bed or by moving to a less congested corner of the room. The patient, who already feels emotionally vulnerable in an ill-fitting hospital gown and amid unfamiliar surroundings, may be so intimidated by being suddenly surrounded by white-coated strangers peering down from all sides that giving accurate or complete answers to their questions is impossible. Whenever possible, interviewers should sit rather than stand and should place the chair at a mutually comfortable distance (which varies among individuals and cultures) and at eye level. In general, at least in dealing with patients of Western cultural background, interviewers should introduce themselves in the "social space" (4 to 12 ft), and carry out the interview in the "personal space" (2 to 4 ft).

Privacy becomes an issue for many patients, particularly when discussing habits, certain bodily functions, or interpersonal relationships, and it may not be possible to complete the interview with family members or others in the room. When privacy cannot conveniently be ensured, the interview may have to be completed later or in a different setting.

Interviewing Skills

Being able to listen and respond appropriately is as important in interviewing as the type and content of the questions asked. Such ability puts the patient at ease, encourages accuracy and completeness, and establishes rapport between clinician and patient. The needed listening and responding skills include confirmation; silence; empathy; summary; confrontation; and restatement, paraphrasing, and interpretation.[16]

Confirmation is a straightforward response to let the patient know that the interviewer is listening and wants to hear more. Examples are "Okay," "All right," or "I understand."

Silence is one of the most difficult skills to master, particularly when interviewers are uncomfortable or unsure of themselves; yet silence is one of the most valuable listening skills. It allows patients time to rethink or expand on their answers and may enable subdued patients to verbalize what is really bothering them. Experienced interviewers develop the ability to remain silent for an effective period of time.

To demonstrate *empathy* interviewers must identify as accurately as possible the emotion that the patient is probably feeling. This differs from paraphrasing (see below), in that the interviewer identifies an emotional state rather than factual content. As an example, when a patient describes a sudden, severe episode of dyspnea, the interviewer might respond, "That must have been frightening for you." A demonstration of empathy is reassuring and indicates that the clinician relates to the patient as a person as well as in a purely objective manner.

Summary communicates to the patient that the interviewer is interested in an accurate understanding of the story being related. This technique consists of concisely restating what the patient has said, particularly when the account of a symptom or illness has been lengthy, confusing, or disjointed. Although it requires effort, briefly summarizing the patient's history will permit correction of any inaccuracies and addition of important details that may have been omitted.

Confrontation means making an observation about the patient's behavior, appearance, or story that the patient has not volunteered. For example, the clinician may say, "You've told me that you will have no trouble getting the physiotherapy treatments done at home, but you've never mentioned anything about your family and no one ever comes with you to the clinic." This maneuver acknowledges an apparent discrepancy and may lead to important clarification or additional information.

Restatement, paraphrasing, and interpretation involve repeating back to the patient something just said in order to clarify or extend the information. By simply restating something the patient has said, the interviewer makes sure that it has been understood correctly and gives the patient an opportunity to comment further. Briefly paraphrasing what the patient says, as with "In other words. . . ," or "It sounds as if. . . ," puts the account into the interviewer's own words and also enables the patient to modify or amplify it. Interpretation goes beyond what the patient actually said in order to clarify the importance of the history to the patient. An example would be to say, "It sounds as though this has been interfering with your activities quite a bit."

Nonverbal Communication

Nonverbal communication is important in any interview, and the clinician should appreciate its potential effects. A patient may convey more important information through body language and facial expression than by the words that are spoken; similarly, the interviewer can facilitate or impede the interview process through nonverbal communication. Posture tells a lot about the clinician: chances for effective communication increase when the clinician is sitting or standing comfortably instead of perching anxiously on the edge of the chair, with arms and legs crossed, fists clenched, or hands covering part of the face. Although there may be cultural exceptions (see Ch. 60), eye contact should be maintained during the interview as much as possible. These and other facets of the nonverbal side of interviewing are important to its ultimate effectiveness.

Questioning Skills

How a question is asked may determine the accuracy and completeness of a patient's answer.[1–3,16] There are five basic types of questions in interviewing: open-ended, focused, closed, compound, and leading. The first of these is usually the most helpful in eliciting a patient's history, and the next two have important uses. The last two types, however, although commonly used, are misleading and counterproductive and should be avoided. Table 44-3 distinguishes among these five types of questions and provides examples of each.

THE MEDICAL HISTORY

This chapter has dealt so far with behavior and communication—what might be thought of as the *art* of patient interaction and history taking. The present section turns to the *science* of the medical history—the factual content, as related by the patient and discovered from other sources, that provides the framework for assessment and management. Although the complete medical history consists of at least

Table 44-3. Types of Questions in Taking a Medical History

Question Type	Description	Comments	Examples
Open-ended	Broad, general question about patient's symptom or illness	Allows patients to give history spontaneously without bias or influence from interviewer; patients direct discussion to whatever they want to cover first; can provide greatest amount of information; should generally be used first in interview	"Tell me about your shortness of breath." "What brings you to the clinic today?"
Focused	Interviewer defines area of inquiry more than in open-ended question or statement	Directs discussion into more specific area but still gives patients latitude in answering	"What treatment have you had for this condition in the past?" "What are the physical requirements of your job?"
Closed-ended	More specific question, which can generally be answered yes or no or by giving objective data such as dates, names, or numbers	Best way to obtain specific data but limits scope of information by restricting patients to individual items requested	"Have you ever had tuberculosis?" "How many puffs from your inhaler do you use in a given day?"
Compound	Two or more separate questions asked at once, without giving patients chance to respond to them individually	May confuse patients; prevents patients from giving answers to all components; induces patients to focus on last question in series. *Should not be used.*	"Tell me about yourself—how old are you, where do you live, and what do you do for a living?" "Have you ever smoked cigarettes, used drugs, worked with asbestos, or been exposed to tuberculosis?"
Leading	Interviewer phrases question so as to lead patient in a particular direction in answering	Reflects interviewer's bias; tends to produce inaccurate, unreliable answer. *Should not be used.*	"You're feeling better today, aren't you?" "You've never used drugs, have you?"

eight different components (Table 44-4), those most important in respiratory care are the present illness, the general history, the patient's personal habits and life-style, and the occupational and environmental history.

In taking a history, as well as in communicating with other professionals, it is important to understand the different terms used to describe illnesses and their manifestations (Table 44-5). Symptoms, signs, findings, syndromes, and diseases all bring patients to the clinician. The primary difference among them is the degree to which they indicate a distinct pathophysiologic entity, and the clinician needs to appreciate this distinction.

Disease is the most specific category: for example, when a patient is diagnosed as having cystic fibrosis, this not only implies a degree of certainty about what is wrong with that patient but also indicates the exclusion of other conditions that share features with it. A syndrome is next in exactness in that it can be produced by more than one disease. Bronchiectasis, for example, comprises a collection of clinical, laboratory, and pathologic findings that may occur in several distinct diseases (e.g., cystic fibrosis, tuberculosis, and Cartagener's syndrome). At the other end of the specificity scale, when patients present with symptoms (for example, dyspnea and productive cough), signs (finger clubbing), or abnormal findings (sputum cultures positive for *Staphylococcus aureus* or *Pseudomonas aeruginosa*), there may be several possible etiologies.

Not included in Table 44-5 is a definition for *illness*. This term refers to the impact of any one of the categories in the table on the patient's life. Some patients with cystic fibrosis are not ill; others are chronically but not acutely ill, and still others have a disabling illness that profoundly limits their ability to function. Illness relates to the degree to which a patient is impaired physiologically or psychologically by an abnormality or disease process. The distinction between im-

Table 44-4. Elements of the Medical History

- Patient identification
- Chief complaint
- History of present illness
- Past medical history
- Family history
- Personal habits and life-style
- Occupational and environmental history
- Review of systems

Table 44-5. Terms Used in Describing an Illness and Its Manifestations

Term	Definition	Examples
Symptom	A phenomenon experienced by an individual as a departure from normal or usual function, sensation, or appearance; a subjective abnormality perceived by the patient's own senses	Dyspnea; chest pain; leg swelling
Sign	An observable or measurable bodily manifestation that serves to indicate the presence of a malfunction or disease; a subjective or objective abnormality perceived by the examiner's senses	Tachypnea; dullness to percussion; pedal edema
Finding	An observation or manifestation of disease as a result of a procedure or test; an objective (or subjective) result of an investigative maneuver (e.g., a laboratory or radiographic finding)	↓ FEV_1/FVC; right lower lobe infiltrate; leukocytosis
Syndrome	A set of symptoms, signs, and/or findings that characteristically occur together (which may signify a specific disease process or be found in more than one disease)	COPD; pneumonia; acute respiratory failure
Disease	A particular pathologic condition or process whose pathophysiology or cause is known or that occurs consistently enough to be assumed to have a single, specific pathophysiology or cause	Alpha-1-antitrypsin deficiency; pneumococcal pneumonia

FEV_1, forced expiratory volume in 1 second; FVC, forced vital capacity; COPD, chronic obstructive pulmonary disease.

pairment and disability is more medicolegal than clinical, as discussed in Chapter 49.

Present Illness

The present illness is the clinical problem of primary concern at the moment. It may or may not be what caused the patient to seek medical attention (i.e., the chief complaint). In respiratory care the history of the present illness usually centers on one or more of the cardinal symptoms and signs of cardiorespiratory disease (Table 44-6). Dyspnea is the most common symptom in both respiratory and cardiovascular disease; the other cardinal symptoms are cough, sputum production, hemoptysis, and chest pain. The main cardiorespiratory signs are stridor, cyanosis, clubbing, and edema. Wheezing is both a symptom and a sign.

Other symptoms and signs may be clues to respiratory disorders. Fever and night sweats suggest infection (especially when accompanied by chills) or other inflammatory disorder. Hoarseness may accompany a viral upper respiratory infection but is also a frequent presenting complaint in patients with lung cancer (from invasion of the recurrent laryngeal nerve by tumor, producing vocal cord paralysis). Apneic episodes while asleep, particularly in a man with a history of loud snoring, raises the suspicion of sleep apnea syndrome. Morning headache may be a symptom of nocturnal hypoventilation with hypercapnia. Weight loss, although nonspecific, is an important sign in patients with histories suggesting tuberculosis, lung cancer, or depression.

Symptoms are experienced by a patient, whereas signs may be detected by either patient or examiner. Accordingly, the patient is the ultimate authority on a symptom, and the clinician's task is to record it as accurately as possible without altering the patient's meaning. In general, the patient's own words are best, even when they are unsophisticated. "Heaviness in the chest" does not mean "chest pain" unless the patient says it does. In addition, the clinician should avoid using medical terms that carry the force of a diagnosis (e.g., angina), unless they are justified. To label a chest symptom angina pectoris requires the presence of several historical factors and the exclusion of a number of others.

Not included in Table 44-6 is the imprecise term *respiratory distress*. This is more a collection of signs (e.g., tachypnea, agitation, use of accessory ventilatory muscles) than a symptom, and is largely subjective on the part of the observer. Patients who complain of dyspnea (a symptom) may or may not manifest tachypnea (a sign), while tachypneic patients may or may not be dyspneic; the clinician may or may not consider respiratory distress to be present.

Hyperventilation is a term from physiology rather than from physical diagnosis and refers to increased alveolar ventilation ($\dot{V}_A$) in relation to CO_2 production, as manifested by a $PaCO_2$ below normal (i.e., less than 36 to 37 mmHg at sea level). Similarly, *hyperpnea* refers to increased total minute ventilation, irrespective of $\dot{V}_A$ and $PaCO_2$. Thus, someone may be hyperpneic without hyperventilating (e.g., during normal exercise), both may be present without dyspnea, and dyspnea may be present without either of them; tachypnea may be present with all or none; patients may complain of dyspnea who do not appear to be in respiratory distress, and someone judged to be in respiratory distress may or may not admit to dyspnea.

A complete history is the most important assessment tool in medicine. Obtaining it requires knowledge, creativity, and perseverance—not unlike the attributes required by a great detective in solving a case. In fact, there are many similarities between the methods of Sherlock Holmes and the armamentarium of a skilled history taker.[17,18] Like Conan Doyle's acclaimed sleuth, the clinician must pursue every possible angle in investigating a symptom or sign (Table 44-7).

Systematically questioning the patient about all aspects of the presenting complaint—what, where, when, and how—will clarify the problem and direct further investigation. In

Table 44-6. Cardinal Symptoms and Signs of Cardiopulmonary Disease

Symptom/Sign	Description
Dyspnea	Shortness of breath; the subjective sensation that one's breathing is inadequate or insufficient; an uncomfortable awareness of the act of breathing
Cough	A sudden noisy expulsion of air from the lungs, brought about through reflex action, for the purpose of clearing the airways; a normal event that becomes a symptom when it is frequent or bothersome to the patient
Nonproductive	Unaccompanied by sufficient sputum to expectorate or swallow consciously
Productive	Sputum, blood, or other material is produced when the patient coughs; expectorated sputum may be either *purulent* (having the appearance of pus) or *nonpurulent*
Hemoptysis	The coughing up of blood from the respiratory tract below the level of the larynx, as distinguished from the expectoration of blood originating in the nose, mouth, or elsewhere in the upper respiratory tract
Chest pain	Any uncomfortable sensation referable by the patient to the thoracic area; it may be *pleuritic* (brought on or worsened by breathing or coughing) or *nonpleuritic* (not influenced by the act of breathing)
Wheezing	A high-pitched, musical sound produced when a patient breathes, originating in narrowed airways, which may occupy either a portion or all of the respiratory cycle
Stridor	A harsh, high-pitched sound, usually on inspiration, typically associated with partial laryngeal obstruction
Cyanosis	A bluish discoloration of skin and mucous membranes due to the presence of increased quantities of reduced (deoxygenated) hemoglobin; under appropriate lighting, typically seen with arterial hypoxemia (in the absence of anemia) or sluggish circulation (e.g., in congestive heart failure or impeded venous return); cyanosis may be either *peripheral* (fingertips, toes) or *central* (mucous membranes)
Clubbing	Diffuse bulbous enlargement of the terminal phalanges of the fingers and toes, due to buildup of fibroelastic soft tissue in the nail bed; usually asymptomatic and of unknown mechanism, it occurs in lung cancer, intrathoracic suppuration (e.g., bronchiectasis, cystic fibrosis, lung abscess, empyema), interstitial lung disease, cyanotic congenital heart disease, and other conditions
Edema	Presence of abnormally large amounts of fluid in the intercellular tissue spaces of the body; may be either *pitting*, as commonly seen with increased hydrostatic pressure (e.g., in congestive heart failure) or *nonpitting*, as occurs with increased capillary permeability (e.g., in an area of soft tissue infection); in pitting edema, pressing a fingertip against the edematous tissue for a few seconds forces fluid away and leaves a depression or "pit" when the finger is withdrawn

the course of learning the answers to the 10 questions in Table 44-7 an interviewer gathers a substantial data base. This is true regardless of the experience of the clinician with the condition presented by the patient. A student who has never before seen a patient with bronchiectasis should still be able to completely describe the illness and formulate a logical approach to its further assessment.

In the investigation of a symptom or sign it is helpful to be quantitative wherever possible: "8 on a scale of 10" is better than "very severe"; "2 to 3 minutes" is better than "not very long"; "able to walk one-half block" is preferable to "can't walk very far."

General History

The general history consists of the past medical history, the family history, and the review of systems (Table 44-4).

Table 44-7. What, Where, When, and How: 10 Questions to Ask a Patient about a Pain or Other Symptom

1. **What does it feel like?**
   Have the patient use own words in describing the character of the symptoms (e.g., dyspnea or pain).
2. **Where is it?**
   If the symptom is a pain, ask the patient to localize it as precisely as possible.
3. **Where else does it go?**
   Inquire about radiation of the pain to other parts of the body.
4. **How bad is it?**
   If possible, have the patient quantitate the symptom, for example, by using a hypothetical scale of 1 to 10, with 10 being the worst discomfort ever experienced.
5. **How long does it last?**
   Again, quantitate as much as possible. Does the pain come and go or is it constant? Is it always the same?
6. **When does it occur?**
   Ask about associations with time of day, physical activity, body position, emotion or stress, and any relationship to eating or drinking.
7. **What brings it on or makes it worse?**
   What would the patient do who wanted to bring on the pain or make it worse?
8. **What relieves it or makes it better?**
   Ask about any medication or activity that the patient has noted improves the symptom.
9. **How does it affect you?**
   What activities are prevented or limited by the symptom? Quantitate if possible. Ask the patient to compare present limitations with past performance or present capabilities with those of peers.
10. **What else is associated with it?**
    Inquire about other phenomena (e.g., fever, diaphoresis, dyspnea) that occur with the symptom in question.

The *past medical history* includes a description of all important past illnesses, surgical operations, serious injuries, childhood illnesses, and allergies. This part of the medical history can be very important to the respiratory care clinician, for example, when a patient scheduled for elective surgery has a past history of asthma. Examples of other items in the past medical history that are important in respiratory care include previous lung resection, rib fractures or other chest trauma, recurrent pneumonias, aspiration of a foreign body, therapy for tuberculosis, and use of corticosteroids or other immunosuppressive agents.[7]

A patient's *family history* can be important in two ways. Some pulmonary diseases are inherited; others such as tuberculosis are not genetically transmitted but may be acquired from affected family members. Other noncommunicable diseases such as asthma and emphysema are more prevalent in some families than in the general population although the precise mechanisms involved are not understood.

Although a thorough *review of systems* is unnecessary for many types of clinical interaction, this part of the medical history is important in any complete workup. It consists of a systematic inquiry into health problems that may not have been covered in the history of present illness or the past medical history. The interviewer proceeds through the different systems (eyes, ears, head and neck, respiratory, cardiovascular, etc.), asking focused or closed-ended questions about symptoms in each. While time-consuming, the review of symptoms may uncover important information that both the patient and the interviewer would otherwise overlook.

Personal Habits and Life-style

Among the aspects of an individual's history that greatly influence the incidence and risk of respiratory disease are personal habits and life-style. Current or past cigarette smoking, the major cause of chronic obstructive pulmonary disease (COPD) and lung cancer, should be quantitated in the same fashion as other components of the history. Cigarette smoking is quantitated in pack-years: smoking one pack per day for 20 years gives 20 pack-years of exposure, which would be roughly the same in terms of impact on health as smoking one-half pack per day for 40 years or two packs per day for 10 years. Although more difficult to quantitate, the type of cigarette (e.g., brand, filtered or unfiltered) is also important. Because of increasing awareness of "passive smoking" as a possible factor in lung disease, nonsmokers should be asked whether they have lived or worked with smokers.

Other aspects of this part of the medical history include the use of alcohol and illicit drugs. Among the latter, it is important to inquire about both smoked (e.g., marijuana or cocaine) and injected (e.g., methylphenidate or heroin) substances. Such matters as diet, sleep, and other habits may also reveal important information in patients with respiratory disease.

Occupational and Environmental History

Inhalation of or exposure to other substances in the environment may produce a wide variety of respiratory illnesses, as discussed in more detail in Chapter 38. Individuals may incur such exposure in the course of work or recreation or simply by living in a particular building or area. However, this association is often not apparent and will not be made on the basis of superficial questioning. Many patients with occupational or environmentally induced illness will give a negative response if asked, "Have you ever been exposed to dusts or other inhaled agents that might injure your lungs?" Taking a complete occupational and environmental history is comprehensive and time-consuming, but such an exercise may furnish invaluable information about the cause of a patient's illness. Table 44-8 summarizes the key elements of the occupational and environmental history,[19] and Table 44-9 gives examples of the more common exposures and the pulmonary diseases associated with them.[20,21]

Table 44-8. Key Elements of an Occupational and Environmental History

Present illness (for each element of problem list)
Symptoms related to work
Other employees similarly affected
Current exposure to dusts, fumes, chemicals, biologic hazards
Prior first report of work injury
Work history
Describe all prior jobs, typical work day, change in work process
Work site
Ventilation; medical and industrial hygiene surveillance; employment examinations; protective measures
Union health and safety requirements; moonlighting; days missed work last year; prior worker compensation claims
Past history
Exposure to noise, vibration, radiation, chemicals, asbestos
Environmental history
Present and prior home and work locations
Jobs of other household members
Hazardous wastes/spills exposure
Air pollution exposure
Hobbies (e.g., painting, sculpture, welding, woodworking)
Home insulation/heating
Home and work cleaning agents
Pesticide exposure
Use of seat belts
Firearms at home or work
Review of systems
Specific emphasis
Shift changes; boredom; reproductive history

(From Becker,[19] with permission.)

PHYSICAL EXAMINATION

A physical examination of the patient is carried out in order to detect the physical signs of disease and to identify the effects of treatment. It is performed in the intimate space (less than 2 ft), where eye contact is inappropriate. The examination should be performed only after rapport has been established with the patient. Each examination is modified according to the patient's history, the purpose of the examination, and in light of initial findings during the examination. Certain abnormalities will prompt further investigation. The techniques that can be incorporated into the examination are described here.

Vital Signs

Collectively the vital signs provide a clinical picture of the patient's health status; for this reason they are used not only as an initial diagnostic tool but also to identify the patient's response to therapy. The four basic vital signs are body temperature, heart rate, respiratory rate, and blood pressure. Clinicians also often report the patient's mental alertness (sensorium) along with the vital signs.

Body Temperature

Normal mean body temperature is approximately 37°C (98.6°F), with a daily variation of about 0.5°C (1°F). When

Table 44-9. Common Occupational or Environmental Exposures Associated with Pulmonary Disease

Occupation or Activity	Exposure	Disease
Asbestos mining/milling/manufacture; pipe fitting; shipbuilding/ship fitting; insulation; construction; demolition; living with someone employed in any of the above	Asbestos	Lung cancer; asbestosis; malignant mesothelioma; nonmalignant inflammatory pleural effusion
Hard-rock mining; quarrying; stone cutting; abrasive industries; foundry work; sandblasting	Crystalline quartz (silica)	Silicosis
Coal mining	Coal dust	Coal workers' pneumoconiosis
Farming; grain handling	Grain dust	Chronic bronchitis; COPD
Farming; animal attendants	Moldy hay (spores of thermophilic actinomycetes [fungus])	Hypersensitivity pneumonitis (farmers' lung)
Cotton/flax/hemp workers; textile industry	Cotton dust	Byssinosis
Pigeon breeding; bird handling	Proteins derived from parakeets, budgerigars, pigeons, chickens, turkeys (avian droppings or feathers)	Hypersensitivity pneumonitis (e.g., pigeon-breeders' lung, etc); bird-fanciers' lung
Woodworking; lumber industry	Wood dust; *Alternaria* (fungus)	Hypersensitivity pneumonitis; woodworker's lung, etc.
	Western red cedar; oak; others	Occupational asthma

body temperature is within the normal range, all metabolic functions occur in a more optimal manner. When the body temperature falls outside the normal range, the metabolic rate changes accordingly, and the demands on the cardiopulmonary system also change. For example, as the body temperature increases, the metabolic rate also increases, resulting in more O_2 consumption and CO_2 production at the cellular level (roughly 8 to 10 percent increase for every degree Celsius deviation above normal). This requires the cardiopulmonary system to work harder to meet this additional demand. An elevation of the body temperature can occur as the result of disease or of normal activities such as exercise. An elevated body temperature due to disease is referred to as a fever and the patient is said to be febrile, as often occurs when the patient has an infection. Hypothermia is said to be present when the patient's body temperature is below the normal range. While not common, it may be present when the patient has been exposed to cold environmental temperatures or has suffered head injuries that affect the hypothalamus.

Body temperature is most often measured orally but can also be measured in the axilla or rectally. The oral temperature measurement is the most acceptable for the awake adult patient. The oral temperature is not affected significantly by O_2 administration via nasal cannula, simple mask, or entrainment mask.[22,23] It is not necessary therefore, to take rectal temperatures or to remove the O_2 from patients receiving it via mask or cannula to obtain an accurate oral reading. The inhalation of a heated mist may slightly increase the oral temperature reading, and similarly, cool mist may slightly decrease it.[24]

Heart Rate

The heart rate or pulse rate in the adult is normally 60 to 100 bpm. The pulse should be evaluated for strength and rhythm in addition to rate. A pulse rate above 100 bpm, termed *tachycardia,* often occurs in response to hypoxemia, fear, fever, anemia, exercise, and hypotension. Tachycardia is also a common side effect of many medications such as bronchodilators, and for this reason the pulse should be evaluated before, during, and after treatment with aerosolized bronchodilators.

Bradycardia, a pulse rate below 60 bpm, is not as common as tachycardia but may occur with hypothermia, some heart diseases, and in particularly fit, athletic individuals. Excessively slow pulse rates may result in lower circulating blood pressure and flow.

Pulse strength is usually a reflection of the strength of the left ventricular contraction. It is evaluated and recorded on a scale of 0 to 3+, where 0 indicates absent; 1+, weak and thready; 2+, normal; and 3+, bounding.

Respiratory Rate

In the adult the normal respiratory rate at rest ranges from 10 to 20 breaths per minute and averages 16 in men and 18 in women. A fast breathing rate, or tachypnea, is normal with exercise but also occurs with fever, hypoxemia, acidosis, anxiety, or pain. Along with the rate, the depth of breathing should be estimated. Bradypnea, a slower than normal respiratory rate, may be seen in patients with head injuries, lesions of the central nervous system, or drug overdose. Bradypnea may be a sign that the metabolic needs of the patient have been reduced or that the respiratory system is failing to meet the bodily needs. Further investigation is often needed to assess which is the case.

The respiratory rate is counted by watching the patient's abdomen or chest wall move in and out with breathing. The breathing rate should be counted without the patient's knowledge since the rate may be altered voluntarily by the patient. If the examiner's fingers are maintained over the radial pulse after the pulse rate has been determined, during which time the patient's breathing rate is counted, the patient will have the impression that the examiner is still counting the pulse rate.

Blood Pressure

The arterial blood pressure is the force exerted against the walls of the arteries as blood moves through the vessels. Systolic blood pressure is a measure of the peak force exerted during left ventricular contraction, and diastolic blood pressure measures the force occurring during relaxation of the ventricles. The difference between systolic and diastolic pressures is referred to as the *pulse pressure.*

Normal systolic pressure in the adult ranges from 95 to 140 mmHg, with 120 mmHg the average; normal diastolic pressure ranges from 60 to 90 mmHg, with 80 mmHg the average; and normal pulse pressure ranges from 35 to 40 mmHg. If the pulse pressure drops below 30 mmHg, the peripheral pulse may be difficult to identify. Hypertension (blood pressure above 140/90 mmHg) may occur when the left ventricle is contracting with increased force or when peripheral vascular resistance is elevated. Hypotension (blood pressure below 95/60 mmHg) may occur with hypovolemia, left ventricular failure, or peripheral vasodilation. Hypotension often indicates that blood flow throughout the body is less than normal and the perfusion of vital organs may be in question. For this reason hypotension, especially for prolonged periods, must be avoided.

The usefulness of a blood pressure evaluation may be reduced because the pressure measurement may not correlate with blood flow. Normal or even elevated blood pressure does not indicate adequate cardiac output, although if blood pressure is significantly reduced, perfusion is probably reduced also.

During inspiration the ventilatory muscles create a negative intrathoracic pressure, which encourages venous return. At the same time, blood flow out of the thorax is reduced, especially during maximal breathing efforts. The reduction in blood flow away from the chest during inspiration may cause a slight, temporary drop in systolic blood pressure. If this fluctuation is significant (greater than 10 mmHg) at rest, paradoxical pulse is present. This is a common finding when severe airway obstruction is present and results in more active breathing efforts.[25] Paradoxical pulse may be identified by palpating the peripheral pulses while noting the changes in pulse amplitude during breathing. It can also be more accurately determined with a sphygmomanometer (blood pressure cuff).

Sensorium

As mentioned, the sensorium is often assessed when vital signs are evaluated since it provides further evidence of the patient's general condition. An alert patient who is oriented to the correct time, place, and person is said to be "oriented × 3" and has a normal sensorium. An abnormal sensorium suggests that the patient may have poor oxygenation of the brain as a result of either respiratory or circulatory failure or both. An abnormal sensorium may also occur with administration of narcotics and with a wide variety of disease states.

Lung Topography

Before describing the techniques of chest examination, topographic (surface) landmarks will be reviewed since these provide the examiner with the ability to identify the positions of underlying structures and are helpful in describing the location of abnormalities. This knowledge will help the examiner to develop a mental picture of the position of the respiratory system within the chest.

Imaginary Lines

For the sake of reference, several imaginary vertical lines are described. The midsternal line, located in the middle of the sternum, divides the anterior chest into the two equal halves (Fig. 44-1). The left and right midclavicular lines parallel the midsternal line and run downward from the midpoint of the left and right clavicles, respectively.

On the lateral chest three vertical lines are recognized: the anterior axillary line is drawn downward from the origin of the anterior axillary fold along the anterolateral aspect of the chest; the midaxillary line divides the lateral chest wall into two equal halves; and the posterior axillary line runs downward along the posterolateral wall of the thorax parallel to the midaxillary line (Fig. 44-2).

On the posterior chest wall a useful landmark is the midspinal line, also called the vertebral line, which runs down the spinous processes of the vertebrae. Another vertebral line on the posterior chest is the scapular line, which parallels the midspinal line and runs downward through the inferior angle of the scapula with the patient's arms in a relaxed position at the sides (Fig. 44-3).

Thoracic Cage Landmarks

On the anterior chest wall the most useful landmark is the manubriosternal junction or sternal angle, a visible ridge formed by the junction of the manubrium and the body of the sternum (Fig. 44-4). The superior border of the second rib articulates with the sternum at this junction. The examiner can begin to palpate and count ribs and rib interspaces from this point. The intercostal spaces are numbered to correspond to the number of the rib immediately above the space (e.g., the second intercostal space lies between the second and third ribs). The manubriosternal junction is also significant as a reference point since it identifies the location of several important structures within the thorax that lie at the same level: (1) the bifurcation of the trachea; (2) the upper level of the atria of the heart; and (3) the fifth thoracic vertebra.

On the posterior chest the spinous processes of the vertebrae are useful landmarks. The spinous process of C7 usu-

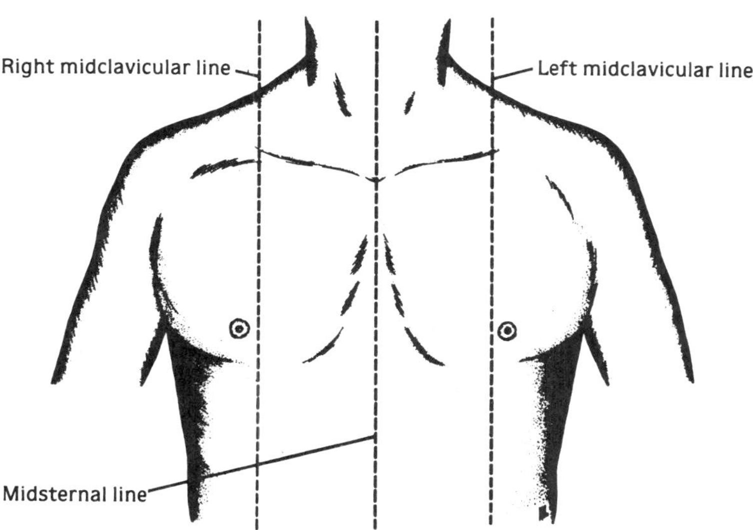

Figure 44-1. Imaginary lines on anterior chest. (From Wilkins et al.,[1] with permission.)

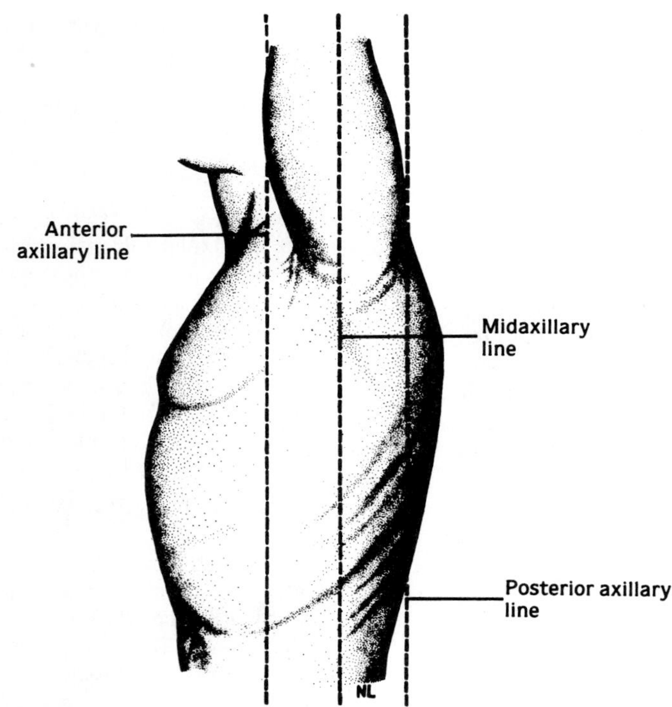

Figure 44-2. Imaginary lines on lateral chest. (From Wilkins et al.,[1] with permission.)

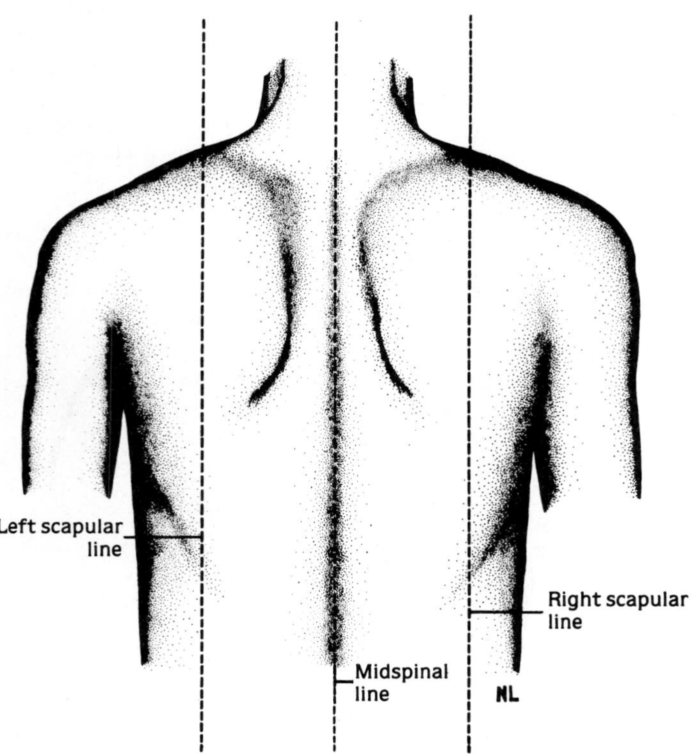

Figure 44-3. Imaginary lines on posterior chest. (From Wilkins et al.,[1] with permission.)

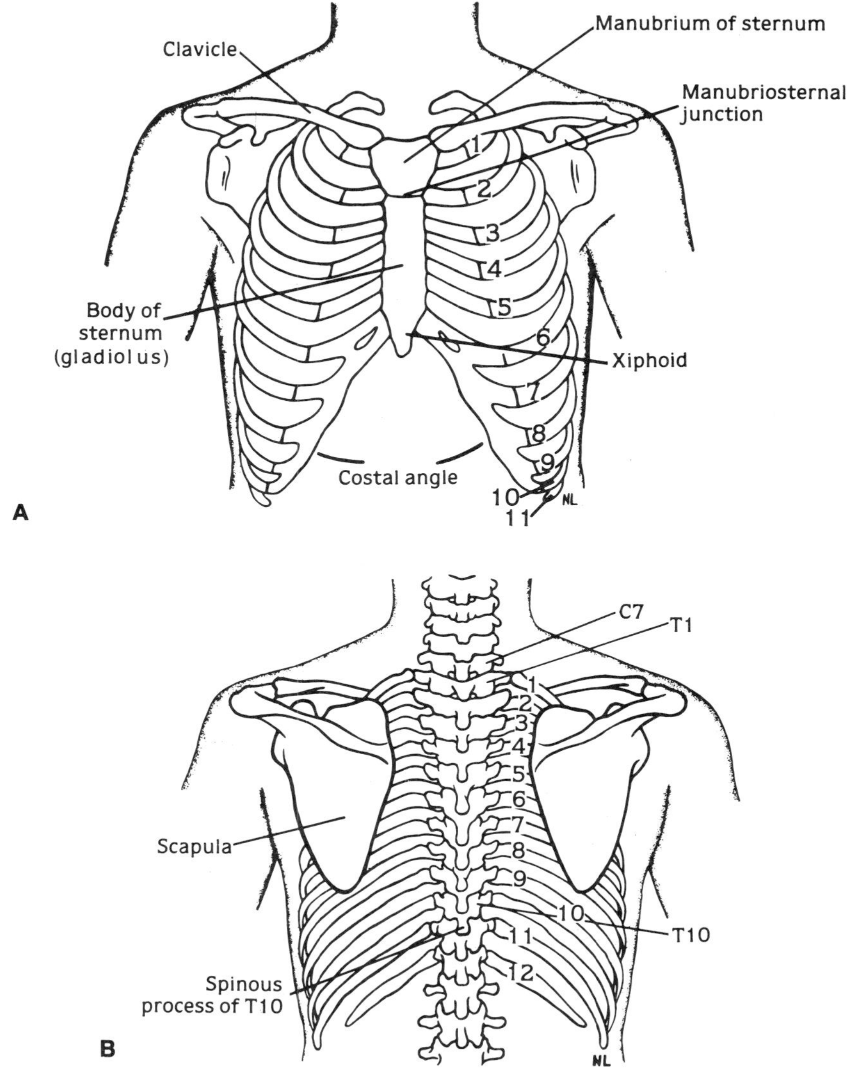

Figure 44-4. Thoracic cage landmarks on (**A**) anterior and (**B**) posterior chest. (From Wilkins et al.,[1] with permission.)

ally can be identified with the patient's head extended forward and downward. It is the most prominent spinous process at the base of the neck, and immediately below is the spinous process of T1. These reference points can be used by the examiner to identify other thoracic vertebrae and posterior ribs.

Lung Fissures

The oblique fissure is found in both lungs and is located in approximately the same position in each. On the anterior chest it runs from the sixth rib and the midclavicular line laterally and upward through the fifth rib at the midaxillary line (Fig. 44-5). It extends around through the posterior chest to approximately T3. On the posterior chest the oblique fissure separates the upper lobe from the lower lobe. The right lung also has a horizontal fissure, which separates the right upper lobe from the right middle lobe and runs from the fourth rib at the sternal border around to the fifth rib at the midaxillary line.

Lung Borders

The superior border of the lung extends 2 to 4 cm above the medial third of the clavicle on the anterior chest and to T1 on the posterior chest. The inferior border of the lung varies with ventilation but is typically found at the sixth rib on the anterior chest, at the eighth rib on the lateral chest, and at T10 on the posterior chest at rest (Fig. 44-5).

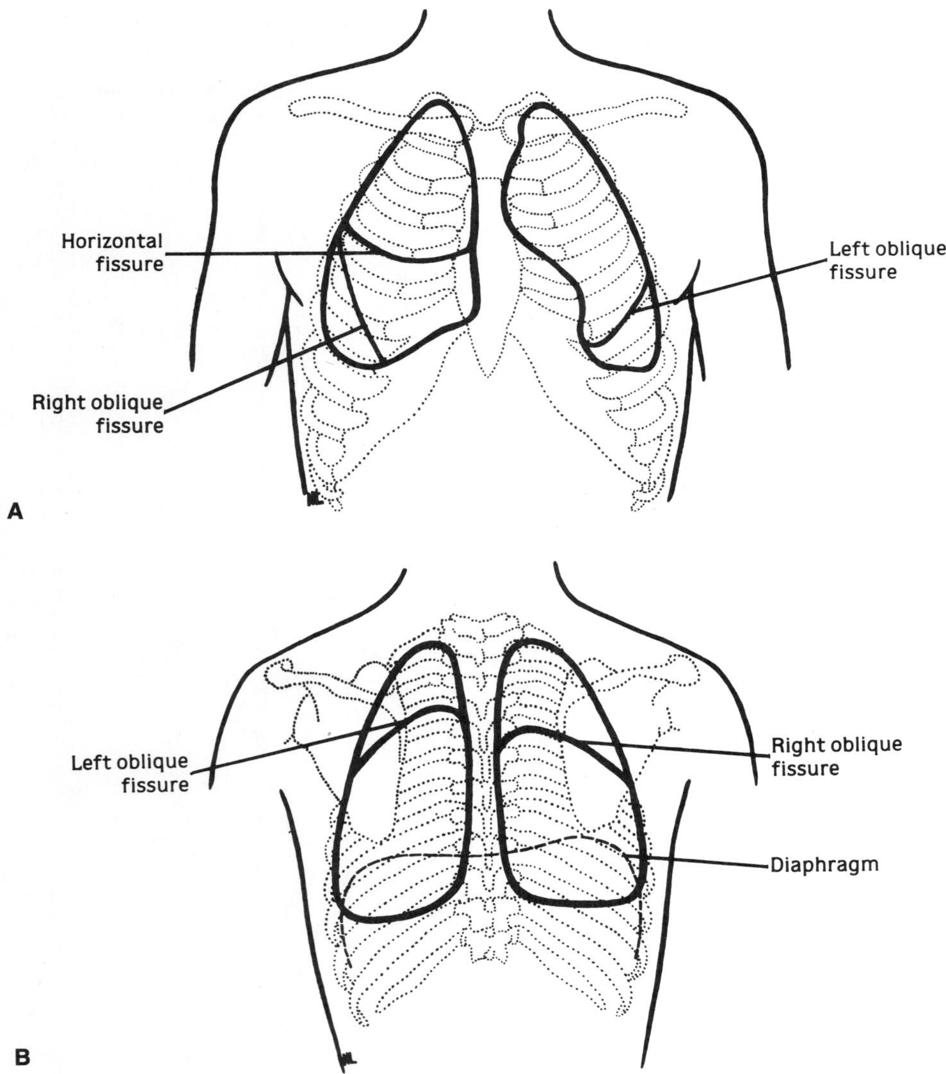

Figure 44-5. Topographic position of lung fissures and borders on **(A)** anterior and **(B)** posterior chest. (From Wilkins et al.,[1] with permission.)

Inspection

Inspection of the patient is an ongoing process, which begins with the initial introduction and continues throughout the examination. It is a series of observations that identify general and specific indications of the patient's health status. A well lit room with the patient sitting comfortably is ideal for adequate inspection. The patient's breathing pattern, chest configuration, digits, and neck should be inspected.

Breathing Pattern

The patient's respiratory rate and pattern of breathing should be evaluated. Rapid and shallow breathing is associated with restrictive lung disease. The examiner should note the timing of the inspiratory and expiratory phases. A prolonged expiratory time is common with obstruction of intrathoracic airways (e.g., asthma), while obstruction of the upper airway (e.g., epiglottitis) often leads to a prolonged inspiratory time. It is important to assess the amount of effort that the patient appears to be putting forth to breathe. Normally, inspiratory effort is minimal and exhalation is passive. Increases in the effort of breathing are identified by noting the degree of accessory muscle usage. As the work of breathing increases, the patient will use the accessory muscles to a greater degree. This is common in pulmonary disorders that increase airway resistance or decrease lung or chest wall compliance.

As the patient's respiratory effort increases, the more significant drop in pleural pressure during inspiration may result in *retractions,* which are identified when the skin overlying the chest wall sinks inward at specific points during inspiration. This usually occurs at the points of least resistance, generally between the ribs (intercostal retractions), above the clavicles (supraclavicular retractions), or below the lower margin of the ribs (subcostal retractions). When the diaphragm fatigues in patients with increased work of breathing, the abdomen may sink inward during inspiration as the thorax expands; this is *paradoxical respiration*.

Chest trauma may cause multiple rib fractures in one or more places. *Flail chest* occurs when a portion of the chest wall becomes independently movable (typically when three or more ribs are each broken in two places). The affected portion of the chest wall will then move inward with inspiration and outward with exhalation (i.e., the chest wall will move paradoxically).

The symmetry of chest expansion during breathing is important to evaluate. Unilateral lung defects that hinder the expansion of one side (e.g., pneumonia or lobar atelectasis) will cause an inspiratory lag, which is identified when one side of the chest is observed to expand more slowly and to a lesser extent than the other side.

Chest Configuration

The normal adult thorax is broader from side to side than from front to back. An increased anteroposterior (AP) diameter is common with emphysema and the patient is said to be "barrel-chested" in such cases (Fig. 44-6 and Table 44-10). The barrel chest configuration is nonspecific and also occurs in individuals without emphysema. Minor variations in thoracic configuration include a funnel-shaped depression of the lower portion of the sternum (pectus excavatum) and the reverse condition in which the sternum protrudes outward (pectus carinatum or pigeon breast).

A severe restrictive defect can result when the spinal column is deformed. An abnormal lateral curvature of the spine is known as *scoliosis;* an abnormally increased AP curvature of the spinal cord is called *kyphosis;* and a combination of the two is referred to as *kyphoscoliosis* (Fig. 44-7). Kyphoscoliosis often causes severe reduction in the lung volumes. The opposite of kyphosis is lordosis.

Digits

Inspection for the signs of respiratory disease requires inspection of more than the thorax. The digits are inspected for evidence of cyanosis, a bluish discoloration of the skin that indicates an increased amount of reduced hemoglobin in the circulating blood. The transparency of the fingernails allows initial detection of cyanosis in this area. Cyanosis also

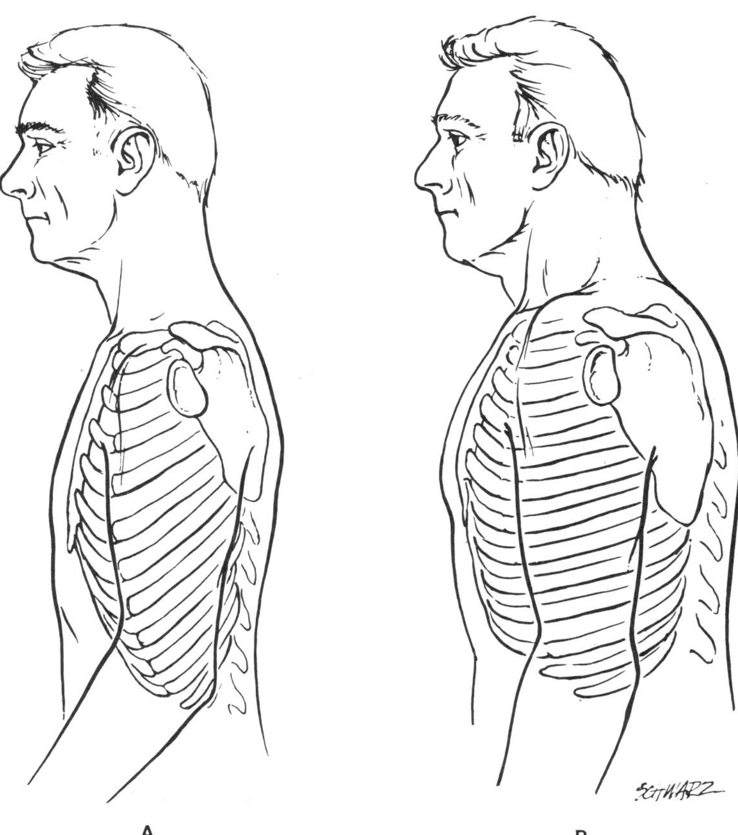

Figure 44-6. **(A)** Normal and **(B)** increased AP diameter. In Figure B note the horizontal position of the ribs and the hypertrophy of the sternomastoid muscle. (From Wilkins et al.,[1] with permission.)

Table 44-10. Expected Physical Findings in Various Disease States

Disease or Disorder	Inspection	Palpation	Percussion	Auscultation
COPD (generalized obstructive defect)	Increased AP diameter; kyphosis; widened intercostal spaces; use of accessory respiratory muscles	Decreased movement of rib cage on deep inspiration; absent apex cardiac impulse; decreased vocal fremitus	Increased resonance (generalized); hemidiaphragms low with little detectable movement	Diminished breath sounds, especially at bases; may have inspiratory crackles or rhonchi; may have expiratory wheezes, especially on forced exhalation
Interstitial pulmonary fibrosis (generalized restrictive defect)	Normal external appearance; reduced chest excursion; tachypnea	Normal to decreased overall movement; vocal fremitus normal or increased	Normal; hemidiaphragms may be high with reduced movement	Breath sounds accentuated with prominent inspiratory crackles ("Velcro" rales)
Lobar pneumonia (localized restrictive defect)	Reduced expansion on affected side with inspiration (due to splinting)	Increased vocal fremitus over involved lung	Dullness to percussion over involved lung	Bronchial breath sounds; inspiratory crackles over affected area; whispered pectoriloquy; E-to-A change
Lobar atelectasis (localized restrictive defect)	Reduced movement on affected side	PMI and trachea may be deviated toward affected side	No change, or elevated hemidiaphragm with reduced movement	Diminished breath sounds
Pneumothorax (compressed lung with surrounding air)	Normal or reduced movement on affected side	PMI and trachea may be deviated away from affected side (if under tension)	Increased resonance over affected side (if large)	Diminished breath sounds
Pleural effusion (compressed lung with surrounding fluid)	Normal; reduced expansion if very large	Vocal fremitus absent over effusion; PMI and trachea may be deviated away from affected side (if very large)	Dullness over affected side; flat percussion note if effusion is very large	Diminished or absent breath sounds; may have bronchial breath sounds and/or E-to-A change just above fluid if effusion is small or moderate in size

is identified readily around the lips and earlobes. The intensity of cyanosis increases with the quantity and degree of desaturated hemoglobin—patients with a high hemoglobin concentration (erythrocytosis) develop cyanosis at a lesser degree of hypoxemia, whereas those with anemia may not be cyanotic even though severe hypoxemia is present.

The digits are also inspected for evidence of digital clubbing, which is manifested by a painless enlargement of the terminal phalanges of the fingers and toes (Fig. 44-8). It usually takes months or years to develop and is associated with a variety of conditions, including carcinoma of the lung, diffuse interstitial fibrosis, and cystic fibrosis (see Ch. 61).

Neck

The neck should be inspected for evidence of jugular venous distension (JVD), which occurs when the right ventricle fails, often as a result of chronic elevation of pulmonary vascular resistance (PVR). This elevation is present in patients with chronic pulmonary disease that causes hypoxemia, and if it is prolonged, the right ventricle will begin to fail, resulting in backup of blood into the veins of the neck (Fig. 44-9). The degree of JVD depends on the severity of right heart failure, and the ability to identify it depends on the patient's neck anatomy. Patients with obese, short, or muscular necks are difficult to evaluate for JVD.

Jugular venous pressure can be estimated by identifying the level of the column of blood in the jugular veins. With the head of the bed elevated at a 45-degree angle, the level of the column of blood descends to a point no more than a few centimeters above the sternal angle with normal venous pressure. When JVD is present, however, the neck veins may be distended as high as the angle of the jaw, even with the patient sitting upright. Exact quantification of the jugular pressure in terms of centimeters above the sternal angle is difficult. A simple grading scale of normal, increased, and markedly increased is acceptable.

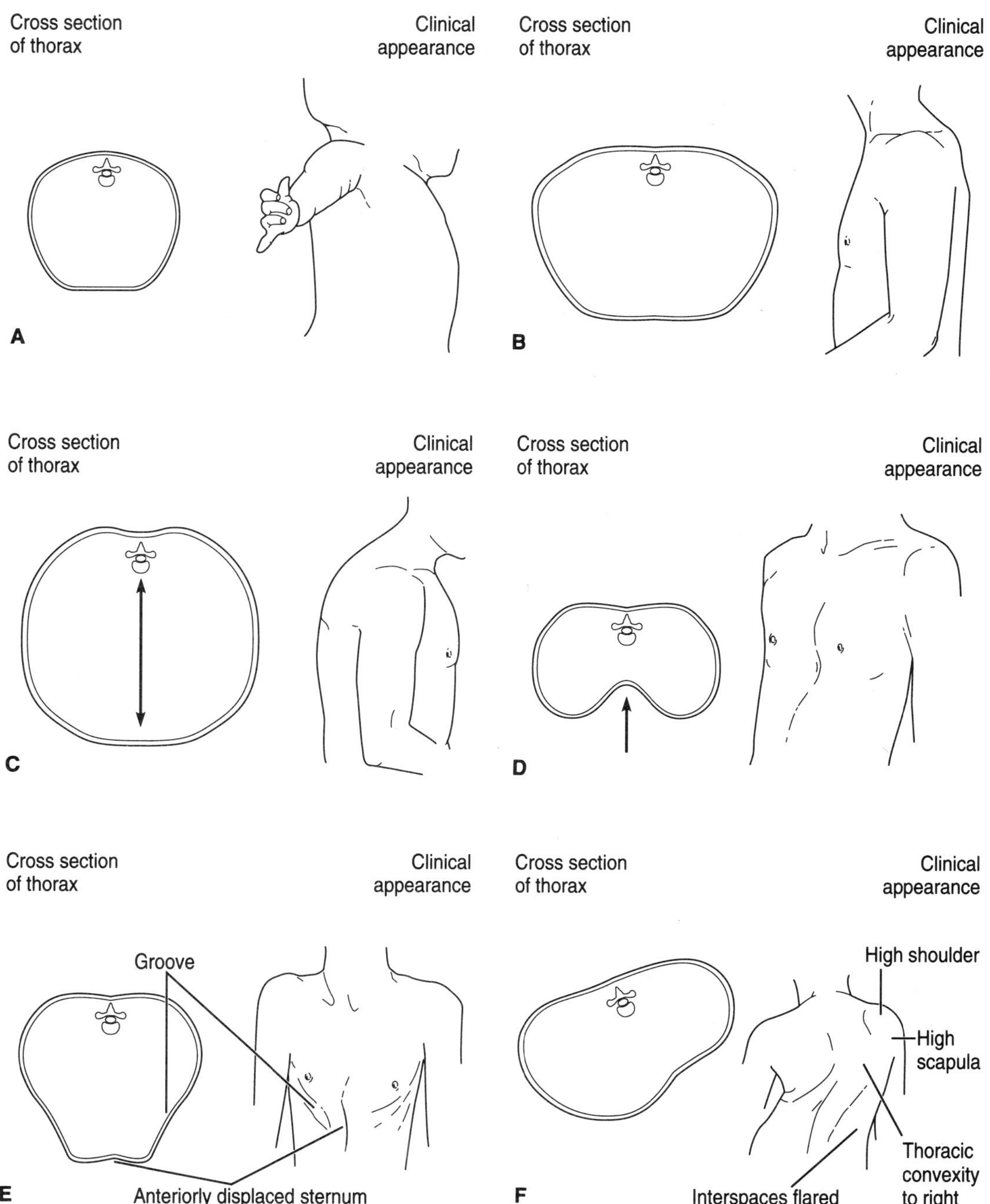

Figure 44-7. **(A)** The chest of the normal infant is approximately round or barrel-shaped in cross section. **(B)** In the normal adult chest the ratio of anteroposterior to lateral diameter ranges from 1:2 to 5:7. **(C)** A barrel chest is associated with pulmonary emphysema or normal aging. The ratio of anteroposterior to lateral diameter approximates 1:1. **(D)** Pectus excavatum (funnel chest) is characterized by a depression in the lower portion of the sternum. Compression of the heart and great vessels may cause murmurs. **(E)** In pectus carinatum the sternum is displaced anteriorly, increasing the anteroposterior diameter. Grooves in the chest wall accentuate the deformity. **(F)** In thoracic kyphoscoliosis the spine is curved and the thorax shows corresponding deformities. Distortion of the underlying lungs may make interpretation of lung findings very difficult. (Modified from Bates,[2] with permission.)

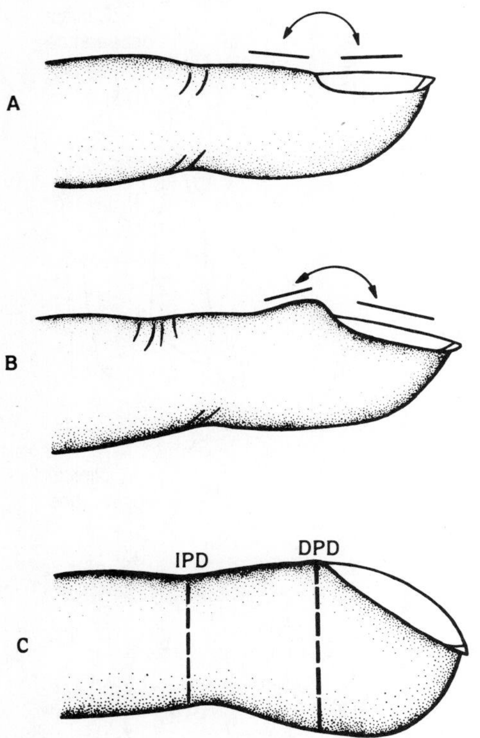

Figure 44-8. **(A)** Normal digit configuration. **(B)** Mild digital clubbing. **(C)** Severe digital clubbing; depth of finger at base of nail (DPD) is greater than depth of interphalangeal joint (IPD) with clubbing. (From Wilkins et al.,[1] with permission.)

Palpation

Chest

Palpation is the best method for evaluation of the degree and symmetry of chest expansion with breathing. Chest expansion is assessed with the examiner standing behind the patient and the examiner's hands placed over the patient's posterolateral chest so that the thumbs meet at the midline approximately at T8. The patient is instructed to exhale slowly and completely during the above-described positioning of the examiner's hands. Once the patient has exhaled fully, the examiner's fingertips should be secured on the patient's lateral chest wall and the patient asked to inhale maximally. The examiner then notes the distance that each thumb moves from midline. Normally, each thumb tip moves an equal distance of about 3 to 5 cm.

Chest expansion will be reduced bilaterally with both obstructive and restrictive lung diseases. Unilateral decreases in expansion are common with pneumonia, lobar atelectasis, pneumothorax, and large pleural effusions.

Palpation of the thorax is of value to assess general changes in lung pathology through the evaluation of vocal fremitus (i.e., the vibrations originating at the vocal cords during phonation). These vibrations travel down the tracheobronchial tree and through the lung parenchyma to the chest wall. When they are felt on the chest wall, they are said to produce *tactile fremitus*. To assess tactile fremitus the patient is asked to repeat the word "ninety-nine" while the examiner systematically palpates the thorax. The examiner should use the volar aspect of the fingers or the ulnar

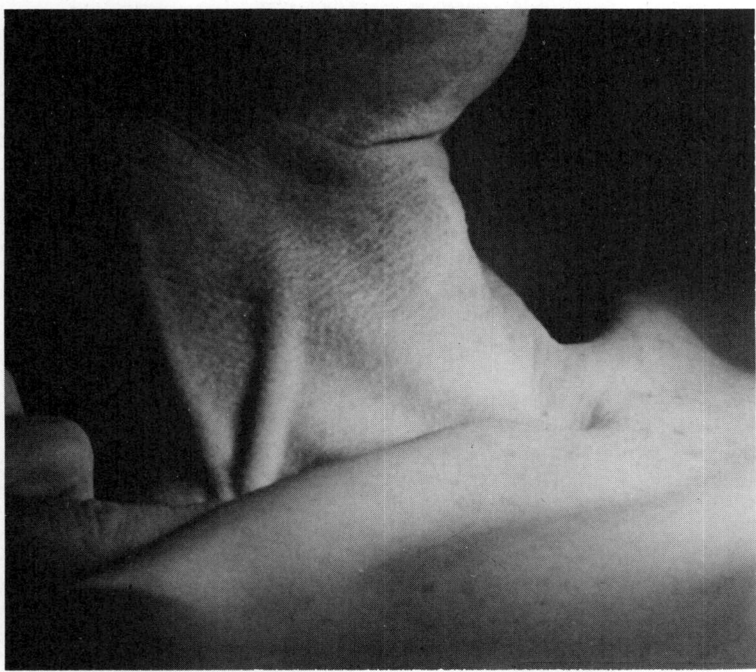

Figure 44-9. Photograph showing jugular venous distension. (From Wilkins,[40] with permission.)

aspect of the hand. Fremitus should be evaluated over all lung segments and the comparative increase or decrease in vibrations noted.

Tactile fremitus increases when the lung increases in density, resulting in a more direct transmission of vocal vibrations. This occurs with pneumonia, fibrosis, and lung tumors. Tactile fremitus are decreased or absent when the vocal vibrations are transmitted poorly through the lung, pleura, or chest wall, as may be the case with emphysema, pleural effusion, pneumothorax, or obesity. Auscultation and percussion (described below) over any area of suspected abnormality will help the examiner confirm the presence and degree of changes in underlying pathology.

The extremities are palpated to assist in assessment of the patient's overall perfusion. Reduced cardiac output is associated with cool extremities and poor capillary refill. Capillary refill is evaluated by pressing on the fingernail for a brief period and then noting the speed at which the circulation under the fingernail returns. Normally, capillary refill occurs in less than 2 to 3 seconds, but with reduced cardiac output more than 3 seconds may be needed.

The neck should be palpated to assess the tracheal position. Normally the trachea is located in the midline when the patient is facing forward, but lateral deviation of the trachea can occur with pneumothorax, mediastinal tumors, or massive atelectasis of an upper lobe. Tension pneumothorax and mediastinal tumors will push the trachea away from the affected side and upper lobe atelectasis will shift it toward the affected side.

Precordium

The area of the chest wall overlying the heart, referred to as the *precordium,* is palpated in an effort to detect the presence and position of normal and abnormal pulsations. Pulsations on the precordium are affected by the intensity of ventricular contraction and by the thickness of the chest wall and the quality of the tissue through which the pulsations must travel. The normal apical impulse is produced by the contraction of the left ventricle during systole and usually is felt near the midclavicular line in the fifth intercostal space on the left side of the patient's chest, a location referred to as the point of maximum impulse (PMI).

The PMI may be difficult to detect with left ventricular failure or obesity or when there is an abnormal buildup of fluid or air between the heart and the chest wall, as can occur with pleural effusion or with pneumothorax. The PMI may be shifted to the left or right with shifts in the mediastinum, which can occur with lobar collapse or tension pneumothorax. In patients with emphysema who have low, flat diaphragms, the PMI is often located in the epigastric area.

Percussion

Percussion over the chest wall is performed to help evaluate the relative amounts of air and solid material in the underlying lung and to determine the relative boundaries of the lung. The procedure most often used is the mediate or indirect technique, which creates vibrations that penetrate, and thus permit evaluation of the lung to a level 5 to 7 cm below the chest wall surface.

Indirect percussion requires the examiner to place the middle finger of the left hand (if the examiner is right-handed) firmly against the patient's chest in the intercostal space parallel to the ribs. The palm and other fingers may be held slightly off the chest so that only the middle finger is making contact. The examiner now uses the tip of the middle finger of the right hand to strike the chest with quick, sharp blows. The striking motion is best generated by appropriate wrist action with the forearm held still. Percussion over the lung fields should be performed in a systematic way, with comparison of both sides (Fig. 44-10).

Percussion over normal air-filled lung will produce a drum-like sound, described as normal resonance. When the percussion note is louder and lower-pitched than normal, the resonance is said to be increased; this occurs with emphysema or pneumothorax. When the percussion note is softer and higher-pitched than normal, it is described as being flat or dull; this sound is identified over areas of pneumonia, atelectasis, lung tumor, or pleural effusion.

The relative position and range of motion for the diaphragm can be identified by percussion, preferably on the posterior chest wall. The examiner strikes the chest wall over the lower lung field, moving downward until a definite change (from resonance to flat) in the percussion note is identified. This procedure is performed at maximal expiration and again at maximal inspiration to determine the degree of diaphragm excursion. Movement of the diaphragm is reduced with some neuromuscular disorders or when emphysema causes it to take a low, flat position.

Auscultation

Auscultation is the process of listening to sounds produced within the body, typically with use of a stethoscope (Fig. 44-11). The modern stethoscope, consisting of a chest piece with a bell or diaphragm (or both) connected with rubber tubing to the earpieces, is designed to allow clear transmission of sound from the patient to the ears of the examiner and at the same time to exclude the majority of extraneous noises.

The diaphragm is used most often during auscultation of the lungs since it is designed for detecting typical lung sound frequencies. The earpieces should point forward slightly to allow a more comfortable fit; the tubing should generally not exceed 20 in. in length, since longer tubing may compromise sound transmission; and the inner diameter of the tubing should be 4 mm (3/16 in.) or greater. Double tubing is acoustically superior to a single tube. The technique of auscultation is described following the discussion of lung sounds.

Lung sounds can be divided into two basic types: breath sounds and adventitious lung sounds. Breath sounds are normal noises, which can be heard with the aid of a stethoscope over the chest wall during breathing. Adventitious lung

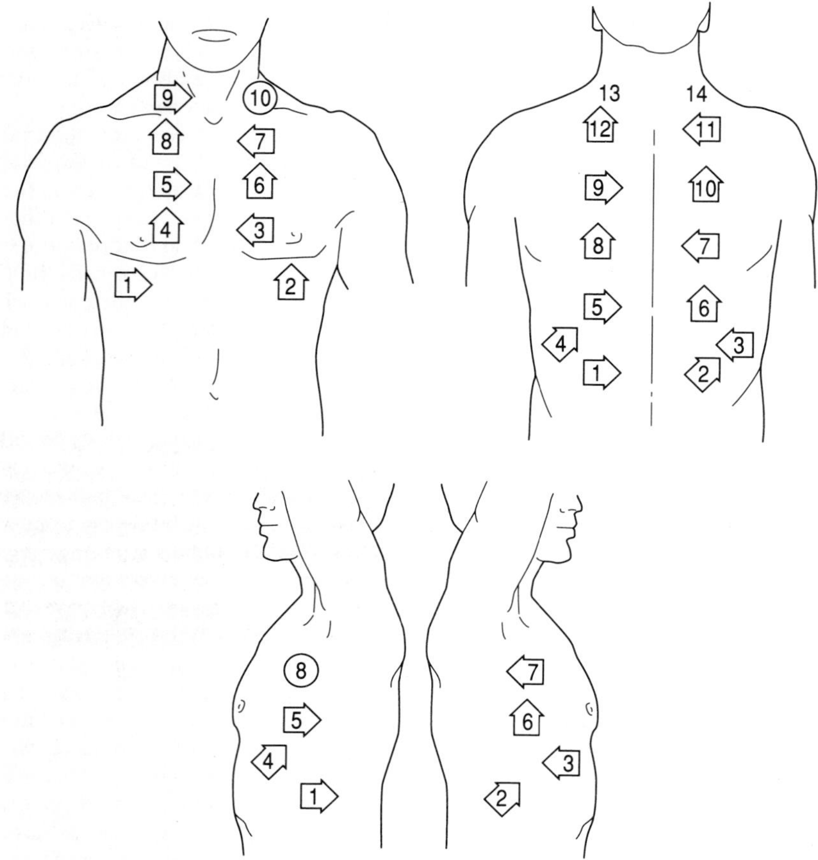

Figure 44-10. Systematic method for percussion and auscultation.

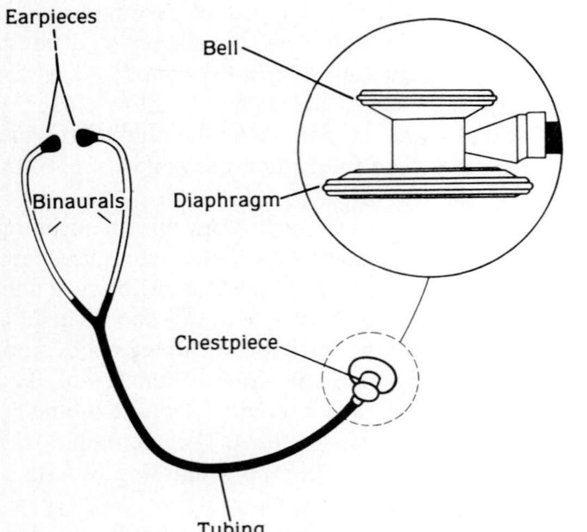

Figure 44-11. Diagram of stethoscope. (From Wilkins et al.,[1] with permission.)

sounds are abnormal noises superimposed on the breath sounds and usually indicate that respiratory disease is present.

Breath Sounds

The normal breath sounds are divided into three different types: bronchial, bronchovesicular, and vesicular. Bronchial breath sounds are relatively loud and high-pitched and have approximately equal inspiratory and expiratory components, with a slight pause between these components (Fig. 44-12). This type of sound is heard when auscultating directly over the trachea and is produced by turbulent flow of air through the upper airway with breathing. These sounds may be referred to as bronchial, tracheal, tracheobronchial, or tubular breath sounds.

Auscultation directly over the main stem bronchi results in identification of bronchovesicular breath sounds, which are softer and lower-pitched than the bronchial breath sounds and do not contain a pause between the inspiratory and expiratory components (Fig. 44-12). They are identified on the anterior chest near the main stem bronchi in the first

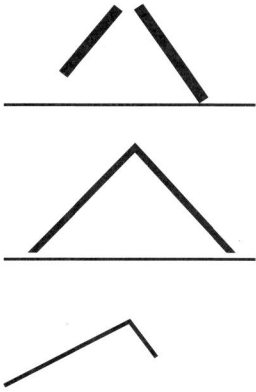

Figure 44-12. Characteristics of normal breath sounds illustrated with diagrams. Upstroke represents inspiration and downstroke represents expiration. (From Wilkins et al.,[41] with permission.)

and second intercostal spaces and on the posterior chest between the scapulae (Fig. 44-13). Bronchovesicular breath sounds also are believed to be produced by turbulent flow in the central airways. This sound is reduced in intensity and pitch as a result of the filtering of the sound that occurs as it passes through the lung and chest wall tissue between the central airways and the surface of the chest. This is in contrast to the bronchial breath sound heard directly over the larynx or upper portion of the trachea, which is not filtered.

Relatively soft, low-pitched sounds, described as vesicular breath sounds, are heard during auscultation over the lung. Vesicular breath sounds are primarily inspiratory sounds, the expiratory portion being heard only during the initial third of exhalation. While the inspiratory component of the vesicular breath sound is believed to be produced more distally than the expiratory component, the vesicular breath sound is believed to primarily represent filtered bronchial breath sounds.

Normal air-filled lung contains millions of alveoli, which act as a sound filter, altering the sounds due to turbulent flow in the central airways as they pass through the lung. Flow in the peripheral airways is laminar and probably does not contribute significantly to sound production, but it may help in the transmittal of the breath sounds to the chest wall surface during inhalation. The expiratory component of the vesicular breath sound is believed to be produced in the larger airways, where airstreams converge rapidly.[26,27] Since airflow is directed toward the upper airway away from the chest wall during exhalation, the expiratory component of the vesicular breath sound fades away as the patient exhales during auscultation over the chest wall.

When the vesicular breath sound becomes louder than expected, it is described as harsh. If it also takes on a prominent expiratory component, it is described as bronchial or tubular; this occurs when the peripheral lung units become denser (more consolidated), as in pneumonia. Consolidated lung does not filter central airway sounds but allows them to pass through the lung more directly. As a result, harsh or bronchial-type breath sounds are heard over areas of lung consolidation.

If the vesicular breath sound is softer than expected, it is described as diminished or reduced, or in extreme cases as absent. Breath sounds are reduced or absent either when the sound production is diminished, as with shallow breathing, or when sound transmission through the lung or chest wall is inhibited. Sound transmission is reduced when the lung becomes less dense (hyperinflated), as with emphysema, or when the airways are obstructed by mucus or other physical obstruction. With pleural effusion, pneumothorax, or obesity, sound transmission through the pleura or chest wall is blocked, and breath sounds will be absent or reduced over the affected area.

Adventitious Lung Sounds

On the basis of acoustical recordings, adventitious lung sounds can be classified into two different types, continuous and discontinuous.[28,29] Continuous adventitious lung sounds are musical-type sounds with a consistent pitch and may be very short (200 msec) or as long as several seconds. They are described as wheezes when high-pitched and as rhonchi when low-pitched (Table 44-11). Since the term *rhonchi* has been used in the past to describe a variety of abnormal lung sounds, some clinicians prefer to refer to low-pitched continuous adventitious lung sounds as *low-pitched wheezes*.

Wheezes are believed to result from narrowing of the air-

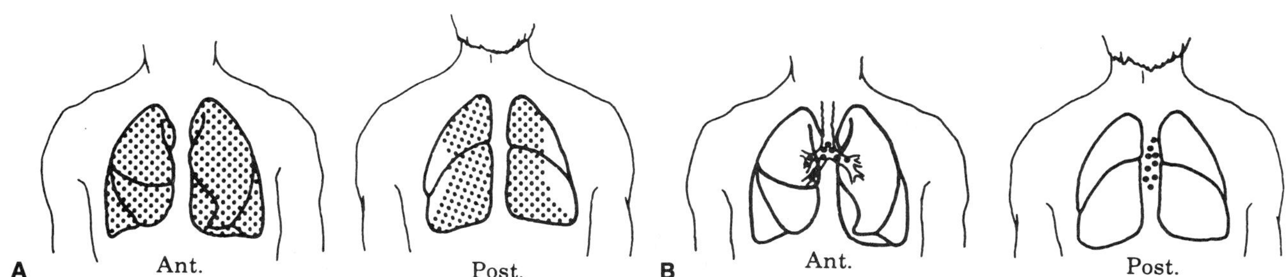

Figure 44-13. Location on chest wall where (A) vesicular and (B) bronchovesicular breath sounds are heard. (From Wilkins et al.,[41] with permission.)

Table 44-11. Terminology and Classification of Adventitious Lung Sounds

Sound	Classification	Other Terms	Timing	Waveform
Crackles	Discontinuous	Rales	Usually inspiratory	
Wheezes	High-pitched continuous	Sibilant rales Musical rales	Usually expiratory	
Rhonchi	Low-pitched continuous	Sonorous rales Low-pitched wheeze	Usually expiratory	

ways. As the airway lumen decreases, airflow increases to allow adequate ventilation, and this in turn causes a drop in the lateral wall pressure, which draws the opposite sides of the airway wall into a closed position (Fig. 44-14). Airflow is thereby interrupted temporarily and the lateral wall pressure increases, returning the airway to a partially open position, so that airflow again increases. This sequence repeats itself in a rapid manner, resulting in vibration of the airway walls between a partially obstructed and a closed position.[30,31] It is important to note that rapid airflow through the obstructed airways is needed to produce this continuous adventitious lung sound. Slower flow rates, as when the patient fatigues, will not cause the airway walls to vibrate. A decrease in respiratory effort therefore may result in a paradoxical absence of wheezing.

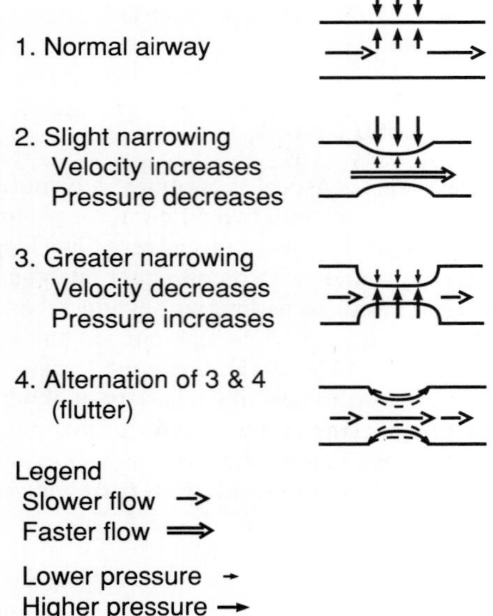

Figure 44-14. Proposed mechanism for wheeze illustrated. (1) Normally the airway wall is stable since there is a balance between internal and external forces. (2) As the airway lumen decreases, the air velocity increases to maintain a constant mass flow rate. This causes a decrease in the lateral wall pressure, allowing external forces to further collapse the airway. (3) When airway collapses to a more closed position, air velocity decreases and internal pressure increases. The airway now returns to a more open (but still narrowed) position. Air velocity increases again and the cycle repeats itself rapidly, causing airway walls to vibrate. (From Murphy and Holford,[43] with permission.)

Three characteristics of the patient's wheezing should be evaluated: pitch, intensity, and the proportion of the respiratory cycle occupied by wheezing. The pitch of the wheeze is determined by the relationship between the flow rate and the degree of airway obstruction. More rapid flow with a similar degree of airway obstruction or more significant obstruction at the same flow rate causes the wheeze to increase in pitch. A change in the wheezes from high to low pitch therefore may indicate less airway obstruction or a decreased respiratory effort. While the intensity of the patient's wheezing does not accurately predict the severity of airway obstruction, loud wheezing does generally indicate moderate to severe obstruction.[32] Louder wheezes occur when the patient's respiratory effort is greater, and although they may be associated with significant airway obstruction, they indicate that airflow is occurring. More severe airway obstruction is suggested when the wheezing occupies a major portion of the respiratory cycle (e.g., pan-inspiratory and -expiratory) as compared with wheezing heard only during the later portion of exhalation. Improvement in expiratory flow rate, as may occur with bronchodilator therapy, is associated with a reduction in the proportion of the respiratory cycle occupied by wheezing.[33]

A high-pitched continuous sound heard over the upper airway of a patient with upper airway obstruction is referred to as *stridor*. Stridor is a sign of a potentially life-threatening disorder and signifies that the patient should be carefully monitored. Resources to place an artificial airway must be available if the patient's ventilatory status is threatened.

Discontinuous adventitious lung sounds are intermittent, crackling, or bubbling sounds of short duration. They are nonmusical sounds that primarily occur during inspiration. They are frequently referred to as *rales,* but since this term has been used in the past to describe both continuous and discontinuous adventitious lung sounds, the Pulmonary Nomenclature Committee of the American Thoracic Society has recommended use of the term *crackles* to describe the discontinuous adventitious sounds.[34] While many clinicians agree with the recommendation, the term rales also remains in common use.[35–38]

Crackles are produced by two basic mechanisms, movement of excessive airway secretions with breathing and sudden opening of small airways.[31,38] Crackles that result from excessive airway secretions are typically coarse and occur with inhalation and exhalation. They often clear with coughing or therapeutic aspiration of the patient's airway. Crackles due to the sudden opening of small airways are produced by the rapid equalization of pressure between patent and collapsed airways. These crackles are inspiratory sounds and are associated with restrictive pulmonary disorders such as atelectasis, pneumonia, and pulmonary fibrosis. With postoperative atelectasis, the crackles occur late in inspiration and often clear with several deep breaths. The crackles associated with pulmonary fibrosis do not disappear with deep breathing.

Qualifying Adjectives

Qualifying adjectives are used to document specific characteristics of any adventitious lung sounds heard during auscultation. Some of the more popular adjectives, such as wet, dry, and sonorous, have no logical basis and are interpreted differently by different clinicians. More accurate terms that have a scientific basis consistent with waveform analysis should be used. Such terms include high-pitched, low-pitched, fine, medium,[39] and coarse.

An important description that should always be included in the documentation of abnormal lung sounds is their timing during the respiratory cycle. Abnormal sounds should be described as inspiratory, expiratory, or both. In addition, the specific timing during inspiration or expiration (e.g., late inspiratory) is of diagnostic value in many cases.

Auscultation Technique

Whenever possible, the patient should be sitting upright in a relaxed position for auscultation. Room noises must be at a minimum. The examiner should ask the patient to take slightly deeper than normal breaths through the open mouth. The stethoscope should be moved back and forth from one side to the other to compare the breath sounds in similar positions on each side. At each position one full respiratory cycle should be evaluated.

While auscultating, the examiner should concentrate first on inspiration, especially noting its length and any adventitial components (e.g., crackles or wheezes). Next the examiner should evaluate expiration for similar characteristics. The expiratory component of the breath sound is especially important to evaluate, since one of the initial signs of pulmonary congestion is an increase in the intensity and length of expiration. This change is often subtle and therefore is easily missed. The examiner should attempt to identify the underlying breath sounds even when adventitious lung sounds are present.

The examiner should not use the stethoscope over clothing, since this makes the breath sounds more difficult to hear. Auscultation over chest hair can pick up a crackling sound that is easily interpreted as an adventitious lung sound. When auscultation over chest hair cannot be avoided, wetting the hair will minimize this phenomenon. The tubing should not touch any objects during auscultation since this will produce artificial noise.

Auscultation of all areas of the anterior, lateral, and posterior chest wall surface will avoid missing abnormalities. It is suggested that the dependent areas be auscultated first in bedridden patients, since the dependent segments are more prone to atelectasis in such patients and as a result late inspiratory crackles are a frequent finding over these lung areas. If nondependent areas are auscultated first, the initial deep inspiratory efforts may cause the atelectasis to temporarily clear, so that subsequent auscultation of the dependent regions will not reveal the early signs of atelectasis and appropriate treatment will be delayed.

Auscultation of Voice Sounds

When the examiner suspects that the patient's lung has undergone certain pathologic changes (e.g., lung consolidation), auscultation of voice sounds can be useful. This procedure requires a cooperative patient who can repeat "1-2-3" or "99" while the examiner auscultates over the chest. Vocal resonance is created as the vibrations of phonation travel down the tracheobronchial tree and throughout the lung. Normally, the air-filled lung filters the voice sound so that it is heard as a low-pitched mumble over the chest wall with a stethoscope. If the lung parenchyma becomes denser, as with the consolidation that occurs in pneumonia, vocal resonance increases and the voice sound is heard more clearly. This increase in vocal resonance is known as *bronchophony*. A decrease in vocal resonance occurs when the lung becomes less dense, as with the hyperinflation of emphysema.

When the voice sound increases in intensity and also takes on a nasal or bleating characteristic, it is described as *egophony*. This sound, generally found over areas of the chest where bronchophony is present, is identified by asking the patient to say "ee." If egophony is present, the "ee" will be heard as "ay" over the area of consolidation. When consolidation is present, whispered voice sounds are transmitted more directly through the consolidated area than through normal air-filled lung. When the whispered sounds are heard with more clarity, they are described as *whispered pectoriloquy*.

THE MEDICAL RECORD

The content of the medical record varies in different health care settings. In hospitals it generally consists of an admission history and physical examination; any operative or procedure notes; narrative progress notes; the results of all laboratory tests, physicians' orders, notes from nursing, respiratory care, and other services; and other data, including administrative and often financial information. In most cases bedside flowsheets, ventilator records, and other "charts" also ultimately become part of the permanent medical record. The medical record is also a legal document, and any information recorded in it becomes a permanent part, regardless of who records it.

Because a patient's medical record contains confidential information, only individuals directly involved in that patient's care have legitimate access to it. Its contents should not be shared with anyone who is not also involved in that patient's care. In particular, information about patients should not be discussed in the hallways or elevators or outside of the work setting (Table 44-1).

In the 1990s information is recorded in patients' charts in many ways—through dictation, by longhand in narrative notes, via data recording on flowsheets or on bedside checklists, or via computer at the bedside or elsewhere. Clinicians making additions to the medical record must identify themselves on the record, both by name and by role: "Mary Williams, R.R.T., Shift Supervisor," or "Richard Sanchez, M.D., Medicine R3." Notes should be concise, use appropriate medical terminology, and be legible. There is no justification for writing sarcastic, critical, or humorous remarks in the chart; personal opinions and disagreements with others participating in the patient's management should be discussed verbally in person and not displayed for all to see in the permanent (legal) medical record.

Nothing may be erased or removed from a patient's medical record. Corrections or addenda to previous notes or data can be made only under certain circumstances defined by the hospital, and when they are made clear identification of the person making the notation, along with the date on which the addition is made, is required.

THE ORAL PRESENTATION

The ability to communicate clinical information verbally to other health care professionals is an important prerequisite for good multidisciplinary patient care. Oral presentations vary from single-sentence orienting statements to complete recitations of history, physical examination, laboratory findings, and treatment, which may take 5 minutes or longer. Regardless of its length, an oral case presentation has the purposes of concisely presenting the patient's history, physical findings, and/or laboratory findings and demonstrating the clinician's understanding of that patient's illness, along with communication of the management plan or response to treatment.

An oral presentation is not an exercise in medical obfuscation or arcane terminology. The common language of medicine is used by all members of the health care team: respiratory care practitioners should be able to summarize patients' histories to attending physicians, just as primary physicians or consulting pulmonologists should be able to describe their findings and recommended care plan to respiratory therapists.

A complete, traditional oral case presentation consists of the following seven sequential parts: (1) identifying sentence, including chief complaint or reason for admission/consultation; (2) history of present illness; (3) other active medical problems; (4) medications, allergies, habits, and pertinent social history; (5) physical examination; (6) laboratory data; and (7) assessment, plan, or course to date.

The *identifying sentence* is used not only to begin a complete oral presentation but also to introduce follow-up or progress reports and to remind the listener of which patient is being discussed. The following examples illustrate its usual contents and the order in which the facts are presented:

> Mr. Swensen is a 68-year-old retired engineer with long-standing COPD who was admitted last night because of increased dyspnea, cough, and purulent sputum of 2 days' duration.
>
> Mrs. Rossi is a 45-year-old housewife with a long history of asthma and obesity who is scheduled for an elective cholecystectomy tomorrow morning and whom we have been asked to see for pre- and postoperative respiratory care.
>
> Jeffrey Jackson is a 17-year-old high school senior who sustained a closed head injury, multiple long bone fractures, and a left lung contusion last night when his motorcycle went out of control and struck a parked car.

The identifying sentence should include the patient's relevant active medical problems (no more than four) listed by diagnosis. The symptoms, signs, and findings justifying these diagnoses will be elaborated in subsequent parts of the presentation; here the purpose is to orient the listener to the patient's overall status or the reason for consultation. Diagnoses, laboratory values, and other aspects of the history not directly bearing on the current admission or visit should be omitted.

The *history of present illness* is the largest and most important part of an oral presentation. A main goal of learning clinical assessment skills is to be able to include everything that is relevant while omitting that which is irrelevant, and this admittedly takes practice. The results of the clinician's pursuit of the present illness during the taking of the history (see earlier section) are presented here. The following example illustrates a possible continuation of the presentation begun with the first identifying sentence above:

> Mr. Swensen has a long history of COPD characterized by one-block dyspnea on exertion, a forced expiratory volume in 1 second earlier this year of 0.8 L, and continuous home O_2 therapy for the last 2 years. He was in his usual state of health until 2 days prior to admission when he noted the gradual worsening of shortness of breath, associated with malaise and a change in his sputum from its usual white to yellow. . .

The presenting symptoms or event should be described in detail, as discussed earlier (Table 44-7). Pertinent negatives should be included: in this example they might include the absence of hemoptysis, chills, or exposure to anyone who was ill.

Other active medical problems might include such things as diabetes or cirrhosis that the presenter considers relevant or possibly relevant to the present problem. Remote or unrelated diagnoses or operations (e.g., malaria in 1965, history of cataract extraction, or long-standing psoriasis) should be omitted.

The patient's *medications, allergies, habits, and pertinent social history* should include a complete list of all current prescription and nonprescription medications, any drug allergies (including a description of the type of reaction), and relevant habits such as smoking, alcohol consumption, and other substance use. Pertinent items in a patient's social history might include such items as living wills or advance directives for health care or membership in churches or groups whose tenets may affect health care (e.g., Jehovah's Witnesses).

The description of the *physical examination* should begin with an introductory sentence, such as "The patient was a chronically ill-appearing elderly man in obvious respiratory distress, sitting on the edge of the bed and able to say only a few words in a single breath." This should always be followed by the vital signs (temperature, pulse, blood pressure, respiratory rate). For purposes of the oral presentation only relevant positive and negative physical findings should be given. In the example being used here, these would include a complete description of the chest examination, with comments on the presence or absence of cyanosis, peripheral edema, and the use of accessory ventilatory muscles.

Although the presenter may know a wide array of *laboratory results* on the patient being discussed, only those relevant to the present illness should be cited. Laboratory results should always be presented in the same order. An example for a general medical patient might be: hemogram, electrolytes, other relevant blood chemistries, urinalysis, chest x-ray, electrocardiogram, and other pertinent tests, including arterial blood gases and results of sputum stains and cultures. In respiratory care the order might be: chest x-ray, arterial blood gas levels, results of sputum stains and cultures, and other pertinent results. Arterial blood gas results should always be recited (and written down) in the same order: inspired O_2 fraction or supplementation, pH, PCO_2, PO_2, HCO_3^-.

The *assessment, plan, or course to date* should be a brief summarizing statement to indicate how the presenter puts the case together and to bring the listener up to date on what has happened since admission. Assessments should be as definite as possible without drawing unwarranted conclusions or making specific diagnoses whose criteria have not yet been fulfilled. Examples based on the hypothetical patient introduced earlier might be

> In summary, Mr. Swensen presents with an acute exacerbation of his COPD. He is being treated with intravenous corticosteroids, inhaled beta agonists, intravenous aminophylline, and oral antibiotics along with nasal O_2 to keep his PaO_2 between 55 and 60 mmHg.

or

> In summary, Mr. Swensen presented with right upper lobe pneumococcal pneumonia. . . (later, once x-ray and culture results have become available)

Experienced presenters avoid several mistakes or pitfalls in oral presentations. The most common of these is not to include enough information in the history of present illness. Another is the imprecise or confusing use of temporal reference points. Time should be related to the time of admission, not to the calendar: "Three days prior to admission" is better than "Last Wednesday." Still another mistake is to interject editorial comments or value judgments into the presentation; the history should be a faithful representation of the patient's own story, and the physical examination and laboratory data should be objective and precise. Finally, the distinctions among symptoms, signs, syndromes, and diseases summarized in Table 44-5 should be observed during oral presentations. Only terms justifiable by the evidence at hand are appropriate, and the use of a specific diagnosis when one has not yet been made can lead to inappropriate treatment and confusion.

References

1. Wilkins RL, Sheldon RL, Krider SJ: Clinical Assessment in Respiratory Care. 2nd Ed. Mosby-Year Book, St. Louis, 1990
2. Bates B: A Guide to the Physical Examination and History Taking. 4th Ed. JB Lippincott, Philadelphia, 1987
3. Hillman RS, Goodell BW, Grundy SM et al: Clinical Skills: Interviewing, History Taking, and Physical Diagnosis. McGraw-Hill, New York, 1981
4. DeGowin EL, DeGowin RL: Bedside Diagnostic Examination. 4th Ed. Macmillan, New York, 1981
5. Murray JF: History and physical examination. pp. 431–451. In Murray JF, Nadel JA (eds): Textbook of Respiratory Medicine. WB Saunders, Philadelphia, 1988
6. Szidon JP, Fishman AP: Approach to the pulmonary patient with respiratory signs and symptoms. pp. 313–366. In Fishman AP (ed): Pulmonary Diseases and Disorders. 2nd Ed. McGraw-Hill, New York, 1988
7. Briggs DD Jr: Essential points of the history and physical examination. pp. 1981–1986. In Kelley WN (ed): Textbook of Internal Medicine. JB Lippincott, Philadelphia, 1989
8. Neff TA: Essential points of the history and physical examination. pp. 1807–1810. In Kelley WN (ed): Textbook of Internal Medicine. 2nd Ed. JB Lippincott, Philadelphia, 1992
9. Pierson DJ: Respiratory care as a science. Respir Care 1988; 33:27–37
10. Sorbello JG: Who is a true professional? AARC Times 1987; 11:22–26 et passim
11. George V, Dundes A: The gomer. A figure of American hospital folk speech. J Am Folklore 1978;91:568–581
12. Shen S: The House of God. Richard Marek Publishers, New York, 1978
13. Dirtball. JAMA 1982;247:3059–3060 and 1983;249:279–280
14. Tumulty PA: What is a clinician and what does he do? N Engl J Med 1970;283:20–24
15. Tumulty PA: The Effective Clinician. WB Saunders, Philadelphia, 1973
16. Gordon MJ, Leversee JH, Pierson DJ (eds): Syllabus for Human Biology 513, 522, and 535: Introduction to Clinical Medicine I. University of Washington School of Medicine, Seattle, 1989
17. Fitzgerald FT, Tierney LM: The bedside Sherlock Holmes. West J Med 1982;137:169–175
18. Miller L: Sherlock Holmes's methods of deductive reasoning applied to medical diagnostics. West J Med 1985;142:413–414
19. Becker CE: Key elements of the occupational history for the general physician. West J Med 1982;137:581–582
20. Speizer FE: Environmental lung diseases. pp. 1056–1063. In Wilson JD, Braunwald E, Isselbacher KJ et al (eds): Harrison's Principles of Internal Medicine. 12th Ed. McGraw-Hill, New York, 1991

21. Hunninghake GW, Richerson HB: Hypersensitivity pneumonitis. pp. 1053–1056. In Wilson JD, Braunwald E, Isselbacher KJ et al (eds): Harrison's Principles of Internal Medicine. 12th Ed. McGraw-Hill, New York, 1991
22. Hasler ME, Cohen JA: The effect of oxygen administration on oral temperature assessment. Nurs Res 1982;31:265–268
23. Lim-Levy F: The effect of oxygen inhalation on oral temperature. Nurs Res 1982;31:150–152
24. Yonkman CA: Cool and heated aerosol and the measurement of oral temperature. Nurs Res 1982;31:354–357
25. Rebuck AS, Pengelly LD: Development of pulsus paradoxus in the presence of airway obstruction. N Engl J Med 1973;288:66–69
26. Kraman SS: Does laryngeal noise contribute to vesicular lung sounds? Am Rev Respir Dis 1981;124:292–294
27. Kraman SS: Vesicular (normal) lung sounds: How are they made, where do they come from, and what do they mean? Semin Respir Med 1985;6:183–191
28. Robertson JA, Coope R: Rales, rhonchi and Laennec. Lancet 1957;2:417–422
29. Murphy RLH, Holford SK, Knowler WC: Lung sound characterization by time-expanded waveform analysis. N Engl J Med 1977;296:968–971
30. Waring WW, Beckerman RC, Hopkins RL: Continuous adventitious lung sounds: Site and method of production and significance. Semin Respir Med 1985;6:201–209
31. Forgacs P: The functional basis of pulmonary sounds. Chest 1978;73:399–405
32. Marini JJ, Pierson DJ, Hudson LD, Lakshminarayan S: The significance of wheezing in chronic airflow obstruction. Am Rev Respir Dis 1979;120:1069–1072
33. Baughman RP, Loudon RG: Quantification of wheezing in acute asthma. Chest 1984;86:718–722
34. Report of the ATS-ACCP Ad Hoc Subcommittee on Pulmonary Nomenclature. ATS News 1977;3:5–6
35. Wilkins RL, Dexter JR, Smith JR: Survey of adventitious lung sound terminology in case reports. Chest 1984;85:523–525
36. Wilkins RL, Dexter JR, Murphy RLH, DelBono EA: Lung sound nomenclature survey. Chest 1990;98:886–889
37. Wilkins RL, Dexter JR: Comparing RCPs to physicians for the description of lung sounds: Are we accurate and can we communicate? Respir Care 1990;35:969–976
38. Murphy RLH: Discontinuous adventitious lung sounds. Semin Respir Med 1985;6:210–219
39. Murphy RLH, Desmeules M, Del Bono EA: Objective correlations of medium crackles, abstracted. Chest 1987;92:152s
40. Wilkins RL, Hodgkin JE: History and physical examination of the respiratory patient. pp. 211–232. In Burton GG, Hodgkin JE, Ward JJ (eds): Respiratory Care: A Guide to Clinical Practice. 3rd Ed. JB Lippincott, Philadelphia, 1991
41. Wilkins RL, Hodgkin JE, Lopez B: Lung Sounds: A Practical Guide. CV Mosby, St. Louis, 1988
42. Arnall D, Ryan M: Screening for pulmonary system disease. pp. 73–103. In Boissonnault WG (ed): Examination in Physical Therapy Practice: Screening for Medical Disease. Churchill Livingstone, New York, 1991
43. Murphy RLH, Holford SK: Lung sounds. Basics Respir Dis. 1980;8:1–6

Chapter 45

Assessment of Lung Volumes

Michael G. Snow

CHAPTER OUTLINE

Lung volumes describe anatomic and physiologic limits, and the relationship between volumes and capacities is determined by pathophysiology. These limits and relationships are altered by obstructive and restrictive processes, which can produce both permanent and transient changes. Individual processes cause characteristic patterns of change, which permit assessment of degree of dysfunction and response to therapy.

The relationship between volumes and capacities in the lungs is depicted in Figure 45-1. Volumes are specific indivisible components, while capacities are functional groupings which include two or more volumes. Assessment is primarily based on the relationships among total lung capacity (TLC), vital capacity (VC), functional residual capacity (FRC), and residual volume (RV). The volume-capacity relationships are defined in Table 45-1.

Without the effects of lung elastic recoil and the ventilatory muscles, the chest wall would expand to approximately 70 percent of the TLC (see Ch. 9). Further expansion must overcome both lung elastic recoil and chest wall recoil. The lungs, on the other hand, tend to contract toward RV owing to elastic recoil. TLC is a function of inspiratory muscle strength as well as of pressure-volume relationships of the lungs and chest wall. It decreases slightly or remains constant with aging and increases during acute asthma.[1–6]

At some point the static recoil forces of the lungs and chest wall balance to define the FRC. FRC can be modified by the aggregate tone of the inspiratory and expiratory muscles and by airway resistance, thoracic cage shape, lung elastic recoil, and abdominal pressure. In conditions in which the lungs are separated from the chest wall, such as pneumothorax or pleural effusion, lung volume decreases and chest wall volume increases until the forces balance once more.

The primary determinants of VC are inspiratory muscle strength, lung elastic recoil, and chest wall mechanics. RV is determined by expiratory muscle strength, airway patency, and chest wall mechanics. The pattern of changes in absolute lung volumes can be used to infer the disease process in restrictive and obstructive disease.

OVERVIEW

VC and its subcomponents can be measured directly with a simple spirometer. RV is usually measured indirectly from FRC since it is the only lung volume or capacity that is largely unaffected by the subject's effort or cooperation. Measurement of FRC or direct measurement of TLC is generally accomplished by one of three primary methods: gas dilution, body plethysmography, and radiography. Each of these methods is discussed in detail.

FRC measurement has been thoroughly reviewed, and recommendations are available.[7] The methodologic recommendations of the Epidemiological Standardization Project (ESP) have been widely adopted by manufacturers.[8] More

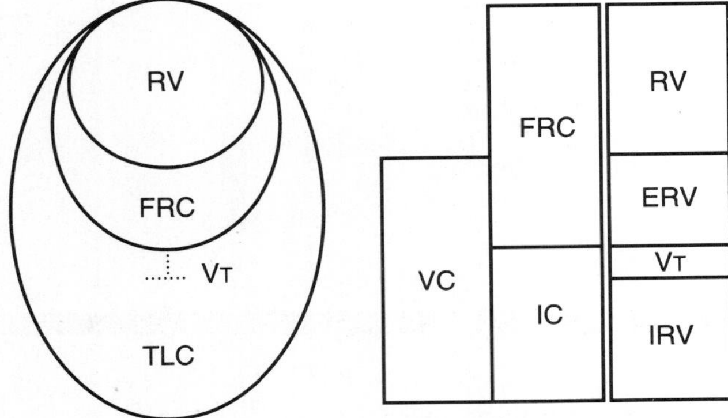

Figure 45-1. Graphic relationship between basic lung volumes and lung capacities. See text and Table 45-1 for details.

recently, the Intermountain Thoracic Society (ITS)[9] and the American College of Chest Physicians (ACCP)[10] have also published recommendations on methodology.

Several studies have compared the different methodologies.[11–14] In general, there is very good agreement among the various dilutional techniques and also between plethysmographic and radiographic techniques. Since dilutional methods only measure the volume of gas that contributes to the dilution, they tend to underestimate actual lung volume relative to both plethysmographic and radiographic methods in patients with air trapping and airflow obstruction. The clinical comparison between results from the different methods in a given patient is a useful means for assessing abnormalities in the distribution of ventilation.[15]

Recently there has been controversy in the literature regarding the accuracy of plethysmography in asthmatics, which has caused some authors to doubt the presence of overinflation during acute bronchial constriction. It is clear from both dilutional and radiographic evidence that TLC and FRC are both increased in asthma. This difference is useful as a way of quantifying the degree of underventilation in poorly ventilated lung areas.

Table 45-1. Lung Volumes and Capacities

Total lung capacity (TLC)	The total amount of air contained within the thoracic cage after a complete inspiration
Vital capacity (VC)	The amount of air that may be exhaled following a complete inspiration
Residual volume (RV)	The amount of air contained within the throracic cage after a complete exhalation
Functional residual capacity (FRC)	The amount of air contained within the thoracic cage after a normal tidal exhalation. This capacity contains both ERV and RV and is the point reached after a passive exhalation
Expiratory reserve volume (ERV)	The amount of air that may be exhaled from FRC
Inspiratory capacity (IC)	The amount of air that may be inspired from FRC
Inspiratory reserve volume (IRV)	The amount of air that may be inspired after a normal tidal inspiration
Tidal volume (V_T)	The amount of air inspired during quiet breathing

GAS DILUTION TECHNIQUES

Closed-Circuit Helium Dilution

Dilutional methods involve washing in an inert gas such as argon (A), neon (N), or more commonly helium (He). The subject is connected to a breathing circuit of known volume and inert gas concentration. The inert gas contained in the breathing circuit is mixed with the volume of air contained in the lungs at the time of switch-in. After equilibrium is reached between the subject and the circuit, the gas concentration provides an indication of the volume added to the circuit by the subject.

The most common implementation of closed-circuit He dilution has been the method developed by Herrald and McMichael.[16] In this technique, the subject rebreathes He from a spirometer while O_2 is added to maintain a constant system volume. An alternative approach, developed by Meneely et al.,[17,18] involves adding a bolus of O_2 sufficient to compensate for the O_2 consumed during the 3- to 7-minute rebreathing period associated with testing. In this method the system volume is constantly decreasing. Both techniques require switch-in at end-expiration and incorporate a correction for the switch-in error and He absorption. Figure 45-2 illustrates a rebreathing circuit.

Equipment

Essentially the circuit consists of a spirometer, a He analyzer, water and CO_2 scrubbers, a blower, and an O_2 source. He analyzers are typically thermal conductivity detectors, although mass spectrometers can also be used if the gas lost through the sampling port is returned to the circuit. Different gases have distinct thermal characteristics. The He analyzer compares the thermal conductivity of the sample gas with that of room air. Changes in thermal conductivity are assumed to result from changes in He concentration, which is a safe assumption if CO_2 and water are removed from the sample prior to analysis.

The CO_2 and water absorbers must be in-line and must not introduce leaks. Since CO_2 absorbers produce water, the water absorber must be placed between the CO_2 absorber and the He analyzer. Typically, the absorbers provide a color change to indicate when the absorber is exhausted. The absorbers should be checked prior to use with each patient.

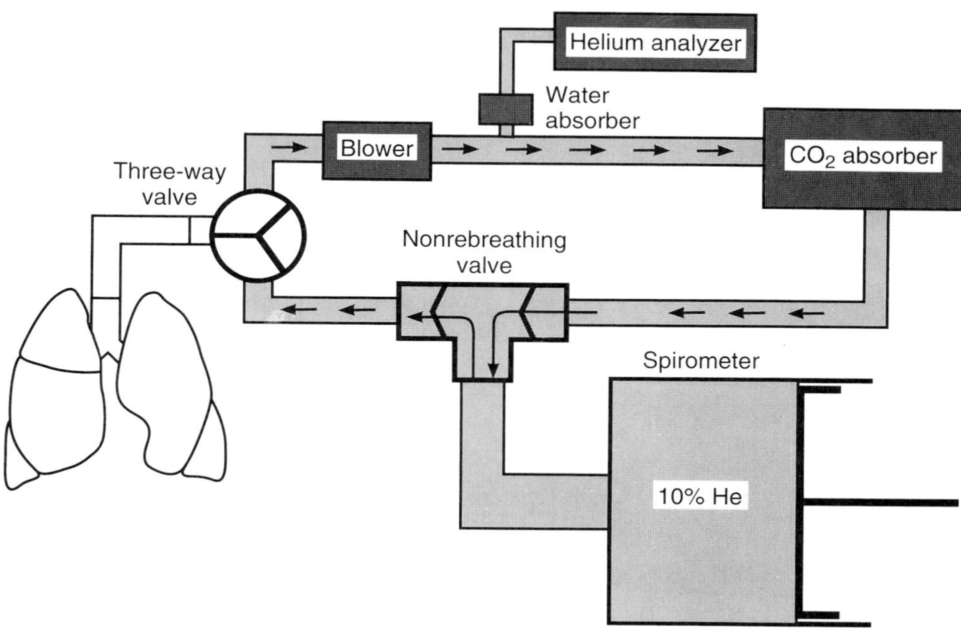

Figure 45-2. Schematic depiction of the closed-circuit He dilution technique for the determination of FRC or TLC. (From Snow,[7] with permission.)

The function of the blower is to keep the gas in the system uniformly mixed by continuously circulating the gas. Inadequate blower speeds compromise equilibration time estimates. Appropriate settings vary among spirometers and should be optimized for the system. The O_2 source is used to maintain a constant volume within the system by adding O_2 to match the patient's O_2 consumption. It is important to note that all gas passing through the He analyzer must be returned to the circuit.

For calculation of FRC the initial and final He concentration and the system volume must be known. The calculation of FRC is shown in Table 45-2.

Advantages and Disadvantages

The primary advantages of He rebreathing methodology are the minimal requirements for patient cooperation, the relatively low cost of the components, and that the analyzer need only be linear. The linearity of the He analyzer should be checked periodically by serial dilutions using a calibration syringe. Disadvantages include inability to measure poorly ventilated airspaces without prolonged rebreathing, difficulty in differentiating leaks from maldistribution, and difficulties relating to adequately cleaning the system.

Changes in O_2 or N_2 concentration will also introduce small errors. Meneely's study,[17,18] noted that changes in N_2 concentration result in slight errors in the He readings. A 100-mL or 1 percent change in O_2 volume caused a 25-mL change in calculated FRC. Assuming a 2500-mL bolus to accommodate up to 10 minutes of rebreathing, the resultant maximum error would be 250 mL. Small amounts of He are actually absorbed during the rebreathing. Meneely[17,18] suggested a correction of 200 mL to the final calculated FRC. Other investigators have suggested 100 mL.[19,20]

Additionally, the use of a chemical absorber to remove CO_2 can lead to underestimation of expiratory volumes, such as the expiratory reserve volume (ERV) or the VC, unless

Table 45-2. Determination of Lung Volume by Helium Dilution

Method 1
Calculate $V_{\text{dead space}}$ as follows

$$V_{\text{dead space}} = \frac{(He_{\text{final}})(V_{\text{He added}})}{He_{\text{initial}} - He_{\text{final}}}$$

After equilibration FRC is calculated as

$$FRC = \frac{(He_{\text{initial}} - He_{\text{final}})(V_{\text{dead space}} + V_{\text{added}})}{He_{\text{final}}}$$

Method 2
Alternatively, system volume can be calculated before and after the patient is connected to the system; the difference between the two calculations is the FRC

$$V_{\text{system}} = \frac{V_{\text{He added}}}{He_{\text{initial}}}$$

After equilibration

$$V_{\text{total}} = \frac{V_{\text{He added}}}{He_{\text{final}}} \quad \text{OR} \quad FRC = V_{\text{total}} - V_{\text{system}}$$

With either method the volume of the valve and connective tubing, which did not contain He at the start of the test, must be subtracted prior to reporting the results corrected. At least one manufacturer automatically adds a 5 percent correction to expiratory volumes. While some correction may be justified, the actual factor depends on the concentration of CO_2, the expiratory flow rate, and the efficiency of the absorber. An empirical determination of the appropriate correction factor should be made for manual systems.

FRC measurements are usually converted from ambient temperature and pressure, saturated (ATPS) to body temperature and pressure, saturated (BTPS). However, this correction has not been universally made, and methodology should be a factor when selecting reference values.

Open-Circuit Nitrogen Washout

The N_2 washout method uses a breathing mixture of high O_2 content to wash out the resident N_2. Since N_2 constitutes approximately 80 percent of the lung gases, collection of all the exhaled gas and determination of the volume of N_2 permits calculation of lung volume provided that the initial N_2 concentration in the lungs, the N_2 concentration in the exhaled volume, and the total exhaled volume are known. It is, of course, essential that all the N_2 in the collection bag come from the patient and not from inadequate flushing or leaks. This technique, initially described by Darling et al.[23] and Emannuel and associates,[24] is illustrated in Figure 45-3.

Numerous variations on the original method have been described. Most modern N_2 washout systems integrate N_2 concentration and expiratory flow on a breath-by-breath basis, as described by Brunner et al.[25] Basically, this involves integrating flow and N_2 and producing a cross-product equivalent to the N_2 leaving the lungs. This technique eliminates the need for a volume collection device and can provide a real time display of the measurement. Procedurally there are no differences between the two methods. The patient must be switched in at end expiration, and washout continues until N_2 has been flushed from the lung, which typically takes 2 to 7 minutes.

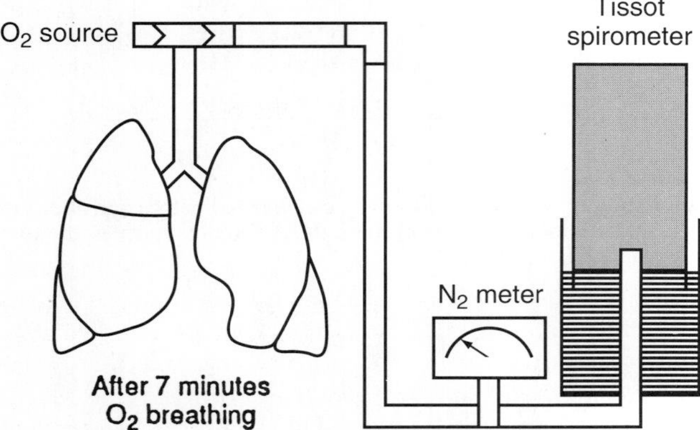

Figure 45-3. Schematic depiction of the open-circuit N_2 washout technique for the determination of FRC or TLC. Measurements are performed after patient breathes O_2 for 7 minutes. (From Snow,[7] with permission.)

Equipment

Equipment necessary to perform a N_2 washout test includes a N_2 analyzer, a collection circuit, a nonrebreathing valve, and an O_2 source. The computerized version substitutes a flow sensor for the collection circuit.

N_2 analysis is based on the principle that the intensity of emission within a spectral band of a gas discharge is proportional to the concentration of the component gas. The method uses a vacuum pump to introduce a gas sample into a low-pressure chamber within an electric field. When a high voltage is applied, ionization of the gas occurs, resulting in emission of radiant energy in the infrared, visible, and ultraviolet spectra. Each gas species appears in a particular band of wavelengths that contributes to the composite emission. Many gases emit in more than one wavelength. Selecting the wavelength to measure is largely based on avoiding interference and maximizing signal strength. By filtering out all but the desired wavelength, the N_2 concentration can be determined. This technique has been applied to other respiratory gases as well.[26]

Advantages and Disadvantages

The primary advantages of the N_2 washout method are the minimal cooperation required from the patient and the simplicity and ease of cleaning of the breathing circuit. Leaks can be easily detected visually. Additionally, a variety of indices for distribution of ventilation and determination of dead space are available from the N_2 washout data.[27,28] The primary disadvantages include inability to measure poorly ventilated airspaces and concerns about the suppression of hypoxic drive in patients by the use of elevated O_2 concentrations. An additional disadvantage is the relative complexity of the analyzer, which requires significant real time signal processing. This can cause subtle problems, which may be difficult to resolve.

When differential pressure flowmeters are used in conjunction with N_2 washout, viscosity corrections must be applied to the flow signal. Additionally, correction must be made for the phase delay difference between flow and N_2 analysis; this can be accomplished by measuring the actual delay associated with N_2 analysis and mathematically aligning the two signals prior to evaluating the cross-product integral.[29]

Single-Breath Techniques

Single-breath techniques for measuring TLC have been used with success.[21] The patient simply takes a single full inspiration of the test gas, and the concentration of the test gas in the exhaled sample reflects the dilution of the inspired concentration by the RV. This method, essentially the same as the alveolar volume measurement in single-breath diffu-

Table 45-3. Determination of Lung Volume by Single-Breath Techniques

For single-breath He dilution, the TLC can be determined as

$$TLC = (V_{inspired}) \left(\frac{He_{initial}}{He_{final}}\right)$$

Single-breath N_2 washout TLC would calculate as

$$TLC = (V_{inspired}) \left(\frac{N_{2\ initial}}{N_{2\ final}}\right)$$

sion, has been subject to criticism for underestimating TLC in patients with chronic obstructive pulmonary disease (COPD). Extrapolation techniques developed by Burns and Scheinhorn[22] in 1984 to correct the measured volume for the degree of airway obstruction may expand the use of this technique. Calculations of TLC from single-breath measurements are shown in Table 45-3.

OTHER METHODS

Body Plethysmography

DuBois et al.[30] described the modern application of body plethysmography, which is based on Boyle's law, according to which a volume of gas varies inversely with the pressure applied to it if temperature is held constant. In this application a patient sits within a sealed chamber. In the absence of respiratory efforts, the pressure within the chamber is ambient barometric pressure. As the patient inspires, the thoracic cage expands, creating an increased pressure in the surrounding chamber and causing the chamber volume to contract in compensation. If the volume of air in the patient's thoracic cage is fixed, pressure changes within the lungs caused by respiratory efforts can be correlated with changes in the chamber volume to calculate the thoracic gas volume. This approach requires the measurement of mouth pressure and plethysmograph volume changes. Mathematically, this can be stated as shown in Table 45-4.

Table 45-4. Determination of Lung Volume by Body Plethysmography

$$PV = P'V' \text{ (if temperature is held constant)}$$

$$P' = (P + \Delta P) \quad \text{and} \quad V' = (V - \Delta V)^{a}$$

$$PV = (P + \Delta P)(V - \Delta V)$$

$$V = P\left(\frac{\Delta V}{\Delta P}\right)$$

P, barometric pressure; V, thoracic gas volume to be measured; P′, associated changes in alveolar pressure; V′, associated changes in thoracic gas volume.

[a] The product of barometric pressure and thoracic gas volume are equal to the product of the pressure plus the change in pressure and the volume minus the change in volume. Solving the equation, for thoracic gas volume equals the product of barometric pressure and the ratio of the change in volume to the change in pressure.

In practice, this means occluding a shutter at the end of a tidal breath and having the subject softly pant or inspire against the shutter while sitting within a rigid cabinet. This has the effect of voluntarily compressing and decompressing the volume trapped within the thoracic cage. This volume change creates an inverse change in plethysmograph volume and a resultant change in alveolar pressure; the slope of the relationship between the volume change and the pressure change can be used to calculate the thoracic gas volume.

Equipment

Most plethysmograph cabinets are designed to minimize patient anxiety. Ease of entry, the patient's sense of control regarding ability to get out of the cabinet, and clear visual lines are design goals. Ease of entry is accomplished by a variety of schemes, generally by making the door as large as possible. Most modern cabinets provide a means for the patient to exit from the cabinet without operator assistance.

The plethysmograph cabinet must be rigid to minimize artifacts and to prevent damping of the signal. In general, since the box volume change is simply that produced by chest wall movement during small respiratory excursions, the smaller the cabinet, the greater the signal. This is particularly important in pediatric testing. This goal conflicts, however, with the need to avoid patient anxiety when entering an enclosed cabinet. As a result, most cabinet designs incorporate large surfaces of transparent acrylic for the walls and doors. Care must be taken to ensure that the acrylic surfaces are sufficiently rigid.

Rapid thermal equilibration is another requirement. Until the cabinet interior warms to approximately body temperature, testing cannot commence. Smaller cabinets offer faster equilibration but must be designed to avoid condensation on the acrylic surface, which would reduce visibility. Adequate cabinet venting will minimize the condensation problem.

Plethysmographs are designed to detect volume change within the cabinet by one of three methods (Fig. 45-4): volume measurement, pressure measurement, and flow integration. These type designations are descriptive of the methods used to monitor changes in cabinet internal volume associated with respiration. For the purpose of lung volume measurement, pressure is by far the most common.

Advantages and Disadvantages

The advantages of the pressure method include relatively low cost, high tolerance for leaks, and excellent sensitivity, frequency response, and reliability. With the pneumotachometer connected to the shutter, an integrated flow signal for performing spirometry is available.

Several studies have purported to show errors in the measurement of alveolar pressure in subjects with severe obstruction.[31–36] In most of the studies esophageal pressure was measured on the assumption that it would reflect alveolar pressure. However, alveolar pressure can only be

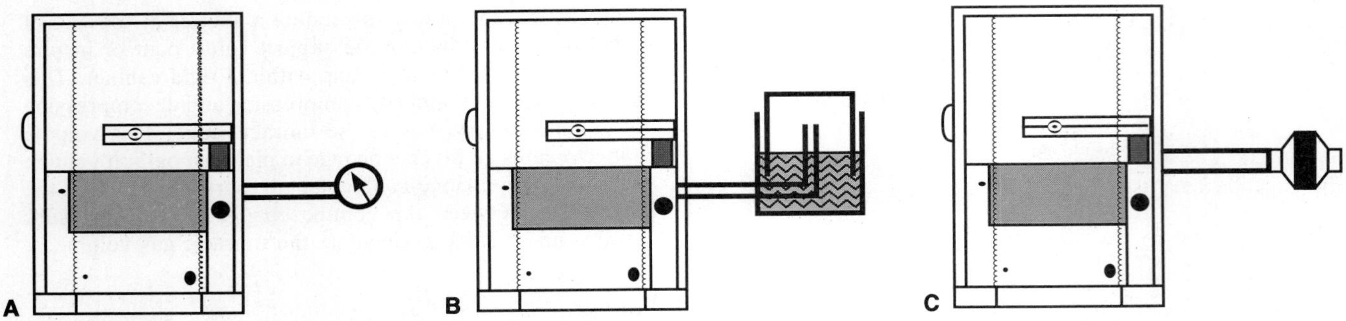

A B C

Figure 45-4. Schematic depiction of the three variations for the determination of total thoracic lung volume by body plethysmography. (**A**) pressure, (**B**) volume, (**C**) flow. (From Snow,[7] with permission.)

measured by this technique if there is no change in lung volume and if panting frequency is controlled. One explanation postulates preferential distribution of gas into highly compliant extrathoracic airways as opposed to more rigid intrathoracic airways. This explanation, however, would clearly involve lung volume changes and thus would invalidate the assumption that esophageal pressure reflects alveolar pressure. Failure of the studies to control panting frequency is an additional problem, since pleural pressure contains both an elastic and a resistive element. A convincing demonstration of the frequency dependency of the elastic contribution of pleural pressure was provided by Hida et al.[37]

Simulated obstructions using bronchial provocation or tracheal balloons do not behave in the same manner as does the diffuse obstruction typical of lung disease. Histamine has been shown to produce laryngeal narrowing as well as airway spasm. Narrowing of the trachea and larynx is as likely a cause for incomplete transmission of alveolar pressure to the mouth as is shunting of gas into more compliant extrathoracic airways.

There is substantial evidence that plethysmographic lung volumes correlate well with radiographic techniques in both normal subjects and those with severe obstruction.[38,39] Several studies have reported that use of controlled, low-frequency panting in plethysmographic tests eliminated the discrepancy for alveolar pressure determinations between mouth pressure and esophageal pressure.[32,34,40,41]

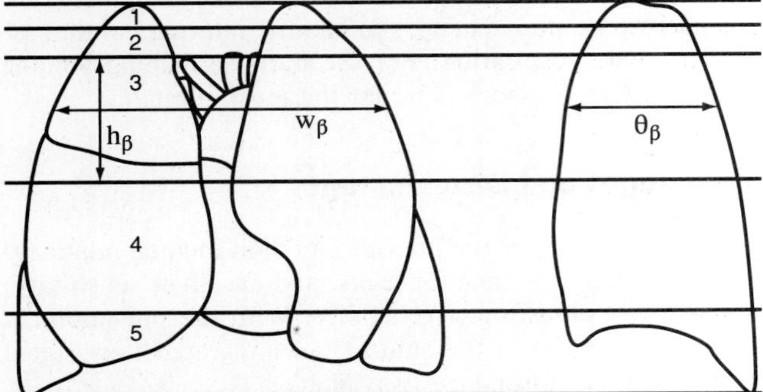

Figure 45-5. Illustration of the method of Barnhard et al.[42] for determination of TLC from radiographs. The lateral and posteroanterior radiographs are divided into a series of ellipsoids, the volumes of which are calculated and summed. (From Snow,[7] with permission.)

Radiographic Techniques

A standard posteroanterior chest radiograph, with or without a lateral view, can be used to measure TLC. The volume contained within the lungs can be calculated by measuring the height, width, and depth and accounting for the irregular shape of the lung. Determination of the lung boundaries on the chest radiograph and subtraction of nonlung volumes are required to accurately complete the measurement. Barnhard et al.[42] introduced the most widely used technique for estimating TLC from standard chest radiographs by an elliptical method (Fig. 45-5). Although their method provides significant improvement over previous methods, the amount of calculation time required has precluded widespread use. Various alternative techniques have been proposed that use different assumptions for outlining the lung and computer-assisted determinations.[43–48]

The major advantages of the radiographic technique are that it uses existing radiographic equipment and is not affected by air trapping or maldistribution of ventilation. Previous chest radiographs can provide a retrospective capability for assessing lung volumes over the course of a patient's illness. Also, the technique provides a complement to dilutional methods when assessing poorly communicating lung units and a cross-check on the reliability of plethysmographic results. Concerns have been raised regarding the potential errors that may result if the subject does not fully inspire prior to the radiograph. This was evaluated by Crapo et al.[49] who found minimal differences between TLC determined with normal instruction and with extra coaching, which has minimized concern regarding adequate inflation during the procedure.

References

1. Woolcock AJ, Read J: The static properties of the lungs in asthma. Am Rev Respir Dis 1968;98:788–794
2. Woolcock AJ, Colman MH, Blackburn CRB: Factors affecting normal values for ventilatory lung function. Am Rev Respir Dis 1972;106:692–709

3. Woolcock AJ, Read J: Lung volumes in exacerbations of asthma. Am J Med 1966;41:259–273
4. Martin J, Powell J, Shore S et al: The role of respiratory muscles in the hyperinflation of bronchial asthma. Am Rev Respir Dis 1980;121:441–447
5. Peress L, Sybrecht G, Macklem PT: The mechanisms of increase in total lung capacity during acute asthma. Am J Med 1976;61:165–169
6. Muller N, Bryan AC, Zamel N: Tonic inspiratory muscle activity as a cause of hyperinflation in histamine-induced asthma. J Appl Physiol 1980;49:869–874
7. Snow MG: Determination of functional residual capacity. Respir Care 1989;34:586–596
8. Ferris BG: Epidemiology standardization project. Am Rev Respir Dis 1978;118:105–111
9. Intermountain Thoracic Society Handbook. 2nd Ed. Intermountain Thoracic Society, Salt Lake City, 1984
10. ACCP Scientific Section Recommendations: The determination of static lung volumes. Chest 1984;86:471–474
11. Cobeel LJ: Comparison between measurement of functional residual capacity and thoracic gas volume in chronic obstructive pulmonary disease. Prog Respir Res 1969;4:194–204
12. Reichel G: Differences between intrathoracic gas measured by the body plethysmograph and functional residual capacity determined by gas dilution methods. Prog Respir Res 1968;4:188–193
13. Hickam JB, Frayser R: A comparative study of intrapulmonary gas mixing and functional residual capacity in pulmonary emphysema, using helium and nitrogen as the test gases. J Clin Invest 1958;37:567–573
14. Tierney DF, Nadel JA: Concurrent measurements of functional residual capacity by three methods. J Appl Physiol 1962;17:871–873
15. Fallat RJ, Snow MG: Distribution of ventilation. pp. 87–107. In Wilson A (ed): Pulmonary Function Testing Indications and Interpretations. Grune & Stratton, Orlando, 1985
16. Herrald FJC, McMichael J: Determination of lung volume, a constant volume modification of Christies's method. Proc R Soc Lond 1939;126:491–501
17. Meneely GR, Ball CO, Kory RC et al: A simplified closed circuit helium dilution method for the determination of residual volume of the lungs. Am J Med 1960;28:824–831
18. Meneely GR, Kaltreider NL: The volume of the lung determined by helium dilution: Description of the method and comparison with other procedures. J Clin Invest 1949;28:129–139
19. Zarins LP: Closed circuit helium dilution method of lung volume measurement. pp. 129–139. In Clausen JL (ed): Pulmonary Function Testing: Guidelines and Controversies. Academic Press, San Diego, 1982
20. Goldman HI, Becklake MR: Respiratory function tests; normal values at median altitudes and the prediction of normal results. Am Rev Respir Dis 1959;79:457–467
21. Hathirat S, Renzetti AD, Mitchell M: Measurement of total lung capacity by helium dilution in a constant volume system. Am Rev Respir Dis 1970; 102:760–770
22. Burns CB, Scheinhorn DJ: Evaluation of single-breath helium dilution total lung capacity in obstructive lung disease. Am Rev Respir Dis 1984;130:580–583
23. Darling RC, Cournand A, Richards DW: Studies on the intrapulmonary mixture of gases. III. An open circuit method for measuring residual air. J Clin Invest 1940;19:609–618
24. Emmanuel G, Briscoe WA, Cournand A: A method for the determination of the volume of air in the lungs: Measurement in chronic pulmonary emphysema. J Clin Invest 1961;20:329–337
25. Brunner JX, Wolff G, Cumming G, Langenstein H: Accurate measurement of N_2 volumes during N_2 washout requires dynamic adjustment of delay time. J Appl Physiol 1985;59:1008–1012
26. Fraser RB, Turney SZ: New method of respiratory gas analysis: Light spectrometer. J Appl Physiol 1985;59:1001–1007
27. Bouhuys A: Pulmonary nitrogen clearance in relation to age in healthy males. J Appl Physiol 1963;18:297–300
28. Cutillo AG, Perondi R, Turiel M et al: Informative value of simple multibreath nitrogen washout measurements for clinical and research purposes. Respiration 1985;47:81–89
29. Mitchell RR: Incorporation gas analyzer response time in gas exchange computations. J Appl Physiol 1979;47:1118–1122
30. DuBois AB, Botelho SY, Bedell GN et al: A rapid plethysmographic method for measuring thoracic gas volume: A comparison with a nitrogen washout method for measuring functional residual capacity in normal subjects. J Clin Invest 1956;35:322–326
31. Brown R, Ingram RH, McFadden ER: Problems in plethysmographic assessment of total lung capacity in asthma. Am Rev Respir Dis 1978;118:685–692
32. Rodenstein DO, Stanescu DC: Reassessment of lung volume measurement by helium dilution and body plethysmography in chronic airflow obstruction. Am Rev Respir Dis 1982;126:1040–1044
33. Rodenstein DO, Stanescu DC, Francis C: Demonstration of failure of body plethysmography in airway obstruction. J Appl Physiol 1982;52:949–954
34. Shore SA, Huk O, Mannix S, Martin JC: Effect of panting frequency on the plethysmographic determination of thoracic gas volume in chronic obstructive pulmonary disease. Am Rev Respir Dis 1983;128:54–59
35. Shore S, Milic-Emili J, Martin JG: Reassessment of body plethysmographic technique for the measurement of thoracic gas volume in asthmatics. Am Rev Respir Dis 1982;126:515–520
36. Stanescu DC, Rodenstein DO, Cauberghs M, Van de Woestijne KP: Failure of body plethysmography in bronchial asthma. J Appl Physiol 1982;52:939–948
37. Hida W, Suzuki S, Sasaki H et al: Effect of ventilatory frequency on regional transpulmonary pressure in normal adults. J Appl Physiol 1981;51:678–685
38. Lloyd HM, String ST, Dubois AB: Radiographic and plethysmographic determination of total lung capacity. Radiology 1965;86:7–14
39. Nicklaus JM, Watanabe S, Mitchell MM, Renzetti AD: Roentgenographic, physiologic and structural estimations of total lung capacity in normal and emphysematous subjects. Am J Med 1967;42:547–552
40. Desmond KJ, Demizio DL, Allen PD et al: An alternate method for the determination of functional residual capacity in a plethysmograph. Am Rev Respir Dis 1988;137:273–277
41. Habbib MP, Engel LA: Influence of the panting technique on the measurement of thoracic gas line. Am Rev Respir Dis 1978;117:265–271
42. Barnhard HF, Pierce JA, Joyce JW, Bates JH: Roentgenographic determination of total lung capacity. Am J Med 1960;28:51–60
43. Barrett WA, Clayton PD, Lambson CR, Morris AG: Computerized roentgenographic determination of total lung capacity. Am Rev Respir Dis 1976;113:239–244
44. Miller RD, Offord KP: Roentgenologic determination of total lung capacity. Mayo Clin Proc 1980;55:694–699
45. Nicklaus TM, Stowell DW, Christiansen WR, Renzetti AD: The accuracy of the roentgenologic diagnosis of chronic pulmonary emphysema. Am Rev Respir Dis 1966;93:889–899
46. Pierce RJ, Brown DJ, Holmes M et al: Estimation of lung volume from chest roentgenographs. Thorax 1979;34:726–734
47. Seeley GW, Mazzeo J, Borgstrom M et al: Radiologic total lung capacity measurement. Eur J Radiol 1986;6:262–265
48. Teklu B, Gray WM, Mills RJ, Moran F: A critical appraisal of a rapid radiographic method of determining total lung capacity. Scott Med J 1986;31:99–102
49. Crapo RO, Montague T, Armstrong J: Inspiratory lung volume achieved on routine chest films. Invest Radiol 1979;14:137–140

Chapter 46

Assessment of Airflow

Michael G. Snow
Richard K. Beauchamp

CHAPTER OUTLINE

Airflow assessment from various breathing maneuvers is widely used as a noninvasive indicator of the mechanical properties of the lungs to provide information on the integrated functional performance of the elastic and resistive forces, pressure-volume relationship, and patency of the airways. Fundamental concepts regarding the assessment of airflow are presented.

DETERMINANTS OF AIRFLOW

Although airflow assessment can usually detect airway dysfunction, it is generally nonspecific, since a variety of factors may affect it. These factors are expressed in Poiseuille's law

$$\text{Flow} = \frac{(\Delta P)(\pi)(r^4)}{(8)(L)(\eta)} \qquad (1)$$

where ΔP is the pressure difference between the lungs and mouth (driving pressure), r is the radius of the airways, L is the length of the airways, and η is the viscosity of the gas. While the effects of airway length and gas viscosity are generally negligible, the driving pressure and the radius of the airway are the primary determinants of airflow. Driving pressure is a function of expiratory force (patient effort), lung elasticity, and frictional resistance. The radius or caliber of the airway, along with a variety of frictional forces, is the primary component of airway resistance.

Flow also can be characterized as a function of pressure and resistance. Using the analogy of Ohm's law for electrical circuits we have

$$\text{Flow} = \frac{\Delta P}{R_{AW}} \qquad (2)$$

where ΔP is the driving pressure and R_{AW} is the airway resistance. As can be seen, flow is inversely related to airway resistance.

The equation can be rearranged to solve for airway resistance as

$$R_{AW} = \frac{\Delta P}{\text{flow}} \quad (3)$$

Flow can be measured easily and driving pressure can be measured intermittently by occluding a shutter at the airway. The only assumption is that mouth pressure equals alveolar pressure when the shutter is occluded. Airway resistance is a measure of the caliber of the airways and, since it can be measured during shallow panting or quiet breathing, it does not require maximal effort. Accordingly, it is a valuable index for monitoring airway changes and for distinguishing between decreases in flow due to dynamic factors, such as those occurring in emphysema, and decreases due to intrinsic airway narrowing, such as those seen in asthma and bronchitis.

Airflow occurs when the driving pressure exceeds the elastic and resistive properties of the lungs that oppose flow. During quiet breathing, diaphragmatic contraction creates a subatmospheric pressure differential relative to the pressure at the mouth as the lung is distended. Essentially, the lungs and the airways are stretched. When this effort is sufficient to overcome the airway resistance, inspiratory flow occurs. During passive exhalation, these same elastic forces in the absence of inspiratory effort cause the lung to recoil. In other words, the lungs, having been stretched, will tend to return to their resting level. As the pressure differential exceeds the resistance, exhalation occurs.

Forced expiratory efforts create a much more complex interrelationship of pressures and flows. The primary determinants of forced expiratory flow are expiratory force, lung recoil, bronchial obstruction, and bronchial stability. During a forced expiration from total lung capacity (TLC) the lungs are again distended. Pleural pressure increases around the alveoli and the airway. This pressure is proportional to effort and, during the initial phase, to elastic recoil, causing a general compression on the alveoli and airway. As lung volume decreases, the contribution from elastic recoil also decreases until airway narrowing occurs. From this point, elastic recoil and airway structural support work to oppose airway collapse. Figure 46-1 illustrates this concept. Emphysematous changes reduce lung elastic recoil and impair the ability of the airways to remain open during sustained expiratory effort. As airway radius is altered by mucosal swelling and/or hypersecretion (as in bronchitis), bronchospasm (as in asthma), or airway compression (as in emphysema), airway resistance increases and airflow decreases.

Airflow is susceptible to pathophysiologic changes associated with airway dysfunction. Understanding how these changes limit airflow is essential to obtaining meaningful assessments of airflow. Careful evaluation of the patterns of abnormality reflected by airflow assessment can provide objective clinical information for monitoring acutely ill and chronically dysfunctional patients, for evaluation of the degree of disability, and for documentation of response to therapy and/or environmental agents and thus can aid in developing a differential diagnosis.

BASIC SPIROMETRY

Patient Performance

Unlike the situation with most laboratory tests, patient performance is critical to obtaining valid measures of air-

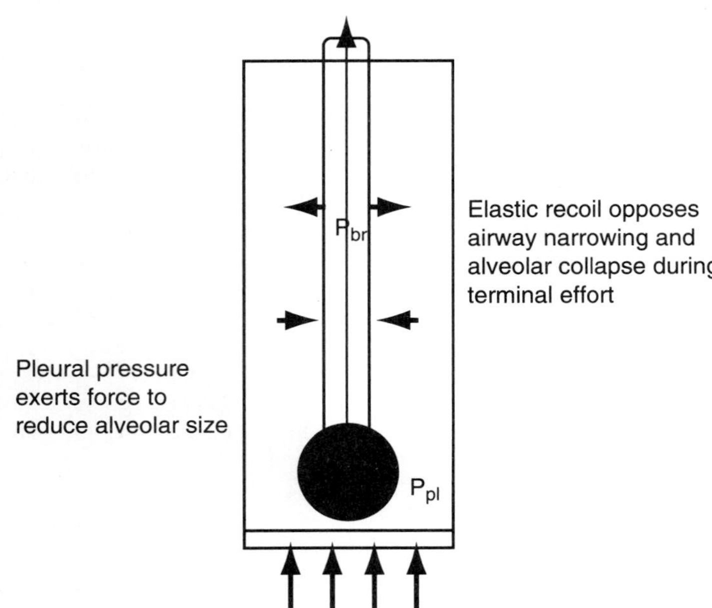

Elastic recoil opposes airway narrowing and alveolar collapse during terminal effort
P_{br}
Pleural pressure exerts force to reduce alveolar size
P_{pl}

Figure 46-1. Schematic representation of factors determining airflow during forced expiration. P_{pl}, pleural pressure; P_{br}, bronchial pressure. See text for discussion.

flow. The patient must learn a particular sequence of breathing maneuvers and perform these maneuvers with maximal effort. This process can be confusing and quite tiring to elderly or debilitated patients, something that places a limit on the number of repetitions that can be obtained. Even in younger asthmatic patients, repeated efforts can lead to increased bronchospasm, which will alter test results. A limit of the total number of efforts is usually set by the laboratory. The guidelines published by the American Thoracic Society (ATS) for the performance of spirometry[1] suggest eight efforts as a maximum. Additionally, sufficient time must be provided between efforts for debilitated patients. The amount of time between efforts will vary depending on the patient, but as a general rule, the patient should be breathing as easily before subsequent efforts as prior to the first effort.

Accordingly, it is critical that the entire process be thoroughly explained prior to testing to minimize unnecessary efforts. Certain common elements are necessary to proper instruction of patients, and include the following:

1. Explanation of the use of the mouthpiece and noseclips
2. What is being measured (i.e., amount of air being exhaled and how fast)
3. What the patient must do (inhale fully and exhale forcefully, smoothly, and completely)
4. Likely outcomes (i.e., several efforts to obtain most reproducible test)
5. Supplementing the explanation of the procedure with an actual demonstration will usually elicit better patient understanding

Explaining the use of the mouthpiece and noseclips helps to allay patient anxiety about the procedure. Many patients are nervous about the testing, and it is important to reassure them that the test is noninvasive (no needles) and only requires them to breath room air.

Forced Vital Capacity

The general procedure for performing forced vital capacity (FVC) or flow-volume maneuvers with combined inspiratory and expiratory curves consists of the following procedural steps:

1. Have the patient begin breathing quietly on the mouthpiece with noseclip positioned.
2. Instruct the patient to inspire fully.
3. After ensuring complete inspiration, encourage the patient to exhale forcefully and completely. This should be accompanied with enthusiastic coaching.
4. The patient should continue to exhale until no observable volume change is detected for at least 2 seconds.
5. Instruct the patient to inspire forcefully and completely, again with appropriate coaching.
6. After the patient has inspired completely, remove the noseclips and have the patient return to quiet breathing.
7. Evaluate the effort and repeat the maneuver at least three times. The two best acceptable efforts should agree within 5 percent for both FVC and forced expiratory volume in 1 second (FEV_1).

Some laboratories separate the inspiratory and expiratory procedures in order to permit the patient to focus each effort. This approach is based on the premise that some patients may have difficulty coordinating the composite maneuver and better individual efforts may be obtained. Regardless of whether the maneuver is combined or fragmented, the instructions are similar. After a complete forceful expiration, it is desirable for the patient to inspire fully even if not as fast as possible. Many severely obstructed patients, with decreased elastic recoil, collapse their airways during forced exhalation, and the act of inspiring fully will help to reopen the airways. After forced inspiration it is only necessary for the patient to return to quiet breathing.

Calculated Variables

Numerous variables are calculated from the FVC curve. These include either relationships between various maneuvers, such as FVC/vital capacity (FVC/VC); exhaled volume assessed at a specific time of exhalation (forced expiratory volume in a given time period [FEV_x]); flow rates at a specific point in time or specific interval (forced expiratory flow at time x or interval x [FEF_x]); or ratios between measurements (e.g., FEV_1/FVC).

Vital Capacity

VC, whether forced or slow, may be defined as the amount of air that can be exhaled from a complete inspiration. Calculation of VC simply requires identifying the points of maximum inspiration and maximum exhalation, the difference between which is the VC. A variety of subdivisions are typically made from the VC maneuver. These include tidal volume (V_T), expiratory reserve volume (ERV), inspiratory capacity (IC), and inspiratory reserve volume (IRV). Figure 46-2 illustrates these subdivisions.

Forced Expiratory Volumes

A forced expiratory volume (FEV) is the maximum volume exhaled during a timed interval.[2,3] The specific FEV identifies the volume exhaled from the start of exhalation to the specified time. For example, as shown in Figure 46-3, FEV_1 indicates the volume expired during the first second of effort. Several timed volumes are typically reported. The most commonly used are $FEV_{0.5}$, FEV_2, FEV_3, and FEV_6.

The onset of exhalation is determined by a process called *back-extrapolation*, an example of which is illustrated in Figure 46-4. By convention, the time at which the forced max-

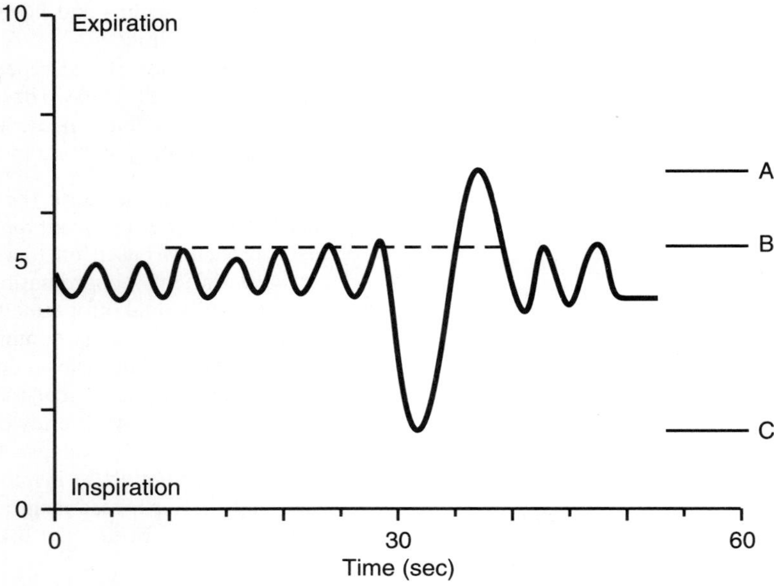

Figure 46-2. Components of the slow vital capacity (SVC). The idealized end-expiratory level is shown by the dotted line. The VC is the volume between A and C, the inspiratory capacity (IC) is the volume between B and C, and the expiratory reserve volume (ERV) is the volume between A and B. (From Beauchamp,[32] with permission.)

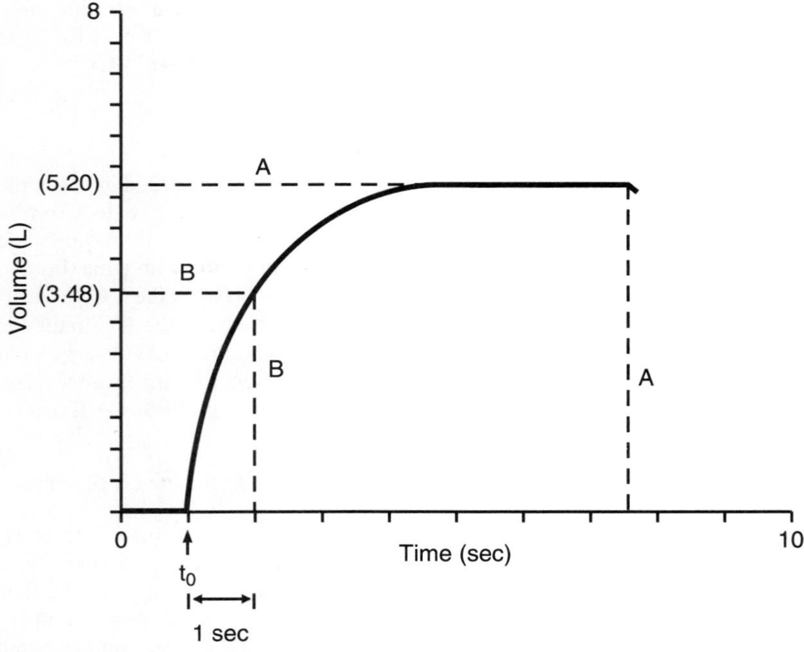

Figure 46-3. Measurement of FVC and FEV_t in the volume-time format. FVC is the maximum volume, shown here by dotted line A (5.20 L in this example). FEV_t is determined as the volume expired at the specified time (t) from t_0 (see Fig. 46-4). Shown here, by dotted line B, is measurement of FEV_1, which is the volume expired at 1 second from t_0 (3.48 L in this example). (From Beauchamp,[32] with permission.)

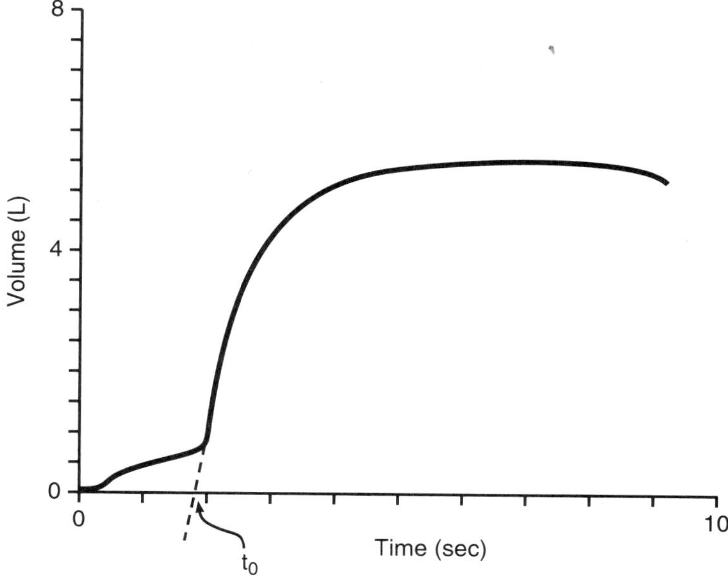

Figure 46-4. Determination of time zero (t_0) at which to begin measurement of time for FEV_t measurements. A line (dotted line) is drawn through the steepest portion of the volume-time curve; the point at which this line intercepts the time line (x-axis) is t_0. (From Beauchamp,[32] with permission.)

imum expiratory flow rate (FEFmax) was reached is identified and a tangent is drawn.[4] From maximal inspiration a line is drawn to intersect with the tangent and this intersection is used as the start time for the calculation of timed volumes. The back-extrapolation volume, usually expressed as a percentage of the FVC, is an indication of hesitation or false starting and according to ATS guidelines should not exceed 5 percent. However, in a patient with a large FVC (e.g., greater than 6 L) it may be difficult to achieve FEFmax in less than 5 percent even with a maximal effort.

Forced Expiratory Flow

Forced expiratory flow (FEF) is an expression of either instantaneous flow at a particular point in the FVC (e.g., FEF_{50}) or average flow over a specific interval (e.g., FEF_{25-75}). Instantaneous flow is measured from the flow-volume curve, and the numerical designation indicates the percentage of volume exhaled from the beginning of exhalation. For example, FEF_{60} indicates the instantaneous flow after 60 percent of the FVC has been exhaled. Figures 46-5 and 46-6 illustrate FEF calculation. By contrast, FEF reported over an interval such as FEF_{25-75} is usually taken from a volume-time tracing, although computerized systems can derive it from the flow-volume curve. By definition, FEF_{25-75} refers to the average flow measured from 25 to 75 percent of the FVC. Other commonly used intervals include $FEF_{200-1200}$, which refers to the average flow between 200 and 1200 mL of the FVC, and FEF_{75-85}.

Forced Inspiratory Volume and Flow

Forced inspiratory flow (FIF) is computed just as is FEF but from the inspiratory side of the curve. By convention, the percent refers to the percentage of inspired volume from the beginning of inspiration.

Ratios

Frequently, it is useful to refer the timed volumes to the FVC or slow VC (SVC), as with FEV_1/FVC. The ratio identified is implicit and displayed as a percentage (e.g., 75 percent). In the United States it is most common to use the FVC as reference, whereas in Europe it is more common to refer to the SVC. Other ratios that are frequently encountered include the FEF_{25-75}/FVC or the FEF_{75-85}/FVC. These ratios can refer to either the absolute value for each variable or to the percent of the predicted value. For example

	Observed Value	Percent of Predicted Value
FVC	4.8	100
FEF_{25-75}	2.4	60
FEF_{25-75}/FVC	50%	60

The ratio calculated by using absolute values is 50 percent, but when the percent of predicted value is used, the ratio is 60 percent. In the presence of restriction without underlying obstruction, the assumption is that the FEF_{25-75} will de-

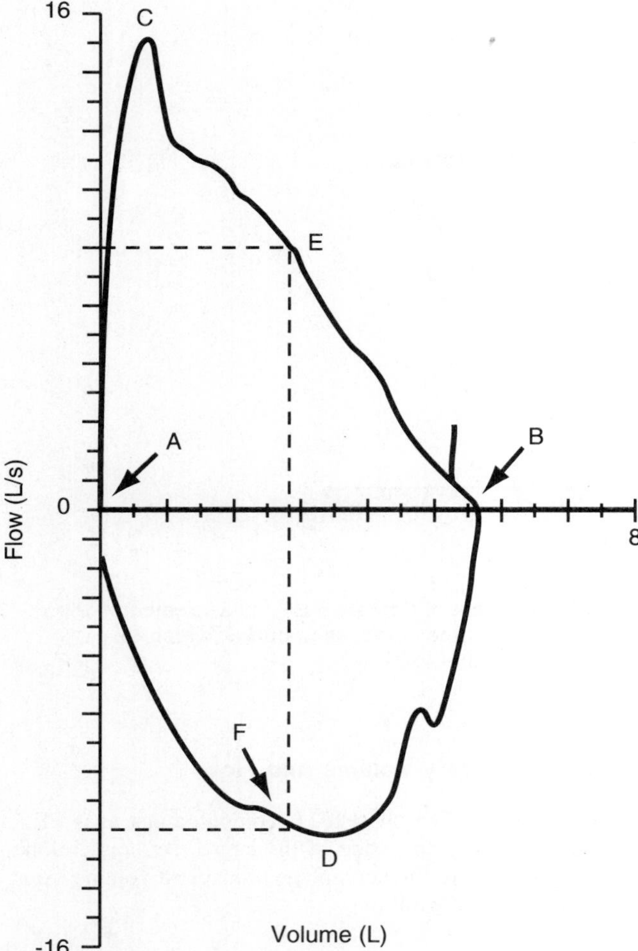

Figure 46-5. Determination of flow-volume parameters. The FVC is the volume between A and B (5.60 L in this example). The FIVC is the volume between B and A; the FVC and the FIVC are equal in this example but will often differ in clinical subjects. The FEFmax (PEF[R]) is represented by point C (15.2 L/s in this example), the FIFmax (PIF[R]) by point D (10.3 L/s in this example). FEF_x is determined by locating point x (a percent of FVC) and reading the flow at this point. In this example line EF is drawn through 50 percent of the FVC; point E is the FEF_{50} (7.8 L/s in this example), and point F is the FIF_{50} (10.1 L/s in this example). (From Beauchamp,[32] with permission.)

crease proportionally with the FVC. Therefore, a disproportionate decrease would indicate an additional obstructive process. Table 46-1 defines the common terms.

Assessment of Patient Effort

Because maximal flows are determined by proper patient performance, it is essential that the patient be appropriately coached. Failure to obtain patient cooperation and maximal effort can render the results worthless. The ATS recommendations also address effort analysis.[1] Evaluation of effort from FVC or flow-volume curves centers around five main points:

1. Maximal inspiration
2. Maximal exhalation without hesitation or false starts
3. Smooth, continuous exhalation
4. Adequate duration of expiratory effort
5. Reproducibility of subsequent efforts

Failure to inspire or exhale fully can cause underestimation of FVC, FEV_1, and all instantaneous flows. To some extent maximal inspiration can be assessed by the reproducibility of the test results. Additionally, it is important to observe the patient's inspiratory effort as well as review the display for sustained effort near TLC. Expiratory effort can be evaluated by observing the terminal portion of the curve. There should not be an abrupt transition from expiratory to inspiratory flow; rather expiratory flow should taper gradually, with no observable volume change for at least 2 seconds. Also, the duration of the expiratory effort, which should be at least 6 seconds, provides an indication of a complete exhalation.

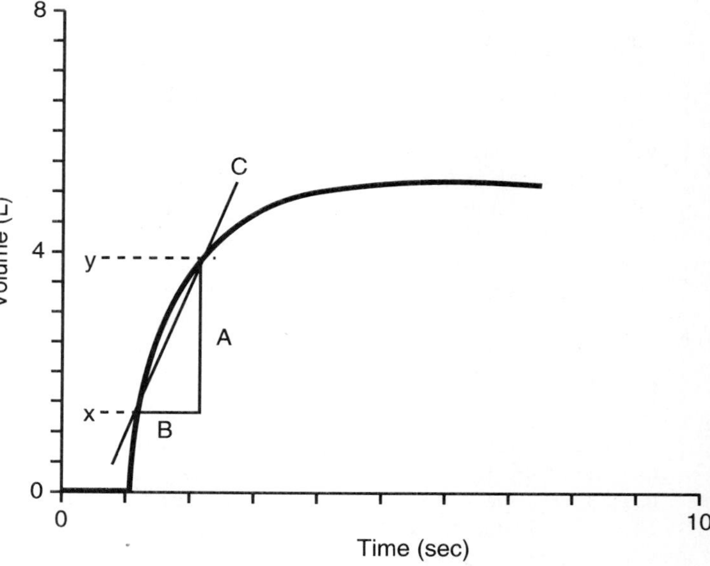

Figure 46-6. Measurement of FEF_{x-y}. The first step is to locate the points specified by x and y. The case illustrated here is FEF_{25-75}; x is 25 percent of FVC (1.3 L in this case), y is 75 percent of FVC (3.9 L). FEF_{x-y} is then calculated either as (1) the volume represented by x − y (A) divided by the time required to expire the volume (B), or (2) the slope of a line (C) drawn through points x and y. Method 2 has the twofold advantage of always allowing one to use 1 second for B, so that A is the value for FEF_{x-y} without any division being necessary, and of allowing one to expand A and B in cases in which one or both may be too small to resolve accurately (e.g., with very high or very low flows). (From Beauchamp,[32] with permission.)

Table 46-1. Spirometry Definitions

FVC	Difference between the lowest and highest volumes obtained during the maneuver.
FIVC	Maximal difference between the highest volume obtained and the lowest volume obtained during maximal inspiration.
FEVC	Maximal difference between the lowest volume obtained and the highest volume obtained during maximal expiration.
FEFmax	Highest measured flow during expiration.
FEV_x	Highest instantaneous expiratory flow is found, a tangent is drawn, and the intersection with minimum measured volume on the maneuver (maximal inspiration) is used for back-extrapolation.
FEF_x	The flow corresponding to the specified percentage is reported by performing a linear interpolation between the surrounding data points.
FIV_x	Highest instantaneous inspiratory flow is found, a tangent is drawn and the intersection with the minimum measured volume on the maneuver (maximal inspiration) is used for back-extrapolation.
FEF_{x-y} **FIF_{x-y}**	The flow data (expiratory or inspiratory) between the selected volume points is averaged and a linear interpolation is made between the data surrounding the selected points.

The initial portion of the exhalation should show an abrupt and unhesitating start. Any hesitation or false start in this initial period can result in underestimation of FEFmax and FEV_1. Back-extrapolation volume must be less than 5 percent of the FVC. During exhalation the display should be smooth and continuous until complete. There should be no coughing during the first second of exhalation.

Observing the patient's second full inspiration provides an important clue to good effort. This inspiration should match the initial one. Failure to achieve the same inspiratory volume or inspiring more the second time indicates either a lack of understanding or inadequate effort.

Finally, the results between subsequent efforts should agree. A minimum of three acceptable efforts should be obtained that meet the above criteria. The two largest FVC and FEV_1 values should be within 5 percent or 100 mL, whichever is greater. FEFmax should agree within 10 percent of the largest value obtained from previous maneuvers. Reproducibility criteria should only be applied to acceptable efforts.

Effort analysis for flow-volume curves should include the same criteria proposed for volume-time tracings. Reproducibility can easily be assessed by overlaying individual efforts. The curves should match when superimposed if the efforts are consistent. Moreover, the FEFmax is perhaps the most sensitive indicator of patient effort. Submaximal effort in a patient with dynamic airway compression can actually result in a higher FEV_1.[5] Consistent FEFmax values and overlapping flow-volume curves are strong evidence for maximal effort.

MAXIMAL VOLUNTARY VENTILATION

The maximal voluntary ventilation (MVV) may be defined as the largest total volume of air that can be moved during a 10- to 15-second interval as a result of repeated voluntary effort. The results are reported as liters per minute at body temperature and pressure, saturated (BTPS). The MVV provides a simple overall test of breathing capacity. A normal result largely rules out significant obstructive or neuromuscular disease. The test is entirely nonspecific since it integrates the results of respiratory muscle strength and control, elastic and resistive properties of the airways, and patient motivation. Subtle abnormalities in these subcomponents may not be detected. However, the test is probably more sensitive to changes secondary to neuromuscular disease, particularly those affecting muscle endurance or coordination, than FVC alone. This makes MVV measurements a useful tool for detecting trends.

The maneuver consists of having the patient breathe deeply and rapidly for 10 to 15 seconds. The total volume moved will be a function of the volume of each breath and the respiratory rate. The respiratory rate selected by the patient provides an indication of the primary response to exertion. The volume moved per breath should be greater than the V_T usually approaching the FEV_1. The highest value is usually obtained with volumes approaching 60 percent of the FVC and rates of 60 to 90 per minute.

Calculations can be made by two techniques. The most common approach is to compute the average volume per breath during the measurement interval and multiply this value by the respiratory rate. Alternatively, the sum of all expiratory volumes can be used and extrapolated from the collection interval to 1 minute. An example of these calculations is shown in Figure 46-7.

Generally, the MVV is calculated for 12 seconds and extrapolated to 60 seconds. An alternative approach is to also calculate a 6-second value and report this as a percent of the 12-second value. With good effort, there should be no significant difference between these values in normal patients. Patients with severe obstruction would show reduced values for both calculations, while patients with neuromuscular disease or less than maximal effort will produce different results. This provides a useful tool for differentiating between underlying pathology and patient motivation without adding to the complexity or duration of the test.

BEDSIDE SPIROMETRY

Spirometry performed at the bedside is probably the easiest method for assessing lung mechanics in spontaneously breathing patients. FEV_1 is widely accepted as an indicator of significant problems in gas exchange, while an adequate VC is frequently used as a criterion for predicting successful weaning from mechanical ventilation. Bedside spirometry is also valuable for assessing response to respiratory therapy, preoperative risk, and postoperative complications.

Performance of bedside spirometry parallels that of spi-

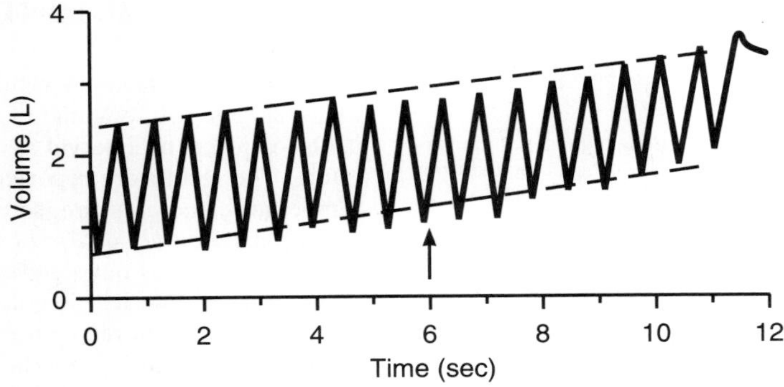

Figure 46-7. Calculation of MVV by averaging excursions. For MVV maneuvers with fairly linear end-expiratory and end-inspiratory levels, the MVV can be computed by drawing lines (the dotted lines shown here) through the end-expiratory and end-inspiratory points, taking the volume at the median time (shown here by the arrow), multiplying that volume by 60 times the number of excursions, and dividing the product by the number of seconds for which excursions were counted. (From Beauchamp,[32] with permission.)

rometry in the laboratory. However, certain aspects of effort analysis are even more critical when the testing is performed at the bedside. Patient position or posture can have significant impact on the results and must be noted. Additional notation must be made of patient cooperation, since a patient's medication can affect mental status and therefore the patient's understanding of the instructions. Caution should be used in interpreting the FEV_1/FVC ratio, since many factors can contribute to underestimation of the FVC and thereby to an erroneous assessment of the degree of airflow obstruction.

Bedside spirometry also places significantly different requirements on equipment than does testing in the pulmonary function laboratory. In addition to accuracy requirements, movement from bed to bed requires portability, which makes size a paramount concern. Instrument warmup time and calibration requirements are also important considerations.

PEAK FLOW

Assessment of peak expiratory flow (PEF) using portable peak flowmeters has been recommended for home use by asthmatic patients to provide an indication of airway status and the need for self-administration of bronchodilators. Although strong correlation exists between PEF and FEV_1 in asthmatic persons, significant discrepancies can occur owing to the relatively greater effort dependence of PEF than of FEV_1.[6,7] This is because the two measurements reflect different determinants; PEF reflects not only the intrinsic resistance of the large airways but also the effect of dynamic compression to a greater degree than does FEV_1. Various studies comparing results between PEF and FEV_1 in patients being assessed for bronchial hyperreactivity[8,9] have led to the conclusion that PEF was less useful than FEV_1. The standard error of PEF measurements is significantly greater than that of FEV_1, which suggests that PEF should be substituted for FEV_1 measurements only after careful consideration and with thorough patient instruction.

Procedurally, the patient should be instructed to inspire fully and exhale as forcefully as possible. At least two determinations should be made to assess reproducibility, and these should agree within 10 percent. It is not necessary for the patient to exhale completely. If the results do not agree, repeat efforts should be made. In general, the maximal value should be selected.

It frequently is asserted that measurement of PEF is easier than measurement of FEV_1. In fact, if measurement of FVC is unnecessary, the patient effort is the same. The primary advantage of PEF measurements is the cost associated with the measurement device, and this may, in fact, be the deciding factor, but the decision should be carefully made after weighing the differences in sensitivity, specificity, and standard error.

The type of peak flowmeter can have a profound effect on the results. In recent tests of available spirometers, no turbine devices passed the minimal criteria.[10] This study also showed significant differences between types of devices on the same flow patterns. These results indicate a need for caution when establishing action limits for unsupervised patients.

AIRWAY RESISTANCE

Airway resistance is most commonly measured by the plethysmographic or interrupter method, both of which have been well described by numerous investigators.[11–16] Plethysmographic determinations can be made with either panting or quiet breathing, while the interrupter method is used only during quiet breathing.

Plethysmographic measurements are made most commonly in the United States by the panting technique. This requires the patient to pant gently for a few seconds at a rate of two or three times per second. Subsequently, a shutter is closed and the pressure is recorded as the patient continues to pant. The pants should only move small volumes, as the panting is designed to minimize the effect of temperature and humidity differences between inspiratory and expiratory gases. Other reasons for panting include phase alignment of the pressure signals and minimization of the oropharyngeal component of resistance.

"Quiet breathing" measurements in a body plethysmograph represent something of a misnomer. The method usually involves breathing at a slightly higher than normal respiratory rate, 30 to 60 breaths per minute. While not actually requiring panting, the method does require some patient cooperation. Results from quiet breathing are generally somewhat higher than from panting measurements. It should also be noted that quiet breathing measurements in a body plethysmograph require subtle changes in software and hardware relative to panting measurements, which may not be available for all plethysmographs.

In either case, the flow and pressure signals are displayed as a function of plethysmographic volume changes, creating two separate curves for flow versus volume and pressure versus volume; the ratio of the two slopes represents the airway resistance. The resistance of the breathing circuit must be considered. Calculations basically are made as follows:

$$R_{AW} = \frac{\text{slope (flow/volume)}}{\text{slope (pressure/volume)}} \qquad (4)$$

The interrupter method is based on the assumption that brief interruptions in quiet breathing produce a balance of pressure. The airways are occluded for short periods (less than 0.1 second) three to five times per second. During occlusion, the mouth pressure should reflect transpulmonary pressure if measured from the plateau that occurs after an initial overshoot. The measurement therefore reflects the total resistance of the respiratory system, including the airway resistance component. This technique requires little patient cooperation and is also appropriate for patients in the intensive care setting. An illustration of panting and quiet breathing measurements is shown in Figure 46-8.

BRONCHODILATOR RESPONSE

Much of respiratory care is aimed at dilating narrowed airways through drug therapy. The efficacy of a bronchodilator is most commonly gauged, at least in the United States, by differences in airflow measurements before and after its administration. Such comparisons may be made either following an individual aerosolized or parenteral dose of the bronchodilator or after a course of oral medication.

The percent change from the predrug to postdrug values is computed as

$$\left(\frac{\text{Postdrug} - \text{predrug}}{\text{predrug}}\right)(100) = \text{percent change} \qquad (5)$$

The FEV_1 is by far the most often used index for bronchodilator response, but the other airflow variables can be useful as well. There is significant variation among the changes proposed by various authors as being required for significance. The very legitimate point is sometimes made that any single value for a given degree of improvement is probably inappropriate. By way of illustration, a 15 percent improvement in someone whose predrug value is 25 percent of predicted probably has very different implications than a 15 percent improvement in someone whose predrug value was 75 percent of predicted. Nevertheless, this approach remains the most widely used. The most important consideration is that changes must be viewed in context rather than individually.

There are two other points to be made concerning assessment of bronchodilator response by airflow measurements. The first is that in the case of acute response assessment, it is essential to wait a sufficient time after administration of the bronchodilator to realize the physiologic effect of the drug. While many subjects may show symptomatic improvement within a few minutes, the peak physiologic response may not occur until 15 minutes afterward

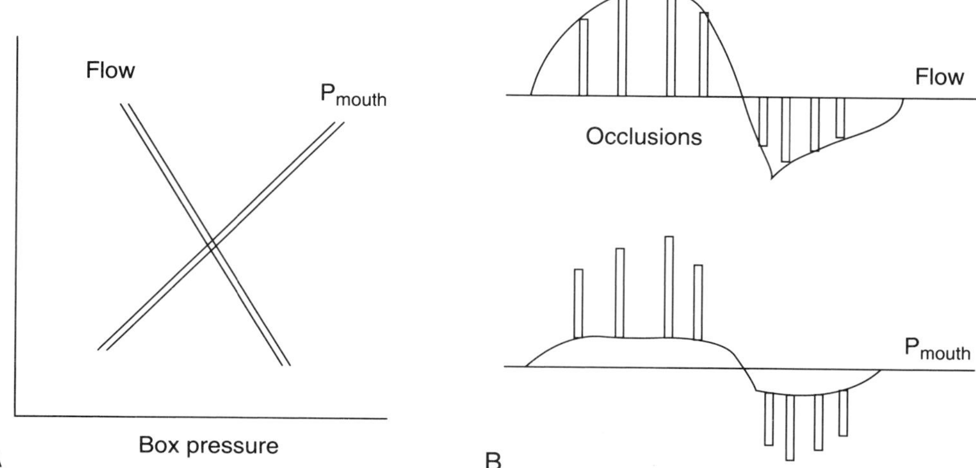

Figure 46-8. Graphic depictions of **(A)** panting and **(B)** interrupter methods of determining airway resistance. See text for discussion.

with the faster-acting agents (such as isoproterenol), up to 30 minutes later with agents such as metaproterenol, and 30 to 60 minutes later with some of the slower-acting agents (such as albuterol or ipratropium). This point is commonly ignored by most texts and, as a result, many institutions inappropriately test almost immediately after administration of an aerosolized drug.

The second point is that despite the widespread use of forced expiratory airflow variables to assess response, there is a potentially significant problem with this approach. When bronchodilation does occur, the same decrease in bronchial muscle tone that caused the bronchodilation can leave the airways more susceptible to dynamic compression during the FVC maneuver. As a result, the true degree of bronchodilation may not be reflected in the airflow indices, and some patients may even appear to worsen although there has been significant bronchodilation. This problem has led some (more commonly in Europe) to recommend concomitant use of airway resistance measurements and nonforced breathing when assessing response to bronchodilators.

This problem is further exacerbated by reliance on single variables, such as the FEV_1/FVC ratio. Significant improvement in FVC may result in a substantial decrease in the FEV_1/FVC ratio. In fact, the single greatest response may be in FVC as a result of the patient's ability to sustain the expiratory effort longer. Again, the primary conclusion should be the need to carefully consider the total picture rather than individual variables.

A corollary of this last point is a phenomenon known as *paradoxical response*. In rare cases, a particular bronchodilator may actually cause airway narrowing in individual patients. The mechanisms for this occurrence are outside the scope of this chapter, but it is obviously important to recognize this phenomenon when it occurs so that the patient is not placed on a drug that would do more harm than good. Unfortunately, when only airflow indices are measured and they become worse after treatment, it is difficult to distinguish the effect of increased collapsibility as described above from a true intrinsic narrowing of the airways. On the other hand, if airway resistance measurements are also made, improvement therein would indicate bronchodilation while the decreased flows would indicate increased dynamic compression. An increase in airway resistance as well as decreased airflow indices would document a true paradoxical response.

BRONCHIAL PROVOCATION TESTING

A converse application of airflow measurement is *bronchial provocation testing* (also called airways challenge testing) to determine the presence of airway hyperreactivity, as discussed in more detail in Chapter 56. In this type of testing, a subject is exposed to one of a number of stimuli that may provoke bronchospasm. Such testing is generally performed as a means of diagnosing the presence of covert asthma, and the stimuli used include exercise, cold air, isocapnic hyperventilation, antigens, environmental irritants, and most commonly, the drug methacholine.

Airflow measurements are used for bronchial provocation testing in much the same way as for bronchodilator response determinations, except that the expected change is in the opposite direction. Luckily, in this case there is somewhat better agreement as to what constitutes a positive response.[17,18]

Methods for assessing response to provocation generally consist of administering the stimuli and performing serial measurements of airflow or airway resistance/conductance. Inhaled provocation agents such as methacholine should be administered over multiple breaths rather than as a single breath. Typically, saline or some other isotonic solution is administered as an initial dose. Maximum response usually occurs within 4 to 10 minutes. The patient is usually followed for 30 to 60 minutes or until a significant response is achieved. Careful monitoring of inhaled agents permits construction of a dose-response curve, which identifies clinically significant provocative doses. Methacholine challenge has become increasingly popular owing to its ease of use and its reproducibility. It is by far the most common method.

INSTRUMENTATION

The type of instrumentation used for airflow assessment can substantially influence the results obtained. Beyond the flow sensor itself, signal processing techniques and software can make marginal sensors adequate and good flow sensors inaccurate. It is important to understand the advantages and limitations of each type of instrumentation in order to select the right equipment for the application.

Various methods exist to identify inadequate equipment, but unfortunately, accepting the manufacturer's assurances is not always sufficient. In 1990 a study of 62 commercially available spirometers,[10] conducted as a follow-up to the original (1980) evaluation by the ATS, showed that not much improvement over the widespread inaccuracies identified in 1980 in existing spirometers had occurred in the intervening 10 years. Only 56.5 percent of the spirometers tested in the 1990 study met the guidelines. This is despite the claim of nearly every manufacturer that its system meets all standards established by the ATS, the Occupational Safety and Health Administration (OSHA), and the National Institute for Occupational Safety and Health (NIOSH).

Instruments for assessing flow generally fall into one of two categories, flow sensors and volume displacement devices. Various types of differential pressure pneumotachographs (pneumotachs) and hot-wire devices are all broadly classified as flow sensors, while water seal, pistons, bellows, and turbines fall within the category of volume displacement devices.

Flow Sensors

A variety of technologies have been used to measure flow. Each technology has specific advantages, and disadvantages but none has proved to be universally acceptable across the application spectra. Most currently used flow sensors can be categorized as differential-pressure devices, turbines, or hot-wire devices.

Pneumotachometers

Differential-pressure flow sensors fall into two categories, laminar or turbulent flow devices. Laminar flow devices, such as the Lilly or Fleisch type of pneumotachograph (Fig. 46-9), typically employ a fixed resistive element, such as screens or parallel capillary tubes, to produce pressure drops proportional to the flow.

Screen pneumotachographs measure flow as a function of the differential pressure generated across a fixed resistance screen placed within the airflow path.[20] Commonly, additional screens are placed upstream and downstream to protect and laminarize airflow across the center screen. These screen-type pneumotachographs, originally described by Lilly and Silverman, are the most common type of differential pressure pneumotachograph used in pulmonary laboratory systems. The device is typically heated to minimize moisture buildup on the screens.

The advantage of screen pneumotachograph lies principally in the relatively smaller effect of the upstream and downstream geometry of the breathing tube and its connectors as compared with the Fleisch-type devices. The primary disadvantage is the significant resistance that the device imposes on the patient, particularly during exercise testing. Also, the screens are subject to occlusion by moisture and particulate matter during long-term monitoring. For improved resolution, two sizes are available with differing peak flow capabilities.

Fleisch-type pneumotachographs measure differential pressure generated across an array of parallel capillary tubes.[21] These tubes serve to distribute the flow across a wide surface area but are prone to inaccuracies if the wave shape is not controlled by tapering connectors upstream and downstream. This sensitivity to airway geometry and the phase lag between flow and pressure are the primary disadvantages to this type of device. Commonly, several different sizes are used to accommodate wide ranges of flow. Like the screen-type device, Fleisch pneumotachographs are typically heated.

Laminar-flow devices have several associated problems. Since a linear relationship between pressure and flow is only achieved when the flow is laminar, the device is sensitive to the geometry of the upstream and downstream flow path. Also, the pressure response to changes in flow may lag the actual event, depending on the design of the device. This phase relationship between the change in pressure and the actual flow signal can be critical for applications requiring phase delay corrections.[22,23]

Turbulent-flow sensors make no attempt to maintain laminar flow profiles and thus are less affected by circuit geometry.[22] In one device a variable orifice is used,[24] and flow is measured by sensing the differential pressure across a variable resistance element. The resistance of the device varies with the rate of flow so that differential pressure can be measured as directly proportional to flow. By carefully selecting the shape and elasticity of the variable resistance element, specific ranges of respiratory flows can be accurately measured. However, the device cannot cover the entire physiologic range necessary.

Turbulent flow sensors without resistive elements measure changes in differential pressure as a function of the square of the flow rate. Perhaps the most common example of a nonresistive flow sensor is the Pitot tube, which measures airflow as a function of the difference between the impact pressure or velocity pressure and the static pressure. Multiple Pitot tubes or transverse Annubar elements sample average upstream and downstream pressures from a series of interconnected tubes. The square law relationship has previously limited the application of these devices since most pressure transducers have insufficient dynamic characteristics to cover the necessary clinical range. However, matched pressure transducers with overlapping ranges can provide the dynamic range required. An example of two turbulent flow devices is shown in Figure 46-10.

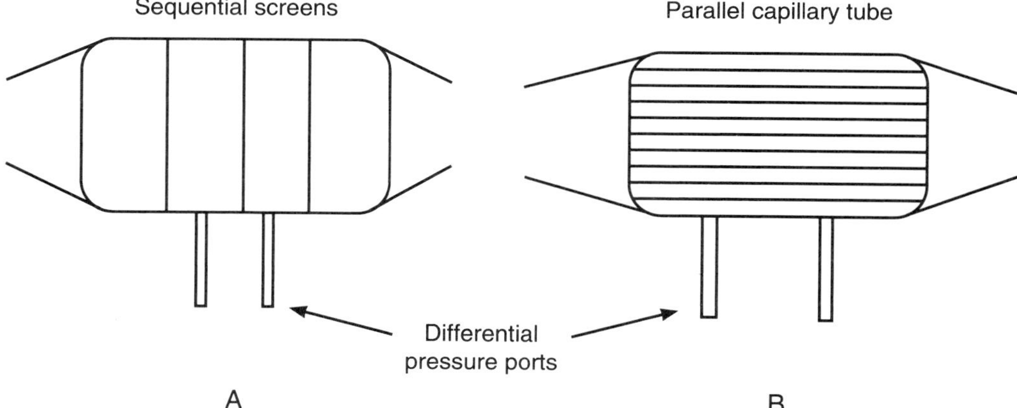

Figure 46-9. Schematic diagrams of **(A)** Lilly- and **(B)** Fleisch-type pneumotachographs. See text for discussion.

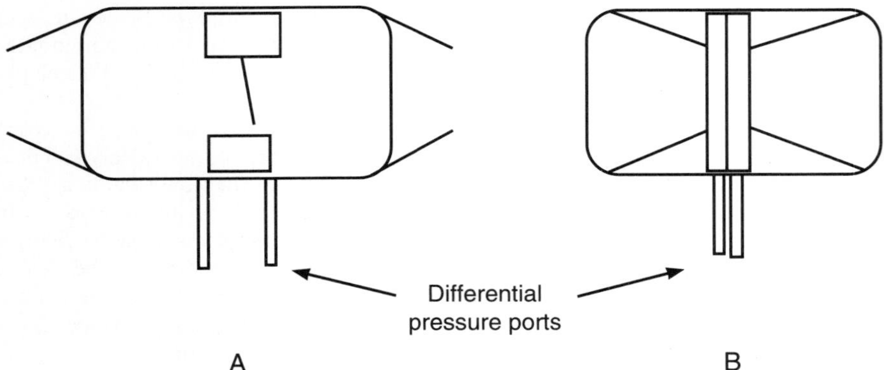

Figure 46-10. Schematic diagrams of (**A**) variable orifice flap and (**B**) multiple Pitot tube turbulent flow measuring devices. See text for discussion.

Hot-Wire Devices

Hot-wire devices rely on the effect of convective cooling as the airstream passes over a heated wire or thermistor. The flow rate is computed as a time function of gas temperature and composition, humidity, and specific heat. Basically, the amount of heat extracted is proportional to the mass of the gases flowing over the surface of the heated wire.[25] With use of heated wires in a constant-temperature device, the presence of saliva or water in the circuit can trigger a failure, since high voltage is applied to compensate for the heat removed from the wire. Automatic shutoff circuits can protect the heated wire but can cause calibration errors until the unit is dried. Heated wires are also sensitive to the presence of moisture in the circuit. An additional problem is the instability caused by adhesion of foreign materials, such as sputum and insufficiently rinsed cleaning solutions, to the heated wire. An example of a hot-wire device is shown in Figure 46-11.

Volume Displacement Devices

Modern volume displacement spirometers, as the name implies, measure volume changes by displacement of a piston, bellows, or cylinder. The amount of displacement for any given volume can be predicted from the cross-sectional area. The displacement can be vertical, as in water-seal spirometers and some rolling seals, or horizontal, as is common in rolling seals and bellows. Nearly all systems are currently available with some form of automation. The output signal is generated either by a potentiometer or a digital encoder. This signal, proportional to changes in volume, is differentiated to a flow signal.

As a group, devices of this type offer simple, reliable detection of volume changes such as static lung volumes. However, the need to measure dynamic lung volumes such as FVC and of flow-volume curves places stricter requirements on the measuring device. These requirements have led to a

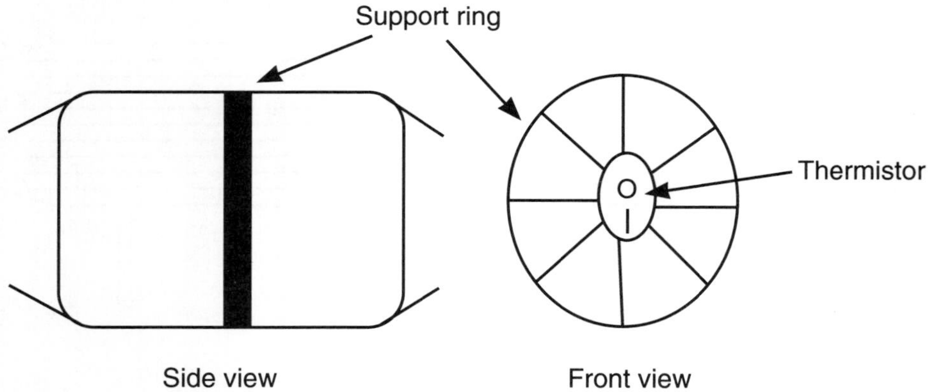

Figure 46-11. Schematic diagram of hot-wire flow-measuring device. See text for discussion.

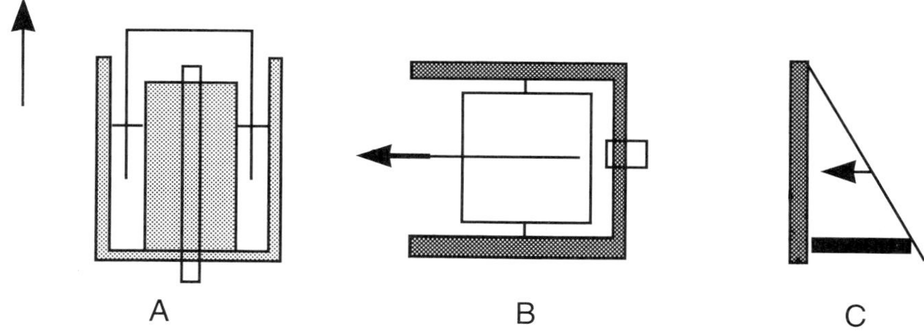

Figure 46-12. Schematic diagrams of **(A)** water seal, **(B)** rolling seal, and **(C)** bellows-type volume displacement spirometers. See text for discussion.

plethora of individual variations to reduce inertia, back pressure, and resistance.

The original volume displacement spirometer was described in 1846 by Hutchinson.[26] Basically, it consisted of a metal cylinder inverted in a container of water. A breathing tube connected the patient with the interior of the cylinder, so that during expiration the cylinder would rise proportionally to the exhaled volume. The device could be designed to accommodate small volumes for FVC measurements or large volumes for exercise testing. In many ways this concept is continued in current water seal spirometers, although many details have been modified.[27] Examples of various volume displacement spirometers are shown in Figure 46-12.

Earlier models were chain-compensated to minimize back pressure and permit the starting volume to be easily set. The recorder pen was connected to the chain, so that as cylinder volume increased, the pen would move downward. However, the chain tended to flex during FVC maneuvers, which caused the device to underestimate peak flows. Other problems with early models were caused by the inertia of the cylinder (a function of the cylinder weight), which would cause the device to be slow to start and to continue after the flow started to decrease. This problem resulted in underestimation of FEFmax and overestimation of FEF_{25-75}.

Most water-seal spirometers use direct linkage to the pen and lightweight plastic cylinders. Linear motion can be read directly from a kymograph or detected by a potentiometer or digital encoder. As a group, water-seal spirometers are mechanically reliable and simple to use. The primary disadvantages specific to these devices are their weight and the relative difficulty of cleaning or decontaminating them.

Dry rolling-seal spirometers offer the same basic advantage of simplicity but without the weight associated with water seals. This device, which is basically a piston with a Silastic or rubber gasket to prevent air leakage, measures volume changes as linear displacements. This type of device is differentiated by the orientation of the piston. Horizontal pistons generally have better performance characteristics since the weight of the piston is not a force acting to empty the device. In recent tests by an independent laboratory, 50 percent of vertical dry rolling-seal spirometers were unable to meet the ATS guidelines, while no horizontal devices were unacceptable.

Similar to rolling seal spirometers, wedge- or bellows-type devices determine volume by measuring displacement. By design, the bellows provides a wide surface area for displacement, which limits the vertical or horizontal movement. This feature has the effect of minimizing resistance or back pressure but also places more emphasis on the resolution of the displacement sensor. In general, this type of device has the same advantages and disadvantages as the rolling seal spirometer.

Turbine devices actually measure volume by equating a predetermined number of revolutions, which are counted by optically interrupting a light beam, to a known volume. The rate of rotation is linearly proportional to flow, or flow can be differentiated from the volume signal. Resolution for turbine-type devices typically ranges from 2 to 10 mL. Changes in gas density or viscosity are a second-order effect and are usually insignificant. Of greater concern is the turbine response time—owing to the effects of inertia, friction, and viscous drag, turbines exhibit a characteristic delay prior to response, which must be corrected. These characteristics may change with normal use or cleaning so that the devices may require periodic recertification. Turbines are more frequently used in exercise gas exchange studies, in which flow can be measured unidirectionally, than in spirometry.

COMPUTERIZATION

Most spirometers and flow sensors provide an analog output proportional to flow and volume, whereas computers require a digital signal for analysis and computation. The translation process, referred to as *analog-to-digital (A-D) conversion*, can take place with varying resolution, which defines the minimum volume or flow change that can be detected. The most common resolutions are 8-, 12-, or 14-bit precision.

If a sensor provides a +/− 10-volt signal proportional to a 20-L/s range, then 8-bit precision would divide the signal into 256 parts, and maximum resolution would be 196 mL/s. This requires the signal to change by at least this amount prior to the computer sensing any change. The same example for 12-bit precision provides for 4096 parts, or a resolution of approximately 10 mL/s. Higher A-D precision provides even finer resolution. For measurement of flow or volume at least 12-bit resolution is required. Higher resolution is acceptable but will greatly add to the cost of the system and likely will not change clinical decisions.

As important as the precision is the sampling rate, or samples per second. Measurement of flow requires the ability to handle rapidly changing signals. For example, in normal patients during forced expiratory maneuvers, flow can change from zero to 12 L/s in a fraction of a second, but inadequate sampling rates can significantly underestimate this change. Forced expiratory efforts have frequency components as high as 25 Hz. The Nyquist sampling theory states that the sampling rate should be at least twice the highest frequency component of the test signal. On this basis, the ATS guidelines suggest a minimum sample rate of 50 samples per second.[1] This should be considered a lower limit only; most commercially available devices sample at a rate of 100 samples per second or greater.

Most flow sensing devices do not present a completely linear output relative to flow. In some, such as turbulent flow sensors, the output is related to the square of the flow rate. More often the nonlinearity is a result of small inaccuracies in the pressure transducers or in the flow characteristics of the sensor itself. Almost all systems provide for linearity correction, which in most modern systems is performed by the computer software.

Measured flow signals are corrected for nonlinearity by using a look-up table as described by Yeh.[28] The look-up table consists of a series of factors to correct actual measured flows. These corrections are unique for each sensor and are usually derived from testing performed by the manufacturer prior to shipment. Repairs to the electronic components will potentially change the sensor characteristics and may require a new look-up table. Corrections for gas viscosity and/or density, temperature, and humidity can also be applied to the shape table. Flows are corrected by multiplying the measured flow by the associated shape table value.

INSTRUMENT PERFORMANCE GUIDELINES

Various governmental agencies and professional groups have promulgated instrument performance guidelines, which are intended to provide some assurance that the results presented are meaningful. In some cases these guidelines have the force of law.[29]

Accepted disability standards now require that all devices measuring flow or volume for disability evaluations have certain common characteristics. These primarily relate to display and reporting. The volume scale must provide at least 10 mm/L while the time scale must provide at least 20 mm/s. Presumably, these standards are intended to guarantee the ability to manually check the calculated values. At least three efforts must be recorded.

ATS recommendations, originally proposed in 1979, were updated in 1987. These recommendations specify range, accuracy, and performance criteria for instruments, as well as effort analysis.

QUALITY ASSURANCE

Meaningful clinical use of spirometry or flow results is possible only when the clinician has confidence in the reliability of the results. The process of ensuring accurate and reliable results is known as quality assurance. Effective quality assurance requires several steps, including a clear procedure manual, selection of valid reference values, a regular equipment maintenance program, appropriate control signals, and testing methodology.

Procedure Manual

Foremost is a clear understanding of the procedure and appropriate performance. Regardless of the instrument's accuracy, all results ultimately reflect the capability of the technologist performing the test. Much of the testing requires subjective assessment of maximal effort, and without a clear understanding of the procedure and rigorous application of the laboratory performance standards results between technologists will inevitably vary. The procedures must be specific in detail and must outline all setup, performance, and evaluation steps necessary to ensure good results. A well written procedure will list the necessary equipment, appropriate calibration, a brief outline of the rationale of and contraindications to the procedure, and effort analysis criteria.

Equipment Maintenance

Regular equipment maintenance is essential to accurate measurements. Failure to follow the appropriate procedures on preventive maintenance, cleaning, and repair can cause substantial errors in measurement. Preventive maintenance requirements differ between devices; some devices require only minimal attention while others may require action after each patient. The type of device also dictates what techniques can be used for cleaning. Volume displacement spirometers typically cannot be immersed for decontamination. Gas sterilization is usually not appropriate for any diagnostic device since aeration requirements would preclude use for a fixed amount of time. Accordingly, many laboratories have instituted policies of using disposable barrier filters, which are changed between patients.

Test Signals

Appropriate test signals are necessary to adequately challenge the device. Flow standards are particularly difficult to produce. While rotameters can provide an accurate constant flow, they are not very useful for volume displacement spirometers, which usually contain 7 to 12 L. Also, patients seldom provide a constant flow. Computerized syringes and explosive decompression cartridges are available to provide flow results, but their cost can be prohibitive. Also, the decompression cartridges, while useful for volume displacement devices, frequently use CO_2 as the carrier gas, which will lead to errors with the Fleisch or screen type of pneumotachograph.

A standard 3-L syringe can be invaluable for the purpose of checking instrument performance over the clinical range. The syringe can provide an absolute standard for volume and accordingly can indirectly check the linearity of flow devices and the frequency response of volume displacement devices. Since flow sensors integrate flow to obtain volume, errors in flow measurement will cause subsequent errors in integrated volume. Use of the syringe to simulate common patient flow-volume curves provides an independent check of flow measurement. At different peak flows the flow sensor should record the same FVC. By varying the peak flow from 0.5 to 12.0 L/s and determining that the FVC measurements did not vary by more than 3 percent (90 mL for a 3-L syringe), it is possible to assure that the device is performing accurately.

An example of this type of testing is shown in Figure 46-13. Notice that despite being injected over a wide range of flows, the measured FVC is well within the 3 percent tolerance. It is also important to note that this technique will not check response to temperature or gas species changes.

A common approach to providing appropriate test signals is to use the concept of "staff normals." Basically, this means testing an individual, generally a staff member. By selecting an individual or group of individuals who will be available over an extended time, it is possible to establish a set of known values with control limits. This approach offers the advantages of testing the device with a physiologic signal subject to all the gas temperature and species variations common to the patient. It provides an excellent tool for monitoring trends as well as for evaluating predicted values. In practice, the staff normal need not actually be normal. In fact, it is frequently advantageous for the individual to be abnormal since this will further test the system as it will be used. However, it should be recognized that more reproducible efforts provide better quality assurance.

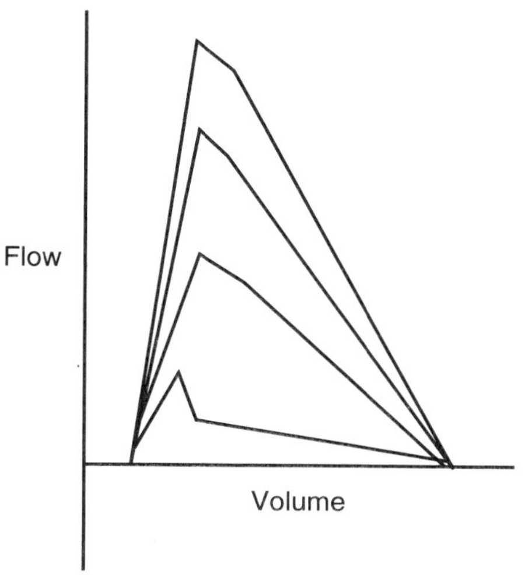

Figure 46-13. An example of linearity testing for a volume-measuring device using a 3-L calibrated syringe. Note that the variation in volume is less than 3 percent over all trials.

Test Sampling

Whatever test signal is selected or available, the most important point to remember is to frequently challenge the device. Syringe checks should be made daily, while staff normals should be tested at least once per week. The actual schedule will vary depending on the scheduled use of the device. Busy laboratories may test several times a day while lightly scheduled laboratories may only test weekly or with each patient. In general, the test scheduling should be based on the number of tests you would want to perform before discovering that the device was not working adequately.

SELECTION OF REFERENCE VALUES

Numerous studies have been published describing reference or predicted values. Unfortunately, these values vary widely. Figure 46-14 shows a sample predicted FVC value for a 20-year-old man, 70 inches tall. As can be seen, selection of the appropriate predicted equation can be critical. Depending on the selection, the predicted FVC value can range from 4.1 to 4.8 L. Representative predicted values for a healthy 20-year-old man are shown in Table 46-2.

A variety of factors can be responsible for such a wide range. Selection of normal subjects, geographic location, testing methodology, and equipment type all exert some influence. Some authors have been extremely stringent in identifying subjects as normal, while others simply have required that the subject be free of symptoms. The most reasonable conclusion is simply that the predicted equations should match the patient population. Accordingly, each laboratory should verify the selection of predicted equations with 20 to 30 normal subjects.

Testing methodology can play a significant role in predicted variances, a fact that is frequently overlooked. Some older studies did not correct predicted values to BTPS, whereas others simply calculated the results differently. Kory et al.[30] started timing for the FEV_1 after 200 mL was expired. Knudson et al.'s 1976 study selected the expiratory flows from different efforts, creating a composite curve with the maximal values.[31] Other examples exist, but again the conclusion to be drawn is that the equations selected must closely parallel methodology and equipment.

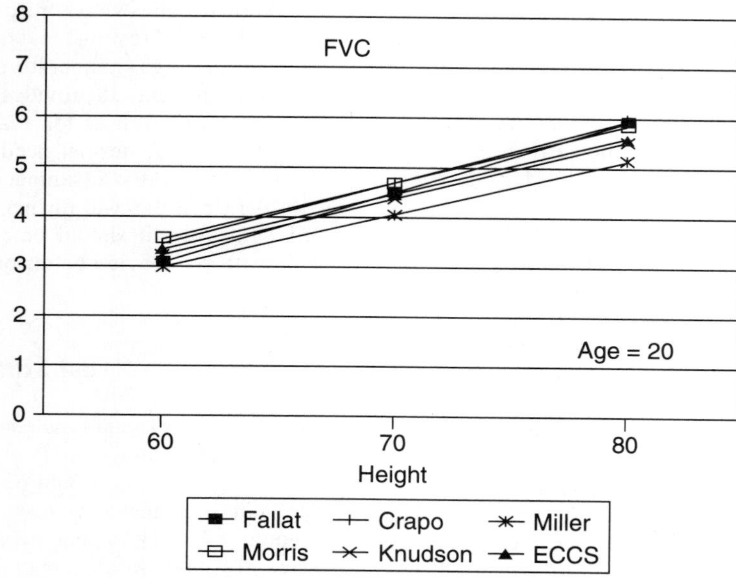

Figure 46-14. Regression lines from six different prediction equations. Note that variance of up to 1.0 L may exist depending on the equation selected.

SETTING LIMITS OF ABNORMALITY

Once a given subject's predicted values are computed, the variation of the actual measured values from those predicted is normally determined in one of two ways. The first and newer approach is calculation of the number of standard deviations (SD) as

$$\frac{(\text{Actual value} - \text{predicted value})}{\text{SD}} = \text{no. of SD} \qquad (6)$$

For most airflow indices, a value of −1.65 or less is considered abnormal. This margin of the predicted value minus 1.65 SD is often termed the lower limit of normal, or the 95 percent confidence interval (CI).

The second, more conventional, approach is calculation of the percent of predicted as

$$\frac{\text{Actual value}}{\text{predicted value}}(100) = \%\text{ of predicted value} \qquad (7)$$

In general, airflow values less than 80 percent of predicted are considered abnormal, although wide ranges are advocated by some authors for variables perceived as having greater inherent variability.

There is considerable controversy as to which of these approaches is preferable in defining the border between normality and abnormality. However, once a value is determined to be abnormal, the percent of predicted serves almost universally as the basis for grading the degree of abnormality. Table 46-3 summarizes a grading scheme for abnormality in the primary airflow indices (not including ratios).

Given this basis for determining and grading abnormality in individual airflow variables, it becomes possible to use airflow measurements to identify various patterns of abnormality. Although specific structural and functional changes are described in more detail in other chapters, they are treated briefly here because an understanding of the usefulness of various airflow indices is essential to obtaining valid results. There are two primary patterns of airflow abnormality within which all mechanical pulmonary disorders are grouped, namely obstructive ventilatory defects and restrictive ventilatory defects.

Obstructive ventilatory defects are characterized by a general decrease in flow rates (as opposed to volumes) and are defined and graded primarily on the basis of the FEV_1/FVC ratio; it is not uncommon practice to use an absolute limit

Table 46-2. Example of Predicted Values for 20-Year-Old Man—Height, 70 in.; Weight, 150 lb[a]

FVC	5.40 L
FEV_1	4.37 L
FEV_1/FVC	80.86%
FEFmax	9.40 L/s
FEF_{200-12}	9.01 L/s
FEF_{25-75}	4.42 L/s
FEF_{10}	9.03 L/s
FEF_{25}	7.52 L/s
FEF_{40}	5.99 L/s
FEF_{50}	4.78 L/s
FEF_{60}	3.66 L/s
FEF_{75}	2.08 L/s
FEF_{90}	0.65 L/s
MVV	188.06 L/min

[a] These are representative values only. Actual predicted values vary substantially depending on author and methods.

Table 46-3. Criteria for Grading Severity of Obstructive Ventilatory Defects

Degree of Severity	Recommended Approach[a]		Standard Approach
	FEV_1/FVC_5	FEF_{25-75}	$FEV_1/FVC(\%)$
Normal	≥pred	≥80% pred	>90(pred)
Minimal	≥pred	<80% pred	
Mild	65–pred		60–90(pred)
Moderate	50–64		46–59
Severe	<50		<45

Pred, predicted value.

The recommended approach is the one we personally favor. The standard approach is an example of the more widely employed grading system.

for normality of this ratio. This is an odd concept for several reasons. It is well established that even in normal subjects FEV_1 declines with age at a faster rate than does FVC (approximately 30 versus 20 mL/yr), and thus it is self-evident that one value for the ratio cannot be appropriately applied to all ages. While FEV_1/FVC ratios less than 75 percent in an adolescent are often associated with clinical disease, values well under 75 or even 70 percent are the rule in perfectly healthy octogenarians being tested for screening purposes. Preferably age-specific predicted values for the FEV_1/FVC ratio should be used. Such values are available from a number of regression equations that specifically predict the ratio itself, as distinct from the separate FEV_1 and FVC values, or they may be calculated by simply dividing the predicted FEV_1 by the predicted FVC.

Abnormalities in the FEV_1/FVC ratio are generally associated with frank obstruction. However the ratio, while very specific for obstruction, is not very sensitive, and subjects often exhibit evidence of an obstructive abnormality, either by more sensitive physiologic measures or clinically, when the FEV_1/FVC ratio is within normal limits. The more sensitive physiologic measures include some that are also derived from airflow measurements, such as the FEF_{25-75}, FEF_{50}, FEF_{75}, and mean transit time. Among many but certainly not all authors, abnormalities in these variables with a normal FEV_1/FVC ratio are held to represent at least minimal obstruction. An overall grading scheme of obstructive ventilatory defects is shown in Table 46-4.

When the more sensitive measures are used, it is very often argued that larger allowances must be made in percent of predicted values before a finding is labeled abnormal. The principal reason for this suggestion is that studies have often shown a greater variability (coefficient of variation) for these indices than for the FEV_1 and FVC. In our experience, these variables do not seem to necessarily exhibit any greater degree of inherent variability. Furthermore, at least in the case of the FEF_{25-75}, when the measured value is below 80 percent of predicted, that finding is usually part of a pattern of abnormalities (airway resistance, RV/TLC ratio, distribution indices, etc) indicative of minor obstructive dysfunction.

Restrictive ventilatory defects are characterized by a decrease in volume (as opposed to flow). A true restrictive defect is actually defined and graded on the basis of abnormalities in TLC, as discussed in the chapter on lung volume measurements. However, restriction is suggested by airflow measurements that show reduction in FVC without a reduction in flow. When restriction is graded on the basis of the FVC in lieu of a determination of TLC, the levels of severity are as outlined in Table 46-4.

At least two important points must be made regarding the foregoing description of restriction; failure to understand these two points commonly leads to incorrect interpretations. First, a reduced FVC was said to suggest restriction when it is present without a reduction in flow. It must be understood that flow is a time function of volume (i.e., flow equals volume per unit time), so that in most cases flow will decrease when volume is decreased. Therefore, normal flows are flows that are proportional to the reduced volume. For example, if 80 percent of predicted is the lower limit of normal for FEF_{25-75} and the FVC is reduced to 60 percent of predicted, then 48 percent of predicted (0.8×0.6) should become the lower limit of normal for FEF_{25-75}.

The second point is that volume can also be reduced in obstructive disorders secondary to collapse of airways (see Fig. 21-5B). Accordingly, a reduced FVC per se does not suggest restriction, but it does so only in the absence of obstruction or when the decrease is out of proportion to the degree of obstruction. Determining the proportionality between a reduction in FVC and the degree of obstruction when both are present is certainly problematic, and several approaches have been proposed. In our experience the best approach seems to be use of the ratio of FEF_{25-75} percent predicted to FVC percent predicted. In our work values less than 0.36 are almost never associated with a reduction in TLC, while values over 0.5 very often do occur with a reduced TLC. This, or any other, approach categorically fails in neuromuscular disease and tends to fail in cases of lung resection. In all cases it assumes complete terminal effort by

Table 46-4. Degrees of Abnormality in Airflow Indices Based on Percent of Predicted Values[a]

Degree of Abnormality	Group A[b] (%)	Group B[b,c] (%)
Normal	≥80	≥60
Mild	65–79	51–59
Moderate	50–61	41–50
Severe	≤49	≤40

[a] There are many minor variations of the breakpoints between these ranges. The values shown here are based on our own experience and distillation of the literature.

[b] Group A includes FVC, FEV_1, FEFmax, and according to some authors FEF_{25} and FEF_{50}. Group B includes FEF_{75}, FEF_{25-75}, and according to some authors FEF_{25} and FEF_{50}, and all other FEF levels.

[c] We personally apply the group A criteria to all variables for reasons given in the text.

the subject, as incomplete exhalation will spuriously decrease FVC and increase FEF_{25-75}.

As implied by the preceding discussion, in addition to obstructive and restrictive defects there are combined ventilatory defects. A combined obstructive and restrictive ventilatory defect would be defined in the context of airflow measurements alone (without static lung volumes) as an obstructive defect with a FVC that is reduced out of proportion to the degree of obstruction.

A final point concerning the two primary types of airflow disorder is that airflow measurements by themselves are generally not very useful in identifying the specific pathology causing the obstruction and/or restriction. There are, however, two exceptions worth noting. In the case of severe obstruction, a normal FVC is much more likely when the obstruction is due to emphysema than when it is due to intrinsic airways disease (e.g., bronchitis). Second, in the case of restriction, an exception to the principle that flow decreases as volume decreases occurs in that group of diseases, primarily interstitial processes, that result in relatively increased flows as a result of increased lung elastic recoil. In these diseases the FEF_{25-75}/FVC relationship will often be increased (e.g., to above 1.2).

INFECTION CONTROL AND DECONTAMINATION

There are basically three methods for preventing the spread of infectious diseases by pulmonary function equipment: thorough disinfection of equipment, generally by using glutaraldehyde solutions; use of disposable patient contact circuits; and use of barrier filters. Most commonly, some combination of the three approaches is used.

Disinfection is historically most common but, since most cleaning agents are selective in their effectiveness against different contaminants, most institutions do not rely solely on this approach. The use of disposable components offers a very effective solution, but all patient contact breathing circuits may not be available as disposables. The other disadvantages of disposables are increased cost and environmental concerns regarding medical waste and biodegradability.

Barrier filters function by forcing airflow through a pathway that removes contaminants by forcing impaction with the filter medium. Removal efficiency is a function of the pore size and geometric design of the filter medium. Pore size cannot be the sole criterion since the filter's resistance to airflow is inversely proportional to pore size. Accordingly, the geometry of the filter medium is structured to allow use of filtration methods other than direct interception, such as inertial impaction and diffusional interception. Barrier filters are widely used but also raise concerns regarding cost and environmental impact. To the extent that disinfection is not performed, there is a trade-off of costs. Other concerns regarding barrier filters include the additional resistance and dead space.

References

1. Standardization of Spirometry—1987 Update. Am Rev Respir Dis 1987;136:1285–1298
2. Tiffeneau R, Pinelli A: Régulation bronchique de la ventilation pulmonaire. J Fr Med Chir Thorac 1948;2:221–244
3. Gaensler EA: Analysis of the ventilatory defect by timed capacity measurements. Am Rev Respir Dis 1951;64:256–278
4. ATS Statement: SnowBird Workshop on Standardization of Spirometry. Am Rev Respir Dis 1979;119:831–838
5. Krowka MJ, Enright PL, Rodarte JR, Hyatt RE: Effect of effort on measurement of FEV_1. Am Rev Respir Dis 1987;136:829–833
6. Meltzer AA, Smolensky MG, D'Alonzo GE et al: An assessment of peak expiratory flow as a surrogate measurement of FEV_1 in stable asthmatic children. Chest 1989;96:329–333
7. Berube D, Cartier A, L'Archeveque J et al: Comparison of peak expiratory flow rate and FEV_1 in assessing bronchomotor tone after challenges with occupational sensitizers. Chest 1991; 99:831–836
8. Murray AB, Ferguson AC: A comparison of spirometric measurements in allergen bronchial challenge testing. Clin Allergy 1981;11:87–93
9. Hetzel MR, Clark TJH: Comparison of normal and asthmatic circadian rhythms in peak expiratory flow rate. Thorax 1980; 35:732–738
10. Nelson SB, Gardner RM, Crapo RO, Jensen RL: Performance evaluation of contemporary spirometers. Chest 1990;97:288–297
11. DuBois AB, Botehlho SY, Comroe JH: A method for measuring airway resistance in man using a body plethysmograph: Values in normal subjects and in patients with respiratory disease. J Clin Invest 1956;35:327–335
12. Frank NR, Mead J, Whittenberger JL: Comparative sensitivity of four methods for measuring changes in respiratory flow resistance in man. J Appl Physiol 1971;31:934–938
13. Briscoe WA, DuBois AB: The relationship between airway resistance, airway conductance and lung volumes in subjects of different age and body size. J Clin Invest 1958;37:1279–1285
14. Fisher AB, DuBois AB, Hyde RW: Evaluation of the forced oscillation technique for the determination of resistance to breathing. J Clin Invest 1968;47:2045–2057
15. Goldman M, Knudson RJ, Mead J et al: A simplified measurement of respiratory resistance by forced oscillation. J Appl Physiol 1970;28:113–116
16. Jackson AC, Milhorn HT, Normal JR: A reevaluation of the interrupter technique for airway resistance measurement. J Appl Physiol 1974;36:264–268
17. Cropp GJA, Bernstein IL, Boushey HA Jr et al: Guidelines for bronchial inhalation challenges with pharmacologic and antigenic agents. ATS News 1980(spring):11–19
18. Chai H, Farr RS, Froehlich LA et al: Standardization of bronchial inhalation challenge procedures. J Allergy Clin Immunol 1975;56:323–327
19. Gardner RM, Hankinson JL, West BJ: Evaluating commercially available spirometers. Am Rev Respir Dis 1980;121:73–82
20. Silverman L, Whittenberger JL: Clinical pneumotachograph. Methods Med Res 1950;2:104–112
21. Fleisch A: Pneumotachograph: Apparatus for recording respiratory flow. Arch Ges Physiol 1925;209:713–722
22. Finucane KE, Egan BA, Dawson SV: Linearity and frequency response of pneumotachographs. J Appl Physiol 1972;32:121–126
23. Kafer ER: Errors in pneumotachography as a result of transducer design and function. Anesthesiology 1973;38:275–279
24. Elliott SE, Shore JH, Barnes CW et al: Turbulent airflow meter for long term monitoring in patient-ventilator circuits. J Appl Physiol 1977;42:456–460
25. Yoshiya I, Shimada Y, Tanaka K: Evaluation of a hot-wire respiratory flowmeter for clinical applicability. J Appl Physiol 1979; 47:1131–1135

26. Hutchinson J: On the capacity of the lungs, and on the respiratory functions with a view of establishing a precise and easy method of detecting diseases by the spirometer. Med Chair Soc Trans 1846;29
27. Wells HS, Stead WW, Rossing TD, Ognanovicax J: Accuracy of an improved spirometer for recording fast breathing. J Appl Physiol 1959;14:451–459
28. Yeh MP, Gardner RM, Adams TD, Yanowitz FG: Computerized determination of pneumotachometer characteristics using a calibrated syringe. J Appl Physiol 1982;53:280–285
29. Code of Federal Regulations: Cotton dust. Appendix D. Occupational Safety and Health Administration 1980; 1910.1046:808–832
30. Kory RC, Callahan R, Boren HG: The Veterans Administration–Army Cooperative Study of Pulmonary Function. I. clinical spirometry in normal men. Am J Med 1961;30:243–258
31. Knudson RJ, Slatin RC, Lebowitz MD, Burrows B: The maximal expiratory flow-volume curve. Am Rev Respir Dis 1976; 113:587–601
32. Beauchamp RK: Pulmonary function testing procedures. pp. 51–82. In Barnes TA (ed): Respiratory Care Practice. Year Book Medical Publishers, Chicago, 1988

Chapter 47

Assessment of Gas Exchange and Acid-Base Balance

Robert M. Kacmarek

CHAPTER OUTLINE

At the basis of the application of respiratory care is the assessment of gas exchange and acid-base balance, both of which have been routinely quantified invasively. However, recent advances in technology have made the noninvasive assessment of gas exchange feasible. This chapter concentrates on both the invasive and the noninvasive assessment of gas exchange from both a clinical and a technical perspective. The reader is also referred to Chapters 1, 13, and 28 for additional background on basic chemistry and physiologic mechanisms associated with acid-base and electrolyte balance, as well as common causes of acid-base disturbances.

NORMAL VALUES

Normal values for any laboratory variable are based on data accumulated from a large series of subjects representative of the group for which the normal values are being defined. Table 47-1 presents normal values for commonly used arterial blood gas (ABG) variables, both measured and derived. Absolute normals and ranges, where identified, are listed. However, the clinician must be cautioned about considering values outside of the ''normal'' ranges as clinically unacceptable. Values for a given patient may fall outside of these defined ranges without indicating an acute clinical

Table 47-1. Normal Laboratory Values for Common Arterial Blood Gas Variables

Variable	Absolute Normal	Range
pH	7.40 units	7.35–7.45
PCO_2	40.0 mmHg	35–45 mmHg
PO_2	97.0 mmHg	≥80 mmHg
HCO_3^-	24.0 mEq/L	22–28 mEq/L
Base excess	0.0 mEq/L	±2 mEq/L
Hb content	14.0 g	12–15 g
$HbO_2\%$	97.5%	≥95%
O_2 content	19.8 Vol%	≥16 Vol%
HbCO%	0.0%	≤2.0%

Hb, hemoglobin; $HbO_2\%$, oxyhemoglobin saturation in percent; HbCO%, carboxyhemoglobin saturation in percent.

problem, for example, in the patient with chronic hypoxemia or compensated respiratory acidosis.

Ranges defined as clinically acceptable for arterial pH, $PaCO_2$, and by Shapiro et al.[1] are listed in Table 47-2.These are not intended to supersede those in Table 47-1 but to represent ranges beyond which clinical intervention is normally required.

As with any laboratory variable it is important for the clinician to consider individual values in relation to the patient's actual clinical presentation and history. One should not necessarily accept a single value as indicative of a clinical abnormality without detailed knowledge of a patient's physical presentation and history.

LAW OF MASS ACTION AND HENDERSON-HASSELBALCH EQUATION

The basis for interpretation of arterial blood gases is the *law of mass action*, from which the Henderson-Hasselbalch equation is derived. According to this law (also referred to as the *law of electrolyte dissociation* or *law of chemical equilibrium*), when a weak electrolyte is placed into solution, only a small percentage of it dissociates, the vast majority of its molecules remaining undissociated. When the product

Table 47-2. Clinically Acceptable Acid-Base Ranges for Arterial Blood

Variable	Range
pH	7.30–7.50 units
PCO_2	30–50 mmHg

Table 47-3. Determination of the Dissociation Constant for a Weak Acid Electrolyte[a]

$$HA \rightleftharpoons H^+ + A^-$$

If 5% of a 0.01 mol/L solution of HA dissociates in solution, the solution contains:

0.0095 mol/L HA

0.0005 mol/L H^+

0.0005 mol/L A^-

$$\frac{[H^+][A^-]}{[HA]} = K$$

$$\frac{(0.0005 \text{ mol/L})\ (0.0005 \text{ mol/L})}{(0.0095 \text{ mol/L})} = 0.0000263$$

$$K = (2.63)(10^{-5})$$

HA, weak acid; A^-, conjugate base; H^-, hydrogen ion; K, dissociation constant.

[a] See text for details.

Table 47-4. Derivation of the Henderson-Hasselbalch Equation for the Weak Acid Buffer HA

Determination of the dissociation constant for HA

$$\frac{[H^+][A^-]}{[HA]} = K \qquad (1)$$

Rearranging Equation 1 and solving for H^+

$$[H^+] = \frac{K[HA]}{[A^-]} \qquad (2)$$

Taking the negative logarithm of Equation 2,

$$-\log [H^+] = -\log K - \log \frac{[HA]}{[A^-]} \qquad (3)$$

Rearranging,

$$-\log \frac{[HA]}{[A^-]}$$

$$-\log [HA]\,(-) - \log [A^-]$$

$$-\log [HA] + \log [A^-] \qquad (4)$$

$$+\log [A^-] - \log [HA]$$

$$+\log \frac{[A^-]}{[HA]}$$

pH is defined as

$$-\log [H^+] \qquad (5)$$

pK is defined as

$$-\log K \qquad (6)$$

Substituting Equations 4, 5, and 6 into Equation 3

$$pH + pK + \log \frac{[A^-]}{[HA]} \qquad (7)$$

Table 47-5. Henderson-Hasselbalch Buffer Equations for Weak Acid and Basic Buffers

Weak acid $HA \rightleftharpoons A^- + H^+$

$$pH = pK + \log \frac{[A^-](\text{conjugate base})}{[HA](\text{undissociated acid})}$$

Weak base $BOH \rightleftharpoons B^+ + OH^-$

$$pOH = pK + \log \frac{[B^+](\text{conjugate acid})}{[BOH](\text{undissociated base})}$$

pOH is defined as $-\log [OH^-]$

of the molar concentrations of the dissociated species is divided by the molar concentration of the undissociated weak electrolyte, a dissociation constant for that weak electrolyte is determined (Table 47-3). This equilibrium relationship holds at the specific temperature that it was determined. Variation in temperature does alter the dissociation relationship.

The Henderson-Hasselbalch equation (the basis for blood gas interpretation) is derived from the law of mass action. As indicated in Table 47-4, it can be derived for any weak acid or basic electrolyte and expresses the buffer relationship for that electrolyte. It must be remembered that a buffer is a substance that when placed in solution, first of all determines the pH of the solution and second minimizes pH change. Buffers are capable of maintaining the pH of a given solution since dissociation of the buffer results in the formation of a conjugate base or conjugate acid (Table 47-5). As a result, for a weak acid buffer the undissociated acid functions as an acid (Table 47-6) while the dissociated conjugate base functions as a base. Thus, the addition of acid or base can be buffered, minimizing pH change.

As noted in Table 47-4, the pK in the Henderson-Hasselbalch equation equals the negative logarithm of the dissociation constant. This value is critical to the optimal function of a given buffer since it defines the pH about which the buffer functions most effectively. Buffers only function at maximum capability within a narrow pH range (about 1.0 pH unit) about the pK valve. As the pH moves outside this range, the buffer's effectiveness is markedly decreased. Within the body numerous buffer systems (Table 47-7) are functional, and all operate within their optimal pH range except for the HCO_3^-/H_2CO_3 buffer system.

Table 47-6. Buffering by Weak Acid Buffers

$$pH = pK + \log \frac{[A^-]}{[HA]}$$

Addition of acid is buffered by the conjugate base A^-

$$A^- + \underset{\text{added acid}}{H^+} = HA$$

Addition of base is buffered by the undissociated acid HA

$$HA + \underset{\text{added base}}{OH^-} = H_2O + A^-$$

Although more acid or base is formed, the pH change is minimal within the functional range of the buffer.

Table 47-7. Primary Body Buffer Systems

Bicarbonate/carbonic acid[a]	HCO_3^-/H_2CO_3
Dibasic/monobasic phosphate	$HPO_4^{-2}/H_2PO_4^-$
Ammonia/ammonium ion	NH_3/NH_4^+
Hemoglobin/hemoglobin ion	Hb/HHb^+
Serum protein/protein ion	$Prot^-/HProt$

[a] Poor chemical buffer but essential physiologic buffer.

THE BICARBONATE-CARBONIC ACID BUFFER SYSTEM

The HCO_3^-/H_2CO_3 buffer system is a poor chemical buffer in blood because the pK of this system is 6.1 (Table 47-8), while the pH of arterial blood is about 7.4. Since the difference between the ideal system pH (6.1) and the actual system pH (7.4) is so great, the chemical buffering capability of the system is lost. In spite of this, the HCO_3^-/H_2CO_3 system is essential for normal bodily functions and is commonly referred to as a physiologic buffer, since large quantities of acid in the form of CO_2 can be added or eliminated by altering ventilation. This ability is based on the reversibility of the hydration reaction of CO_2:

$$CO_2 + H_2O \rightleftharpoons H_2CO_3 \rightleftharpoons H^+ + HCO_3^- \quad (1)$$

It should be noted that the right-hand side of this equation

Table 47-8. The Bicarbonate-Carbonic Acid Buffer System

Basic Henderson-Hasselbalch equation:

$$pH = pK + \log \frac{[HCO_3^-]}{[H_2CO_3]}$$

$$pK = 6.1$$

$$[HCO_3^-] = 24.0 \text{ mEq/L}$$

$$[H_2CO_3] = 1.2 \text{ mEq/L}$$

$$pH = 7.4$$

Ratio between HCO_3^-/H_2CO_3 at a normal pH of 7.4 is $^{20}/_1$

$$[H_2CO_3] = (0.0301)(PCO_2)$$

Basic equation used to calculate $[HCO_3^-]$:

$$pH = 6.1 + \log \frac{[HCO_3^-]}{(0.0301)(PCO_2)}$$

Table 47-9. Acute Effect of PCO_2 Change on pH and Bicarbonate Concentration

PCO_2 (mmHg)	pH (units)	$[HCO_3^-]$ (mEq/L)
80	7.20	28
60	7.30	26
40	7.40	24
30	7.50	22
20	7.60	20

includes the components of the buffer system. If metabolic acid is added to the system, Equation 1 shifts to the left, with formation of more CO_2 and H_2O. The increased CO_2 produced is rapidly exhaled. It is for this reason that administration of $NaHCO_3$ is capable of neutralizing a metabolic acidosis. If CO_2 could not be eliminated via the lung, the metabolic acidosis would simply become a respiratory acidosis as HCO_3^- was added. The converse would occur if metabolic base were added to the system. The added base would react with the H^+, causing Equation 1 to shift to the right and thus decrease the CO_2 level. As this occurs, the level of ventilation decreases, allowing CO_2 to increase to its normal level. Table 47-9 lists pH and HCO_3^- changes associated with each 10 mmHg PCO_2 change. These changes are acute chemical changes without any compensation by the kidney.

The reversibility of the CO_2 hydration reaction accounts for the respiratory system's ability to compensate for metabolic acid-base disturbances. This compensation can occur very rapidly but is usually incomplete—that is, the greater the magnitude of the metabolic disturbance, the less likely is the pH to normalize (at a value of 7.35 to 7.45) during compensation.

Compensation for acute respiratory acid base disturbance is performed by the kidney (Table 47-10). Normally the kidney secretes H^+ and reabsorbs HCO_3^-. As indicated in Figure 47-1, carbonic anhydrase, contained within renal tubular cells, accelerates the reaction of CO_2 and water as it occurs in red blood cells. The HCO_3^- from this reaction is reabsorbed into the peritubular plasma, and the H^+ is actively transported into the lumen of the kidney tubule.[2] As H^+ is secreted, Na^+ is reabsorbed into the blood. The H^+ entering the kidney tubule is buffered by the HCO_3^- present in the glomerular filtrate, which contains HPO_4^{-2} and NH_3 in addition to HCO_3^- (Figs. 47-2 and 47-3).

Under normal acid-base conditions, most of the secreted H^+ is buffered by HCO_3^-. However, if PCO_2 increases, renal tubular formation of H^+ and HCO_3^- also increases, which results in absorption of greater quantities of HCO_3^- to normalize the acidic pH and the larger quantities of secreted H^+. The increased secretion of H^+ is buffered by HPO_4^{-2} and NH_3. The exact opposite occurs if PCO_2 decreases. First of all, less CO_2 enters the renal tubular cells, and thus less HCO_3^- ion is reabsorbed and less H^+ is secreted. As a result, the plasma HCO_3^- concentration decreases, allowing the pH to decrease to within normal range. Since only about 4 to 5 percent of the cardiac output perfuses the kidneys' tubules, compensation by the kidneys takes 24 to 48 hours or longer; however, it usually proceeds to completion. Thus the pH is normalized to a greater extent during renal compensation for respiratory abnormalities than during respiratory compensation for metabolic disorders.

Standard versus Actual Bicarbonate

HCO_3^- ion concentration is always a calculated value, based on pH and PCO_2 via the Henderson-Hasselbalch equation (Table 47-8). Depending on which PCO_2 and pH values (arterial or venous) are used to calculate the HCO_3^- concentration, it is referred to as *standard* or *actual* HCO_3^-. The actual HCO_3^- is calculated from the measured arterial pH and $PaCO_2$, while the standard HCO_3^- is usually calculated from venous blood in which the blood is equilibrated to a PCO_2 of 40 mmHg, after which the pH is measured. Thus, standard HCO_3^- is always determined at a PCO_2 of 40 mmHg. As a result, the actual HCO_3^- and standard HCO_3^- may markedly differ. In interpreting blood gas data, the actual HCO_3^- should always be used.

Table 47-10. Arterial PCO_2 and Serum HCO_3^- Changes during Chronic Compensation

42	Acid-Base Disorder	Compensatory Change	Example	
45	Metabolic acidosis	1.0–1.5 mmHg decrease in PCO_2 for each mEq/L decrease in HCO_3^-	HCO_3^- PCO_2	25 → 10 40 → 25
47	Metabolic alkalosis	0.5–1.0 mmHg increase in PCO_2 for each mEq/L increase in HCO_3^-	HCO_3^- PCO_2	25 → 35 40 → 50
49	Respiratory acidosis	4 mEq/L increase in HCO_3^- for each 10 mmHg increase in PCO_2	PCO_2 HCO_3^-	40 → 60 25 → 33
51	Respiratory alkalosis	2.5 mEq/L decrease in HCO_3^- for each 10 mmHg decrease in PCO_2	PCO_2 HCO_3^-	40 → 20 25 → 20

(Modified from Effros,[5] with permission.)

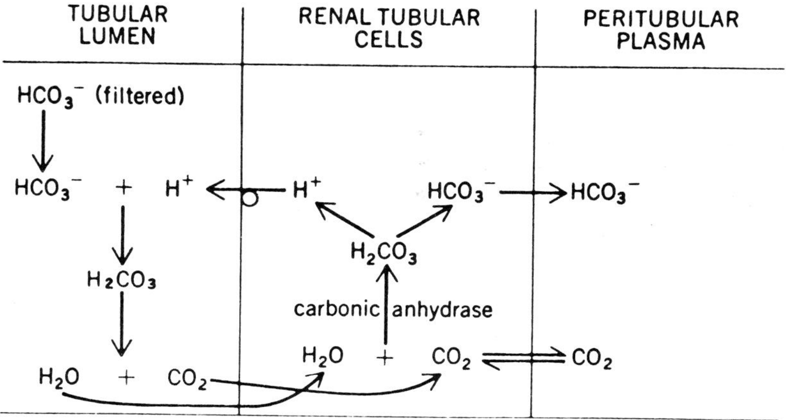

Figure 47-1. The normal mechanism for the reabsorption of filtered HCO_3^-. For every HCO_3^- ion reabsorbed, one H^+ ion is secreted. O indicates that movement of H^+ is via an active transport mechanism. (From Vander,[2] with permission.)

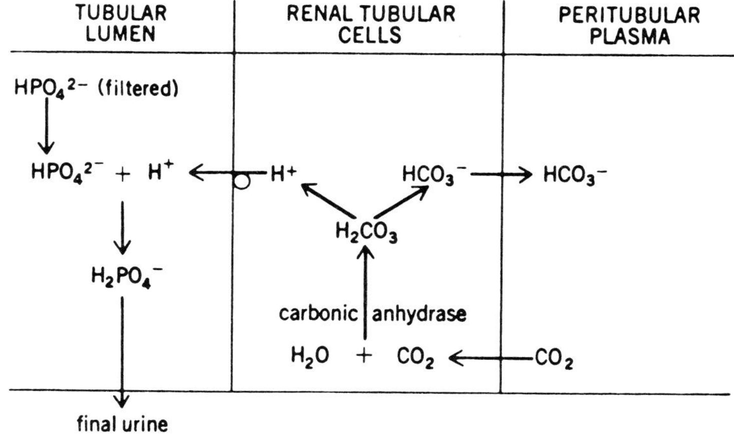

Figure 47-2. The use of HPO_4^{-2} as a buffer of secreted H^+. This system is active primarily in the presence of excess PCO_2, resulting in secretion of a larger than normal quantity of H^+. With each H^+ ion secreted, a HCO_3^- ion is reabsorbed, thus increasing total extracellular HCO_3^- concentration. (From Vander,[2] with permission.)

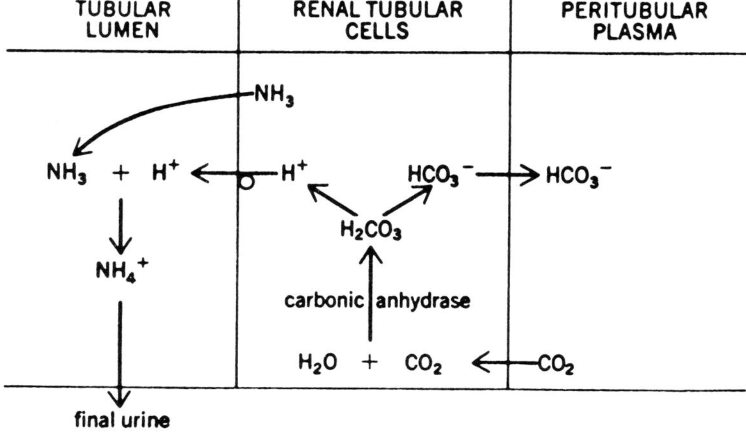

Figure 47-3. The reaction of secreted H^+ with NH_3. This system is active primarily in the presence of excess PCO_2. The additional H^+ formed is buffered, and HCO_3^- is reabsorbed, increasing the total extracellular HCO_3^- concentration. (From Vander,[2] with permission.)

Base Excess and Base Deficit

The PCO_2 is the primary indicator of the magnitude of respiratory acid-base disturbances, while the base excess/base deficit (BE/BD) is the primary indicator of metabolic acid-base disorders. HCO_3^- concentration is a secondary indicator of metabolic disorders, since it only accounts for about 50 to 60 percent of the body's buffering capability, while hemoglobin and plasma proteins account for an additional 30 percent and the remaining buffering capability is provided by miscellaneous buffers present in the blood in small quantities (Table 47-7). When considering the body's buffering of acid or base, the total buffering capacity is usually taken to be a combination of the primary buffers, namely HCO_3^-/H_2CO_3 and all protein buffers (Table 47-11). Equations 1 and 2 in Table 47-11 illustrate the buffer equations for HCO_3^- and $Prot^-$. It should be noted that if respiratory acid (CO_2) is added to the system, the hydration of CO_2 (Table 47-11, Equation 3) shifts to the right, increasing the H^+ concentration, which forces the $Prot^-$ buffer reaction to shift to the left (Table 47-11, Equation 4). As a result, no change in total body base occurs. Equations 5 and 6 of Table 47-11 indicate the effect of decreasing respiratory acid. Here, the decrease in CO_2 causes H^+ to react with HCO_3^- shifting the reaction to the left. This results in a decrease in H^+, and causes the $Prot^-$ buffer reaction to shift to the right. Again, there is no change in total body base.

As shown in Equations 7 to 10 of Table 47-11, a grossly different effect results when metabolic acid or base is added. Metabolic acid shifts both Equation 7 and Equation 8 to the left, decreasing total body base, while metabolic base shifts both Equation 9 and Equation 10 to the right, increasing total body base. This occurs because regardless of the metabolic acid or base added, the H^+ concentration in both sets of equations (7 and 8 or 9 and 10) is affected.

Table 47-11. Function of HCO_3^-/H_2CO_3 and HProt/$Prot^-$ Buffers in Various Acid-Base Disorders

$$CO_2 + H_2O \rightleftharpoons H_2CO_3 \rightleftharpoons H^+ + HCO_3^- \quad (1)$$

$$HProt \rightleftharpoons H^+ + Prot^- \quad (2)$$

Respiratory acidosis would cause

$$\uparrow CO_2 + H_2O \rightarrow H_2CO_3 \rightarrow \uparrow H^+ + HCO_3^- \quad (3)$$

$$HProt \leftarrow \downarrow H^+ + Prot^- \quad (4)$$

Respiratory alkalosis would cause

$$\downarrow CO_2 + H_2O \leftarrow H_2CO_3 \leftarrow \downarrow H^+ + HCO_3^- \quad (5)$$

$$HProt \rightarrow \uparrow H^+ + Prot^- \quad (6)$$

Neither respiratory acidosis or alkalosis results in a change in the total base (HCO_3^- plus $Prot^-$)

Metabolic acidosis would cause

$$CO_2 + H_2O \leftarrow H_2CO_3 \leftarrow \uparrow H^+ + HCO_3^- \quad (7)$$

$$HProt \leftarrow \uparrow H^+ + Prot^- \quad (8)$$

Metabolic alkalosis would cause

$$CO_2 + H_2O \rightarrow H_2CO_3 \rightarrow \downarrow H^+ + HCO_3^- \quad (9)$$

$$HProt \rightarrow \downarrow H^+ + Prot^- \quad (10)$$

Both metabolic acidosis and alkalosis result in an alteration in total base (a decrease or increase in HCO_3^- plus $Prot^-$).

The combination of all body base is referred to as the *total buffer base* (BB), which normally equals 54 ± 2 mEq/L. Base excess or base deficit is determined by comparing the actual BB with the normal BB.

$$BE/BD = \text{actual BB} - \text{normal BB} \quad (2)$$

The normal BE/BD is ±2 mEq/L.

CLASSICAL INTERPRETATION OF ARTERIAL BLOOD GASES

Interpretation of ABGs is approached in precise steps: (1) evaluating the pH as normal, increased, or decreased; (2) determining whether the PCO_2 is normal, increased, or decreased and whether the change in PCO_2 has caused the alteration in pH noted; and (3) assessing oxygenation state.

Evaluation of Acid-Base Status

Four general categories of acid-base disturbances exist: respiratory acidosis, respiratory alkalosis, metabolic acidosis, and metabolic alkalosis. Under each of these headings three subdivisions are possible: uncompensated or acutely developed; partially compensated, with the pH moving back toward normal as a result of attempted compensation by the respiratory system or kidney; and compensated, with normalization of the pH by either the kidney or the respiratory system. In addition, a combined respiratory and metabolic acidosis or combined respiratory and metabolic alkalosis may develop.

The mathematical interrelationship among pH, PCO_2, and HCO_3^- and the basis for all acid-base interpretation is

$$pH \approx \frac{HCO_3^-}{PCO_2} \quad (3)$$

that is, the *pH* and the *PCO_2* are *always inversely related*, while the *pH* and *HCO_3^-* are *always directly related*. Table 47-12 lists the level of change in pH, PCO_2, HCO_3^-, and BE/BD associated with each of the specific acid-base disturbances. It should be noted that although ranges for a compensated metabolic alkalosis are presented, it is rare to see this acid-base state clinically—in other words it is unlikely that PCO_2 would increase into the 45 to 60 mmHg range in order to fully compensate for a metabolic alkalosis. The normal drive to ventilate would usually inhibit this change. ABG values suggesting this interpretation may actually represent a superimposed acid-base disturbance (see below). Figure 47-4 presents an algorithm for use in interpretation of ABGs from a classical perspective. However, it is important that all laboratory data, especially ABGs, be interpreted in the light of a patient's history and clinical presentation.

The first step in interpreting the acid-base status depicted

Table 47-12. Classical Method of Arterial Blood Gas Interpretation

Status	pH (units)	PCO_2 (mmHg)	HCO_3^- (mEq/L)	BE (mEq/L)
Respiratory acidosis				
Uncompensated	<7.35	>45	Normal	Normal
Partially compensated	<7.35	>45	>28	> +2
Compensated	7.35–7.40	>45	>28	> +2
Respiratory alkalosis				
Uncompensated	>7.45	<35	Normal	Normal
Partially compensated	>7.45	<35	<22	< −2
Compensated	7.40–7.45	<35	<22	< −2
Metabolic acidosis				
Uncompensated	<7.35	Normal	<22	< −2
Partially compensated	<7.35	<35	<22	< −2
Compensated	7.35–7.40	<35	<22	< −2
Metabolic alkalosis				
Uncompensated	>7.45	Normal	>28	> +2
Partially compensated[a]	>7.45	>45	>28	> +2
Compensated[a]	7.41–7.45	>45	>28	> +2
Combined respiratory and metabolic acidosis	<7.35	>45	<22	< −2
Combined respiratory and metabolic alkalosis	>7.45	<35	>28	> +2

[a] In general, partially compensated or compensated metabolic alkalosis is rarely seen clinically because of the body's mechanism to prevent hypoventilation.

(From Kacmarek et al.,[62] with permission.)

by an ABG determination is to evaluate the pH (i.e., to determine if it is normal, increased, or decreased). If the pH is above or below the normal range, the task is to determine whether the abnormality results from a PCO_2 change. If it is not, the abnormality is metabolic in origin. One must then determine whether the condition is acute (uncompensated) or partially compensated. If it is uncompensated, then either the PCO_2 or HCO_3^- is normal, whereas if the correct interpretation is that the condition is partially compensated, both the PCO_2 and HCO_3^- are abnormal. A normal pH reflects either a normal acid-base status or a completely compensated abnormality. One can never interpret any laboratory data with 100 percent accuracy without clinical information about the patient, but as a general rule for compensated states if the pH is between 7.41 and 7.45, the correct interpretation is compensated alkalosis, and if the pH is between 7.35 and 7.40, the interpretation is compensated acidosis.

Many complex acid-base interactions may exist that require knowledge of a patient's previous baseline ABG values to ensure correct interpretation. This is particularly true in patients with chronic respiratory acidosis (Table 47-13). An acute acid-base disturbance may be superimposed on the chronic state, grossly altering interpretation, as noted in Table 47-13. Accurate interpretation of ABGs always requires knowledge of the patient's baseline ABG data.

Evaluation of Oxygenation Status

As indicated in Table 47-1, an acceptable level of PO_2 is 80 mmHg or higher. ABG data with PO_2 levels less than 80 mmHg should be interpreted as indicating arterial hypoxemia, which is generally correct for individuals less than 60 years of age. However, as discussed in Chapter 19, lung function decreases with increasing age, as does PO_2. Some authors[1] use a 1 mmHg decrease below 80 as an acceptable limit of normal PO_2 for every year over 60. More precise estimates of lower limits of acceptable PO_2 have been determined by Sorbini et al.[3] and Mellemgaard.[4] The following regression equations are used to determine minimally acceptable PO_2 at sea level[3]:

$$\text{Predicted } PaO_2 = 109 - (0.43 \times \text{age}) \pm 4 \text{ (for ages 14–84 supine)}^3 \quad (4)$$

$$\text{Predicted } PaO_2 = 104.2 - (0.27 \times \text{age}) \pm 6 \text{ (for ages 15–75 seated)}^4 \quad (5)$$

As noted, the guidelines for interpreting PO_2 are determined at sea level, and therefore adjustments must be made when evaluating PO_2 levels at increased altitude. In addition to evaluating PO_2, a complete evaluation of oxygenation state requires an evaluation of SaO_2 and O_2 content, as defined in Table 47-1.

With altitude, the maximum PO_2 without hyperventilation decreases, as predicted by Dalton's law of partial pressure. For example, in Denver at an altitude of 5000 ft, when the barometric pressure is 623 mmHg, the PCO_2 is 40 mmHg, and the inspired O_2 fraction (F_{IO_2}) 0.21, then the P_{AO_2} is 73 mmHg. Considering a normal alveolar-arterial gradient [$P(A\text{-}a)O_2$] of 5 to 10 mmHg, a normal PaO_2 is about 65 mmHg. Thus, hypoxemia is considered to be present when the PaO_2 falls below 50 to 55 mmHg.

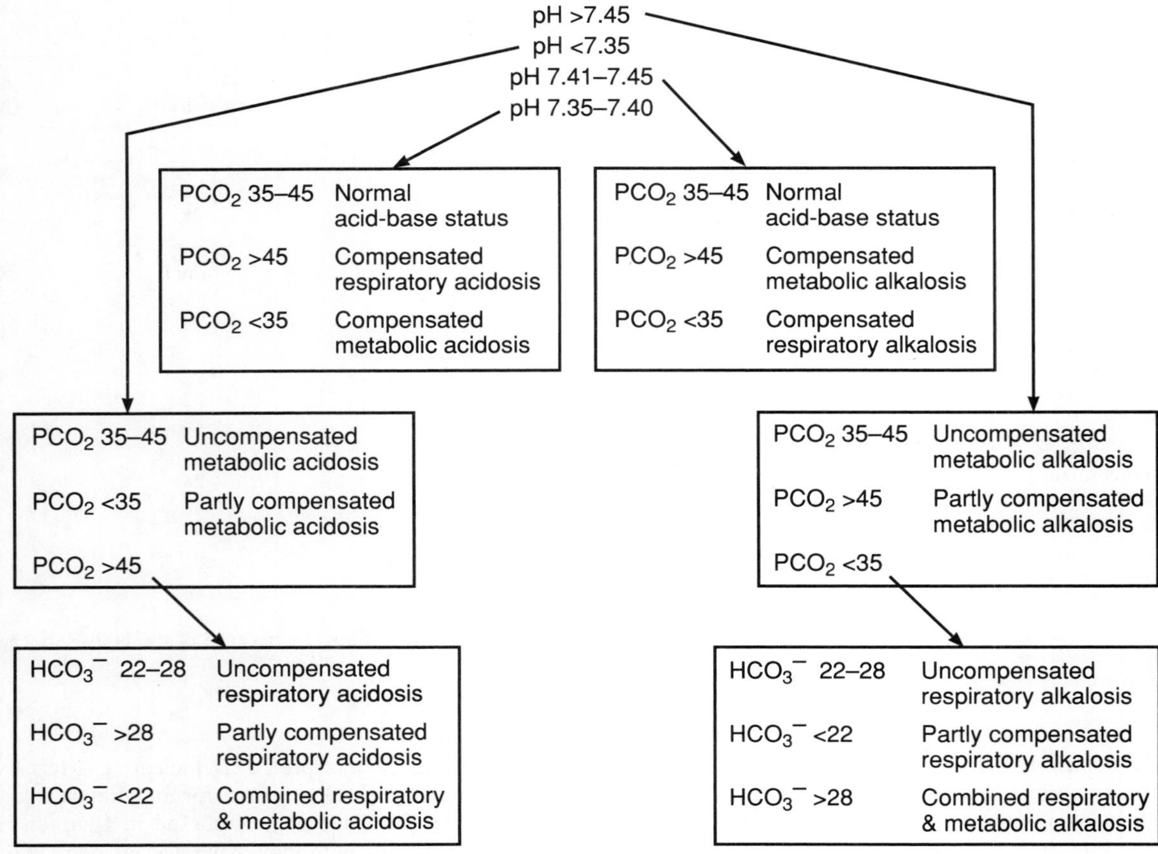

Figure 47-4. Algorithm: classical interpretation of acid-base balance.

CLINICAL GUIDELINES FOR INTERPRETING ARTERIAL BLOOD GASES

Table 47-2 lists ranges for pH and PCO_2 that are considered acceptable in clinical settings. It is important not to infer from these values that a PCO_2 of 49 mmHg and a pH of 7.31, although in the normal range, have not deviated sufficiently from usual normal values to merit intervention in all clinical settings. Table 47-14 lists the level of change in pH, PCO_2, HCO_3^-, and BE/BD that are associated with each of the specific acid-base disturbances. The terminology used for interpretation has been changed by Shapiro et al.[1] with reference to respiratory abnormalities. Respiratory acidosis is referred to as *ventilatory failure* with only two subdivisions, acute or chronic, and respiratory alkalosis is referred to as *alveolar hyperventilation*, again either acute or chronic. The terms ventilatory failure and alveolar hyperventilation are used to better reflect the actual physiologic abnormality noted in the ABG data. Figure 47-5 presents an algorithm for use in clinical approaches to interpretation of ABG data.

CAUSES OF ACID-BASE DISTURBANCES

Detailed discussion of metabolic causes of acid-base disturbance is presented in Chapter 28. Tables 47-15 and 47-16 from Effros[5] list the primary reasons for the development of respiratory acidosis and alkalosis. As noted, respiratory aci-

Table 47-13. Acute Respiratory Alkalosis Superimposed on Compensated Respiratory Acidosis

	pH	PCO_2	HCO_3^-
Baseline acid-base status	7.38	60	33
An acute pulmonary insult may result in increased or decreased ventilation from this level.			
Increased ventilation	7.48	47	31

[a] Evaluation of these values without knowledge of the patient's history would lead to a diagnosis of partially compensated metabolic alkalosis. However, when the patient's actual baseline is considered, the proper interpretation is uncompensated or acute respiratory alkalosis superimposed on a compensated respiratory acidosis.

Table 47-14. Clinical Method of Arterial Blood Gas Interpretation

Status	pH (units)	PCO_2 (mmHg)	HCO_3^- (mEq/L)	BE (mEq/L)
Ventilatory failure (respiratory acidosis)				
Acute	<7.30	>50	Normal	Normal
Chronic	7.30–7.40	>50	>28	>+2
Alveolar hyperventilation (respiratory alkalosis)				
Acute	>7.50	<30	Normal	Normal
Chronic	7.40–7.50	<30	<22	<−2
Metabolic acidosis				
Uncompensated	<7.30	Normal	<22	<−2
Partially compensated	<7.30	<30	<22	<−2
Compensated	7.30–7.40	<30	<22	<−2
Metabolic alkalosis				
Uncompensated	>7.50	Normal	>28	>+2
Partially compensated[a]	>7.50	>50	>28	>+2
Compensated[a]	7.41–7.50	>50	>28	>+2
Combined ventilatory failure and metabolic acidosis	<7.30	>50	<22	<−2
Combined alveolar hyperventilation and metabolic alkalosis	>7.50	<30	>28	>+2

[a] In general, partially compensated or compensated metabolic alkalosis is rarely seen clinically because of the body's mechanism to prevent hypoventilation.

(From Kacmarek et al.,[62] with permission.)

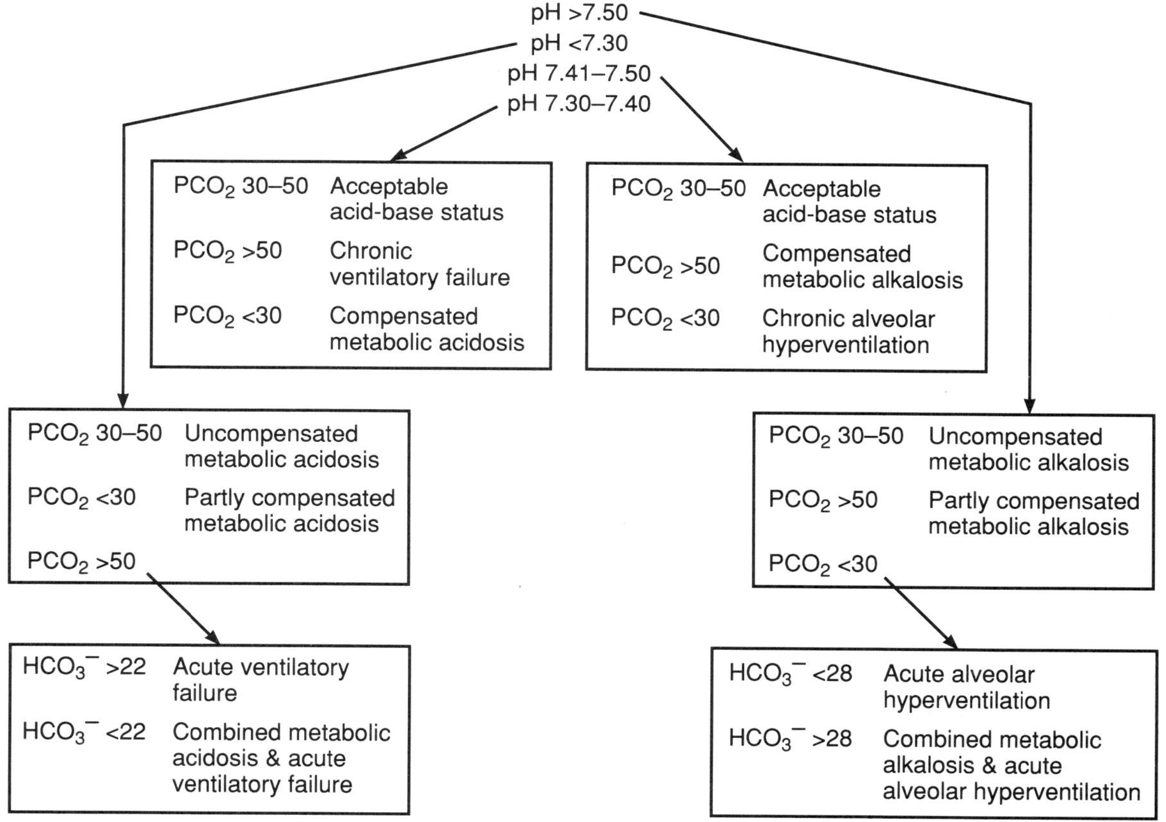

Figure 47-5. Algorithm: clinical interpretation of acid-base balance.

Table 47-15. Primary Causes of Respiratory Acidosis

Central depression
- Drugs: opiates, sedatives, anesthetics
- O_2 therapy in chronic obstructive lung disease (COPD)
- Obesity-hypoventilation syndrome
- Central nervous system disorders

Neuromuscular disorders
- Neurologic: multiple sclerosis, poliomyelitis, phrenic nerve injuries, high cord lesions, Guillain-Barré syndrome, botulism, tetanus
- End-plate: myasthenia gravis, succinylcholine chloride, curare, aminoglycosides, organophosphorus compounds
- Muscle: hypokalemia, hypophosphatemia, muscular dystrophy

Airway obstruction
- COPD
- Acute aspiration, laryngospasm

Chest wall restriction
- Pleural: effusions, empyema, pneumothorax, fibrothorax
- Chest wall: kyphoscoliosis, scleroderma, ankylosing spondylitis, extreme obesity

Severe pulmonary restrictive disorders
- Pulmonary fibrosis
- Parenchymal infiltration: pneumonia, edema

(From Effros,[5] with permission.)

dosis is a result of depression of ventilatory drive or mechanical limitation to ventilation, while respiratory alkalosis is normally a result of hypoxemia, central nervous system stimulation, or mechanical ventilation.

ESTIMATING BASE EXCESS/BASE DEFICIT

Since the BE/BD is a calculated value based in part on another calculated value (HCO_3^- content), gross estimates of the BE/BD can be easily made based on the actual $PaCO_2$ and arterial pH. It is assumed that the BE/BD is based totally on the HCO_3^- level. The first step is to determine the variance in the PCO_2 from a normal value of 40 mmHg. Second, the acute change in pH predicted by the PCO_2 change (step 1) is determined. For every 10 mmHg PCO_2 decrease, the pH should increase by 0.05 units, and for every 10 mmHg PCO_2 increase, the pH should decrease by 0.10 units. A baseline pH of 7.40 is assumed. Third, the BE/BD is estimated as two-thirds of the difference between the actual pH and the predicted pH (move the decimal point in the difference between pH values two places to the right). A base deficit is present if the measured pH is less than predicted, while a base excess is present if it is greater than predicted (Table 47-17).

Table 47-16. Primary Causes of Respiratory Alkalosis

Primary central nervous system disorders
- Hyperventilation syndrome, anxiety
- Cerebrovascular disease
- Meningitis, encephalitis

Hypoxemia

Pulmonary disease
- Interstitial fibrosis
- Pneumonia
- Pulmonary embolism
- Pulmonary edema (some patients)

Septicemia, hypotension

Hepatic failure

Drugs
- Salicylates
- Nicotine
- Xanthines
- Progestational hormones

High altitude

Mechanical ventilators

(From Effros,[5] with permission.)

QUANTIFYING EXTRACELLULAR BICARBONATE DEFICIT

HCO_3^- ion is administered to normalize the pH in severe metabolic acidosis or sustained mechanical alveolar hyperventilation. An estimate of the HCO_3^- concentration needed to normalize the pH in extracellular fluid may be obtained if the BD is known and an estimate of extracellular fluid volume can be made. Generally, extracellular fluid volume is estimated as equal to 25 percent of body weight in kilograms. Thus, the extracellular HCO_3^- deficit can be determined by the equation:

$$HCO_3^- \text{ deficit (mEq/L)} = \frac{\text{(BD)(kg weight)}}{4} \qquad (6)$$

Since this is a calculated estimate based on other estimated or calculated values, generally half the calculated deficit is administered after which the pH is reassessed and the HCO_3^- requirement recalculated.

HCO_3^- is usually not administered to treat a metabolic acidosis unless a base deficit of at least 10 mEq/L is present with a pH less than 7.20 or cardiovascular instability is present with a pH less than 7.25 to 7.30.

Table 47-17. Estimates of Base Excess/Base Deficit

Actual ABG: pH 7.15, PCO_2 30 mmHg

1. Estimate pH based on actual PCO_2
   For every 10 mmHg PCO_2 decrease, pH increases 0.05 unit
   For every 10 mmHg PCO_2 increase, pH decreases 0.10 unit

   PCO_2 30, predicted pH 7.45
2. Determine difference between actual and predicted pH

   $7.15 - 7.45 = -0.30$
3. Eliminate decimal and multiply by ⅔

   $(2/3)(-30) = -20$
4. Actual pH greater than predicted, BE is present
   Actual pH less than predicted, BD is present

   BD = −20 mEq/L

ASSESSMENT OF INTRAPULMONARY SHUNT

As discussed in Chapter 10, the intrapulmonary shunt is an expression of the percentage of the total cardiac output that perfuses nonventilated alveoli. From a pathophysiologic perspective, shunting results from the combined effect of true shunting (no ventilation) and ventilation/perfusion ($\dot{V}/\dot{Q}$) mismatch (i.e., low $\dot{V}/\dot{Q}$ areas). However, the contribution of low $\dot{V}/\dot{Q}$ areas on the calculated shunt can be decreased by administration of O_2, whereas true shunting cannot be eliminated or minimized unless the pathophysiologic cause is reversed.

Total intrapulmonary shunt is frequently referred to as *physiologic shunt* since it encompasses all aspects of shunting (anatomic shunt, capillary shunt, and $\dot{V}/\dot{Q}$ mismatch). The anatomic shunt ($\dot{Q}s$) equals the portion of the cardiac output ($\dot{Q}_T$) that passed from the right to left side of the heart, bypassing the lung. Capillary shunt refers to areas perfused but not ventilated while $\dot{V}/\dot{Q}$ mismatch refers to areas of the lung in which perfusion is in excess of ventilation. Table 47-18 lists the major causes of each aspect of the physiologic shunt. The total physiologic shunt is determined by the shunt equation (Tables 47-19 and 47-20), which as noted in Table 47-20, is a comparison of O_2 contents—ideal end-capillary (CcO_2), arterial (CaO_2), and mixed venous ($C\bar{v}O_2$).

In order to accurately calculate $\dot{Q}s/\dot{Q}_T$, a number of assumptions must be valid. First, the P_AO_2 must be high enough (about 150 mmHg) to saturate blood perfusing the ideal alveolar-capillary unit. This is to allow calculation of CcO_2, since this value cannot be directly measured. The PO_2 of ideal end-capillary blood is equal to the P_AO_2 calculated by the alveolar gas equation:

$$P_AO_2 = (P_b - PH_2O)(F_IO_2) - (PaCO_2)\left(F_IO_2 + \frac{1 - F_IO_2}{R}\right) \quad (7)$$

where P_b is barometric pressure (see Ch. 1 for details). Once P_AO_2 is calculated and since the SaO_2 is assumed to be 100 percent, all that is necessary to calculate CcO_2 is hemoglobin (Hb) content.

Ideally, a pulmonary artery sample must be obtained to determine $C\bar{v}O_2$. A central venous sample may be used; however in this case mixing of blood from the superior and inferior vena cava may be incomplete, leading to erroneous results. If $C\bar{v}O_2$ cannot be obtained, the modified shunt equation may be used (Table 47-21). However, for this equation to accurately reflect $\dot{Q}s/\dot{Q}_T$ the patient must be paralyzed, nonseptic, nonfebrile, and hemodynamically stable. The modified shunt equation is based on the arteriovenous O_2 content difference $[C(a\text{-}v)O_2]$ in stable, nonfebrile, paralyzed patients being equal to 3.5 Vol% instead of the normal 5 to 6 Vol% in healthy individuals. This assumption can only rarely be made in the acutely ill patient.

Finally, the resulting $\dot{Q}s/\dot{Q}_T$ is dependent on F_IO_2. Historically, $\dot{Q}s/\dot{Q}_T$ was determined at an F_IO_2 of 1.0, at which the effects of low $\dot{V}/\dot{Q}$ regions are eliminated, either by increasing the PaO_2 sufficiently to oxygenate capillary blood or by causing N_2 washout atelectasis in those regions with very low $\dot{V}/\dot{Q}$. As a result, calculated $\dot{Q}s/\dot{Q}_T$ may differ depending on F_IO_2. The difference in values calculated at the

Table 47-18. Components of the Total Physiologic Shunt

Anatomic shunt, normally about 2–5% of cardiac output
- Normal components, veins emptying into the left side of heart
  - Bronchial
  - Pleural
  - Thebesian
- Abnormal causes of anatomic shunt
  - Vascular pulmonary tumors
  - Arteriovenous anastomosis
  - Congenital cardiac anomalies
  - Severe liver disease

Capillary shunt, normally zero, is that portion of the cardiac output perfusing nonventilated alveoli
- Atelectasis
- Consolidating pneumonia
- Complete airway obstruction
- Pneumothorax
- Pleural effusion
- Any pathophysiologic process that eliminates ventilation to perfused alveoli

Ventilation/perfusion ($\dot{V}/\dot{Q}$) mismatch (i.e., low $\dot{V}/\dot{Q}$ areas)
- Normally low $\dot{V}/\dot{Q}$ areas exist in the bases when $\dot{V}/\dot{Q}$ is less than 1.0
- Low $\dot{V}/\dot{Q}$ areas caused by
  - Retained secretions
  - Bronchospasm
  - Partial airway obstruction
  - Regional increases in fibrotic tissue
  - Decreased tidal volume
  - Mucosal edema

Table 47-19. Definition of Terms Used in Shunt and Dead Space Equations

Term	Definition
$\dot{V}O_2$	Volume of O_2 consumed per minute
$\dot{Q}s$	Shunted cardiac output
$\dot{Q}c$	Capillary cardiac output
$\dot{Q}_T$	Total cardiac output
CcO_2	Capillary O_2 content
CaO_2	Arterial O_2 content
$C\bar{v}O_2$	Mixed venous O_2 content
P_AO_2	Alveolar O_2 partial pressure
PaO_2	Arterial O_2 partial pressure
V_T	Tidal volume
V_D	Dead space
V_A	Alveolar volume
F_ACO_2	Fractional concentration of CO_2 in alveolar gas
$F\bar{E}CO_2$	Mean fractional concentration of CO_2 in mixed expired gas
$PaCO_2$	Arterial CO_2 partial pressure
$P\bar{E}CO_2$	Partial pressure of mean exhaled CO_2
F_DCO_2	Fractional concentration of dead space CO_2

Table 47-20. Derivation of the Shunt Equation from the Fick Equation

$$\dot{V}O_2 = \dot{Q}_T(CaO_2 - C\bar{v}O_2) \quad (1)$$

Replacing $\dot{Q}_T$ with $\dot{Q}c$ (the portion of the cardiac output perfusing well ventilated alveoli) and replacing CaO_2 with CcO_2 (see Table 47-19),

$$\dot{V}O_2 = \dot{Q}c(CcO_2 - C\bar{v}O_2) \quad (2)$$

Total cardiac output equals shunted cardiac output plus capillary cardiac output

$$\dot{Q}_T = \dot{Q}c + \dot{Q}s \quad (3)$$

Solving Equation 3 for $\dot{Q}c$,

$$\dot{Q}c = \dot{Q}_T - \dot{Q}s \quad (4)$$

Substituting into Equation 2 the equivalent of $\dot{V}O_2$ from Equation 1,

$$\dot{Q}_T(CaO_2 - C\bar{v}O_2) = \dot{Q}c(CcO_2 - C\bar{v}O_2) \quad (5)$$

Substituting into Equation 5, the equivalent of $\dot{Q}c$ from Equation 4,

$$\dot{Q}_T(CaO_2 - C\bar{v}O_2) = (\dot{Q}_T - \dot{Q}s)(CcO_2 - C\bar{v}O_2) \quad (6)$$

Rearranging Equation 6,

$$\dot{Q}_TCaO_2 - \dot{Q}_TC\bar{v}O_2 = \dot{Q}_TCcO_2 - \dot{Q}_TC\bar{v}O_2 - \dot{Q}sCcO_2 + \dot{Q}sC\bar{v}O_2 \quad (7)$$

Eliminating $-\dot{Q}_TC\bar{v}O_2$ from both sides of Equation 7,

$$\dot{Q}_TCaO_2 = \dot{Q}_TCcO_2 - \dot{Q}sCcO_2 + \dot{Q}sC\bar{v}O_2 \quad (8)$$

Rearranging Equation 8,

$$\dot{Q}sCcO_2 - \dot{Q}sC\bar{v}O_2 = \dot{Q}_TCcO_2 - \dot{Q}_TCaO_2 \quad (9)$$

Simplifying Equation 9,

$$\dot{Q}s(CcO_2 - C\bar{v}O_2) = \dot{Q}_T(CcO_2 - CaO_2) \quad (10)$$

Rearranging Equation 10,

$$\dot{Q}s/\dot{Q}_T = \frac{CcO_2 - CaO_2}{CcO_2 - C\bar{v}O_2} \quad (11)$$

Table 47-21. Derivation of the Modified Shunt Equation from the Classic Shunt Equation

$$\dot{Q}s/\dot{Q}_T = \frac{CcO_2 - CaO_2}{CcO_2 - C\bar{v}O_2} \quad (1)$$

The denominator of Equation 1 encompasses the capillary, arterial and venous O_2 contents:

$$CcO_2 - C\bar{v}O_2 = (CcO_2 - CaO_2) + (CaO_2 - C\bar{v}O_2) \quad (2)$$

The assumption is made when using the modified shunt equation that $CaO_2 - C\bar{v}O_2$ equals 3.5 Vol% (see text)

$$CcO_2 - C\bar{v}O_2 = (CcO_2 - CaO_2) + 3.5 \quad (3)$$

Substituting Equation 3 into Equation 1 gives the modified shunt equation

$$\dot{Q}s/\dot{Q}_T = \frac{CcO_2 - CaO_2}{(CcO_2 - CaO_2) + 3.5} \quad (4)$$

actual F_IO_2 (or 0.5) and an F_IO_2 of 1.0 permits estimation of the extent of $\dot{V}/\dot{Q}$ mismatch.

Clinical Use of the Shunt Calculation

The shunt calculation has been used to titrate O_2 therapy and PEEP levels (see Ch. 76), to assess spontaneous breathing capabilities, to assess specific cardiopulmonary abnormalities, and as a means of determining the cause of hypoxemia. Hypoxemia is primarily a result of pulmonary abnormalities but its severity can be markedly increased by a decrease in cardiac output. Since the numerator of the shunt equation ($CcO_2 - CaO_2$) reflects pulmonary pathology and the denominator ($CcO_2 - C\bar{v}O_2$) reflects nonpulmonary pathology [because the denominator contains the $C(a\text{-}v)O_2$], hypoxemia primarily from pulmonary problems results in an increase in $\dot{Q}s/\dot{Q}_T$ while hypoxemia of nonpulmonary pathology only minimally affects $\dot{Q}s/\dot{Q}_T$.

The greater the $\dot{Q}s/\dot{Q}_T$, the less likely it is that spontaneous ventilation can be sustained. Shunt fractions greater than 20 to 30 percent are associated with such marked increases in work of breathing that ventilatory failure frequently occurs if sustained spontaneous ventilation is attempted. The shunt fraction can also be used to quantify the extent of a right-to-left congenital cardiac anomaly and the effect of unilateral pulmonary disease. $\dot{Q}s/\dot{Q}_T$ values calculated for different positions can identify the contribution of position to hypoxemia.

Other Methods of Estimating Shunt

Three other relationships have been used to estimate shunt fraction (Table 47-22): $P(A\text{-}a)O_2$, arterial/alveolar ratio (PaO_2/PAO_2), and PaO_2/F_IO_2 ratio. Each of these relationships is much easier to determine than is $\dot{Q}s/\dot{Q}_T$, but they have limited accuracy, although they do provide gross estimations of oxygenation capabilities. More importantly, however, they reflect the effect of change in management on oxygenation state. The major limitation of $P(A\text{-}a)O_2$ is its variability with changes in F_IO_2, while the PaO_2/F_IO_2 ratio

Table 47-22. Methods of Calculating or Estimating Shunt

Index	Normal Value	Abnormal Value	Limitations
$\dot{Q}s/\dot{Q}_T$	2–5%	>10%	Invasive
$P(A\text{-}a)O_2$	7–14 mmHg (RA) 31–56 mmHg (1.0)	100–150 at F_IO_2 1.0	Varies with F_IO_2
PaO_2/PAO_2	>0.75	<0.75	—
PaO_2/F_IO_2	450–500	<300–350	Varies with $PaCO_2$ and F_IO_2

RA, room air; 1.0, 100% O_2.

is inversely affected by $PaCO_2$ as well as by increased FIO_2. Of the three parameters, PaO_2/PAO_2 appears to be the most reliable, since it is not affected by FIO_2 or $PaCO_2$, and in our opinion is as useful as $\dot{Q}S/\dot{Q}T$ for evaluating the effect of alterations in management of critically ill patients.

DEAD SPACE TO TIDAL VOLUME RATIO

Normally about 20 to 40 percent of tidal volume (VT) is wasted ventilation. This is primarily due to the volume of the upper respiratory tract and conducting airways where no gas exchange occurs, referred to as anatomic *dead space*. This volume is equal to about 1 mL/lb ideal body weight. In addition, the total physiologic dead space (VD) is composed of alveolar dead space, ventilated but unperfused lung units, and areas of high $\dot{V}/\dot{Q}$ (Table 47-23). Total physiologic dead space is normally calculated by the Enghoff modification of the Bohr equation (Tables 47-19 and 47-24). This requires an arterial blood sample and a collection of exhaled gas. Since the mean exhaled PCO_2 ($P\bar{E}CO_2$) is required and ventilation during spontaneous breathing varies considerably, about 40 L is usually collected for analysis of $P\bar{E}CO_2$. During controlled mechanical ventilation a 5-L sample is usually adequate.

The VD/VT ratio is helpful in determining if patients receiving mechanical ventilation are capable of breathing spontaneously. Normally mechanical ventilation increases VD/VT, with levels up to 50 percent considered normal. However, because of the large minute ventilation required and the correspondingly increased work load, patients with VD/VT ratios greater than 60 percent are rarely capable of sustaining spontaneous breathing. This VD/VT level frequently translates into minute ventilations greater than 15 L/min. Although not definitive, increased VD/VT also assists in the diagnosis of dead space-producing disease, particularly pulmonary embolism.

VD/VT ratios are always increased if there is a disparity between minute ventilation and expected $PaCO_2$ (Table 47-25). The normal $PaCO_2$ of 40 mmHg is generally associated with an alveolar ventilation of about 5.0 L in adults. When minute ventilation is doubled and $PaCO_2$ is still 40 mmHg, a marked increase in dead space exists.

Table 47-23. Components of the Total Physiologic Dead Space

Anatomic dead space
- The portion of total ventilation that does not contact the alveolar epithelium
- Normally equals 1 mL/lb ideal body weight
- Increased as a result of
  - Positive pressure ventilation
  - Mechanical dead space

Alveolar dead space
- Ventilated but unperfused alveoli
- Normally equals minute component of VD/VT
- Increased as a result of
  - Pulmonary emboli
  - Emphysema
  - Adult respiratory distress syndrome (ARDS)

High $\dot{V}/\dot{Q}$ areas
- Normally all lung areas where $\dot{V}/\dot{Q}$ is >1.0
- Increased as a result of
  - Rapid shallow breathing
  - Positive pressure ventilation
  - Decreased cardiac output
  - Alveolar septal wall destruction

Table 47-24. Derivation of the Dead Space to Tidal Volume Equation

Tidal volume is equal to dead space volume plus alveolar volume:

$$V_T = V_D + V_A \qquad (1)$$

Total exhaled CO_2 is equal to VT times concentration of CO_2 in exhaled gas:

$$(V_T)(F\bar{E}CO_2) = \text{total } CO_2 \text{ exhaled} \qquad (2)$$

Equation 2 can be divided into CO_2 exhaled from dead space and alveoli

$$(V_T)(F\bar{E}CO_2) = (V_A)(F_ACO_2) + (V_D)(F_DCO_2) \qquad (3)$$

Since CO_2 concentration in dead space gas is zero, Equation 3 can be rewritten as

$$(V_T)(F\bar{E}CO_2) = (V_A)(F_ACO_2) \qquad (4)$$

Since $V_A = V_T - V_D$, Equation 20 can be rewritten as

$$(V_T)(F\bar{E}CO_2) = (V_T)(F_ACO_2) - (V_D)(F_ACO_2) \qquad (5)$$

Rearrangement and simplification of Equation 21 gives the Bohr equation

$$V_D/V_T = \frac{F_ACO_2 - F\bar{E}CO_2}{F_ACO_2} \qquad (6)$$

Since concentration of CO_2 can be replaced with partial pressure of CO_2, Equation 6 can be rewritten as the Enghoff modification of the Bohr equation

$$V_D/V_T = \frac{PaCO_2 - P\bar{E}CO_2}{PaCO_2} \qquad (7)$$

BLOOD GAS ELECTRODES

The assessment of ABGs requires careful and accurate measurement of PO_2, PCO_2, and pH. All modern blood gas

Table 47-25. Normal Minute Volume–$PaCO_2$ Relationship

$\dot{V}_A$ (L/min)	$PaCO_2$ (mmHg)
1.25	60
2.50	50
5.00	40
10.00	30
20.00	20

analyzers measure pH with a Sanz electrode, PCO_2 with a Severinghaus electrode, and PO_2 with a Clark electrode.

Sanz Electrode

The function of the pH electrode is based on the use of a special glass capable of generating an electrical potential when solutions of differing pH are placed on either side of it. Thus, if a solution of known pH (6.80) is separated from a solution of unknown pH, a measurable voltage is established across the glass. The conversion of the potential difference across the glass to the pH of the unknown solution is described by the Nernst equation[1]:

$$pH_u = pH_k + \frac{(Eu - Ek)}{(2.3026T)} \frac{(F)}{R} \tag{8}$$

where pH_u is the unknown pH, pH_k is the known pH, Eu − Ek is the potential difference across the glass, T is absolute temperature, F is the Faraday constant, and R is the molar gas constant.

The basic design of the modern pH electrode is illustrated in Figure 47-6. Essentially the electrode is divided into a measuring electrode composed of silver/silver chloride (Ag/AgCl) and a reference electrode composed of mercurous chloride (HgCl). The reference electrode establishes a constant voltage while the measuring electrode evaluates the voltage established across the pH-sensitive glass. The two half-cells are connected by a potassium chloride (KCl) bridge completing the electrical circuit. During calibration a solution of pH 7.384 is normally placed in the measuring chamber; this results in a potential difference of 33.5 mV. A zero-voltage calibration is usually performed with a solution of pH 6.80. This two-point calibration is normally sufficient since the potential difference across the electrode is linear in the physiologic range. The accuracy of the Sanz electrode is about ±0.02 pH units.

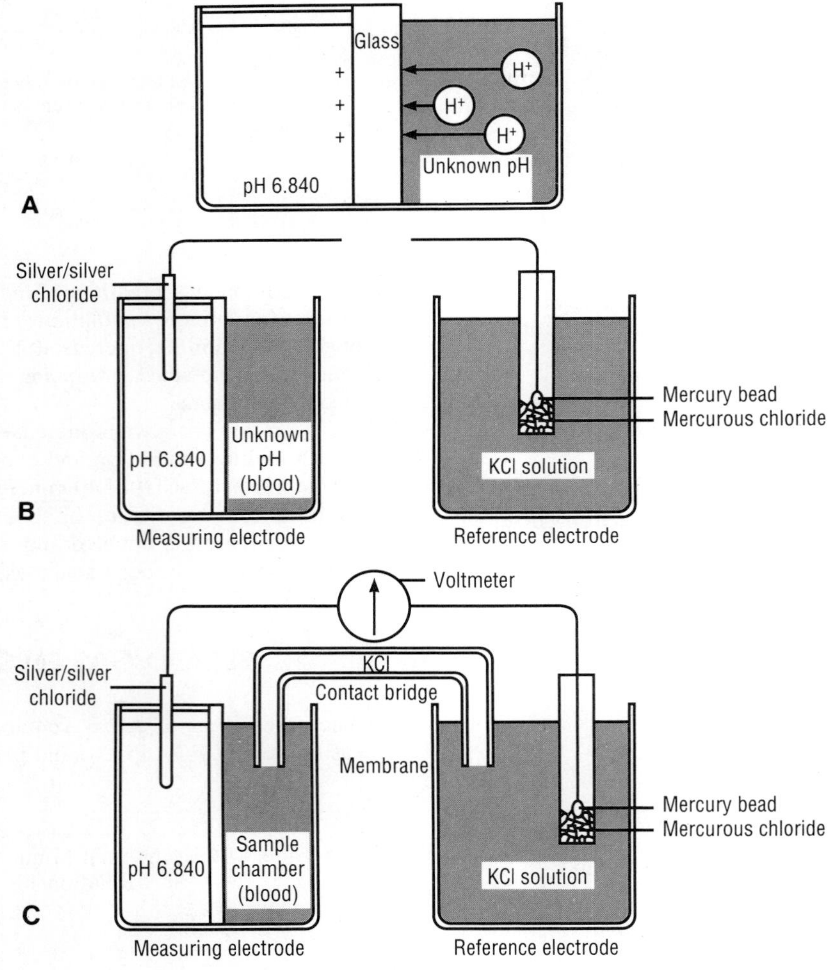

Figure 47-6. Basic principles of the pH electrode. **(A)** Voltage developed across pH-sensitive glass when H^+ concentration is unequal in the two solutions; **(B)** chemical half-cell is used as the measuring electrode and another half-cell is the reference electrode; **(C)** schematic of overall electrode. (From Shapiro et al.,[1] with permission.)

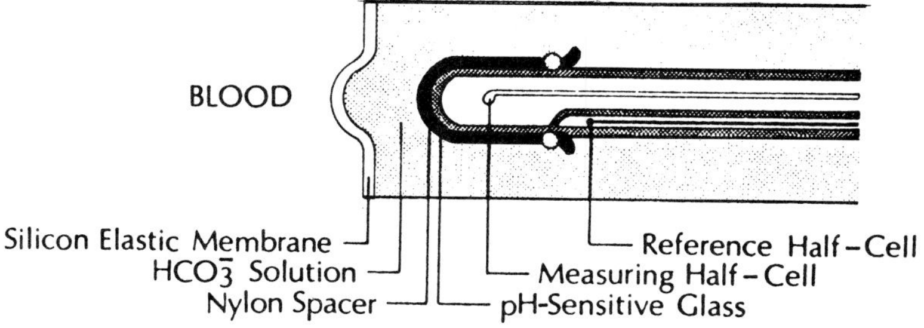

Figure 47-7. Schematic illustration of the modern PCO_2 electrode. See text for details. (From Shapiro et al.,[1] with permission.)

Severinghaus Electrode

The Severinghaus electrode is essentially a modification of the Sanz electrode.[6] Blood drawn into the electrode is separated from the measuring half-cell by a silicone elastic membrane, which allows CO_2 to diffuse into a HCO_3^--buffered solution separated from the measuring electrode by a nylon spacer (Fig. 47-7). CO_2 is unable to diffuse across the nylon spacer, but H^+ can. As CO_2 moves into the electrode, it is hydrated, with formation of H^+ and HCO_3^-. The H^+ moves to the pH-sensitive glass, establishing an electrical potential across the glass. The potential is subsequently converted to PCO_2 in millimeters of Hg. Generally the analysis of PCO_2 is linear over a 10- to 90-mmHg PCO_2 range. A two-point calibration with gas containing zero CO_2 and about 5 percent CO_2 is usually performed. The accuracy of the electrode is about ± 2 mmHg.

Clark Electrode

The Clark electrode (Fig. 47-8) consists of a Ag anode immersed in a KCl electrolyte solution and a platinum (Pt) cathode. The Ag anode participates in an oxidation reaction with the Cl^- in solution, producing electrons. In the presence of O_2 the electrons reaching the cathode are used in the reduction of O_2 and water to OH^-:

$$O_2 + 2H_2O + 4 \text{ electrons} \rightarrow 4OH^- \quad (9)$$

The magnitude of the decrease in current is indirectly proportional to the O_2 concentration. An external polarizing voltage of about -0.6 to -0.7 V is required to minimize reduction of other gases at the cathode.

The actual tip of the electrode is covered by a polypropylene membrane permeable to O_2. Careful calibration of this electrode is required to establish linearity, drift, re-

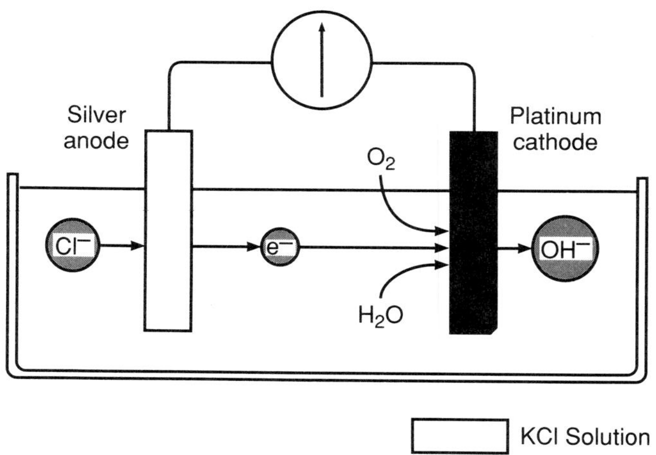

Figure 47-8. The basic principle of the polarographic electrode. The Cl^- ion reacts with the silver anode to form silver chloride (AgCl) in an oxidation reaction, which produces electrons; O_2 reacts with platinum and water, with a gain of electrons (a reduction reaction); and the flow of electrons (current) is measured. The greater the O_2 concentration in solution, the greater the current generated. (From Shapiro et al.,[1] with permission.)

sponse time, zero current level, and flow sensitivities. Generally, the electrode's response is linear over the clinical range of PO_2 change. The Clark electrode's accuracy at PO_2 levels of 40 to 100 is about ±2 mmHg. Accuracy decreases outside of this range.

OXIMETRY

The term used to define the analysis of the percentage of the total hemoglobin chemically bound to various substances is *oximetry*. All oximeters are essentially spectrophotometers, that is, instruments capable of converting light intensity into electric current. They function by determining the intensity of light of specific wavelengths transmitted through a sample of blood. The probability of light of a single wavelength being absorbed by a substance is described by the Beer-Lambert law,[7] which states essentially that the intensity of light absorbed while passing through a substance is directly related to the thickness (or concentration) of the substance:

$$L_n (I_0/I) = K'Cl \qquad (10)$$

where L_n is the natural logarithm, l is the path length, I_0 is the initial and I the final intensity of the light passing through the sample, K′ (the extinction coefficient) is a constant that depends on the properties of the substance, and C is the concentration of the absorbing substance. Transmitted light can be converted to absorbed light by the equation:

$$A = -\log T \qquad (11)$$

where A is light absorbed and T (which is equivalent to I_0/I) is light transmitted.

A co-oximeter is a laboratory instrument capable of measuring the concentration of oxyhemoglobin, reduced hemoglobin, carboxyhemoglobin, and methemoglobin in a sample of blood. During actual operation the co-oximeter measures the absorption of light at four different wavelengths, one specific for each form of hemoglobin evaluated. The only significant hemoglobin species not measured by the co-oximeter is fetal hemoglobin. If adult values for the extinction coefficient are used in the presence of oxygenated fetal hemoglobin, a 4 to 7 percent error in carboxyhemoglobin reading results, while with reduced fetal hemoglobin this error is 0.2 to 1.5 percent.[9] Most co-oximeters are capable of compensating for fetal hemoglobin.

PULSE OXIMETRY

The most common method of assessing oxygenation noninvasively is the pulse oximeter. Like the co-oximeter, it is a spectrophotometer, normally using only two wavelengths of light (Fig. 47-9), one in the infrared range at a wavelength of 940 nm and one in the red range at 660 nm.[10] Oxyhemoglobin absorbs more in the infrared range, while reduced hemoglobin absorbs more in the red range. Comparison of

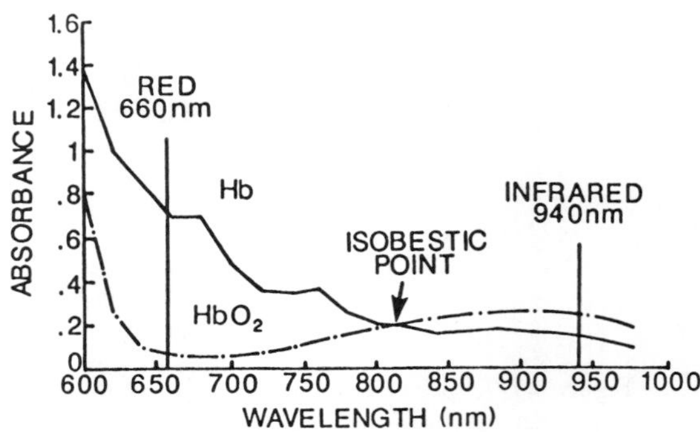

Figure 47-9. Spectrum of optical absorption of oxyhemoglobin and reduced hemoglobin in the visible and near infrared wavelength range. The ratio of transmitted to absorbed light at preset red and infrared wavelengths emitted by the oximeter determines the oxyhemoglobin saturation by pulse oximeter (SpO_2) value. The isobestic point is the wavelength of equal absorption by reduced hemoglobin and oxyhemoglobin. (From Szaflarski and Cohen,[10] with permission.)

absorption at these two wavelengths allows quantification of percentages of oxygenated and reduced hemoglobin. In order to limit error by absorption from venous blood, tissue, bone, and skin pigmentation, the pulse oximeter compares absorption during systole and diastole, the difference in absorption being taken as reflective only of the absorption of arterial blood. As a result, most oximeters include a plethysmographic waveform of arterial pulse or indicate each heartbeat. A well designed pulse oximeter does not display a saturation reading unless a pulse is recognizable.

Accuracy

Pulse oximeters are not periodically calibrated before use. Their data displays are based on empirical calibration developed from studies of volunteers[11] (Fig. 47-10). These calibration curves are limited by the range of saturation that the volunteers could achieve. As a result, the accuracy of most oximeters decreases at saturations below 70 to 75 percent; generally, the accuracy of pulse oximeters is ±4 percent at saturations above 70 percent and ±6 percent at saturations below 70 percent[12,13] (95 percent confidence interval). As a result it is important to realize that pulse oximeters should be used to only monitor change in saturation and not as an absolute indication of actual saturation.

Performance Limitations

Numerous factors encountered at the bedside may further limit the accuracy of pulse oximeters (Table 47-26). The most significant of these is their inability to distinguish dyshemoglobins, most importantly carboxyhemoglobin (COHb) and methemoglobin (MetHb), from oxyhemoglobin. Thus, in the presence of dyshemoglobin a higher than actual SpO_2 (O_2 saturation obtained with pulse oximeter) may be dis-

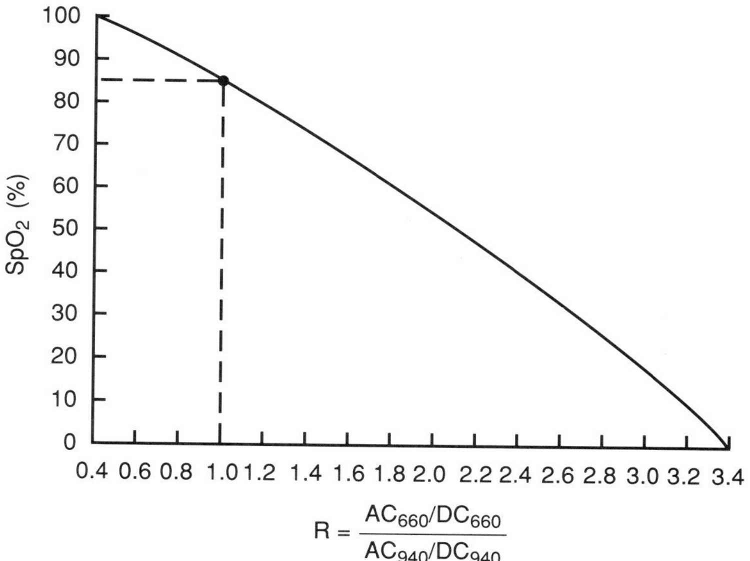

Figure 47-10. Illustration of a pulse-added calibration curve. Dividing the AC (pulsatile systolic absorption) signal by the DC (nonpulsatile diastolic absorption) signal for both wavelengths and then reducing the resulting fractions yields a theoretical calibration curve that is insensitive to light intensity. Actual calibration curves are based on experimental data and therefore may differ from theoretical values. (From Welch et al.,[11] with permission.)

played.[14,15] This is a particular problem in the emergency department with smoke inhalation victims. Inappropriate assumptions about oxygenation status are made if one does not consider the effect of carboxyhemoglobin. The effect of MetHb is more complex than that of COHb since MetHb absorbs in the red region, as does reduced Hb, and in the infrared region, as does oxyhemoglobin.[16,17] Experimental data[13] imply that SpO_2 would be falsely low at high concentrations of methemoglobin for SpO_2 values above 85 percent and falsely high for SpO_2 values below 85 percent.

Table 47-26. Clinical Factors Affecting the Accuracy of Pulse Oximetry

Factor
Presence of dyshemoglobins
Carboxyhemoglobin
Methemoglobin
Presence of fetal hemoglobin
Motion
Vascular dyes
Methylene blue
Indigo carmine
Indocyanine green
Ambient light
Fluorescent
Infrared
Xenon lamps
Dark skin pigmentation
Nail polish

Motion may also cause an erroneous display of SpO_2.[18,19] Any factor artificially affecting the instrument's assessment of the arterial pulse may distort the reading. If the motion is identified as causing an increased pulse, falsely high or low readings may be displayed. Newer units allowing for pulse beat-to-beat recognition and synchronization with cardiac monitors greatly reduces this problem.

Certain vascular dyes—methylene blue, indigo carmine, and indocyanine green—decrease the SpO_2 reading.[20,21] The most significant effect is seen with methylene blue, since it is a major absorber in the red region.

Pulse oximeters attempt to adjust for ambient light, but specific light sources, such as fluorescent lamps,[22] infrared lamps,[23] and xenon lamps[24] can cause erroneous signals. Care should be taken to shield the peripheral probe from all light sources to prevent interference.

Since pulse oximeters must recognize a distinct pulse, they are unreliable in low perfusion states.[13] Ideally, no data should be displayed if the instrument is unable to identify a distinct pulse. Consequently, pulse oximeters are useless during cardiac arrest or cardiopulmonary bypass. For conditions in which peripheral perfusion is poor, the earlobe is the best site for accurate monitoring.[25]

The greater the melanin concentration in the skin, the less accurate is a pulse oximeter. As a result, careful assessment of oximeter readings is required in patients with dark skin pigmentation.[11,26] Nail polish, particularly dark colors such as black, blue, and green, also lowers oximeter readings.[27]

Clinical Use

Pulse oximeters first established themselves as a standard of care in the operating room[28] because of the frequency of hypoxemia episodes affecting morbidity and mortality.[29] This standard has moved into most recovery rooms[30] as well as into neonatal intensive care units (ICUs). It is difficult to argue against the use of pulse oximeters in these areas since oxygenation state is very labile in these populations. However, care must be exercised in the neonatal ICU not to hyperoxygenate newborns. As noted earlier, the accuracy of pulse oximeters is ±4 percent at the high end; as a result, an SpO_2 of 96 percent may actually mean an SaO_2 of 100 percent and reflect a PaO_2 of well over 100 mmHg, thus posing an increased risk of retinopathy of prematurity. As a result, unless regular ABG determinations are performed to correlate SpO_2 and PaO_2, SpO_2 readings in the neonatal ICU should be kept below 95 percent to avoid unrecognized hyperoxia.

In pediatric and adult ICUs, pulse oximetry should ideally be used in every patient with a labile oxygenation status. This includes both spontaneously breathing patients and those receiving mechanically ventilation. However, we would caution against relying heavily on SpO_2 monitoring during weaning, since ventilation, more than alterations in oxygenation, signals failure during weaning. Simply monitoring pulse oximetry may prevent adequate assessment of ventilation and acid-base balance, especially if increased F_IO_2 levels are set during weaning trials.

Pulse oximetry is also useful in selected patients with labile oxygenation states outside of the ICU. We have found oximetry particularly useful in children with congenital cardiac anomalies who present with respiratory distress or in patients with chronic obstructive pulmonary disease (COPD) or cystic fibrosis who present in an acute exacerbation in which F_IO_2 is difficult to titrate.

SpO_2 monitoring is also useful during pulmonary rehabilitation and for the monitoring of home O_2 therapy but should not be used to determine need for O_2 therapy. As noted in Figure 47-11, the correlation of PaO_2 and SaO_2 in the range documenting the need for home O_2 therapy is poor.[31] Patients may be refused reimbursement for home O_2 therapy because the SpO_2 is 90 percent; however, actual PaO_2 may be below 55 mmHg. In addition to the various patient factors that affect the position of the oxyhemoglobin dissociation curve, it should be remembered that the accuracy of the oximeter is ±4 percent. Once the need for O_2 has been established and the correlation between SpO_2 and PaO_2 for a given patient determined, SpO_2 provides a useful monitor.

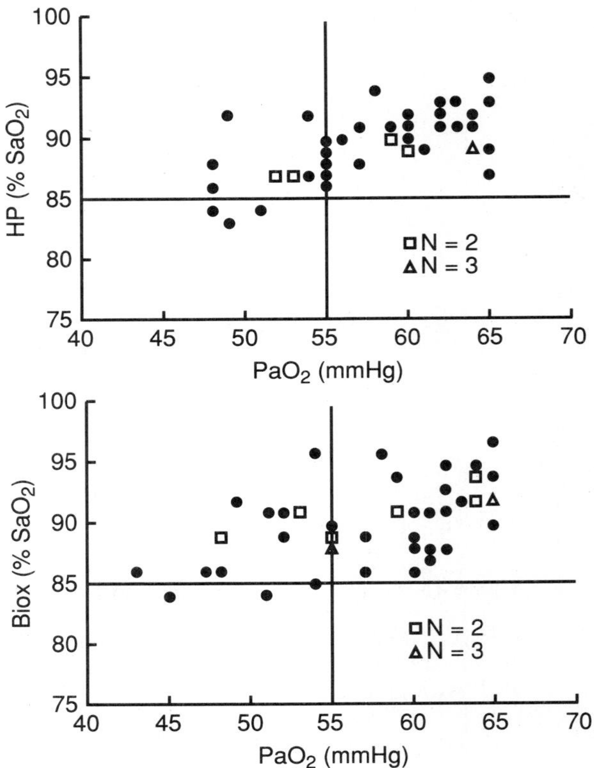

Figure 47-11. The relationship between resting PaO_2 and percentage of SaO_2 on a Biox 11A (bottom) ear oximeter. The vertical line at 55 mmHg indicates the U.S. Medicare threshold level for reimbursement for long-term O_2 therapy. (Modified from Carlin et al.,[31] with permission.)

TRANSCUTANEOUS BLOOD GAS MONITORING

Transcutaneous O_2 and CO_2 electrodes are essentially miniature Clark and Severinghaus electrodes that are capable of measuring arterialized capillary blood gas data by enhancing diffusion across the skin. Figure 47-12 depicts the layers of the skin. The outermost layer, the stratum corneum serves as a barrier to prevent significant fluid loss and as a tough exterior shield. However, heating this layer to about 42°C disrupts its structure, melting its lipid matrix and enhancing diffusion some 1000-fold.[32] The epidermis does not create a diffusion barrier but is highly active metabolically. This activity may affect blood gases, causing an increased transcutaneous PCO_2 ($TcPCO_2$) and decreased transcutaneous PO_2 ($TcPO_2$). The dermis is highly vascular, being composed of connective tissue, lymphatic vessels, and nerves as well as blood vessels. About 33 percent of all blood flow circulates to the skin via the dermis.[33]

Surface heating by a transcutaneous monitor dilates blood vessels in the dermis, hyperperfusing this area. This results in increased O_2 delivery to the epidermis, which allows gases from arterialized capillary blood to reach the transcutaneous monitor. However, heating does increase metabolism, causing overestimation of PCO_2 and slight underestimation of PO_2.

The Electrodes

As indicated, the $TcPO_2$ electrode is a modified Clark electrode, which functions in exactly the same way as any blood gas electrode. To ensure that capillary blood is arterialized,

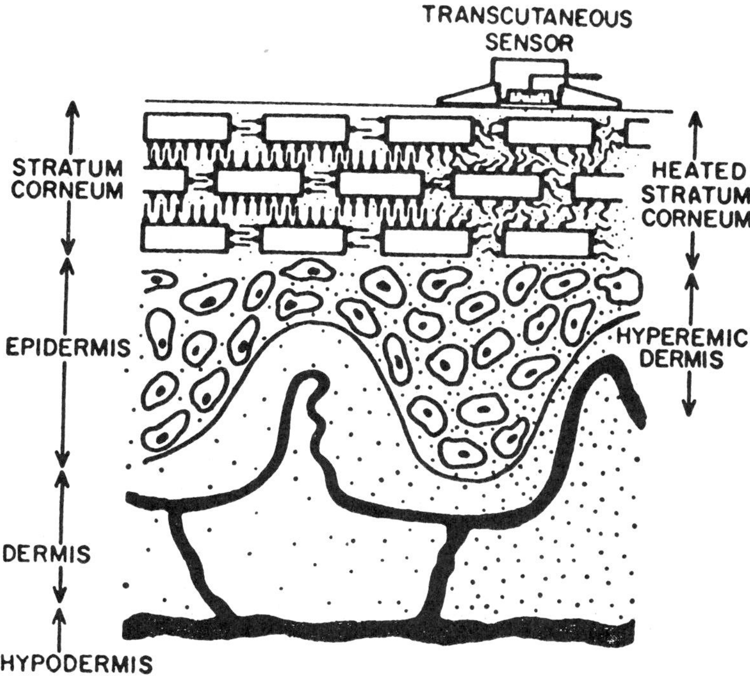

Figure 47-12. Schematic cross section of a transcutaneous electrode and skin: stratum corneum, epidermis, dermis, and hypodermis. The irregular structure of the stratum corneum beneath the electrode represents melted lipid. The dots represent O_2. (From Van Duzee,[33] with permission.)

these electrodes heat the skin to 42.5°C to 45°C.[34] As a result, frequent site changes are required to avoid surface burns. In neonates site changes must occur every 2 to 3 hours to prevent blister formation.[35] The $TcPCO_2$ electrode is a modified Severinghaus electrode. To ensure diffusion of CO_2, these electrodes require a skin temperature of 42°C.[35] As noted in Figure 47-13, many of today's transcutaneous electrodes are dual $TcPO_2/TcPCO_2$ electrodes. As a result, skin surface temperature is maintained in the range required for $TcPO_2$ monitoring, and electrodes need repositioning every 2 to 3 hours.

Electrode Placement

Electrode placement is the key to reliable data. Regardless of the age of the patient, the transcutaneous monitor must be placed on a relatively well perfused, flat area. Placement

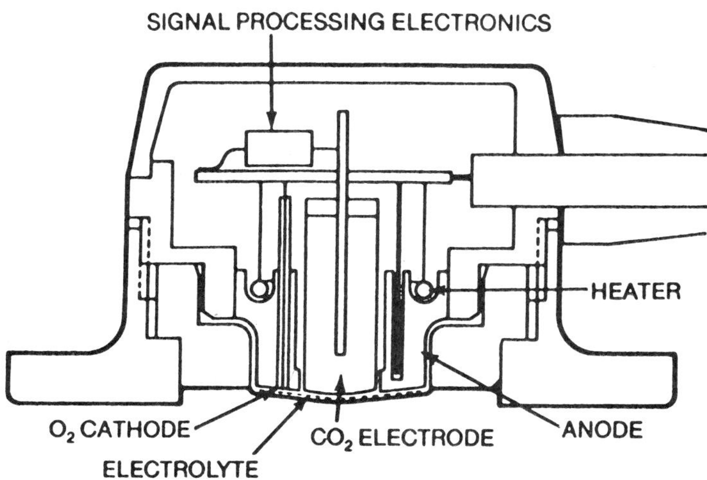

Figure 47-13. Schematic diagram of the O_2/CO_2 transcutaneous sensor. (From Mahutte et al.,[41] with permission.)

Table 47-27. Acceptable Transcutaneous Probe Placement Sites

Fetal	Neonatal	Pediatric	Adult
Scalp	Abdomen Chest Lower back Thigh Upper right chest[a]	Abdomen Lower back Chest	Chest Abdomen Lower back Shoulder[b] Limb[c]

[a] Assessment of ductal flow.
[b] Assessment of efficacy of cardiopulmonary resuscitation.
[c] Assessment of peripheral perfusion.

over bony areas (scapula, spinal cord, etc.) or hair is not recommended. Primary placement sites are listed in Table 47-27.

With neonates the abdomen, inner thigh, chest, and lower back are primary sites.[34] If preductal and postductal $TcPO_2$ values are to be compared because of suspected persistent fetal circulation, two $TcPO_2$ monitors are frequently employed,[36] one placed in the upper right chest (preductal) and the other normally placed on the left side of the body. Since the right innominate artery leaves the aorta before the ductus arteriosus enters, in the presence of a patent ductus arteriosus the postductal $TcPO_2$ will be lower than preductal $TcPO_2$.

The electrodes must be attached to the skin in a manner to prevent room air from contacting the electrode surface. This is accomplished by the use of a double-sided adhesive disk. Care must be exercised to prevent folds in the disk. A few drops of either deionized water or manufacturer-supplied contact gel are placed in the center of the disk to enhance contact between the skin and the electrode.[37] Once appropriate contact is established, an equilibration time of about 10 to 20 minutes is required before valid data are provided.

Clinical Use

A number of factors affect the clinical utility of transcutaneous blood gas monitoring and its ability to represent true arterial blood values (Table 47-28). It was initially introduced in the neonatal ICU but has since been used for all age groups. The $TcPCO_2$ monitor appears to provide a relatively accurate estimate of $PaCO_2$ in all age groups; however, $TcPO_2$ appears to be useful only in neonates, particularly if PaO_2 is below 80 mmHg.[38] The most extensive study of the accuracy of transcutaneous monitoring was conducted by Palmisano and Severinghaus,[38] who performed a multicenter study of 756 samples from 251 patients in all age groups. Figures 47-14 and 47-15 illustrate the results of this study. $TcPCO_2$ correlated well with $PaCO_2$ across all age groups, with good agreement between the two values. However, in many instances $TcPCO_2$ either over- or underestimated $PaCO_2$ and therefore can only be considered a gross estimate of $PaCO_2$. $TcPO_2$, as noted in Figure 47-14, agreed less favorably with PaO_2 values in all age groups when PaO_2 was above 80 mmHg but was predictive of PaO_2 below 80 mmHg in neonates. As a result, $TcPO_2$ can only be recommended for use in the neonatal age group and should only be relied on as a predictor of O_2 changes when PO_2 is below 80 mmHg. The introduction of pulse oximetry has greatly reduced the number of $TcPO_2$ monitors currently in use; however, there are still a large number of neonatal units in which $TcPO_2$ is commonly used. Table 47-29 lists the advantages and disadvantages of $TcPO_2$ and pulse oximetry in neonates.

$TcPCO_2$ has been and is being used in all age groups and accurately reflects $PaCO_2$ changes regardless of age. Its accuracy is not affected by changes in hematocrit, treatment with tolazoline, or the presence of scleredema[39] but does, however, decrease at higher $PaCO_2$ levels.[35] In addition, Hand et al.[40] reported that the correlation between $PaCO_2$ and $TcCO_2$ was negatively affected by the presence of acidosis. A number of studies[41–43] have demonstrated that $TcPCO_2$ is useful in determining trends in $PaCO_2$ at all age levels. It must, however, be remembered that the $TcPCO_2$ is a qualitative, not a quantitative reflection of the $PaCO_2$ change. Although theoretically useful in adults, the technical problems associated with $TcPCO_2$ monitoring have limited its use in adult populations.

Table 47-28. Primary Factors Affecting Transcutaneous and Arterial Relationships

	O_2	CO_2
Patient factors	Skin thickness Perfusion Blood pressure Vasodilators Age	Acidotic conditions Perfusion
Electrode factors	Calibration Membrane condition Contact Probe placement Temperature	

CAPNOMETRY

The measurement of CO_2 at the patient's airway during ventilation is referred to as *capnometry*, while the graphic display of exhaled CO_2 concentration as a waveform is *capnography*.[44] The most common capnometers used in clinical medicine are based on the CO_2 absorption spectrum, which has a peak in the infrared region at 4.26 μm[46] (i.e., the greater the light absorption in this area, the higher the CO_2 concentration). However, the accuracy of capnometers is affected because the absorption peaks for CO and N_2O are close to that of CO_2 and because pressure broadening (due to collisions between CO_2 and other gas molecules) affects the infrared energy absorption of CO_2.[46,47]

Two general types of capnometers are currently in use, mainstream and sidestream.[48] Mainstream units analyze for CO_2 content directly at the endotracheal tube, whereas sidestream analyzers draw a gas sample from the airway and

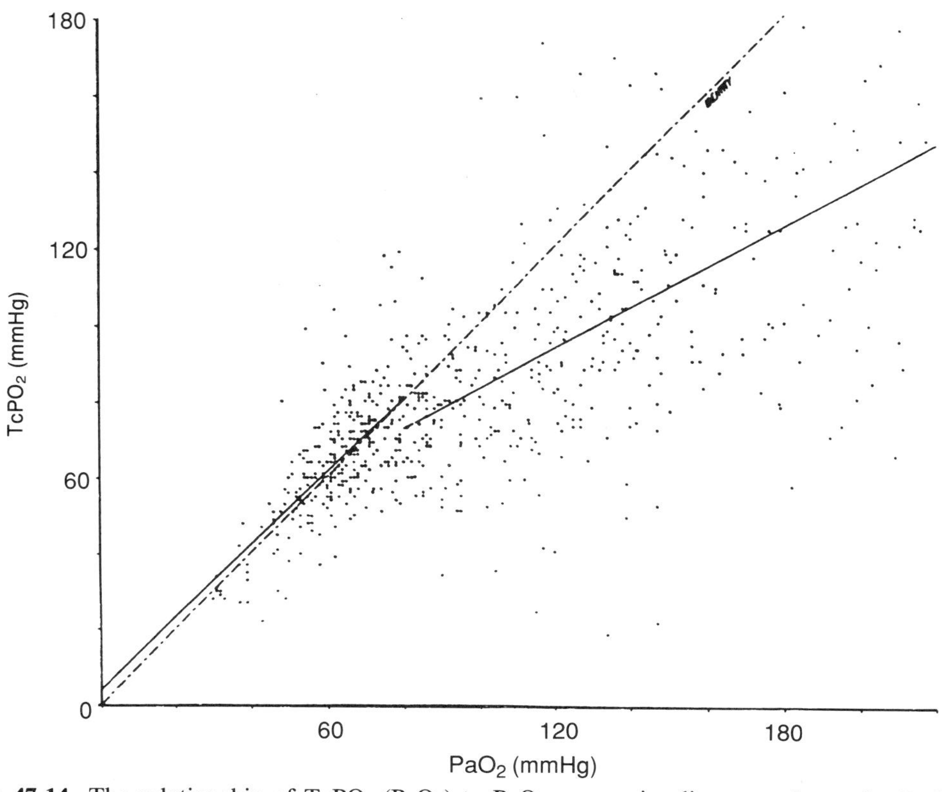

Figure 47-14. The relationship of $TcPO_2$ (PsO_2) to PaO_2; regression lines are shown for PaO_2 below and above 80 mmHg; N = 723. (From Palmisano and Severinghaus,[38] with permission.)

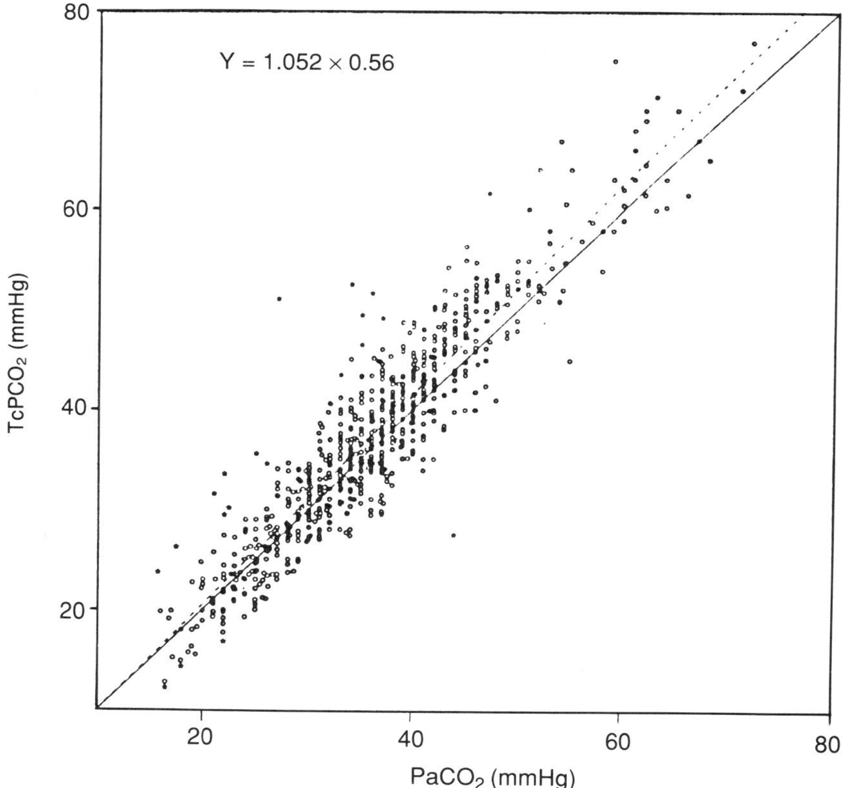

Figure 47-15. The relationship of $TcPCO_2$ ($PsCO_2$) to $PaCO_2$; the solid line is the line of identity; N = 723. (From Palmisano and Severinghaus,[38] with permission.)

Table 47-29. Pulse Oximetry versus $TcPO_2$ Monitoring in Neonates

	Pulse Oximetry	$TcPO_2$
Advantages	Rapidly operational	More accurately reflects PaO_2 change in 40–80 mmHg range
	Does not cause skin burns	Less affected by altered peripheral perfusion
	Does not require calibration	Able to be calibrated
Disadvantages	Insensitive to PO_2 changes resulting in SaO_2 changes in the 90% saturation range	Warming time 15–20 minutes
	Greatly affected by peripheral perfusion	Probe site must be changed every 2–3 hours
		Causes surface burns
	Cannot be calibrated	Must be calibrated

analyze for CO_2 content at a location remote from the airway itself.[44,48] Generally, the mainstream analyzers are more cumbersome and increase the torque on the artificial airway; moreover they do not function if CO_2 is present in the inspired gas. Sidestream analyzers have a phase delay since gas must be drawn from the airway to the measuring chamber for analysis. Table 47-30 compares the advantages and disadvantages of mainstream and sidestream analyzers.

Table 47-30. Mainstream versus Sidestream Capnometers

	Mainstream	Sidestream
Advantages	V_T unaffected	May be used with nonintubated patients
	No phase delay	No bulky sensor at airway
	Fast response	Disposable sample line
Disadvantages	Bulky sensor at airway	Phase delay
	Requires sterilization	Slow response to CO_2 changes
	Sensor requires heating to prevent condensation	Requires water trap
	Secretions and humidity may block sensor window	Secretions may block sampling tubing

Figure 47-16 depicts the overall operation of a typical nondispersive double-beam, positive-filter sidestream capnometer. Light passes via a chopper through a reference and sample cell onto the CO_2-filled detection chamber.[44] The presence of CO_2 in the sample cell decreases the amount of radiation entering the lower half of the detection chamber. As a result, unequal absorption in the two parts of the detection chamber is translated into CO_2 concentration in the sample cell.[48] The chopper is used in both sidestream and mainstream capnometers for the following reasons: (1) it allows a common source and detector to be used with the

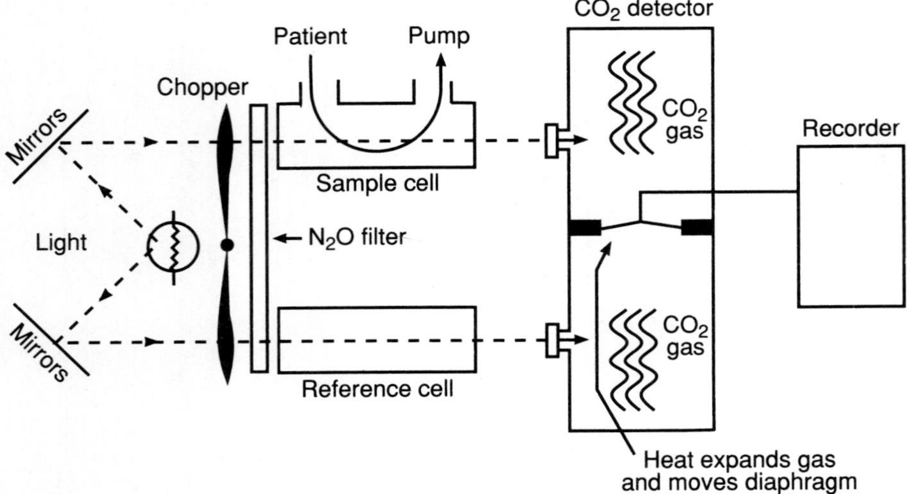

Figure 47-16. Schematic diagram of nondispersive double-beam positive-filter capnometer. See text for details. (From Gravenstein et al.,[44] with permission.)

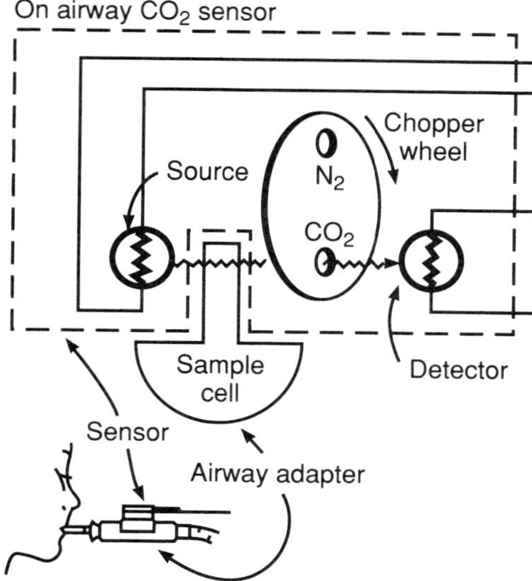

Figure 47-17. Schematic diagram of single-beam, negative-filter capnometer. See text for details. (From Gravenstein et al.,[44] with permission.)

double-beam capnometer; (2) it provides an alternating signal from the reference and sample cells; and (3) it produces a null signal (no signal from the reference and sample cell), which helps to eliminate drift and interference.[44]

A single-beam negative-filter mainstream capnometer is depicted in Figure 47-17. The infrared signal passes through the sample cell and then through a cell contained in the chopper onto the CO_2 detector.[44] Actually, two cells are present in the chopper, one containing CO_2 and the other N_2. As a result, the detector receives two signals, the ratio between which is used to determine CO_2 concentration.[48]

Mass spectrometry is also used to determine exhaled CO_2 concentrations[49,50]; Figure 47-18 illustrates a typical instrument. Most mass spectrometers function by aspirating the sample gas into a vacuum chamber, where the gas is ionized.[48] The charged particles are then accelerated into a dispersion chamber, where they are separated according to mass on a collection plate, on which the composition of the gas is continuously analyzed.[44] Mass spectrometers are used in large-system gas analysis both for monitoring anesthesia and in critical care—that is, 8, 16, or more patients are monitored by a single system. In addition to CO_2, many other gases, including anesthetics, can be monitored with these systems.[49,50] Because of cost and operational difficulty, infrared capnometers individualized to each patient are more commonly used in ICUs to ensure proper operation. All capnometers require regular calibration.

The Normal Capnogram

The percent CO_2 inhaled and exhaled during normal breathing is depicted in Figure 47-19 as the normal capnogram. The section between points A to B represents inspiration, for which CO_2% is zero, while the B to C section represents primarily gas leaving the conducting airway. Here CO_2% is initially zero, but rapidly increases as dead space gas, mixed with alveolar gas, is exhaled. The C to D section represents primarily gas leaving alveoli; here the CO_2% varies little between C and D. Usually a distinct plateau exists at D. This CO_2 level is referred to as the end-tidal CO_2 ($ETCO_2$) and is normally expressed as a partial pressure ($PETCO_2$). The D to E section represents the rapid decline in CO_2% as inspiration begins.

Relationship of Arterial to End-Tidal PCO_2

The $PETCO_2$ represents the $PACO_2$ and is a composite result of the total $\dot{V}/\dot{Q}$ relationships of the lung. If the $\dot{V}/\dot{Q}$

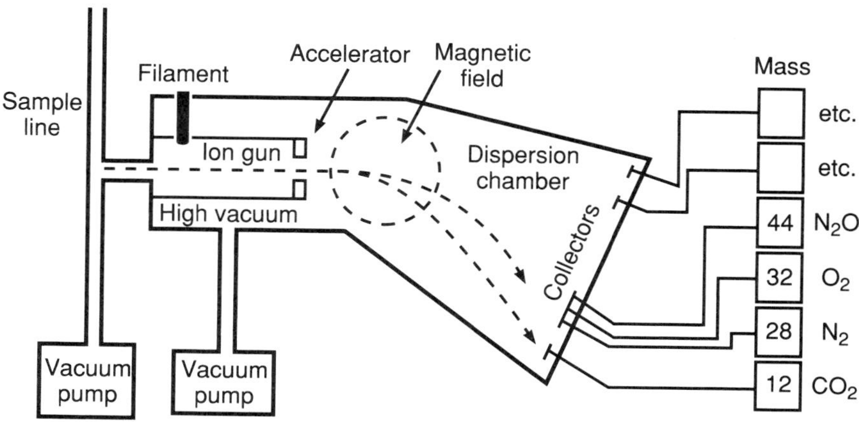

Figure 47-18. Schematic diagram of mass spectrometer. See text for details. (From Gravenstein et al.,[44] with permission.)

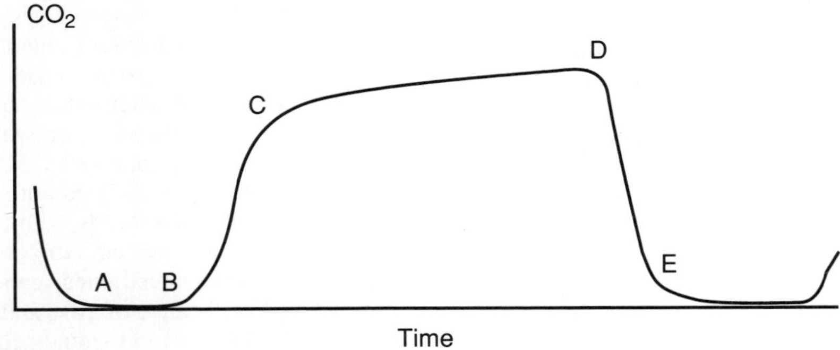

Figure 47-19. Normal capnogram. See text for details. (From Swedlow,[61] with permission.)

relationship is normal, the P_ACO_2 ($P_{ET}CO_2$) will approximate the $PaCO_2$. If the $\dot{V}/\dot{Q}$ is decreased (i.e., ventilation decreased or perfusion increased), the P_ACO_2 ($P_{ET}CO_2$) increases, approaching the level of the $P\bar{v}CO_2$.[48] However, if ventilation increases relative to perfusion (dead space, high $\dot{V}/\dot{Q}$ areas), the P_ACO_2 ($P_{ET}CO_2$) falls below the $PaCO_2$ and begins to approach the P_ICO_2.[48] Clinical situations in which $P_{ET}CO_2$ may be increased or decreased are outlined in Table 47-31. Of primary clinical significance are those circumstances in which $PaCO_2$ rises while $P_{ET}CO_2$ stays the same or decreases (Table 47-32). It is in these situations that $P_{ET}CO_2$ may provide very misleading information regarding overall cardiopulmonary status. Normally, $P_{ET}CO_2$ is about 5 mmHg lower than $PaCO_2$.

Table 47-31. Causes of Alterations in $P_{ET}CO_2$

Increased $P_{ET}CO_2$
Increased CO_2 production and delivery to the lungs
Fever
Sepsis
Bicarbonate administration
Increased metabolic rate
Seizures
Decreased alveolar ventilation
Respiratory center depression
Muscular paralysis
Hypoventilation
COPD
Equipment malfunction
Rebreathing
Exhausted CO_2 absorber (anesthesia system)
Leak in ventilator circuit
Decreased $P_{ET}CO_2$
Decreased CO_2 production and delivery to the lungs
Hypothermia
Pulmonary hypoperfusion
Cardiac arrest
Pulmonary embolism
Hemorrhage
Hypotension
Increased alveolar ventilation
Equipment malfunction
Ventilator disconnect
Esophageal intubation
Complete airway obstruction
Poor sampling
Leak around endotracheal tube cuff

(From Hess,[48] with permission.)

Clinical Use

One of the most common serious complications of endotracheal intubation is caused by inadvertent esophageal intubation. Capnometry allows for immediate recognition of an esophageal intubation. The use of a standard capnometer is cumbersome for this purpose, but recent advances in capnometry make evaluation simple.[51–53] MacLeod et al.[51] and Anton et al.[52] have reported 100 percent sensitivity of the Fenem FEF CO_2 detector in intubations for conditions other than cardiac arrest, while VuKmir et al.[53] have reported similar results with the Minicap III (Mine Safety Appliances Co.) miniaturized infrared qualitative CO_2 detector. Both the FEF and the Minicap III are designed to identify the presence of CO_2 qualitatively, with no attempt made to precisely quantify CO_2 levels. The FEF is a disposable adapter attached to the endotracheal tube, which changes color in the presence of CO_2, while the Minicap III is a miniaturized infrared analyzer. Although both operate well if CO_2 is present, their use during intubations for cardiopulmonary resuscitation requires caution because the presumption that no CO_2 means esophageal intubation may be false if circulation is not established. In addition, the presence of carbonated beverage in the abdomen prevents recognition of an esophageal intubation. Data provided by Garnett et al.[54] indicate that CO_2 should be monitored for at least 20 to 30 seconds to ensure

Table 47-32. Causes of Increased $PaCO_2$-$P_{ET}CO_2$

Pulmonary hypoperfusion
High-rate, low tidal volume ventilation
Positive pressure ventilation
Cardiac arrest
Pulmonary embolism

(From Hess,[48] with permission.)

that all gastric CO_2 is washed out in the case of an esophageal intubation in the presence of ingested carbonated beverage.

The capnometer, although expensive, is an excellent monitor of ventilator disconnection. Most of the newer capnometers have alarm capabilities, indicating significant change in $P_{ET}CO_2$ or the absence of CO_2. The use of capnometers for this purpose has been established as a standard of care in the operating room by the American Association of Anesthesiologists.[28] The use of capnometers for this purpose in the ICU is much more limited, since ICU ventilator alarm packages are capable of rapidly identifying ventilator disconnections.

Monitoring of gas exchange during weaning trials is difficult and can only be accomplished periodically. As a result, many have used capnometry to monitor changes in $PaCO_2$ during weaning.[55–60] Most reports of the relationship between $PaCO_2$ and $P_{ET}CO_2$ during weaning demonstrate good correlations and agreement; however, close examination of data indicates that in many individual circumstances $P_{ET}CO_2$ incorrectly predicted the direction of change in $PaCO_2$. Healey et al.,[55] in an evaluation of the use of $P_{ET}CO_2$ during weaning of postoperative patients, found that $P_{ET}CO_2$ incorrectly predicted the change in $PaCO_2$ in 25 percent of their cases. Hess et al.,[56] in a series of postsurgical cardiac patients, noted that $P_{ET}CO_2$ and $PaCO_2$ moved in opposite directions in 43 percent of the comparisons (Fig. 47-20). Similar data have been reported by Niehoff et al.[57] These discrepancies are a result of marked variations in $\dot{V}/\dot{Q}$ relationships during weaning. As a result, we recommend against the routine use of $P_{ET}CO_2$ during weaning, since it may give rise to the assumption that $PaCO_2$ has remained constant when it is in fact increasing. Until we are able to precisely differentiate the specific patients for whom $P_{ET}CO_2$ is always predictive of directional change in $PaCO_2$, the use of capnometers during weaning must be considered experimental.

Capnograph Waveforms

As noted in Figure 47-19, a very distinct capnogram is normally produced, so that variations in waveform can be used to identify specific abnormalities. Figure 47-21, from Swedlow,[61] illustrates some common waveform variations. All the waveforms in Figure 47-21 are presented at both slow speed and normal speed; slow speed allows for trend analysis, while high speed allows for identification of specific abnormalities. Figure 47-21A illustrates the fluctuations resulting from cardiac contraction, which are normally only noticeable during hypovolemia. Figure 47-21B illustrates hyperventilation, still maintaining the end-expiratory plateau. Figure 47-21C illustrates hypoventilation, while Figure 47-21D illustrates rebreathing of CO_2, a potential problem in anesthesia systems (it should be noted that the inspired CO_2 is greater than zero). Figure 47-21E illustrates ventilator disconnection or apnea; Figure 47-21F illustrates cardiovascular decompensation as seen at the onset of cardiac arrest or rapidly developing profound shock; Figure 47-21G illustrates a cleft in the waveform, indicative of diaphragmatic spasm; and Figure 47-21H illustrates low $P_{ET}CO_2$, without a plateau indicative of ineffective tidal volumes or poor samplings. The information provided by analysis of the capno-

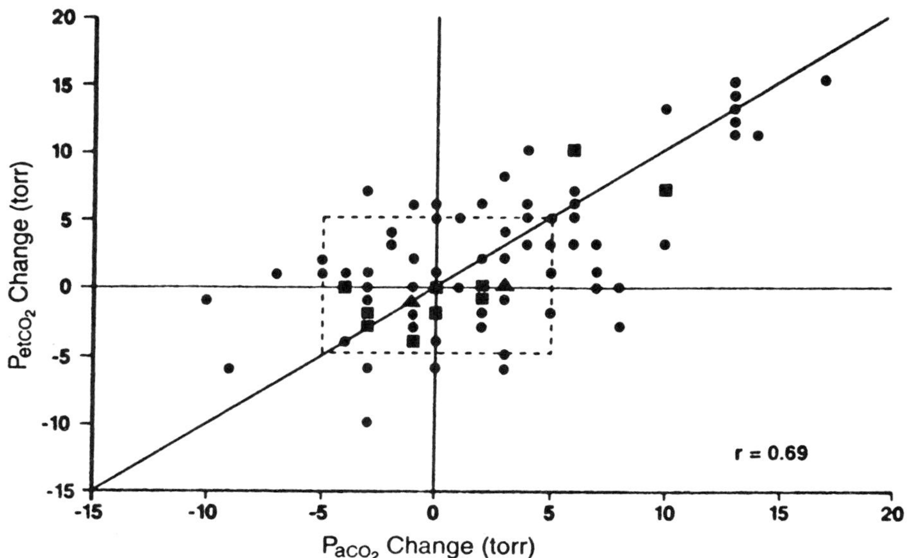

Figure 47-20. The relationship between the change in $P_{ET}CO_2$ and the change in $PaCO_2$ in 113 data sets from a series of postsurgical cardiac patients. The diagonal line is the line of identity. Solid squares represent two data points with the same value. Those values within the data box represent a change of ±5 mmHg. Note that data points in the left upper and right lower quadrants represent data sets in which $PaCO_2$ and $P_{ET}CO_2$ changed in opposite directions. (From Hess et al.,[56] with permission.)

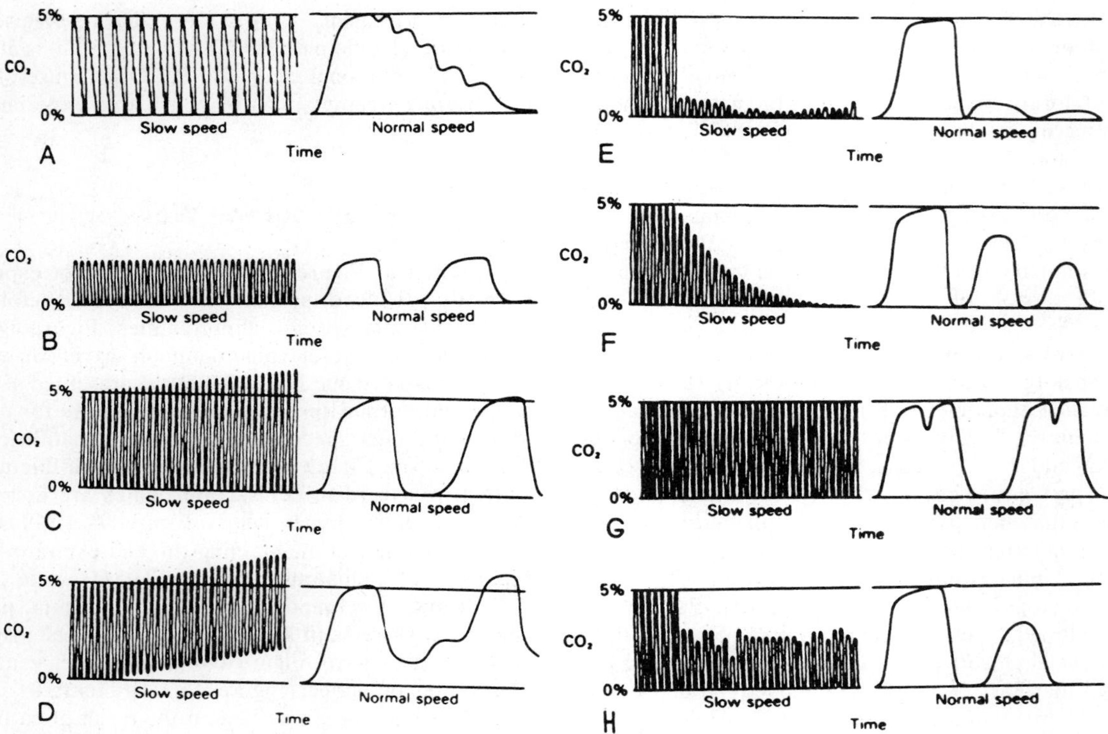

Figure 47-21. Variations in normal capnograms in specific clinical settings. See text for details. (From Swedlow,[61] with permission.)

gram is generally much more variable than the actual $P_{ET}CO_2$ level in patients monitored in the ICU.

References

1. Shapiro BA, Harrison RA, Cane RD, Templin R: Clinical Application of Blood Gases. 4th Ed. Mosby-Year Book, St. Louis, 1989
2. Vander AJ: Renal Physiology. 3rd Ed. McGraw-Hill, New York, 1985
3. Sorbini CA, Grassi V, Sotinas E: Arterial oxygen tension in relation to age in healthy subjects. Respiration 1968;25:3–9
4. Mellemgaard K: The alveolar arterial oxygen difference: Its size and components in normal man. Acta Physiol Scand 1966;67:10–15
5. Effros RM: Acid-base balance. pp. 129–148. In Murray JF, Nadel JA (eds): Textbook of Respiratory Medicine. WB Saunders, Philadelphia, 1988
6. Severinghaus JW, Bradley AG: Electrodes for blood PO_2 and PCO_2 determinations. J Appl Physiol 1958;13:515–520
7. Millikan GA: An oximeter: An instrument for measuring continuously oxygen saturation of arterial blood in man. Rev Sci Instrum 1942;13:434–444
8. Hemmingway AH, Taylor CB: Laboratory tests of oximeter with automatic compensation for vasomotor changes. J Lab Clin Med 1944;29:987–991
9. Severinghaus JW, Honda Y: History of blood gas analysis. VI. Oximetry. J Clin Monit 1986;2:270–280
10. Szaflarski NL, Cohen NH: Use of pulse oximetry in critically ill adults. Heart Lung 1989;18:444–455
11. Welsh JP, DeCesare R, Hess D: Pulse oximetry: Instrumentation and clinical applications. Respir Care 1990;35:584–601
12. Kelleher JF: Pulse oximetry. J Clin Monit 1989;5:37–62
13. Tremper KK, Barker SJ: Pulse oximetry. Anesthesiology 1989; 70:98–108
14. Raemer DB, Elliott WR, Topulos GP, Philip JH: The theoretical effect of carboxyhemoglobin on the pulse oximeter. J Clin Monit 1989;5:246–249
15. Barker SJ, Tremper KK: The effect of carbon dioxide inhalation on pulse oximeter signal detection. Anesthesiology 1987;67:599–603
16. Watch MF, Connor MT, Hing AV: Pulse oximetry in methemoglobinemia. Am J Dis Child 1989;143:845–847
17. Rieder HV, Frei FJ, Binden AM, Thomson DA: Pulse oximetry saturation. Anaesthesia 1989;44:326–327
18. Pologe JA: Pulse oximetry: Technical aspects. Int Anesthiol Clin 1987;25:137–154
19. Tyler IL, Tantisira B, Winter PM, Motoyama EK: Continuous monitoring of arterial oxygen saturation with pulse oximetry during transfer to the recovery room. Anesth Analg 1984;64:1108–1112
20. Scheller MS, Unger RJ, Kelner MJ: Effects of intravenously administered dyes on pulse oximetry readings. Anesthesiology 1986;65:550–552
21. Sidi A, Paulus DA, Rush W et al: Methylene blue and indocyanine green artificially lower pulse oximetry reading of oxygen saturation: Studies in dogs. J Clin Monit 1987;3:249–256
22. Amar D, Neidswski J, Wald A, Pinck AD: Fluorescent light interferes with pulse oximetry. J Clin Monit 1989;5:135–136
23. Block FE: Interference in a pulse oximeter from a fiberoptic light source. J Clin Monit 1987;3:210–211
24. Costarino AT, Davis DA, Keon TP: False normal saturation reading with the pulse oximeter. Anesthesiology 1987;67:830–831
25. Evans ML, Geddes LA: An assessment of blood vessel vasoactivity using photoplethysmography. Med Instrum 1988;22:29–32

26. Ries AL, Prewitt LM, Johnson JJ: Skin color and ear oximetry. Chest 1989;96:287–290
27. Cote CJ, Goldstein EA, Fuchsman WH, Hoaglin DC: The effect of nail polish on pulse oximetry. Anesth Analg 1989;67:683–686
28. American Society of Anesthesiologists: Standards for basic intra-operative monitoring. ASA Newsletter 1986;50:12
29. Cooper JB, Newbower RS, Kitz RJ: An analysis of major errors and equipment failures in anesthesia management: Considerations for prevention and detection. Anesthesiology 1984;60:34–42
30. Smith DC, Canning JJ, Crul JF: Pulse oximetry in the recovery room. Anaesthesia 1989;44:345–348
31. Carlin BW, Clausen JL, Ries AL: The use of cutaneous oximetry in the prescription of long-term oxygen therapy. Chest 1988; 94:239–241
32. Tremper KK, Waxman K, Shoemaker WC: Effects of hypoxia and shock on transcutaneous PO_2 values in dogs. Crit Care Med 1979;7:526–531
33. Van Duzee BF: Thermal analysis of human stratum corneum. J Invest Dermatol 1975;65:404–408
34. Martin RJ: Transcutaneous monitoring: Instrumentation and clinical applications. Respir Care 1990;35:577–583
35. Martin RJ, Beoglos A, Miller MJ et al: Increasing arterial CO_2 tension: Influence on transcutaneous carbon dioxide tension measurements. Pediatrics 1988;81:684–687
36. Huch R, Huch A, Lubbers DW: Transcutaneous measurement of blood PO_2: Method and application in perinatal medicine. J Perinat Med 1973;1:183–186
37. Patel BT, Delpy DT, Hillson PJ, Parker D: A topical metabolic inhibitor to improve transcutaneous estimation of arterial oxygen tension in adults. J Biomed Eng 1989;11:381–383
38. Palmisano BW, Severinghaus JW: Transcutaneous PCO_2 and PO_2: A multicenter study of accuracy. J Clin Monit 1990;6:189–195
39. Brustler I, Enders A, Versmold HT: Skin surface PCO_2 monitoring in newborn infants in shock. J Pediatr 1982;100:454–457
40. Hand IL, Shepart EK, Krauss AN, Auld PAM: Discrepancies between transcutaneous and end-tidal carbon dioxide monitoring in critically ill neonates with respiratory distress syndrome. Crit Care Med 1989;17:556–559
41. Mahutte CK, Michaels TM, Hassell KT, Trueblood DM: Evaluation of a simple transcutaneous PO_2–PCO_2 sensor in adult patients. Crit Care Med 1984;12:1063–1066
42. Phan CQ, Tremper KK, Lee SE, Barker SJ: Noninvasive monitoring of carbon dioxide: A comparison of the partial pressure of transcutaneous and end tidal carbon dioxide with the partial pressure of arterial carbon dioxide. J Clin Monit 1987;3:149–154
43. Healey CJ, Fedullo AJ, Swinburne AJ, Wahl GW: Comparison of noninvasive measurements of carbon dioxide tension during withdrawal from mechanical ventilation. Crit Care Med 1987; 15:764–768
44. Gravenstein JS, Paulus DA, Hayes TJ: Capnography in Clinical Practice. Butterworths, Boston, 1989
45. Collier CR, Affeldt JE, Farr AF: Continuous rapid infrared CO_2 analysis. J Lab Clin Med 1955;45:526–539
46. Severinghaus JW, Larson CP, Eger EI: Correction factors for infrared carbon dioxide pressure broadening by nitrogen, nitrous oxide and cyclopropane. Anesthesiology 1961;22:429–432
47. Ammann ECB, Galvin RD: Problems associated with the determination of carbon dioxide by infrared absorption. J Appl Physiol 1968;25:333–335
48. Hess D: Capnometry and capnography: Technical aspects, physiologic aspects, and clinical applications. Respir Care 1990; 35:557–576
49. Ayres SM: Use of mass spectrometry for evaluation of respiratory function in the critically ill patient. Crit Care Med 1976; 4:219–222
50. Riker JB, Haberman B: Expired gas monitoring by mass spectrometry in a respiratory intensive care unit. Crit Care Med 1976; 4:223–229
51. MacLeod BA, Heller MB, Gerard J et al: Verification of endotracheal tube placement with colorimetric end-tidal CO_2 detection. Ann Emerg Med 1991;20:267–270
52. Anton WR, Gordon RW, Jordan TM et al: A disposable end-tidal CO_2 detector to verify endotracheal intubation. Ann Emerg Med 1991;20:271–275
53. VuKmir RB, Heller MB, Stein KL: Confirmation of endotracheal tube placement: A miniaturized infrared qualitative CO_2 detector. Ann Emerg Med 1991;20:726–729
54. Garnett AR, Gervin CA, Gervin AS: Capnographic waveforms in esophageal intubation: Effect of carbonated beverages. Ann Emerg Med 1989;18:387–390
55. Healey CJ, Fedullo AJ, Swinburne AJ, Wahl GW: Comparison of noninvasive measurements of carbon dioxide tension during withdrawal from mechanical ventilation. Crit Care Med 1987; 15:764–767
56. Hess D, Schlottag A, Levin B et al: An evaluation of the usefulness of end-tidal PCO_2 to aid weaning from mechanical ventilation following cardiac surgery. Respir Care 1991;36:837–843
57. Niehoff J, DelGuercio C, LaMorte W et al: Efficacy of pulse oximetry and capnometry in postoperative ventilatory weaning. Crit Care Med 1988;16:701–705
58. Withington DE, Ramsey JG, Saoud T, Bilodeau J: Weaning from ventilation after cardiopulmonary bypass: Evaluation of a non-invasive technique. Can J Anaesth 1991;38:15–19
59. Weinger MB, Brimm JE: End-tidal carbon dioxide as a measure of arterial carbon dioxide during intermittent mandatory ventilation. J Clin Monit 1987;3:73–79
60. Smith RA, Novak RA, Venus B: End-tidal CO_2 monitoring utility during weaning from mechanical ventilation. Respir Care 1989;34:972–975
61. Swedlow DB: Capnometry and capnography: The anesthesia disaster early warning system. Semin Anesth 1986;5:194–202
62. Kacmarek RM, Mack C, Dimas S: The Essentials of Respiratory Care. 3rd Ed. Mosby-Year Book, St. Louis, 1990

Chapter 48

Assessment of Pulmonary Capillary Surface Area (Diffusing Capacity)

Richard K. Beauchamp

CHAPTER OUTLINE

Of the many changes that can occur in the structure and function of the lung as a result of disease, perhaps none is more significant than alteration of the alveolar-capillary interface. Changes in the surface area or permeability of this gas exchange membrane can have important diagnostic, therapeutic, and prognostic implications. This chapter describes the clinical methodology for determining the status of the alveolar-capillary membrane.

While the ultimate purpose of the alveolar-capillary interface is exchange of the respiratory gases, routine measurements of O_2 or CO_2 exchange, such as arterial blood gases, do not provide a direct determination of alveolar-capillary integrity. A number of other factors affect the lung-to-blood differences of these gases. In order to determine the discrete function of the alveolar-capillary interface, it is necessary to isolate the process of gas transfer across the membrane. This process is commonly termed *diffusion*.

Even when the process of diffusion is isolated, however, the transfer of the respiratory gases, particularly O_2, is somewhat difficult to quantitate. The reason for this difficulty can be seen in the mathematical expression of the factors that determine diffusion of a gas ($\dot{V}_{GAS}$) across a liquid-interface membrane. A simplified version of that expression tells us that

$$\dot{V}_{GAS} \propto \left(\frac{A}{T}\right)(P_1 - P_2)\left(\frac{SC}{\sqrt{MW}}\right)$$

where A is the surface area of the membrane, P_1 is the pressure (tension) of the diffusing gas on the membrane side, P_2 is the pressure in the liquid, SC is the solubility coefficient of the particular gas in the particular liquid, MW is the molecular weight of the gas, and T is the thickness of the membrane.

As shown, diffusion of a gas is determined in part by the pressure difference ($P_1 - P_2$) of the gas on the two sides of the membrane (i.e., the lungs and the blood). In the case of O_2, which is present on both faces of the membrane, this difference changes constantly and nonlinearly, making it difficult to measure. To measure diffusion easily, then, it is necessary to introduce a gas into the lungs that is diffusive across the alveolar-capillary membrane but is not normally present on the capillary side. Such a gas is CO.

In many ways CO (in very low concentrations) is an ideal gas for quantitating lung diffusion. Not only is it easily transferred across the lung-blood barrier and not normally present in any significant amount in the blood, but it also has a very high affinity for hemoglobin, indeed some 210 times that of O_2. This characteristic is important because the partial pressure of the gas on the "receiving" side of the membrane must remain low to avoid evolution of a backpressure, which would slow further diffusion. As a result of its high affinity, virtually all CO transferred to the blood combines readily with hemoglobin, thereby preventing development of a backpressure in the plasma. By contrast, O_2 does develop such a backpressure, and its transfer then relies on "new" blood moving into the capillaries. Therefore, CO transfer is *diffusion*-limited, while O_2 transfer is largely *perfusion*-limited. Accordingly, CO has long been used to measure diffusion in the lung. These measurements of the *d*iffusing capacity of the *l*ung for *CO* are generally referred to by the acronym DLCO.

TECHNIQUES FOR MEASURING DLCO

Historically, a number of techniques and variations thereof have been employed to determine DLCO. The two that are in routine clinical use today and that are discussed here are the single-breath ($DLCO_{SB}$) and steady-state ($DLCO_{SS}$) methods. A number of other methods exist but are used only occasionally in research and rarely, if ever, for clinical testing.

Single-Breath Method

The single-breath method is by far the most widely used technique for determining DLCO and is the primary focus of this chapter. In the basic test sequence for the $DLCO_{SB}$, subjects

1. Exhale to residual volume (RV)
2. Inhale rapidly to total lung capacity (TLC) from a gas source (reservoir bag or demand valve) containing a small fraction of CO (usually 0.3 percent), an inert "tracer" gas (usually 10 percent He or 0.5 percent neon), 20 to 21 percent O_2, and the balance N_2
3. Hold their breath for approximately 10 seconds, preferably by relaxing against a closed shutter rather than by sustaining an inspiratory effort
4. Exhale rapidly, during which a sample of the expired gas is collected after a volume sufficient to clear both anatomic and mechanical dead space has been exhaled

This procedure is illustrated schematically in Figure 48-1. The expired sample is analyzed, and the concentrations of CO and inert gas determined. In addition, the volume of gas inspired in step 2 and the exact duration of breath holding are measured. The $DLCO_{SB}$ is then calculated as follows:

The alveolar CO concentration (CO_A) is computed first as

$$CO_A(CO_i)\left(\frac{TG_E}{TG_i}\right) \quad (1)$$

where CO_i is the source gas (initial) concentration of CO, TG_E is the concentration of tracer gas in the expired sample, and TG_i is the source gas (initial) concentration of tracer gas:

Then $DLCO_{SB}$ is computed as

$$DLCO_{SB} = \left(\frac{60}{BHT}\right)\left[[(V_A[STPD]) \ln\left(\frac{CO_A}{CO_E}\right) \Big/ (P_b - 47)\right] \quad (2)$$

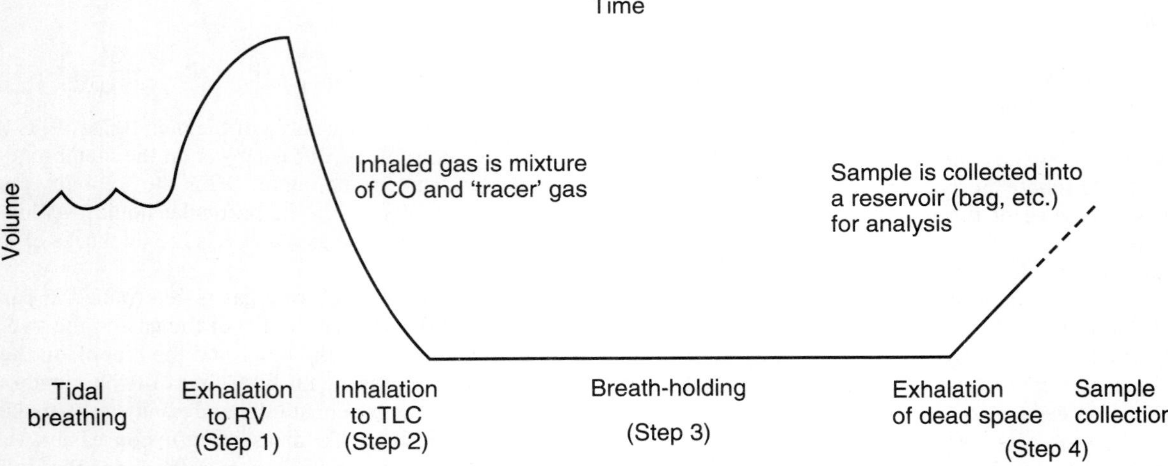

Figure 48-1. Schematic representation of the single-breath DLCO maneuver, showing the four steps described in the text. The ordinate is volume, the abscissa, time.

where BHT is the breath holding time in seconds; $V_{A[STPD]}$ is alveolar volume, standard temperature and pressure in milliliters; ln is the natural logarithm; CO_E is the concentration of CO in the expired sample; and P_b is the barometric pressure in millimeters of Hg.

In order to understand what is actually represented by D_LCO_{SB} measurements, it is necessary to understand the function of several of the terms in these equations. Two of the terms serve to standardize the D_LCO_{SB} value. The ratio 60/BHT standardizes the D_LCO_{SB} value to the amount of CO transferred in one full minute. As the volume of CO transferred increases with increasing duration of breath holding (although the *rate* of transfer decreases), tests with different breath hold durations would otherwise not be comparable. The second standardizing term is the barometric pressure (corrected for water vapor) in Equation 2, which accounts for differences in the driving (partial) pressure of CO inside the lung at any given CO concentration. On the basis of these two factors, D_LCO_{SB} values are expressed in milliliters of CO transferred per minute per millimeter of Hg driving pressure.

The purpose of the term TG_E/TG_i in Equation 1 is to determine the CO concentration at the beginning of breath holding (which is then compared with the concentration exhaled to determine the amount diffused). Although the concentration of *inspired* CO (i.e., the source gas) will be known, the *alveolar* concentration in the lungs once the gas is inhaled will be different as a result of the dilutional effect of the RV. By including a physiologically inert gas in the CO mixture, the magnitude of this dilution can be computed by determining the ratio of the inspired concentration to the expired concentration of this tracer gas.

In Equation 2 the natural logarithm of the beginning to the ending CO ratio (CO_A/CO_E) is taken because it is generally accepted that the disappearance of CO from the lungs is an exponential function, although this assumption has been questioned.[1]

The most complex, and controversial, of the terms in the calculation of D_LCO_{SB} is $V_{A[STPD]}$ in Equation 2. This term represents the volume in the lungs during breath holding (essentially TLC), expressed at its STPD value. There are several issues involved in understanding the complexity of and the controversy associated with this term. The first concerns the very purpose for its inclusion in the equation, which, at least implicitly, is that lung volume provides an estimate of the surface area available for diffusion. Intuitively it would seem to make sense that surface area increases as lung volume increases. However, it has now been shown that much of the change in surface area as the lung expands occurs through enlargement of the interalveolar pores,[3] so that the *functional* alveolar surface area remains relatively constant.

A second issue is the method by which V_A should be determined. The D_LCO_{SB} maneuver itself provides a measure of V_A based on the dilution of the tracer gas, calculated as

$$V_A = (IVC - V_D)(TG_I/TG_E) \tag{3}$$

where IVC is the inspired volume (forced inspired volume) and V_D is the combined mechanical and anatomic dead space.

As is widely recognized, this method may yield artificially low values in the presence of maldistribution of inspired gas, as often occurs in various lung disorders. Accordingly, it is sometimes suggested that TLC values derived from more exacting methods—N_2 washout, He equilibration, or plethysmography—be used in place of the single-breath dilution value. However, a number of studies[4–8] have demonstrated no significant difference between the single-breath V_A and volumes measured by other methods in normal subjects, restricted subjects, and subjects with mild to moderate obstruction. Significant differences do tend to occur in subjects with more pronounced obstruction, but a correction factor[9] has now been described that allows for accurate single-breath V_A volumes even in those subjects. In any case the single-breath V_A is currently the most commonly used value.

The third, and most important, issue concerning the inclusion of V_A in the computation of D_LCO_{SB} is the experimental relationship between the two. While there are far too many articles on this subject to cite, there is profound disagreement in the medical and physiologic literature about this relationship (although most clinical texts fail to reflect this controversy). Some studies have demonstrated a linear relationship (D_LCO_{SB} increases in proportion to V_A), others a quantitative but nonlinear relationship (D_LCO_{SB} increases as V_A increases, but not proportionally or changes over only a portion of the volume range), and still others no relationship (D_LCO_{SB} does not change with changes in V_A). One study[10] has even demonstrated that D_LCO is different at a given lung volume depending on whether the volume was reached by inhaling from a lower volume or exhaling from a higher volume. Furthermore, in the studies that do show increases in D_LCO_{SB} with increases in V_A, it is unclear to what extent that relationship is simply a mathematical perturbation[2] (as V_A is a factor in the D_LCO_{SB} equation). This issue certainly cannot be resolved here, but it should be obvious that the rationale for inclusion of V_A is controversial at best.

These and other considerations about the role of V_A have led to a number of alternative diffusion indices that remove its effect from the computed D_LCO value. The most obvious and common approach has been to divide D_LCO by the same V_A value (here in liters) that went into its calculation (or, more simply, to leave V_A out of the calculation in the first place). This index is called variously D_LCO/V_A (or D_L/V_A), transfer coefficient, specific diffusing capacity, and K_{CO}, among other terms. A second approach has been to rearrange the factors in the D_LCO_{SB} equation so as to express the diffusion process by a time function (measured in seconds). This index is termed tau (τ) or the RC time constant, and is calculated as

$$\tau = \left(\frac{60}{D_LCO}\right)\left[\frac{V_A}{(P_b - 47)}\right] \tag{4}$$

These volume-corrected measures may be viewed in one of two ways. First, they may be viewed as the true measure of diffusion in the lung in lieu of the standard D_LCO value.

This approach assumes constant diffusion at all levels of lung expansion, at least above functional residual capacity (FRC). While this concept is difficult for many to accept, there is rather compelling morphologic evidence for it.[11] Alternatively, and as is more common, these volume-corrected measures may be viewed in addition to the standard D_LCO value as a means of differentiating values due merely to altered volume from those due to actual gas transfer abnormalities. As V_A is factored directly into the calculation of D_LCO, almost all abnormalities that reduce lung volume, by definition, reduce D_LCO, but only a few actually alter alveolar-capillary permeability, the detection of which is generally the purpose of diffusion measurements in restrictive abnormalities. Both logic and the consensus in published studies tell us that if a decreased D_LCO is normalized by removing volume as a factor, decreased volume was the source of the abnormality, whereas a diffusion measurement that remains abnormal after adjustment for lung volume represents a true diffusion defect. Despite the rather self-evident nature of this contention, it has been recently and aggressively challenged.[12] It will also be appreciated that increases in V_A can cause spurious results. If diffusion in each lung unit is at only a portion of its normal value but a larger than normal V_A (hyperinflation) enters the equation, the resulting D_LCO_{SB} may appear normal.

Steady-State Method

In the steady-state method the subject breathes normally from a source gas containing 0.1 to 0.2 percent CO until a constant rate of CO uptake is established and then continues to breathe normally for several more minutes as exhaled gas is collected. The expired gas is analyzed for CO concentration (and incidentally for O_2 and CO_2), and D_LCO_{SS} is calculated as follows:

1. The total CO uptake in milliliters per minute ($\dot{V}CO$) is computed as

$$\dot{V}_{CO} = (\dot{V}_E)\,[CO_I\,(N_{2I}/N_{2E}) - CO_E] \qquad (5)$$

   where, $\dot{V}_E$ is minute volume (tidal volume × respiratory rate), corrected to STPD, CO_i is the source gas (initial) concentration of CO, N_{2I} is the inspired N_2 concentration N_{2E} is the expired N_2 concentration of nitrogen (which is taken to be the fraction not occupied by O_2 and CO_2), and CO_E is the mixed expired concentration of CO
2. P_ACO (in millimeters of Hg) is calculated in one of the ways described below
3. D_LCO_{SS} is then calculated as

$$D_LCO_{SS} = \dot{V}\frac{\dot{V}CO}{(P_ACO - P\bar{c}CO)} \qquad (6a)$$

   where, $P\bar{c}CO$ is the mean capillary pressure of CO. As in the case of D_LCO_{SB}, $P\bar{c}CO$ is usually considered to be zero, at least for purposes of calculation, so that the above equation becomes

$$D_LCO_{SS} = \dot{V}CO/P_ACO \qquad (6b)$$

   yielding, like D_LCO_{SB}, a value in milliliters per minute per millimeter of Hg.

There are several variations of the steady-state method, based on the way P_ACO is determined. The three most common are

1. The *end-tidal method,* in which end-tidal CO values are taken as a measure of alveolar CO
2. The *measured dead space (Filley) method,* in which an arterial blood sample is taken to determine $PaCO_2$; and the subject's dead space/tidal volume ratio (V_D/V_T) is then computed by the standard Bohr equation

$$V_D/V_T = (PaCO_2 - P_ECO_2)/PaCO_2 \qquad (7)$$

   and used to derive the P_ACO from the mixed expired values by the equation

$$P_ACO = (P_b - 47)\left[\frac{(CO_E - V_D/V_T)(CO_I)}{(1 - V_D/V_T)}\right] \qquad (8)$$

3. The *assumed dead space method,* in which P_ACO is determined as just described but with use of an assumed value for V_D/V_T (negating the need for measurement of $PaCO_2$.

The method by which P_ACO is determined can have a marked effect on the accuracy of D_LCO_{SS} in different contexts. Much has been written on the comparative usefulness of the various D_LCO_{SS} methods, but space limitations preclude a detailed review here. The interested reader is referred to the overview by Bates et al.,[13] which, while somewhat dated on some points of detail, is still one of the best on this subject.

Single-Breath versus Steady-State Methods

Much has also been written on the comparative advantages and disadvantages of the single-breath and steady-state methods and the relationship between values obtained by the two. Again, this issue cannot be reviewed here in its entirety, but the principal points of comparison are outlined in Table 48-1.

The reason for the higher values by the single-breath method has been long debated. Proposed explanations include the larger lung volume and assumed greater surface area during D_LCO_{SB} determinations (see earlier discussion), the better distribution of a full inspiration, and the effects of

Table 48-1. Comparison of Steady-State and Single-Breath Methods for Determination of DLCO

Steady-State	Single-Breath
Generally easier for the subject to perform, as no special breathing maneuvers are required	Far less susceptible to development of CO back pressure and to effects of $\dot{V}/\dot{Q}$ abnormalities
Adaptable to use during exercise and other applications where breath holding is not feasible	Tends to be more reproducible
	Generally yields higher values (than steady-state methods) in a given subject

the more negative intrathoracic pressures during a $DLCO_{SB}$ maneuver; however, the actual mechanism is not known.

One last advantage of the single-breath approach, which is not inherent to the method but is significant nonetheless, is that it has been more widely studied, is better understood, and, as discussed below, has now been well standardized.

FACTORS AFFECTING DLCO

Measurements of DLCO are affected by a number of methodologic and physiologic factors, which must be appreciated if such measurements are to be applied meaningfully (Table 48-2).

Methodologic Factors

Some methodologic factors have already been broached in the discussion of testing techniques, but there are a number of factors beyond those directly reflected in the test sequences. In the case of the single-breath method, the American Thoracic Society (ATS) has proposed guidelines,[14] now widely accepted, which have effectively standardized most of the methodologic vagaries of the $DLCO_{SB}$. These guidelines are mandatory reading for anyone performing this type of testing. Of the many factors discussed in the ATS statement, we will elaborate on three of the most critical.

Table 48-2. Some of the Factors Affecting $DLCO_{SB}$

- Methodologic factors
  - Inspiratory and expiratory time
  - Breath-holding time measurement method
  - Dead space washout and expired sample size
- Physiologic factors
  - Body habitus (accounted for by predicted values)
  - Alveolar-capillary interface surface area
  - Alveolar-capillary membrane permeability
  - Hemoglobin concentration
  - Carboxyhemoglobin concentration
  - Pulmonary capillary blood volume
  - Intrasubject diurnal variation
  - Subject's position (posture) during testing
  - Intrathoracic pressure
  - Recent alcohol consumption
  - Subject's anxiety
  - O_2 concentration

The first factor is the rapidity of inspiration and expiration of the test gas as described in steps 2 and 4, respectively, of the $DLCO_{SB}$ maneuver. This factor is critical because the standard equation by which $DLCO_{SB}$ is calculated is valid only during breath holding, so that the $DLCO_{SB}$ maneuver really assumes instantaneous filling and emptying. Of course, even healthy subjects cannot make large lung volume changes instantaneously, and patients with obstructive disorders may take several seconds to effect such volume changes. An alternate approach to calculation of $DLCO_{SB}$ using separate equations appropriate to inspiration, breath holding, and expiration has been proposed[11] but has not been widely adopted. In lieu of such an approach, it is imperative that the time of inspiration and expiration (including sample collection) be minimized. The ATS guidelines recommend that the time to 90 percent of inspiration not exceed 2.5 seconds in subjects with a forced expiratory volume in 1 second/forced vital capacity (FEV_1/FVC) ratio greater than 0.50, or 4 seconds in subjects with an FEV_1/FVC ratio less than 0.50; in all subjects, expiratory time (sample collection) should not exceed 3 seconds.

The second factor is the calculation of BHT, for which several methods have been proposed. The start of BHT is alternately timed from the beginning of inspiration, 50 percent of inspired volume, 33 percent of inspiratory time, and various other points, while the end of BHT may be measured from the beginning of sample collection, the midpoint of sample collection, and various other points. The particular interval chosen can have rather dramatic effects on the computed $DLCO_{SB}$. Differences in $DLCO_{SB}$ have been demonstrated[15] even in normal subjects on the basis of different BHT calculation methods, and in persons with obstruction the differences may be 20 percent or more.[8,16]

The third methodologic factor concerns the final expiration of test gas, how much volume is allowed for clearing the dead space, and how much volume is collected as a sample for analysis. Current general practice, as well as the specific ATS recommendation, is to allow between 0.75 and 1.0 L for washout and then to collect 0.5 to 1.0 L of sample. However, it has been shown that in as many as 26 percent of subjects a volume greater than 1 L is actually required to clear dead space.[8] The appropriateness of the recommended sample volume is debatable as well. On the one hand, a larger sample tends to be more representative of the true alveolar mix, while the prolonged time required for a patient with pulmonary obstruction to exhale a larger sample tends to falsely raise $DLCO_{SB}$ for the reasons discussed above. One elegant study[17] has concluded that the former problem is of greater consequence, and that collecting significantly smaller samples (85 mL in that study) improves the accuracy of $DLCO_{SB}$ measurements.

Overall, differences in the above factors can cause considerable interlaboratory (and even intralaboratory) differences in $DLCO_{SB}$; it has been shown that computational differences alone can account for 41 percent variations.[18] Therefore, it is imperative that (1) these factors be rigorously controlled and (2) normal ("predicted") values be taken from a study in which the methodology matches that being used for testing.

In the case of $DLCO_{SS}$, the various techniques are subject to different methodologic aberrations. The end-tidal method is susceptible to large errors if end-tidal gas is not representative of alveolar gas, as may occur at rest if a subject's VT is not large enough to clear the mechanical dead space, and as is common during exercise. The assumed dead space method is obviously subject to errors resulting from incorrect estimation of dead space. Such errors are most likely to occur in subjects with significant lung disease, in whom estimated VD/VT is least reliable, and are of less consequence during exercise, when VD/VT falls. The measured dead space method is potentially very sensitive to errors in $PaCO_2$ determinations.

Physiologic Factors

In normal subjects diffusion varies with age, body size, and sex, these variations being accounted for in the predicted values with which DLCO measurements are compared. Unfortunately, the population studies from which predicted values have been derived suffer from the same sources of variability we have been discussing, leading to wide discrepancies. Table 48-3 provides examples of the ranges of normal DLCO values. Aside from these sources of natural variation, the two principal physiologic factors that affect DLCO and that provide the primary basis for its clinical usefulness are

Table 48-3. Sample Predicted Values for DLCO Illustrating the Range of Normal for Various Subject Groups

	$DLCO_{SB}$ (mL/min/mmHg) Low	$DLCO_{SB}$ (mL/min/mmHg) High	$DLCO_{SS}$ (mL/min/mmHg)
Short, elderly woman (Ht, 60 in.; age, 60 yr)	14.1	24.2	11.2
Short, elderly man (Ht, 65 in.; age, 60 yr)	17.1	29.2	12.1
Tall, young woman (Ht, 70 in.; age, 20 yr)	24.1	41.4	22.7
Tall, young man (Ht, 77 in.; age, 20 yr)	41.5	49.6	26.5

[a] The low and high values for $DLCO_{SB}$ illustrate the range of values that may be predicted for a *single* subject by different published studies. The variation in these values should make obvious the need to select a predictive equation taken from a study in which the testing methodology matches as closely as possible that which will be used to test subjects.

changes in the surface area and changes in the permeability of the alveolar-capillary membrane. The net effects of these are discussed elsewhere. This section deals with a number of secondary physiologic factors, which, unless otherwise indicated, apply to the $DLCO_{SB}$ only.

The first such factor is the amount of hemoglobin in contact with CO in the lungs. Most discussions of DLCO include an obligatory explanation that what is actually measured by DLCO determinations is at least a two-phase process, which includes not only the actual diffusion across the membrane but, as discussed in the introduction to this chapter, also the reaction with red blood cells. The former is termed the *membrane diffusion* (DM) component, and the latter the *capillary blood volume* (Vc) component. Each of these processes represents a resistance to CO uptake, so that their relationship to the total uptake is usually expressed by an electrical analogue of reciprocals

$$\frac{1}{DLCO} = \frac{1}{DM} + \frac{1}{\theta Vc} \qquad (9)$$

where, θ is the volume of CO that will combine with 1 mL of blood in 1 minute.

The obvious implication of this relationship is that DLCO will be altered in the presence of a change in either "available" hemoglobin content or pulmonary capillary blood volume. In fact, it is common practice to correct DLCO values for the patient's measured hemoglobin and carboxyhemoglobin, using several available formulae. Likewise, it is fairly well understood that conditions that increase blood volume, such as pulmonary vascular congestion, can increase DLCO, while pulmonary embolic disease or other causes of decreased blood volume can reduce DLCO. (It is important to understand that this effect is a function of blood *volume,* not blood *flow.*) A less obvious implication is that DLCO will also be increased by intrapulmonary hemorrhage, which places hemoglobin in direct contact with the alveolar CO.

The second physiologic factor is diurnal variation. It has been demonstrated that DLCO decreases throughout the day, although there is disagreement as to the rate. Studies have demonstrated rates between 0.4 and 2.2 percent[19,20] per hour. A third factor is the subject's position. Both $DLCO_{SB}$[21] and $DLCO_{SS}$[22] have been shown to be higher with the subject supine than with the subject seated.

Measurements of $DLCO_{SB}$ are also probably affected by increases in intrathoracic pressure, although here again the evidence is contradictory. To the extent that there is an effect, this factor has at least two ramifications: (1) $DLCO_{SB}$ will be affected if the subject either pulls or pushes against the shutter during breath holding; and (2) $DLCO_{SB}$ may be spuriously increased in subjects with high inspiratory airway resistance as a result of the attendant higher pressures generated during the maximal inspiration of test gas. In support of the second point, a number of studies have demonstrated increases in $DLCO_{SB}$ associated with asthma.[23,24] Two additional factors have been demonstrated in only one study each but are of sufficient interest to note. One is that $DLCO_{SB}$ is decreased by recent alcohol (ethanol) consumption[25]; the other, and more intriguing, is that $DLCO_{SB}$ is increased by the subject's anxiety.[26]

The seventh and last factor discussed here is O_2. We have saved this factor for last because it has unique implications in the use of DLCO to assess the alveolar-capillary membrane. As O_2 and CO compete for hemoglobin binding sites, increasing alveolar O_2 will reduce DLCO. On the basis of a classic article by Roughton and Foster,[27] this fact has been exploited to differentially measure the DM and Vc components of diffusion (Equation 9). The basic idea is that if DLCO is measured at two levels of O_2 and each value is plotted as 1/DLCO against its corresponding $1/\theta$ value, Equation 9 can be solved to quantitate DM and Vc, as illustrated in Figure 48-2. This effect of O_2 has another practical implication, which is that when DLCO is measured at an altitude significantly different than sea level, it is necessary to augment the O_2 component of the test gas such that a PAO_2 of approximately 150 mmHg is achieved, in order to make the values comparable with standard measurements.

Having now delineated a number of factors that do affect DLCO, we would like to discuss one factor that does *not* affect DLCO in the way widely believed. That factor is ventilation/perfusion ($\dot{V}/\dot{Q}$) mismatching, which is commonly viewed as affecting all diffusion measurements. While $DLCO_{SS}$ determinations may be affected by $\dot{V}/\dot{Q}$ inequality, $DLCO_{SB}$ determinations are not, despite contentions to the contrary in many clinical texts. A number of features in the $DLCO_{SB}$ maneuver mitigate against such an effect. A full discussion is beyond the scope of this chapter, but there is one very simple bit of empirical evidence that makes the point. As PaO_2 is determined largely by $\dot{V}/\dot{Q}$ matching, any subject with a low PaO_2 should have a low $DLCO_{SB}$ if, in fact, $\dot{V}/\dot{Q}$ inequality were a factor. Such is clearly not the case. Indeed, one of the most common applications of diffusion measurements is to distinguish subjects with bronchitis, who may have very low $\dot{V}/\dot{Q}$ ratios and low PaO_2 but normal $DLCO_{SB}$, from subjects with emphysema, who have high $\dot{V}/\dot{Q}$ ratios and *relatively* well preserved resting PaO_2 but low $DLCO_{SB}$.

DIFFUSING CAPACITY OF OXYGEN

This chapter opened with an explanation of why CO is used to determine diffusion across the alveolar-capillary membrane when, in fact, it is the diffusion of O_2 in which we are interested. We will close the chapter by returning to that point. Once diffusion of CO has been determined, it is generally held that O_2 diffusion (DLO_2) can then be inter-

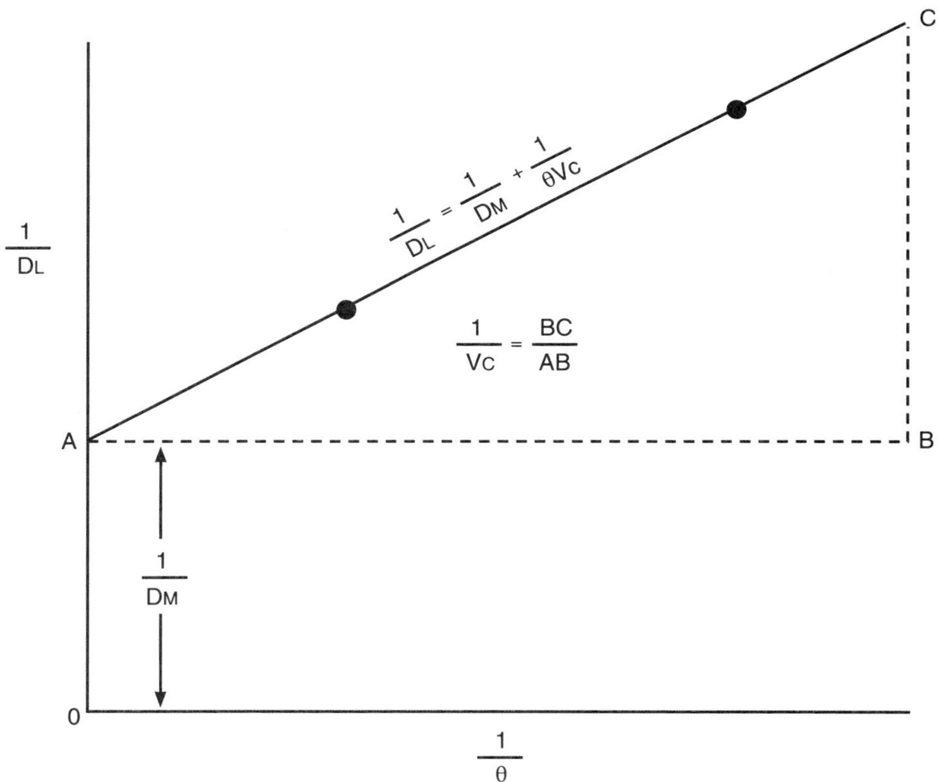

Figure 48-2. Illustration of method for determining DM and Vc. The two solid circles are actual DLCO measurements at differing levels of alveolar O_2, plotted as their reciprocals (1/DL). The slope of the line drawn through these points is then the reciprocal of capillary blood volume (1/Vc), and the Y-intercept of the line is the reciprocal of membrane diffusing capacity (1/DM).

polated as follows:

$$D_{L}O_2 = (D_{L}CO)(1.23) \quad (10)$$

where 1.23 represents the relationship between the solubility coefficients of CO and O_2 in blood and their molecular weights.

However, this relationship is not always demonstrable experimentally. Marks et al.[28] have shown that such interpolated values are, *on average,* very close to directly measured DLCO values (which can be measured directly with great difficulty), but this agreement is fortuitous; the interpolated values in this study either underestimate or overestimate the direct $D_{L}O_2$ in most individual subjects. Miller and Johnson[29] have also demonstrated discrepancies between measured and interpolated $D_{L}O_2$ at rest but better correlation during exercise. Thus, it is unclear whether DLCO can be translated into a quantitative measure of O_2 diffusion, but the need to do so has really become moot as DLCO itself has become the established index of diffusion.

References

1. Forster RE, Fowler WS, Bates DV, van Lingen B: The absorption of carbon monoxide by the lungs during breathholding. J Clin Invest 1954;33:1135–1145
2. Forster RE: The single-breath carbon monoxide transfer test 25 years on: 1—Physiological considerations, editorial. Thorax 1983;38:1–9
3. Takaro T, Price HP, Parra SC: Ultrastructural studies of apertures in the interalveolar septum of the adult human lung. Am Rev Respir Dis 1979;119:425–434
4. McGrath MW, Thomson ML: The effect of age, body size and lung volume change on alveolar-capillary permeability and diffusing capacity in man. J Physiol 1959;146:572–582
5. Hamer NAJ: The effect of age on the components of the pulmonary diffusing capacity. Clin Sci 1962;23:85–93
6. Mitchell MM, Renzetti AD: Application of the single-breath method of total lung capacity measurement to the calculation of the carbon monoxide diffusing capacity. Am Rev Respir Dis 1968;97:581–584
7. Ferris BG: Epidemiology standardization project. Am Rev Respir Dis, suppl. 1978;118:62–72
8. Graham BL, Mink JT, Cotton DJ: Overestimation of the single-breath carbon monoxide diffusing capacity in patients with airflow obstruction. Am Rev Respir Dis 1984;129:403–408
9. Burns CB, Scheinhorn DJ: Evaluation of single-breath helium dilution total lung capacity in obstructive lung disease. Am Rev Respir Dis 1984;130:580–583
10. Cassidy SS, Murugappan R, Rose GL, Johnson RL: Hysteresis in the relation between diffusing capacity of the lung and lung volume. J Appl Physiol 1980;49:566–570
11. Graham BL, Mink JT, Cotton DJ: Improved accuracy and precision of single-breath CO diffusing capacity measurements. J Appl Physiol 1981;51:1306–1313
12. Kanengiser LC, Rapoport DM, Epstein H, Goldring RM: Volume adjustment of mechanics and diffusion in interstitial lung disease: Lack of clinical relevance. Chest 1989;96:1036–1042
13. Bates DV, Macklem PT, Christie RV: Respiratory Function in Disease. 2nd Ed. WB Saunders, Philadelphia, 1971, pp. 75–91
14. Crapo RO (chairman): Single breath carbon monoxide diffusing capacity (transfer factor): Recommendations for a standard technique. Am Rev Respir Dis 1987;136:1299–1307
15. Leech JA, Martz L, Liben A, Becklake MR: Diffusing capacity for carbon monoxide: The effects of different derivations of breathhold time and alveolar volume and of carbon monoxide back pressure on calculated results. Am Rev Respir Dis 1985;132:1127–1129
16. Colp C, Goldman DE: Diffusing capacity measurement in patients with airway obstruction. Chest 1986;90:925
17. Jones RS, Meade F: A theoretical and experimental analysis of anomalies in the estimation of pulmonary diffusing capacity by the single breath method. Q J Exp Physiol 1961;46:131–143
18. Morris AH, Crapo RO: Standardization of computation of single-breath transfer factor. Bull Eur Physiopathol Respir 1985; 21:183–189
19. Frey TM, Crapo RO, Jensen RL, Elliott CG: Diurnal variation of the diffusing capacity of the lung: Is it real? Am Rev Respir Dis 1987;136:1381
20. Cinkotai FF, Thomson ML: Diurnal variation in pulmonary diffusing capacity for carbon monoxide. J Appl Physiol 1966; 21:539–542
21. Ogilvie CM, Forster RE, Blakemore WS, Morton JW: A standardized technique for the clinical measurement of the diffusing capacity of the lung for carbon monoxide. J Clin Invest 1957;36:1–17
22. Sundstrom G: Influence of body position on pulmonary diffusing capacity in young and old men. J Appl Physiol 1975;38:418–423
23. Keens TG, Mansell A, Krastins IRB et al: Evaluation of the single breath diffusing capacity in asthma and cystic fibrosis. Chest 1979;76:41–44
24. Stewart RI: Carbon monoxide diffusing capacity in asthmatic patients with mild airflow limitation. Chest 1988;94:332–336
25. Peavy HH, Summer WR, Gurtner G: The effects of acute ethanol ingestion on pulmonary diffusing capacity. Chest 1980;77:488–492
26. Cinkotai FF, Thomason ML, Guyatt AR: Effect of apprehension on pulmonary diffusing capacity in man. J Appl Physiol 1966;21:534–538
27. Roughton FJW, Forster RE: Relative importance of diffusion and chemical reaction rates in determining rate of exchange of gases in the human lung, with special reference to true diffusing capacity of pulmonary membrane and volume of blood in the lung capillaries. J Appl Physiol 1957;11:290–302
28. Marks A, Cugell DW, Cadigan JB, Gaensler EA: Clinical determination of the diffusion capacity of the lungs: Comparison of methods in normal subjects and patients with "alveolar-capillary block" syndrome. Am J Med 1957;22:51–73
29. Miller JM, Johnson RL: Effect of lung inflation on pulmonary diffusing capacity at rest and exercise. J Clin Invest 1966;45:493–500

Chapter 49

Clinical Exercise Testing and Assessment of Disability

Robert B. Schoene

CHAPTER OUTLINE

Chapter 15 laid the foundation of normal exercise physiology for understanding the pathophysiology of exercise limitation. The purpose of this chapter is threefold: (1) to provide a general approach to the preparation for and administration of a clinical exercise test, (2) to review the interpretation of results for patients with various pathophysiologic disorders, and (3) to describe the determination of impairment and consequently disability.

The pulmonary physician has extended the role of the cardiologists who for years have done treadmill stress testing for patients with chest pain. Now a number of pathophysiologic disorders fall under the aegis of the pulmonary clinician. In the context of the discussion in Chapter 15, the pulmonary physician and cardiopulmonary technologist have reassumed the role of the physiologist and can now extend the diagnostic capabilities of the pulmonary function laboratory.

Although a specific diagnosis is often not made, the pulmonary physiologic exercise test can be helpful in guiding the clinician to an extended and more specific workup. Testing is undertaken most commonly to evaluate dyspnea, disability, exercise-induced asthma, chest pain, subjective decrease in exercise tolerance, and aerobic fitness. In all cases a careful history and physical examination, selected blood tests, pulmonary function tests, and an electrocardiogram (ECG) are needed to ascertain the indications for exercise testing, to direct interpretation and further workup, and to determine safety for the patient. Obviously, if the patient has significant cardiovascular disease or unstable chest pain, the risk/benefit ratio for the patient would be too high and the test should be deferred. Additionally, the procedure and its risks should be carefully explained to all patients to allay their fears and encourage them to give their best effort.

ADMINISTRATION OF EXERCISE TESTS

Each laboratory should (1) have the facility to administer exercise tests to a wide range of patients and athletes; (2)

be familiar with the responses that are obtained on its system; (3) be able to troubleshoot problems; and (4) be able to individualize the test to a patient's physical ability or handicap. For instance, some patients may be able to walk on a treadmill better than they can ride a stationary bicycle, while others may have disabling arthritis and only be able to use an arm ergometer. The most reliable form of ergometer is a stationary cycle. Specified work loads can be delivered to the patient so that each test on a given subject and between subjects is comparable. A number of very sophisticated cycle ergometers are available which can incrementally and automatically increase the work load, but any basic belted-resistance ergometer with precalibrated work loads will suffice. If the clinician is more familiar with the treadmill, this can also provide an acceptable way to increase the patient's work.

There are many types of exercise protocols,[1] but the most commonly used are either a stepwise increase of work loads for specified periods of time to exhaustion or the progressively increasing work load to exhaustion of the ramp test. Most clinicians feel that pushing the patient to tolerance or exhaustion is safe and gives valuable information at the upper levels. This is essential in evaluation of athletes. If one chooses stepwise increases of work loads, the increments of the work loads must not be so small that the test takes too long or so great that the patient cannot achieve more than one or two stages. The clinician should aim for a test of anywhere between 7 and 15 minutes' duration, and after 1 or 2 minutes of unloaded cycling, work load increments of 100 kpn/min or 15 watts/min to exhaustion usually encompass the abilities of most patients. Obviously, for an elite athlete these work load increments would be too small. A minute or less at each work load does not allow the patient to achieve a steady state, which usually requires at least 3 to 5 minutes at any power output, but for clinical purposes the information obtained from a steady-state test does not add much to an incremental test to exhaustion. Most importantly, to obtain the best results patients must be made aware of what is going to be done and what is expected of them. Most patients need to be encouraged as they approach exhaustion, but most make a good effort, and therefore the results are valid.

Equipment

Aside from the ergometer, several pieces of equipment are necessary to obtain accurate data. First, the laboratory should be equipped with a functional cardiac defibrillator and resuscitation cart. Pertinent to the issue of safety as well as to the evaluation of the cardiac and pulmonary response, the patient should be monitored with an ECG, which gives a clear tracing on an oscilloscope and can also give hard copy on a rhythm strip. Some clinicians may also be interested in 12-lead ECGs during exercise to evaluate ischemic changes of the ST segments more thoroughly.

Measurements of ventilation are also mandatory, and this can be achieved in several ways. Exhaled gas samples over a precise period of time (usually 1 to 3 minutes) can be collected in a meteorologic balloon or Douglas bag and its volume measured either with a Tissot spirometer or a gasometer. More commonly, pneumotachographs or turbine spirometers are utilized, but they must be carefully and frequently calibrated with a known volume of gas in a calibration syringe at different flow rates. With pneumotachographs flow is measured over a screen with fixed resistance, and volume is integrated from the flow signal. Turbine spirometers are also available, and as their technology improves, they are gaining increasing popularity.

From the volume of exhaled gas, fractions of O_2 and CO_2 can be measured to determine O_2 consumption ($\dot{V}O_2$) and CO_2 production ($\dot{V}CO_2$). These measurements must be made with accurate and fast sampling O_2 and CO_2 analyzers. Many commercially available exercise systems designed since about the mid-1970s are computerized and can make determinations of minute ventilation and metabolic rate either over fixed periods of time through a gas mixing chamber or on a breath-by-breath basis with gases sampled at the mouth valve. Careful and thorough calibration is necessary before each test regardless of the system. Accuracy depends on precise timing of the gas samples through a high-flow sample line and rapid response analyzers or mass spectrometers and integration of that phase delay with the volume measurements from the pneumotachograph or turbine spirometer.

It is also helpful to use a noninvasive oximeter for measurement of arterial O_2 saturation during exercise. This capability not only provides a second line of safety but also gives important insight into the physiology of gas exchange. An ear probe is probably more satisfactory for exercise, since finger probes tend to become dislodged or to give inaccurate data if blood flow is restricted by gripping of the handle bars or safety railings. There is also less time delay with the earlobe oximeter than there is with the more distal finger probes.

If measurements of physiologic dead space are important in certain patients, an arterial line is the only way to obtain accurate measurements of $PaCO_2$, which is needed for the dead space calculation. Additionally, an arterial line provides the ability to measure the alveolar-arterial O_2 difference [$P(A\text{-}a)O_2$], which is important for ascertaining the integrity of gas exchange. Furthermore, accurate measurements of pH and perhaps lactate concentrations are helpful for determining whether the patient reached a metabolic acidosis at high levels of exercise.

Finally, one of the most important components in this entire system is a capable, meticulous, and enthusiastic technician who has an understanding of and appreciation for the physiology of exercise.

Aerobic Fitness

Although it is not within the purview of this chapter to review the exercise physiology of the elite athlete, it is important for the pulmonary physiology laboratory to be prepared to evaluate athletes of all levels since other physicians or coaches may refer athletes to them. Precise physiologic measurements are very important in this group of individuals. Athletes may be referred for testing of their aerobic fitness to determine potential in many of the aerobic sports such as running, swimming, rowing, and Nordic skiing[2] (Fig. 49-1). There is virtually no overlap in maximum O_2 consumption ($\dot{V}O_2max$) between the normal or even good athlete and the potentially elite athlete. Athletes are also often referred to the laboratory for evaluation of training effects, and both submaximal and maximal values are extremely important. For instance, submaximal heart rates at a specific work load will be lower after a period of training, while $\dot{V}O_2max$ with the same maximum heart rate but higher stroke volume should be greater[3] (Fig. 49-2).

Exercise-Induced Asthma

Exercise-induced asthma is encountered in as many as 20 percent of competing athletes.[3] On the positive side, it is a treatable disorder, since many Olympic caliber athletes have been treated with bronchodilators, and most of the routine therapeutic interventions have been determined to be legal for use by athletes by the United States and International Olympic committees. Several exercise protocols are used to try to induce airway reactivity, but all of them are based on spirometer measurements prior to an exercise test and 5 to 30 minutes after the test.[4] A drop of 15 to 20 percent or more in the forced expiratory volume in the first second (FEV_1) is indicative of an abnormal airway response to exercise[5] (Fig. 49-3). One of the more popular protocols is to have the patient exercise for at least 6 minutes at 80 percent of the

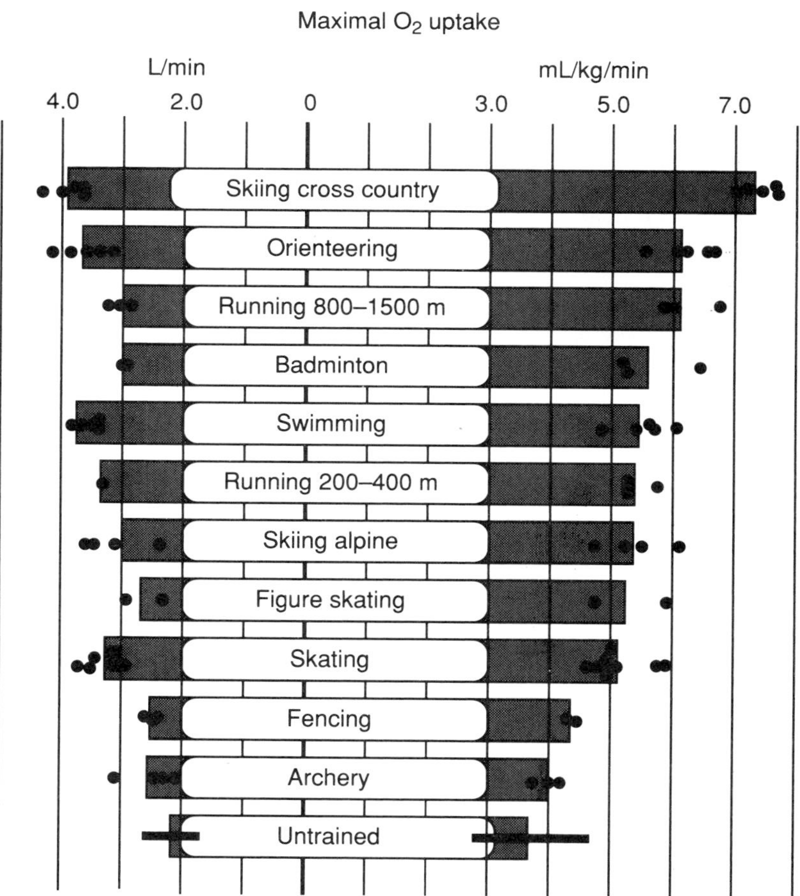

Figure 49-1. Maximum $\dot{V}O_2$ values in a number of individuals, ranging from sedentary controls to highly trained Nordic skiers. There is virtually no overlap between elite athletes and normal control subjects. (From Astrand and Rodahl,[2] with permission.)

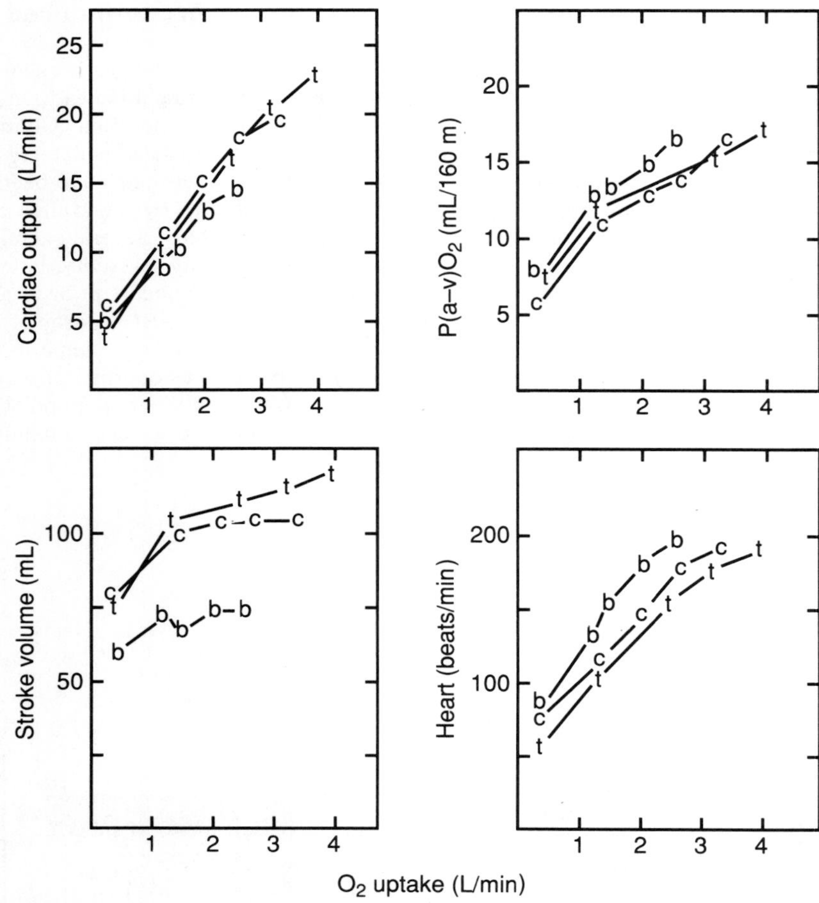

Figure 49-2. The components of $\dot{V}O_2$ that are affected by training. Data on cardiac output, arteriovenous O_2 content difference, stroke volume, and heart rate at increasing levels of $\dot{V}O_2$ are shown for three groups of individuals (c, control subjects, b, bed rest, and t, training). Training results in a higher $\dot{V}O_2$max, which is largely achieved by an increase of stroke volume with lower heart rates at submaximal levels of $\dot{V}O_2$. (From Astrand and Rodahl,[2] with permission.)

predicted maximum heart rate. A progressive work test to exhaustion is also usually sufficient to induce airway reactivity. Interestingly, running on a treadmill is more effective than the bicycle ergometer in inducing bronchospasm.

PULMONARY RESPONSE

If a patient has exercise limitation, it is important to determine whether that limitation is secondary to cardiac and/or pulmonary impairment. A systematic approach to evaluation of the physiologic data will allow an accurate evaluation and thus often leads to the use of more specific diagnostic tests (Fig. 49-4).

Even though dyspnea is one of the most common symptoms for which a patient is referred, its etiology is not always pulmonary. In order to determine if a patient has a pulmonary limitation to exercise, it is important to determine the patient's own predicted maximum expired minute ventilation ($\dot{V}$Emax) prior to the test. From spirometry and a maximum voluntary ventilation (MVV) maneuver, the clinician can determine the level of $\dot{V}$E that a patient should achieve in terms of maximum ventilation. Patients therefore act as their own standard. There are several methods to determine the predicted $\dot{V}$Emax. If the patient can perform a good MVV maneuver, 70 to 80 percent of that value should equal what the patient can achieve during a maximal exercise test. It should be kept in mind that the MVV is really an unnatural maneuver of high-tidal volume (VT), high-frequency breathing, whereas normal maximum ventilation is achieved with greater biomechanical efficiency and less energy expenditure, with VT approximately 60 percent of vital capacity (VC) and respiratory rate anywhere from 40 to 70 breaths per min-

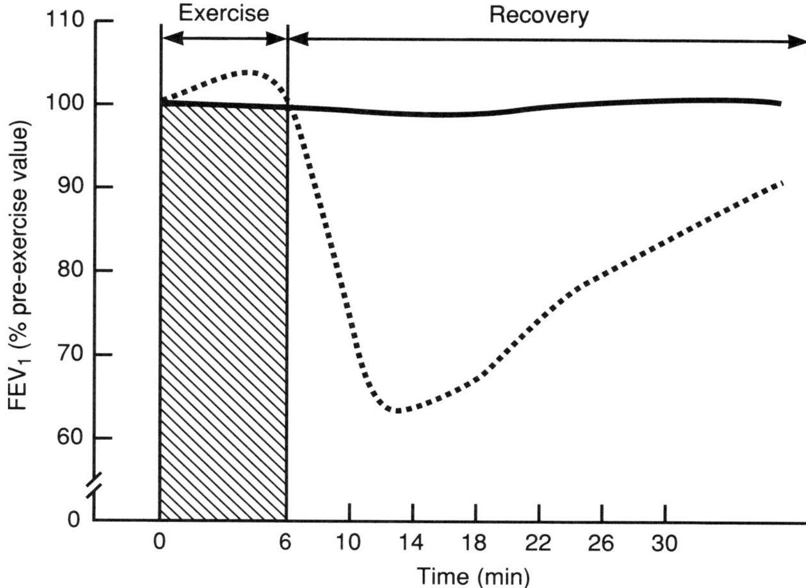

Figure 49-3. Responses to exercise of airflow (FEV_1, percent of control value) in normal subjects (solid line) and subjects with exercise-induced bronchospasm (dashed line). (From McKenzie,[5] with permission.)

ute. An equally valid technique to predict a patient's $\dot{V}_{Emax}$ is to take 70 percent of 40 times the FEV_1 or 80 percent of 35 times the FEV_1.

The difference between the patient's predicted $\dot{V}_{Emax}$ and the actual measured $\dot{V}_{Emax}$ is called the *ventilatory reserve* (Fig. 49-5A). Patients who have a ventilatory reserve that is 20 percent or more of their predicted $\dot{V}_{Emax}$ either do not have a ventilatory limitation to exercise and/or did not exert themselves to a symptom-limited level of work. Patients who have no ventilatory reserve or actually exceed their predicted $\dot{V}_{Emax}$ are said to have reached a mechanical ventilatory limitation. There may be other concomitant factors limiting exercise, but these patients have at least in part stopped exercise because of ventilatory limitation.

The *ventilatory pattern* throughout exercise may also give insight into patients' mechanics of ventilation and thereby into their underlying pathophysiology. Patients with *restrictive disease* characteristically have low-V_T, high-frequency patterns of ventilation, which may also be accompanied by hyperventilation. The low V_T, however, may be a normal or high percentage of the vital capacity. In patients with moderate to severe restrictive disease who make a good effort, a true ventilatory limitation at the end of exhaustive exercise is associated with hypercapnia and respiratory acidosis.

Patients with *obstructive pulmonary disease* may exhibit a variety of respiratory patterns. Some may show a relatively high-V_T, low-frequency ventilation, which is imposed on them by air trapping (Fig. 49-5B). These patients characteristically also develop a hypercapnic respiratory acidosis at the latter stages of exercise and thus have ventilatory limitation. Some patients may exhibit a tachypneic, low-V_T pattern, but they too, if they push themselves, will develop hypercapnia relative to their baseline state. Many are too sick to make an effort on the test, the result of which is not adequate for evaluation.

The pattern and level of alveolar ventilation that is found is also in large part secondary to the patient's inherent *ventilatory drives*. For instance, most patients with even mild restrictive disease have high ventilatory drives, which are thought to be secondary to the stimulation of the J (stretch) receptors in the lung. Patients with obstructive airway disease may have a whole spectrum of ventilatory drives, from the classic obese hypoventilator, who rarely is dyspneic, to the hyperventilator who will have a compensated respiratory alkalosis and be quite dyspneic.

Ventilatory Equivalent

A great deal of insight can be obtained from evaluation of the ventilatory equivalent ($\dot{V}_E/\dot{V}O_2$ or $\dot{V}_E/\dot{V}CO_2$) throughout exercise (Fig. 49-5C). As defined in Chapter 15, the ventilatory equivalent is the amount of ventilation dedicated to a given metabolic rate. The units of measure (liters per minute) cancel out, and a value of 20 ± 2 is normal for all levels of rest and exercise at and below the ventilatory or anaerobic threshold. Since $\dot{V}_E$ consists of alveolar ventilation ($\dot{V}_A$) and dead space ventilation ($\dot{V}_D$), the ventilatory equivalent is the reflection of both components as dictated by the metabolic rate ($\dot{V}O_2$ or $\dot{V}CO_2$) and the need to maintain CO_2 homeostasis at or below the ventilatory or anaerobic threshold, as well as a reflection of the metabolic demand, ventilatory drive, and $\dot{V}_D$.

In normal subjects $\dot{V}_E/\dot{V}O_2$ increases above 30 and beyond

Clinical Exercise Test Interpretation

Name: ______________________ Hospital #: ________ Test Date: ________

Age: ____________ Height: ____________ Weight: ____________

Interpreter: ______________________ Hospital: ____________

Patient profile: ______________________

Referral source: ______________________

PFT's: (done on______________)

a. Spirometry: (Including MVV) ______________________

b. Lung volumes: ______________________

c. Diffusing capacity: ______________________

d. Impression: ______________________

Exercise Protocol : ______________________

Reason for stopping exercise: ______________________

Overall performance and cooperation: ______________________

Work rate: (Maximum predicted: ______________) ______________

Oxygen consumption: ($\dot{V}O_2$; Maximum predicted: ______ml/min, or ______ml/kg/min.)

Dyspnea : (Borg or visual analogue scale) ______________________

Ventilatory response:

a. Ventilation: (Maximum predicted ventilation: ________L/min.) ____________

b. Pattern (rate, V_T, V_T/IC): ______________________

c. Ventilatory equivalent: ($\dot{V}_E/\dot{V}O_2$) ______________________

d. Bohr Dead space: ($V_D/V_T = (Pa_{CO_2} - P\bar{E}_{CO_2})/Pa_{CO_2}$) ______________________

Gas exchange:

a. Respiratory exchange ratio: ($R = \dot{V}CO_2/\dot{V}O_2$) ______________________

b. Oxygenation saturation: (%) ______________________

c. Alveolar-arterial oxygen difference: (Torr) ______________________

Cardiac response:

a. Heart rate: (Maximum predicted: ________bpm) ______________________

b. O2 pulse: ($\dot{V}O_2$/HR; Predicted: >________ml/beat) ______________________

c. Ischemic changes: ______________________

d. Blood pressure response: ______________________

Anaerobic/ventilatory threshold: ______________________

Lactate levels: (mmol/ml)______________________

Impression: ______________________

Signed: ______________________

Figure 49-4. Example of a clinical exercise report form detailing what such a report should contain.

the anaerobic or ventilatory threshold. Below these levels some accomplished endurance athletes and some patients who have hypoventilation will exhibit ventilatory equivalents from approximately 18 to 20 and have a mildly elevated $PaCO_2$.[6,7] The more common finding in patients is a high ventilatory equivalent throughout exercise. Clinically this is accompanied by inordinate dyspnea and is secondary to increased ventilatory drive and/or increased $\dot{V}_D$. Sometimes the ventilatory equivalents in these patients can be as high as the 40 to 50 range, which is distinctly abnormal and indicative of inefficient ventilation.

In the exercise laboratory the distinction between these two underlying mechanisms may have both practical and physiologic importance. The pathophysiology of these two mechanisms must also be distinguished from psychogenic hyperventilation, which is associated with a respiratory alkalosis and irregular breathing pattern.

Dead Space Ventilation

$\dot{V}_D$ consists of both anatomic and physiologic dead space, the latter being defined by ventilation/perfusion ($\dot{V}/\dot{Q}$) relationship areas with ventilation and no perfusion (Fig. 49-

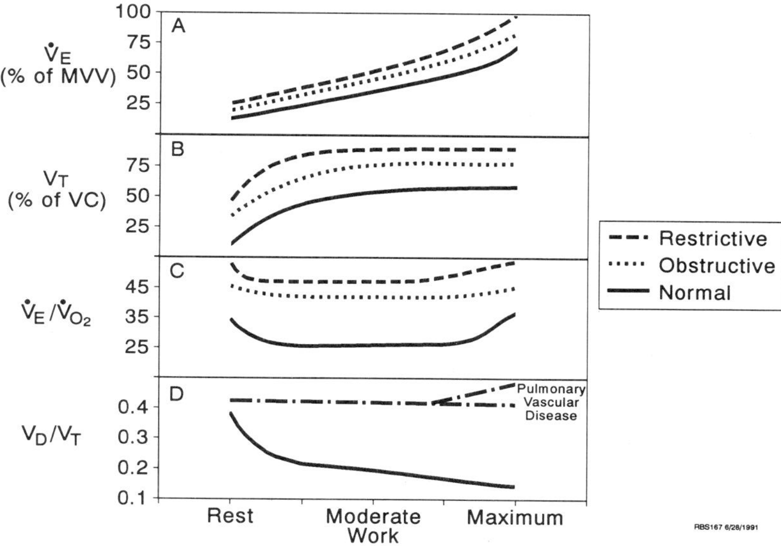

Figure 49-5. Ventilatory response to exercise: schematic examples of typical exercise responses in different clinical conditions. **(A)** Patients with pulmonary disease tend to reach the limit of the lungs' mechanical capability at the end of exhaustive exercise (MVV), while normal subjects have about 20 percent reserve. **(B)** Patients with pulmonary disease use a higher percentage of their VC at all levels of work. **(C)** Most patients with pulmonary disease breathe less efficiently and with a higher dead space tidal volume ratio (V_D/V_T) during exercise, which contributes to a higher ventilatory equivalent ($\dot{V}_E/\dot{V}O_2$). **(D)** V_D/V_T decreases rapidly during exercise in normal subjects. Higher cardiac output results in recruitment of the pulmonary vasculature. Patients with pulmonary vascular compromise cannot achieve the same level of cardiac output and tend not to be able to decrease V_D/V_T.

5D). Because of gravitational forces the apices of the lung at rest have areas of high $\dot{V}_A/\dot{Q}$ and $\dot{V}_D$. The overall V_D/V_T ratio at rest in normal subjects may be as high as 0.4. Exercise improves $\dot{V}_A/\dot{Q}$, so that an increase in cardiac output results in an improvement of perfusion to the previously under or nonperfused areas of the lung, which is disproportionate to the increase in ventilation, and thus $\dot{V}_D$ decreases. This phenomenon requires the increased blood flow from increased cardiac output to be able to recruit the previously nonperfused pulmonary capillaries. Patients with compromise of the pulmonary vasculature (e.g., pulmonary vasculitis or chronic recurrent pulmonary emboli) do not decrease V_D/V_T and may in fact increase it during progressive exercise. These findings are distinctly abnormal and should lead the clinician to investigate possible pulmonary vascular involvement in patients with high ventilatory equivalents who are inordinately dyspneic during exercise.

Respiratory Exchange Ratio

The progression of the respiratory exchange ratio (R), defined as $\dot{V}CO_2/\dot{V}O_2$, throughout exercise from 0.8 to greater than 1.0 provides important information on the patient's ability to perform exercise, increase metabolic rate, and undergo gas exchange as measured with exhaled gases. Indirectly, the patient's effort can thereby be determined. A normal progression of R from 0.8 to 1.1 or greater usually indicates a reasonable effort to exhaustion. When R exceeds 1.0, this point corresponds roughly with the onset of the ventilatory or anaerobic threshold and the development of metabolic acidosis. A number of patterns of the progression of R may be encountered in different patient populations. For instance, patients with ventilatory limitation often will not reach an R of 1.0 or greater. On the other hand, some patients with hyperventilation even at lower levels of exercise may have R above 1.0, never go higher than that, and still not incur a metabolic acidosis. They may stop their exercise because of dyspnea or ventilatory limitation.

Gas Exchange

O_2 saturation can easily be measured with oximeters although some finger probes may give erroneous results during exercise because they become dislodged or because of a decrease in perfusion to the fingers due to gripping of the handlebars. Arterial O_2 saturation (SaO_2) does not decrease with exercise at sea level in normal subjects. If a patient has a decrease in SaO_2 during exercise, this is an important finding, which suggests abnormal gas exchange and/or inadequate $\dot{V}_A$ (Fig. 49-6A and B). For instance, patients with obstructive disease may develop relative hypercapnia at the end of exercise, which may result in worsening hypoxemia secondary to hypoventilation. Additionally, such patients may accentuate areas of low ventilation and perfusion, which results in a decrease in SaO_2. Many patients with interstitial disease or pulmonary vascular disease may also exhibit a

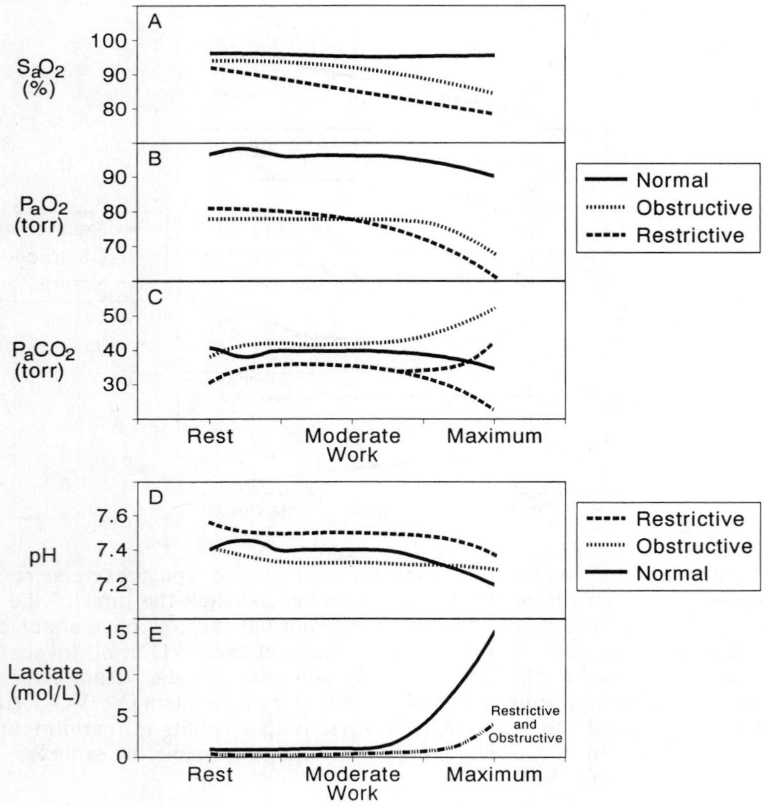

Figure 49-6. (A–E) Arterial blood gases and serum lactic acid concentrations during progressive work. There is variation between individuals in all states, but these patterns are typical of most patients.

decrease in SaO_2 throughout exercise, which is a reflection of worsening $\dot{V}/\dot{Q}$ match.

The measurement of arterial blood gases throughout exercise with or without measurement of lactate concentrations provides important insight into gas exchange and extent of exercise. The development of a metabolic acidosis with a decrease in pH and base excess and an increase in serum lactate concentration are important markers to determine the degree of effort above the anaerobic/ventilatory threshold (Fig. 49-6C–E). The measurement of $PaCO_2$ is also important because its increase in the latter stages of exercise is one of the important determinants of inadequate $\dot{V}_A$ and respiratory limitation to exercise. A $PaCO_2$ value is also necessary to calculate V_D/V_T from the Bohr dead space equation. The measurement of PaO_2 also can both corroborate the measurement of SaO_2 and allow one to evaluate the $P(A\text{-}a)O_2$, of which an increase above normal is a reflection of abnormal gas exchange.[8]

CARDIAC RESPONSE

Heart Rate

As in the measurement of ventilatory reserve, the difference between predicted maximum heart rate and achieved maximum heart rate will give information regarding the cardiac reserve (Fig. 49-7A). Unless the patient has some form of heart block or is receiving some medication (digitalis or beta-blockers) that will decrease the chronotropic response, the presence of a cardiac reserve (i.e., a heart rate greater than 20 percent below the predicted maximum rate), is indicative of a noncardiac limitation to exercise.[1] On the other hand, a patient who reaches a predicted maximum heart rate at a level of work or O_2 consumption that is below that patient's predicted maximum can be said to have a cardiac limitation to exercise, whether it be atherosclerotic cardiovascular disease, cardiomyopathy, or cardiac valvular disease.

Oxygen Pulse

The O_2 pulse ($\dot{V}O_2$/heart rate) (Fig. 49-7B) is an indirect measurement of stroke volume. Most individuals reach an O_2 pulse in the mid-teens, although this depends on age and body size. Most patients with cardiac limitation will, as mentioned, reach a predicted maximum heart rate at a work load lower than predicted maximum and in addition will have a lower than predicted maximum O_2 pulse. This is a reflection of an impaired stroke volume and the heart's attempt to maintain cardiac output by increasing heart rate.

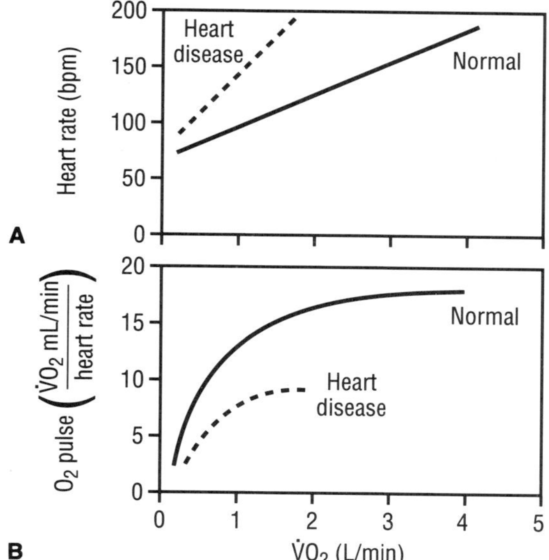

Figure 49-7. **(A & B)** Cardiac response to progressive work in normal subjects and in patients with cardiac impairment. As a patient is limited to a low $\dot{V}O_2$max by a low stroke volume (O_2 pulse), compensation is attempted by invoking a chronotropic response.

Cardiac Ischemia or Dysrhythmia

It is also important to observe the ECG for ischemic changes and to monitor the patient for symptoms such as chest pain. Most pulmonary exercise systems have two- or three-lead ECGs, which are adequate to determine heart rate and rhythm and in some cases ischemia. Excellent 12-lead ECG monitors are also available (which can provide accurate reading of ischemic changes). Regardless of which system is used, the clinician should keep a careful eye on the ECG to observe for abnormal rate or rhythm or ischemic changes throughout the exercise test.

Blood Pressure Response

A widening of the pulse pressure, with an increase in systolic and a decrease in diastolic pressure, is normal during exercise. Pathologic findings throughout exercise may involve an abnormal blood pressure response. Some patients with essential or other forms of hypertension may have an accelerated blood pressure response in the early stages of exercise such that the clinician should prudently observe the patient or stop the test. Systolic blood pressure above 200 mmHg in the early stages of exercise is abnormal, although such levels may be reached at high levels of work even in normal individuals. Patients whose systolic blood pressure decreases during exercise have cardiac disease or autonomic insufficiency, and their exercise test should be stopped. It is particularly important that patients who show an initial increase and then a decrease in blood pressure should terminate exercise, since they may have severe aortic stenosis, other valvular disease, or cardiomyopathy.

Peripheral Vascular Disease

The patient with peripheral vascular disease may be exercise-limited secondary to the symptoms of claudication in the lower extremities. A hallmark of this condition is severe calf or sometimes thigh pain, which resolves shortly after termination of exercise. This finding will provide important insight into the cardiovascular status of the patient and therefore provide some diagnostic direction.

Miscellaneous

A number of other conditions may be reflected characteristically by certain types of responses during exercise. For instance, patients with obesity or musculoskeletal disease may not be able to exercise to a metabolic rate that will provide much insight into their exercise limitations. However, in such cases an adequate history and physical examination may obviate the need for an exercise test. Neuromuscular diseases and psychosomatic disorders may also produce characteristic responses, which are important for the clinician to recognize.

DISABILITY EVALUATION

Impairment versus Disability

Pulmonary function and cardiopulmonary exercise testing have come to play a critical role in the evaluation of a patient's vocational capabilities. The legal and medical professions have attempted to derive standards that will allow accurate determination of a patient's physiologic and vocational ability or disability. The approach to these evaluations should be fair and in the patient's best interest; however, in the evaluation of conditions potentially related to occupational exposures the arena has become adversarial, and the patient often gets lost in the battle. It is therefore essential for the clinician to play the role of an objective expert in determining the patient's state of health or disease.

It is thus very important for the physician to distinguish between impairment and disability. Most experts agree that the term *impairment* is a medical one, which refers to the determination of dysfunction of one or more biologic systems of the body. For example, severe arthritis can impose a musculoskeletal impairment on a patient's ability to work and exercise, while emphysema or coronary artery disease can impair a patient's function from a pulmonary or cardiac standpoint, respectively. Careful musculoskeletal or physiologic testing will allow the clinician to make equitable determinations of impairment in those situations.

On the other hand, *disability* can be defined as limitation in performing specific vocational tasks imposed on a person by one or more physical or physiologic impairments. In light of these distinctions, by using the objective evaluation of physical and physiologic status and the home and work environment in which the patient functions, the clinician can formulate an evaluation of a patient's "whole body" disability. The American Medical Association (AMA) has published a book, *Guides to the Evaluation to Permanent Impairment,*[9] which outlines, system by system, levels of impairment such that clinicians and legal agencies can formulate specific classes to determine disability. For the respiratory system a simple table has been designed (Table 49-1), which gives four classes of impairment from none to severe, based on the patient's resting spirometry and diffusing capacity (DLCO) or maximum O_2 consumption. Other evaluations, based on maximum O_2 consumption, have been designed to assign individuals to specific categories of work tasks, ranging from sedentary to highly physical ones.

Elements of the Disability Evaluation

Although these determinations are credible and helpful guidelines for the clinician, they are just that—guidelines. The art of disability evaluation really lies in a thorough clinical and physiologic evaluation done by an experienced clinician. A careful *history* still remains the vital element, since it is only from this that the interviewer can determine the patient's past and present life-style, occupational experience from youth, exposure to potential environmental toxins, family and social environment, and hopes and dreams for future avocations and vocations.

The general *physical examination* is also important for determining the presence of obvious cardiopulmonary as well as musculoskeletal diseases. The *laboratory examination* should be a general screening one (i.e., it should include a complete blood count, blood chemistries, urinalysis, carboxyhemoglobin level, ECG, and chest x-ray). The ECG provides information regarding past myocardial events, but the resting ECG is not particularly helpful for predicting cardiac ischemia. The chest x-ray is crucial for determining if there is obvious cardiac disease such as congestive heart failure; however, the presence of long-standing, obstructive or interstitial pulmonary disease is also important. The ILO classification for interstitial disease is used to determine the presence of fibrotic lung disease, and the presence of pleural thickening helps the clinician to determine the presence or absence of asbestos exposure as an etiology of the interstitial changes. On the other hand, it is important to understand that there is little correlation between the severity of abnormalities on the chest x-ray and either resting or exercise pulmonary function.

Resting pulmonary function tests are helpful particularly if they are abnormal, but subtle, mild abnormalities may manifest themselves as more overt impairment during exercise. Spirometry is essential to determine obstructive disease but can only suggest the presence of restrictive disease. Although the measurement of lung volumes by either dilution or plethysmographic techniques is not part of the official AMA guidelines for the determination of impairment, the presence of restrictive disease cannot be accurately determined without lung volume measurements. The presence of even mild restrictive disease can be significant. Although the DLCO measurement is nonspecific and is quite variable even in the same patient, a consistently low DLCO denotes a decrease in surface area for gas exchange, whether from the vascular, blood, or airspace compartment.

It is also important to know and understand the normal standards that each laboratory is using. In the same patient, therefore, the absolute values and their trends are key, but

Table 49-1. Classes of Respiratory Impairment[a]

	Class 1	Class 2	Class 3	Class 4
	0%, No Impairment of the Whole Person	10–25%, Mild Impairment of the Whole Person	30–45%, Moderate Impairment of the Whole Person	50–100%, Severe Impairment of the Whole Person
FVC	≥80% AND	60–79% OR	51–59% OR	≤50% OR
FEV_1	≥80% AND	60–79% OR	41–59% OR	≤40% OR
FEV_1/FVC	≥70% AND	60–69% OR	41–59% OR	≤40% OR
DLCO *or* $\dot{V}O_2$max	≥80% *or* >25 mL/kg/min	60–79% *or* 20–25 mL/kg/min	41–59% *or* 15–20 mL/kg/min	≤40% *or* <15 mL/kg/min

[a] Percentages equal percent of predicted.
(From Engelberg,[9] with permission.)

in order to place the patient in the context of a normal population, standards must be used.

ROLE OF EXERCISE TESTING IN DISABILITY EVALUATION

Not all patients require cardiopulmonary exercise testing to determine degrees of impairment or disability. Many times the data discussed above are quite adequate for those purposes. Additionally, some patients cannot exercise because of either cardiopulmonary or musculoskeletal disease. The clinician therefore must be selective. In the light of these considerations, however, the cardiopulmonary exercise test can provide critical data that otherwise would not have been apparent in the routine evaluation.

First, a great deal can be discerned from the patient's attitude and performance on an exercise test. The patient's enthusiasm or lack thereof, the patient's intent, and the patient's overall emotional health profile can in most cases be determined merely by the clinician's subjective evaluation. Most patients do not want to be sick or impaired, and therefore their exercise data can in most cases be interpreted as a valid reflection of their attitude and physical ability. There are some patients, on the other hand, who clearly want to be judged as having a disability imposed on them for purpose of compensation and therefore can be considered to be malingering. An astute clinician can almost always determine this by both subjective and objective criteria based on the exercise test.

Second, subtle abnormalities determined by resting pulmonary function tests or from historical information can become much more overt during exercise. For instance, mild restrictive disease as determined at rest and during exercise may be signaled by an inordinate tachypnea, which may be reflected in a high ventilatory equivalent; this, as mentioned above, may be secondary to increased $\dot{V}_D$ and/or increased respiratory drive. A certain level of impairment and subsequent disability can be assigned to a patient who reaches a normal predicted $\dot{V}O_2max$ if the patient has paid a high price to achieve this level by an extraordinary ventilatory response. Many patients will make a good effort to reach a maximum level but may not have reached that level of $\dot{V}O_2$ in a normal way. It is therefore extremely important for the clinician to understand the normal physiology, as previously discussed.

Third, unsuspected disease states, particularly cardiac impairment, may become apparent during an exercise test. Fourth, often both obstructive and restrictive disease can be present, and it is difficult if not impossible in many cases to determine which of those two entities is contributing to exercise limitation if a respiratory limitation has been reached.

References

1. Wasserman K, Hansen JE, Sue DY, Whipp BJ (eds): Protocols for exercise testing. pp. 36–37, 58–71. In Principles of Exercise Testing and Interpretation, Lea & Febiger, Philadelphia, 1987
2. Astrand P, Rodahl K: Textbook of Work Physiology: Physiological Basis of Exercise. 3rd Ed. McGraw-Hill, New York, 1986, pp. 414, 440
3. Deal EC Jr, McFadden ER Jr, Ingram RH et al: Roll-over respiratory heat exchange in production of exercise-induced asthma. J Appl Physiol 1979;46:467–475
4. Cropp GJA: The exercise broncho provocation test: Standardization of procedures and evaluation of response. J Allergy Clin Immunol 1979;64:627–633
5. McKenzie DC: The asthmatic athlete: A brief review. Clin J Sport Med 1991;1:110–114
6. Martin BJ, Sparks KE, Zwillich CW, Weil JV: Low exercise ventilation in endurance athletes. Med Sci Sports Exerc 1979;11: 181–185
7. Schoene RB, Robertson HT, Pierson DJ, Peterson AP: Respiratory drives in exercise in menstrual cycles of athletic and nonathletic women. J Appl Physiol 1981;50:1300–1305
8. West JB: Ventilation/Perfusion in Gas Exchange. Blackwell Scientific Publications, Oxford, 1965, p. 8
9. Engelberg AL: Guides to the Evaluation of Permanent Impairment. 3rd Ed. American Medical Association, Chicago, 1988, pp. 107–144

Chapter 50

Assessment and Monitoring of Cardiovascular Function

Herbert P. Wiedemann

CHAPTER OUTLINE

> It seems likely to me that the charts of pulse rates will be supplemented before long by charts of blood pressure taken at regular intervals as a matter of routine.

Although the above 1903 prediction by Richard Cabot[1] was soon realized, it is unlikely that he or any other practitioner of the early 1900s could have conceptualized the methods of cardiovascular monitoring that are now applied routinely in the intensive care unit (ICU).

This chapter reviews the major procedures and techniques used for monitoring the circulation of patients in the ICU and operating room. The focus is on two frequently used invasive monitoring techniques: (1) peripheral artery cannulation, and (2) pulmonary artery catheterization. However, emerging noninvasive techniques for the monitoring of blood pressure and cardiac function are discussed as well. The goal of this chapter is to provide the reader with practical advice regarding the skillful and timely application of monitoring devices, avoidance of complications, and accurate physiologic interpretation of the resulting data.

For the reader interested in a more comprehensive treatment of the material covered in this chapter, additional sources of information are available.[2–6]

PERIPHERAL ARTERY CATHETERIZATION

Indications

Peripheral artery catheterization is commonly and routinely performed in the ICU and operating room. Cannulation of a peripheral artery allows for (1) continuous monitoring and graphic display of systemic arterial blood pressure, and (2) repeated analysis of arterial blood gases. Peripheral artery catheterization is therefore warranted in most patients with actual or potential hemodynamic or respiratory instability.

In view of evolving noninvasive monitoring techniques, however, the need for arterial cannulation should be carefully considered. For example, noninvasive monitoring of gas exchange (e.g., pulse oximetry, transcutaneous measurements of PO_2 and PCO_2, capnography), as discussed in Chapter 11, may obviate the need for peripheral artery cannulation in some hemodynamically stable patients (e.g., during weaning from mechanical ventilation). When necessary, such noninvasive respiratory monitoring can be supplemented by occasional "single stick" direct samples of arterial blood, without resorting to the placement of an arterial line for that purpose. By contrast, the presence of hemodynamic instability represents a strong indication for the placement of a peripheral artery catheter, since currently available technologies for the noninvasive assessment of blood pressure (discussed subsequently below) are not sufficiently reliable in this setting.

Arterial Pressure Monitoring: Methodology and Normal Waveforms

The arterial pressure waveform varies as the pressure wave moves from the proximal aorta toward the periphery[5–7] (Fig. 50-1). As the arterial pressure wave moves distally from the aorta, the systolic pressure gradually increases and the diastolic pressure gradually decreases, whereas the mean pressure remains relatively constant. In adults the systolic pressure can increase by as much as 20 mmHg from the central aorta to the major branches, such as the femoral artery. For clinical purposes the differences observed among the brachial, radial, and femoral arteries are usually not significant. However, the systolic pressure in the dorsalis pedis artery of the foot may be up to 25 mmHg higher than the systolic pressure in the radial artery, especially in children.[8]

The contour of the arterial pressure waveform varies at different anatomic sites according to the particular combination of "incident" waves (those that travel from the aorta toward the periphery) and "reflected" waves (those that bounce back from the peripheral vasculature).[7] The incident waves are a function of left ventricular stroke volume and compliance of the arterial tree, whereas the reflected waves are a function of peripheral vascular resistance.

The waveform display that appears on the electric monitor is produced by a complex system that represents fluid motion in the vascular system by an electrical signal.[5,9] The key component of this system is the transducer, an electromechanical device that changes energy generated by pulsatile flow into an electric current (Fig. 50-2). The transducer consists of a fluid-filled chamber applied against a stiff, low-compliance pressure-sensing diaphragm. The resulting mechanical movement is converted into an electrical signal by a component called a wheatstone bridge. Periodically, transducers should be calibrated directly with a mercury manometer.

In order to provide meaningful pressure measurements, the transducer needs to be leveled.[5] Arterial pressure is usually referred to the left ventricle. Thus, at the level of the left ventricle with the stopcock open (to atmospheric pressure), the transducer output should read zero. Subsequent readings should all be obtained with the transducer at the level of the left ventricle; a transducer set too low will record pressures that are falsely high, whereas a transducer set too high will indicate pressures that are falsely low. Precise leveling is especially important when recording pressures from

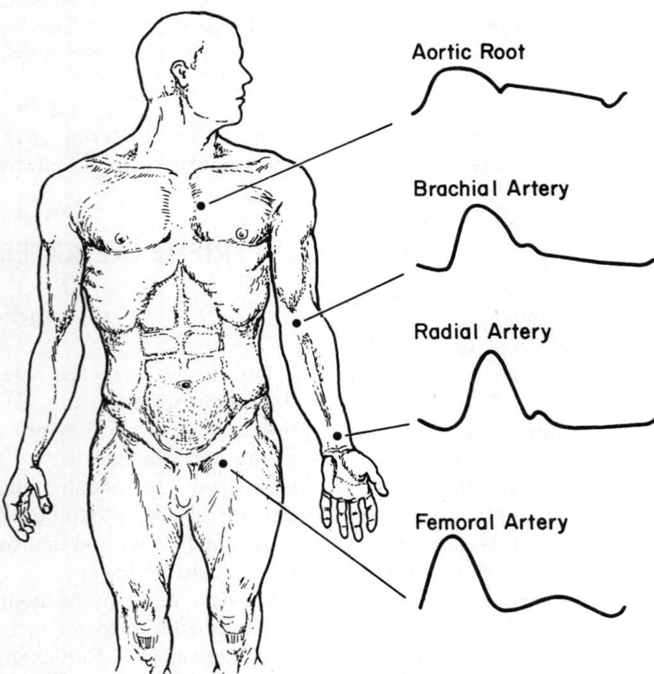

Figure 50-1. The normal arterial waveform recorded from different parts of the arterial tree. (From Marino,[6] with permission.)

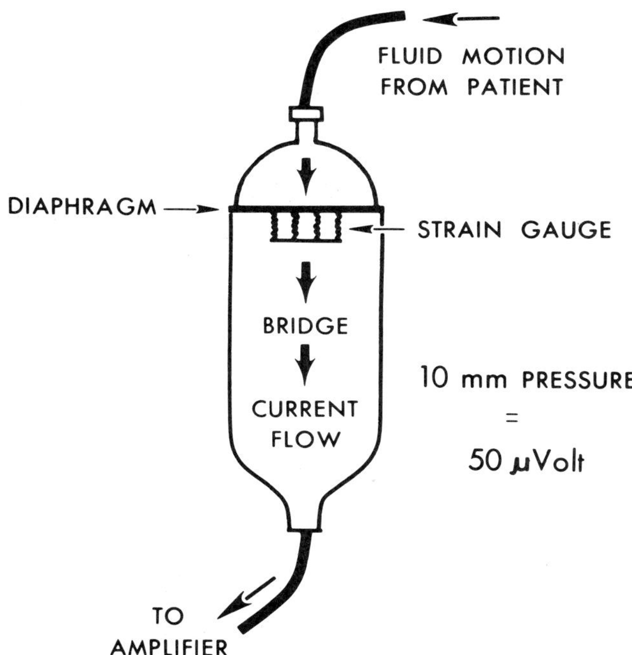

Figure 50-2. Diagrammatic representation of a pressure transducer. The energy generated by the pulsatile flow against the transducer diaphragm is transformed into an electric current. (From Civetta,[9] with permission.)

the pulmonary artery (see under Pulmonary Artery Catheterization), which is a low-pressure system.

It is also important to recognize that inappropriate damping of the transmission system may cause waveform distortion.[5,6,9] Applying a brief flush test to the catheter-tubing system can be useful in determining if the recording system is distorting the pressure waveform.[6] Most transducer systems are now equipped with a one-way valve, which can be used to deliver a flush from a pressurized source. The results of a flush test in three different situations are illustrated in Figure 50-3. The response at the end of the flush assesses the resonant frequency of the recording system; signal distortion is minimal when the natural resonant frequency of the recording system is 25 Hz, or five times greater than the frequency of the incoming waveform (the major frequency in the arterial pulse is approximately 5 Hz).[10] The resonant frequency of the recording system is calculated by first measuring the distance between two of the few oscillating waveforms that occur at the end of a flush. When using standard strip-chart recording paper divided into 1-mm segments, the resonant frequency (f) of the recording system can be determined by dividing this distance into the paper speed (25 mm/s). Figure 50-3A, therefore, represents a system that is not distorting the incoming waveform. However, the flush test in Figure 50-3B reveals the presence of an underdamped system. The distortion caused by such a system produces systolic amplification of the incoming signal. For example,

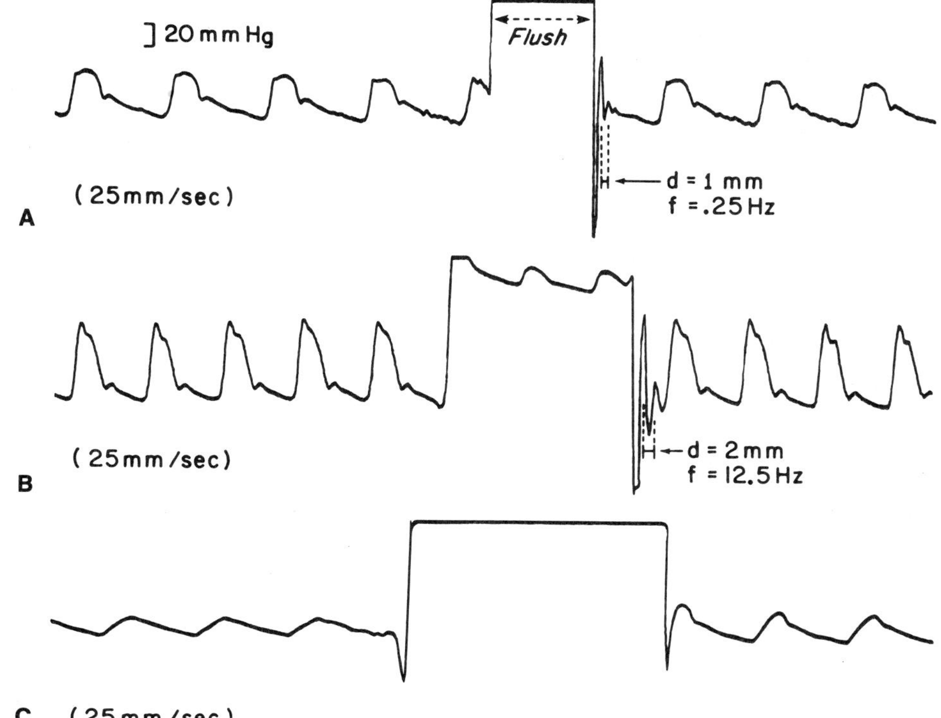

Figure 50-3. The flush test to determine distortion of the arterial pressure waveform. (**A**) Normal test; (**B**) underdamped system; (**C**) overdamped system. See text for further discussion. (From Marino,[6] with permission.)

a recording system with a resonant frequency of 8 Hz can cause a 27 percent increase in the systolic pressure recorded from the brachial artery.[11] The flush test in Figure 50-3C demonstrates no resulting oscillations, indicating that the system is overdamped and will underestimate the actual arterial pressure.

Air bubbles in the system constitute the greatest source of errors in measuring vascular pressure.[5] Large bubbles tend to cause overdamping of the system, whereas small bubbles may promote ringing or hyperresonance (the latter causes a falsely elevated systolic pressure). Frequent attention to the potential problem of damping is essential. When an inappropriately damped system is discovered, the apparatus (including all stopcocks) should be flushed thoroughly to release any trapped air bubbles. If the problem persists, the arterial catheter may need to be repositioned or changed.

Insertion Sites and Technique

The best sites for catheter insertion are the radial and femoral arteries.[2,5,6] The radial artery is usually the first choice because of its accessibility and generally good collateral circulation via the ulnar artery. Prior to insertion, the status of this collateral circulation should be assessed by an Allen's test, in which both the ulnar and radial arteries are occluded by pressure at the wrist; after the hand becomes pale and cool, releasing only the ulnar occlusion should restore adequate circulation (normal color of the fingers) within about 5 to 7 seconds. Cannulation of the brachial artery is often avoided since it represents the sole blood supply to the forearm and hand. (The larger size of the femoral artery obviates a similar concern regarding the potential impact of femoral artery catheterization on leg circulation.) The dorsalis pedis artery is relatively undesirable because of distortion in the pulse waveform at this site, as discussed earlier.

Catheterization of a peripheral artery is usually achieved via percutaneous insertion of an 18- or 20-gauge catheter. The transfixation method of catheter insertion (posterior wall deliberately punctured first) and the direct threading technique are equally acceptable[12] (Fig. 50-4).

Complications

With proper technique (Table 50-1), peripheral artery cannulation is generally safe.[2,13] The major potential complications include infection[14–16] and ischemia.[17–22] Ischemia may result from either thrombosis (local occlusion) or distal embolization. The incidence of catheter-related septicemia can be reduced to less than 1 percent with adherence to proper technique and precautions.[16] Of note, the infection rate is no higher with femoral artery catheters than with radial artery catheters.[23]

Subclinical and reversible arterial occlusion is common, with up to one-fourth of arteries remaining angiographically occluded 1 week after catheter removal.[18–21] The occlusion is permanent in about 3 percent of cases.[24] Risk factors for development of arterial occlusion include larger catheter size (18 gauge is worse than 20 gauge), smaller wrist size (women

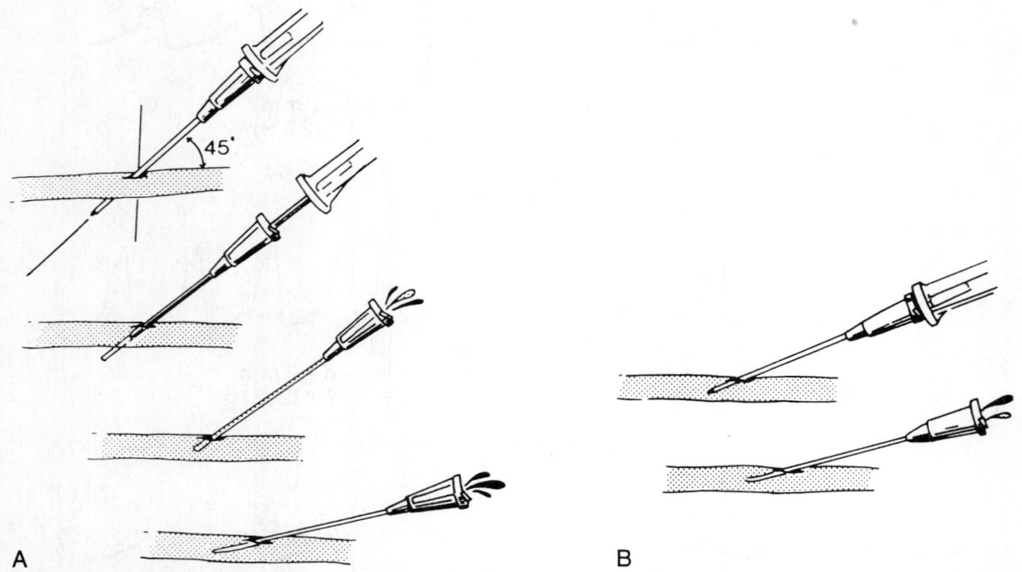

Figure 50-4. Two methods of arterial cannulation. (**A**) In the transfixation technique, the posterior wall of the artery is penetrated before the inner needle is withdrawn, and the outer plastic cannula is then withdrawn slowly until blood flows freely from the end. The cannula can then be advanced farther up the arterial lumen. (**B**) Direct insertion is also possible, but the tip must be positioned so that the cannula is entirely within the arterial lumen before advancing it over the needle. There is no difference in the incidence of local thrombosis or distal ischemia. (From Marini,[69] with permission.)

Table 50-1. Recommended Technique for Inserting and Maintaining Systemic Arterial Lines

Do an Allen test prior to radial artery cannulation. Ischemic complications will be lowest if ulnar artery refill time is less than 5 seconds.
Use sterile technique for insertion (antiseptic preparation, gloves, drapes).
Percutaneous insertion is preferred over surgical cutdown.
Use 20-gauge catheter if wrist circumference is small.
Use continuous flush system with a nondextrose solution (normal saline) containing heparin.
Transducer should have disposable dome.
Assess daily Catheter site for evidence of inflammation Distal extremity for evidence of ischemia
Limit cannulation to 4 to 5 days at one site.
Remove catheter for Distal ischemia Local infection Persistently damped pressure tracing Difficulty with blood withdrawal

(Modified from Matthay,[68] with permission.)

and children), repeated attempts before successful cannulation (ideally a site should be abandoned after two unsuccessful attempts), and duration of cannulation (risk increases after 3 to 4 days).[19–22,25] Ulnar refill time, determined by the Allen's test prior to insertion, may also be a factor. Preferably, palmar blush due to filling via the ulnar artery should appear within 5 to 7 seconds; if instead 15 seconds is used as an acceptable upper limit, distal ischemia may be more frequent (about 10 percent incidence).[20] However, one large prospective study found no instances of ischemic damage to the hands when the Allen's test demonstrated poor collateral flow.[26] Despite the relatively high incidence of angiographically demonstrable occlusion following catheterization, clinically significant thrombosis or embolism is rare.[17–20] In over 12,000 consecutive placements (including radial, brachial, and dorsalis pedis arteries) necrosis of fingers or toes occurred in only 15 (less than 0.2 percent).[17] Similarly, Gardner et al.[18] found that 3 of 531 patients (0.6 percent) required emergency thrombectomies for distal ischemia. Clinical risk factors for acute distal ischemia include systemic hypotension, severe peripheral vascular disease, and the use of vasopressor drugs.[17,18]

PULMONARY ARTERY CATHETERIZATION

Routine bedside catheterization of the pulmonary artery became feasible in 1970 with the introduction of the balloon-tipped catheter by Swan and colleagues.[27] Since the inflatable balloon at the tip allows the catheter be directed by blood flow, fluoroscopy is usually not necessary for proper placement. Many modifications of the original pulmonary artery catheter, often referred to as the Swan-Ganz catheter, are now available. An important modification of the original design is the placement of a thermistor near the distal tip, which allows for measurement of cardiac output by the thermodilution technique. Figure 50-5 depicts the most frequently used pulmonary artery catheter.

The properly positioned catheter allows for the direct acquisition of three important physiologic variables (Table 50-2):(1) cardiac output; (2) intravascular pressures (right heart chambers, pulmonary artery, and pulmonary artery occlusion or wedge pressure); and (3) mixed venous oxygenation. Representative normal values are provided in Table 50-3. In

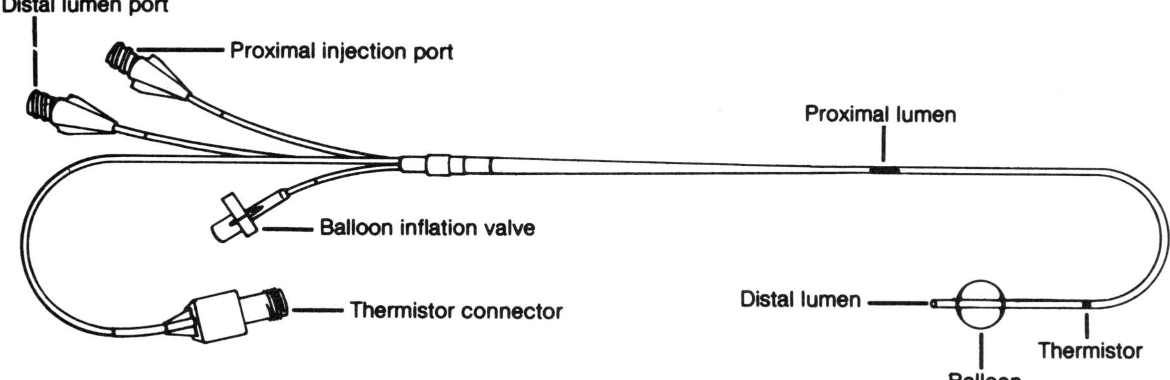

Figure 50-5. Typical triple-lumen pulmonary artery catheter. When the catheter is properly positioned and the balloon is deflated, the distal lumen records pulmonary artery pressure. When the balloon is inflated enough to occlude the segmental pulmonary artery, the distal lumen measures wedge pressure. The proximal lumen is 30 cm from the catheter tip and lies in the right atrium. A thermistor located just proximal to the balloon is used for cardiac output studies; the thermistor senses a temperature change shortly after a cold bolus of fluid exits from the proximal lumen. (From Matthay,[70] with permission.)

Table 50-2. Directly Measured Physiologic Variables Obtained with Pulmonary Artery Catheterization

Cardiac output
Intravascular pressures
Right atrial pressure
Right ventricular pressure
Pulmonary artery pressure
Pulmonary artery wedge pressure
Mixed venous oxygenation

addition, a large number of important calculated physiologic parameters can be derived from these primary measurements (Table 50-4).

Indications

Use of the pulmonary artery catheter should be reserved for those patients in whom the diagnosis or a reasonable initial therapeutic strategy remains uncertain following a careful clinical and noninvasive assessment or for patients who are so unstable that the proposed treatment requires invasive monitoring. Clinical settings in which pulmonary artery catheters are frequently used include complicated myocardial infarction or congestive heart failure; the adult respiratory distress syndrome (ARDS), especially if positive end-expiratory pressure (PEEP) of 15 cmH_2O or higher is required); septic shock; pulmonary embolism with hypotension; and major cardiac or vascular surgery (Table 50-5).

Table 50-3. Normal Values for Variables Commonly Assessed with a Pulmonary Artery Catheter

Variable	Normal Range
Cardiac output	Varies with patient size (see cardiac index, Table 50-4)
Right atrial pressure	0–8 mmHg
Right ventricle	
Systolic	15–30 mmHg
Diastolic	0–8 mmHg
Pulmonary artery	
Systolic	15–30 mmHg
Mean	9–16 mmHg
Diastolic	4–12 mmHg
Pulmonary artery occlusion pressure (PAOP) or pulmonary artery wedge pressure (PAWP)	2–12 mmHg
Mixed venous PO_2 ($P\bar{v}O_2$)	36–42 mmHg
Mixed venous oxygen saturation ($S\bar{v}O_2$)	75%

Table 50-4. Physiologic Data Derived from Invasive Monitoring

	Normal Range
Cardiac index ($L/min/m^2$) $CI = \frac{CO}{BSA}$	2.4–4.4
Systemic vascular resistance (dynes × s × cm^{-5}) $SVR = \frac{MAP - CVP}{(CO)}(79.9)$	900–1400
Pulmonary vascular resistance (dynes × s × cm^{-5}) $PVR = \frac{MPAP - PAWP}{CO}(79.9)$	150–250
Stroke volume (mL) $SV = \frac{CO}{HR}$	
Stroke volume index (mL/m^2) $SVI = \frac{SV}{BSA} = \frac{CI}{HR}$	30–65
Left ventricular stroke work index (g × m/m^2) LVSWI = (SVI)(MAP − PAOP)(0.0136)	43–61
Right ventricular stroke work index (g × m/m^2) RVSWI = (SVI)(MPAP − CVP)(0.0136)	7–12
O_2 content (mL/dL blood) $CaO_2 = Hb(SaO_2)(1.36) + [(PO_2)(0.003)]$	~19.5
Arteriovenous O_2 content difference (mL/dL) $avDO_2 = CaO_2 - C\bar{v}O_2$	3–5
O_2 Delivery (mL/min) O_2 delivery = $(CO)(CaO_2)(10)$	800–1200
O_2 consumption (mL/min) $VO_2 = (CO)(CaO_2 - C\bar{v}O_2)(10)$	180–280
Pulmonary shunt (venoarterial admixture) (%) $\frac{Qs}{Q_T} = \frac{CcO_2 - CaO_2}{CcO_2 - CvO_2}$	<3–5%

BSA, body surface area; CaO_2, arterial O_2 content; CcO_2, pulmonary capillary O_2 content (assumed equal to P_AO_2; CI, cardiac index; CO, cardiac output; $C\bar{v}O_2$, mixed venous O_2 content; CVP, central venous pressure; Hb, hemoglobin concentration; HR, heart rate; LVSWI, left ventricular stroke work index; MAP, mean arterial pressure; MPAP, mean pulmonary artery pressure; PAWP, pulmonary artery wedge pressure; PVR, pulmonary vascular resistance; Qs/Q_T, pulmonary shunt; RVSWI, right ventricular stroke work index; SaO_2, arterial O_2 saturation; SV, stroke volume; SVI, stroke volume index; SVR, systemic vascular resistance.

(Modified from Sprung,[4] with permission.)

Insertion and Normal Waveforms

Central venous access can be achieved via percutaneous insertion of the catheter through the subclavian, internal jugular, external jugular, femoral, or antecubital vein.[2,4,5,13] In ICUs and operating rooms, the internal jugular route is usually selected as offering the best compromise between ease of insertion and avoidance of major complications.

Table 50-5. Some Indications for Pulmonary Artery Catheterization

To distinguish between noncardiogenic and cardiogenic pulmonary edema
Adult respiratory distress syndrome: Manage PEEP and volume therapy
Myocardial infarction complicated by
Hypotension unresponsive to volume challenge
Hemodynamic instability requiring vasoactive drugs or mechanical assist devices
Suspected cardiac tamponade (equalization of end diastolic pressures)
Suspected mitral regurgitation (giant v waves)
Suspected ruptured interventricular septum (step-up in right heart O_2 saturation)
Unresponsive congestive heart failure
Resolving doubts about volume and cardiovascular status in complex illnesses (e.g., sepsis, pulmonary embolism)
Diagnosis and monitoring of pulmonary hypertension
Major cardiac surgery

(Modified from Goldenheim and Kazemi,[3] with permission.)

The catheter is advanced with continuous monitoring of both the electrocardiogram (ECG) (for arrhythmia detection) and the pressure recorded from the distal orifice. A sudden increase in the respiratory fluctuation of recorded pressures signals that the catheter tip has reached a central intrathoracic vein. The balloon is then inflated with air to the full recommended volume (1.5 mL for the 7 French catheter; 0.8 mL for the 5 French catheter) for subsequent flow-directed passage through the right atrium and right ventricle and into the pulmonary artery. Representative normal pressure tracings seen during passage of the catheter are shown in Figure 50-6. The catheter is advanced until a pulmonary artery "wedge" tracing is obtained. This occurs when the balloon occludes the pulmonary artery segment; the pressure tracing from the distal orifice of the catheter then reflects left atrial pressure (Fig. 50-7).

During flotation of the catheter, it is important to have the balloon fully inflated in order to prevent protrusion of the catheter tip. A protruding tip may cause endovascular damage and increase the risk of ectopy during passage through the right ventricle.[28] In addition, a fully inflated balloon will ensure a proximal wedge position, which is important for accurate thermodilution cardiac output determinations and mixed venous blood gas measurements. A catheter tip that is too distal and located in a small pulmonary artery may result in falsely high measurements of cardiac output and mixed venous PO_2 ($P\bar{v}O_2$).[4] Finally, distal positioning of the catheter tip increases the chance of pulmonary infarction.

Because measurement of the pulmonary artery wedge pressure (PAWP) is a major application of the pulmonary artery catheter and provides the basis for important diagnostic and therapeutic decisions, it is essential that a valid PAWP be obtained. Adherence to the following criteria will help ensure a valid PAWP[2,13,29]: (1) A tracing characteristic of a left atrial waveform should be seen; a highly "damped" tracing devoid of oscillations except those due to ventilation-induced pressure changes is not acceptable. The PAWP waveform should disappear promptly with balloon deflation, yielding a pulmonary artery tracing, and return rapidly after balloon reinflation. (2) The mean PAWP should be lower than or equal to the pulmonary artery diastolic pressure (the PAWP may transiently exceed pulmonary artery diastolic pressure in severe mitral regurgitation). (3) Catheter obstruction should be ruled out by the ability of a saline flush solution to flow through the distal lumen. (4) Blood gas analysis of blood withdrawn from the distal port should reflect systemic PaO_2 and $PaCO_2$ rather than the PO_2 and PCO_2 of mixed venous blood. Although this last criterion is usually not routinely tested, it may be of help in confusing situations. The validity of this criterion is supported by recent information that highly oxygenated blood is usually withdrawn from a true wedge position even in areas of radiographic infiltrates or in patients with large intrapulmonic shunts.[30]

Inability to obtain a valid PAWP tracing could be due to a catheter tip that is not located in zone 3 of the lung (Fig. 50-8). If the catheter tip is located in zone 2, the pulmonary artery tracing may appear normal until the balloon is inflated. Since alveolar pressure exceeds pulmonary capillary pressure in zone 2, the vessel distal to the inflated balloon will then collapse, causing PAWP to reflect alveolar pressure rather than left atrial pressure. Because most pulmonary blood flows through zone 3, the flow-directed catheter usually migrates into this region during initial insertion.[31] However, the size of the lung zones may change in response to subsequent physiologic alterations. For example, diuresis or ventilation with high levels of PEEP will reduce the size of zone 3 via a decrease in pulmonary venous pressure or an increase in alveolar pressure, respectively. Thus, a catheter tip originally correctly positioned in zone 3 may subsequently be in zone 2. In order to obtain a valid wedge position, it may be necessary to refloat the catheter under these new physiologic conditions.

When a proper wedge tracing cannot be obtained, pulmonary artery diastolic pressure is sometimes used to estimate PAWP. In individuals with a normal heart rate and normal pulmonary vascular resistance, the relationship between these values is close. However, with significant tachycardia (heart rates above 120 per minute) or pulmonary hypertension, pulmonary artery diastolic pressure will often exceed PAWP by large amounts.[32] Thus, in many circumstances (e.g., ARDS, pulmonary embolism) accurate estimation of PAWP from the pulmonary artery diastolic pressure is not possible.

The normal waveforms depicted in Figure 50-6 may be altered significantly by pathophysiologic conditions. For example, right ventricular infarction may reduce the pressure generated by this chamber to such a degree that right atrial, right ventricular, and pulmonary artery waveforms and pressures are nearly identical (Fig. 50-9). Severe mitral value insufficiency leads to a wedge tracing with a large left atrial v wave, which may mimic the pulmonary artery waveform. These and other situations may cause significant confusion unless the clinician anticipates the possibility of aberrant waveforms through an awareness of the clinical setting.

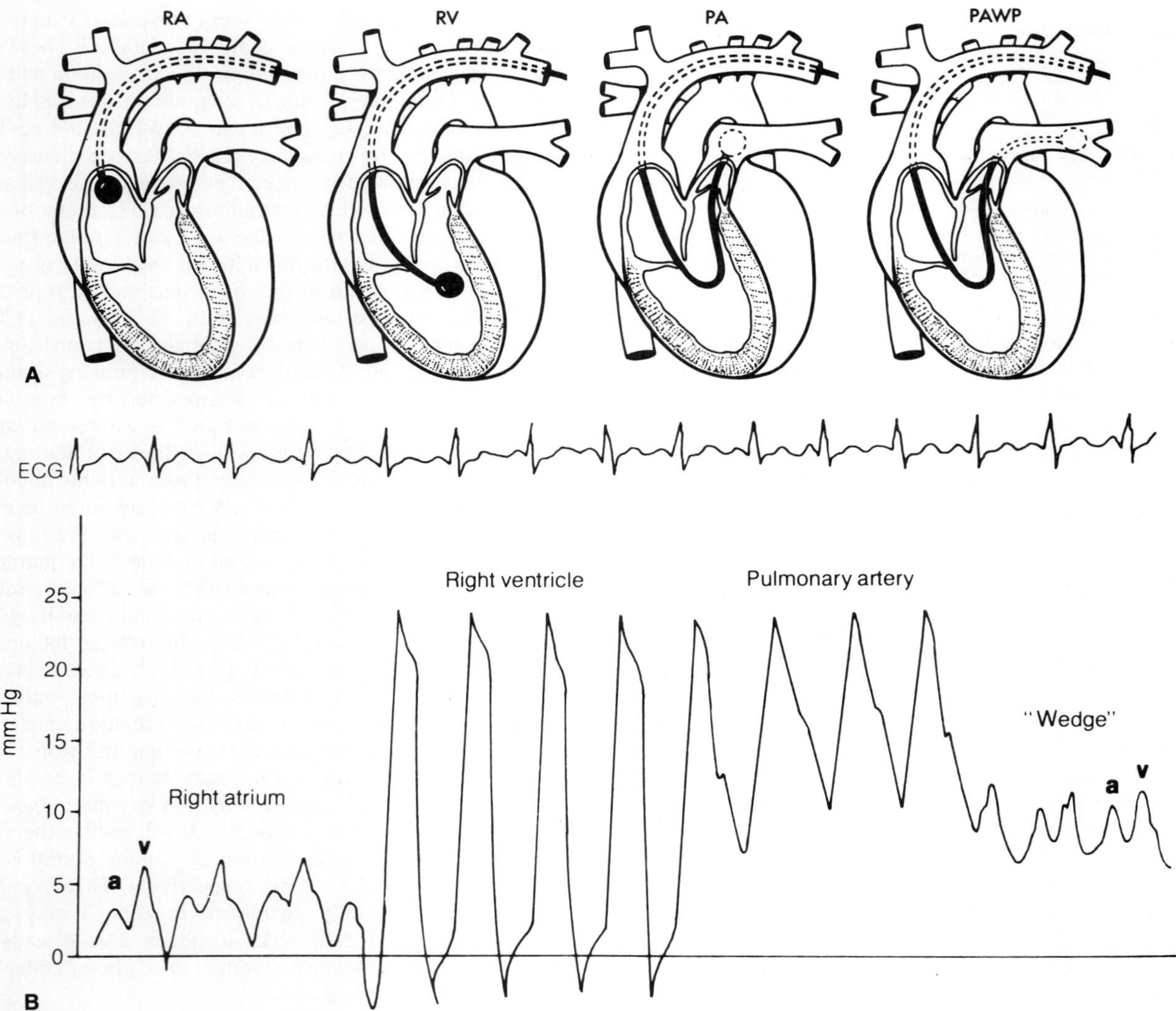

Figure 50-6. (A & B) Representative recording of normal pressures and waveforms as a Swan-Ganz catheter is passed through the right side of the heart into the pulmonary artery. The first waveform is a right atrial tracing with characteristic a and v waves. The right ventricular, pulmonary artery, and pulmonary artery wedge tracings follow in sequence. Note that the wedge tracing shows a and v waves transmitted from the left atrium. In addition, the wedge pressure (mean) is less than pulmonary artery diastolic pressure. The wedge tracing is not always this distinct, but a very damped tracing or a mean wedge pressure greater than pulmonary artery diastolic pressure usually indicates some mechanical problem in the system (e.g., air bubble in the connecting tubing, catheter tip "overwedged," balloon inflated over distal orifice, or catheter tip in zone 1 or zone 2). (Fig. A from Martin[71]; Fig. B from Matthay,[68] with permission.)

Since intravascular pressure measurements such as PAWP are calibrated relative to atmosphere, these readings will reflect transmural vascular pressures (pressure difference across the wall of the vessel or heart chamber) only if the pleural and atmospheric pressures are equal. (The importance of correctly assessing transmural pressure and the interpretation of PAWP during PEEP therapy are addressed more fully in the subsequent discussion of the relationship between PAWP and left ventricular preload.) Since pleural pressure most closely approximates atmospheric pressure at end expiration, vascular pressure readings should be obtained at this time. In patients with rapid, labored breathing, this may present a problem because of the large deflection in vascular pressures and the short expiratory time. In such instances a printout of the actual pressure tracing on a strip chart recorder may be required; end expiration can be identified visually, and the vascular pressure during the brief end-expiratory phase can be directly measured. By contrast, reliance on most currently available electronic digital displays can provide misleading information, since the displayed pressure represents an average value obtained during a scanning period that exceeds the end-expiratory pause.[32]

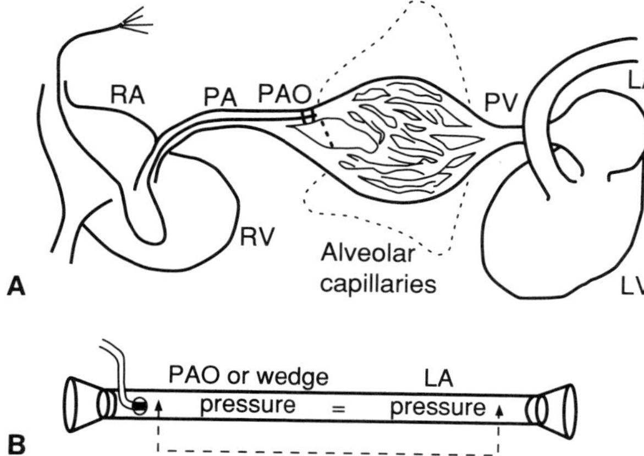

Figure 50-7. (**A**) Simplified representation of the pulmonary artery catheter in the wedge or pulmonary artery occlusion (PAO) position. With the balloon inflated, no flow exists. (**B**) By analogy to a "closed pipe" system, equal pressure readings are found for the wedge pressure, pulmonary venous (PV) pressure, and left atrial (LA) pressure. This simple model ignores the continuous flow of blood from nonoccluded pulmonary arteries to the PV and LA. These "flowing" columns are open to the "static" column at the level of the PV system. Thus, mechanical obstruction to flow through the PV system (e.g., tumor) near the left atrium will cause the wedge pressure to overestimate the LA pressure. (From Sprung et al.,[29] with permission.)

Thermodilution Cardiac Output

With a thermistor-tipped pulmonary artery catheter and a bedside microprocessor, measurement of cardiac output is an easy, rapid, and safe procedure that can be performed many times in a single day if necessary. Thermodilution measurements correlate well with the Fick or dye dilution techniques, which are much more difficult to perform.[33] To measure cardiac output by the thermodilution technique, 10 mL of room temperature or iced saline solution is injected as rapidly as possible into the proximal catheter port. The fluid bolus exits the catheter in the right atrium and travels into the pulmonary artery, where the thermistor detects the resulting change in temperature over time. The bedside microprocessor quickly calculates and displays the cardiac output. The use of a 0°C injectate solution (ice water temperature) carries a theoretical advantage over a room temperature (22°C) solution, since the contrast with core body temperature is greater with the former (better signal/background ratio). However, room temperature injectate is entirely acceptable except in significantly hypothermic patients; if core body temperature is 6 to 11°C (10 to 20°F) below normal, ice temperature solution is mandatory.[34,35]

Phasic changes in intrathoracic pressure and venous return induced by spontaneous or mechanical ventilation may cause significant variability in single measurements. To minimize this problem as well as other causes of variability, it is standard practice to average three consecutive measure-

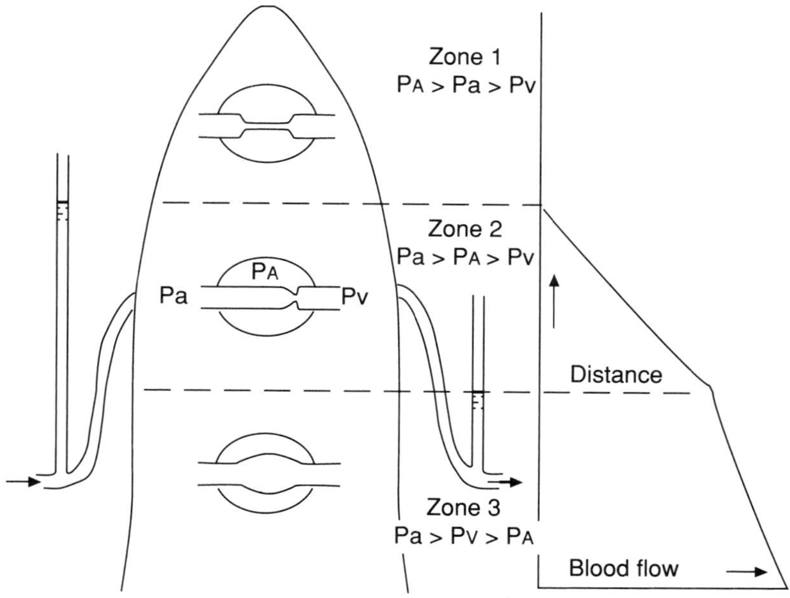

Figure 50-8. Zones of the lung, based on the relationship among pulmonary artery (Pa) pressure, alveolar pressure (PA), and pulmonary venous pressure (Pv). The zones are not constant. For instance, a decrease in Pv (e.g., diuresis) or an increase in PA (e.g., PEEP therapy) will convert some zone 3 area into zone 2 or zone 1. The pulmonary wedge pressure reflects Pv (and thus left atrial pressure) only if the tip of the Swan-Ganz catheter lies in zone 3 before balloon inflation. If the balloon is inflated in zone 2, the occluded vessel will collapse, since PA will be greater than Pv. Without a continuous column of the blood between the catheter tip and the left atrium, the wedge pressure cannot reflect left atrial pressure. (From West et al.,[72] with permission.)

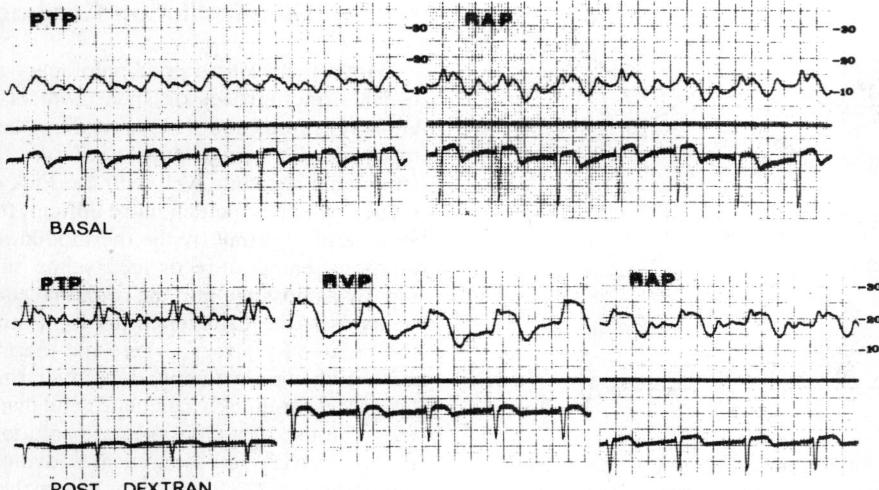

Figure 50-9. Pressure tracings from the pulmonary trunk (PTP), right ventricle (RVP), and right atrium (RAP) in a patient with acute right ventricular infarction are shown. The tracings were obtained before and after volume expansion. Owing to a decrease in generation of right ventricle pressure, the tracings may be quite similar. This may lead to confusion during bedside right heart catheterization. (From Coma-Canella et al.,[73] with permission.)

ments, all obtained at end expiration, to constitute a single determination. Cardiac output determinations performed in this manner have an accuracy and reproducibility that are usually very acceptable for clinical use. However, the thermodilution technique may not be accurate in the presence of significant tricuspid valve regurgitation (which causes an underestimation of cardiac output),[36] intracardiac shunts, or a too distally placed catheter.

Mixed Venous Oxygen Saturation

Mixed venous blood is sampled through the distal orifice of the pulmonary artery catheter with the balloon deflated (the 7 French catheter has a 2.5-mL dead space, which must first be eliminated by discarding the initial sample). In patients receiving mechanical ventilation and a very high inspired O_2 concentration, a rapid rate of blood withdrawal may lead to a falsely elevated mixed venous O_2 saturation ($S\bar{v}O_2$) due to contamination of the sample with pulmonary capillary blood.[37,38] A slow rate of blood withdrawal (less than 3 mL/min) will eliminate this possibility. Severe mitral valve regurgitation may also cause a falsely elevated $S\bar{v}O_2$ due to retrograde pulmonary capillary blood flow.

Clinically, mixed venous oxygenation is used to monitor changes in cardiac output and to assess tissue oxygenation. In normal individuals and many patients, as O_2 delivery (cardiac output × arterial O_2 content) decreases, increased extraction of O_2 from circulating blood allows tissue O_2 consumption to remain stable (i.e., O_2 consumption is independent of O_2 delivery) but causes the $S\bar{v}O_2$ to decrease. Thus, a decrease in cardiac output will be reflected by a corresponding decline in $S\bar{v}O_2$. Furthermore, as $P\bar{v}O_2$ approaches 27 to 30 mmHg (normal, 39 mmHg) blood lactate levels usually increase, indicating that tissue oxygenation is reaching a critically low level. These interpretations of mixed venous oxygenation are most valid in patients with "simple" hemodynamic problems, such as isolated myocardial dysfunction.

In more complex illnesses, including sepsis and ARDS, interpretation of mixed venous oxygenation is much more complex. In sepsis, peripheral "shunting" of arterial blood past tissue beds may lead to maintenance of a high mixed venous oxygen level despite tissue O_2 deprivation indicated by high blood lactate levels. Furthermore, in some ARDS patients O_2 consumption varies with O_2 delivery, even at normal or high cardiac outputs, which suggests an abnormal "supply dependence" of O_2 consumption.[39–41] This phenomenon may be related in part to abnormalities in the systemic capillary circulation, which prevent normal tissue O_2 extraction. The result is that mixed venous oxygenation may remain high and relatively stable despite large, and presumably clinically important, decreases in cardiac output, O_2 delivery, and O_2 consumption. In view of this, monitoring solely the mixed venous oxygenation in patients with sepsis or ARDS is inadequate. The clinician also needs to monitor several other parameters, including cardiac output, arterial O_2 saturation (SaO_2), and lactate levels in order to be informed about changes in hemodynamic status of these patients.[42]

Pulmonary artery catheters that provide a continuous measurement of the $S\bar{v}O_2$ through use of fiberoptic reflectance oximetry are currently available. Although the continuous monitoring of mixed venous oxygenation may provide a helpful "early warning system" for detecting adverse hemodynamic trends, its value in this regard is limited by the factors outlined in the preceding discussion. Reliance on stable or normal mixed venous oxygenation may provide a

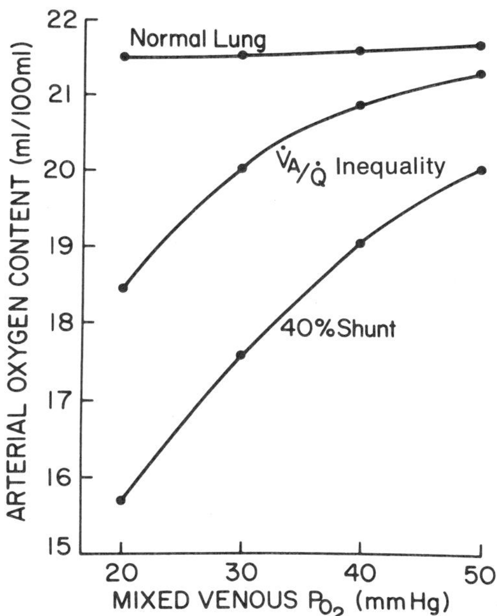

Figure 50-10. The effect of changing the $P\bar{v}O_2$ on the CaO_2 in a patient with normal lungs, one with marked ventilation-perfusion inequality, and one with a large shunt. Each theoretical patient was assumed to be breathing 50 percent O_2, and cardiac output and minute ventilation were held constant. (From Dantzker,[74] with permission.)

false sense of security in patients with illnesses such as ARDS or sepsis.

Left-to-right intracardiac shunts will cause elevated mixed venous oxygenation. This fact may be helpful in diagnosing atrial or ventricular septal defects; during passage of the catheter, blood samples will show an abnormal "step-up" in O_2 saturation as the tip is passed into the right atrium or right ventricle.

Mixed venous oxygenation influences SaO_2 when there is a high degree of shunt through the lungs (e.g., in ARDS) (Fig. 50-10), but this is often overlooked. Although clinicians often reflexively attribute a decrease in SaO_2 to a worsening of lung function, such a decrease may in fact be due to nonrespiratory factors that cause a reduction in mixed venous oxygenation (e.g., anemia, increased O_2 consumption, low cardiac output). If such factors are corrected, SaO_2 may improve even if lung disease does not.

Pulmonary Artery Wedge Pressure

Measurement of PAWP is an important use of the pulmonary artery catheter. PAWP allows the clinician to make important assumptions regarding left ventricular preload and pulmonary capillary hydrostatic pressure. As already discussed, wedge pressure produced by balloon occlusion of a pulmonary artery correlates well with venous pressure at or near the left atrium. Because little pressure difference normally exists among the large pulmonary veins, left atrium, and left ventricle during end diastole, PAWP usually is a good approximation of intracavitary left ventricular end-diastolic pressure (LVEDP).

Relationship to Left Ventricular Preload

According to the Frank-Starling principle, left ventricular preload determines the force of cardiac contraction for any given level of myocardial contractility. Therefore, a measurement of left ventricular function (e.g., cardiac output), in conjunction with an assumption regarding the state of left ventricular preload, allows the clinician to draw important conclusions regarding left ventricular contractility. Since PAWP is frequently used to assess left ventricular preload, it is important to understand the relationship between the two, which are sometimes incorrectly assumed to be identical.

Preload refers to stretch of myocardial fibers and therefore is best thought of as being represented by left ventricular end-diastolic *volume* (LVEDV). The LVEDV is determined by the transmural ventricular distending *pressure* (intracavitary pressure, or PAWP, minus juxtacardiac pressure) and ventricular *compliance* (pressure-volume relationship). The relationship between PAWP and left ventricular preload is shown in Figure 50-11, which illustrates how a given PAWP may be associated with varying degrees of left ventricular filling in critically ill patients with altered juxtacardiac pressure (e.g., mechanical ventilation and PEEP) or ventricular compliance (e.g., myocardial ischemia, pericardial effusion).

Failure to understand the PAWP-LVEDV relationship may lead to misdiagnosis and institution of inappropriate therapy. For example, a hypotensive patient on high PEEP levels may have a relatively normal PAWP, which may erroneously be interpreted to indicate the presence of adequate left ventricular preload. Assuming therefore that intrinsic cardiac dysfunction exists, the clinician may use inotropic or vasopressor agents. However, in this example, left ventricular filling volume may in fact be low, since PAWP is greater than left ventricular transmural distending pressure when pleural pressure is elevated (Fig. 50-11A); perhaps a volume infusion trial would be the most appropriate initial therapy for this patient.

How can the clinician compensate for the effect of PEEP on PAWP measurements? Pleural pressure at end expiration cannot be assumed to be equal to PEEP, since lung and chest wall compliance will affect the relationship between these pressures. In patients with poor lung compliance (e.g., ARDS), the change in pleural pressure will usually be about one-fourth of the applied PEEP.[32] Temporarily disconnecting PEEP in order to measure PAWP is not recommended. The resulting new measurement will be of questionable value since hemodynamics will be altered (e.g., an acute increase in venous return).[43,44] In addition, abrupt removal of PEEP may cause dangerous hypoxemia, and this may not be fully and rapidly reversible with reinstitution of PEEP.[45,46] Although a reasonably accurate estimation of juxtacardiac pressure can be achieved with an esophageal balloon, this is impractical for routine ICU use. For most purposes it is

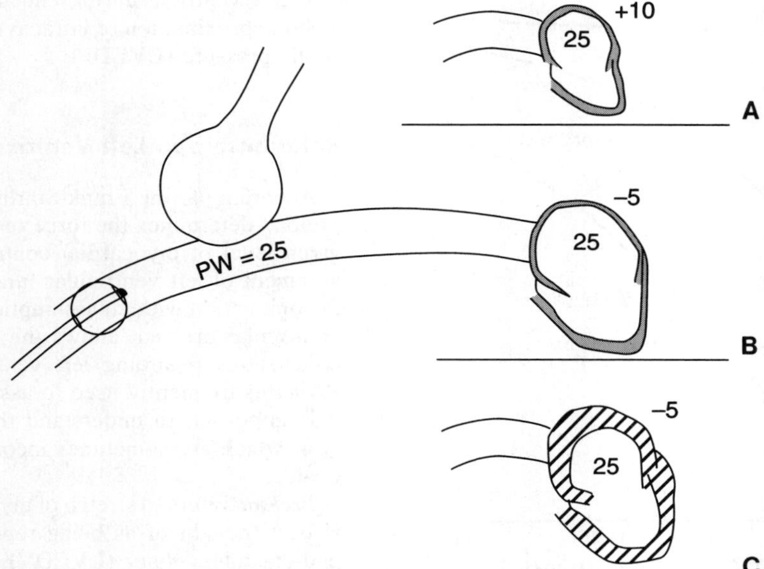

Figure 50-11. Relationship of pulmonary artery wedge pressure (PW) to left ventricular preload (left ventricular volume or "stretch") in three situations, illustrating the importance of considering pleural (juxtacardiac) pressure and ventricular compliance along with PW when making assumptions about left ventricular preload. The PW is elevated in each example and reflects the intracavitary left ventricular end-diastolic pressure. **(A)** The pleural pressure is increased, as might occur with PEEP therapy. Transmural left ventricular pressure is approximately normal, as is the preload. **(B)** The pleural pressure is normal. Transmural left ventricular pressure is elevated, and preload is increased. **(C)** The ventricle is stiff, as might occur with myocardial ischemia. Although PW and pleural pressure are identical to those in Figure B, the preload in this instance is normal. (From O'Quin and Marini,[32] with permission.)

sufficient to be cognizant of the qualitative influence of PEEP and to make the necessary mental adjustment in interpretation of PAWP, as outlined in the preceding paragraph. Most important, serial changes in PAWP that occur with therapeutic interventions should be correlated with other hemodynamic and clinical parameters (e.g., blood pressure, cardiac output, arterial blood gases, urine output) to determine empirically the optimum PAWP for a given patient.

Relationship to Pulmonary Capillary Hydrostatic Pressure

The other major clinical utility of PAWP is that it provides an assessment of pulmonary capillary pressure, which is the filtration pressure favoring the development of pulmonary edema (Fig. 50-12). This information often allows for the distinction between cardiogenic ("hydrostatic") and noncardiogenic ("leaky capillary") origins of lung edema fluid. Thus, the presence of pulmonary edema with a normal PAWP suggests capillary injury (e.g., ARDS), whereas pulmonary edema with a high PAWP supports a cardiogenic cause such as congestive heart failure (but does not rule out coexisting lung injury). In most clinical settings PAWP provides a reasonable assessment of pulmonary capillary pressure. However, these values are not equivalent, and the

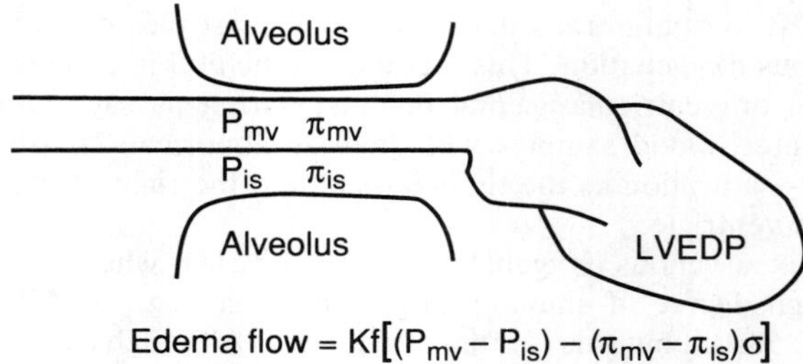

Figure 50-12. Relation of forces governing the fluid flux between the pulmonary capillary microvasculature (mv) and the pulmonary interstitium (is). P refers to hydrostatic pressure, and π refers to oncotic pressures. Kf is the permeability constant of the vessel wall and σ is the reflection coefficient. The latter indicates the relative effectiveness of the membrane in preventing the passage of proteins as compared with water. In "leaky capillary" edema, the σ value is low, and thus hydrostatic forces become much more important than oncotic forces in determining net fluid flux. The PAWP provides an indirect assessment (for important qualifications see text) of both Pmv and LVEDP. (From Prewitt et al.,[75] with permission.)

common practice of referring to PAWP as "pulmonary capillary wedge pressure" should be discouraged.[2,47]

Complications

The potential adverse effects of pulmonary artery catheterization are now well recognized from over two decades of experience[2,48] (Table 50-6). Ventricular arrhythmias often occur during insertion of the catheter but are usually transient and self-limited. In critically ill patients the incidence of ventricular tachycardia (three or more consecutive premature ventricular contractions) is about 20 to 50 percent, but sustained ventricular tachycardia requiring therapy occurs in only 1 to 2 percent of such patients. Risk factors for ventricular tachycardia include hypocalcemia, myocardial infarction or ischemia, hypotension, and hypokalemia. However, the two most significant risk factors are hypoxemia (PO_2 less than 60 mmHg) and acidosis (pH below 7.20).[49] In such high-risk patients the use of prophylactic lidocaine during catheter insertion should be considered.

During the initial years of Swan-Ganz catheter use, pulmonary infarction was one of the most common serious complications; its incidence was found to be greater than 7 percent in the mid-1970s.[2] However, more recent experience suggests that the incidence of pulmonary infarction is now at most 1 percent. The difference may be due to better understanding of techniques that minimize this complication. For instance, the risk of thrombus developing on the catheter tip is now reduced by continuous flushing with heparin solutions. Equally important is avoidance of persistent wedging of the catheter tip. Distal migration of the catheter can be prevented by maintaining it in a position such that nearly the full recommended balloon inflation volume is required to produce a wedge tracing. Furthermore, the balloon should never be inflated for longer than is necessary to obtain a wedge pressure reading (15 to 20 seconds).

The incidence of pulmonary artery rupture is about 0.2 percent. This is a serious complication, with approximately a 50 percent mortality. The major risk factor for pulmonary artery rupture is pulmonary artery hypertension. Proper technique can minimize the risk of this serious complication. The balloon should always be inflated slowly and with continuous pressure monitoring; inflation should cease as soon as a wedge tracing is obtained. Hand flushing of the catheter while it is in a wedge position should be avoided.

Table 50-6. Complications of Balloon Flotation Right Heart Catheterization

- Arrhythmias
  - Transient premature ventricular contractions (PVCs)
  - Sustained ventricular tachycardia
  - Ventricular fibrillation
  - Atrial fibrillation
  - Atrial flutter
- Right bundle branch block
- Pulmonary infarction
- Pulmonary artery rupture
- Catheter-related infections
- Balloon rupture
- Catheter knotting
- Endocardial damage
  - Valve cusps
  - Chordae tendineae
  - Papillary muscles
- Complications at insertion site
  - Pneumothorax
  - Arterial puncture
  - Venous thrombosis or phlebitis
  - Air embolism

NONINVASIVE CARDIOVASCULAR MONITORING

Despite its widespread application and apparent value in the management of critically ill patients, invasive cardiovascular monitoring has certain major drawbacks, the most important of which is the inherent physical risk to the patient. In addition, the application of invasive monitoring techniques tends to be time-consuming and labor-intensive. Coincident with a growing appreciation of some of the disadvantages of invasive monitoring, new technological developments are raising the prospects that practical and reliable methods of noninvasive cardiovascular monitoring may become available in the near future.[50] The following section reviews the emerging—and still evolving—methods by which blood pressure and cardiac output can be measured noninvasively.

Arterial Blood Pressure

In the ambulatory patient, blood pressure is commonly assessed by use of an inflatable arm cuff and auscultation of the Korotkoff sounds over the brachial artery.[51] However, the technique of manual sphygmomanometry is not practical in the ICU, where continuous or very frequent monitoring is necessary. An even more important limitation of this technique is the inaccuracy that occurs in patients with compromised hemodynamic status; the arm cuff method can underestimate the true systolic pressure by an average of 64 mmHg in patients with heart failure and 34 mmHg in hypotensive patients.[52] In view of its limitations, the manual ausculatory method of blood pressure measurement has largely been abandoned in the ICU, where blood pressure is usually directly measured via indwelling arterial catheters. However, emerging technologies may ultimately allow for accurate automated, noninvasive blood pressure measurements in ICU patients. Development of automated noninvasive monitors has generally proceeded along one of two lines, (1) the oscillometric method[53] and (2) the Penaz method.[54]

The majority of automated noninvasive monitors use some variant of the oscillometric method. The first commercially viable device became available in 1976 under the trade name Dinamap (an acronym for "device for indirect noninvasive mean arterial pressure"). The principles that govern this oscillometric method have been recently reviewed in detail.[53] In brief, the process depends on the detection of oscillations and quantification of their amplitudes during automated stepwise decrements (usually 5 mmHg intervals) of cuff pressure. Various algorithms have been used to convert these data into arterial pressures, and further refinements continue to be tested. Generally, the systolic blood pressure is the cuff pressure at which the amplitude of oscillation increases rapidly and the diastolic pressure is that at which such amplitude decreases rapidly. The mean arterial pressure is generally the lowest cuff pressure with the greatest oscillation amplitude.

The oscillometric technique has certain inherent problems and limitations. Significant hypotension and low pulse pressure may reduce the amount of oscillation to such a degree that only mean arterial pressure is measurable, and in extreme situations even mean pressures may be unattainable. Motion artifact represents another important problem, especially when such motion is rhythmic, as may occur during patient shivering (or seizures) or during transport in ambulances and helicopters. Under such circumstances, the algorithm-based measurements are confounded and machine performance deteriorates. Often, however, stabilization of the limb around which the cuff is placed will allow for accurate results.

The method of Penaz is used in the Finapress device, an automated monitor that provides continuous blood pressure and arterial waveform display with the use of a finger cuff.[55] The Penaz method utilizes the volume-clamp principle. Circumferential pressure applied by a finger cuff is varied in order to maintain constant arterial size (as assessed by a photoplethysmograph); under such circumstances, the cuff pressure equals arterial pressure. A rapidly responding servomechanism continuously adjusts finger cuff pressure to maintain zero transmural arterial pressure and thereby continuously derives arterial pressures (systolic, mean, diastolic) and heart rate.

Both the Dinamap and Finapress devices have been studied in various clinical settings, although head-to-head comparisons of the two devices are few. Experience with the Dinamap is far greater, since this device was introduced much earlier. Furthermore, the Finapress is currently in a more dynamic phase of its development, with comparatively more rapid improvements in the finger cuff and calculation algorithms occurring recently.

According to standards recommended by the Association for the Advancement of Medical Instrumentation, blood pressure devices should be accurate to within a mean error of less than 5 mmHg, with a standard deviation of less than 8 mmHg when compared with an arterial catheter.[53] Neither the Dinamap nor the Finapress device reliably meets these standards in critically ill patients.[56–63] For example, Venus et al.[56] evaluated the Dinamap in 43 critically ill patients requiring extensive hemodynamic monitoring in the ICU. The Dinamap underestimated systolic blood pressure by a mean of 8.7 ± 16.4 mmHg and overestimated diastolic blood pressure by a mean of 8.7 ± 10.6 mmHg. In patients undergoing general anesthesia, Epstein et al.[62] found that the Finapress was markedly inaccurate in 20 percent of the study population.

In short, present techniques for automated noninvasive measurement of blood pressure do not meet standards for ideal clinical performance when used in critically ill patients with hemodynamic instability. Further technological advances may allow for more reliable indirect automated blood pressure measurements.

Cardiac Output

Techniques for measuring cardiac output noninvasively are undergoing active development and investigation. Although not yet ready for routine clinical application, two methodologies appear to offer the greatest potential for such use in the relatively near future: (1) Doppler ultrasound, and (2) thoracic electrical bioimpedance.

A full description of these methodologies is beyond the scope of this chapter. In brief, the various Doppler ultrasound techniques rely on the principle that ultrasound waves directed at flowing blood are back-scattered by moving erythrocytes at a "shifted" frequency proportional to the velocity of the erythrocytes moving along the axis of the ultrasound beam. The bioimpedance methodologies employ the relationship between current, voltage, and impedance as defined by Ohm's law. Alternating current of high frequency and low amplitude is passed through the thorax between two or more surface electrodes. A measured change in impedance between two electrodes is related to cyclic changes in thoracic blood volume; an increase in blood volume results in a fall in impedance.

The interested reader is referred to recent investigations into the clinical applicability of these technologies for measuring cardiac output noninvasively.[50,64–67]

References

1. Cabot R: Physical Diagnosis of Diseases of the Chest. William Wood, New York, 1903
2. Wiedemann HP, Matthay MA, Matthay RA: Cardiovascular-pulmonary monitoring in the intensive care unit (Parts 1 & 2). Chest 1984;85:537–549, 656–668
3. Goldenheim PD, Kazemi H: Cardiopulmonary monitoring of critically ill patients. N Engl J Med 1984;331:717–720, 776–780
4. Sprung CL (ed): The Pulmonary Artery Catheter: Methodology and Clinical Applications. University Park Press, Baltimore, 1983
5. Sladen A (ed): Invasive Monitoring and Its Complications in the Intensive Care Unit. Mosby-Year Book, St. Louis, 1990
6. Marino PL (ed): The ICU Book. Lea & Febiger, Philadelphia, 1991
7. O'Rourke MF, Yaginuma T: Wave reflections and the arterial pulse. Arch Intern Med 1984;144:366–371

8. Park MK, Robotham JL, German VF: Systolic pressure amplification in pedal arteries in children. Crit Care Med 1983;11:286–289
9. Civetta JM: Pulmonary artery catheter insertion. pp. 21–71. In Sprung CL (ed): The Pulmonary Artery Catheter: Methodology and Clinical Applications. University Park Press, Baltimore, 1983
10. The 1984 report of the Joint National Committee on Detection, Evaluation, and Treatment of High Blood Pressure. Arch Intern Med 1984;144:1045–1057
11. Kroeker EJ, Wood EH: Comparison of simultaneously recorded central and peripheral arterial pressure pulse during rest, exercise, and tilted position in man. Circ Res 1955;3:623–628
12. Jones RM, Hill AB, Nohrwold ML, Bolles RE: The effect of method of radial artery cannulation on postcannulation blood flow and thrombus formation. Anesthesiology 1981;55:76–78
13. Wiedemann HP: Intensive care monitoring and mechanical ventilation. pp. 616–630. In Stein JH (ed): Textbook of Internal Medicine. Little Brown, Boston, 1990
14. Band JD, Maki DG: Infections caused by arterial catheters used for hemodynamic monitoring. Am J Med 1979;67:735–741
15. Weinstein RA, Stamm WE, Kramer L: Pressure monitoring devices: Overlooked sources of nosocomial infection. JAMA 1976;236:936–938
16. Shinozaki T, Deane R, Mazuzan JE et al: Bacterial contamination of arterial lines: A prospective study. JAMA 1983;249:223–225
17. Shapiro BA: Monitoring gas exchange in acute respiratory failure. Respir Care 1983;28:605–607
18. Gardner RM, Schwartz R, Wong HC, Burke JP: Percutaneous indwelling radial-artery catheters for monitoring cardiovascular function. N Engl J Med 1974;290:1227–1231
19. Davis FM, Stewart JM: Radial artery cannulation. Br J Anaesth 1980;52:41–47
20. Bedford RF: Radial artery function following percutaneous cannulation with 18 and 20-gauge catheters. Anesthesiology 1977;47:37–39
21. Bedford RF: Long-term radial artery cannulation: Effects on subsequent vessel function. Crit Care Med 1978;6:64–67
22. Bedford RF: Wrist circumference predicts the risk of radial arterial occlusion after cannulation. Anesthesiology 1978;48:377–378
23. Thomas F, Burke JP, Parker J et al: The risk of infection related to arterial vs. femoral sites for arterial cannulation. Crit Care Med 1983;11:807–812
24. Weiss BM, Gattiker RI: Complications during and following radial artery cannulation: A prospective study. Intensive Care Med 1986;12:424–428
25. Russell JA, Joel M, Hudson RJ et al: Prospective evaluation of radial and femoral artery catheterization sites in critically ill adults. Crit Care Med 1983;11:936–939
26. Slogoff S, Keats AS, Arlund C: On the safety of radial artery cannulation. Anesthesiology 1983;59:42–47
27. Swan HJC, Ganz W, Forrester JS et al: Catheterization of the heart in man with the use of a flow-directed balloon-tipped catheter. N Engl J Med 1970;283:447–451
28. Sprung CL: Complications of pulmonary artery catheterization. pp. 73–101. In Sprung CL (ed): The Pulmonary Artery Catheter: Methodology and clinical applications. University Park Press, Baltimore, 1983
29. Sprung CL, Rackow EC, Civetta JM: Direct measurements and derived calculations using the pulmonary artery catheter. pp. 105–140. In Sprung CL (ed): The Pulmonary Artery Catheter: Methodology and Clinical Applications. University Park Press, Baltimore, 1983
30. William WH, Olsen GN, Allen WG et al: Use of blood gas values to estimate the source of blood withdrawn from a wedge flow-directed catheter in critically ill patients. Crit Care Med 1982;10:636–640
31. Kronberg GM, Quan SF, Schlobohm RM et al: Anatomic locations of the tips of pulmonary-artery catheters in supine patients. Anesthesiology 1979;51:467–469
32. O'Quin R, Marini JJ: Pulmonary artery occlusion pressure: Clinical physiology, measurement, and interpretation. Am Rev Respir Dis 1983;128:319–326
33. Stetz CW, Miller RG, Kelly GE, Raffin TA: Reliability of the thermodilution method in the determination of cardiac output in clinical practice. Am Rev Respir Dis 1982;126:1001–1004
34. Shellock FG, Riedinger MS, Bateman TM, Gray RJ: Thermodilution cardiac output determination in hypothermic postcardiac surgery patients: Room vs. ice temperature injectate. Crit Care Med 1983;11:668–670
35. Elkayam U, Berkley R, Azen S et al: Cardiac output by thermodilution technique: Effect of injectate's volume and temperature on accuracy and reproducibility in the critically ill patient. Chest 1983;84:418–422
36. Gigarroa RG, Lange RA, Williams RH et al: Underestimation of cardiac output by thermodilution in patients with tricuspid regurgitation. Am J Med 1989;86:417–420
37. Douglas ME: So much, so little. Chest 1980;78:418–419
38. Suter PM, Lindauer JM, Fairly HB, Schlobohm HM: Errors in data derived from pulmonary artery blood gas values. Crit Care Med 1975;3:175–181
39. Danek SJ, Lynch JP, Weg JG, Dantzker DR: The dependency of oxygen uptake on oxygen delivery in the adult respiratory distress syndrome. Am Rev Respir Dis 1980;122:387–395
40. Mosenifar Z, Goldbach P, Tashkin DP, Campisi DJ: Relationship between O_2 delivery and O_2 consumption in the adult respiratory distress syndrome. Chest 1983;84:267–271
41. Schumacker PT, Samsel RW: Oxygen supply and consumption in the adult respiratory distress syndrome. Clin Chest Med 1990;11:715–722
42. Wiedemann HP: Monitoring priorities in the adult respiratory distress syndrome. J Intensive Care Med 1987;2:179–180
43. Zarins CK, Virgilio RW, Smith DE, Peters RM: The effect of vascular volume on positive end-expiratory pressure-induced cardiac output depression and wedge-left atrial pressure discrepancy. J Surg Res 1977;23:348–360
44. Downs JB, Douglas ME: Assessment of cardiac filling pressure occurring in continuous positive-pressure ventilation. Crit Care Med 1980;8:285–292
45. DeCampo T, Civetta JM: The effect of short-term discontinuation of high-level PEEP in patients with acute respiratory failure. Crit Care Med 1979;7:47–49
46. Luterman A, Horovitz JH, Carrico CJ et al: Withdrawal from positive end-expiratory pressure. Surgery 1978;83:328–332
47. Wiedemann HP: Wedge pressure in pulmonary veno-occlusive disease. N Engl J Med 1986;315:1233
48. Boyd KD, Thomas SJ, Gold J, Boyd AD: A prospective study of the complications of pulmonary artery catheterizations in 500 consecutive patients. Chest 1983;84:245–249
49. Sprung CL, Pozen RG, Rozanski JJ et al: Advanced ventricular arrhythmias during bedside pulmonary artery catheterization. Am J Med 1982;72:203–208
50. Shoemaker WC, Appel PL, Kram HB et al: Multicomponent noninvasive physiologic monitoring of circulatory function. Crit Care Med 1988;16:482–490
51. The 1988 report of the Joint National Committee on Detection, Evaluation, and Treatment of High Blood Pressure. Arch Intern Med 1988;148:1023–1038
52. Cohn JN: Blood pressure measurement in shock. Mechanism of inaccuracy in auscultatory and palpatory methods. JAMA 1967;199:118–122
53. Ramsey M: Blood pressure monitoring: Automated oscillometric devices. J Clin Monit 1991;7:56–67
54. Penaz J: Photoelectric measurement of blood pressure, volume and flow in the finger. Digest 10th Int Conf Med Biol Eng 1973; 104
55. Boehmer RD: Continuous, real-time, noninvasive monitoring of blood pressure: Penaz methodology applied to the finger. J Clin Monit 1987;3:282–287
56. Venus B, Mathru M, Smith RA, Pham CG: Direct versus indirect blood pressure measurements in critically ill patients. Heart Lung 1985;14:228–231

57. Gravlee GP, Brockschmidt JK: Accuracy of four indirect methods of blood pressure measurement, with hemodynamic correlations. J Clin Monit 1990;5:284–298
58. Epstein RH, Kaplan S, Leighton BL et al: Evaluation of a continuous noninvasive blood pressure monitor in obstetric patients undergoing spinal anesthesia. J Clin Monit 1989;5:157–163
59. Kurki TS, Smith NT, Sanford TJ, Head H: Pulse oximetry and finger blood pressure measurement during open heart surgery. J Clin Monit 1989;5:221–228
60. Kermode JL, Davis NJ, Thompson WR: Comparison of the Finapress blood pressure monitor with intra-arterial manometry during induction of anesthesia. Anesth Intensive Care 1989; 17:470–486
61. Gibbs NM, Larach DR, Derr JA: The accuracy of Finapress noninvasive mean arterial pressure measurements in anesthesized patients. Anesthesiology 1991;74:647–652
62. Epstein RH, Huffnagle S, Bartkowski RR: Comparative accuracies of a finger blood pressure monitor and an oscillometric blood pressure monitor. J Clin Monit 1991;7:161–167
63. Gorback MS, Quill TJ, Lavine ML: The relative accuracies of two automated noninvasive arterial pressure measurement devices. J Clin Monit 1991;7:13–22
64. Singer M, Clark J, Bennett ED: Continuous hemodynamic monitoring by esophageal Doppler. Crit Care Med 1989;17:447–452
65. Castor G, Molter G, Itelms J et al: Determination of cardiac output during positive and expiratory pressure: Noninvasive electrical bioimpedance compared with standard thermodilution. Crit Care Med 1990;18:544–546
66. Wong DH, Mahutte CK: Two-beam pulsed Doppler cardiac output measurement: Reproducibility and agreement with thermodilution. Crit Care Med 1990;18:433–437
67. Notterman DA, Castello FV, Steinberg C et al: A comparison of thermodilution and pulsed Doppler cardiac output in critically ill children. J Pediatr 1989;115:554–560
68. Matthay MA: Invasive hemodynamic monitoring in critically ill patients. Clin Chest Med 1983;4:233–249
69. Marini JJ: Respiratory Medicine and Intensive Care for the House Officer. Williams & Wilkins, Baltimore, 1981
70. Matthay MA: Intensive hemodynamic monitoring in acute respiratory failure. J Respir Dis 1981;2:40–53
71. Martin L: Pulmonary Physiology in Clinical Practice: The Essentials for Patient Care and Evaluation. CV Mosby, St. Louis, 1987
72. West JB, Dollery CT, Naimark A: Distribution of blood flow in isolated lung: Relation to cascular and alveolar pressures. J Appl Physiol 1964;19:713–724
73. Coma-Canella I, Lopez-Sendon J, Camallo C: Low output syndrome in right ventricular infarction. Am Heart J 1979;98:613–620
74. Dantzker DR: Gas exchange in the adult respiratory distress syndrome. Clin Chest Med 1982;3:57–67
75. Prewitt RM, Matthay MA, Ghignone M: Hemodynamic management in the adult respiratory distress syndrome. Clin Chest Med 1983;4:251–268

Chapter 51

Assessment of Metabolic and Nutritional Status

Dean R. Hess
Janine Mundroff

CHAPTER OUTLINE

An important relationship exists between respiratory function and nutritional status[1–9]—measurements of breathing can be used to assess nutritional status, and nutritional support affects breathing (Fig. 51-1). This chapter discusses the relationships between breathing, metabolism, and nutritional support.

DEFINITIONS

Carbohydrates are composed of sugars and these molecules can consist of a single sugar unit (monosaccharides), two sugar units (disaccharides), or many sugar units (polysaccharides). A common simple sugar is glucose (also called dextrose). Common disaccharides are sucrose (glucose plus fructose), lactose (glucose plus galactose), and maltose (glucose plus glucose). Polysaccharides are storage forms of glucose, and include glycogen, which is found in animals, and starch, which is found in plants.

Proteins are large molecules made up of amino acids. There are 20 amino acids that are commonly used to build protein molecules, 9 of which are essential amino acids that cannot be synthesized within the body and thus must be supplied in the diet.

Lipids (fats) are a heterogeneous group of water-insoluble biochemicals. Fatty acids are an integral part of many lipids and can be either saturated (all single bonds) or unsaturated (at least one double bond). Fatty acids combine with glycerol to produce triglycerides, which are the storage form of fatty acids in adipose tissue. Several fatty acids, namely, linoleic and linolenic acids, are essential lipids and must be provided in the diet.

The nucleic acids include DNA and RNA, which are important in the storage and transfer of genetic information, adenosine triphosphate (ATP), which serves for the storage of energy, and cyclic adenosine monophosphate (AMP), which provides intracellular control. Biochemical functions of carbohydrates, lipids, proteins, and nucleic acids are listed in Table 51-1.

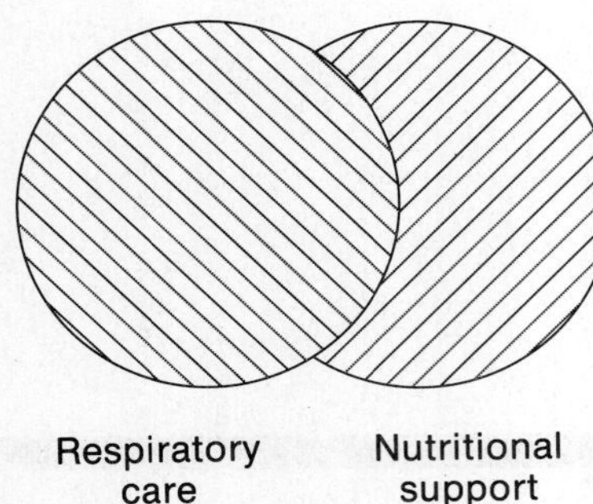

Figure 51-1. Overlap between respiratory care and nutritional support.

Vitamins are organic molecules, which are present in trace amounts within the cell. They are vital for life and are essential in the diet because they cannot be synthesized endogenously. Vitamins can be classified as water-soluble (thiamine, riboflavin, biotin, folic acid, ascorbic acid, vitamin B_{12}) or fat-soluble (vitamins A, D, E, K). Organic vitamins and inorganic minerals (magnesium, phosphorus, calcium, sodium, chloride, and potassium) serve as coenzymes of many intracellular reactions. Minerals are also essential in the diet.

CELLULAR RESPIRATION

The biochemical reactions that occur in the cell are referred to as *metabolism* or *metabolic pathways*. The most important product of these reactions is energy, which is stored in the ATP molecule. One type of metabolism, *catabolism*, is responsible for breaking down molecules into simpler units, while another type, *anabolism*, is responsible for building molecules from simpler materials. The metabolic pathways most important to respiratory care are the reactions of cellular respiration, which are the energy-producing reactions of the cell. These include glycolysis, the Krebs cycle (tricarboxylic acid), and the electron transport chain.

Table 51-1. Biologic Functions of Carbohydrates, Lipids, and Proteins

Carbohydrates	
	Energy
	Structure
Lipids	
	Energy
	Structure (membranes)
	Hormones (steroids)
	Surfactant
Proteins	
	Enzymes
	Structure
	Hormones
	Carrier molecules (hemoglobin)
	Antibodies
	Colloid osmotic pressure
	Buffer
	Muscle contraction
Nucleic acids	
	Genetic information
	Energy transfer
	Intracellular controls

Glycolysis is a series of nine reactions in which glucose (a six-carbon molecule) is broken into two molecules of pyruvic acid (a three-carbon molecule). As a result of these reactions, a small amount of ATP and a small amount of reduced nicotinamide adenine dinucleotide (NAD) are produced (Fig. 51-2). The small amount of energy produced by glycolysis is insufficient to support life. One of the intermediate reactions in glycolysis is also responsible for the production of 2,3-diphosphoglyceric acid (2,3-DPG), which is important in O_2 transport (see Ch. 11).

In the presence of O_2 (aerobic metabolism), the pyruvic acid produced from glycolysis is oxidized to produce acetyl coenzyme A (CoA) in a reaction also yielding CO_2 and reduced NAD. In the absence of O_2 (anaerobic metabolism), pyruvic acid is reduced to lactic acid, the production of which explains the metabolic acidosis that occurs under conditions of decreased O_2 delivery to cells. In fermentation, yeast cells are able to reduce pyruvic acid to ethyl alcohol and CO_2 (Fig. 51-3).

Acetyl CoA is oxidized in a cyclic series of six reactions known as the Krebs cycle (Fig. 51-4), which produces CO_2, a small amount of ATP, a small amount of reduced flavin adenine dinucleotide (FAD), and a large amount of reduced NAD. As with glycolysis, the amount of ATP produced by the Krebs cycle is not sufficient to support life.

The reduced NAD and reduced FAD produced by glycolysis, pyruvic acid oxidation, and the Krebs cycle enter a series of reactions known as electron transport (Fig. 51-5), which is responsible for the production of most of the ATP. At the end of the electron transport chain, O_2 serves as the final electron receptor and is reduced to water. Cyanide poisoning inhibits one of the enzymes required for electron transport, resulting in decreased ATP production, decreased O_2 consumption, and ultimately death.

Each of the reactions of cellular respiration is catalyzed by a specific enzyme. Glycolysis occurs within the cyto-

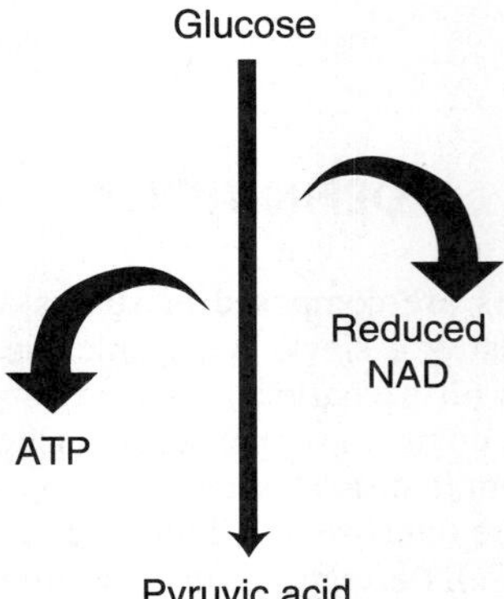

Figure 51-2. Schematic diagram of glycolysis.

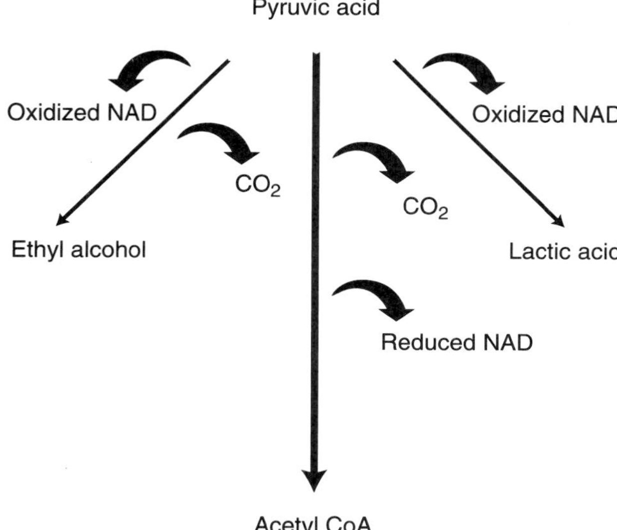

Figure 51-3. Schematic diagram of oxidation of pyruvic acid.

plasm of the cell, whereas the Krebs cycle and electron transport occur in the mitochondria. The net result of the oxidation of glucose is the production of 38 ATP molecules from the same number of adenosine diphosphate (ADP) molecules:

$$\text{Glucose} + 38\ \text{ADP} + 38\ \text{HPO}_4^{-2} + 6\ \text{O}_2 \rightarrow 6\ \text{CO}_2 + 38\ \text{ATP} + 44\ \text{H}_2\text{O} \quad (1)$$

The cardiopulmonary system must deliver the required O_2 to the cells and the produced CO_2 to the ambient atmosphere.

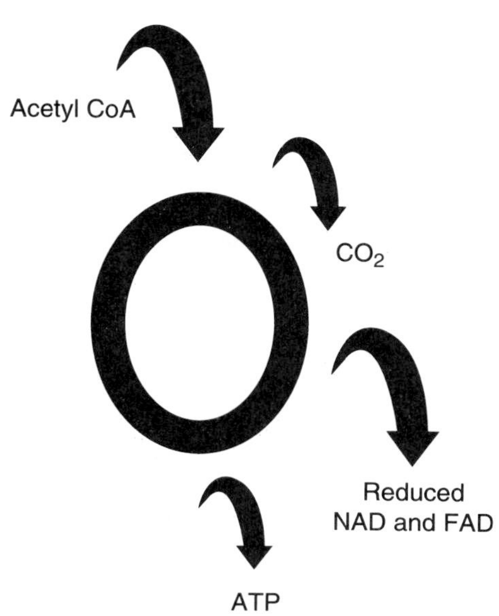

Figure 51-4. Schematic diagram of Krebs cycle.

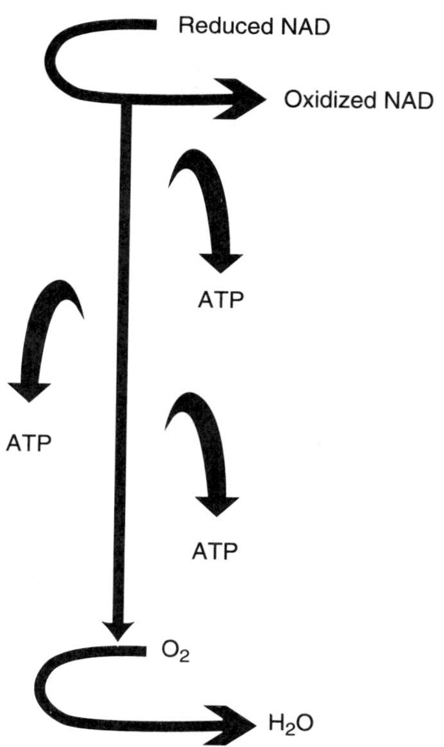

Figure 51-5. Schematic diagram of electron transport chain and oxidative phosphorylation.

Acetyl CoA can also be produced from the metabolism of fats and proteins as well as glucose. The process whereby fats are broken down to acetyl CoA is called *beta oxidation*, and the process whereby proteins are broken down to acetyl CoA is called *deamination*. Thus, acetyl CoA serves a central role in tissue metabolism.

The production of glycogen from glucose is called *glycogenesis*, and the breakdown of glycogen to glucose is called *glycogenolysis*. The storage and metabolism of glycogen occurs primarily in the liver and muscle. If glucose intake is excessive, the excess can be converted to lipid (fat) in a process known as *lipogenesis*. Glucose can also be produced from fat and protein, a process known as *gluconeogenesis*.

When insulin concentrations are low (as with diabetes or fasting), acetyl CoA can be converted in the liver to acetoacetate, which can then be converted to beta-hydroxybutyrate or acetone. These three chemicals are ketone bodies, and they can be used by cells as a source of acetyl CoA. This is particularly important in the brain, where as much as half of the glucose requirement can be replaced with ketone bodies. Ketone bodies are strong acids that produce a metabolic acidosis as they are transported in the circulation. Their presence explains the metabolic acidosis that occurs with uncontrolled diabetes.

OXYGEN CONSUMPTION, CARBON DIOXIDE PRODUCTION, AND ENERGY EXPENDITURE

There is a relationship between the energy produced from metabolism, the amount of O_2 consumed, and the amount of CO_2 produced. This relationship is dependent on the specific substrate that is metabolized.[1,10,11] Carbohydrate (CHO) is metabolized according to the reaction

$$1 \text{ g CHO} + 0.83 \text{ L } O_2 \rightarrow 0.83 \text{ L } CO_2 + 0.6 \text{ g } H_2O + 4.17 \text{ kcal} \quad (2)$$

The amount of CO_2 produced when carbohydrate is metabolized is equal to the amount of O_2 consumed. The CO_2 production rate ($\dot{V}CO_2$) divided by the O_2 consumption rate ($\dot{V}O_2$) is referred to as the respiratory quotient (RQ). For carbohydrate metabolism the RQ is 1.0. Very little nutritional support is derived from a 5 percent dextrose solution (a common intravenous sugar solution), since 1 L of this solution provides only 170 kcal of energy (3.4 kcal/g of dextrose).

When fat is metabolized, the following reaction occurs:

$$1 \text{ g fat} + 2.02 \text{ L } O_2 \rightarrow 1.43 \text{ L } CO_2 + 1.07 \text{ g } H_2O + 9.3 \text{ kcal} \quad (3)$$

For the metabolism of fat, the RQ is 0.71. Note that much more energy is produced from the metabolism of fat than from the metabolism of glucose.

Protein (PRO) is metabolized according to the following reaction:

$$1 \text{ g PRO} + 0.97 \text{ L } O_2 \rightarrow 0.78 \text{ L } CO_2 + 0.41 \text{ g } H_2O + 0.16 \text{ g urea} + 4.3 \text{ kcal} \quad (4)$$

The RQ for protein is 0.81, and urea is produced as a byproduct. Urea is excreted in the urine, and its measurement as urinary nitrogen provides an indicator of protein metabolism:

$$(\text{Urinary nitrogen}) (6.25) = \text{protein metabolism} \quad (5)$$

With lipogenesis, the following reaction occurs:

$$2.82 \text{ g glucose} + 0.078 \text{ L } O_2 \rightarrow 1 \text{ g fat} + 0.68 \text{ L } CO_2 + 0.61 \text{ g } H_2O \quad (6)$$

The RQ associated with lipogenesis is thus 8.7. With ketogenesis, the following reaction occurs:

$$0.72 \text{ g fat} + 0.437 \text{ L } O_2 \rightarrow 1 \text{ g ketones} + 0.111 \text{ L } CO_2 \quad (7)$$

The RQ for this reaction is 0.25.

Normally, the whole body RQ is between 0.7 and 1.0, depending on the principal substrate being metabolized. With a balanced diet, the RQ is about 0.8 to 0.85. Carbohydrate metabolism raises the RQ toward 1.0, and fat metabolism lowers it toward 0.7. With lipogenesis the whole body RQ may be greater than 1.0 but seldom exceeds 1.2. With ketogenesis the whole body RQ may be less than 0.7 but is seldom less than 0.65.

It should be apparent that there is a definite relationship between energy expenditure, $\dot{V}O_2$, and $\dot{V}CO_2$. The principal function of the cardiopulmonary system is to provide the O_2 to the cells needed for energy production and to clear the CO_2 produced. An increase in metabolic rate (i.e., energy expenditure) results in increased $\dot{V}O_2$ and $\dot{V}CO_2$, which requires an increase in ventilation.

EFFECTS OF STARVATION

The metabolic effects of starvation (fasting) are important to appreciate. Although they are not intentionally starved, many chronically and critically ill patients receive inadequate nutritional support and thus suffer the effects of starvation.

The initial response to starvation is an increase in glycogen and fat metabolism.[1] Glycogenolysis provides glucose, which is necessary for brain cell metabolism. However, glycogen stores are limited and are depleted after 4 to 5 days of fasting. Lipolysis from adipose tissue triglycerides produces ketones, which can also be metabolized by brain cells. Gluconeogenesis also occurs, primarily as a result of the breakdown of muscle and visceral proteins. By the third day of fasting, ketogenesis and gluconeogenesis are proceeding at maximal rates. Because of limited fat stores in the body, complete starvation usually cannot continue for more than 60 days before death occurs. With starvation, however, there is a decrease in metabolic rate, which slows the rate at which nutritional stores are depleted.

The following are effects of starvation on respiratory function[2,4,5,12–17]:

Respiratory muscle function: Catabolism of muscle protein causes weakening of respiratory muscles. This can result in respiratory muscle fatigue in spontaneously breathing patients and difficulty in weaning ventilated patients.

Decreased surfactant production: Surfactant production is reduced, which decreases lung compliance and increases the work of breathing.

Respiratory drive: The respiratory response to hypoxia is decreased.

Pulmonary defense mechanisms: Immune response is impaired; the cause of death from starvation is often pneumonia.

Decreased colloid osmotic pressure: A decrease in circulating albumin decreases colloid osmotic pressure, thereby increasing lung water and contributing to pulmonary edema.

Decreased replication of pulmonary epithelium: Malnutrition may contribute to laryngeal ulceration with prolonged intubation.

CALORIMETRY

Calorimetry is used to measure energy expenditure. In direct calorimetry heat production is measured, but because this method confines the subject to a small chamber for long periods of time, it is impractical for patient care. In indirect calorimetry energy expenditure is calculated from measurements of $\dot{V}O_2$ and $\dot{V}CO_2$, which are converted to energy expenditure in kilocalories per day by the Weir equation:

$$\text{Energy} = [(\dot{V}O_2)(3.941) + (\dot{V}CO_2)(1.11)](1440) \quad (8)$$

Indirect calorimetric data also allow calculation of the RQ. Indirect calorimeters use either an open circuit or a closed circuit method. The subject of indirect calorimetry has been reviewed in detail, and many evaluations of calorimeters have been published.[1,2,11,18–33]

The open circuit method measures the concentrations and volumes of inspired and expired gases to determine $\dot{V}O_2$ and $\dot{V}CO_2$. The following equations are used to calculate $\dot{V}O_2$ and $\dot{V}CO_2$:

$$\dot{V}O_2 = (\dot{V}_I)(F_IO_2) - (\dot{V}_E)(F_EO_2) \quad (9)$$

$$\dot{V}CO_2 = (\dot{V}_E)(F_ECO_2) - (\dot{V}_I)(F_ECO_2) \quad (10)$$

where $\dot{V}_I$ is the inspired volume, F_IO_2 is the inspired O_2 fraction, and $\dot{V}_E$, F_EO_2, and F_ECO_2 are, respectively, the expired volume and expired O_2 and CO_2 fractions. Since F_ICO_2 is less than 0.03 percent when breathing room air (and should be zero in a ventilator circuit), the term $(\dot{V}_I)(F_ICO_2)$ is deleted.

One of the difficulties encountered with indirect calorimetry is the measurement of $\dot{V}_I$. If $\dot{V}_I$ is assumed to equal $\dot{V}_E$, an error of 15 to 20 percent in $\dot{V}O_2$ may result (if RQ is 0.8). The Haldane transformation permits calculation of $\dot{V}_I$ from the measured $\dot{V}_E$ by means of the nitrogen fraction in inspired (F_IN_2) and expired gas (F_EN_2).
Since

$$\dot{V}_I = \frac{F_EN_2}{F_IN_2}(\dot{V}_E) \quad (11)$$

then

$$\dot{V}O_2 = \left[\frac{F_EN_2}{F_IN_2}(F_IO_2) - F_EO_2\right](\dot{V}_E) \quad (12)$$

The N_2 concentration is usually determined by measurement of the other gases in the sample:

$$F_IN_2 = 1 - (F_IO_2 - F_ICO_2) \quad (13)$$

$$F_EN_2 = 1 - (F_EO_2 - F_ECO_2) \quad (14)$$

the resulting final equation for $\dot{V}O_2$ is:

$$\dot{V}O_2 = \left[\frac{(1 - F_EO_2 - F_ECO_2)(F_IO_2)}{(1 - F_EO_2)} - F_EO_2\right](\dot{V}_E) \quad (15)$$

Most manufacturers of indirect calorimeters use this equation to calculate $\dot{V}O_2$.

$\dot{V}O_2$ and $\dot{V}CO_2$ can be measured by collecting expired gas and then measuring the F_EO_2 of the gas collected in the bag, $\dot{V}_E$ from the volume of gas collected in the bag and the F_IO_2 of the inspired gas. Energy expenditure can then be calculated from the Weir equation. With this method gas collection time is limited by the volume of the bag, which can result in relatively short collection times and incorrect estimates of caloric requirements. Therefore, it is important to measure $\dot{V}_E$, F_IO_2, and F_EO_2, very accurately; O_2 analyzers and volume monitors commonly used in bedside respiratory care are not accurate enough for this application.

Open Circuit Method

The key components of an open circuit calorimeter are the O_2 and CO_2 analyzers, a volume measuring device, and a mixing chamber. The analyzers must be capable of measuring small changes in gas concentrations (0.001 percent), and the volume monitor must be capable of accurately measuring volumes from 0.05 to 1.0 L. Since most O_2 analyzers in indirect calorimeters use the polarographic principle, changes in pressure (such as those that occur during mechanical ventilation) affect the measurement of F_IO_2. A pressure transducer is used to correct the analyzer for pressure changes.

The open circuit method can be used with spontaneously breathing subjects and those requiring mechanical ventilation. Figure 51-6 shows the movement of gas through an open circuit calorimeter. Expired gas from the patient is directed into the mixing chamber, at the end of which a vacuum pump aspirates a small sample of gas for measurement of O_2 and CO_2. A pressure transducer within this circuit ensures pressure-compensated measurements. After analysis, this sample is returned to the mixing chamber. Periodically the analyzer also measures F_IO_2. The entire volume of gas then exits through a volume monitor, which uses a thermistor for temperature correction of the volume. A microprocessor controls the calorimeter and performs the necessary calculations.

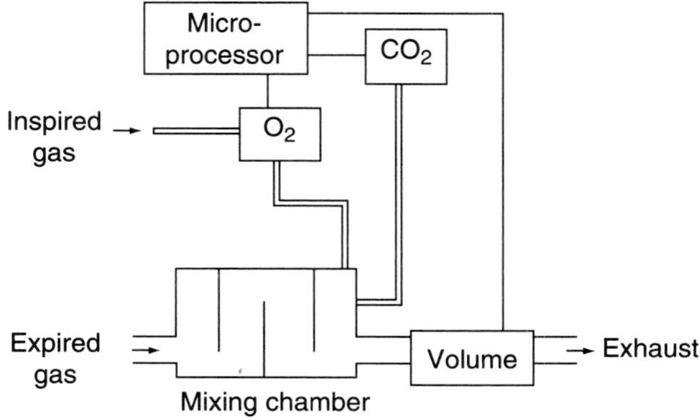

Figure 51-6. Schematic diagram of open circuit indirect calorimeter.

Several points must be observed in order for the open circuit technique to work properly.

The F_IO_2 must be stable to within ± 0.005 percent: An air-O_2 blender is often used to prevent fluctuations caused by the instability of gas mixing systems in mechanical ventilators.[34]

The F_IO_2 must be less than 0.60: Open circuit calorimeters tend to measure $\dot{V}O_2$ inaccurately at high F_IO_2.[35]

The entire system must be leak-free: Loss of gas from the system results in incomplete gas collection, and addition of gas from the atmosphere dilutes the collected gas. Accurate measurements are impossible in patients with uncuffed airways, those with pleural air leaks, or those undergoing renal dialysis; measurements also cannot be accurate if a sidestream capnograph is in line.

Inspired and expired gases must be completely separated: This can be a problem with continuous flow systems.

Closed Circuit Method

The closed circuit method differs from the open circuit method in the measurement of $\dot{V}O_2$. The measurement of $\dot{V}CO_2$ is identical for both systems. The key components of the closed circuit calorimeter are a volumetric spirometer, a mixing chamber, a CO_2 analyzer, and a CO_2 absorber. The spirometer is filled with a known volume of O_2 and is connected to the patient. As the patient rebreathes from the spirometer, O_2 is consumed and CO_2 is produced. The CO_2 is removed from the system by the CO_2 absorber before the gas is returned to the spirometer. The decrease in the volume of the system equals $\dot{V}O_2$.

The closed circuit calorimeter is illustrated in Figure 51-7. Gas from the patient flows into the mixing chamber, and a sample is aspirated for analysis of F_ECO_2. From the mixing chamber, gas flows through a CO_2 absorber (such as barium hydroxide) and then to the spirometer. The volume of the spirometer is electronically monitored to measure V_T. The difference between end-expiratory volumes is calculated by a microprocessor to determine $\dot{V}O_2$. If the patient is being mechanically ventilated, a bag-in-the-box system is used as a part of the inspiratory limb of the calorimeter. The bellows is pressurized by the ventilator, which results in ventilation of the patient. Measurement time is limited by F_IO_2 and the volume of the spirometer. When the volume in the spirometer decreases to a critical level, the measurement is interrupted to refill the spirometer.

Leaks from the closed circuit system, due to an uncuffed airway, a bronchopleural fistula, or a sidestream capnograph will result in erroneously high $\dot{V}O_2$ measurements. Another problem with this technique is related to ventilatory support, involving increased compressible volume and decreased trigger sensitivity. Generally, this approach should not be used with low-rate intermittent mandatory ventilation systems. The major advantage of the closed over the open circuit method is its ability to make measurements at high F_IO_2 levels (up to 1.0). A modified version of the closed circuit method for measuring $\dot{V}O_2$ is the replenishment technique, which determines the amount of O_2 necessary to maintain a constant volume in the spirometer, thereby eliminating the need for a large spirometer and interruptions to refill the spirometer.

The Vital Stat VVR calorimeter is a $\dot{V}O_2$ monitor that uses the replenishment technique. Because $\dot{V}CO_2$ is not measured, this device is technically not a calorimeter. As shown in Figure 51-8, the major components of the VVR are a bellows, a CO_2 absorber, and an ultrasonic sensor. Prior to testing the system is primed with O_2, and the position of the bellows is determined by the ultrasonic sensor. The patient rebreathes from the bellows, and CO_2 is removed by the CO_2 absorber. After a programmed number of breaths, the ultrasonic sensor determines the new position of the bellows. Since O_2 is consumed, the end-expiratory level of the bellows is raised. Calibrated pulses of O_2 are added to the bellows until the original level is reached. The number of O_2 pulses multiplied by their volume equals $\dot{V}O_2$. The problems and advantages of this system are the same as those of other closed circuit systems.

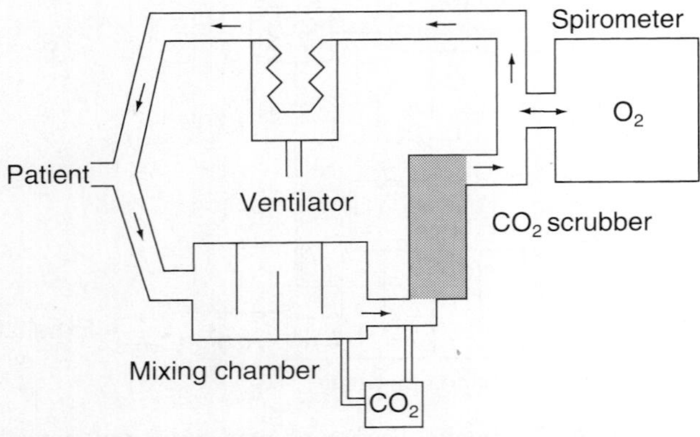

Figure 51-7. Schematic diagram of closed circuit indirect calorimeter.

General Measurement Considerations

When measuring resting energy expenditure (REE) by indirect calorimetry, one must consider both the duration of each measurement and the number of measurements required to produce an estimate of 24-hour REE. Ideally, 24 hours of continuous indirect calorimetry would produce the best estimate, but 24-hour measurements of $\dot{V}O_2$ and $\dot{V}CO_2$ are usually not possible. Two 15-minute measurements at 12-hour intervals produce a reasonable estimate of REE.[1] For many critically ill patients it is impossible to obtain measurements for longer than 15 to 30 minutes more often than once in a given day. It is important, however, to recognize that shorter and less frequent measurements produce less correct estimates of total energy expenditure.

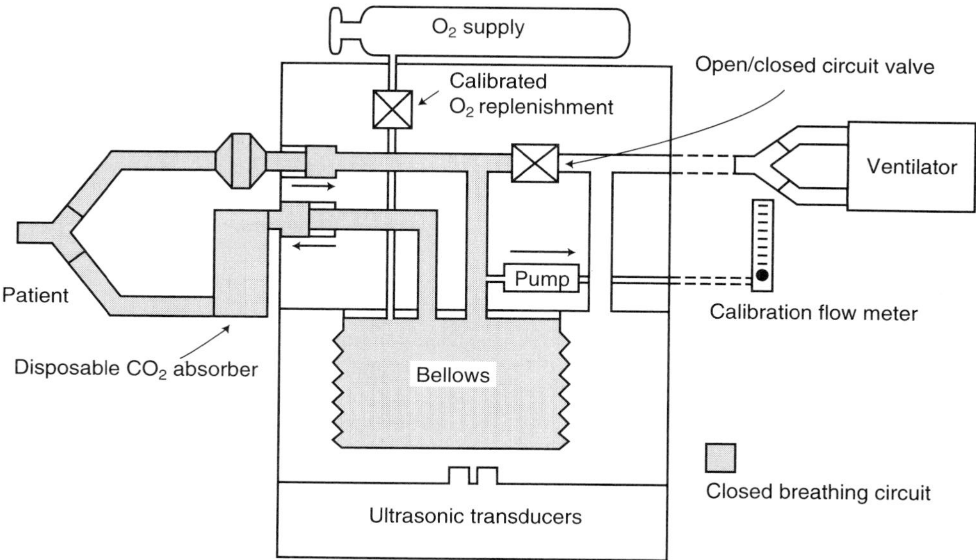

Figure 51-8. Schematic diagram of VVR calorimeter.

During indirect calorimetry patients should be undisturbed, motionless and at rest in the supine position, and aware of their surroundings (unless comatose).[36–40] The patient should either be receiving continuous nutritional support or have fasted for several hours before the measurement. Before indirect calorimetry is performed, there should have been no changes in ventilation for at least 90 minutes, no factors that affect $\dot{V}O_2$ for at least 60 minutes (change in fever, motion, etc.), and stable hemodynamics for at least 2 hours.[41] The validity of the measurements should be assessed by direct observation rather than by relying on a steady-state indicator from the calorimeter. To obtain valid indirect calorimetry results is a labor-intensive process.

REE is similar but not equivalent to basal energy expenditure (BEE). BEE is measured in a neutral thermal environment after 12 hours of fasting. Because REE is measured with the patient at rest, calories must be added to correct for patient activity. There may be considerable fluctuation in REE throughout the day and from day to day.[42] However, measurements are equally valid whether they are made in the morning or in the afternoon.[43]

The patient can be connected to the indirect calorimeter in several ways. For mechanically ventilated patients the calorimeter is connected in line with the ventilator so that the patient's ventilation is not interrupted. A mask, mouthpiece, or canopy can be used with spontaneously breathing patients. A canopy is often preferred because it is more comfortable for the patient and interferes less with the patient's steady state. However, use of a mouthpiece or a mask may give comparable results.[44]

To obtain reliable results, periodic quality control procedures should be conducted according to the recommendations of the equipment manufacturer. Comprehensive evaluation procedures involving the burning of alcohol (which has a known RQ of 0.67) have also been described in the literature.[45]

In critically ill patients who have a pulmonary artery (Swan-Ganz) catheter in place, $\dot{V}O_2$ can be calculated from the difference between arterial and mixed venous O_2 content $[C(a\text{-}\bar{v})O_2]$ and cardiac output (CO):

$$\dot{V}O_2 = (CO)\ (\text{in L/min}) \times [C(a\text{-}\bar{v})O_2]\ (\text{in mL/dL}) \quad (16)$$

This method (Fick equation) is acceptable but can only be used if a thermodilution pulmonary artery catheter is in place.

Caloric expenditure can be calculated from $\dot{V}O_2$ alone, $\dot{V}CO_2$ alone, or both $\dot{V}O_2$ and $\dot{V}CO_2$. Calculation of energy expenditure from $\dot{V}O_2$ or $\dot{V}CO_2$ alone requires an estimation of RQ. Although this is acceptable for clinical estimates of REE, it is often desirable to know RQ in order to evaluate substrate metabolism (carbohydrate versus fat). When REE is estimated from $\dot{V}O_2$ or $\dot{V}CO_2$ alone, the following equations can be used[46,47]:

$$REE = (\dot{V}O_2)(\text{in L/min})(4.83\ \text{kcal/L})(1440\ \text{min/d}) \quad (17)$$

$$REE = (\dot{V}CO_2)(\text{in L/min})(5.52\ \text{kcal/L})(1440\ \text{min/d}) \quad (18)$$

NUTRITIONAL ASSESSMENT

To identify patients with nutritional deficits, a thorough nutritional assessment is performed. Dietary history and intake are evaluated, including diet restrictions, use of food supplements, chewing and swallowing difficulty, smell and taste perception, limitations on meal preparation and food procurement, and any special needs regarding eating arrangements. Aspects of the clinical examination relative to nutritional assessment include pertinent medical history, physical signs suggestive of malnutrition, the presence of dyspnea during eating, and bowel function. Psychosocial aspects, such as changes in behavior, may also indicate a nutritional deficit.

Anthropometric Data

Anthropometric data are useful in the nutritional assessment. These include height, weight, ideal body weight (desirable weight for height), and weight change. Upper arm anthropometry, such as triceps skinfold thickness and midarm muscle circumference, may also be useful. Skinfold thickness is an indicator of body fat, and the midarm muscle circumference is an indicator of somatic protein reserve. From height and weight, the basal energy requirements can be estimated by the Harris-Benedict equation:

$$\text{BEE} = 66 + [(13.7)(W)] + [(5)(H)] - [(6.8)(A)] \text{ for males} \quad (19)$$

$$\text{BEE} = 655 + [(9.66)(W)] + [(1.8)(H)] - [(4.7)(A)] \text{ for females} \quad (20)$$

where W is ideal body weight in kilograms, H is height in centimeters, and A is age in years. The total daily energy (TDE) need as calculated from the Harris-Benedict equation is increased by an activity factor (AF) and an injury stress factor (IF) to determine the caloric needs of a patient[48]:

$$\text{TDE} = \text{BEE} + \text{AF} + \text{IF} \quad (21)$$

The AF is 20 percent of BEE if the patient is confined to bed and 30 percent of BEE if the patient is ambulatory. Typical IF values are 10 to 30 percent of BEE for major trauma, 25 to 60 percent of BEE for sepsis, and 50 to 110 percent of BEE for burns (Fig. 51-9).

Although the Harris-Benedict equation is useful for estimating the caloric requirements of many patients, indirect calorimetry has been shown to be superior in patients who are critically ill and have numerous nutritional stress factors.[49–52] However, indirect calorimetry is labor-intensive and expensive and should be reserved for selected patients (Table 51-2); it should not be used unless the physicians, dietitians, and clinicians caring for the patient understand its role in patient management.[53]

Biochemical Data

Biochemical data are also useful in the assessment of nutritional status,[54,55] as described below.

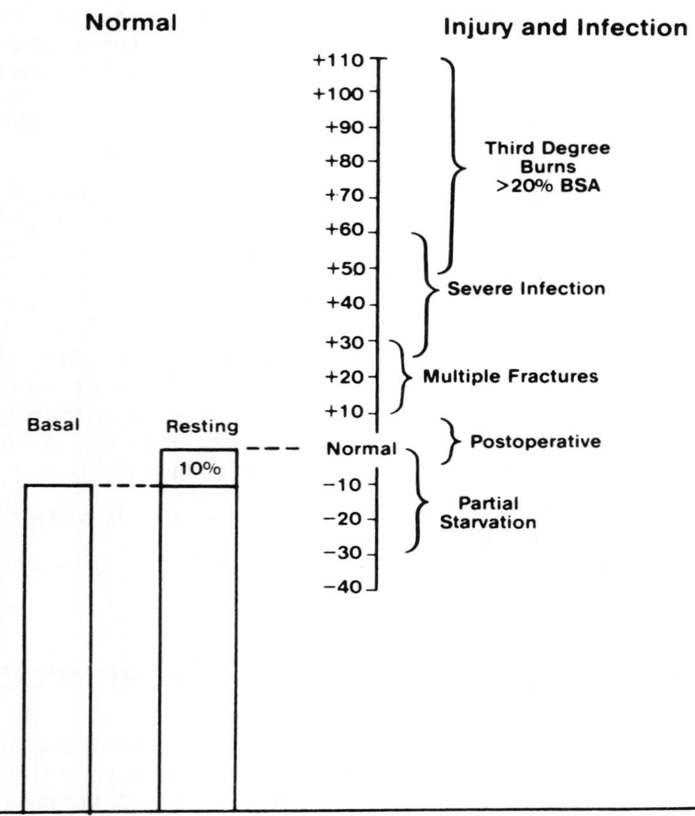

Figure 51-9. The effects of injury, sepsis, and nutritional depletion on REE. (From Elwyn,[48] with permission.)

Table 51-2. Indications for Indirect Calorimetry
Nutritional stress factors (trauma, sepsis, burns, etc.)
Difficulty weaning from mechanical ventilation
Pediatric patients in whom caloric requirements are uncertain
Obese patients in whom caloric requirements are uncertain
Malnourished patients in whom caloric requirements are uncertain
Patients who fail to respond appropriately to nutritional support

Serum Albumin

Circulating albumin is important as a carrier protein (for zinc, magnesium, calcium, fatty acids), in the maintenance of oncotic pressure, and as a buffer. Albumin levels correlate with the degree of malnutrition, decreased levels being associated with increased risk of morbidity and mortality. Because albumin has a half-life of about 20 days, albumin levels reflect chronic rather than acute protein depletion. Albumin is not a definitive indicator of visceral protein status. It can be decreased not only by malnutrition but also by infection, postoperative status, metabolic stresses, inadequate protein intake, and fluid imbalances (overhydration, ascites, edema). Albumin levels are decreased with kwashiorkor, a condition of severe protein deficiency. Normal albumin levels are 3.5 to 5 g/dL.

Transferrin

Transferrin is a carrier protein for iron. It is a more sensitive indicator of acute changes in nutritional status than is albumin because it has a half-life of about 8 to 10 days. As compared with albumin, it is a more useful indicator of visceral protein stores in patients with liver disease. In addition to visceral protein depletion, conditions that can decrease transferrin levels include chronic infections, acute catabolic states, uremia, nephrotic syndrome, increased iron stores, liver disease, overhydration, and kwashiorkor. Transferrin levels can be increased by hepatitis, pregnancy, iron deficiency anemia, dehydration, and chronic blood loss. Normal levels are 200 to 400 mg/dL.

Thyroxine-Binding Prealbumin (Transthyretin)

Prealbumin is a carrier protein for retinol-binding protein and is a transport protein for thyroxine. It is a sensitive indicator of visceral protein status, especially in acute stages of protein-energy malnutrition. A major advantage of prealbumin as an indicator of nutritional status is its short half-life, about 2 to 3 days. It has limited use as an assessment parameter during acute demands for protein synthesis. A number of factors in addition to malnutrition can decrease the prealbumin level, including acute catabolic states, surgery, altered energy and nitrogen balance, infection, hepatic necrosis, hyperthyroidism, and dialysis. Its level may be increased by renal failure and steroid therapy. Normal prealbumin levels are 15 to 35 mg/dL.

Retinol-Binding Protein

Retinol-binding protein transports the alcohol of vitamin A (retinol). It is highly sensitive to changes in nutritional status, having only a 12-hour half-life. It has limited use as an assessment parameter in renal failure because it is filtered by the glomerulus and metabolized by the kidney. In addition to malnutrition, conditions in which it is decreased include acute catabolic states, vitamin A deficiency, liver disease, hyperthyroidism, and postsurgical status. Levels may increase with vitamin A supplementation or renal failure. The normal retinol-binding protein level is 3 to 6 μg/dL.

Total Lymphocyte Count

Total lymphocyte count (TLC) is an indicator of immune function and reflects both B cells and T cells. It is calculated from the white blood cell (WBC) count as

$$\text{TLC} = \frac{(\%\ \text{lymphocytes})\ (\text{WBC})}{100} \tag{22}$$

The TLC is useful as a screening parameter in noncritically ill patients and correlates with albumin in predicting postsurgical mortality and morbidity. The TLC is not an absolute indicator of nutritional state. It is increased by infection and leukemia and decreased by cancer, metabolic stress, surgery, and steroid therapy. Normal TLC is 1500 to 3500 cells/mm^3.

Delayed Hypersensitivity Reactivity Skin Testing

Delayed hypersensitivity reactivity skin testing is a measure of cell-mediated immunity. In addition to evaluation of nutritional status, it is useful as an indicator of postsurgical sepsis and mortality. The technique requires skill in reading the induration produced and has varied effects due to various antigen concentrations. It is not useful in the presence of infection, cancer, hepatic necrosis, renal failure, trauma, immunosuppressive diseases such as the acquired immunodeficiency syndrome (AIDS), or immunosuppressive drugs.

Nitrogen Balance

The nitrogen balance determines the amount of nitrogen (protein) required to maintain nitrogen equilibrium and reflects anabolism or catabolism and distribution of protein. It is determined as follows:

$$\text{N balance} = \text{nitrogen intake} - \text{nitrogen output}$$

$$\text{N balance} = (\text{protein intake}/6.25) - (\text{UUN} + 4) \tag{23}$$

where UUN is the urine urea nitrogen. The determination of nitrogen balance requires accurate 24-hour urine collection, accurate assessment of protein intake, and a creatine clearance greater than 50 mL/min. Nitrogen balance is normally positive but becomes negative with inadequate caloric and/or protein intake and metabolic stress.

NUTRITIONAL SUPPORT

As shown in Figure 51-10, too low or too high a caloric intake can result in respiratory muscle fatigue and lead to respiratory failure. The recommended number of kilocalories for maintenance therapy is 1 to 1.3 times the REE or 25 to 35 kcal/kg body weight. For repletion therapy the recommended level is 1.4 to 1.6 times the REE or 35 to 45 kcal/kg. About 50 percent of total kilocalories should be provided as carbohydrate. Excessive carbohydrate can increase RQ, metabolic rate, and ventilatory requirements, which can result in respiratory distress.[56–64] Maximal glucose utilization (tolerance) is about 5 mg/kg/min or 7.23 g/kg body weight. Protein/amino acid intake should be 1.2 to 1.9 g protein/kg body weight for maintenance therapy (100 to 150 kcal/g N) and 1.6 to 2.5 g protein/kg for repletion therapy (8 to 120 kcal/g N). Excessive amino acid intake can stimulate the ventilatory drive.[17] The recommended fat (lipid) intake is 30 percent of total kilocalories. Fat intake as intralipids may result in a decrease in PaO_2 in patients with the adult respiratory distress syndrome (ARDS).[64] Infusion of fat emulsions has also been associated with a reduction in pulmonary diffusion capacity.[65] However, PaO_2 may improve slightly following infusion of intravenous fat emulsions in patients with normal lung function, in COPD patients, and in patients with infectious lung disease.[66]

Daily requirements for vitamins and minerals as listed in Table 51-3 are important.[2,54,55] In patients with pulmonary disease, it is particularly important to provide adequate phosphorus intake to maintain adequate 2,3-DPG levels and respiratory muscle contractility. Respiratory failure is associated with severe hypophosphatemia. Hypophosphatemia and hypocalcemia can result in decreased diaphragmatic strength. Hypomagnesemia is associated with abnormalities of myocardial and skeletal muscle function. Respiratory muscle strength improves when magnesium levels are restored to normal.

Nutritional support can be either enteral (i.e., using the gut) or parenteral (i.e., using a vein). A decision tree for selection of the type of nutritional support[9] is shown in Figure 51-11.

As a general rule, the gut should be used for nutritional support if it is functional. If oral intake is not possible, a nasoenteral (gastric, duodenal, or jejunal) tube can be used. For long-term enteral nutrition, a gastrostomy or jejunostomy tube is preferred. When initiating enteral feeding, a continuous infusion is usually better tolerated than intermittent administration. Enteral feedings are usually started at 25 to 50 mL/h full strength solutions. If this is tolerated, the rate of administration is gradually increased to the desired level. Complications of enteral feedings include improper placement of the tube (into the bronchial tree), nausea and vomiting, aspiration, and diarrhea.[67,68] If large-volume intermittent feedings are used, the patient should be maintained in a head-up position for 1 to 2 hours after each feeding, and chest physiotherapy should not be performed during

Table 51-3. Daily Maintenance Doses for Vitamins, Minerals, and Trace Elements in Adults

Nutrient	Enteral	Parenteral
Vitamin A	800–1000 μg RE	660 μg RE
Vitamin D	5–10 μg	5 g
Vitamin E	8–10 μg TE	10 mg TE
Vitamin C	50–60 mg	100 mg
Vitamin K	70–140 μg	0.7–2 μg
Folic acid	400 μg	400 μg
Niacin	13–19 mg NE	40 mg NE
Riboflavin	1.2–1.6 mg	3.6 mg
Thiamine	1–1.5 mg	3 mg
Pyridoxine	1.8–2.2 mg	4 mg
Cyanocobalamin	3 μg	5 μg
Pantothenic acid	4.7 mg	15 mg
Biotin	100–200 μg	60 μg
Potassium	1875–5625 mg	60–100 mEq
Sodium	1100–3300 mg	60–100 mEq
Chloride	1700–5100 mg	—
Fluoride	1.5–4 mg	—
Calcium	800–1200 mg	600 mg
Phosphorus	800–1200 mg	600 mg
Magnesium	300–400 mg	10–20 mEq
Iron	10–18 mg	1–7 mg
Zinc	15 mg	2.5–4 mg
Iodine	150 μg	70–140 μg
Copper	2.3 mg	0.5–1.5 mg
Manganese	2.5–5 mg	0.15–0.8 mg
Chromium	0.05–0.2 mg	10–15 mg
Selenium	0.05–0.2 mg	40–120 μg
Molybdenum	0.15–0.5 mg	20–30 μg

RE, retinol equivalence; TE, tocopherol equivalence; NE, niacin equivalence.
(Adapted from Skipper,[55] with permission.)

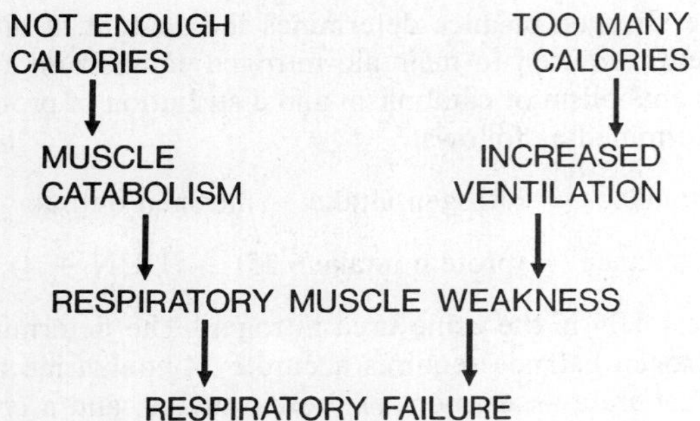

Figure 51-10. Nutrition and respiration. The effect of too low and too high a caloric intake on respiratory function.

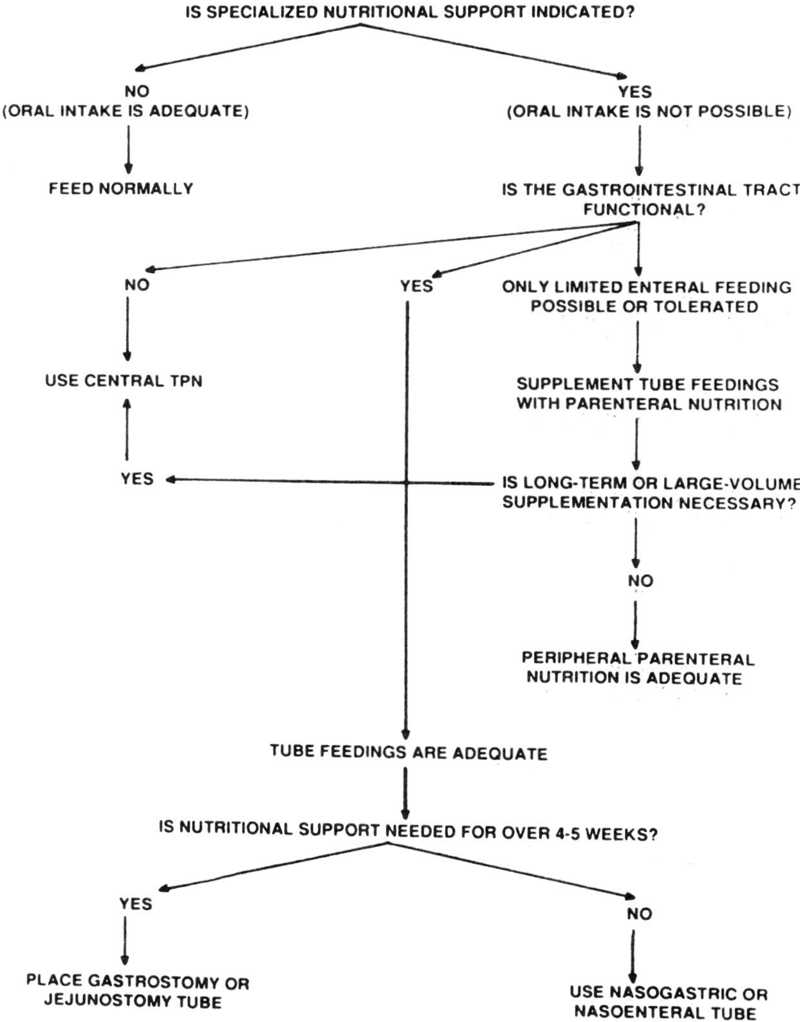
IS SPECIALIZED NUTRITIONAL SUPPORT INDICATED?
NO
(ORAL INTAKE IS ADEQUATE)
YES
(ORAL INTAKE IS NOT POSSIBLE)
FEED NORMALLY
IS THE GASTROINTESTINAL TRACT FUNCTIONAL?
NO
YES
ONLY LIMITED ENTERAL FEEDING POSSIBLE OR TOLERATED
USE CENTRAL TPN
SUPPLEMENT TUBE FEEDINGS WITH PARENTERAL NUTRITION
YES
IS LONG-TERM OR LARGE-VOLUME SUPPLEMENTATION NECESSARY?
NO
PERIPHERAL PARENTERAL NUTRITION IS ADEQUATE
TUBE FEEDINGS ARE ADEQUATE
IS NUTRITIONAL SUPPORT NEEDED FOR OVER 4-5 WEEKS?
YES
NO
PLACE GASTROSTOMY OR JEJUNOSTOMY TUBE
USE NASOGASTRIC OR NASOENTERAL TUBE

Figure 51-11. Decision tree for selection of the type of nutritional support (From Berger and Adams,[9] with permission.)

this time. While moving the patient (as with chest physiotherapy) and providing airway care, it is important for the clinician to be certain that the feeding tube does not become dislodged.

The compositions of some commonly used tube feeding formulas are listed in Table 51-4.

If enteral feedings are not possible, parenteral nutrition is provided. For short-term, small-volume nutritional support, peripheral parenteral nutrition can be used; otherwise central parenteral nutritional support is recommended. Parenteral nutritional formulas typically include dextrose and amino acids, as well as other nutrients such as vitamins. Lipids also are administered as part of parenteral nutritional support. The composition of typical parenteral nutritional formulations are shown in Table 51-4. Because of its expense, parenteral nutrition should be used judiciously. Complications include pneumothorax (during central line placement), phlebitis and thrombosis, and infection.

Nutritional support should begin early in the patient's hospital course (within 1 to 3 days of admission). Failure to provide this support may produce the results of starvation discussed above. It should be recognized that many patients have been ill for some time before admission to the hospital and may thus be calorically depleted at admission.

Chronic Obstructive Pulmonary Disease

Weight loss and malnutrition are common findings in patients with chronic obstructive pulmonary disease (COPD),[69–78] particularly those with emphysema. Malnutrition in COPD is associated with reduced respiratory muscle function, increased severity of disease, and reduced rate of survival. Protein-calorie malnutrition is a common finding. Possible mechanisms for this malnutrition and weight loss include impaired gastrointestinal function, altered dietary in-

Table 51-4. Composition of Common Nutritional Formulas

Formula	Calories (kcal/L)	Fat (g/L)	Carbohydrate (g/L)	Protein (g/L)	Osmolality (mOsm/L)
Enteral					
Ensure	1057	37	144	37	450
Ensure-Plus	1497	53	200	55	600
Ensure-Plus HN	1502	50	200	63	650
Isocal	1060	44	132	34	300
Isocal HCN	2019	91	225	75	690
Magnacal	2000	80	250	70	590
Osmolite	1061	37	145	37	300
Vivonex Standard	1017	1.5	231	20	550
Vivonex TEN	1000	2.8	206	38	630
Jevity	1061	36.9	152	44.5	310
Peptamen	1000	39	127	40	262
Pulmocare	1500	92	106	63	490
Parenteral (York Hospital)					
Peripheral					
Standard	720		50	21.25	780
Special	670		50	42.5	900
Central (without lipids)	850		250	42.5	1925
Intralipid					
10%	1100	100			260
20%	2000	200			260

(Adapted from Berger and Adams,[9] with permission.)

take, breathlessness that limits the ability to ingest sufficient amounts of food, and hypermetabolism.

Nutritional repletion of patients with COPD must be carefully initiated and monitored. When COPD patients are hospitalized, nutritional support should begin soon after admission. COPD patients may become more dyspneic and uncomfortable than usual, secondary to the increased respiratory demand caused by increased nutrient intake. Because of limited tolerance of large fluid loads, close attention to fluid balance is a necessity. Therefore, a slow increase in caloric and fluid intake over the first week of nutritional repletion is required. Respiratory rate, blood gases, exercise tolerance, and body weight should be monitored during repletion.

Table 51-5 lists some nutritional guidelines for the care of patients with COPD. Providing a high fat, adequate protein, low carbohydrate diet may improve the nutritional status of COPD patients without resulting in increased CO_2 retention. However, provision of an adequate caloric total may be more important than specific formulas.

Table 51-5. Diet Suggestions for Pulmonary Disease Patients

Make food preparation easy
Rest before eating
Eat in a quiet, relaxed atmosphere
Take meals early in the day
Avoid foods that produce gas or bloating
Eat small, frequent meals
Substitute low cholesterol fats for high carbohydrate foods
Avoid overfeeding of protein, but provide enough for protein balance
Restrict fluids and/or sodium as needed

Trauma, Sepsis, and Burns

Patients with trauma, sepsis, and burns are metabolically stressed.[79,80] This stress is characterized by hypermetabolism, hypercatabolism, skeletal muscle proteolysis, and lipolysis. In hypermetabolic conditions, there is often a high rate of muscle catabolism without an adaptation to lipid utilization. Such patients are often insulin-resistant and are hyperglycemic owing to increased glucose production as well as decreased glucose utilization (insulin resistance). The increased glucose production results from glycogenolysis and gluconeogenesis as well as lipolysis. The nutritional depletion of these patients is primarily the result of hypermetabolism and hypercatabolism rather than starvation. Because nutritional stores can be quickly depleted following injury, it is important to begin nutritional support soon after admission (within 1 to 3 days), even though the patient's nutritional status may have been normal before the injury.

Pediatric Patients

There are several specific concerns regarding the nutritional support of infants and children.[2] Neonates and small infants lack energy stores such as fat reserves and have a higher metabolic rate in relation to body weight than the adult (Table 51-6). Much of the additional energy requirement is that needed for growth. Because caloric requirements predicted from adult nomograms are inaccurate and are often excessive, it may be best to determine caloric requirements by indirect calorimetry in children. The protein per kilogram requirements of children are higher than those

Table 51-6. Calorie and Protein Requirements of Children

Age	Calorie (kcal/kg)	Protein (g/kg)
Birth–6 mo	120	2.0–3.0
6 mo–1 yr	110	2.0–2.75
1–3 yr	100	1.8–2.2
4–6 yr	90	1.4–1.6
7–10 yr	80	1.1–1.3
Boys		
11–14 yr	65	0.9–1.0
15–18 yr	50	0.8–1.0
Girls		
11–14 yr	55	0.9–1.0
15–18 yr	40	0.8–1.0

of the adult. Children also have a higher water requirement per unit of body weight than do adults, and they require more calcium and phosphorus to support growth of the skeleton. Although children have higher protein and water requirements per kilogram of body weight, their absolute protein and water requirements are less than those of adults.

References

1. Bursztein S, Elwyn DH, Askanazi J, Kinney JM: Energy Metabolism, Indirect Calorimetry, and Nutrition. Williams & Wilkins, Baltimore, 1989
2. Weissman C (ed): Nutrition and respiratory disease. Probl Respir Care 2(4), 1989
3. Orme JF, Clemmer TP: Nutrition in the critical care unit. Med Clin North Am 1983;67:1295–1304
4. Rochester DF, Esau SA: Malnutrition and the respiratory system. Chest 1984;85:411–415
5. Pingleton SK, Harmon GS: Nutritional management in acute respiratory failure. JAMA 1987;257:3094–3099
6. Benotti PN, Bistrian B: Metabolic and nutritional aspects of weaning from mechanical ventilation. Crit Care Med 1989;17:181–185
7. Pingleton SK: Nutritional support in the mechanically ventilated patient. Clin Chest Med 1988;9:101–112
8. McCauley K, Weaver TE: Cardiac and pulmonary diseases: Nutritional implications. Nurs Clin North Am 1983;18:81–96
9. Berger R, Adams L: Nutritional support in the critical care setting, parts 1 and 2. Chest 1989;96:139–150, 372–380
10. Silberman H, Silberman AW: Parenteral nutrition, biochemistry, and respiratory gas exchange. JPEN J Parenter Enteral Nutr 1986;10:151–154
11. Damask MC, Schwarz Y, Weissman C: Energy measurements and requirements of critically ill patients. Crit Care Clin 1987;3:71–96
12. Lewis MI, Belman MJ: Nutrition and the respiratory muscles. Clin Chest Med 1988;9:337–348
13. Barrocas A, Tretola R, Alsonso A: Nutrition and the critically ill pulmonary patient. Respir Care 1983;28:50–61
14. Doekel RC, Zwillich CW, Scoggin CH et al: Clinical semi-starvation. Depression of hypoxic ventilatory drive. N Engl J Med 1976;295:358–361
15. Askanazi J, Weissman C, Rosenbaum SH et al: Nutrition and the respiratory system. Crit Care Med 1982;10:163–172
16. Kahan BD: Nutrition and host defense mechanisms. Surg Clin North Am 1981;61:557–570
17. Zwillich CW, Sahn SA, Weil JV: Effects of hypermetabolism on ventilation and chemosensitivity. J Clin Invest 1977;60:900–906
18. Nelson ND, Anderson HB, Garcia H: Clinical evaluation of a new metabolic monitor suitable for use in critically ill patients. Crit Care Med 1987;10:951–957
19. Deckert RE, Wesley JR, Schafer LE et al: A water-sealed indirect calorimeter for measurement of oxygen consumption, carbon dioxide production, and energy expenditure in infants. JPEN J Parenter Enteral Nutr 1988;12:256–259
20. Keppler T, Deckert RE, Arnoldi DK et al: Evaluations of the Waters MRM-6000 and Biergy VVR closed-circuit indirect calorimeters. Respir Care 1989;34:28–35
21. Takala J, Keinanen O, Vaisanen P, Kari A: Measurement of gas exchange in intensive care: Laboratory and clinical evaluation of a new device. Crit Care Med 1989;17:1041–1047
22. Livinson MR, Groeger JS, Miodownik S et al: Indirect calorimetry in the mechanically ventilated patient. Crit Care Med 1987;15:144–147
23. Long CL, Schaffer N, Schiller WR, Blakemore WS: Metabolic response to injury and illness: Estimation of energy and protein needs from indirect calorimetry and nitrogen balance. JPEN Parenteral Enteral Nutr 1979;3:452–456
24. Bursztein S, Saphar P, Glaser P et al: Determination of energy metabolism from respiratory functions alone. J Appl Physiol 1977;43:117–119
25. Westenskow DR, Cutler CA, Wallace WD: Instrumentation for monitoring gas exchange and metabolic rate in critically ill patients. Crit Care Med 1984;12:183–187
26. Gazzaniga AB, Polachek JR, Wilson AV, Day AT: Indirect calorimetry as a guide to caloric replacement during total parenteral nutrition. Am J Surg 1978;136:128–133
27. Hunker FD, Bruton CW, Hunker EM et al: Metabolic and nutritional evaluation of patients supported with mechanical ventilation. Crit Care Med 1980;8:628–632
28. Head CA, Grossman GD, Jordan JC et al: A valve system for accurate measurement of energy expenditure in mechanically ventilated patients. Respir Care 1985;30:969–973
29. Head CA, McManus CB, Seitz S et al: A simple and accurate indirect calorimetry system for assessment of resting energy expenditure. JPEN J Parenter Enteral 1984;8:45–48
30. Raurich JM, Ibanez J, Marse P: Validation of a new closed circuit indirect calorimetry method compared with the open Douglas bag method. Intensive Care Med 1989;15:274–278
31. Braun U, Zundel J, Freiboth K et al: Evaluation of methods for indirect calorimetry with a ventilated lung model. Intensive Care Med 1989;15:196–202
32. Branson RD, Hurst JM, Davis K, Palsfort R: A laboratory evaluation of the Biergy VVR calorimeter. Respir Care 1988;33:341–347
33. Branson RD: The measurement of energy expenditure: Instrumentation, practical considerations and clinical application. Respir Care 1990;35:640–659
34. Browning JA, Linberg SE, Turney SZ, Chodoff P: The effects of a fluctuating F_{IO_2} on metabolic measurements in mechanically ventilated patients. Crit Care Med 1982;10:82–85
35. Ultman JS, Bursztein S: Analysis of error in the determination of respiratory gas exchange at varying F_{IO_2}. J Appl Physiol 1981;50:210–216
36. Weissman C, Kemper M, Damask MC et al: Effect of routine intensive care interactions on metabolic rate. Chest 1984;86:815–818
37. Weissman C, Kemper M, Elwyn DH et al: The energy expenditure of the mechanically ventilated critically ill patient. An analysis. Chest 1986;89:254–259
38. Damask MC, Askanazi J, Weissman C et al: Artifacts in measurement of resting energy expenditure. Crit Care Med 1983;11:750–752
39. Klein P, Kemper M, Weissman C et al: Attenuation of the hemodynamic responses to chest physiotherapy. Chest 1988;93:38–42
40. Weissman C, Kemper M, Damask MC et al: Effect of routine

intensive care interactions on metabolic rate. Chest 1984;86:815–818

41. Henneberg S, Soderberg D, Groth T et al: Carbon dioxide during mechanical ventilation. Crit Care Med 1987;15:8–13
42. Vermeij DG, Feenstra BWA, van Lanschot JB, Bruining HA: Day-to-day variability of energy expenditure in critically ill surgical patients. Crit Care Med 1989;17:623–626
43. Zurlo F, Frascarolo P, Enzi G et al: Variability of resting energy expenditure in healthy volunteers during fasting and continuous enteral feeding. Crit Care Med 1986;14:535–557
44. McAnea OJ, Harvey LP, Katzeff HL, Daly JM: Indirect calorimetry: Comparison of hood and mask systems for measuring resting energy expenditure in healthy volunteers. JPEN J Parenter Enteral Nutr 1986;10:555–557
45. Damask MC, Weissman C, Askanazi J et al: A systematic method for validation of gas exchange measurements. Anesthesiology 1982;57:213–218
46. McCamish MA, Dean RE, Ouellette TR: Assessing energy requirements of patients on respirators. JPEN J Parenter Enteral Nutr 1981;5:513–516
47. Hess D, Daugherty A, Large E, Agarwal NN: A comparison of four methods of determining caloric requirements of mechanically ventilated trauma patients. Respir Care 1986;31:1197–1203
48. Elwyn DH: Nutritional requirements of surgical patients. Crit Care Med 1980;8:9–20
49. van Lanschot JJB, Feenstra BWA, Vermeij CG, Bruining HA: Calculation versus measurement of total energy expenditure. Crit Care Med 1986;14:981–985
50. Mann S, Westenskow DR, Houtchens BA: Measured and predicted caloric expenditure in the acutely ill. Crit Care Med 1985;13:173–177
51. Weissman C, Kemper M, Askanazi J et al: Resting metabolic rate of the critically ill patient: Measured versus predicted. Anesthesiology 1986;64:673–679
52. Rodriquez JL, Askanazi J, Weissman C et al: Ventilatory and metabolic effects of glucose infusions. Chest 1985;88:512–518
53. Campbell SM, Kudsk KA: "High tech" metabolic measurements: Useful in daily clinical practice? JPEN J Parenter Enteral Nutr 1988;12:610–612
54. Shronts EP: Nutrition Support Dietetics. American Society of Parenteral and Enteral Nutrition (ASPEN), Rockville, MD, 1989
55. Skipper A: Dietician's Handbook of Enteral and Parenteral Nutrition. Aspen Publishers, Gaithersburg, MD, 1989
56. Delafosse B, Bouffard Y, Viale JP: Respiratory changes induced by parenteral nutrition in postoperative patients undergoing inspiratory pressure support ventilation. Anesthesiology 1987;66:393–396
57. Laaban JB, Lemaire F, Baron JF et al: Influence of caloric intake on the respiratory mode during mandatory minute ventilation. Chest 1985;87:67–72
58. MacFie J, Holmfield JHM et al: Effect of the energy source on changes in energy expenditure and respiratory quotient during total parenteral nutrition. JPEN J Parenter Enteral Nutr 1983;7:1–5
59. Nordenstrom J, Askanazi J, Elwyn DH et al: Nitrogen balance during total parenteral nutrition. Glucose vs. fat. Ann Surg 1983;197:27–33
60. Dark DS, Pingleton SK, Kerby GR: Hypercapnia during weaning. A complication of nutritional support. Chest 1985;88:141–143
61. Askanazi J, Nordenstrom J, Rosenbaum SH et al: Nutrition for the patient with respiratory failure: Glucose vs. fat. Anesthesiology 1981;54:373–377
62. van dem Berg B, Stam H: Metabolic and respiratory effects of enteral nutrition in patients during mechanical ventilation. Intensive Care Med 1988;14:209–211
63. Al-Saady NM, Blackmore CM, Bennett ED: High fat, low carbohydrate, enteral feeding lowers $PaCO_2$ and reduces the period of ventilation in artificially ventilated patients. Intensive Care Med 1989;15:290–295
64. Venus B, Smith RA, Patel C, Dandoval E: Hemodynamic and gas exchange alterations during intralipid infusion in patients with adult respiratory distress syndrome. Chest 1989;95:1278–1281
65. Greene LHL, Hazlett D, Demaree R: Relationship between intralipid-induced hyperlipidemia and pulmonary function. Am J Clin Nutr 1976;29:127–135
66. Hwang T, Huang S, Chen M: Effects of intravenous fat emulsion on respiratory failure. Chest 1990;97:934–938
67. Pesola GE, Hogg JE, Yonnios T et al: Isotonic nasogastric tube feedings: Do they cause diarrhea? Crit Care Med 1989;17:1151–1155
68. Harris MR, Huseby JS: Pulmonary complications from nasoenteral feeding tube insertion in an intensive care unit: Incidence and prevention. Crit Care Med 1989;17:917–919
69. Braum SR, Dixon RM, Keim NL et al: Predictive clinical value of nutritional assessment factors in COPD. Chest 1984;85:353–357
70. Schols A, Mostert R, Soeters P et al: Inventory of nutritional status in patients with COPD. Chest 1989;96:247–249
71. Wilson DO, Rogers RM, Wright EC, Anthonisen NR: Body weight in chronic obstructive pulmonary disease. Am Rev Respir Dis 1989;139:1435–1438
72. Efthimiou J, Fleming J, Gomes C, Spiro SG: The effect of supplementary oral nutrition in poorly nourished patients with chronic obstructive pulmonary disease. Am Rev Respir Dis 1988;137:1075–1082
73. Golstein SA, Thomashow BM, Kvetan V et al: Nitrogen and energy relationships in malnourished patients with emphysema. Am Rev Respir Dis 1988;138:636–644
74. Knowles JB, Fairbarn MS, Wiggs BJ et al: Dietary supplementation and respiratory muscle performance in patients with COPD. Chest 1988;93:977–983
75. Hunter AMB, Carey MA, Larsh HW: The nutritional status of patients with chronic obstructive pulmonary disease. Am Rev Respir Dis 1981;124:376–381
76. Openbreir DR, Irwin MM, Rogers RM et al: Nutritional status and lung function in patients with emphysema and chronic bronchitis. Chest 1983;83:17–22
77. Driver AG, McAlevy, Smith JL: Nutritional assessment of patients with chronic obstructive pulmonary disease and acute respiratory failure. Chest 1982;82:568–571
78. Fiaccadori E, Del Canale S, Coffrini E et al: Hypercapnic-hypoxemic chronic obstructive pulmonary disease (COPD): Influence of severity of COPD on nutritional status. Am J Clin Nutr 1988;48:680–685
79. Bynoe RP, Kudsk KA, Fabian TC, Brown RO: Nutrition support in trauma patients. Nutr Clin Pract 1988;3:137–144
80. Adams M, Luterman A: Nutritional support of the burn patient. Trauma Q 1989;5:45–55

Chapter 52

Assessment and Monitoring of Ventilatory Muscle Function

Robert M. Kacmarek

CHAPTER OUTLINE

The evaluation of ventilatory muscle function and the determination of dysfunction constitute an essential aspect of the assessment of the cardiopulmonary system. In a previously healthy young adult with neuromuscular or neurologic disease who experiences progressive ventilatory difficulty, ventilatory muscle dysfunction is relatively easy to identify and monitor. However, in the elderly patient with severe chronic obstructive pulmonary disease (COPD), who normally functions at a compromised level, it is difficult to quantify progressive muscular dysfunction until marked changes in clinical presentation and gas exchange are noted. This chapter details the methods, both laboratory and clinical, used to assess and monitor dysfunction of ventilatory muscles.

MEASUREMENT OF PRESSURES

As detailed in Chapter 5, a number of distinct pressures related to ventilatory muscle capabilities are measurable and can be monitored to assess ventilatory muscle function. Maximum inspiratory pressure (MIP) and maximum expiratory pressure (MEP) are the easiest and most frequently measured pressures, both in the laboratory and at bedside. Since MIP evaluates inspiratory muscle capability, its measurement should occur at the optimal (shortest) length of the inspiratory muscles or at residual volume (RV) level[1] to ensure maximum force generation, while MEP measurements are performed at total lung capacity (TLC) level.[2] As muscular dysfunction progresses, lower levels of MIP or MEP can be expected. Ventilatory failure has been associated with MIP measurements of less than 20 cmH_2O.[3,4]

MIP measurements provide a global assessment of inspiratory muscle function. Specific assessment of diaphragmatic function is best accomplished by the evaluation of transdiaphragmatic pressure (P_{di}),[5] which is equal to gastric pressure minus esophageal pressure and is measured with esophageal and gastric balloons. This measurement, although difficult to perform, provides a better assessment of diaphragm function and the presence of fatigue, especially if measured in conjunction with direct stimulation of the phrenic nerve.[6] When P_{di} measurements are made during phrenic nerve stimulation at various frequencies, a force-frequency curve can be developed, which can be used to detect peripheral fatigue.[7] Although this measurement accurately assesses diaphragmatic function, because of its invasiveness it is rarely performed at the bedside.

In the intensive care unit (ICU), MIP is used to assess ventilatory muscle strength, since inspiratory muscle dys-

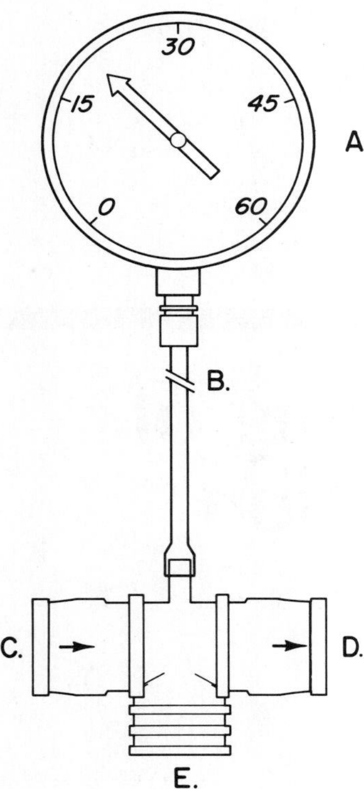

Figure 52-1. Apparatus used to determine MIP in patients with artificial airways. A, manometer; B, connecting tubing; C, inspiratory one-way valve with port for thumb occlusion; D, expiratory one-way port; E, 22-mm ID port for attachment to artificial airway. (From Kacmarek et al.[8] with permission.)

function is more commonly a cause of ventilatory failure than expiratory muscle dysfunction. Figure 52-1 depicts the apparatus we use to evaluate MIP. One-way valves are used to allow exhalation but not inspiration during the measurement. This ensures that the lung is at minimal volume and thus that the diaphragm is at its maximum fiber length during measurement.[8] In addition, measurement of MIP in the ICU should last 20 seconds to ensure that the patient is stressed to a level that results in maximal contraction.[9] A single measurement of one breath, as performed in the pulmonary function laboratory, normally results in a grossly diminished measurement. During MIP measurement the patient's electrocardiogram (ECG) and oxyhemoglobin saturation should be monitored, and the measurement should be discontinued if dysrhythmias or desaturation occur.

MEP is measured in the pulmonary function laboratory by having the patient exhale as forcefully as possible from TLC. However, this determination is of little use in the ICU and is rarely performed outside of the laboratory setting. Table 52-1 lists normal and abnormal levels of MIP, MEP, and P_{di}.

Table 52-1. Respiratory System Pressure Measurement

Measurement	Normal Value (cmH_2O)		Markedly Abnormal (cmH_2O)
	Males	Females	
MIP[1,2]	100–140	70–110	≤25
MEP[1,2]	200–250	130–170	≤50
P_{di}[3] (maximal)	90–110	70–90	≤30

LUNG VOLUMES

Ventilatory muscle weakness may also be assessed by evaluating lung volume, specifically, vital capacity (VC),[10] which is defined as the maximum volume that can be exhaled after a complete inspiration. As a gross estimate, VC in normal, healthy young adults is equal to about 70 to 90 mL/kg ideal body weight.[11] Decreases in VC always indicate a dimi-

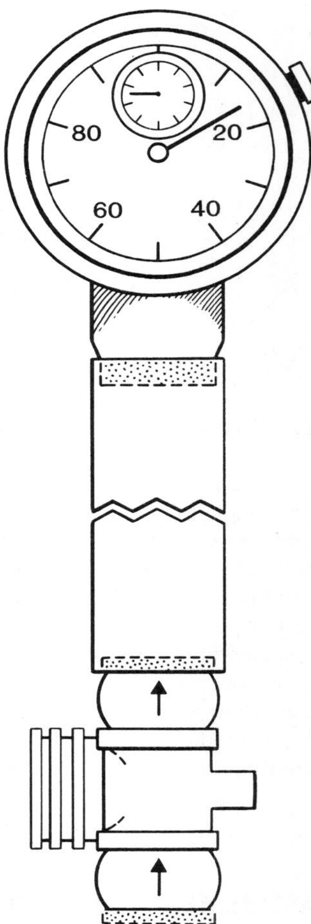

Figure 52-2. Apparatus used to determine VC in patients with artificial airways. A Wright respirometer is attached to a 6-inch flex tube, which in turn is attached to a T piece fitted with two one-way valves to allow unidirectional gas flow into the patient, with exhalation directed through the respirometer. (From Kacmarek et al.,[13] with permission.)

nution in ventilatory reserve, that is, a decrease in the ability to respond to stressful stimuli.[12] The closer the VC is to the tidal volume (V_T), the less is the ventilatory reserve and the greater is the ventilatory muscle dysfunction. Decreased VC can be directly attributed to dysfunction of the diaphragm and other inspiratory muscles. In the critically ill patient VC can be assessed by the use of any bedside spirometer (Fig. 52-2). As in the pulmonary function laboratory, patients are coached to take as deep a breath as possible and then to exhale as completely as possible. We customarily perform three measurements of VC, recording the largest. The major difficulty with the determination of VC in critically ill patients is their lack of cooperation; VC is a voluntary maneuver, requiring maximum patient effort. In those individuals with an artificial airway who are unable to cooperate with the measurement, we have found that measurement of the first exhaled volume following a 20-second MIP measurement produces a good estimate of the VC (Fig. 52-3). In fact, in a series of cooperative medical ICU patients, the MIP-induced exhaled volume was equal to the VC if 80 mL was added to the exhaled volume measurement.[13]

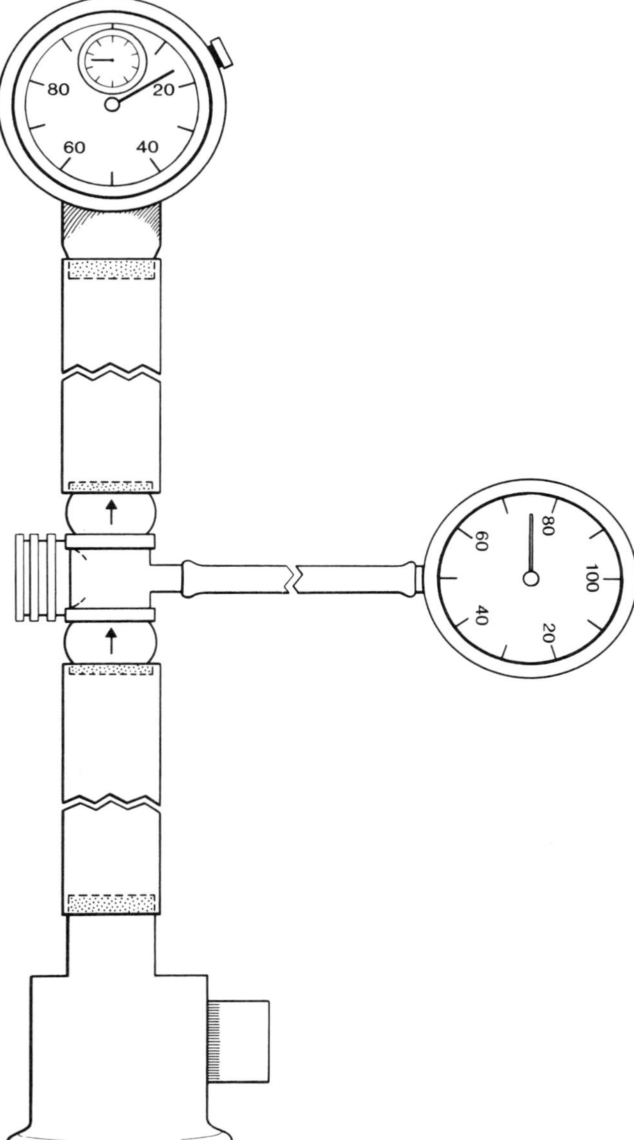

Figure 52-3. Apparatus used to determine MIP-induced exhaled volume in uncooperative patients with artificial airways. The basic setup is the same as for MIP determination (see Fig. 52-1), with the addition of a 6-inch flex tube and a Wright respirometer attached to the expiratory one-way valve outlet. After the MIP measurement the occlusion at the inspiratory port is released, allowing inspiration. The first exhalation is recorded. (From Kacmarek et al.,[13] with permission.)

It is difficult to identify a specific VC that is associated with ventilatory muscle failure or fatigue in the presence of underlying chronic lung disease. However, most would agree that a VC below 10 to 15 mL/kg ideal body weight in the normally healthy individual correlates well with an inability to sustain spontaneous ventilation for prolonged periods.[10]

DIAPHRAGMATIC ELECTROMYOGRAMS

One of the most reliable methods of assessing ventilatory muscle function is the evaluation of the electromyographic (EMG) activity of the diaphragm.[14] The EMG records the electrical activity of a muscle during contraction. If the electrical activity is divided into high and low frequencies, a ratio between these frequencies (H/L ratio) can be determined. In normally functioning muscle, the H/L ratio is greater than 80 percent.[15] Ratios below 80 percent indicate muscle fatigue.[15]

Another way to evaluate diaphragmatic function by using EMGs is to compare the integrated EMG activity (E_{di}) with the P_{di} or the P_{di}/E_{di} ratio.[16] As this ratio decreases, muscle dysfunction increases. Normally, an increase in electrical activity to the diaphragm results in a larger P_{di}. When this does not occur, dysfunction of the contractile process must be present. The lower the P_{di}/E_{di} ratio, the greater the probability of fatigue of the diaphragm.[14]

Although the assessment of EMG activity and P_{di} provide reliable indications of diaphragmatic function, their use has been relegated to the laboratory or to research studies. It is rare for these techniques to be used at the bedside. Assessment at the bedside is usually based on evaluation of the other variables discussed in this chapter.

TESTS OF ENDURANCE

In Chapter 26 sustained maximum voluntary ventilation (MVV) was described as that percentage of the MVV that can be maintained over time.[17] Normally, 60 percent of the MVV can be sustained for about 30 minutes. One method of estimating the capacity of ventilatory muscles to respond to increased stress is to have patients perform an MVV maneuver. If patients are capable of doubling their minute ventilation, the probability that sustained spontaneous ventilation can be maintained is high.[18] Although seemingly easy to perform at the bedside, MVV studies do require patient cooperation and as a result are unreliable, since it is difficult to elicit the level of cooperation required to properly perform an MVV maneuver in the ICU. As with VC determination, suboptimal performance is normally the rule. As a result, these studies are rarely performed in the ICU.

VENTILATORY PATTERN

Of all the various tests used to assess ventilatory muscle dysfunction, in my opinion assessment of ventilatory pattern may be the most reliable. The single factor that most correlates with failure to sustain spontaneous ventilation in studies of patients being weaned from ventilatory support is respiratory rate.[19–21] Since respiratory rate frequently correlates directly with ventilatory work, the need for high respiratory rates is frequently a prelude to ventilatory muscle dysfunction. Many have indicated that respiratory rates over 35 per minute cannot be sustained and signal the development of fatigue.[10,11]

VT is less precise than respiratory rate but does provide some insight into ventilatory muscle dysfunction.[21] As the VT decreases, the ability to sustain spontaneous ventilation must be questioned, although many patients are capable of maintaining adequate gas exchange for hours in spite of a VT at physiologic dead space levels (150 to 200 mL). However, ventilatory patterns defined by small VT levels, especially if respiratory rate is high, normally indicate ventilatory muscle dysfunction. Tobin and associates[21,22] have used the respiratory rate/VT ratio (f/VT) as an indicator of muscular dysfunction. Normally, the f/VT is about 40 to 60 breaths/min/L.[21] Values over 100 are indicative of dysfunction and poor probability of sustained spontaneous ventilation[21] (see Ch. 86).

Recruitment of accessory muscles also signals significant ventilatory muscle stress. If the need for accessory muscle use is continual, the probability of fatigue is increased, especially if this need is associated with alterations in respiratory rate and VT volume and with ventilatory muscle dissynchrony.

Dissynchrony of abdominal and chest wall movement is also an indicator of ventilatory muscle dysfunction.[20,22] During normal breathing, whether quiet or stressed, the sequence of abdominal and chest wall movement is (1) the abdomen protrudes as the diaphragm contracts; (2) the lateral chest wall expands as a result of diaphragm and external intercostal contraction; and (3) the upper chest wall expands because of external intercostal contraction. *Thoracoabdominal dissynchrony*, or *discoordinate breathing*, is defined as a variation from the normal pattern. The two patterns associated with diaphragmatic fatigue are paradoxical breathing and respiratory alternans.[20]

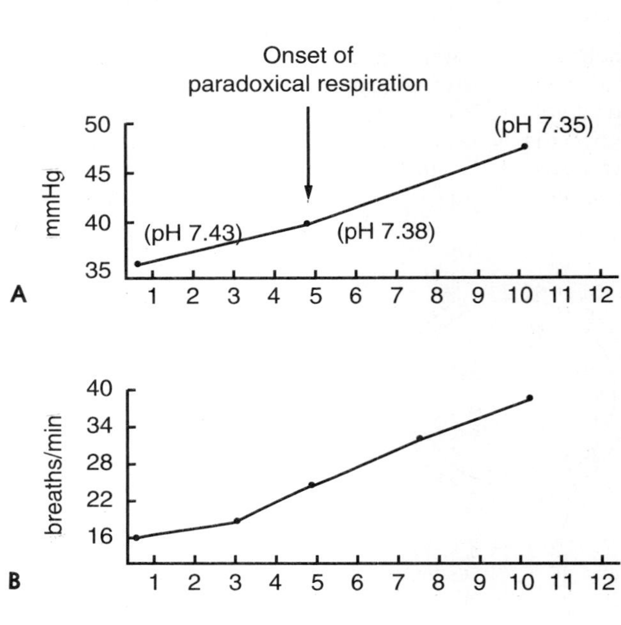

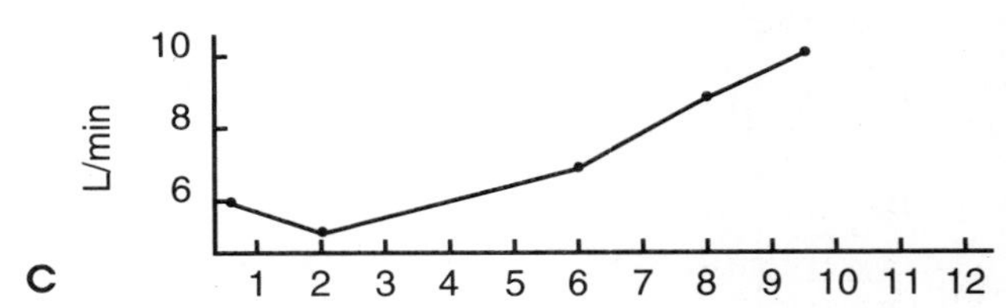

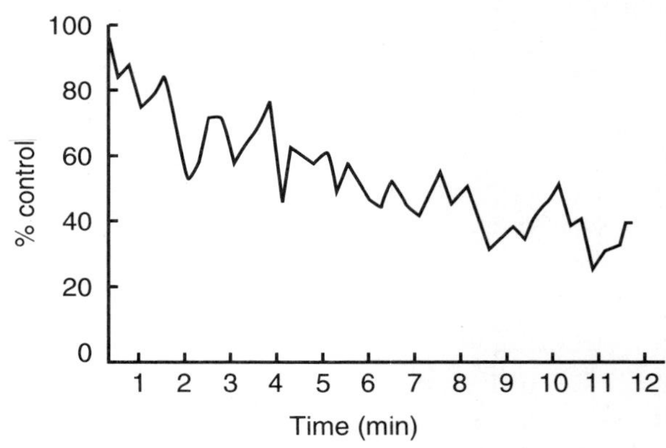

Figure 52-4. Sequence of changes in **(A)** $PaCO_2$, **(B)** respiratory rate, **(C)** minute ventilation, and **(D)** H/L frequency distribution of the diaphragmatic EMG in a patient during a 20-minute attempt at discontinuation from ventilatory support. The $PaCO_2$ initially fell, and the patient became alkalemic. Paradoxical abdominal movements were not noted until after there had been substantial increases in respiratory rate and minute ventilation. Hypercapnia and respiratory acidosis did not develop until after abdominal paradox and respiratory alternans were noted. Just before mechanical ventilation was reinstituted, there was a sharp fall in respiratory frequency and minute ventilation. The H/L ratio of the diaphragm indicated a fatiguing load after 1 minute of spontaneous ventilation. (From Cohen et al.,[20] with permission.)

Table 52-2. Signs of Severe Respiratory Muscle Dysfunction in Order of Occurrence

Decreased H/L ratio of EMG
Respiratory alternans
Paradoxical breathing
Accessory muscle use
Increased respiratory rate
Increased minute ventilation
Increased $PaCO_2$
Decreased pHa

Associated with these changes is a stimulation of the cardiovascular system (e.g., increase pulse and blood pressure).
(From Cohen et al.,[20] with permission.)

Paradoxical breathing is best defined as an inward movement of the abdomen during inspiration. This is commonly seen in patients with diaphragmatic paralysis and indicates that the diaphragm is not contracting properly. Inward movement of the abdomen may also be seen in severe COPD, with marked hyperinflation, resulting in a flattened diaphragm. Here, contraction causes a decrease in the diameter of the lateral rib cage and may show inward abdominal movement. Although the reason for inward abdominal movement is the flattened diaphragm, many patients with this condition also demonstrate dysfunctional diaphragmatic muscles. Respiratory alternans is an alternation between a normal respiratory pattern and paradoxical breathing.

The sequence in which clinical signs of ventilatory muscle fatigue presents is still controversial. Cohen et al.[20] (Fig. 52-4) noted respiratory alternans or paradoxical breathing in a series of patients whom they were attempting to wean from mechanical ventilation before changes in respiratory rate, minute ventilation, $PaCO_2$ or pH were noted. These authors noted paradoxical breathing whenever the H/L ratio of the diaphragmatic EMG indicated fatigue. As may be seen from Figure 52-4, respiratory rate markedly increased before $PaCO_2$. In general, $PaCO_2$ is a late sign of muscle fatigue (Table 52-2). By the time the $PaCO_2$ increases, fatigue is well established. As a result, clinical signs of fatigue should always be used to monitor the presence of muscle dysfunction, not $PaCO_2$, which should be used to substantiate the diagnosis. In other words, during weaning trials decisions to terminate the trial are best based on alterations in ventilatory pattern, not on changes in blood gases. If spontaneous breathing trials are pushed until large changes in $PaCO_2$ are noted, marked ventilatory muscle dysfunction may occur.

TENSION-TIME INDEX

Bellemare and Grassino,[23] in 1982, presented a unifying view of diaphragmatic fatigue by evaluating tension developed during diaphragmatic contraction in relation to the amount of time contraction was maintained, referred to as the *tension-time index* (TT_{di}) of the diaphragm (Fig. 52-5). On the time axis the ratio of inspiratory time (TI) to total

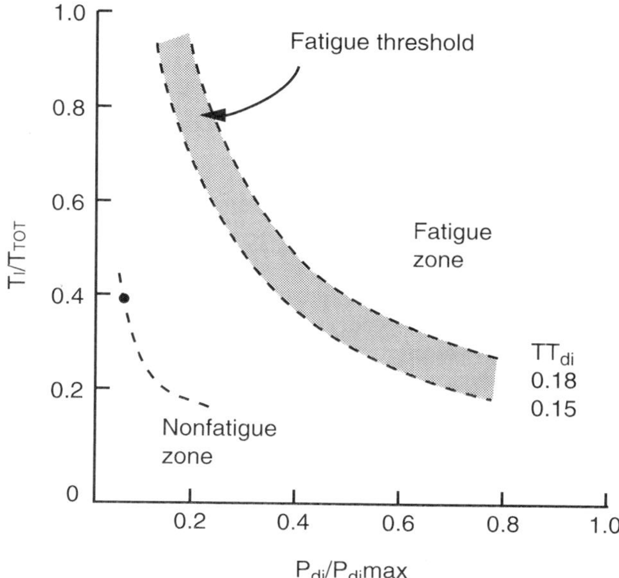

Figure 52-5. Tension-time index for the human diaphragm (TT_{di}). The inspiratory time/total ventilatory cycle time ratio (T_I/T_{TOT}) plotted against the ratio of transdiaphragmatic pressure during normal breathing to the maximum P_{di} possible ($P_{di}/P_{di}max$). The fatigue threshold represents a TT_{di} that can be sustained for 1 hour or longer and has a value of 0.15 to 0.18 in the normal human diaphragm. The TT_{di} threshold can be achieved with a large variety of P_{di} and T_I/T_{TOT} values. Patterns in the "fatigue zone" will result in fatigue in less than 1 hour; patterns in the nonfatigue zone can be sustained indefinitely. The circle represents TT_{di} during resting breathing in normal subjects. (From Grassino et al.,[24] with permission.)

ventilatory cycle time (T_{TOT}) is plotted. Normally, T_I is about 30 to 40 percent of T_{TOT}. The greater the percentage T_I is of T_{TOT}, the shorter the recovery time postcontraction, and the greater the probability of fatigue.[23] The tension axis shows the ratio of the P_{di} required during a tidal breath to the maximum P_{di} obtainable ($P_{di}max$). As may be seen from Figure 52-5, $P_{di}/P_{di}max$ ratio is normally about 5 to 15 percent. The greater the tidal P_{di} or the lower the $P_{di}max$, the less reserve available to the muscle and the greater the probability of fatigue.[24] For normal, healthy individuals, a tension-time index of about 0.035 is obtained from the T_I/T_{TOT} versus $P_{di}/P_{di}max$.[23] If this index exceeds 0.15, the probability of fatigue is greatly increased, and if it exceeds 0.18, fatigue will occur if the ventilatory pattern is maintained. The 0.15 to 0.18 range is referred to as the *fatigue threshold*.[24]

The T_I/T_{TOT} ratio has a much more limited range than the $P_{di}/P_{di}max$ ratio. T_I/T_{TOT} normally does not exceed 0.5, but $P_{di}/P_{di}max$ may approach 1.0 during severe ventilatory fatigue. Although P_{di} is rarely measured in the ICU, MIP measurement provides a global evaluation of the inspiratory muscles, of which the diaphragm is primary, especially in the patient with an artificial airway. Thus, at the bedside the

TT_{di} can be at least qualitatively assessed by comparing respiratory rate with MIP, since the T_I/T_{TOT} ratio increases as respiratory rate increases, as does the tension required for each V_T. It has been our clinical impression that fatigue and ventilatory failure are directly related to respiratory rate and indirectly related to MIP.

BEDSIDE ASSESSMENT

Evaluation of ventilatory muscle function can be accurately performed in the laboratory. However, assessment at the bedside is much more difficult and much less precise. Bedside monitoring of respiratory rate, ventilatory pattern, and MIP, in our opinion, provides the most reliable clinical data to guide evaluations of ventilatory muscle function. $PaCO_2$ and pHa, although definitive for the presence of acute fatigue, are poor monitors of the development of fatigue, since, as noted by Cohen et al.,[20] increases in $PaCO_2$ and decreases in pHa normally occur after fatigue develops (provided ventilatory drive is intact).

References

1. Black LF, Hyatt RE: Maximal respiratory pressures: Normal valves and relationship to age and sex. Am Rev Respir Dis 1969;99:696–702
2. Nickerson BG, Keens TG: Measuring ventilatory muscle endurance in humans as sustainable inspiratory pressure. J Appl Physiol 1982;52:768–772
3. Sahn SA, Lakshminarayan S: Bedside criteria for discontinuation of mechanical ventilation. Chest 1973;63:1002–1005
4. Feeley TW, Hedley-Whyte T: Weaning from controlled ventilation and supplemental oxygen. N Engl J Med 1975;292:903–906
5. Gibson GJ, Clark E, Pride NB: Static transdiaphragmatic pressures in normal subjects and in patients with chronic hyperinflation. Am Rev Respir Dis 1981;124:685–689
6. Aubier M, Farkas G, DeTroyer A et al: Detection of diaphragmatic fatigue in man by phrenic stimulation. J Appl Physiol 1981;50:538–544
7. Moxham J, Morris AJR, Spiro SG et al: Contractile properties and fatigue of the diaphragm in man. Thorax 1981;34:164–168
8. Kacmarek RM, Cycyk-Chapman MC, Young-Palazzo PJ, Romagnoli DM: Determination of maximal inspiratory pressure: A clinical study and literature review. Respir Care 1989;34:868–878
9. Marini JJ, Smith TC, Lamb V: Estimation of inspiratory muscle strength in mechanically ventilated patients: Measurement of maximal inspiratory pressure. J Crit Care 1988;1:32–38
10. Shapiro BA, Kacmarek RM, Cane R et al: Clinical Application of Respiratory Care. 4th Ed. Mosby-Year Book, St. Louis, 1990
11. Kacmarek RM, Mack C, Dimas S: The Essentials of Respiratory Care. 3rd Ed. Mosby-Year Book, St. Louis, 1990
12. Feeley TW, Hedley-Whyte T: Weaning from controlled ventilation and supplemental oxygen. N Engl J Med 1975;292:903–906
13. Kacmarek RM, Foley K, Cheever P, Romagnoli D: Determination of ventilatory reserve in mechanically ventilated patients: A comparison of techniques. Respir Care 1991;36:1085–1092
14. Roussos C, Moxham J: Respiratory muscle fatigue. In Roussos C, Macklem P (eds): The Thorax. Marcel Decker, Philadelphia, 1985
15. Gross D, Grassino A, Ross WRD, Macklem PT: Electromyogram pattern of diaphragmatic fatigue. J Appl Physiol 1979;46:1–7
16. Aubier M, Trippenback T, Roussos C: Respiratory muscle fatigue during cardiogenic shock. J Appl Physiol 1981;51:499–508
17. Rochester DF, Arora NS, Braun NMT et al: The respiratory muscles in chronic obstructive pulmonary disease (COPD). Bull Eur Physiopathol Respir 1979;15:951–960
18. Sahn SA, Lakshminarayan S: Bedside criteria for discontinuation of mechanical ventilation. Chest 1973;63:1002–1005
19. Pierson DJ: Weaning from mechanical ventilation in acute respiratory failure. Concepts, indications and techniques. Respir Care 1983;28:646–662
20. Cohen C, Zagelbaum G, Gross D et al: Clinical manifestations of inspiratory muscle fatigue. Am J Med 1982;73:308–316
21. Tobin MJ, Perez W, Guenther SM et al: The pattern of breathing during successful and unsuccessful trials of weaning from mechanical ventilation. Am Rev Respir Dis 1986;134:1111–1118
22. Tobin MJ, Perez W, Guenther SM et al: Does rib cage abdominal paradox signify respiratory muscle fatigue? J Appl Physiol 1987;63:851–860
23. Bellemare F, Grassino A: Effect of pressure and timing of contraction on human diaphragm fatigue. J Appl Physiol 1982;53:1190–1195
24. Grassino A, Bellemare F, Laporta D: Diaphragm fatigue and the strategy of breathing in COPD. Chest 1984;85:51S–54S

Chapter 53

Assessment and Management of Airway Protection, Obstruction, and Secretion Clearance

Robert M. Kacmarek
David J. Pierson

CHAPTER OUTLINE

Although they are central to many facets of intensive respiratory care, assessment and management of the airways tend to be neglected subjects. There are literally hundreds of studies on the initiation and discontinuation of mechanical ventilation and many more on the specifics of ventilator management, but almost none on assessment of the adequacy of airway protection and secretion clearance, primarily because of the inherent difficulties of quantifying these important functions. As a result the clinician must depend on common sense and empirically derived guidelines for most aspects of airway management.

For all practical purposes, management of acute respiratory failure with mechanical ventilation requires endotracheal intubation or tracheotomy, and discontinuation of invasive management means removal of the tubes placed during these procedures. Failure to intubate and ventilate in time may result in death or irreversible brain damage from hypoxia or respiratory acidosis; inappropriate delay in extubation prolongs the patient's jeopardy from nosocomial pneumonia and airway damage and invites self-extubation.

The subject of this chapter is thus both crucially important and largely lacking in objective data to guide the clinician. In view of this, our intent is to provide a logical approach to ensuring the adequacy of airway patency and secretion clearance, which is based on physiology and buttressed by practical experience. We first examine the need for establishing an artificial airway, considering the mechanisms by which such a need might arise, and then discuss how to determine that a given patient no longer needs an endotracheal tube and how to carry out extubation in the safest, most successful manner. The rest of the chapter deals with the tracheostomized patient. It discusses how to predict the adequacy of upper airway function following decannulation and describes the various appliances that may be used in a stepwise progression from use of a standard cuffed tracheostomy tube to complete decannulation.

ASSESSMENT OF THE NEED FOR INTUBATION

The four primary reasons for endotracheal intubation or tracheotomy are (1) to provide positive-pressure ventilation; (2) to bypass or prevent upper airway obstruction; (3) to prevent aspiration; and (4) to facilitate secretion clearance. In addition, artificial airways are necessary in some patients to ensure consistent and precise delivery of O_2. Chapter 81 discusses determination of the need for ventilation, and Chapters 75 and 76 discusses oxygenation. As for the other primary indications listed, while extreme examples are not hard to envision, bedside methods for objective assessment are sorely needed but generally lacking.

Table 53-1 lists a number of clinical settings in which intubation may be required to prevent aspiration or to maintain patency of the airway. However, when confronted with a patient with any of the listed conditions, the clinician must still decide whether the upper airway is compromised enough, the bulbar weakness severe enough, or the airway secretions copious enough to warrant intubation. No exact criteria could be listed that would cover all patients. Still, consideration of several types of clinical information can help in the decision process. Whether establishment of an artificial airway is desirable will depend on

The severity of the problem threatening the airway (e.g., impending upper airway obstruction, potential aspiration, obstructing secretions)

The patient's underlying respiratory status (e.g., airflow obstruction, severe restriction, vascular impairment, disordered ventilatory regulation)

The nature, severity, and expected duration of the acute episode (e.g., transient fluid overload versus gram-negative pneumonia)

The availability of alternative measures to intubation (e.g., pharmacologic reversal of the effect of narcotics or neuromuscular blocking agents)

The first two of the above-listed factors are especially important; also key is the coexistence of two or more of the items listed in Table 53-1. Mild impairment of consciousness, for example, in a patient with partial upper airway obstruction or underlying bulbar weakness, can mandate immediate intubation, whereas any of these three factors by themselves may not.

Table 53-1. Clinical Settings in Which Intubation May Be Required to Prevent Aspiration or Maintain Airway Patency

Impaired consciousness (loss of reflexes protecting airway)
- Primary
  - Drug overdose, head trauma, brain tumor, cerebrovascular accident, central nervous system infection
- Secondary
  - Administration of sedatives, narcotic analgesics, inhalational anesthetics

Upper airway obstruction (physical impingement on airway lumen)
- Trauma to face or neck
- Infections
  - Peritonsillar abscess, acute epiglottitis, croup
- Foreign body
- Neoplasm
- Postsurgical swelling
- Laryngeal edema
  - Angioedema, anaphylaxis, postextubation
- Instrumentation
  - Sengstaken-Blakemore tube, endoscopy, operative procedures on upper airway

Neuromuscular weakness
- Amyotrophic lateral sclerosis
- Guillain-Barré syndrome
- Cerebrovascular accident
- Myasthenia gravis
- Lambert-Eaton syndrome
- Administration of muscle relaxants (e.g., pancuronium bromide)

Excessive volume of potential aspirate
- From upper respiratory tract
  - Blood (e.g., massive epistaxis)
- From lower respiratory tract
  - Sputum, blood, sloughed airway epithelium (e.g., in acute inhalation injury)
- From gastrointestinal tract
  - Vomitus, blood (e.g., massive hematemesis)

ASSESSMENT FOR EXTUBATION

The familiar "weaning parameters" (ventilation requirement, spontaneous vital capacity, maximum inspiratory force) that have been used for predicting a patient's ability to ventilate without assistance have no counterparts for extubation. In large measure this is because ventilatory needs and capabilities are relatively easy to quantitate at the bedside, while there is no convenient measurement to predict reliably whether patients can protect their airways, avoid aspirating, and adequately clear secretions. Lacking objective measurements and a body of literature, the clinician must nonetheless decide when extubation can safely be carried out. Table 53-2 presents a set of criteria for extubation based on the possible reasons for intubation and a logical plan for assessing them.

Weaning and extubation are often lumped together. In fact, in a number of published reports it is impossible to tell whether ventilator weaning, extubation, or both were being studied. And while many patients can simply be extubated once the ventilator is no longer needed, this is clearly not the case for others. It is safest to think of weaning and extubation as separate processes and to assess patients separately for each. First, the patient must no longer need the ventilator for alveolar ventilation and oxygenation. In general, a trial of spontaneous ventilation with the endotracheal tube still in place is the safest approach, since if the patient is unexpectedly incapable of generating the required minute ventilation or quickly demonstrates signs of ventilatory muscle fatigue and respiratory distress, reintubation will not be required.

The work of spontaneous breathing through a small-di-

Table 53-2. Clinical Assessment for Extubation

Ability to maintain adequate ventilation and oxygenation
- Patient does not need mechanical ventilation (e.g., meets criteria for weaning)
- F_{IO_2} requirement achievable by mask or nasal cannula

No immediate need for future intubation or mechanical ventilation
- Impending procedures requiring intubation and mechanical ventilation (e.g., surgery, angiography, CT scan)
- Developing medical problem that may increase need for airway protection and mechanical ventilation (e.g., alcohol withdrawal, upper gastrointestinal bleeding)

Ability to spontaneously clear secretions
- Maximum inspiratory/expiratory pressures
- Generation of adequate forced airflow
- Ability to cough (intact glottic function)[a]
- Underlying pulmonary status

Ability to maintain adequate peak lung inflation (i.e., to prevent atelectasis)
- Spontaneous inspiratory vital capacity

Ability to protect airway and avoid aspiration (see Table 53-1)
- Intact gag reflex
- Mental status, sensorium, ability to cooperate with care

[a] Difficult to assess with endotracheal tube in place.

ameter endotracheal tube (see Ch. 72, Fig. 72-7) can be substantially greater than would be the case following extubation, particularly if the minute ventilation is high. Because of this, a few patients may "fail" a T-piece trial who can nonetheless be successfully extubated. If this situation is suspected, empirical extubation with its risk of emergency reintubation can be avoided by using low-level pressure support during the T-piece trial to effectively neutralize the endotracheal tube's additional resistance and its attendant increase in the work of breathing. Table 53-3 shows approximate levels of pressure support required to counteract this added resistance without providing the patient with additional ventilatory support; these levels depend on the size of the endotracheal tube and the patient's minute ventilation. The table has been adapted from a bench study,[1] which empirically determined these levels during a square-wave inspiratory flow pattern.

In reality, inspiratory flow changes continuously, so that the pressure support levels shown can only be regarded as general approximations. However, Table 53-3 is used routinely at Harborview Medical Center to determine pressure

Table 53-3. Pressure Support Required to Overcome Tube Resistance during T-Piece Trials or Low-Rate IMV

Endotracheal Tube Diameter (mm)	Patient's Minute Ventilation (L/min)		
	12	16	20
6	11	17	47
7	5	8	20
8	5	5	9

IMV, intermittent mandatory ventilation.

support levels during T-piece trials when patients have very small endotracheal tubes or are considered marginal weaning candidates because of respiratory muscle weakness or general frailty. Such patients are then extubated directly from this level of pressure support.

Once clinicians have determined that patients no longer need ventilatory assistance, judgments must be made about their ability to spontaneously clear secretions, to maintain peak lung inflation that is adequate to prevent development of atelectasis, and to protect the airway from aspiration. Table 53-2 lists general guidelines for these judgments, although most must be made subjectively rather than by specific measurements. Assessment of the presence and strength of a patient's gag reflex is especially difficult in the presence of an endotracheal tube, and the usual maneuver, which uses a tongue blade, must be considered only the grossest of tests. Finally, the patient's mental status and ability to cooperate with airway care and bronchial hygiene following extubation are also important.

Successful extubation must surely be associated with some combination of level of consciousness, amount and character of secretions, vigor of cough, and underlying pulmonary function. Studies prospectively examining these and other possible predictors in well defined patient groups would be of great help to the clinician.

EXTUBATION PROTOCOL

Once the decision to extubate has been made, a number of specific steps should be followed before and during extubation (Table 53-4), the first of which is assistance with removal of secretions from the lower respiratory tract. This frequently includes chest physiotherapy, aerosolized bronchodilator therapy, and vigorous tracheal suction. Following suctioning of the lower respiratory tract, the oral pharynx and larynx should be meticulously suctioned to remove all secretions that have pooled above the cuff of the endotracheal tube. If these secretions are not removed, the probability of their aspiration during extubation is high.

After the clinician has made sure that bronchial hygiene and secretion removal are complete, the patient's cuff is deflated and the endotracheal tube removed while positive pressure is applied to the airway with a manual ventilator.

Table 53-4. Extubation Procedure

Bronchial hygiene therapy
- Aerosolized bronchodilator
- Chest physiotherapy
- Suctioning of lower airway

Suctioning of oral pharynx and larynx
Removal of airway-securing tape
Cuff deflation
Extubation with positive pressure via manual ventilator
Cough
Assessment of upper airway obstruction
Administration of aerosolized racemic epinephrine
Assessment of ability to protect the airway

Manual ventilation will force secretions remaining above the cuff into the mouth during the extubation procedure. Once extubated, the patient should be encouraged to cough to clear any secretions aspirated during the procedure.

ASSESSMENT OF THE AIRWAY FOLLOWING EXTUBATION

In evaluating the patient in the immediate postextubation period, two primary concerns predominate, namely, obstruction of the airway and the ability of the patient to protect the airway from aspiration. With both endotracheal and tracheostomy tubes, postextubation or postdecannulation obstruction and aspiration may occur. However, in tracheostomized patients, detailed assessment of the patient's ability to perform these functions can be carried out prior to decannulation. This is not the case with endotracheal intubation. Careful and detailed postextubation evaluation is critical in all extubated patients, and is especially important when the period of intubation has been several days or longer.

Obstruction

The most critical problem following endotracheal extubation is obstruction at the level of the larynx. Obstruction may occur as a result of the development of laryngospasm or laryngeal edema. Laryngospasm is the primary concern in the first few minutes postextubation. In some patients the extubation procedure causes stimulation of the superior laryngeal nerve, resulting in sustained activation of the glottic closure reflex.[2] This reflex normally results in sphincter closure of the upper airway at three levels[3]:

1. Approximation of the aryepiglottic folds by contraction of the thyroarytenoid muscles results in a functional closure of the epiglottis (Fig. 53-1).
2. Contraction of the thyroarytenoid muscles also brings together the false vocal cords. Although there is a functional closure at this level, the false vocal cords do little to prevent the ingress of air or foreign material into the lung but play a predominant role in preventing the egress of air from the lung[4] (Fig. 53-2).
3. The most formidable barrier to the ingress of air and foreign material into the lower respiratory tract is provided by the true vocal cords, formed in part by the inferior division of each thyroarytenoid muscle.[5] Because the true vocal cords are shelf-like, with slightly upturned free borders, they are capable of resisting pressures of up to 140 mmHg from above.[5] As a result, the development of laryngospasm may be life-threatening.

Laryngospasm occurs primarily during intubation of the well oxygenated and ventilated patient in the operating room and during elective extubation. The hypoxemia and hypercarbia present during acute intubations outside of the operating room result in direct depression of adductor motor response and relaxation of the airway closure reflex,[3] minimizing the probability of laryngospasm in this setting.

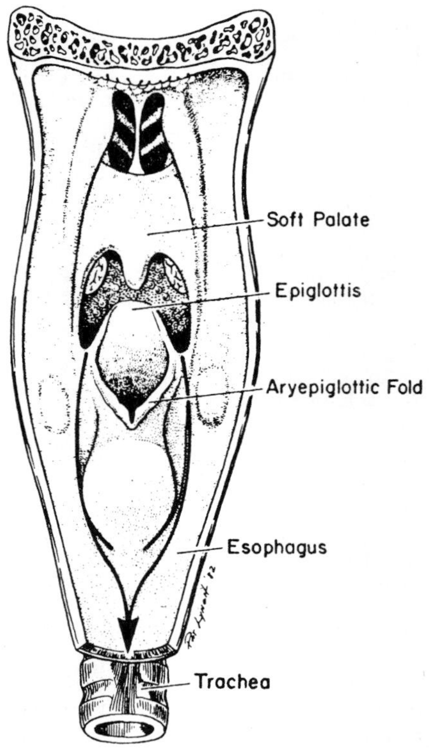

Figure 53-1. View of the larynx and pharynx from posterior to anterior. Arrows depict the route of food during swallowing. The epiglottis and the aryepiglottic folds direct food around the laryngeal opening. In addition, the bolus of food itself helps to close the epiglottis over the laryngeal opening. (From Sasaki and Isaacson,[3] with permission.)

The presence of laryngospasm postextubation is easily established. The patient presents with (1) marked audible inspiratory and expiratory stridor; (2) significant respiratory distress; and (3) in some cases complete airway obstruction. If laryngospasm is prolonged, cardiopulmonary failure may develop. When confronted with this scenario, the clinician should rapidly oxygenate the patient with 100 percent O_2 via a manual ventilator, with the head, neck and jaw properly placed to ensure maximum airway opening. Although the spasm markedly increases resistance to ventilation, continuous positive pressure should be applied, followed by small tidal volume ventilation as the airway opens.[6] In severe cases intravenous muscle relaxants may be necessary.[7]

Postextubation laryngeal edema is normally less acute than laryngospasm, with its progression frequently insidious. As with marked laryngospasm, however, reintubation may be necessary if the condition becomes severe. Most patients experience some laryngeal edema postextubation, manifested by loss of voice, hoarseness, sore throat, and minor

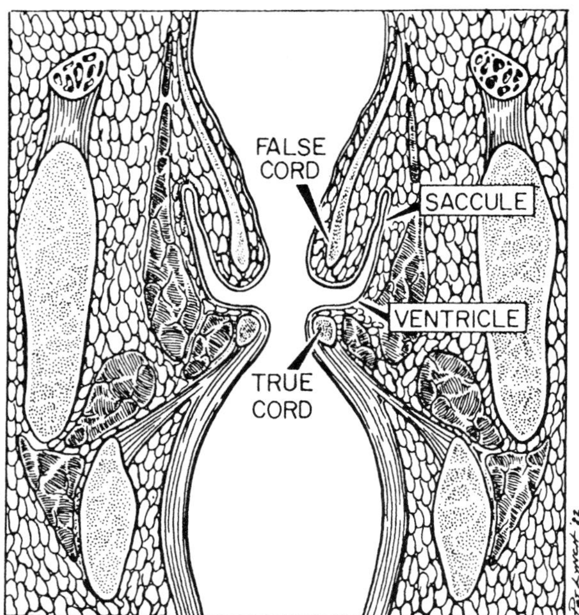

Figure 53-2. Frontal section through the larynx, indicating the valvular structures of the false and true vocal cords. (From Sasaki and Isaacson,[3] with permission.)

inspiratory stridor on auscultation of the lateral neck. This usually resolves in a matter of hours or days with administration of a continuous cool aerosol. Many clinicians also administer periodic racemic epinephrine (Vaponephrine) aerosols for their vasoconstricting effect.[6,8,9] Others have recommended the use of 1 mg of dexamethasone sodium phosphate (Decadron) aerosol postextubation,[6] although its effect is questionable, since steroids generally require 12 to 24 hours to produce effects. In the patient who has required reintubation because of laryngeal edema, a 48-hour course of systemic steroid therapy should precede attempted extubations.

In infants presenting with stridor postextubation, Kemper et al.[10] have improved gas exchange and prevented reintubation by administration of He-O_2 mixtures. Because of the low density of helium and the small tidal volumes of infants, the use of this less dense gas may markedly decrease the resistance to gas flow across the larynx. The efficacy of He-O_2 mixtures has not been demonstrated in adults.

Aspiration

Postextubation aspiration occurs as a result of a disruption of the normal swallowing (deglutition) mechanism because of disuse, trauma, or neurologic dysfunction.[11,12] Deglutition is performed in four distinct stages: oral preparation, the oral stage, the pharyngeal stage, and the esophageal stage.[13] Each stage is essential for normal swallowing (Fig. 53-3). Problems in any stage may result in aspiration. The oral preparatory stage, in which food is broken down and mixed with saliva, requires coordinated jaw motion, lip closure, and tongue movement, as well as a widening of the nasal airway and a narrowing of the oropharyngeal inlet to allow normal breathing via the nose. If appropriate coordination is lacking, food may be scattered about the mouth, allowing passage into the pharynx at a later time and aspiration. Poor closure of the soft palate may allow food to fall into the open airway.

In the oral stage, food is formed into a bolus and is moved by the tongue in a peristaltic manner into the pharynx. If coordination of the oral stage is lacking, food may fall into the valleculae, eventually continuing into the airway.

The pharyngeal stage of swallowing is the most complex, requiring coordination of the following activities to prevent aspiration[11,13]: (1) velopharyngeal closure (closure of the nasopharynx); (2) laryngeal closure (as discussed above); (3) laryngeal elevation and anterior movement of the larynx under the tongue to allow access to the esophagus; and (4) relaxation of the cricopharyngeus muscle. This coordinated activity allows the bolus to pass into the valleculae and then through the pyriform sinuses into the entrance of the esophagus.[14] Inappropriate performance of any of these activities may result in aspiration. Finally, the esophageal stage involves the active peristaltic movement of food through the esophagus.

Postextubation assessment of swallowing can be performed at the bedside by having the patient attempt to swallow progressively more difficult substances—ice chips initially, followed by clear liquids, soft solids, and finally normal food. If the patient chokes and coughs while attempting to swallow, the trial should be stopped and repeated at a later time. It is essential to place patients in the sitting position during swallow evaluation and to instruct them to exaggerate each stage of swallowing to ensure proper mechanical function. Those failing repetitive trials require formal evaluation by a speech therapist and possibly video fluoroscopy (barium swallow). Speech therapy can frequently identify swallowing disorders by palpation of the external laryngeal area[15] (Fig. 53-4). Results of this assessment may be sufficient to determine exercises that would improve swallowing or may signal the need for a barium swallow to fully identify the mechanical malfunction.

In patients intubated endotracheally, problems are frequently at the level of the true or false vocal cords as a result of trauma or possibly as a result of disuse of the muscles associated with swallowing. In many patients simple muscle reconditioning may eliminate the problem; in others dysfunction may require tracheotomy or other surgical intervention. In post-tracheotomy patients, the primary dysfunction is an inability to lift the larynx during the pharyngeal stage of swallowing.[15–19] This can be corrected with exercise or surgical manipulation of the tracheostomy site.

ASSESSMENT FOR DECANNULATION IN THE PATIENT WITH A TRACHEOSTOMY

Provided that a patient with a tracheostomy can breathe spontaneously, the clinician weighing the decision to decannulate must make sure that the patient can clear secretions, has no upper airway obstruction inhibiting ventilation, and can protect the lower airway. Assessment of these variables is much easier in the presence of a tracheostomy tube than with an endotracheal tube, since alternate tracheal appliances can be used to gradually allow the patient to ventilate via the upper respiratory tract.

Aspiration

The performance of a tracheotomy and the presence of a tracheostomy tube can markedly affect the pharyngeal stage of swallowing.[12,13] The severity of this impairment is related to the specific surgical procedure used in the tracheotomy. The skin incision and subsequent tracheal ring incision may be performed by one of two methods, using either a horizontal or a vertical incision. The horizontal incision is cosmetically more acceptable and as a result is more frequently performed. This type of incision may interfere with swallowing, especially if a Bjork flap[18] (the suturing of the inferiorly based flap of tracheal mucosa, including the anterior cartilage of one or two tracheal rings, to the lower end of the skin incision) is performed, since it prevents the larynx from rising and moving forward during swallowing.[12,13] The Bjork flap essentially anchors the trachea and larynx to the anterior neck. On the other hand, a vertical incision with the removal of sections of one or two tracheal cartilages allows the larynx to move in a more coordinated manner during swallowing.[12,13]

Aspiration may occur in patients with tracheostomies for two other reasons. First, the tube itself or the cuff may compress the anterior wall of the esophagus, causing food or secretions to stagnate above the level of the cuff in the esophagus.[19,20] These may overflow into the airway with movement or forced inspiration. Second, because large-volume, low-pressure cuffs are normally used, folds in the inflated cuff can cause channels through the cuff where secretions can be aspirated, especially during head movement.[21] This is particularly prevalent in mechanically ventilated patients.

In spite of these factors that increase the incidence of aspiration, many patients with tracheostomies are able to swallow normally.[14] Patients at greatest risk for dysphagia and aspiration are those who have received prolonged mechanical ventilation and sedation, in whom disuse and muscle weakness add to the factors listed above.

Airway protection in tracheostomized patients can easily be assessed at the bedside by having the patient perform the methylene blue test.[6,12,22] This test is performed by mixing methylene blue dye with ice chips or water, deflating the

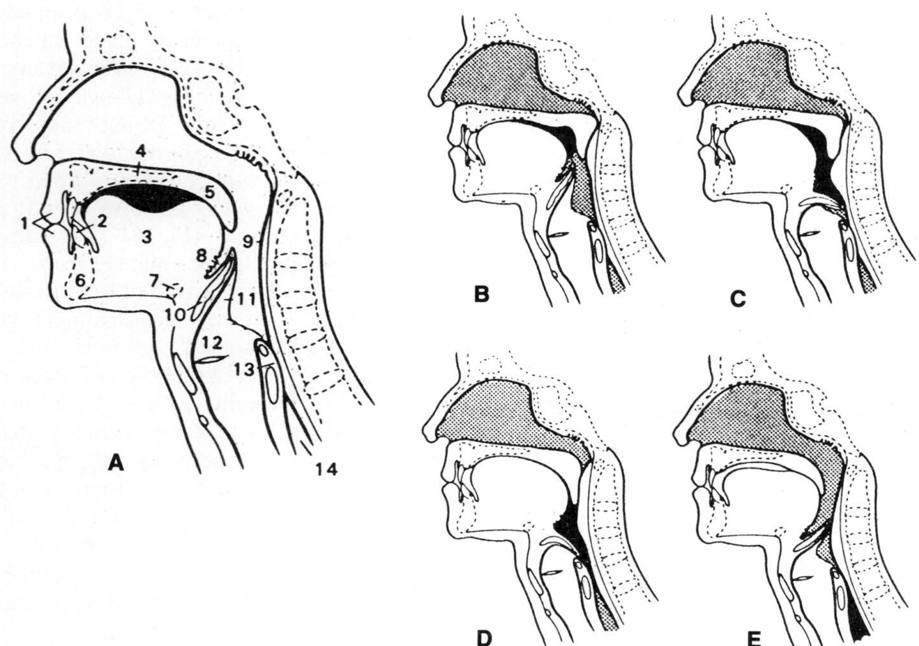

Figure 53-3. The normal sequence of swallowing. **(A)** Oral preparation of the material. **(B)** Initiation of swallow reflex with soft palate elevation as bolus enters oropharynx. **(C)** Pharyngeal peristalsis moves bolus into valleculae as larynx elevates and epiglottis tilts to protect the airway. **(D)** Cricopharyngeus muscle relaxes as bolus enters the esophagus. **(E)** Oral, pharyngeal, and laryngeal structures return to rest position as bolus moves through the esophagus. 1, lips; 2, teeth; 3, tongue; 4, hard palate; 5, soft palate; 6, mandible; 7, hyoid bone; 8, valleculae; 9, posterior pharyngeal wall; 10, epiglottis; 11, aryepiglottic fold; 12, vocal cords; 13, cricopharyngeus muscle; 14, esophagus. (From Weisinger and Goldsmith,[13] with permission.)

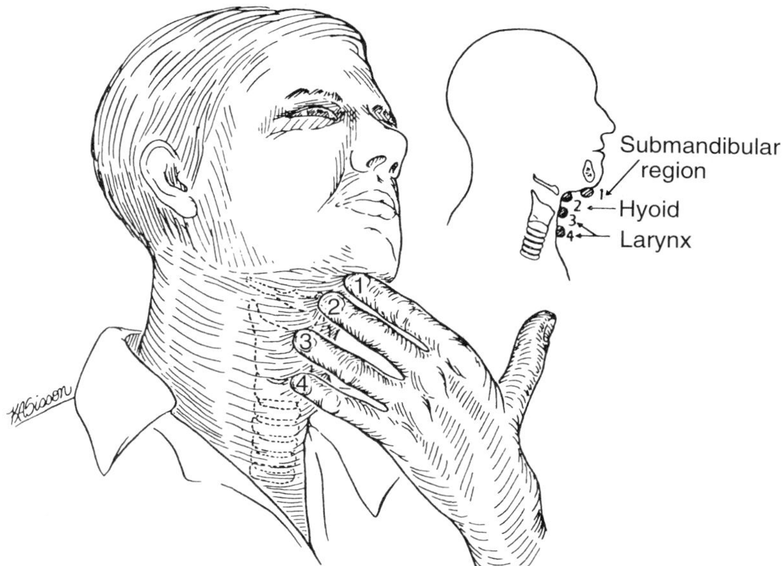

Figure 53-4. Positioning of fingers during bedside evaluation of swallowing. The index finger (1) at the submandibular area immediately behind the mandible assesses tongue movement. The second finger (2) evaluates movement of the hyoid bone, while the third (3) and fourth (4) fingers can define laryngeal movement. No pressure is exerted on the tissue; a light touch is used to identify and assess strength of movement. (From Logemann,[14] with permission.)

cuff of the tracheostomy tube, and having the patient swallow. The clinician must remember to ensure that the patient is properly positioned during the evaluation and exaggerates the steps in swallowing. If the patient's airway reflexes are intact, aspiration should elicit coughing. However, even if coughing does not occur, the airway should be suctioned for the presence of methylene blue. Those who fail the methylene blue test may need to be scheduled for a barium swallow to identify the cause of the dysphagia. Although many patients may aspirate a small amount of methylene blue while the tracheostomy tube is in place, they are usually capable of swallowing normally after the tube is removed. We frequently decannulate patients when minor aspiration is noted. In others, speech therapy and the use of other tracheal appliances (see below) may gradually improve swallowing efficiency.

Secretion Removal

Many patients require a tracheostomy tube to facilitate secretion removal after they are capable of ventilating and protecting their airways. The patient's ability to mobilize secretions is normally assessed by the ability to take a deep breath (vital capacity over 15 mL/kg) and to forcefully exhale, moving secretions to the trachea.[6] In patients in whom this ability is questionable, fenestrated tracheostomy tubes or tracheal buttons (see below) can be used to maintain the airway. These devices also force the patient to breathe from the upper airway and allow the patient to cough but also allow the clinician to suction the airway.

Obstruction

As a result of prolonged use of an artificial airway and trauma to the pharynx and larynx, some patients with tracheostomies are incapable of maintaining a patent upper airway and require gradual weaning from their artificial airway to ensure return of normal upper airway function. Fenestrated tracheostomy tubes, small-sized uncuffed tracheostomy tubes, tracheal buttons, and Passy Muir valves can facilitate this transition.

AIRWAY APPLIANCES

In addition to standard tracheostomy and endotracheal tubes, a number of other tracheal appliances are available for use in the gradual or phased removal of a tracheostomy tube from the patient having difficulty with secretion removal, airway protection, or upper airway obstruction.

Fenestrated Tracheostomy Tubes

The fenestrated tube is a standard cuffed tracheostomy tube with a precut fenestration (perforation) in the outer cannula, an unfenestrated inner cannula, and an outer cannula plug (Fig. 53-5). Patients with questionable upper airway obstruction or ability to mobilize secretions may benefit from the interim use of a fenestrated tube.[14,22] When the inner cannula is removed, the cuff deflated, and the outer cannula

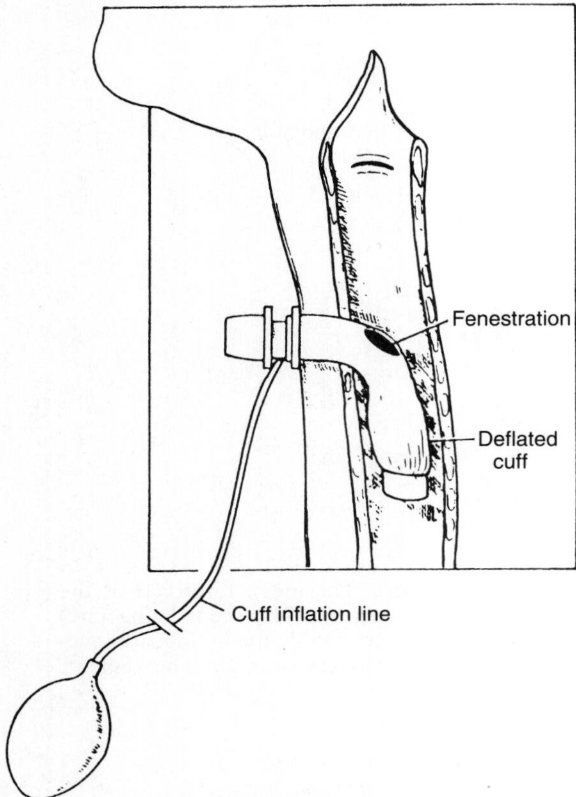

Figure 53-5. Fenestrated tracheostomy tube with cuff deflated and inner cannula removed as it sits in the airway. (From Wilson,[22] with permission.)

plugged, patients are forced to breathe through the upper airway and are capable of coughing by occluding the glottis and generating intrathoracic pressure. When patients are capable of tolerating a plugged fenestrated tube for about 2 days without the need of frequent tracheal suctioning, they normally can be decannulated.

Fenestrated tubes should only be used in patients who can protect their airways. These tubes must be properly sized from overexposed lateral neck radiographs or by use of "pipe cleaners" (Fig. 53-6) at the bedside.[14,22] It is imperative that the fenestration not touch the wall of the trachea. If it does, granulation tissue may rapidly grow into the fenestration, causing bleeding during insertion of the inner cannula or obstruction. As a result of the potential for development of granulation tissue and for obstruction by secretions, fenestrated tubes should not be plugged for longer than 16 hours. During the night the plug is removed, the inner cannula inserted, and a heated aerosol applied to the airway. An additional problem noted in some patients is inability to tolerate the increased resistance to gas flow from the fenestrated tube even when the cuff is deflated. In these patients a Passy Muir valve (see below) may be used until a small-sized tracheostomy tube or tracheal button can be placed or the patient can be decannulated.

Care must always be exercised when an airway is plugged to ensure that ventilation can be maintained via the upper airway. Assessment should include auscultation, evaluation of speech and cough, and evaluation of ventilatory pattern. If any difficulty is noted, the tube should be immediately unplugged.

Tracheal Buttons

Figure 53-7 illustrates an Olympic tracheal button. These buttons, which fit through the tracheal stoma, come in dif-

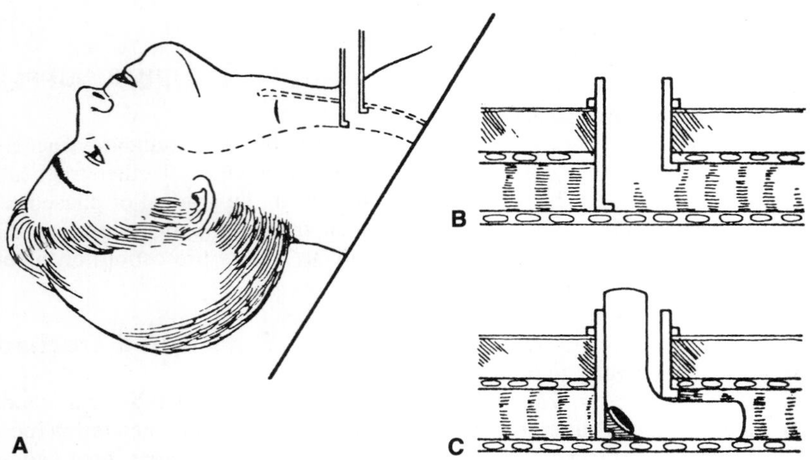

Figure 53-6. Measurement for proper placement of a fenestrated tracheostomy tube. **(A)** Hyperextended head for proper visualization of the stoma. **(B)** Anterior and posterior wall to skin measurements, using sterile "pipe cleaners." **(C)** Measurements used to determine proper location of fenestration on outer cannula of tracheostomy tube. (From Wilson,[22] with permission.)

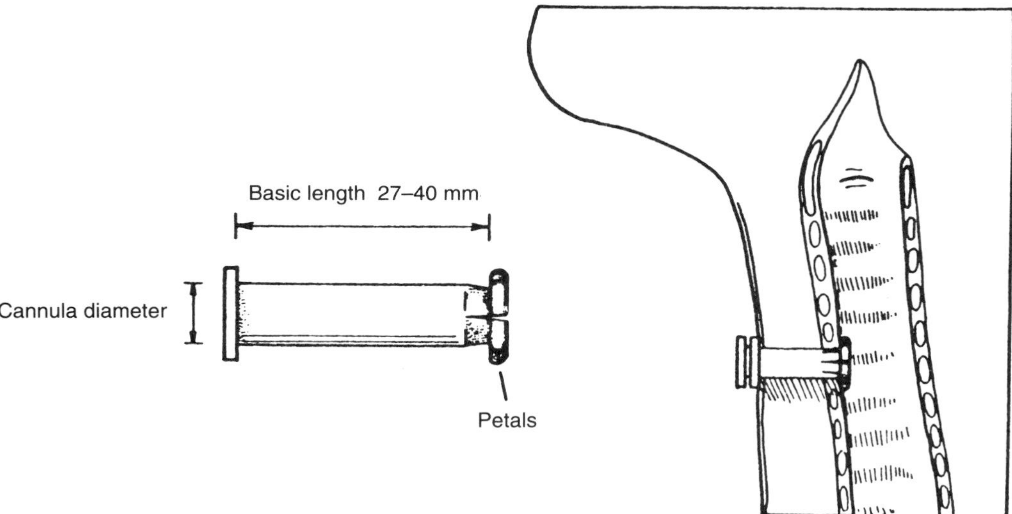

Figure 53-7. Dimensions and actual positioning of an Olympic tracheostomy button. (From Wilson,[22] with permission.)

ferent lengths and have two parts, the outer cannula and the inner plug. Prior to insertion the depth of the stoma between the skin surface and the anterior wall of the trachea must be measured with a hooked pipe cleaner so that a button of appropriate length may be selected.[22] If the button length exceeds the stomal depth, the inner petals of the button may obstruct the airway.[22]

To insert the button the inner plug is removed and the button positioned so that the petals (Fig. 53-7) are inside the tracheal wall. Insertion of the plug into the button causes the petals to expand, securing the button in place. Once secured, the button should be rotated 180 degrees and the petals visualized with a flashlight to ensure that no tissue adheres to the petals. Subsequently, buttons should be rotated every 4 hours to prevent tissue adhesion.

Tracheal buttons are used if questions regarding ability to clear secretions, upper airway obstruction, or the need to ventilate still exist. The button maintains the stoma open, allows for tracheal suctioning, and can easily be replaced by a tracheostomy tube if necessary. This appliance is usually the last step in a difficult decannulation.

Table 53-5. Plugging of Fenestrated or Small Tracheostomy Tube and Use of Passy Muir Valve

- Perform bronchial hygiene therapy
- Suction lower respiratory tract
- Suction above cuff via oral pharynx
- Deflate cuff while manually ventilating
- Remove any mobilized secretions
- Remove inner cannula of fenestrated tracheostomy tube
- Plug inner cannula or small tracheostomy tube or attach Passy Muir valve
- Assess ability to ventilate
    - Ability to cough
    - Ability to speak
    - Auscultate chest
    - Ventilatory pattern
- Do not leave bedside until assured patient can ventilate adequately

Small Tracheostomy Tubes

In patients who are experiencing difficulty with fenestrated tracheostomy tubes and who still require an artificial airway for frequent suctioning or obstruction but are generally capable of breathing via the upper airway, a small (4 mm ID) uncuffed tracheostomy tube can be placed. Depending on the patient's ability to ventilate, these tubes can be plugged or can have a Passy Muir valve attached. These tubes, like fenestrated tubes, should only be plugged for a 16-hour period. Heated aerosol should be applied during the night. The patient's ability to breathe via the upper airway must be carefully evaluated immediately after plugging (Table 53-5).

Passy Muir Valves

In those patients in whom inspiratory upper airway obstruction is a persistent problem or in whom resistance to flow-through, a fenestrated tube, or a small tracheostomy tube is encountered, a Passy Muir valve (Fig. 53-8) can be attached to a fenestrated or a small tracheostomy tube. The Passy Muir valve is a one-way valve, allowing inspiration only and forcing exhalation via the upper airway, although inspiration can occur both from the upper airway and via the valve. The use of this valve assists in gradual recovery of upper airway muscle tone and allows for a smooth transition from a normal cuffed tracheostomy tube to a plugged small tracheostomy tube or a fenestrated tube.

In patients requiring O_2 therapy, careful assessment of the method of application must be made when a Passy Muir

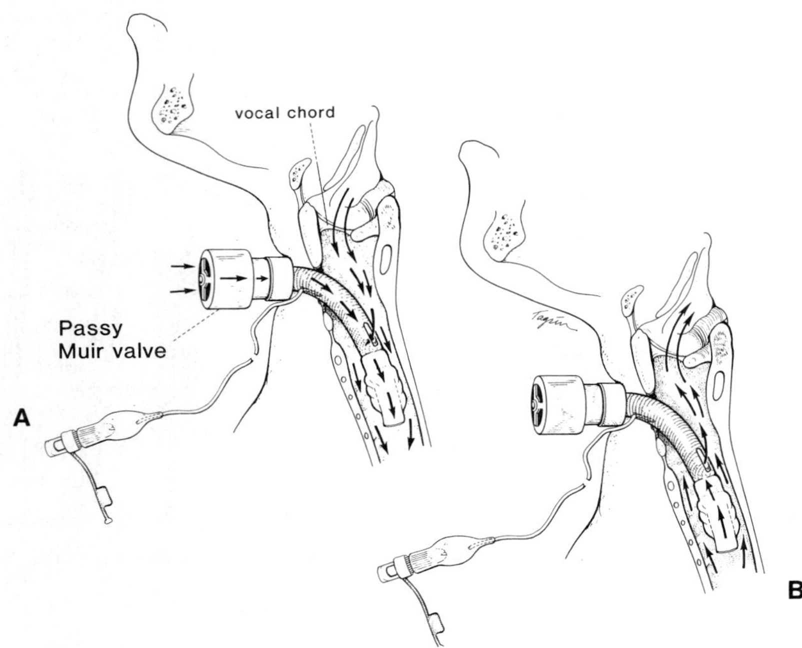

Figure 53-8. Passy Muir valve. This valve attaches to a standard 15-mm tracheostomy adapter. It allows inspiration (**A**) via the valve, but exhalation (**B**) must occur via the upper airway.

valve is used. Some patients require delivery of O_2 via the valve, whereas in others a nasal cannula or other facial appliance can be used. Blood gas or oximetry comparison during O_2 administration by either route must be performed daily. Frequently, patients initially require O_2 administration via the Passy Muir valve but progress to upper airway administration as they regain normal upper airway function. During initial use of the valve, constant observation should be maintained to ensure patient tolerance. As noted with fenestrated tracheostomy tubes, the patient's ability to ventilate must be carefully assessed and the continued maintenance of this ability must be ensured before the clinician leaves the bedside.

References

1. Robinson C, Bishop MJ, Ritz RH: Guidelines for choosing the appropriate level of pressure support with a Servo 900C to overcome imposed work of breathing, abstracted. Respir Care 1988;33:936
2. Suzuki M, Sasaki CT: Laryngeal spasm: A neurophysiologic redefinition. Ann Otol Rhinol Laryngol 1977;86:150–156
3. Sasaki CT, Isaacson G: Functional anatomy of the larynx. Otolaryngol Clin North Am 1988;21:595–612
4. Lindsay JR: Laryngocele ventricularis. Ann Otol Rhinol Laryngol 1940;49:661–669
5. Brunton TL, Cash T: The valvular action of the larynx. J Anat 1883;17:363–369
6. Shapiro BA, Kacmarek RM, Cane RA et al: Clinical Application of Respiratory Care. 4th Ed. Mosby-Year Book, St. Louis, 1990, pp. 181–200
7. Applebaum EL, Bruce DL: Tracheal Intubation. WB Saunders, Philadelphia, 1976, p. 62
8. Blanc VF, Tremblay NAG: The complications of tracheal intubation: A new classification with a review of the literature. Anesth Analg 1974;53:202–213
9. Kacmarek RM, Dimas S, Mack C: The Essentials of Respiratory Care. 3rd Ed. Mosby-Year Book, St. Louis, 1990, pp. 422–430
10. Kemper KJ, Ritz RH, Benson MS et al: Helium-oxygen mixture in the treatment of postextubation stridor in pediatric trauma patients. Crit Care Med 1991;19:356–362
11. Logemann JA: Swallowing physiology and pathophysiology. Otolaryngol Clin North Am 1988;21:613–623
12. Nask M: Swallowing problems in tracheotomized patients. Otolaryngol Clin North Am 1988; 21:701–709
13. Weisinger W, Goldsmith T: Artificial ventilation: Its impact on communication and swallowing. Probl Respir Care 1988;1:204–216
14. Logemann J: Evaluation and Treatment of Swallowing Disorders. College Hill Press, 1983, pp. 115–130
15. Bonanno PC: Swallowing dysfunction after tracheostomy. Ann Surg 1971;174:29–38
16. Butcher BR: Treatment of chronic aspiration as a complication of cerebrovascular accident. Laryngoscope 1982;92:681–697
17. Feldman SA, Deal CW, Urguhart W: Disturbances of swallowing after tracheostomy. Lancet 1966; 30:954–958
18. Bjork VO: Partial resection of the only remaining lung with the aid of respirator treatment. J Thorac Cardiovasc Surg 1960;39:179–188
19. Groher ME: Mechanical disorders of swallowing. pp. 61–84. In Groher ME (ed): Dysphagia: Diagnosis and Management. Stoneham, Butterworth, London 1984
20. Stauffer JL, Olson DE, Petty TL: Complications and consequences of endotracheal intubation and tracheostomy. Am J Med 1981;70:65–72
21. Fleming S: Treatment of mechanical swallowing disorders. pp. 157–172. In Groher ME (ed): Dysphagia: Diagnosis and Management. Stoneham, Butterworth, London, 1984
22. Wilson D: Airway appliances and management. pp. 80–90. In Kacmarek RM, Stoller JK (eds): Current Respiratory Care. BC Decker, Toronto, 1988

Chapter 54

Preoperative Evaluation of Respiratory Function

Jay A. Johannigman
James M. Hurst

CHAPTER OUTLINE

The importance of the preoperative evaluation of the surgical patient gains perspective when one considers the potential scope of the problem. In the 1990s hundreds of thousands of patients will undergo some form of major surgery. Estimates of pulmonary complications in the postoperative period range from 6 to 35 percent.[1–3] Over the years a number of discrete pulmonary risk factors that may influence the postoperative outcome have been identified. One of the goals of this chapter is to delineate these risk factors, along with specific interventions that may favorably alter their impact. In addition, specific maneuvers for the assessment of patients undergoing lung resection are considered. The value of preoperative intervention as well as the various regimens utilized is discussed in hopes of providing a framework from which all patients who are at risk may be evaluated.

PATHOPHYSIOLOGIC CHANGES RESULTING FROM SURGERY

Prior to any discussion of risk factors, it is important to review the fundamental physiologic changes that surgery effects. Upper abdominal and thoracic surgery result in a significant decrease in both vital capacity (VC) and functional residual capacity (FRC) within the first 24 postoperative hours. After upper abdominal surgery, VC may be decreased by as much as 50 to 60 percent while FRC is reduced by about 30 percent,[4] as depicted in Figure 41-1. The degree of postoperative risk directly correlates with the reductions in lung volume. The etiology of the reductions in VC and FRC is most certainly multifactorial. Postoperative pain alters the mechanics of respiration, and accordingly, upper abdominal and thoracic incisions have the greatest impact. Treatment of incisional pain with narcotic analgesia carries its own inherent risks because it eliminates sighing and thereby promotes atelectasis. Although postoperative pain is certainly important, it is not the sole factor responsible for the observed changes.

Even if pain is eliminated by the institution of epidural anesthesia, there remains a demonstrable decrease in VC and FRC.[5,6] This observation has led investigators to suggest a role for primary diaphragmatic dysfunction following upper abdominal surgery. Ford et al.[7] used magnetometer measurements of abdominal and rib cage excursions as well as transdiaphragmatic pressures to document a significant decrease in diaphragmatic function following upper abdominal incisions. Institution of epidural anesthesia to eliminate postoperative pain did not alter these changes. Dureuil et al.[8] demonstrated that diaphragmatic muscular contractility is preserved in the postoperative period, suggesting that the observed dysfunction may be the result of altered neural input via the phrenic nerve. They speculated that suppression of the phrenic nerve may be the result of inhibitory reflexes arising from sympathetic, vagal, or abdominal receptors. Along these same lines, Dureuil et al.[8] demonstrated an improvement in postoperative diaphragmatic dysfunction following administration of aminophylline. Aminophylline is known to produce an increase in phrenic nerve activity in anesthetized animals; therefore, this agent may partially reverse postoperative reflex phrenic nerve inhibition.

A second important physiologic change occurring in the postoperative period is a decrease in closing volume (CV),[9] which is the lung volume at which airway closure is first detectable. Loss of FRC, elimination of sighing (by narcotic analgesics), and the change to a postoperative breathing pattern of small frequent breaths combine to lower the end-tidal point to a level below CV. Alveolar collapse rapidly occurs in this setting and results in the pattern of atelectasis so often observed in the postoperative period. This predilection is accentuated in smokers, who characteristically have a higher CV because of diseased airways, and therefore puts them at an even greater risk of atelectatic changes.

CLINICAL RISK FACTORS

Given this background of primary physiologic changes that occur with surgical intervention, it is important to evaluate the patient for the presence of known risk factors (Table 54-1). Some of these risk factors cannot be appreciably altered (age, cardiac disease, surgical site), but many risk factors may be favorably influenced during the preoperative evaluation period.

Smoking

When considering the impact of smoking as a risk factor for surgery, it is important to distinguish the chronic parenchymal changes caused by smoking from the short-term, potentially reversible effects. The long-term effects that result in chronic obstructive pulmonary disease (COPD) and abnormal pulmonary function tests (PFTs) are discussed in a later section.

Table 54-1. Risk Factors for Perioperative Pulmonary Complications

Smoking history
Preexisting pulmonary disease
Age
Anesthetic time >3.5 hr
Obesity
Cardiac disease
Upper abdominal surgery
Nasogastric tubes

Patients who smoke are encouraged to stop prior to their operation. This recommendation is based on a number of prospective and retrospective studies that have documented increased morbidity in smokers.[10,11] If chronic parenchymal changes and sputum production resulting from cigarette smoking are separately controlled, it becomes more difficult to identify the short-term benefits to the patient of cessation of smoking. Warner et al.[10] specifically examined this issue in a retrospective study of 500 patients undergoing coronary artery bypass grafting (CABG). Their results demonstrated a threefold decrease in the incidence of postoperative pulmonary complications in patients who had stopped smoking at least 8 weeks prior to their operation. Patients who had ceased smoking for more than 8 weeks did not have a statistically significant increase in pulmonary complications as compared with patients who had never smoked. By contrast, there was no significant improvement in the incidence of respiratory problems in patients who abstained from smoking for less than 8 weeks when compared with those who never stopped. Warner et al.[10] cite supportive evidence from studies demonstrating that improvement in ciliary and small airway function and decrease in sputum production occur slowly over a period of weeks after smoking is stopped. Separate studies by Buist et al.,[11] Bode and colleagues,[12] and Mitchell et al.[3] all documented that improved mucociliary clearance is a slow process, showing little demonstrable improvement in periods less than 2 months. Unfortunately, the stress that often accompanies a surgical procedure makes it a difficult time for most patients to stop. Bode et al.[12] found that only 20 percent of patients stopped smoking preoperatively, although all had been advised to do so.

Cessation of smoking is associated with a reduction of carboxyhemoglobin levels within 12 hours, but Gracey et al.[13] were unable to demonstrate any postoperative advantage to this reduction. Thus, it would appear that a patient must abstain from smoking for at least 2 months if any definite advantage is to be gained.

Preexisting Pulmonary Disease

Patients with preexisting pulmonary disease have long been recognized to be at increased risk of postoperative complications. PFTs are of value in this setting because they provide a means to objectively quantify existing pulmonary abnormalities. Over the years almost every conceivable parameter obtained via spirometry has been championed as predictive of postoperative morbidity. What is clear from a review of the literature is that patients who exhibit abnormal preoperative pulmonary function are at increased risk following abdominal or thoracic surgery. Of the various parameters that may be obtained, forced expiratory flow in 1 second (FEV_1), forced vital capacity (FVC), peak expiratory flow rate (PEFR), and FEV_1/FVC ratio appear to be the most useful in predicting perioperative risk. Table 54-2 provides

Table 54-2. Pulmonary Function Testing Suggesting Increased Risk of Postoperative Pulmonary Complications

FVC	<70% predicted
FEV_1	<70% predicted
PEFR	<200 L/min
FEV_1/FVC	<65%

a listing of spirometric indicators of increased risk of postoperative respiratory complications.

Several authors have emphasized the significance of preoperative arterial hypercapnia ($PaCO_2$ above 45 mmHg).[14–16] In one report all four patients with a $PaCO_2$ above 45 had complications, and two of the four died.[16] By contrast, hypoxemia in the absence of hypercapnia was inconsistently identified as a marker for increased risk. These authors suggest that preoperative arterial blood gas levels be obtained in those patients who display significantly abnormal pulmonary function.

Age

It is difficult to determine the risk attributable to age independently of the associated changes that accompany the aging process. The literature varies in its assessment of age as an independent risk factor but appears to support the contention that advanced age alone should not govern the decision for or against surgery. A much more useful concept is to recognize the distinction of chronologic age from physiologic age. Marx et al.[17] determined that mortality was lowest in patients aged 1 to 30 and that this risk rose progressively from age 30 to age 80. Analysis revealed that overall poor physical status rather than advanced age was the most important risk factor in determining mortality. The studies suggest that age is useful in predicting preoperative risk primarily because of its usual association with other physiologic changes. If other more specific physiologic parameters such as pulmonary function are unknown, age may serve to provide a reasonable estimation of risk.

Anesthesia

It is generally accepted that there is no difference in risk between spinal and general anesthesia. As one might expect, the technique of regional anesthesia is associated with fewer pulmonary complications. The one circumstance that does relate to an increased postoperative complication rate is the duration of anesthesia. Several studies have emphasized that anesthesia time longer than 3.5 hours is associated with increased postoperative pulmonary complications.[18–20]

Obesity

The predilection for the development of postoperative complications that is noted in obese patients relates to the underlying pulmonary dysfunction characteristic of this patient population. Burwell et al.[21] demonstrated a marked decline in FRC among patients who exceeded their ideal body weight by more than 30 percent. The observed reduction in FRC is most probably the result of a reduction in chest wall compliance. This loss of FRC is further potentiated by assumption of the supine position, which accentuates ventilation/perfusion mismatching, thereby increasing hypoxemia. Massively obese patients may also hypoventilate as a result of mechanical limitations, respiratory muscle dysfunction, impaired ventilatory regulation, or postoperative incisional pain. The resultant effect of these many abnormalities is to create a situation in which the obese patient's tidal volume (V_T) is at an FRC below CV. When this occurs, alveoli are unventilated and rapidly collapse, leading to atelectasis. Latimer et al.[22] noted the development of macroatelectasis in 53 percent of obese patients as compared with 9 percent of those of normal weight.

Cardiac Disease

It is difficult to assess the additional risk, if any, that isolated cardiac dysfunction imposes in the perioperative period because of the intimate relationship between the cardiac and respiratory systems. The presence of cardiovascular disease (angina, myocardial infarction, or congestive heart failure) was not found to influence the incidence of postoperative pulmonary complications in Wightman's series.[2] By contrast, Mittman[23] found that an electrocardiogram (ECG) with "nonspecific abnormalities" identified a subset of patients who subsequently suffered a 46 percent incidence of fatal postoperative cardiorespiratory complications. It is not clear what role pulmonary complications alone contributed to this mortality rate. Goldman et al.[24] included pulmonary edema as a postoperative complication and described an incidence of 2.5 percent in patients over 40 years of age. Patients with jugular venous distension, a third heart sound, or a previous history of pulmonary edema were most likely to develop this complication. Patients who manifest findings of significant cardiac dysfunction, as well as trauma patients who receive large amounts of fluids during resuscitation, should be followed closely for the development of pulmonary edema in the postoperative period.

Location and Nature of Surgery

Many investigators have noted a higher incidence of postoperative complications following upper abdominal versus lower abdominal or extremity surgery. As discussed previously, this may be a result of the diaphragmatic dysfunction resulting from upper abdominal incisions. In addition to these differences, there are data suggesting that the type of incision may affect the development of complications. Numerous studies[19,23,25] have documented a decreased incidence of pulmonary complications with the use of a horizontal rather than a vertical laparotomy incision. In a study by Mitchell et al.,[3] the presence of a nasogastric tube 24 hours postoperatively was the factor most frequently associated with the development of postoperative respiratory morbidity. The authors suggested that the presence of a nasogastric tube may predispose to esophageal reflux, pulmonary aspiration, or reduced efficiency of the cough mechanism, thereby contributing to decreased sputum clearance.

THORACIC SURGERY FOR PULMONARY RESECTION

The evaluation of the patient about to undergo lung resection requires not only consideration of the effects considered above but also a prediction of the function that will remain following the removal of one or more functional segments of the lung. In spite of the recent advances in chemotherapy and radiation therapy, surgical intervention continues to offer the best chance of cure for patients with pulmonary neoplasms. The degree of functional and respiratory compromise, as well as postoperative mortality, that one deems acceptable must be weighed against the knowledge that without surgical resection the majority of pulmonary neoplasms are universally fatal.[26] Traditionally, spirometry has been the cornerstone on which all therapeutic decisions were based. If the results of spirometry are inconclusive or marginal, further evaluative testing is indicated. All candidates scheduled for lung resection should be evaluated as if pneumonectomy were required. This will provide the surgeon with the greatest amount of information and allow for the greatest breadth of options at the time of operation.

Spirometry has traditionally been used to predict postoperative morbidity and mortality following lung resection. Although there is a degree of correlation between preoperative spirometric abnormalities and postoperative dysfunction, specific indicators have been difficult to establish. A generally accepted algorithm is depicted in Figure 54-1.

FVC is the parameter most routinely evaluated preoperatively because it is easily measured, is readily reproducible, and provides a reasonable estimate of risk. It is generally agreed that a FVC of less than 50 percent or an absolute value of less than 1.75 to 2.0 L is indicative of an increased postoperative risk.[23] FEV_1 provides an estimate of the degree of airflow obstruction. Most reports identify a predicted postoperative FEV_1 of less than 800 to 1000 mL as the cutoff point beyond which there is significant increase in postoperative morbidity and mortality.[17] Patients with a predicted postoperative FEV_1 below this level should not necessarily be excluded from consideration for surgery but most certainly require further evaluation (see below). Maximum voluntary ventilation (MVV) is regarded as a valuable test by many clinicians because it combines estimation of airway disease with an indication of the ability of the patient to cooperate and complete a physiologic stress test. MVV provides an intangible estimate of the patient's ability to respond to a measured stressor. Most authors indicate that a MVV below 50 percent of the predicted value places the patient in a category of high risk.[17,23] Midexpiratory flow measurements such as the maximum midexpiratory flow rate

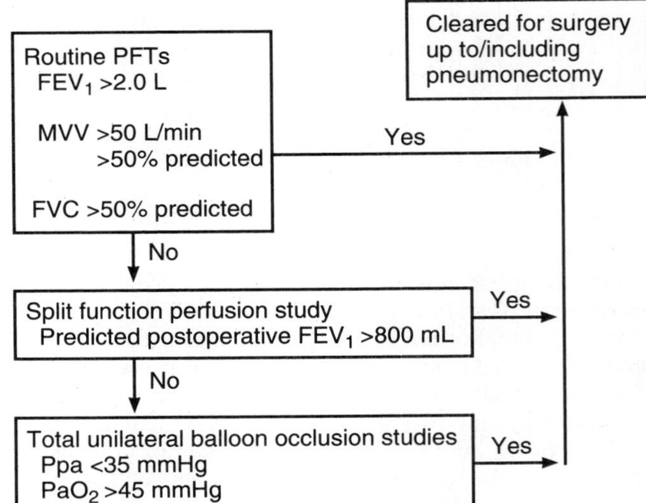

Figure 54-1. Algorithm for determining appropriateness of pulmonary resectional surgery based on results of tests of pulmonary function. (Adapted from Boysen,[20] with permission.)

(MMEFR) and forced expiratory flow between 25 and 75 percent of the exhaled volume (FEF_{25-75}) are indicative of the small airway dysfunction present in COPD. Values below 50 percent for either of these tests predict a higher risk for a variety of surgical procedures, including pulmonary resection.[13,17]

For those patients in whom resectional surgery is contemplated but whose spirometric tests place them in a high-risk category, further testing is indicated. Although a number of different tests have been employed over the years, the most popular tests in current use include radionuclide studies, exercise testing, maximum O_2 consumption ($\dot{V}O_2max$) determination, and unilateral pulmonary artery occlusion.

Radionuclide Studies

When a patient is considered for resection, it is critical to arrive at an accurate estimate of the pulmonary function that will be retained following surgery. A surgical resection that reduces FEV_1 to 800 mL or less will result in a significant degree of pulmonary disability, which may seriously jeopardize the patient's quality of life.[27] A number of radionuclide techniques have been developed in the hope of providing an accurate prediction of postresection FEV_1; the most commonly employed of these are xenon radiospirometry and technetium macroaggregate lung scanning. Both these techniques allow for quantification of the functional contribution of segmental portions of the lung, and both have been shown to display a high degree of correlation in predicting postpneumonectomy FVC and FEV_1. Wernly et al.[28]

tested a number of different formulas and found a reliable prediction to be given by

Postoperative FEV_1

$$= (\text{Preoperative } FEV_1)\left(\frac{\text{no. of functional segments to be resected}}{\text{total no. of segments in both lungs}}\right)$$

Lung scanning may be completed with negligible risk to the patient and is readily available at most institutions. The high accuracy of this technique makes it very useful in the preoperative evaluation of the lung resection candidate.

Exercise Testing

Reichel[29] has made the most complete analysis of exercise testing as a means of preoperative evaluation of the thoracotomy patient. His study used a modified cardiac treadmill protocol, which required the patient to negotiate seven stages of treadmill elevation at 2 minutes per stage. Among the 12 patients who were capable of completing the 14-minute protocol, there were no deaths and no complications. In seven patients unable to complete 4 minutes of the protocol, three died and three suffered complications. Many surgeons traditionally use a "rule of thumb" equivalent to this test by asking patients to negotiate two flights of stairs as a rough correlate of their ability to withstand operation and resection.

Maximum Oxygen Consumption

Two recent studies have suggested that exercise testing to measure $\dot{V}O_2max$ is an accurate means of identifying those patients who possess sufficient physiologic reserves to undergo pulmonary resection. The procedure uses a bicycle ergometer for this determination. Smith et al.[30] demonstrated that only 1 of 10 patients with a $\dot{V}O_2max$ of more than 20 mL/kg/min suffered a complication, while all 6 patients with a $\dot{V}O_2max$ of less than 15 mL/kg/min had cardiopulmonary complications or died. In a series reported by Eugene et al.,[31] a significant relationship was documented between $\dot{V}O_2max$ and postoperative mortality: a $\dot{V}O_2max$ less than 1 L/min was associated with a 75 percent mortality, while there were no deaths if $\dot{V}O_2max$ was above this value. Both groups of authors concluded that determination of $\dot{V}O_2max$ at peak exercise is a very valuable noninvasive means of preoperative assessment.

Pulmonary Vascular Resistance

Many investigators have suggested that postoperative alterations in pulmonary vascular resistance play an important role in the development of cardiorespiratory complications. Temporary unilateral pulmonary artery occlusion was developed as a technique for evaluating the changes that may occur in the pulmonary vascular bed following resection. Its use is advocated in patients who fall into a high-risk category and may otherwise be denied resectional surgery on the basis of routine spirometry. The technique consists of measurement of pulmonary artery pressures and PaO_2 at rest and during maximum exercise while the pulmonary artery supplying the lung to be resected is temporarily occluded by a balloon-tipped catheter. The information gained from these studies has led to an increased understanding of the interplay between pulmonary circulation, right heart function, and pulmonary capillary bed compliance and the morbidity and mortality following lung resection. Because of the technical difficulty of the procedure and the relative risks involved, its use is limited to that of a final avenue of investigation to determine whether a patient is fit for the proposed operative resection.

PREOPERATIVE EVALUATION

In the process of preoperative evaluation three questions must be addressed: (1) Should testing be carried out and which tests should be done? (2) Which patients should be tested? (3) Of what value are the results?

The cornerstone of the preoperative evaluation remains the history and physical examination (Table 54-3). The patient should be closely questioned for a history of smoking habits and known lung disease. The history should also include the presence of cough, sputum production, dyspnea, wheezing, and exercise tolerance. The physical examination should place special emphasis on the respiratory system and include evaluation of the presence and character of breath sounds, the shape of the chest and respiratory musculature, and the presence of rales or wheezing. Additional information may be obtained by having the patient complete a forced expiratory VC test while the examiner listens for the presence or absence of wheezing and rales. The chest x-ray, ECG, and sputum evaluation remain adjunctive procedures, which complement rather than replace the physical examination.

Pulmonary function testing remains the most controversial

Table 54-3. Preoperative Evaluation

History
Smoking
COPD
Cough, sputum, dyspnea, wheezing
Physical examination
Breath sounds
Chest wall excursion
Rales/wheezes/rhonchi
Bedside forced expiratory VC/wheezing
Laboratory tests
Chest x-ray, ECG, arterial blood gas levels
Sputum

Table 54-4. Candidates for Preoperative Pulmonary Function Tests

Smoking history
COPD history
Wheezing/dyspnea on exertion
Exercise intolerance
Abnormal physical examination
Abnormal chest x-ray

approach to determining the presence of respiratory disease. A number of investigators[16,25,31] have suggested that spirometry is of little value in quantitating the increased risk of serious postoperative pulmonary complications in COPD patients. A much larger body of data suggests that preoperative pulmonary function testing offers important information in predicting postoperative morbidity. While not all published reports are in agreement, most suggest that the preoperative PFT remains an important part of the evaluative process. The specific test results that should be examined vary depending on the author, but the most commonly cited function tests are those listed in Table 54-2.

If preoperative PFT is of value, which patients are candidates? Patients in whom there is a reasonable expectation of pulmonary dysfunction should be tested, including (1) those with a positive smoking history; (2) those with a history of symptoms of respiratory disease (wheezing, exertional dyspnea, etc); (3) those with an abnormal physical examination; and (4) those with an abnormal chest x-ray (Table 54-4).

If it is possible to define and test a high-risk patient population, is it also possible to use this identification to favorably alter the postoperative course? Stein and Cassara[9] were among the first to examine this question in 1970. In this study patients who were identified as being at increased risk on the basis of preoperative PFTs, (PEFR, FVC, FEV_1, and PCO_2) were divided into two groups, one who received intensive perioperative chest therapy and a control group. The two groups were evenly matched with respect to age and pulmonary function abnormalities. The results demonstrated a significant reduction in postoperative pulmonary complications, from 60 to 22 percent, in those who received chest therapy. Since this time, a number of other reports, including those of Gracey et al.,[13] Tarkan et al.,[15] and Stein et al.,[1] have supported a similar conclusion regarding postoperative intervention. In an earlier extensive study by Thoren,[18] similar findings had also been obtained.

The incidence of pulmonary complications in patients with COPD may be reduced by such adjuncts as deep breathing maneuvers and chest physiotherapy. Bronchospasm should be eliminated before surgery and may require the use of bronchodilators and steroids during the perioperative period. The addition of aminophylline may provide the benefit of improved diaphragmatic function, particularly for those patients undergoing upper abdominal procedures. Antibiotics should be initiated if a productive cough is present. It is useful to monitor pulmonary function during the preoperative period. Gracey et al.[13] have shown that those who show an improvement in function have a more favorable outcome. Finally, it is of paramount importance for the clinician to develop a relationship with the patient before surgery. The process of preoperative patient education and instruction in the techniques of deep breathing, coughing, and the use of incentive spirometry is likely to be more effective than attempting to teach these principles in the presence of postoperative pain and analgesics. Unfortunately, the ever pressing concern for limitation of hospital stay has in many cases eliminated the once routine practice of preoperative admission.

The goal of respiratory care is to provide the safest perioperative course for the patient undergoing surgery. Recognition of the risk factors associated with pulmonary dysfunction, and hence increased postoperative risk, allows identification of patients who will require special attention. In the words of Mendenhall,[32] "It is far easier to avoid postoperative respiratory failure than it is to treat this problem in addition to the problems of the surgery itself once the respiratory insufficiency has occurred."

Author's Note

This chapter was written in the author's private capacity. No official support or endorsement by the United States Air Force is intended or should be inferred.

References

1. Stein M, Koota GM, Simon M, Frank HA: Pulmonary evaluation of surgical patients. JAMA 1962;181:765–770
2. Wightman JAK: A prospective survey of the incidence of postoperative pulmonary complications. Br J Surg 1968;55:85–91
3. Mitchell C, Garrahy P, Peake P: Postoperative respiratory morbidity: Identification and risk factors. Aust NZ J Surg 1982;52:203–209
4. Luce JM: Clinical risk factors for postoperative pulmonary complications. Respir Care 1984;29:484–495
5. Ali J, Weisel RD, Layug AB et al: Consequences of postoperative alterations in respiratory mechanics. Am J Surg 1974;128:376–382
6. Bromage PR, Camporesi E, Chestnut D: Epidural narcotics for postoperative analgesia. Anesth Analg 1980;59:473–480
7. Ford GT, Whitelaw WA, Rosenal TW et al: Diaphragm function after upper abdominal surgery in humans. Am Rev Respir Dis 1983;127:431–436
8. Dureuil B, Desmonts JM, Mankikian B et al: Effects of aminophylline on diaphragmatic dysfunction after upper abdominal surgery. Anesthesiology 1985;62:242–246
9. Stein M, Cassara EL: Preoperative pulmonary evaluation and therapy for surgery patients. JAMA 1970;211:787–790
10. Warner MA, Divertie MB, Tinker JH: Preoperative cessation of smoking and pulmonary complications in coronary artery bypass patients. Anesthesiology 1984;60:380–383
11. Buist AS, Sexton GJ, Nagy JM et al: The effect of smoking cessation and modification on lung function. Am Rev Respir Dis 1976;114:115–122
12. Bode FR, Dosman J, Martin RR et al: Reversibility of pulmonary function abnormalities in smokers. Am J Med 1975;59:43–52
13. Gracey DR, Divertie MB, Didier EP: Preoperative pulmonary preparation of patient with chronic obstructive pulmonary disease. Chest 1979;76:123–129
14. Tisi GM: Preoperative evaluation of pulmonary function. Am Rev Respir Dis 1979;199:293–310
15. Tarkan S, Moffit EA, Sessler AD et al: Risk of anesthesia and surgery in patients with chronic bronchitis and chronic obstructive pulmonary disease. Surgery 1973;74:720–726
16. Milledge JD, Nunn JF. Criteria of fitness for anaesthesia in pa-

tients with chronic obstructive lung disease. Br Med J 1975;3:670–673
17. Marx GF, Mates CV, Orkin LR: Computer analysis of postanaesthetic deaths. Anesthesiology 1973;39:54–58
18. Thoren L: Postoperative pulmonary complication: Observations on their prevention by chest physiotherapy. Acta Chir Scand 1954;107:193–205
19. Vaughn RW, Wise L: Choice of abdominal operative incision in the obese patient. Ann Surg 1975;181:829–835
20. Boysen PG: Assessment for lung resection. Respir Care 1984;29:506–515
21. Burwell CS, Robin ED, Whaley RD, Bickelman AG: Extreme obesity associated with alveolar hypoventilation—a pickwickian syndrome. Am J Med 1956;27:811–818
22. Latimer RG et al: Ventilatory patterns and pulmonary complications after upper abdominal surgery determined by preoperative and postoperative computerized spirometry and blood gas analysis. Am J Surg 1971;122:622–632
23. Mittman C: Assessment of operative risk in thoracic surgery. Am Rev Respir Dis 1961;84:197–207
24. Goldman L, Caldera DL, Nussbaum AR et al: Multifactorial index of cardiac risk in noncardiac surgical procedures. N Engl J Med 1977;297:845–850
25. Williams CD, Brenowitz JB: Prohibitive lung function and major surgical procedures. Am J Surg 1976;132:763–766
26. Bousky SF, Billig DM, North LB, Helgason AH: Clinical course related to preoperative and postoperative pulmonary function in patients with bronchogenic carcinoma. Chest 1971;59:383–391
27. Boysen PG, Block AJ, Olsen GN et al: Prospective evaluation for pneumonectomy using the 99m technetium quantitative perfusion lung scan. Chest 1977;72:422–425
28. Wernly JA, De Meester TR, Kirchner PT et al: Clinical value of quantitative ventilation-perfusion lung scans in the surgical management of bronchogenic carcinoma. J Thorac Cardiovasc Surg 1980;30:535–543
29. Reichel J: Assessment of operative risk of pneumonectomy. Chest 1972;62:570–576
30. Smith TP, Kinasewitz GT, Tucker WY et al: Exercise capacity as a predictor of post-thoracotomy morbidity. Am Rev Respir Dis 1984;129:730–734
31. Eugene J, Brown SE, Light RW et al: Maximum oxygen consumption: A physiologic guide to pulmonary resection. Surg Forum 1982;33:260–262
32. Mendenhall JT: Evaluation and management of pulmonary insufficiency in surgical patients. Surg Clin North Am 1968;48:773–778

Chapter 55

Assessment of Respiratory Function During Sleep

Eugene C. Fletcher

CHAPTER OUTLINE

Monitoring sleep and its many behavioral aspects is common practice in sleep disorders centers throughout the world. A fully equipped and staffed sleep disorders center is an integrated multidisciplinary service[1] and is managed by a certified polysomnographer (Ph.D. or M.D.) who has completed 2 or more years of training in the specialty of sleep disorders. Such training is not just in the use of sleep laboratory equipment but in the diagnosis and treatment of a variety of sleep disorders such as insomnia, hypersomnia, respiratory abnormalities during sleep, and disorders of sexual function.[2] The consulting staff of such a laboratory will include psychiatrists, neurologists, pulmonologists, urologists, otolaryngologists, neonatologists, and members of other disciplines needed to diagnose and treat a variety of problems.

A number of community hospitals have established sleep laboratories because of the common occurrence of respiratory disorders during sleep and the high demand for local diagnostic centers for such disorders. Thus, there has been a rapid growth of cardiopulmonary sleep laboratories, which specialize in respiratory disorders during sleep. As pointed out in a joint publication by the American College of Chest Physicians and the Association of Sleep Disorders Centers, the medical director of such laboratories needs to be familiar with noncardiopulmonary sleep-related problems so as to be able to make appropriate referrals.[3] The purpose of this chapter is to concentrate on the requirements for adequate cardiopulmonary sleep studies based on the view that a sleep laboratory must be more than just a "place to diagnose sleep apnea."

RATIONALE FOR A SPECIALIZED SLEEP DISORDERS CENTER

In severe symptomatic cases, simple bedside observation by a knowledgeable clinician can establish the diagnosis of sleep apnea. Why then do we need sleep laboratories, polygraphs, oximeters, and expensive consultants? Here are a few reasons. Obstructive sleep apnea is not the only cause of excessive daytime somnolence (EDS). Another common cause is nocturnal myoclonus (restless legs syndrome), which must be diagnosed by appropriate pretibial electromyographic (EMG) leads.[4] The treatment is, of course, radically different from that of obstructive sleep apnea. Narcolepsy, another clinical syndrome that is frequently confused with sleep apnea,[5] consists of irresistible daytime hypersomnolence associated with several other symptoms, including cataplexy (the sudden loss of skeletal muscle tone in response to strong emotions such as laughter or anger), sleep paralysis (the inability to voluntarily move when just waking up or falling asleep), or hypnogogic hallucinations (vivid, life-like dreams at sleep onset). Narcolepsy is diagnosed by the occurrence of at least two of four rapid eye movement (REM) periods within 15 minutes of sleep onset during the daytime Multiple Sleep Latency Test (MSLT). The definitive diagnosis of narcolepsy is important to the clinician interested in respiratory disorders during sleep, since narcolepsy is included in the differential diagnosis of disorders associated with daytime hypersomnolence but is treated differently from sleep apnea.

In those patients with EDS whose spouses give classic histories of apnea symptoms and have observed cessation of breathing during sleep, what is the role of formal polysomnographic study and why can the diagnosis not be made with a simple apnea monitor on the hospital ward?[6] The answer is that it is simply not enough to know that the patient does or does not have sleep apnea. To aid the physician in selecting the appropriate therapy, one must have some method of quantifying the apneas in terms of number and duration. This must be corrected for the amount of sleep time, which can only be documented with use of the electroencephalograph (EEG). The physician must be assured not only that the patient slept adequately but that a variety of stages were experienced, including REM sleep, in which apneic episodes should be most frequent and of longest duration and deepest desaturation. Quantification of oxyhemoglobin saturation (SaO_2) must be available, as several studies have shown an association of the extent of daytime symptoms, as well as nocturnal arrhythmias, with the level of nocturnal SaO_2 (see Ch. 27). Establishment of a direct correlation between apnea and nocturnal cardiac arrhythmias could have a profound effect on treatment modalities. Finally, if the clinician contemplates anything other than a 100 percent curative procedure (e.g., tracheotomy), a basal level of apnea severity is needed to be able to later assess the success or lack of success of the selected therapy. Such therapeutic approaches would include the use of weight loss, drugs, and uvulopalatopharyngoplasty. All in all, the cardiopulmonary sleep laboratory is important in establishing a diagnosis as well as in providing adequate information to allow optimum treatment.

ELEMENTS OF THE CARDIOPULMONARY SLEEP STUDY

This chapter is not intended to give the reader the detailed information needed to set up and run a polysomnographic sleep study. Excellent technical manuals are available on all aspects of polysomnography, including equipment, lead connections, and scoring of the studies.[7,8] Only essential materials and techniques are described in this section. The basic tool for the polysomnographer is the polysomnograph (Fig. 55-1). Its multiple amplifiers allow recording of the low-voltage EEG electro-oculographic (EOG), EMG, and electrocardiographic (ECG) potentials to aid in the staging of sleep.

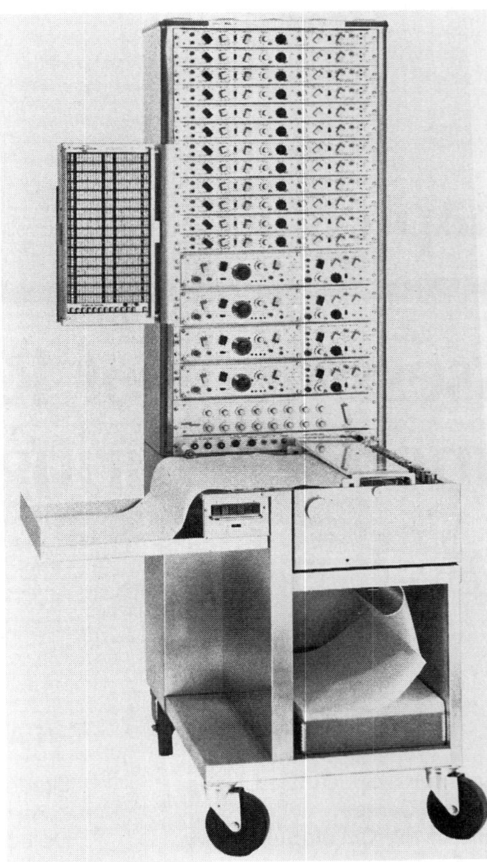

Figure 55-1. One of several commonly used polysomnographs for monitoring all parameters of the cardiopulmonary sleep study. The top 12 amplifiers monitor the low-voltage signals, such as the EEG and EOG signals. The higher-gain amplifiers receive raw signals from pressure amplifiers or processed signals from such devices as the ear oximeter. (Courtesy of Grass Instruments, Quincy, MA).

Other amplifiers receive signals from sensing devices for airflow and chest/abdominal wall motion (Fig. 55-2) and from ear or finger pulse oximeters.

Detection of Sleep Stage

Various montages for monitoring EEG signals are favored by different laboratories, but the most frequently used are the C_3 and C_4 leads placed just to the left and right of midline over the vertex (Fig. 55-3). These are referred to leads placed over the contralateral mastoid areas or on the earlobes (A_1 and A_2). Eye movements are monitored by leads placed over the outer canthus or temporal area of each eye. Two EMG leads are placed over or beneath the chin to detect tonic and phasic genioglossus muscle activity (particularly useful as an aid in detecting REM sleep). Single or multiple chest leads

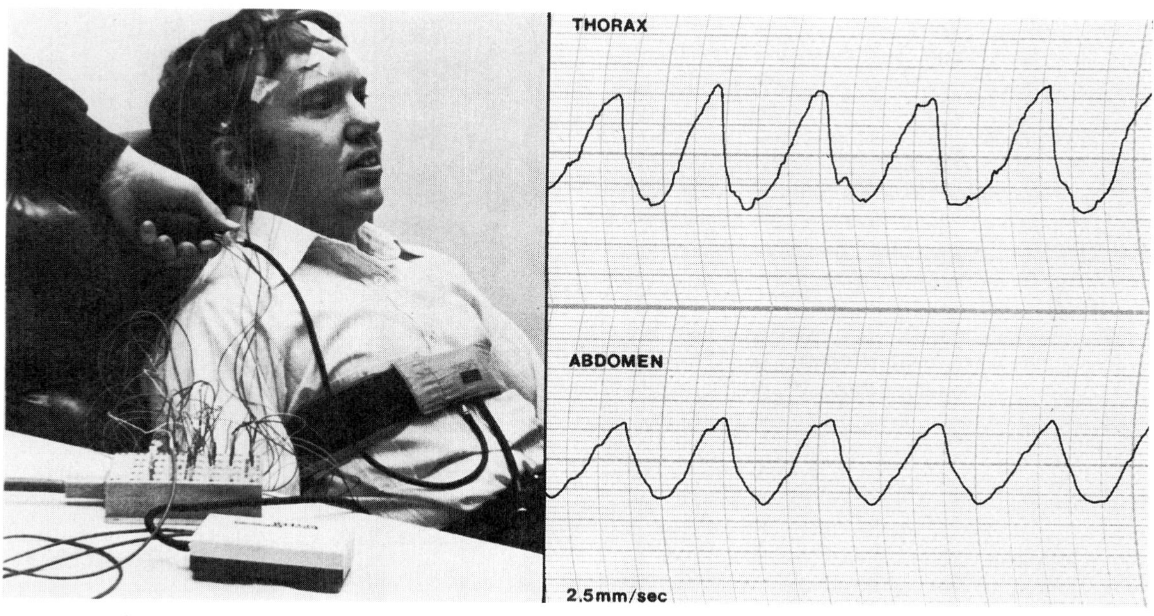

Figure 55-2. The pneumobelt, a simple, inexpensive monitor of chest and abdomen movement. Inflated cuffs are attached to belts around the chest and abdomen. Expansion of the chest increases pressure in the bladder, which is transmitted to a pressure transducer and amplified by the polysomnograph. (Courtesy of Grass Instruments, Quincy, MA).

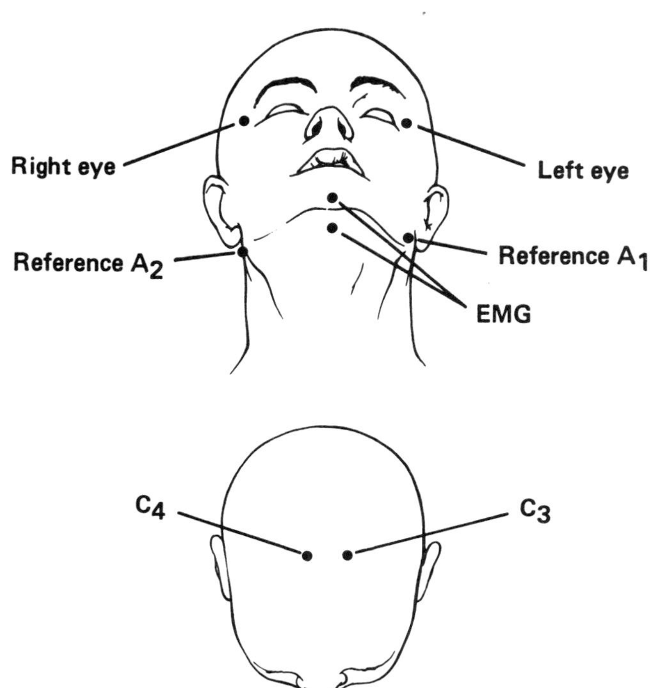

Figure 55-3. A common montage for placement of EEG, EOG, and EMG leads. Cortical activity is monitored by the C_4 and C_3 leads referred to the opposite ear or mastoid area (A_2, A_3). Leads over the outer canthi of the eyes monitor eye movement. Genioglossus muscle activity is monitored by leads over the chin. (From Fletcher,[38] with permission.)

may be used to monitor cardiac rhythm throughout the night to allow reporting of rate and rhythm. A pretibial electrode is frequently used to detect nocturnal myoclonus.

Detection and Quantitation of Airflow

In my opinion a monitor of expiratory airflow over the mouth and nose is essential in most sleep studies. Some laboratories avoid sensors over the face by calibrating abdominal and chest inductance plethysmographs (Respitrace, Ardsley, New York) so that absence of airflow is inferred by a ''zero sum'' signal from the inductance vests. However, such laboratories must be set up for computer calibration of this device and must have technicians experienced enough to ensure that the device remains properly calibrated in all sleep positions throughout the night.[9]

Two commonly used airflow sensing devices are heat-sensitive thermistors and the rapid-response end-tidal CO_2 analyzer (capnograph). The thermistor, which detects changes in temperature between room and expired air, is the most commonly used flow detector. The capnograph continuously samples air from a face mask or nosepiece and measures expired PCO_2. Inspiration causes a fall in PCO_2 as the sampling line picks up room air, while expiration causes an upward deflection as exhaled CO_2 is picked up by the sensing device (Fig. 55-4). It is important to monitor airflow from the mouth and both nares, as small volumes of air should be detected in order to differentiate apnea from hypopnea.

Another device for monitoring expiratory airflow is the

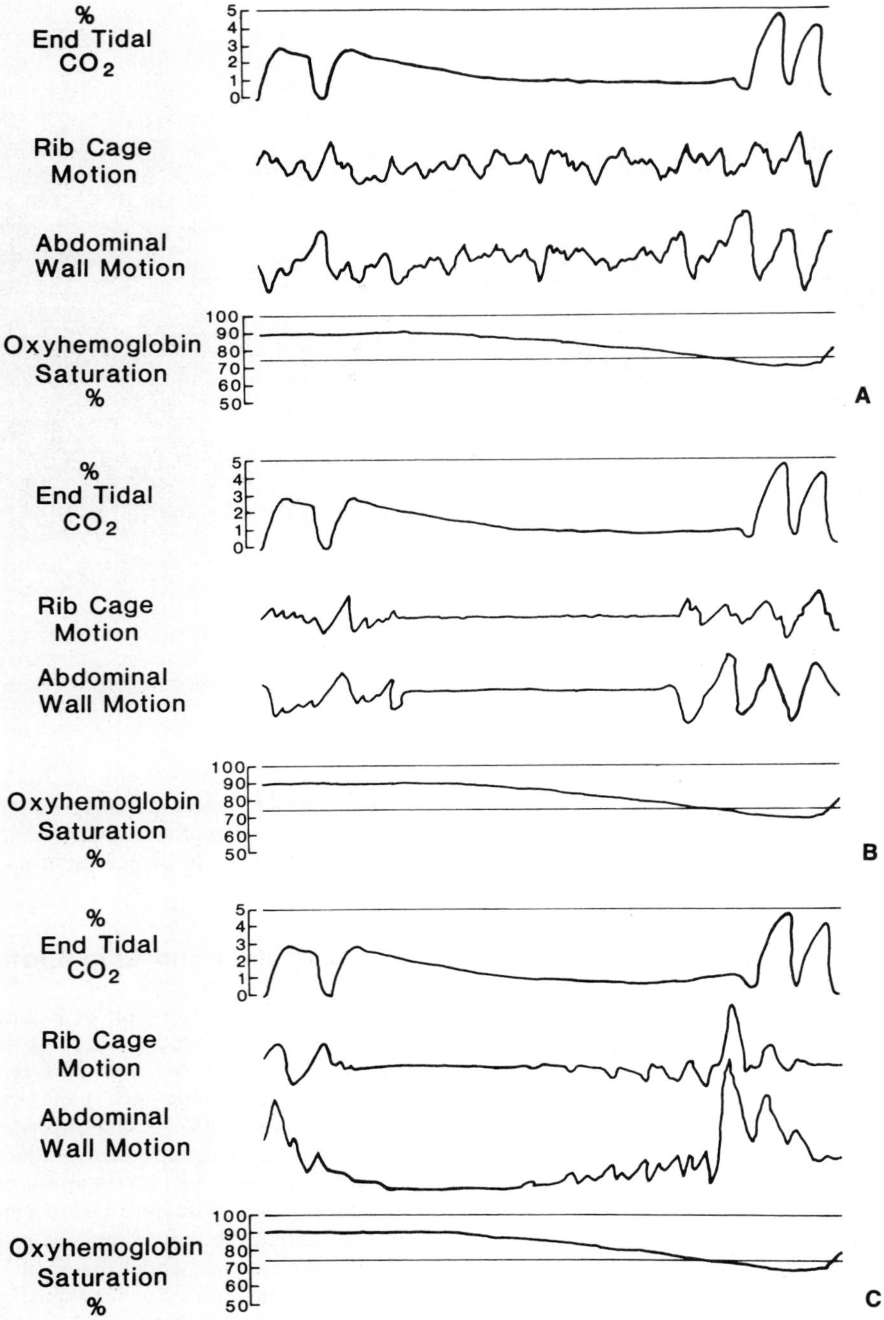

Figure 55-4. **(A)** Example of obstructive apnea. One normal breath appears, followed by an apneic period lasting about 30 seconds. Obstruction is evidenced on the rib cage and abdominal wall motion channels by continued movement revealing efforts to overcome the upper airway obstruction. The apnea is terminated by a supranormal size breath, and normal respiration follows. The fall in SaO_2 is slightly delayed owing to the circulation time required for desaturated blood to reach the earpiece of the oximeter. **(B)** Example of central apnea. There is no apparent chest or abdomen movement during the apnea, which reflects lack of central controller output to the respiratory muscles. **(C)** Example of mixed apnea. The first half of the apnea is central in origin, with no obvious respiratory effort. The second half shows a gradual increase in respiratory effort, with a final large effort overcoming the obstruction.

pneumotachograph, now practical as an airflow monitor since lightweight, easier to use models have been developed.[10] The drawback to this device is that if tidal volume is to be measured accurately, a tight-fitting mask must be worn over the mouth and nose, which may be uncomfortable for the patient. Such techniques are more applicable to the research laboratory. More recent technology monitors airflow by use of tracheal microphones provided with appropriate amplifiers and filters to detect fine air movements.[11,12]

There are three general types of apnea, defined on the basis of respiratory controller output. *Obstructive apnea* results from anatomic or functional obstruction to inspiratory airflow. To document obstructive apnea, one must demonstrate the absence of airflow at the nose and mouth in the presence of continued respiratory effort, manifested either by paradoxical chest wall/abdominal wall motion or by the generation of negative inspiratory pleural pressure (Fig. 55-4A). *Central apnea* is seen less commonly than obstructive apnea, although almost all apnea patients exhibit some of each apnea type (Fig. 55-4B). To document central apnea one must demonstrate the absence of airflow along with the *absence* of respiratory effort. Mixed apnea is commonly seen accompanying obstructive apnea (Fig. 55-4C). The first portion of the mixed apnea is of a central nature with absence of airflow and respiratory effort. During the second portion the polysomnogram shows gradual onset of respiratory muscle effort, often building to a crescendo, until the apnea is broken. The central portion always precedes the obstructive portion, and the obstructive portion may constitute such a small part of the apnea that at first glance the apnea appears to be purely central in nature.

Detection of Ventilatory Muscle Activity

There are many methods available for detecting respiratory effort. The most sensitive is to measure negative deflections in esophageal pressure by a balloon-tipped catheter swallowed prior to sleep.[13,14] Newer, smaller catheters with miniature transducers located in the catheter tip are available, which make this procedure much more tolerable to the patient[15] (Fig. 55-5). This method is particularly useful in morbidly obese patients, in whom chest and abdominal wall movements may not be well detected so that there is a question of differentiating obstructive from central apnea. Such devices detect virtually any respiratory effort in any size patient. One disadvantage, aside from discomfort to the patient, is that additional technical skill is required to calibrate and insert the catheter.

Other noninvasive techniques for measuring of respiratory effort, which are accurate enough for the usual clinical study and very acceptable to the patient, are diaphragmatic and intercostal muscle EMG,[16] and use of mercury strain gauges,[17] pneumatic belt devices, magnetometers,[18] and the Respitrace inductance vests mentioned earlier.[19–22] With the exception of the intercostal EMG, these devices rely on physical movement of the abdomen and/or chest wall to produce a change in an amplified electrical signal. They are relatively simple to use and in most clinical laboratories are used in a semiquantitative mode, that is, they are not reliable for exact quantification of tidal volume. With proper computer-assisted calibration, the Respitrace can be brought to within 15 percent accuracy of measured expired volume.[19]

Monitoring Oxygenation

Ear and finger pulse oximetry is now widely used to measure SaO_2 during sleep. The early oximeters such as the Hewlett-Packard 47201A were extremely accurate and easy to calibrate but were uncomfortable because of the large size of the earpiece and the necessity to heat the ear to "arterialize" capillary circulation. This oximeter measures eight wavelengths of light transmitted through the capillary bed of

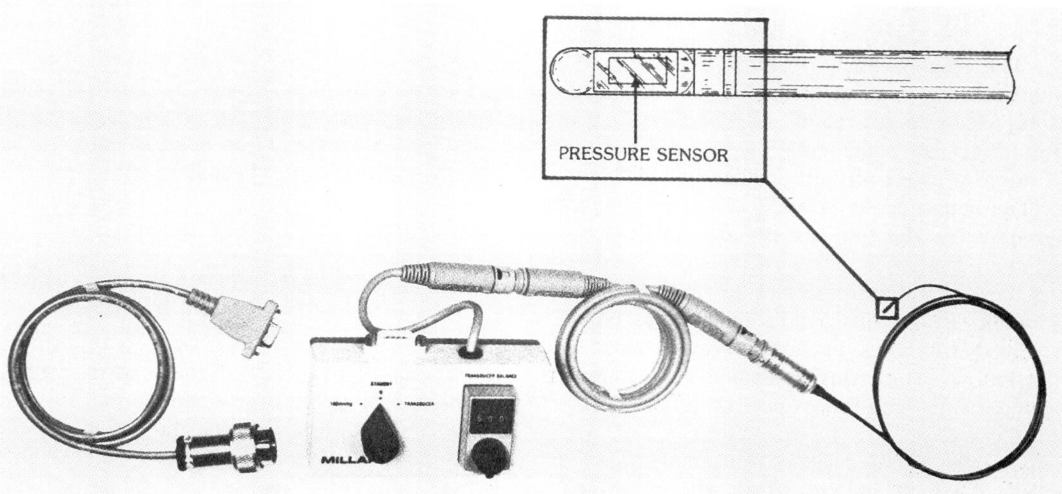

Figure 55-5. Pressure monitoring system that can be used to monitor esophageal and hence intrathoracic pressure. Since the pressure transducer is located in the tip of the catheter, there is no bulky balloon. The catheter is soft and pliable, so that most patients tolerate it and sleep with little difficulty.

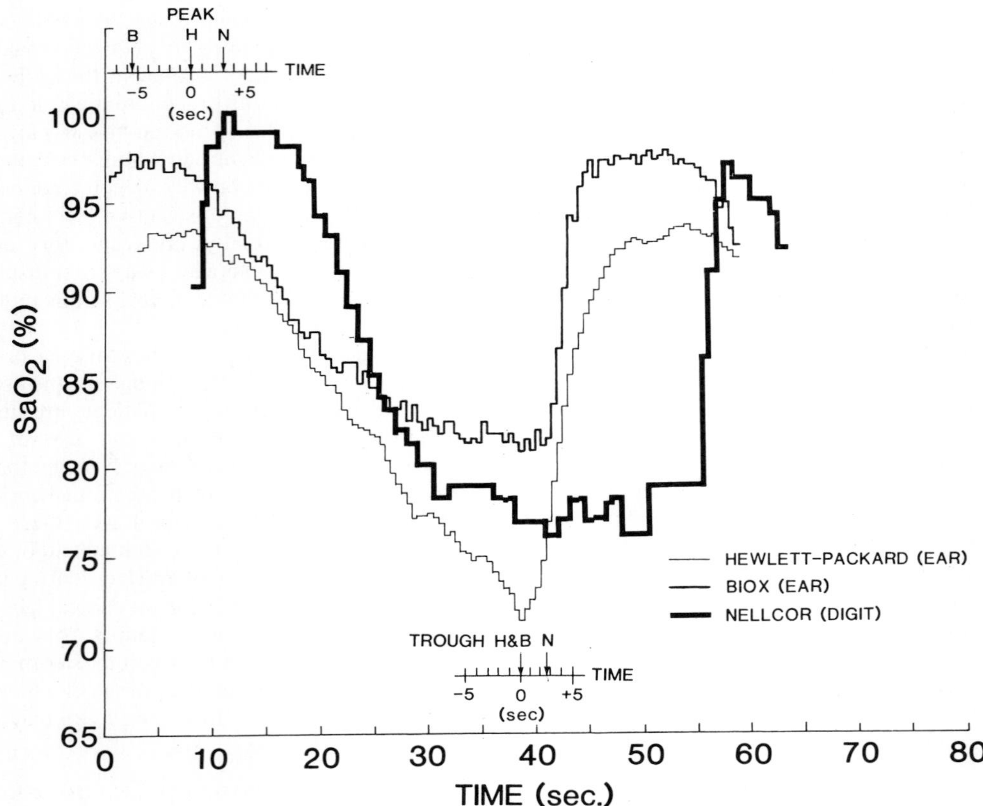

Figure 55-6. Comparison of dynamic response to changing SaO_2 in three oximeters, namely, Hewlett-Packard (H-P), Biox III (ear), and Nelcor (digit). The H-P ear oximeter is described in the text and in this comparison is used as the standard. Note that the Biox peaks at the high saturation about 5 seconds before the H-P but corresponds in time to the H-P trough. The Nelcor oximeter registers both the peak and the trough later than does the H-P. Differences in the dynamic response may be due to differences in circulation time, oximeter software, and methods of measurement among the machines. Also note the differences in absolute SaO_2 levels among the three machines. (From West et al.,[39] with permission.)

the earlobe. The Hewlett-Packard 47201A oximeter is no longer manufactured or serviced and has been replaced by newer models, which do not require heating the skin above 37°C, are less affected by pigmentation, and are in general more comfortable because of their smaller size and ease of application. The newer pulse oximeters employ photoelectric plethysmography and two wavelengths of light transmitted through a pulsatile capillary bed. To avoid excessive instability of the signal due to fluctuations in the pulse and sensor movement, the output signal is computed as a moving time average of saturations, usually ranging from a 3- to a 5-second window. Numerous published clinical evaluations and comparisons with co-oximetered blood are available[23–30] (Fig. 55-6).

Brief mention must also be made of transcutaneous O_2 and CO_2 monitoring.[31] This technique, which relies on the physical transfer of these gases across the skin, where they are picked up by a sensing electrode and analyzed, has been very successful in monitoring neonates and children, probably because of better transfer of gases across pediatric skin and the lack of need to monitor rapid changes.[32] The technique is not well adapted to adults because of the difficulty in finding suitable areas of skin in which gas transfer is adequate and also because of the need in adults to monitor rapidly changing levels of oxygenation from apnea.

ELEMENTS OF THE SLEEP STUDY REPORT

The final product of all the sophisticated equipment used in the cardiopulmonary sleep laboratory is the report. This report should first mention the patient's sleep architecture, including relative and absolute time spent in each sleep stage, number of awakenings, latency to sleep onset, and sleep efficiency. A complete description of the breathing pattern should follow, with the number and types of apnea and their relative distribution, the mean and longest duration, the mean and lowest saturation, modifications in frequency of apnea due to body position change, and effect of sleep stage on apnea severity. In some laboratories on-line computer sampling systems are used continuously to monitor such events as saturation. Thus, these laboratories are able to report the time spent in O_2 saturations between 80 and 90 percent, 70 and 80 percent, and so forth, which can be quite helpful in assessing the effects of treatment modalities.[33] It is not difficult to appreciate that scoring the study of a patient with 400 to 500 apneas per night would be quite difficult and time-consuming, and many efforts have been made to devise automated scoring techniques and shortcuts in scoring. Sampling methods that assess only 50, 25, or 12.5 percent of the apneas have been demonstrated to yield accurate information and to closely approximate the results of full record scoring.[34]

SPECIALIZED STUDIES

An older technique for measuring oxygenation during sleep was to draw frequent blood gases through an indwelling arterial line. This, of course, is highly subject to sampling error and is reserved for special research situations in which acute changes in blood pressure or PaO_2 must be monitored. An example of such a situation would be the monitoring of the response in CO_2 retention brought about by using supplemental O_2 in apnea patients with baseline hypercarbia.[35] With proper technique, the well-placed arterial line does not interfere with sleep and allows the patient sufficient movement capability. Other specialized studies, such as the sampling of blood catecholamines, can be frequently performed during the night without disturbing the patient.

Monitoring of pulmonary artery pressure by central flotation catheters is a highly specialized technique reserved for sleep research laboratories. Although such studies have limited application, the information produced by them has added greatly to our understanding of the effect of nocturnal sleep disturbances on both sleep and awake cardiopulmonary function. Acute elevations in pulmonary artery pressure have been shown to accompany the transient hypoxemia of apnea and the longer, deeper desaturations of REM-related hypoxemia in chronic lung and chest wall diseases. Such techniques have little clinical applicability.[36,37]

References

1. Standards for Accreditation: Association of Sleep Disorders Centers Accreditation Package. Association of Sleep Disorders Centers, Rochester, MN, 1987, Section III pp. 1–17
2. Association of Sleep Disorder Centers: Diagnostic classification of sleep and arousal disorders. (1st Ed.) Sleep 1979;2:1–137
3. Block AJ, Cohn MA, Conway WA et al: Indications and standards for cardiopulmonary sleep studies. Sleep 1985;8:371–379
4. Coleman RM: Periodic movements in sleep (nocturnal myoclonus) and restless legs syndrome. p. 265–295. In Guilleminault C (ed): Sleeping and Waking Disorders: Indications and Techniques. Addison-Wesley, Menlo Park, CA, 1982
5. Roth B: Narcolepsy and hypersomnia. pp. 29–59. In Williams RL, Karacan I (ed): Sleep Disorders: Diagnosis and Treatment. John Wiley & Sons, New York, 1978
6. Rutherford R, Popkin J, Nguyen HK et al: Reliability of respiratory sleep studies versus polysomnography in the investigation of suspected obstructive sleep apnea. Am Rev Respir Dis 1987;135:A48
7. Carskadon MA: Basics for polygraphic monitoring of sleep. pp. 1–16. In Guilleminault C (ed): Sleeping and Waking Disorders: Indications and Techniques. Addison-Wesley, Menlo Park, CA, 1982
8. Rechtschaffen A, Kales A (eds): A Manual of Standardized Terminology, Techniques and Scoring System for Sleep Stages of Human Subjects. NIH Publication 204 National Institutes of Health, Washington, DC, 1968
9. Morel DR, Forster A, Suter PM: Noninvasive ventilatory monitoring with bellows pneumographs in supine subjects. J Appl Physiol 1983;55:598–606
10. Sullivan WJ, Petters GM, Enright PL: Pneumotachographs: Theory and clinical applications. Respir Care 1984;29:736–49
11. Krumpe PE, Cummiskey JM: Use of laryngeal sound recordings to monitor apnea. Am Rev Respir Dis 1984;122:797–801
12. Peirick J, Shepard JW Jr: Automated aponea detection by computer: analysis of tracheal breath sounds. Med Bio Eng Comput 1983;21:632–635
13. Lemen R, Benson M, Jones JG: Absolute pressure measurements with hand-dipped and manufactured esophageal balloons. J Appl Physiol 1974;37:600–603
14. Milic-Emili J, Mead J, Turner JM, Glauser EM: Improved technique for estimating pleural pressure from esophageal balloons. J Appl Physiol 1984;19:207–211
15. Geddes LA: Blood pressure transducers. pp. 46–47. In Geddes LA (ed): Cardiovascular Devices and Their Applications. John Wiley & Sons, New York, 1984
16. Sanders MH, Holzer BC, Reynolds CF: A tale of two polysomnographic techniques. Sleep Res 1984;13:212
17. BHL Electronics: SR-4 Strain Gauge Handbook. Electronics, Waltham, MA, 1980
18. Sharp JT, Druz WS, Foster JR et al: Use of the respiratory magnetometer in diagnosis and classification of sleep apnea. Chest 1980;77:350–353
19. Gonzalez H, Haller B, Watson HL, Sackner MA: Accuracy of respiratory inductive plethysmograph over wide range of rib cage and abdominal compartmental contributions to tidal volume in normal subjects and in patients with chronic obstructive pulmonary disease. Am Rev Respir Dis 1984;130:171–174
20. Hudgel DW, Capehart M, Johnson B et al: Accuracy of tidal volume, lung volume, and flow measurements by inductance vest in COPD patients. J Appl Physiol 1984;56:1659–1665, 1984
21. Chadha TS, Watson H, Birch S et al: Validation of respiratory inductive plethysmography using different calibration procedures. Am Rev Respir Dis 1982;125:644–649
22. Loveridge B, West P, Anthonisen NR, Kryger MH: Single-position calibration of the respiratory inductance plethysmograph. J Appl Physiol 1983;55:1031–1034
23. Douglas NJ, Brash HM, Wraith PK et al: Accuracy, sensitivity to carboxyhemoglobin, and speed of response of the Hewlett-Packard 47201A ear oximeter. Am Rev Respir Dis 1979;119: 311–313
24. Kagle DM, Alexander CM, Berko RS et al: Evaluation of the Ohmeda 3700 pulse oximeter: Steady-state and transient response characteristics. Anesthesiology 1987;66:376–380
25. Mackenzie N: Comparison of a pulse oximeter with an ear oximeter and an in-vitro oximeter. J Clin Monit 1985;1:156–160
26. Stradling JR: The accuracy of the Hewlett-Packard 47201A ear oximeter below 50% saturation. Bull Eur Physiopathol Respir 1982;18:791–794
27. Chapman KR, Liu FLW, Watson RM, Rebuck AS: Range and accuracy of two-wavelength oximetry. Chest 1986;89:540–542
28. Rebuck AS, Chapman KR, D'Urzo A: The accuracy and response characteristics of a simplified ear oximeter. Chest 1983;83:860–864
29. Tytler JA, Seeley HF: The Nellcor N-101 pulse oximeter. Anaesthesia 1986;41:302–305
30. George CF, West P, Kryger MH: The accuracy and response

dynamics of transmittance and pulse oximeters in sleep apnea. Am Rev Respir Dis 1987;135:A50
31. Burki NK, Albert RK: Noninvasive monitoring of arterial blood gases. A report of the ACCP section on respiratory pathophysiology. Chest 1983;83:666–670
32. Schoemaker WC, Vidyasagar D (eds): Transcutaneous O_2 and CO_2 monitoring of the adult and neonate. Crit Care Med 1981;9:689–760
33. Slutsky AS, Strohl KP: Quantification of oxygen saturation during episodic hypoxemia. Am Rev Respir Dis 1980;121:893–895
34. Steyer BJ, Quan SF, Morgan WJ: Polysomnography scoring for sleep apnea. Am Rev Respir Dis 1985;131:592–595
35. Alford NJ, Fletcher EC, Nickeson D: Effects of acute oxygen in patients with sleep apnea and chronic obstructive lung disease. Chest 1986;898:30–38
36. Fletcher EC, Levin DC: Effect of acute and chronic oxygen on cardiopulmonary hemodynamics during sleep in patients with COPD. Chest 1984;85:6–14
37. Coccagna G, Mantovani M, Brignani F et al: Continuous recording of the pulmonary and systemic arterial pressure during sleep in syndromes of hypersomnia with periodic breathing. Bull Eur Physiopathol Respir 1972;8:1159–1172
38. Fletcher EC: History, techniques, and definitions in sleep related respiratory disorders. pp. 1–20. In Fletcher EC (ed): Abnormalities of Respiration during Sleep: Diagnosis, Pathophysiology, and Treatment. Grune & Stratton, Orlando, FL, 1986
39. West P, George CF, Kryger MH: Dynamic in vivo response characteristics of three oximeters: H-P 47201A, Biox III, and Nellcor N-100. Sleep 1987;10:263–271

Chapter 56

Airway Challenge Testing

Michael T. Kochansky
Dean R. Hess

CHAPTER OUTLINE

Since about the middle of the twentieth century very few changes have taken place in the basic diagnostic procedures that are used to assess pulmonary function. Growth in pulmonary diagnostics has consisted primarily of better understanding of the physiology of pulmonary disease and computerization of existing pulmonary function techniques. One important exception to this has been the clinical introduction of *airway challenge testing*.

Airway challenge testing, sometimes called *bronchial provocation testing*, is the use of a bronchoconstricting agent to induce bronchial reactivity under laboratory conditions. Originally this testing was performed on patients who were experiencing transient asthma-like symptoms but who had no prior documentation of asthma. The test was very useful in confirming newly developed cases of asthma that were not clinically apparent.

Variant forms of asthma have been recognized. An example is a condition called *chronic cough asthma*, which is a form of bronchial hyperreactivity characterized by chronic persistent cough, usually following a viral respiratory infection.[1] Cough is often the only symptom, and the patient may have normal spirometry. The airway challenge test can determine whether the cough is secondary to bronchial hyperreactivity. The largest number of patients referred for airway challenge testing may fall into this category.

A feature common to all forms of asthma is bronchial hyperreactivity. It is this feature that allows one to "challenge" the bronchi with an appropriate constricting agent and to confirm the diagnosis of asthma or bronchial hyperreactivity. Indications for airway challenge testing are

- Asthma-like symptoms in otherwise normal subjects
- Asthma-like symptoms in atopic, nonasthmatic subjects
- Chronic persistent cough of unknown etiology
- Occupationally associated asthma-like symptoms
- Exercise-induced asthma-like symptoms
- Assessment of the therapeutic value of medications in known asthmatic patients

Challenge testing has widespread applicability. Failure to perform such a test in some of these situations may result in misdiagnosis or mismanagement of the patient. However, the converse is not necessarily true.

Although a positive challenge test is an indication of nonspecific bronchial hyperreactivity, it does not conclusively demonstrate the cause of the patient's hyperreactivity. As

Table 56-1. Methods of Airway Challenge Testing

Cholinergic drugs or mediating substances
Methacholine, carbachol, histamine
Specific allergens
Grains, pollens
Other
Exercise, exercise/cold air, isocapnic hyperventilation of cold air, isocyanates or various other chemicals, fumes

Table 56-2. Recommended Times to Refrain from Medications before Airway Challenge Testing

24 hours
Beta-adrenergic agents, alpha-adrenergic blockers, anticholinergic agents, cromolyn sodium
48 hours
Decongestants, antihistamines
96 hours
Hydroxyzine

seen in Table 56-1, there are many forms of challenge testing, of which the most common and safest are the methacholine challenge and the exercise challenge. Cold air challenge is also receiving attention as a safe and reproducible test but is still not widely used.[2]

DRUG CHALLENGES

Acetyl-beta-methylcholine (Methacholine, Mecholyl, Provocholine) is the beta-methyl homologue of acetylcholine. An important difference is that its duration of action and selectivity are somewhat greater than those of acetylcholine. Methacholine chloride is a parasympathomimetic (cholinergic) bronchoconstrictor that is administered in aerosol form. Bronchial smooth muscle, having significant parasympathetic (cholinergic) innervation, responds promptly to administration of the drug. Aerosolization localizes the response to the bronchial muscle, and because methacholine is more slowly hydrolyzed by acetylcholinesterase than is acetylcholine, the response can be easily measured. Considerable research with methacholine since the mid-1960s attests to its safety for widespread clinical use.[3–11] Adverse reactions to methacholine are rare, but a distinct contraindication to performing the test is a history of cholinergic hypersensitivity (cholinergic urticaria).[12]

Carbachol chloride has been studied to a lesser extent than methacholine. Its stimulatory action and results are similar, but its use is limited because it is not widely available.[13] *Histamine phosphate* also may be given by inhalation, following a protocol similar to that with methacholine. Although many researchers have shown responses similar to that of methacholine, others believe that methacholine is better in differentiating between asthmatic and normal subjects.[8,10]

PREREQUISITES FOR TESTING

Methacholine, carbachol, and histamine challenges are all safe enough to be performed on an outpatient basis. Induction of bronchoconstriction may be promptly reversed by an aerosolized bronchodilator. To ensure test validity, however, there are several important prerequisites for testing. Patients should be tested in an asymptomatic state and should not be taking medications. Specific minimum recommended times to refrain from various medications prior to the test are listed in Table 56-2. Corticosteroids have little or no effect on reactivity and do not need to be held.[14] Patients also should refrain from using over-the-counter drugs such as cold preparations. Additionally, patients should refrain from caffeine and smoking on the day of the test. Patients who are receiving beta-adrenergic blocking drugs should be tested with caution, since their response to the challenge agent may be enhanced and prolonged.

TESTING PROCEDURE

After verifying normal reproducible spirometry, the patient may first be given five breaths of a control substance such as physiologic saline solution. However, some laboratories prefer not to administer the saline control. If repeat spirometry is still normal after the control, the patient proceeds with the methacholine challenge. One of three protocols is used: the single-strength multiple breath test, the variable dilution technique, or the timed tidal breathing technique.

Single-Strength Multiple Breath Test

The single-strength multiple breath test is perhaps the simplest semiquantitative test. A single concentration of methacholine (5 mg/mL) is used for the duration of the test. Increasing doses are given by increasing the number of breaths until a maximum number of breaths is reached or a positive test is apparent. With all techniques, the most common criterion for determining a positive response is a 20 percent drop in the absolute value of the forced expiratory volume in 1 second (FEV_1) from the baseline FEV_1 in less than about 200 cumulative dose units (cdu) of the drug (1 cdu is defined as one breath of a 1 mg/mL solution). In the single-strength test this would be 40 breaths of a 5 mg/mL solution.[6]

If the patient exhibits a 20 percent decrease in FEV_1 at any time during the test, the reversal drug is administered. Confirmation of bronchodilator reversal by spirometry is also necessary. The dose-response graph in Figure 56-1 shows the results of a positive test by this technique. Such results are usually expressed in terms of the provocative dose required to produce a 20 percent fall in FEV_1 (PD_{20}) or of the equivalent concentration (PC_{20}) when using the variable dilution technique.

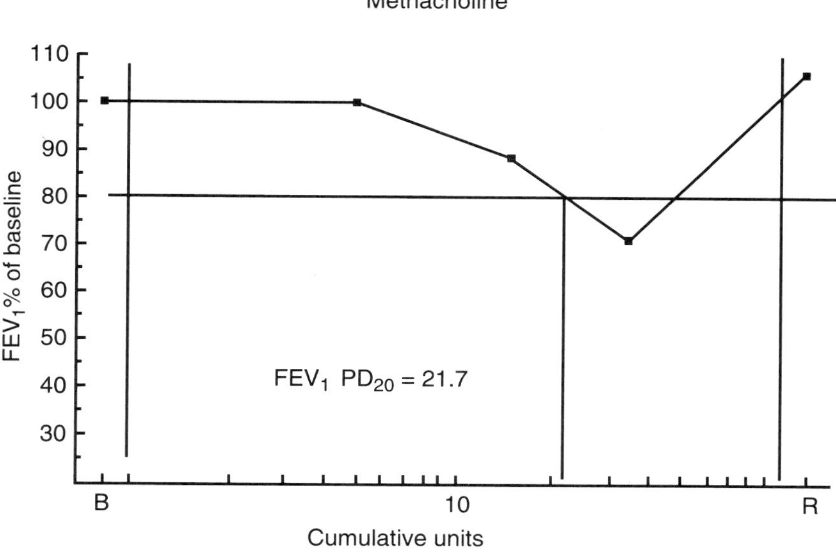

Figure 56-1. Dose-response graph of a positive methacholine challenge test. B, baseline; R, reversal.

Variable Dilution Technique

The variable dilution technique is the recommended standard method[15,16]; however, it requires more time and equipment than the single-strength test. The procedure is to administer five breaths each of increasing concentrations of methacholine (0.025 mg/mL, 0.25 mg/mL, 2.5 mg/mL, 10 mg/mL, and 25 mg/mL) until a positive response is encountered or until the end of this dosing sequence. The total dosage after this test is 188.88 cumulative dose units. This test requires six different nebulizers, one for each dilution and one for the reversal agent. It also requires preparation of the different solutions either in the laboratory or the hospital pharmacy.

Timed Tidal Breathing Technique

The *timed tidal breathing technique* is a very simple method, but its results are not easily quantitated. It involves administering the agent during a 2-minute period of tidal breathing, followed by spirometry testing to determine response. The number of these 2-minute periods varies among laboratories. This technique is not as widely used as the others because the amount of the drug administered is not easily measured. There is also debate about exactly when the patient should be tested if symptoms occur before the scheduled total exposure time has elapsed. The induction of symptoms alone does not necessarily suggest a positive response. With all techniques, an aerosolized bronchodilator should be administered even if the patient does not exhibit a positive response to the test.

With both the single-strength and the variable dilution techniques, some laboratories prefer to use a medication dosimeter (Fig. 56-2). This device actuates the nebulizer for a precise time interval while the patient inhales. Although in theory it seems to help quantify the delivered dose of the agent, most laboratories do not use this device. The most common practice is to have the patient inhale the agent from functional residual capacity to total lung capacity (inspiratory capacity) by using a disposable nebulizer such as that used for bronchodilator administration.

EXERCISE AND COLD AIR CHALLENGE

Although patients with bronchial hyperreactivity may be stimulated into bronchospasm with exercise, there are many individuals who only have bronchoconstriction during or immediately following exercise. The cause of this reaction is not clear, but current research is showing that respiratory heat loss and/or respiratory water loss are the probable causative factors.[17]

It is often difficult to reproduce the conditions necessary to bring about exercise-induced bronchoconstriction in the laboratory. Exercise on a bicycle ergometer or treadmill may not be as productive as free running.[18] As a result, researchers have been searching for other methods of testing that correlate with exercise-inducing conditions.[19–21] Breathing subfreezing air during exercise and isocapnic hyperventilation of cold air are two of these methods.

Isocapnic hyperventilation of cold air allows the patient to hyperventilate subfreezing air from a cooling device while CO_2 is titrated into the circuit to maintain a normal $PaCO_2$. Beside being safe and reproducible, this technique may produce positive test results in some patients who do not re-

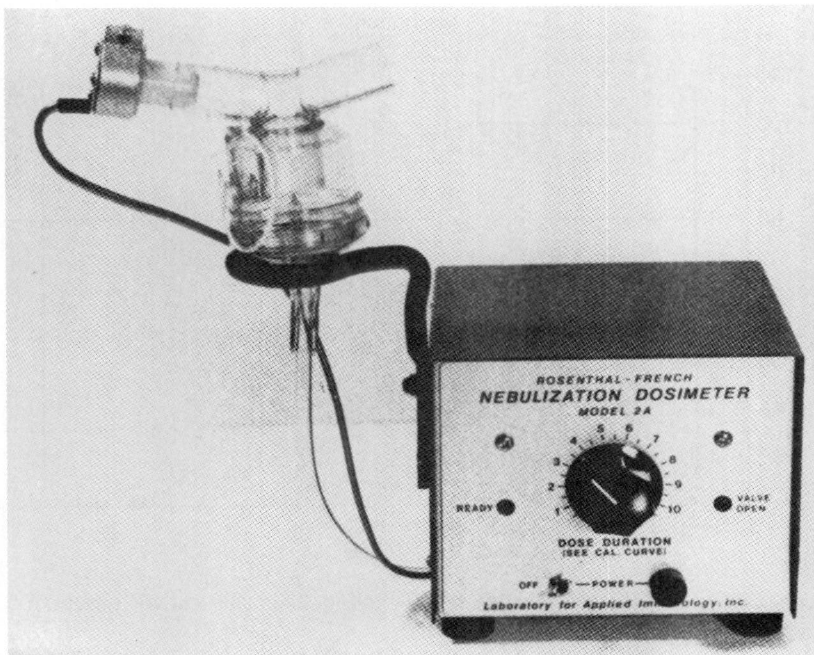

Figure 56-2. Rosenthal nebulization dosimeter. (Courtesy of Richard Rosenthal, M.D., Laboratory for Applied Immunology, Fairfax, VA.)

spond to methacholine. The somewhat simpler method of breathing chilled air from a cooling device during exercise may also be used. With both methods the prerequisites for drug challenges should be followed prior to the test.

OTHER FORMS OF AIRWAY CHALLENGE TESTING

While the tests described thus far are safe and reproducible, there are others that warrant a considerable amount of caution. Use of a specific grain, pollen, or other allergen presents a new set of problems to the laboratory. It is difficult to determine a safe concentration by inhalation. While some patients may tolerate moderate concentrations, others may respond severely to extremely small amounts. When using these agents it is also common for the patient to have an immediate reaction as well as a late reaction, or sometimes only a late reaction. Late reactions may occur as much as 12 to 18 hours after inhalation of the substance, so it is advisable for the patient to be admitted to the hospital for the study.[22]

The reactions also may be substantially more severe than those seen with cholinergic agents. They may even require subcutaneous or intravenous bronchodilators for reversal. Because of these potential problems, these challenge tests are probably best left to research institutions or clinicians with a considerable degree of experience in the more common forms of airway challenge testing.

New irritants and sensitizing agents are being recognized regularly, especially in industrial work environments.[23] In the future there may be more testing in the work environment to identify causes of occupational asthma. The work environment itself is a challenge agent for some individuals.

Airway challenge testing is the newest form of pulmonary function testing to find a permanent place in the testing schemes of laboratories. At this time it is still in its infancy.

References

1. Corrao W, Braman S, Irwin R: Chronic cough as the sole presenting manifestation of bronchial asthma. N Engl J Med 1979;300:633–637
2. Deal E, McFadden E, Ingram R et al: Airway responsiveness to cold air and hyperpnea in normal subjects and in those with hay fever and asthma. Am Rev Respir Dis 1980;121:621–628
3. Parker C, Bilbo R, Reed C: Methacholine aerosol as a test for bronchial asthma. Arch Intern Med 1965;115:452–458
4. Townley R, Dennis M, Itkin I: Comparative action of acetyl-beta-methylcholine, histamine, and pollen antigens in subjects with hay fever and patients with bronchial asthma. J Allergy Clin Immunol 1965;36:121–137
5. Itkin I: Bronchial hypersensitivity to mecholyl and histamine in asthma subjects. J Allergy Clin Immunol 1967;40:245–256
6. Townley R, Ryo U, Kolotkin B, Kang B: Bronchial sensitivity to methacholine in current and former asthmatics and allergic rhinitis patients and control subjects. J Allergy Clin Immunol 1975;56:429–442
7. Conner G, Sparrow D, Segel M, Weiss S: Smoking, atopy, and methacholine airway responsiveness among middle-aged and elderly men. Am Rev Respir Dis 1989;140:1520–1526
8. Spector S, Farr R: A çomparison of methacholine and histamine inhalations in asthmatics. J Allergy Clin Immunol 1975;56:308–316

9. Lam S, Wong R, Yeung M: Nonspecific bronchial reactivity in occupational asthma. J Allergy Clin Immunol 1979;63:28–34
10. Chatham M, Bleeker E, Smith P et al: A comparison of histamine, methacholine, and exercise airway reactivity in normal and asthmatic subjects. Am Rev Respir Dis 1982;126:235–240
11. Townley R, McGeady S, Bewtra A: The effect of beta adrenergic blockade on bronchial sensitivity to acetyl-beta-methacholine in normal and allergic rhinitis subjects. J Allergy Clin Immunol 1976;57:358–366
12. Van Assendelft A: Syncope caused by methacholine in a patient with exercise-induced anaphylaxis (letter). Chest 1989;96:1442–1443
13. Orehek J, Gayrard P, Smith AP et al: Airway responses to carbachol in normal and asthmatic subjects. Am Rev Respir Dis 1977;115:937–943
14. Easton J: Effect of an inhaled corticosteroid on methacholine airway reactivity. J Allergy Clin Immunol 1981;67:388–390
15. Rosenthal R: Workshop proceedings on bronchoprovocation techniques for the evaluation of asthma. J Allergy Clin Immunol 1979;64:563–568
16. Chai H, Farr R, Froehlich L et al: Standardization of bronchial inhalation challenge procedures. J Allergy Clin Immunol 1975;56:323–327
17. Strauss R, McFadden E, Ingram R et al: Influence of heat and humidity on the airway obstruction induced by exercise in asthma. J Clin Invest 1978;61:433–440
18. Shapiro G, Pierson W, Furukawa C, Bierman C: A comparison of the effectiveness of free-running and treadmill exercise for assessing exercise-induced bronchospasm in clinical practice. J Allergy Clin Immunol 1979;64:609–611
19. Aquilina A: Comparison of airway reactivity induced by histamine methacholine, and isocapneic hyperventilation in normal and asthmatic subjects. Thorax 1983;38:766–770
20. O'Byrne P, Ryan G, Morris M et al: Asthma induced by cold air and its relation to nonspecific bronchial responsiveness to methacholine. Am Rev Respir Dis 1982;125:281–285
21. Heaton R, Henderson A, Costello J: Cold air as a bronchial provocation technique. Reproducibility and comparison with histamine and methacholine inhalation. Chest 1984;86:810–814
22. Spector S, Farr R: Bronchial inhalation challenge with antigens. J Allergy Clin Immunol 1979;64:580–586
23. Tarlo S, Broder I: Irritant-induced occupational asthma. Chest 1989;96:297–300

Chapter 57

Diagnostic Imaging

Justin P. Smith
David J. Pierson

CHAPTER OUTLINE

This chapter is a user's guide to diagnostic imaging of the chest. The bulk of the chapter is devoted to the role of conventional radiography for the evaluation of pulmonary abnormalities. We discuss how chest radiographs are made, the radiographic anatomy of the chest, the description of the abnormalities seen on a chest radiograph, a systematic method for evaluation of chest radiographs, and the radiographic characteristics of common pulmonary disorders. This chapter concludes with examples of the other forms of diagnostic imaging of the chest, including computed tomography (CT), fluoroscopy, pulmonary angiography, radionuclide studies, diagnostic ultrasound, and magnetic resonance imaging (MRI). The reader is encouraged to consult the general radiology texts[1–6] and the specialized references indicated throughout the chapter for elaboration on these topics.

CONVENTIONAL RADIOGRAPHY OF THE CHEST

Principles and Techniques

The radiographic appearance of the chest, normal or abnormal, depends on the patient's phase of respiration, position (supine, semiupright, or upright), and orientation with respect to the x-ray tube (anteroposterior [AP] or posteroanterior [PA]).

Figure 57-1A shows a PA upright radiograph taken in the main x-ray department with a dedicated chest x-ray machine with a grid and a 6-ft tube-screen distance. Figure 57-1B shows an AP supine radiograph of the same subject taken with the bedside x-ray machine at a 4-ft tube-screen distance—conditions that are typical for radiographs taken in the intensive care unit (ICU). How do the images differ (Table 57-1)? On the AP supine film the heart and superior mediastinum are considerably wider than on the PA upright film. The pulmonary vessels are less distinct and the hemidiaphragms higher on the AP supine film. Overall, the AP supine film shows greater contrast than does the PA upright film. Radiography, the process of making radiographs, is the key to understanding these differences.

Generation and Manipulation of X-Rays

Chest radiography involves several steps[7,8] (Fig. 57-2). The primary x-ray beam is generated by the interaction of a beam of electrons with a tungsten anode target. X-rays are

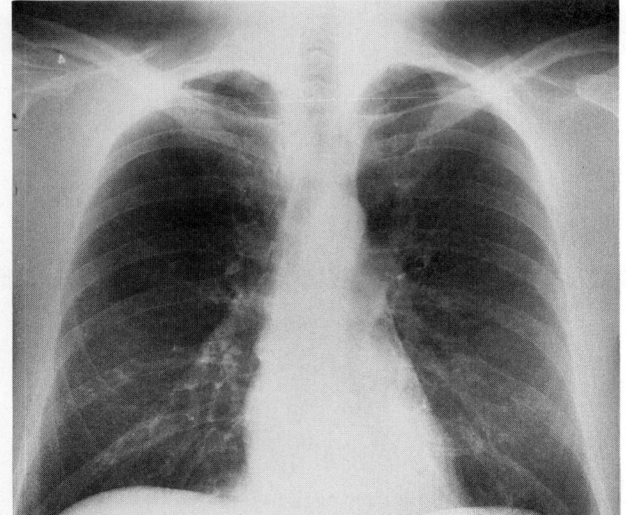

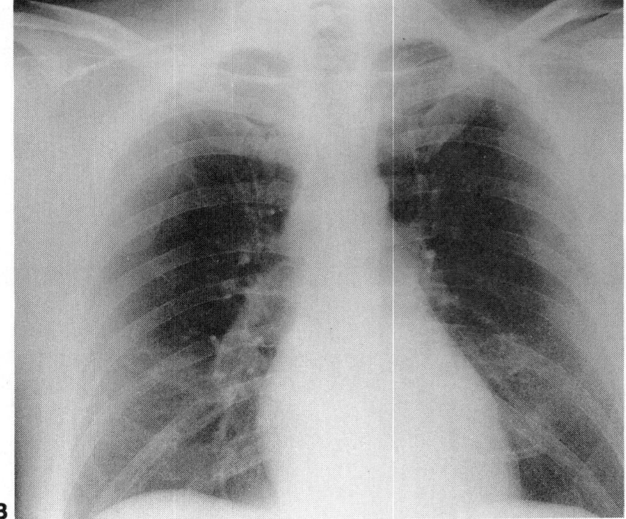

Figure 57-1. Chest radiographs of a 47-year-old, 6 ft 4 in. healthy man, comparing PA upright technique with AP supine technique. (**A**) PA upright 72-in. tube–subject distance: because of the patient's height, the supraclavicular region and the costophrenic sulci could not be included on the same film. (**B**) AP supine 48-in. tube–subject distance. As compared with the PA upright radiograph, the AP supine chest shows cephalization of flow, distension of the azygos vein, magnification of the heart, decreased lung volume, and increased opacity at the lung bases.

produced when the electrons bombarding the target undergo three possible interactions with tungsten atoms: pair production, photoelectic effect, and Compton scattering. Once the x-rays have been generated, they must be shaped to dimensions appropriate for an exposure (collimation) and filtered to remove the low-energy x-rays that would increase the patient's radiation dose without increasing the radiograph's diagnostic content.

As the collimated and filtered x-ray beam passes through the patient, a portion of the primary beam becomes scattered, forming secondary radiation. If the scattered radiation were allowed to reach the film, the contrast of the resulting radiograph would decrease. To limit the scattered radiation that reaches the film, a grid is placed between the patient and the film cassette.

X-radiation is inefficient in exposing film as compared with visible light. The ability of the primary x-ray beam to expose the film is increased 1000-fold by converting the x-rays emerging from the patient into visible light by means of the phosphors in the film cassette. As a result, radiographs are exposed almost entirely by visible light rather than by x-rays.

Table 57-1. How the AP Supine 48-Inch Chest Differs from the PA Upright 72-Inch Chest[a]

Relative to the normal PA upright chest, the AP supine chest shows
Cephalization of flow
Distension of the azygous vein
Magnification of the heart
Decreased depth of inspiration owing to the pressure of the abdominal contents on the diaphragm; shallower inspiration creates increased density of pulmonary vessels at the lung bases, which can be mistaken for pneumonia or pulmonary edema

[a] See Figure 57-1.

Anteroposterior versus Posteroanterior Projections

Divergence of the x-ray beam over distance distorts the patient's anatomy. The greater the distance between the patient and the film cassette, the greater the magnification of the patient's radiographic anatomy.

For the AP examination the patient's back is against the film cassette, and for the PA examination the patient's chest is against the cassette. Because the heart lies in the anterior chest, the PA examination brings the heart closer to the cassette than does the AP examination. Because the heart is farther from the film during an AP exposure, divergence of the beam magnifies the heart relative to the PA position[9] (Fig. 57-1).

Bedside radiographs are taken at a 48- rather than a 72-in. distance from x-ray tube to film cassette because of the lack of overhead space in the average ICU and because the 48-in. exposure conserves the batteries of the mobile x-ray machine. The price, however, is poorer spatial resolution. As a result the bedside radiograph is not as accurate as the upright 72-in. PA radiograph for evaluating the mediastinum, for determining heart size, for detecting subtle masses in the lung parenchyma, or for identifying thoracic fractures.

Radiographic Contrast

Differences in the absorption of the x-ray beam by tissues lead to different degrees of light and dark on a radiograph.

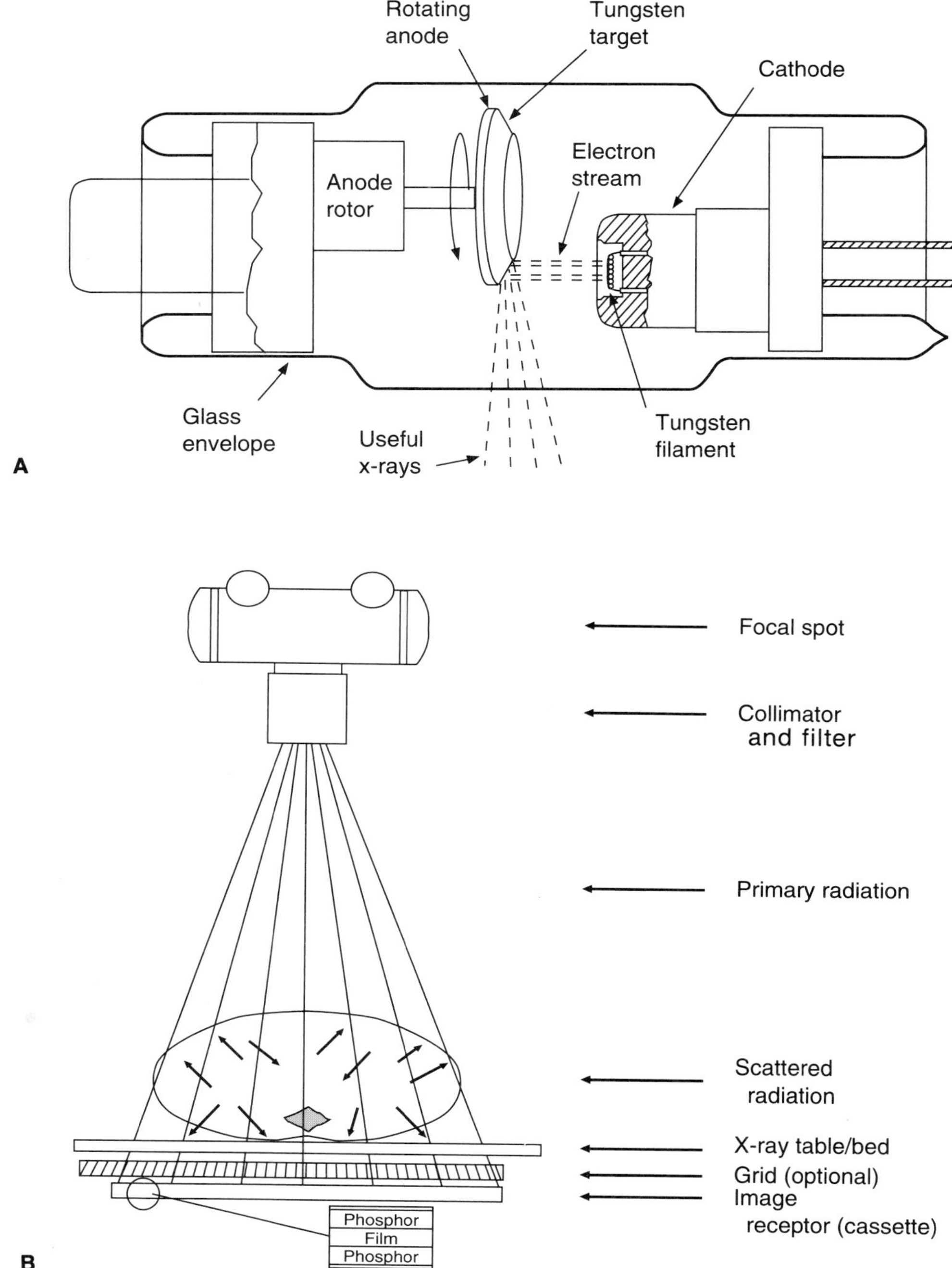

Figure 57-2. X-ray image generation. (**A**) Electrons "boil off" the incandescent cathode filament and are driven to the rotating anode target by a high voltage (70-150 kV). When the electrons strike the target (focal spot) they interact with the target atoms to create x-rays. The size of the emerging x-ray beam is set by the collimator and an aluminum filter removes undesirable, low-energy x-rays from the beam. (**B**) The primary beam passes through the patient and is attenuated to different degrees by different tissues. The emerging beam enters the film cassette and causes the two phosphor screens on either side of the film to emit visible light (fluoresce), which exposes the film. A grid may be placed between the patient and the film cassette to decrease scattering. Scattering of the x-ray beam by dense tissue (such as the abdomen) decreases the contrast resolution of the study.

Radiographs with high contrast show large differences in the degrees of absorption of various tissues. High-contrast chest radiographs show very dark lungs and very light ribs (Figure 57-3A). Radiographs with high contrast are useful for detecting fractures or abnormalities of bone such as tumors, but they can hide subtle abnormalities of the lung parenchyma such as metastases.

Radiographs with low contrast emphasize the small differences in absorption between soft tissues and are used to evaluate the soft tissues (Fig. 57-3B). Low-contrast radiographs appear relatively gray, without the extremes of dark and light seen in the high-contrast radiographs. Low-contrast radiographs are produced by x-ray beams having relatively high energy and high-contrast radiographs by beams having

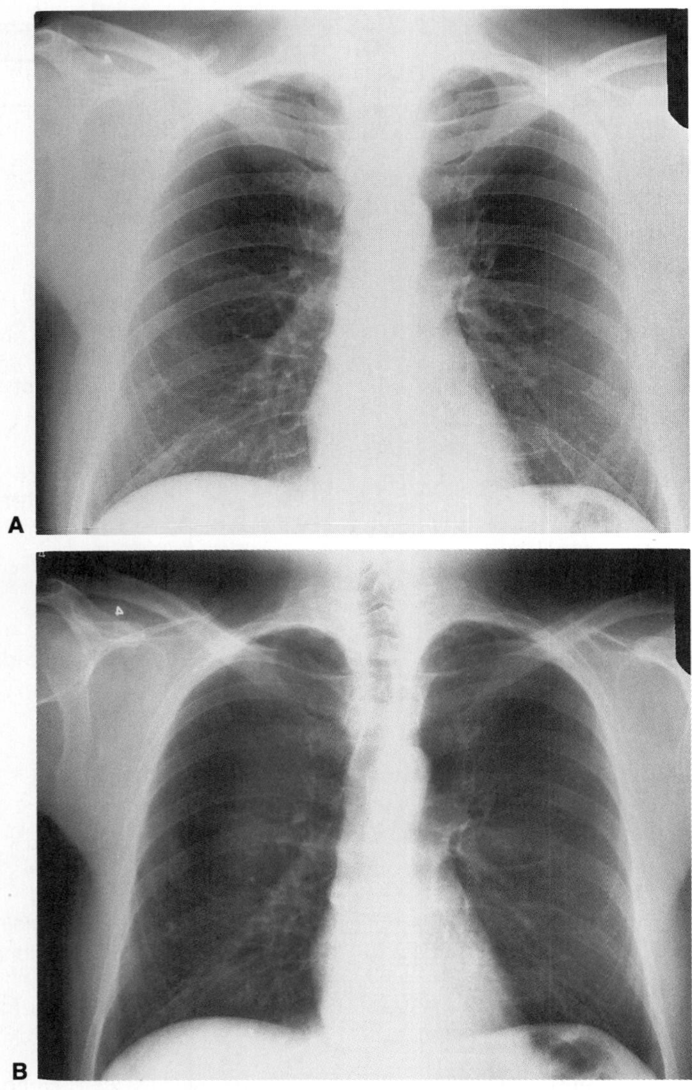

Figure 57-3. Chest radiographs of the same normal subject shown in Figure 57-1, illustrating differences in high- and low-contrast radiographic technique. Both radiographs are PA upright 72-in. exposures using the same mAS value. The contrast of a chest radiograph is determined by the energy of the photons that make the exposure rather than by the number of photons that make the exposure. A high-contrast radiograph is made with a relatively low kilovoltage and a low contrast radiograph is made with a relatively high kilovoltage. (**A**) High-contrast (72 kV). Note that the rib margins are more sharply defined and the pulmonary vessels in the left lower lobe are more distinct. High-contrast technique is useful for evaluating the bony structures and for detecting calcification in a parenchymal nodule. (**B**) Low-contrast technique (150 kV). The rib margins and lower lobe pulmonary vessels are less distinct than with the high-contrast technique (Fig. A). Low-contrast technique is useful for detecting subtle differences among soft tissues, as in evaluating for metastases or infection.

relatively lower average energy. The energy of the beam is determined by the kilovoltage potential (kVp) of the x-ray machine.

Photons interact with tissue by transferring either all or part of their energy to the tissues. The greater the amount of primary beam reaching the cassette, the darker the film. This is why tissues that absorb only a small fraction of the beam, such as lung, appear darker than do tissues that absorb most of the primary beam, such as the upper abdomen.

The greater the scattering the less the contrast of the film.[8] This is why chest and abdominal radiographs of obese patients lack the range of contrast shown by radiographs of lean individuals. A radiograph is said to be *underpenetrated* when the number of x-ray photons generated is insufficient to adequately expose the film and *overpenetrated* when the number of photons generated is excessive. The milliamperage setting of the x-ray machine determines the number of x-ray photons that will be generated. The underpenetrated film appears too light and the overpenetrated film appears too dark (Fig. 57-4).

Radiation Safety

All x-ray machines generate scattered radiation into the space surrounding the patient (Table 57-2). Only a miniscule fraction of the photons that leave the patient will scatter into the room, but these photons may be absorbed by anyone standing near the patient. There are two ways of lowering the dose to a bystander from scattered radiation, by increasing distance and by increasing shielding. Scattered radiation from the patient diminishes as the square of the distance between the patient and the bystander increases.[10] For example, if the clinician is standing 2 ft from the center of the CT ring and moves to a position 4 ft away, the dose to the clinician will be reduced by 75 percent. The other way of decreasing the exposure to bystanders is to use shielding. By wearing a lead apron and thyroid shield the exposed bystander can reduce the exposure by as much as 90 percent. Standing behind a portable lead shield can reduce the exposure by an additional 90 percent.

Table 57-2. Absorbed Dose of Ionizing Radiation from Various Imaging Studies

Study	Absorbed Dose (mSv)[a]
72-in. upright PA chest	0.1–0.5
48-in. bedside supine chest	0.3–1.0
Chest fluoroscopy (per minute)	50–100
Chest CT	25–50
Barium enema	180–300
MRI	0
Diagnostic ultrasound	0

[a] mSv, milliSievert; 1 mSv, 100 millirem.

We should minimize our exposure to occupational radiation, but it is important to keep the actual risk of such exposure in perspective.[11] The likelihood of injury from an accident while commuting to work is far greater than the cumulative risk of injury from occupational or diagnostic radiation exposure. It is also important to remember that we are constantly exposed to several sources of low-level radiation: indoor radon, terrestrial gamma-rays, ingested natural radionuclides, and cosmic rays.

Radiographic Anatomy

Figure 57-5 shows an example of normal radiographic anatomy.

Extrathoracic Objects and the Chest Wall

Items external to the chest add their shadows to the patient's radiograph. Occasionally subtle shadows caused by external structures can mimic disease. Nipples are easy to recognize when they are bilaterally symmetrical, but when the patient is slightly rotated, one of the nipples can become less visible because it presents a wider cross section to the x-ray beam. The other nipple then appears as a unilateral chest mass and could trigger an unnecessary workup for a pulmonary mass. The patient who has undergone mastectomy will have unilateral hyperlucency on the side of the mastectomy; alternatively, the side of the chest with a breast may appear abnormally opaque and raise the suspicion of a parenchymal lesion.

The faint outline of O_2 tubing superimposed over the lung apex can mimic a pneumothorax; on the other hand, the corrugated tubing connected to an endotracheal tube can obscure an apical pneumothorax. A skin fold can simulate a pneumothorax but can be distinguished from a true pneumothorax by two findings: (1) the interface between air in the pleural space and the lung parenchyma should be a thin white line in a true pneumothorax but will appear as a broad linear area of increased opacity with a skin fold; and (2) the line representing the visceral pleura of a pneumothorax will not extend beyond the chest wall, whereas the opacity representing the margin of skin fold will often extend beyond the anatomic boundary of the thoracic cavity. If there is any doubt as to whether a pneumothorax is present, the study should be repeated promptly, and special care should be taken to avoid introducing skin folds when the film cassette is placed under the patient.

Studying the ribs will answer several questions: Is the patient rotated relative to the film? Is the patient kyphotic or lordotic? What was the depth of inspiration at the time the exposure was made? The bedside chest radiograph should be taken with the patient positioned so that the x-ray beam is perpendicular to the plane of the chest. A lordotic view (Fig. 57-6A) arises when the x-ray beam is no longer perpendicular to the plane of the chest but has instead become parallel to the ribs. Figure 57-6B shows how kyphotic distortion is caused by the patient leaning forward into the x-ray beam.

Figures 57-1A and 57-7 were taken within minutes of each

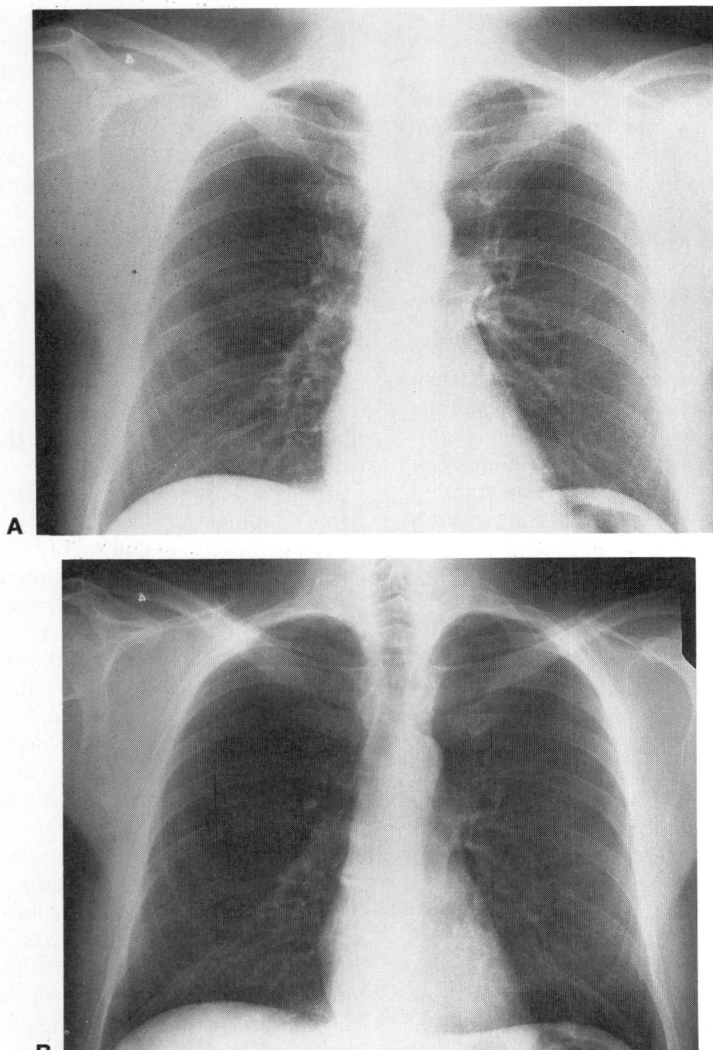

Figure 57-4. Radiograph of same normal subject as in Figure 57-1, illustrating differences between underpenetrated and overpenetrated radiographs. The overall lightness or darkness of a chest radiograph is determined by the number of x-ray photons reaching the film cassette. With a low mAS technique, few photons reach the cassette, and the resulting exposure is underpenetrated. With a high mAS exposure, a large number of photons reach the cassette, resulting in an overexposed radiograph. The energy of the photons is relatively unimportant in determining whether an exposure will be overpenetrated or underpenetrated. Two films showing high and low contrast can be distinguished from films showing over- and underexposure because in the under- and overexposed radiographs the pulmonary vessels and ribs will have the same degree of sharpness. (**A**) Underpenetrated AP supine 48-in. exposure. As compared with Figure 57-1, the pulmonary vessels can be followed far into the periphery and the overall appearance of the film is light. (**B**) Overpenetrated AP supine 48-in. exposure. In an underpenetrated exposure, the pulmonary vessels do not appear to travel as far toward the periphery as they are seen to in the normal exposure shown in Figure 57-1B.

other and show the same healthy individual, yet they are strikingly different. Figure 57-1A was taken at maximal inspiration and Figure 57-7 shows maximal expiration. If inspiration and expiration can have such a pronounced effect on a normal chest, it is not hard to see how the phase of respiration and the depth of inspiration can complicate the appearance of the diseased chest. If six or more anterior ribs are showing above the medial right hemidiaphragm, the depth of inspiration is adequate.

Rotation of the patient can be recognized by the position of the heads of the clavicles relative to the midline. Patients are rotated to the left when their anterior aspect is turned toward their left, which causes the left clavicular head to move away from the midline (Fig. 57-8). Patients are rotated

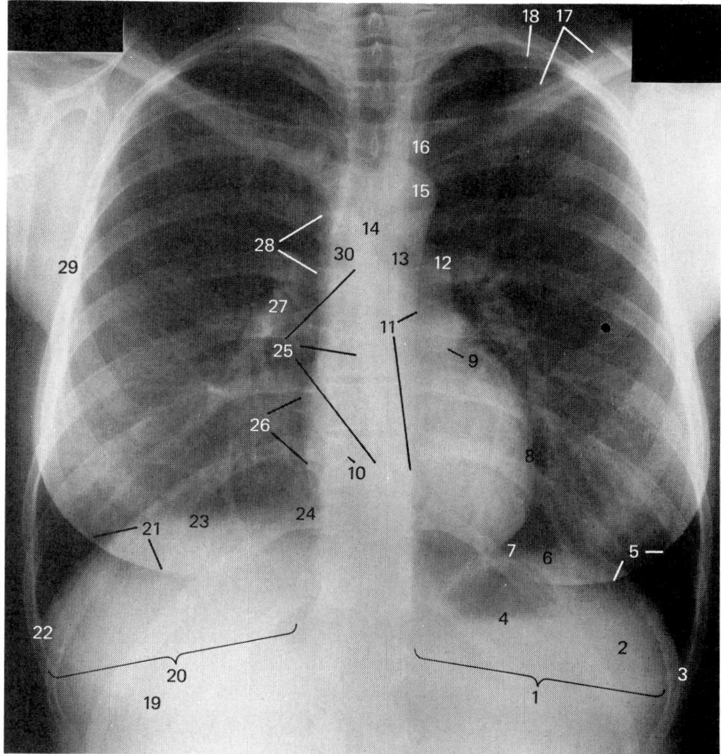

Figure 57-5. Normal radiographic anatomy, as seen on an upright PA 72-in. chest radiograph of a normal woman.

1, lung projecting below the left diaphragm dome, recognizable because of images of blood vessels extending well toward the periphery;
2, spleen;
3, left costophrenic angle;
4, air in the stomach;
5, margin of the left breast;
6, left hemidiaphragm;
7, left cardiophrenic angle;
8, edge of the left ventricle;
9, transverse process of a lower vertebra behind the heart and beneath the medial end of the corresponding rib;
10, pedicle of a lower vertebra seen end-on;
11, left lateral margin of the descending thoracic aorta;
12, left pulmonary artery;
13, left main bronchus;
14, carina of the trachea;
15, aortic arch (note its impression on the adjacent trachea; the "aortic knob" is the posterior turn of the aortic arch, which is seen as a prominent image on a PA view);
16, left subclavian artery;
17, supraclavicular soft tissue companion shadow;
18, companion shadow of the second rib;
19, liver;
20, lung projecting below the right diaphragm dome, recognizable because of images of blood vessels extending well toward the periphery;
21, margin of the right breast;
22, right costophrenic angle;
23, right hemidiaphragm;
24, right cardiophrenic angle;
25, azygoesophageal pleural reflection, prespinal; medial edge of the right lung;
26, edge of the right atrium (right heart border);
27, interlobar branch of the right pulmonary artery (the branch beyond the origin of the pulmonary artery trunk that is the main supply of the upper lobe);
28, superior vena cava;
29, minor interlobar fissure;
30, right main bronchus.
(From Blank,[6] with permission.)

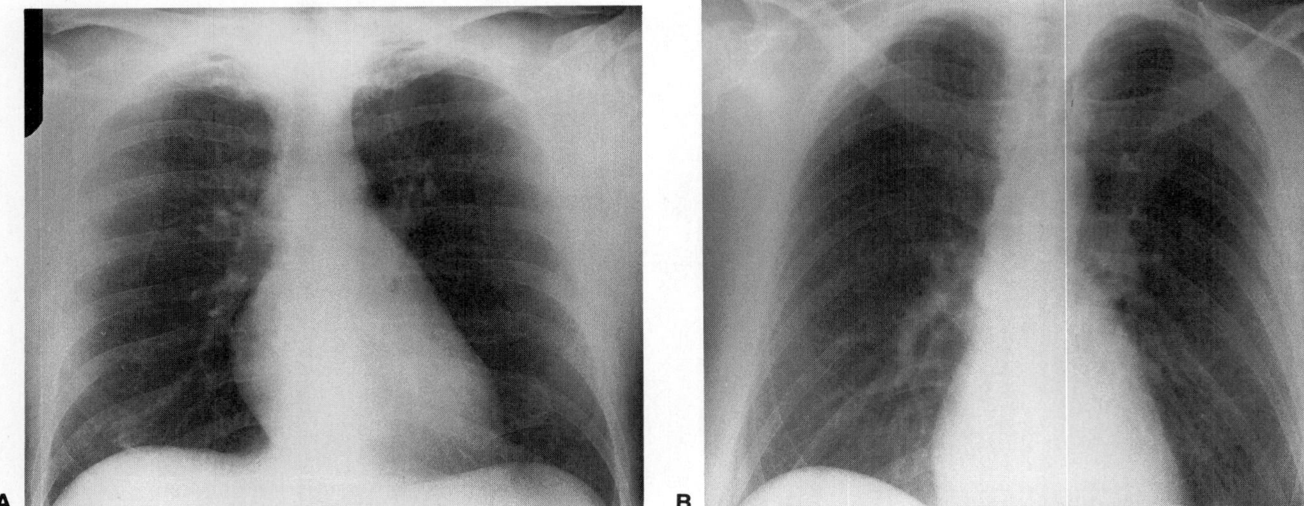

Figure 57-6. AP supine 48-in. chest radiographs of the same normal subject shown in Figure 57-1, illustrating the differences that occur when the patient is lordotic or kyphotic with respect to the film cassette. With a lordotic exposure, the clavicles are almost completely superimposed on the first rib. With a kyphotic exposure, the clavicles are projected over the midthorax. (**A**) Lordotic exposure. Because the ribs are parallel to the x-ray beam, the lung apices are well seen, owing to the minimal obstruction by overlapping ribs. However, because the lordotic view magnifies structures in the upper chest, the mediastinum can appear widened and the aortic arch can appear indistinct, which can lead to the incorrect diagnosis of aortic injury in a trauma patient. Magnification of pulmonary vessels in the upper chest can simulate cephalization of flow and pulmonary venous hypertension. Occasionally the ends of ribs will be so prominent that they will mimic pulmonary nodules. (**B**) Kyphotic exposure. In contrast to the lordotic exposure shown in Figure A, the lung apices are projected over the midlungs when the patient is kyphotic. The hila become quite prominent and can assume a mass-like appearance, simulating adenopathy.

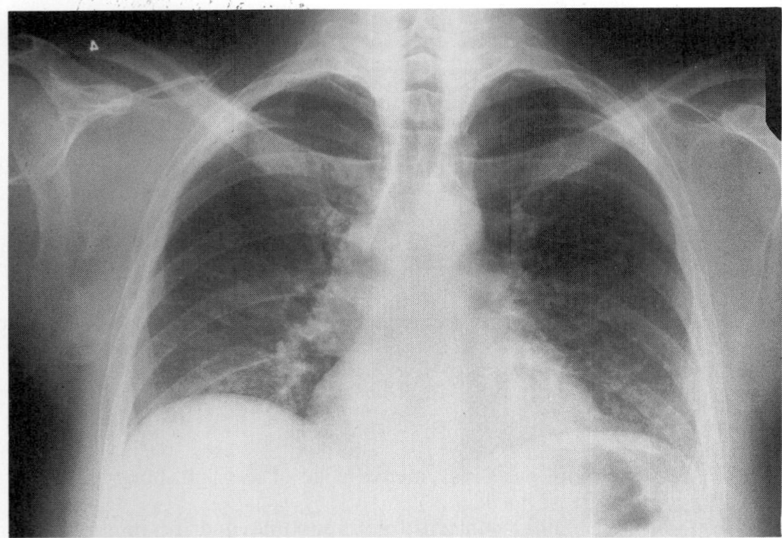

Figure 57-7. PA upright chest radiograph at full expiration (residual volume) of the same normal individual and at the same sitting shown in Figure 57-1A. Notice the small lung volumes, the relatively large heart, and the crowding of the pulmonary vasculature in the lower lobes, which simulates perihilar infiltrates.

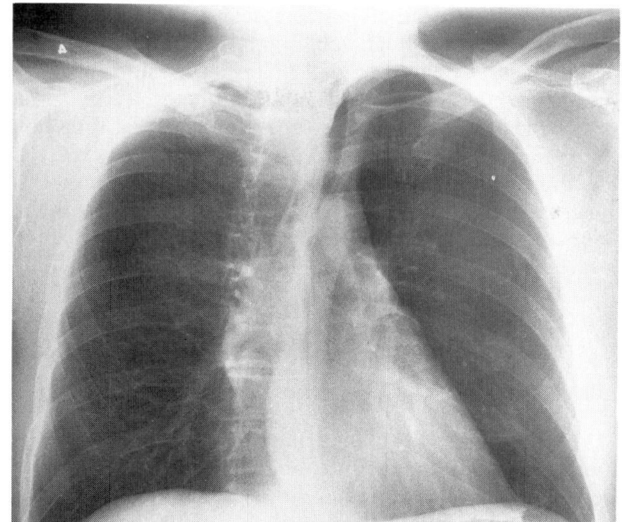

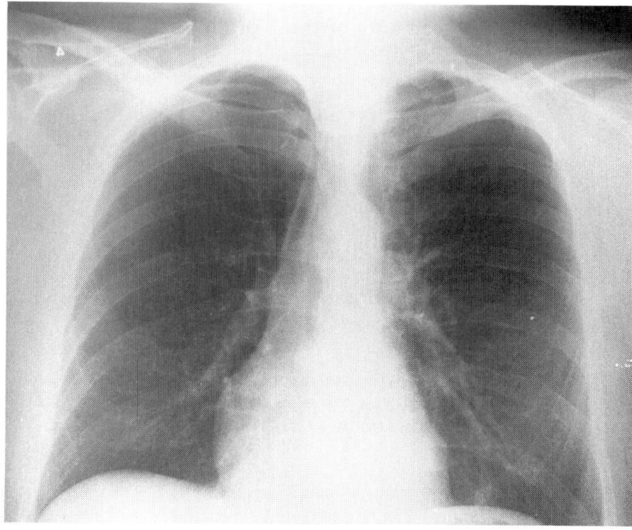

Figure 57-8. Upright PA chest radiographs showing leftward and rightward rotation of the same normal individual shown in Figure 57-1. It is important to emphasize that films described as showing rightward rotation, means that patients are rotated toward their right side (and vice versa for leftward rotation). This convention holds true whether a PA upright chest radiograph or an AP supine bedside radiograph is viewed. **(A)** Leftward rotation: The patient is rotated anteriorly toward his left arm. With leftward rotation, the left clavicular head moves away from the midline, the heart appears larger, the left hilum appears smaller, and the aortic arch appears larger. These changes are the same whether the film is a PA upright or an AP supine radiograph. **(B)** Rightward rotation: The patient is rotated anteriorly toward his right side. The head of the right clavicle moves away from the midline, the heart appears smaller and more opaque because it is now viewed down its long axis, the left hilum appears larger, and the aortic arch appears smaller. These changes are the same whether the film is taken using AP supine technique or PA upright technique.

to the right when their anterior aspect is rotated toward their right, which causes the right clavicular head to move away from the midline. Identifying which clavicular head is displaced away from the midline will indicate the direction that the patient is rotated for either the PA upright or the AP supine radiograph.

Pleura and Lung Parenchyma

In the normal person the pleural space is radiographically invisible because it contains only a minute amount of fluid. When pleural fluid accumulates, however, the pleural space becomes radiographically apparent. The earliest finding of pleural effusion on a PA upright chest film is blunting of the costovertebral sulci. As little as 75 to 100 mL of fluid may be detected in this way under ideal radiographic conditions. To blunt the lateral costophrenic sulci requires at least 175 to 200 mL.

Pleural effusions are usually undetectable on supine bedside examinations until the volume reaches 75 to 100 mL, when blunting of the sulci appears. In the supine patient fluid will layer along the posterior wall of the chest. If the layering is symmetrical, it can be very difficult to detect even much larger effusions on the supine examination. Lateral decubitus views are far more sensitive than supine views in detecting effusions (see subsequent section). Under ideal conditions, as little as 10 mL of fluid can be detected by noting the appearance of a slight thickening of the inferolateral juxtapleural stripe.[12]

Healthy lung parenchyma shows only the white branching pulmonary arteries and veins against a black background. Occasionally the normal chest will show a very faint network of fine lines representing the interstitium. This network becomes much more prominent in the presence of interstitial lung disease. The perihilar bronchi appear as white "doughnuts" adjacent to their companion pulmonary arteries, which appear as white dots of comparable diameter.

The lobes of the lungs are separated by fissures lined by the pleura. The fissures are important radiographic landmarks; alterations in their positions indicate where an abnormality is located in the parenchyma. For example, elevation of the minor fissure (between the right upper and middle lobes) can be caused by partial upper lobe collapse. Depression of the minor fissure could indicate hyperexpansion of the upper lobe or collapse of the middle lobe. Thickening of a fissure can indicate a pleural effusion, a scarring process, or a tumor.

Heart and Mediastinum

The mediastinum is the portion of the intrathoracic cavity that lies outside the pleural spaces. For the purpose of evaluating radiographs, the mediastinum is divided into three

Table 57-3. Contents of the Normal Mediastinum

Anterior mediastinum
Location
Everything forward of and superior to the heart shadow in the lateral projection
Contents
Thymus gland
Substernal extensions of thyroid and parathyroid glands
Lymphatic vessels and lymph nodes
Aortic arch and its major branches
Innominate veins
Areolar connective tissue
Middle mediastinum
Location
Extends from lower sternal border posteriorly along diaphragm to anterior vertebral border and vertically to the anterior mediastinum at approximately T4
Contents
Heart
Pericardium
Trachea and main bronchi
Hila
Lymph nodes
Phrenic and vagus nerves
Posterior mediastinum
Location
Consists of the space seen on the lateral projection within the margins of the vertebrae, from the diaphragm cephalad to the first rib
Contents
Esophagus
Descending aorta
Azygos and hemiazygos veins
Thoracic duct
Lymph nodes
Vagus nerves and sympathetic chains
Areolar connective tissue

compartments: anterior, middle, and posterior[13] (Table 57-3).

Lower Neck, Thoracic Spine, and Upper Abdomen

Almost every chest film, whether AP or PA, upright or supine, will include portions of the lower neck and upper abdomen, and all properly exposed chest films will show the thoracic spine. Figure 57-9 shows a new thin lucent stripe along the left heart border in a 20-year-old man with chest pain. The lucent line could indicate a medial pneumothorax or a pneumomediastinum. Because the lucent line extends into the neck, the diagnosis is pneumomediastinum, since the mediastinum is continuous with the fascial planes of the neck. Gas from a pneumothorax is contained in the pleural space and cannot extend beyond the thorax. Although it is still possible for the stripe to represent a pneumomediastinum even if it does not extend into the neck, this simple observation can avoid the need for additional studies.

The trachea lies in the midline of the neck and its appearance depends on the patient's phase of respiration. The vocal cords project at the level of the fifth cervical vertebral body.

The fundus of the stomach is seen as a lucent area just inferior to the left hemidiaphragm. This portion of the radiograph is evaluated to determine the position of enteral tubes, such as a nasogastric suction catheter, a feeding tube, or a Sengstaken-Blakemore tube. If an enteral tube enters the patient's oropharynx but it is not seen in the left upper quadrant of the abdomen, the clinician should carefully inspect the course of the esophagus for the tube tip. If the tube is not visible within the esophagus, the tube may be coiled in the patient's posterior oropharynx.

Describing the Findings on a Chest Radiograph

The more accurately clinicians describe the findings, the more accurately they will be able to reach a diagnosis. The description should begin with the location of the major ab-

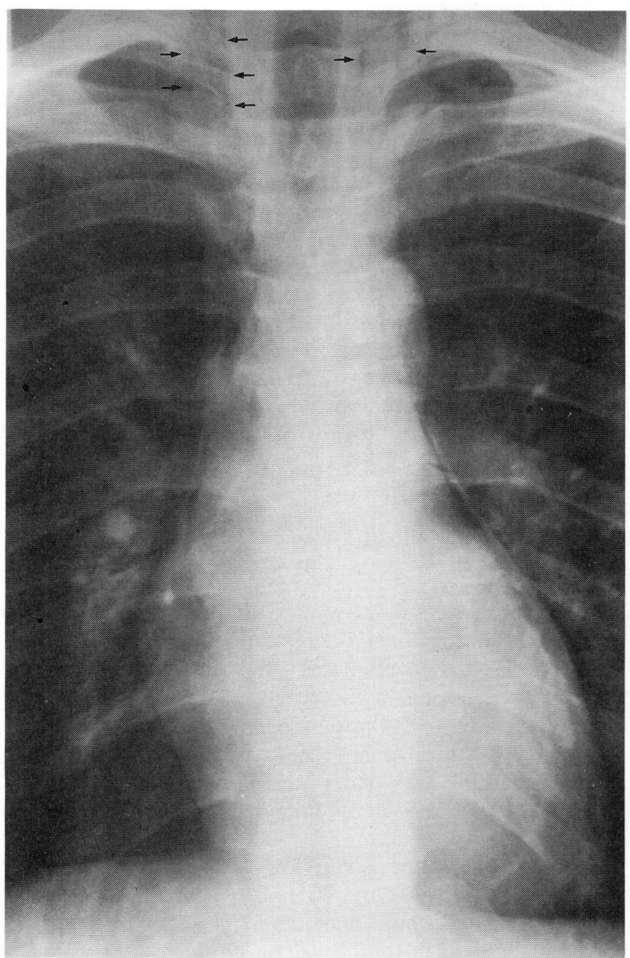

Figure 57-9. Pneumomediastinum. The linear opacities extending from the level of the origin of the great vessels into the neck represent visceral pleura that has been separated from the parietal pleura of the mediastinum by intrapleural air. (From Blank,[6] with permission.)

normality and its radiographic characteristics. Next the viewer should comment on the other radiographic findings that might be associated with the major abnormality. These pertinent positive and negative findings will help the viewer narrow the possible causes of the main abnormality. For example, diffuse indistinctness of the pulmonary vessels could be caused by infection, congestive heart failure, or noncardiac pulmonary edema. If the heart is not enlarged, chronic heart failure becomes much less likely.

Clinicians should favor descriptive terms over those that imply a diagnosis. It is one thing to describe abnormal linear opacities extending from the hilum to the apex; it is a different matter to call the abnormality "scarring." Scarring is one cause of linear opacity, but so is recurrent cancer. If the linear opacities are unchanged when we compare the patient's radiograph obtained 4 years previously with the current study, we are entitled to draw the conclusion that the opacities represent scarring. To say "linear opacities" is to describe a finding—to say "scarring" is to state a conclusion.

Practical Analysis of the Bedside Radiograph: the "BaSICCs"

How should a chest radiograph be studied?[14–16] Some prefer to begin at the lateral margin of the chest and to move medially, studying each successive structure that their eyes encounter. Others prefer to begin at the center and to work outward. Some of the most skilled readers will say they just look at the film. All these methods have their strengths and weaknesses. The method that we offer is tailored to the ICU bedside chest radiograph and can be remembered by the mnemonic "BaSICC": *Ba*ckground, *S*urvey, *I*dentify, *C*ompare, and *C*onclude (Table 57-4).

Background

Background refers to the work that we must do before we can turn our attention to the diagnostic information shown by the radiograph. Evaluation of the background consists of two steps. First, does the film represent the patient we think it does? If it is from the proper patient, are the date and time correct? Second, review the technical factors affecting the study. What is the patient's position—supine, semiupright, upright, or lateral decubitus? Have all areas of the chest been included, or is the radiograph missing a lateral costophrenic sulcus? Is the exposure just right to penetrate opaque areas of lung but not so penetrating as to "burn out" lung markings? What is the patient's depth of inspiration?

Survey

Surveying the radiograph consists of noting what foreign materials are shown and determining the correctness of their positions. Many foreign materials are commonly seen on ICU chest films.

Table 57-4. The BaSICC Approach to the Bedside Chest Radiograph

Ba (background)
- Confirm the date and time of the study and the patient's name
- Confirm technical factors
  - Position of the patient for the study: supine, semiupright, upright
  - Is the film marked to indicate right and left?
  - Are all areas of the chest included?
  - Is the degree of penetration correct?
  - What is the patient's depth of inspiration?

S (survey)
- Survey chest for extrinsic devices and judge the correctness of their positions: lines, tubes, catheters, pacer wires

I (identify)
- Identify specific abnormalities of the chest wall, pleurae, lungs, mediastinum, heart, abdomen, neck, and bones

C (compare)
- Compare the current chest radiograph with the next most recent radiograph and with an older radiograph; comparing the current study with an old study show subtle changes that might be missed by comparison with yesterday's examination

C (conclude)
- Draw conclusions from the collected data; are there any new developments, and if so, what are their implications; is the patient better or worse?

Identify

Next we identify specific abnormalities of the various tissue compartments of the chest. Beginning from the chest wall, we study the subcutaneous tissues, bones, pleural space, lungs, diaphragm, airways, mediastinum, heart, abdomen, and neck, looking for the specific abnormalities of each compartment (Table 57-3). An organized approach is particularly important when evaluating chest radiographs obtained immediately postintubation (Table 57-5), postoperatively,[20] or following trauma.[21]

Compare and Conclude

Having thoroughly studied the chest as described above, we are ready to compare the present chest radiographs with the patient's recent chest films to look for progression or

Table 57-5. Checking the Postintubation Chest Radiograph

The tip of the tube should be a minimum of 3 cm from the carina to avoid bronchial intubation

The cuff should be below the level of the vocal cords, which is usually at the level of C4

Exclude pneumothorax and shift of the mediastinum

Are there new areas of atelectasis that could indicate aspiration?

Is the tip of nasogastric/feeding tube in the stomach, or has it migrated into the esophagus?

resolution of disorders or the appearance of new problems. Before concluding that pathologic changes have occurred in the time between two radiographs, we must make sure that the technical factors and the patient's position are similar. Finally, we can summarize our findings in a conclusion. For example, in the conclusion we can say that there has been enlargement of the apical pneumothorax over the past 3 days or that the degree of congestive heart failure (CHF) is less.

Radiographic Appearance of Chest Disease

Air Bronchograms and the Silhouette Sign

Suppose the lung becomes filled with fluid, as could happen as a result of pneumonia, interstitial edema, or hemorrhage. The contrast between air-filled bronchi and adjacent fluid-filled lung becomes greater, causing the lucent segmental bronchi to appear on the radiograph. This is an air bronchogram (Fig. 57-10).

The other common cause of air bronchograms is atelectasis. Because atelectasis indicates airless lung associated with volume loss, atelectatic lung will cause more attenuation of the x-ray beam than will aerated lung. This differential absorption of the x-ray beam explains why bronchi within atelectatic lung, like those within fluid-filled lung, show air bronchograms.

If the bronchi become obstructed by a mucus plug, secretions are retained, which leads to greater attenuation of the x-ray beam and thus decreases the contrast between the bronchi and the surrounding atelectatic lung. When the bronchi are completely filled and the differential contrast is very small, the air bronchograms disappear. The presence or absence of an air bronchogram indicates the likelihood of success for procedures to drain the bronchi.

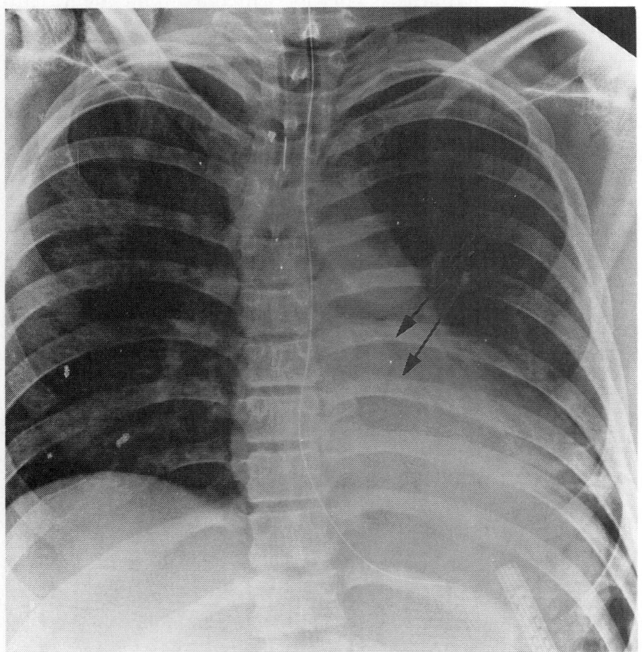

Figure 57-10. Left lower lobe atelectasis showing an air bronchogram (arrow). (From Pierson,[42] with permission.)

In the normal patient there is high contrast between the aerated right middle lobe and the fluid-filled right heart. When the attenuation caused by the middle lobe increases, as when pneumonia fills the alveoli with fluid, the contrast between the heart and the middle lobe diminishes. The less the contrast between two adjacent structures, the more difficult it becomes to identify their common border.

On the other hand, the right lower lobe lies posterior to the right heart border and does not border the right heart. When the right lower lobe fills with fluid or develops atelectasis, its attenuation of the x-ray beam will increase and approach the attenuation of the fluid-filled heart. No matter how similar the attenuations of the heart and the right lower lobe become, the right heart border will remain sharply defined. This is because the posterior lobe and the heart do not share a common border. The presence or absence of a distinct border between two structures is an important guide to the location of abnormalities in the chest (Fig. 57-11A & B). If the border between the right heart and the lung is distinct, the pneumonia involves the lower lobe; if the border is indistinct or absent, the pneumonia is in the middle lobe. The loss of distinctness of a common border is called the silhouette sign.

In a similar way the silhouette sign will distinguish a left lower lobe pneumonia from a lingular pneumonia. The lingula lies adjacent to the left heart border, and the left lower lobe lies posterior to the left heart. When pneumonia involves the lingula, the left heart border will be indistinct, and when it involves the lower lobe, the border between the heart and the lung will be distinct.

These same rules apply to the localization of areas of atelectasis.[22] When the right middle lobe collapses, the right heart border becomes indistinct, but when the right lower lobe collapses, the right heart border remains distinct. The left lung shows the same pattern: when the lingula collapses, the left heart border becomes indistinct, and when the left lower lobe collapses, the left heart border remains distinct (Fig. 57-12).

Table 57-6 compares the typical findings in lobar atelectasis, pneumonia, and pleural effusions, three acute conditions commonly confused in ICU patients.

Atelectasis

Atelectasis appears as a linear or curvilinear opacity, most commonly found at the lung bases (Fig. 57-11A). The margins of the airless atelectatic lung are relatively sharply defined as compared with the often indistinct margins seen in pneumonia or interstitial edema. Atelectasis is seldom parallel to the pleural margins, and so a stripe of increased opacity along the pleural margin is far more likely to represent an effusion than atelectasis.

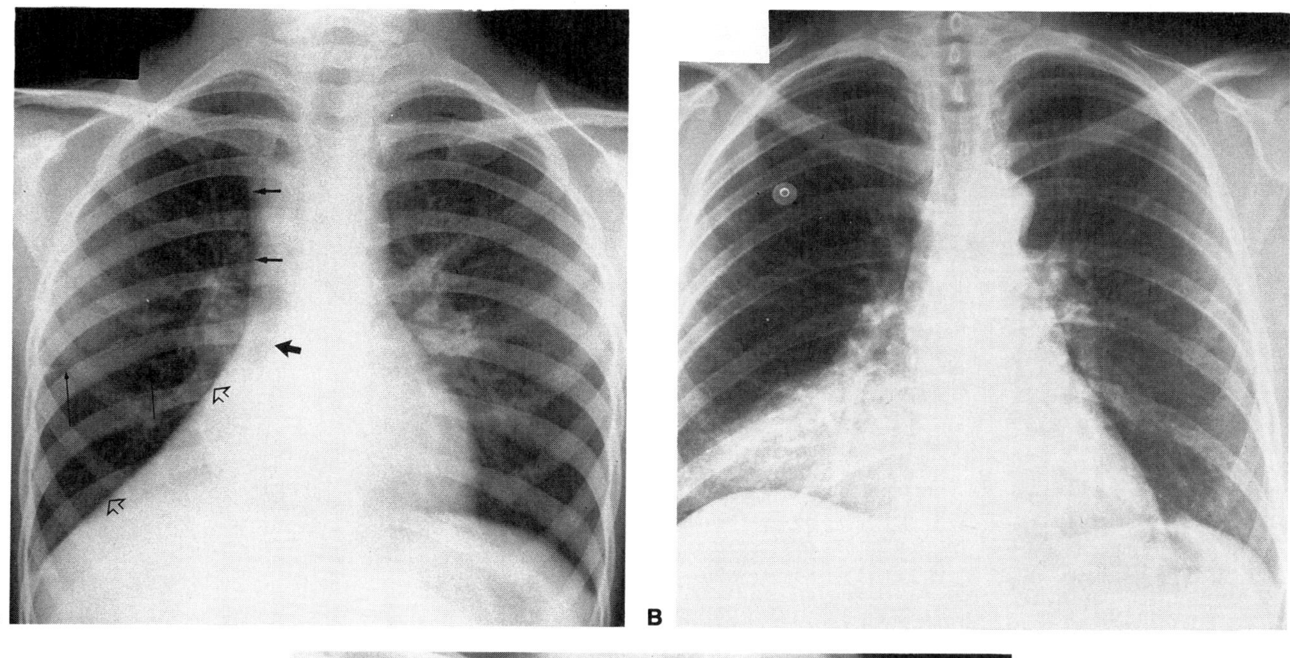

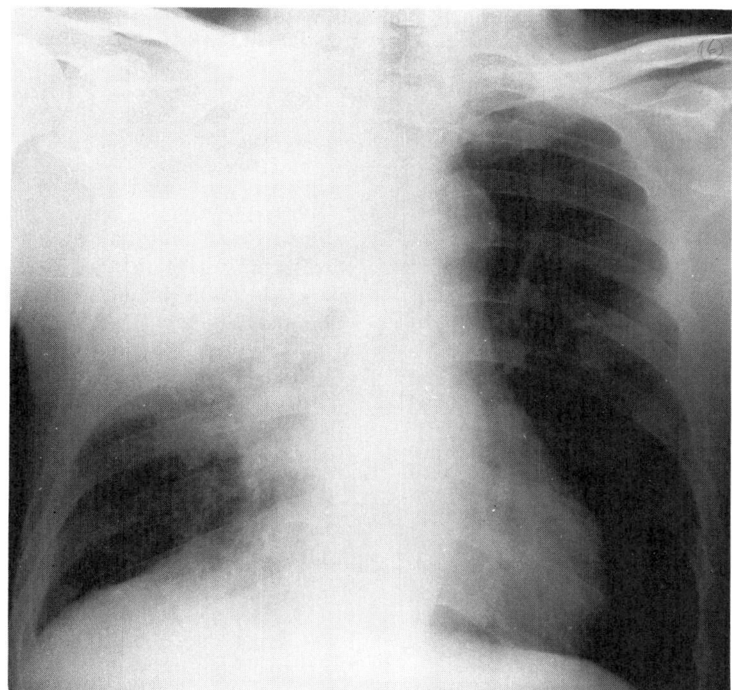

Figure 57-11. Disorders involving each of the three lobes of the right lung. (**A**) Right lower lobe atelectasis. The diaphragm is effaced, but the right border of the heart is not effaced as it would be with right middle lobe atelectasis or pneumonia. (**B**) Right middle lobe pneumonia. The diaphragm is distinctly seen, but the right border of the heart is effaced. These features distinguish a right middle lobe process from one involving the right lower lobe. A snap from the patient's gown projects over the right upper lung. (**C**) Right upper lobe pneumonia. (From Blank,[6] with permission.)

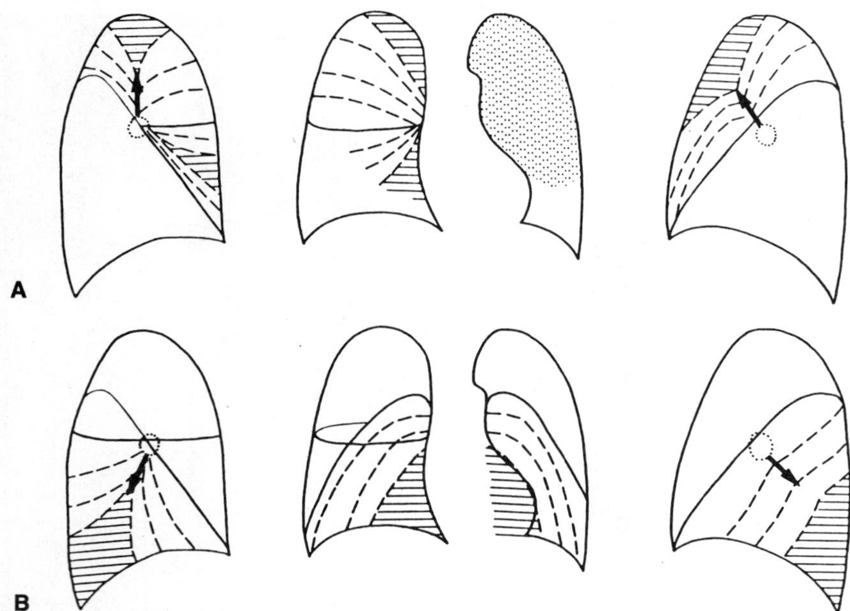

Figure 57-12. The radiographic patterns of atelectasis involving the various lobes of the lungs. (**A**) Upper and middle lobe patterns of atelectasis. The right upper lobe and right middle lobe tend to collapse medially, creating increased opacity at these aspects of the right lung. The left upper lobe collapses anteriorly, which leads to diffusely increased opacity over the mid- and upper portion of the left lung, as seen on the frontal radiograph. When the right upper lobe collapses, the right hilum is elevated, and when the left upper lobe collapses, the hilum is displaced superiorly and anteriorly, as shown (arrows). (**B**) Lower lobe patterns of atelectasis. The lower lobe of each lung tends to collapse posteriorly and medially. As a result, the hila are retracted inferiorly and posteriorly, as shown (arrows). (From Taveras et al.,[4] with permission.)

Pneumonia

The radiographic appearance of pneumonia is diverse.[23] Focal bacterial pneumonia can densely opacify a segment or lobe without causing volume loss (Fig. 57-11B and C). Diffuse pneumonia can be subtle, manifested only by increased visibility of the interstitial pattern. Such an appearance could indicate a viral or early mycoplasmal pneumonia in an otherwise healthy outpatient or could be the first sign of *Pneumocystis carinii* pneumonia in a patient with the acquired immunodeficiency syndrome (AIDS). When severe, the diffuse pneumonia is indistinguishable from the uniformly opacified appearance of the lungs in the adult respiratory distress syndrome (ARDS) or cardiogenic pulmonary edema.

Table 57-6. Comparison of the Chest Radiographic Findings in Atelectasis, Pneumonia, and Pleural Effusion

Atelectasis
The margins tend to be relatively sharply defined and linear
Atelectasis tends to occur in the outer third of the lung
Areas of lung adjacent to atelectatic regions may be hyperlucent because of volume loss in the atelectatic area
Atelectasis tends to respect segmental and lobar boundaries
Pneumonia
The margins are indistinct unless the disease is strictly lobar or segmental
The distribution tends to be patchy rather than linear (as is seen with atelectasis)
Pneumonia tends to preserve the volume of the involved lung (atelectasis tends to cause volume loss)
Pleural effusion
The effusion tends to diffusely increase the opacity of the involved hemithorax; this effect is most noticeable at the bases
Effusions often layer when the patient is placed in a decubitus position
Effusions mimic pleural thickening

Cardiogenic and Noncardiogenic Pulmonary Edema

Dilation of the left ventricle is the first radiographic sign of chronic CHF (Fig. 57-13). On the upright PA radiograph the heart is enlarged if its width is greater than half the width of the chest. There is a catch, however. Although dilation is the first sign of CHF, it can be difficult to accurately judge heart size from the bedside AP radiograph unless a rigorous approach is taken.[9] Serial examinations may also be helpful. This difficulty arises because the AP exposure magnifies the heart size to a much greater degree than does the PA view.

As CHF worsens, increased interstitial fluid overwhelms the capacity of the interstitium to remove it and leads to interstitial edema. Radiographically, mild interstitial edema is seen as peribronchial cuffing, an apparent thickening of the bronchial walls seen best in the larger perihilar bronchi. Like most signs in radiology, cuffing is not unique to interstitial edema and can also be seen with bronchitis and reactive airways disease. With bronchitis or reactive airways disease, the heart size remains normal, but with CHF the heart is enlarged.

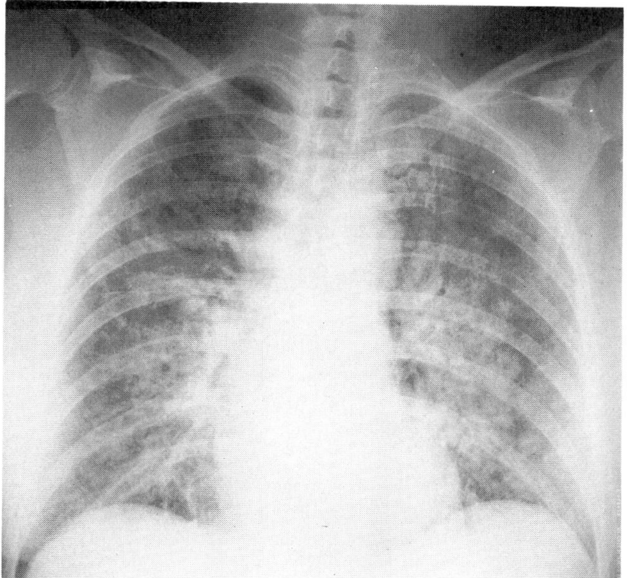

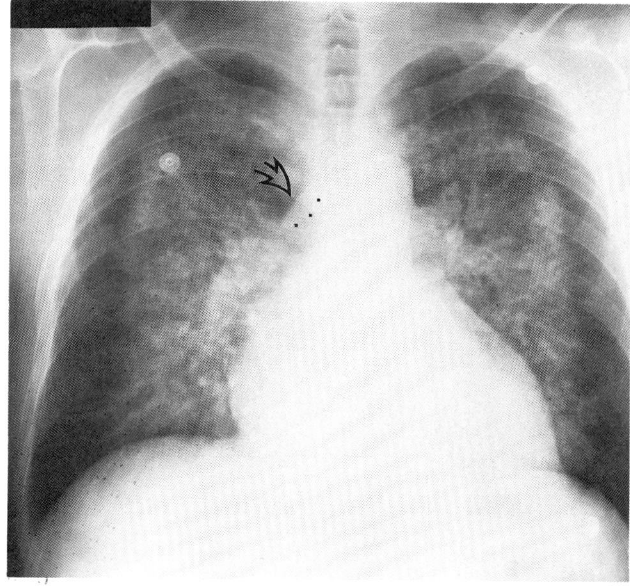

Figure 57-13. Pulmonary edema. (**A**) Noncardiogenic pulmonary edema, with which the heart is not enlarged. The classic perihilar patchy opacities that are characteristic of pulmonary edema are seen with both cardiogenic and noncardiogenic forms. (**B**) Cardiogenic pulmonary edema. The heart is enlarged and the azygous vein is distended (arrow). A snap from the patient's gown projects over the right upper lung. (From Blank,[6] with permission.)

As left ventricular failure worsens, the amount of abnormal interstitial fluid increases, and the margins of the pulmonary vessels become blurred or indistinct (Fig. 57-14). This change is most easily identified by comparing the radiograph in question with an earlier film taken when the patient was not acutely ill. Fluid begins to accumulate in the fissures and in the costophrenic and costovertebral sulci, making them more prominent. Fluid that accumulates in the subpleural septa thickens them, and they appear radiographically as lines perpendicular to the pleural surface, measuring approximately 1 cm and usually seen at the lateral aspects of the lower lungs; these are called *Kerley B lines*.

Finally, fluid from the engorged interstitium floods out into the alveoli, creating the radiographic appearance of diffuse airspace disease, also known as an alveolar pattern (Fig. 57-13A). This diffuse parenchymal opacity completely obscures the pulmonary vessels and makes the cardiac borders indistinct. This is the radiographic picture of pulmonary edema.

From just a single AP bedside radiograph it would be difficult to distinguish advanced pulmonary edema from ARDS or from diffuse pneumonia in a patient with an enlarged heart (Fig. 57-13B). The best guide to what the underlying process represents is a review of the patient's serial chest films rather than an over-reading of a single examination.

Pleural Effusion

Pleural effusions will tend to layer along the dependent portions of the chest if they are able to flow without restriction. In the supine patient effusions will layer along the posterior chest wall causing diffusely increased opacity of the involved hemithorax (Fig. 57-15A). This subtle increase in opacity may be the only hint of an effusion and could be mistaken for an intraparenchymal process such as infection or edema.

The appearance of the pulmonary vessels can help to distinguish a posterior effusion from an intraparenchymal process. If the vessels show normal, sharp margins, the opacifying process is most likely to be a posterior effusion. It should be kept in mind that partial collapse of a lobe can increase the opacity of the involved hemithorax while preserving the normal appearance of the vessels in the overlying lung. If the vessels are indistinct, the process is more likely to be intraparenchymal.

A more accurate way of determining whether an effusion is present is to obtain lateral decubitus views. In these views the patient is positioned with right or left flank on the bed, the film cassette is placed against the back, and the exposure is made perpendicular to the plane of the bed (Fig. 57-15B). If there is clinical concern for a right pleural effusion, the patient is placed with the right flank against the bed, and the resulting exposure is called a *right lateral decubitus* view or a *right side down decubitus* view. Pleural fluid will flow to the dependent region and layer along the lateral chest wall. If the pleural effusion is loculated because of old scarring or acute inflammatory adhesions, the fluid will not flow into the dependent region. By obtaining both decubitus views the underlying lung parenchyma can be evaluated even in the presence of large effusions.

Pneumothorax

In the characteristic radiographic appearance of a pneumothorax the visceral pleura appears as a thin, discrete white

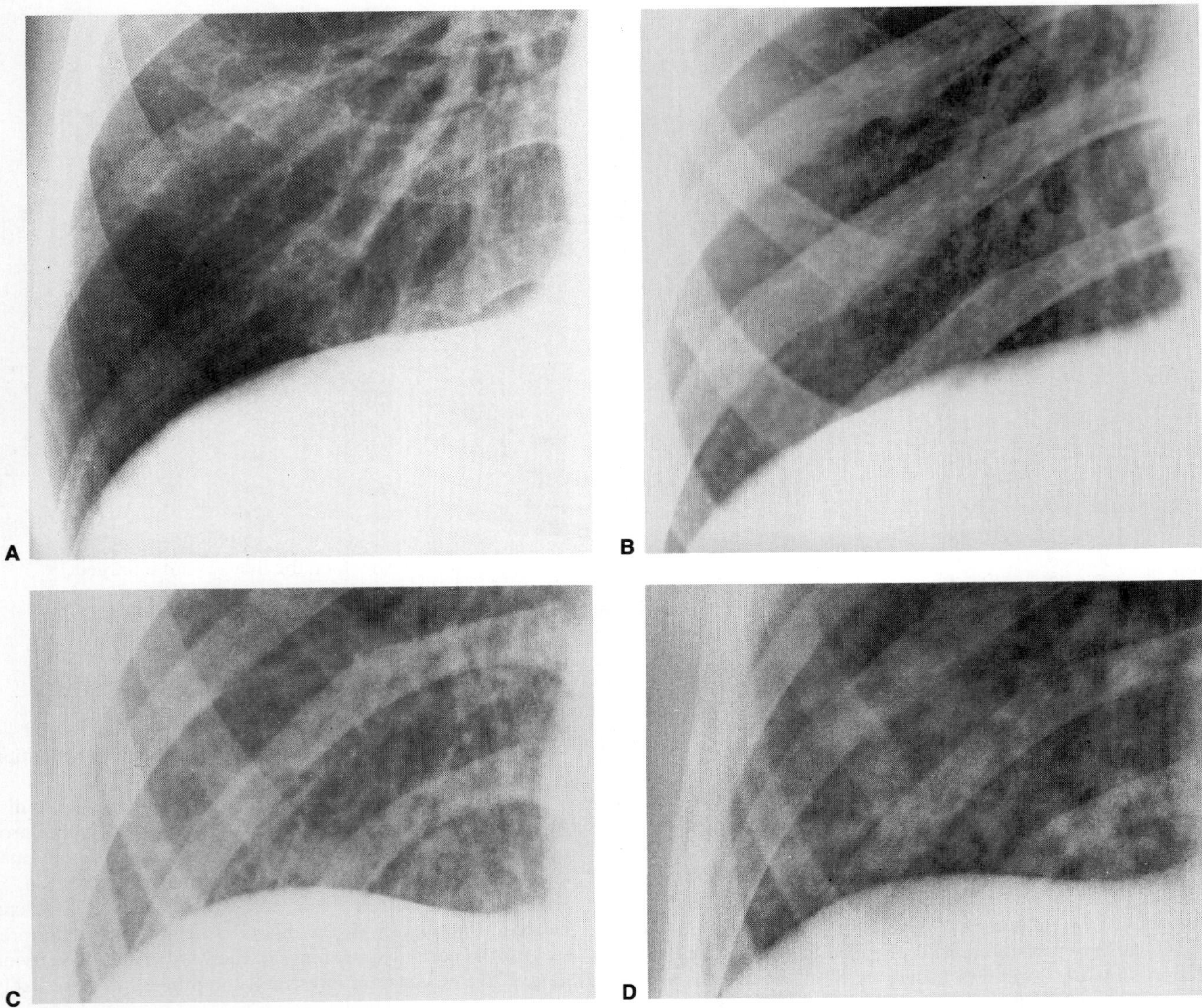

Figure 57-14. Pulmonary edema and pneumonia decrease the distinctness of the pulmonary vessels; this is illustrated by four examples of decreasing clarity of these vessels in the right lower chest. The advantage of assessing the degree of disease by the loss of sharpness of the vessel margins is that this finding is relatively independent of exposure technique. (**A**) Normal chest. Notice the sharpness of the margins of the pulmonary vessels. (**B**) A febrile patient with acute myelogenous leukemia. The pulmonary vessels are less distinct than in Figure A but are not definitely abnormal, as in Figure C. This is an example of very mild interstitial edema. (**C**) The same patient shown in Figure B, 24 hours later. Although there are differences in exposure, the pulmonary vessels are less distinct than in Figure B and are clearly abnormal. (**D**) The same patient shown 2 days after Figure B. The vessels are almost indistinguishable from the interstitial and alveolar diseased area caused by pneumonia. (From Blank,[6] with permission.)

line separated from the chest wall (parietal pleura) by a lucent region that does not contain pulmonary vessels or interstitium. Although this definition seems self-evident, patients have received chest tubes for treatment of a skin fold mimicking a pneumothorax (Fig. 57-16).

When there is suspicion of a pneumothorax, the radiograph should be taken with the patient in deep expiration. During expiration the volume of the lungs is decreased, but the volume of the pneumothorax should remain unchanged; this will cause a pneumothorax to be more evident than during inspiration although its volume is the same at inspiration and expiration. One should beware of concluding that pneumothorax is larger or smaller than on a prior film without considering that the change might be caused by differences

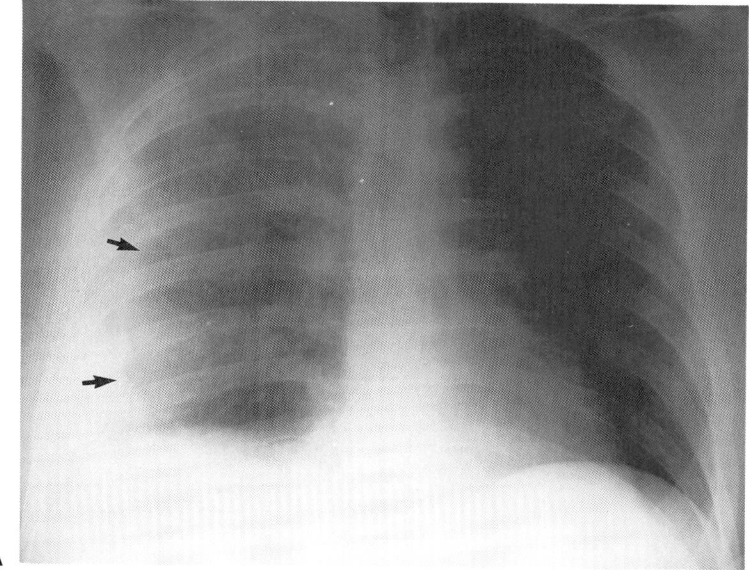

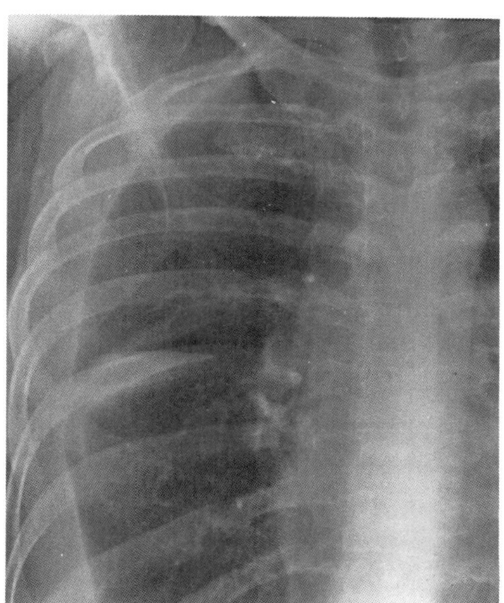

Figure 57-15. The appearance of pleural fluid on the supine and lateral decubitus bedside radiograph. (**A**) AP supine view shows a large pleural effusion that layers posteriorly and laterally and extends into the subdiaphragmatic region. The effusion is large enough to displace the lung medially from the lateral rib margins. The indistinct area of increased opacity in the portion of the lung immediately medial to the fluid along the lateral chest wall is caused by the posterior effusion. Often, smaller effusions will manifest only by subtly increased opacity of the hemithorax rather than by the obvious band at the lateral wall seen here. (**B**) Right side down decubitus view. The patient is positioned with the right side down to allow the pleural effusion to drain into the dependent portion of the lung. This results in a sharp interface between the pleural effusion and the aerated lung. The lateral decubitus view is more sensitive than the supine view for detecting pleural effusions because it allows the viewer to detect a small pleural effusion by noting displacement of the lungs from the lateral rib margins. The pleural fluid extends into the lateral aspect of the right minor fissure. (From Blank,[6] with permission.)

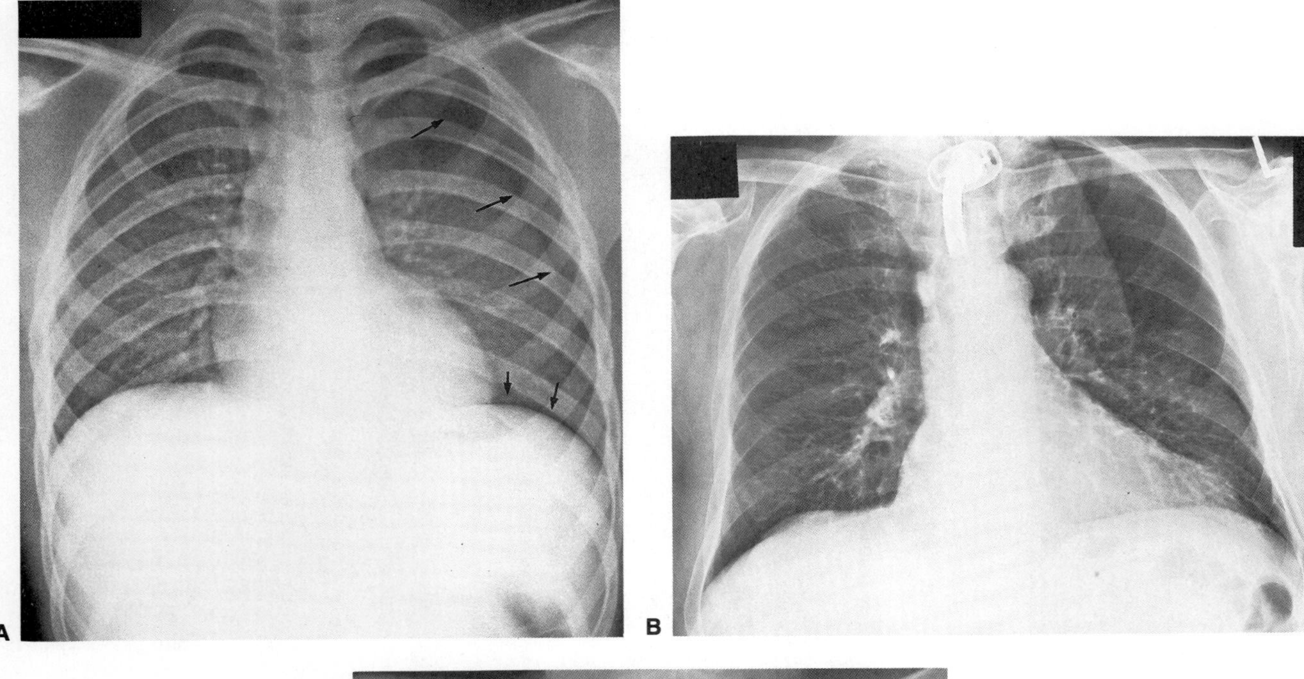

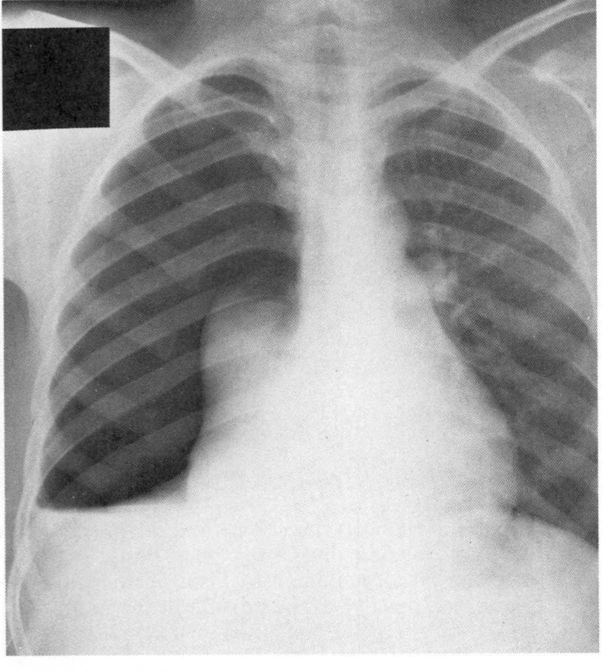

Figure 57-16. Pneumothorax and its mimics. (**A**) PA upright view taken at maximum expiration, showing a left partial pneumothorax. (**B**) Artifact mimicking pneumothorax. The curved opacity over the upper left portion of the medial left hemithorax is caused by a skin fold rather than by pneumothorax. Two observations allow pneumothorax to be distinguished from a skin fold: (1) with a pneumothorax the margin between aerated lung and free air in the pleural space is a sharp line representing the visceral pleura, whereas with a skin fold, the margin of what appears to be a pneumothorax is not sharp, but broad and indistinct, as would be expected; and (2) the pulmonary vessels extend peripherally to the opacity caused by the skin fold but do not extend beyond the visceral pleura with a pneumothorax. (**C**) Complete right pneumothorax. The right lung has collapsed against the right heart border and superficially resembles right lower lobe collapse (see Fig. 57-11A). The fluid level at the right base represents a hydropneumothorax. (From Blank,[6] with permission.)

in the degree of expiration. An easy and accurate way to measure the size of a pneumothorax is to measure the distance between the visceral pleura and the chest wall at the same phase of respiration. Calculating a volume for the pneumothorax is an unnecessary step, which does not improve accuracy. A chest radiograph should be obtained following central line placement or thoracentesis but may not be necessary following fiberoptic bronchoscopy.[24]

A tension pneumothorax occurs when the expanding volume of air in the pleural space accumulates under positive pressure sufficient to impair venous return and compromise cardiac output. A simple pneumothorax does not compromise cardiac output although it may cause substantial right-to-left intrapulmonary shunt. As the volume of gas within the pleural space increases, the mediastinal contents become displaced toward the contralateral side, and the ipsilateral hemidiaphragm is displaced inferiorly.

OTHER IMAGING TECHNIQUES

Questions that the chest film cannot answer can be resolved by the appropriate companion study.[25] Most of the companion studies we use are designed to overcome the fundamental limitation of the chest radiograph—projection of the complicated three-dimensional anatomy of the chest onto the two-dimensional chest film. CT, MRI, diagnostic ultrasound, and fluoroscopy allow us to study the chest in three dimensions. In addition, each of these modalities has characteristics that make it particularly useful for selected indications. Although CT and MRI are considered safe, they do pose potential risks that clinicians should consider:

1. The gantry table moves during the examination. Make sure that there is sufficient ventilator tubing to avoid unintentional disconnection.
2. Position the ventilator so that it can be monitored during the examination. Many MR imagers create substantial noise, which could mask a ventilator's disconnect alarm.
3. Know how to slide the gantry out of the imager should an emergency occur. Virtually all CT scanners and MR imagers have an emergency release button on their gantries for this purpose.
4. Make sure that the conscious intubated patient can communicate by at least a hand motion to warn observers of a problem during the study.
5. The strong magnetic field of MR imagers can exert a potentially dangerous torque on ferromagnetic surgical materials. Patients who have ferromagnetic cerebral aneurysm clips, ferromagnetic heart valves, or pacemakers should not be scanned by MRI.
6. During MRI wires that are attached to the patient for monitoring (e.g., electrocardiograph or pulse oximeter wires) must not be allowed to form loops. Unlike a straight wire, a loop can absorb radiofrequency energy during imaging and can severely burn the patient by induction.

Computed Tomography

CT offers three major advantages as compared with the conventional chest film. It images the chest in three dimensions, provides submillimeter spatial resolution, and demonstrates subtle differences in tissue contrast. By using CT one can accurately evaluate the hila and mediastinum.[26] In the critically ill patient CT is superb for locating small pulmonary cavitary lesions, occult pneumothorax, and subtle loculated pleural fluid collections.[27] Using thin-section CT one can study the bronchial tree for bronchiectasis and the interstitium for chronic diffuse interstitial disease[28] (Fig. 57-17). For pediatric CT or for patients who will require serial CT studies of the chest, recent developments have led to the use of low-dose chest CT that delivers as little as one-tenth of the radiation associated with conventional chest CT.

Physics of Computed Tomography

In CT a narrow fan-shaped x-ray beam is passed through a thin section of the patient's body, and the intensity of the beam is measured at the opposite side (Fig. 57-18). The x-ray tube is rotated a few degrees and another exposure is made. In this way CT scanners produce over 1 million data for each cross-sectional image of the patient's body. A mathematical technique called the modified Radon transformation converts these raw data into a single cross-sectional image.[29] Two parameters, window and level, are used to adjust the appearance of the image and can be set to emphasize the mediastinum, the lung parenchyma, or the bones of the chest.

When the clinical problem requires high resolution but does not require analysis of a large contiguous region, thin sections of 1- to 3-mm thickness are used.[30] Thin sections are required for evaluating the interstitium for chronic diffuse interstitial disease and for evaluating bronchial abnormalities. Contiguous 10-mm sections are used when the problem requires evaluation of a large area of the chest, as when evaluating the mediastinum, hila, and great vessels and searching for pulmonary metastases, empyemas, subtle diffuse infection, or occult pneumothorax.[31] Chest CT is used to guide needles in biopsying suspicious parenchymal lesions as small as 1 cm in diameter.

Nuclear Medicine

The basic principle of nuclear medicine is to find a drug that has a specific affinity for a particular organ and then attach a radioactive atom to the drug. The attachment of a radioactive atom to a nonradioactive drug is called *labeling*. Because radioactive atoms give off gamma rays, they are easily detected. The radiolabeled drug combines the specificity of the drug with the detectability of the radioactive atom.

The radiolabeled drug (also known as a *tracer*) is distributed in proportion to function in the affected organ; areas of high accumulation indicate greater physiologic activity.

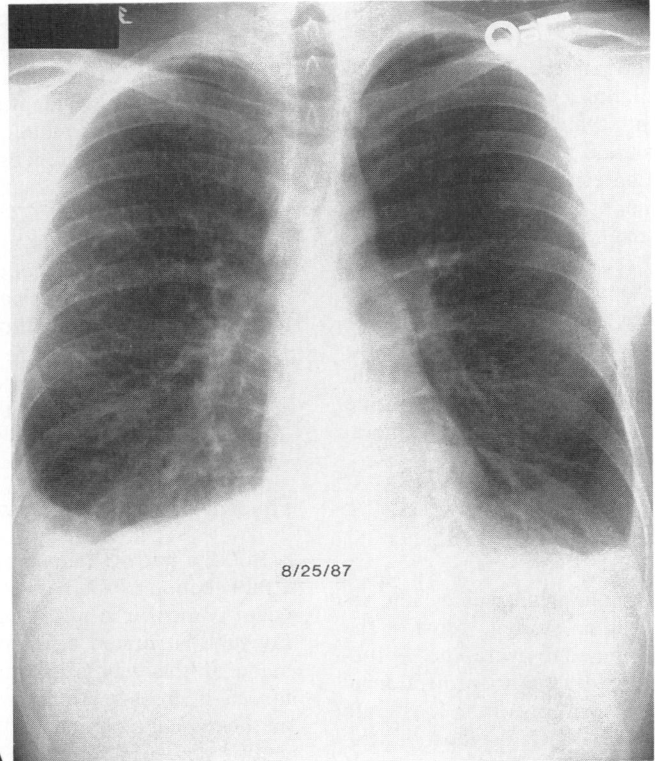

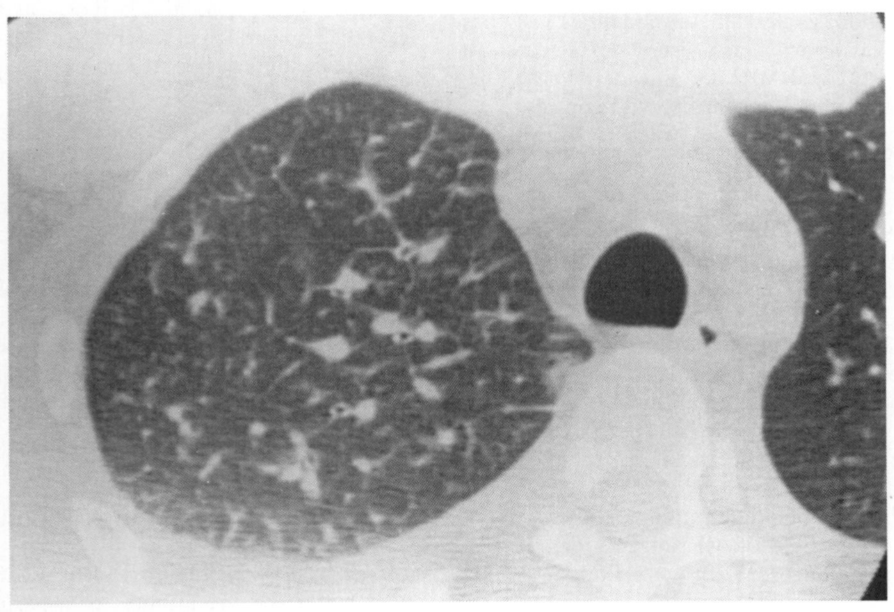

Figure 57-17. A 33-year-old man with a history of asthma and sinusitis who developed pleuritis, pulmonary infiltrates, pleural effusions, and peripheral eosinophilia. (**A**) PA upright chest radiograph showing bilateral pleural effusions, abnormal interstitial opacities in the lower lobes and right middle lobe, and abnormally prominent bronchovascular markings. (**B**) A high-resolution chest CT (HRCT) section through the right upper lobe, showing abnormal enlargement of the pulmonary arteries compared to their companion bronchi. Although the bronchi are of normal caliber, their walls are abnormally thickened. The small patchy opacities seen in the parenchyma are thought to be a manifestation of eosinophilic pneumonia. (*Figure continues.*)

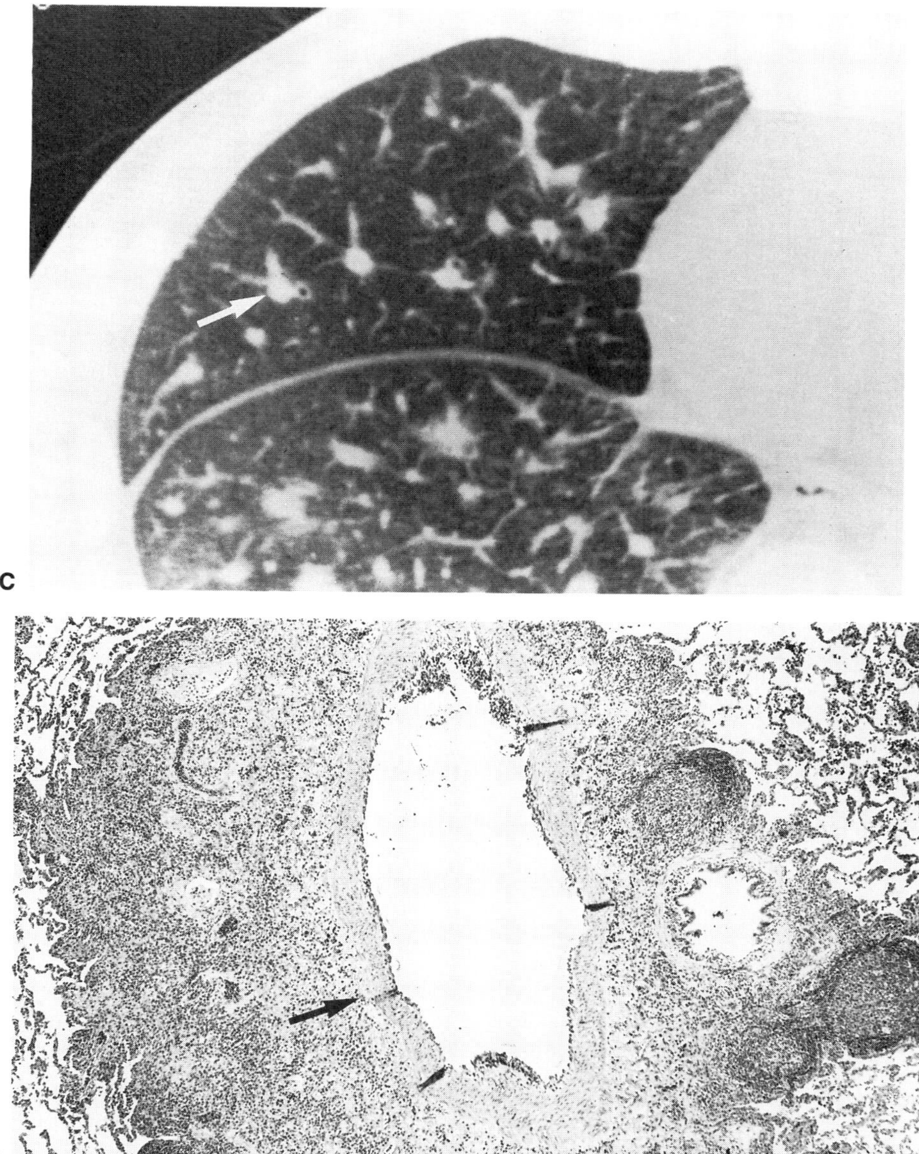

Figure 57-17 (*Continued*). (**C**) An HRCT section through the right lower and middle lobes. There is thickening of the major fissure and of the subpleural interlobular septa. The pulmonary arteries are abnormally large compared to their companion bronchi and have a stellate appearance that is thought to be the result of inflammation (arrow). (**D**) Biopsy specimen from the right lower lung. (×10.) The arterial wall is greatly thickened relative to the adjacent bronchioles by eosinophil-rich inflammatory infiltrate (arrow). The lymphatic channels are dilated, and the walls of the bronchioles are thickened. Combined with the clinical presentation, these histologic findings indicate Churg-Strauss syndrome with necrotizing vasculitis. (From Buschman et al.,[44] with permission.)

The film record of the distribution of activity reflects the underlying physiologic process. The gamma camera detects the gamma rays and records their spatial location.[32] Because areas of greater tracer accumulation emit more gamma rays, these areas will appear darker on film than will areas of lesser accumulation.

Two examinations account for most of the nuclear medicine studies performed on ICU patients: the ventilation/perfusion ($\dot{V}/\dot{Q}$) scan and the gated blood pool study of the heart. These studies provide physiologic rather than anatomic information, and therefore it is unimportant that their spatial resolution is low compared with that of a chest radiograph.

The gated blood pool study estimates the percentage of left ventricular volume that is ejected during systole.[33] The

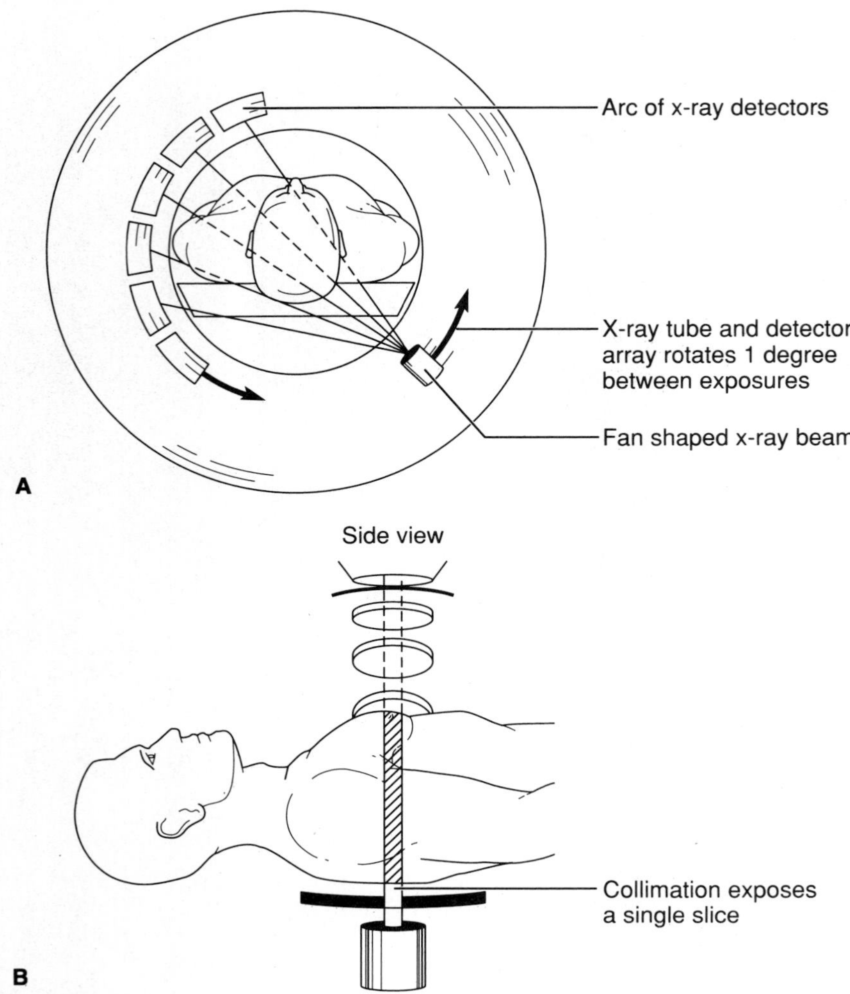

Figure 57-18. Generation of CT images of the head and body. The patient is placed supine on the CT table (gantry), which is advanced, slice by slice, into the scanning plane under computer control. When the body part to be studied is centered in the CT ring, a fan-shaped beam of x-rays travels from the x-ray tube to an arc of x-ray detectors on the opposite side. A brief exposure is made, and then the x-ray tube and detectors are rotated a few degrees and another exposure is made. This sequence of exposure and rotation by a few degrees is performed over 180 to 398 degrees for each anatomic slice. The resulting data are transferred to the computer, where they are reconstructed to form an image of the single section.

values that are considered normal depend on the individual laboratory but are typically above 60 percent. As the left ventricle fails, the ejection fraction decreases. Values below 25 percent indicate severe myocardial impairment.

Ventilation/Perfusion Scans

The $\dot{V}/\dot{Q}$ scan identifies regions of lung that are ventilated but not perfused[34] (Fig. 57-19). This condition is referred to as a $\dot{V}/\dot{Q}$ mismatch and is characteristically seen with pulmonary embolism. The $\dot{V}/\dot{Q}$ scan is performed in two phases. To show the distribution of ventilation to the lungs, the patient inhales a small amount of a gaseous tracer, which is either a true gas, such as Xenon 133 or 127, or a fine mist of technetium 99m in water. The particles deposit in the alveoli and distal airways. Imaging begins when the ventilatory tracer is at its maximum concentration in the lungs. The greater the ventilation to a segment, the greater the amount of tracer activity that will accumulate in that segment, and the darker the segment will appear on film.

After the ventilation scan is performed, the patient is given a venous injection of the perfusion tracer Tc 99m macroaggregated albumin (MAA). These radiolabeled microscopic particles of denatured albumin become lodged in the pulmonary capillary bed, the amount deposited being proportional to the flow of pulmonary arterial blood into each lung segment. The greater the blood flow, the greater the amount of radiolabeled MAA that becomes lodged in the segment,

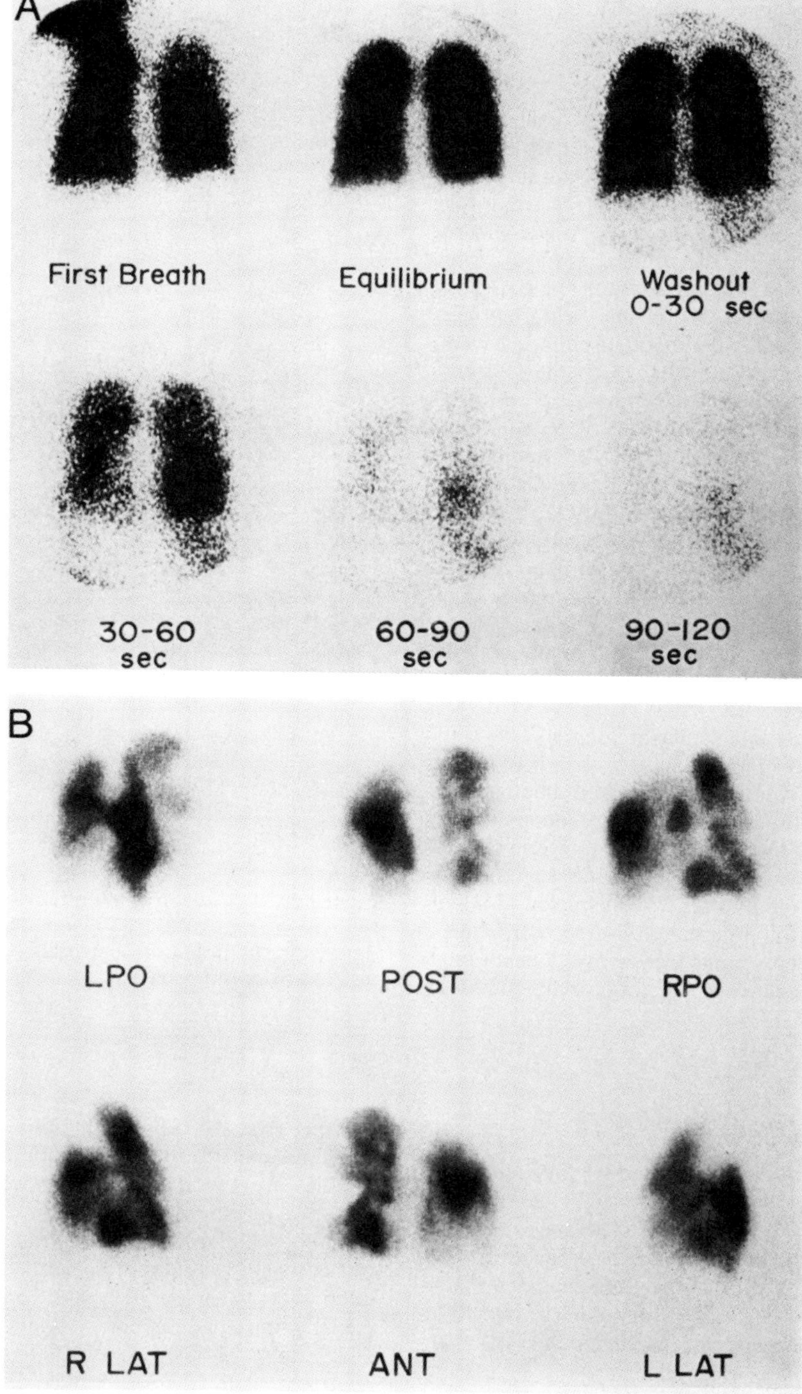

Figure 57-19. Ventilation/perfusion scanning. (**A**) Normal xenon ventilation. (**B**) Perfusion images that show multiple bilateral segmental and subsegmental defects. The presence of multiple segmental and subsegmental perfusion defects with normal distribution of ventilation in a patient who has no significant radiographic abnormalities indicates a high probability of pulmonary embolism. (From George et al.,[43] with permission.)

and the darker it will appear on the film. This is why areas of normal perfusion appear black on the perfusion image. Segments of the lung that have decreased pulmonary blood flow will appear lighter on the perfusion scan.

How is the information given by the $\dot{V}/\dot{Q}$ scan used to estimate the likelihood that a patient has pulmonary emboli? There is substantial overlap between the appearance of abnormal perfusion caused by emboli and the abnormal perfusion caused by pre-existing lung disease. To account for this source of uncertainty in the interpretation of $\dot{V}/\dot{Q}$ scans, the scans are classified by the likelihood that the pattern is caused by emboli. The most useful result is a normal perfusion scan, which reduces the likelihood of pulmonary embolism to 4 percent or less.[35] At the other end of the spectrum is the high-probability scan. Patients who have no perfusion to two or more segments that are normally ventilated have over a 90 percent chance (a high probability) of having pulmonary emboli.[36] These outcomes are unambiguous and the answers provided by the $\dot{V}/\dot{Q}$ scan are definitive.

The diagnostic value of the $\dot{V}/\dot{Q}$ scan is lessened when the patient has chronic lung disease. Chronic obstructive pulmonary disease (COPD) creates a pattern of numerous small subsegmental defects in ventilation and perfusion. The alterations in perfusion and ventilation caused by nonembolic disease can mimic those caused by pulmonary emboli. Hilar adenopathy and pneumonia can cause larger $\dot{V}/\dot{Q}$ defects such as segmental or even lobar mismatching.

When the $\dot{V}/\dot{Q}$ scan is of intermediate probability, further evaluation is needed to confirm or exclude pulmonary emboli. Because most emboli arise in the deep venous system of the lower extremities, thrombosis in these deep veins (as determined by contrast venography) in a patient who has an intermediate probability study is highly suspicious for pulmonary embolism.[36] On the other hand, if the lower extremities show no signs of deep venous thrombosis, further evaluation of the pulmonary arteries to detect thrombi within the lungs may be required.

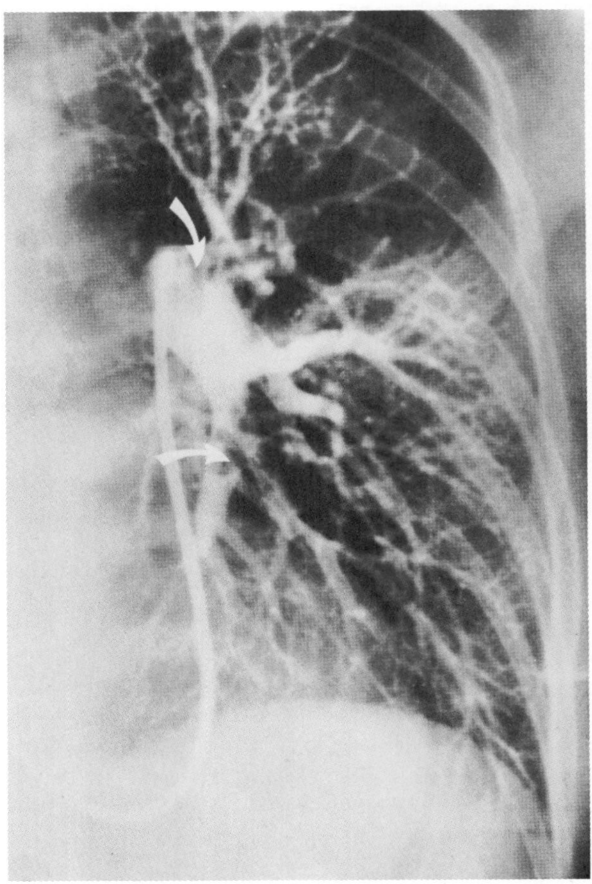

Figure 57-20. Selective pulmonary angiogram on same patient as in Fig. 57-19, showing multiple intraluminal filling defects in the pulmonary arteries (arrows). (From George et al.,[43] with permission.)

Pulmonary Angiography

A pulmonary angiogram is performed by introducing a catheter into the inferior vena cava through the common femoral vein in the groin. The catheter is advanced through the right heart and into the pulmonary artery that shows the largest perfusion defect. If possible, the tip of the catheter is positioned in the lobar branch of the pulmonary artery that supplies the hypoperfused segment. Contrast material is then injected during rapid filming. An embolus appears as a filling defect within the artery (Fig. 57-20). Because the angiogram shows the embolus directly, it is considered the most accurate test for emboli, but because it is an invasive examination it is reserved for the resolution of ambiguous results.

Fluoroscopy

If the x-ray beam passing through the patient's body is allowed to illuminate a video image intensifier rather than a film cassette, the result is fluoroscopy. Fluoroscopy permits real-time observation of the patient's internal anatomy.

What are the indications for chest fluoroscopy? When there is a question about phrenic nerve dysfunction (e.g., in a patient who has sustained injury to the cervical spine) fluoroscopy shows the motion of the hemidiaphragms. The injured side will show decreased or paradoxical motion, especially during a momentary "sniff" maneuver. Another indication is the need to evaluate the cause of chronic or recurrent aspiration pneumonia. One of the major causes of chronic aspiration is esophageal dysfunction, which can be caused by disordered motility or by a structural abnormality such as a Zenker's diverticulum. The best way to image these abnormalities is an esophagram. The patient is placed in a supine or an oblique prone position and asked to take a small mouthful of dilute barium sulfate suspension. The patient is told to swallow, and the passage of the bolus through the esophagus is watched under fluoroscopy. The normal esophagus shows a coordinated wave of contraction propelling the bolus into the stomach; aspiration should not occur. The esophagram is also used to evaluate the possibility of esophageal injury in patients who have sustained chest trauma.

A common use of chest fluoroscopy is to further evaluate the patient whose chest radiograph shows a possible lung nodule.[37] By watching the motion of the abnormality as the patient is slowly rotated, the presence of an abnormality can be confirmed and its location determined. Percutaneous and transbronchial lung biopsies are often guided by fluoroscopy, which confirms correct positioning of the biopsy needle or forceps and permits immediate inspection for pneumothorax.

Magnetic Resonance Imaging

MRI may be as important a medical advance as was the discovery of x-rays. MRI uses no ionizing radiation, has the high resolution of CT, and can image the body along any geometric plane (Fig. 57-21). MRI has the advantage of being able to create extremely high contrast images to depict subtle abnormalities better than can CT. Although CT and MRI are similar in their ability to show cross-sectional anatomy, the methods they use to accomplish this are different. The CT image depends on the linear attenuation coefficient of the tissues. The MR image depends on the biochemistry of the tissues and thus gives more information about tissue physiology than can CT.

Because the MR imager generates an intense magnetic field, ferromagnetic objects brought close to the magnet will be strongly attracted to it, possibly with harmful effects. For example, patients who have ferromagnetic cerebral aneurysm clips or ferromagnetic prosthetic cardiac valves should not undergo MRI because the strong magnetic field can cause displacement of these devices. Patients with cardiac pacemakers should avoid MRI because the strong magnetic field can interfere with the normal function of the pacemaker. Large ferromagnetic objects such as ventilators or hospital beds can interfere with the stability of the magnetic field if they are brought close to the magnet, resulting in degradation of the images. Nonferromagnetic ventilators, stretchers, intravenous solution poles, and other equipment have been developed to overcome this problem.

In general, most abnormalities of the chest are better evaluated by CT than by MRI, for two reasons—motion and spatial resolution. Regarding motion, because the exposure for chest CT is about 2 seconds per section, most patients are able to hold their breath during the scan. On the other hand, an MRI examination of the chest requires 5 to 10 minutes. The minimum spatial resolution of CT is 0.5 mm routinely, whereas MRI is limited to 3 to 4 mm in the chest. The susceptibility of MRI to motion will become less objectionable as new fast scanning and motion-compensated sequences are introduced into clinical practice.

MRI is superior to CT and ultrasound for depicting complex congenital heart disease, marrow diseases, adenopathy, and lesions of the chest wall. MRI can be particularly helpful for studying the mediastinum and hila.[38] For example, it can be difficult for CT to determine whether an enlarged hilum is caused by abnormal soft tissue or by unusual prominence of the pulmonary artery. Flowing blood in the hila has mod-

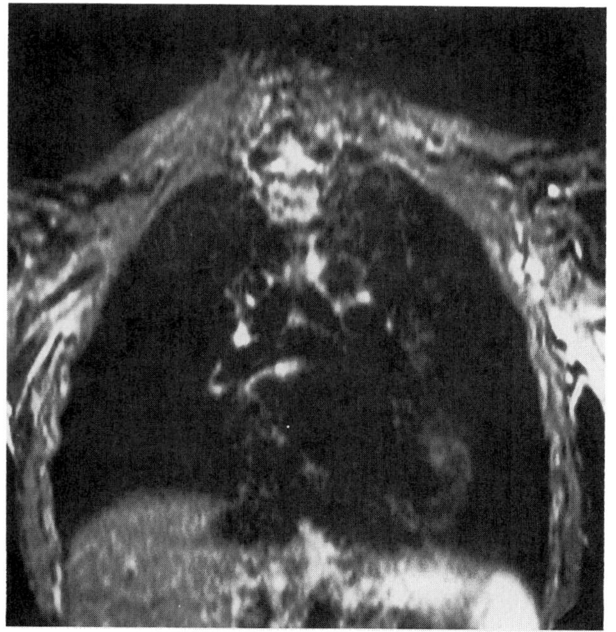

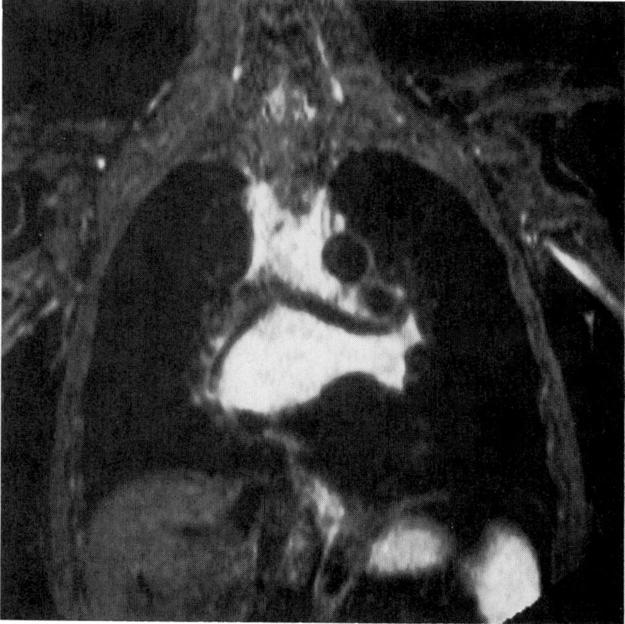

Figure 57-21. MRI of the chest in the coronal plane in a normal individual and in a patient with mediastinal lymphadenopathy, using a STIR (short inversion time recovery) sequence technique. (**A**) Normal chest. (**B**) Hodgkin's lymphoma with extensive mediastinal lymphadenopathy that is made conspicuous (white) by the STIR sequence. The STIR sequence is an invaluable tool for staging lymphomas and other malignancies because of its extreme sensitivity for detecting lymphadenopathy and involvement of the bone marrow.

erately high attenuation on CT and can be mistaken for abnormal tissue, but flowing blood in the pulmonary arteries creates an MRI signal of very low intensity. The absence of a signal from flowing blood means that the pulmonary arteries in the hila will appear black. The surrounding tissues, normal or pathologic, have much greater signal intensity and will appear gray-white. CT is clearly superior for demonstrating the lung interstitium, bronchi, and abnormalities of cortical bone; MRI and CT are about equal for evaluating the mediastinum.

The Physics of Magnetic Resonance Imaging

To create an MR signal the protons of the tissue must be placed in a strong magnetic field,[39] which creates a new energy level, representing an excited state that is initially empty, in the protons. Once the magnetic field has created the new higher energy level, the MR imager delivers a brief pulse of radio waves to the entire tissue. This pulse raises the energy of a small fraction of protons, boosting them from the ground state into the new excited state.

The MR imager measures how quickly excited protons lose energy. The amount of energy that can be stored in the excited state of a proton is the same for all protons; what differs among protons is how quickly they lose the energy by relaxing to the ground state. Protons in different environments—fat, muscle, bone marrow, cerebrospinal fluid, or tumor—lose energy at different rates.

The process of unraveling the signals from innumerable relaxing protons and reweaving them into a cross-sectional image is called *reconstruction* and is accomplished by Fourier transformation.[40]

Bronchography

Bronchography is an older technique, which formerly was extensively used to visualize abnormalities of the tracheobronchial tree. As CT and fiberoptic bronchoscopy have become the preferred methods of evaluating the chest, the role of bronchography has become increasingly restricted. Thin-section (1 to 2 mm) CT is now the preferred imaging technique for evaluating bronchiectasis. The CT examination is fast and no contrast material, intrabronchial or intravenous, is needed.

To create a bronchogram, the patient must inhale an oil-based contrast material, which coats the tracheobronchial

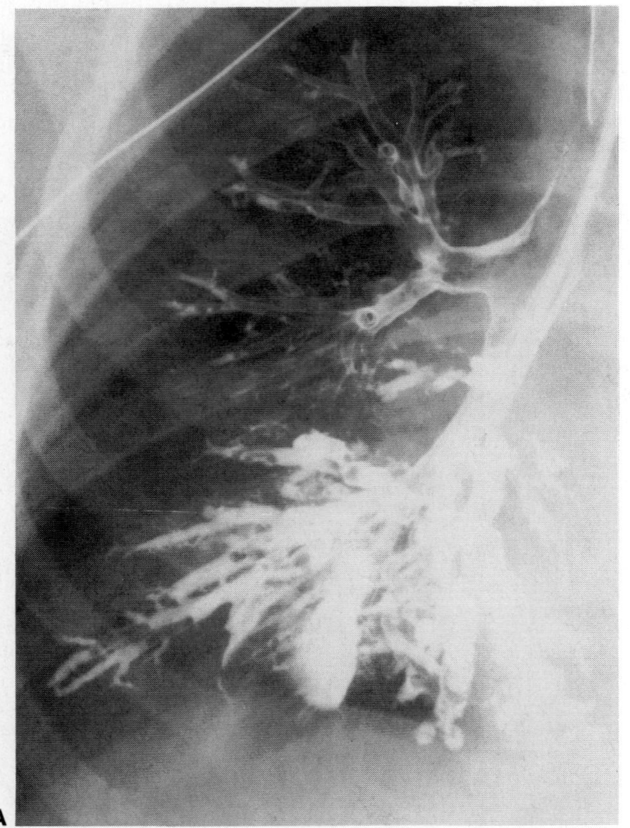

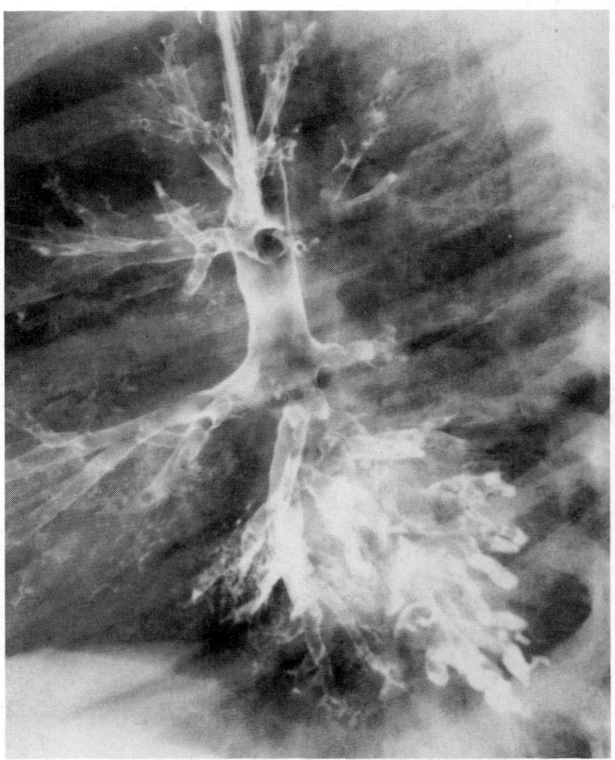

Figure 57-22. Use of bronchography to demonstrate bronchiectasis in the right lung, in both (**A**) AP and (**B**) lateral projections. There is gross distortion of the basilar segmental bronchi, which show loss of tapering, extensive marginal irregularities, saccular dilatations, and nonfilling of small branches. (From Blank,[6] with permission.)

tree. Inhaling this material is unpleasant, and the material can cause a chemical pneumonitis. The coated bronchi are first studied by fluoroscopy and then radiographs of the lungs are taken in several projections (Fig. 57-22). Of the few remaining indications for bronchography, its most frequent use is to localize regions of bronchiectasis in patients who are being evaluated for curative resection.

Diagnostic Ultrasound

The use of ultrasound in medicine evolved from sonar used during World War II for detecting underwater objects such as enemy submarines. Diagnostic ultrasound produces images by sending out a train of pulses of high-frequency sound, which are reflected to varying degrees by internal organs.[41] The ultrasound scanner is portable, uses no ionizing radiation, and provides real-time video images of the structures immediately beneath the ultrasound transducer. The ultrasound transducer is lightweight and small, allowing examination of the chest of even an immobile patient receiving mechanical ventilation.

The role of diagnostic ultrasound in evaluating the chest is limited because ultrasound will not pass through bone or air-filled spaces. Ultrasound plays an important role in localizing small effusions for thoracentesis. The ultrasound probe can be fitted with a needle guide, which will allow precise placement of the aspiration needle under direct real-time visualization. Ultrasound is particularly helpful for locating the internal jugular veins and the subclavian veins to facilitate central line placement in the ICU.

References

1. Reed JC: Chest Radiology: Plain Film Patterns and Differential Diagnoses. 3rd Ed. Mosby–Year Book, St. Louis, 1991
2. Felson B: Chest Roentgenology. WB Saunders, Philadelphia, 1973
3. Fraser RG, Pare JAP, Pare PD et al: Diagnosis of Diseases of the Chest. 3rd Ed. WB Saunders, Philadelphia, Vol. 1, 1988; Vol. 2, 1989; Vol. 3, 1990; Vol. 4, 1991
4. Taveras JM, Ferrucci JT, Buonocore E et al (eds): Radiology: Diagnosis-Imaging-Intervention. JB Lippincott, Philadelphia, 1990
5. Eisenberg RL: Clinical Imaging: An Atlas of Differential Diagnosis. 2nd Ed. Aspen, Rockville, MD, 1991
6. Blank N: Chest Radiographic Analysis. Churchill Livingstone, New York, 1989
7. Webster EW: X-ray generation. Ch. 2. In Taveras JM, Ferrucci JT, Buonocore E et al (eds): Radiology: Diagnosis-Imaging-Intervention. Vol. 1. JB Lippincott, Philadelphia, 1987
8. Webster EW: Absorption and scattering of x-rays and gamma rays. Ch. 3. In Taveras JM, Ferrucci JT, Buonocore E et al (eds): Radiology: Diagnosis-Imaging-Intervention. Vol. 1. JB Lippincott, Philadelphia, 1987
9. Milne EN, Burnett K, Aufrichtig D et al: Assessment of cardiac size on portable chest films. J Thorac Imaging 1988;3:64–72
10. Hale J: X-ray protection. Ch. 14. In Taveras JM, Ferrucci JT, Buonocore E et al (eds): Radiology: Diagnosis-Imaging-Intervention. Vol. 1. JB Lippincott, Philadelphia, 1990
11. Little JB: Biologic effects of low-level radiation exposure. Ch. 13. In Taveras JM, Ferrucci JT, Buonocore E et al (eds): Radiology: Diagnosis-Imaging-Intervention. Vol. 1. JB Lippincott, Philadelphia, 1990
12. Stark P: The pleura. In Taveras JM, Ferrucci JT, Buonocore E et al (eds): Radiology: Diagnosis-Imaging-Intervention. Vol. 1. JB Lippincott, Philadelphia, 1990
13. Proto AV: Mediastinal anatomy: Emphasis on conventional images with anatomic and computed tomographic correlations. J Thorac Imaging 1987;2:1–48
14. Elliott LP: The plain film approach using differential diagnostic vascular-anatomical sets. Ch. 13. In Taveras JM, Ferrucci JT, Elliott LP, Buonocore E (eds): Radiology: Diagnosis-Imaging-Intervention. Vol. 2. JB Lippincott, Philadelphia, 1990
15. Elliott LP: Roentgenologic approach to heart disease stage I—extracardiac analysis. Ch. 10. In Taveras JM, Ferrucci JT, Elliott LP, Buonocore E et al (eds): Radiology: Diagnosis-Imaging-Intervention. Vol. 2. JB Lippincott, Philadelphia, 1990
16. Elliott LP: Stage II—physiologic stage of analysis. Ch. 11. In Taveras JM, Ferrucci JT, Buonocore E et al (eds): Radiology: Diagnosis-Imaging-Intervention. Vol. 2. JB Lippincott, Philadelphia, 1990
17. Milne EN: A physiological approach to reading critical care unit films. J Thorac Imaging 1986;1:60–90
18. Newman B, Bowen A, Oh KS: A practical approach to the newborn chest. Curr Probl Diagn Radiol 1990;19:41–84
19. Henry DA, Jolles H, Berberich JJ, Schmelzer V: The post-cardiac surgery chest radiograph; a clinically integrated approach, J Thorac Imaging 1989;4:20–41
20. Green CE, Elliott LP: Radiology of the post-operative chest. Ch. 126. In Taveras JM, Ferrucci JT, Buonocore E et al (eds): Radiology: Diagnosis-Imaging-Intervention. Vol. 2. JB Lippincott, Philadelphia, 1990
21. Tocino I, Armstrong JD III: Trauma to the lung. Ch. 50. In Taveras JM, Ferrucci JT, Buonocore E et al (eds): Radiology: Diagnosis-Imaging-Intervention. Vol. 1. JB Lippincott, Philadelphia, 1988
22. Mintzer RA, Sakowicz BA, Blonder JA: Lobar collapse: Usual and unusual forms. Chest 1988;94:615–620
23. Miller WT: Pulmonary infections. Ch. 49. In Taveras JM, Ferrucci JT, Buonocore E et al (eds): Radiology: Diagnosis-Imaging-Intervention. Vol. 1. JB Lippincott, Philadelphia, 1990
24. Milam MG, Evins AE, Sahn SA: Immediate chest roentgenography following fiberoptic bronchoscopy. Chest 1989;96:477–479
25. Ferrucci JT: Imaging algorithms for radiologic diagnosis. Ch. 36. In Taveras JM, Ferrucci JT, Buonocore E et al (eds): Radiology: Diagnosis-Imaging-Intervention. Vol. 1. JB Lippincott, Philadelphia, 1990
26. Lee JKT, Sagel SS, Stanley RJ (eds): Computed Body Tomography with MRI Correlation. 2nd Ed. Raven Press, New York, 1989
27. Snow N, Bergin KT, Horrigan TP: Thoracic CT scanning in critically ill patients: Information obtained frequently alters management. Chest 1990;97:1467–1470
28. Zerhouni E: Computed tomography of the pulmonary parenchyma. An overview. Chest 1989;95:901–907
29. Pelc NJ, Colsher JG: Principles of x-ray computed tomography. Ch. 30. In Taveras JM, Ferrucci JT, Buonocore E et al (eds): Radiology: Diagnosis-Imaging-Intervention. Vol. 1. JB Lippincott, Philadelphia, 1990
30. Genereux GP: The Fleischner lecture: Computed tomography of diffuse pulmonary disease. J Thorac Imaging 1989;4:50–87
31. Golding RP, Knape P, Strack van Schijndel RJ et al: Computed tomography as an adjunct to chest x-rays of intensive care unit patients. Crit Care Med 1988;16:211–216
32. Zimmerman RE: Radionuclide imaging systems. Ch. 20. In Taveras JM, Ferrucci JT, Buonocore E et al (eds): Radiology: Diagnosis-Imaging-Intervention. Vol. 1. JB Lippincott, Philadelphia, 1990
33. Alazraki N: Nuclear imaging of the cardiovascular system. Ch. 6. In Elliott LP, Buonocore E (eds): Radiology: Diagnosis-Imaging-Intervention. Vol. 2. JB Lippincott, Philadelphia, 1990
34. Alderson PO, Biello DR: Radionuclide studies of the pulmonary

vasculature. Ch. 72. In Taveras JM, Ferrucci JT, Buonocore E et al (eds): Radiology: Diagnosis-Imaging-Intervention. Vol. 1. JB Lippincott, Philadelphia, 1990
35. Bone RC: Ventilation-perfusion scan in pulmonary embolism: The emperor is incompletely attired (editorial). JAMA 1990;263:2794–2795
36. PIOPED Investigators: Value of the ventilation/perfusion scan in acute pulmonary embolism: Results of the prospective investigation of pulmonary embolism diagnosis. JAMA 1990;263:2753–2759
37. Caskey CI, Templeton PA, Zerhouni EA: Current evaluation of the solitary pulmonary nodule. Radiol Clin North Am 1990;28:511–520
38. Swensen SJ, Ehman RL, Brown LR: Magnetic resonance imaging of the thorax. J Thorac Imaging 1989;4:19–33
39. Partain CL, Jones JP: Physics of magnetic resonance. Ch. 32. In Taveras JM, Ferrucci JT, Buonocore E et al (eds): Radiology: Diagnosis-Imaging-Intervention. Vol. 1. JB Lippincott, Philadelphia, 1990
40. Shepard JO: Radiology of the bronchial tree. Ch. 67. In Taveras JM, Ferrucci JT, Buonocore E et al (eds): Radiology: Diagnosis-Imaging-Intervention. Vol. 1. JB Lippincott, Philadelphia, 1990
41. Goodsitt MM: Ultrasound instrumentation and the A,B,M's of ultrasound. Ch. 29. In Taveras JM, Ferrucci JT, Buonocore E et al (eds): Radiology: Diagnosis-Imaging-Intervention. Vol. 1. JB Lippincott, Philadelphia, 1990
42. Pierson DJ: Acute respiratory failure. In Sahn SA (ed): Pulmonary Emergencies. Churchill Livingstone, New York, 1982, p. 120
43. George RB, White RW, Matthey RA (ed): Chest Medicine. Churchill Livingstone, New York, 1987
44. Buschman DL, Waldron JA Jr, King TL Jr: Churg-Strauss pulmonary vasculitis. Am Rev Respir Dis 1990;142:458–461

Chapter 58

Pulmonary Diagnostic Procedures

Noel T. Johnson
David J. Pierson

CHAPTER OUTLINE

Pulmonary medicine relies more and more on specialized diagnostic procedures. Increasingly, performing these procedures and processing the specimens that they produce are activities requiring more than one person. This requirement underscores the need for smooth coordination and teamwork in respiratory care. This chapter describes the main pulmonary diagnostic procedures and provides practical guidance intended for both operators (usually physicians) and assistants (often respiratory care practitioners or technicians). The approach used assumes that diagnostic yield, safety, and efficiency will be improved if everyone involved in a given diagnostic procedure understands its purpose, the equipment and materials used, the protocol to be followed, and the optimum handling of specimens. For a more extensive review of the topics discussed in this chapter, along with comprehensive references to the relevant literature, the reader should consult the section on diagnostic evaluation in Murray and Nadel's *Textbook of Respiratory Medicine*.[1]

SPUTUM ANALYSIS

The word *sputum* is derived from the Latin *spuere* ("to spit"). It is used in medical jargon to denote material that is coughed up (expectorated) from the lower respiratory tract—that is, below the vocal cords.[2] This material is largely a mixture of tracheobronchial secretions, consisting mainly of mucins, proteins, electrolytes, and water. Sputum may also contain cellular elements such as leukocytes from areas of inflammation and cells shed from the respiratory epithelium, including ciliated columnar cells, goblet cells, clara cells, basal cells, and pulmonary macrophages. Sputum may contain inhaled or aspirated material, including dust and microorganisms, as well.

This definition of sputum is commonly broadened to include matter that is aspirated from the lower airway via endotracheal tubes, nasotracheal suction, and transtracheal puncture. Specifically excluded from this definition are secretions from the nasal cavity and saliva from the oral cavity. Thus, an ideal sputum specimen contains only lower respiratory tract material.

Inspection with Unaided Eye

Macroscopic examination of the sputum specimen as it is obtained allows only a few generalizations regarding the implications of its appearance for the diagnosis of lung disease. There are virtually no findings that permit presumptive diagnosis of specific microbes based solely on visual examination with the unaided eye. The "sulfur granules" found in infection with *Actinomyces israelii* may be a notable and unusual exception. These appear as yellow granules up to 2 mm in size when examined against a dark background, but they can only rarely be identified in sputum.[3]

Bacterial infections of the lower respiratory tract are generally associated with thickening and opacification of the sputum. In addition, there may be yellow or green discoloration. The greenish hue is imparted by peroxidases released from granulocytes in the sputum.[2] If there is pulmonary hemorrhage associated with the infection, there may be red to brown discoloration, depending on latency from hemorrhage to expectoration. These changes, however, are nonspecific, and color may not be reliably used to identify the microbial pathogen. Yellow sputum due to the presence of bile pigments may also be seen in patients who are jaundiced, and, rarely, in the presence of a biliary-bronchial fistula.

Microscopic Examination

Microscopic examination of the sputum is the foundation upon which the diagnosis of the lung infection is built. Stains of sputum enable us to identify specific groups of microbial pathogens that cause infections of the lung. They also serve as an index of the specimen's acceptability for routine bacteriologic culture.[4] Common microbial pathogens are easily seen on a Gram stain. This stain separates stainable organisms into gram-positive (bluish staining) and gram-negative (reddish staining) categories, each of which connotes distinct treatment considerations for initial, empiric antimicrobial therapy. It is also frequently possible to make presumptive identification of the common fungus *Candida albicans* or the higher bacteria *Nocardia* and *Actinomyces* with the Gram stain and occasionally to diagnose pneumonia caused by *Pneumocystis carinii.*

A Gram-stained sputum devoid of stainable microorganisms but with an abundance of leukocytes also has diagnostic implications. This finding is consistent with infections caused by viruses, *Coxiella* (Q fever), *Legionella* (legionnaire's disease), mycobacteria (tuberculosis), *Mycoplasma*, or chlamydial species. None of these organisms are easily identified with the Gram stain.

By using the Ziehl-Neelsen stain, up to 40 percent of cases of active pulmonary tuberculosis can be identified by examination of sputum. The small, acid-fast (red) staining organisms of *Mycobacterium tuberculosis* are readily demonstrated by this technique, provided that they are present in the sputum sample in adequate numbers. In the appropriate clinical setting a diagnosis can be made and therapy started while awaiting confirmation by culture methods. Cultures for *M. tuberculosis* are essential for definitive identification in suspected cases and to exclude the possibility of nontuberculous mycobacteria. These bacteria will also stain acid-fast, but they engender different treatment and public health considerations. When specifically looking for fungal pathogens or *P. carinii*, the methenamine silver stain is commonly employed. Both fungal pathogens and the *P. carinii* appear blackened and have characteristic shapes.

Sputum analysis can also be helpful in the diagnosis of lung cancer. The expectorated sputum may reveal malignant cells when stained by the Papanicolaou method. Submission of five properly collected samples for sputum cytology may detect three-quarters of primary lung tumors and half of metastatic ones.[5] Current practice, however, has come to favor fiberoptic bronchoscopy (in areas where it is readily available) as a front-line diagnostic mode over sputum cytology. In addition to expediency, fiberoptic bronchoscopy has a higher diagnostic yield than sputum cytology.[6]

Sputum cytology is commonly requested, however, as an adjunctive diagnostic mode following fiberoptic bronchoscopy. Postbronchoscopy sputum cytology may occasionally be positive even when all other bronchoscopic samples are negative.[7] The value of the postbronchoscopy sputum may lie in disrupting and recovering material from tumor tissue that are beyond the reach of the flexible bronchoscope.

Certain findings in the sputum have previously been used as supportive evidence of asthma. Eosinophils, characteristic granules called Charcot-Leyden crystals, or large compact clusters of ciliated columnar cells known as Creola bodies may all support the diagnosis of asthma. However, because the diagnosis of asthma is generally made on the basis of clinical findings and spirometry, sputum examination finds little role in this setting.

Cultures

For the most part, sputum bacterial cultures should be interpreted only in the context of the Gram stain findings. For example, the sputum Gram stain may show a preponderance of gram-positive cocci while the culture grows only gram-negative bacilli. In such a case it is likely that the more efficient gram-negative organism, originally present in smaller numbers (and possibly a contaminant), has overwhelmed the growth of the gram-positive organism (the more likely pathogen). It is not uncommon for the sputum culture in blood-culture-positive pneumococcal pneumonia to fail to grow the organism despite the appearance of characteristic gram-positive cocci in chains on a sputum smear.[8] The fastidious bacterium *Haemophilus pneumoniae* also occasionally fails to grow on sputum culture despite the appearance of characteristically small, pleiomorphic, gram-negative rods on the sputum smear. Anaerobic lung infection may be suspected when a proper sputum specimen contains mixed bacterial flora and routine aerobic culture fails to grow an organism. Sputum culture growth may be inhibited by the effects of local anesthetics such as lidocaine (for example, sputum obtained via bronchoscopy).[9] Thus, sputum cultures are of limited value when interpreted outside the context of Gram stain findings. When culture results are consistent with the findings on a quality Gram-stained sputum, more specific antimicrobial therapy based on antibiotic susceptibility testing may be used.

Sputum culture is essential in the diagnosis of tuberculosis. It distinguishes between *M. tuberculosis* and other, nontuberculous mycobacteria, and also permits antibiotic susceptibility testing. Special culture medium is required, and "culture for tuberculosis or AFB (acid-fast bacilli)" is specifically requested in such cases.

Expectorated sputum as well as that obtained via instrumentation of the pharynx (e.g., by nasotracheal suction) has the opportunity to mix with the secretions and bacteria of the pharynx. This contamination must be kept to a minimum if the sample is to be truly representative of the lung. Each specimen so obtained must be carefully inspected under the microscope for evidence that it represents an area of inflammation and is free of upper airway contamination. Cellular markers are used to indicate the adequacy of the sputum specimen. Leukocytes serve as evidence of inflammation, and squamous epithelial cells serve as evidence of upper airway contamination. The latter cells are continually shed from the pharyngeal epithelium and are not generally found in the airway below the vocal cords in patients with normal laryngeal function. They may be found in the lower airway, however, when aspiration occurs. Specimens without evidence of inflammation or with evidence of contamination should be discarded while another specimen is obtained.[10] Grading criteria have been devised to establish a standard methodology for distinguishing adequate specimens (primarily lower airway secretions) from inadequate ones (those contaminated with upper airway secretions). Thus far no universal convention has been widely adopted.

As noted, the ideal sputum specimen contains only matter from the lower respiratory tract. Table 58-1 describes one grading scheme that separates samples into acceptable and unacceptable categories. The goal of this grading process is to determine how well the specimen represents material from the site of infection. Slides are examined in areas where the preparation is only one or two cells in depth. This scheme was devised by using data from the agreement between bacterial cultures of paired transtracheal aspirates and sputa. Numbers of squamous epithelial cells are a more powerful predictor of agreement than are numbers of leukocytes.[11]

The ideal (lower airway) specimen is replete with leukocytes and devoid of squamous epithelial cells (Fig. 58-1A). Further evidence of a lower airway specimen is provided by the presence of macrophages in the sample (Fig. 58-1C). These cells are found mainly in the alveoli and thus are the hallmark of a "deep" specimen.[12] Ciliated pseudocolumnar epithelial cells are found in both the upper and lower respiratory tract and are therefore unhelpful in distinguishing upper from lower airway secretions.

SPUTUM COLLECTION

Expectoration

The best opportunity to collect sputum is when the patient coughs spontaneously and has adequate sputum production.

Table 58-1. Scheme for Grading Acceptability of Sputum Samples for Staining and Culture

Class	Squamous Epithelial Cells per Low-Power Field	Leukocytes per Low-Power Field	Interpretation	Acceptable for Culture?
Good	<10	>25	Minimal oral contamination; inflammation present	Yes
Fair	10–25	>10	Minimal oral contamination	Yes
Unsatisfactory	>25	<10	Regarded as saliva, not sputum	No

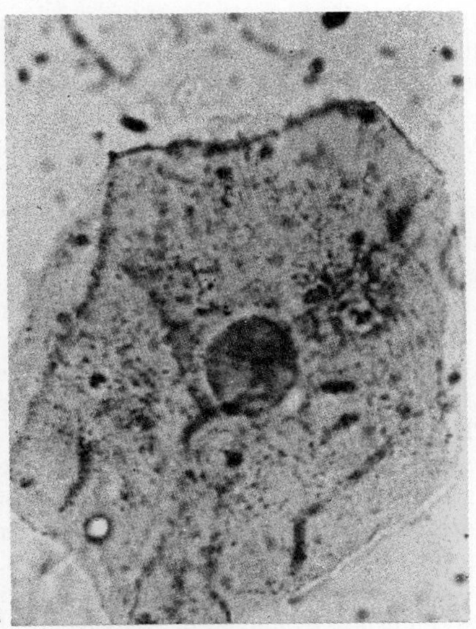

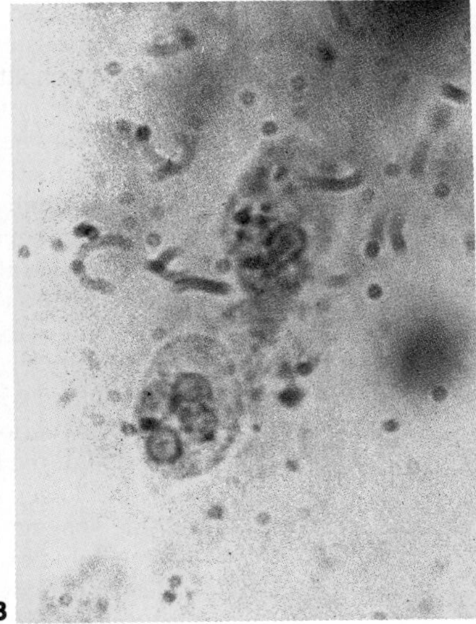

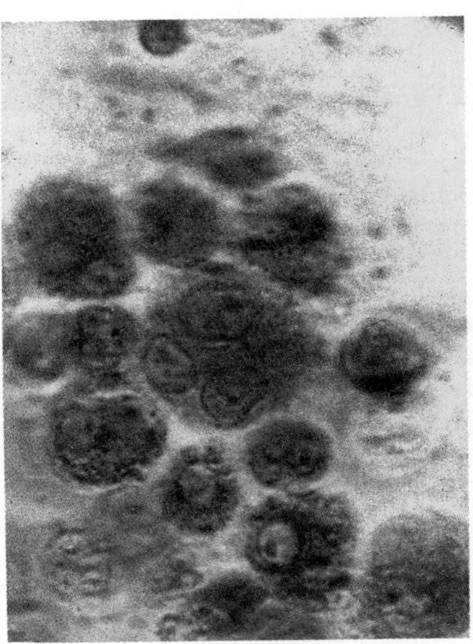

Figure 58-1. Cells commonly found in sputum, as seen on wet-mount preparations. (**A**) Squamous epithelial cells from the upper respiratory tract are helpful in sputum grading to assess the degree of contamination by upper airway secretions. (**B**) Polymorphonuclear leukocytes indicate that the sputum specimen is representative of an area of inflammation. (**C**) Macrophages are an indicator of a deep cough specimen, as these cells are found primarily in the lower airways and alveoli. (From Chodosh,[54] with permission.)

A practical procedure for sputum collection is summarized below:

1. Provide patient with a sterile sputum cup labeled with patient's name.
2. Have patient rinse mouth with water.
3. Obtain specimen immediately if possible and transport to the laboratory for processing for requested tests.
4. If the patient is unable to cough up a specimen at the time the specimen cup is delivered, leave specimen container at bedside and instruct patient in proper sputum collection technique—the patient must
   a. Rinse out mouth prior to coughing up specimen
   b. Avoid collection after meals if possible
   c. Understand that a specimen from the lungs is needed, not a specimen of saliva or nasal secretions
   d. Notify the nurse immediately after the specimen is obtained so that it may be transported to the laboratory for processing without delay
5. Outpatient sputum collection should be obtained at the time the cup is dispensed if bacterial infection is suspected.
6. Outpatient sputum collection for tubercle bacilli or carcinoma is carried out in the patient's home. The patient is instructed to collect the specimens on arising in the morning if possible and to keep the container in the refrigerator. A preservative such as Carbowax is included in cups dispensed for carcinoma detection to preserve the epithelial cells. The samples are brought back to the hospital on the day they are obtained or on the last day of a multiple-day collection.

Generally, a sterile sputum cup is left at the bedside of hospitalized patients or given to ambulatory patients along with instructions on its use. Patients are instructed in good expectoration technique (mouth rinsing beforehand to dilute oral flora and food particles) and timing (first morning sputum, not after meals). Instructions are also given for disposition of the specimen once it is obtained. Hospitalized patients are instructed to call the nurse once the specimen is obtained so that it can be processed directly and ambulatory patients are instructed to bring the specimen to the laboratory as soon as possible after collection. Adequate instruction of patients is essential to provide them with an adequate understanding of what is required for a good specimen. Leaving written instructions with patients following oral instruction may enhance compliance.

Sputum Induction

Sputum induction is used to increase the volume of sputum produced. A protocol for sputum induction is summarized below:

1. Observe body secretion precautions (see Ch. 97).
2. Explain the procedure to the patient.
3. Provide sputum cup for collection of specimen.
4. Have patient rinse mouth with water.
5. Administer two puffs of bronchodilator aerosol (optional); (helpful in asthmatic patients and in those with frequent cough, as the hypertonic saline aerosol will cause increased coughing and/or bronchospasm in such individuals).
6. Place 30 mL of 3% NaCl in ultrasonic nebulizer.
7. Have patient breathe from nebulizer via mouthpiece until either an acceptable sputum speci-

men is collected (for diagnosis of *P. carinii* pneumonia, a sample of at least 15 mL should be submitted to the laboratory) or the patient is unable to tolerate the procedure.
8. If initially unsuccessful, this protocol may be repeated after several hours.

Sputum induction is used when larger samples are desired, for expediency of sample collection, or when specimens are difficult to obtain because of scant secretions.[13] Aerosolized hypertonic saline (e.g., 3 to 30 mL of 3 percent NaCl) is commonly used in a hand-held, compressor-powered nebulizer for inhalation. The use of an ultrasonic nebulizer (as in the above list) maximizes delivery of aerosol to the patient. The saline may serve to increase secretions by irritant effect (stimulating mucus hypersecretion) and/or by osmotic pressure (drawing water out of the mucous membrane of the airway) and also may stimulate more coughing.

Nasotracheal Suction

Nasotracheal suction (NTS) is generally reserved for sputum collection when the patient is unresponsive or unable to cough spontaneously. Not only is this procedure noxious to the patient, but also it affords additional opportunity for sputum contamination via passage of the catheter through the nasopharynx. Nasotracheal suction does have an advantage over orotracheal suction in ease of access to the lower airway, since the anatomy of the nasopharynx naturally flexes the straight catheter toward the trachea, generally causing less gagging and less laryngeal trauma.

Recently, NTS has been used for sputum collection in patients with documented or suspected infection with the human immunodeficiency virus (HIV) who are suspected of having *P. carinii* pneumonia.[14] The procedure is better tolerated if an anxiolytic agent and topical lidocaine nasal and pharyngeal anesthesia are administered prior to the procedure, as in fiberoptic bronchoscopy.

Transtracheal Aspiration

Transtracheal aspiration (TTA) is the percutaneous aspiration of tracheal secretions through the cricothyroid membrane (Fig. 58-2). Its advantage over expectoration and NTS lies in avoidance of upper airway contamination. In addition, TTA serves to procure a relatively uncontaminated lower respiratory specimen in patients unable or disinclined to cough. This procedure can be useful in diagnosing anaerobic lung infections[15]; all specimens passing through the pharynx are contaminated with the abundant anaerobic flora there and are thus useless in the diagnosis of anaerobic lung disease.

TTA requires a skilled practitioner and a cooperative (or motionless) patient.[16] It is not recommended in critically ill patients who may require positive-pressure ventilation or in those with bleeding diatheses. Local anesthesia with intradermal and subcutaneous lidocaine is administered over the

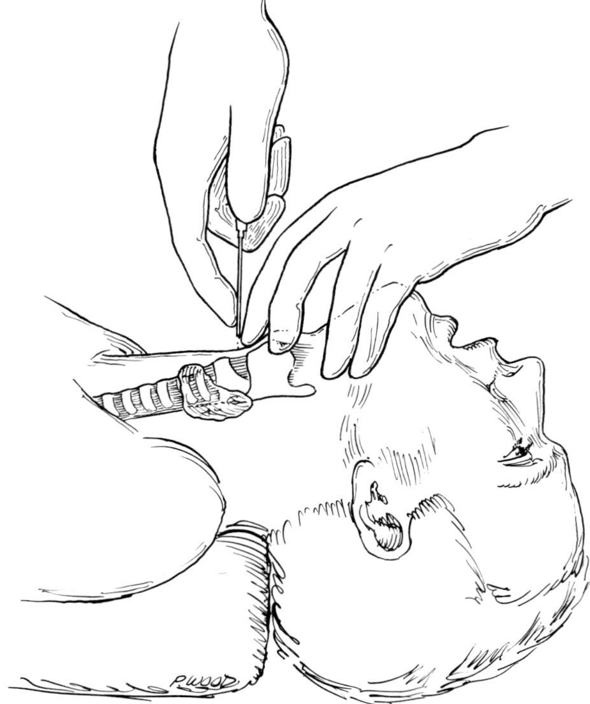

Figure 58-2. Technique of transtracheal aspiration. After administration of local anesthetic a large-bore needle is passed percutaneously through the cricothyroid membrane into the tracheal lumen. A short catheter is then passed through the needle, and lower respiratory tract secretions are aspirated by use of a syringe.

cricothyroid membrane. A large-bore needle is then carefully passed percutaneously through the overlying skin and cricothyroid membrane into the trachea. Tracheal penetration is signaled by the ability to aspirate air from an attached syringe. A small plastic catheter is then threaded through the large-bore needle, and tracheal secretions are aspirated and processed immediately for Gram stain and culture. Expertise with and use of this method tend to be regional; while commonly employed in some centers, it is not used at all in many areas.

Tracheal Tube Suctioning

In patients with nasotracheal, orotracheal, or tracheostomy tubes a suction catheter is simply passed down the lumen of the tube for a deep suction specimen with use of sterile technique. Intubated patients aspirate oral secretions despite the presence of an inflated tube cuff; this aspiration tendency is probably related to glottic dysfunction induced by the tube and an incomplete seal between the trachea and the cuff of the tube. Results from specimens obtained in this manner thus need to be interpreted with this in mind. The presence of squamous epithelial cells in these specimens is a clue to possible upper respiratory contamination. Additionally, the suction catheter is passed along the length of the tube, which affords opportunity for contamination with organisms colonizing the tube.

Standard suction catheters preferentially slide down the right main stem bronchus because of the more obtuse angle it makes with the trachea. For tracheostomy patients in situations in which a left-sided specimen or left-sided secretion clearance is desired, a specially shaped suction catheter has been developed, which reliably enters the left main stem bronchus instead (Bronchitrac-L). This catheter can be used with oral endotracheal tubes as well; successful left main stem cannulation rates vary from 44 to 65 percent depending on head position and endotracheal tube tip distance from the carina.[17]

Bronchoscopic Collection

Sputum samples obtained by bronchoscopy through the nose, mouth, or artificial airway for microbial analysis can be expected to be contaminated with microorganisms from those portals unless a protected specimen catheter is used. In this method a specimen brush is passed through the bronchoscope in a protective sheath. The specimen brush is then passed beyond the sheath by extruding a wax plug from its tip (Fig. 58-3), and proximal contamination is thereby avoided.[18] Organisms captured by this method can be relied on to reflect the microbiology of distal lung infection. In addition, quantitative cultures from such specimens are useful in ruling out pneumonia.[19] The protected specimen catheter technique can yield clinically useful information in addition to that obtained from standard endotracheal suctioning, provided that the patient has not been receiving antibiotics.

SPUTUM HANDLING AND PROCESSING

Sample Quantity

The volume of sample needed depends on the numbers of pathogenic organisms or pathologic cells present in the pulmonary secretions. Generally, for usual bacterial lung infections accompanied by a productive cough, a small quantity of adequately gathered purulent sputum (e.g., a teaspoonful) is sufficient for Gram stain and culture.

To make the diagnosis of mycobacterial infection (e.g., tuberculosis) multiple specimens are often necessary. Because the bacilli may be relatively sparse, a larger sample size and multiple samples reduce sampling error. Customarily, three specimens are requested when the diagnosis of mycobacterial infection is considered.[20] Multiple positive cultures for nontuberculous mycobacteria implicate that organism as having a causal role in lung infection.[21] Nontuberculous mycobacteria are commonly saprophytic rather than disease-causing and might be suspected as being saprophytic if only one out of three specimens were positive.

Timing of Collection

Morning is generally the best time of day to collect sputum. The recumbent position and sleep allow pooling of secretions produced during the night, especially if nocturnal coughing is minimal. Collecting sputum shortly after eating is undesirable, as such specimens may show inordinate contamination with food particles; this may be avoided by rinsing the mouth with water prior to expectoration to wash out food particles as well as other upper respiratory secretions.

Gastric aspiration via a nasogastric tube is occasionally used to collect culture specimens in cases of suspected pulmonary tuberculosis, especially in small children and others who do not or cannot voluntarily produce sputum.[20] Such specimens need to be collected immediately upon awakening, before the thought of breakfast causes the stomach to empty. Gastric specimens are appropriate for culture but not for staining, owing to the frequent presence of nontuberculous acid-fast organisms in the stomach.

Containment

When sputum is collected for microbiology stain and culture, a sterile plastic cup with a screw-on top is generally used for both collection and transport. Bacteriostatic saline should not be used in the transport or collection of specimens for microbiologic evaluation; when diluent is necessary, as with transtracheal or endotracheal tube suctioning, normal saline (0.9 percent NaCl) without preservatives is used. When testing for sputum cytology, a small amount (e.g., 20 mL) of 50 percent ethyl alcohol and 2 percent Carbowax is furnished in the bottom of a wide-mouthed, screw-top jar to preserve cell integrity while awaiting transport or analysis. For cytologic examination in outpatients, sputum is collected for three to five mornings in a single container and may be processed as a single, pooled specimen.

Specimen Handling and Transport

Generally, all specimens should be handled as if they are capable of transmitting infection, in accordance with the principles discussed in Chapter 97. Gloves should be worn when contact with sputum is unavoidable or anticipated. Hands should be washed after handling sputum containers. All specimens should be taken expeditiously to the laboratory for analysis. Best results are obtained when the specimens are delivered and processed immediately.[22] At worst, specimens should at least be transported to the laboratory on the same day that they are collected. Anaerobic cultures need to be placed immediately in a special O_2-poor environment, such as a CO_2 incubator. If anaerobic infection is suspected, specimens can be transported to the laboratory in an air-free syringe similar to that used for transport of blood gas specimens. A special anaerobic transport medium is also available. Specimens for viral culture (usually bronchoscopic specimens) are placed immediately in viral transport medium.

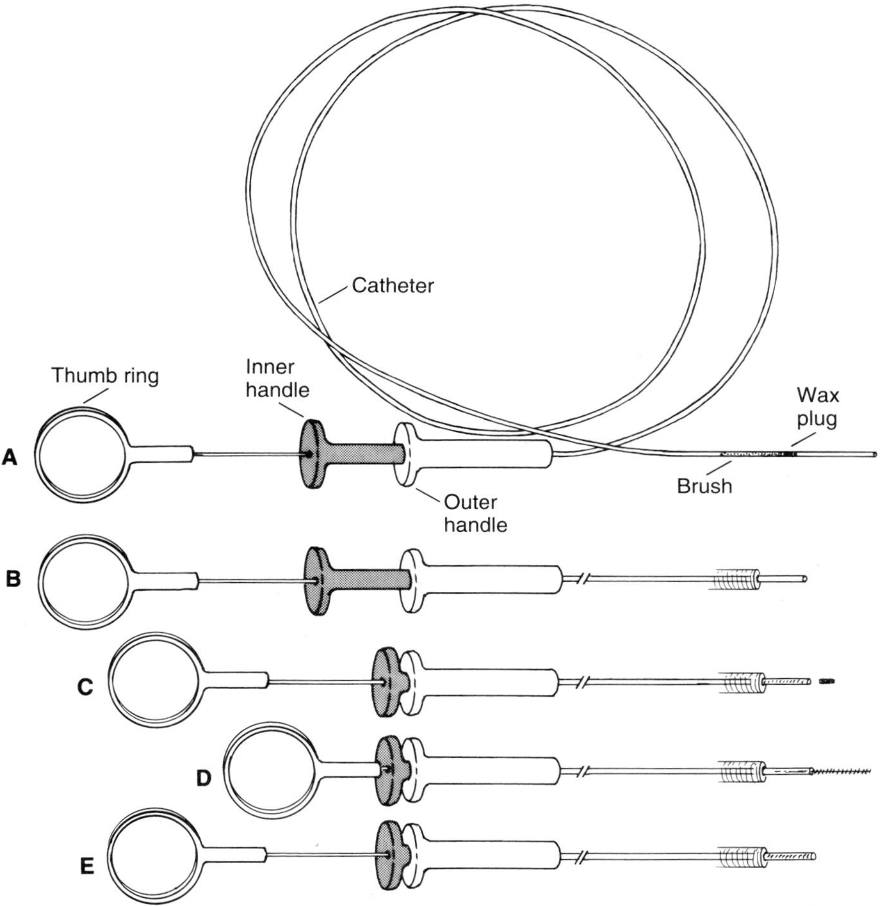

Figure 58-3. Protected specimen brush assembly for obtaining an uncontaminated microbiologic specimen from the distal airways via the fiberoptic bronchoscope. (**A**) Microbiology brush assembly. (**B**) Assembly advanced into bronchoscope beyond tip in target area. (**C**) Handles squeezed together and snapped into place; this expels the wax plug and locks inner catheter into position. (**D**) Thumb ring depressed; this positions brush outside catheter; brushing action gathers sample. (**E**) Brush retracted into catheter to prevent contamination and entire assembly removed from bronchoscope (not shown).

Stains Commonly Ordered for Sputum Analysis

It is the nature of pulmonary infections that numerous different microbial pathogens can cause similar radiographic patterns. As such, an expedient diagnosis requires an orderly approach based on a reasonable differential diagnosis. Consideration is given to travel history, nutritional state, immune status, underlying lung disease, local epidemiology, and age when formulating this differential diagnosis. A battery of tests is then ordered based on the likelihood of each of the possibilities under consideration. This battery commonly includes one or more of the sputum stains depicted in Table 58-2.

BRONCHOSCOPY AND BRONCHOSCOPIC PROCEDURES

Since Ikeda's introduction of the flexible fiberoptic bronchoscope in 1966, the fiberoptic instrument has come to replace rigid bronchoscopy in all but a few applications such

Table 58-2. Stains Commonly Ordered on Sputum or Other Respiratory Specimens

Stain or Test	Agent or Abnormality Sought
Gram stain	"Usual" bacteria
Methenamine-silver stain	*P. carinii*; fungi
Ziehl-Neelsen stain; auramine stain	Mycobacteria
Direct fluorescent antibody (DFA) test	*Legionella* species; cytomegalovirus
Papanicolaou stain	Abnormal exfoliative cytology (e.g., malignant cells)

as laser bronchoscopy. This section therefore deals mainly with flexible fiberoptic bronchoscopy. A more detailed and more extensively illustrated discussion of this topic can be found in a standard text on the subject.[23] As compared with the rigid bronchoscope, the flexible bronchoscope permits increased visualization, comfort, cost savings, and safety in most clinical settings.

Indications for Bronchoscopy

Bronchoscopy is generally undertaken with one or more of several broad goals in mind: to inspect the airways, to remove obstructions, and to take samples of lower respiratory tract fluids or lung tissue for diagnostic purposes. Examples of these and some other less common uses of bronchoscopy are listed in Table 58-3. Indications for the use of bronchoscopy may be found in consensus guidelines promulgated by the American Thoracic Society[24] and are not reviewed extensively here.

Description of the Bronchoscope

The fiberoptic bronchoscope consists of a rigid hand piece and a long flexible tube, which is advanced into the lungs (Fig. 58-4). The flexible portion is usually 55 to 60 cm long in instruments for use in adult patients. Most bronchoscopes in current use transmit images via fiberoptics. Newer types of flexible bronchoscopes have a video charge-coupled device (CCD) chip in the tip to capture and transmit images electronically with improved resolution. The hand piece contains a viewfinder lens (not present in video bronchoscopes); a thumb-lever for cable-actuated flexion and extension of the bronchoscope tip; a finger-operated suction valve opposite the thumb lever; an instrument port for passing catheters and forceps or for instillation of liquid through the "working channel"; and a metal nipple for connection to a suction source. The viewing angle from the tip of the bronchoscope may be up to 100 degrees (120 degrees with the video bronchoscope), and the tip may be angulated in an arc of up to 280 degrees. There is also an extension of flexible fiberoptic cable that connects to the light source.

The external diameter of the flexible portion of the bronchoscope may vary from 3.4 to 5.9 mm. The working channel to which suction is applied and through which instruments are passed varies from 1.2 to 2.6 mm in diameter. Larger bronchoscopes generally have the advantage of larger working channels for suction and instrumentation. They are better

Table 58-3. Bronchoscopy: Indications and Therapeutic Applications

Diagnostic uses

- Inspection of the lower airways
  - Mass, infiltrate, or other radiographic abnormality
  - Hemoptysis
  - Unexplained cough
  - Recurrent pneumonia or atelectasis
  - Localized wheezing
  - Symptoms or laboratory findings suggesting upper airway obstruction
  - Paralysis of recurrent laryngeal or phrenic nerve
  - Staging of known lung cancer
  - Positive sputum cytology without radiologic abnormality
  - Suspected tracheobronchial injury
  - Suspected bronchopleural fistula following lung surgery
  - Follow-up examination after therapeutic procedures (see below)
- Bronchography (injection of contrast dye through bronchoscope to visualize airways radiographically)
  - Suspected bronchiectasis
  - Assessment of anatomy following surgery, laser treatment of obstructing tumor, or other procedure.
- Acquisition of specimens for staining, culture, and/or pathologic examination
  - Bronchoalveolar lavage (e.g., diagnosis of *P. carinii* pneumonia; assessment of interstitial lung disease)
  - Bronchial washings (e.g., sputum-negative suspected tuberculosis)
  - Protected catheter specimen brush (e.g., pneumonia undiagnosed by other methods)
  - Forceps biopsy or brushing of airway lesions or bronchial wall under direct vision
  - Transbronchial biopsy or brushing of distal airways and/or lung parenchyma under fluoroscopic guidance
  - Transbronchial needle aspiration or biopsy (e.g., to sample adjacent lymph nodes for metastasis)

Therapeutic uses

- Facilitation of endotracheal intubation (passage of endotracheal tube over bronchoscope passed through vocal cords)
- Removal of airway secretions (e.g., acute lobar atelectasis refractory to chest physiotherapy)
- Removal of aspirated foreign bodies or other loose material from proximal bronchial tree
- Therapeutic bronchial or whole-lung lavage (e.g., in pulmonary alveolar proteinosis)
- Palliative therapy of malignant tumors causing tracheal or bronchial obstruction
  - Brachytherapy (direct application of radiation therapy)
  - Laser phototherapy (vaporization of tumor tissue)
  - Fulguration using heater probes or bipolar electrodes

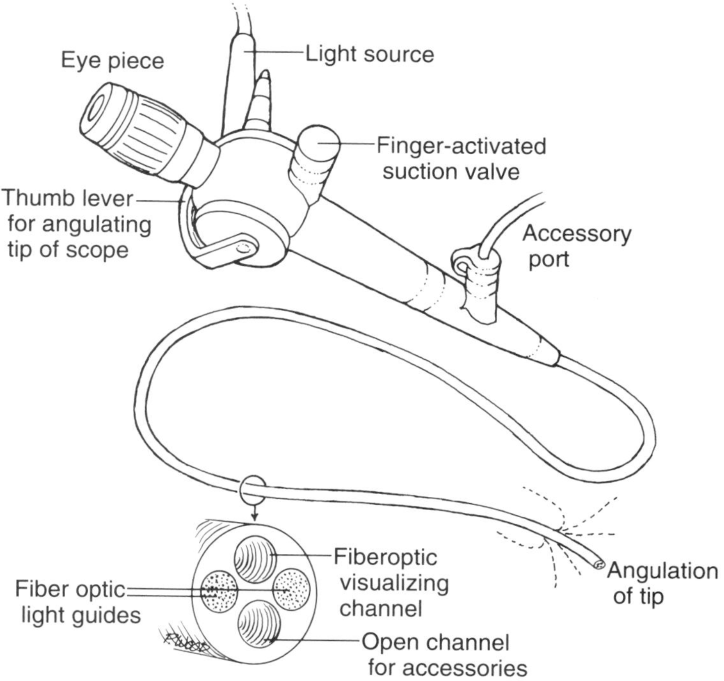

Figure 58-4. Diagram of a fiberoptic bronchoscope, showing essential features. Some models have fewer channels, depending on the diameter and intended application of the bronchoscope.

fitted for therapeutic applications such as electrocautery, endobronchial laser therapy, foreign body removal, and suctioning of thick secretions. In some cases they also have improved optics. However, larger bronchoscopes sacrifice some accessibility to, and maneuverability in, more distal airways, especially in the upper lobes. They are also more difficult to pass through the nose and are more likely to interfere with ventilation when bronchoscopy is performed on intubated patients, especially those with narrow-bore tracheal tubes. Ideally, both large and small bronchoscopes should be available in a given institution.

Preparation for Bronchoscopy

Ideally, patients are kept from eating or drinking for 6 hours prior to bronchoscopy to allow for adequate gastric emptying. The anesthetic procedure entails some gagging and attendant threat of emesis and concomitant aspiration, and an empty stomach hedges against the risk of pulmonary aspiration.

If biopsy is anticipated, a history relevant to bleeding disorders must be obtained prior to bronchoscopy. Patients considered to be at increased risk for bleeding complications should then be evaluated by obtaining an activated partial thromboplastin time (APTT) and a prothrombin time (PT). The appropriate use of hemostatic screening tests for prebronchoscopic evaluation are as follows[25]:

Evidence of liver disease on physical examination

History of malabsorption or malnutrition

Clinical history unavailable prior to procedure

Active bleeding or evidence of abnormal bleeding on physical examination

History of abnormal, excessive, or spontaneous bleeding, including hemoptysis

Recent or current use of therapeutic heparin or warfarin

Suspected or proved thromboembolism

Suspected or proved disseminated intravascular coagulation

There is little correlation between the results of nonselective screening and the occurrence of procedure-related bleeding.[26] Moreover, the most sensitive single test for bleeding disorders is to obtain a thorough history.[27]

The patient should be told what to expect during the bronchoscopy. The anesthetic procedure and side effects of the premedications should be explained. For example, lidocaine "will make your mouth numb and it will feel hard to swallow"; atropine "will make your mouth very dry"; and meperidine, morphine, midazolam, or diazepam "will make you feel drowsy." Outpatients should be told to bring another responsible person to take them home following the procedure because the effects of sedative medications may linger.

Patients should be told that the procedure will make them cough and that coughing is understandable and expected but should be consciously suppressed as much as possible.

Several aspects of preparation for bronchoscopy are summarized as follows:

1. **Scheduling**
   A. Confirm scheduling with person who will perform procedure and other personnel as applicable
   B. Confirm if there is need for fluoroscopy and schedule accordingly
2. **Instruct the patient in bronchoscopy logistics**
   A. Confirm bronchoscopy date, time, and place with the patient
   B. Review prebronchoscopy instructions with the patient
      i. Nothing by mouth after midnight for morning bronchoscopy
      ii. Light breakfast if scheduled for afternoon bronchoscopy
      iii. If patient is taking insulin, ask the physician for changes in dosing for bronchoscopy
      iv. Instruct patient to take other usual medications
      v. If the bronchoscopy is to be done on an outpatient basis, a driver must be available to take the patient home afterward
   C. Instruct the patient to take nothing by mouth for several hours after bronchoscopy to reduce risk of aspiration
3. **Set-up and hook-up monitoring apparatus**
   A. Pulse oximetry
   B. Blood pressure monitoring
   C. Electrocardiographic (ECG) monitor (single lead)
   D. Respiration monitor (visual or palpable)
4. **Bronchscopy cart**
   Confirm that it is completely stocked (see Table 58-4) and draw up commonly used medications and saline
5. **Confirm that patient has signed a consent form**
6. **Start a heparin lock for intravenous sedation if this is to be used**

Site and Equipment

Where the bronchoscopy takes place should be decided after consideration of the individual patient's needs. Outpatient bronchoscopies are performed in a special procedure/endoscopy room in many hospitals and clinics; some facilities have designated bronchoscopy suites. Inpatients may be transported to the procedure room, or bronchoscopy may be performed at the bedside. Staffing, availability of monitoring equipment, and ease of transport of bronchoscopy equipment are factored into the selection of the bronchoscopy site.

For bronchoscopy requiring fluoroscopy, the procedure should be performed on a fluoroscopy table, and in most institutions this is done in the radiology department, to which bronchoscopy supplies are transported via cart. When fluoroscopy is not needed, the patient may sit in a dental-type chair or lie on a cart in the bronchoscopy suite.

Table 58-4. Contents of the Basic Bronchoscopy Cart[a]

For operator and assistant
Masks
Gloves
Gowns
For airway management
Endotracheal tubes
Bronchoscope adapter for endotracheal tube
Yankauer-type suction catheters
Suction pump
Suction tubing
Bite block
Adhesive tape
Water-soluble lubricant
Syringes, needles, and solutions
10- and 20-mL syringes, Luer-Lok
10- and 20-mL syringes, non-Luer-Lok
Needles, sharp tip
Needles, blunt-tip
Saline
Nonbacteriostatic saline
For obtaining specimens
Bronchoscope accessories
Specimen cups
Sputum traps
For handling specimens
Microscope slides
Viral and anaerobic transport media
Carbowax
Formalin
Miscellaneous items
Bronchoscope light source
Denture cups
Emesis basins
Sunglasses, radio
Medicine cups
Cotton 4 × 4s and 2 × 2s
For patient support and monitoring
Pulse oximeter
Oxygen cannulae
ECG leads
Cardiac monitor
For anesthesia and sedation
Jackson forceps
Cotton balls
Heparin locks or caps
Intravenous catheters or "butterflies"
Alcohol wipes
Bandaids
Sterile swabs
Atomizer and accessories
Medications
Epinephrine 1:1000
Heparin lock flush solution
Sedatives (e.g., meperidine [Demerol], codeine, morphine, diazepam [Valium], midazolam [Versed])
Topical anesthetics (e.g., lidocaine [1, 2, & 4%], cocaine [4 or 10%], Cetacaine [solution of benzocaine and tetracaine], lidocaine jelly)
Paperwork
Consent forms
Specimen labels
Laboratory specimen forms
Radiology requisitions
Bronchoscopy charge slips
Physician's order forms

[a] "Crash" cart should be available in addition to listed items.

Regardless of the site, O_2 and resuscitation equipment and supplies (a crash cart) should be readily available. A viewbox should be present for prebronchoscopy review of the patient's radiographs and in case questions arise during the procedure that require referral to these radiographs. Table 58-4 provides a checklist of equipment and supplies included on the typical bronchoscopy cart.

Monitoring the Patient

Pulse oximetry and single-lead ECG monitoring during bronchoscopy have become standard of care (Fig. 58-5). Cardiac dysrrhythmias and O_2 desaturation are common during bronchoscopy,[28] and appropriate monitoring makes early recognition and management of these and other problems possible. Intermittent blood pressure monitoring and visual or palpable respiratory monitoring provide additional safety. Palpable respiratory monitoring is accomplished by placing the fingers of the hand on the lower sternum and the heel of the hand gently on the epigastric area to sense both chest and abdominal respiratory movements.

The bronchoscopist, although ultimately responsible for the safety of the patient, may easily become absorbed in bronchoscopic visualization and operations. The bronchoscopy assistant should assume responsibility for monitoring for untoward effects and discreetly notify the physician as they occur, taking care not to unduly alarm the patient. The bronchoscopy assistant should be familiar with and be able to recognize common cardiac dysrrhythmias.

Venous Access

We find it most efficient to establish venous access via a "heparin lock" prior to bronchoscopy if an intravenous line is not already in place. Administration of sedation and atropine intravenously in the bronchoscopy suite avoids absorption problems that are occasionally encountered with oral or intramuscular administration of medications. It also ensures ready venous access for fluids should the patient become hypotensive during the procedure, permits intravenous treatment of cardiac dysrhythmias when clinically indicated, and allows for rapid administration of naloxone (Narcan) for rapid reversal of narcotics when necessary.

Use of Systemic Drugs

Atropine

Atropine is a cholinergic blocking agent used to deter the outpouring of airway secretions normally encountered with instrumentation of the airway and also to prevent hypotension associated with vagal stimulation. Atropine makes it easier to keep the bronchoscope tip clear of secretions and to preserve visibility of airway anatomy; it also inhibits oral secretions that may otherwise be aspirated owing to the temporarily dysfunctional glottis. Atropine may be given in doses of 0.4 to 1.0 mg IV or IM.

Sedation

Bronchoscopy can be an anxiety-provoking, noxious procedure and is much better tolerated when patients are under sedation. Narcotics and minor tranquilizers are most commonly used for this purpose.[29] Frequently used narcotics are meperidine (Demerol) and morphine; minor tranquilizers most often employed are diazepam (Valium) and midazolam (Versed). These drugs are all capable of causing respiratory depression and should be given with caution; their admin-

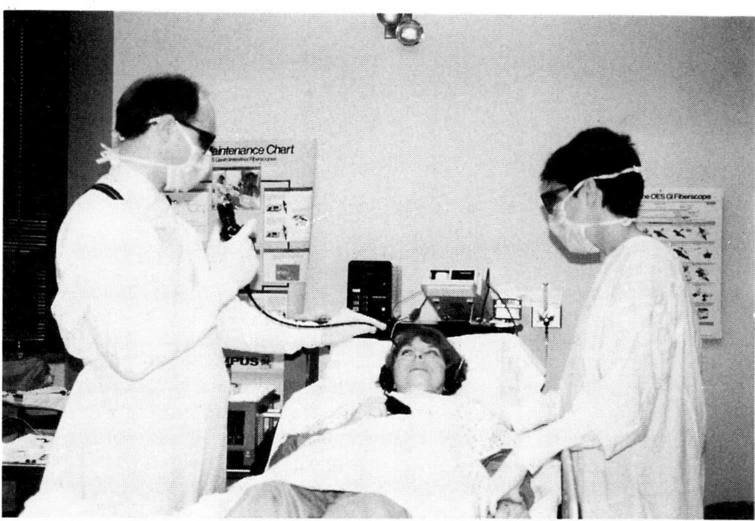

Figure 58-5. Proper bronchoscopy set-up. Note the body secretion precautions (masks, gloves, gowns, and glasses). Sunglasses and radio or tape headphones may be used as an adjunct to sedative medication. The oximetry and ECG monitors are easily visible to both the bronchoscopy technician and the physician.

istration should be followed by respiratory monitoring. Narcotics have the advantage of rapid reversibility by administration of naloxone (0.4 to 0.8 mg), as well as a marked depressant effect on the cough reflex. The minor tranquilizers have the advantage of a retrograde amnestic effect so that patients seldom recall the unpleasant details of the procedure.

With venous access, sedation may be titrated rapidly by giving periodic doses of narcotics and/or minor tranquilizers. The sedative effect of these drugs occurs within minutes of intravenous administration. Among the narcotics, meperidine is commonly given in 25-mg increments and morphine in 2 to 5 mg increments. Of the available benzodiazepines, diazepam is usually given in increments of 2 to 5 mg. Midazolam is more rapid in onset and shorter in duration of action; it is administered in 0.5 to 2 mg increments. Midazolam may be preferable to other agents for outpatient procedures when extended patient monitoring is not practical.

Airway Anesthesia

In patients without airway intubation, adequate anesthesia of the upper respiratory tract is essential. The powerful gag reflex, mediated by the nerves innervating the mucosa of this area, must be suppressed if the patient is to tolerate bronchoscopy. In addition, if use of the nasal route is contemplated, this area requires anesthesia to reduce the considerable local discomfort caused by passage of the bronchoscope.

The complex innervation of the upper airway is illustrated in Figure 58-6. With such an extensive and diverse nerve

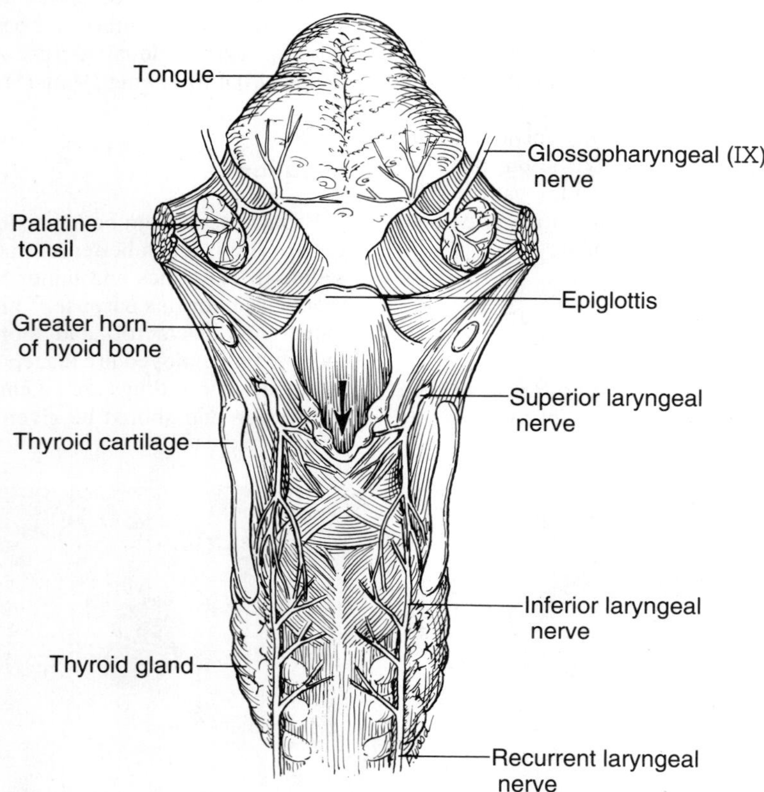

Figure 58-6. Schematic representation of the region of the oropharyngeal airway as seen from behind, showing the innervation of the upper airway. The lingual nerve supplies the anterior two-thirds of the tongue with general sensation. The glossopharyngeal nerve (cranial nerve IX) enters the root or pharyngeal part of the tongue and supplies this area with general sensation. The internal branch of the superior laryngeal nerve supplies sensation to the laryngeal mucosa as far down as the vocal folds. The recurrent laryngeal nerve is the principal motor nerve of the larynx and supplies all the laryngeal muscles except the cricothyroid muscle (which is supplied by the external branch of the superior laryngeal nerve). The recurrent laryngeal nerve also supplies innervation to the mucous membrane below the level of the vocal folds. The nasal mucosa (not shown) is supplied with sensory fibers from the nasal nerves, which then join the maxillary branch of the trigeminal nerve (cranial nerve V) as well as the olfactory nerve (cranial nerve I).

supply to the mucosa of the larynx and below, it follows that anesthesia here cannot be readily accomplished with regional nerve blocks. Rather, an attempt is made to anesthetize the entire mucosal surface of the larynx by topical application of lidocaine or similar anesthetic substances.[30] Considerable regional and personal variation exists in customary methods for anesthesia of the nasal and oral mucosa. Methods are based on prior training and personal experience.

Nasal Anesthesia

If the transnasal bronchoscopy route is to be attempted, the "best-flow" nostril should first be identified. This is a subjective assessment of best airflow through a nostril when the contralateral nostril is occluded. The chosen best-flow nostril is numbed by occluding the contralateral side with cotton and asking the patient to sniff while instilling atomized 4 percent lidocaine into the nostril. A pump-type atomizer may be used to transform the lidocaine into a fine mist. The atomizer may also be connected to an air or O_2 source with an in-line finger suction valve from suction tubing. The finger suction valve is intermittently occluded when atomization is desired. Nasal anesthesia by sniffing atomized lidocaine is continued until the patient consistently notes the transit of the lidocaine to the back of the throat. Alternatively, 10 mL of viscous lidocaine or lidocaine jelly can be injected via a syringe. The nostril is then stoppered with cotton to prevent prenasal backflow while attention is given to oral and laryngeal anesthesia.

Topical cocaine may also be used here for its additional vasoconstrictive effects, which shrink the mucosa, widening the nasal passage and reducing the likelihood of epistaxis. Occasionally, the best-flow nostril may not permit passage of the bronchoscope. In this case passage through the other nostril may be attempted after additional local anesthesia. If this fails as well, a bite block should be slipped over the bronchoscope and the latter passed into the trachea via the mouth. The bite block is then slipped into place to protect the bronchoscope from bite injury.

Oral and Laryngeal Anesthesia

Following nasal anesthesia the patient should gargle with 5 mL of 4 percent lidocaine and then spit it into an emesis basin. The patient should then extrude the tongue, whereupon it is grasped with a cotton 4×4. As the patient takes small panting breaths through the mouth, the posterior pharyngeal mucosa is sprayed with atomized lidocaine. The patient is intermittently allowed to spit into an emesis basin. This sequence is repeated until gagging subsides. The atomizer tip is then directed downwards and placed far back in the throat. Lidocaine is sprayed down toward the vocal chords while the patient pants. Coughing suggests the passage of lidocaine past the vocal cords and may indicate the approach of optimal anesthesia. Alternatively, or prior to use of the atomizer, lidocaine may be administered by updraft or ultrasonic nebulizer.[31] Cotton balls may be wrapped around the tip of a Jackson forceps, soaked in lidocaine, and positioned in the pyriform recesses of either lateral pharyngeal wall for additional anesthesia. These are left in place for about 2 minutes on each side with gentle lateral pressure.

Lidocaine jelly or water-soluble lubricant is used on the distal end of the bronchoscope (but not the tip) to lubricate its passage through the nose or mouth. When the bronchoscope has been passed to just above the vocal cords, it is common to inject about 5 mL of 1 or 2 percent lidocaine onto the cords and beyond to bolster the local anesthesia in this sensitive area.

Transnasal versus Transoral Bronchoscopy

Transnasal bronchoscopy involves more initial discomfort but probably results in less gagging sensation than the transoral approach, possibly because it avoids draping the instrument over the tongue and epiglottis. The nasal passage also more firmly holds the barrel of the bronchoscope and stabilizes it so that the tip is less easily dislodged by movements. However, the route selected remains largely a matter of operator preference.[32,33]

Bronchoscopy during Mechanical Ventilation

Bronchoscopy on intubated patients who are receiving mechanical ventilation poses unique logistic problems for the bronchoscopy team. Such patients may have oxygenation problems and require high levels of supplemental O_2 to achieve adequate blood oxygenation.[34] Because bronchoscopy is associated with desaturation, the inspired O_2 fraction ($F_{I}O_2$) should be set on 1.0 for the duration of the procedure, and oximetry monitoring is especially critical.

Patients receiving positive end-expiratory pressure (PEEP) therapy should be maintained at their current level throughout the procedure to avoid inadvertent discontinuation of PEEP and resultant hypoxemia. The PEEP level should be monitored closely during the entire procedure. Auto-PEEP may arise during the bronchoscopy owing to an increase in the expiratory time from partial obstruction of the airway by the bronchoscope. A special bronchoscopy adapter on the end of the tracheal tube (Fig. 58-7) allows passage of the bronchoscope without loss of airway pressure.

Successful bronchoscopy hinges on fluent passage of the bronchoscope through the endotracheal tube while allowing adequate ventilation. The ideal setting is the use of a large endotracheal tube with a small bronchoscope. The smallest bronchoscope available should be obtained for these cases. If the endotracheal tube is 7.5 mm or less in diameter, consideration should be given to changing the endotracheal tube prior to the procedure or preparing for this contingency if unable to pass the bronchoscope and/or maintain ventilation. An 8.5-mm endotracheal tube is ideal for this situation.

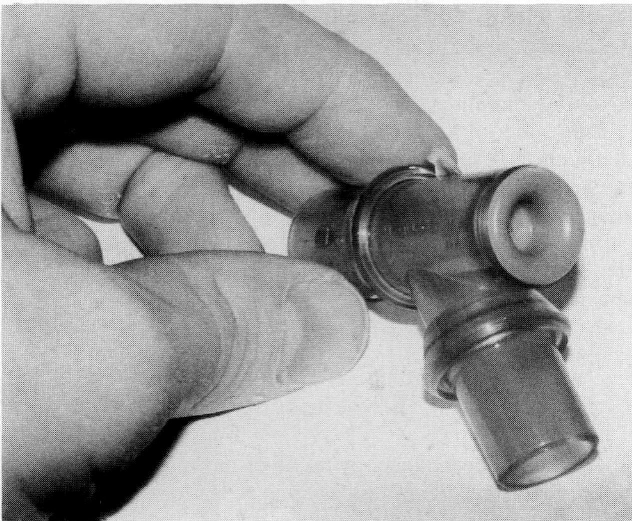

Figure 58-7. Endotracheal tube adapter for bronchoscopy during mechanical ventilation. The diaphragm through which the bronchoscope passes prevents loss of PEEP during the procedure.

The peak pressure alarms on the ventilator should be offset to a higher range because the peak pressure will consistently rise, reflecting the increased resistance to inspiratory airflow with the bronchoscope in place. Such an increase in peak inspiratory pressure does not in itself signify an increased risk of air trapping and barotrauma. However, exhaled tidal volumes should be monitored closely because the expiratory airflow obstruction created by the bronchoscope will increase the tendency for air trapping as the time constant for expiratory airflow increases.

Bronchoscopic Biopsies

Despite the small diameter of the flexible fiberoptic bronchoscope, a variety of biopsy and aspiration procedures can be performed through the instrument by using specialized appliances developed for this purpose (Fig. 58-8). These include both plastic and stainless steel needles, brushes for both cytology specimens and bacterial cultures, several types of forceps, and snares for capturing aspirated teeth and other foreign objects in the airways. A detailed and well illustrated review of these methods is available elsewhere[35] and is not repeated in this overview.

The bronchoscopy assistant has a vital role in biopsy procedures. Usually, the bronchoscopist will pass the forceps, position it, and ask the assistant to work the jaws by depressing and withdrawing the plunger. Following biopsy, the assistant generally clears the forceps of the tissue, places the tissue in the appropriate specimen container, and hands the forceps back to the bronchoscopist if so desired. Following biopsy the bronchoscopist may request a saline wash (injection of 5 to 10 mL) or instillation of topical epinephrine to stop bleeding. A dilute solution of epinephrine (1:1000, 1 mL in 10 mL saline, mixed in a 10-mL syringe) may be mixed for this purpose when biopsies are anticipated.

When we perform transbronchial biopsies we ask the assistant to classify the specimens as ''floaters'' or ''sinkers'' on the basis of their buoyancy. Floaters float for 15 seconds or more, whereas ''sinkers'' float for less than 15 seconds or sink directly to the bottom; as a rule the floaters consist predominantly of alveolar tissue whereas the sinkers consist predominantly of bronchial tissue. As such, the buoyancy of the biopsy material may be used as a rough index of its adequacy or alveolar tissue content. A transbronchial biopsy is a blind sampling of parenchymal tissue; fluoroscopy during this procedure gives an indication of the proximity of the biopsy forceps to the pleura, where pneumothorax is more likely. However, transbronchial biopsies can be done with-

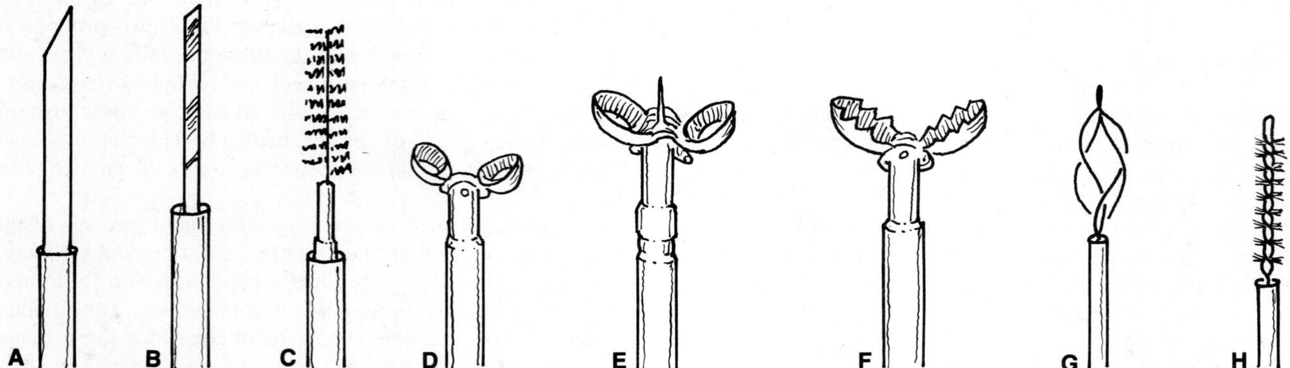

Figure 58-8. Examples of aspiration and biopsy appliances available for passage through the fiberoptic bronchoscope and into the lower respiratory tract. **(A)** plastic needle, **(B)** stainless steel needle, **(C)** brush, **(D)** fenestrated forceps, **(E)** fenestrated forceps with needle, **(F)** piranha forceps, **(G)** basket, **(H)** microbiology brush.

out the use of fluoroscopy in diffuse lung disease, and this has been shown to be as safe as fluoroscopic methods.[36]

If biopsy of a peripheral lung mass is to be attempted, fluoroscopy is requested to ensure that the bronchoscope is within the area where biopsy is desired when the specimen is taken. This is difficult to assess without fluoroscopy because endobronchial anatomy may be remarkably well preserved despite the presence of extremely large masses.

Stiff-needle transbronchial biopsies are performed to stage carcinoma or to diagnose masses that abut and indent the proximal airways but are not exophytic.[37] Soft-needle biopsies are performed in distal airways for masses without exophytic endobronchial manifestations. The soft plastic needle, unlike the stiff steel needle, can be passed through the angulated bronchoscope. Aspiration biopsy is similar with both needles. The bronchoscopist advances the needle's outer sheath until it is visualized at the bronchoscope tip; the assistant then advances the needle out of the catheter and the bronchoscopist stabs the needle into the biopsy site. The assistant then places traction on the plunger of the syringe attached to the distal needle hub. If resistance is met, needle entry into the putative tumor or lymph node is assumed, and the bronchoscopist makes multiple, rapid, short-amplitude, in-out movements with the needle while traction is maintained. Traction is then released, the needle is withdrawn, and the catheter assembly is withdrawn from the bronchoscope. This material is injected into Saccamano fixative and centrifuged into a pellet, and a smear is then made on a microscope slide for fixation and staining.

Bronchoalveolar Lavage

Bronchoalveolar lavage (BAL) is a modified bronchial wash, which entails occlusion of a distal airway with the bronchoscope tip ("wedging") and multiple sequential instillations and aspirations of saline.[38] The purpose is to sample the cytology of the alveolar surface for diagnostic purposes and occasionally to remove pathologic fluids, as in pulmonary alveolar proteinosis.[39,40]

A variety of techniques may be used for BAL.[41] One commonly employed approach is to instill five 20-mL aliquots and pool the aspirated material. Aliquots are rapidly injected with a 20-mL syringe into the working channel of the bronchoscope with use of either a non-Luer-Lok syringe or a Luer-Lok syringe with a blunt-tip needle. The fluid is aspirated immediately after instillation by gentle suction. A large (50-mL) sputum trap is attached to the suction nipple, which is then connected to suction. Fluid is then aspirated by working the finger suction valve after each instillation of saline. A 50 to 70 percent return, or 50 to 70 mL of fluid, is generally recovered. The sputum trap may need to be changed after several instillations if the recovery is good. Adequacy of alveolar sampling is indicated by the turbidity and foaminess of the recovered fluid. In general, the best method is that recommended by the individual laboratory processing the specimens, as these methods are likely to be the basis for their normative reference data.[42]

During lavage patients may experience a cool sensation in the chest with each instillation of liquid. They also may experience transient sensations of asphyxia and undergo O_2 desaturation. When cellular analysis of the lavage fluid is required, the sample is placed immediately on ice to retard cell lysis during transport.

A textbook dealing solely with the rationale, indications, and methodology of BAL was published in 1988 and may be consulted for more detailed discussion of these topics.[43]

Complications of Fiberoptic Bronchoscopy

In experienced hands, fiberoptic bronchoscopy is generally a safe and well tolerated procedure. When reasonable precautions are taken and careful monitoring is practiced, there are very few complications causing substantial morbidity. Table 58-5 lists these complications and estimates of their incidence.[44]

Rigid Bronchoscopy

The rigid bronchoscope has a light source on the distal end and an extremely large working channel as compared with the fiberoptic bronchoscopes.[45] The large working channel permits good visualization of the proximal airways, passage of large instruments, and ventilation if required. Laser airway procedures are commonly carried out by using a flexible bronchoscope through the lumen of a rigid bronchoscope. The large working channel is advantageous for removal of foreign bodies as well. Disadvantages include the necessity for general anesthesia and the inability to access the distal bronchial tree and upper airway. Access to both flexible and rigid bronchoscopy provides a complete armamentarium of investigational and therapeutic capability for disorders of the airways.

Table 58-5. Complications of Fiberoptic Bronchoscopy

Complication	Incidence (%)
Pneumonia	0.6
Pneumothorax	0.4
Airway obstruction	0.4
Respiratory arrest	0.2
Death	0.1
Vasovagal reaction	2.4
Fever	1.2
Cardiac dysrhythmia	0.9
Bleeding	0.7
Nausea and vomiting	0.2
ECG abnormality	0.2
Psychotic reaction	0.1
Aphonia	0.1

PERCUTANEOUS LUNG ASPIRATION AND BIOPSY

Fine-Needle Aspiration

In fine-needle aspiration a long narrow-bore needle is used to puncture and aspirate diagnostic material from chest masses.[46] It is usually employed with masses that are bronchoscopically inaccessible (e.g., extremely peripheral or in the mediastinum) or that have been subjected to bronchoscopy without a diagnosis. This procedure is performed under fluoroscopic or ultrasound guidance.[47] Common complications include hemoptysis and pneumothorax, although these are usually readily managed without serious morbidity.

Cutting Needle Biopsy

A cutting needle is used for retrieval of a large fragment of tissue as opposed to the cellular aspirate obtained in fine-needle biopsy. This technique is more likely to cause hemorrhage and pneumothorax than fine-needle aspiration and therefore is generally reserved for biopsy of chest masses that directly abut the chest wall.[48]

DIAGNOSTIC PROCEDURES INVOLVING THE PLEURA

Thoracentesis

Thoracentesis is the aspiration of fluid from the pleural space, usually after radiologic detection. As discussed in Chapter 92, examination of this fluid is necessary in most clinical situations in which its presence is discovered. Although it is usually performed for diagnostic reasons, thoracentesis is also used as a therapeutic procedure in conditions such as metastatic breast cancer, in which the presence of a large effusion causes severe symptoms. In the latter instance a large volume of pleural fluid (1 to 2 L or more) is removed, whereas diagnostic thoracentesis usually removes less than 100 mL of pleural fluid.

After the operator selects the area for needle entry, this area is cleaned and local anesthesia is administered first intradermally and then subcutaneously with lidocaine. A thoracentesis needle (usually 2 in. or longer) is attached to a syringe and introduced just over the inferior rib and into the pleural space. It is important to insert the needle just above rather than just below the rib in order to avoid lacerating the blood vessels and nerves that run along the inferior margins of the ribs. Penetration into the pleural space is heralded by the appearance of fluid in the syringe as steady suction is applied by withdrawing the plunger.[49]

Complications are unusual with thoracentesis, especially when performed by experienced personnel.[50,51] Pneumothorax and pleural hemorrhage, however, are occasionally encountered, and thus post-thoracentesis chest x-rays and monitoring are standard. Rarely, the liver or spleen may be inadvertently penetrated owing to judgment error in selection of sampling site.

Needle Biopsy of the Pleura

Closed-needle biopsy of the parietal pleura is commonly performed in cases of unexplained inflammatory (exudative) pleural effusions, most often to rule out (or in) malignancy

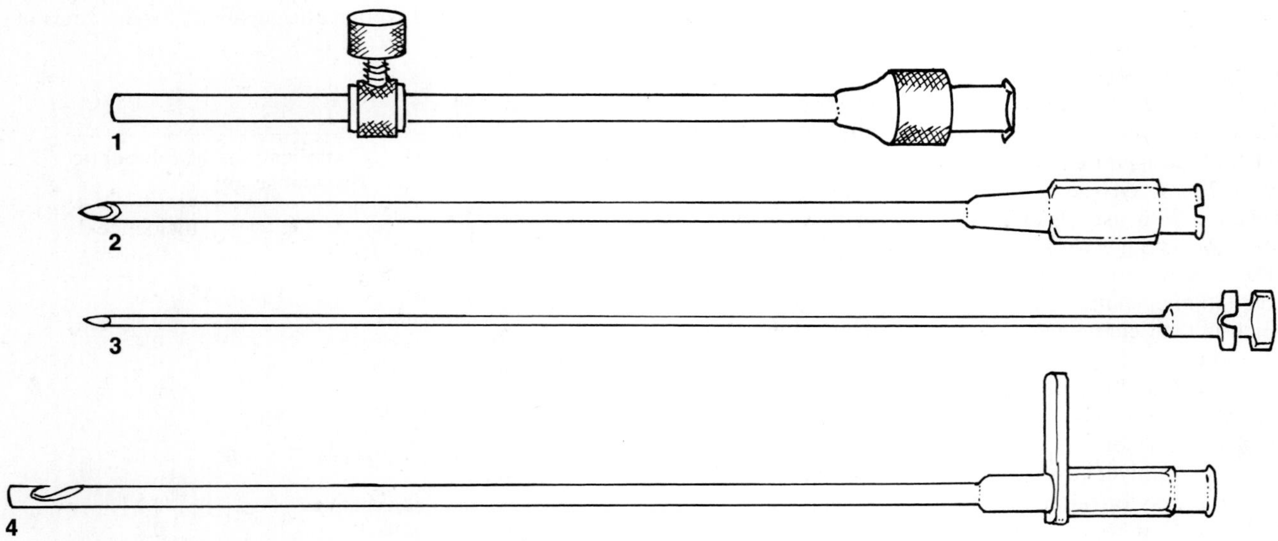

Figure 58-9. Components of the Cope pleural biopsy needle: 1, sheath with depth indicator set at 1 in.; 2, hollow needle (inserts into sheath); 3, obturator (inserts into needle or hook); 4, hook (inserts into sheath).

or tuberculosis.[50] Two types of biopsy needle, Cope and Abrams, are commonly used, as illustrated in Figures 58-9 through 58-12. These two needles are similar in efficacy and ease of operation, and selection is based largely on the prior training, experience, and personal preference of the operator. The Abrams needle may yield slightly more pleural tissue per pass, but this advantage may be offset by its higher price and the necessity to completely withdraw the needle following each biopsy pass.[52] The Cope needle is equipped with an introducer sheath, which may be left in place between biopsy passes.

Anesthetic technique and needle placement are the same

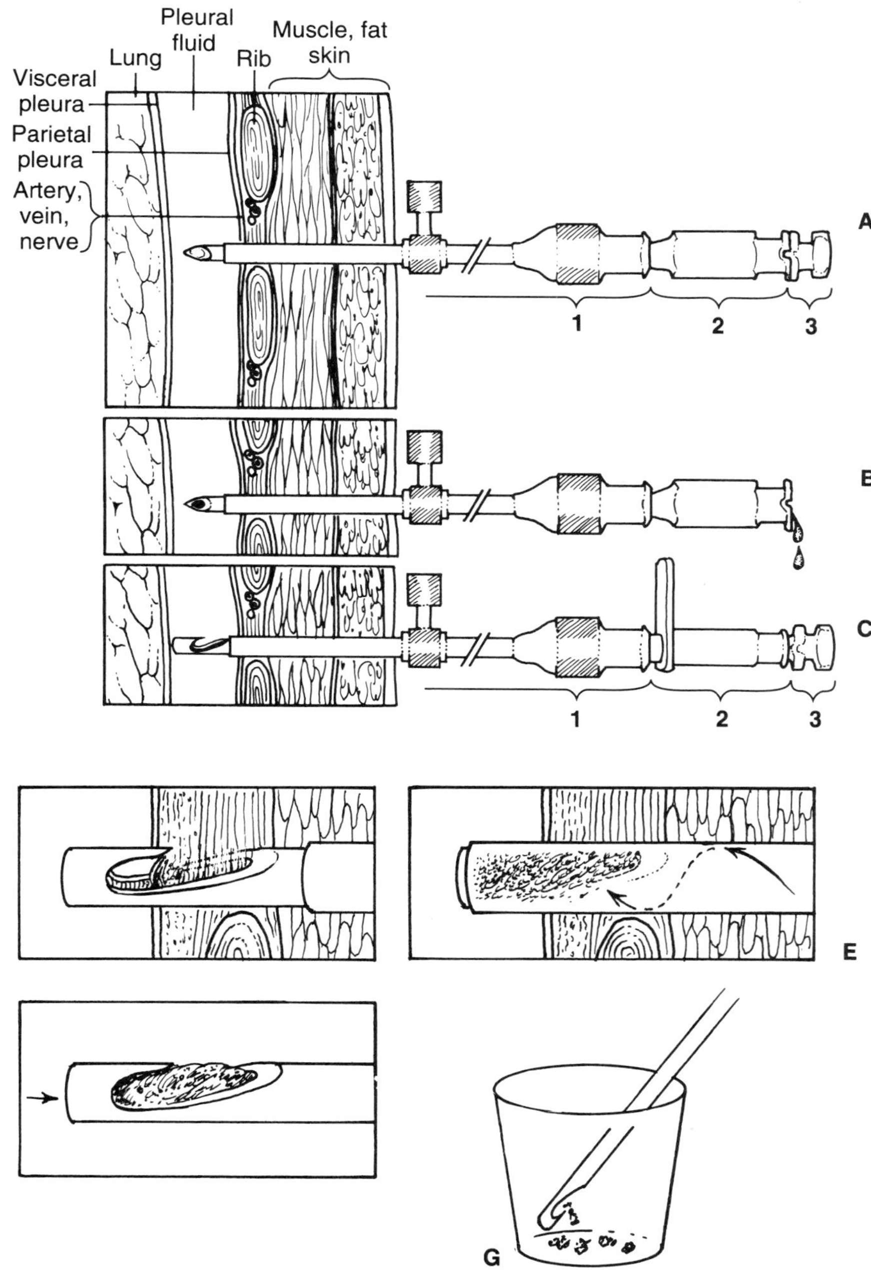

Figure 58-10. Technique of closed biopsy of the parietal pleura using the Cope needle. (**A**) Insertion over rib into pleural space. (**B**) Obturator removed; fluid runs out confirming placement of needle tip. (**C**) Hook with obturator inserted into sheath, replacing hollow needle. (**D**) Hook grasps fragment of pleura. (**E**) Hook held steady; sheath (outer cutting cannula) advanced to secure sample. (**F**) Hook with biopsy sample withdrawn. (**G**) Several samples taken.

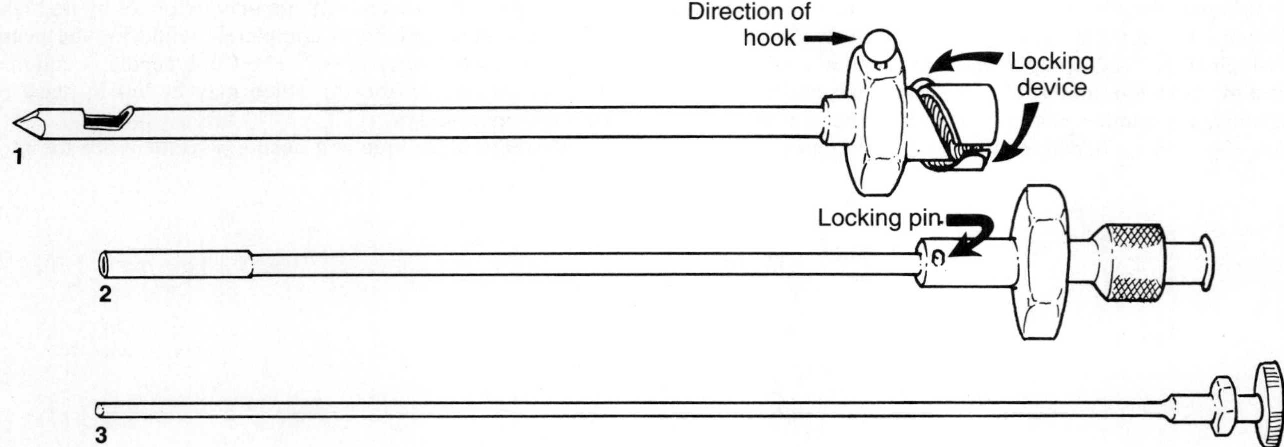

Figure 58-11. The Abrams pleural biopsy needle: 1, sheath-hook (biopsy trochar); 2, hollow needle; 3, obturator.

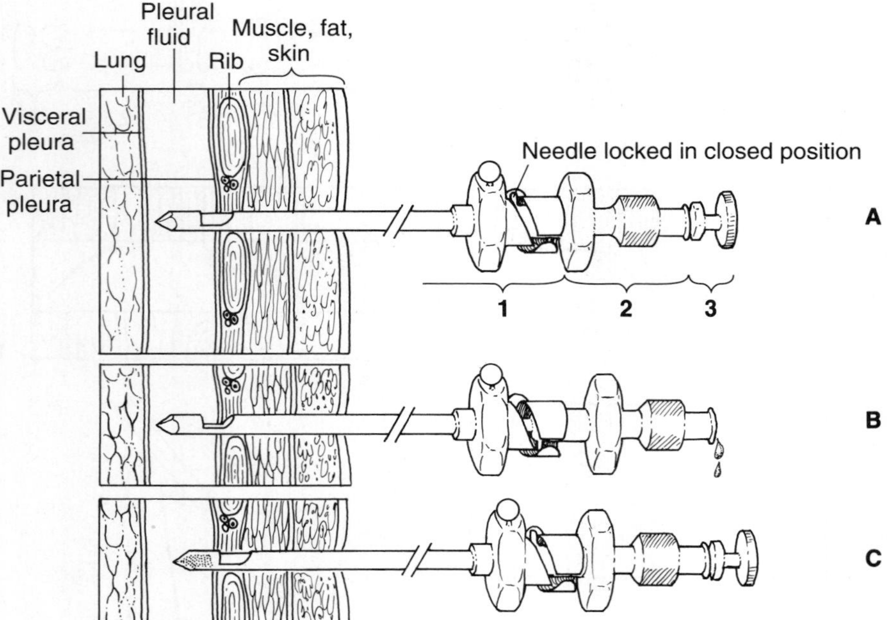

Figure 58-12. Technique of pleural biopsy using the Abrams needle. (**A**) Sheath, hollow needle, and obturator inserted over rib into pleural fluid space. (**B**) Obturator removed; hollow needle turned to open position; fluid runs out, confirming placement of needle tip. (**C**) Obturator reinserted; hook retracted with lateral pressure to trap specimen inside tip of hook; hook placed in closed/locked position. (**D**) Entire assembly with specimen withdrawn; procedure repeated to take several specimens (not shown).

as for thoracentesis, except that because of larger needle bore, a nick is made in the skin with a #11 scalpel blade following local infiltration of lidocaine. Biopsy technique with both needles requires the operator to press the needle's side aperture against the parietal pleural surface to ensnare a small portion of tissue. The pleural fragment is then pinched off by the action of one needle shaft advanced across the distal tissue-containing side aperture of the other needle shaft.

Pleuroscopy

Pleuroscopy (thoracoscopy) allows direct visualization of both visceral and parietal pleurae without having to perform a thoracotomy.[53] The pleuroscope is inserted through an intercostal incision. Pleural biopsy can be performed under direct visualization, which allows directed sampling of any abnormal-appearing tissue. This procedure may be chosen to investigate exudative pleural effusions when multiple needle biopsies of the pleura have failed to yield a diagnosis and is especially helpful when malignant mesothelioma or other malignancy is suspected.

References

1. Murray JF, Nadel JA (eds): Textbook of Respiratory Medicine. Section G: Diagnostic Evaluation. WB Saunders, Philadelphia, 1988, pp. 431–733
2. Chodosh S: Sputum examination. pp. 411–426. In Fishman AP (ed): Pulmonary Diseases and Disorders. 2nd Ed. McGraw-Hill, New York, 1988
3. Harvey JC, Cantrell JC, Fisher AM: Actinomycosis: Its recognition and treatment. Ann Intern Med 1957;46:868–885
4. Bartlett JG, Brewer NS, Ryan KJ: Laboratory diagnosis of lower respiratory tract infections. pp. 1–15. In Washington JA, II (ed): Cumitech 7. American Society for Microbiology, Washington, DC, 1978
5. Erozan YS: Cytopathologic diagnosis of pulmonary neoplasms in sputum and bronchoscopic specimens. Semin Diagn Pathol 1986;3:188–195
6. Rosenthal DL: Cytopathology of Pulmonary Diseases. Karger, Basel, 1988
7. Risse EKJ, van't Hoff MA, Lavrini RN, Vooijs PG: Relationship between patient characteristics and sputum cytologic diagnosis of lung cancer. Acta Cytol 1987;31:159–165
8. Barret-Conner E: The nonvalue of sputum culture in the diagnosis of pneumococcal pneumonia. Am Rev Respir Dis 1974;103:843–848
9. Wimberly N, Willey S, Sullivan N, Bartlett JG: Antibacterial properties of lidocaine. Chest 1979;76:37–40
10. Chodosh S: Examination of sputum cells. N Engl J Med 1970;282:854–857
11. Geckler DW, Gremillion DH, McAllister CK, Ellenbogen C: Microscopic and bacteriologic comparison of paired sputa and transtrancheal aspirates. J Clin Microbiol 1977;6:396–399
12. Courcol RJ, Ramon P, Voisin C, Martin GR: Presence of alveolar macrophages as a criterion for determining the suitability of sputum specimens for bacterial culture. Eur J Clin Microbiol Infect Dis 1984;3:122–125
13. Luce JM: Sputum induction in the acquired immunodeficiency syndrome, editorial. Ann Intern Med 1986;133:515–518
14. Larson RP, Ingalls-Severn KJ, Wright JR et al: Diagnosis of *Pneumocystis carinii* pneumonia by respiratory care practitioners: Advantages of a nasotracheal suctioning method over sputum induction. Respir Care 1989;34:249–253
15. Hahn HH, Beaty HN: Transtracheal aspiration in the evaluation of patients with pneumonia. Ann Intern Med 1970;72:183–187
16. Bartlett JG: The technique of transtracheal aspiration. J Crit Illness 1986;1:43–49
17. Panacek EA, Albertson TE, Rutheford WF, Fisher CJ: Selective left endobronchial suctioning in the intubated patient, abstracted. Chest, suppl. 1988;92:106S
18. Higuchi JH, Coalson JJ, Johanson WG: Bacteriologic diagnosis of nosocomial pneumonia in primates. Am Rev Respir Dis 1982;125:53–57
19. Chastre J, Viau F, Brun P et al: Prospective evaluation of the protected specimen brush for the diagnosis of pulmonary infections in ventilated patients. Am Rev Respir Dis 1984;130:924–929
20. Kubica GP, Gross WM, Hawkins JE et al: Laboratory services for mycobacterial diseases. Am Rev Respir Dis 1975;112:773–787
21. American Thoracic Society, medical branch of the American Lung Association, and Centers for Disease Control: Diagnostic standards and classification of tuberculosis and other mycobacterial diseases. Am Rev Respir Dis 1981;123:343–358
22. Jefferson H, Dalton HP, Escobar MR, Allison MJ: Transportation delay and the microbiological quality of clinical specimens. Am J Clin Pathol 1975;64:689–693
23. Du Bois RM, Clarke SW: Fiberoptic Bronchoscopy in Diagnosis and Management. Grune & Stratton, Orlando, 1987
24. American Thoracic Society, medical section of the American Lung Association: Guidelines for fiberoptic bronchoscopy in adults. Am Rev Respir Dis 1987;136:1066
25. Erban SB, Kinman JL, Schwartz JS: Routine use of the prothrombin and partial thromboplastin times. JAMA 1989;262:2428–2432
26. Suchman AL, Mushlin AI: How well does the activated partial thromboplastin time predict postoperative hemorrhage? JAMA 1986;256:750–753
27. Williams WJ: Clinical manifestations of disorders of hemostasis. pp. 69–72. In Williams WJ, Bentler E, Ebler AJ, Lichtman MA (eds): Hematology. McGraw-Hill, New York, 1986
28. Suratt PM, Smiddy JF, Bruber B: Deaths and complications associated with fiberoptic bronchoscopy. Chest 1976;69:747–751
29. Shelley MP, Wilson P, Normal J: Sedation for fiberoptic bronchoscopy. Thorax 1989;44:769–775
30. Kirkpatrick MB: Lidocaine topical anesthesia for flexible bronchoscopy, editorial. Chest 1989;96:965–967
31. Gove RI, Wiggins J, Stableforth DE: A study of the use of ultrasonically nebulised lignocaine for local anesthesia during fibreoptic bronchoscopy. Br J Dis Chest 1985;79:49–59
32. Harrell JH: Transnasal approach for fiberoptic bronchoscopy. Chest, suppl. 1978;73:704–706
33. Sanderson DR, McDougal JC: Transoral bronchofiberscopy. Chest, suppl. 1978;73:701–703
34. Olopode CO, Prakash UBS: Bronchoscopy in the critical care unit. Mayo Clin Proc 1989;64:1255–1263
35. Kitamura S: Clinical Applications of Fiberoptic Bronchoscopy. Mosby–Year Book, St. Louis, 1990, pp. 110–121
36. Anders GT, Johnson JE, Bush BA, Matthews JI: Transbronchial bronchoscopy without fluoroscopy. Chest 1988;94:557–564
37. Gay PC, Brutinel WM: Transbronchial needle aspiration in the practice of bronchoscopy. Mayo Clin Proc 1989;64:158–162
38. Reynolds HY: Bronchoalveolar lavage. Am Rev Respir Dis 1987;135:250–263
39. Claypool WD, Rogers RM: Update on the clinical diagnosis, management, and pathogenesis of pulmonary alveolar proteinosis (phospholipidosis). Chest 1984;85:550–558
40. American Thoracic Society, medical section of the American Lung Association: Clinical role of bronchoalveolar lavage in

adults with pulmonary disease. Am Rev Respir Dis 1990; 142:481–486
41. Crystal RG, Reynolds HY, Kalica AR: Bronchoalveolar lavage: The report of an international conference. Chest 1986;90:122–131
42. The BAL Cooperative Group Steering Committee: Bronchoalveolar lavage constituents in healthy individuals, idiopathic pulmonary fibrosis, and selected comparison groups. Am Rev Respir Dis 1990;141:S169–S202
43. Linder J, Rennard SI: Bronchoalveolar Lavage. ASCP Press, Chicago, 1988
44. Pereira V, Kovnat DM, Snider GL: A prospective cooperative study of complications following fiberoptic bronchoscopy. Chest 1978;73:813–816
45. Stradling P: Diagnostic Bronchoscopy. Churchill Livingstone, Edinburgh, 1976
46. American Thoracic Society, medical section of the American Lung Association: Guidelines for percutaneous transthoracic needle biopsy. Am Rev Respir Dis 1989;140:255–256
47. Conces DJ, Schwenk R Jr, Doering PR, Glant MD: Thoracic needle biopsy: Improved results using a team approach. Chest 1987;91:813–816
48. Pang JA, Tsang V, Hom BL, Metreweli C: Ultrasound-guided tissue-core biopsy of thoracic lesions with Trucut and Surecut needles. Chest 1987;91:823–828
49. Bone RC: The technique of diagnostic and therapeutic thoracentesis. J Crit Illness 1990;5:371–379
50. American Thoracic Society, medical section of the American Lung Association: Guidelines for thoracentesis and needle biopsy of the pleura. Am Rev Respir Dis 1989;140:257–258
51. Godwin JE, Sahn SA: Thoracentesis: A safe procedure in mechanically ventilated patients. Ann Intern Med 1990;113:800–802
52. Morrone N, Algranti E, Barreto E: Pleural biopsy with Cope and Abrams needles. Chest 1987;92:1050–1057
53. Oldenburg RA Jr, Newhouse MT: Thoracoscopy: A safe, accurate diagnostic procedure using the rigid thoracoscope and local anesthesia. Chest 1979;70:45–50
54. Chodosh S: Sputum evaluation—why, when, how and by whom. pp. 129–131. In Brody JS, Snider GL (eds): Current Topics in the Management of Respiratory Diseases. Vol. 2. Churchill Livingstone, New York, 1985

Chapter 59

Assessment of Respiratory Function in Infants and Children

Robert L. Chatburn
Juliann M. DiFiore

CHAPTER OUTLINE

The measurement of pulmonary function in infants and children can provide important information for both clinical and research purposes. Alterations in forced expiratory volume in 1 second (FEV_1), flow-volume curves, resistance, and compliance can show the effect and duration of the patient's response to different therapies, such as the administration of bronchodilators. Measurement of tidal volume (V_T) and airway pressure can be useful for optimal management of mechanical ventilation. Such measurements can, for example, help to prevent overdistension of the lung and increased risk of pulmonary barotrauma.

Pulmonary function measurements are probably underutilized at this time owing to the difficulty in obtaining accurate results. Most traditional pulmonary function evaluations require some type of patient cooperation, which makes measurement very difficult in very young patients. For example, adult values for vital capacity (VC) can be measured by having the patient inspire and expire with a maximal effort. An infant could hardly cooperate with such a maneuver. Therefore, methods such as the crying vital capacity (CVC) and chest squeezing techniques have been developed to estimate this parameter. Even if measurements can be made, there is a paucity of data for defining "normal" or expected parameter values in infants. Given the different techniques used, it is difficult to standardize these data.

This chapter presents a brief overview of the study of pulmonary function in general. The available techniques presently being used for infant pulmonary function testing are described, along with a few of the advantages and disadvantages of each.

MODELS OF PULMONARY PHYSIOLOGY

The study of respiratory system function can be divided into two main activities, research and clinical application.

Research primarily involves gathering of information in order to describe how the respiratory system works both normally and abnormally. In particular, research involves the use of inductive reasoning (i.e., reasoning from specific observations to general concepts) in an attempt to develop *models* of respiratory function. These models serve to organize data and present compact statements of information. They are used to clarify understanding and to help predict the behavior of the respiratory system.

Physiology Models

There are two sets of models that are of particular interest in pulmonary research, *physiology models* and *pathology models*.[1] Physiology models are the products of basic research. They relate measurable variables, such as volume, pressure, flow, temperature, and chemical concentration, and their purpose is to describe the underlying physical and physiologic processes in the respiratory system. They are often graphical or verbal in nature but are most useful when expressed in mathematical form as algebraic equations. Examples include oxyhemoglobin dissociation curves and nomograms; gas exchange models incorporating the concepts of alveolar ventilation, anatomic dead space, and diffusing capacity; and kinetic models that give rise to parameters such as total lung capacity (TLC), residual volume (RV), and functional residual capacity (FRC).

One of the most useful models in pulmonary mechanics is that of a single flow conducting tube (representing the airways) connected to a single elastic compartment (representing the lungs and chest wall), as shown in Figure 59-1A. The model can be expanded by adding another elastic component to represent the chest wall (Fig. 59-1B). Graphical models such as those in Figure 59-1 can be used as the basis of mathematical models simply by specifying the location of measurable variables and then defining the relations among them. For example, we can measure pressure at the airway opening, on the body surface, in the pleural space, and—with a little ingenuity—in the alveolar region. If we can relate these pressure changes to changes in volume and flow (using an algebraic equation), we can then estimate resistance and compliance. A common mathematical model relating pressure, volume, and flow (sometimes referred to as the *equation of motion of the respiratory system*) has the form[2]

$$\text{Pressure} = \frac{\text{lung volume}}{\text{compliance}} + (\text{resistance})(\text{flow})$$

From this model it follows that compliance equals Δvolume/Δpressure and resistance equals Δpressure/Δflow (Δ indicates the change in the variable). Whether these parameters describe the lungs, the chest wall, or the entire respiratory system depends on how the pressure measurements are made.[1]

In practice, the equation of motion is used to derive estimates of compliance and resistance from measurements of pressure, volume, and flow under two sets of experimental conditions. Under *static* conditions the variables are measured at two moments in time when the respiratory system is held motionless (e.g., at end expiration and end inspiration). Such measurements may be made with an inspiratory pause during mechanical ventilation, which yields so-called plateau pressure, or by training the patient to perform the required breathing maneuvers. However, in dealing with small children and infants it is often more convenient to calculate *dynamic* estimates of compliance and resistance by analyzing data points obtained during continuous ventilation

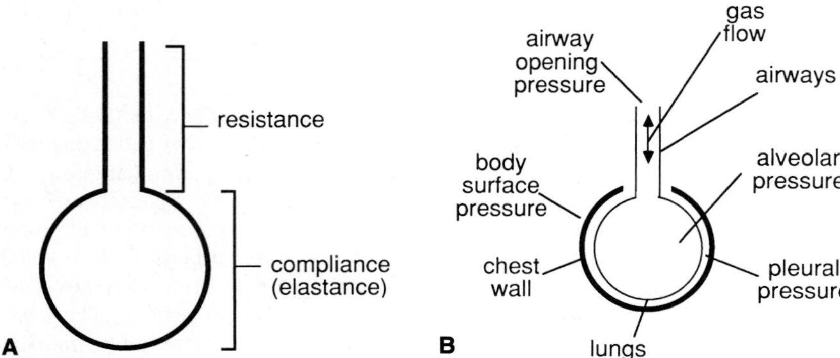

Figure 59-1. **(A)** A single-compartment model of the respiratory system, in which the airways are represented by a flow-resistive conduit and the lungs and chest wall are represented by an elastic compartment. **(B)** More detail can be achieved by adding another compartment such that the lungs can be distinguished from the chest wall. The system can be described mathematically by first specifying measurable variables (e.g., the equation of motion). The separate components of the model (i.e., airway, lungs, and chest wall) are thus *imaginary* structures, whose physical extents are mathematically defined by the points in space between which the pressures are measured. For example, the airway is defined as anything that exists between the airway opening and the alveoli (which might include an endotracheal tube); the lungs are anything that exists between the alveoli and the pleural space; and the chest wall is anything that exists beween the pleural space and the body surface.

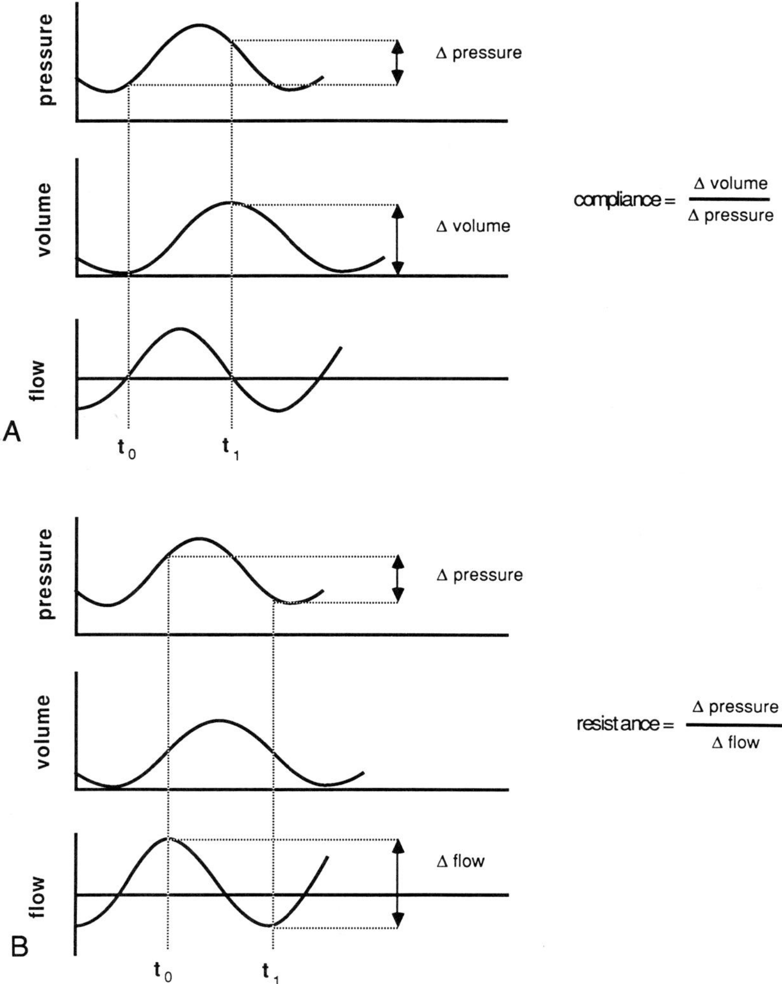

Figure 59-2. **(A)** Data analysis for the calculation of dynamic pulmonary compliance based on esophageal pressure changes and volume changes measured between two points in time (t_0 and t_1) when flow at the airway opening is zero. **(B)** Data analysis for the calculation of pulmonary resistance based on pressure and flow changes between two points in time (t_0 and t_1) when lung volumes are equal.

(either spontaneous or mechanical). For normal lungs at normal frequencies, static and dynamic estimates yield similar values. Dynamic compliance is generally lower in lungs that have a nonhomogeneous distribution of mechanical properties, a finding that may indicate pathology.

The term *dynamic compliance* has been a source of confusion among clinicians. Some authors writing on the mechanics of breathing have erroneously used the term to mean the value calculated from the total pressure change required to deliver a VT.[3–9] Thus, during mechanical ventilation this value would be calculated as VT divided by the difference between peak inspiratory pressure (PIP) and positive end-expiratory pressure (PEEP). However, this pressure difference not only reflects the force necessary to overcome elastic recoil but also includes the component of pressure required to overcome flow resistance, because PIP occurs during inspiratory flow. Therefore, the index calculated with PIP is not compliance, dynamic or otherwise, and has been more appropriately called the *dynamic characteristic*[10,11]:

$$\text{Dynamic characteristic} = \frac{V_T}{\text{PIP} - \text{PEEP}}$$

The correct definition of dynamic compliance, as used by those familiar with classic physiology,[2,12–19] is the ratio of VT to the pressure difference measured between two points in time when flow at the airway opening (but not necessarily in the lungs) is zero (Fig. 59-2). Dynamic compliance is intended to be an estimate of static compliance. However, flow can be zero at the airway opening but still exist between lung units that have different time constants, a condition known as *pendelluft*. In this situation dynamic compliance will be less than static compliance.[2,12]

Static compliance is calculated as the ratio of VT to the

pressure difference measured between two points in time when flow throughout the lungs has ceased. During mechanical ventilation this is achieved by instituting an inspiratory pause of sufficient duration. Once inspiratory flow has stopped (and flow within the lungs decays to zero), airway pressure drops from PIP to a steady-state plateau pressure (P_{plt}), which reflects the true elastic recoil pressure:

$$\text{Static compliance} = \frac{V_T}{P_{plt} - \text{PEEP}}$$

Further clouding the issue, some authors have added the term *effective*, as in *dynamic effective compliance*[20] or *effective compliance, dynamic*.[21] The term *effective* is redundant as a qualifier because any calculation of respiratory system compliance is an effective value. That is, the multiple compliances in the actual respiratory system are lumped together into a single imaginary component whose "effect" is that of a single compliant chamber with a given value of compliance.

It is important for clinicians to be clear on these issues, not only to be able to interpret studies published in physiology journals but to understand their own technology. For example, the Bennett 7200 ventilator has the capability of measuring both static and dynamic mechanics, leaving the clinician in a quandary about which to choose.[22] There are also dedicated pulmonary function evaluation systems that use a variety of methods, such as least-squares regression analysis (a dynamic technique) or the "interrupter" adaptation of the static method. It therefore becomes necessary to understand the distinction between and clinical significance of static versus dynamic mechanics and their related algorithms.[2]

Pathology Models

Once models of physiologic processes are developed, they can be used as descriptors of disease. The focus of clinical research is to relate physical processes to functional categories or diseases by the creation of pathology models. Such models describe characteristics of specific populations of patients who have in common certain signs and symptoms of pulmonary function, either normal or abnormal. Pathology models are often described in terms of the probability (either explicit or implicit) that a particular pattern of parameters can be associated with a given disease or category of function, such as "restricted" or "obstructed." If one or more of the variables measured on a patient in the pulmonary function laboratory are out of the normal range, the model does not fit the clinical picture of normal pulmonary function and may be one of, say, chronic obstructive pulmonary disease (COPD).

Pulmonary Function Testing

Pulmonary function testing is the clinical application of physiology and pathology models. Using patient information in the form of history, physical signs, blood samples, and so on, clinicians first match the pattern of initial observations with those of their experience (memory) to postulate a pathology model. A clinician might, for example, hypothesize "this patient's lungs are obstructed." The pathology model the clinician has in mind may then predict that the patient's airway resistance is high, maximal voluntary ventilation (MVV) is decreased, and so forth. Next, the patient is sent to the pulmonary function laboratory to take part in a series of experiments (often misleadingly referred to as pulmonary function *tests*). There, breathing maneuvers are performed and variables are measured. The variables are used to estimate the parameters of the physiology models (e.g., calculation of airway resistance from plethysmography data or FEV_1 from a flow-time curve). Finally, the clinician compares the data from the pulmonary function studies (i.e., the values of the physiology model parameters) with the reference values for normal and diseased patients. If the patient's pulmonary function data and clinical characteristics are consistent with those of the reference population on which the pathology model is based, the patient is assumed to belong to that population.

For the most part, the study of pediatric pulmonary function has not reached the stage of actual pulmonary function testing, as described above. For this discussion the pediatric population is defined as those patients who are too small to undergo testing with equipment designed for adults. This includes children under 5 or 6 years of age, particularly babies, and most especially premature infants. As with other areas of pediatric medicine, pulmonary research has lagged behind research in adults. Appropriate pathology models are simply not available. For example, bronchopulmonary dysplasia, a condition similar to adult emphysema, is usually not characterized in terms of pulmonary function measurements as is emphysema but rather is commonly diagnosed on the basis of supplemental O_2 requirement at a given age (e.g., 28 days). Many established techniques have had to be adapted or approximated to fit pediatric patients. Measuring devices need to be more sensitive to handle the smaller signals. However, the most significant limiting factor is simply that pediatric patients do not cooperate—obtaining parameters such as FEV_1 or MVV is virtually impossible. Therefore when reviewing the pediatric pulmonary literature, one mostly finds descriptions of basic research regarding compliance and resistance measurements, with the occasional appearance of data on lung volumes. What follows is a description of the most common procedures used in studies of pediatric pulmonary function.

EXPERIMENTAL TECHNIQUES

Lung Volumes

Because some diseases are characterized by changes in lung volume, its measurement can be of diagnostic value.[23] However, lung volumes are most often used to index other volume-dependent parameters such as resistance and compliance. For example, compliance is dependent not only on the elastic properties of the lungs but on the volume at which the measurements are made. Thus, the calculation of specific compliance (compliance/FRC) allows comparison of the elastic properties of different size lungs. It also helps to distinguish an increase in compliance due to resolution of pathology from that due to the opening of atelectatic areas.

Functional Residual Capacity

By definition, the FRC includes only the volume of gas in communication with open airways. Thus, the use of indicator dilution techniques is appropriate. Both the closed-system He dilution technique, and N_2 washout have been used with newborns.[24,25] It has been speculated that because atelectasis is the principal pathologic lesion of respiratory distress syndrome (RDS), measurements of FRC should be an excellent reflection of its severity.[26] In these patients FRC is generally below 1.0 mL/cm body length and returns to the normal range for gestational age at about 2 weeks of age. FRC has also been shown to correlate inversely with $P(A\text{-}a)O_2$ and shunt fraction.[26]

With the He technique, the patient's airway is connected to a bag with a known volume containing a known concentration of He. The dilution caused by the addition of the FRC volume to the system causes the He concentration to drop. If the distribution of ventilation in the lungs is normal, the He concentration stabilizes in the bag at a lower value within 30 to 60 seconds. FRC is then estimated by an equation based on a simple mass balance:

$$FRC = \frac{[(V_i)(He_i)] - [(V_f)(He_f)]}{He_F}$$

where V_i and V_f are the initial and final volumes of the bag and He_I and He_F are the initial and final He concentrations.

The underlying assumption of this technique is that no helium is lost from the system; thus any leaks, such as from around masks or uncuffed endotracheal tubes, will cause errors. Schwartz et al.[27] have described a mathematical analysis that corrects for changes in He concentration due to endotracheal tube leaks. If the patient's distribution of ventilation is impaired, the equilibration time may be extended to the point that hypercapnia and hypoxia may occur. The necessity of adding O_2 and absorbing CO_2 further complicates the procedure.

In the N_2 washout technique, the infant breathes 100 percent O_2 in an open system. After washout of N_2 from the lungs, FRC is calculated from measurements of the volume of exhaled gas collected in a spirometer and the N_2 concentration in end-tidal gas and in the spirometer.

One improvement on this technique involves the continuous measurement and integration of N_2 concentration in exhaled gas that has passed through a mixing chamber.[28] A further improvement, described by Richardson et al.,[29] uses a computerized sampling system, which requires that the patient take only four breaths of 100 percent O_2. With this technique, FRC can be determined in less than 1 minute, allowing repeated measurements in critically ill infants and reducing the risk of toxic effects of O_2 (e.g., retinopathy and absorption atelectasis).

Despite the improvements that have been made, both the He and the N_2 washout techniques still only approximate FRC because they include the dead space volume of the equipment being used.

Thoracic Gas Volume

Thoracic gas volume (TGV), including all the gas in the thorax regardless of communication with open airways, has been measured by plethysmography. This involves placing the infant's body inside the plethysmograph (with the head or face exposed to the atmosphere) and measuring the pressure both at the airway opening and inside the plethysmograph.[30,31] When the airway is occluded at end expiration, subsequent inspiratory efforts cause an increase in the volume of the thorax, which causes a decrease in the pressure measured at the airway opening. At the same time, the expansion of the thorax causes a decrease in the internal volume of the plethysmograph and hence an increase in pressure. These pressure changes are multiplied by a known calibration factor to convert to changes in volume, then used to calculate TGV. Unfortunately, this technique is cumbersome to use and is impractical for critically ill infants.

Crying Vital Capacity

In 1936 Deming and Hanner[32] first suggested that the volume of a crying exhalation might approximate the VC, an index commonly used in adult pulmonary function studies. Since that time several studies have shown that a CVC maneuver is a quick, easy, inexpensive, and relatively safe method of evaluating the pulmonary status of both normal and sick neonates.[33–35] The so-called reverse plethysmography technique has often been used to provide a sensitive measurement of exhaled volume. Infants are stimulated to cry by "flicking" the soles of their feet, and exhaled volumes are recorded for 20 to 30 seconds. Two to four of the largest volumes are analyzed. If they differ by more than 4 mL, the series is discarded; if not, their mean value is taken as the CVC. CVC values have been indexed to chest circumference and body length for comparison of different size infants. Serial measurements have shown that babies with transient tachypnea of the newborn (TTN) have lower CVC values than normal babies, and neonates with RDS have even lower values (3.23, 2.6, and 1.9 mL/cm chest circumference at 10 days, for normal, TTN, and RDS, respectively). Thus, CVC has been proposed as an adjunctive observation to distinguish TTN from RDS.[34] In addition, preliminary data suggest that in infants weighing more than 1200 g or having a gestational age of 30 weeks or more, successful extubation can be achieved at CVC of 0.5 mL/cm body length.[35]

Forced Expiration

A forced expiratory maneuver can be simulated in neonates by wrapping an inflatable cuff around the chest and abdomen and pressurizing it at the end of inspiration.[36] The cuff is inflated rapidly from about 40 to 80 mmHg, either by hand or by using a solenoid valve triggered by a computer. Normal values for this technique (referred to by some as "squeezing the wheeze") have yet to be described, and the results need to be indexed to FRC or weight so that comparisons of different size infants can be made. When more fully developed, it may be a valuable tool in assessing small airways disease.

Ventilatory Patterns

Measurement of the size and timing of V_T is useful in the calculation of minute ventilation and lung mechanics and in identifying abnormal breathing patterns. A variety of techniques have been described, but most of them are used only under experimental conditions.

Plethysmography

The plethysmograph is first calibrated by pumping known volumes of gas in and out of the chamber at rates similar to the respiratory rates to be measured. An object (usually a water bag of the same weight as the infant) must be placed inside the chamber to simulate the infant's mass during calibration. During use of the instrument, its calibration may be inadvertently changed if its internal temperature increases significantly or if leaks develop. An alternative procedure to avoid these problems is to connect the chamber to atmosphere through a pneumotachometer.[37]

The disadvantage of plethysmography is the need to remove the infant from a controlled environment, which precludes its use in critically ill patients. In addition, it is difficult to maintain a seal around the infant's face. On the other hand, connections to the airway are not required, which avoids the addition of system (e.g., mask) dead space and resistance and allow repeated measurements with minimal disturbance of the infant[38] (Fig. 59-3).

Pneumotachography

Pneumotachometers are the most widely used devices for measuring V_T in infants (Fig. 59-4). They are essentially flow resistors designed to produce a pressure drop when exposed to a given flow.[39] The pressure drop is measured with a differential pressure transducer and calibrated to read out in units of flow; the flow signal can be electronically integrated to produce a volume signal.[40] An appropriately sized pneumotachometer must be selected for the anticipated flow rates to ensure linearity of the pressure-flow relation (and hence calibration) and to minimize the added dead space. (A linear relation between two variables is one in which the measured values lie on an approximately straight line when graphed.) Rebreathing can be avoided if the device is flushed with a continuous background flow of fresh gas. Dead space has also been reduced by building the pneumotachometer into the face mask[41] (Fig. 59-4C); however, a face mask may alter the patient's ventilatory pattern.[42] To avoid this, Courtney et al.[43] have developed a head box technique, which avoids contact with the infant's face and is better tolerated than a face mask.

Impedance Pneumography

Impedance pneumography is used in many apnea monitors for newborns and is based on measurement of electrical impedance of the thorax. During the ventilatory cycle, the

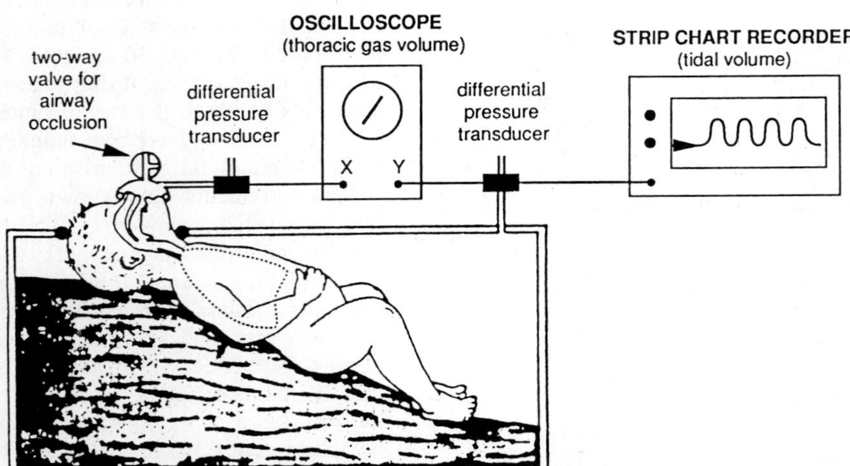

Figure 59-3. An infant body plethysmograph used to measure V_T. Changes in chest volume create changes in pressure that are detected by the pressure transducer. The plethysmograph is calibrated with a syringe of known volume so that the pressure changes can be read as volume measurements.

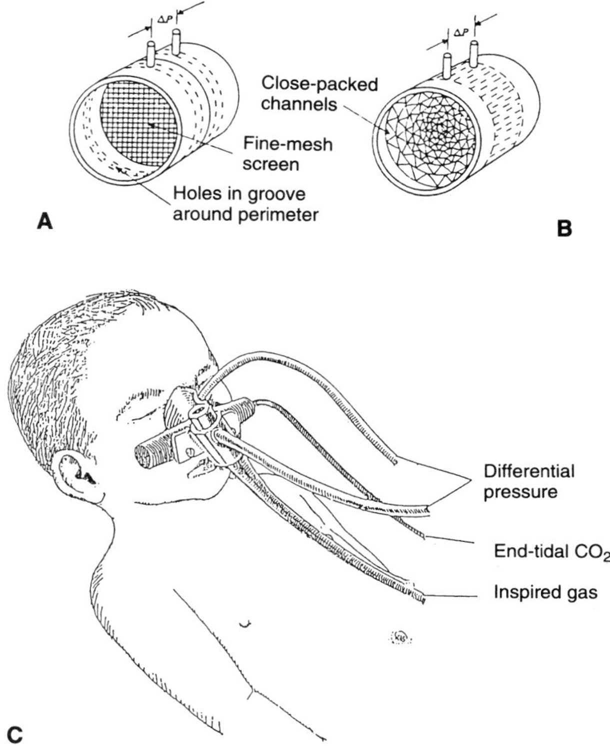

Figure 59-4. (A & B) Two types of pneumotachometer; Figure A, Silverman or screen type; Figure B, Fleisch or capillary-tube type. (C) Experimental setup for measuring V_T with a pneumotachometer incorporated into a face mask.

gas/tissue ratio changes, which changes the electrical impedance (i.e., high gas/tissue ratio corresponds to high impedance). Devices have been described that can measure V_T with only a 10 percent error.[44] Factors that affect accuracy include fluid retention, air leak, pneumonia, and atelectasis, all of which affect thoracic impedance. The major advantage of this technique is that it only requires the placement of an electrode on each side of the chest. Its disadvantage is that it must be calibrated repeatedly by use of another volume measurement technique.

Inductive Plethysmography

Respiratory inductive plethysmography is a recent noninvasive method first described in 1985, which can be used in newborns.[45] The transducer used in this technique consists of coils of insulated wire sewn into elastic bands, which encircle the rib cage and abdomen. When driven by high-frequency electrical oscillations, the coils exhibit self-inductance, which changes as a function of ventilatory movements. Although the system requires careful calibration against another volume-measuring device (e.g., a pneumotachometer), it can measure small V_T levels with errors of less than 10 percent.[46]

Strain Gauges

Mercury-in-rubber strain gauges, placed around the infant's chest and abdomen, can also be used to measure changes in volume, although this method is less quantitative than other methods. Its one advantage, besides being noninvasive and easy to apply, is that it can be used to distinguish between paradoxical and nonparadoxical chest wall motion (Fig. 59-5). This can be shown by observing a phase shift (approaching 180 degrees) between the chest and abdomen signals. Any measurements of esophageal pressure during paradoxical chest wall motion should be interpreted with caution.[47]

One disadvantage of mercury strain gauges as well as of impedance pneumonography and inductive plethysmography is that they cannot distinguish between obstructive and nonobstructive breaths and hence may indicate a falsely high V_T and minute ventilation.

Hot-Wire Anemometer

The hot-wire anemometer consists of a heated wire placed across the channel of a cylinder and is used in a fashion similar to a pneumotachometer. Electrical heating is supplied, and the wire temperature is monitored. Gas flow across the wire produces a cooling effect, which can be calibrated to provide an indication of flow rate. The Bear Neonatal Volume Monitor, introduced in 1988, has made continuous monitoring of V_T a practical reality for critically ill neonates.[48,49] It incorporates a unique design using two heated wires, which allow measurement of bidirectional flow. As a consequence, the device can calculate both inspiratory and expiratory volumes and thus give an indication of the amount of gas leaking around an uncuffed endotra-

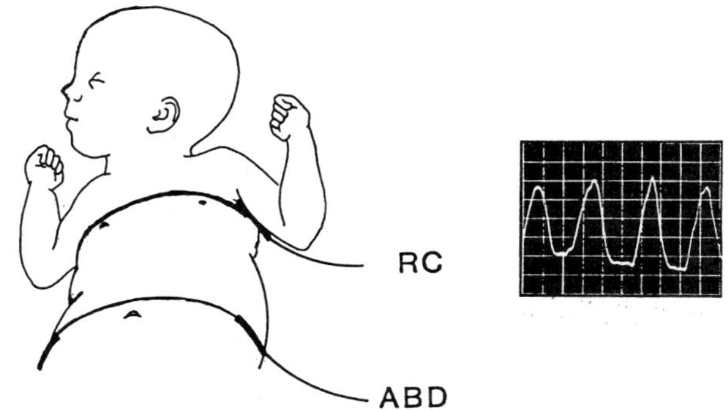

Figure 59-5. An example of strain gauges placed around an infant's rib cage and abdomen for measurement of neonatal chest wall movements. Each strain gauge gives a signal proportional to the change in rib cage or abdomen circumference during breathing, as shown in the sample waveform. The two signals can be used to determine whether the baby is breathing paradoxically (signals out of phase) or nonparadoxically (signals in phase).

cheal tube. It is accurate over a flow range of 0.15 to 20.58 L/min and can measure volumes from 1 to 100 mL. One disadvantage is that it introduces 1 to 2 mL of dead space. Of greater concern is that it cannot discriminate between spontaneous and mechanical breaths, displaying an "average" V_T, which can be misleading.

Reference values would be helpful when using any of the above techniques to measure ventilation. The normal range reported in the literature for minute ventilation is about 200 to 300 mL/kg/min; normal V_T ranges from 5 to 7 mL/kg.

Mechanics of Breathing

Most pulmonary function studies in neonates revolve around the various methods of determining compliance and resistance. These methods can be grouped into two broad categories: the classical techniques based on the analysis of pressure, volume, and flow tracings obtained during spontaneous breathing or mechanical ventilation; and specialized techniques based on unusual maneuvers such as forced oscillations or multiple occlusions.

Ideally, mechanical properties should be indexed to lung volume so that values from different size patients are comparable. In lieu of volume measurements, researchers have used body weight, chest circumference, and body length. Because body weight can vary widely over a short time and because it is difficult to measure in ventilated infants, *birth weight* is a more accurate description of size in the first days of life.[50] At present, there is no consensus about which indexing procedure is best.

Classical Techniques

During spontaneous breathing, the pressure driving the respiratory system is generated by the ventilatory muscles. Unfortunately, this pressure cannot be measured; therefore, total respiratory system mechanics cannot be measured during normal breathing. However, it is possible to measure transpulmonary pressure (i.e., the difference between airway opening pressure and pleural pressure), so that dynamic lung mechanics can be evaluated.[51] Furthermore, pleural pressure can be approximated by esophageal pressure so that the procedure is less invasive. Esophageal pressure is measured with either a small balloon-tipped[52] or a water-filled catheter, each of which has its own advantages and disadvantages.[23,53,54] Some studies, however, indicate that esophageal pressure does not accurately reflect pleural pressure in some infants.[47,55] If the rib cage moves paradoxically during inspiration, pleural pressure is not distributed evenly within the thorax, and lung parameters cannot be accurately assessed. This happens frequently in premature infants, during rapid eye movement (REM) sleep in term infants, and in older infants with COPD.

Flow measurements are usually made with a pneumotachometer, which also provides the signal for volume measurements. The pneumotachometer can be connected either to a face mask or to an endotracheal tube. Once simultaneous tracings of pressure, volume, and flow have been obtained, lung compliance and resistance are computed by calculating the ratios of volume change to pressure change and pressure change to flow change, respectively, as specified by the equation of motion.

Two basic techniques have been used to evaluate dynamic compliance and resistance during both inspiration and expiration. The first is the subtraction technique of Mead and Whittenberger,[51] which separates the elastic from the resistive components of the transpulmonary pressure signal (Fig. 59-2). This method has been used to calculate resistance at either a given volume (usually half the maximal volume) or a given flow. The second method is a least-squares regression technique. A computer is used to sample discrete values of pressure, volume, and flow during a ventilatory cycle, and a statistical analysis is performed to fit the equation of motion to the data. Besides its ability to discriminate between inspiratory and expiratory mechanics, this technique can function in real time. An example of a commercial device using this method is the PEDS system marketed by MAS Inc. (Hatfield, PA), which incorporates a microcomputer with custom software and data acquisition hardware for bed-

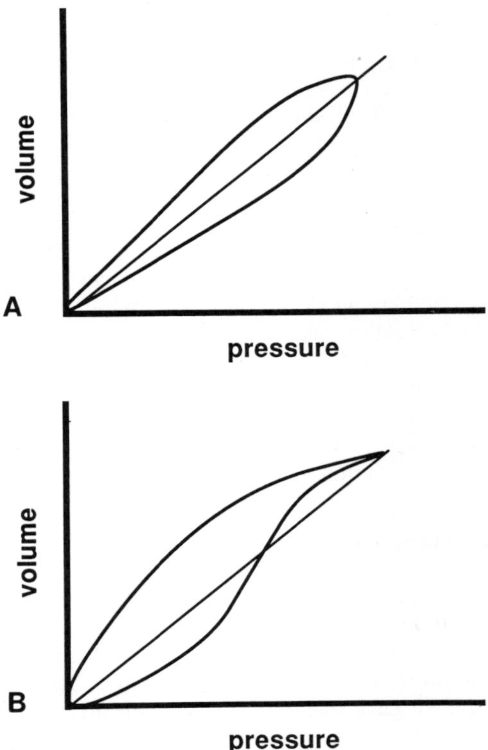

Figure 59-6. Pressure-volume curves for **(A)** linear and **(B)** nonlinear compliance throughout the breath. Nonlinear compliance values are thought to be predictive of pulmonary fibrosis and overdistension of the lung during mechanical ventilation, although nonlinear compliance values have been observed in normal preterm infants.

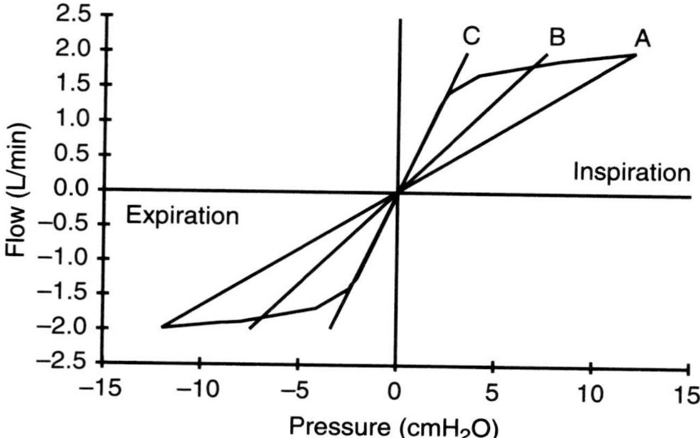

Figure 59-7. A simulated pressure-flow curve where pressure equals Δvolume/compliance and resistance equals Δpressure/Δflow. Slopes A, B, and C are defined as follows: A, resistance at peak flow or one-half maximal volume (Mead-Whittenberger technique); B, resistance calculated by fitting the equation of motion to the data by least-squares regression (with r = 0.95); C, resistance in the linear or flow-independent portion of the pressure-flow curve. Corresponding values of resistance for each technique are as follows: A, 365 $cmH_2O/L/s$; B, 226 $cmH_2O/L/s$; C, 103 cm $H_2O/L/s$. This illustrates that caution must be used when comparing different techniques.

side evaluation of the respiratory status of full-term and premature infants.

The assumption inherent in the above techniques is that compliance is linear and constant throughout the breath. A constant compliance is assumed in the algorithms used by commercial systems such as the PEDS and Star Calc devices. Both allow display of pressure-volume curves in which one can observe the points of end inspiration and expiration. If a straight line cannot be drawn between these two points while staying within the pressure-volume loop, compliance is not linear (i.e., independent of volume), violating the assumption of both the Mead-Whittenberger and least-squares techniques (Fig. 59-6).

The least-squares technique used by current commercially available computer systems also assumes that resistance is constant within a breath and is independent of flow. This relationship can only be verified by observing the pressure-flow curves. Technique comparisons based on a single breath would show that the highest value of resistance is calculated by the Mead-Whittenberger technique at half maximal volume, followed by the least-squares technique, and finally the Mead-Whittenberger technique in the linear (flow-independent) portion of the pressure-flow curve (Fig. 59-7).

Special Techniques

Most specialized techniques have been developed to evaluate total respiratory system mechanics. This is because transrespiratory system pressure can only be measured if the system is forced by an external driving pressure (e.g., a mechanical ventilator) or if the pressure generated by the ventilatory muscles can somehow be indirectly evaluated.

An estimate of transrespiratory system pressure can be obtained during spontaneous breathing by instituting an inspiratory hold maneuver and waiting until the ventilatory muscles relax. The resulting static pressure can then be used to calculate total respiratory system compliance if the preceding V_T is known. This *occlusion* technique[56] relies on the observation that infants have a powerful Hering-Breuer reflex and will normally relax when their airway is occluded at a lung volume above end-expiratory volume.[57] In practice, several measurements of static pressure are made at different V_T levels by occluding the airway at different times in the inspiratory phase; a linear regression line is then fitted to the data points, and a value for compliance is obtained from the slope. Compliance is not determined from a single occlusion because infants often maintain an end-expiratory volume that exceeds FRC.[58,59] Even with multiple determinations of volume and pressure, the technique assumes that end-expiratory volume remains constant, a condition that may not hold true in the nonintubated infant, especially during REM sleep.[60]

Mortola et al.[59,61] have applied a modified version of the occlusion technique[62] to include respiratory system resistance and time constant determinations in their studies of breathing dynamics (the time constant is calculated as resistance times compliance[1]). By calculating the slope of the flow-volume curve after release of an end-inspiratory occlusion, they obtained an estimate of the respiratory system time constant; with the time constant and compliance known, resistance was easily calculated.

A further refinement has been added by LeSouef et al.,[63] who reasoned that the volume obtained by extrapolating the passive flow-volume curve to zero flow was the true volume above FRC at which the occlusion occurred. Dividing this volume by the occlusion pressure gives compliance. Thus, a single occlusion maneuver could be used to estimate respiratory system compliance, resistance, and time constant (Fig. 59-8). Because this maneuver necessitates only a short disruption of ventilation, it is more applicable to sick infants, particularly during mechanical ventilation. The limitation of this technique is that it is only valid if a linear flow-volume relation is obtained. Otherwise, it can be inferred that the respiratory system cannot be characterized by a single constant value for compliance and resistance.

One reason for a nonlinear flow-volume relation would be that expiration is not passive. To further ensure passive expiration and increase the range of V_T for which pulmonary mechanics are calculated, Grunstein et al.[64] created a modification of the occlusion technique, which they described as *expiratory volume clamping*. This is achieved by using a two-way valve to prevent expiration for three to five tidal volumes, which produces a corresponding increase in pressure and lung volume with each inspiration. After the cumulative increases in V_T have occurred, the expiratory valve is opened and data are gathered for the calculation of passive mechanics, as previously described. Using this technique,

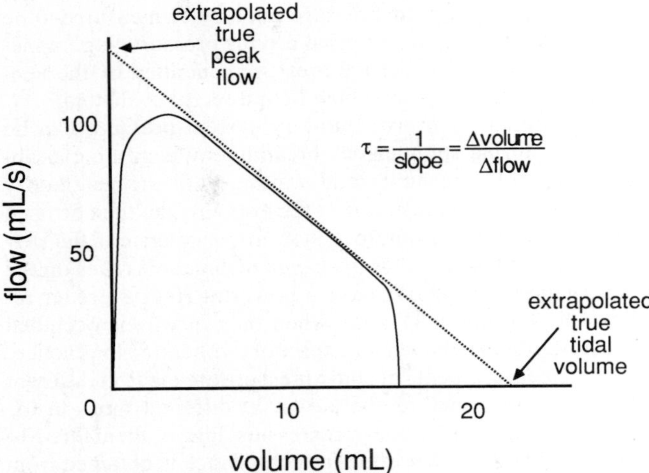

Figure 59-8. An example of the expiratory phase of the flow-volume curve. This example shows inspiration occurring before complete expiration has been achieved. Therefore a line is extrapolated back to zero flow and zero volume to calculate the V_T. The reciprocal of the slope of the extrapolated line is the time constant (τ) of this breath. (Modified from LeSouëf et al.,[63] with permission.)

Grunstein et al.[64] found a decrease in both compliance per kilogram and conductivity per kilogram (conductivity is the reciprocal of resistance) in preterm infants with chronic lung disease as compared with full-term normal infants, which suggests airway obstruction.

When the occlusion technique is carried to its logical extreme, we arrive at the *interrupter* technique.[65] In this method expiratory flow is interrupted multiple times by a computer-controlled valve. The initial spike in pressure is combined with the instantaneous flow rate immediately prior to the occlusion in order to calculate respiratory system resistance. This initial pressure slowly decays to a plateau, reflecting tissue stress relaxation and redistribution of gases between lung units (pendelluft).[66,67] The plateau pressure is used with the associated volume measurement to calculate respiratory system compliance (Fig. 59-9). Multiple determinations of resistance and compliance reveal nonlinearities within a single breath, but this method is subject to the same limitations mentioned for the occlusion technique.

SPECIFIC CLINICAL APPLICATIONS

Although not common yet, the evaluation of pulmonary mechanics has been applied in several areas related to pediatrics. Unfortunately, there is no clear consensus regarding values considered "normal" for infants. Values reported in the literature can vary depending not only on the age and size of the subjects but on the technique used. In general, however, values for total resistance range from 30 to 80 $cmH_2O/L/s$, and those for compliance range from 1 to 3 $mL/cmH_2O/kg$ for normal (nonintubated) infants from newborn to 2 years of age. Compliance for infants with RDS can range from 0.2 to 0.9 $mL/cmH_2O/kg$.[68] There is little information about the effect of intubation on total respiratory system resistance in premature infants. One study has shown that for a small group of infants recovering from RDS, pneumonia, or TTN, total respiratory system resistance averaged 128 $cmH_2O/L/s$ for those with 3.0-mm ID endotracheal tubes and 73 $cmH_2O/L/s$ for those with 3.5-mm ID tubes.[69] After extubation, the resistance for these two groups dropped to 75 and 37 $cmH_2O/L/s$, respectively. Based on these data, the 3.0-mm tube had an effective resistance of about 53 $cmH_2O/L/s$ while the 3.5-mm tube had an effective resistance of about 36 $cmH_2O/L/s$. The compliance for these infants was about 1.1 $mL/cmH_2O/kg$ and did not change after extubation. The time constant before extubation averaged 0.17 seconds; after extubation it was about 0.09 seconds, owing to the decrease in resistance.

Many of the following studies report changes in respiratory mechanics in groups of infants with different treatments or illnesses. For example, Miller et al.[70] have shown a decrease in both total pulmonary and supraglottic resistance in response to nasal continuous positive airway pressure (CPAP) in healthy preterm infants, with 60 percent of the decrease occurring in the supraglottic airway. They concluded that the decrease in resistance, as a result of mechanical splinting of the airway, may be the primary mechanism by which CPAP reduces obstructive apnea.

Some studies have tried to use mechanical parameters as a basis for predicting severity of bronchopulmonary dysplasia (BPD). Dreizzin et al.[68] measured static compliance in preterm infants with RDS weaned from mechanical ventilation. This group of infants was found to have higher compliance values than acutely ill infants requiring ventilation and O_2 therapy and infants who subsequently developed BPD. The authors concluded that compliance may be predictive of BPD.

Graff et al.[71] measured dynamic compliance in preterm infants with RDS during the first 3 days of life. They found a lower compliance in those infants who subsequently developed BPD than in those who did not. Furthermore, they used a threshold of 0.45 mL/cmH_2O as a predictor of survival. Of 47 infants whose compliance was above this threshold, 45 survived, while 11 of 13 infants below this level died.

Once the patient has BPD and survived, the next logical step is to facilitate intervention. Tay-Uyboco et al.[72] hypothesized that infants recovering from severe BPD have airway constriction, which could be reversed with administration of O_2. They found that pulmonary resistance decreased and compliance increased when the inspired O_2 fraction (F_IO_2) was increased from 0.21 to 1.0. However, these findings could not be reproduced by Carlo et al.[73]

Respiratory mechanics in conjunction with other parameters have been applied to weaning infants from mechanical ventilation. Fox et al.[74] found that infants with a combination of low birth weight, low gestational age, and high pulmonary resistance at the time of pre-extubation were more likely to require reintubation.

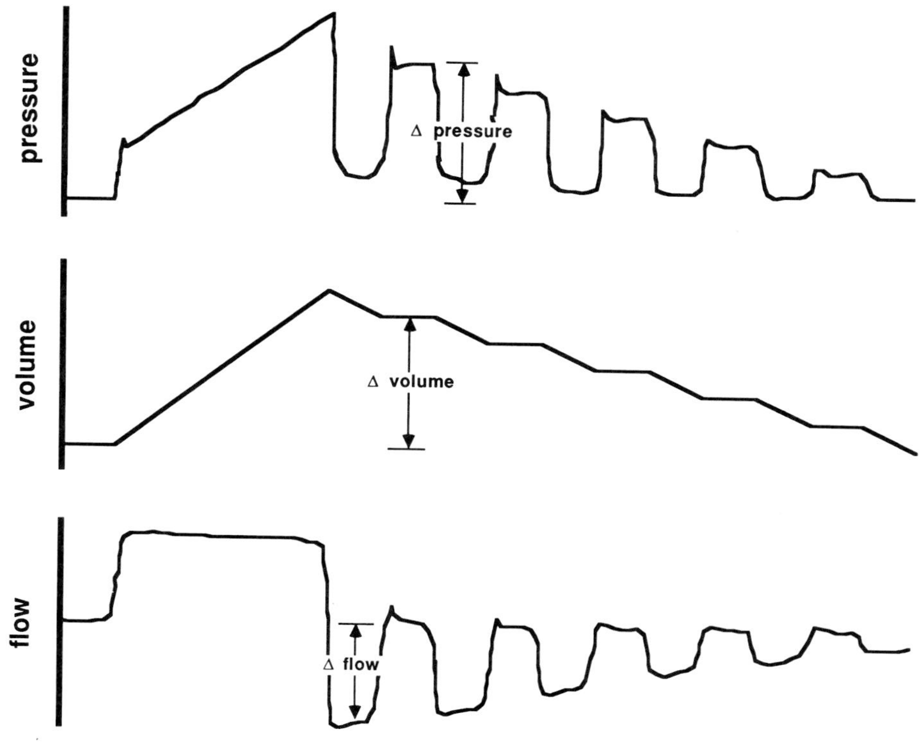

Figure 59-9. An example of one breath with multiple occlusions used for the calculation of static compliance and resistance by the interrupter technique. Static compliance is defined as Δvolume/Δpressure and resistance by Δpressure/Δflow for each occlusion. In this example five values of compliance and resistance can be calculated and compared with volume throughout the breath to reveal any nonlinear relationship.

Pediatric pulmonary function studies have not yet reached the level of sophistication seen in the adult arena. This has been largely due to the difficulty in obtaining pulmonary function measurements. However, with the appearance of commercially available and user-friendly data acquisition systems, this situation is changing. Perhaps the most fruitful short-term benefits will come from the application of such devices to the optimization of mechanical ventilation. The computer-aided ventilation system offered by Siemens is an example. Such advances are particularly needed for neonatal mechanical ventilation. Continuous measurement and analysis of volume and flow data could help bring time-cycled, pressure-limited ventilation techniques out of the realm of art and into the light of science. Some researchers have already begun to identify clinically useful patterns that, for example, would help to avoid lung overdistension.[75] Yet much work needs to be done, particularly in gathering data on specific populations of patients, such as those with RDS or pneumonia and those who might be ready for extubation. A sufficient number of different physiologic parameters have been created and measurement techniques developed for pediatric patients. What is needed now are the relevant clinical observations, treatment procedures, and probable outcomes to form the pathology models on which all pulmonary function interpretations are based.

References

1. Primiano FP Jr, Chatburn RL: The use of models in pulmonary physiology. pp. 39–57. In Chatburn RL, Craig KC (eds): Fundamentals of Respiratory Care Research. Appleton & Lange, East Norwalk, CT, 1988
2. Chatburn RL: Dynamic respiratory mechanics. Respir Care 1986;31:703–711
3. Chatburn RL, Primiano FP Jr, Lough MD: Mechanical ventilation. pp. 159–223. In Chatburn RL, Lough MD (eds): Handbook of Respiratory Care. 2nd Ed. Yearbook Medical Publishers, Chicago, 1990
4. Martz KV, Joiner JW, Shepherd RM: Management of the Patient-Ventilator System. CV Mosby, St. Louis, 1984
5. Nilsestuen JO: Applied mathematics for respiratory care. pp. 550–572. In Barnes TA (ed): Respiratory Care Practice. Year Book Medical Publishers, Chicago, 1988
6. Riggs JH: Respiratory Facts. FA Davis, Philadelphia, 1989
7. Harper RW: A Guide to Respiratory Care. JB Lippincott, Philadelphia, 1981
8. Rarey KP, Youtsey JW: Respiratory Patient Care. Prentice-Hall, Englewood Cliffs, NJ, 1981, pp. 228–229
9. DiPietro JS, Mustard MN: Clinical Guide for Respiratory Care Practitioners. Appleton & Lange, East Norwalk, CT 1987, p. 102
10. Bone RC: Diagnosis of causes for acute respiratory distress by pressure-volume curves. Chest 1976;70:740–746
11. Bone RC, Graverstein N, Kirby RR: Monitoring respiratory and hemodynamic function in the patient with respiratory failure.

pp. 301–336. In Kirby RR, Smith RA, Desautels DA (eds): Clinical Applications of Ventilatory Support. Churchill Livingstone, New York, 1990

12. Otis AB, McKerrow CB, Bartlett RA et al: Mechanical factors in the distribution of pulmonary ventilation. J Appl Physiol 1956;8:427–443
13. Mead J, Lindren I, Gaensler EA: The mechanical properties of the lungs in emphysema. J Clin Invest 1955;34:1005–1016
14. Zamel N: Normal lung mechanics. pp. 115–127. In Baum GL, Wolinsky E (eds): Textbook of Pulmonary Diseases. 4th Ed. Little Brown, Boston, 1983
15. Grodins FS, Yamashiro SM: Respiratory Function of the Lung and its Control. Macmillan, New York, 1978, p. 36
16. Cook CD, Sutherland JM, Segal RB et al: Studies of respiratory physiology in the newborn infant. III. Measurements of mechanics of respiration. J Clin Invest 1957;36:440–448
17. Nunn JF: Applied Respiratory Physiology. 2nd Ed. Butterworths, London, 1978, pp. 91–93
18. Miller WF, Scacci R, Gast LR: Laboratory Evaluation of Pulmonary Function. JB Lippincott, Philadelphia, 1987, p. 20
19. Mead J: Mechanical properties of lungs. Physiol Rev 1961;41:281–330
20. Freeman C, Cicerchia E, Demers RR, Saklad M: Static compliance, static effective compliance, and dynamic effective compliance as indicators of elastic recoil in the presence of lung disease. Respir Care 1976;21:323–326
21. Hodgkin JE: Specialized pulmonary function tests. pp. 205–233. In Burton GG, Gee GN, Hodgkin JE (eds): Respiratory Care. JB Lippincott, Philadelphia, 1977
22. Chatburn RL: Estimates of true compliance versus dynamic characteristic, letter. Respir Care 1987;32:1161
23. Bancalari E: Pulmonary function testing and other diagnostic laboratory procedures. pp. 195–233. In Thibeault DW, Gregory GA (eds): Neonatal Pulmonary Care. 2nd Ed. East Norwalk, CT. Appleton & Lange, 1986
24. Kraus AN, Auld PAM: Measurement of functional residual capacity in distressed neonates by helium rebreathing. J Pediatr 1970;77:228–232
25. Nelson NM, Prod'hom LS, Cherry RB et al: Pulmonary function in the newborn infant. I. Methods: Ventilation and gaseous metabolism. Pediatrics 1962;30:963–974
26. Tori CA, Krauss AN, Auld PA: Serial studies of lung volume and $\dot{V}A/\dot{Q}$ in hyaline membrane disease. Pediatr Res 1973;7:82–88
27. Schwartz JG, Fox WW, Shaffer TH: A method for measuring functional residual capacity in neonates with endotracheal tubes. IEEE Trans Biomed Eng 1978;25:304–307
28. Gerhard T, Hehre D, Bancalari E: A simple method of measuring functional residual capacity in the newborn by N_2 washout. Pediatr Res 1985;19:1165–1169
29. Richardson P, Galway W, Olsen S, Bunnell JB: Computerized estimates of functional residual capacity in infants. Ann Biomed Eng 1981;9:243–255
30. Klaus M, Tooley WH, Weaver KL et al: Lung volume in the newborn infant. Pediatrics 1962;30:111–116
31. Stocks J, Levy NM, Godfrey S: A new apparatus for the accurate measurement of airway resistance in infancy. J Appl Physiol 1977;43:155–159
32. Denning J, Hanner JP: Respiration in infancy: Study of rate, volume and character of respiration in healthy infants during neonatal period. Am J Dis Child 1936;51:823–831
33. Sutherland JM, Radcliff JW: Crying vital capacity. Am J Dis Child 1961;101:93–100
34. Chiswick ML, Milner RDG: Crying vital capacity. Measurement of neonatal lung function. Arch Dis Child 1976;51:22–27
35. Andreou A, Keh E, Bhat R, Vidyasagar D: Critical care problems in the newborn: CVC in infants on assisted ventilation. Prognostic indicator and ability to wean. Crit Care Med 1980;8:291–293
36. Taussig LM, Landau LI, Godfrey S et al: Determinants of forced expiratory flows in newborn infants. J Appl Physiol 1982; 53:1220–1227
37. Ahlstrom H: Studies on pulmonary mechanics in infants: Methodological aspects. Scand J Respir Dis 1974;55:129–140
38. Polgar G, Lacourt G: A method for measuring respiratory mechanics in small newborn (premature) infants. J Appl Physiol 1972;32:555–559
39. Sullivan WJ, Peters GM, Enright PL: Pneumotachographs: Theory and clinical application. Respir Care 1984;29:736–749
40. Ligas JR: Instrumentation. pp. 281–303. In Chatburn RL, Craig KC (eds): Fundamentals of Respiratory Care Research. Appleton & Lange, East Norwalk, CT, 1988
41. Anderson JV Jr, Martin RJ, Lough MD, Martinez A: An improved nasal mask pneumotachometer for measuring ventilation in neonates. J Appl Physiol 1982;53:1307–1309
42. Fleming PJ, Levine MR, Goncalves A: Changes in respiratory pattern resulting from the use of a facemask to record respiration in newborn infants. Pediatr Res 1982;16:1031–1034
43. Courtney SE, Weber KR, Hopson JF et al: Use of a head box for pneumotachography in neonates, abstracted. Respir Care 1988;33:890
44. Itoh A, Ishida A, Kikuchi N et al: Non-invasive ventilatory volume monitor. Med Biol Eng Comput 1982;20:613–619
45. Warren RH, Alderson SH: Calibration of computer assisted (Respicomp) respiratory inductive plethysmography in newborn infants. Am Rev Respir Dis 1985;131:564–567
46. Warren RH, Anderson SH: The accuracy of respiratory inductive plethysmography in measuring breathing patterns of sedated piglets receiving controlled mechanical ventilation. Respir Care 1988;33:846–851
47. Heaf DP, Turner H, Stocks J, Helms P: The accuracy of esophageal pressure measurements in convalescent and sick intubated infants. Pediatr Pulmonol 1986;2:5–8
48. MacDonald K, Wirtshafter D, McEvoy C, Franceschini R: The use of a hot-wire anemometer in the differential diagnosis of neonatal endotracheal tube (ETT) obstruction, abstracted. Respir Care 1988;33:886
49. Post DJ, Kita R, Myers TF, Paveza G: Neonatal volume monitoring: A new device, abstracted. Respir Care 1988;33:890
50. England SJ: Current techniques for assessing pulmonary function in the newborn and infant: Advantages and limitations. Pediatr Pulmonol 1988;4:48–53
51. Mead J, Whittenberger JL: Physical properties of human lungs measured during spontaneous respiration. J Appl Physiol 1953;5:779–796
52. Beardsmore CS, Helms P, Stocks J et al: Improved esophageal balloon technique for use in infants. J Appl Physiol 1980;49: 735–742
53. Gerhardt T, Jensen LP. Physiologic monitoring and pulmonary function. In Carlo WA, Chatburn RL (eds): Neonatal respiratory care. Year Book Medical Publishers, Chicago, 1988
54. Bryan AC, Wohl MEB: Respiratory mechanics in children. pp. 179–191. In Geiger SR, Macklem PT, Mead J, Fishman AP (eds): Handbook of Physiology. Section 3: The Respiratory System. Vol. 3. Mechanics of Breathing, Part 1. American Physiological Society, Bethesda, 1986
55. LeSouëf PN, Lopes JM, England SJ et al: Influence of chest wall distortion on esophageal pressure. J Appl Physiol 1983;55:313–318
56. Olinsky A, Bryan AC, Bryan MH: A simple method of measuring total respiratory system compliance in newborn infants. S Afr Med J 1976;50:128–130
57. Cross KW, Klauw M, Tooley WH, Weisser K: The response of the new-born baby to inflation of the lung. J Physiol 1960;151:551–565
58. Korsch PC, Stark AR: Dynamic maintenance of end-expiratory lung volume in full-term infants. J Appl Physiol 1984;57: 1126–1133
59. Mortola JP, Milic-Emili J, Nowaraj A et al: Muscle pressure and flow during expiration in infants. Am Rev Respir Dis 1984;129:49–53
60. Bryan AC, England SJ: Maintenance of an elevated FRC in the newborn: Paradox of REM sleep. Am Rev Respir Dis 1984; 129:209–210

61. Mortola JP, Fisher JT, Smith B et al: Dynamics of breathing in infants. J Appl Physiol 1982;52:1209–1215
62. McIlroy MB, Tierney DF, Nadel JA: A new method for measurement of compliance and resistance of lungs and thorax. J Appl Physiol 1963;18:424–427
63. LeSouëf PN, England SJ, Bryan AC: Passive respiratory mechanics in newborns and children. Am Rev Respir Dis 1984;129:552–556
64. Grunstein MM, Springer C, Godfrey S et al: Expiratory volume clamping: A new method to assess respiratory mechanics in sedated infants. J Appl Physiol 1987;62:2107–2114
65. Gottfried SB, Rossi A, Calferley PMA et al: Interrupter technique for measurement of respiratory mechanics in anesthetized cats. J Appl Physiol 1984;56:681–690
66. Bates JHT, Rossi A, Milic-Emili J: Analysis of the behavior of the respiratory system with constant inspiratory flow. J Appl Physiol 1985;58:1840–1888
67. Jackson AC, Milhorn HT, Norman JT: A re-evaluation of the interrupter technique of airway resistance measurement. J Appl Physiol 1974;36:264–268
68. Dreizzin E, Migdal M, Praud JP et al: Passive compliance of total respiratory system in preterm newborn infants with respiratory distress syndrome. J Pediatr 1988;112:778–781
69. LeSouëf PN, England SJ, Bryan AC: Total resistance of the respiratory system in preterm infants with and without an endotracheal tube. J Pediatr 1984;104:108–111
70. Miller MJ, DiFiore JM, Strohl KD, Martin RJ: The effects of nasal CPAP on supraglottic and total pulmonary resistance in preterm infants. J Appl Physiol 1990;68:141–146
71. Graff MA, Novo RP, Diaz M et al: Compliance measurements in RDS: The prediction of outcome. Pediatr Pulmonol 1986;2:332–336
72. Tay-Uyboco JS, Kwaitkowski K, Cates DB et al: Hypoxic airway constriction in infants of very low birth weight recovering from moderate to severe bronchopulmonary dysplasia. J Pediatr 1989;115:456–459
73. Carlo WA, Siner BS, DiFiore JM, Martin RJ: Oxygen saturation and pulmonary resistance in infants with bronchopulmonary dysplasia. Pediatr Res 1990;27:1189A
74. Fox WW, Schwartz JG, Shaffer TH: Successful extubation of neonates: Clinical and physiological factors. Crit Care Med 1981;9:823–826
75. Fisher JB, Mannel MC, Coleman M et al: Identifying lung overdistention by using volume-pressure loops. Pediatr Pulmonol 1988;5:10–14

Chapter 60

Psychosocial Assessment of the Patient with Chronic Respiratory Disease

Tammy H. Abuan
David J. Pierson

CHAPTER OUTLINE

Patients with chronic respiratory disease are affected by many separate yet interrelated aspects of their illness, all of which together determine clinical severity and overall impact on function. For example, in a patient with disabling chronic obstructive pulmonary disease (COPD), several processes interact to determine the degree to which the illness impairs that person's ability to function (Fig. 60-1). To the list in Figure 60-1 could be added several other processes, including disadvantageous breathing patterns, adverse effects of drugs, metabolic and electrolyte abnormalities, concomitant disease in other organ systems, and anxiety and depression. Any one of these may be the factor that most severely compromises the patient's function; even ideal management of the others can fail to help the patient if this one element is ignored.

This book emphasizes the importance of a logical approach to patient care based on pathophysiology. The best management requires first a thorough understanding of the pathophysiology of a patient's illness, followed by assessment appropriate to that pathophysiology, the setting of realistic treatment goals, and finally individualization of specific management modalities to the pathophysiology and severity of the disorder. Although most of this book is concerned with the biomedical aspects of organ dysfunction, these principles are equally applicable to the psychosocial aspects of illness and its management. For example, appropriate management of a patient with severe COPD can lead to better family and social relationships, improved sleep, better appetite, and improved sexual function and can radically improve the patient's quality of life, even if no improvement in pulmonary function is possible. In order for this to happen, however, the clinician must deal with more than just the biomedical aspects of the illness. Assessment and management of COPD and other chronic respiratory illnesses must

Airway obstruction
Excessive secretions
Hypoxemia and cor pulmonale
Ventilatory muscle dysfunction
Physical deconditioning
Nutritional deficiencies
Psychosocial factors

→ Inability to function

Figure 60-1. Processes that interact in a patient with COPD and help determine clinical severity and overall impact on the patient's ability to function.

take place in the context of the patient's own life experience rather than in some stereotypical, cookbook fashion intended for the hypothetical, generalized patient.

Let us consider the following individuals, each with severe COPD, with identical findings on spirometry (forced expiratory volume in 1 second [FEV_1], 1.0 L) and arterial blood gas measurement (PaO_2, 54 mmHg):

> A 61-year-old, divorced former farm worker with no immediate family, living alone in a small rural community, supported by a modest pension, with a recent history of depression and excessive drinking
>
> A 54-year-old aerospace engineer with a comfortable income, who lives with his wife in a large suburban home, has several hobbies including international travel, and enjoys excellent medical insurance coverage
>
> A 66-year-old, non-English-speaking woman who has recently emigrated to this country to join her son, who lives with his wife and four children in low-income housing in a large city and works as a grocery clerk

In these hypothetical individuals, despite the same disease process and physiologic impairment, attempts at management that did not take into consideration their specific psychosocial problems, needs, and resources could not hope to be optimally successful.

Webster's *New World Dictionary* defines psychosocial as "of or pertaining to the psychological development of the individual in relation to his social environment."[1] The psychosocial assessment of an individual then attempts to elicit information that pertains to that individual's personality, thinking processes and emotions, all of which are intimately linked to the ability to cope with a chronic illness. Patients come to us with certain complaints or symptoms that affect their well-being and quality of life. The clinician's goal is to treat the whole patient, not simply the sick or injured part. We need to understand the patient's life outside the hospital or clinic setting in order to achieve effective care, set appropriate and attainable goals, and ultimately improve the patient's quality of life. Psychosocial assessment will help the clinician to attain these goals.

Table 60-1. Components of the Psychosocial Assessment

Demographics
Economic and employment factors
Education
Religion and spiritual factors
Cultural factors
Health beliefs
Current stresses
Interpersonal support systems
Interactional support systems
Psychiatric and substance use history
Premorbid functional level
Current functional level (impact of illness)
Value systems
Understanding and perceptions of the illness
Previous experiences with the health care system
Adaptation to change and stress
External psychosocial resources

There are many individual components to the psychosocial assessment (Table 60-1). This chapter summarizes these components, provides examples of many of them, and indicates how to best use the information obtained in caring for patients with chronic respiratory disease.

DEMOGRAPHICS

Commonly elicited demographics include name, age, sex, race or ethnic identification, and marital status. Additional questions should pursue information about the patient's family and friends, such as whom the patient can rely on for help; who relies upon the patient; and whether the patient's living arrangements are adequate for someone with chronic respiratory disease. This information can be obtained in casual conversation, with the clinician showing genuine interest in the patient. Giving the appearance of wanting to quickly "fill in the blanks" will not help to build a trusting and open relationship between patient and caregiver.

ECONOMIC AND EMPLOYMENT FACTORS

In the same manner in which the caregiver has obtained demographic data, information about the patient's occupation and sources of income needs to be elicited. Is the patient still able to work or too disabled by the disease? Does the patient have a pension, collect welfare, rely on the income of family members? Is there medical insurance, and does the patient have the resources to pay for prescriptions and treatments that might be helpful? If the clinician caring for our 61-year-old farm worker finds him to be a candidate for home O_2 therapy, will that fit into the constraints of his "modest pension" and remote rural domicile?

EDUCATION

Caregivers often spend a lot of time teaching patients about the nature of their disease and its treatment and prognosis. If this teaching is done at a level beyond the patient's ability to understand, then everyone will end up frustrated and confused. On the other hand, if the information presented is at such an elementary level as to insult the patient, resentment and anger can override any positive effect the teaching may have had. Consider again the 61-year-old farm worker. Is he literate? Did he graduate from high school? The answers to these questions may help determine how to approach this patient with information about his COPD. Brochures from the local lung association about quitting smoking may be of little benefit to a man who cannot read. Conversely, a man who has worked with farm animals for 45 years may have a more sophisticated understanding of anatomy and physiology than our 54-year-old aerospace engineer. Determining all patients' educational background, in combination with their employment history, will help the clinician present information to them in an appropriate manner.

RELIGIOUS AND SPIRITUAL FACTORS

Religious and spiritual beliefs are an inherent part of each person. Members of the same religion may interpret and apply religious doctrine in completely different ways. Catholics are taught by the Church that birth control is never an option, but a 34-year-old mother of three who has a new diagnosis of idiopathic pulmonary fibrosis may decide that this does not apply to her current situation (and her priest may concur!). Jehovah's Witnesses and Christian Scientists may or may not strictly adhere to their religious teachings. Asking patients what religion they belong to—and also how their beliefs may affect their health care—will provide patients with the opportunity to discuss their wishes.

CULTURAL FACTORS AND HEALTH BELIEFS

In the same way that religious beliefs affect patients' attitudes toward their disease and its treatment, cultural background can have an enormous impact on how illness is regarded by both patient and family. Asian and Middle Eastern immigrants often regard Americans as being too direct.[2,3] When working with a patient from one of these cultural groups, the caregiver will accomplish more by taking the time to exchange pleasantries with the patient and family members for a few minutes before jumping into specific questions about illness and treatment. Native-born Americans from English-speaking backgrounds need to keep in mind that many cultural groups consider casualness (e.g., the use of first names) to be rude and insulting behavior. It is preferable simply to introduce oneself to a patient and ask "How should I address you?" Mispronunciation of names can also cause offense. Nonverbal communication (body language) varies between cultures also, so that sitting on patients' beds or touching their bodies (in what may be intended as a caring manner) may be interpreted as unwarranted intimacy.[4]

When the patient speaks English as a second language (or not at all), interpreters become invaluable. There are problems, however, that need to be considered. Does the interpreter have adequate knowledge of medical terms both to understand the clinician's questions and to elicit the needed information from the patient? The clinician may need to provide careful explanations to the interpreter about the kind of information needed from the patient. Interpreters who are adolescent or adult children of the patient are usually effective.

Health practices in various cultural groups may include the use of alternative healers (folk healers, faith healers, herbalists) or the use of home remedies. Medical personnel are seen as skilled technicians, whose role is to assist in the treatment of the disease, not to take over. The responsibility for the patient's healing remains with the patient and the patient's family.[5] Recall our 66-year-old woman who recently came to this country and lives with her son and his family: eliciting information from her and her son about her cultural background will provide the clinician with much needed help in determining what her goals are and how to best meet them.

CURRENT STRESSES

The patient with chronic respiratory disease has many potential stresses that are directly related to the illness. Loss of employment due to disability, loss of physical independence, and decreases in self-esteem, sexual potency, social interactions, and feelings of self-worth are all reported frequently among patients entering pulmonary rehabilitation programs.[6] Unfortunately these patients usually have other problems as well. Perhaps they are coping with an impending or recent divorce or are concerned about an adolescent daughter's illegitimate pregnancy. Granted, not every patient's concerns will be so dramatic, but by being aware of these problems and talking about them the clinician helps patients to focus on the immediate complaint that brought them to the clinician.

SUPPORT SYSTEMS

Interpersonal Support Systems

On whom can the patient count for help and support? Not every patient has a loving family, who will selflessly provide care for as long as is necessary. Are there friends, neighbors, or co-workers who will lend a hand? Religious groups often are a source of tremendous comfort and support. The severity of each patient's illness will determine how much support from others is necessary. Patients going home on mechanical ventilation will require long-term, active support (see Ch. 101), whereas patients with exertional dyspnea may be able to care for themselves at home by pacing most activities and may need help only with shopping.

Interactional Support Systems

Patients who do not have a close-knit circle of family and friends may be able to find much-needed support in societal groups. Social support is a buffer from the stresses of chronic illness. Patients feel cared for and become a member of a network of communication and mutual obligation,[7] in which they are able to give as well as receive support and strength. Interactional support groups can also provide needed relief for family members. The American Lung Association sponsors lung clubs for patients with chronic lung diseases. These groups offer nonconfrontational support, sharing of problems and solutions, and access to information. Other examples of societal support systems include social or special interest clubs (e.g., Elks lodge, knitting group), volunteer organizations, and neighbors.

PSYCHIATRIC AND SUBSTANCE USE HISTORY

Although many patients will have no history of psychiatric illness; depression, general dissatisfaction with life, and anxiety are the most common emotional reactions to COPD.[7–9] When these symptoms become severe enough to interfere with sleep or with the patient's daily routine, some type of pharmacotherapy may be needed. Because excessive sedation and bronchoconstriction are side effects of some antidepressant medications, these drugs must be used cautiously in pulmonary patients.

Most COPD patients will have a history of cigarette smoking, and some may still be smoking. Guilt over past and/or present smoking is an understandable emotion. Patients who have quit smoking deserve our praise, and those who continue to smoke need encouragement to quit (see Ch. 102). Continued substance abuse of any kind needs to be addressed openly with the patient.

FUNCTIONAL LEVEL

Prior to developing chronic respiratory disease, was the patient's life different? The former farm worker probably led a vigorous life, while the aerospace engineer's life was more sedentary. How did the patient cope with stresses or challenges? Perhaps the farm worker dealt with pressures by exerting himself physically, while the engineer smoked more cigarettes when feeling stressed.

The impact of a chronic respiratory illness on functional levels and coping behaviors varies from patient to patient. The former farm worker's vigorous life and coping behaviors have both been dramatically curtailed by dyspnea. The aerospace engineer's sedentary life-style has not required major adjustments due to dyspnea, but his coping behavior of cigarette smoking must change, and this will, at least temporarily, increase stress.

ATTITUDES AND PERCEPTIONS

Quality of life must be assessed from the patient's point of view, not the caregiver's, in order to avoid drawing inappropriate conclusions regarding what is and what is not acceptable.[10,11] What activities does the patient value, and are these possible in view of current limitations? The components of the psychosocial assessment (Table 60-1) should provide the information needed to answer these questions. There are many formal tools with which to measure the patient's emotional adjustment to chronic illness[12–20] (Table 60-2), but they are lengthy and in most cases are better suited to the research setting than to everyday clinical practice.

What is the patient's understanding of the diagnosis? Does the patient understand that the condition is chronic and not curable and have accurate perceptions regarding the prognosis? A patient whose perceptions are realistic is likely to follow through with long-term care plans and chronic medication regimens. Setting attainable goals will provide both

Table 60-2. Psychosocial Assessment Tools

Instrument	Comments	Reference
Sickness Impact Profile	Impact of physical disability on daily activities	12
Profile of Mood States	Self-report of affect	13
Quality of Well-Being	Comprehensive outcome measure of health status and life quality	14
Minnesota Multiphasic Personality Inventory	Multidimensional assessment of personality characteristics	15
McMaster Health Index Questionnaire (MHIQ)	Self-report of physical, social and emotional functioning	16
State-Trait Anxiety Inventory	Self-report of anxiety	17
Beck Depression Inventory	Self-report of depression	18
Meaning of Illness Questionnaire (MIQ)	Self-report of stress, impact of illness, and response to illness	19
COPD Self-Efficacy Scale	Self-report of situational dyspnea	20

patient and caregiver with a much needed sense of accomplishment.

The aerospace engineer is likely to have had several exposures to the health care system over his lifetime. He has enjoyed the benefits of health insurance, and while he may never have had a problem more serious than heartburn, in all likelihood he and members of his family have experienced long- and short-term health care and hospitalizations. The recent immigrant to the United States, however, is unlikely to have had experience with such a sophisticated and confusing health care system. Both she and her family may well be baffled by the process of seeing a primary care physician, a pulmonary specialist, pulmonary function technicians, respiratory therapists, pharmacists, social workers, and so on. Patients who have had prior experience with a chronic illness (either personally or in a family member) will be more likely to have realistic expectations about their care.

Adaptive ability is defined as the patient's ability to adapt to existing environments.[21] Is the patient a person with a history of adapting easily to change or a person who resists change? Living with chronic respiratory disease will require change and adaptation for each patient, if not at the time of diagnosis then later as the disease progresses. Caregivers should discuss ways in which patients can adapt to their limitations and should combine treatment instructions with positive expectations, not threats of dire consequences.[21]

PSYCHOSOCIAL RESOURCES IN THE COMMUNITY

Resources available to patients vary tremendously from one community to the next. Generally, smaller, more remote areas have less to offer than larger towns and cities. The hospital social worker is a valuable contact person, who will be able to help with financial concerns as well as direct patients to the most appropriate and available resources. Examples of types of social resources that may be available in the community are listed in Table 60-3.

Table 60-3. Examples of Psychosocial Resources in the Community[a]

Visiting nurses
Chore service (e.g., for help with housework)
Meals on wheels
Home health aides (help with bathing, etc.)
Adult daycare programs
Hospices
Nursing homes
Group homes
Support groups (e.g., lung clubs)
Smoking cessation programs
Pulmonary rehabilitation programs
Counseling (e.g., for depression, marital counseling)
Substance abuse programs
Welfare caseworkers
Emergency services (e.g., food banks, shelters)

[a] Specific resources vary in different communities, but these illustrate the range of available resources in an urban area.

HOW TO USE PSYCHOSOCIAL INFORMATION IN PATIENT CARE

Patients with chronic respiratory disease are often difficult for the clinician to treat. Patients (and their families) may feel that they are being cheated by life and be less likely to express appreciation to the caregivers.[21] The interest that a caregiver demonstrates when talking about such a patient's background, family, and concerns improves the relationship between them. Realistic goals for patients like this may include relief or alleviation of symptoms, minimizing the effect of the disease on the patients' lives, and helping them to live meaningful lives (according to their own definition) by maximizing their individual potential.[21–24] The psychosocial assessment will provide the information needed to achieve these goals. Helping patients to accept the diagnosis and prognosis and making plans for future hospitalizations and terminal care will be easier when the clinician's goal is to care for (not cure) patients with chronic respiratory disease.

References

1. Webster's New World Dictionary of the American Language. 2nd College Ed. World Publishing, New York, 1970, p. 1147
2. Anderson JN: Health and illness in Filipino immigrants. West J Med 1983;139:811–819
3. Lipson JG, Meleis AI: Issues in health care of Middle Eastern patients. West J Med 1983;139:854–861
4. Hartog J, Hartog EA: Cultural aspects of health and illness behavior in hospitals. West J Med 1983;139:910–916
5. Clark MM: Cultural context of medical practice. West J Med 1983;139:806–810
6. Make BJ, Paine R: Pulmonary rehabilitation for COPD patients. Hosp Pract 1987;22:26–27, 31–34
7. Hunter SM, Hall SS: The effect of an educational support program on dyspnea and the emotional status of COPD clients. Rehabil Nurs 1989;14:200–202
8. Williams SJ: Chronic respiratory illness and disability: A critical review of the psychosocial literature. Soc Sci Med 1989;28:791–803
9. Sandhu HS: Psychosocial Issues in chronic obstructive pulmonary disease. Clin Chest Med 1986;7:629–642
10. Hudson LD: Quality of life in patients with pulmonary disease. 2nd International Colloquium on Progress in Pulmonary Medicine: New Perspectives on Bronchospastic Disorders and the Quality of Life, Deauville, France, June 17–23, 1989
11. Jones PW, Baveystock CM, Littlejohns P: Relationships between general health measured with the sickness impact profile and respiratory symptoms, physiological measures, and mood in patients with chronic airflow limitation. Am Rev Respir Dis 1989;140:1538–1543
12. Bergner M, Bobbit RA, Pollard WE: The Sickness Impact Profile: Validation of a health status measure. Med Care 1976;14:57–67
13. McNair DM, Lorr M, Droppleman LF: EDITS Manual for the Profile of Mood States. Educational and Industrial Testing Service, San Diego, 1971
14. Fanshel F, Bush JW: A health status index and its applications to health services outcomes. Operations Res 1970;18:1021–1066
15. Dahlstrom WG, Welsh GS, Dahlstrom LE: An MMPI Handbook. Rev. Ed. University of Minnesota, Minneapolis, 1972
16. Chambers LW, MacDonald LA, Tugwell P: The McMaster health index questionnaire as a measure of the quality of life for patients with rheumatoid disease. J Rheumatol 1982;9:780–784

17. Speilberger CD, Gorsuch RL, Lushene RE: Manual for the State-Trait Anxiety Inventory. Consulting Psychologist Press, Palo Alto, CA, 1970
18. Beck AT, Rush AJ, Shaw BF: Cognitive Therapy of Depression. Guilford Publications, New York, 1979
19. Browne GB, Byrne C, Roberts J et al: The meaning of illness questionnaire: Reliability and validity. Nurs Res 1988;37:368–373
20. Wigal JW, Creer TL, Kostes H: The COPD self-efficacy scale. Chest 1991;99:1193–1196
21. Dudley DL, Sitzman J: Psychosocial and psychophysiologic approach to the patient. Semin Respir Med 1979;1:59–83
22. McDonald GJ: A home care program for patients with chronic lung disease. Nurs Clin North Am 1981;16:259–273
23. Davido J: Pulmonary rehabilitation. Nurs Clin North Am 1981;16:275–283
24. Renfroe KL: Effect of progressive relaxation on dyspnea and state anxiety in patients with chronic obstructive pulmonary disease. Heart Lung 1988;17:408–413.

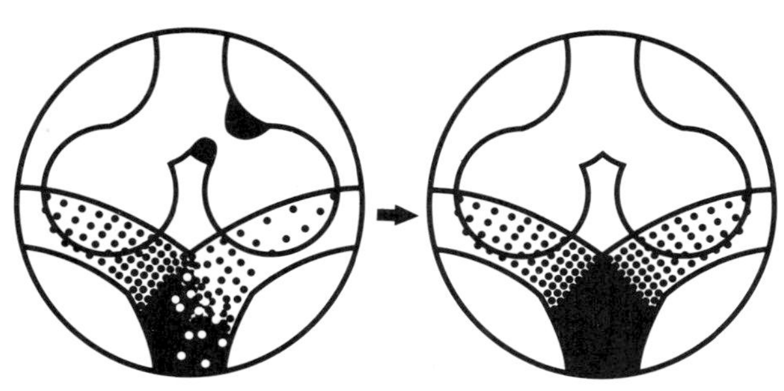

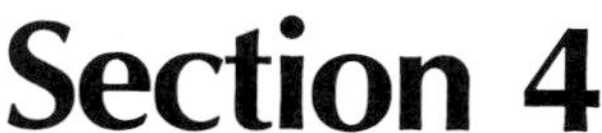

Section 4

Clinical Approach to the Patient with Respiratory Disease

Chapter 61

Cardinal Symptoms and Signs in Respiratory Disease

Nirmal B. Charan
Paula Carvalho

CHAPTER OUTLINE

Respiratory disorders clinically manifest with a great variety of symptoms and signs. Certain manifestations will be more indicative of local disease, whereas others will signify more generalized pulmonary disorders. In addition, a given symptom or sign may be associated with entirely different clinical syndromes. For example, exertional dyspnea quite frequently occurs in patients with widespread pulmonary fibrosis as well as in those with anemia. Subtle variations in symptoms may also characterize distinctive disorders. A persistent nonproductive cough in a patient with orthopnea and pedal edema has different implications than a nonproductive cough in a heavy smoker with recent weight loss.

It is also essential to consider the complete clinical picture when evaluating a patient, as certain interrelationships between symptoms and signs will characterize distinct disease processes. For instance, the mechanism for hemoptysis in a patient with dyspnea and mitral stenosis is different than that in a patient with Goodpasture's syndrome. The clinician must therefore be able to interpret the symptoms and signs of pulmonary disease in the context of the patient's pre-existing physical status and must consider the predisposition, onset, and progression of disease in order to arrive at the correct diagnosis. This chapter discusses the features and implications of 12 symptoms, signs, and/or clinical presentations with which clinicians involved in respiratory care should be familiar.

COUGH

Cough is a complex reflex that normally results from stimulation of the bronchial mucosa in the region between the larynx and the second-order bronchi. In healthy people it is a normal response to aspiration of inhaled or aspirated particles or, in rare instances, to pressure in the external auditory canal. Cough can also be a harbinger of serious disease in that it may result from a new growth in the airway or an inflammatory pleural process.

Pathophysiology

Two sites for cough receptors in the lung have been postulated, one in the airway epithelium and the other in the deeper airway structures.[1] It has been suggested that the mucosal receptors respond to stimuli that directly contact the airway, whereas receptors in the deeper structures respond to mechanical distortion of the airways. There is a dense distribution of receptors at the tracheal bifurcation and at points of bronchial branching. Quantitatively, airway receptors are more concentrated in the larger, proximal airways than in the smaller, distal branches of the tracheobronchial tree.[1] Cough receptors are also thought to exist in the paranasal sinuses, pleurae, diaphragm, and pericardium, as cough may be associated with disease processes affecting these structures.[2] Irritation of the external auditory canal can also produce cough by vagal stimulation.[3]

Cough stimuli are of three common types: mechanical stimuli, such as that resulting in airway distortion by extrabronchial masses, pulmonary fibrosis, or lobar atelectasis; inflammatory stimuli, such as inhaled particles and fumes from cigarette smoke; and psychogenic cough, which is a diagnosis of exclusion. Cough can be voluntary or involuntary. The first step in the cough mechanism is inspiration of a variable amount of gas above functional residual capacity (FRC). The advantage of inhaling larger amounts of air is the resulting optimized length-tension relationship of the expiratory muscles, whose function is thereby improved. The glottis closes and intrapleural pressure increases because of thoracic and abdominal expiratory muscle contraction. As the pleural pressure increases, the alveolar gas is compressed and lung volume decreases. The glottis then opens suddenly, and air is forcefully expelled through the airways. When the glottis opens, pressure in the central intrathoracic airways drops toward atmospheric levels, but the alveolar and pleural pressures continue to rise. This combination of high intrapleural and intra-alveolar pressures results in high expiratory flow rates, and the burst of air removes particulate matter from the airways.

A pressure drop occurs in the airways between the alveoli and the mouth because of the frictional heat gain and the acceleration of gas molecules (Bernoulli principle). Airway pressure then becomes smaller than pleural pressure at a point between the trachea and the peripheral airways, and these airways become compressed as a result of high intrapleural and intra-alveolar pressures. Flow in these segments is limited by dynamic airway compression, the location at which the flow-limiting mechanism operates being known as the *equal pressure point*. This point is normally located near the carina at high lung volumes but shifts to the peripheral airways as lung volumes decrease and the airways narrow. Dynamic compression of the intrathoracic airways is essential to an effective cough, as the linear velocities of gas are higher in the narrowed segment, which results in more efficient movement of secretions from the airway wall. The lung volume at which the cough mechanism takes place ultimately determines the cough effectiveness. Only particles downstream (toward the mouth) from the equal pressure point can be removed. A series of uninterrupted coughs moves the equal pressure point from the large, proximal airways to the smaller, distal airways as lung volumes become smaller with each cough. This mechanism allows cleansing of the deeper part of the lungs.

Causes

Acute Infection

Viral respiratory infections account for the majority of episodes of cough in all age groups. Cough is thought to be triggered by stimulation of receptors in the paranasal sinuses, larynx, pharynx, and tracheobronchial tree. Cough occurring with viral infection is usually paroxysmal, may be productive or nonproductive, and is associated with other symptoms such as sore throat and rhinorrhea. A viral illness may lead to a chronic cough syndrome associated with hyperreactive airways.[4] Postviral cough is usually transient but may be prolonged for weeks and may be exacerbated by exercise and by cold air.

Bacterial infection of the upper respiratory tract may cause cough by stimulating receptors in the sinuses and retropharynx. Sinus tenderness, headache, and fever are generally also present. Bronchopneumonia usually presents initially as acute bronchitis. Patients with normal airway function generally are not susceptible to bacterial tracheobronchitis; however, patients with chronic obstructive pulmonary disease (COPD) are commonly infected with *Streptococcus pneumoniae* and *Haemophilus influenzae*.[5] In these patients excess secretions that overwhelm the mucociliary clearance mechanism may produce cough by direct stimulation of the tracheobronchial receptors. Mycoplasmas and *Legionella* spp. often cause tracheobronchitis, resulting in a paroxysmal cough productive of scant, often blood-tinged sputum.[2]

Chronic Infection

Bronchiectasis is an uncommon condition in the postantibiotic era; however, it was second only to tuberculosis in the 1950s. Bronchiectasis may result from infections such as tuberculosis or from viral infections occurring before 5 years of age. Cough is the most common symptom in bronchiectasis and is productive of copious amounts of mucopurulent sputum, often more than a cupful a day. Tuberculosis or chronic fungal infections may present with a persistent cough and blood-tinged sputum. Tuberculosis of the larynx is associated with painful swallowing, in addition to cough and radiographic evidence of pulmonary involvement.

Cough in patients with COPD is a result of chronic bronchitis due to direct irritation of receptors by cigarette smoke, increased secretions, and decreased mucociliary clearance. A productive cough is usually present in these patients and is by definition present for more than 3 consecutive months and for at least 2 years.[6]

Asthma

Cough in asthma may be associated with wheezing and dyspnea or may be the only symptom. In the latter cases cough is described as intractable, paroxysmal, and nonproductive. In asthma cough may induce bronchospasm and vice versa. When comparative pulmonary function tests were performed in a series of asthmatic patients with cough or with dyspnea,[7] the patients with cough had a moderately severe obstructive pattern and increased airway resistance, apparently because of increased resistance to flow in the proximal airways, where cough receptors are more numerous; in the patients with dyspnea, obstruction was present in the small airways, where cough receptors are rare. In asthmatic patients cough and bronchospasm may cause further distortion of the airways, which then causes more coughing and bronchoconstriction.

A type of cough-variant asthma also exists in which pulmonary function tests are normal unless provoked with methacholine or other bronchoconstricting agents. A response to methacholine is not necessarily diagnostic of asthma, but nevertheless bronchodilator therapy is appropriate.[2]

Tumors

Cough occurs in the majority of patients with lung cancer but is the earliest presenting sign in less than 20 percent of patients.[8] Bronchogenic carcinoma is associated with nonproductive or productive cough for weeks, and hemoptysis is often present. The nature of the cough in alveolar cell carcinoma may be the same as in bronchogenic carcinoma, but occasionally copious amounts of watery sputum may be produced.[9]

Miscellaneous Causes

Aortic aneurysms may cause a brassy cough, and mediastinal tumors may result in cough associated with dyspnea due to compression of the bronchi or trachea.[2] Cough in patients with idiopathic pulmonary fibrosis is likely caused by distortion of the airways and may be worsened by deep breathing. Cough in these patients is usually chronic and nonproductive.[10]

Drug-induced cough has been reported with beta-blockers,[11] angiotensin-converting enzyme inhibitors,[12] and amiodarone.[13] Left ventricular failure may cause cough, which may be aggravated by lying down and is often associated with dyspnea.[14] Psychogenic cough is a diagnosis of exclusion; cough in this circumstance is nonproductive and does not occur while sleeping. Aspiration may cause cough in patients with swallowing difficulties or in those with esophageal disorders.

Approach to Diagnosis and Management

The history and physical examination (see Ch. 44) offer the correct diagnosis in the majority of cases of cough. Pulmonary function tests and, if necessary, airway challenge testing are important to demonstrate fixed, reversible, or inducible airflow obstruction. Chest and sinus radiographic examinations and laryngoscopy are useful; however, a study by Poe et al.[15] indicates that bronchoscopy has a low diagnostic yield. In patients with suspected aspiration, a barium swallow may be useful.

Treatment of cough has to be aimed at the specific cause. Asthma is managed with inhaled or oral beta-agonist drugs, and theophylline preparations are also effective. Corticosteroids and aerosolized cromolyn are also useful in cough-variant asthma. Antihistamines and decongestants are used in rhinitis, and antibiotic courses are vital for management of both upper and lower respiratory tract bacterial infections. Antitussives may be used for a chronic cough if it is not serving a beneficial effect. Mucolytic agents are thought by some to have a role in management of chronic bronchitis.[16]

HEMOPTYSIS

Hemoptysis refers to the coughing up of blood from the respiratory tract below the level of the larynx and can be due to many causes.[17]

Pathophysiology

The lungs receive a dual blood supply: the pulmonary circulation is a low-pressure system, whereas the bronchial circulation is a high-pressure system arising from the systemic vasculature.[18] These circulations are connected by numerous bronchopulmonary anastomoses. Hemorrhage from the bronchial arteries tends to be more severe because of the pressure gradient from the systemic to the pulmonary circulation.[18] Conditions that may result in bronchial arterial bleeding include tuberculosis, bronchiectasis, bronchial arteriovenous malformations, tumor, and mitral stenosis.

In tuberculosis, hemoptysis is more common in inactive disease, in which it results from rupture of small vessels,

Table 61-1. Relatively Frequent Causes of Hemoptysis

Causes
Pulmonary
Infectious
Bronchitis
Tuberculosis
Pneumonia
Cystic fibrosis
Parasites
Bronchiectasis
Lung abscess
Mycetoma
Fungal infections
Noninfectious
Bronchogenic carcinoma
Foreign body
Trauma
Bronchoscopy
Idiopathic pulmonary hemosiderosis
Cocaine-induced
Acute lupus pneumonitis
Bronchial adenoma
Coagulation defects
Post-needle biopsy
Goodpasture's syndrome
Wegener's granulomatosis
Cardiovascular
Pulmonary embolism with infarction
Left ventricular failure
Mitral stenosis
Arteriovenous malformation

unsupported because of extensive fibrosis and parenchymal destruction, that become dilated. Bronchiectasis is associated with exuberant proliferation of the bronchial circulation and formation of large bronchopulmonary anastomoses, which may bleed.[18] Primary neoplasms of the lung are supplied by the bronchial circulation, and hemoptysis may result from tumor invasion of hypervascular mucosa. Hypertrophied bronchial veins are associated with mitral stenosis and can rupture as a result of elevated intravascular pressures. In left ventricular failure, hemoptysis results from rupture of pulmonary capillaries and veins. The inflamed, vascular mucosa in tracheobronchitis may bleed. Other mechanisms for hemoptysis include pulmonary infarction and vasculitis.

Causes

Hemoptysis can be a prominent symptom of many pulmonary diseases (Table 61-1). However, the more important causes of hemoptysis are infection, neoplasms, trauma, and cardiovascular disease. Cocaine abuse and bleeding disorders, including anticoagulant use, are also discussed.

Infection

Infection is the most common cause of hemoptysis. Bronchitis and bronchiectasis are responsible for hemoptysis in 20 to 40 percent of cases. Pneumonia may cause hemoptysis, and some organisms such as *Pseudomonas* and *Aspergillus* invade the pulmonary vasculature and cause in situ thrombosis, infarction, and bleeding. Chronic granulomatous infections such as tuberculosis, lung abscess, and parasitic infections such as amebiasis and *Paragonimus westermani* infestation account for a large proportion of hemoptysis cases.

Neoplasm

Hemoptysis in patients over 40 years of age is often due to bronchogenic carcinoma. Bronchial adenomas are slow-growing vascular tumors, which may bleed profusely, and benign tumors such as bronchial carcinoids often cause bleeding, which is difficult to stop. Tumors metastatic to the lung do not often cause hemoptysis, as few impinge on the airways.

Trauma

Direct or penetrating chest trauma is often followed by hemoptysis. Inhalation of smoke or toxins can also cause bleeding due to necrosis of the bronchial epithelium.[19] After lung resection, a hemothorax may drain into the airways; this condition requires immediate surgical intervention.

Cardiovascular Disease

Pulmonary venous hypertension, such as that found with left ventricular failure or mitral stenosis, may result in periodic hemoptysis. Under these conditions hemosiderin is often present inside alveolar macrophages. Bronchial venous bleeding may also result from mitral stenosis, as bronchial veins proliferate and markedly hypertrophy in this disorder. Hemoptysis can also result from pulmonary thromboembolic disease, especially when lung infarction occurs,[20] and is then generally accompanied by pleuritic chest pain and a small pleural effusion.

Cocaine Abuse

Pulmonary complications of cocaine abuse are becoming increasingly recognized. Free-base cocaine ("crack") is obtained by extraction from the solvent layer of a mixture of cocaine hydrocholoride, an alkaline solution (baking soda), and a solvent (ether or alcohol), which yields the drug in nearly pure form. This form of cocaine, when injected intravenously or smoked in a water pipe, rapidly reaches high levels in the bloodstream. Up to 25 percent of free-base users have hemoptysis, as well as cough, dyspnea, and chest pain.[21] Pulmonary hemorrhage with respiratory failure has also been reported after inhaling free-base cocaine.

Miscellaneous

Bleeding disorders such as thrombocytopenic purpura and hemophilia, as well as anticoagulant use, may be associated with hemoptysis. Hemoptysis is life-threatening in condi-

Table 61-2. Most Likely Causes of Hemoptysis in Certain Patient Groups

Healthy Nonsmoker (under age of 40)	"Healthy" Cigarette Smoker	COPD	Granulomatous Lung Disease (e.g., Tuberculosis)	Chronic Alcoholism
Bronchitis	Bronchitis	Lung cancer	Bronchiectasis	Tuberculosis
Pneumonia	Lung cancer	Bronchitis	Tuberculosis	Lung abscess
Pulmonary infarction	Pneumonia	Bronchiectasis	Lung cancer	Necrotizing pneumonia
Bronchial adenoma			Aspergillosis	Lung cancer
Arteriovenous malformation			Bronchitis	Foreign body
				Bronchiectasis
				Chest trauma

tions such as Goodpasture's syndrome or idiopathic pulmonary hemosiderosis. Sarcoidosis, cystic fibrosis, and broncholithiasis are other disorders that may predispose to hemoptysis.

Approach to Diagnosis

Although the list of possible causes of hemoptysis is extensive, two or three most likely etiologies can usually be identified in an individual patient, by the history and clinical circumstances. The most likely causes in five commonly encountered patient groups are listed in Table 61-2. Other considerations that influence the probability of various diagnoses include geographic factors, such as the increased likelihood of tuberculosis in developing countries, paragonimiasis in Southeast Asia, or coccidioidomycosis in the southwestern United States; population base; coexisting disease, such as pulmonary infarction in postsurgical patients and in patients with congestive heart failure or coagulopathy and opportunistic infection in patients who have undergone organ transplantation and those receiving chemotherapy; and associated symptoms, such as cancer and tuberculosis in patients with anorexia and weight loss, pneumonia and bronchiectasis in patients with fever and purulent sputum or pulmonary infarction in patients with phlebitis and pleuritic chest pain.

The history and physical examination as well as a chest radiograph usually provide the diagnosis in many cases of hemoptysis. Standard laboratory tests, including coagulation studies and urinalysis, may reveal thrombocytopenia, coagulopathy, or renal disease. Leukocytosis may signify infection, and hyponatremia may be present with carcinoma, pneumonia, or tuberculosis. Abnormal renal function and urinalysis can be suggestive of Goodpasture's syndrome or Wegener's granulomatosis. Sputum examination and tuberculin skin testing with an anergy panel are part of the evaluation. An electrocardiogram (ECG) may show evidence of acute right ventricular strain, suggestive of pulmonary embolism.

The etiology and site of bleeding may be identified by fiberoptic bronchoscopy. This procedure is used mainly to evaluate the airways for malignancy, as lesions may be present in up to 16 percent of patients with normal chest x-rays.[22] Bronchoscopy is recommended in patients with mild to moderate hemoptysis and risk factors such as age over 40, long smoking history, weight loss, and persistent cough.[23] Patients with massive hemoptysis require urgent rigid bronchoscopy to localize the site of bleeding.

Selective bronchial arteriography (SBA) may assist in localizing the site of bleeding that was not found by bronchoscopy. This procedure may be complicated by myelitis, as the spinal arteries communicate with the bronchial arteries via the intercostal trunks in approximately 5 percent of patients.[24]

Other diagnostic tests, such as ventilation/perfusion ($\dot{V}/\dot{Q}$) scans and pulmonary angiography, may be indicated if pulmonary embolism with infarction is suspected. Bronchography is no longer commonly used but is primarily helpful in evaluating for bronchiectasis. Computed tomography (CT) of the chest with contrast injection may detect pulmonary masses or vascular abnormalities such as aneurysms.

Despite all diagnostic procedures, hemoptysis remains unexplained in 5 to 10 percent of patients. Such *"essential hemoptysis"* usually carries a good prognosis.

Approach to Management

Management of hemoptysis depends on the amount and rate of bleeding (Table 61-3). Mild hemoptysis (less than 25 mL in 24 hours) may be treated conservatively, with management of the predisposing problem. Patients with moderate hemoptysis (25 to 500 mL in 24 hours) may require hospitalization and bed rest. Antibiotics, if indicated, O_2, bronchodilators, and suctioning may be necessary. If the decision is made to manage hemoptysis nonsurgically, positioning the patient with the site of bleeding downward may prevent aspiration of blood into the nonbleeding lung. Careful postural drainage may also be employed. The management of massive hemoptysis (more than 500 mL in 24 hours) is an emergency, as death by asphyxiation may occur. Air-

Table 61-3. Classification of Hemoptysis by Volume of Blood Expectorated

Mild	<25 mL in 24 hours
Moderate	25–500 mL in 24 hours
Massive	>500 mL in 24 hours

way protection is essential, and intubation with a single or double-lumen endotracheal tube may be necessary. Selective bronchial artery injection with coagulant material has been used with some success,[25] and combined balloon occlusion of a small pulmonary artery and bronchial arterial embolization may be used in cases in which hemoptysis persists because of a bronchial-pulmonary anastomosis.[26] Surgical resection of the area of lung containing the bleeding site may be needed if the site has been localized and if medical therapy fails. In some cases pneumonectomy may be necessary.

CYANOSIS

The term *cyanosis* denotes the blue skin and mucous membrane color that occurs when increased amounts of desaturated hemoglobin are present. It implies arterial hypoxemia but is not necessarily a reliable sign of its presence. Cyanosis depends on the amount of reduced hemoglobin present in the blood and may be pronounced in conditions of decreased blood flow, such as congestive heart failure, and in polycythemia, in which increased amounts of hemoglobin are present. When hemoglobin levels are low, as in severe anemia, cyanosis is not apparent despite a low O_2 content. Cyanosis may be purely a peripheral phenomenon or may be associated with cardiac disease, pulmonary disease, or methemoglobinemia.

Causes

Peripheral Cyanosis

Peripheral cyanosis is often found in normal individuals and is due to simple vasoconstriction, which may be easily corrected by warming the hands and feet. Peripheral cyanosis may also be present in patients with decreased cardiac output and accompanying peripheral vasoconstriction as O_2 is extracted from the peripheral capillaries and reduced hemoglobin becomes evident.

Cardiac Disease

The presence of cyanosis in infants, young children, and young adults is generally caused by right-to-left shunts of cyanotic congenital heart disease. In older adults, however, cardiac-related cyanosis is usually associated with congestive heart failure or cyanotic cor pulmonale.

The distribution of cyanosis (which is usually accompanied by clubbing) is diagnostically important: in congenital heart disease, identical cyanosis and clubbing of both hands and feet indicate an intracardiac right-to-left shunt. Differential cyanosis and clubbing, such as that present in the feet but not in the hands, represents a right-to-left shunt through a patent ductus arteriosus with an intact ventricular septum. In this congenital abnormality, pulmonary vascular resistance is higher than systemic resistance, and mixed venous blood from the pulmonary artery flows through the ductus and enters the aorta at or distal to the left subclavian artery, causing cyanosis of the lower extremities. In another form of differential cyanosis and clubbing, the hands are affected more than the feet; this occurs when the aorta arises from the right ventricle, resulting in cyanosed hands, and the pulmonary trunk is right ventricular or biventricular, and originates just above a patent ventricular septal defect. In this condition oxygenated blood from the left ventricle enters the pulmonary trunk and then flows through a patent ductus arteriosus (again, because pulmonary vascular resistance exceeds systemic) into the descending aorta and to the lower extremities, which results in relatively noncyanotic feet.

Pulmonary Disease

Lung disorders, such as COPD, pneumonia, and pulmonary vascular disease, may cause arterial hypoxemia secondary to $\dot{V}/\dot{Q}$ inequalities. In addition, patients with interstitial disease may develop cyanosis because of hemoglobin desaturation with exercise.

Methemoglobinemia

Methemoglobinemia is an hereditary or drug-induced condition that may result in cyanosis. The hemoglobin molecule is unable to bind O_2 or CO_2, as ferrous iron is oxidized to ferric iron. The PaO_2 is normal. Methemoglobinemia is generally asymptomatic unless concentrations of methemoglobin exceed 25 percent, after which point headaches and dizziness may occur. Intravenous methylene blue is used for the treatment of symptomatic patients.

WHEEZING

Wheezes are defined as continuous sounds that are longer than 250 ms and high-pitched, with dominant frequency of 400 Hz or more. Wheezes may be audible to the unaided ear at some distance from the patient or by auscultation over the chest.

Pathophysiology

Wheezes are produced by the movement of air through narrow airways. When airway caliber is so narrow that opposite walls nearly touch one another, there is an increase in air velocity, which in turn causes a decrease in air pressure in that narrow segment of the airway (Bernouilli's principle). This causes further collapse of the airway. When the lumen has been reduced so much that the flow rate decreases, the process reverses and the pressure in the airway begins to increase, reopening the lumen of the airway. These repeated cyclic changes in lumen size result in generation of continuous sound. Forgacs[27] observed that the pitch of a wheeze is relatively independent of gas density. This means that the wheezes are not produced in the same way as the note of a pipe organ, in which a column of air vibrates and the pitch of the tone depends on both the length of the pipe and on the density of the gas in the pipe. By contrast, the pitch of a wheeze depends on the velocity of airflow and the degree of airway narrowing rather than on the length of the airway. Thus, wheezing is always associated with airway narrowing, but airway narrowing may not necessarily be accompanied by wheezing because airflow is needed to produce sound. If severe airway obstruction has caused airflow to decrease markedly, wheezing may not be heard.

Whether wheezes have one pitch or many depends on whether sound is being generated by a single narrowed bronchus or by many bronchi. Thus, if a major bronchus is obstructed (e.g., by a foreign body), only one pitch may be heard. Furthermore, wheezes may be inspiratory, expiratory, or both. If the narrowing affects a large bronchus and the stenosis is comparatively rigid, as when a tumor occludes the bronchus, the wheeze may be present during both inspiration and expiration. If the constricted airway is not rigid, a wheeze may intensify or change in pitch during inspiration and expiration because of change in airway caliber. This may happen in patients with asthma; with the onset of an asthmatic attack, when the bronchospasm is mild, wheezes may be heard only during expiration because airway diameter is narrower during expiration, but as bronchospasm increases in severity, wheezes may be heard during both inspiration and expiration. It must also be emphasized that the transmission of wheezing sounds through the airways is better than the transmission of the sound through the lung parenchyma to the chest wall and therefore listening over the trachea may at times reveal wheezing when auscultation of the chest is not that remarkable.

Wheezes have also been classified as random (monophonic) or simultaneous (polyphonic). The random-onset wheezes can be inspiratory or expiratory and may start and end at different times. These wheezes are classically heard in asthma. Simultaneous-onset wheezes are expiratory sounds consisting of several harmonically unrelated musical tones that tend to start and end simultaneously. They can be heard in a normal individual during a forceful expiration as the end of the vital capacity is approached. They are also heard in patients with COPD, in whom they are produced by dynamic compression of airways.

Differential Diagnosis

There are many diseases that can result in narrowing of the airway and thus are associated with wheezing (Table 61-4).

Asthma is the most common cause of diffuse wheezing. The conditions that lead to airway narrowing and hence wheezing in asthma include reversible bronchoconstriction, edema of the bronchial mucosa, mucus secretion, and smooth muscle hypertrophy. It has been suggested that the wheeze duration as a portion of respiratory cycle duration and the frequency of the sound are associated with the degree of bronchospasm, whereas the intensity of wheeze sound is not.[28] It appears that with increasing severity of asthma, the duration of the wheeze in relation to the total respiratory cycle increases as does the frequency of the sound. However, the changes in sound frequency may be difficult to appreciate with auscultation alone.

Table 61-4. Differential Diagnosis of Wheezing

Upper Respiratory Tract
Angioedema
Foreign body
Large goiter
Infection
Tracheal stenosis
Tumor
Lower Respiratory Tract
Adenopathy pressing on bronchus
Asthma
Aspiration
Bronchiolitis
COPD
Foreign body
Vascular
Adult respiratory distress syndrome (ARDS)
Pulmonary edema
Pulmonary embolism
Extrathoracic
Carcinoid
Factitious
Vasculitis

Asthma-like wheezing has also been described in approximately one-third of patients who aspirate large amounts of gastric contents.[29] The wheeze is due to airway mucosal edema resulting from low pH and intraluminal obstruction. Chronic aspiration due to reflux of gastric acid can also cause wheezing and an asthma-like syndrome. In fact, reflux of acid into the lower esophagus without actual aspiration has been shown to cause wheezing. Wheezing resulting from foreign body aspiration depends on the size and shape of the object as well as the site of obstruction. In these situations wheezing is usually localized.

The mechanism of wheezing seen in patients with pulmonary edema, known as *cardiac asthma,* is less clear. It has been suggested that airway narrowing may occur because of development of mucosal edema, extrinsic compression of the airways by interstitial fluid, and a decrease in the transmural distending pressure that normally holds the airways open.[30] Patients with cardiac asthma usually do not response to inhaled bronchodilators, which suggests that bronchospasm is not associated with cardiac asthma.

Wheezing is an uncommon finding in patients with acute pulmonary embolism. It has been suggested that mediators released during platelet aggregation may occasionally cause significant bronchoconstriction and hence wheezing.

Diagnosis and Treatment

Although the characteristics of wheezing may correlate with the severity of airway obstruction, the diagnosis of airway obstruction should be confirmed by spirometry.[31] In the emergency department measurement of peak expiratory flow rate using a simple peak flowmeter can be very useful in assessment of the patient and monitoring of the response to bronchodilator therapy. Patients who wheeze because of asthma generally show a marked reversibility of airway obstruction with bronchodilators. Some patients who have a history of occasional wheezing but normal pulmonary function tests may need to be challenged with methacholine to document hyperreactivity of the airways. Assessment of flow-volume loops may be helpful in differentiating between extrathoracic and intrathoracic airway obstruction. A chest radiograph may provide useful information in patients who do not have a history of obstructive airway disease. Patients suspected of having a foreign body in the airways may need bronchoscopy to visualize the airways.

Treatment depends on the disease process responsible for wheezing. Bronchodilator therapy is the mainstay of treatment for patients with obstructive airway disease. Some patients with severe disease may need corticosteroid therapy.

STRIDOR

Inspiratory sounds may result from the narrowing of the glottis or subglottic region. Severe narrowing may cause stridor, a high-pitched inspiratory "crowing" sound accompanied by supraclavicular inspiratory retraction. It should be noted that slowly progressive upper airway obstruction may produce only a few symptoms until the degree of obstruction becomes very severe. Inspiratory wheezes without expiratory wheezes are sometimes suggestive of upper airway obstruction.

Epiglottitis, laryngeal edema, bilateral vocal cord paralysis, tracheal stenosis, foreign bodies, goiter, and tumors are some of the common causes of stridor. Flow-volume loops, radiologic examinations, and direct laryngoscopy and bronchoscopy will usually reveal the actual diagnosis. The treatment depends on the cause of airway obstruction. If a patient has severe laryngeal obstruction, an urgent tracheotomy may need to be performed.

DYSPNEA

The word *dyspnea* denotes disordered breathing (being derived from the Greek roots *dys*, abnormal or disordered, and *pnoia,* breath). Although dyspnea is probably the most common respiratory symptom, it is difficult to define.

Breathing is normally an unconscious act, and therefore a simplified definition of dyspnea is "an uncomfortable awareness of breathing." This respiratory sensation is usually described as *breathlessness* or *shortness of breath* by lay people. The severity and intensity of dyspnea may range from an awareness of breathing during exertion to an incapacitating state of intolerable respiratory distress even at rest. However, dyspnea, like pain, is subjective, and it involves both the perception of and the reaction to the sensation by the patient.

Pathophysiology

The exact pathophysiologic mechanisms leading to dyspnea are not well understood. Potential mechanisms can be divided into four major categories involving disturbances of chemosensitivity, pulmonary receptors, respiratory muscle receptors, and outgoing respiratory motor commands.[32]

Although both hypoxia and hypercarbia can cause severe dyspnea, it is not clear whether dyspnea is due to chemoreceptor stimulation or due to the accompanying increase in respiratory motor output activity and the resulting increase in ventilation. In experimental studies an increase in end-tidal PCO_2 ($P_{ET}CO_2$) by about 10 mmHg has been shown to produce dyspnea in normal healthy volunteers. However, dyspnea may occur and may be intense even in the presence of normal blood gases.

Dyspnea may occur when there is an increase in ventilation above the normal resting level, as happens physiologically with exercise. Dyspnea can also occur when there is an increase in elastic or resistive forces during active respiration. Initially, Campbell and Howell[33] postulated that dyspnea occurs when there is length-tension inappropriateness of the respiratory muscles. In essence, this means that if the change in length of the respiratory muscle is inappropriate for the tension produced relative to the subject's previous experience, the sensation of dyspnea ensues. Later, Campbell[34] modified this concept to include "mechanical inappropriateness," including phasic distortion in the chest. Thus, this theory takes into account that dyspnea is a complex sensation, which occurs in a given subject because the breathing apparatus is not performing as it ought to for a given respiratory drive.

Causes

Acute and chronic diseases of the lung are common causes of dyspnea. Common causes of acute dyspnea are listed below:

- Anxiety
- Chest trauma
  - Fractured ribs
  - Pulmonary contusion
    - Hemothorax
- Hemorrhage into the lung (e.g., Goodpasture's syndrome)
- Asthma
- Infections
- Acute bronchitis
- Pneumonia (bacterial, viral, fungal)
- Pneumothorax
- Pulmonary edema
- Pulmonary embolism

Table 61-5. Causes of Chronic Dyspnea

Respiratory
- Airway disease
  - Upper airway obstruction (e.g., carcinoma of the larynx)
  - Asthma
  - COPD
  - Bronchiectasis
  - Cystic fibrosis
  - Endobronchial obstruction (e.g., carcinoma, foreign body)
- Parenchymal lung diseases
- Interstitial lung disease (e.g., sarcoidosis, pulmonary interstitial fibrosis)
- Malignancy
- Chronic lung infections (mycobacterial disease, fungal infections, lung abscess)
- Pulmonary vascular disease
  - Arteriovenous malformations
  - Chronic pulmonary embolism
  - Pulmonary vasculitides
  - Pulmonary venous hypertension
- Pleural diseases
  - Pleural effusions
  - Pleural fibrosis
  - Malignancy (e.g., mesothelioma)
  - Diseases of the chest wall
- Deformities (e.g., kyphoscoliosis)
  - Severe thoracic burns
- Restrictive diaphragmatic movements (e.g., pregnancy, ascites)
- Diseases of the respiratory muscles
  - Myopathies
  - Multiple sclerosis
  - Motor neuron disease
  - Neuropathies (Guillain-Barré syndrome)
  - Myasthenia gravis

Cardiovascular
- Left ventricular failure
- Mitral valve disease
- Congenital heart disease
- Deconditioning

Anemia

Anxiety/psychogenic (hyperventilation syndrome)

Chronic dyspnea is probably the most common respiratory complaint. By itself it is not diagnostic of any lung disease, but there are a number of diseases (Table 61-5) in which dyspnea is a prominent symptom.

Hyperventilation Syndrome

Hyperventilation is an increase in alveolar ventilation that reduces $PaCO_2$, to subnormal levels. The mechanisms responsible for initiating and sustaining hyperventilation in patients without obvious pulmonary disease are unknown. Stressful situations are known to cause disturbance in the pattern of breathing even in normal subjects. It is possible that patients with the so-called hyperventilation syndrome have an over-responsiveness of the respiratory center to stress and have a hypocapnic "set point." Once hyperventilation is established, it is easy to maintain it; it has been found that a single deep inspiration and expiration can lower $PaCO_2$ by 7 to 16 mmHg. Therefore, only an occasional deep sigh superimposed on normal respiration can maintain the hyperventilation state.

Hyperventilation as a primary finding has numerous potential causes including the following:

- Neurologic disease
- Salicylate intoxication
- Hepatic failure
- Severe pain
- Asthma
- Interstitial lung disease
- Pulmonary vascular disease
- Psychogenic (e.g., anxiety)
- High altitude

Conditions such as interstitial lung diseases can cause hyperventilation because of excessive stimulation of lung receptors; the hyperventilation observed in high altitude is probably due to hypoxia, and salicylates cause hyperventilation by stimulating the respiratory centers. Patients with psychogenic hyperventilation syndrome often present to the emergency department complaining of severe dyspnea. This condition may affect as many as 10 percent of the general population at some point in their lives, and 50 to 90 percent of such patients complain of dyspnea. Characteristically they describe the sensation of dyspnea as an inability to take deep breaths, a sense of suffocation, or pressure in the chest. Individuals with hyperventilation syndrome also tend to sigh frequently.

Approach to Diagnosis

Patterns of dyspnea are at times sufficiently characteristic to warrant a separate designation. Episodes of dyspnea that wake patients from a sound sleep are called *paroxysmal nocturnal dyspnea*. These patients usually wake during the night with a sensation of suffocation from which they obtain some relief by sitting at the edge of the bed or walking around. This pattern of dyspnea is characteristically seen in patients with left ventricular cardiac failure. Onset or worsening of dyspnea on assuming a supine position is called *orthopnea;* this condition is found in patients with heart disease but may also occur in those with chronic lung disease and diaphragmatic muscle weakness. The inability to assume a supine position (instant orthopnea) is particularly characteristic of paralysis of both hemidiaphragms. The term *platypnea* denotes dyspnea that occurs in the upright position in patients with advanced portal cirrhosis and congenital vascular shunts in the lung. *Trepopnea* is a rare form of dyspnea that develops in either the right or left lateral decubitus position and may occur with a large unilateral pleural effusion, unilateral lung disease and unilateral obstruction of the airway. Recently it has been suggested that the terms *dyspnea* and

Table 61-6. Procedures and Tests That May Be Useful in Evaluating Patients with Dyspnea

History and physical examination (see Ch. 44)
Chest radiograph (see Ch. 57)
Pulmonary function tests, including lung volumes and diffusing capacity (see Chs. 45–48)
Cardiac assessment: ECG and echocardiogram (see Ch. 50)
Assessment of pulmonary vascular tree (i.e., ventilation/perfusion scan and angiogram (see Ch. 57)
Exercise testing (see Ch. 49)
Assessment of respiratory drive (see Ch. 66)
Assessment of diaphragmatic function (see Ch. 52)

breathlessness encompass multiple sensations, that these can be distinguished by patients, and that they may point toward certain disease processes.[35]

Patients who complain of dyspnea may need to have some or all of the tests shown in Table 61-6.

Approach to Treatment

There are currently no specific therapeutic modalities for the treatment of dyspnea as such, and management should be aimed primarily at the underlying disease process. However, several drugs seem to decrease the sensation of dyspnea. It has been reported that diazepam may provide some relief from breathlessness in patients with COPD.[36] This effect could not be confirmed in other studies, however, and diazepam has serious potential side effects in patients with COPD.[37] Similarly, dihydrocodeine was shown in a 1981 study to be helpful in relieving dyspnea and improving exercise tolerance in patients with COPD,[38] and in 1989, oral morphine was shown to decrease the sensation of breathlessness and improve the exercise tolerance in COPD patients.[39] However, since these drugs can have serious side effects in these patients, their use should still be considered investigational.

EDEMA

Edema is an accumulation of excessive fluid in the interstitial space, which may have a number of causes. Clinically, edema is either *pitting* or *nonpitting*. In pitting edema, pressure with a finger over the edematous area for 5 to 30 seconds leaves a depressed area. The cause of this pitting is translocation of edema fluid away from the area beneath the pressure point into the other tissue space. After the finger is removed, the fluid slowly flows back to its original space. In nonpitting edema the fluid can not be mobilized to other areas. The usual cause for this is coagulation of the proteins, particularly fibrinogen, in the tissue. For example, in infection or trauma large quantities of fluid may collect, but coagulation of the proteins entraps the fluid in the form of gel and thus prevents it from migrating. *Brawny edema* is the term used for edema that is due to the swelling of the tissue cells that may occur with cell trauma. This type of edema is also nonpitting.

Pathophysiology

Several mechanisms contribute to the formation of edema. *Increased capillary pressure* can occur as a result of any clinical condition that causes either venous obstruction or arteriolar dilatation. For instance, large venous clots in the inferior vena cava or deep venous thrombosis of the legs can cause edema of the legs. Obstruction of venous return to the heart may occur in pulmonary hypertension because of either chronic left heart failure or various lung diseases (cor pulmonale). *Decreased plasma proteins* result in a fall in plasma colloid oncotic pressure, which in turn reduces fluid reabsorption from the extravascular compartment. Because lymphatics are responsible for removal of fluid from the interstitium, *lymphatic obstruction* (e.g., by cancer, surgery, or radiation therapy) also results in edema formation. *Increased capillary permeability* is another important cause of edema. Capillaries become permeable when there is damage to the capillary endothelium, and this causes leakage of protein-rich fluid into the interstitium. The edema that occurs following burns is an example of increased capillary permeability.

Diagnosis and Treatment

It is important to diagnose the cause of edema. The patient's history may provide a clue. For example, edema of the leg about a week after surgery may suggest deep vein thrombosis. Ankle edema that becomes noticeable at the end of the day and subsides at rest may be a sign of early right heart failure due to pulmonary hypertension. Nephrotic syndrome and hypernephroma may occasionally cause thrombosis in the inferior vena cava and hence bilateral leg edema. Superior vena cava obstruction due to lung cancer or mediastinitis may present with arm and facial swelling along with distended neck veins.

The chest x-ray may reveal signs of pulmonary hypertension. Laboratory investigations such as impedance plethysmography or radiocontrast venography may reveal the site of venous obstruction. Measurement of serum albumin is indicated in proper clinical settings. An echocardiogram may be needed in some patients to evaluate cardiac function.

The treatment of edema depends on its cause. Anticoagulation therapy may be indicated in deep vein thrombosis for prevention of further clotting. Congestive heart failure may be treated by diuretics and other therapy aimed at decreasing intravascular volume. Very rarely, a patient may need intravenous infusion of albumin in an attempt to increase serum colloidal oncotic pressure.

CLUBBING

Digital clubbing is defined as a focal enlargement of the connective tissue in the terminal phalanges of the digits, especially on the dorsal surface. It is usually bilateral and symmetrical and involves both fingers and toes. Hippocrates is credited with the first recorded description of clubbing of the digits in 400 BC among patients with empyema, and therefore, clubbing is also called *hippocratic fingers*.

Normally the soft tissue that separates the base of the fingernail from the distal phalanx is less than 2 mm thick but in severe cases of clubbing, this thickness may increase to 4 or 5 mm. The connective tissue bed is enlarged by an increase in blood volume and interstitial edema. Generally there is no inflammation, although a mild infiltration of lymphocytes, eosinophils, and plasma cells is often present. Later, the edema is replaced by a thick mesh of collagen. In severe clubbing a mild periostitis of the terminal phalanges is often present. The shape and structure of the bone are usually normal.

Diagnosis

There are two diagnostic signs of clubbing, "floating" nails and alteration in the unguophalangeal angle. Both these signs occur because of the proliferation of the tissue between the nail plate and the bone. The floating nail can be demonstrated by applying gentle pressure to the end of the nail as if to move the nail toward and away from the bone. Normally the nail does not move, but in clubbing the tissue underlying the nail compresses easily, and therefore, the nail seems to float. The proximal edge of the fingernail is also palpable through the soft tissue just proximal to the cuticle.

Obliteration of the hyponychial angle is noted by inspecting the profile of the terminal digit. Normally the angle between the nail plate and the proximal part of the digit is 180 degrees or less, but with clubbing it increases to more than 180 degrees (Fig. 61-1). Convexity of the nail appears after the above two signs; it is not a diagnostic sign of clubbing and may occur without clubbing. Normally, the nail on its long axis has a very long radius, but as the clubbing develops, the radius becomes shorter.

Recently the ratio of the distal phalangeal depth (DPD) to the interphalangeal depth (IPD) has been used as an objective criterion for the determination of digital clubbing (Fig. 61-1). In normal people this ratio averages 0.895 and is independent of age, sex, and race. A ratio greater than unity is significant.

Clubbing may develop very rapidly—for example, it may begin within 7 to 10 days after the development of lung abscess. As the clubbing advances, the convexity of the nail plate becomes extreme and the finger becomes bulbous. Various terms including *drumstick fingers, parrot's beak,* and *serpent's head,* have been used to describe this advanced clubbing (Fig. 61-2). Differences in type of clubbing have no known clinical significance.

Causes and Differential Diagnosis

Clubbing occurs in several distinct clinical syndromes, which have been referred to collectively as *dysacromelias* (Table 61-7). In a 1980 report clubbing was described in about half of patients suffering from hypersensitivity pneumonitis due to pigeon breeder's disease, and its presence has been thought to be a predictor of clinical deterioration.[40]

No specific treatment for clubbing is known.

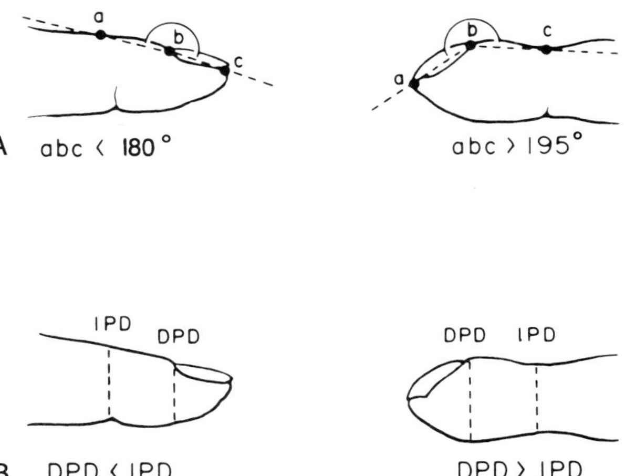

Figure 61-1. Measurements used in the identification of finger clubbing. (**A**) Hyponychial angle. The hyponychial angle is formed by the junction of a line connecting the dorsal surface of the distal interphalangeal joint and the cuticle with a line joining the cuticle and the hyponychium. In young healthy adults this angle is 180 degrees (left); with clubbing it increases above 195 degrees (right). (**B**) Phalangeal depth ratio. In clubbing the enlargement of the soft tissue at the base of the fingernail also increases the depth of the fingertip measured at the cuticle relative to the depth of at the distal interphalangeal joint. The ratio of the distal phalangeal depth (DPD) to the interphalangeal depth (IPD) is normally less than 1 (left), but with clubbing, it exceeds 1.0 (right). (Adapted from Hansen-Flaschen and Nordberg,[41] with permission.)

Table 61-7. Conditions Frequently Associated with Clubbing

Pulmonary
Bronchiectasis
Empyema
Pulmonary alveolar proteinosis
Interstitial pulmonary fibrosis
Bronchogenic carcinoma
Lung abscess
Pneumoconiosis
Cystic fibrosis
Cardiac
Cyanotic heart disease
Subacute bacterial endocarditis
Gastrointestinal
Ulcerative colitis
Hepatic cirrhosis
Regional enteritis
Gastrointestinal cancers

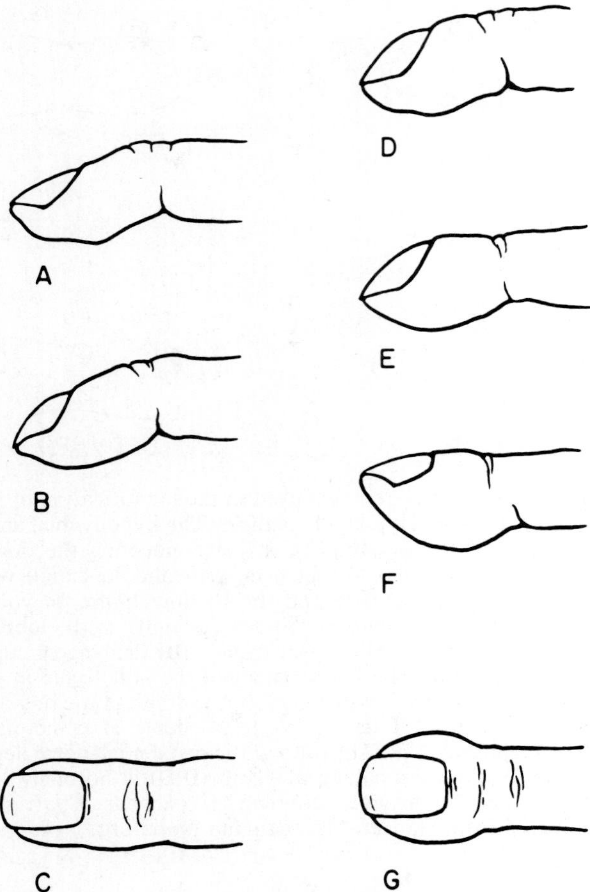

Figure 61-2. Variations of finger clubbing as compared with normal: (**A**) Normal, (**B**) increased curvature of nail; (**C**) normal (from above); (**D**) mild clubbing; (**E**) *parrot's beak* type; (**F**) watchglass type; (**G**) drumstick type. In the parrot's beak type the swelling is localized to the proximal portion of the distal digit. A uniform enlargement of the connective tissue in the base of the nail may result in a watchglass type of clubbing. Marked circumferential enlargement of the soft tissue at the midportion of the distal digit can give the finger a drumstick appearance. (Adapted from Hansen-Flaschen and Nordberg,[41] with permission.)

HYPERTROPHIC OSTEOARTHROPATHY

Hypertrophic osteoarthropathy refers to a collection of clinical findings[41] that include clubbing of fingers and toes, chronic proliferative periostitis associated with subperiosteal new bone formation, arthritis, and signs of autonomic dysfunction such as flushing, blanching, and profuse sweating. The association between clubbing and bone and joint disease was first established by Bamberger in 1889 and Marie in 1890, and therefore this condition is at times referred to as the *Marie-Bamberger syndrome*.

In hypertrophic osteoarthropathy the periosteum is edematous and contains focal accumulations of lymphocytes and plasma cells; the vascularity of the periosteum is increased; the walls of the arterioles may be thickened; and the activity of osteoclasts and osteoblasts is increased. New bone forms along the periosteum at the same time that the underlying cortex is thinned. Bone reabsorption may extend to the newly formed periosteal bone, leaving a thinly trabeculated space beneath the surface. Thus, multiple lamellae of new bone separated by trabeculated space are formed. These changes commonly occur along the peripheral epiphyses of the long bones and are particularly prominent at points of insertion of muscles and tendons.

Causes and Associations

Hypertrophic osteoarthropathy is classified as either primary or secondary. The primary syndrome, also called *pachydermoperiostosis,* may be hereditary or idiopathic. The hereditary form is transmitted as a mendelian dominant trait with incomplete penetrance; its onset is usually after puberty and its course is self-limited to one to two decades. It is more common in men than in women. The main complaint is usually hyperhidrosis of the palms and soles. In some patients gynecomastia, feminine distribution of body hair, striae, and acne vulgaris may develop. Bone and joint symptoms are uncommon.

The secondary form is more common and occurs with a variety of intrathoracic, cardiac, and gastrointestinal diseases.[41] However, more than 90 percent of cases result from the diseases in the thorax and as a result the syndrome is often referred to as *hypertrophic pulmonary osteoarthropathy* (HPO). Among the intrathoracic diseases associated with HPO are bronchogenic carcinoma, bronchiectasis, lung abscess, empyema, and interstitial fibrosis. Recently, HPO has been described in a patient with the acquired immunodeficiency syndrome (AIDS). About 10 percent of patients with intrathoracic malignancies have all or part of the syndrome; however, it seems to be relatively less common with the small cell lung cancer than with other cell types. Clubbing develops in about half of patients with mesothelioma, but other features of the syndrome occur less often. It has also been suggested that HPO is more common in benign pleural mesothelioma than in malignant mesothelioma or disease metastatic to the pleura. It should be noted that HPO may precede the clinical diagnosis of bronchogenic carcinoma by as much as 2 years.

Clinical Manifestations and Diagnosis

Symptoms of HPO range from mild arthralgia to severe deep-seated pain. The ankles and wrists are the joints most commonly involved, followed by the metacarpophalangeal joints and knees, with the elbows and shoulders involved least often. Aggravation of bone pain with dependency of the limb is a unique feature of this syndrome. Episodic sweating and sensations of warmth may occur, and there may be some increase in thickness of the skin overlying areas of periostitis.

The manifestations of HPO resemble those of rheumatoid arthritis and many patients are misdiagnosed as having the latter disease. In patients presenting with symmetric polyarticular pain, swelling, and stiffness, the presence of clubbing may be the clue to a correct diagnosis of HPO.

Hypertrophic osteoarthropathy is distinguished radiographically from other causes of bone pain and swelling in the extremities by the characteristic periosteal changes along the long bones. Periostitis appears as a thin sclerotic line separated from the underlying cortex by a radiolucent line. Multilaminated new bone formation may be seen in some cases; in others, the periosteal new bone becomes thicker and merges with the cortex, so that no intervening radiolucent line is visible. The radius, ulna, tibia, and femur are the most commonly affected bones.

A bone scan with technetium 99m-polyphosphate may show an increase in radioactivity at the distal end of the long bones and is the most sensitive test. Hypertrophic osteoarthropathy can be differentiated from focal metastatic disease by finding the concentration of the radionuclide in pericortical and periarticular regions. Bone scan may detect evidence of periostitis in patients who have no other clinical or radiographic manifestation of HPO.

Treatment

The most effective treatment of HPO is the curative treatment of the primary condition. Thus, resection of a primary or metastatic lung tumor may be undertaken for relief of bone and joint pain. Resection of a tumor sometimes decreases the symptoms even if the resection does not offer a cure. It should be noted that the presence of HPO by itself does not contraindicate surgery for lung cancer. Aspirin or other anti-inflammatory agents, including steroids, often provide symptomatic relief. Surgical or chemical vagotomy or radiation therapy can also provide relief in some patients.

ABNORMAL BREATHING PATTERNS

An observation of the pattern of breathing of a patient may give valuable information regarding the disease process. Ventilation is adjusted to meet changes in external conditions and internal demands by regulating systems that limit variations in $PaCO_2$ and PaO_2 by feedback control mechanisms. Thus, changes in ventilation alter the levels of PaO_2 and $PaCO_2$, and these changes reach the respiratory centers and readjust the neural output to the respiratory muscles according to a desired reference value, which readjusts the ventilation.

The term *eupnea* describes a normal breathing pattern. The relationship between ventilation and $PaCO_2$ is set by the respiratory center. In adults the normal respiratory rate at rest is about 14 to 18 breaths per minute; in the newborn, it is about 40 to 45. The term *tachypnea* (fast breathing) is used if the respiratory rate is higher than normal. Tachypnea occurs with fever, exertion, congestive heart failure, pain, acute respiratory distress due to any cause, thyrotoxicosis, metabolic acidosis, restrictive lung disease, asthma, and acute respiratory failure. The term *bradypnea* describes a pattern of breathing in which the respiratory rate is slow but the rhythm is regular and breaths may be deeper than normal. Bradypnea may be seen in uremia, diabetic coma, and central nervous system depression due to any cause (e.g., morphine overdose or excessive alcohol consumption). *Kussmaul breathing* usually occurs in diabetic ketoacidosis and is described as deep, regular breathing at a slow, normal, or fast rate. It may also be seen in uremia.

Periodic Breathing

The most common type of periodic breathing is *Cheyne-Stokes breathing,* which is characterized by slowly waxing and waning respiration, the cycle repeating every 45 seconds to 3 minutes. It is caused by two factors, delay in blood flow from the lungs to the brain and increased feedback gain in the respiratory center. When circulation from lungs to brain is slowed, as in congestive heart failure, the changes in blood PCO_2 caused by changes in ventilation are not detected by the brain for several seconds. Therefore, blood PCO_2 continues to rise or fall to abnormal levels before appropriate corrections are made in the ventilation. Cycle length increases when circulation time is prolonged.

Gain, defined as a change in ventilation for a given change in $PaCO_2$, may increase owing to structural damage of the respiratory center. It is possible for gain to increase while the sensitivity of the respiratory center decreases. For example, in a given patient a $PaCO_2$ of 40 mmHg may cause no ventilation, which represents greatly decreased sensitivity, but in the same patient a $PaCO_2$ of 45 mmHg may increase ventilation to normal, which represents very high gain, and consequently respiration may oscillate back and forth between apnea and breathing. Therefore, Cheyne-Stokes breathing with overall depressed breathing is an ominous sign. Cheyne-Stokes breathing may also occur during hypoxia because when a person becomes very hypoxic, the gain of the O_2 deficiency mechanism for controlling respiration increases as much as 5- to 10-fold. When this extra gain is added to the gains of the CO_2 and pH mechanisms, Cheyne-Stokes breathing occurs. The presence of hypoxia could explain the Cheyne-Stokes breathing seen in mountain climbers, particularly at night during sleep, because the diminished respiration during sleep exacerbates the condition.

In *Biot's breathing,* in contrast to Cheyne-Stokes breathing, the tidal volumes between periods of apnea are uniform. Biot's breathing is sometimes seen in meningitis. It is possible that Cheyne-Stokes breathing and Biot's breathing are produced by the same mechanism.

Apneustic Breathing

Apneustic breathing was first described in 1888 by Marckwald,[42] who noted prolonged inspiratory pauses occurring following upper brain stem transection in vagotomized rabbits. The term *apneusis* (derived from the Greek word for breath holding) is used to describe these inspiratory pauses. Although apneustic breathing has been studied extensively in animals, it appears to be a very rare clinical entity.[43]

CUTANEOUS SIGNS IN PULMONARY DISEASE

The skin may be involved in a number of diseases that affect the lung.[44] Some of the cutaneous lesions are of diagnostic value.

Urticaria

Urticaria is often seen as edematous papules with a fine *peau d'orange* type of surface and is usually surrounded by macular erythema. Itching is the predominant symptom. Urticaria may be seen as a manifestation of many bacterial and fungal lung infections, as well as in cystic fibrosis.

Erythema Multiforme

Erythema multiforme often presents as transient edematous papules, which become fixed in about 24 hours and begin to develop central clearing, at which time changes in the size, shape, and color of the lesion occur. The most characteristic appearance of the lesion is that of a target, iris, or bull's eye. The condition, in which there is always involvement of the palms, soles, or both, differs from urticaria in that itching is not a prominent symptom. When bullous erythema multiforme is associated with mucocutaneous ulcerations, it is given the eponym *Stevens-Johnson syndrome*. Like urticaria, erythema multiforme is seen most commonly with the bacterial pneumonias caused by organisms such as *Streptococcus* spp., *Pseudomonas, Legionella,* and *Haemophilus influenzae*. *Mycoplasma pneumoniae* is probably one of the most common identifiable organisms causing erythema multiforme. Recurrent erythema multiforme complicated by severe oral ulceration has been reported to occur with severe episodes of *Mycoplasma pneumoniae* infection. Erythema multiforme has also been seen in association with pulmonary blastomycosis.

Erythema Nodosum

Erythema nodosum is a form of panniculitis and only secondarily involves the skin. It usually involves the anterior tibial region and may start with pain. After a few days erythema appears on the same location and is followed by development of exquisitely tender nodules on the shins. Pain can be intense, making walking difficult, and constitutional symptoms such as fever, malaise, and loss of appetite may also occur. Lesions resolve in a few weeks and may leave a purple discoloration. Erythema nodosum may occur in patients with pulmonary coccidioidomycosis or histoplasmosis. The presence of erythema nodosum with hilar adenopathy usually indicates sarcoidosis or fungal infections in the lung.

Cutaneous Signs in Vasculitis

The clinical indicator of cutaneous vasculitis is palpable purpura. Deep fungal infections may also manifest with vasculitis of the small cutaneous vessels; blastomycosis is associated with vasculitis of the skin and the lung; and bacterial and mycobacterial diseases may also be associated with vasculitis of cutaneous vessels. Vasculitis is most commonly seen with the collagen-vascular diseases, such as systemic lupus erythematosus and scleroderma. In the latter the skin becomes diffusely edematous and then progresses to a generalized tightening. Telangiectasias are usually present on the face, lips, arms, palms, and periungual areas. Cutaneous lesions may be present in the form of ulcerating nodules and vasculitic ulcers in half of patients with Wegener's granulomatosis. Conjunctivitis, uveitis, and episcleritis can all result from the vasculitic process. The Churg-Strauss syndrome is also complicated by cutaneous disease in 70 percent of patients. Palpable purpura, urticaria, vasculitic ulcers, and nodules may be present.

Cutaneous Signs in Malignancy

Erythema gyratum repens is a rare skin eruption consisting of undulating erythematous bands with the appearance of wood grain. The undulating pattern changes on a daily basis. This cutaneous finding is associated with pulmonary malignancy in 30 percent of cases and may appear several years prior to the diagnosis. The eruption usually resolves when the primary tumor is treated.

Kaposi's sarcoma is a multicentric vascular neoplasm. This disease ranges from the classic form, an indolent cutaneous disorder, occurring most often in elderly men in southern and eastern Europe, to the disseminated form associated with AIDS. In classic Kaposi's sarcoma the cutaneous lesions occur first on the lower extremities as asymptomatic bluish-red macules and papules. Plaques and nodules subsequently develop on the trunk, head, and neck, as well as on internal organs, but the visceral disease is usually asymptomatic. The median survival in these patients is 8 to 10 years and most die of unrelated causes.

Kaposi's sarcoma is now most commonly seen in patients with AIDS. AIDS-associated Kaposi's sarcoma is quite different from the classic form, in that cutaneous lesions are small, generally nonulcerated, and usually disseminated, with some sparing of the lower extremities. Extensive lymphadenopathy and visceral involvement are also seen, and the disease often has a rapidly progressive fulminant course.

OCULAR MANIFESTATIONS IN PULMONARY DISEASE

Eye involvement occurs in various diseases that also involve the lungs.[45] Conjunctival follicles and lacrimal gland enlargement commonly occur in sarcoidosis, but these rarely produce symptoms. Anterior uveitis (iridocyclitis) is a feature of sarcoidosis, ankylosing spondylitis, Behçet's disease, and the Stevens-Johnson syndrome; it is also rarely seen in patients with *Mycoplasma pneumoniae* infections. Posterior uveitis may occur with histoplasmosis, sarcoidosis, and Behçet's disease. Optic nerve involvement with acute visual loss may rarely be seen with sarcoidosis. Wegener's granulomatosis may involve the eyes, producing lid edema, nasolacrimal duct obstruction, proptosis, conjunctival chemosis, and scleritis. Uveitis and retinal vasculitis occur in the limited form of Wegener's granulomatosis. In miliary tuberculosis one may find choroidal tubercles. Certain connective tissue disorders, such as systemic lupus erythematosus, rheumatoid arthritis, scleroderma, and Sjögren's syndrome, may involve both the lungs and the eyes and may present with scleritis, episcleritis, retinal artery occlusion, or keratoconjunctivitis sicca.

References

1. Sant'Ambrogio G, Remmers JE, DeGroot WJ et al: Localization of rapidly adapting receptors in the trachea and mainstem bronchus of the dog. Respir Physiol 1978;33:359–366
2. Braman SS, Corrao WM: Cough: Differential diagnosis and treatment. Clin Chest Med 1987;8:177–188
3. Wolff AP, May M, Nuelle D: The tympanic membrane: A source of the cough reflex. JAMA 1973;223:1269
4. Hall WS, Hall CB: Clinical significance of pulmonary function tests: Alterations in pulmonary function following respiratory viral infections. Chest 1977;76:458–465
5. Irwin RS, Erickson AD, Pratter MR et al: Current cigarette smoking in chronic obstructive bronchitis predicts tracheobronchial colonization. J Infect Dis 1982;145:234–241
6. American Thoracic Society, Medical Section of the American Lung Association: Standards for the diagnosis and care of patients with chronic obstructive pulmonary disease (COPD) and asthma. Am Rev Respir Dis 1987;136:225–244
7. McFadden ER Jr: Exertional dyspnea and cough as preludes to acute attacks of bronchial asthma. N Engl J Med 1975;292:555–559
8. Hyde L, Hyde CI: Clinical manifestations of lung cancer. Chest 1974;65:299–306
9. Szidon JP, Fishman AP: Approach to the pulmonary patient with respiratory signs and symptoms. pp. 313–366. In Fishman AP (ed): Pulmonary Diseases and Disorders. 2nd Ed. McGraw-Hill, New York, 1988
10. Crystal RG, Fulmer JD, Roberts WC et al: Idiopathic pulmonary fibrosis: Clinical, histologic, radiographic, physiologic, scintigraphic, cytologic, and biochemical aspects. Ann Intern Med 1976;85:769–788
11. Vedal S, Anantharaman A, Israel RH: Hidden asthmatic: Identification required for propranolol usage. NY State J Med 1980;80:648–649
12. Sesoko S, Kaneko Y: Cough associated with the use of captopril. Arch Intern Med 1985;145:1524
13. Rakita L, Sobol SM, Mostow N, Vrobel T: Amiodarone pulmonary toxicity. Am Heart J 1983;106:906–916
14. Wenzel SA: The effect of cardiac disorders on the lungs. p. 53. In Cooper KA (ed): Pulmonary Manifestations of Systemic Disease. Futura Publishing, New York, 1990
15. Poe RH, Israel RH, Utell MJ, Hall WJ: Chronic cough: Bronchoscopy or pulmonary function testing? Am Rev Respir Dis 1982;126:160–162
16. Petty TL: The National Mucolytic Study: Results of a randomized, double-blind, placebo-controlled study of iodinated glycerol in chronic obstructive bronchitis. Chest 1990;97:75–83
17. Winter SM, Ingbar DH: Massive hemoptysis: Pathogenesis and management. Intensive Care Med 1983;3:171–188
18. Deffebach ME, Charan NB, Lakshminarayan S, Butler J: State of the art: The bronchial circulation: Small, but a vital attribute of the lung. Am Rev Respir Dis 1987;135:463–481
19. Wald PH, Balmes JR: Respiratory effects of short-term, high-intensity toxic inhalations: Smoke, gases, and fumes. Intensive Care Med 1987;2:260–278
20. Dalen JE, Haffajee CI, Alpert JS et al: Pulmonary embolism, pulmonary hemorrhage, and pulmonary infarction. N Engl J Med 1977;296:1431–1435
21. Cregler LL, Mark H: Medical complications of cocaine abuse. N Engl J Med 1986;315:1495–1500
22. Smiddy JF, Elliott RC: The evaluation of hemoptysis with fiberoptic bronchoscopy. Chest 1973;64:158–162
23. Weaver LJ, Solliday N, Cugell DW: Selection of patients with hemoptysis for fiberoptic bronchoscopy. Chest 1979;76:7–10
24. Cohen AM, Doershuk CF, Stern RC: Bronchial artery embolization to control hemoptysis in cystic fibrosis. Radiology 1990;175:401–405
25. Roberts AC: Bronchial artery embolization therapy. J Thorac Imaging 1990;5:60–72
26. Ferris EJ: Pulmonary hemorrhage. Vascular evaluation and interventional therapy. Chest 1979;80:710–714
27. Forgacs P: The functional basis of pulmonary sounds. Chest 1978;73:399–405
28. Baughman RP, Loudon RG: Quantitation of wheezing in acute asthma. Chest 1984;86:718–722
29. Bynum LJ, Pierce AK: Pulmonary aspiration of gastric contents. Am Rev Respir Dis 1976;114:1129–1136
30. Hogg JC, Agarwal JB, Gardiner AJS et al: Distribution of airway resistance with developing pulmonary edema in dogs. J Appl Physiol 1972;32:20–24
31. Shim CS, Williams HM: Relationship of wheezing to the severity of obstruction in asthma. Arch Intern Med 1983;143:890–892
32. Tobin MJ: Dyspnea: Pathophysiologic basis, clinical presentation, and management. Arch Intern Med 1990;150:1604–1613
33. Campbell EJM, Howell JBL: The sensation of breathlessness. Br Med Bull 1963;19:36–40
34. Campbell EJM: Comments during discussion of symposium. pp. 221–222. In Pengelly LD, Rebuck AS, Campbell EJM (ed): Loaded Breathing. Churchill Livingstone, Edinburgh, 1974
35. Simon PM, Schwartzstein RM, Weiss JW et al: Distinguishable types of dyspnea in patients with shortness of breath. Am Rev Respir Dis 1990:142:1009–1014
36. Mitchell-Heggs P, Murphy K, Minty K et al: Diazepam in the treatment of dyspnea in the "pink puffer" syndrome. Q J Med 1980;49:9–20
37. Woodcock AA, Gross ER, Geddes DM: Drug treatment of breathlessness: Contrasting effects of diazepam and promethazine in pink puffers. Br Med J 1981;283:343–346
38. Woodcock AA, Gross ER, Geller A et al: Effects of dihydrocodeine, alcohol, and caffeine on breathlessness and exercise tolerance in patients with chronic obstructive lung disease and normal blood gases. N Engl J Med 1981;305:1611–1616
39. Light RW, Muro JR, Sato RI et al: Effects of oral morphine on breathlessness and exercise tolerance in patients with chronic obstructive pulmonary disease. Am Rev Respir Dis 1989;139:126–133

40. Sansores R, Salas J, Chapela R et al: Clubbing in hypersensitivity pneumonitis: Its prevalence and possible prognostic role. Arch Intern Med 1990;150:1849–1851
41. Hansen-Flaschen J, Nordberg J: Clubbing and hypertrophic osteoarthropathy. Clin Chest Med 1990;8:287–298
42. Marckwald M: The Movements of Respiration and Their Innervation in the Rabbit. Translated by Haig TA. Blackie & Son, London, 1888
43. Mador JM, Tobin MJ: Apneustic breathing: A characteristic feature of brainstem compression in achondroplasia? Chest 1990;97:877–883
44. Alper J, Kegel M: Skin signs in pulmonary disease. Clin Chest Med 1990;8:299–312
45. Tsiaras WG, Gridley M: Ophthalmic manifestations of pulmonary disease. Clin Chest Med 1987;8:313–328

Chapter 62

Clinical Approach to the Patient with Obstructive Lung Disease

David J. Pierson

CHAPTER OUTLINE

This chapter serves as a bridge between those chapters describing the physiologic and clinical characteristics of obstructive lung diseases and those discussing practical and technical aspects of assessment and management. Its main goal is to provide a logical, physiologically based framework for the clinician—a system in which the individual components of respiratory care fit together coherently and logically. In no area of respiratory care are empiricism and individual preference more prominent. This chapter's approaches are by no means the only ones the clinician will encounter, but effort has been made to make them internally consistent, rational, and in keeping with the fundamental themes of logic and scientific method presented throughout this book.

Four general elements constitute the clinical approach taken in this chapter: (1) conceptual separation of obstructive lung disease into several distinct types or syndromes, and assignment of a given patient's illness to whichever of these is most appropriate clinically; (2) clinical assessment of the individual components and their functional severity in that individual; (3) an overall philosophy for management; and (4) specific application of each component of management for that individual.

The obstructive lung diseases form a family of overlapping disorders, as described in Chapter 22. Most important among these, at least in terms of overall impact on respiratory care, are asthma and chronic obstructive pulmonary disease (COPD). These disorders, or syndromes, are conceptually distinct even though they share numerous features. Each has two classic subtypes—"extrinsic" and "intrinsic" asthma and "type A" and "type B" COPD. Many authorities now dispute the existence of these idealized subtypes in terms of pathogenesis, but an appreciation of them can be conceptually useful to the clinician, even though they are almost never encountered in "pure" form.

Separation of the obstructive disorders into distinct syndromes can be useful in assessing prognosis and adjusting management to the individual patient, and some clinicians have found an algorithmic approach to be helpful in this setting.[1,2] Figure 62-1 depicts such an algorithm and illustrates how this approach can be used to characterize a given patient by using specific clinical features.

Several questions need to be answered for the patient suspected of having obstructive lung disease. Does the patient indeed have obstructive lung disease? Many individuals are mistakenly so labeled on the basis of symptoms, radiographic findings, or other inappropriate information. If obstructive disease is present, what type or syndrome best fits this individual's clinical picture? How severe is it, both physiologically and in terms of its impact on function? What laboratory workup should be undertaken, keeping in mind both the need to characterize the illness and the imperative to be cost-effective? For this patient, what should be the goals of assessment? Clinical, administrative, and legal evaluations have different purposes and different components. What should be the specific goals of management in this patient? Finally, which elements of therapy should be included? There can be no uniform, ''cookbook'' routine for the patient with obstructive lung disease, and each of these questions must be answered individually, with management adjusted

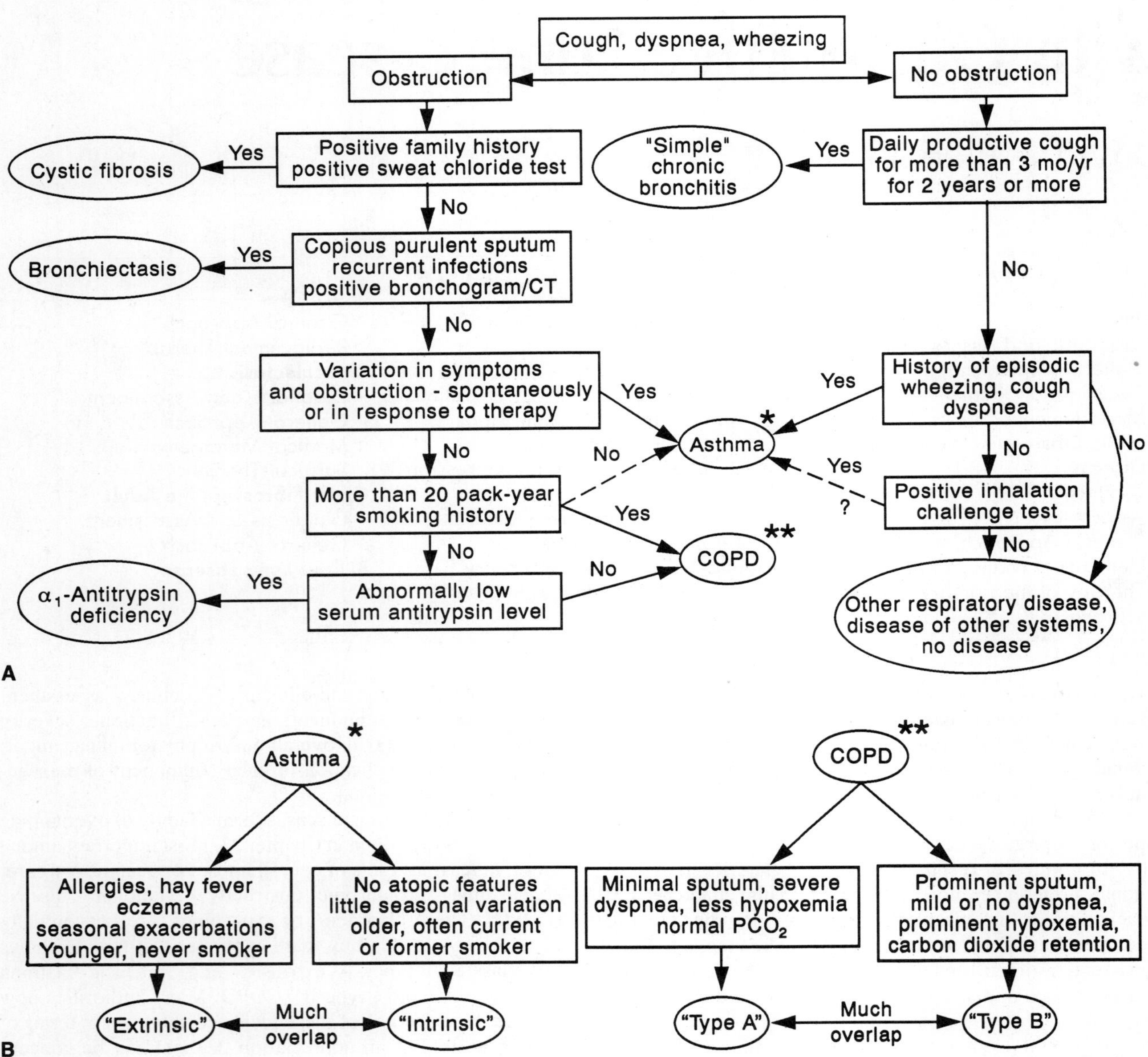

Figure 62-1. **(A & B)** Algorithm for classifying patients with suspected obstructive lung disease into clinical categories or syndromes. (Modified from Pierson,[1] with permission.)

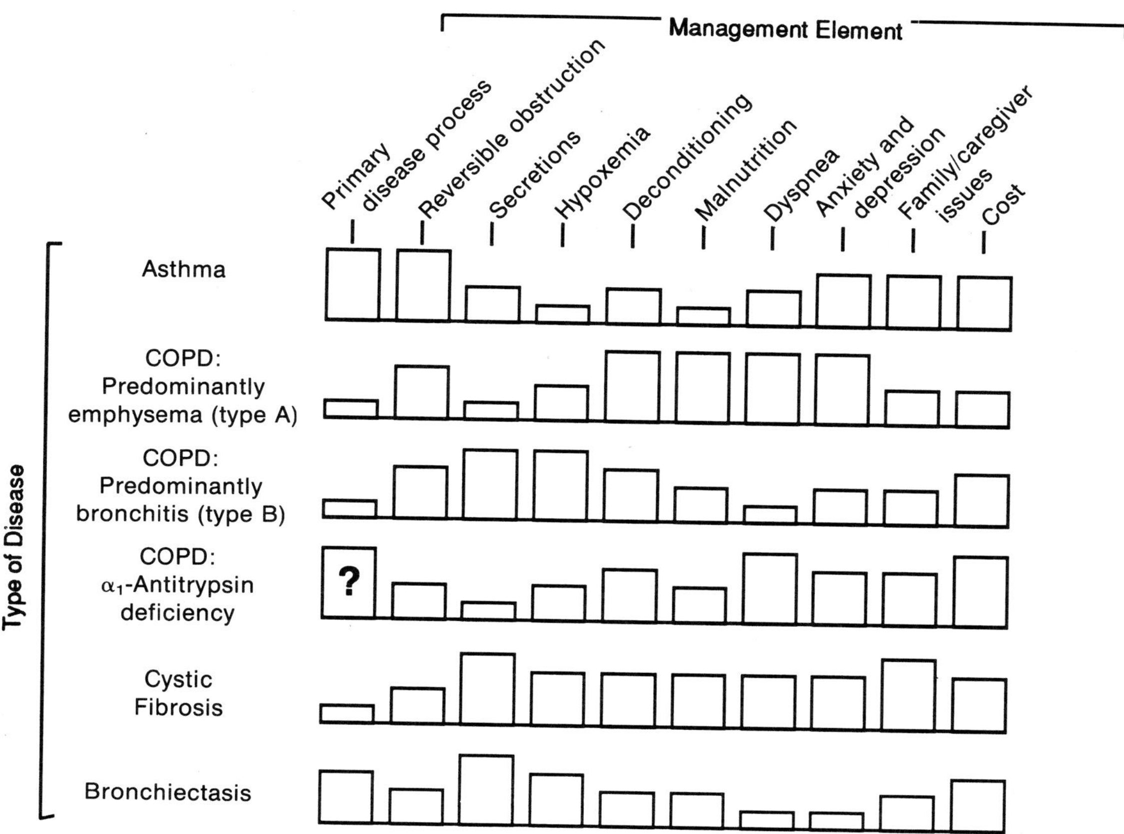

Figure 62-2. General importance of 10 different elements of management in 6 subtypes of obstructive lung disease, as indicated by the relative heights of individual bars. In alpha-1-antitrypsin deficiency, replacement therapy is extremely expensive and of uncertain benefit, hence the question mark. For further explanation see text. (Adapted from Pierson,[1] with permission.)

to that patient's unique situation. Nonetheless, a number of general principles do apply, as discussed below for each of the general disease categories.

Patient management in the different clinical types of obstructive lung disease may be divided into distinct components, which vary in importance. Figure 62-2 illustrates this conceptually, showing the general importance of 10 different elements of management in asthma, COPD, cystic fibrosis, and bronchiectasis.[1] Although this scheme is an oversimplification and not all clinicians would agree with the relative weights assigned in each category, it shows some of the major differences between different clinical types of obstructive disease and emphasizes the importance of properly diagnosing and assessing each patient.

The following sections present a clinical approach for each main category of obstructive lung disease. Some aspects of management (for example, bronchodilator therapy) are important in several categories. Approaches to cor pulmonale, long-term O_2 therapy, and acute respiratory failure in patients with obstructive lung disease are covered in Chapters 63 and 64; aspects specific to obstructive disease in children are discussed in Chapter 88.

ASTHMA

Diagnosis and Assessment

Everyone knows what asthma is but no one can give a really good definition. As pointed out in Chapter 22, the many published definitions for asthma tend to be awkwardly worded and cumbersome, as they try to encompass all the features of what is perhaps the respiratory system's most variable and inconsistent condition. In COPD, asthma (or the "asthmatic component") can be thought of as that portion of the patient's airflow obstruction that can be reversed by bronchodilators and other asthma medications. For the patient whose only respiratory disorder is asthma, perhaps the best definition is "episodic wheezing dyspnea," that is, the main symptoms are wheezing and/or dyspnea (usually also with cough and commonly with chest tightness), and these symptoms wax and wane in severity. Although other diseases can produce this picture, in an otherwise healthy person it is usually due to asthma.

Physicians vary with respect to how much objective documentation they require in making the diagnosis of asthma,

Table 62-1. Assessment of the Severity of Acute Asthma

PEFR		FEV_1		
Absolute Value (L/min)[a]	% of Predicted Value	Absolute Value (L)[a]	% of Predicted Value	Severity
>200	>60	>2.0	>60	Mild to moderate
80–200	30–60	1.0–2.0	30–60	Moderately severe
<80	<25–30	<1.0	<25–30	Severe

[a] Representative values for an average-sized adult patient. (Adapted from Pierson[3] with permission.)

particularly in a patient who is not actually having symptoms when seen. Most would accept the combination of audible wheezing, airflow obstruction (i.e., reduced ratio of forced expiratory volume in the first second to forced vital capacity [FEV_1/FVC]), and improvement after inhaled bronchodilator (a more than 15 percent increase in FVC or FEV_1 or a more than 25 percent increase in the forced expiratory flow between 25 and 75 percent of the vital capacity [FEF_{25-75}]) in an otherwise healthy patient with an appropriate history. The more severe or atypical the symptoms, the worse the obstruction, or the less the response to initial treatment, the more extensive should be the workup. In recent years some clinicians have turned to bronchial provocation with methacholine or other stimuli in an attempt to induce airflow obstruction if this is not initially present, but most would accept the clinical circumstance of episodic symptoms relieved by inhaled bronchodilator even if airflow is normal in the doctor's office.

In the acute asthma attack, on the other hand, objective assessment of severity is important for both prognosis and management. Good bedside indicators of a severe attack include tachypnea, severe dyspnea, inability to remain recumbent, and inability to speak in whole phrases or sentences; disturbances of mental state (irritability, uncooperativeness, confusion, drowsiness); gross chest overexpansion, absence of wheezes, and use of accessory respiratory muscles; pulsus paradoxus higher than 15 mmHg; severe sinus tachycardia, hypertension, or hypotension; and ineffective cough, diaphoresis, exhaustion, or dehydration.[3] The most reliable indicator of an attack's severity, however, is an objective measurement of airflow, using either spirometry or a hand-held peak-flow meter.[4,5] Table 62-1 classifies acute asthma into three categories according to the initial results of peak expiratory flow rate (PEFR) or FEV_1 measurement.[3]

General Approach

In the past most clinicians managed asthma mainly according to the patient's symptoms: asthma was regarded primarily as a problem of bronchospasm, and measures to prevent or reverse bronchospasm comprised the mainstay of therapy. However, since the early 1980s asthma has come to be regarded as an inflammatory rather than primarily a bronchospastic disorder, and the basic approach has switched from control of symptoms to control of underlying airway inflammation.[6,7]

The goal of management for most patients with asthma is to prevent or suppress airway inflammation, and primary therapy consists of long-term, continuous topical anti-inflammatory therapy. In most instances this consists of inhaled corticosteroids such as beclomethasone or triamcinolone. Beta-adrenergic bronchodilators such as albuterol and terbutaline are now used as sole therapy only in patients with mild, intermittent asthma. Many leading clinicians, rather than using these bronchodilators as primary therapy, in most cases now track the patient's use of bronchodilators as a monitor of the effectiveness of primary therapy (usually inhaled corticosteroids). Systemic steroids are reserved for severe acute attacks or for unremitting chronic symptoms that cannot be controlled with less hazardous therapy; every effort is made to reduce or eliminate the long-term use of prednisone and other systemic steroids.

Steps in Management

According to the general approach indicated above, asthma is managed in a series of progressive steps, as dictated by disease severity and response to treatment.[6,8] This stepwise approach is illustrated in Table 62-2. Mild, intermittent asthma is treated symptomatically by using beta agonists as needed. Patients with daily symptoms are treated prophylactically with inhaled corticosteroids or, in the case of younger patients whose disease has prominent atopic features, with cromolyn; in these patients beta agonists and other bronchodilators are used as needed for symptom control in addition to their role in regular prophylactic therapy.

Doses and dosing intervals currently recommended by U.S. manufacturers and the Food and Drug Administration for beta-adrenergic drugs administered by metered dose inhaler (MDI) are substantially lower than those routinely used in Europe and elsewhere for many years. Currently available agents (e.g., albuterol, terbutaline, pirbuterol) are much safer in higher doses than their less beta-2-specific predecessors (e.g., epinephrine, isoproterenol, isoetharine). When required by symptoms or as guided by peak flow measurements to maximize the therapeutic effect in a given patient, a regimen such as albuterol, four to six puffs or more every 4 to 6 hours is acceptable and should be considered standard therapy.[5,9]

Some authorities[6,10] advocate the use of higher-dose inhaled steroids prior to starting second-line asthma drugs such as theophylline or ipratropium. This therapy is facilitated by

Table 62-2. Successive Steps in Asthma Management

Step	Clinical Setting	Rationale and Goals	Drugs Used[a]	Example of Initial Prescription[b]
I	Mild, infrequent, or seasonal symptoms	Symptomatic therapy: control of disease manifestations	Inhaled beta agonist	Albuterol MDI, 2 puffs q4–6h prn
			OR	OR
			Inhaled anticholinergic	Ipratropium bromide MDI, 2 puffs q4–6h prn
II	Frequent symptoms requiring daily or near daily medication	Prophylaxis: anti-inflammatory control of disease process itself	Inhaled corticosteroid	Triamcinolone acetonide MDI, 2–4 puffs tid–qid
			OR	OR
			Inhaled cromolyn[c]	Cromolyn MDI or turbohaler, 2 puffs qid
		Symptomatic therapy: control of disease manifestations	Inhaled beta agonist	Albuterol MDI, with spacer if necessary, 2–6 puffs q4–6h prn
			Inhaled anticholinergic	Ipratropium bromide MDI, 2 puffs q2–6h prn
			Oral theophylline	Theophylline SA 300 mg hs or bid[d]
			OR	OR
			Oral beta agonist	Albuterol SA, 4 mg hs or bid
III	Symptoms uncontrolled with steps I and II; frequent office and/or emergency department visits with acute attacks; hospitalization because of asthma	Systemic treatment of inflammation: minimize disability; prevent emergency visits; prevent hospitalization; reduce likelihood of potentially fatal asthma	Oral corticosteroid	Acute therapy (short course): Prednisone 20–40 mg qAM for 3–5 days, then tapered to 0 over 4–7 days
				Long-term therapy for unremitting symptoms: prednisone at lowest AM dose that maintains acceptable control; attempt to switch to qod dosing; attempt to reduce oral dose by adding inhaled steroid 4 puffs tid to qid
		Symptomatic therapy	(as in step II)	

[a] If allergic features are present, environmental control should also be instituted.
[b] Doses shown are examples of initial doses for average-sized adult patient.
[c] Cromolyn may be especially effective in younger patients whose asthma has prominent allergic features.
[d] Serum theophylline level should be measured if drug is used daily.

use of the more concentrated topical steroid formulations available by MDI in Europe and is unfortunately very expensive when currently available U.S. preparations are used. Accessory devices (e.g., spacers) should generally be used with inhaled steroids to decrease the incidence of oral candidiasis.[9]

Patients whose asthma is still uncontrolled following steps I and II as shown in Table 62-2 require systemic corticosteroids (step III), which carry a substantial risk for serious toxicity when used frequently or long-term (see Ch. 20). Systemic corticosteroids administered in the form of short bursts to control acute exacerbations are relatively free of adverse effects, especially if they are not required more than a few times per year. However, the likelihood of serious side effects increases substantially when these agents are taken daily for more than a few weeks. In such cases therapy with other agents should be maximized (e.g., by more intensive administration of beta agonists[9] or titration of theophylline to a target serum level), and attempts should always be made to reduce the daily dose to the minimum level that maintains acceptable symptom control.

Some clinicians use so-called steroid-sparing drugs to try to reduce daily corticosteroid dosage in patients who require such therapy chronically. Troleandomycin (TAO), an antibiotic related to erythromycin, has long been used for this purpose. Studies confirm that when TAO is given concomitantly with prednisolone (but not prednisone), the daily steroid requirement diminishes in many patients[11]; long-term steroid side effects may also be reduced, although the proof for this is less convincing.[12] Since the late 1980s there has been considerable interest in the potent anti-inflammatory agent methotrexate as a steroid-sparing agent.[13,14] Regular, long-term administration of methotrexate may reduce corticosteroid requirements in some patients, but this dangerous drug requires close monitoring, and its adverse effects are potentially life-threatening. Because of this it cannot be recommended for asthma patients outside the research setting.

Management of Acute Asthma

Initial steps in the assessment and management of acute asthma[3,15] are listed in Table 62-3. Short-term, high-dose systemic corticosteroids constitute the most important component of management and are important determinants of the duration of an attack and its likelihood of recurrence. However, steroids have little clinical effect for at least several hours, so that the mainstay of initial management is beta-adrenergic bronchodilators, administered promptly and intensively.

The generation-old approach of giving subcutaneous epinephrine has recently given way to aggressive administration of more beta-2-specific agents by aerosol, particularly in adult patients. If the patient can be given bronchodilator by aerosol (e.g., albuterol two to eight puffs q15–30min for three to four doses, then q2–4h for 24 hours, then q4–6h) it is doubtful whether parenteral administration offers any advantage.[16] Under appropriate observation and medical supervision patients can safely be given as many as 20 puffs or more of albuterol or other beta-2 agonist per dose via MDI during attacks of acute severe asthma.[9] In Sweden and elsewhere it is not uncommon to administer doses even higher than this without producing an increase in side effects.[16]

Table 62-3. Approach to the Patient with an Acute Asthma Attack

Assessment
1. Brief, directed history and physical examination
2. Assessment of severity of airflow obstruction (PEFR or FEV_1)
3. Arterial blood gas measurement[a] if
   A. Patient is somnolent, confused, or uncontrollably agitated
   B. PEFR or FEV_1 is <25–30% of predicted value
   C. Patient fails to improve clinically after steps 4–8 below

Management
4. Oxygen, 2–4 L/min by nasal cannula or 28–35% by venturi mask[b]
5. Beta-adrenergic bronchodilator by inhalation (e.g., albuterol, terbutaline), via metered-dose inhaler[c]
6. Beta-agonist bronchodilator administered subcutaneously (e.g., terbutaline, epinephrine) if patient cannot take medication by inhalation[d]
7. Systemic corticosteroid, intravenous or oral
8. Aminophylline IV, if assessment indicates severe attack, if patient has not improved markedly with steps 4–6, and if no contraindication is present
9. Fluids, IV or PO, 1 L in initial 2 hours, 2–4 L in 24 hours

[a] Pulse oximetry is not sufficient in this setting.

[b] Patients with asthma complicating COPD should initially receive lower doses (e.g., 1 L/min or 24%), with response verified by repeat arterial blood gases.

[c] Use spacer device if patient cannot coordinate inhalation; switch to nebulizer if initial therapy with MDI is ineffective.

[d] Use with caution in the presence of cardiovascular disease or if the patient is over age 40.

Table 62-4. Seven Cardinal Principles in the Assessment and Management of Acute Asthma

1. Repeated asthma attacks in a given individual tend to be similar and to respond similarly to therapy
2. The longer an asthma attack lasts, the more severe it becomes, and the more severe an attack, the longer it will last
3. The event or factors precipitating an asthma attack will influence its duration (e.g., an attack accompanying a viral upper respiratory tract infection will not resolve until the infection resolves)
4. Regardless of what precipitated the attack, therapy will be essentially the same (e.g., even an attack of psychogenic origin will require bronchodilators and other standard therapy)
5. Individual elements of therapy should be added rather than alternated (e.g., if corticosteroids are indicated by the severity of the attack, beta agonists and other previously initiated therapies should still be continued until the patient improves)
6. Unless toxicity occurs, therapy should not be cut back until the patient improves (e.g., the corticosteroid dose should not be tapered until the attack breaks, even if the dose has been administered for several days)
7. Airway function should be assessed and monitored objectively (e.g., via PEFR or FEV_1) in addition to the use of symptoms and physical signs

(Adapted from Pierson,[3] with permission.)

Most American clinicians still administer aminophylline in addition to the therapy described above for severe acute asthma. However, use of this less effective, more toxic bronchodilator must be monitored closely throughout the acute episode. Theophylline will not be required by most asthmatic patients once the acute attack has resolved.

Table 62-4 lists seven cardinal principles, based more on clinical experience than on hard data, that should be taken into consideration during the assessment and management of an acute attack of asthma.

CHRONIC OBSTRUCTIVE PULMONARY DISEASE

COPD is the "bread and butter" of respiratory care. Except in settings restricted to neonates and children, the clinician encounters COPD in every aspect of clinical practice—in the hospital (ward, intensive care unit, emergency department), in the office or clinic, in the pulmonary function laboratory, and in home care—and patients with this condition account for a large proportion of the practices of pulmonologists, internists, and family physicians. In addition, COPD is one of the major causes of mortality, morbidity, and excessive health care costs among patients hospitalized for surgery and other reasons. A solid understanding of the clinical features of COPD is a basic requirement for the clinician, and a reasoned, logical approach to patients with this disorder is indispensable for optimum, cost-effective assessment and management.

Diagnosis

As discussed in Chapter 20, COPD is a syndrome caused by a collection of separate disease processes. Chief among these are emphysema, chronic bronchitis, and a component of asthma, and all three are present to some extent in the majority of patients.[17] This pathophysiologic definition is not very helpful to the clinician in terms of diagnosis, however, and for practical purposes COPD may be defined as the coexistence of two essential features: chronic dyspnea and/or productive cough and airflow obstruction.[18] Because airflow obstruction is defined by the presence of a reduced FEV_1/FVC ratio, it follows that COPD cannot be definitively diagnosed without spirometry. As a result, because spirometry remains underused as a screening procedure in individuals with respiratory symptoms, the diagnosis is often missed, and patients may not receive medical attention until the disease is far advanced.

COPD is also one of the most misdiagnosed conditions in medicine, and once an individual is given the label, it tends to stick, correct or not. The diagnosis cannot be made from a chest x-ray; although there are radiographic signs suggestive of emphysema, these may correlate poorly with symptoms or spirometry, and some patients with severe airflow obstruction have normal chest radiographs. All chronic respiratory disease is not COPD, although the term tends to become a catchall for patients with long-standing pulmonary conditions. Many patients labeled as having COPD really have silicosis, for example, or old tuberculosis, or chronic congestive heart failure—clearly these conditions should be assessed and managed differently from COPD. In addition, it is all too common to make this diagnosis for anyone with a chronic productive cough, especially if that patient is a smoker; only 10 to 20 percent of such individuals actually have airflow obstruction, however, so that again, the term COPD is incorrect.

Some patients seem to be affected mainly by the emphysematous aspect of COPD; these individuals have severe dyspnea on exertion but little or no sputum. Others seem predominantly bronchitic, with cough and sputum but little dyspnea. The concepts of type A and type B COPD (and their extremes, the "pink puffer" and the "blue bloater") arise from this observation (Fig. 62-1). However, these theoretical COPD subtypes are of little diagnostic value, since in reality there is a broad, continuous spectrum of patients, and "pure" classic A's and B's are almost never encountered in real life. Such subdiagnoses are also of no help in present-day management, as one of the basic characteristics of management is the adaptation of its various elements to the specific needs of each individual patient.[18]

As defined here by the coexistence of chronic respiratory symptoms and airflow obstruction, COPD encompasses several other diagnoses that should be identified when present. Airflow obstruction and symptoms of relatively recent onset (e.g., less than 1 year), particularly in a nonsmoker, are characteristic of asthma, which can first appear clinically in middle age or even in the elderly. Such "pure" asthma should be separated from the asthmatic component in the usual case of COPD because symptoms and airflow obstruction in the former may be entirely reversible with aggressive therapy. By contrast, the asthmatic component in most COPD cases is only modestly reversible at best.

When the diagnosis of COPD is entertained in a patient younger than those generally seen (i.e., under age 40 to 45), particularly in a nonsmoker, both *cystic fibrosis* and *alpha-1-antitrypsin deficiency* should be considered (Fig. 62-1). Most commonly, *bronchiectasis* and *bullous lung disease* are generalized conditions not amenable to surgical resection and hence can be thought of as clinical subsets of COPD. However, occasional individuals with each of these processes have predominantly localized disease, in which case cure or dramatic improvement with surgery are possible.

Assessment

When the diagnosis of COPD is first made in patients with clinically significant disease, a relatively thorough workup should be undertaken in order to fully characterize the physiologic impact of the disease and to exclude other, concomitant cardiopulmonary disorders. Table 62-5 summarizes the components of this initial complete evaluation, along with the possible implications of the results of each.[1]

A complete medical history and physical examination provide the best assessment of the impact of the illness on the patient's life-style. Spirometry identifies and quantitates the obstruction, and the initial response to inhaled bronchodilator may provide some indication of how much potential there is for physiologic improvement. Determination of lung volumes, especially residual volume (RV), functional residual capacity (FRC), and total lung capacity (TLC), permits

Table 62-5. Clinical Assessment of the Patient with COPD

Type of Assessment	Tests Performed	Implication of Results
Office evaluation	Complete history; physical examination; chest x-ray	Functional status; concomitant disease
Spirometry; bronchodilator response	FEV_1; FVC; FEV_1/FVC; FEF_{25-75}	Severity of obstruction; reversibility
Lung volumes	RV; FRC; TLC	Hyperinflation; concomitant disease
Diffusing capacity	D_{LCO}	Reversibility; concomitant disease
Arterial blood gases	PO_2; PCO_2; pH	Hypoxemia; hypercapnia
Exercise study	$\dot{V}O_2max$; V_D/V_T; PO_2; PCO_2; heart rate	Clarification of functional limitations

$\dot{V}O_2$ max, maximum O_2 consumption; V_D/V_T, dead space/tidal volume ratio.

(From Pierson,[1] with permission.)

quantitation of the degree of hyperinflation, which may be an important determinant of overall functional impairment; this procedure also helps to rule out concomitant restrictive disease.

Because the diffusing capacity for carbon monoxide (DLCO) correlates better with the severity of anatomic emphysema than any other test of pulmonary function,[19] it may be of help in estimating the potential reversibility of obstruction and hence gauging the vigor with which to attempt this. For example, consider two patients with the same degree of airflow obstruction as indicated by FEV_1 or FEV_1/FVC, whose DLCO values are 50 and 90 percent of predicted. It should be recalled from Chapter 48 that the DLCO is primarily a measure of available pulmonary capillary surface area. Because emphysema destroys both alveoli and capillaries, airflow obstruction in the first patient (DLCO 50 percent of predicted) may well be explainable by emphysema and hence be irreversible. On the other hand, the second patient's obstruction may be due primarily to asthma, which does not destroy capillaries and hence reduce the DLCO, and may therefore be markedly reversible with bronchodilators or corticosteroids.

Hypoxemia and hypercapnia cannot be predicted or quantitated reliably by symptoms or physical signs. For this reason, every patient with COPD of at least moderate severity should have an arterial blood gas measurement as part of the initial complete evaluation. If the patient's symptoms or functional impairment seem out of proportion to the results of these tests, cardiopulmonary exercise testing may be the best means for further evaluation, as described in Chapter 49. Exercise testing is also important in assessment for pulmonary rehabilitation, as described in Chapter 98.

Once physiologically characterized by this initial workup, patients with COPD may be followed primarily by simple office assessment consisting of history, physical examination, and spirometry. Because the course and prognosis of the disorder are better predicted by the severity of obstruction (i.e., FEV_1) than by any other laboratory value[17] (Fig. 62-3), there is little to be gained by routinely repeating the other tests listed in Table 62-5. New or changing symptoms or more rapid deterioration than expected over several months may prompt more thorough re-examination.

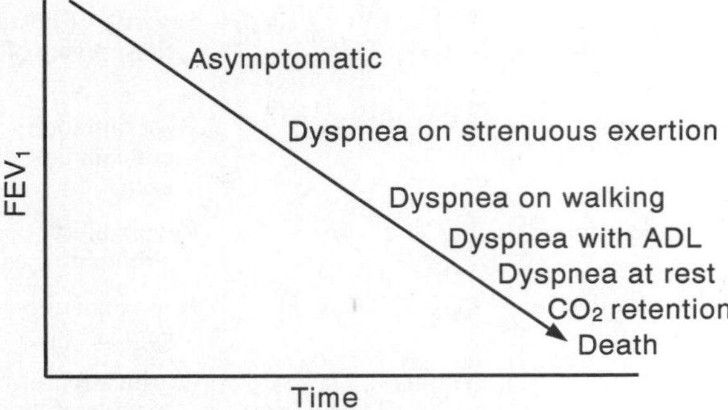

Figure 62-3. Clinical severity of COPD in relation to progressive reduction in FEV_1 over time. The FEV_1 correlates better with prognosis and functional impairment than does any other physiologic measurement. ADL, activities of daily living.

Although the FEV_1 is the best objective monitor of airway function in COPD, it can vary markedly in a given patient over time. This is illustrated by Figure 62-4, which shows repeat FEV_1 determinations after 6 or 7 years in 60 individuals with initially abnormal FEV_1/FVC and/or chronic respiratory symptoms.[20,21] Because of this variability, the clinical course of COPD in a given patient should be followed mainly by symptoms, signs, and functional status, with FEV_1 measurement at regular intervals (e.g., every year) as a supplementary assessment.

General Approach and Philosophy

Management of the patient with disabling COPD is different from treatment of an otherwise healthy person for pneumococcal pneumonia or a fractured femur. Appreciation of this difference is crucial to the overall success of the endeavor and also to the interaction of the caregiver with the COPD patient. Medical students are traditionally taught in the "cure" mode—the patient presents with a constellation of findings, the physician sorts through them, the correct diagnosis is made, and the indicated treatment is carried out, resulting in cure or at least dramatic improvement in the patient's condition. Nursing students, on the other hand, have been taught throughout history in the "care" mode—to care for the patient who is sick, even if they could do little to affect the natural history of the illness. Physicians accustomed to interacting with patients in the cure mode may be frustrated and discouraged as they encounter patients with severe COPD. Such patients often complain bitterly of dyspnea and other symptoms and remain dyspneic despite all the efforts of caregivers; most will never be able to go back to their previous life-styles. It is important for everyone participating in the management of COPD to appreciate this distinction between cure and care for the sake of both patient and caregiver.

As will be discussed, there are a few patients in whom intervention can make a huge difference, not only in symptoms but also in prognosis, but for most patients little physiologic improvement will occur despite the best efforts of everyone involved. This does not mean, as some physicians have told patients over the years, that "nothing can be done." It means that the focus of management must be different. Rehabilitation is defined as the restoration of patients to the fullest potential of which they are capable, with consideration of physiologic, mental, emotional, social, and vocational function. Management of the patient with severe COPD involves all these elements, and meaningful functional improvement can be achieved in virtually every patient.

Figure 62-5 depicts a general relationship between the objective function of a particular organ system and the overall functional status of the individual. This relationship applies to the kidney, the liver, or the brain but is especially relevant to the respiratory system in the case of COPD. As physiologic capacity declines (e.g., as FEV_1 decreases) there is little impact on the individual's ability to carry on normally until a substantial reduction has occurred. With 60 or 70 percent of one's initial maximum FEV_1 it is still possible to carry

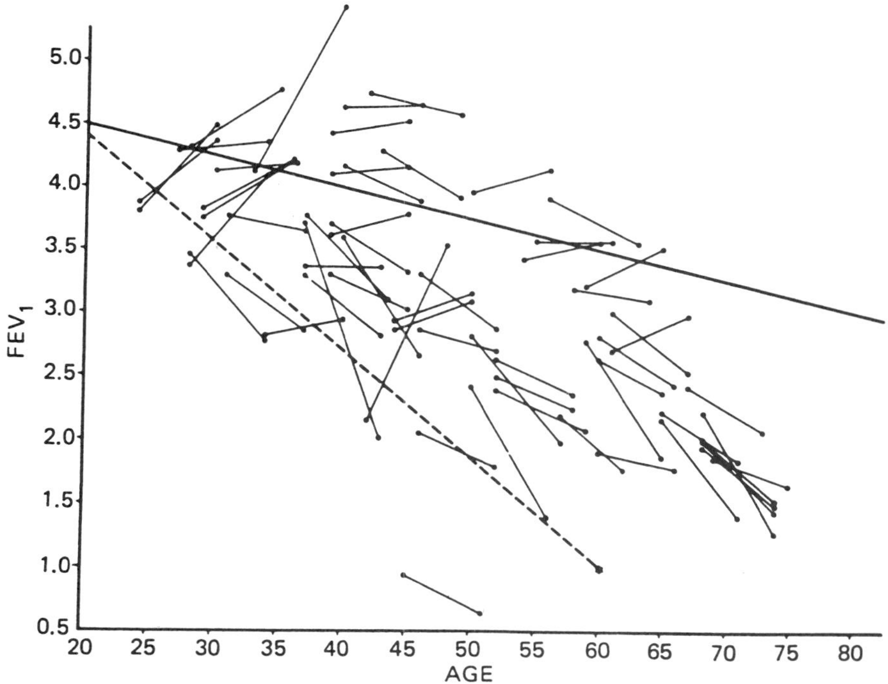

Figure 62-4. Variability in FEV_1 when repeated only once after an interval of 6 or 7 years, illustrating the importance of serial (e.g., yearly) measurements in following any individual patient. Data were obtained on 60 individuals with FEV_1/FVC ratios <60% or chronic respiratory symptoms when initially tested. (Data from Petty et al.[20]) Although most measurements lie roughly on the expected deterioration curve for COPD (60–90 mL annual loss, dashed line), some fall on the "normal" curve for nonsmokers without COPD (30 mL/yr, solid line), and some even increase. (Adapted from Petty,[21] with permission.)

out most normal activities. However, as further physiologic deterioration occurs, the impact on the activities of daily living becomes proportionally greater and greater, so that by the time the FEV_1 reaches 1.0 L, in most patients overall function has been profoundly impaired. In this range of impairment, even a small increase in organ function (the horizontal axis) can make a large difference in life-style (the vertical axis). This is the reasoning behind efforts to achieve maximal pulmonary function in all patients with severe COPD, even those who appear to have "pure" emphysema, and the more severe the obstruction, the more important it is to try.

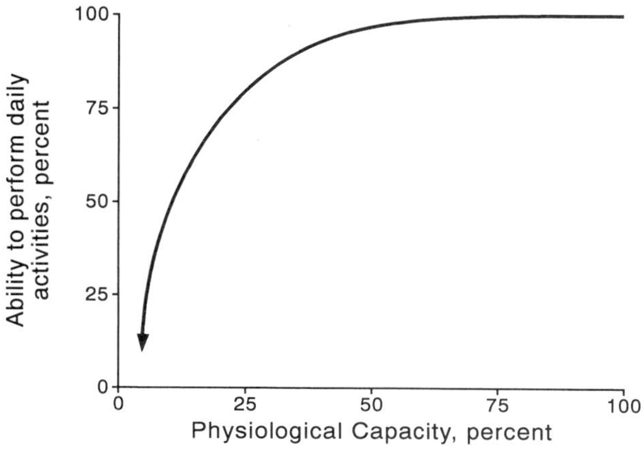

Figure 62-5. Overall relationship between organ system function (e.g., FEV_1, horizontal axis) and functional impact on the individual (vertical axis). In severe airflow obstruction, even small physiologic changes can have important clinical impact.

In view of the limitations imposed by the disease, Table 62-6 lists the goals that the clinician should reasonably expect to achieve in managing the patient with severe COPD. Virtually every patient can achieve better control of symptoms and improved exercise tolerance with appropriate management.[22,23] Psychological improvement, along with better appetite and sleep, should be possible in every case. Improvement in sexual function, an often overlooked but important part of the COPD patient's life, can also be achieved

Table 62-6. Management of the Patient with Severe COPD: Realistic Goals

- For all patients
  - Symptom reduction
  - Improved exercise tolerance
  - Psychological improvement
  - Reduced hospitalization
- For selected patients
  - Improved pulmonary function
  - Increased survival

if special effort is made.[24,25] Several studies have shown that comprehensive management can reduce the need for hospitalization,[26,27] and thereby providing an attendant reduction in monetary cost.[27,28]

For two subsets of patients, other important outcomes can be achieved by appropriate management (Table 62-6). These are individuals with a large reversible (asthmatic) component, whose functional level can be improved markedly by vigorous therapy (see subsequent section), and those patients suitable for long-term O_2 therapy, whose survival and quality of life can be increased if this therapy is used appropriately (see Ch. 63).

Elements of Management

Comprehensive care for the patient with severe COPD consists of an array of empirically derived therapies used together. As shown in Figure 62-2, these individual elements of management vary in importance in the different forms of obstructive lung disease. Each element's importance also varies among patients within a given diagnostic category, so that management must always be individualized. Table 62-7 lists seven important categories of management as most often prescribed by physicians and indicates whether the therapeutic efficacy of each main modality within a given category has been shown convincingly. These and other elements of management vary considerably in the ease with which their intended effects can be achieved in COPD, either because of the inherent difficulty of the therapy or because of failure of many patients to adhere to the prescribed regimen (Table 62-8).

The following sections highlight the general approach to COPD management within each of the major categories of therapy.

Therapy of the Primary Disease Process

Every person who smokes should quit, but smoking cessation is especially important for that subset of smokers who are susceptible to development of COPD. As discussed in Chapter 37 and diagrammed in Figure 37-2, stopping smoking can halt or reduce the rate of subsequent functional loss and thus determine to a major degree the patient's later clinical course. The still functional individual whose FEV_1 is 60 or 70 percent of predicted at the time of quitting may never live long enough to become completely disabled by COPD; survival in even the already disabled patient may be extended by smoking cessation (see Fig. 37-2). In addition, the COPD patient who stops smoking can also expect decreased sputum production and a reduced risk of dying from lung cancer and coronary artery disease.

Should COPD patients change their jobs or move to another part of the country in order to prevent progression of the disease? In most instances, no. There are instances in which occupational or environmental exposures contribute to the development of obstructive lung disease (see Ch. 38), but these are uncommon, and most such exposures aggravate rather than cause COPD. Cigarette smoking is by far the most important etiologic factor, and smoking cessation should be a primary goal in the care of every patient with COPD.

Reversible Airway Obstruction (the Asthmatic Component)

Bronchodilators

Every patient with COPD should be treated with bronchodilators, at least on a trial basis. Even those in whom

Table 62-7. Management of COPD: Available Modalities

Category of Therapy	Modalities of Proven Benefit in Appropriate Patient Populations	Modalities Whose Efficacy Is Uncertain
Prevention	Smoking cessation[a] Influenza vaccine	Pneumococcal vaccine
Bronchodilatation	Anticholinergics Beta agonists Theophylline	
Suppression of inflammation	Systemic corticosteroids	Inhaled corticosteroids Cromolyn sodium
Therapy for infection	Antibiotics (for pneumonia or other specific infection)	Antibiotics (for acute exacerbation)
Therapy for secretions	Systemic hydration Chest physiotherapy	Mucolytics, expectorants
Exercise rehabilitation	Systemic conditioning (walking, cycling)	Respiratory muscle exercises
Therapy for hypoxemia	Long-term O_2 therapy[a]	Almitrine, protriptyline, progesterone

[a] Can extend survival.

Table 62-8. Management of COPD: Relative Difficulty of Different Components

Relatively easy
Making diagnosis
Quantitating physiologic abnormalities
Prescribing medications
Relatively difficult
Achieving improvement in acutely reversible components of disease
Asthma
Infection
Excessive secretions
Counseling patients on behavioral change
Addressing sensitive issues: depression; anxiety; sexuality; prognosis; code status
Very difficult
Achieving behavioral change
Smoking cessation
Life-style
Occupational exposure
Impossible
Reversing existing anatomic damage
Complete return to previous life-style (most patients)

laboratory testing shows no acute reversibility on inhalation of beta-adrenergic agonists may benefit clinically, although there is controversy over how to define "benefit." Some clinicians continue any medication that the patient says improves symptoms; others withhold any agent that does not improve the patient's FEV_1.

Beta-Adrenergic Agonists and Anticholinergics

Beta-adrenergic agonists (e.g., albuterol) and anticholinergics (e.g., ipratropium bromide) are the most effective bronchodilators in COPD (see Ch. 20), and should be used as first-line drugs. They should be given via MDI, with addition of a spacer device if the patient has difficulty coordinating activation with inhalation.[9] Especially with the beta agonists, the best dose for a given patient should be determined individually, preferably by using spirometry and constructing a dose-response curve.[5] Considerably more than the two puffs traditionally used in the United States may be required.[29,30]

If enough puffs of a beta agonist are given, there is no need to use a nebulizer.[9] No type of nebulizer is inherently superior to the MDI if the patient can use the latter, although many patients have been taught that nebulizers "work better" and hence prefer them. Administration of bronchodilators via intermittent positive-pressure breathing (IPPB) offers no advantage over simpler, less costly methods.[31]

Long-acting oral preparations of beta agonists taken at bedtime can occasionally be helpful for patients with prominent nocturnal dyspnea despite intensive inhaler use. In general, however, oral bronchodilators cause more systemic side effects and are unnecessary if appropriate aerosol dosage is used.[32]

Theophylline

Theophylline's place in the therapeutic armamentarium has slipped from initial therapy to a second- or third-line drug,[33,34] and some clinicians believe that it should not be used at all in COPD.[35] As discussed in Chapter 20, the various formulations of theophylline have a low therapeutic index, that is, the ratio of therapeutic to adverse effects is unfavorable. Theophylline is a weak bronchodilator in comparison with the beta agonists and anticholinergics, and its potential for serious toxicity is considerably greater. Many patients say they feel better while taking theophylline, often in the absence of changes in FEV_1. Whether this represents a placebo effect or some legitimate pharmacologic action (e.g., on the respiratory muscles or ventilatory control system) is unclear.

It seems reasonable to try theophylline in patients with severe disease who cannot or will not take inhaled medications or who remain severely symptomatic despite maximal therapy with beta agonists and anticholinergics. A sustained-action theophylline preparation taken at bedtime helps to reduce nocturnal symptoms in some patients and is an alternative to beta agonists for this use. However, blood levels should always be monitored when theophylline is used regularly, and the target range should probably be 10 to 15 rather than 15 to 20 μg/mL. Subtle side effects (abdominal discomfort, insomnia, nervousness) are more common with long-term theophylline use than many clinicians appreciate.

Corticosteroids

Corticosteroids are important drugs, whose use in COPD should be considered in two distinct settings with separate rationales, indications, and administration regimens.[18,36] Short-term administration (i.e., up to 1 to 2 weeks) is relatively safe and constitutes the most effective available drug therapy for acute exacerbations; long-term therapy with systemic corticosteroids is fraught with many, sometimes serious, adverse effects and is justifiable in only a few patients.

Short-term Administration

The efficacy of high-dose, short-term administration of corticosteroids in acute exacerbations of COPD was shown in a study by Albert and colleagues.[37] This often quoted study demonstrated more rapid improvement in pulmonary function in patients who received methylprednisolone 0.5 mg/kg IV every 6 hours for 3 days as compared with placebo, all other aspects of therapy being equal and maximal[37] (Fig. 62-6). Patients with features of asthma and those with pneumonia or other coexisting disease were excluded, so that the participants in this study are probably similar to COPD patients with acute exacerbations as encountered elsewhere by the clinician.

Whether the dose used in the study by Albert et al.[37] is optimal is not known, but methylprednisolone 2 mg/kg/d in divided doses has become a standard for hospitalized patients, with rapid tapering after 3 to 4 days. Corticosteroids are well absorbed after oral administration, and this route

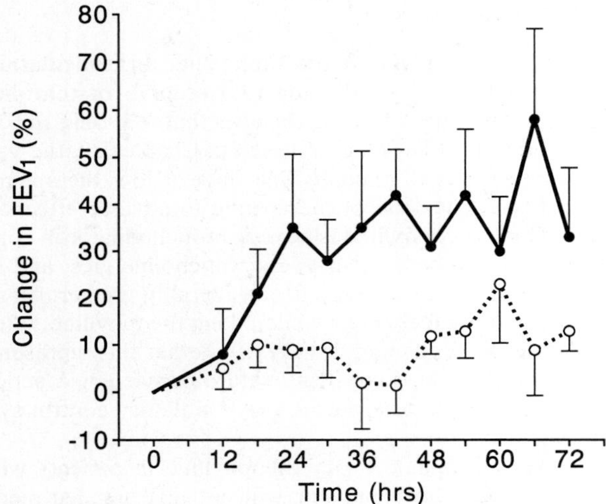

Figure 62-6. Effect on FEV_1 of systemic corticosteroid therapy (solid line) as compared with placebo (dashed line) in 44 patients with acute exacerbations of COPD. Patients who received corticosteroid treatment in addition to bronchodilators and other therapy improved faster than those who did not. (Adapted from Albert et al.,[37] with permission.)

would probably work just as well as the intravenous route, although this question has not been studied. Whether the daily dose should be divided or given once in the morning is also unknown. Outpatients with less severe exacerbations are given the drug by mouth, typically prednisone 40 mg (or equivalent) once daily on arising for 3 to 4 days, with gradual discontinuation over the next 5 to 7 days.

Long-term Administration

Whereas therapy for an acute exacerbation can be given empirically and without testing pulmonary function, neither of these liberties can be taken in long-term administration of corticosteroids.[18,36] This is because osteoporosis, hyperglycemia, increased susceptibility to infection, and other serious adverse effects are common with prolonged use, rendering such therapy medically unjustifiable unless there is objective evidence of efficacy. Because corticosteroids often produce euphoria and a general sense of well-being, particularly in the initial weeks, the patient's subjective response cannot be used as sole determinant for continuing therapy. Instead, a structured trial should be carried out at a time when the patient's disease is clinically stable[18]; the steps in such a trial are outlined in Table 62-9.

Every patient with severe, disabling COPD should probably undergo such a trial. This is because it is not possible to predict with accuracy which patients will experience physiologic improvement and hence increased functional capacity with steroid administration.[36,38–40] Even when atopic features and other possible correlates of steroid responsiveness are absent, 10 to 20 percent of patients with severe COPD will have a clinically significant response to a steroid trial, that is, an improvement in FEV_1 of at least 30 percent. Figure 62-7 is taken from one[39] of several studies[36,38–40] that have demonstrated this phenomenon. It shows the changes from baseline FEV_1 that occurred in 46 COPD patients while they took either placebo or methylprednisolone 32 mg/d for 2 weeks, in random sequence, in addition to their regular therapy. Although there is a variability in these patients' FEV_1 values of up to 30 percent without corticosteroids, 6 of the 46 showed a dramatic (more than 50 percent) improvement from methylprednisolone that did not occur with placebo.

In this minority of patients who demonstrate a substantial steroid response, care should be taken to determine the lowest daily or every-other-day dose of prednisone or equivalent that maintains the improvement. In the other 80 to 90 percent, short-term corticosteroid treatment may still be used during acute exacerbations, but long-term daily administration is not indicated.

Because of the frequency and severity of adverse effects, special measures should be taken to minimize such effects whenever systemic corticosteroids are given chronically. Table 62-10 lists a number of such measures, arranged in the form of a series of "do's" and "don't's."

In contrast to the situation with asthma, inhaled corticosteroids have not been shown to be effective in COPD. It would be reasonable to attempt to switch to inhaled steroids in patients who have experienced dramatic improvement with systemic therapy, although whether this can be done has not been studied. Inhaled steroids should not be used to initiate corticosteroid therapy in COPD.

Table 62-9. Clinical Trial of Systemic Corticosteroid Therapy for Patients with Severe, Clinically Stable COPD[a]

1. Maximize other therapy first
   - A. Inhaled beta-adrenergic bronchodilator (e.g., albuterol)
   - B. Inhaled anticholinergic bronchodilator (e.g., ipratropium bromide)
   - C. Chest physical therapy (as appropriate for patient's secretions and breathing pattern)
   - D. Optional: oral theophylline, titrated to serum level 10–15 μg/mL
2. Explain proposed steroid trial to patient
   - A. Potential adverse effects
   - B. Criteria to be used to continue or stop therapy
3. Assess airflow objectively: spirometry before and after inhaled bronchodilator
4. Add prednisone 40 mg (or equivalent), once daily on arising, for 2–3 weeks
5. Repeat spirometry before and after inhaled bronchodilator
6. If pulmonary function has objectively improved (e.g., >30% increase in FEV_1), continue prednisone, attempting to taper to lowest effective dose
   - A. Alternate-day administration, or
   - B. Replacement with inhaled steroid (e.g., triamcinolone; beclomethasone)
7. If pulmonary function has not improved objectively, taper and discontinue prednisone over 1 week, as previously discussed with patient; subjective improvement alone is insufficient to justify risks of prolonged systemic steroid therapy

[a] In general, appropriate only for patients with severe disease (e.g., FEV_1/FVC <60% and marked impairment in life-style); should be done only when patient is at stable, baseline clinical status, with no current or recent acute exacerbation, respiratory infection, etc.

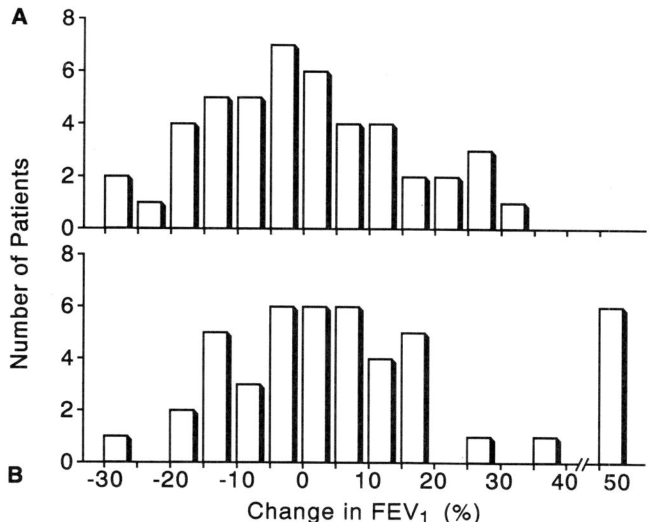

Figure 62-7. (**A**) Placebo, (**B**) corticosteroids. Response to a 2-week trial of systemic corticosteroids as compared with placebo in 46 clinically stable patients with severe COPD. Change in FEV_1 from baseline measurements is shown on the horizontal axis. FEV_1 varies widely in such patients, but in six of them it improved >50% on steroids. The six who responded could not be separated from the others in advance. (Adapted from Mendella et al.,[39] with permission.)

Infection in COPD

Patients with COPD should receive yearly vaccination against influenza, which will reduce the incidence of clinical infection and hence morbidity and mortality.[41] Although administration of pneumococcal vaccine would be highly desirable, whether it actually protects COPD patients from pneumococcal pneumonia is uncertain.[41] Because it has low morbidity and need only be given once, vaccination is nonetheless reasonable in such patients. The role of infection in acute exacerbations and the role of antimicrobials in management are discussed later in this chapter.

Management of Airway Secretions

Clearance of airway secretions can be a problem for the patient with COPD for two reasons: more than the normal quantity of mucus is present in the airways, and the usual clearance mechanisms are impaired. For some patients, frequent coughing and the need to raise secretions is a major subjective concern, leading to severe social impairment. Excessive secretions can also worsen airflow obstruction and hypoxemia. Excessive secretions, like bronchospasm, should be viewed as a potentially reversible aspect of COPD, and when treatment for secretions per se is indicated, it should be pursued vigorously.

Patients whose illness most closely fits with type A COPD (i.e., is assumed to be primarily emphysema) often cough little and expectorate no secretions at all. On the other hand, the copious secretions and frequent expectoration that are typical of type B COPD are not in themselves indications for specific therapy, as individuals with these symptoms may be able to raise their secretions adequately without help.

A wide variety of measures can be applied in the management of airway secretions[42] (Table 62-11). Which ones to use and with how much vigor must be determined empirically for most patients. Adequate systemic hydration and appropriate therapy for bronchospasm and airway inflammation should obviously be sought in all patients. Most individuals

Table 62-10. Practical "Do's and Don't's" of Long-Term Corticosteroid Therapy

Do	Don't
Use lowest effective dose[a]	Rely on steroids alone to control disease
Increase dose to cover stress	Withdraw steroids rapidly
Continually attempt to wean patient from steroids[b]	Allow patient to increase dosage irresponsibly
Administer daily single dose of steroid in the morning	Administer daily single dose of steroid at bedtime
Attempt to switch patient to alternate-day dosage regimen	Administer steroids oftener than once daily when patient is clinically stable
Use inhaled rather than oral steroids in asthma	Use steroids in combination preparations
Control weight gain by diet	Permit liberal use of salt in diet
Administer antacids and/or H2 blockers if patient has symptoms of peptic disease	Administer peptic ulcer therapy in absence of symptoms or history of disease
Use most suitable and least expensive steroid preparation	Use steroids with marked mineralocorticoid effect, especially in patients with hypertension, edema, obesity, or known cardiac, renal, or hepatic disease
Carry out routine medical follow-up	Allow patients to go for long periods without medical supervision
Consider administration of prophylactic antituberculous therapy in patients with positive tuberculin skin tests	Vaccinate against smallpox; use caution in administering other immunizations

[a] Side effects are minimal if daily corticosteroid dose is less than 6 mg prednisone or its equivalent (see Table 20-4).
[b] No patient should be considered "steroid-dependent" until such attempts have failed several times.
(Modified, from Ziment,[76] with permission.)

Table 62-11. Strategies for the Management of Excessive Airway Secretions

Preservation of natural mucokinetic mechanisms
Normal quantity and consistency of secretions
Appropriate sol-gel relationship
Activity and coordination of cilia
Airway patency
Adequate airflow
Use of mechanical factors
Stimulation, encouragement, and teaching of patient
Cough stimulation
Postural drainage
Chest percussion
Suctioning (nasotracheal, endotracheal)
Administration of pharmacologic agents
Hypoviscosity agents and diluents (e.g., water)
Bronchomucotropic agents (e.g., iodides)
Mucolytics (e.g., acetylcysteine)
Detergents and surfactants (e.g., sodium bicarbonate)
Bronchodilators (e.g., albuterol)

(Adapted from Ziment,[42] with permission.)

with severe, disabling airflow obstruction should receive a trial of chest physical therapy, as described in Chapter 70. If such measures are going to help, this should be apparent after a few treatments, and an elaborate ritual of humidification, breathing exercises, postural drainage, and chest percussion should not automatically be prescribed in open-ended fashion. Patients generally discontinue therapies they deem ineffective, and discouragement with a lack of obvious benefit can lead them to be noncompliant with other aspects of management as well.

Mucolytics and expectorants are more commonly prescribed in parts of Europe than in the United States. As pointed out in Chapter 20, objective evidence for the efficacy of these agents in clinical patient care is generally lacking. The majority of COPD patients can be managed satisfactorily without addition of drugs for secretions to what is often an already lengthy list of medications.

Approach to Management of Acute Exacerbations

Most patients with COPD experience episodes of increased dyspnea, cough, and sputum production, usually accompanied by a change in sputum color (from clear to yellow or from yellow to green, occasionally with streaks of blood). Such episodes often follow an upper respiratory infection, although whether they themselves represent infections remains unclear. In many patients they also occur at times of heavy air pollution, a change in the weather, or temporary discontinuation of bronchodilators. It is not possible to identify a specific cause for most acute exacerbations.

A careful history and physical examination are usually all that is necessary for evaluation. Chest radiographs are not helpful unless there are symptoms or signs suggesting pneumonia or pneumothorax. Sputum cultures and Gram stains seldom contribute additional information. Studies have shown that patients with COPD are usually colonized with *Streptococcus pneumoniae* and *Haemophilus influenzae*, both during flare-ups and when clinically stable, so that demonstrating their presence adds nothing; other organisms are not usually found. Arterial blood gases should be measured as part of the clinical assessment if the patient appears seriously ill; pulse oximetry, which assesses only oxygenation and not PCO_2 or pH, should not be used as the sole assessment of gas exchange and acid-base status in this setting.

In contrast to the situation with corticosteroids, most carefully controlled studies have failed to substantiate the common impression that antibiotic therapy is helpful in acute exacerbations of COPD.[43] If there is a positive effect of antibiotic therapy in this setting, it is not a dramatic one.[44] If drugs are prescribed for the treatment of infection, agents should be selected to cover the organisms most likely to be present (i.e., *S. pneumoniae* and *H. influenzae*). Amoxicillin, ampicillin, a tetracycline, or trimethoprim-sulfamethoxazole are good choices; erythromycin and penicillin are less appropriate, and there is no need to use newer, more expensive, broader-spectrum agents. Therapy is generally given for 5 to 10 days.

As discussed previously, corticosteroids appear to be the most effective agents in acute exacerbations. Bronchodilator therapy should be continued and may need to be intensified during these times. Patients with cor pulmonale may have increased right-sided heart failure during acute exacerbations, which should be treated appropriately (see Ch. 63). Although unnecessary at other times, therapy for excessive airway secretions may be required during exacerbations. Sedatives, hypnotics, and drugs to reduce dyspnea should be used cautiously, even if tolerated by the patient while clinically stable. These and other aspects of management in severe acute exacerbations are discussed further in Chapter 64.

Dyspnea, Anxiety, and Depression

Some patients are incapacitated by dyspnea as the primary manifestation of their disease. Such patients typify the type A or pink puffer concept as discussed in Chapter 22. If the distress is commensurate with the severity of airflow obstruction (e.g., FEV_1 less than 1.0 L), treatment directed at the dyspnea itself may be worthwhile. However, if the shortness of breath is out of proportion to the patient's airflow obstruction, an appropriate workup for concomitant cardiac dysfunction, pulmonary vascular disease, or restrictive pulmonary disorder should be carried out.

Anxiety is common in patients with severe COPD, and some experience panic attacks that can be severely disabling. Before anxiolytic agents such as benzodiazepines are prescribed for such patients, an attempt at behavioral modification through breathing retraining or pursed-lips breathing (see Ch. 98) can be helpful. Such measures, which slow and deepen inefficient breaths, can enable patients to better tolerate their airflow obstruction even if this cannot be improved by other therapy.

Although clinicians have been taught for a generation never to administer sedatives, particularly opiates, to patients with severe COPD, there are circumstances in which such drugs can be used safely and with striking benefit. Potential candidates are patients in whom dyspnea is severe despite all other appropriate therapy, who are clinically stable, and who do not have hypoxemia or hypercapnia (see Ch. 66). Under such conditions, the cautious addition of codeine 15 to 30 mg or oxycodone 5 mg (typically in a combination preparation also containing acetaminophen or aspirin) twice or three times daily to the patient's other medications can produce substantial relief of dyspnea.[45] Codeine and its derivatives tend to be more effective in treating dyspnea than are benzodiazepines or barbiturates. Constipation can be a troublesome side effect, and the medication must be used cautiously (and the dose not increased) during acute exacerbations.

Antianxiety agents (e.g., benzodiazepines) are helpful in a few patients with dyspnea related to anxiety, but these drugs are vastly overused. Insomnia, a common complaint in patients with COPD, is exceedingly difficult to treat, particularly if it becomes chronic. However, if accompanied by other features of depression, insomnia may respond to bedtime administration of doxepin, 75 to 150 mg, or triazolam 0.125 to 0.25 mg.[46] Depression is common in COPD and can be an unrecognized, debilitating problem.[47] As with other disabling chronic diseases, suicide is more common in patients with COPD than in the general population. A worsening of signs of depression and, particularly, any expression of suicidal thoughts should prompt the clinician to discuss the issue directly with the patient and family members, with referral for professional help if warranted.

Nutrition

Malnutrition, anorexia, and weight loss occur frequently in patients with severe COPD and become increasingly problematic in the later stages of the disease.[48,49] Although these phenomena surely contribute to the patient's decline, it is uncertain whether measures directed specifically at reversing them, in addition to good general care, are of benefit. Intensive nutritional supplementation in the research setting has achieved weight gain in some patients, along with increased respiratory muscle strength.[50] However, in practice it can be exceedingly difficult to effect a real increase in caloric intake in the face of poor appetite and severely restricted physical activity.[49,51]

Attempts should be made to provide a balanced diet that is appealing to the patient. Protein-calorie supplementation with between-meal milk shakes and commercially available drinks may help but can decrease the patient's appetite at mealtime. Sodium intake should be reduced in patients with congestive heart failure, but the practical benefit of special dietary formulations with reduced carbohydrate calories for pulmonary patients is yet to be shown.

Family and Caregiver Issues

Patients with severe COPD may fail to improve despite accurate diagnosis and the prescription of appropriate therapy. As in other chronic disabling conditions, an individual's prognosis, response to therapy, and quality of life depend on nonmedical as well as medical factors. The patient's family support system, living situation, socioeconomic status, and other psychosocial factors (see Ch. 60) are crucial elements in the overall effectiveness of management. As discussed in more detail in Chapters 98 and 101, prognosis and the overall success of management will be determined as much by these nonmedical factors as by any other.

For some patients, certain types of care such as long-term O_2 therapy and home ventilatory assistance will be impossible, not for medical or even financial reasons but because of family and social factors. Success with other less technology-dependent elements of management, such as chest physical therapy and taking prescribed medications in the right doses and at the right times, may require considerable effort and creativity on the part of the management team. For some patients transportation to the physician's office, laboratory, or pharmacy can be an obstacle; for others, assistance with household chores or activities of daily living is necessary. These are only examples of the wide array of family and caregiver issues of which the clinician must be aware in order to accomplish the best possible patient care.

For severely impaired patients it is vital that the physician or someone else on the management team actually visit the home and become acquainted with those on whom the patient depends. Family dynamics, the physical arrangement of the living environment, and other key factors cannot be properly appreciated without a home visit. Fortunately, home care is expanding rapidly in the 1990s, and levels of in-home management that were previously impossible or inconvenient to attain are now routinely available in many areas.

Terminal Management

Because COPD is a progressive, fatal disease, the clinician must contend with the terminal phase and death of the patient.[48] Dealing with these aspects of the illness is difficult for many health professionals, but not to do so may subject the patient to unnecessary suffering and deprive both patient and family of much needed planning, support, and other care.

Although the rates of functional and physiologic deterioration vary, all patients nonetheless suffer a progression in the manifestations of COPD, as depicted in Figure 62-3. Once a patient is in the late stages of the illness (e.g., homebound, requiring assistance in activities of daily living, perhaps requiring repeated admissions to the hospital), it is important that consideration be given to terminal management. It is never possible to predict survival precisely in terms of weeks or months, and this should be communicated to all concerned, but patients and families are usually grateful for a general discussion of prognosis and what can be expected at the end of life. They should be assured that appropriate treatment (e.g., for dyspnea or pain) will continue and that caregivers will not abandon them.

When the time comes, many patients prefer to die at home among family members and in familiar surroundings rather than in the hospital. If this is the case, it should be discussed in advance so that the others in the home will know what to do if the patient suddenly deteriorates. Once the telephone number 911 is called and the patient is rushed to the hospital emergency department, it can be extremely difficult to prevent intubation, mechanical ventilation, and admission to the intensive care unit.

Withholding intubation and other life-prolonging measures is generally counter to the purposes of emergency departments and their staffs. However, under certain circumstances the most medically appropriate and humane action is "Don't just do something—stand there!"[52] Not to proceed with all available therapy requires certainty that this is appropriate. To help resolve this issue, Petty[52] offers four questions for deciding whether to institute resuscitative measures when faced with a patient in extremis or in cardiopulmonary arrest, who is known or suspected to have end-stage COPD or some other terminal condition:

1. Do I know the patient's underlying disease process and its course and prognosis?
2. Do I know the patient's quality of life in the context of the disease process?
3. Do I have anything more to offer the patient by resuscitative efforts designed to gain more time?
4. Do I wish to gain more time through resuscitative efforts to resolve these other questions?[52]

It may not be possible to know the answers to the first three of these questions in the heat of the moment, and intubation must proceed in response to the fourth question. Figure 62-8 depicts two hypothetical settings in which these questions might be asked. Point B indicates terminal, irreversible respiratory failure as a result of the inexorable progression of disease, for which intubation and mechanical ventilation can offer no meaningful benefit. Point A, however, represents an acute, potentially reversible deterioration in a patient who could be returned to a reasonable functional level with appropriate treatment. It would be reasonable to intubate the patient at point A, or if insufficient information is at hand to know where a patient should be placed on this curve. Intubation and other life-sustaining therapy would not be appropriate for the patient at point B.

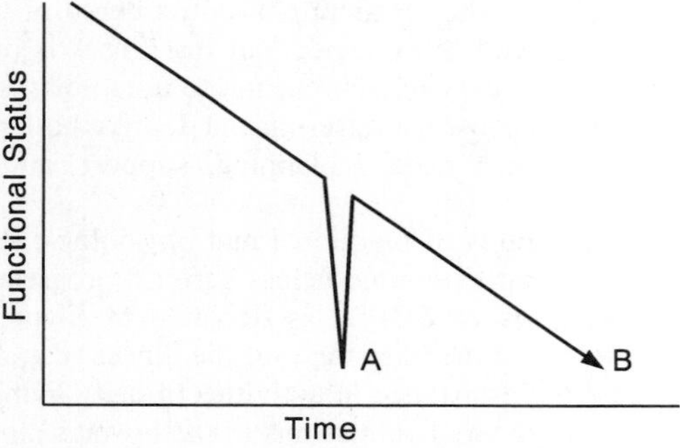

Figure 62-8. Two possible points in the course of a COPD patient's illness in which intubation and other life-support measures might be considered. At point A the patient suffers an acute deterioration while still retaining a reasonable degree of function; this level of function should again be attainable after the acute episode. Respiratory failure at point B represents the end stage of the patient's underlying disease; little functional improvement could be hoped for here. For further discussion see text.

ALPHA-1-ANTITRYPSIN DEFICIENCY

The clinical features of the lung disease, predominantly emphysema, associated with congenital homozygous deficiency of alpha-1-antitrypsin (AAT) (alpha-1-protease inhibitor) constitute a subset of COPD.[53,54] This disease differs from COPD as seen in other patients mainly in our knowledge of its etiology, the specifics of diagnosis, some relatively unimportant aspects of the clinical presentation, the need for family intervention and genetic counseling, and the potential for treating the primary disease process.

Diagnosis and Assessment

Patients with clinically significant COPD who present in their forties or earlier, especially if they are nonsmokers, should be considered for the diagnosis of AAT deficiency, and serum AAT level should be measured. New standards fix the normal range for serum AAT at 150 to 350 mg/dL (20 to 48 μmol/L).[53] If a result below the lower limit of this range is obtained, the test should be repeated. The threshold protective level is believed to be 35 percent of normal (i.e., 80 mg/dL or 11 μmol/L); more than 95 percent of individuals in the severely deficient category most often associated with progressive emphysema have levels of 2.5 to 7 μmol/L.[53]

General Approach

Management of COPD in patients with AAT deficiency includes all the components of comprehensive care discussed earlier in this chapter and covered in more detail in Section 5 of this book. The avoidance or cessation of smoking is especially important in these individuals. Two additional management elements are augmentation (replacement) therapy[55–57] and lung transplantation. Only preliminary experience is available with lung transplantation for end-stage emphysema associated with AAT deficiency,[58] but replacement therapy is currently available and in use in the United States.[59]

Replacement Therapy

Partially purified AAT (Prolastin) was approved by the U.S. Food and Drug Administration in 1987 for the treatment of AAT deficiency. Replacement therapy is currently recommended for patients with obstructive lung disease whose serum AAT levels are less than the threshold protective level of 80 mg/dL (11 μmol/L).[53] It is administered intravenously at a dose of 60 mg/kg each week and costs approximately $25,000 annually in 1991 for a 70-kg patient.[53] Such administration produces an increase in both serum and lung AAT levels,[57,59] although it is too early to tell whether this affects the rate of loss of FEV_1 or any other manifestation of the disease. It may be possible to deliver the replacement protein directly into the lower airway.[60]

BRONCHIECTASIS

Bronchiectasis, defined as abnormal dilatation of bronchi greater than 2 mm in diameter, can be either focal or diffuse. When focal, it is most often the result of localized bronchial obstruction (e.g., by a foreign body) or distortion following an infection. Much more commonly bronchiectasis is a diffuse, generalized process, which occurs either as a feature of COPD or in association with a variety of immunodeficiency states or congenital conditions (e.g., cystic fibrosis, AAT deficiency, immotile cilia syndrome).[61] The three pathologic-radiologic types originally described by Reid[62] (cylindrical, varicose, and saccular) are conceptually but not clinically helpful because they produce the same general clinical picture.[61]

Diagnosis and Assessment

Bronchiectasis produces a classic combination of symptoms, including chronic cough, purulent expectoration of often copious and foul-smelling sputum, recurrent episodes of fever, weakness, and weight loss.[63] Clinical severity correlates loosely with the quantity of sputum produced; patients with severe disease produce over 150 mL in 24 hours, and many expectorate much more than this. The sputum typically separates into three layers. Recurrent hemoptysis is common and can be massive. Finger clubbing is also common. Most patients manifest airflow obstruction on pulmonary function testing, and mild restriction may also be present. The DLCO may be decreased, but this is variable. Most patients are mildly hypoxemic until late in the disease, at which time both severe hypoxemia and progressive hypercapnia may be seen.

The diagnosis is suggested clinically on the basis of the features listed above (Fig. 62-1). Until recently, confirmation required bronchography[63]; computed tomography (CT) has now largely replaced this procedure,[64] although some surgeons still rely on bronchography prior to any contemplated resectional surgery.

General Approach

Except when it is purely localized or a feature of an immunodeficiency state or congenital condition, bronchiectasis may be thought of as one end of the spectrum of chronic bronchitis in COPD. That is, bronchiectasis is most often diffuse and a feature of the broader COPD syndrome. Management generally differs only in degree from that of COPD in other settings and is guided by the clinical features presented by the individual patient.

Medical Management

Antibiotics are the mainstay of management and in most cases should be prescribed according to the results of aerobic and anaerobic cultures.[61,65] When the sputum contains only mixed or "normal" flora, amoxicillin, ampicillin, a tetracycline, or trimethoprim-sulfamethoxazole should be used. Several approaches to the use of these agents exist—most clinicians prescribe them only during acute exacerbations, but some prefer to give them on a regular, recurring basis, such as 2 weeks in each month. Efficacy is judged by clinical response rather than by serial cultures, chest radiographs, or other laboratory studies.

Chest physical therapy is especially helpful in some patients with bronchiectasis, although this is variable.[65] A regimen of bronchodilator inhalation, humidification, postural drainage, and chest percussion should be tried and should be continued if it appears to facilitate expectoration. Some patients benefit considerably from such a regimen during acute exacerbations but less so when clinically stable. Mucolytic drugs such as acetyl cysteine are prescribed by some clinicians for patients with bronchiectasis, although most do not find them helpful.

Surgical Therapy

Medical management will control the clinical manifestations of bronchiectasis in most patients. In most cases either the distorted bronchi are distributed widely throughout both lungs or the patient has such severe generalized airflow obstruction that surgery is not an option. Resection is technically feasible, however, when lung function is good and the abnormal bronchi are confined to one or a few pulmonary segments. Still, despite claimed improvement following surgery in some series,[66] no randomized studies have been carried out using intensive medical management as a control.

Surgery should probably be reserved for patients with focal abnormalities who are unwilling or unable to comply with medical management.[61,65] Life-threatening hemoptysis is another potential indication for surgical intervention, although advances in interventional radiology (i.e., angiography with arterial embolization) provide another option, particularly for patients with very poor pulmonary function.

CYSTIC FIBROSIS IN THE ADULT

The relation of lung disease in cystic fibrosis (CF) to the genetic defect in this disease is uncertain; pulmonary manifestations consist mainly of the consequences of recurrent bacterial infections and unremitting airway inflammation.[67–69] The clinical picture is dominated by the manifestations and consequences of bronchiectasis. Common complications as the lung disease progresses include clubbing and hypertrophic pulmonary osteoarthropathy, recurrent hemoptysis (which can be massive and fatal), pneumothorax, lobar atelectasis, and finally cor pulmonale. Early in the clinical course the airways usually become infected with *Staphylococcus aureus*, which is typically succeeded some time later by mucoid strains of *Pseudomonas aeruginosa*, which are virtually impossible to eradicate.

Diagnosis and Assessment

Whereas in infancy CF can present with either gastrointestinal involvement (intestinal obstruction, malabsorption, failure to thrive) or lung disease, in older children and adults the initial manifestations are nearly always pulmonary.[67,68] Typical circumstances leading to the diagnosis in young adults are recurrent pneumonia, chronic productive cough, and lobar atelectasis. Some patients have features of asthma and are followed for years with this diagnosis before the correct one is made. Symptoms or radiographic findings of bronchiectasis are perhaps most common and should always prompt suspicion of CF when they occur in a young white adult (CF occurs once in every 2000 live births in whites, once in 17,000 in blacks, and once in 90,000 in Orientals).[68]

The diagnosis of CF is made when chronic obstructive lung disease and/or pancreatic insufficiency occurs in a patient with an elevated sweat chloride level (above 60 mEq/L) on at least two determinations.[70] A positive family history for CF is helpful but often absent in adults. The sweat test (technically, quantitative pilocarpine iontophoresis) yields chloride concentrations higher than 60 mEq/L in over 98 percent of individuals with CF, whereas only 4 percent of healthy adults show this result.[68]

Abnormalities in pulmonary function often follow a characteristic sequence in patients with CF, and this may guide both assessment and prognosis.[67,68] All tests may be normal for years. The initial abnormality is usually detected in tests of small airway function, for example by a reduction in FEF_{25-75} or frequency dependence of compliance. Next, air trapping becomes evident in the form of an increased ratio of RV/VC. Later airflow obstruction becomes overt and FEV_1 falls, and in the late stages of the disease FVC also diminishes. Gas exchange is usually well preserved until late; the alveolar-arterial O_2 partial pressure difference [P(A-a) O_2] and DLCO are often normal despite marked reduction in FEV_1. Hypoxemia and especially hypercapnia are characteristically late findings.

General Approach

The cornerstones of management[68] are (1) vaccination and other measures to prevent viral infections; (2) vigorous treatment of bacterial infections with antibiotics (often parenteral) as determined by the sensitivities of bacteria on sputum culture[69,71]; and (3) assistance with the clearance of respiratory secretions,[72] usually by means of regular chest percussion and postural drainage. Close follow-up and long-term continuity of care are especially important.

Hemoptysis occurs in the majority of patients with CF. In some it may be massive (more than 500 mL in 24 hours), and in these instances it can be fatal. However, hemoptysis is generally managed conservatively, and patients with this complication do no worse than those who do not experience it. Pneumothorax, common in older patients with CF, is considered an adverse prognostic sign. Because of the frequency of recurrence many authorities now recommend pleurodesis after the first episode, with surgical intervention if this fails. Another frequent complication is acute lobar atelectasis, although this may produce little clinical deterioration. Bronchoscopy is not considered any more effective in re-expanding the collapsed lung tissue than chest physiotherapy, and the latter is preferable.

Late in the illness long-term O_2 therapy is commonly initiated, often during night-time hours,[73] although this practice is based on extrapolation of studies in COPD rather than on data from CF patients, and its efficacy is unknown.[69] Bilateral lung transplantation has recently been used with success in CF,[74,75] and this therapy, though expensive, is likely to become more widespread. On the distant horizon is gene therapy, which becomes a feasible goal now that the nature of the genetic defect is better understood.

BULLOUS LUNG DISEASE

Bullae consist of areas of massive focal dilatation of respiratory air spaces; these may result from coalescence of adjacent areas of emphysema, from localized panacinar emphysema, or from a ball-valve effect in the airways supplying an emphysematous area.[17] Bullae usually occur in the apices of the lungs and are more common in cigarette smokers. Most often bullae are features of widespread, diffuse emphysema, although they can occur as an isolated phenomenon.

When they become very large, bullae may compress adjacent, more normal lung tissue and cause both dyspnea and deranged gas exchange. Surgical removal can produce dramatic improvement if the function of the rest of the lung is good. However, more often bullae are detected radiographically in patients with severe COPD, in whom symptoms and physiologic abnormalities are more likely due to the diffuse underlying pathology than to the bullae themselves.

Individuals with large bullae are at increased risk of pneumothorax if subjected to sudden changes in atmospheric pressure. Such persons should not engage in scuba diving or other activities in which rapid barometric pressure changes occur. Travel in pressurized aircraft is of less concern because the pressure changes gradually.

Occasionally bullae become partially filled with fluid, as detected by an air-fluid level on upright chest radiograph. This may be due to hemorrhage, accumulation of (noninfected) fluid near a region of pneumonitis, or frank infection of the bullous cavity. In the last situation management can be difficult and frustrating because of the severity of underlying lung dysfunction and the high incidence of bronchopleural fistula accompanying tube thoracostomy. Bullae filled with noninfected fluid generally do not require any special management.

References

1. Pierson DJ: An algorithmic approach to obstructive pulmonary disease. J Respir Dis, Suppl. 6, 1990;11:S30–S34
2. Stuhlbarg MS, Gerbert B, Kemeny ME et al: Outpatient treatment of chronic obstructive pulmonary disease—a practitioner's guide. West J Med 1985;142:842–846
3. Pierson DJ: Asthma. pp. 141–146. In Luce JM, Pierson DJ (eds): Critical Care Medicine. WB Saunders, Philadelphia, 1988
4. Rebuck AS, Read J: Assessment and management of acute asthma. Am J Med 1971;51:788–798
5. Newhouse MT, Dolovich MB: Control of asthma by aerosols. N Engl J Med 1986;315:870–874
6. Barnes PJ: A new approach to the treatment of asthma. N Engl J Med 1989;321:1517–1527
7. Barnes PJ: New concepts in the pathogenesis of bronchial hyperresponsiveness and asthma. J Allergy Clin Immunol 1989;83:1013–1026
8. Bone RC: Step care for asthma, editorial. JAMA 1988;260:543
9. Concensus conference on aerosol delivery. Respir Care 1991; 36:916–1044
10. Barnes PJ: Effect of corticosteroids on airway hyperresponsiveness. Am Rev Respir Dis, Suppl. 1990;141:S70–S76
11. Zeiger RS, Schatz M, Sperling W et al: Efficacy of troleandomycin in outpatients with severe, corticosteroid-dependent asthma. J Allergy Clin Immunol 1980;66:438–446
12. Harris R, German D: The incidence of corticosteroid side effects in chronic steroid-dependent asthmatics on TAO (troleandomycin) and methylprednisolone. Ann Allergy 1989;63:110–111
13. Mullarkey MF, Blumenstein BA, Andrade WP et al: Methotrexate in the treatment of corticosteroid-dependent asthma. A double-blind crossover study. N Engl J Med 1988;318:603–607
14. Mullarkey MF, Lammert JK, Blumenstein BA: Long-term methotrexate treatment in corticosteroid-dependent asthma. Ann Intern Med 1990;112:577–558
15. Reed CE, Hunt LW: The emergency visit and management of asthma. Ann Intern Med 1990;112:801–802
16. Swedish Society of Chest Medicine: High-dose inhaled versus intravenous salbutamol combined with theophylline in severe acute asthma. Eur Respir J 1990;3:163–170
17. Snider GL: Chronic bronchitis and emphysema. pp. 1069–1106. In Murray JF, Nadel JA (eds): Textbook of Respiratory Medicine. WB Saunders, Philadelphia, 1988
18. Pierson DJ: Chronic obstructive pulmonary disease and bronchiectasis. pp. 96–106. In Rakel RE (ed): Conn's current therapy 1985. WB Saunders, Philadelphia, 1985
19. Gelb AF, Gold WM, Wright RR et al: Physiologic diagnosis of subclinical emphysema. Am Rev Respir Dis 1973;107:50–63
20. Petty TL, Pierson DJ, Dick NP, et al: Follow-up evaluation of a prevalence study for chronic bronchitis and chronic airway obstruction. Am Rev Respir Dis 1976;114:881–890
21. Petty TL: Early diagnosis. pp. 221–238. In Petty TL (ed): Chronic Obstructive Pulmonary Disease. Marcel Dekker, New York, 1978
22. Lertzman MM, Cherniack RM: Rehabilitation of patients with chronic obstructive pulmonary disease. State of the art. Am Rev Respir Dis 1976;114:1145–1168
23. Fishman DJ, Petty TL: Physical, symptomatic, and psychosocial improvement in patients receiving comprehensive care for chronic airway obstruction. J Chronic Dis 1971;24:755–785
24. Della Bella L: Sexuality and the pulmonary patient. pp. 239–261. In Hodgkin JE, Zorn EG, Connors GL (eds): Pulmonary Rehabilitation: Guidelines to Success. Butterworth-Heinemann, Stoneham, MA, 1984
25. Selecky PA: Sexuality and the COPD patient. pp. 215–226. In Hodgkin JE, Petty TL (eds): Chronic Obstructive Pulmonary Disease: Current Concepts. WB Saunders, Philadelphia, 1987
26. Hudson LD, Tyler ML, Petty TL: Hospitalization needs during an outpatient rehabilitation program for chronic airway obstruction. Chest 1976;70:607–610
27. Burton GG, Gee G, Hodgkin JE, Dunham JL: Cost effectiveness in respiratory care: An overview and some possibly early solutions. Hospitals 1975;49:61–71
28. Dunham JL, Hodgkin JE, Nicol J, Burton GG: Cost effectiveness of pulmonary rehabilitation programs. pp. 389–402. In Hodgkin JE, Zorn EG, Connors GL (eds): Pulmonary Rehabilitation: Guidelines to Success. Butterworth-Heinemann, Stoneham, MA, 1984
29. Vathenen AS, Britton JR, Ebden P et al: High-dose inhaled albuterol in severe chronic airflow obstruction. Am Rev Respir Dis 1988;138:850–855
30. Gross NJ: Ipratropium bromide. N Engl J Med 1988;319:486–494
31. The Intermittent Positive Pressure Breathing Trial Group: Intermittent positive pressure breathing therapy of chronic obstructive lung disease: A clinical trial. Ann Intern Med 1983;99:612–620
32. Svedmyr N: Clinical advantages of the aerosol route of drug administration. Respir Care 1991;36:922–930
33. Rossing TH: Methylxanthines in 1989. Ann Intern Med 1989;110:502–504
34. Drazen JM, Gerard C: Reversing the irreversible. N Engl J Med 1989;320:1555–1556
35. Rice KL, Leatherman JW, Duane PG et al: Aminophylline for acute exacerbations of chronic obstructive pulmonary disease. A controlled trial. Ann Intern Med 1987;107:305–309
36. Hudson LD, Monti CM: Rationale and use of corticosteroids in chronic obstructive pulmonary disease. Med Clin North Am 1990;74:661–690
37. Albert RK, Martin TR, Lewis SE: Controlled clinical trial of methylprednisolone in patients with chronic bronchitis and acute respiratory insufficiency. Ann Intern Med 1980;92:753–758
38. Petty TL, Brink GA, Miller MW, Corsello PR: Objective functional improvement in chronic airway obstruction. Chest 1970;57:216–223
39. Mendella LA, Manfreda J, Warren CPW, Anthonisen NR: Steroid response in stable chronic obstructive pulmonary disease. Ann Intern Med 1982;96:17–21
40. Shim C, Stover DE, Williams MH: Response to corticosteroids in chronic bronchitis. J Allergy Clin Immunol 1978;62:363–367
41. American Thoracic Society, Medical Section of the American Lung Association: Prevention of influenza and pneumonia. Am Rev Respir Dis 1990;142:487–488
42. Ziment I: Drugs used in respiratory therapy. pp. 456–492. In Burton GG, Hodgkin JE (eds): Respiratory Care. A Guide to Clinical Practice. 2nd Ed. JB Lippincott, Philadelphia, 1985
43. Tager I, Speizer FE: Role of infection in chronic bronchitis. N Engl J Med 1975;292:563–571
44. Anthonisen NR, Manfreda J, Warren CPW et al: Antibiotic therapy in exacerbations of chronic obstructive pulmonary disease. Ann Intern Med 1987;106:196–204
45. Woodcock AA, Gross ER, Gellert A et al: Effects of dihydrocodeine, alcohol, and caffeine on breathlessness and exercise tolerance in patients with chronic obstructive lung disease and normal blood gases. N Engl J Med 1981;305:1611–1616
46. Timms RM, Dawson A, Hajdukovic RM, Mitler M: Effect of triazolam on arterial oxygen saturation in patients with chronic obstructive pulmonary disease. Arch Intern Med 1988;148:2159–2163
47. Dudley DL, Sitzman J: Psychosocial and psychophysiologic approach to the patient. Semin Respir Med 1979;1:59–83
48. Petty TL: Dealing with the final stages of disease. pp. 279–293. In Hodgkin JE, Petty TL (eds): Chronic Obstructive Pulmonary Disease: Current Concepts. WB Saunders, Philadelphia, 1987

49. Wilson DO, Rogers RM, Hoffman RM: Nutrition and chronic lung disease. Am Rev Respir Dis 1985;132:1347–1365
50. Wilson DO, Rogers RM, Sanders MH et al: Nutritional intervention in malnourished patients with emphysema. Am Rev Respir Dis 1986;134:672–677
51. Lewis MI, Belman MJ, Dorr-Uyemura L: Nutritional supplementation in ambulatory patients with chronic obstructive pulmonary disease. Am Rev Respir Dis 1987;135:1062–1068
52. Petty TL: Don't just do something—stand there! Arch Intern Med 1979;139:920–921
53. Snider GL: Pulmonary disease in alpha-1-antitrypsin deficiency. Ann Intern Med 1989;111:957–959
54. Idell S, Cohen SB: Alpha-1-antitrypsin deficiency. Clin Chest Med 1983;4:359–376
55. Crystal RG, Brantly ML, Hubbard RC, et al: The alpha 1-antitrypsin gene and its mutations. Clinical consequences and strategies for therapy. Chest 1989;95:196–208
56. Wewers MD, Casolaro MA, Sellers SE et al: Replacement therapy for alpha 1-antitrypsin deficiency associated with emphysema. N Engl J Med 1987;316:1055–1062
57. Alpha-1-antitrypsin deficiency: Usage of alpha-1-proteinase inhibitor concentrate in replacement therapy. Am J Med 1988; 84(6A):1–90
58. Cooper JD, Patterson GA, Grossman R, Maurer J: Double-lung transplant for advanced chronic obstructive lung disease. Am Rev Respir Dis 1989;139:303–307
59. American Thoracic Society, Medical Section of the American Lung Association: Guidelines for the approach to the patient with severe hereditary alpha 1-antitrypsin deficiency. Am Rev Respir Dis 1989;140:1494–1497
60. Hubbard RC, Brantly ML, Sellers SE et al: Anti-neutrophil elastase defenses of the lower respiratory tract in alpha 1-antitrypsin deficiency directly augmented with an aerosol of alpha 1-antitrypsin. Ann Intern Med 1989;111:206–212
61. Luce JM: Bronchiectasis. pp. 1107–1125. In Murray JF, Nadel JA (eds): Textbook of Respiratory Medicine. WB Saunders, Philadelphia, 1988
62. Reid LM: Reduction in bronchial subdivison in bronchiectasis. Thorax 1950;5:233–247
63. Crofton J: Diagnosis and treatment of bronchiectasis. Br Med J 1966;1:721–723, 783–785
64. Pang JA, Hamilton-Wood C, Metreweli C: The value of computed tomography in the diagnosis and management of bronchiectasis. Clin Radiol 1989;40:40–44
65. Stockley RA: Bronchiectasis—a management problem? Br J Dis Chest 1988;82:209–219
66. Annest LS, Kratz JM, Crawford FA: Current results of treatment of bronchiectasis. J Thorac Cardiovasc Surg 1982;83:546–550
67. Boat TF: Cystic fibrosis. pp. 1126–1152. In Murray JF, Nadel JA (eds): Textbook of Respiratory Medicine. WB Saunders, Philadelphia, 1988
68. Davis PB: Cystic fibrosis. pp. 1899–1902. In Kelley WN (ed): Textbook of Internal Medicine. JB Lippincott, Philadelphia, 1989
69. Fick RB, Jr, Stillwell PC: Controversies in the management of pulmonary disease due to cystic fibrosis. Chest 1989;95:1319–1327
70. Rosenstein BJ: Interpreting sweat tests in the diagnosis of cystic fibrosis. J Respir Dis 1990;11:519–528
71. Michel BC: Antibacterial therapy in cystic fibrosis. Chest 1988;94:129s–140s
72. Schoni MH: Autogenic drainage: A modern approach to physiotherapy in cystic fibrosis. J R Soc Med, suppl. 16, 1989;82:32–37
73. Zinman R, Corey M, Coates AL et al: Nocturnal home oxygen in the treatment of hypoxemic cystic fibrosis patients. J Pediatr 1989;114:368–377
74. Geddes DM, Hodson ME: The role of heart and lung transplantation in the treatment of cystic fibrosis. J R Soc Med, Suppl. 16, 1989;82:49–53
75. Pasque MK, Cooper JD, Kaiser LR et al: Improved technique for bilateral lung transplantation: Rationale and initial clinical experience. Ann Thorac Surg 1990;49:785–791
76. Ziment I: Respiratory Pharmacology and Therapeutics. WB Saunders, Philadelphia, 1978, p. 230

Chapter 63

Clinical Approach to the Patient with Chronic Hypoxemia or Cor Pulmonale

David J. Pierson

CHAPTER OUTLINE

Chronic arterial hypoxemia occurs in patients with several types of respiratory disease and may lead to cor pulmonale, as described in Chapter 24. While both hypoxemia and cor pulmonale may be regarded as secondary to the primary respiratory disorder, both are major determinants of functional status, complications, and overall survival. Accurate assessment and appropriate management are therefore important if patients with these conditions are to benefit maximally from current respiratory care.

Table 63-1 outlines the general settings for and therapeutic rationale in chronic hypoxemia and cor pulmonale due to respiratory disease and indicates the chapters in which treatment for each disorder is discussed in more detail. The present chapter focuses primarily on chronic obstructive pulmonary disease (COPD), which is by far the most frequent cause of these conditions in adult patients and is the setting in which most scientific study has been done. The concepts presented vary in the degree to which they apply in other diseases, and the reader should refer to the other chapters cited in the table for more information.

Pulmonary hypertension, cor pulmonale, and the clinical conditions in which they occur are described in more detail in Chapter 24. For the patient with COPD, the information presented here should be integrated into an overall approach to assessment and management, as described in Chapter 62. Technical aspects of O_2 therapy and its practical application in hypoxemia are covered in detail in Chapters 75 and 99. This chapter deals only with chronic, stable hypoxemia; the approach to hypoxemia in the setting of acute illness in patients with COPD involves important differences, as discussed in Chapter 64. Finally, the approach described here applies primarily to adult patients, and this should be considered by the clinician when dealing with infants and small children.

EFFECTS OF OXYGEN THERAPY IN CHRONIC HYPOXEMIA

Present knowledge of the effects of long-term O_2 therapy (LTOT) in COPD comes primarily from two studies carried

Table 63-1. Treatment Rationale for Chronic Hypoxemia and Cor Pulmonale in Different Clinical Settings

Disorder	Physiologic Category	Principal Mechanism of Hypoxemia	Main Need for Relief of Hypoxemia	Primary Therapy for Hypoxemia	Chapters in Which Therapy Is Discussed
COPD	Obstructive (generalized, lower airway)	$\dot{V}/\dot{Q}$ mismatching	Increased F_{IO_2}	Long-term O_2 therapy	62, 63, 99
Cystic fibrosis	Obstructive (generalized, lower airway)	$\dot{V}/\dot{Q}$ mismatching	Increased F_{IO_2}	Long-term O_2 therapy[a]	62, 88, 99
Obstructive sleep apnea	Obstructive (localized, upper airway)	Alveolar hypoventilation	Relief of obstruction	Nasal CPAP; uveopalatopharyngoplasty; tracheotomy	67
Primary alveolar hypoventilation (e.g., pickwickian syndrome)	Regulation of ventilation	Alveolar hypoventilation	Increased ventilatory drive	Respiratory stimulants (e.g., progesterone)	66
Neuromuscular disease (e.g., muscular dystrophy)	Restrictive	Alveolar hypoventilation; respiratory muscle fatigue	Decrease in work of breathing; rest respiratory muscles	Long-term mechanical ventilation	101
Chronic mountain sickness	?Regulation of ventilation (environmental)	Low P_{IO_2}	Increased P_{IO_2}	Long-term O_2 therapy[a]; relocation to lower altitude	16, 99

CPAP, continuous positive airway pressure; F_{IO_2}, inspired O_2 fraction; P_{IO_2}, inspired O_2 partial pressure.
[a] There is less scientific evidence of effectiveness in these conditions than in COPD.

out during the 1970s in the United States (Nocturnal Oxygen Therapy Trial Group [NOTT])[1] and Great Britain.[2] These large-scale, comprehensive studies demonstrated that LTOT can substantially lengthen survival in appropriately selected patients. Figure 63-1 shows their combined survival data.[1–3]

The study by the British Medical Research Council (MRC)[2] included only patients with a history of right-sided heart failure. These patients were randomly assigned to receive LTOT (15 h/d) or no O_2. In the NOTT study[1] patients were not required to have had overt right-sided heart failure and were randomly assigned to receive LTOT 24 h/d versus only 12 h/d, including the hours of sleep. Patients on continuous O_2 therapy were also provided with liquid O_2 units for use during ambulation.

As shown in Figure 63-1, for appropriately selected patients with COPD (see next two sections), LTOT for 12 or 15 h/d significantly lengthens survival, and continuous (24 h/d) administration provides an additional substantial increase. Most patients assigned to continuous O_2 in the NOTT study actually used their O_2 for less than 20 h/d, so that it is reasonable to expect an even greater survival benefit with true 24 h/d use.

Survival in patients with COPD is most closely related to the severity of airflow obstruction as measured by forced expiratory volume in 1 second (FEV_1). Individuals with untreated chronic hypoxemia have a substantially increased mortality rate, but relief of hypoxemia with LTOT can effectively eliminate this excess mortality. Figure 63-2 illus-

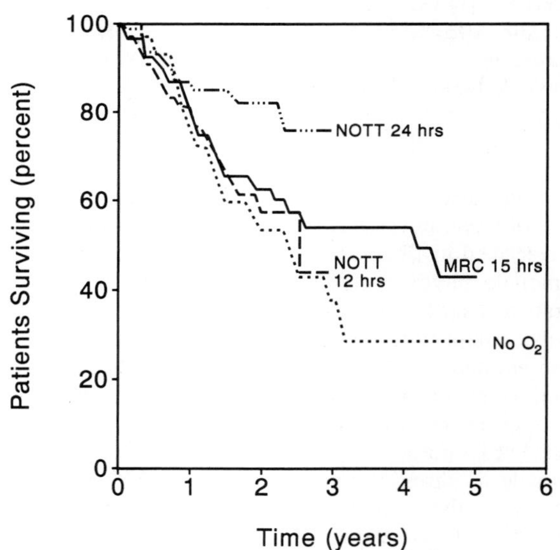

Figure 63-1. Effects of LTOT on survival in hypoxemic COPD. Results of the British (MRC)[2] and American (NOTT)[1] multicenter studies are combined, showing that LTOT at 12 to 15 h/d improves survival in comparison with no O_2, but that LTOT 24 h/d (actually, on average 19 h/d[1]), including ambulatory O_2 therapy, provides a substantial additional benefit. (Modified from Flenley,[3] with permission.)

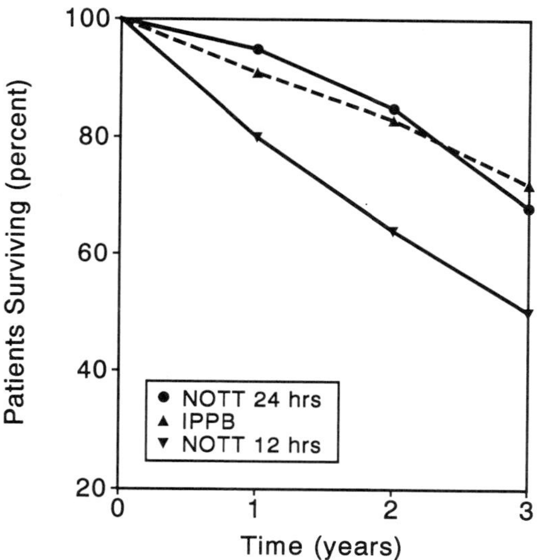

Figure 63-2. Effects of LTOT at night (NOTT 12 hours) and continuously (NOTT 24 hours) on survival in hypoxemic patients with severe COPD, as compared with survival of nonhypoxemic COPD patients matched for the same degree of airflow obstruction, as measured by FEV_1 (intermittent positive-pressure breathing, dashed line). (Adapted from Anthonisen et al.,[5] with permission.)

trates this by comparing the survival of the 12-hour and 24-hour NOTT patients with that of a group of nonhypoxemic patients with comparable airflow obstruction.[4,5]

Although alveolar hypoxia is the primary cause of pulmonary hypertension in COPD (see Figure 24-4), LTOT is not associated with a return of pulmonary artery pressures to normal levels.[6,7] In part, this may be because structural changes (e.g., capillary obliteration by emphysema) contribute to the pulmonary hypertension in COPD; hypoxic pulmonary vasoconstriction may also become less reversible after it has been present for months or years.

Increased survival is not the only potential benefit of LTOT. Improved exercise tolerance is potentially achievable in all patients and can be a crucial factor in improving quality of life by enabling patients to return to a more active life-style. Hospitalization needs may be decreased, which not only conserves health care resources but also reduces this important cause of morbidity in patients with COPD. Neuropsychological abnormalities, which are well documented in chronically hypoxemic individuals,[8,9] are improved by LTOT.[9–11] Sleep patterns may be improved, as may sexual function and other components of quality of life.

INDICATIONS FOR LONG-TERM OXYGEN THERAPY

Present understanding of the benefits from and indications for LTOT[12–14] comes primarily from the NOTT and MRC studies.[1,2,15] In both, patient selection was based on all available scientific data plus the clinical experience and judgment of the most expert clinicians in the United States and Great Britain. Because of the scope and expense of these investigations, it is unlikely that other large-scale studies will emerge to modify this understanding in the near future.

Table 63-2 lists the current indications for LTOT of which there are basically four: an appropriately documented diagnosis; appropriate use of other modalities of therapy; documentation of the hypoxemia; and demonstration that the hypoxemia is chronic. Economic, personal, and social factors may render LTOT impossible or impractical despite the presence of these four indications, as also shown in Table 63-2. When LTOT is prescribed, sufficient O_2 should be administered to raise PaO_2 above 60 mmHg or to increase arterial O_2 saturation (SaO_2) to 90 percent or higher.

The validity of the indications shown in Table 63-2 is most certain for patients who are hypoxemic while awake and at rest, as these are the conditions used in the NOTT and MRC

Table 63-2. Indications for Long-Term Oxygen Therapy

1. Diagnosis of COPD[a]
2. Clinical stability
3. Other aspects of medical management (e.g., bronchodilator therapy, diuretics, chest physiotherapy, reconditioning exercises) optimized according to individual needs of patient
4. Documentation of hypoxemia, while awake and at rest[b]
   A. PaO_2 <55 mmHg,[c] *or*
   B. PaO_2 55–59 mmHg,[c] *plus* evidence of significant end-organ dysfunction due to chronic hypoxia, as shown by one or more of the following:
      i. P-pulmonale (P waves 3 mm or more in leads II, III, or a VF of electrocardiogram)
      ii. Clinical right-sided heart failure (pedal edema)
      iii. Erythrocytosis (hematocrit over 55%)
5. Demonstration that hypoxemia is chronic by follow-up assessment with patient breathing room air, made at least 3–4 weeks after above criteria are met, by either
   A. Persistence of above PaO_2 findings, *or*
   B. SaO_2 <89% for condition A above[d]
   C. SaO_2 89% for condition B above[d]
6. Appropriate social and economic resources (see Ch. 60)
7. Physical and psychological capability of patient to use apparatus appropriately and safely
8. Willingness of patient to comply with prescribed regimen

[a] These indications may also apply to patients with other chronic pulmonary conditions (e.g., interstitial pulmonary fibrosis, cystic fibrosis, kyphoscoliosis), although this has not yet been proved.

[b] If the patient does not meet these arterial oxygenation criteria at rest while awake but does so during exercise or while asleep, long-term O_2 therapy is indicated during those circumstances but not continuously.

[c] Although arterial oxyhemoglobin saturation measurements using pulse or ear oximetry are currently acceptable for reimbursement purposes in the United States, these do not provide sufficient physiologic assessment for *initiation* of therapy. They may be used in follow-up, as shown under item 5.

[d] If criteria are not met according to results of oximetry at follow-up, arterial blood gas measurements should be obtained.

studies. Hypoxemia occurring only during exercise and/or sleep is assumed also to be an indication for LTOT, although not all experts agree. One study has found that COPD patients who do not meet the oxygenation criteria while awake but desaturate substantially while asleep have more severely deranged hemodynamics and end-organ function than do patients with equivalent airflow obstruction and daytime oxygenation but without nighttime desaturation.[16] Whether this means that nighttime LTOT would improve survival in these or other patients remains unproven.

Data supporting the use of LTOT in conditions other than those discussed above are also largely lacking. For example, although it is often prescribed for patients with cystic fibrosis and severe hypoxemia, no randomized study has been done to determine whether LTOT prolongs life or provides other objective benefits in this patient population. LTOT may actually worsen the condition of patients with obstructive sleep apnea by reducing the hypoxic stimulus for arousal, prolonging the periods of apnea, and worsening respiratory acidosis. For chronic hypoxemia and cor pulmonale in other settings, the use of LTOT must rest on extrapolation of data from the NOTT and MRC studies as well as on the anecdotal experience and judgment of clinicians experienced in managing patients with these conditions.

The requirement for documentation that the hypoxemia is *chronic* is especially important in order to ensure that this expensive, intrusive therapy is prescribed only for patients who need it.[13,15,17] Patients are commonly referred for LTOT prior to establishment of a comprehensive care regimen or while recovering from an acute exacerbation, a setting in which physiologic recovery can take longer than subjective improvement. This was confirmed in the NOTT study, in which 45 percent of all patients initially meeting the hypoxemia criteria were found to have PaO_2 values of 60 mmHg or higher after 3 to 4 weeks of observation.[15] In a multicenter French study,[18] improvement continued in some patients for as long as 90 days, and about 20 percent of individuals who still met the hypoxemia criteria at 1 month failed to do so at 3 months.

In view of the above, it is appropriate to think of outpatient O_2 therapy in two distinct categories: short-term O_2 therapy (up to 30 to 90 days) and LTOT.[13,19] Initiation or continuation of O_2 therapy may be warranted for patients with symptomatic hypoxemia when first seen or on discharge from the hospital. However, in such cases a repeat assessment should be carried out after an appropriate interval.[13,15,20]

Once begun, LTOT in the setting of severe COPD will generally be required for the remainder of the patient's life. After the initial observation period when LTOT is first prescribed, the subsequent finding of a PaO_2 value exceeding 60 mmHg while breathing air may be a sign of physiologic improvement and should not prompt the clinician to discontinue the therapy.[6,21]

PATIENT SELECTION FOR LONG-TERM OXYGEN THERAPY

Although current U.S. Medicare reimbursement policy accepts pulse or ear oximetry readings as a substitute for PaO_2, only the latter should be used in initially evaluating patients for LTOT[13,22] (Table 63-3). SaO_2 is increased for any given PaO_2 value in the presence of alkalosis; for this and other reasons, oximetry may fail to detect hypoxemia that would merit LTOT.[22,23] In addition, because it assesses oxygenation but not alveolar ventilation or acid-base status, the use of oximetry in lieu of arterial blood gases prevents full evaluation of gas exchange and clinical stability.

Table 63-4 illustrates the importance of determining $PaCO_2$ and alveolar-arterial O_2 partial pressure difference $[P(A\text{-}a)O_2]$ as well as PaO_2 in evaluating a patient for LTOT. In the hypothetical circumstances shown, using current U.S. Medicare reimbursement criteria, sample 1 would qualify the patient for LTOT according to both PaO_2 and SaO_2, sample 2 would meet the criteria by PaO_2 but not by SaO_2 unless the patient had edema, P-pulmonale, or polycythemia, and sample 3 would preclude reimbursement for LTOT altogether.

Exercise testing (see Ch. 49) should be considered for patients with severe exercise limitation who are not hypoxemic while at rest breathing air. Although a severely reduced CO diffusing capacity (DLCO) correlates with an increased likelihood of desaturation during exercise,[24,25] the former is not sensitive or specific enough to eliminate the need for exercise testing. The finding of significant desaturation with exercise, along with improvements in both symptoms and exercise performance with supplemental O_2, indicates a trial of LTOT during ambulation and other exertion. Patients with COPD

Table 63-3. Arterial Blood Gas Measurements versus Pulse Oximetry in Chronic Respiratory Disease

Arterial Blood Gases Required	Pulse Oximetry Acceptable or Preferable
Initial diagnosis and assessment of patients with unexplained respiratory symptoms	Titration of O_2 dose in clinically stable patients At rest During exercise
Selection of patients for long-term O_2 therapy	Assessment of oxygenation during sleep
Formal diagnostic exercise testing	Clinical monitoring of patients during routine follow-up In office or clinic In patient's home
Assessment during acute exacerbation	Monitoring of O_2 therapy during recovery phase of acute exacerbation
Adjustment of initial O_2 dose during acute exacerbation	

Table 63-4. Arterial Blood Gas and Oximetry Results Determined Three Times on the Same Occasion from a Hypothetical Patient, Assuming Three Different Levels of Alveolar Ventilation

	Sample 1	Sample 2	Sample 3
PaO_2 (mmHg)	48	54	60
SaO_2 (%)	83	89	93
$PaCO_2$ (mmHg)	52	47	42
Arterial pH	7.38	7.43	7.48
$P(A\text{-}a)O_2$ (mmHg)	42	42	42

who are not hypoxemic while awake but who show signs of hypoxia-related end-organ dysfunction should be evaluated for desaturation during sleep. If the latter is documented, these patients are candidates for LTOT administered during the hours of sleep.

Although hemodynamic measurements obtained through right heart catheterization are useful for research and can more clearly delineate a patient's physiologic state by quantifying pulmonary hypertension, such invasive studies are not necessary in the selection of individual patients for LTOT. In the NOTT study,[1] which did not include right heart catheterization in initial patient assessment, increased survival and other benefits occurred both in patients with a history of overt right heart failure (suggesting advanced, prolonged pulmonary hypertension) and in those without such manifestations.

As implied by items 6 through 8 in Table 63-2, factors other than strictly medical ones are also important in the selection of patients for LTOT. A psychosocial assessment as described in Chapter 60 should be carried out in every patient being considered for initiation of LTOT. The factors listed for patient selection for home mechanical ventilation in Table 101-3 also generally apply to the clinician's decision of whether to prescribe LTOT.

POTENTIAL ADVERSE EFFECTS AND HAZARDS OF LTOT

Table 63-5 summarizes several potential adverse effects of LTOT.[26] From the clinician's standpoint the threat of alveolar hypoventilation and CO_2 retention due to suppression of the patient's hypoxic ventilatory drive is often the most worrisome of these. However, although this complication is both frequent and potentially life-threatening in acute ven-

Table 63-5. Potential Adverse Effects of Oxygen Therapy in COPD

Adverse Effect	Mechanism	Comment
Persistent hypoxemia	Failure to prescribe LTOT when indicated; patient noncompliance; not prescribing enough O_2 to raise $PaO_2 > 60$ mmHg	More important problem overall than the other potential adverse effects listed
CO_2 retention	Depression of hypoxic ventilatory drive (changes in $\dot{V}/\dot{Q}$ matching)	Rarely a problem in stable patients; avoidable in acute exacerbations if PaO_2 is initially kept <60–65 mmHg
Increased $P(A\text{-}a)O_2$	Absorption atelectasis	An acute effect of breathing 100% O_2; not a problem in LTOT
Pulmonary O_2 toxicity	Free-radical lung injury, producing hyaline membranes, interstitial fibrosis, and neovascularization	Histologic changes sometimes found at autopsy after years of therapy; not clinically detectable during life
Fire; explosion	Smoking while using O_2; carelessness; inadequate patient education and supervision; substance abuse	Life-threatening burns can occur, although most are minor; not a problem with sensible use of equipment
Frostbite	Skin contact with cold surfaces or frost associated with liquid O_2 systems	Easily avoidable with proper instruction, equipment maintenance, and care
Nasal irritation (drying, congestion, crusting, bleeding)	Mechanical effects of nasal cannula and continuous flow of O_2	May respond to creams and other topical measures; transtracheal O_2 administration eliminates problem
Contact dermatitis; abrasions of nose, ears, or cheeks	Physical irritation from cannulae or tubing; rarely allergic reaction	May respond to switching to different brand of tubing; transtracheal O_2 administration eliminates problem
Adverse psychosocial effects	Reluctance to be seen wearing O_2 cannula; impaired social function; reduced ambulation	May respond to reassurance and counseling; more cosmetically pleasing delivery device may help (e.g., tubing concealed in eyeglass frames); transtracheal oxygen administration eliminates problem

tilatory failure (see Ch. 64), it is not commonly observed in stable outpatients.[26–30] As shown in Figure 63-3, if only enough O_2 is administered to raise PaO_2 into the 60 to 80 mmHg range, any increase in $PaCO_2$ should be modest and not enough to cause clinically significant acidemia.[27]

Fire is a possibility whenever O_2 is in use, because although O_2 itself does not burn, it supports combustion and makes inflammable articles burn more vigorously.[31] Burns do occasionally occur in patients who smoke or use open flames near their cannulae while the O_2 is flowing, but these are not usually life-threatening. Along with frostbite from mishandling of liquid O_2 units and physical injuries caused by O_2 cylinders and regulators, burns are preventable with proper education and patient compliance. Some patients experience irritation of the nose or skin, and a few cases of allergy to O_2 tubing have been reported[26] (also see Ch. 99 and Table 99-4). In most cases minor adjustments will eliminate these problems, although they can be a reason for noncompliance with prescribed O_2 use.

Easily the most significant "adverse effect" associated with LTOT is the clinician's failure to correct the patient's hypoxemia by not prescribing LTOT when indicated,[32] not adjusting the prescription to the patient's specific requirements, or not instructing the patient properly or the patient's failure to use the O_2 as directed. The other problems listed in Table 63-5 should not be of sufficient magnitude to prevent the appropriate use of this important therapy.

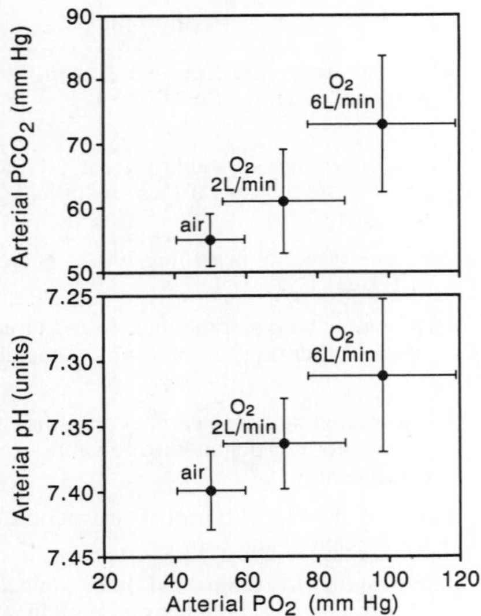

Figure 63-3. Effects of low-flow O_2 administration on $PaCO_2$ and pHa in 16 hypercapnic patients with severe but stable COPD. Although on average some additional CO_2 retention did occur when PaO_2 was raised to approximately 65 mmHg with nasal O_2 at 2 L/min, this was not enough to cause a clinically important fall in pHa. With nasal O_2 at 6 L/min, which raised PaO_2 well above 80 mmHg in most of the patients, some of them did develop significant respiratory acidosis. (Adapted from Nolte,[27] with permission.)

POSSIBLE PHARMACOLOGIC ALTERNATIVES TO OXYGEN IN CHRONIC HYPOXEMIA

Although mismatching of ventilation and perfusion ($\dot{V}/\dot{Q}$) is the main cause for chronic hypoxemia in patients with severe COPD, there is usually also a component of alveolar hypoventilation as manifested by hypercapnia. If such patients could be induced to increase alveolar ventilation, for example by a respiratory stimulant drug, their hypoxemia might be improved and the need for LTOT eliminated or delayed by months or years. However, clinical experience with respiratory stimulants such as progesterone and acetazolamide has been disappointing for reasons that are easily understood if the patients' severe airflow obstruction is taken into account. Increasing the drive to breathe in someone for whom any augmentation of overall ventilation requires a substantial increase in the work of breathing can be predicted to increase the sensation of breathlessness, and this is what generally happens with classical respiratory stimulant drugs.[33]

However, since the early 1980s there has been considerable interest in almitrine bismesylate, a peripheral chemoreceptor stimulant that also appears to improve $\dot{V}/\dot{Q}$ matching in the lung, as a possible pharmacologic substitute for O_2.[34–38] At doses too low to cause substantial increases in overall ventilation, almitrine can raise PaO_2 by 5 to 10 mmHg even in individuals with severe obstruction. In one double-blind, placebo-controlled study, almitrine administered at a dose of 50 mg twice daily for 1 year to patients with an average PaO_2 of 54.3 mmHg caused a sustained increase in PaO_2 that averaged 8 mmHg, while there were much smaller changes in $PaCO_2$ and minute ventilation.[38] Thus, if PaO_2 alone had been used as a criterion for initiating LTOT, the drug could have deferred this move for at least the duration of the study. Other investigators have documented similar improvements in oxygenation and have also shown saturation to be increased during sleep.[37]

Despite almitrine's apparent promise as at least a temporary substitute for LTOT, it has not found wide clinical application in countries in which it is available. In part this may be due to several adverse effects, which include peripheral neuropathies, weight loss, and progression of pulmonary hypertension despite improvement in hypoxemia.

A recent study has shown the nonsedating tricyclic antidepressant protriptyline to be effective in raising PaO_2 levels in patients with severe COPD, both while awake and during sleep.[39] Both the mechanism and the clinical significance of these observations are unknown, and further studies will be required before this agent can be recommended routinely in hypoxemic patients with COPD.

POLYCYTHEMIA (ERYTHROCYTOSIS) IN CHRONIC HYPOXEMIA

As described in Chapter 16, one of the normal adaptive responses to sustained hypoxia is an increase in hemoglobin,

Table 63-6. Potential Treatments for Chronic Cor Pulmonale Due to Pulmonary Disease

Strategy	Available Therapy	Comment
Increase P_{IO_2}	LTOT	Goal: maintain PaO_2 >60 mmHg (SaO_2 >90%)
Increase alveolar ventilation	Almitrine bismesylate	Can raise PaO_2 5–10 mmHg; may not decrease PVR
	Progesterone; other respiratory stimulants	Ineffective in presence of severe airflow obstruction; may increase dyspnea
Decrease PVR (reduce RV afterload)	Vasodilator drugs	Limited clinical effectiveness
Reduce blood volume (reduce RV preload)	Diuresis	Limited effectiveness in presence of uncorrected hypoxemia
	Phlebotomy	Only for hematocrit >55–58; rarely needed with LTOT
Increase RV contractility	LTOT	Increases myocardial O_2 supply
	Digitalis	Only effective in presence of LV disease; increased propensity for toxicity with hypoxemia, respiratory acidosis, hypokalemia

LV, left ventricular; P_{IO_2}, inspired O_2 tension; PVR, pulmonary vascular resistance; RV, right ventricular.

mediated by erythropoietin, a protein originating in the kidneys that helps to regulate the balance between overall O_2 supply and demand. The increased red blood cell mass increases the hematocrit, which increases blood viscosity progressively at levels exceeding 50 to 55 percent. Intravascular sludging at hematocrit levels over 60 to 65 percent increases the risk of cerebrovascular accidents and also may impair cardiac output by increasing pulmonary vascular resistance. Phlebotomy was once a common procedure in treating patients with hypoxemic COPD and secondary polycythemia. Although symptoms tended to be improved,[40,41] this procedure produced inconsistent physiologic effects.[42,43]

By removing the hypoxic stimulus for increased erythropoietin production, LTOT has essentially eliminated the need for phlebotomy in COPD. Persistent or recurrent polycythemia in patients for whom LTOT has been prescribed usually indicates noncompliance or equipment malfunction; if these are not present, the patient should be evaluated for primary hematologic causes of a raised hematocrit.

APPROACH TO THE PATIENT WITH CHRONIC COR PULMONALE

The symptoms and signs of chronic cor pulmonale are nonspecific, and diagnosis of this condition is often made quite late in a patient's clinical course.[44–46] Once identified, cor pulmonale might theoretically be amenable to several avenues of treatment[45,47] (Table 63-6). However, aside from relieving the alveolar hypoxia that is the main pathophysiologic cause of the condition, most therapies have not lived up to this theoretical promise. Supplemental O_2 therapy is thus the most important treatment. Although P_{AO_2} varies throughout the lung and is essentially unmeasurable, raising PaO_2 to at least 60 mmHg or SaO_2 to more than 90 percent is a generally accepted goal.

A wide variety of vasodilator drugs have been tried in cor pulmonale complicating severe COPD. These include hydralazine and other direct vasodilators, alpha-1-blockers (e.g., prazosin), calcium channel blockers (e.g., verapamil or nifedipine), and angiotensin-converting enzyme inhibitors (e.g., captopril).[46] Despite their theoretical advantages, because of side effects and disappointing clinical efficacy none of these drugs can be recommended in the management of patients.

Diuretics are commonly used when edema and other signs of fluid overload are present but must be used cautiously, particularly in the presence of hypercapnia and uncorrected hypoxemia. Digitalis and other cardiac glycosides are ineffective except when left ventricular disease is also present; patients with hypoxemia, respiratory acidosis, and diuretic-induced hypokalemia and/or metabolic alkalosis are particularly at risk for serious digitalis toxicity.

References

1. Nocturnal Oxygen Therapy Trial Group: Continuous or nocturnal oxygen therapy in hypoxemic chronic obstructive lung disease. Ann Intern Med 1980;93:391–398
2. Report of the Medical Research Council Working Party: Long-term domiciliary oxygen therapy in chronic hypoxic cor pulmonale complicating chronic bronchitis and emphysema. Lancet 1981;1:681–686
3. Flenley DC: Long-term oxygen therapy. Chest 1985;87:99–103
4. The Intermittent Positive Pressure Breathing Trial Group: Intermittent positive pressure breathing therapy of chronic obstructive lung disease. Ann Intern Med 1983;99:612–620
5. Anthonisen NR, Wright EC, Hodgkin JE, Intermittent Positive Pressure Breathing Trial Group: Prognosis in chronic obstructive pulmonary disease. Am Rev Respir Dis 1986;133:14–20
6. Weitzenblum E, Sautegeau A, Ehrhart M et al: Long-term oxygen therapy can reverse the progression of pulmonary hypertension in patients with chronic obstructive pulmonary disease. Am Rev Respir Dis 1985;131:493–498

7. Weitzenblum E, Oswald M, Mirhom R et al: Evolution of pulmonary hemodynamics in COLD patients under long-term oxygen therapy. Eur Respir J, suppl. 7, 1989;2:669s–673s
8. Grant I, Heaton RK, McSweeny AJ et al: Neuropsychologic findings in hypoxemic chronic obstructive pulmonary disease. Arch Intern Med 1982;142:1470–1476
9. Block AJ: Neuropsychological aspects of oxygen therapy. Respir Care 1983;28:885–888
10. Krop HD, Block AJ, Cohen E: Neuropsychologic effects of continuous oxygen therapy in chronic obstructive pulmonary disease. Chest 1973;64:317–322
11. Borak J, Sliwinski P, Piasecki Z, Zielinski J: Psychological status of COPD patients on long term oxygen therapy. Eur Respir J 1991;4:59–62
12. Petty TL: Who needs oxygen therapy? Am Rev Respir Dis 1985;131:930–931
13. Pierson DJ: Indications for oxygen therapy. Probl Respir Care 1990;3:549–562
14. Fulmer JD, Snider GL: ACCP-NHLBI national conference on oxygen therapy. Chest 1984;86:234–247
15. Timms RM, Kvale PA, Anthonisen NR et al: Selection of patients with chronic obstructive pulmonary disease for long-term oxygen therapy. JAMA 1981;245:2514–2515
16. Fletcher EC, Luckett RA, Miller T et al: Pulmonary vascular hemodynamics in chronic lung disease patients with and without oxyhemoglobin desaturation during sleep. Chest 1989;95:157–166
17. Further recommendations for prescribing and supplying long-term oxygen therapy. Am Rev Respir Dis 1988;138:745–747
18. Levi-Valensi P, Weitzenblum E, Pedinelli J-L et al: Three-month follow-up of arterial blood gas determinations in candidates for long-term oxygen therapy. Am Rev Respir Dis 1986;133:547–551
19. O'Donohue WJ Jr, Petty TL, Gracey DR et al: New problems in supply, reimbursement and certification of medical necessity for long-term oxygen therapy. Am Rev Respir Dis 1990;142:721–725
20. Levi-Valensi P, Aubry P, Rida Z et al: Selection of patients for long-term oxygen therapy. Eur Respir J, suppl. 7, 1989;2:624s–629s
21. O'Donohue WJ Jr: Effect of oxygen therapy on increasing arterial oxygen tension in hypoxemic patients with stable chronic obstructive pulmonary disease while breathing ambient air. Chest 1991;100:968–972
22. Pierson DJ: Pulse oximetry versus arterial blood gas specimens in long-term oxygen therapy. Lung, suppl. 1990;168:782–788
23. Carlin BW, Clausen JW, Ries AL: The use of cutaneous oximetry in the prescription of long-term oxygen therapy. Chest 1988;94:239–241
24. Kelley MA, Panettieri RA Jr, Krupinski AV: Resting single-breath diffusing capacity as a screening test for exercise-induced hypoxemia. Am J Med 1986;80:807–812
25. Owens GR, Rogers RM, Pennock BE, Levin D: The diffusing capacity as a predictor of arterial oxygen desaturation during exercise in patients with chronic obstructive pulmonary disease. N Engl J Med 1984;310:1218–1221
26. Pierson DJ: The toxicity of low-flow oxygen therapy. Respir Care 1983;28:889–897
27. Nolte D: Nutzen und Gefahren der Sauerstofftherapie bei chronischer Ateminsuffizienz. Wien Med Wochenschr 1976;126:325–329
28. Geisler LS: Risiken der Sauerstofftherapie bei chronischer CO_2-Retention. Med Welt 1971;22:1593–1595
29. Morse JO, Kettel LJ, Diener CF, Burrows B: Effects of long-term, continuous oxygen therapy in patients with severe chronic hypercapnia. Am Rev Respir Dis 1973;107:1064–1066
30. Neff TA, Petty TL: Tolerance and survival in severe chronic hypercapnia. Arch Intern Med 1972;129:591–596
31. West GA, Primeau P: Non-medical hazards of long-term oxygen therapy. Respir Care 1983;28:906–912
32. Pierson DJ: The physician's role in the costs of long-term oxygen therapy. Respir Care 1987;32:339–344
33. Pierson DJ: Respiratory stimulants: Review of the literature and assessment of current status. Respir Care 1973;18:549–554
34. Bell RC, Mullins RC III, West LG et al: The effect of almitrine bismesylate on hypoxemia in chronic obstructive pulmonary disease. Ann Intern Med 1986;105:342–346
35. Tweney J, Howard P: Almitrine bismesylate. Z Erkr Atmungsorgane 1987;168:197–215
36. Voisin C, Howard P, Ansquer JC: Vectarion international multicentre study. Bull Eur Physiopathol Respir, suppl. 1987;23:169s–182s
37. Gothe B, Cherniack NS, Bachand RT Jr et al: Long-term effects of almitrine bismesylate on oxygenation during wakefulness and sleep in chronic obstructive pulmonary disease. Am J Med 1988;84:436–444
38. Watanabe S, Kanner RE, Cutillo AG et al: Long-term effect of almitrine bismesylate in patients with hypoxemic chronic obstructive pulmonary disease. Am Rev Respir Dis 1989;140:1269–1273
39. Series F, Cormier Y: Effects of protryptyline on diurnal and nocturnal oxygenation in patients with chronic obstructive pulmonary disease. Ann Intern Med 1990;113:507–511
40. Weisse AB, Moschos CB, Frank MJ et al: Hemodynamic effects of staged hematocrit reduction in patients with stable cor pulmonale and severely elevated hematocrit levels. Am J Med 1975;58:92–98
41. Chetty KG, Brown SE, Light RW: Improved exercise tolerance of the polycythemic lung patient following phlebotomy. Am J Med 1983;74:415–420
42. Segel N, Bishop JM: The circulation in patients with chronic bronchitis and emphysema at rest and during exercise with special reference to the influence of changes in blood viscosity and blood volume on the pulmonary circulation. J Clin Invest 1966;45:1555–1568
43. Dayton LM, McCullough E, Scheinhorn DJ, Weil JV: Symptomatic and pulmonary response to acute phlebotomy in secondary polycythemia. Chest 1975;68:785–790
44. Fishman AP: Pulmonary hypertension and cor pulmonale. pp. 998–1048. In Fishman AP (ed): Pulmonary Diseases and Disorders. 2nd Ed. McGraw-Hill, New York, 1988
45. Palevsky HI, Fishman AP: Chronic cor pulmonale: Etiology and management. JAMA 1990;263:2347–2353
46. Klinger JR, Hill NS: Right ventricular dysfunction in chronic obstructive pulmonary disease. Evaluation and management. Chest 1991;99:715–723
47. Rubin LJ: Pulmonary hypertension secondary to lung disease. pp. 291–320. In Weir EK, Reeves JT (eds): Pulmonary Hypertension. Futura Publishing, Mount Kisco, NY, 1984

Chapter 64

Clinical Approach to the Patient with Acute Ventilatory Failure

David J. Pierson

CHAPTER OUTLINE

GENERAL CONSIDERATIONS

Chapter 29 develops the concept of acute respiratory failure based on sudden interference with one or more of three basic functions, namely, ventilation of the alveoli, oxygenation of the arterial blood, and oxygenation of the tissues. Although these three are inseparably intertwined, any given case of acute respiratory failure tends to develop primarily because of derangement in one of them. The second and third mechanisms are often grouped together into the broad category of oxygenation failure (gas exchange failure or lung failure), whereas the different causes of acute ventilatory failure can be thought of as *pump failure*, whether the main cause of this is diminished ventilatory drive, dysfunction of the thorax or ventilatory muscles, or disease of the conducting airways[1] (Fig. 64-1). This chapter deals with the clinical approach to ventilatory failure in the acute setting. Chronic ventilatory failure that is not an immediate threat to a patient's life is discussed in Chapter 63 and the clinical approach to acute oxygenation failure in Chapter 65.

Definitions and Overall Approach

Because P_ACO_2 and $PaCO_2$ can be thought of as the same, hypercapnia (a PCO_2 higher than normal) and alveolar hypoventilation are clinically synonymous. Convention has defined ventilatory failure (ventilatory insufficiency) as a $PaCO_2$ of 50 mmHg or higher. This condition may be considered *chronic* (compensated) when the arterial pH is close to normal (e.g., above 7.30) regardless of the absolute value of $PaCO_2$ and *acute* when the pH is below 7.25 to 7.30. Thus, *acute ventilatory failure* is the clinical state produced when $PaCO_2$ rises sufficiently and rapidly enough to produce an immediate threat to the patient's life; the life-threatening nature of the change (indicated by an unphysiologic pH) is what distinguishes acute from chronic hypercapnia.

Acute respiratory failure in any clinical setting can best be approached by separating it into the main elements influencing the clinician's approach to management, namely (1) oxygenation, (2) ventilation, (3) airway protection, and (4) secretion clearance.[2] A given patient may need assistance

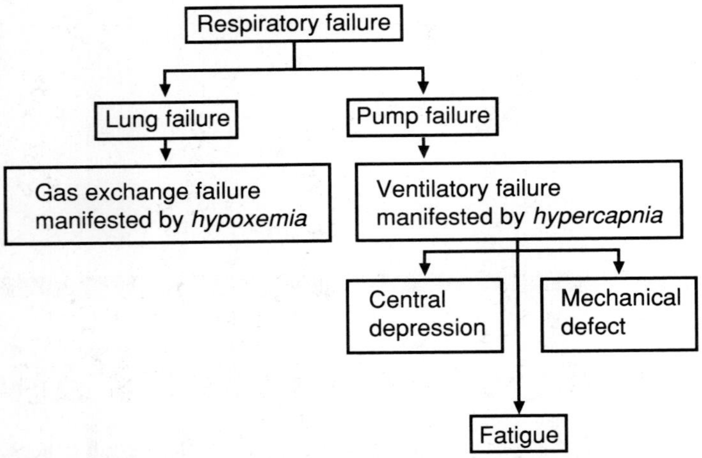

Respiratory failure

Lung failure

Gas exchange failure manifested by *hypoxemia*

Pump failure

Ventilatory failure manifested by *hypercapnia*

Central depression

Mechanical defect

Fatigue

Figure 64-1. Conceptual scheme separating acute respiratory failure into either lung failure (acute oxygenation failure) or pump failure (acute ventilatory failure). (From Roussos,[1] with permission.)

with any or all of these elements regardless of the primary type of acute respiratory failure, and an approach to management based on the needs of the specific patient rather than in a generalized fashion based on rote can help to optimize efficacy, efficiency, and safety.

The clinical approach to airway protection and secretion clearance is discussed in Chapters 53 and 72, and therapy primarily directed at improving oxygenation is discussed in Chapter 65 as well as in Chapter 75. However, therapy affecting alveolar ventilation necessarily influences oxygenation as well, as discussed in Chapter 29 and illustrated in Figure 64-2. Although there is no defect in O_2 transfer from alveolus to capillary in acute ventilatory failure, a fall in alveolar ventilation reduces alveolar access to O_2 and results in hypoxemia to a degree approximately equivalent to the increase in $PaCO_2$. It can readily be seen, however, that correction of hypoxemia in this setting is primarily a problem of restoring adequate ventilation.

Indications for Mechanical Ventilation

The possible indications for mechanical ventilation are summarized in Table 64-1 according to six general categories of physiologic dysfunction.[3,4] Although hypoxemia as a primary reason for initiating ventilatory support is uncommon in acute ventilatory failure, the other categories are both frequent and interrelated in this setting. Understanding the physiologic processes involved is important even if the objective assessments listed in Table 64-1 are arbitrary and sometimes difficult to obtain in nonintubated patients. More specific examples of indications in the most common clinical settings for acute ventilatory failure are given in subsequent sections of this chapter.

A main determinant of the clinician's approach to acute ventilatory failure is whether the patient has underlying lung disease. This chapter first considers acute life-threatening hypoventilation in otherwise healthy individuals, in whom management focuses primarily on supporting ventilation until normal pump function returns. It then discusses means for approaching the more complex issue of acute ventilatory failure as a complication of obstructive pulmonary disease.

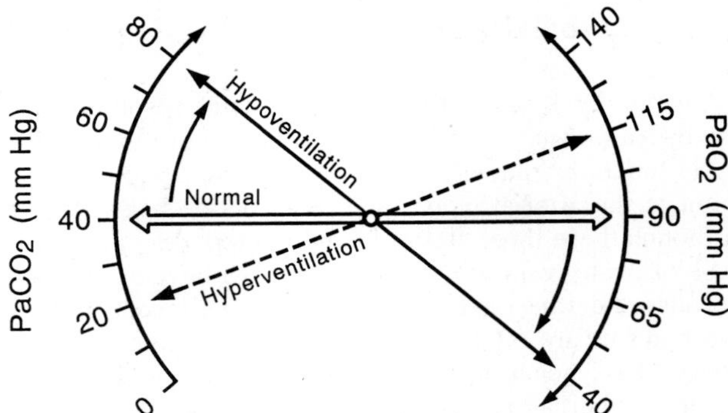

Figure 64-2. Relationship of $PaCO_2$ to PaO_2 in acute ventilatory failure. So long as the alveolar-to-arterial PO_2 difference [$P(A\text{-}a)O_2$] is normal, an increase in $PaCO_2$ due to alveolar hypoventilation will be associated with a roughly equivalent decrease in PaO_2, depending on the respiratory quotient (RQ). If RQ is 0.8, the PaO_2 will fall 12.5 mmHg for every 10 mmHg increase in $PaCO_2$.

Table 64-1. Indications for Mechanical Ventilation

Physiologic Mechanism	Best Clinical Indicators	Normal Range	Values Suggesting Need for Mechanical Ventilation
Inadequate alveolar ventilation	$PaCO_2$ (mmHg)	36–44[a]	Acute increase from normal or from patient's baseline
Inadequate lung expansion	V_T (mL/kg)	5–8	<4–5
	VC (mL/kg)	60–75	<10–15
	Respiratory rate (breaths/min)	12–20	>35
Ventilatory muscle weakness	MIF (cmH_2O)	80–100	<20–30
	MVV (L/min)	120–180	<2 × resting $\dot{V}_E$ requirement
	VC (mL/kg)	60–75	<10–15
Excessive work of breathing	$\dot{V}_E$ required to keep $PaCO_2$ normal (L/min)	5–10	>15–20
	V_D/V_T (%)	25–40	>60
Unstable ventilatory drive	Breathing pattern; clinical setting	—	—
Hypoxemia	$P(A\text{-}a)O_2$ on FiO_2 = 1.0 (mmHg)	25–65	>350
	PaO_2/FiO_2 ratio (mmHg)	350–400	<200

V_T, tidal volume; VC, vital capacity; MIF, maximum inspiratory force; MVV, maximum voluntary ventilation; $\dot{V}_E$, minute ventilation; V_D, dead space; $P(A\text{-}a)O_2$, alveolar to arterial PO_2 difference; FiO_2, inspired O_2 fraction.

[a] Normal values at sea level.

ACUTE VENTILATORY FAILURE IN THE ABSENCE OF UNDERLYING LUNG DISEASE

Short-Term Suppression of Ventilatory Drives

Clinical Settings

Acute ventilatory failure due to short-term depression of ventilatory drives occurs most commonly in the postoperative state and following accidental or suicidal drug overdose. Patients in these settings usually have normal underlying respiratory function and can be expected to recover quickly and completely once the drugs wear off; ventilatory support is generally needed for 1 to 2 days or less.

Problems

Here the primary defect is a loss of the normal drive to breathe, manifested by acute respiratory acidosis, but the latter is not the only problem. Loss of the normal gag reflex and of glottic function predisposes patients to aspiration of oropharyngeal or gastric contents, with subsequent asphyxia or pneumonia. Depression of the cough reflex and mucociliary function further impairs airway clearance. Even when patients are able to maintain normal alveolar ventilation in the presence of respiratory depressants, their normal sigh function is generally lost, and they fail to adequately expand their lungs, predisposing them to atelectasis.

Indications for Mechanical Ventilation

Most of the indicators listed in Table 64-1 apply well to these patients, although they generally have bradypnea rather than tachypnea. The most direct indications that such patients should be intubated and placed on ventilatory support are arterial pH below 7.30 and V_T below 5 mL/kg, unless the drug can promptly and completely be reversed, as with naloxone in the case of narcotic overdose. The patient who is so lethargic as to be unarousable with verbal stimuli or gentle prodding probably cannot provide adequate airway protection. Patients may need to be intubated in order to ensure airway protection and adequate ventilation during transport or for gastric lavage. Persons who overdose with tricyclic antidepressant drugs may be at increased risk for development of the adult respiratory distress syndrome (ARDS), particularly if they have aspirated, and such patients should be observed closely even after initial awakening.[5]

Ventilator Management

Patients with depressed ventilatory drive should be managed with full, not partial, ventilatory support. This is especially important when the patient's mental or neurologic status is fluctuating. Thus, if intermittent mandatory ventilation (IMV) is selected, the mandatory rate should be sufficient to provide all the patient's ventilatory needs. Stand-alone inspiratory pressure support and other spontaneous breathing modes should not be used in this setting until the patient has awakened fully. Because a main purpose of ventilatory support is the prevention and treatment of atelectasis, a large V_T (12 to 15 mL/kg) should be used unless the patient has significant underlying lung disease. The inspired O_2 fraction (FiO_2) should be sufficient to produce a PaO_2 above 70 mmHg, and the pH should be kept in the normal range. Ventilatory drive may fluctuate after apparent awakening in overdose patients, and extubation should not be attempted until they are completely and consistently awake.

Ventilatory Failure in Acute Neuromuscular Disease

Clinical Settings

Any of the neuromuscular disorders listed in Table 30-1 can be encountered.[6,7] Those most commonly seen in usual clinical settings are cervical spinal cord injury and acute inflammatory polyneuropathy (e.g., Guillain-Barré syndrome). Myasthenia gravis, botulism, organophosphate poisoning, and polymyositis may also be encountered as causes of acute ventilatory failure.

Problems

In these cases ventilatory drive is intact (and often accentuated), and underlying lung function tends to be normal, but the pump is dysfunctional so that patients cannot fully expand their lungs. Even if alveolar ventilation can be maintained, at least transiently, atelectasis will likely develop because of inadequate surfactant generation and progressively falling lung compliance. In addition, such patients cannot cough effectively because of accessory ventilatory muscle weakness, and they often cannot fully protect the airway against aspiration. Development of frank respiratory acidemia is a late sign.

Indications for Mechanical Ventilation

The most sensitive indicators for mechanical ventilation are those signifying progressive ventilatory muscle weakness: tachypnea, decreasing vital capacity (VC), and loss of maximum inspiratory force (MIF). Respiratory rate, VC, and MIF should be measured frequently in patients with acute muscle weakness, and ideally they should be charted graphically at the bedside. Intubation and initiation of ventilatory support should be carried out if the rate is consistently in the mid- to high 30s, if VC falls progressively to 10 to 15 mL/kg, or if MIF reaches 20 to 25 cmH_2O. The clinician should not wait for life-threatening respiratory acidemia (e.g., arterial pH below 7.30).

In patients who are paralyzed but alert, nasotracheal tubes tend to cause less discomfort than orotracheal tubes. If it can be predicted that airway access will be needed for longer than a few days or if secretion management is a major problem, this is a setting in which it is wise to perform a tracheotomy earlier rather than later. Tracheostomy tubes tend to be more comfortable for patients than either nasotracheal or orotracheal tubes (see Ch. 53).

Ventilator Management

Patients with compliant lungs who are awake and dyspneic tend to prefer large V_T levels (12 to 15 mL/kg) and rapid inspiratory flow rates (70 to 100 L/min). They may be more comfortable with a mild respiratory alkalosis (e.g., $PaCO_2$ 30 to 35 mmHg); external dead space may be added in an attempt to counteract this effect, but this is seldom done today, and renal compensation usually occurs within 2 to 3 days. Any ventilator mode can be used successfully, but it must be individually adjusted to the patient's comfort, and this may require repeated adjustments. Dyspneic patients tend not to be comfortable on low-rate IMV unless inspiratory pressure support is added. If ventilatory support is going to be required long-term (see Ch. 101), the least complicated mode consistent with patient tolerance should be used.

Mortality in neuromuscular respiratory failure is due primarily to infectious complications. Therefore scrupulous, ongoing attention to airway care and prompt treatment of clinical infections are of paramount importance. Nutritional support is a crucial element in successful management and should be addressed early and vigorously[8] (see Ch. 51).

ACUTE VENTILATORY FAILURE IN CHRONIC OBSTRUCTIVE PULMONARY DISEASE

The patient with severe chronic obstructive pulmonary disease (COPD) and acute ventilatory failure (so-called acute-on-chronic ventilatory failure)[9–13] presents the clinician with a challenging situation, not only from a medical point of view but from the psychosocial and ethical standpoints as well. Such individuals have a progressive, debilitating illness, which must ultimately prove fatal, and it is natural for health care professionals to wonder whether aggressive medical intervention should be undertaken. Would intubation and intensive care unit (ICU) management be likely to be successful? Would it be in the patient's best interests? Would it be a justifiable use of available medical resources? Would the patient ever be able to be weaned from the ventilator?

It may be appropriate not to pursue vigorous treatment, but only if three conditions are met: the persons caring for the patient at that moment should be thoroughly familiar with that patient's history and should have available the appropriate medical records; the patient's own wishes should be known; and acute-on-chronic ventilatory failure at this time should represent an irreversible, terminal physiologic situation for this patient. This last condition requires that the clinician know where this particular patient is on the COPD natural history curve shown in Figure 62-3. In Figure 62-8 are represented two different points on this curve: a patient in acute ventilatory failure at point B (e.g., with a forced expiratory volume in 1 second [FEV_1] of 0.5 L and chronic CO_2 retention) would not be expected to benefit from aggressive therapy, whereas for someone at point A it would be inappropriate not to attempt to reverse the acute episode. As is discussed later in this chapter, the prognosis for such an individual after successful treatment of the acute episode may be the same as if that episode had not occurred.

Unfortunately, patients with acute-on-chronic ventilatory failure often present emergently, and the clinicians who must decide immediately on a course of management do not have access to complete information on their underlying pulmonary function, previous responses to treatment, or wishes for aggressive care. In such situations there can be no alternative to aggressive management. The clinical approach that follows is designed for such a circumstance and assumes that all medically appropriate therapy should be pursued.

General Approach

The great majority of episodes of acute-on-chronic ventilatory failure can be reversed successfully and the patient's previous level of health restored.[9,11,14–16] When this is not the case, it is often because of coexisting medical problems or complications of management.[17,18] Successful management requires awareness and active avoidance of a number of such complications, as summarized in Table 64-2. Most of the principles summarized in the table are related to avoiding endotracheal intubation and the adverse events that commonly follow this procedure.

Clinical Assessment and Triage

Consider the following sequence: a patient with known severe COPD presents to a hospital's emergency department with respiratory distress; he is initially hypoxemic and moderately hypercapnic, but feels better after 1 hour of bronchodilator therapy and supplemental O_2 and is admitted to a medical floor, where he appears to be stable; 4 hours later, at 2:00 AM, he is found in extremis, a "code" is called, and he is emergently intubated and transferred to the ICU.

This not uncommon scenario allows two important points to be made: (1) it may be difficult on initial assessment to appreciate how ill such a patient is; and (2) because respiratory arrest does not occur suddenly in a manner analogous to ventricular fibrillation, close observation of such a patient for progressive respiratory distress can permit early recognition of clinical deterioration and avoidance of the morbidity and mortality associated with "crash" intubations. Initially admitting this hypothetical patient to an ICU or special respiratory unit (Table 64-2) would have facilitated more accurate assessment of illness severity, permitted closer monitoring, and led either to avoidance of the need for intubation or to performance of the procedure under more elective, controlled conditions. Figure 64-3 presents a general scheme for initial triage of a patient with COPD who presents acutely with increased respiratory symptoms.

One physical sign that acute ventilatory failure may be imminent is abdominal paradox, or asynchronous breathing, as diagrammed in Figure 64-4. This pattern of ventilatory motion is associated with other evidence of ventilatory muscle fatigue,[1] as described in Chapter 52. A well documented sequence precedes the onset of overt ventilatory failure in such circumstances[1]; it begins with a reduction in the high/low power spectrum ratio of the diaphragmatic electromyogram, which is followed by tachypnea, and then by the development of abdominal paradox. The asynchronous chest and abdominal movements may persist, or they may alternate with a more normal pattern (respiratory alternans). Only after those phenomena have occurred does a rise in $PaCO_2$ begin, to be followed eventually by bradypnea and decreasing minute ventilation.[1,19]

Patients with signs of pump failure, or with the other findings listed in Figure 64-3, should be admitted initially to an ICU if possible. It may be obvious after a few hours that ICU care is unnecessary, and the patient can be transferred to an acute care floor. However, it is better that this order, rather than the reverse sequence described in the example cited earlier, be followed.

Oxygen Therapy

One reason for admitting the patient to the ICU is to avoid both over- and underoxygenation (Table 64-2), either of which can substantially increase morbidity. Administration of too much O_2 to an acutely ill COPD patient can worsen hypercapnia and acidemia. This phenomenon, known to clinicians for many years, has a more complex genesis than previously believed.[9,20] The traditional explanation is that the patient's ventilation may be stimulated primarily by hypoxic ventilatory drive and that abruptly removing this stimulus leads to hypoventilation (Fig. 64-5). More recent studies have shown, however, that the hypercapnia secondary to acute hyperoxia in such patients is not generally accompanied by a decrease in minute ventilation, suggesting that alterations in ventilation/perfusion ($\dot{V}/\dot{Q}$) matching or other mechanisms may be involved.[21] Whatever its mechanism, alveolar hypoventilation is a significant danger if PaO_2 is raised above 60 to 65 mmHg in some acutely ill COPD patients, and initial O_2 therapy should be carried out in such a manner as to avoid this[22] (Table 64-3).

Persistence of acute hypoxemia should also be avoided. As illustrated by the hemoglobin-O_2 dissociation curve (Fig. 64-6), PaO_2 values below 50 mmHg are associated with sharply reduced blood oxygenation. A PaO_2 below 50 mmHg in an acutely ill patient should always be treated, and patients should never be allowed to remain hypoxemic below this level for fear of worsening respiratory acidosis.[22]

Figure 64-7 shows the rationale behind a target PaO_2 level of 55 to 65 mmHg for the acutely ill COPD patient: it relieves serious hypoxemia while avoiding CO_2 retention in all but exceptional patients. The target PaO_2 range should initially be approached from below, starting with the lowest level of O_2 supplementation (e.g., 1 L/min by nasal cannula or 24 percent by mask) and increasing this sequentially, rather than risking a worsening of hypercapnia from initially overestimating the patient's O_2 requirement.

Because both ventilation and oxygenation must be monitored during the initial hours of therapy, pulse oximetry should not be used as a substitute for arterial blood gas analysis in acute ventilatory failure. Once the patient's condition has stabilized and the responses of both PaO_2 and $PaCO_2$ to supplemental O_2 have been documented, pulse oximetry can help to decrease the number of arterial punctures required.

Table 64-2. Approach to the Patient with Acute-on-Chronic Ventilatory Failure: "10 Commandments" for the Clinican

Commandment	Rationale	Management Approach
1. Thou shalt not unwisely admit thy patient to a regular medical floor	Avoid potentially serious consequences of initially underestimating severity of acute exacerbation and/or degree of physiologic compromise Decrease likelihood of acute decompensation and need for emergent intubation during initial hours in hospital	See Fig. 64-3 When in doubt, admit patient to ICU; err on side of closer observation during first 24 hours
2. Thou shalt not *over*-oxygenate thy patient	Avoid worsening respiratory acidosis through suppression of hypoxic ventilatory drive and/or exacerbation of $\dot{V}/\dot{Q}$ mismatching with excessive O_2 administration Avoid need for emergent intubation	See Table 64-3 Start with low-flow O_2 (e.g., nasal cannula at 1–2 L/min) Keep $PaO_2 < 60$–65 mmHg initially Approach target PaO_2 from below Use arterial blood gases, not just pulse oximetry, to titrate initial O_2 doses
3. Thou shalt not *under*-oxygenate thy patient	Correct potentially life-threatening acute hypoxemia	See Table 64-3 Always provide enough O_2 to raise $PaO_2 > 50$ mmHg
4. Thou shalt not under-treat with corticosteroids and bronchodilators	Aggressively treat reversible component of airway obstruction Avoid prolongation of acute exacerbation and predisposition to complications	Assume that every patient has an "asthmatic" component Give systemic corticosteroids, adequate doses of inhaled beta-agonist, and inhaled anticholinergic, with or without theophylline (see Ch. 62)
5. Thou shalt not unwisely sedate thy patient	Avoid suppressing ventilatory drives Avoid unnecessary intubation	Aggressively treat the *reasons* for patient distress (bronchospasm, airway inflammation, diaphragm fatigue), not the distress itself
6. Thou shalt not intubate thy patient needlessly	Avoid unnecessary therapy (intubation should be required in <10% of cases) Avoid complications of endotracheal tubes and mechanical ventilation Avoid weaning problems	See Commandments 1 to 5 and Table 64-5
7. Thou shalt not allow thy patient to become alkalemic during mechanical ventilation	Avoid arrhythmias, muscle weakness, and other acute complications of alkalosis Avoid weaning problems See Table 64-6	Correct respiratory acidemia gradually Use physiologic pH, not normal $PaCO_2$, as therapeutic goal (target pH 7.30–7.40) See Table 64-7
8. Thou shalt not make thy intubated patient struggle to breathe	Relieve patient discomfort Avoid prolongation of ventilatory muscle fatigue Avoid weaning problems	Provide full (not partial) ventilatory support Avoid prolonged low-rate IMV Add pressure support if low-rate IMV is used Keep total respiratory rate <30 breaths/min See Chs. 83 & 87
9. Thou shalt not prolong ventilator weaning unnecessarily	Avoid ventilator- and endotracheal tube-related complications Minimize ICU and hospital stays Relieve patient discomfort	Attempt weaning as soon as possible (need for ventilatory support is usually <1–2 days) Avoid excessive sedation See Chs. 86 & 87
10. Thou shalt not starve thy patient	Avoid/treat acute malnutrition Avoid weaning problems	Initiate nutritional support within 1–2 days if intubated Use nutritional consultation service if available Avoid excessive carbohydrate loads but provide patient's basic caloric needs (e.g., 2000 kcal/d) See Ch. 51

$\dot{V}/\dot{Q}$, ventilation/perfusion ratio.

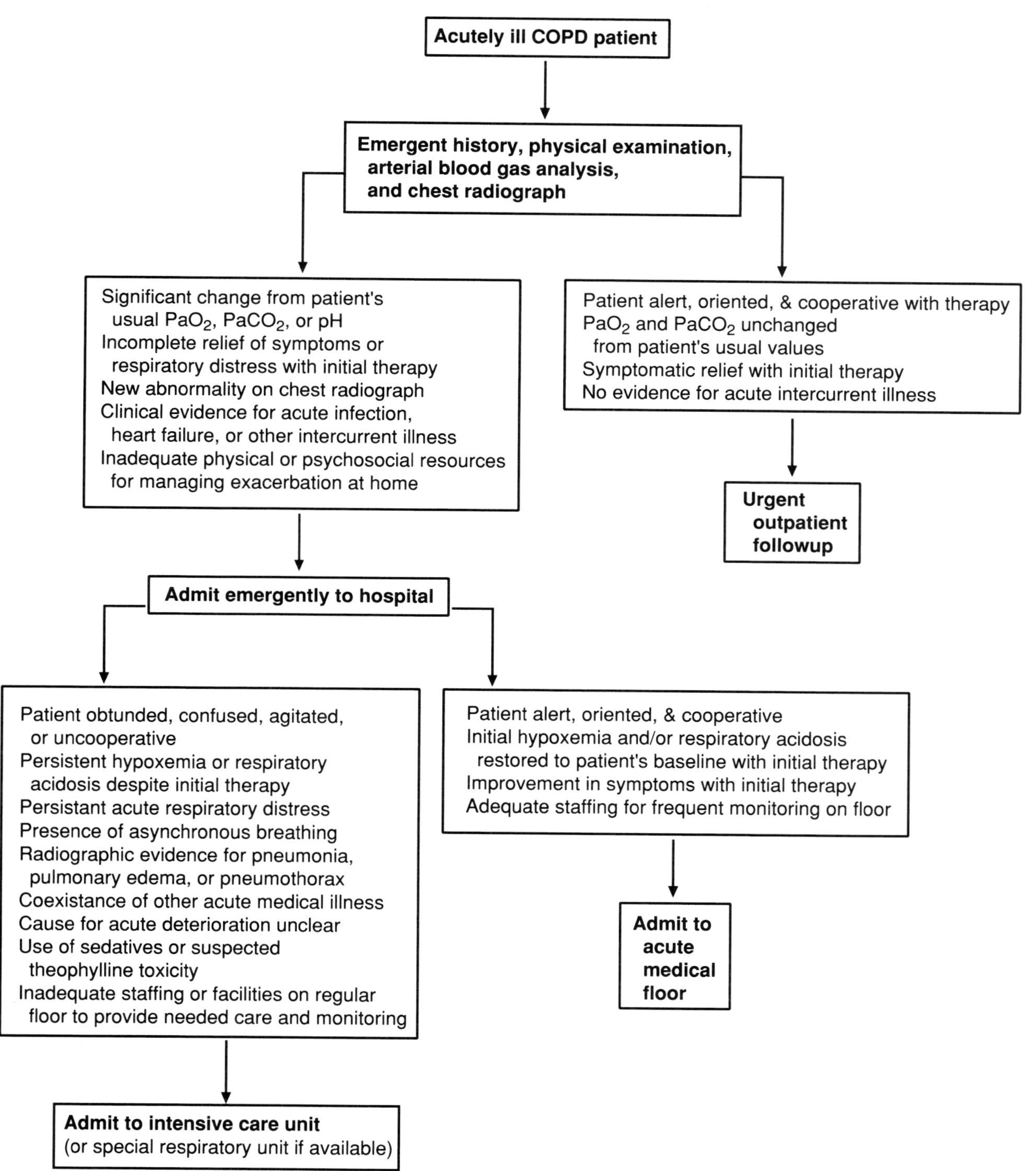

Figure 64-3. Clinical algorithm for triage of an acutely ill patient with COPD presenting emergently to a hospital emergency department or physician's office. For further details see text.

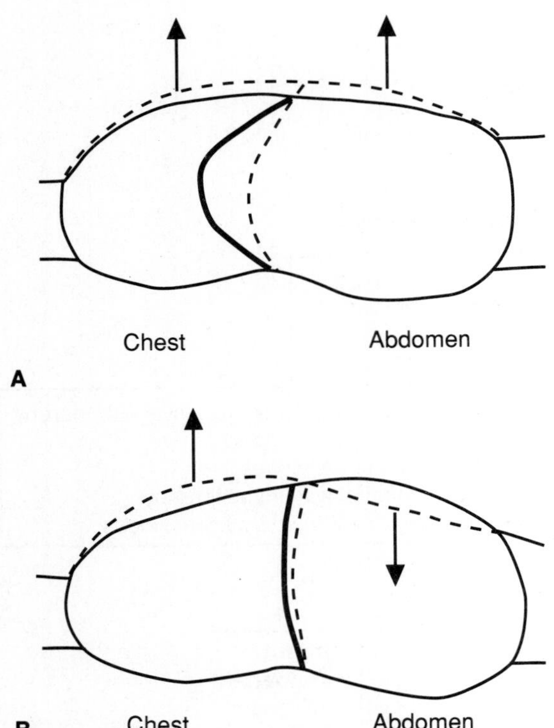

Figure 64-4. Asynchronous breathing or *abdominal paradox,* indicating severe mechanical inefficiency and probably fatigue of the ventilatory muscles. **(A)** Normally, descent of the diaphragm expands the thorax and displaces the abdominal contents, causing both chest and abdomen to expand outward. **(B)** In the presence of diaphragmatic weakness or fatigue, the abdomen is sucked inward during inspiration as the chest expands, producing a rocking, back-and-forth ventilatory pattern. This pattern is both mechanically inefficient and a harbinger of acute ventilatory failure.

Table 64-3. Guidelines for Oxygen Therapy in Acute Exacerbations of COPD

Increase O_2 flow rate or F_IO_2 gradually until PaO_2 rises into target range
>50 mmHg
<65 mmHg, during initial hours of therapy or until patient stabilizes
Assess response using arterial blood gases, not just pulse oximetry
During initial hours of therapy
If $PaCO_2$ trends upward on serial measurements
If respiratory symptoms worsen
If patient's mental status changes
Keep O_2 administration constant, not intermittent
Nasal cannula (more likely to stay on patient)
Venturi-type mask (requires motivated patient and close monitoring)

However, an arterial specimen should be examined whenever a patient becomes more dyspneic, develops unexplained tachycardia or changes in blood pressure, or experiences a change in mental status, even if the oximeter does not indicate desaturation.

Nasal cannulas tend to be better tolerated by acutely ill patients than venturi-type O_2 masks. As a result, the former tend to stay in place more consistently. As discussed in Chapter 75, the true F_IO_2 is not known with either technique, which emphasizes the need for arterial blood gas confirmation of the effects of therapy. Patients receiving O_2 by either device should be closely monitored during the initial hours of therapy.

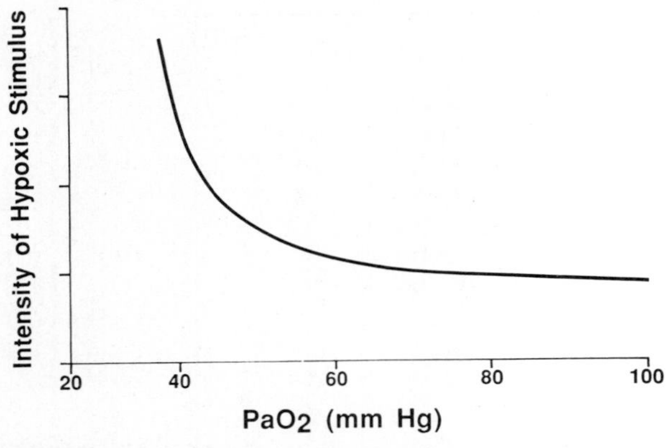

Figure 64-5. General relationship between PaO_2 and hypoxic ventilatory drive. As PaO_2 falls below about 65 mmHg, hypoxic drive begins to increase its contribution to the stimulus to breathe. In some patients with acutely exacerbated COPD, particularly those with hypercapnia, abruptly raising PaO_2 above 55 to 60 mmHg results in progressive respiratory acidosis, in part because of removal of this hypoxic stimulus to ventilation.

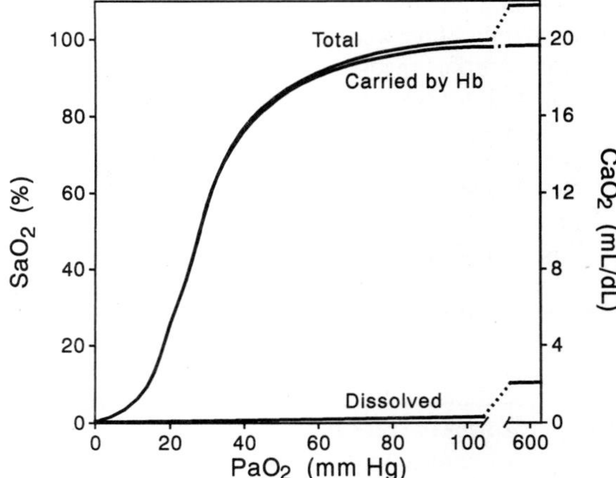

Figure 64-6. Relationship between PaO_2 and blood oxygenation, measured both by oxyhemoglobin saturation (SaO_2) and blood O_2 content (CaO_2). As PaO_2 falls below 50 mmHg, there is an increasing fall in both SaO_2 and CaO_2. Raising PaO_2 to at least 50 mmHg (SaO_2 82 to 85 percent and CaO_2 to approximately 17 mL/dL) prevents severe hypoxemia, and at 65 mmHg arterial oxygenation is largely complete.

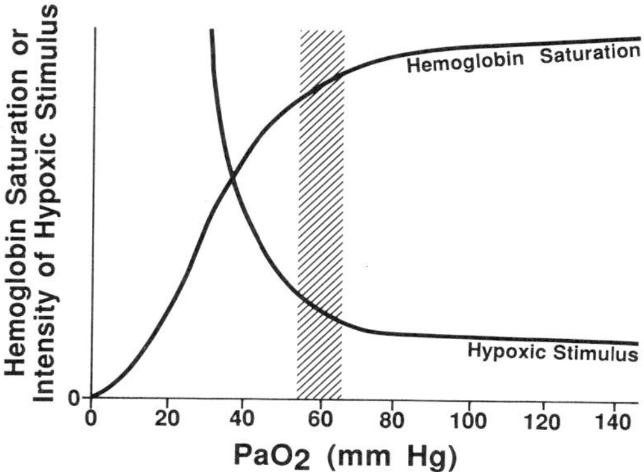

Figure 64-7. Combining Figures 64-5 and 64-6 yields a PaO_2 "target range" of 55 to 65 mmHg (shaded area), which should prevent further serious CO_2 retention while effectively relieving potentially life-threatening hypoxemia. Initial O_2 therapy in acute exacerbations of COPD should be administered so as to approach this target PaO_2 from below, avoiding even transient elevation above 65 mmHg.

Use of Medications

As discussed in Chapter 62, the clinician should assume that the airflow obstruction of every patient with acute ventilatory failure complicating COPD has a significant reversible component and should administer drugs to improve this. To try to achieve the greatest possible improvement as quickly as possible, bronchodilator and anti-inflammatory therapy should be given intensively from the moment of admission. Fortunately, the most effective agents currently in use have relatively few adverse effects with short-term administration.

Corticosteroids and Bronchodilators

Systemic corticosteroids (e.g., methylprednisolone, 0.5 mg/kg IV q 6h) increase the rate of spirometric improvement during the initial days of acute exacerbations.[23,24] Whether this dose or administration schedule is optimal has never been determined, nor has it been established that the drug needs to be given parenterally, but therapy for several days as described is generally free of side effects. Administration of a beta-adrenergic agent (e.g., albuterol) and an anticholinergic (e.g., ipratropium), both by inhalation, completes the standard regimen.

Giving bronchodilators by metered-dose inhaler (MDI), using an auxiliary device (spacer) if necessary, is more cost-effective and no less efficacious than using a nebulizer, provided a sufficient number of puffs are used.[25] Typical initial orders might be for albuterol four to eight puffs every 1 to 2 hours, doubling the number of puffs if necessary, and a reduction in the frequency of administration within a few hours, plus ipratropium four puffs every 4 hours. Corticosteroids are probably ineffective in COPD when given via aerosol, particularly during acute exacerbations.

Theophylline remains an important part of the therapeutic armamentarium but is no longer a first-line drug. It is a less effective bronchodilator than the inhaled beta-adrenergic and anticholinergic agents, and its use must be monitored carefully because of its narrow therapeutic window. Intravenous loading and maintenance infusions of theophylline are described in Chapter 20.

Antibiotics

In contrast to the situation with corticosteroids, most carefully controlled studies have failed to substantiate the common impression that antibiotic therapy is helpful in acute exacerbations of COPD,[26] and if there is a positive effect of antibiotic therapy in this setting, it is not a dramatic one.[27] Pneumonia or other specific bacterial infections should be treated as described in Chapter 68. However, even in the absence of evidence for specific infection, an antibiotic is often added to the management regimen for exacerbations severe enough to prompt acute hospitalization. If drugs are prescribed for the treatment of infection, agents should be selected to cover the organisms most likely to be present; *Streptococcus pneumoniae* and *Haemophilus influenzae*. Amoxicillin, ampicillin, a tetracycline, or trimethoprim-sulfa are good choices; erythromycin and penicillin are less appropriate, and there is no need to use newer, more expensive, broader-spectrum agents. Therapy is generally given empirically for 5 to 10 days.

Sedatives

Patients and other members of the management team may implore the physician to prescribe a sedative or tranquilizer "to help the patient get some rest." Unfortunately, any agent that calms the patient or otherwise decreases respiratory distress must also depress ventilatory drive; there is no "safe" sedative in this circumstance. Administration of sedating drugs to patients in acute ventilatory failure is all too often followed by somnolence, worsened respiratory acidosis, and the need for emergent intubation.

The rationale for withholding all sedating agents acutely can be understood by recalling the reasons for the patient's distress and fatigue, which include increased work of breathing (from bronchospasm, airway inflammation, and excessive secretions), ventilatory muscle fatigue, and acute malnutrition. Reducing the patient's distress will not change any of these factors but will inevitably decrease the patient's efforts to maintain alveolar ventilation. Instead, therapy must focus on reducing the work of breathing, improving tissue oxygenation, and restoring adequate nutritional status. If such therapy is successful, the patient's distress will lessen over a period of hours, and rest will become more feasible as the effort to breathe diminishes.

Endotracheal Intubation

As mentioned earlier, a primary goal of management in acute-on-chronic ventilatory failure should be to avoid in-

Table 64-4. Reasons to Avoid Intubation in Patients with COPD

Unnecessary in great majority of cases
Impairment of airway clearance
Interference with mucociliary function
Reduction in effectiveness of cough
Exposure of lower respiratory tract to infection
Bacterial colonization
Nosocomial pneumonia
Predisposition to complications associated with mechanical ventilation

tubation and mechanical ventilation. There are two main reasons for this (Table 64-4): intubation is generally unnecessary, and it predisposes to additional complications and morbidity. The outcome of an episode of ventilatory failure is likely to be the same with or without intubation. In fact, one well performed older study found that patients who received mechanical ventilation after failure of other aggressive management had a worse prognosis than either those in whom this was avoided or those in whom intubation and mechanical ventilation were part of initial management.[28]

Despite intentions to avoid it, intubation becomes necessary in some cases. Table 64-5 lists the circumstances in which this generally occurs. The last indication in the table, progressive respiratory acidosis, is the least certain, and the arterial pH value below which survival is less likely without intubation and mechanical ventilation is unknown. Flenley[29] advocated intubation for patients who deteriorate despite appropriate bronchodilator and other therapy, as well as controlled O_2 administration once their pH fell below 7.26, and this appears to be a reasonable threshold.[30] However, as long as the patient remains awake and cooperative, other therapy can continue and the need for intubation need not be regarded as an emergency.

Mechanical Ventilation

Once a patient with severe COPD has been intubated and placed on a ventilator, a primary goal should be weaning as soon as possible.[4] Unless pneumonia or other complicating medical process is present, patients with acute ventilatory failure in the setting of an acute COPD exacerbation seldom require ventilatory support for more than 1 to 2 days. However, during the period of mechanical ventilation they are subject to a variety of iatrogenic and other ventilator-associated complications,[17,18] and this increases the urgency of weaning.

One complication that commonly develops on initiation of ventilatory support is acute alkalemia due to overventilation, as illustrated in Table 64-6. Patients with underlying chronic ventilatory insufficiency (far left column in the table) who develop acute-on-chronic ventilatory failure (second column of Table 64-6) should receive only enough ventilatory support to bring arterial pH back into the physiologic range (i.e., above 7.30 but below 7.40). If the ventilator is set to provide "normal" alveolar ventilation ($PaCO_2$ 40 mmHg), the underlying metabolic alkalosis will result in acute alkalemia (third column in Table 64-6), which may threaten the patient's life as much as the initial acidosis. Additionally, if such overventilation is not corrected promptly, over the next 2 to 3 days the patient's kidneys will excrete the "extra" HCO_3^-, leading to the "normal" acid-base status depicted in the far right column in Table 64-6. At this point the patient will likely fail attempts at weaning and develop acute respiratory acidosis because of having been maintained at a level of ventilation incompatible with the mechanical limitations imposed by the underlying airway obstruction. Successful weaning at this point will require re-establishment of the original compensated respiratory acidosis, which will likely require several more days to accomplish.

Table 64-7 provides general guidelines for ventilatory management in patients with severe COPD. It is important to adjust the ventilator so that the patient can actually rest if this is the intention (Table 64-2). Partial ventilatory support, as with low-rate IMV without added pressure support, is unlikely to achieve this goal, and the patient may remain tachypneic and restless.[31]

Outcome and Long-Term Prognosis

The large majority of COPD patients survive an episode of acute ventilatory failure, even if they are elderly[32] and even if ventilatory support is required.[16,33] Mortality in numerous older studies ranged between 20 and 40 percent, but

Table 64-5. Indications for Intubation in Acute Exacerbations of COPD

Apnea; agonal respiration
Obtundation; lethargy
Uncontrollable agitation
Progressive respiratory acidosis despite aggressive therapy (e.g., arterial pH < 7.25–7.30 and falling)

Table 64-6. Acute Alkalosis Complicating Mechanical Ventilation in Acute-on-Chronic Ventilatory Failure

	Baseline Stable State	Acute Ventilatory Failure	Initial Values on Ventilator	New Stable State after 2–3 Days at Same Settings
pH (units)	7.38	7.24	7.56	7.40
PCO_2 (mmHg)	56	86	40	40
HCO_3 (mEq/L)	33	36	34	24

Table 64-7. Guidelines for Ventilatory Management in Patients with COPD

Management Element	Comments
Ventilator mode	AMV, IMV, or PSV appropriate if used correctly AMV: use high inspiratory flow rate; minimize triggering effort; sedate patient if necessary IMV: monitor patient's total rate as index of comfort (should be <30/min); sedate patient if necessary PSV: may be more comfortable for some patients; patient's ventilatory drive must remain intact (minimize sedation); adjust inspiratory pressure to keep rate < 30/min
Inspired O_2 fraction	Sufficient to keep $SaO_2 > 90\%$ during full ventilatory support Hypoxemia typically due to $\dot{V}/\dot{Q}$ mismatching and easy to correct Keep PaO_2 55–65 mmHg (SaO_2 85–90%) during partial ventilatory support and when attempting weaning
Tidal Volume	Lower than usual for other patients (e.g., 7–10 mL/kg, especially if severely hyperinflated) Avoid larger volumes because of risk of increasing auto-PEEP and likelihood of alveolar rupture
Inspiratory flow rate	Use high flows (e.g., 70–100 L/min) Maximize expiratory time Decrease patient's air hunger Decrease inspiratory work of breathing
Rate (minute ventilation)	Sufficient to keep arterial pH 7.30–7.40 (avoid alkalemia) Absolute $PaCO_2$ value less important Monitor patient for auto-PEEP
Positioning	Keep patient upright or semiupright as much as possible to improve efficiency of ventilatory muscles
Weaning	Attempt as soon as possible (usually possible within 1–2 days) Avoid prolonged low-rate IMV without added pressure support Add 5–8 cmH_2O pressure support during trial of spontaneous ventilation prior to extubation if patient's endotracheal tube is 7.5-mm ID or less May elect to extubate patient without trial of spontaneous ventilation (see weaning guidelines in Ch. 86)

AMV, assisted mechanical ventilation (assist/control); PSV, pressure support ventilation.

in all series published since 1975, survival has exceeded 90 percent,[14–16] which probably reflects advances in ventilator care and monitoring.

Figure 64-8 shows survival after an episode of acute ventilatory failure.[33] The majority of such patients should still be living 2 years following the acute episode, according to a comparison study by Martin et al.[33] Episodes of acute ventilatory failure may not have a major adverse impact on overall survival in COPD, which is more closely related to FEV_1 than to any other factor. Figure 64-9 illustrates this point by comparing the course of 44 consecutive patients initially presenting in acute ventilatory failure with the course of patients from two other reported series, categorized according to FEV_1.[33]

ACUTE VENTILATORY FAILURE IN ASTHMA

General Approach

The approach to assessment and management of the patient with acute severe asthma is discussed in Chapter 62 and summarized in Table 62-3. Management of acute ventilatory failure relies on maximizing therapy with corticosteroids, bronchodilators, and other agents. Maximum dosages, particularly of corticosteroids, have generally not been established, and clinical wisdom suggests that the steroid dose should be increased every 1 to 2 days as long as the patient has not improved. There is evidence that hospitalized asthmatics who are seen by pulmonary specialists do better than those managed entirely by their primary physicians.[34]

Mechanical Ventilation

Are the indications for intubation and mechanical ventilation in acute asthma different from those in COPD and other disorders? In general the answer is no. However, some clinicians, particularly in Europe, feel that the arterial pH cutoff used in other conditions is too high, and favorable outcomes have been achieved without intubation despite pH values that dropped to 7.20 or below. As with COPD, as long as a patient remains alert and cooperative with therapy, the need for intubation is probably not emergent, particularly if the arterial blood gases stabilize and begin to improve.

Because status asthmaticus is an obstructive process characterized by marked pulmonary hyperinflation, ventilator tidal volumes should be smaller than those used in most other settings (e.g., not more than 8 to 10 mL/kg). Because of high resistance in the intrathoracic airways, peak inspiratory pressures are often very high in ventilated asthmatics, but these do not imply a markedly increased likelihood of barotrauma as is the case in ARDS.[35] Decreasing peak inspiratory pressure by reducing inspiratory flow rate is not feasible because of the need for a long expiratory time, and high inspiratory flows should be used. Peak airway pressures decrease as bronchospasm, airway inflammation, and hyperinflation improve.[36]

Darioli and Petter[37] in 1984 and Menitove and Goldring[38] in 1983 reported successful management of refractory status asthmaticus by using deliberate hypoventilation, with HCO_3^- infusion to restore physiologic arterial pH. With this technique $PaCO_2$ is allowed to rise as high as 90 mmHg,

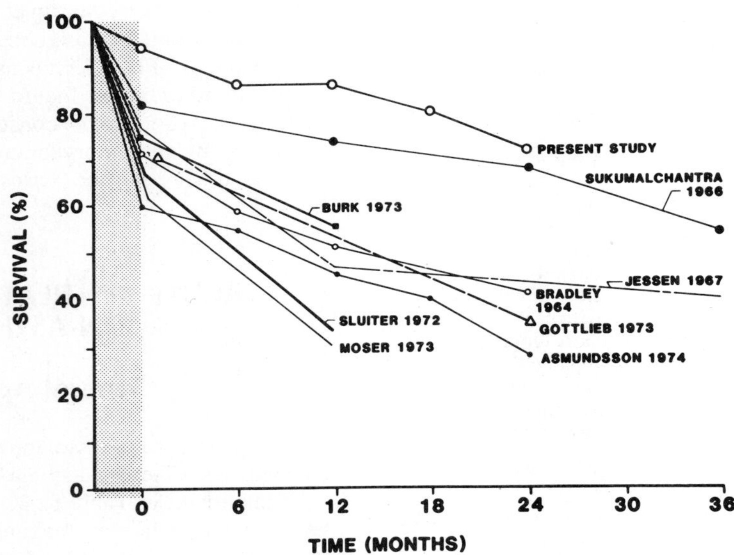

Figure 64-8. In-hospital mortality from and survival following episodes of acute ventilatory failure complicating COPD, based on comparison of the findings of nine reported series of patients. The shaded area at left represents in-hospital mortality, which was 20 to 40 percent in older studies but has been less than 10 percent in studies published since 1975. "Present study" indicates Martin et al.'s study. (From Martin et al.,[33] with permission.)

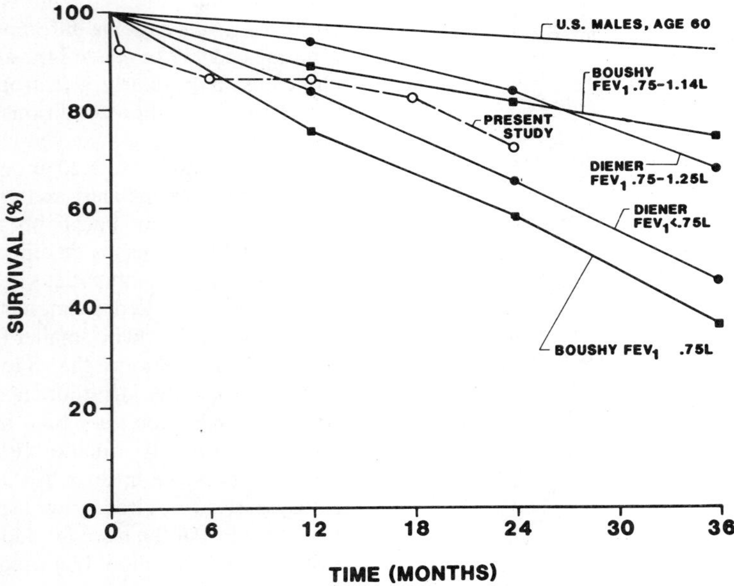

Figure 64-9. Survival curves for patients with COPD following hospitalization for acute ventilatory failure (Martin et al.'s "present study," dashed line), compared with that of COPD patients in two long-term follow-up series who had not suffered acute ventilatory failure. As discussed in Chapter 22 and illustrated in Figure 22-9, mortality in COPD increases with increasing severity of airflow obstruction, as measured by FEV_1. However, survival is not appreciably worse among patients who have had a bout of acute ventilatory failure. The solid line at the top represents expected survival for U.S. men at age 60 years. (From Martin et al.,[33] with permission.)

which decreases ventilatory requirements, while the asthma attack can be improved through pharmacologic therapy. Although very high survival rates have been reported with use of this technique,[37] other investigators have achieved comparable results with conventional ventilator management.[17,39,40]

References

1. Roussos C: Respiratory muscle fatigue and ventilatory failure. Chest, suppl. 1990;97:89s–96s
2. Pierson DJ: Acute respiratory failure. pp. 75–126. In Sahn SA (ed): Pulmonary Emergencies. Churchill Livingstone, New York, 1982
3. Pierson DJ: Indications for mechanical ventilation in acute respiratory failure. Respir Care 1983;28:570–578
4. Pierson DJ: Exacerbation of chronic bronchitis and emphysema: Ventilatory management. pp. 267–272. In Kacmarek RM, Stoller JK (eds): Current Respiratory Care. BC Decker, Philadelphia, 1988
5. Vincent JM, Blair AD, Romaneschi KB et al: ARDS following drug overdose: Incidence with tricyclic antidepressant ingestion, abstracted. Am Rev Respir Dis 1985;131(4, Pt 2):A52
6. Bennett DA, Bleck TP: Diagnosis and treatment of neuromuscular causes of acute respiratory failure. Clinical Neuropharmacol 1988;11:303–347
7. Bergofsky EH: Respiratory failure in disorders of the thoracic cage. Am Rev Respir Dis 1979;119:643–669
8. Pingleton SK, Harmon GS: Nutritional management in acute respiratory failure. JAMA 1987;257:3094–3099
9. Derenne JP, Fleury B, Pariente R: Acute respiratory failure of chronic obstructive pulmonary disease. Am Rev Respir Dis 1988;138:1006–1033
10. Hudson LD: Acute respiratory failure in patients with chronic obstructive pulmonary disease. pp. 155–172. In Bone RC, George RB, Hudson LD (eds): Acute Respiratory Failure. Churchill Livingstone, New York, 1987
11. Petty TL: Acute respiratory failure in chronic obstructive pulmonary disease. pp. 558–565. In Shoemaker WC, Ayres S, Grenvik A et al (eds): Textbook of Critical Care Medicine. 2nd Ed. WB Saunders, Philadelphia, 1989
12. Schmidt GA, Hall JB: Acute on chronic respiratory failure. Assessment and management of patients with COPD in the emergent setting. JAMA 1989;261:3444–3453
13. Rosen RL, Bone RC: Treatment of acute exacerbations of chronic obstructive pulmonary disease. Med Clin North Am 1990;74:691–700
14. Hudson LD: Prognosis: Immediate and long-term sequelae of acute respiratory failure. Respir Care 1983;28:663–670
15. Hudson LD: Respiratory failure: Etiology and mortality. Respir Care 1987;32:584–593
16. Hudson LD: Survival data in patients with acute and chronic lung disease requiring mechanical ventilation. Am Rev Respir Dis 1989;140:S19–S24
17. Pingleton SK: Complications of acute respiratory failure. Am Rev Respir Dis 1988;137:1463–1493
18. Pierson DJ: Complications of mechanical ventilation. Current Pulmonol 1990;11:19–46
19. Cohen C, Zagelbaum G, Gross D et al: Clinical manifestations of inspiratory muscle fatigue. Am J Med 1982;73:308–316
20. Aubier M, Murciano D, Fournier M et al: Central respiratory drive in acute respiratory failure of patients with chronic obstructive pulmonary disease. Am Rev Respir Dis 1980;122: 191–199
21. Aubier M, Murciano D, Milic-Emili J et al: Effects of the administration of O_2 on ventilation and blood gases in patients with chronic obstructive pulmonary disease during acute respiratory failure. Am Rev Respir Dis 1980;122:747–754
22. Pierson DJ: Indications for oxygen therapy. Probl Respir Care 1990;3:549–562
23. Albert RK, Martin TR, Lewis SW: Controlled clinical trial of methylprednisolone in patients with chronic bronchitis and acute respiratory insufficiency. Ann Intern Med 1980;92:753–758
24. Hudson LD, Monti CM: Rationale and use of corticosteroids in chronic obstructive pulmonary disease. Med Clin North Am 1990;74:661–690
25. Special Issue: Consensus conference on aerosol delivery. Respir Care 1991;36:916–1044
26. Tager I, Speizer FE: Role of infection in chronic bronchitis. N Engl J Med 1975;292:563–571
27. Anthonisen NR, Manfreda J, Warren CPW et al: Antibiotic therapy in exacerbations of chronic obstructive pulmonary disease. Ann Intern Med 1987;106:196–204
28. Sluiter HJ, Blokzuil EJ, van Dijl W et al: Conservative and respirator treatment of acute respiratory failure in patients with chronic obstructive pulmonary disease. Am Rev Respir Dis 1972;105:932–943
29. Flenley DC: Problems before, during, and after mechanical ventilation in chronic bronchitis and emphysema. Schweiz Med Wochenschr 1985;115:186–189
30. Muir JF, Levi-Valensi P: When should patients with COPD be ventilated? Eur J Respir Dis 1987;70:135–139
31. Bartlett RH: A critical carol. Being an essay on anemia, suffocation, starvation, and other forms of intensive care, after the manner of Dickens. Chest 1984;85:687–693
32. Pierson DJ, Neff TA, Petty TL: Ventilatory management of the elderly. Geriatrics 1973;28:86–95
33. Martin TR, Lewis SW, Albert RK: The prognosis of patients with chronic obstructive pulmonary disease after hospitalization for acute respiratory failure. Chest 1982;82:310–314
34. Bucknall CE, Robertson C, Moran F, Stevenson RD: Differences in hospital asthma management. Lancet 1988;1:748–750
35. Pierson DJ: Alveolar rupture during mechanical ventilation: Role of PEEP, peak airway pressure, and distending volume. Respir Care 1988;33:472–484
36. Mansel JK, Stogner SW, Petrini MF, Norman JR: Mechanical ventilation in patients with severe asthma. Am J Med 1990;89:42–48
37. Darioli E, Petter C: Mechanical controlled hypoventilation in status asthmaticus. Am Rev Respir Dis 1984;129:385–387
38. Menitove SM, Goldring RM: Combined ventilator and bicarbonate strategy in the management of status asthmaticus. Am J Med 1983;94:898–901
39. Higgins B, Greening A, Crompton G: Assisted ventilation in severe acute asthma. Thorax 1986;41:464–467
40. Santiago SN, Klaustermeyer WB: Mortality in status asthmaticus: A nine-year experience in a respiratory intensive care unit. J Asthma 1980;2:75–79

Chapter 65

Clinical Approach to the Patient with Acute Oxygenation Failure

Kenneth P. Steinberg
David J. Pierson

CHAPTER OUTLINE

Chapter 29 discusses three basic mechanisms of acute respiratory failure: ventilatory failure, failure to oxygenate the arterial blood, and failure of tissue oxygenation (see Table 29-3). Oxygenation failure can also be divided conceptually into four categories: hypoxemia, reduced arterial O_2 content (CaO_2), decreased O_2 transport, and impaired tissue O_2 utilization. Table 65-1 lists these four categories, recalling the physiologic mechanisms that can produce them, along with familiar clinical examples of each, and also indicates the clinical usefulness of supplemental O_2 therapy in these settings.[1] It can be seen that O_2 therapy is helpful primarily for hypoxemia, and further that O_2 is not the primary treatment for all forms of acute oxygenation failure.

Physiologically, there are five potential mechanisms for hypoxemia (Table 29-5): low inspired O_2 pressure ($P_{I}O_2$), alveolar hypoventilation, ventilation/perfusion ($\dot{V}/\dot{Q}$) mismatch, right-to-left shunt, and diffusion limitation. Because diffusion limitation is not considered an important mechanism for hypoxemia as encountered in respiratory care, only the first four of these mechanisms are discussed here (Table 65-1).

This chapter provides the clinician with a framework with which to understand and approach the management of patients with hypoxemia. Primary emphasis is given to bedside recognition of the physiologic mechanism(s) of hypoxemia, and particularly to measures for correcting this hypoxemia when it is due to right-to-left intrapulmonary shunt. Although localized disease processes producing shunt are covered briefly at the end, diffuse shunt as encountered in the adult respiratory distress syndrome (ARDS) is the main focus of this discussion.

This chapter forms a bridge between earlier chapters that

Table 65-1. Effectiveness of Supplemental Oxygen Therapy in Different Types of Tissue Hypoxia

Type of Defect	Mechanism of Tissue O_2 Deficiency	Clinical Examples	Supplemental O_2 Helpful
Hypoxemia	Low P_IO_2	High altitude; patient not receiving prescribed O_2	Yes
	Aveolar hypoventilation	Narcotic overdose; severe COPD; sleep apnea	Yes[a]
	$\dot{V}/\dot{Q}$ mismatch	COPD; asthma; diffuse lung disease	Yes
	Right-to-left shunt	Generalized Cardiogenic pulmonary edema; ARDS	Yes[b]
		Localized Lobar pneumonia; acute atelectasis	Yes[b]
Decreased CaO_2	Hypoxemia	See above	
	Insufficient functional hemoglobin	Anemia; CO poisoning	No[c]
Decreased O_2 transport	Decreased CaO_2	See above	
	Decreased $\dot{Q}_T$	Cardiogenic shock; hemorrhagic shock; excessive PEEP	No
Decreased tissue O_2 utilization	Inadequate delivery of O_2 to hypoxic tissue bed	See above	
	Inability of tissues to use O_2	Cyanide poisoning	No

ARDS, adult respiratory distress syndrome; COPD, chronic obstructive pulmonary disease; PEEP, positive end-expiratory pressure; P_IO_2, inspired O_2 tension; $\dot{V}/\dot{Q}$; ventilation perfusion; $\dot{Q}_T$, cardiac output.
[a] Primary therapy is to increase alveolar ventilation.
[b] Improvement often minimal; other measures (PEEP, position changes, correction of primary problem) usually required.
[c] No clinically significant benefit from raising PaO_2 >80–90 mmHg; if immediately available, hyperbaric O_2 therapy may temporarily reverse tissue hypoxia in selected circumstances.
(From Pierson,[1] with permission.)

describe the physiologic mechanisms (Ch. 29) and clinical manifestations (Chs. 31, 32, and 35) of acute oxygenation failure and those in subsequent sections that deal with practical aspects of therapy. Important among the latter are Chapters 75 (Supplemental Oxygen and Other Medical Gas Therapy), 76 (Positive End-Expiratory Pressure Therapy), and 83 (Clinical Management of Mechanical Ventilation). The reader should refer to these other discussions of the various aspects of oxygenation failure and its management as needed to appreciate the unified approach presented in this book. Because most of the discussion in the present chapter pertains to management of ARDS, the manifestations and natural history of this syndrome should be reviewed (Ch. 35). Physiologic and clinical aspects of acute ventilatory failure are discussed in Chapters 29 and 30, and an integrated approach to the management of this second main category of respiratory failure is presented in Chapter 64. Failure of systemic O_2 transport and failure of tissue O_2 use are discussed in Chapters 33 and 34, respectively.

THERAPEUTIC IMPLICATIONS OF THE DIFFERENT PHYSIOLOGIC MECHANISMS OF HYPOXEMIA

When initially assessing a patient with hypoxemia, it is important to try to identify the mechanisms or mechanisms causing it, because this can determine the approach, type, and response to therapy.[1,2] Each of the five causes of hypoxemia responds differently to O_2 therapy, and understanding the mechanism of a patient's hypoxemia allows the clinician to anticipate the amount of O_2 that may be required. It may also help the clinician to predict the possibility of being unable to correct the hypoxemia with O_2 therapy alone. Finally, it guides the clinician in considering additional or alternate therapies that may help to reverse the patient's hypoxemia. These additional therapies (discussed later) may include positive end-expiratory pressure (PEEP), novel ventilatory strategies such as independent lung ventilation (ILV), and changes in the patient's body position.

Low Inspired Oxygen Pressure

Situations in which the P_IO_2 is reduced include being at higher altitudes where atmospheric pressure is lower than it is at sea level, being in an enclosed space without fresh air, or being trapped near a fire where there is a rapid consumption of ambient O_2 (see Ch. 31). In the intensive care unit (ICU), low P_IO_2 is generally due to a reduction in inspired O_2 fraction (F_IO_2) during supplemental O_2 therapy that occurs either by intentional adjustment or technical mishap.

The most clinically important etiology of this problem is the failure of the system being used to augment a patient's F_IO_2. In this regard, a patient receiving supplemental O_2 therapy could become hypoxemic if the tubing became disconnected or occluded, or if the O_2 supply became depleted. Patients wearing nasal cannulae and face masks often remove them intermittently or wear them incorrectly[2] and this can lead to hypoxemia. Another common problem with face masks is air entrainment around a poorly fitted mask on a patient whose inspiratory flow rate exceeds that of the supplemental O_2 (see Ch. 75). In this setting, the patient can entrain a substantial amount of air around the mask, diluting the set F_{IO_2}, and thus receiving an F_{IO_2} less than the intended amount. Finally, for patients on ventilators, machines can malfunction and tubing can become disconnected,[3] again causing lower F_{IO_2} levels than desired, which leads to hypoxemia. These causes of hypoxemia seem trivial and obvious, but they should always be thought of when evaluating a hypoxemic patient in the hospital setting.[4]

Alveolar Hypoventilation

Alveolar hypoventilation is dealt with in Chapter 64, which discusses in detail the approach to ventilatory failure. In the presence of a normal alveolar-arterial O_2 tension difference [$P(A\text{-}a)O_2$], PaO_2 falls in the presence of hypoventilation by an amount approximately equal to the rise in $PaCO_2$ (see Fig. 29-2). Often both hypoventilation and $\dot{V}/\dot{Q}$ mismatch are present, as in severe chronic obstructive pulmonary disease (COPD) with acute exacerbation, in which case the contribution of alveolar hypoventilation to the hypoxemia can be estimated from the severity of hypercapnia. Using the alveolar gas equation, $P(A\text{-}a)O_2$ should always be estimated when hypoxemia is present; when alveolar hypoventilation is the sole cause of hypoxemia the $P(A\text{-}a)O_2$ is normal (i.e., not greater than 20 mmHg in the young or 30 mmHg in the elderly).

Primary treatment for hypoxemia due to alveolar hypoventilation is to restore normal alveolar ventilation, since by definition this will relieve the hypoxemia (Table 65-2).[1] Supplemental O_2 administration is highly effective in raising PaO_2 when hypoxemia is caused by this mechanism, and should also be used when immediate restoration of normal ventilation cannot be accomplished. In patients with acute-on-chronic ventilatory failure, the administration of supplemental O_2 is more complicated and may be associated with worsening of respiratory acidosis (see Ch. 64 for details).

Proper positioning of a patient can also improve ventilation in the appropriate situations. In patients with diaphragmatic paralysis or a large abdominal cavity, sitting up or being in reverse Trendelenberg's position may improve ventilatory mechanics and hence improve gas exchange.

Minimizing the use of sedative, analgesic, and paralytic drugs may improve ventilatory drive and mechanics. These agents are used frequently in the ICU and also in postoperative patients. Many patients metabolize these drugs slowly and the effects can be sustained for longer periods than might be expected. In patients who have received or overdosed on narcotics, use of a narcotic antagonist such as naloxone can often reverse life-threatening hypoventilation.

Ventilation to Perfusion Mismatch

Probably the most common physiologic mechanism for hypoxemia in the hospital setting is $\dot{V}/\dot{Q}$ mismatching. This mechanism is characteristic for obstructive lung disease (e.g., COPD, acute asthma) and for most diffuse restrictive processes (e.g., pulmonary fibrosis, moderate congestive heart failure). Because low P_{IO_2} in the ICU setting is usually readily detectable, and any component of hypoxemia due to alveolar hypoventilation can be identified by reference to the $PaCO_2$, the clinician's main task is to differentiate between $\dot{V}/\dot{Q}$ mismatch and shunt as the main mechanism for hypoxemia with an increased $P(A\text{-}a)O_2$. Such distinction is valuable not only diagnostically but also therapeutically because of its implications for the ease with which the hypoxemia can be corrected using supplemental O_2.

Figure 29-4 illustrates why hypoxemia resulting from $\dot{V}/\dot{Q}$ mismatch generally corrects with only a modest increase in F_{IO_2}—at least in terms of restoring normal CaO_2: P_{AO_2} need only be raised sufficiently to exceed the rate of O_2 removal from that alveolus. In clinical practice this can usually be accomplished using nasal O_2 or O_2 via mask at an F_{IO_2} less than 0.50. By contrast, hypoxemia due to right-to-left shunt

Table 65-2. Response to Oxygen Therapy with Different Physiologic Mechanisms of Hypoxemia

Physiologic Mechanism	ABG Values Before Therapy (mmHg)	Therapy Administered	ABG Values with Therapy (mmHg)
Alveolar hypoventilation (e.g., narcotic drug overdose)	PaO_2 = 50 $PaCO_2$ = 70	Increase alveolar ventilation (no supplemental O_2)	PaO_2 = 80 $PaCO_2$ = 40
$\dot{V}/\dot{Q}$ mismatch (e.g., acute asthma attack)	PaO_2 = 55 $PaCO_2$ = 34	Nasal O_2, 2 L/min	PaO_2 = 80 $PaCO_2$ = 38
Right-to-left shunt (e.g., acute pulmonary edema)	PaO_2 = 44 $PaCO_2$ = 34	Nasal O_2, 2 L/min	PaO_2 = 46 $PaCO_2$ = 34
		OR	
		100% O_2 by mask	PaO_2 = 52 $PaCO_2$ = 35

ABG, arterial blood gas.
(From Pierson,[1] with permission.)

responds only slightly to O_2 supplementation (see Fig. 29-5): regardless of how high the PO_2 is raised in airways that lead to collapsed or occluded alveoli, the capillary blood perfusing such alveoli still "sees" no O_2 and exits the lung still desaturated.

Accordingly, the clinical response to initial O_2 supplementation as reflected in the PaO_2 can be used as an indicator not only of the predominant physiologic derangement but also of the vigor with which the hypoxemia must be treated (Table 65-2). In clinical settings in which $\dot{V}/\dot{Q}$ mismatch can be predicted to be the probable cause of hypoxemia, such as an acute exacerbation of COPD, it is wisest to start with low-flow O_2 therapy (e.g., 2 L/min via nasal cannulae) and to increase this if necessary as guided by initial arterial blood gas (ABG) response (see Ch. 64). However, as discussed below, in settings dominated by shunt (e.g., lobar pneumonia), considerably higher levels of O_2 supplementation likely will be necessary and the response may be only modest.

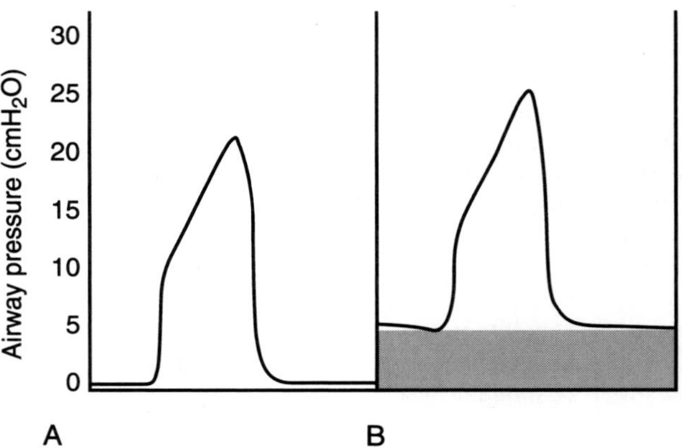

Figure 65-1. The effect of PEEP on airway pressure, as demonstrated in one of the first clinical reports of its use in severe oxygenation failure. Tracheal pressure measurements were made during volume-limited ventilation with an Ohio 560 ventilator. **(A)** Airway pressure increases progressively during inspiration and then falls quickly to zero (ambient). **(B)** With addition of 5 cmH_2O PEEP the same tidal volume (V_T) is delivered but from a starting and ending pressure kept positive to the extent of the added PEEP; both peak and end-expiratory pressures are higher than they were before PEEP was added. (From McIntyre et al.,[15] with permission.)

Right-to-Left Shunt

Hypoxemia that is relatively refractory to treatment with supplemental O_2 typifies the clinical settings characterized by right-to-left shunt. Physiologic studies using the multiple inert gas elimination technique[5–7] demonstrate that this "shunt" is often a mixture of true right-to-left shunt ($\dot{V}/\dot{Q}$ of zero) and very low $\dot{V}/\dot{Q}$ areas in ARDS, but this distinction is unimportant to the clinician in the context of this discussion, since the clinical effects and response to therapy are the same. In such settings the disease may be either diffuse (e.g., ARDS; cardiogenic pulmonary edema) or localized (e.g., lobar pneumonia; acute atelectasis of a lobe or entire lung). In either situation there may be little improvement in PaO_2 with even high-FIO_2 supplemental O_2 therapy. When the shunt results from widespread alveolar collapse and/or flooding with blood, edema fluid, or exudate, mechanically expanding the lungs through the use of PEEP may produce dramatic improvement in PaO_2.

POSITIVE END-EXPIRATORY PRESSURE

Identification and Physiologic Effects

PEEP has become an integral component in the treatment of acute respiratory failure.[8,9] Its use dates to 1938 when it was introduced as a method of treating acute cardiogenic pulmonary edema.[10] Later, it was tried as a means of preventing hypoxemia in pilots flying at high altitude in nonpressurized cabins. The use of PEEP did not become popular, however, until Ashbaugh and Petty documented its efficacy in improving oxygenation in patients with ARDS.[11,12] Since that time, there has been an extensive accumulation of clinical and experimental experience with PEEP.[9,13,14]

To use PEEP effectively, it is important to understand its beneficial and adverse effects. PEEP refers to the application of pressure above atmospheric to the airways during expiration. Thus, PEEP prevents airway pressure from returning to zero at the end of expiration. By preventing the airway pressure from dropping to zero, PEEP results in an increase in lung volume throughout the ventilatory cycle, especially the volume in the lungs at end-expiration (i.e., an increase in functional residual capacity [FRC]). Figure 65-1 illustrates this effect of PEEP on lung volume,[15] which is thought to be the primary mechanism behind all beneficial and adverse physiologic effects of PEEP.[8]

Beneficial Effects

The single most important beneficial effect of PEEP in acute respiratory failure is an improvement in PaO_2 (Fig. 65-2),[15] the main management benefit of which is the clinician's ability to reduce the FIO_2 and thus any risk of O_2 toxicity. This improvement in PaO_2 is thought to be due to the ability of PEEP to increase lung volume and mean alveolar pressure, which in turn re-expands collapsed alveoli and prevents collapse of unstable, low-$\dot{V}/\dot{Q}$ alveoli (Fig. 65-3A & B).[8] By opening previously atelectatic alveoli, PEEP can markedly reduce intrapulmonary shunting and improve $\dot{V}/\dot{Q}$ matching.

In addition to increasing alveolar volume, PEEP can also improve $\dot{V}/\dot{Q}$ matching by redistributing the extravascular lung water (pulmonary edema) that accumulates during ARDS. It used to be thought that PEEP could "squeeze" water out of alveoli and force it back into the bloodstream, and thereby decrease total lung water. More recently, it has

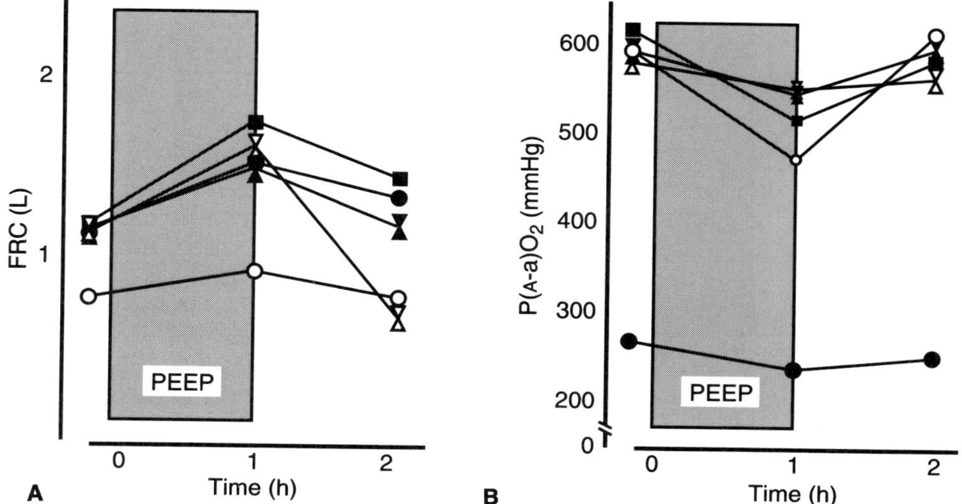

Figure 65-2. Effects of PEEP on lung volume and arterial oxygenation, as shown in one if the earliest clinical reports on the use of this therapy. Data were obtained in 5 patients with severe hypoxemia requiring mechanical ventilation and 100% O_2; diagnoses included both diffuse and localized pulmonary processes. **(A)** Effects of 5 cmH_2O PEEP on FRC. **(B)** Effects of 5 cmH_2O PEEP on P(A-a)O_2 (F_IO_2 = 1.0). (Modified from McIntyre et al.,[15] with permission.)

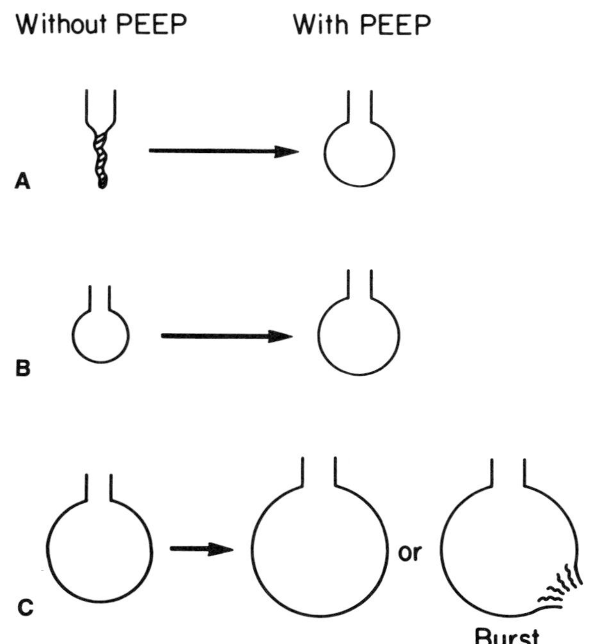

Figure 65-3. Postulated alveolar effects of PEEP. **(A)** If the lung contains alveoli that are collapsed or fluid-filled, PEEP may reinflate them or displace the fluid into the interstitium. **(B)** Alveoli that are at low volume and thus at increased likelihood of collapse may be restored to normal volume with application of PEEP. **(C)** However, alveoli that are normal in size or already enlarged would be expected to be further overinflated by addition of PEEP, possibly leading to rupture (barotrauma). (From Craig et al.,[8] with permission.)

been shown that PEEP may in fact result in a translocation of edema fluid from the alveolar space into the interstitial space.[16] However, because of the simultaneous effect of PEEP on distension of the interstitial spaces and on pulmonary venous and lymphatic pressures, PEEP may actually cause an increase in total lung fluid.[8,16] This increase in total lung water has potentially deleterious consequences. Nevertheless, the reduction in alveolar fluid can reduce the shunt fraction and improve $\dot{V}/\dot{Q}$ ratios.

Work of breathing may be affected by PEEP in a complex fashion. As PEEP improves lung volumes by recruiting collapsed alveoli, lung compliance can improve, which reduces the work load placed on inspiratory muscles in a spontaneously breathing patient. However, overdistension of the lung by PEEP can lead to a decreased compliance (Fig. 65-4) and to inspiratory muscles that are stretched to a degree that places them on a disadvantageous point of their length-tension curve. Both of these factors can lead to an increased inspiratory workload.

Adverse Effects

PEEP can improve hypoxemia and lung–thorax compliance when used appropriately and in properly selected patients. Unfortunately, PEEP also has several possible untoward effects (see Ch. 84). One of the major problems with PEEP is its effect on hemodynamics. In contrast to normal spontaneous ventilation, PEEP causes an increase in pleural and intrathoracic pressures. This pressure increase is transmitted to the heart and great vessels, which results in diminished venous return to the right side of the heart and in an increase in pulmonary vascular resistance (Fig. 65-5).[17]

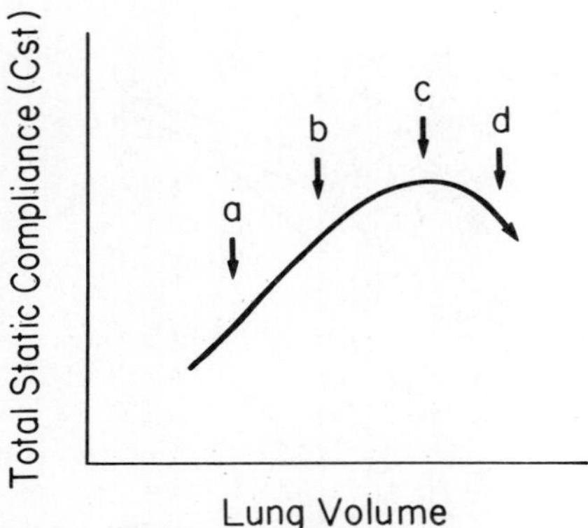

Figure 65-4. Effect of increasing lung volume (i.e., increasing levels of PEEP) on lung compliance (total static compliance [Cst]). Cst is initially low (a), associated with alveolar collapse, edema, and hemorrhage in ARDS, and increases progressively (b and c) as lung volume is increased through progressive increments in PEEP. Overdistension (d) results in a fall in Cst with attendant risk of alveolar rupture and clinical barotrauma. Overall, Cst is probably a poor indicator of this risk, as the sequence illustrated here likely occurs at different volumes in different areas of the lung, but no other practical assessment is presently available. (From Craig et al.,[8] with permission.)

These two factors can result in a decrease in cardiac output ($\dot{Q}_T$) that is occasionally sufficient to produce a drop in arterial blood pressure. Since $\dot{Q}_T$ is essential for adequate tissue O_2 delivery, in such instances the latter may actually fall despite an increase in PaO_2 on application of increasing levels of PEEP.

As mentioned earlier, PEEP raises lung volume and alveolar pressures. This can work to open atelectatic alveoli but PEEP is not always uniformly distributed and some of the extra volume can go to already patent alveoli (Fig. 65-3C).[8] This regional overdistension is probably the main mechanism of alveolar rupture in barotrauma associated with mechanical ventilation (see Ch. 84).[18] Barotrauma from PEEP can take other forms besides alveolar rupture. It has been concluded from some animal models that PEEP, high peak airway pressures, and very large tidal volumes (V_T), when applied to normal lungs, can injure those lungs in a way that pathologically appears very similar to the injury seen in ARDS.[19–22] Patients with ARDS have been shown to develop cystic dilatations in distal airways that could be a manifestation of injury by this mechanism and that may be an equivalent of the bronchopulmonary dysplasia (BPD) seen in neonates who have been mechanically ventilated.[23,24] Although the mechanisms by which the various forms of barotrauma occur in patients managed with PEEP remain uncertain,[18] few clinicians would disagree that this type of adverse effect is common and of much concern in patients who require therapy with PEEP.[4,25]

PEEP can occasionally have an adverse affect on oxygenation by causing a shift in the distribution of blood flow within the lung. As PEEP distends alveoli that are open, the increased volume and pressure in those alveoli causes an increase in the resistance to blood flow past those alveoli. Hence, blood may be redirected to areas of the lung getting proportionately less ventilation, and thus worsen $\dot{V}/\dot{Q}$ mismatching. This effect is usually outweighed by the beneficial effects of PEEP on alveolar recruitment in diffuse lung injury, but may be more important in patients who have unilateral or focal lung diseases.

PEEP often impairs ventilation in that it can increase physiologic dead space. It does this by reducing lung perfusion (reduction in $\dot{Q}_T$) and by increasing the volume in patent alveoli. These effects create areas of high $\dot{V}/\dot{Q}$ ratios, the most extreme form of which is dead space. This can make CO_2 elimination more difficult, especially in patients who already have a very high minute ventilation requirement and in whom minute ventilation cannot readily be further increased.

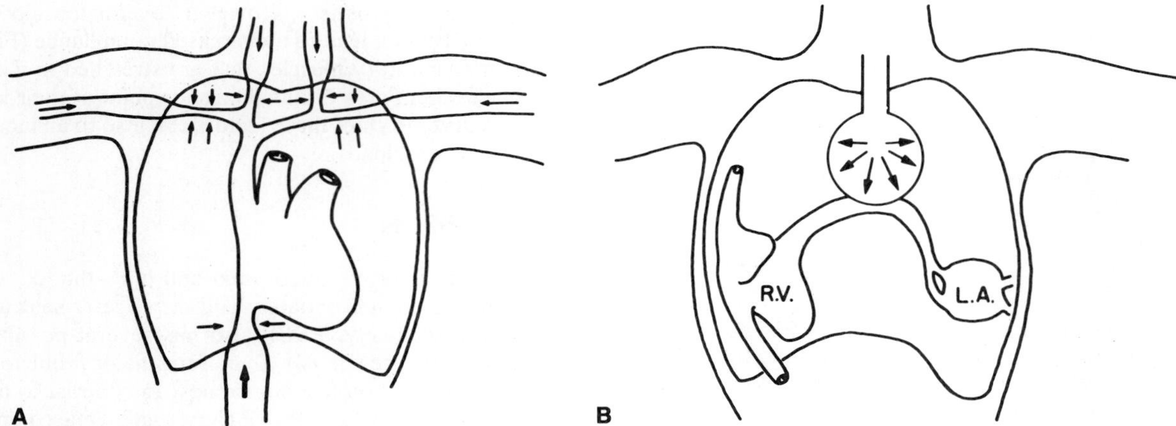

Figure 65-5. Mechanisms of impaired $\dot{Q}_T$ with application of PEEP. **(A)** Impaired venous return, and **(B)** increased pulmonary vascular resistance. Although other mechanisms have been proposed, their existance and clinical importance are uncertain. R.V., right ventricle; L.A., left atrium. (Adapted from Harken et al.,[17] with permission.)

Clinical Effects

From the above discussion it is apparent that PEEP may benefit arterial oxygenation if its attendant increase in FRC reduces shunt and improves $\dot{V}/\dot{Q}$ matching; this would be most likely to occur in acute pulmonary disease that is *diffuse* and also *restrictive* in its effects on pulmonary mechanics.[2] In diffuse obstructive disease such as emphysema any measure that further expands the lungs is deleterious. In localized restrictive disease, such as lobar pneumonia, application of PEEP might well impair $\dot{V}/\dot{Q}$ matching and worsen hypoxemia: if the involved (stiff) area were unaffected while the surrounding (compliant) normal lung tissue were distended, an increase in vascular resistance in the latter might divert more perfusion into the affected area, thereby worsening hypoxemia.

Thus, although its purpose is to increase PaO_2 in cases of severe hypoxemia, PEEP should not be thought of automatically as a general treatment for refractory hypoxemia. Reference to two patients whose chest radiographs appear in Figures 31-2 and 35-2 illustrates this important point. Both patients presented to the emergency department of the same hospital during the same week, and both had very severe hypoxemia that responded poorly to mechanical ventilation with 100 percent O_2. The patient whose radiograph is shown in Figure 35-2 (which shows diffuse bilateral airspace density) had acute noncardiac pulmonary edema secondary to a heroin overdose; when PEEP was applied this patient's PaO_2 increased dramatically, and she promptly recovered. The patient whose radiograph is shown in Figure 31-2, however, had bacteremic right upper lobe pneumonia, with normal lung in the remainder of the chest; this patient's hypoxemia worsened and she developed cardiovascular collapse with the application of PEEP.

As discussed later in this chapter, PEEP may occasionally benefit a patient whose lung disease appears asymmetric on chest radiograph. However, great caution must be used in such settings lest the adverse sequence just described develop. Table 65-3 summarizes the expected effects of PEEP in acute oxygenation failure due to different physiologic mechanisms.[26]

In simplest terms, the clinical application of PEEP should focus on achieving one beneficial effect and avoiding two adverse effects. The beneficial effect, regardless of the philosophic approach used (see Philosophic Approaches to the Use of PEEP in ARDS) is *improved oxygenation*, while the two adverse effects are *impaired cardiac function* and *barotrauma*. Although different approaches may dictate more or less aggressive application of PEEP, and hence require more or less invasive monitoring to assess these effects, the latter comprise the essential aspects of PEEP therapy.

THERAPEUTIC OPTIONS IN ADULT RESPIRATORY DISTRESS SYNDROME

Prevention

Clinical risk factors that predispose an individual to development of ARDS are discussed in Chapter 35. These risk factors include sepsis syndrome, multiple long bone fractures, pulmonary contusion, massive transfusion, aspiration of gastric contents, and drug overdose.[27–30] Once one or more of these risk factors is present in a given patient, what

Table 65-3. Expected Effects of PEEP in Acute Oxygenation Failure of Different Etiologies

Setting	Effect on FRC	Effect on Compliance	Risk of Barotrauma	Effect on Pulmonary Blood Flow	Effect on Gas Exchange	Effect on PaO_2
Pulmonary edema (hemodynamic, increased capillary permeability)						
PEEP used appropriately	Increase toward normal	Increase toward normal	Low	Better matching of perfusion to ventilation	Decreased shunt	Increase
Too much PEEP	Increase above normal	Decrease	High	Increased vascular resistance	Increased dead space	None or decrease
Localized process (lobar pneumonia or lobar atelectasis)						
Involved area	No change	None	Low	None	None	None
Surrounding normal lung	Increase above normal	Decrease	High	Increased vascular resistance	Increased shunt	Decrease
Generalized obstruction (COPD; asthma)	Further increase	Decrease	High	Increased vascular resistance	Increased dead space	None or decrease

(From Pierson,[26] with permission.)

can be done to prevent ARDs from developing? Unfortunately, at present there does not seem to be any way to prevent the syndrome.[30]

Several studies in the 1970s concluded that ARDS could be prevented through the use of "prophylactic" PEEP,[31,32] but deficiencies in study design render each of them unconvincing. A carefully done, controlled study by Pepe and associates,[33] of the early application of 8 cmH_2O PEEP versus no PEEP inpatients at high, documented risk for ARDS, demonstrated no differences in ARDS incidence, mortality, or morbidity. Although its pathogenesis is incompletely understood, ARDS appears to be one manifestation of multiple organ system dysfunction that occurs in response to injury, and at present there is no established way to interfere with its development once the injury has occurred.[30]

Reversal or Modification of Clinical Course

Once ARDS develops, can therapy cure it or ameliorate its course? Here again, unequivocal proof of a favorable effect of any modality is lacking. There has long been controversy as to whether one mode of mechanical ventilation, or one approach to PEEP application, is superior to others in terms of complications and patient survival. In large part because of the difficulty of performing appropriately controlled clinical trials of these therapies, this issue remains one of opinion and personal philosophy rather than of objective data.

Because ARDS is accompanied by a variety of physiologic changes, and numerous biochemical mediators or markers of lung injury have been detected in patients with the syndrome, there has been intense interest in the possibility of reversing or counteracting these through the use of pharmacologic and other agents.[34,35] Table 65-4 lists a number of the agents that have been studied or proposed in this context.[5,36–71]

Therapies that have been or will soon be tried in an attempt to reverse or modify the course of ARDS include agents to combat inflammation, such as corticosteroids, nonsteroidal anti-inflammatory drugs, pentoxifylline, and monoclonal antibodies to specific mediators of inflammation (anti-tumor necrosis factor, anti-interleukin-1, and anti-endotoxin). Another groups of drugs are those that alleviate some of the physiologic consequences of ARDS, thereby making it easier to oxygenate and ventilate the patient. Drugs in this category include surfactant and almitrine. Finally there are a few drugs that could minimize the toxic effects of the therapy for ARDS (i.e., abate the effects of O_2 toxicity). These agents include glutathione, vitamin E, *N*-acetylcysteine, and allopurinol, which could work by binding to and "scavenging" toxic products of O_2 metabolism (superoxide anion, hydrogen peroxide, and the hydroxyl radical).

Despite this long list of possible therapies, none of them is of any proven benefit at this time.[34] Several of the agents listed in Table 65-4 are currently under investigation and may turn out to be effective, but as of 1992 none can be recommended for routine clinical use.

Table 65-4. Pharmacologic and Other Modalities of Potential Value in Treating ARDS

Drugs to correct hypoxemia
- Surfactant replacement (aerosol; direct instillation)[36–38]
  - Bovine surfactant (Survanta)
  - Artificial surfactant (Exosurf)
  - Phospholipid/recombinant protein combination
- Reduction in airway resistance
  - Beta-agonist bronchodilators[39]
- Reduction in lung edema
  - Diuretics[40]
  - Beta agonists (terbutaline)[41]
- Improvement in $\dot{V}/\dot{Q}$ matching
  - Almitrine[42]
  - Hypercapnia (mechanical hypoventilation)[5,43]

Drugs to correct pulmonary hypertension and right heart failure
- Vasodilators
  - Nitroprusside[44]
  - Prostaglandin E_1[45,46]
- Inotropic agents[44]
  - Dobutamine
  - Dopamine
  - Amrinone
- Anticoagulant and fibrinolytic agents
  - Protein C[47]
  - Urokinase[48]

Drugs to reduce alveolar inflammation
- Nonspecific anti-inflammatory agents
  - Corticosteroids[49–53]
  - Ibuprofen[54–57]
  - Zileuton[58]
  - Pentoxyfylline[59]
- Scavengers of products of inflammation
  - *N*-acetylcysteine[58,60]
  - Glutathione
  - Alpha-1-proteinase inhibitor[34]
  - Superoxide dismutase[61]
  - Catalase[61]
- Specific anti-inflammatory agents
  - Anti-endotoxin antibodies[62]
  - Anti-tumor necrosis factor antibodies[63]
  - Interleukin-1 receptor antagonists (IL-1ra)[64]
  - Anti-C5a antibodies[65]
  - Leukocyte adhesion molecule antibodies (anti-CD18; anti-CD11b)

Agents and modalities to prevent secondary infection and sepsis
- Broad spectrum antibiotics[52]
- Kinetic bed therapy[66–68]
- Selective oropharyngeal/gut decontamination[69,70]
- *Pseudomonas* immunoglobulin[71]

PHILOSOPHIC APPROACHES TO THE USE OF PEEP IN ARDS

PEEP is an adjunct to mechanical ventilation whose primary effect is improvement in oxygenation in patients with ARDS. This led some people to believe that PEEP may in some way be curative or therapeutic in ARDS,[72,73] perhaps by reversing alveolar edema by the application of pressure within the alveolus, which pushes the edema fluid back into the bloodstream. If this were true, then the application of PEEP such that lung function were optimized might be expected to afford the best possible therapeutic effect. This theory, which had vigorous advocates in the 1970s and early 1980s,[72–74] has received little support from the hundreds of studies on therapy in ARDS, and retains few adherents today. The body of available data is most supportive of the theory that PEEP works only in a supportive fashion, helping to keep previously atelectatic alveoli open and allowing those alveoli to participate in gas exchange; thus decreasing the intrapulmonary right-to-left shunt and thereby improving oxygenation of the blood.[75]

Maximum versus Minimum PEEP

During the 1970s and early 1980s, two distinct philosophic approaches to the ventilatory management of ARDS emerged, based on belief in or rejection of the concept that PEEP had a primary effect on the course of the illness.[8] These were the *maximum PEEP* and *minimum PEEP* approaches. Adherents to the concept that PEEP ameliorates the actual disease process note that lung function, as measured by shunt fraction ($\dot{Q}_S/\dot{Q}_T$), can be improved to a certain limit, but that it often takes very high levels of PEEP to achieve this. This approach requires invasive monitoring because of the effects of such maximum PEEP on cardiac function; and supporting circulatory function in the face of as much as 40 cmH_2O of PEEP or higher requires the use of vasopressors, volume expansion with whole blood transfusion, and other measures. At the other end of the philosophic spectrum are those clinicians who reject the notion of any "curative" effect of PEEP and instead focus on avoiding its adverse effects. Advocates of the minimum PEEP approach (also referred to as *least PEEP* or *good-enough PEEP*) generally use levels of 10 cmH_2O or less and are usually able to avoid invasive monitoring such as pulmonary artery catheterization.

Table 65-5 summarizes the stances of these two opposing views, along with a middle ground approach used during the 1980s at Harborview Medical Center, dubbed *moderate PEEP*.[8,76] During the 1990s the tide seems to be turning in the direction of minimum PEEP, and many clinicians are seeking to manage ARDS patients with as little fluid administration as possible in light of studies suggesting that this may be associated with better survival and lower morbidity than more aggressive approaches.[40]

Role of Oxygen Toxicity

Central to an approach to the use of PEEP in managing ARDS is the clinician's position on O_2 toxicity. Although there is bountiful evidence that administration of O_2 at high P_{IO_2} is damaging to the lungs of normal human volunteers[77] (Fig. 65-6A) and experimental animals,[78,79] proof that pulmonary O_2 toxicity occurs in critically ill patients who require high F_{IO_2} levels in the treatment of hypoxemia is essentially nonexistent.[80] This distinction is important in view of animal studies suggesting that hypoxemia and pre-existing lung injury may be protective against such damage.

However the clinician interprets the available data on O_2 toxicity, this will strongly influence that person's use of PEEP in managing ARDS. Because PEEP is used primarily to permit a reduction in F_{IO_2}, how much PEEP is required depends on the clinician's "comfort level" of F_{IO_2}. Advocates of maximum PEEP, and many other clinicians seek to avoid exposing their patients to F_{IO_2} levels exceeding 0.40; some will further increase PEEP and employ other maneuvers to lower the F_{IO_2} to 0.30 or even lower, believing that the risk of O_2 toxicity outweighs the risks of these other therapies. Other clinicians will accept an F_{IO_2} of 0.60 or even 0.70, for many days, if its use is necessary to achieve acceptable arterial oxygenation, rather than pushing upward with PEEP beyond 10 or 15 cmH_2O, which increases the likelihood of cardiac impairment and barotrauma.

One interpretation of the risk of O_2 toxicity in hypoxemic

Table 65-5. Clinical Approaches to the use of PEEP in ARDS

	Maximum PEEP	Moderate PEEP	Minimal PEEP
Purpose	To 'normalize' pulmonary function; to reverse pathophysiologic defect in ARDS	To improve O_2 transport while avoiding potential harmful PEEP effects	To lower F_{IO_2} to safe level consistent with adequate blood oxygenation
Goal	$\dot{Q}_S/\dot{Q}_T$ <15%	P/F >200 with fall in $\dot{Q}_T$ <20%	$SaO_2 \geq 90\%$ on nontoxic F_{IO_2}; lowest PWP with adequate $\dot{Q}_T$
Level usually applied	25–40+ cmH_2O	10–20 cmH_2O	<10–15 cmH_2O
Effect on $\dot{Q}_T$ treated with vasopressors and/or transfusion	Yes	No	No
Beneficial effect on ARDS course assumed	Yes	?	No

P/F, PaO_2 divided by F_{IO_2}; PWP, pulmonary (capillary) wedge pressure; SaO_2, arterial oxyhemoglobin saturation (%).
(Adapted from Craig et al.[8] with permission.)

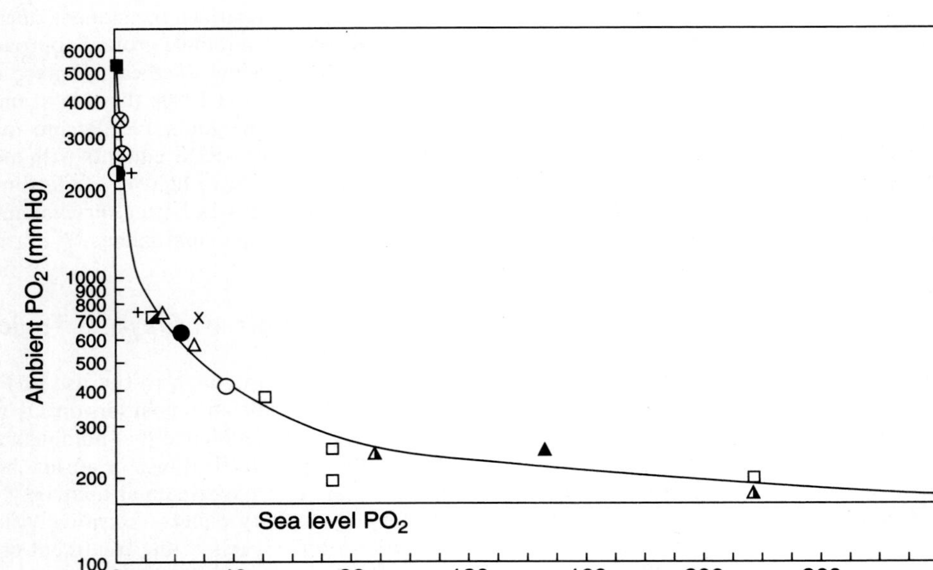

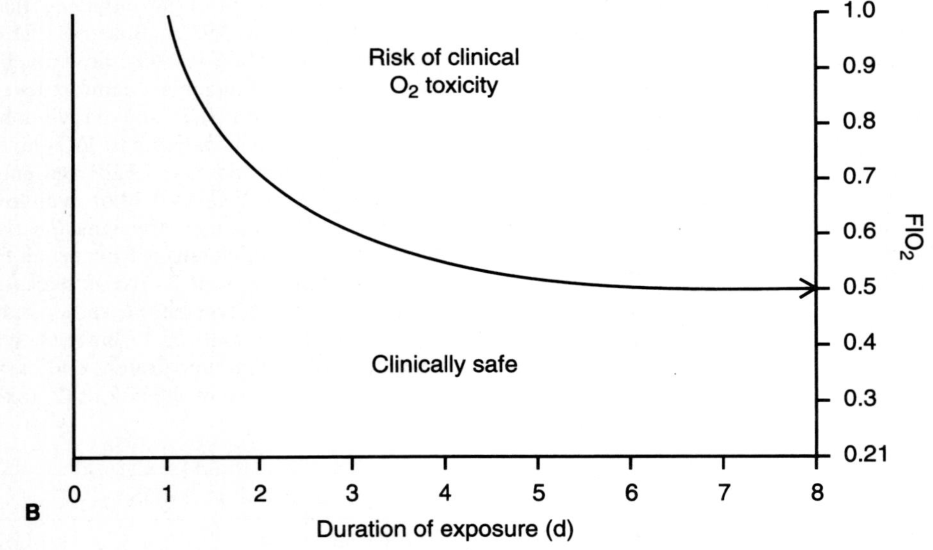

Figure 65-6. Relationship of clinical O_2 toxicity to intensity and duration of exposure. (**A**) Curve drawn on the basis of 17 studies in normal humans using ambient PO_2 levels ranging from 174 to >5000 mmHg, as constructed by Welch et al.[77] Symbols mark the first appearance of toxicity, which for most subjects was the onset of chest tightness or other subjective symptoms. (**B**) Proposed curve relating clinically significant O_2 toxicity to duration of exposure for critically ill patients given supplemental O_2 in the FIO_2 levels encountered in clinical practice. This curve is consistent with our clinical experience but is admittedly hypothetical since there are no relevant experimental data from patients in such circumstances. According to the relationship depicted, exposures above the curve (e.g., FIO_2 = 1.0 for 1 day; FIO_2 = 0.7 for >2–3 days) may risk clinical O_2 toxicity, while exposures below the curve (e.g., FIO_2 = 1.0 for <24 hr; FIO_2 = <0.50 for days to weeks) appear clinically safe. (Fig. A from Welch et al.,[77] with permission; Fig. B from Pierson,[26] with permission.)

patients in the ICU that leans more toward this latter approach is shown in Figure 65-6B.[26] As depicted in Figure 65-6B, exposure to more than 24 hours of 100 percent O_2 should be avoided if possible, but if the FIO_2 can be reduced to 0.70 within about 2 days, and to 0.50 within 5 days, this is probably clinically safe. There is little direct evidence for clinically significant O_2 toxicity at an FIO_2 of 0.50, even if this must be continued for weeks. In fact, when its use is mandated by the patient's critical hypoxemia, and the PaO_2 is kept in a reasonable range (e.g., 50 to 70 mmHg), even 100 percent O_2 for many days may not necessarily result in irreversible lung damage. We have cared for patients with ARDS who required high PEEP levels and 100 percent O_2 for as long as 2 to 4 weeks, who survived and eventually recovered normal or near-normal pulmonary function. Thus, if O_2 toxicity is produced by such exposure, it appears to be reversible, at least in these anecdotal cases.

Different interpretations of the clinical risk of O_2 toxicity lead to very different basic approaches to PEEP therapy in ARDS, and carry with them implications regarding certain other aspects of management. For example, the clinician who regards all FIO_2 levels above 0.40 as toxic will generally need to use higher PEEP levels, and with them more aggressive support and more invasive monitoring, than the clinician who is comfortable administering an FIO_2 of 0.60. At the present time, no one can say for sure which approach is correct, and in our opinion either approach can be used effectively. However, it is necessary for one's management strategy to be consistent in its various components. For example, a clinician who uses PEEP aggressively cannot also opt *not* to use invasive hemodynamic monitoring, because of the likelihood of adversely affecting cardiac output at higher levels of PEEP. Similarly, use of higher levels of PEEP implies fairly liberal fluid administration, so that the clinician who seeks aggressively to lower the FIO_2 to less than 0.40 will probably not also be successful in a "keep the lungs dry" approach to fluid management.

THE PEEP TRIAL IN PATIENT MANAGEMENT

Based primarily on the known physiologic responses to the application of PEEP, some patients will respond well to PEEP and others may not only fail to improve but develop deleterious side effects. Unfortunately, it is often difficult to predict which patients will have what response. Nevertheless, there are some basic guidelines that can help the bedside clinician decide whether a trial of PEEP is warranted.

Good candidates for a trial of PEEP are those who generally have (1) hypoxemia despite an FIO_2 of 0.50 or more; (2) diffuse, acute lung disease; (3) poorly compliant (stiff) lungs; (4) adequate cardiac function and (5) normal or increased intravascular volume.[76] Patients who should be considered poor candidates for PEEP usually have (1) unilateral or localized lung disease; (2) already hyperinflated lungs; (3) normal or elevated lung compliance; (4) poor cardiac function; and (5) intravascular volume depletion or hypotension.

These are helpful parameters to consider when evaluating a patient for the possible use of PEEP. However, they are not absolute; a cautious trial of PEEP should not be withheld from patients who appear to be poor candidates but who have severe, refractory hypoxemia.

Once it is determined that PEEP should be attempted, it should be applied in a systematic, incremental manner with an evaluation made at each level of PEEP to assess its relative beneficial and adverse effects on that individual patient.[8,76,81] Use of this quasi-scientific "PEEP trial" has advantages over the arbitrary or uncontrolled use of this potentially hazardous therapy. It seeks to determine objectively the answers to two questions: Will PEEP benefit this patient, at this point in the clinical course of the illness? If so, how much PEEP should be used? The answers to these questions, and especially to the second of them, depend greatly on the managing clinician's position on the purpose of PEEP (e.g., primary therapy for ARDS versus simply improvement in PaO_2) and what constitutes a "safe" FIO_2. Regardless of the clinical approach being used in a given patient's care and the sought-after end points of the therapy, however, a systematic PEEP trial as described here is the recommended means for adjusting PEEP.

A PEEP trial consists of a series of systematic, incremental increases in PEEP, while keeping all other elements of management constant insofar as this can be done, and assessment of the patient's physiologic response at each level[8,76] (Fig. 65-7). Table 65-6 details the protocol for per-

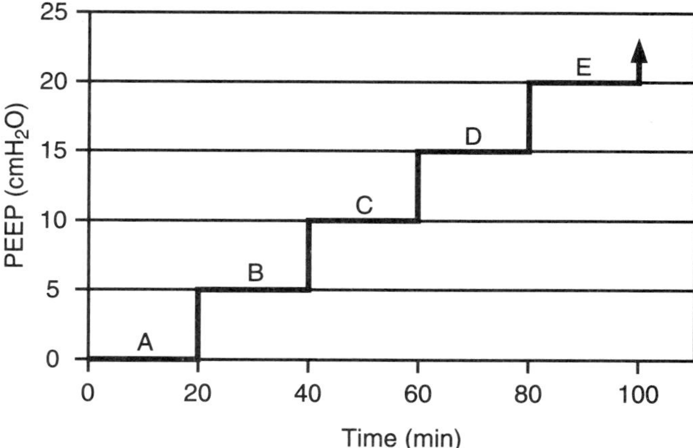

Figure 65-7. The systematic PEEP trial. After initial physiologic measurements are made, and with all other aspects of management unchanged, PEEP is increased sequentially in increments of 5 cmH_2O until the desired therapeutic effect (i.e., improved oxygenation) is achieved or adverse effects (i.e., decrease in either $\dot{Q}_T$ or static respiratory system compliance) occur. An initial PEEP of zero is shown here, but a PEEP trial can be carried out from any starting level of PEEP. The time at each PEEP level should kept short during the trial so that changes in the patient's condition do not confuse the results; increments of 5 cmH_2O are used rather than smaller steps so that the entire trial can be completed within about 2 hours. (From Pierson,[81] with permission.)

Table 65-6. Protocol for the Therapeutic Application of PEEP in Acute Hypoxemic Respiratory Failure: The PEEP Trial

1. Obtain baseline respiratory and hemodynamic data before initiating PEEP and at each level employed in trial[a]
   a. Respiratory data (all patients): F_{IO_2}, PEEP level, corrected V_T, respiratory rate (ventilator; patient), PIP, end-inspiratory static hold pressure, ABG values (PaO_2, pHa, $PaCO_2$)
   b. Additional respiratory data (in extremely ill or unstable patients, or for aggressive management approach): $P\bar{v}O_2$ and $S\bar{v}O_2$, CaO_2 and $C\bar{v}O_2$
   c. Hemodynamic data (all patients): heart rate, blood pressure, continuous ECG monitoring
   d. Additional hemodynamic data (for PEEP >10 cmH_2O, suspected hypovolemia [unexplained tachycardia], or coexistent cardiac disease): $\dot{Q}_T$, pulmonary arterial wedge pressure
2. Change only one variable at a time (i.e., PEEP level)—keep V_T, F_{IO_2}, and other ventilator settings the same at each level; avoid transfusion, position changes, changes in pressor infusions during trial if possible
3. Keep time intervals between PEEP increments short (e.g., 15–30 min) to minimize confounding data from changes in patient's underlying condition
4. Apply PEEP in sequential increments (e.g., 5 cmH_2O); smaller increments may prolong trial; larger increments increase likelihood of adverse effects
5. Monitor for immediate adverse effects at each new PEEP level
   a. Hypotension or >20% fall in $\dot{Q}_T$
   b. Fall in respiratory system compliance
   c. Cardiac arrhythmias or increased intracranial pressure, where appropriate
6. Repeat baseline respiratory and hemodynamic data collection as in step 1 above once patient has stabilized at each new PEEP level (e.g., 15–20 minutes)
7. Evaluate overall cardiorespiratory response at each PEEP level used
   a. Favorable: improved oxygenation; improved compliance
   b. Unfavorable: hypotension; decreased $\dot{Q}_T$; decreased compliance; decreased oxygenation
8. Assess results in light of overall goals for PEEP therapy
   a. If O_2 delivery has improved without adverse effects, leave patient on current PEEP level, reduce F_{IO_2} if possible, and re-evaluate frequently as indicated
   b. If oxygenation is still inadequate or F_{IO_2} is still unacceptably high, and no adverse effects have occurred, increase PEEP sequentially, applying steps 4–7
   c. If O_2 delivery has decreased or compliance has fallen significantly at new PEEP level, return patient to previous PEEP level and re-evaluate
      i. If deterioration is due to decreased PaO_2, reassess indications for PEEP
      ii. If deterioration is due to decreased $\dot{Q}_T$, consider volume loading or administration of pressor drugs
      iii. If compliance has fallen but O_2 delivery has not decreased, consider reducing V_T to reduce risk of alveolar rupture (barotrauma)

$P\bar{v}O_2$, mixed venous P_{O_2}; $C\bar{v}O_2$, mixed venous O_2 content; $S\bar{v}O_2$, mixed venous O_2 saturation; PIP, peak inspiratory pressure.
[a] Measurements and invasiveness depend on overall approach being used as well as degree of illness of the patient (see text).

forming the trial as it has been used at Harborview Medical Center during the past decade.

PEEP trials are most often performed to establish the best PEEP level to use in the initial ventilator management of a patient with ARDS. The patient's gas exchange and pulmonary mechanics may change over time, however, and the PEEP level initially selected may subsequently become suboptimal. The approach given in Table 65-6 can provide valuable management guidance later in the course of the syndrome as well. In a patient already on PEEP who is deteriorating or failing to improve, or when adverse effects such as barotrauma develop that may indicate excessive PEEP, modifying the trial to include both decreases and increases in PEEP level may help to indicate a new, preferable level.

Insofar as possible only the PEEP should be varied during the trial, and the entire trial should be accomplished within about 2 hours, so that changes in the patient's underlying condition can be minimized and the observed effects on PaO_2 and hemodynamics can be truly ascribed to changes in PEEP. If other therapy is varied (e.g., F_{IO_2}, mode, V_T, vasopressor infusion, or transfusion), the "experiment" has more than one variable and its results are more difficult to interpret.

In most circumstances PEEP should be increased in 5-cmH_2O increments rather than in smaller steps; the main disadvantage of the latter is that the total duration will be prolonged, which increases the likelihood of introducing additional variables. Smaller PEEP increments may be necessary in children or in patients who have demonstrated unusual sensitivity to PEEP. Each interval should be short (e.g., 15 to 30 minutes). Because cardiac compromise and alveolar overdistension are the main complications to be avoided and may occur quickly once PEEP is increased, the patient's hemodynamic status and total respiratory system compliance should be assessed within 3 to 5 minutes of each PEEP increment. An arterial blood specimen should be drawn 15 to 30 minutes after the PEEP is increased, as it may take somewhat longer for the beneficial effects of PEEP on arterial oxygenation to occur. As long as cardiac function has not been impaired and compliance has not fallen, the PEEP can be increased by the next 5-cmH_2O increment even if the ABG results have not yet returned from the laboratory.

The trial is continued incrementally until an arbitrary upper limit of PEEP is reached; this depends on the therapy approach that is being used. In the population of adult patients with trauma and other medical-surgical settings for ARDS that is most often managed in our ICUs, and in keeping with the moderate PEEP approach indicated in Table 65-5, we commonly continue PEEP trials to a level of 15 to 25 cmH_2O or until a clearly detrimental response is seen. Once the trial has been completed, the appropriate level of PEEP can be chosen based on an analysis of the PaO_2 change, the O_2 delivery to the tissues, any changes in compliance, the hemodynamic change, and the ability to reduce the F_{IO_2} at each level of PEEP.

In general, invasive hemodynamic monitoring (e.g., use of a pulmonary artery catheter and measurement of $\dot{Q}_T$ changes in response to PEEP) is advisable when any one of the following three conditions exists (see also Table 65-6):

1. Use of PEEP greater than 10 cmH_2O
2. Suspected hypovolemia (e.g., unexplained tachycardia)
3. Coexisting cardiac disease

In each of these circumstances the likelihood of adverse cardiovascular effects is increased, and it is wisest to be able to detect and quantify these directly rather than to rely on noninvasive measures. A fall in $\dot{Q}_T$ of 20 percent or more is regarded as clinically significant and generally indicates excessive application of PEEP, at least for the patient's present inotropic state and circulating blood volume. If none of the criteria listed above is present, and especially if the patient is alert with good renal function and only single-organ (e.g., pulmonary) failure, performance of a PEEP trial without invasive hemodynamic monitoring is acceptable.

The clinical application of PEEP in ARDS is discussed further in Chapter 76, using an approach most consistent with the minimum PEEP philosophy described above. In addition, Table 76-11 gives gas exchange, hemodynamic, and compliance data from representative PEEP trials to illustrate the practical application of the principles summarized here.

PEEP WITHOUT ENDOTRACHEAL INTUBATION

In certain circumstances it may be possible to apply PEEP (in the form of continuous positive airway pressure [CPAP]) in the treatment of acute hypoxemic respiratory failure without endotracheal intubation.[82] Administration of CPAP via whole-face or nasal mask is employed widely in other clinical settings, notably in postoperative lung expansion therapy (see Ch. 73) and the long-term management of obstructive sleep apnea (see Ch. 67). Its application in acute oxygenation failure is limited to a few settings, but can be accomplished successfully if certain precautions are taken. Relatively comfortable, close-fitting CPAP masks are currently available that may be tolerable to acutely ill patients for periods of days. An appropriate candidate for CPAP without intubation is a patient that

1. Has acute pulmonary disease that is diffuse (e.g., *Pneumocystis carinii* pneumonia [PCP]) rather than localized (e.g., lobar pneumonia)
2. Is expected to recover or substantially improve within a few days at most
3. Does not require more than 10 to 15 cmH_2O CPAP (most patients do not tolerate more than 10 cmH_2O for more than a few hours)
4. Does not have coexisting serious disease in other organ systems
5. Can be managed in a setting where appropriate observation and monitoring can be carried out (e.g., ICU or special respiratory unit)
6. Is fully alert and cooperative at all times (to assure effective therapy, and to be able to remove the mask immediately should vomiting occur)
7. Does not require mechanical restraints or heavy sedation

The great majority of patients with ARDS do not meet these criteria: in an institution managing approximately 120 cases of ARDS each year, we have been able to avoid intubation in this fashion in fewer than one ARDS patient annually. However, mask CPAP is much more useful in conditions such as PCP, and can permit avoidance of endotracheal intubation and mechanical ventilation in most instances, even when hypoxemia is severe. In the latter setting mask CPAP can sometimes be tolerated for many days if needed. It is crucial, however, that the patient remain fully cooperative throughout the period that mask CPAP is in use.

PEEP WITHDRAWAL

Once the patient with ARDS improves, both in general status and with respect to arterial oxygenation, PEEP should be gradually withdrawn ("PEEP weaning") rather than abruptly discontinued. However, just as PEEP improves oxygenation by improving $\dot{V}/\dot{Q}$ matching in the presence of atelectatic or unstable alveoli, its premature withdrawal can lead to worsening of both oxygenation and compliance as some of these unstable alveoli again collapse. Accordingly, it is important to be able to predict accurately when PEEP can be safely reduced in an individual patient.

Three studies conducted at Harborview Medical Center have clarified this issue and led to the establishment of a protocol for PEEP weaning that is effective and safe.[83–85] The first, a retrospective study, examined 242 attempts at PEEP reduction by 5-cmH_2O increments in 82 surgical patients.[83] PEEP had been reduced at the discretion of the responsible physician and no specific criteria were used systematically in making the decision to lower the PEEP level. In this series, the PEEP reduction was unsuccessful (PaO_2 fell below 65 mmHg and PEEP had to be increased) in 33 percent of patients. In addition, in most of those patients it took more than 24 hours, and often a higher level of PEEP than was present before the failed reduction attempt, to return to the same level of oxygenation. This is consistent with the idea that unstable alveoli had become atelectatic and less compliant due to premature PEEP withdrawal.

Data from the study[83] just mentioned revealed that several characteristics of the patients who "passed" the PEEP reduction test (i.e., PaO_2 remained above 65 mmHg and PEEP did not need to be raised) were different from those in patients who "failed." A second, prospective study of PEEP weaning[84] was then conducted using the following criteria, based on the findings of the first study:

1. Hemodynamic stability without signs of sepsis
2. PaO_2 80 mmHg or greater on an F_IO_2 of 0.40 (e.g., PaO_2/F_IO_2 [P/F ratio] 200 mmHg or greater)
3. No changes in PEEP level for at least 12 hours

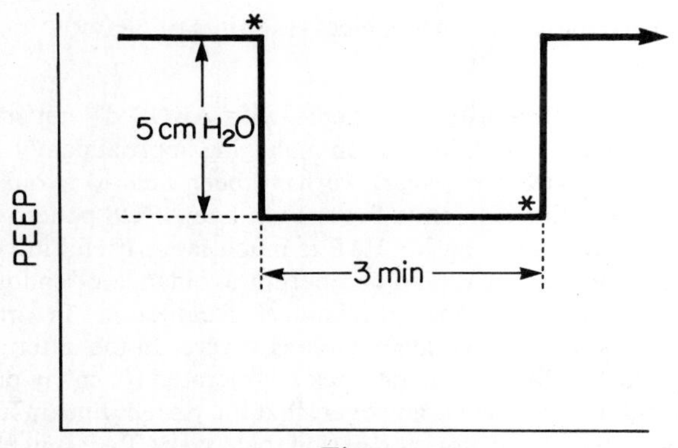

Figure 65-8. The 3-minute PEEP wean trial, to predict accurately and safely whether the present PEEP level can be reduced in a patient recovering from ARDS. Once clinical criteria have been met for PEEP reduction (see Table 65-7), PEEP is lowered by 5 cmH_2O for 3 minutes and then returned to baseline. Specimens for ABG analysis are drawn before and after 3 minutes, just before PEEP reinstitution (time of drawing indicated by asterisks). A fall in PaO_2 of >20–25% of the initial value indicates that the patient is not yet ready to be managed on reduced PEEP. (From Craig et al.,[8] with permission.)

In this study of 89 PEEP reductions in 40 patients with ARDS, the above criteria predicted successful PEEP reduction in 80 percent of attempts.

To this protocol was then added a "3-minute PEEP wean" test, as diagrammed in Figure 65-8. In the third study,[86] once the above three criteria were met, PEEP was reduced by 5 cmH_2O for 3 minutes, an arterial blood specimen was drawn for ABG analysis, and the PEEP was returned to its previous level until the results were available. If oxygenation remained acceptable (i.e., if there was no more than a 20 percent fall in PaO_2 at 3 minutes), the PEEP was again reduced for at least 12 hours before another attempt was considered. In this study, out of 82 PEEP reduction attempts in 47 ARDS patients, 90 percent of the trials were successful, and no patient who "failed" the 3-minute PEEP wean suffered a prolonged deterioration in oxygenation.

These results are consistent with the interpretation that readiness for PEEP weaning can be predicted using readily available clinical criteria, and that reducing PEEP by 5 cmH_2O for only 3 minutes does not lead to deleterious effects in patients who are not yet ready to be managed at the lower PEEP level. Based on the results of these three studies and subsequent clinical experience at our institution, we developed the clinical criteria for PEEP withdrawal listed in Table 65-7. A protocol for PEEP reduction according to these criteria is given in Table 65-8. Table 65-9 provides two examples of the use of this protocol using the clinical criteria discussed above.

Table 65-7. Clinical Criteria for Reducing PEEP in Patients with Acute Hypoxemic Respiratory Failure

Criteria	Success Rate[a] (%)	Reference
1. Clinical judgement alone	67	83
2. Hemodynamic stability for ≥6–12 h No clinical signs of sepsis[b] PaO_2 ≥80 mmHg on FIO_2 ≤0.40	80	84
3. Same as No. 2 above plus successful 3-minute PEEP wean (see Table 65-8)	90	85

[a] Acceptable arterial oxygenation (e.g., PaO_2 ≥65 mmHg) after PEEP reduction by 5 cmH_2O.

[b] Features suggesting sepsis include tachycardia, fever or hypothermia, leukocytosis or leukopenia, high $\dot{Q}T$, and low systemic vascular resistance, with or without positive blood cultures.

SPECIAL CONSIDERATIONS FOR UNILATERAL OR ASYMMETRIC LUNG DISEASE

The patient with acute hypoxemic respiratory failure in the presence of pulmonary disease that involves only one lung, or that is markedly heterogeneous in distribution, poses special management problems. Administration of supplemental O_2 may have little effect. Therapies such as PEEP affect the whole respiratory system, and if the distensibility

Table 65-8. Protocol for Reduction of PEEP in Patients with Hypoxemic Acute Respiratory Failure: The PEEP Wean

1. Patient should meet criteria for reducing PEEP (see Table 65-7)
2. Obtain baseline respiratory and hemodynamic data, including ABG levels[a] (see Table 65-6), as clinically indicated
3. Reduce PEEP level by 5 cmH_2O[b]
4. After 3 minutes, obtain a second specimen for ABG analysis[a] and return PEEP to previous level while awaiting results
5. Compare prereduction and 3-minute PaO_2 values (assuming $PaCO_2$ value is unchanged)
   a. A substantial fall in PaO_2 (e.g., >20%) suggests that the patient's oxygenation may deteriorate and/or be slow to recover if PEEP is reduced at this point; the PEEP level should be maintained at the higher level for another 6–12 hr before a repeat PEEP wean is considered
   b. Satisfactory oxygenation (e.g., no change or <20% drop in PaO_2) on the 3-minute specimen indicates that the PEEP may be decreased by 5 cmH_2O, with repeat assessment (Step 2 above), as clinically indicated during the next several hours

[a] Arterial saturation as measured by pulse oximetry is a poor estimate of the magnitude of change in arterial oxygenation with PEEP reduction unless the PaO_2 falls below 65–70 mmHg. However, pulse oximetry may afford an additional element of safety during PEEP weaning if the initial PaO_2 is in the range of 80 mmHg.

[b] Smaller decrements (e.g., 2.5 cm H_2O) may be appropriate in pediatric patients or in unstable adults, although this will slow the PEEP reduction process unnecessarily for most patients.

Table 65-9. Examples of Successful and Unsuccessful PEEP Reduction[a]

	Example No. 1[b]		Example No. 2[c]	
Elapsed time (min)	0	3	0	3
PEEP (cmH_2O)	15	10	15	10
PaO_2 (mmHg) on F_IO_2 0.40	100	65	100	85
BP (mmHg)	110/60	120/60	110/60	120/60
Crs (mL/cmH_2O)	30	30	30	30

CRS, static compliance of the respiratory system at end-inspiration.

[a] Clinical setting: 42-year-old patient with resolving ARDS after abdominal sepsis, who is clinically stable and now being considered for PEEP reduction (see Table 65-7).

[b] In example no. 1, the PaO_2 is still clinically acceptable after 3 minutes at the lower PEEP level, but has fallen substantially from its baseline value. Based on clinical experience and published studies,[83–85] if the patient were left at the lower PEEP level, further deterioration in oxygenation would be likely, and the PEEP should be kept at the higher level for at least several more hours.

[c] In example no. 2, the fall in PaO_2 after 3 minutes at the lower PEEP level is less than 20%, satisfactory oxygenation will probably continue if the PEEP is left at this lower level.

of one lung is markedly different from that of the other, the more involved lung may be largely unaffected while the more normal lung becomes overdistended.[86] In such circumstances the patient's condition may be harmed rather than helped (Table 65-3).

Causes

Patients who gradually develop unilateral lung disease generally do not demonstrate dramatic physiologic impairment and may not need emergent, aggressive therapy to improve blood oxygenation. However, when acute respiratory failure develops because of a unilateral process, life-threatening hypoxemia may develop. When this occurs in the hospital the most common causes include lobar or multi-lobe pneumonia, aspiration of gastric contents, and massive atelectasis. Several other potential etiologies should also be considered (Table 65-10).

Some of the conditions listed in Table 65-10 (e.g., acute massive atelectasis) are more immediately reversible than others (e.g., pneumonia). The mechanisms of hypoxemia, however, are the same in both groups. Unilateral acute lung disease typically produces right-to-left intrapulmonary shunt, or $\dot{V}/\dot{Q}$ mismatching characterized by very low $\dot{V}/\dot{Q}$ ratios. As discussed above and illustrated in Table 65-2, such hypoxemia usually does not improve very much with the administration of supplemental O_2. Hypoxic pulmonary vasoconstriction may diminish the perfusion to the involved area, but this protective mechanism cannot compensate completely for the defect, and it may be impaired by disease or therapeutic agents in critically ill patients.

Table 65-10. Causes of Unilateral or Markedly Asymmetric Lung Involvement in Patients with Acute Oxygenation Failure

Aspiration
Acute lobar or whole-lung atelectasis
Endobronchial obstruction (e.g., foreign body; mucus plug)
Mainstem bronchus intubation
Massive pleural effusion (e.g., hemothorax)
Pulmonary contusion
Lobar pneumonia
Pulmonary infarction
Pulmonary hemorrhage
Cardiogenic pulmonary edema with lateral decubitus positioning
Re-expansion pulmonary edema
Pulmonary edema (any cause) in absence or attenuation of one main pulmonary artery

Approach to Management

When an immediately remediable process such as a mucus plug or obstructing foreign body is the cause of severe hypoxemia, it may be possible to alleviate the problem by prompt attention to the obstruction. However, while therapy for the primary disease process is important, this may not result in rapid improvement in the patient's hypoxemia. Supportive therapy to improve arterial oxygenation should be initiated immediately, and involves three possible therapeutic approaches, not all of which are applicable in any given situation. These approaches are high-F_IO_2 supplemental O_2 therapy, changes in the patient's body position, and application of PEEP.

Supplemental Oxygen Therapy

High-F_IO_2 supplemental O_2 therapy, as described in Chapter 75, should be the first intervention in severe hypoxemia associated with unilateral lung disease. However, as illustrated in Table 65-2, administration of even 100 percent O_2 to a patient with a large right-to-left intrapulmonary shunt may fail to saturate the hemoglobin in arterial blood fully. This is particularly likely to be the case in whole-lung atelectasis and in lobar or multi-lobe pneumonia. Severe pneumonia is one example of a disorder in which complete correction of hypoxemia may not be possible for several days. In such instances the clinician must keep in mind the other components of oxygenation—blood O_2 content (i.e., hemoglobin concentration) and O_2 delivery (i.e., $\dot{Q}_T$)—and optimize these whenever possible.

Changes in Body Position

Severe hypoxemia resulting from unilateral pulmonary disease may be improved by placing the most involved lung area uppermost.[86–91] This is because, in the presence of a right-to-left shunt, the severity of hypoxemia may fluctuate markedly with the quantity of blood flow to the more severely diseased lung, where the blood "sees" no ventilation and hence no O_2 (see Fig. 29-5). Any maneuver that redirects perfusion to more normal lung zones should reduce the effective shunt and improve arterial oxygenation. A convenient mnemonic for remembering this is, "Down with the good lung!" While it may not be possible to manage patients in one position continuously, avoiding placement of the most involved lung in the dependent position can help to avoid the most severe hypoxemia.

Even in ARDS, which is often thought of as a diffuse, homogeneous process, consolidation is typically densest in the most dependent (i.e., posterior) lung regions[92] (see Fig. 35-3). In the presence of profound, refractory hypoxemia, moving the patient from the supine to the prone position may improve PaO_2 [93,94]—at least until the edema and inflammatory cells gravitate to the newly dependent anterior lung regions. In our experience this maneuver tends to be of only temporary benefit in ARDS, and its heavy toll on nursing and other management makes other approaches (e.g., transfusion, inotropic therapy) more attractive in such instances.

One setting in which placing the good lung down is inadvisable is massive ongoing hemoptysis, in which free-flowing blood may flood the normal lung and cause asphyxia.[89] The same is true for very large lung abscesses that contain large amounts of pus, especially after bronchoscopy and other airway manipulation, and particularly in patients with severe COPD or muscle weakness who might have difficulty clearing their airways if the abscess should rupture and abruptly release its contents.

Positive End-Expiratory Pressure

Patients with severe hypoxemia in the setting of unilateral or markedly heterogeneous lung disease are generally poor candidates for PEEP therapy, as the PEEP would be expected to over-expand more normal, more compliant lung regions and have little effect in those that are most abnormal. In fact, as shown in Table 65-3, if anything, PEEP might be expected to increase pulmonary vascular resistance in the normal lung areas, diverting perfusion to those less well ventilated and thus worsening hypoxemia. Nonetheless, it is sometimes appropriate to perform a careful PEEP trial (Table 65-6; Fig. 65-7) when life-threatening hypoxemia is accompanied by asymmetric consolidation on the chest radiograph. The latter may sometimes represent uneven edema in the early stages of ARDS, with the process really more diffuse than is radiographically apparent, and the patient's oxygenation may improve dramatically on the judicious application of PEEP. However, because of the increased likelihood of cardiovascular impairment and pulmonary overdistension, PEEP by any delivery technique must be used very cautiously, and carefully monitored, in patients with unilateral or asymmetric lung disease.

Independent Lung Ventilation

When severe hypoxemia occurs in the setting of unilateral or markedly asymmetric lung disease, a logical and conceptually attractive approach would be to ventilate the two lungs independently, using a double-lumen endotracheal tube, and to apply PEEP only in the lung in which it is most needed.[95–98] With this approach the normal lung can be ventilated in the standard fashion, avoiding excessive airway pressures or potentially toxic $F_{I}O_2$, while the more severely injured lung can be managed aggressively with PEEP, rested with CPAP with or without low-frequency ventilation, or treated using any of several other reported approaches.[98–105]

As attractive as ILV is in theory, it is fraught with technical difficulties and potentially life-threatening complications, and has never been shown to be truly *necessary*, even in profound hypoxemia. Although current double-lumen endotracheal tubes are made from materials less injurious to airway mucosa and are less prone to crusting and secretion inspissation than their predecessors, such tubes are much more difficult to place than standard single-lumen tubes, and the small internal diameters of the two halves of the tube (see Fig. 72-4) make suctioning less effective. Such tubes are intended primarily for operating room use, and are less well suited to continuous use for days or weeks, as may be necessary in the ICU.

The literature on ILV consists mainly of anecdotal (often single-patient) reports that demonstrate the possibility of this extreme form of ventilator therapy but neglect to point out its pitfalls and fail to convince the reader of its necessity. The few reported multiple-patient series are retrospective, focus on technical application rather than clinical indications, and generally include few data to demonstrate the failure of conventional ventilator management prior to initiation of ILV.

ILV can generally be avoided, even in the presence of uncorrectable hypoxemia in patients with unilateral lung disease, if the clinicians managing such patients focus on systemic O_2 transport and tissue oxygenation rather than just PaO_2. In this respect ILV may be thought of in the same category as extracorporeal membrane oxygenation (ECMO) (see Ch. 78). Both therapies require more technical expertise and are more hazardous and expensive than conventional management; they have not been shown to improve outcomes when compared directly with conventional ventilation in the most desperately ill patients, and they are unnecessary in those who are less critically ill.

References

1. Pierson DJ: Indications for oxygen therapy. Probl Respir Care 1990;3:549–562
2. Pierson DJ: Acute respiratory failure. pp. 75–126. In Sahn SA (ed): Pulmonary emergencies. Churchill Livingstone, New York, 1982
3. Zwillich CW, Pierson DJ, Creagh CE et al: Complications of assisted ventilation: A prospective study of 354 consecutive episodes. Am J Med 1974;57:161–70
4. Pierson DJ: Complications of mechanical ventilation. pp. 19–46. In Simmons DH (ed): Current Pulmonology. Vol. 11. Year Book Medical Publishers, Chicago, 1990
5. Dantzker DR, Brooks CJ, Dehart P et al: Ventilation-perfusion distribution in the adult respiratory distress syndrome. Am Rev Respir Dis 1979;120:1039–1052

6. Craig KC: Determining distributions of ventilation-perfusion ratios with the multiple inert gas elimination technique (MIGET). Respir Care 1981;26:860–870
7. Ralph D, Robertson HT: Respiratory gas exchange in adult respiratory distress syndrome. Semin Respir Med 1981;2:114–122
8. Craig KC, Pierson DJ, Carrico CJ: The clinical application of positive end-expiratory pressure (PEEP) in the adult respiratory distress syndrome (ARDS). Respir Care 1985;30:184–201
9. Kacmarek RM, Petty TL: Historical development of positive end-expiratory pressure (PEEP). Respir Care 1988;33:422–431
10. Barach AL, Martin J, Eckman M: Positive pressure respiration and its application in the treatment of acute pulmonary edema. Ann Intern Med 1938;12:754–795
11. Ashbaugh DG, Petty TL, Bigelow DB, Harris TM: Continuous positive-pressure breathing (CPPB) in adult respiratory distress syndrome. J Thorac Cardiovasc Surg 1969;57:31–40
12. Petty TL, Nett LM, Ashbaugh DG: Improvement in oxygenation in the adult respiratory distress syndrome by positive end-expiratory pressure (PEEP). Respir Care 1971;16:173–176
13. Positive end-expiratory pressure (PEEP). Respir Care 1988;33:419–501, 539–637
14. Pierson DJ, Kacmarek RM: Positive end-expiratory pressure—state of the art after 20 years. Respir Care 1988;33:419–421
15. McIntyre RW, Laws AK, Ramachandran PR: Positive expiratory pressure plateau: Improved gas exchange during mechanical ventilation. Canad Anaesth Soc J 1969;16:477–486
16. Pare PD, Warriner B, Baile EM et al: Redistribution of pulmonary extravascular water with positive end-expiratory pressure in canine pulmonary edema. Am Rev Respir Dis 1983;127:590–593
17. Harken AH, Brennan MF, Smith B, Barsamian EH: The hemodynamic response to positive end-expiratory ventilation in hypovolemic patients. Surgery 1974;76:786–793
18. Pierson DJ: Alveolar rupture during mechanical ventilation: Role of PEEP, peak airway pressure, and distending volume. Respir Care 1988;33:472–484
19. Kolobow T, Moretti MP, Fumagalli R et al: Severe impairment in lung function induced by high peak airway pressure during mechanical ventilation. Am Rev Respir Dis 1987;135:312–315
20. Tsuno K, Prato P, Kolobow T: Acute lung injury from mechanical ventilation at moderately high airway pressures. J Appl Physiol 1990;69:956–961
21. Dreyfuss D, Soler P, Basset G, Saumon G: High inflation pressure pulmonary edema: Respective effects of high airway pressure, high tidal volume, and positive end-expiratory pressure. Am Rev Respir Dis 1988;137:1159–1164
22. Dreyfuss D, Saumon G: Lung overinflation: Physiologic and anatomic alterations leading to pulmonary edema. pp. 433–449. In Zapol WM, Lemaire F (eds): Adult Respiratory Distress Syndrome. Marcel Dekker, New York, 1991
23. Churg A, Golden J, Fligiel S, Hogg JC: Bronchopulmonary dysplasia in the adult. Am Rev Respir Dis 1983;127:117–120
24. Rouby J-J, Lherm T, de Lassale EM et al: Pulmonary barotrauma and bronchopulmonary dysplasia in critically ill patients with acute respiratory failure. Presented at 32eme Congrès de la Société Francaise d'Anesthesie-Réanimation, Paris, September, 1990
25. Pingleton SK: Complications of acute respiratory failure (state of the art). Am Rev Respir Dis 1988;137:1463–1493
26. Pierson DJ: Therapy to improve tissue oxygenation. pp. 207–226. In Luce JM, Tyler ML, Pierson DJ (eds): Intensive Respiratory Care. WB Saunders, Philadelphia, 1984
27. Pepe PE, Potkin RT, Holtman Reus D et al: Clinical predictors of the adult respiratory distress syndrome. Am J Surg 1982;144:124–129
28. Maunder RJ: Clinical prediction of the adult respiratory distress syndrome. Clin Chest Med 1985;6:413–426
29. Maunder RJ, Hudson LD: Clinical risks associated with the adult respiratory distress syndrome. pp. 1–21. In Zapol WM, Lemaire F (eds): Adult Respiratory Distress Syndrome. Marcel Dekker, New York, 1991
30. Hudson LD: The prediction and prevention of ARDS. Respir Care 1990;35:161–173
31. Schmidt GB, O'Neill WW, Kotb K et al: Continuous positive airway pressure in the prophylaxis of the adult respiratory distress syndrome. Surg Gynecol Obstet 1976;143:613–618
32. Weigelt JA, Mitchell RA, Snyder WH III: Early positive end-expiratory pressure in the adult respiratory distress syndrome. Arch Surg 1979;114:497–501
33. Pepe PE, Hudson LD, Carrico CJ: Early application of positive end-expiratory pressure in patients at risk for the adult respiratory distress syndrome. N Engl J Med 1984;311:281–286
34. Maunder RJ, Hudson LD: Pharmacologic strategies for treating the adult respiratory distress syndrome. Respir Care 1990;35:241–246
35. Christman J, Wheeler A, Bernard G: Cytokines and sepsis: What are the therapeutic implications? J Crit Care 1991;6:172–182
36. Gregory TJ, Longmore WJ, Moxley MA et al: Surfactant chemical composition and biophysical activity in adult respiratory distress syndrome. J Clin Invest 1991;88:1976–1981
37. Spragg RG: Abnormalities of lung surfactant function in patients with acute lung injury: Implications for therapy. pp. 381–396. In Zapol WM, Lemaire F (eds): Adult Respiratory Distress Syndrome. New York, Marcel Dekker, 1991
38. Weg JG, Reines H, Balk R et al: Safety and efficacy of an aerosolized surfactant (Exosurf) in human sepsis-induced ARDS, abstracted. Chest 1991;100:137s
39. Wright PE, Bernard GR: The role of airflow resistance in patients with the adult respiratory distress syndrome. Am Rev Respir Dis 1989;139:1169–1174
40. Sznajder J, Wood LDH: Beneficial effects of reducing pulmonary edema in patients with acute hypoxemic respiratory failure. Chest 1991;100:890–891
41. Berthaume Y, Staub NC, Matthay MA: Beta-adrenergic agonists increase lung liquid clearance in anesthetized sheep. J Clin Invest 1987;79:335–343
42. Reyes A, Lopez-Messa JB, Alonso P: Almitrine in acute respiratory failure: Effects on pulmonary gas exchange and circulation. Chest 1987;91:388–393
43. Voelkel NF: Mechanisms of hypoxic vasoconstriction. Am Rev Respir Dis 1986;133:1186–1195
44. Broaddus VC, Berthaume Y, Biondi JW, Matthay MA: Hemodynamic management of the adult respiratory distress syndrome. Intensive Care Med 1987;2:190–213
45. Bone RC, Slotman G, Maunder R et al: Randomized double-blind, multicenter study of prostaglandin E_1 in patients with adult respiratory distress syndrome. Chest 1989;96:114–119
46. Melot C, Lejeune P, Leeman M et al: Prostaglandin E_1 in the adult respiratory distress syndrome: Benefit for pulmonary hypertension and cost for pulmonary gas exchange. Am Rev Respir Dis 1989;139:106–110
47. Taylor FB, Chang A, Esmon CT et al: Protein C prevents the coagulopathic and lethal effects of *Escherichia coli* infusion in the baboon. J Clin Invest 1987;79:918–925
48. Hardaway RM, Williams CH, Marvasti M et al: Prevention of ARDS with urokinase, abstracted. J Trauma 1988;28:1087
49. Bernard GR, Luce JM, Sprung CL et al: High-dose corticosteroids in patients with the adult respiratory distress syndrome. N Engl J Med 1987;317:1565–1570
50. Hooper RG, Kearl RA: Established ARDS treatment with a sustained course of adrenocortical steroids. Chest 1990;97:138–143
51. Hooper RG: ARDS: Inflammation, infections, and corticosteroids. Chest 1991;100:889–890
52. Hooper RG, Kearl RA: Treatment of established ARDS—steroids, antibiotics, and antifungal therapy, abstracted. Chest 1991;100:137s
53. Bone RC, Fischer CJ Jr, Clemmer TP et al: A controlled clinical trial of high dose methylprednisolone in the treatment of severe sepsis and septic shock. N Engl J Med 1987;317:653–658
54. Carey PD, Leeper-Woodford SK, Walsh CJ et al: Delayed cyclo-oxygenase blockade reduces the neutrophil respiratory

burst and plasma tumor necrosis factor levels in sepsis-induced acute lung injury. J Trauma 1991;31:733–741
55. Metz C, Sibbald WJ: Anti-inflammatory therapy for acute lung injury: A review of animal and clinical studies. Chest 1991;100:1110–1119
56. Rinaldo JE, Pennock B: Effects of ibuprofen on endotoxin-induced alveolitis. Am J Med Sci 1986;291:29–38
57. Sprague RS, Stephenson AH, Dahus TE et al: Effects of ibuprofen on the hypoxemia of established ethchlorvynol-induced unilateral acute lung injury in anesthetized dogs. Chest 1987;92:1088–1093
58. Bernard GR, Lucht WD, Niedermeyer ME et al: Effect of *N*-acetylcysteine on the pulmonary response to endotoxin in the awake sheep and upon in vitro granulocyte function. J Clin Invest 1984;73:1772–1784
59. Mandell G, Novak W (eds): Proceedings of a symposium: Pentoxyfylline and neutrophil function. Hoechst-Roussel Pharmaceuticals Inc, Somerville NJ, 1988
60. Berend N: Inhibition of bleomycin lung toxicity by *N*-acetylcysteine in the rat. Pathology 1985;17:108–110
61. Turrens JF, Crapo JD, Freeman BA: Protection against oxygen toxicity by intravenous injection of liposome-entrapped catalase and superoxide dismutase. J Clin Invest 1984;73:87–95
62. The HA-1A Sepsis Study Group: Treatment of gram-negative bacteremia and septic shock with HA-1A human monoclonal antibodies against endotoxin: A randomized double blind placebo-controlled trial. N Engl J Med 1991;324:429–436
63. Exley AR, Cohen J, Buurman W et al: Monoclonal antibodies to TNF_{alpha} in severe septic shock. Lancet 1990;335:1275–1277
64. Ohlsson K, Bjork P, Bergenfeldt M et al: Interleukin-1 receptor antagonist reduces mortality from endotoxin shock. Nature 1990;343:550–552
65. Stevens JH, O'Hanley P, Shapiro JM et al: Effects of anti-C5a antibodies on the adult respiratory distress syndrome in septic primates. J Clin Invest 1986;77:1812–1816
66. Summer WR, Curry P, Haponik EF et al: Continuous mechanical turning of intensive care unit patients shortens length of stay in some diagnosis-related groups. J Crit Care 1989;4:45–53
67. Gentilello L, Thompson DA, Tonnesen AS et al: Effect of a rotating bed on the incidence of pulmonary complications in critically ill patients. Crit Care Med 1988;16:783–786
68. Hess D, Agarwal NN, Myers CL: Positioning, lung function, and kinetic bed therapy. Respir Care 1992;37:181–197
69. Pugin J, Auckenthaler R, Lew DP, Suter PM: Oropharyngeal decontamination decreases incidence of ventilator-associated pneumonia: A randomized, placebo-controlled, double-blind clinical trial. JAMA 1991;265:2704–2710
70. Aerdts S, van Dalen R, Clasener H et al: Antibiotic prophylaxis of respiratory tract infection in mechanically ventilated patients. A prospective, blinded, randomized trial of the effect of a novel regimen. Chest 1991;100:783–791
71. Collins MS, Edwards A, Roby RE et al: *Pseudomonas* immune globulin therapy improves survival in experimental *Pseudomonas aeruginosa* bacteremic pneumonia. Antibiot Chemother 1989;42:184–192
72. Kirby RR, Downs JB, Civetta JM et al: High level positive end-expiratory pressure (PEEP) in acute respiratory insufficiency. Chest 1975;67:156–163
73. MacIntyre NR: Does positive end-expiratory pressure (PEEP) affect the natural history of acute lung injury? . . . Yes! Respir Care 1988;33:487–492
74. Civetta JM, Flor RJ, Smith LO: Aggressive treatment of acute respiratory insufficiency. South Med J 1976;69:749–751
75. Boysen PG: Does positive end-expiratory pressure (PEEP) affect the natural history of acute lung injury? . . . No! Respir Care 1988;33:493–498
76. Maunder RJ, Rice CL, Benson MS, Hudson LD: Managing positive end-expiratory pressure (PEEP): The Harborview approach. Respir Care 1986;31:1059–1066
77. Welch BE, Morgan TE Jr, Clamann HG: Time-concentration effects in relation to oxygen toxicity in man. Fed Proc 1963;22:1053–1056
78. Clark JM, Lambertsen CJ: Pulmonary oxygen toxicity: A review. Pharmacologic Rev 1971;23:37–133
79. Jenkinson SG: Oxygen toxicity in acute respiratory failure. Respir Care 1983;28:614–617
80. Bryan LC, Jenkinson SG: Oxygen toxicity. Clin Chest Med 1988;9:141–152
81. Pierson DJ: Respiratory care as a science. Respir Care 1988;33:27–37
82. Branson RD, Hurst JM, DeHaven CB Jr: Mask CPAP: State of the art. Respir Care 1985;30:846–857
83. Luterman A, Horovitz JH, Carrico CJ et al: Withdrawal from positive end-expiratory pressure. Surgery 1978;83:328–332
84. Weaver LJ, Haisch CE, Hudson LD, Carrico CJ: Prospective analysis of PEEP reduction, abstracted. Am Rev Respir Dis 1979;119(4, pt 2):182
85. Hudson LD, Weaver LJ, Haisch CE, Carrico CJ: Positive end-expiratory pressure: Reduction and withdrawal. Respir Care 1988;33:613–617
86. Faysal HM, Beller TA, Sobonya RE et al: Effect of positive end-expiratory pressure and body position in unilateral lung injury. J Appl Physiol 1982;52:147–154
87. Remolina C, Khan AU, Santiago TV, Edelman NH: Positional hypoxemia in unilateral lung disease. N Engl J Med 1981;304:523–525
88. Syracuse DC, Hyman AI, King TC: Postural influences on arterial blood bases in patients with unilateral pulmonary consolidation. Surg Forum 1979;30:173–174
89. Tyler ML: Complications of positioning and chest physiotherapy. Respir Care 1982;27:458–466
90. Dhainaut J-F, Bons J, Bricard C, Monsallier J-F: Improved oxygenation in patients with extensive unilateral pneumonia using the lateral decubitus position. Thorax 1980;35:792–793
90. Dhainaut JF, Bons J, Bricard C, Monsallier JF: Improved oxygenation in patients with extensive unilateral pneumonia using the lateral decubitus position. Thorax 1980;35:792–793
91. Ibanez J, Paurich JM, Abizanda R et al: The effect of lateral positions on gas exchange in patients with unilateral lung disease during mechanical ventilation. Intensive Care Med 1981;7:231–234
92. Maunder RJ, Shuman WP, McHugh JW et al: Preservation of normal lung regions in the adult respiratory distress syndrome. JAMA 1986;255:2463–2465
93. Douglas WW, Rehder K, Beynen FM et al: Improved oxygenation in patients with acute respiratory failure: The prone position. Am Rev Respir Dis 1977;115:559–566
94. Langer M, Mascheroni D, Marcolin R, Gattinoni L: The prone position in ARDS patients: A clinical study. Chest 1988;94:103–107
95. Carlon GC, Kahn R, Howland WS et al: Acute life-threatening ventilation perfusion inequality: An indication for independent lung ventilation. Crit Care Med 1978;6:380–383
96. Carlon GC, Ray C Jr, Klein R et al: Criteria for selective positive end-expiratory pressure and independent synchronized ventilation of each lung. Chest 1978;74:501–507
97. Glass DD, Tonnesen AS, Gabel JC, Arens JF: Therapy of unilateral pulmonary insufficiency with a double lumen endotracheal tube. Crit Care Med 1976;4:323–326
98. Ray C Jr: Independent lung ventilation. pp. 164–166, In Kacmarek RM, Stoller JK (eds): Current Respiratory Care. BC Decker, Philadelphia, 1988
99. Branson RD, Hurst JM, DeHaven CB: Synchronous independent lung ventilation in the treatment of unilateral pulmonary contusion: A report of two cases. Respir Care 1984;29:361–367
100. Gallagher TJ, Banner MS, Smith RA: A simplified method of independent lung ventilation. Crit Care Med 1980;8:396–399
101. Hillman KM, Barber JD: Asynchronous independent lung ventilation. Crit Care Med 1980;8:390–395

102. Kvetan V, Carlon GC, Howland WS: Acute pulmonary failure in asymmetric lung disease. Crit Care Med 1982;10:14–117
103. Parish JM, Gracey DR, Southern PA et al: Differential mechanical ventilation in respiratory failure due to severe unilateral lung disease. Mayo Clin Proc 1984;59:822–828
104. Popovich J, Sanders OJ, Vij D et al: Differential lung ventilation with a modified ventilator. Crit Care Med 1981;9:490–493
105. Powner DJ, Eross B, Grenvik A: Differential lung ventilation with PEEP in the treatment of unilateral pneumonia. Crit Care Med 1977;5:170–172

Chapter 66

Clinical Approach to Disorders of Ventilatory Control

Robert B. Schoene
David J. Pierson

CHAPTER OUTLINE

Chapters 14 and 25 describe the physiology of the regulation of ventilation and some of the disease states either primarily due to or clinically associated with disordered ventilatory drives. Although a thorough understanding of ventilatory drives and their implications for disease is imperative for optimal treatment of patients with pulmonary disorders, it is usually not necessary to actually measure these drives in the laboratory in order to assess and manage patients effectively. This chapter deals with two main aspects of the control of ventilation in respiratory care: (1) when to suspect a drive disorder and how to evaluate a patient's drives clinically; and (2) what therapeutic interventions are available and when to use them in patients whose primary pathophysiologic process may involve disordered ventilatory drives.

WHEN TO SUSPECT A DISORDER OF VENTILATORY CONTROL

Clinically significant derangements of ventilatory control are generally suspected on the basis of arterial blood gas findings, that is, either an abnormal PCO_2 or an inappropriately high PCO_2 in the presence of hypoxemia. *Hypoventilation* as a result of abnormally low ventilatory drives typically presents with hypoxemia with either an elevated or an inappropriately "normal" PCO_2, as illustrated here:

	PCO_2	
PO_2	Expected	Decreased Drives
70 mmHg	40 mmHg	50 mmHg
50 mmHg	30 mmHg	40 mmHg

Hyperventilation due to abnormally accentuated ventilatory drive could be present when hypocapnia occurs in the absence of hypoxemia. However, in both instances the clinician's first responsibility is to exclude other, more common reasons for hypo- or hyperventilation, as discussed below.

Disordered ventilatory control may occur acutely, but in most instances the disorders under consideration here are chronic.[1–4] Table 66-1 summarizes the symptoms, laboratory findings, potential diagnoses, and possible approaches to

Table 66-1. Clinical Settings for Possible Disorders of Ventilatory Control

Category	Symptoms	Laboratory Findings	Possible Diagnoses	Approach to Therapy
Hypoventilation	Lethargy; headache; hypersomnolence; decreased exercise tolerance; confusion	Acute (uncompensated) respiratory acidosis Hypoxemia	Acute ventilatory failure (see Ch. 30)	See Ch. 64
		Chronic (compensated) respiratory acidosis Hypoxemia Erythrocytosis	COPD (type B) with or without cor pulmonale Other obstructive lung disease (see Ch. 22) Restrictive lung disease (see Ch. 23)	See Chs. 62 & 63
			Sleep-related breathing disorder (see Ch. 27)	See Ch. 67
			Primary disorder of ventilatory control (see Ch. 25)	Consider respiratory stimulant drugs (see Fig. 66-5) Consider long-term mechanical ventilation (see Ch. 101)
Hyperventilation	Dyspnea; anxiety; decreased exercise tolerance	Acute respiratory alkalosis Normoxemia	Acute cardiopulmonary illness "Primary" hyperventilation syndrome	Therapy for primary problem Rule out other disease; consider behavioral therapy and breathing retraining
		Chronic respiratory alkalosis Normoxemia	Restrictive lung disease	Treat primary disease; consider behavioral therapy
			COPD (type A)	See Ch. 62; behavioral therapy; consider codeine or other drive-depressing drug
			Hyperventilation syndrome	Behavioral therapy; breathing retraining

therapy in the disorders that are most frequently encountered clinically. It is important to remember that this category of disorders is more often suspected than confirmed—that is, while diseases of ventilatory drive should be considered in a variety of clinical settings, they are relatively uncommon, and in most instances another, more common explanation will be found.

Quantitative assessment of ventilatory control, using hypoxic ventilatory response (HVR) and hypercapnic ventilatory response (HCVR) or measurement of mouth occlusion pressure ($P_{0.1}$) as an index of central drive, is described in Chapter 14. These formal investigations are seldom necessary in clinical practice and can be both difficult to perform and potentially harmful to patients who may already be hypoxemic and/or acidemic. In fact, it is usually possible to identify the contribution of disordered ventilatory drives to a patient's clinical picture through a careful history, performance of routine pulmonary function tests, and measurement of arterial blood gases.

Abnormally Low Drives (Hypoventilation Syndromes)

Identification of decreased ventilatory drive as a cause for hypoventilation rests primarily on determining the patient's ability to ventilate appropriately. Patients who hypoventilate at rest may do so because they either are not sufficiently stimulated (or lack an appropriate central drive response to such stimulation) or are incapable of increasing ventilation appropriately. This distinction between being unable ("can't breathe") and not being driven ("won't breathe") is diagrammed in Figure 66-1.

When studies of HVR and HCVR are carried out on normal, healthy individuals, a small number of them (5 percent or less) have markedly blunted drives.[5,6] If such an individual developed acute hypoxemia (e.g., in the setting of lobar pneumonia), the usual hyperventilation response might not occur and arterial blood gas analysis might show an inappropriately "normal" PCO_2. Persons with blunted hypoxic drives are probably at increased risk for development of chronic mountain sickness if they live at moderate or high altitude.[4,7,8] Other drives may be similarly affected. If such individuals develop lung disease that increases the work of breathing, they may respond less than would persons with normal ventilatory drives and be at risk for the sequelae of chronic hypoventilation.[9] This is thought by some to be a major determinant of the clinical manifestations of chronic obstructive pulmonary disease (COPD), as diagrammed in Figure 66-2. Individuals with inherently blunted drives may breathe less and be less uncomfortable in the presence of chronic hypoxemia than their counterparts with the same

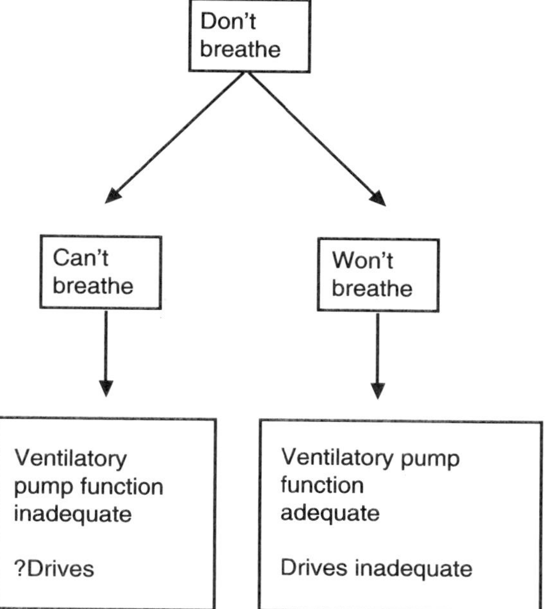

Figure 66-1. Conceptual scheme for differentiating the possible mechanisms in a given patient with hypoventilation. Some patients with hypercapnia (who by definition "don't breathe") are mechanically incapable of increasing their alveolar ventilation (and hence "can't breathe") because of severe airflow obstruction, ventilatory muscle weakness, or other mechanism of pump failure. Others (who "won't breathe") have the mechanical capability of increasing alveolar ventilation and reversing their hypercapnia but do not do so because of decreased ventilatory drives.

degree of airflow obstruction who have stronger ventilatory drives; this distinction may be involved in the development of type B ("blue and bloated") versus type A ("pink and puffing") COPD.

The distinction between "can't breathe" and "won't breathe" can be invoked when assessing a given patient who manifests chronic hypoventilation[10] (Fig. 66-3). Very severe airflow obstruction, such as that indicated by a forced expiratory volume in 1 second (FEV_1) of 0.5 L in an average-sized adult, may render the patient incapable of maintaining a normal $PaCO_2$. On the other hand, a patient with chronic hypercapnia who does not have significant airflow obstruction must have some other explanation for this phenomenon. Even in patients with COPD, airflow obstruction should not be assumed to be the whole explanation for hypoventilation unless the obstruction is severe.

One convenient way to distinguish between patients who "can't breathe" and those who "won't breathe" is to measure arterial blood gases before and after a short period (e.g., 3 minutes) of voluntary hyperpnea. A patient who gives a good effort and is unable to lower the $PaCO_2$ by 10 to 20 mmHg or more may be mechanically unable to sustain normocapnia. On the other hand, individuals with good ventilatory pump function can drop their $PaCO_2$ values to 20 mmHg or lower with 3 minutes of voluntary hyperventilation.

Although insufficient ventilatory drive is often proposed as a reason for unweanability following prolonged ventilatory support in patients with acute respiratory failure, this is rarely the case. As discussed in Chapter 86, most patients fail to wean because of other identifiable respiratory[11] or nonrespiratory[12] factors for which corrective measures can be attempted. In fact, studies of ventilatory drive using $P_{0.1}$ measurements have shown that most "unweanable" patients have increased, not decreased, drives.[13,14] In such individuals inability to sustain spontaneous ventilation is more likely to be due to inadequate ventilatory muscle strength and endurance than to insufficient desire to breathe.

Abnormally High Drives (Hyperventilation Syndrome)

Clinical illness due to abnormally increased ventilatory drives is considerably less common than the hypoventilation syndromes just discussed. Hyperventilation syndrome is frequently diagnosed in patients who are actually suffering from acute or chronic cardiorespiratory disease (Table 66-1). This disorder appears to be a real entity[3,15,16] but one that should be diagnosed only after excluding other causes for dyspnea and hyperventilation.

Unlike $PaCO_2$, a patient's dyspnea cannot be measured directly. The clinician must rely on a careful history and other clinical skills. The first priority should be to search for "usual" physiologic explanations for dyspnea and hyperventilation, such as hypoxemia and abnormal lung-thorax stiffness. While patients with obstructive lung disease may or may not complain of shortness of breath, persons with pulmonary restrictive and/or vascular disorders are usually dyspneic, especially with exercise, and chronic hyperven-

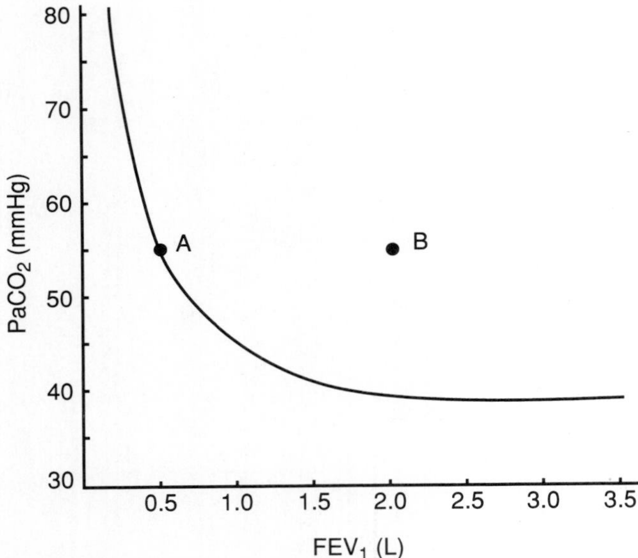

Figure 66-2. General relationship between declining lung function (here represented by forced expiratory volume in 1 second [FEV_1]) and CO_2 retention in COPD. If a given patient with a $PaCO_2$ of 55 mmHg has an FEV_1 of 0.5 L (point A), it is reasonable to ascribe the hypercapnia to the airflow obstruction. However, if the patient's FEV_1 is substantially greater (e.g., 2.0 L, point B), another mechanism such as decreased ventilatory drive should be sought. With respect to Figure 66-1, patient A would fall in the "can't breathe" category, while patient B would be labeled "won't breathe."

tilation is common. Individuals with primary restrictive lung disease such as idiopathic pulmonary fibrosis may experience more severe air hunger than any other diagnostic group the clinician encounters. In patients without hypoxemia or spirometric evidence for obstructive disease it is important to look for decreased lung compliance as an explanation for chronic hyperventilation; it may be necessary to measure this directly (see Ch. 45).

Brodkorb et al.[17] have described a means for distinguishing between hyperventilation syndrome due to increased ventilatory drive and that due to other conditions with normal drives. With this approach, patients are asked to voluntarily hyperventilate for 12 minutes. $PaCO_2$ is measured during the 12-minute test and 12 minutes after its completion, and the end-tidal PCO_2 ($P_{ET}CO_2$) in exhaled gas is monitored throughout by use of a capnometer. These investigators reported that patients with hyperventilation syndrome had lower $PaCO_2$ values during hyperventilation than did a normal control group and that the patients' $P_{ET}CO_2$ readings did not return to normal following voluntary hyperventilation, as did those of the normal control subjects.[17]

Figure 66-4 presents a clinical algorithm for approaching patients with suspected hyperventilation syndrome, which incorporates several of the points just discussed.

APPROACH TO THE MANAGEMENT OF DRIVE DISORDERS

Hypoventilation Syndromes

Disordered ventilatory drive is usually only one of several processes contributing to a patient's illness, and it is im-

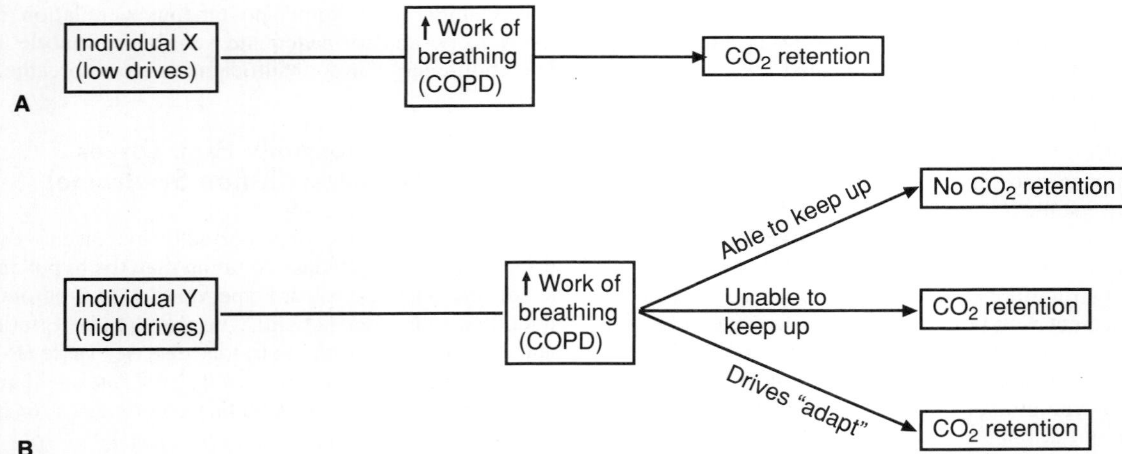

Figure 66-3. Conceptual scheme to explain the genesis of CO_2 retention in COPD as a function of the patient's underlying ventilatory drives in combination with the severity of airflow obstruction and hence the added work of breathing. **(A)** Individual X with weak drives is not stimulated to work harder and maintain normal alveolar ventilation when confronted by the increased demand produced by airflow obstruction. **(B)** Individual Y, whose inherent drive to breathe is strong, may respond to the increased demand in three possible ways: by increasing breathing work in order to keep alveolar ventilation and PCO_2 normal; by trying unsuccessfully to do so and developing hypercapnia despite attempts to prevent it; or by allowing the ventilatory drives to be "reset" and thus tolerating hypercapnia in order to avoid excessive breathing work.

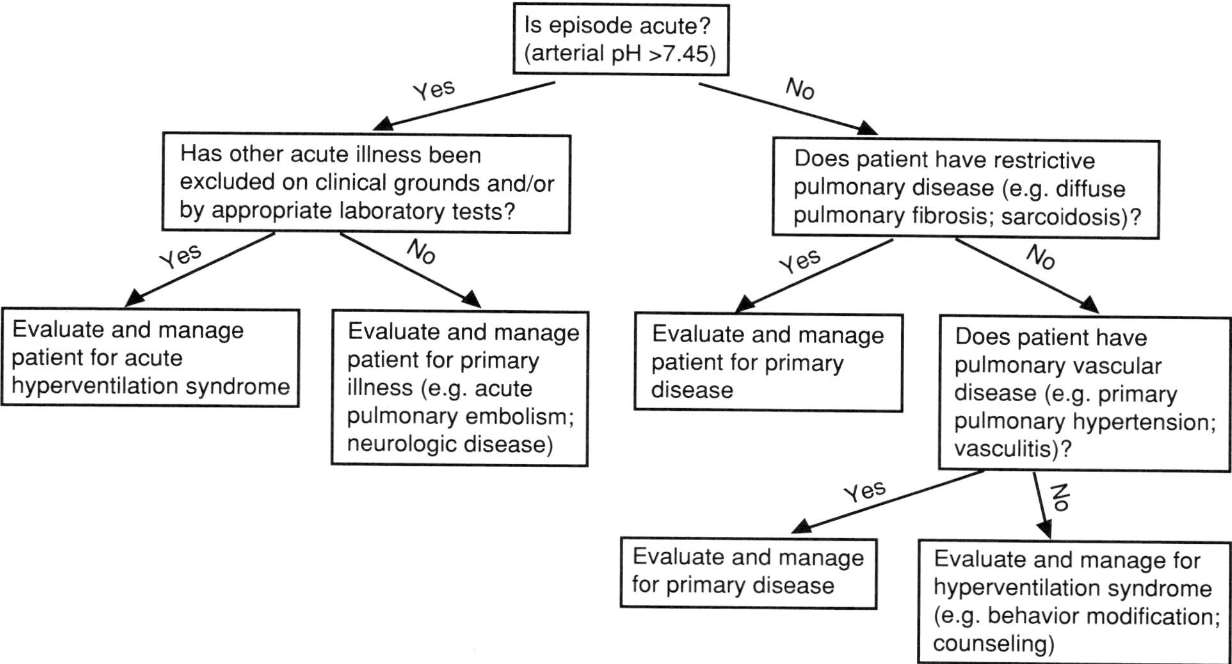

Figure 66-4. Algorithm for clinical assessment of the patient with hyperventilation, as manifested by dyspnea and hypocapnia (decreased $PaCO_2$).

portant that the others be recognized and managed appropriately. Once it has been determined that blunted drive is clinically important in a given patient (i.e., the patient "won't breathe" according to the criteria discussed above) and that any coexisting medical conditions are being managed optimally, consideration should be given to drive augmentation with respiratory stimulant drugs. Progesterone (medroxyprogesterone acetate [Provera]) and acetazolamide (Diamox) are the agents most often used. Figure 66-5 presents an algorithm for selecting patients appropriate for such drive stimulation.

Progesterone is given as a 20-mg tablet tid,[18] and at least 1 to 2 weeks' administration is generally necessary before substantial clinical change occurs. Indicators of a favorable response include decreased $PaCO_2$ and increased PaO_2, eventual improvement in secondary erythrocytosis and signs of cor pulmonale, and improved symptoms of hypersomnolence and lethargy. Many patients experience increased dyspnea while taking progesterone, however, and the drug can cause decreased libido and impotence in men and vaginal bleeding in women.

Acetazolamide is generally more effective than progesterone in decreasing nocturnal dysrhythmic breathing and desaturation in patients with chronic mountain sickness.[19,20] Acetazolamide is administered in 250-mg tablets, commonly bid or tid. Increased ventilation related to establishment of a mild metabolic acidosis is detectable within a few hours. The main side effect, besides increased breathlessness, is an unpleasant taste, especially when drinking carbonated beverages.

Hyperventilation Syndrome

Hyperventilation syndrome merges indistinguishably with neurocirculatory asthenia, panic disorder, symptoms seen in mitral valve prolapse, and noncoronary chest pain.[21] Once other organic disease has been ruled out, breathing retraining and other forms of behavior modification constitute the preferred approach to management. Several investigators have reported substantial clinical improvement in patients with hyperventilation syndrome in response to therapy specifically targeted at having them modify their breathing pattern.[22,23]

The administration of drugs to blunt ventilatory drives in patients with incapacitating dyspnea complicating COPD has been the subject of several studies.[24,25] Such therapy should never be attempted in patients who are acutely ill or clinically unstable, and most authorities feel it is contraindicated in the presence of hypercapnia. For highly selected, clinically stable patients with intolerable dyspnea despite maximal therapy for reversible airflow obstruction and hypoxemia, some clinicians prescribe codeine (15 to 30 mg bid, tid, or qid) or equivalent doses of such analogues as dihydrocodeine

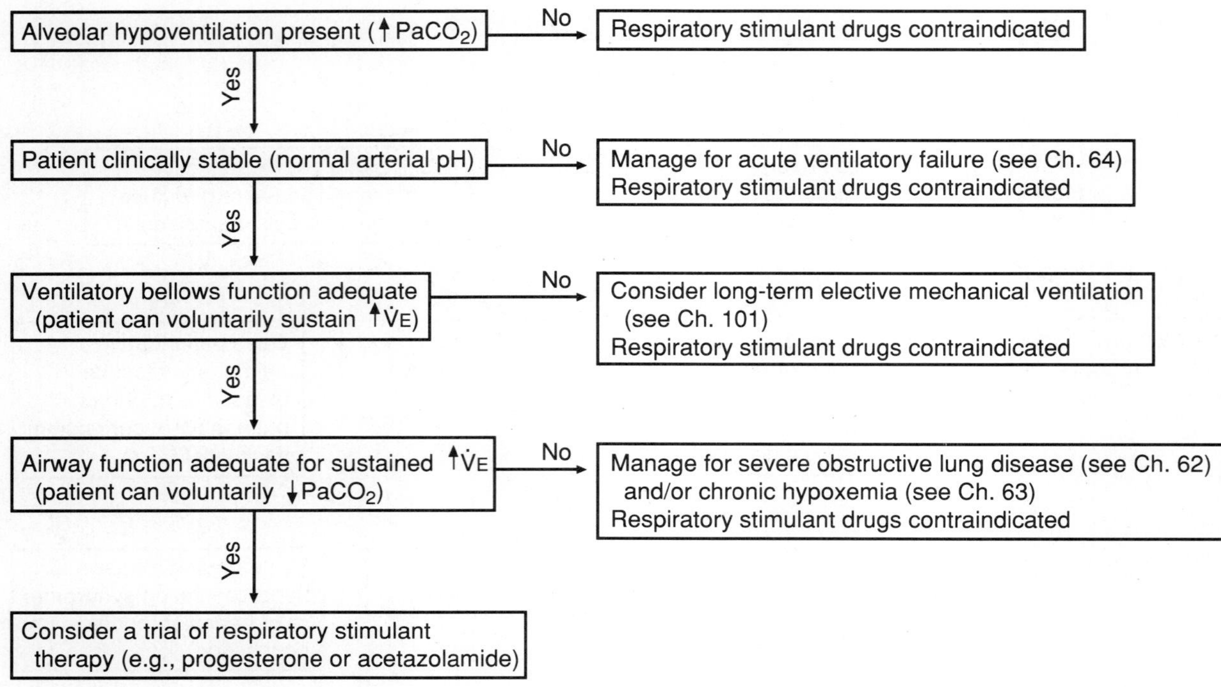

Figure 66-5. Algorithm for selecting patients who might benefit from a respiratory stimulant drug.

and oxycodone. Benzodiazepines such as diazepam (Valium) have been used by some[25] but have generally been less efficacious. The administration of respiratory depressants to patients with chronic illness should always be undertaken with great caution, and the patients should be monitored closely for signs of dangerous respiratory depression.

References

1. Zwillich CW: Diseases of ventilatory control. pp. 1790–1794. In Kelley WN (ed): Textbook of Internal Medicine. 2nd Ed. JB Lippincott, Philadelphia, 1992
2. Phillipson EA: Hypoventilation syndromes. pp. 1831–1840. In Murray JF, Nadel JA (eds): Textbook of Respiratory Medicine. WB Saunders, Philadelphia, 1988
3. Cherniack NS: Hyperventilation syndromes. pp. 1861–1866. In Murray JF, Nadel JA (eds): Textbook of Respiratory Medicine. WB Saunders, Philadelphia, 1988
4. Schoene RB: Diseases of high altitude. pp. 1805–1807. In Kelley WN (ed): Textbook of Internal Medicine. 2nd Ed. JB Lippincott, Philadelphia, 1992
5. Weil JV, Byrne-Quinn E, Sodal IE et al: Hypoxic ventilatory drive in normal man. J Clin Invest 1970;49:1061–1072
6. Rebuck AS, Campbell EJM: Clinical method for assessing the ventilatory response to hypoxia. Am Rev Respir Dis 1974; 109:345–350
7. Schoene RB: Adaptation and maladaptation to high altitude. pp. 1035–1054. In Baum GL, Wolinsky E (eds): Textbook of Pulmonary Diseases. 4th Ed. Little Brown, Boston, 1989
8. Kryger M, McCullough R, Doekel R et al: Excessive polycythemia of high altitude: Role of ventilatory drive in lung disease. Am Rev Respir Dis 1978;118:659–666
9. Park SS: Respiratory control in chronic obstructive pulmonary diseases. Clin Chest Med 1980;1:73–84
10. Fahey PJ, Hyde RW: "Won't breathe" vs "Can't breathe": Detection of depressed ventilatory drive in patients with obstructive pulmonary disease. Chest 1983;84:19–25
11. Yang KL, Tobin MJ: A prospective study of indexes predicting the outcome of trials of weaning from mechanical ventilation. N Engl J Med 1991;324:1445–1450
12. Pierson DJ: Overcoming nonrespiratory causes of weaning failure. J Crit Illness 1990;5:267–283
13. Montgomery B, Holle RHO, Naegley SR et al: Prediction of successful ventilator weaning using airway occlusion pressure in hypercapnic challenge. Chest 1987;91:496–499
14. Sassoon CJ, Te T, Mahutte CK et al: Airway occlusion pressure (P0.1) as a reliable predictor to weaning? Chest 1985;88:38S
15. Lum LC: Hyperventilation and anxiety state. J R Soc Med 1981; 74:1–4
16. Plum F: Mechanisms of "central" hyperventilation. Ann Neurol 1982;11:636–637
17. Brodkorb E, Gimse R, Antonaci F et al: Hyperventilation syndrome: Clinical, ventilatory, and personality characteristics as observed in neurological practice. Acta Neurol Scand 1990; 81:307–313
18. Sutton FD, Zwillich CW, Creagh CE et al: Progesterone for outpatient treatment of pickwickian syndrome. Ann Intern Med 1975;83:476–479
19. Sutton JR, Houston CS, Mansell AL et al: Effect of acetazolamide on hypoxemia during sleep at high altitude. N Eng J Med 1979;301:1329–1331
20. Weil JV, Kryger MH, Scoggin CH: Sleep and breathing at high altitude. pp. 119–136. In Guilleminault C, Dement C (ed): Sleep Apnea Syndromes. Alan R Liss, New York, 1978
21. Tavel ME: Hyperventilation syndrome—hiding behind pseudonyms? [Editorial] Chest 1990;97:1285–1288
22. Grossman P, de Swart JCG, Defares PB: A controlled study of

a breathing therapy for treatment of hyperventilation syndrome. J Psychosom Res 1985;29:49–58
23. Clark DM, Salkovskis PM, Chalkley AJ: Respiratory control as a treatment for panic attacks. J Behav Ther Exp Psychiatry 1985; 16:23–30
24. Woodcock AA, Gross ER, Gellert A et al: Effects of dihydrocodeine, alcohol, and caffeine on breathlessness and exercise tolerance in patients with chronic obstructive lung disease and normal blood gases. N Engl J Med 1981;305:1611–1616
25. Woodcock AA, Gross ER, Geddes DM: Drug treatment of breathlessness: Contrasting effects of diazepam and promethazine in pink puffers. Br Med J 1981;283:343–346

Chapter 67

Clinical Approach to Breathing Disorders During Sleep

Eugene C. Fletcher

CHAPTER OUTLINE

CLINICAL MANIFESTATIONS OF SLEEP-DISORDERED BREATHING

Clinical manifestations of sleep-disordered breathing cover a very wide range, from absolutely no symptoms and perhaps just mildly bothersome snoring or a history of mild essential hypertension, to severe daytime hypersomnolence. Such severe hypersomnolence may occur that the patient is unable to perform the usual mental and physical tasks that those of us with so-called normal breathing during sleep take for granted. Just as the degree of symptomatology may cover a broad spectrum, so may the degree of abnormality of nocturnal respiration. Disordered breathing may range from mild degrees of desaturation induced by central hypopneas or obstructive hypopnea (some forms of snoring) to marked hypoxemia caused by prolonged central and obstructive apnea. In the strict sense, *apnea* is the appearance of a 10-second or longer pause in breathing that occurs during sleep. A loose definition of *sleep apnea* is the presence of 30 or more of these apneas per 7 hours of sleep (more than 5 such episodes per hour).[1] *Sleep apnea syndrome* (SAS), on the other hand, is "a potentially lethal condition characterized by multiple obstructive or mixed apneas during sleep, associated with repetitive episodes of inordinately loud snoring and excessive daytime sleepiness."[2]

The distinction between minimum sleep apnea and sleep apnea syndrome is clinically important, since the latter may require treatment whereas the former almost certainly will not. Nevertheless, in many epidemiologic surveys, especially in older populations, this distinction is unclear.[1,3–5] The following section discusses the most blatant symptoms of SAS, but the reader should keep in mind that a milder variation of signs and symptoms will most frequently constitute the patient's presenting picture. In many circumstances a history of milder symptoms must be diligently sought by the examiner.

The most important signs and symptoms of SAS are listed in Table 67-1. Only the more important aspects of these are discussed, since excellent reviews of this topic have already been published.[6–15]

Snoring

"Olympic class" snoring is a universal symptom of obstructive SAS, and most patients have a history of snoring

Table 67-1. Clinical Manifestations of Sleep Apnea Syndrome

Abnormal sleep behavior
Loud, sonorous snoring
Audible pauses in breathing terminated by loud inspiratory grunts
Excessive and often violent motor activity
Nocturnal enuresis
Somnambulism
Talking during sleep
Feeling of insomnia
Daytime hypersomnolence
Mild napping to inability to stay awake when the situation demands
Hypnagogic hallucinations
Automatic behavior
Personality changes and cognitive dysfunction
Memory, intellect, and reasoning impairment
Anxiety and or depression
Confusion, irritability, aggressiveness, irrational behavior
Physical symptomatology and signs
Morning headaches
Sexual dysfunction and impotence
Chronic tiredness and malaise
Systemic hypertension
Peripheral edema (pulmonary hypertension and cor pulmonale)
Laboratory abnormalities
Polycythemia
Alveolar hypoventilation with hypercarbia and hypoxemia
Abnormal electrocardiogram reflecting arrhythmias and right ventricular hypertrophy

dating back to their late adolescence and early twenties. Snoring associated with SAS is often of a severity that creates marital discord. This, along with excessive and violent thrashing that can be injurious to both patient and spouse, frequently causes them to seek separate beds or separate bedrooms. Speaking to a patient's spouse about nocturnal sleep habits may lead to a tentative diagnosis, and not infrequently a patient will seek a medical opinion with a statement such as "My wife says I stop breathing at night." A rare exception to the rule of snoring is the patient who has so many and such long apneas that the whole night is spent in suspended breathing and grunting (apnea-terminating snorts), allowing little time for snoring in the more traditional sense. Indeed, the whole topic of snoring is now being intensely investigated, since hypoxemia and systemic hypertension may be associated with snoring alone.[16] Some investigators are examining possible cerebrocortical dysfunction associated with snoring.[17]

Insomnia

It is worth mentioning the unlikely symptom of *insomnia* in a patient who is supposedly suffering from a syndrome causing hypersomnolence. It should be remembered that each apnea is terminated by an arousal from electroencephalographic (EEG) sleep, bringing about activation of upper pharyngeal muscles needed to overcome obstruction.[10] Frequently, these arousals are accompanied by excessive motor activity and behavioral awakening of the patient. Occasionally and quite accurately, the patient interprets this frequent arousal and inability to remain asleep as "insomnia," and such a history is not incompatible with severe SAS. On the other hand, nocturnal enuresis and somnambulism are less frequently reported symptoms.

Daytime Hypersomnolence

Daytime hypersomnolence is the main symptom of SAS. There are a large number of anecdotal accounts of the degree of hypersomnolence that may be experienced by apnea patients. One of the earliest descriptions of the pickwickian syndrome was that of a patient who came to the physician because he fell asleep during a poker game and failed to bid a "full house."[18] Rather than such amusing tales about hypersomnolence, however, it is important to seek historical facts that relate to the patient's day-to-day function. Such information will not only help in confirming the presence of daytime somnolence but will determine how aggressive the treatment should be for this patient.

The two most important areas to explore are *vehicular driving* and *behavior in the workplace*. There should be a high degree of motivation to stay awake in both of these situations, in the first for safety reasons and in the second to maintain the patient's income. Falling asleep in either of these settings is a strong historical point. Over 50 percent of apnea patients seeking medical attention give a history of falling asleep at the wheel, and some recent investigations show a high incidence of accidents among such patients.[19] A frequent history among SAS patients is recent job loss or frequent change of jobs.

In some cases of particularly stoic patients, historical information, even from spouses, may not be enough to confirm the presence of excessive daytime somnolence (EDS). The Multiple Sleep Latency Test (MSLT) was developed to avoid the subjective aspect of daytime hypersomnolence and quantitatively measure sleep onset latency. During the day in the sleep laboratory, the patient is wired for EEG monitoring and rests supine in bed. The time to onset of sleep is measured during several nap periods, limited to 20 minutes each. The rapid onset of sleep is indicative of pathologic somnolence.[20,21]

Just as disabling as EDS but often more subtle are the impaired cognitive effects of SAS. Memory deficit, impaired reasoning, and decreased intellect are very common, as are personality changes such as inappropriate behavior, aggressiveness, or depression. A history of frequent job changes, marital discord, or divorce is common. The latter may to a great extent reflect the common finding of sexual dysfunction and impotence. Again, such a history, in combination with findings on the nocturnal polysomnogram, should strongly affect the treatment choice in such patients.

The last four clinical and laboratory findings listed in Table 67-1 are worthy of special mention as they, in combination with marked obesity and hypersomnolence, constitute the pickwickian syndrome, a term that should *not* be used synonymously with sleep apnea syndrome. The pickwickian syndrome is seen in a morbidly obese individual with marked daytime hypersomnolence, plethora (polycythemia), alveolar hypoventilation while awake, and cor pulmonale.[18] No sleep studies were made in the first case described, so that it is uncertain that the original case was caused by obstructive sleep apnea. We now know that patients with severe obesity-hypoventilation syndrome can develop pickwickian-type symptoms and yet have minimal obstructive sleep apnea. In this situation tracheotomy would likely be of little help; drugs (e.g., medroxyprogesterone acetate), supplemental O_2, and certainly weight loss would be first lines of treatment, with perhaps more aggressive therapy taking the form of nocturnal artificial ventilation.

Brief mention must be made of the disturbances in nocturnal arterial O_2 saturation (SaO_2) experienced by patients with chronic lung disease. Early in their disease desaturation seldom leads to daytime symptoms, which, if present, would suggest the need for a sleep study, although a recent study has challenged this concept.[22] When clinically diagnosable cor pulmonale is present, the patient usually has daytime hypoxemia, which can be confirmed by arterial blood gas measurement, and proper supplemental O_2 therapy can be instituted if appropriate. There are exceptions to this; therefore if only mild daytime hypoxemia is present in a lung disease patient with peripheral edema, elevated neck veins, and perhaps signs of pulmonary hypertension on physical examination, electrocardiography (ECG) and chest radiography, one should suspect significant nocturnal oxyhemoglobin desaturation. Appropriate studies in this setting would include some measure of right ventricular function (e.g., gated or single-pass nuclear ventriculography) and a nocturnal oximeter tracing. It should be noted, however, that an oximeter trace alone showing no drop in SaO_2 does not rule out nocturnal hypoxemia, since the presence of rapid eye movement (REM) sleep cannot be confirmed in the absence of the EEG. Therapy of patients with neuromuscular disease involving the chest wall is discussed below.

Before discussing the integrated approach to a patient suspected of having a nocturnal disturbance in breathing, current options for treatment of obstructive sleep apnea are reviewed critically in order to provide the reader with the necessary basic understanding of the variety of treatments now available to the clinician.

TREATMENT OPTIONS IN SLEEP APNEA SYNDROME

Medical Treatment

Weight Loss

Weight loss is still the first line of therapy in overweight patients who have symptomatic obstructive sleep apnea. It is effective when accomplished and involves low risk, but it is probably the least successful approach because of lack of compliance. An interesting case report demonstrates the relationship of apnea frequency and apneic oxyhemoglobin desaturation to body weight in a 111-kg man. At that weight this patient's apnea index (number of apneas per hour) was 60, with a nadir SaO_2 of 40 percent. With gradual weight loss, his apnea index decreased during five studies to 22, 17, 6, and 3 per hour at a final weight of 85 kg, with a nadir SaO_2 of 88 percent.[23] Aids to weight loss such as intestinal bypass have been tried, but objective data on improvement and long-term follow-up are rare. One study reports 2-year follow-up in four morbidly obese men who went from a mean preoperative weight of 231 to 123 kg following jejunoileal bypass: their mean apnea index fell from 78 before to 1.4 after weight loss.[24,25]

When dietary therapy for apnea is considered, one must remember that sudden death due to arrhythmia/asphyxia is always a possibility during the weight loss period. Also, the extreme depression and mental changes brought on by chronic sleep disturbance may preclude successful weight loss because of poor motivation. Under these circumstances, or in the presence of apparently life-threatening arrhythmias during sleep, one should consider nasal continuous positive airway pressure (CPAP) or immediate tracheotomy, in the hope that decannulation or removal of CPAP will be possible if the patient is successful at losing weight.

Mechanical Devices

Apneas are often fewer (on the average 50 percent less) when patients sleep on their sides. There have been reports that taping or sewing a tennis ball into the back of the sleeping garment will decrease the apnea and improve symptoms. Again, compliance could be a major problem, and one would not consider this therapy in severe apnea. Also, if the patient has been having 100 severe apneas per hour, how much benefit can be expected from a 50 percent reduction in apnea index?[26]

Another nonsurgical method of treating apnea is a suction device fitted to the tongue to pull it forward during sleep. A major problem appears to be the discomfort involved in wearing the device. Patients are encouraged to wear it only half of the night. In a recent series of 20 men, only 11 were reported wearing the device after 6 months. Since the device is worn only half of the night and the apnea frequency is reduced by only 50 percent, the treatment cannot be considered curative.[27]

Pharmacologic Agents

Several drugs have been tried with limited success in treating both central and obstructive sleep apnea. In individual patients these may be quite useful if they can be demonstrated by objective parameters (sleep study) to benefit the patient. Acetazolamide (Diamox) has been shown under acute circumstances to reduce central apneas by about 70 percent. Its chronic effect is unproven, and it may worsen obstructive apnea.[28–30] There are conflicting opinions in the literature as to the efficacy of medroxyprogesterone acetate

(Provera) in treating obstructive apnea. It is not considered effective therapy in most obstructive apnea patients, although it may help in some pickwickian-type patients.[30–33]

Protriptyline has received new attention following a recent report.[34] Much of the improvement in apnea frequency was attributed to a reduction in REM sleep time, the period of sleep when apneas are more frequent and more severe. Other experience with the drug has shown a reduction of apnea frequency and duration and an improvement in saturation during all stages of sleep.[35] More data are needed on the chronic effects of protriptyline, such as the incidence of side effects, which include difficulty urinating, impotence, and dry mouth. Such problems make chronic compliance poor.[36–38]

Certain drugs may be harmful to patients with apnea. Patients with sleep apnea should be warned about the danger of drinking alcohol before bedtime. It is no coincidence that snoring worsens after a night of heavy drinking. Taasan et al.[39] in 1981 found that in asymptomatic men, disordered breathing events associated with arterial O_2 desaturation increased from a mean of 207 per night during control to 383 per night after alcohol ingestion. Numerous reports since then have supported this finding, and subsequent studies have demonstrated a physiologic basis for the apnea worsening.[40,41] Alcohol administered to cats caused a marked decrease in electromyographic (EMG) tonic activity of the upper airway pharyngeal muscle constrictors and in respiratory response during tidal respiration. This decrease in tone probably allows negative inspiratory pressure to collapse the upper airway during early inspiration.

Benzodiazepines have been implicated in worsening obstructive apneas and decreasing oxyhemoglobin desaturation during sleep in patients with chronic obstructive pulmonary disease (COPD). To date most of these investigations have involved flurazepam in 30-mg doses. Needless to say, sleeping pills probably are not a good idea in apneics. Many older patients have unrecognized sleep apnea, and sleeping pills in these patients may aggravate the underlying disordered breathing condition.[42–44] Premedication before surgery is relatively contraindicated in known apnea patients since loss of upper airway tone may make intubation more difficult.[45]

Oxygen

O_2 has had the following beneficial effects in the treatment of apnea.[46–48] It decreases the hourly index of obstructive and central apnea by about 20 or 30 percent; improves baseline (nonapneic) SaO_2, as well as the nadir level of desaturation during apnea, by about 5 percent; and improves the quality of sleep in many patients and reduces daytime somnolence in a few, but objective data are scant. The possible harmful effects of O_2 include prolongation of apneas (particularly in those with underlying lung disease) and worsening of end-apneic CO_2 retention. No studies have been done examining the hemodynamic or symptomatic effect of supplemental O_2 administered chronically to apneic patients. A single study has indicated that 30 to 90 nights of use may reduce apnea frequency when the patient is restudied after discontinuation of O_2.[47] This study was hampered in that some patients also lost weight during the chronic use period. If one is considering supplemental O_2 for an apnea patient, it would be wise to conduct a formal sleep study using O_2 to look for possible worsening.[48]

Continuous Positive Airway Pressure

The nonsurgical treatment of obstructive sleep apnea that is now in most frequent use worldwide is nasal CPAP, first described in 1981 by Sullivan et al.[49] The system consists of a tight-fitting mask, which covers the nasal alae but not the mouth, allowing the patient to swallow. A source of high-bias airflow is connected to the mask, forcing air through relatively small tubing and thereby generating positive pressure throughout the respiratory cycle. The amount of pressure is varied by the size of the expiratory valve and the rate of flow of air. During a trial sleep study, variable levels of CPAP, ranging from 5 to 17 cmH_2O are applied, until most of the apneas disappear (Fig. 67-1). The CPAP eliminates apnea by making the normally negative intrapharyngeal pressure *positive* during inspiration. Since negative airway pressure is important in generating the obstruction, conversion to positive pressure allows the pharyngeal constrictors to maintain airway patency (Fig. 67-2).

The disadvantages of this method are that many patients find the continuous "inflated" feeling uncomfortable and that wearing a mask is cumbersome and may cause some compliance problems.[50] Several commercial devices are now available at a cost of about $1300. Many short-term and some long-term studies have demonstrated the efficacy of this device in eliminating apnea and improving daytime hypersomnolence.[50–53] One interesting finding that has emerged from these studies is that if the patient wears the mask for several nights, there is a decrease in the number of apneas on subsequent nights when the mask is not used. However, a return to the original symptomatic apnea state occurs 3 to 4 nights after discontinuing CPAP. Thus, the patient can sleep with CPAP "part time" and still benefit from the therapy.[50]

Surgical Treatment

Tracheotomy is the treatment of choice in patients with severe obstruction in whom weight loss and other medical approaches (particularly compliance with CPAP therapy) have failed. It is surprising to realize how recently this treatment was first described and that it is the only 100 percent curative procedure for obstructive sleep apnea.[54] Unfortunately, it has many problems, not the least of which is patient acceptance. The presence of a tracheostomy requires lifelong cleaning and care of the stoma and tube; can be complicated by infection, granulation tissue, and tracheal obstruction; can affect the voice; may be malodorous; and often results in increased tracheobronchial secretions. However, it does eliminate apnea, oxyhemoglobin desaturation,

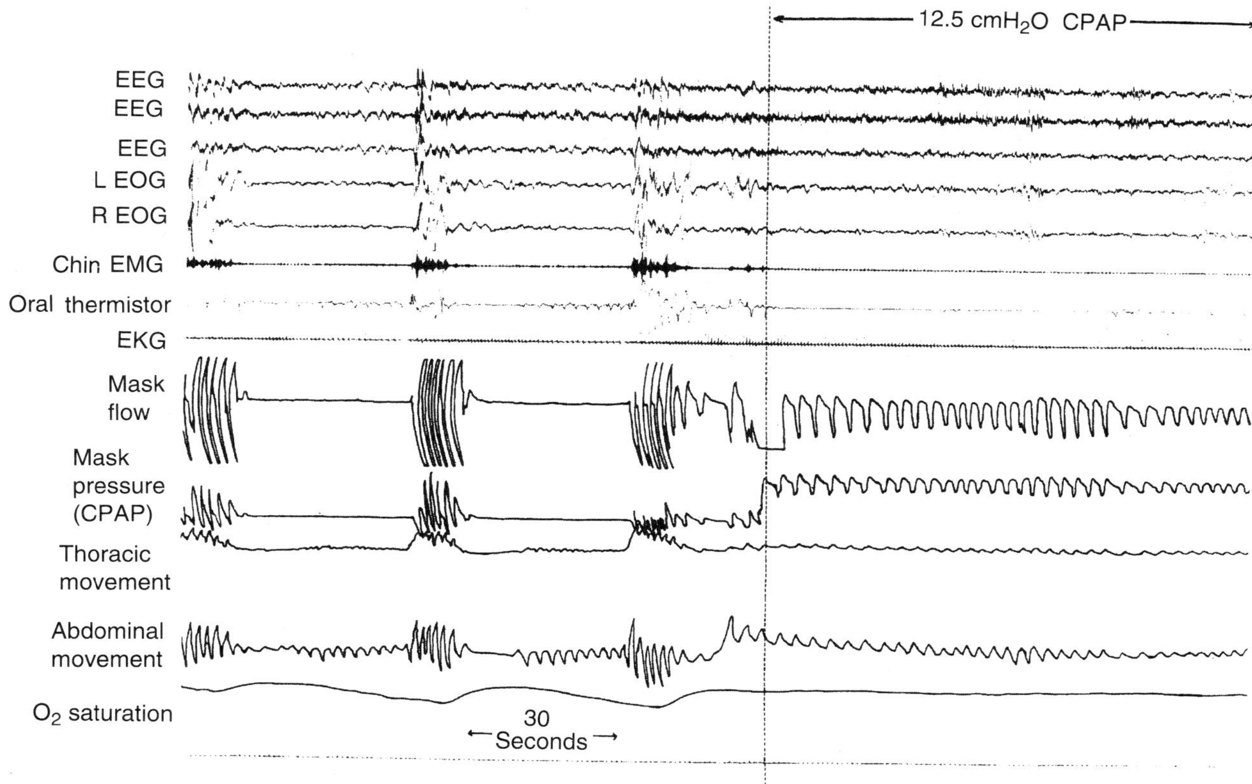

Figure 67-1. Polysomnogram of a patient with sleep apnea in whom nasal CPAP has been applied at the midpoint of the tracing. The top eight channels are EEG (first three channels), L electro-oculogram (EOG), R EOG, Chin EMG, oral thermistor, and EKG. Nasal airflow (mask flow) becomes regular following application of 12.5 cmH_2O CPAP. Also, on the right side of the figure there is disappearance of O_2 desaturation associated with the apneas. (From Rapoport et al.,[98] with permission.)

and arrhythmias and regularizes sleep patterns.[55–57] Before considering tracheotomy, one or more of the following should be present. The patient should have moderate to severe symptoms, including somnolence, cerebral dysfunction resulting in social or economic impairment, evidence of pulmonary hypertension or cor pulmonale, and/or life-threatening arrhythmias during apnea; should be strongly motivated to be cured; and should have the capability of cleaning and caring for the stoma and tube.

Patients most likely to need tracheotomy are the massively obese with frequent apneas (e.g., more than 70/h), severe desaturation (e.g., less than 50 percent SaO_2 during apnea), and definite signs of pulmonary hypertension and cor pulmonale. A more recent use of tracheotomy is as a temporizing measure to protect the airway during anesthesia while other surgical procedures, such as uvulopalatopharyngoplasty (UPPP) or mandibular advancement, are carried out in an attempt to eliminate the apnea. Patients with a tracheostomy who have apnea and intrinsic lung disease should be examined for continued oxyhemoglobin desaturation during REM sleep, which may require supplemental O_2 therapy.[58]

Several reports have shown that septoplasty and other procedures aimed at opening the nasal airways resulted in amelioration or cure of the apnea; however, cases have also been reported in which elimination of the obstruction did not correct the apnea.[59,60] It has been demonstrated that nasal obstruction induces or worsens apnea in asymptomatic individuals.[61,62] One explanation of this is based on the observation that airflow or pressure changes over the nasal mucosa increase the EMG activity of the pharyngeal and genioglossus muscles, while absence of airflow has the opposite effect; thus, reduced airflow through the nasal passages could increase the negative pressure/EMG ratio by reducing EMG activity. An alternative explanation is that simple mechanical obstruction could lead to increased pharyngeal resistance, which would in turn increase the negative pressure/EMG ratio.[63,64]

The application of UPPP to patients with obstructive sleep apnea was first described in 1981 by Fujita.[65] The procedure consists of removal of the tonsils or tonsillar bed, removal of excessive mucosal tissue from the posterior pharynx (the "pharyngeal tuck"), and shortening of the soft palate by removal of its mucosal portion distal to the tensor veli palatini (Fig. 67-3). Success may be defined either by subjective improvement in clinical symptoms or objective elimination

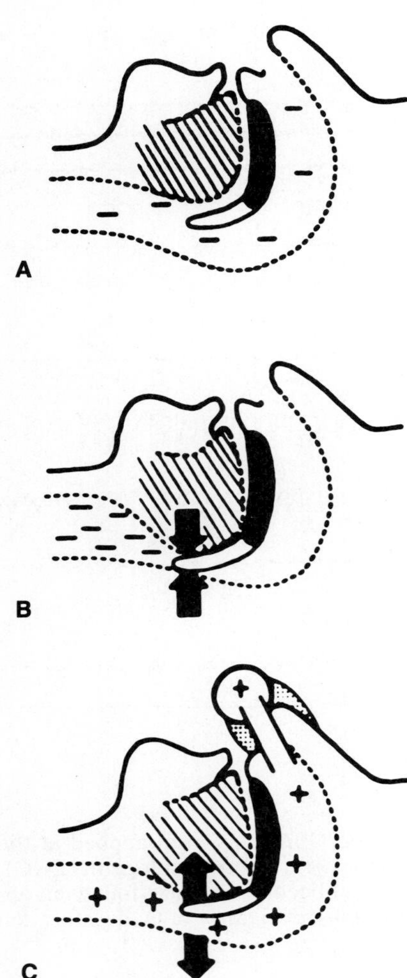

Figure 67-2. Representation of the mechanism of action of nasal CPAP in preventing upper airway closure during inspiration. **(A)** Normal negative inspiratory pressure generated by the thoracic cage and diaphragm. **(B)** Collapse involving the soft palate and genioglossus muscle opposing the posterior pharyngeal wall. **(C)** Effect of CPAP in maintaining positive pressure within the airway throughout inspiration, thus preventing inspiratory collapse. (From Sullivan et al.,[49] with permission.)

or amelioration of apneas as evaluated by polysomnography. The former criterion indicates that UPPP has roughly a 90 percent success rate but, according to the latter criterion, the procedure is successful less than 50 percent of the time. Table 67-2 was compiled from some recent reports in the literature on follow-up sleep studies made 2 to 4 months postoperatively.[65–70] The failure rate in terms of elimination of apnea is quite high for a surgical procedure that may cost $5000 or more and carries some risk. One study reports initial improvement at 3 months postsurgery, with deterioration of apnea parameters in two of four patients studied at 1 year.[70]

Complications of UPPP include the usual anesthetic problems, with special attention to difficult intubation, postsurgical apnea (criteria must be developed for those patients who should have concomitant tracheotomies to protect the airway postoperatively), postoperative nasal speech and nasal reflux, and postoperative hemorrhage and infection. None of the reports on this procedure provide detailed information on complication rates.[65–70] Patients most likely to benefit from UPPP are those with fewer than 30 apneas per hour or those who do not exceed 130 percent of ideal body weight. The probable reason for failure with this procedure is that airway obstruction may not be at the level affected by surgery—that is, it may be occurring in the lower oropharynx and hypopharynx. Of 1000 patients with sleep apnea referred to the Stanford Sleep Disorders Center, 6 percent had mandibular defects and 32 percent had borderline overjets that may contribute to apnea. The latest approach is to find methods to better define the area of obstruction before surgery so that a comprehensive plan can be formulated.

Several studies have been published on the application of maxillofacial surgical procedures to enlarge the airway behind the tongue. This is accomplished in several ways: advancing the mandible, pulling the genioglossus forward, or sectioning the hyoid with splinting of the pieces outward to widen the hypopharyngeal space. Detailed descriptions of these methods are beyond the scope of this chapter, and the reader is referred to other sources for a more complete description of these techniques.[71–76] Surgical procedures aimed at enlarging the upper airway in patients with sleep apnea but no gross anatomic abnormalities must be considered experimental until more data are available on success, morbidity, and long-term outcome.

Nocturnal Mechanical Ventilation

In the early 1970s it would have been ludicrous to talk about home nocturnal ventilation. Four things have occurred to change our concepts in this regard. First, the postpoliomyelitis era saw the development of smaller, more efficient, and more portable ventilators. Positive-pressure ventilators have been developed and refined that allow control of tidal volume, assist/control, intermittent mandatory ventilation, and control of pressure limits and that provide reliable alarms. At present virtually any type of ventilator can be selected to fit individual needs, and home ventilation is a reality[77–79] (see Ch. 101). Second, improved salvage of patients with acute respiratory failure in critical care units has provided a large population of patients with borderline respiratory function. Third, the increased popularity of sleep disorders studies and research into all aspects of nocturnal disordered breathing has alerted us that patients without obvious daytime respiratory failure can be profoundly hypoxemic at night. This may take the form of nocturnal alveolar hypoventilation with continuous nocturnal hypoxemia, REM-related nonapneic desaturation due to hypoventilation and abnormalities of gas exchange (see Ch. 27, Table 27-4), and intermittent central and obstructive apnea. Fourth, it has been recognized that many of these patients need not use continuous artificial ventilation. Intermittent ventilation dur-

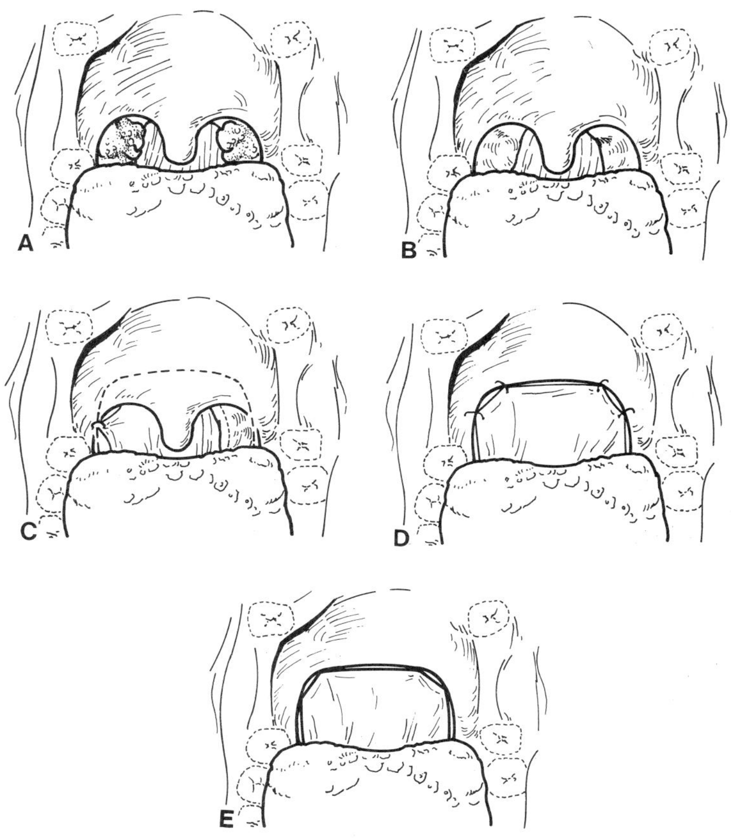

Figure 67-3. Diagram of the surgical steps in uvulopalatopharyngoplasty. **(A)** Oropharyngeal cavity. **(B)** Tonsilar tissue removed. **(C)** Tonsilar fossa closed and membranous portion of the soft palate marked for excision. **(D)** Membranous portion of the soft palate removed and posterior pharyngeal wall stretched and sutured over tonsilar beds. **(E)** Finished procedure. (From Thawley and Shepard,[98] with permission.)

ing the day or night with rest of the respiratory muscles may provide enough correction of blood gas abnormalities to stave off the symptomatic and hemodynamic consequences of chronic respiratory failure.[80]

The combination of these four developments in pulmonary research has led to the use of nocturnal ventilation in a variety of situations in which nocturnal hypoxemia may be the prime factor in worsening of pulmonary vascular hemodynamics, deterioration of daytime blood gases, and the daytime presence of fatigue and hypersomnolence. Such diseases include COPD,[81,82] diaphragmatic paralysis and several types of muscular dystrophy,[83–86] severe kyphoscoliosis,[87,88] alveolar hypoventilation syndromes,[88] and restrictive lung disease.[89]

Two types of ventilators can be used to assist nocturnal ventilation. Negative-pressure ventilators include the iron

Table 67-2. Current Reported Success Rate for Uvulopalatopharyngoplasty

Group	Year	Subjective Improvement	Apneas Decreased 50%	Apneas "Cured"	No Change in Apnea Frequency
Fujita et al.,[65] Detroit	1981	12/12	8/12	4/12	4/12
Zorick et al.,[66] Detroit	1983	27/31	16/31		15/31
Guilleminault et al.,[67] Stanford	1983	31/35		15/35	9/35
Dinner et al.,[68] Cleveland	1984	8/8	2/8	0/8	3/8
Kramer et al.,[69] Univ Miss	1984		9/13		
Thorpy et al.,[70] Einstein	1984	15/15		6/15	
Overall		93/101	35/64	25/70	31/86

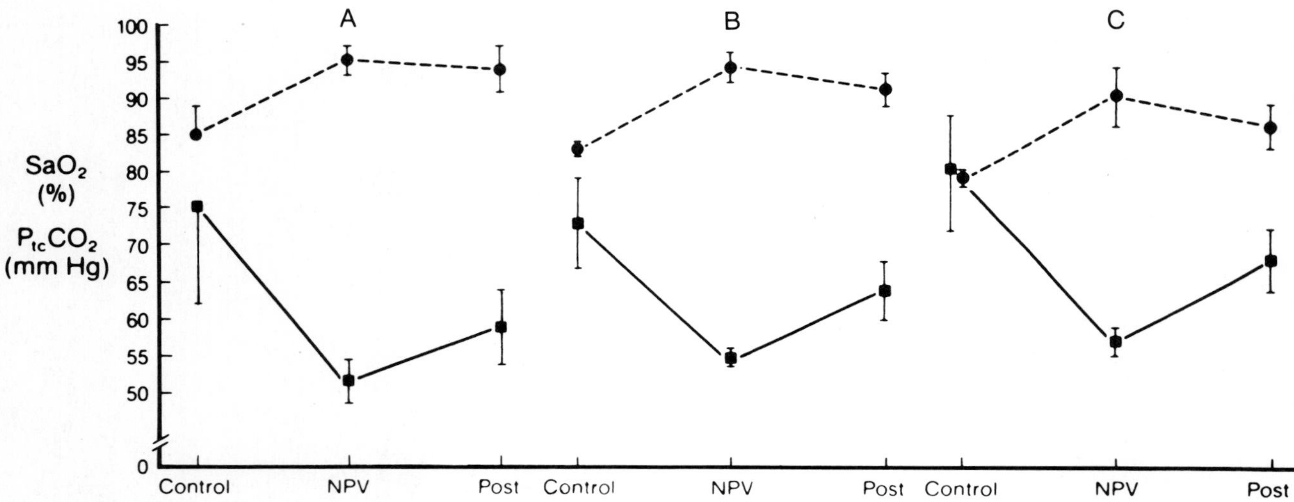

Figure 67-4. Mean nocturnal SaO_2 (dashed lines) and $PaCO_2$ (solid lines) in three patients with interstitial lung disease treated for 8 weeks with nocturnal negative pressure ventilation. The "control" night represents mean SaO_2 and PCO_2 before treatment. The "NPV" night represents a full night of sleep while on therapy during the 8-week period. The "post" night is the first night off of ventilator therapy; **(A)** awake, **(B)** non-REM sleep, and **(C)** during REM sleep. There is normalization of SaO_2 during awake period and both sleep types. Transcutaneous PCO_2 does not completely normalize. The improvement is carried over for the first night off the ventilator. (From Goldstein et al.,[93] with permission.)

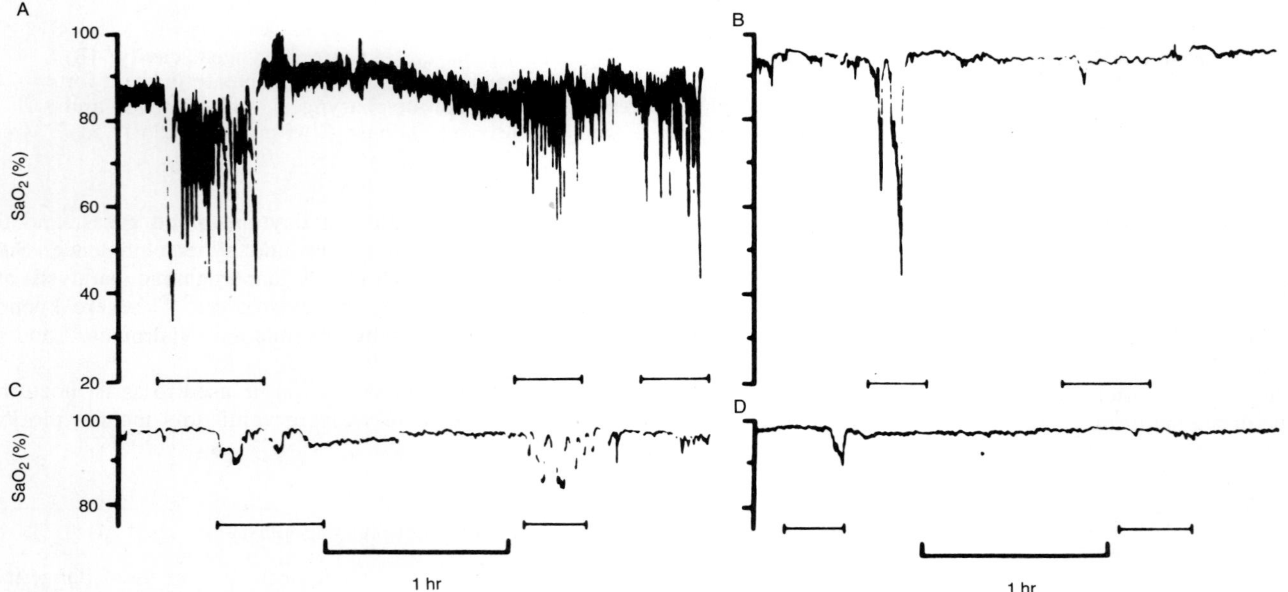

Figure 67-5. Slow-speed oximeter tracings of a patient treated three different ways. **(A)** Baseline SaO_2 without ventilator support shows and frequent 3 to 4 percent oscillations (creating the heavy black line), probably caused by repeated hypopneas, and marked REM desaturation to below 40 percent. **(B)** Another night with the assistance of a cuirass ventilator. Saturation improves and the hypopneas disappear, but REM desaturation is still present. **(C)** Positive-pressure ventilation through a mouth seal still allows some REM desaturation. **(D)** Positive-pressure ventilation through a nose seal (similar to a CPAP mask) virtually eliminates the REM desaturation. (From Ellis et al.,[94] with permission.)

lung of poliomyelitis days, cuirass or shell ventilators, body suits, and custom-made fiberglass shells to fit the thorax. Negative-pressure ventilators have offered numerous problems, not the least of which is poor comfort, convenience, and accessibility. The respirator is not synchronized with the patient's ventilatory effort and for this reason may predispose to the development of obstructive apnea during sleep.[90,91] Similar upper airway obstruction has been seen in patients treated for respiratory failure with diaphragmatic stimulation.[92] Positive-pressure type ventilators offer greater portability, more convenience, and better control. However, tracheotomy has been assumed necessary to gain control of the airway for using positive-pressure ventilation, since face masks have led to difficulty in swallowing, dry mouth, facial pain, air swallowing, and significant air leaks. This has led to renewed interest in noninvasive methods, and recent interesting reports indicate alternative ways to achieve adequate nocturnal ventilation.

Goldstein and colleagues[93] report the use of cuirass or poncho ventilators during sleep in five patients with chronic interstitial lung disease and daytime hypoxemia and hypercarbia. The problem of upper airway obstruction was overcome with the use of protriptyline in one patient and nasal CPAP in the other four. In addition to a marked improvement in daytime symptoms, the notable part of this study was the improvement in chronic daytime blood gases despite no detectable improvement in the underlying lung disease (Fig. 67-4). This improvement in blood gases, which has been observed previously, is an important consideration in deciding when to use home nocturnal ventilation.[83,88]

In an acute study, Ellis and colleagues[94] compared negative-pressure (cuirass) ventilation to positive-pressure ventilation administered by a nasal CPAP mask in five patients with neuromuscular disease. They found fewer complications (better avoidance of airway obstruction) with the positive-pressure ventilator. The CPAP mask appeared to be a comfortable method of administering the positive pressure. As with the previous study, significant improvement in daytime PaO_2 and $PaCO_2$ was noted. Of note is that positive pressure proved superior to negative pressure in improving REM desaturation, a finding that supports the concept that decreases in functional residual capacity and worsening of gas exchange cause this desaturation (Fig. 67-5). A 6-month study in which a similar group and number of patients were given positive-pressure ventilation via CPAP mask has produced similar results.[95]

ORGANIZED APPROACH TO DIAGNOSIS AND TREATMENT OF SLEEP-DISORDERED BREATHING

Limitations of space prevent a complete discussion of the finer points of the workup of sleep-related breathing problems; for such a discussion the reader is referred to other sources.[96] As in any medical problem, the first part of the workup is a detailed history and physical examination. As stated above, the history not only gives the interviewer the necessary constellation of symptoms to justify ordering a formal polysomnogram but also provides a guide to the type of treatment required once a definitive diagnosis is established. For example, mild subjective sleepiness and snoring in a young obese man might be treated with weight loss alone or in combination with the temporary use of a drug such as protriptyline. On the other hand, a history of three automobile accidents, loss of job, and marital discord may mandate an immediate trial of CPAP or tracheotomy with UPPP. Documentation of cor pulmonale or the appearance of nocturnal arrhythmias might indicate the need for immediate tracheotomy.

Important factors influencing the clinician that may be revealed by the physical examination include the presence and degree of obesity, systemic hypertension, and correctable upper airway pathology; signs of cardiac or pulmonary disease that might worsen the cardiovascular sequelae of SAS; signs of systemic diseases such as hypothyroidism and acromegaly, that may *cause* sleep apnea; and signs of congestive heart failure. The presence of surgically correctable upper airway pathology such as nasal polyps or a soft palate tumor would certainly influence therapy. A minimum list of laboratory tests that may help the clinician in determining the severity of end-organ damage from disordered breathing would be an ECG, a chest radiograph, pulmonary function tests in smokers, resting arterial blood gases, and a radionuclide determination of right ventricular ejection fraction.

The formal sleep study is to the polysomnographer what the ECG is to the cardiologist and the chest radiograph is to the pulmonologist. It confirms the diagnosis and establishes severity by giving the number and duration of apneic episodes and the level of nadir saturation, which can be used in a general way to classify the severity of the breathing disorder. No specific criteria can be given to delineate the severity of the apnea based on number of episodes, but a very general classification would consider less than 150 apneas per night and lowest SaO_2 above 80 percent as mild, whereas upward of 350 to 400 apneas per night with lowest SaO_2 less than 50 percent would be considered severe. Of course, symptomatology will heavily shade this classification. Also, the presence of arrhythmias clearly induced by apnea may be an overriding factor in classification of severity.

One of the most important points in deciding what therapy to recommend to a patient is to know when *not* to treat. Basically, all treatments, with the exception of weight loss, carry side effects or are somewhat cumbersome to use (e.g., nasal CPAP); therefore one cannot expect to improve on the asymptomatic state with a treatment or device that creates discomfort. Asymptomatic patients sometimes come to medical attention in the course of workup for other problems, for example, patients with impotence undergoing nocturnal penile tumescence studies. One exception to this rule is the asymptomatic patient with nocturnal malignant arrhythmias, although such patients will usually be symptomatic. Another problem to watch for is "perceived asymptomaticity"; these patients have had daytime hypersomnolence and intellectual dysfunction so long that they are unaware how badly they feel or how well they could feel. In such cases a history from a spouse or the MSLT could be of great advantage.

An additional concept is that of "routine" versus "urgent" treatment groups. Most patients will present with mild to moderate symptoms that may not be life-threatening (routine), and there will be time to try such therapies as drugs and dietary weight loss. From time to time, patients will present with advanced stages of cor pulmonale, severe daytime hypoxemia, or life-threatening arrhythmias. Such patients frequently have concomitant symptomatic cardiac or lung disease and require immediate aggressive therapy, including nasal CPAP or tracheotomy. Following successful institution of such therapy, dietary weight loss or upper airway surgery can be pursued without fear of sudden death during sleep.

With regard to the chronic lung disease patient, the presence of daytime hypoxemia will always indicate the presence of nocturnal hypoxemia, and from this standpoint patients with a daytime PaO_2 of less than 55 mmHg need no formal sleep study. In such cases, the use of supplemental O_2 during sleep will correct the vast majority of nocturnal desaturations. The patient with PaO_2 above 60 mmHg presents a different problem. First, such patients will rarely come to clinical attention because of the lack of symptoms and clinical findings that point to this condition.[97] Second, if they do somehow come to clinical attention, there is no proof that the condition will progress to pulmonary hypertension or that supplemental O_2 during sleep would prevent such progression. The most conservative posture at this time for patients with PaO_2 above 60 mmHg is to reserve nocturnal polysomnography and O_2 treatment for those who exhibit clear-cut signs of otherwise unexplained congestive heart failure.

References

1. Guilleminault C, Dement WC: Sleep apnea syndromes and related sleep disorders. pp. 9–26. In Williams RL, Karacan I (eds): Sleep disorders: Diagnosis and Treatment. John Wiley & Sons, New York, 1978
2. Association of Sleep Disorders Centers: Diagnostic classification of sleep and arousal disorders (1st Ed.) Sleep 1979;2:1–37
3. Berry DTR, Webb WB, Block AJ: Sleep apnea syndrome—a critical review of the apnea index as a diagnostic criterion. Chest 1984;86:529–31
4. Krieger J, Turlot JC, Mangin P, Kurtz D: Breathing during sleep in normal young and elderly subjects: Hypopneas, apneas, and correlated factors. Sleep 1983;6:108–120
5. Bliwise D, Carskadon M, Carey E, Dement W: Longitudinal development of sleep-related respiratory disturbance in adult humans. J Gerontol 1984;39:290–293
6. Guilleminault C, van den Hoed J, Mitler MM: Clinical overview of the sleep apnea syndromes. pp. 1–12. In Guilleminault C, Dement WC (eds): Sleep Apnea Syndromes. Alan R Liss, New York, 1978
7. Strohl KP, Saunders NA, Sullivan CE: Sleep apnea syndromes. pp. 365–394. In Saunders NA, Sullivan CE (eds): Sleep and Breathing. Marcel Dekker, New York, 1984
8. Martin RJ: Sleep-related respiratory disorders associated with daytime somnolence: Sleep apnea and hypoventilation syndromes. pp. 65–118. In Martin RJ (ed): Cardiorespiratory Disorders During Sleep. Futura Publishing, Mount Kisco, New York, 1984
9. Hudgel DW: Clinical manifestations of the sleep apnea syndrome. In Fletcher EC (ed): Abnormalities of Respiration During Sleep: Diagnosis, Pathophysiology, and Treatment. Grune & Stratton, Orlando, FL, 1986
10. Remmers JE, Anch AM, deGroot WJ: Respiratory disturbances during sleep. Clin Chest Med 1980;1:57–71
11. Block AJ: Respiratory disorders during sleep. Parts I & II. Heart Lung 1980;9:1011–1024 and 1981;10:90–96
12. Hudgel DW: Diagnosis and therapy of sleep apnea. J Fam Pract 1981;12:1001–1007
13. Tobin MJ, Cohn MA, Sackner MA: Breathing abnormalities during sleep. Arch Intern Med 1983;143:1221–1228
14. Orr WC, Moran WB: Diagnosis and management of obstructive sleep apnea: A multidisciplinary approach. Parts I & II. Arch Otolaryngol Head Neck Surg 1985;111:583–588
15. Kales A, Vela-Bueno A, Kales JD: Sleep disorders: Sleep apnea and narcolepsy. Ann Intern Med 1987;106:434–443
16. Lugaresi E, Coccagna G, Cirignotta F: Snoring and its clinical implications. pp. 13–21. In Guilleminault C, Dement WC (eds): Sleep Apnea Syndromes. Alan R Liss, New York, 1978
17. Block AJ: Snoring: Noisy or Noxious? Louis Mark Memorial Lecture. 52nd Annual Scientific Assembly, American College of Chest Physicians, San Francisco, 1986
18. Burwell D, Robin ED, Whaley RD, Bickelmann AG: Extreme obesity associated with alveolar hypoventilation: A pickwickian syndrome. Am J Med 1956;21:811–818
19. George CF, Nickerson P, Kryger MH: Sleep apnea patients have increased automobile accidents. Am Rev Respir Dis 1987; 139:A37
20. Mitler MM: The multiple sleep latency test as an evaluation for excessive somnolence. pp. 145–155. In Guilleminault C (ed): Sleeping and Waking Disorders: Indications and Techniques. Addison-Wesley, Menlo Park, CA, 1982
21. Browman CP, Gujavarty KS, Sampson MG, Mitler MM: REM sleep episodes during the maintenance of wakefulness test in patients with sleep apnea syndrome and patients with narcolepsy. Sleep 1983;6:23–28
22. Klink M, Quan SF: Prevalence of reported sleep disturbances in a general adult population and their relationship to obstructive airways diseases. Chest 1987;91:540–546
23. Browman CP, Sampson MG, Yolles SF et al: Obstructive sleep apnea and body weight. Chest 1984;85:435–436
24. Harman EM, Wynne JW, Block AJ: The effect of weight loss on sleep-disordered breathing and oxygen desaturation in morbidly obese men. Chest 1982;82:291–294
25. Peiser J, Lavie P, Ovnat A et al: Sleep apnea syndrome in the morbidly obese as an indication for weight reduction surgery. Ann Surg 1984;199:112–115
26. Jackson E, Schmidt H: Modification of sleeping position in the treatment of obstructive sleep apnea, abstracted. Sleep Res 1982;11:149
27. Cartwright RD, Samelson CF: The effects of a non-surgical treatment for obstructive sleep apnea. The tongue retaining device. JAMA 1982;248:705–709
28. White DP, Zwillich C, Pickett CK et al: Central sleep apnea: Improvement with acetazolamide therapy. Arch Intern Med 1982;142:1816–1819
29. Shore ET, Millman RP: Central sleep apnea and acetazolamide therapy (letter). Arch Intern Med 1983;143:1278
30. Whyte KF, Gould GA, Airlie MAA et al: A placebo controlled trial of protriptyline or acetazolamide in sleep apnea syndrome. Am Rev Respir Dis 1987;135:A36
31. Sutton FD Jr, Zwillich C, Creagh CE et al: Progesterone for outpatient treatment of pickwickian syndrome. Ann Intern Med 1975;83:476–479
32. Orr WC, Imes NK, Martin RJ: Progesterone therapy in obese patients with sleep apnea. Arch Intern Med 1979;139:109–111
33. Strohl K, Hensley MJ, Saunders NA et al: Progesterone administration and progressive sleep apneas. JAMA 1981; 245:1230–1232
34. Brownell LG, West P, Sweatman P et al: Protriptyline in obstructive sleep apnea: A double blind trial. N Engl J Med 1982; 307:1037–1042

35. Fletcher EC, Lavoi M, Zenner G et al: Protriptyline in the treatment of sleep apnea. Am Rev Respir Dis 1984;129:A59
36. Schmidt HS, Clark RW, Hyman PR: Protriptyline: An effective agent in the treatment of narcolepsy-cataplexy syndrome and hypersomnia. Am J Psychiatry 1977;134:183–185
37. Clark RW, Schmidt HS, Schaal SF, et al: Sleep apnea: Treatment with protriptyline. Neurology 1979;29:1287–1292
38. Smith PL, Gheris C, Haponik EF et al: Uvulopalatopharyngoplasty in sleep apnea. Am Rev Respir Dis 1983;127:85A
39. Alford NJ, Fletcher EC, Nickeson D: Effect of acute oxygen in patients with sleep apnea and chronic obstructive lung disease. Chest 1986;89:30–39
40. Martin RJ, Sanders MH, Gray BA et al: Acute and long-term ventilatory effects of hyperoxia in the adult sleep apnea syndrome. Am Rev Respir Dis 1982;125:175–180
41. Smith PL, Haponik EF, Bleecker ER: The effects of oxygen in patients with sleep apnea. Am Rev Respir Dis 1984;130:958–963
42. Taasan VC, Blovic AJ, Boysen PG, Wynne JW: Alcohol increases sleep apnea and oxygen desaturation in asymptomatic men. Am J Med 1981;71:240–245
43. Krol RC, Knuth SI, Bartlett D Jr: Selective reduction of genioglossal muscle activity by alcohol in normal human subjects. Am Rev Respir Dis 1984;129:247–250
44. Bonora M, Shields GI, Knuth SL et al: Selective depression by ethanol of upper airway respiratory motor activity in cats. Am Rev Respir Dis 1984;130:156–161
45. Guilleminault C, Silvestri R, Mondini S et al: Aging and sleep apnea: Action of benzodiazepine, acetazolamide, alcohol, and sleep deprivation in a healthy elderly group. J Gerontol 1984; 39:655–661
46. Mendelson WB, Ganett D, Gillin JC: Flurazepam-induced sleep apnea syndrome in a patient with insomnia and mild sleep-related respiratory changes. J Nerv Ment Dis 1981;169:261–264
47. Dolly FR, Block AJ: Effect of flurazepam on sleep-disordered breathing and nocturnal oxygen desaturation in asymptomatic subjects. Am J Med 1982;73:239–243
48. Fletcher EC, Munafo DA: The role of nocturnal oxygen therapy in obstructive sleep apnea. When should it be used? Chest 1990; 98:1497–1504
49. Sullivan CE, Berthon-Jones M, Issa FG et al: Reversal of obstructive sleep apnea by continuous positive airway pressure applied through the nares. Lancet 1981;1:862–865
50. Sanders MH, Gruendl CA, Rogers RM: Patient compliance with nasal CPAP therapy for sleep apnea. Chest 1986;90:330–333
51. Rajagopal KR, Bennett LL, Dillard TA et al: Overnight nasal CPAP improves hypersomnolence in sleep apnea. Chest 1986; 90:172–176
52. Rapoport DM, Surkin B, Gasay SM et al: Reversal of the "pickwickian syndrome" by long term use of nocturnal nasal airway pressure. N Engl J Med 1982;307:931–933
53. Sullivan CE, Issa FG, Berthon-Jones M et al: Treatment of obstructive sleep apnea with continuous positive airway pressure applied through a nose-mask. Bull Eur Physiopathol Respir 1984;20:49–54
54. Kuhlo W, Doll E, Frame M: Erfolgreiche Behandlung eines Pickwicksyndrome durch eine dauertracheal Kanule. Dtsch Med Wochenschr 1969;94:1286–1290
55. Weitzman ED, Kahn E, Pollack CP: Quantitative analysis of sleep and sleep apnea before and after tracheostomy in patients with the hypersomnia-sleep apnea syndrome. Sleep 1980;3:407–423
56. Guilleminault C, Simmons FB, Motta J et al: Obstructive sleep apnea syndrome and tracheostomy. Arch Intern Med 1981; 141:985–989
57. Conway WA, Victor LD, Magillian DJ Jr et al: Adverse effects of tracheostomy for sleep apnea. JAMA 1981;246:347–350
58. Fletcher EC, Brown DL: Nocturnal oxyhemoglobin desaturation following tracheostomy for sleep apnea. Am J Med 1985; 79:35–42
59. Heimer D, Scharf SM, Lieberman A et al: Sleep apnea syndrome treated by repair of a deviated nasal septum. Chest 1983; 84:184–185
60. Simmons FB, Guilleminault C, Dement WC et al: Surgical management of airway obstructions during sleep. Laryngoscope 1977;87:326–338
61. Suratt PM, Turner BL, Wilhoit SC: Effect of intranasal obstruction on breathing during sleep. Chest 1986;90:324–329
62. Olsen KD, Kern EB, Westbrook PR: Sleep and breathing disturbance secondary to nasal obstruction. Arch Otolaryngol Head Neck Surg 1981;89:804–810
63. Zwillich CW, Pickett C, Hanson FN et al: Disturbed sleep and prolonged apnea during nasal obstruction in normal men. Am Rev Respir Dis 1981;124:158–160
64. McNicholas W, Coffey M, McDonnell T et al: Upper airway obstruction during sleep in normal subjects after selective topical oropharyngeal anesthesia. Am Rev Respir Dis 1987;135: 1316–1319
65. Fujita S, Conway W, Zorick F et al: Surgical correction of anatomic abnormalities in obstructive sleep apnea syndrome: Uvulopalatopharyngoplasty. Arch Otolaryngol Head Neck Surg 1981;89:923–934
66. Zorick F, Roehrs T, Conway W et al: Effects of uvulopalatopharyngoplasty on the daytime sleepiness associated with sleep apnea syndrome. Bull Eur Physiopathol Respir 1983;19:600–603
67. Guilleminault C, Hayes B, Smith L et al: Palatopharyngoplasty and obstructive sleep apnea syndrome. Bull Eur Physiopathol Respir 1983;19:595–599
68. Dinner DS, Luders H, Morris HH, Lesser RP: Polysomnograms before and after uvulo-palato-pharyngoplasty for obstructive sleep apnea. Sleep Res 1984;13:139A
69. Kramer M, Blumenthal B, Schoen L, Weisenberger S: Comparison of ENT examination, CT scan, and lateral neck x-rays in identifying upper airway pathology in sleep apnea. Sleep Res 1984;13:151A
70. Thorpy MJ, Scher A, Spielman AJ: Uvulopalatopharyngoplasty (UPPP) for obstructive sleep apnea: II. Early results. Sleep Res 1984;13:171A
71. Wittig R, Wolford G, Conway W et al: Mandibular advancement as a treatment for sleep apnea syndrome. Sleep Res 1983; 12:296A
72. Riley R, Guilleminault C, Powell N: Mandibular osteotomy and hyoid bone advancement for obstructive sleep apnea: A case report. Sleep 1984;7:79–82
73. Powell N, Guilleminault C, Riley R et al: Mandibular advancement and obstructive sleep apnea syndrome. Bull Eur Physiopathol Respir 1983;19:607–610
74. Spire JP, Kuo PC, Campbell N: Maxillofacial surgical approach: An introduction and review of mandibular advancement. Bull Eur Physiopathol Respir 1983;19:604–606
75. Kaya N: Sectioning of the hyoid bone as a therapeutic approach for obstructive sleep apnea. Sleep 1984;7:77–78
76. Patton TJ, Thawley SE, Waters RC et al: Expansion hyoidplasty: A potential surgical procedure designed for selected patients with obstructive sleep apnea syndrome. Experimental canine results. Laryngoscope 1983;93:1387–1396
77. Shea TA, Becker E: Choosing the mechanical ventilator system. pp. 153–184. In Johnson DL, Giovanni R, Driscoll SA (eds): Ventilation Assisted Care: Planning for Hospital Discharge and Home Care. Aspen Publication, Rockville, MD, 1986
78. Splaingard ML, Frates RC Jr, Jefferson LS et al: Home negative pressure ventilation: Report of 20 years experience in patients with neuromuscular disease. Arch Phys Med Rehabil 1985; 66:239–242
79. Splaingard ML, Frates RC Jr, Harrison GM et al: Home positive pressure ventilation—20 years experience. Chest 1983;84: 376–382
80. Marino W, Braun NMT: Reversal of the clinical sequelae of respiratory muscle fatigue by intermittent mechanical ventilation. Am Rev Respir Dis 1982;125:A85
81. Braun NMT, Marino W: Effect of daily intermittent rest of respiratory muscles in patients with chronic airflow limitation (CAL). Chest, Suppl. 1984;85:595S
82. Rabinovitch B, Pardy RL, Hussain SNA, Macklem PT: The

acute effects of rest on ventilatory muscle function in patients with severe chronic airflow limitation. Physiologist 1983;26:21A
83. Curran FJ: Night ventilation by body respirators for patients in chronic respiratory failure due to late stage Duchenne muscular dystrophy. Arch Phys Med Rehabil 1981;62:270–274
84. Alexander MA, Johnson EW, Petty T, Stauch D: Mechanical ventilation of patients with late stage Duchenne muscular dystrophy: Management in the home. Arch Phys Med Rehabil 1979; 60:289–292
85. Skatrud JL, Iber C, McHugh N et al: Determinants of hypoventilation during wakefulness and sleep in diaphragmatic paralysis. Am Rev Respir Dis 1980;121:587–593
86. Weirs PWJ, Le Coultre R, Dalliga OJ et al: Cuirass respiratory treatment of chronic respiratory failure in scoliotic patients. Thorax 1977;32:221–228
87. Hoeppner VH, Cockcroft DW, Dosman JA, Cotton DJ: Nighttime ventilation improves repiratory failure in secondary kyphoscoliosis. Am Rev Respir Dis 1984;129:240–243
88. Garay S, Turino GT, Goldring R: Sustained reversal of chronic hypercapnia in patients with alveolar hypoventilation syndromes: Long-term maintenance with noninvasive mechanical ventilation. Am J Med 1981;70:269–274
89. Sawicka EH, Branthwaite MA, Spencer GA: Respiratory failure after thoracoplasty: Treatment by intermittent negative pressure. Thorax 1983;38:433–435
90. Glenn WL, Gee JB, Cole DR et al: Combined central alveolar hypoventilation and upper airway obstruction. Am J Med 1978; 64:50–60
91. Scharf SM, Feldman NT, Goldman MD et al: Vocal cord closure: A cause of upper airway obstruction during controlled ventilation. Am Rev Respir Dis 1978;117:391–397
92. Hyland RH, Hutcheon MA, Perl A et al: Upper airway occlusion induced by diaphragm pacing for primary alveolar hypoventilation: Implications for the pathogenesis of obstructive sleep apnea. Am Rev Respir Dis 1981;124:180–185
93. Goldstein RS, Molotiu N, Skrastins R et al: Reversal of sleep-induced hypoventilation and chronic respiratory failure by nocturnal negative pressure ventilation in patients with restrictive ventilatory impairment. Am Rev Respir Dis 1987;135:1049–1055
94. Ellis ER, Bye PTP, Bruderer JW, Sullivan CE: Treatment of respiratory failure during sleep in patients with neuromuscular disease. Am Rev Respir Dis 1987;135:148–152
95. Kerby GR, Mayer LS, Pingleton SK: Nocturnal positive pressure ventilation via nasal mask. Am Rev Respir Dis 1987; 135:738–740
96. Fletcher EC: Sleep apnea treatment algorithm. pp. 141–154. In Fletcher EC (ed): Abnormalities of Respiration During Sleep: Diagnosis, Pathophysiology, and Treatment. Grune & Stratton, Orlando, FL, 1986
97. Fletcher EC, Miller J, Divine GW et al: Nocturnal oxyhemoglobin desaturation in COPD patients with arterial oxygen tensions above 60 torr. Chest 1987;92:604–608
98. Rapoport DM, Garay SM, Goldring RM: Nasal CPAP in obstructive sleep apnea: Mechanisms of action. Bull Eur Physiopathol Respir 1983;19:616–620
99. Thawley SE, Shepard JW Jr: Understanding the sleep apnea syndrome: Causes and treatment. VA Practitioner 1985;Jan: 60–83

Chapter 68

Clinical Approach to Respiratory Infections

Jan V. Hirschmann

CHAPTER OUTLINE

This chapter extends the material in Chapter 36 to provide the clinician with an approach to the patient with respiratory infection. The approach is based on an understanding of basic mechanisms of infectious disease and a familiarity with the characteristics of the specific conditions covered in the earlier chapter. Four main categories of infection are covered here—community-acquired pneumonia, hospital-acquired pneumonia, thoracic empyema, and tuberculosis. For more comprehensive treatment of these and other respiratory infections the reader is referred to recent texts on infectious diseases[1,2] and excellent sections in current textbooks of internal medicine.[3,4]

Not covered here is the approach to infections in the immunocompromised host, including individuals infected with the human immunodeficiency virus (HIV), which is the subject of Chapter 69. Both the approach to and protocols for infection control in respiratory care are covered in Chapter 97.

COMMUNITY-ACQUIRED PNEUMONIA

It is useful to characterize pneumonias as community-acquired or hospital-acquired, because the likely organisms responsible are very different and, therefore so is the therapeutic approach. In both circumstances the major goal is to make a reasonable presumptive diagnosis and institute prompt, appropriate therapy as indicated, since a precise laboratory confirmation of the cause usually requires at least 24 hours and often up to several weeks. As indicated in Chapter 36, the basic information to obtain, in addition to a thorough history and physical examination, includes a complete white blood cell count with differential, sputum for Gram stain and culture, a chest radiograph, blood cultures in patients requiring hospitalization, and arterial blood gas measurements in those with suspected hypoxemia.

Examination of Sputum

Although the white blood cell count and the chest radiographic appearance may be somewhat helpful in differentiating among causes of community-acquired pneumonias, an accurate presumptive diagnosis usually rests on the history and the results of the sputum Gram stain. In pneumonias due to inhalation of airborne pathogens, the major information needed to determine the cause is the history. The actual symptoms, being so similar in pneumonias due to most causes, are not very helpful, but the history of recent exposure to potential sources of infection is paramount. The clinician should inquire carefully about the patient's occupation and hobbies, recent exposure to animals (including birds), illness in the family or close contacts, and recent travel or residence in areas where certain pathogenic soil organisms are known to dwell, such as the southwestern United States for the fungus *Coccidioides immitis*. As indicated in Chapter 36, these pieces of information are critically important because airborne pathogens causing pneumonia are usually not visible on sputum Gram stain, do not grow on conventional media for isolation of bacteria, typically grow slowly on the appropriate special culture media (if isolation is attempted), and are often definitively implicated as the cause of pneumonia only in retrospect by serologic testing.

For pneumonias developing from the aspiration of organisms present in the upper respiratory tract, the most important information in making an accurate presumptive diagnosis derives from careful examination of the sputum Gram stain.[5] A good specimen shows more than 25 neutrophils and fewer than 10 epithelial cells per low-power field ($\times 100$). Indeed, in a good sample the leukocytes should outnumber the squamous epithelial cells by a ratio of more than 5:1. Samples with more numerous squamous epithelial cells (which arise from the upper airway, not the tracheobronchial tree) are too contaminated with upper respiratory secretions to reliably reflect the organisms present in the lung. If the specimen is a good one, as judged by these criteria, the next step is to evaluate the adequacy of staining. The nuclei of neutrophils should be gram-negative (red). Blue nuclei mean that the stain has been inadequately decolorized with the acetone or acid-acetone solution used in the Gram staining process. Since sputum is difficult to decolorize uniformly, most specimens will inevitably have areas in which the neutrophils' nuclei are blue. The examiner should seek another portion in which the nuclei are red; if none exists, the specimen requires restaining.

The examiner should evaluate those areas of the stain in which leukocytes abound and ignore the portions in which squamous epithelial cells are present, since oropharyngeal flora tends to adhere to and cluster around these cells. When scrutinizing areas in which only leukocytes are present, the examiner should determine whether any organism clearly predominates. Most sputum specimens from patients with pneumonia will show more than one type of bacteria, but usually one kind clearly predominates. The examiner infers, usually correctly, that this predominant organism is the cause of the pneumonia, especially if there are at least 10 of these bacteria per oil immersion field ($\times 1000$) in the areas of abundant leukocytes. This density of organisms corresponds to the growth of at least 10^5 colony-forming units (bacteria) per milliliter of sputum on culture.[5] Table 68-1 summarizes the interpretation of Gram stain results.

The sputum Gram stain is very important in evaluating the information from the sputum culture, which is often meaningless or misleading without it. First, it demonstrates, by the criteria mentioned above, whether the specimen emanates from the lower respiratory tract and thus whether it accurately reflects the flora of the pneumonia. Specimens judged as inadequate by these criteria should not be cultured. Second, some pathogens, such as *Streptococcus pneumoniae* or *Haemophilus influenzae*, are fastidious and may be overgrown by other organisms. In fact, if the laboratory does not routinely culture the sputum on chocolate agar, *H. influenzae* will be missed altogether because it does not grow on blood-agar plates or on media, such as MacConkey's or EMB (eosin-methylene blue), used to isolate enteric gram-negative bacilli. The presence of abundant organisms with the typical morphology of pneumococci or *H. influenzae* on Gram stain along with their failure to grow on sputum culture suggests a delay in culturing the specimen, overgrowth by hardier organisms, sampling of a portion of the sputum that did not correspond to the areas of purulence, or some other technical problem. Relying only on the culture results and not the sputum Gram stain in this situation is misleading. Third, some organisms, such as *Moraxella catarrhalis*, may be dismissed as normal, nonpathogenic flora and not be further speciated unless a Gram stain demonstrates gram-negative diplococci as the predominant species. This finding will indicate that the bacteria on culture that look like the nonpathogenic *Neisseria* spp. found in normal subjects may really be a pure growth of *M. catarrhalis*, which also is part of the normal flora but potentially pathogenic. Fourth, the Gram stain may strongly suggest that the pneumonia is due to a mixture of aerobic and anaerobic bacteria because there

Table 68-1. Interpretation of Sputum Gram Stains

Predominant Organism	Probable Identity
Gram-positive, oval-shaped cocci in pairs	*Streptococcus pneumoniae* (pneumococcus)
Gram-positive cocci in chains	Group A or B streptococci
Gram-positive cocci in clusters	*Staphylococcus aureus*
Gram-negative, kidney-shaped cocci in pairs	*Moraxella catarrhalis* or *Neisseria meningitidis*
Gram-negative, pleomorphic coccobacilli	*Haemophilus influenzae*
Gram-negative bacilli, fairly uniform shape and size	Aerobic or facultative gram-negative bacilli (e.g., *Klebsiella, Pseudomonas, Escherichia coli*)
Abundant mixture of gram-positive and gram-negative cocci and bacilli	Mixed aerobic-anaerobic or purely anaerobic organisms, probable large-volume aspiration
Few or no organisms	Consider Prior antimicrobial therapy *Mycoplasma pneumoniae* *Legionella* pneumonia *Chlamydia pneumoniae* Psittacosis Q fever Viral cause Fungal infection Tuberculosis Noninfectious cause of pulmonary inflammation

are abundant organisms, both gram-positive and gram-negative, of varying morphology. Because anaerobic bacteria are always present in expectorated sputum and their isolation from such a specimen requires special techniques and is time-consuming and meaningless, their presence as potential pathogens can be strongly suggested only by the sputum Gram stain unless another kind of specimen is obtained, such as a transtracheal or transthoracic needle aspirate. Finally, the presence of few or no organisms on the sputum Gram stain in association with a culture showing only normal flora should make the clinician suspect several entities (Table 68-1).

The sputum Gram stain has several limitations. Even a good specimen occasionally fails to reflect accurately the flora of the pneumonia. Second, the Gram stain by itself cannot indicate whether a pneumonia is present, since bronchitis without lung parenchymal inflammation will cause purulent sputum, especially in patients with chronic bronchitis, whose tracheobronchial tree is normally colonized with pneumococci and *H. influenzae*. Determination of the presence of pneumonia rests not on the Gram stain but on the physical examination and, predominantly, the chest radiograph. Third, the sputum Gram stain and culture are not appropriate indices of successful antimicrobial therapy and should not be obtained routinely following therapy unless a superinfection is suspected. The sputum of patients receiving appropriate and successful therapy often becomes colonized with other organisms, especially gram-negative bacilli. Their presence on sputum Gram stain and culture is misleading and should not lead to a change in treatment in the absence of clinical evidence of a new pulmonary infection. Finally, many patients, because of weakness, poor cooperation, or the nature of the pneumonia itself, cannot provide a satisfactory sputum sample for examination and culture.

Selection of Antimicrobial Therapy

Once the history, sputum Gram stain, and other helpful information have been obtained, the clinician begins appropriate antimicrobial therapy. The general guideline should be to choose an agent with the narrowest spectrum of activity, the lowest toxicity, and the lowest cost. Some clinicians tend to treat all pneumonias with one or more agents possessing a broad spectrum of antimicrobial activity, such as a second- or third-generation cephalosporin, without carefully considering which organisms are likely to be present and which ones are not. This approach is unwise. Usually an astute clinician, using the information discussed in this chapter and in Chapter 36, can make a reasonable inference about the cause of a pneumonia. Use of an antimicrobial agent that kills much more than just the responsible pathogen is wasteful and potentially dangerous. Such drugs often eradicate the normal upper respiratory flora, which is replaced by organisms (especially gram-negative bacilli) that are resistant to the medication employed. Should pulmonary infection with these organisms develop, treatment is often difficult and mortality is high. Narrow-spectrum antimicrobial therapy causes less change in the resident flora. Widespread use of the broad-spectrum antimicrobials also affects other hospitalized patients in that the indigenous hospital flora becomes resistant to these agents, making infections that develop in other patients more difficult to treat and more often fatal. Furthermore, these medications are usually much more expensive than the narrow-spectrum agents, unnecessarily increasing the cost of medical care. Finally, they are often more toxic, and adverse effects may be more frequent. Aminoglycosides, the second- and third-generation cephalosporins, and other expensive broad-spectrum antibiotics are rarely indicated in community-acquired pneumonia.

Pneumonia due to *S. pneumoniae* (pneumococcus) can be presumptively diagnosed by the appearance of numerous oval (lancet-shaped) gram-positive diplococci on sputum Gram stain. It is best treated with penicillin. If the patient receives outpatient therapy, oral penicillin V or erythromycin (for penicillin-allergic patients) suffices in doses of 250 mg qid. For hospitalized patients procaine penicillin G, 600,000 U IM bid, or aqueous penicillin G, 600,000 U IV q6h, provides adequate therapy for this very susceptible organism even if bacteremia is present. Higher doses are not more effective and, by killing the normal upper respiratory flora, may predispose to superinfections by hospital-acquired gram-negative bacilli. Only for extrapulmonary infections such as endocarditis or meningitis are higher doses (usually 20 to 24 million U/d) indicated. For penicillin-allergic patients, clindamycin or a first-generation cephalosporin such as cefazolin can be used, although cephalosporins, because they are structurally similar to penicillins, should not be used for patients with a history of life-threatening penicillin allergy. Treatment for pneumococcal pneumonia often causes defervescence within 48 to 72 hours, but many patients will be febrile for up to 1 week or more, even without other complications.[6] Treatment for 1 week usually suffices, however, unless extrapulmonary infection is present. The chest radiographic abnormalities usually resolve by 6 weeks but occasionally only resolve later.[7] The mortality rate of pneumococcal pneumonia is less than 5 percent, but with bacteremia it is about 20 percent. Factors other than bacteremia that impose a higher mortality rate are multilobar involvement, old age, serious underlying disease, leukopenia, and infection with pneumococcus type 3.[8]

H. influenzae appears on sputum Gram stain as numerous pleomorphic ("many-shaped") gram-negative organisms ranging from coccoid (nearly round) to bacilli (rod-shaped). The bacilli are slender and variable in size, unlike enteric gram-negative rods such as *Escherichia coli* or *Klebsiella*, which tends to be plump and relatively uniform in length. Moreover, *H. influenzae* does not have the bipolar staining (intense staining at the ends but weak in the middle) sometimes seen with the enteric gram-negative bacilli. *H. influenzae* often appears in the cytoplasm of white blood cells, where it may be mistaken for granules on cursory examination. Both white blood cells and organisms are usually profuse, but the bacteria are often present in great numbers in the pink-staining mucus between white blood cells and may be overlooked without careful, systematic examination of the Gram stain. Most *H. influenzae* isolates from adults are susceptible to ampicillin, which can be given in a dose of 500 mg qid PO for outpatients or 1 g IV q4h for hospitalized patients. Since some strains of *H. influenzae*, especially in children, are ampicillin-resistant, other agents should be used in cases of known resistance, childhood infection, severe illness, or penicillin allergy. Choices include chloramphenicol, a second-generation cephalosporin (such as cefuroxime or cefamandole), tetracycline, and sulfamethoxazole-trimethoprim. Patients with *H. influenzae* pneumonia are commonly febrile longer than those with pneumococcal pneumonia, but by 1 week defervescence usually occurs. However, the chest radiographic abnormalities may require several weeks to resolve.[9]

M. catarrhalis appears as gram-negative, kidney-shaped diplococci on Gram stain. Since most isolates are resistant to penicillin, this agent should not be used for therapy unless the organism is known to be susceptible. Reasonable choices for treatment include a first-generation cephalosporin (e.g., cefazolin), tetracycline, erythromycin, and sulfamethoxazole-trimethoprim. This pneumonia is usually fairly mild, most patients respond rapidly to therapy, and the mortality rate is low.

The appearance of *Neisseria meningitidis* on Gram stain is indistinguishable from that of *M. catarrhalis*, and until the organism is identified, it is prudent to treat the patient as though *M. catarrhalis* were present. When *N. meningitidis* is identified, the drug of choice is penicillin G, although all agents listed above for *M. catarrhalis* are also effective against meningococci. The response to therapy is rapid and the mortality rate low.

Staphylococcus aureus appears on sputum Gram stain as gram-positive cocci in clusters. The treatment of this pneumonia is a penicillinase-resistant penicillin such as nafcillin in a dose of 2 g IV q4–6h. For penicillin-allergic patients, cephalothin or cefazolin is an adequate alternative. Some strains of *S. aureus* are resistant to these agents (methicillin-resistant); the drug of choice is then vancomycin, 1 g IV q12h. Clinical resolution of *S. aureus* pneumonia is typically slow, and complications of lung cavitation and empyema are common. At least 2 weeks of treatment is usually required.

Streptococci other than *S. pneumoniae* (pneumococcus) appear on Gram stain as chains of gram-positive cocci. Treatment should be aqueous penicillin G, 1 million U q6h. For penicillin-allergic patients a cephalosporin or vancomycin will suffice. Empyema formation is a common complication, typically requiring chest tube drainage.

When the normal mouth flora causes pneumonia because of aspiration, the organisms usually appear on sputum Gram stain as numerous gram-negative and gram-positive bacteria of all sizes and shapes. Anaerobic gram-positive cocci in chains (peptostreptococci) are usually much smaller than aerobic streptococci. The gram-negative bacilli are typically pleomorphic and often long and curved or spindle-shaped. Occasionally, small gram-positive cocci in chains will be the only organisms seen. Treatment with aqueous penicillin G in the same doses as for pneumococcal pneumonia is adequate for these mixed aerobic-anaerobic pneumonias. Most clinicians use 6 to 10 million U for necrotizing pneumonia or lung abscess. These lung infections may fail to respond to penicillin; in these cases or when patients are allergic to penicillin or are quite ill, clindamycin 600 mg IV q8h is the drug of choice. Treatment is continued for 3 to 6 weeks.

Facultative or aerobic gram-negative bacilli causing pneumonia are usually plump gram-negative rods of reasonably uniform size, often with bipolar staining (staining especially prominent at both ends). Different species of these organisms cannot be distinguished on Gram stain, although *Pseudomonas* spp. are usually thin and do not show bipolar staining. Accordingly, a clinician must use antibiotics with a wide spectrum of coverage against gram-negative bacilli when a pneumonia due to these organisms is suspected, until the specific cause is identified. This coverage should include agents active against *Pseudomonas aeruginosa*. Several combinations are reasonable, but perhaps the most reliable is an aminoglycoside such as gentamicin, tobramycin, or amikacin plus an antipseudomonal penicillin such as mezlocillin. The regimen can be adjusted when the organism and its susceptibilities are identified. Gram-negative bacillary pneumonia is ordinarily slow to respond to treatment, complications such as empyema and cavitation are common, and mortality is high.

In the pneumonias discussed below the Gram stain of sputum, if attainable, shows white blood cells with few or no organisms. The diagnosis must be suspected on the basis of history or other features. *Legionella* pneumonia is treated with erythromycin, 500 mg to 1 g q6h PO or IV, depending on the severity of illness. Rifampin 600 mg bid PO is often added for critically ill patients. Treatment should be continued for at least 2 weeks. The overall mortality for *Legionella* pneumonia is unknown, but for hospitalized patients it is about 15 percent.

Mycoplasma pneumoniae and *Chlamydia pneumoniae* pneumonias are treated with tetracycline 250 mg qid PO, doxycycline 100 mg bid, or erythromycin 500 mg q6h PO. For parenteral therapy erythromycin 500 mg IV q6h is satisfactory. Treatment is continued for 14 days. Response is usually rapid and the mortality rate very low. Psittacosis and Q fever are best treated by tetracycline 500 mg qid PO. Both usually show a rapid response to therapy, and in both the mortality rate is very low.

Sometimes the patient is unable to expectorate sputum, and no clinical clues suggest a specific diagnosis. In these situations erythromycin is a good choice if the patient is young, since that antibiotic will be effective against *Legionella, M. pneumoniae, C. pneumoniae,* and *S. pneumoniae*. In the older patient erythromycin is also a reasonable choice, but if *Legionella* and *Mycoplasma* seem unlikely, penicillin or a first-generation cephalosporin is a good alternative, especially since mixed aerobic-anaerobic and pneumococcal pneumonias are so likely in that population.

Currently, there is no effective specific treatment of pneumonia due to influenza, only supportive measures to maintain adequate oxygenation and hemodynamic stability. Amantadine, an oral antiviral agent, can reduce the duration and severity of symptoms when given early in the course of *uncomplicated* influenza, but its efficacy with influenza pneumonia is unknown.

The fungal infections most likely to present as acute pneumonia, coccidioidomycosis and histoplasmosis, generally resolve over a few days to weeks without therapy. For very severe disease intravenous amphotericin B may be required in doses of 0.5 mg/kg/d or 1 mg/kg qod. Few patients require such therapy, however.

PNEUMONIA IN HOSPITALIZED PATIENTS

The most likely causes of hospital-acquired pneumonia are facultative or aerobic gram-negative bacilli such as *P. aeruginosa* or *Klebsiella*, mixed aerobic-anaerobic infection from aspiration of large volumes of oropharyngeal contents, *S. aureus*, or *S. pneumoniae*. The basic evaluation includes blood cultures, chest radiography, complete blood count with white blood cell differential, and sputum for Gram stain and culture. The most important information for presumptive diagnosis comes from the sputum Gram stain. Usually, a good specimen will demonstrate a predominant organism, and antibiotic choice can be guided by the considerations discussed in the preceding sections. Often, however, a good specimen is unobtainable, and empiric therapy must be given. Unlike the empiric treatment of community-acquired pneumonia, penicillin, erythromycin, or a first-generation cephalosporin will not suffice because infection with gram-negative bacilli resistant to these agents is so common. Several different antimicrobial regimens are reasonable, but they should all probably include an aminoglycoside such as gentamicin, tobramycin, or amikacin, the choice depending on the antimicrobial susceptibility of gram-negative bacilli in the individual hospital. The agent to be combined with the aminoglycoside can be a first-, second-, or third-generation cephalosporin, an antipseudomonal penicillin such as mezlocillin, or an antistaphylococcal penicillin such as nafcillin or oxacillin. No combination is inherently superior, and the choice revolves around the nature of the individual hospital's flora, the kind of underlying disease in the patient, and the clinician's personal preferences.

A particularly difficult problem in hospitalized patients is accurate diagnosis of the presence of pneumonia and therefore of the necessity of antimicrobial therapy in patients with tracheal intubation in an intensive care unit. Tracheal tubes or tracheotomy impairs some major local defense mechanisms that keep the tracheobronchial tree sterile in normal people—glottic closure, forceful coughing, and effective mucociliary transport. Consequently, following intubation or tracheotomy, the tracheobronchial tree quickly becomes colonized with flora, often the gram-negative bacilli prominent in the hospital environment. These organisms may provoke tracheobronchial inflammation and therefore purulent sputum without causing pneumonia. The presence of purulent sputum alone in the absence of radiographic evidence of pneumonia, even with heavy growth of a potential pathogen, therefore does not warrant treatment with antimicrobial therapy, which typically results only in replacement of the organisms with ones resistant to the antimicrobial used. This alteration in flora is unaccompanied by any clinical benefit to the patient and means that a subsequent pneumonia might be more difficult to treat, since the organism may be resistant to multiple agents.

The diagnosis of pneumonia in intubated patients is difficult not only because purulent sputum is so often present in the absence of pneumonia but also for several other reasons. Pulmonary infiltrates due to a noninfectious cause, such as pulmonary edema, are often present and may be radiographically indistinguishable from a pneumonia. Good radiographic studies are difficult to obtain in intensive care units, since normally only portable radiographic equipment is available, which allows only an anteroposterior view without the benefit of a lateral film, and the lung fields are often partially obscured by wires and other medical monitoring equipment on the patient. Furthermore, patient positioning is frequently suboptimal, and even with good technique the presence of atelectasis and pleural fluid is often difficult to distinguish from parenchymal inflammation. Finally, patients in intensive care units commonly have fevers from sources other than lung infection such as intra-abdominal sepsis or infected intravenous catheter sites.

The presence of a pneumonia can, therefore, be a perplexing diagnosis to establish in intubated patients.[10] The diagnosis of pneumonia is almost certain if, in a patient with a new or progressive pulmonary infiltrate, one or more of the following is also present: (1) cultures of pleural fluid or blood positive for the same organism present in the tracheal aspirate; (2) radiographic cavitation; (3) histopathologic evidence of pneumonia or necrosis; or (4) new fever, leukocytosis, and purulent tracheal aspirate. The diagnosis of pneumonia is probably, but less certainly, correct if at the time of a new or progressive pulmonary infiltrate two of the following are present: (1) purulent tracheal aspirate; (2) a rise in body temperature of at least 1°C to at least 38.3°C; (3) an increase of at least 25 percent in white blood cell count in the peripheral blood. Patients with definite or probable pneumonia tend to have more neutrophils (usually at least 10 per high-power field [$\times 400$]) and bacteria (usually 1 or more organisms per oil field [$\times 1000$]) on sputum Gram stain than patients without pneumonia by the above criteria, but neither of these features clearly separates the two groups.

Using the criteria listed above and other elements of clinical judgment, the clinician determines whether a pneumonia is present, often with a great deal of residual uncertainty. Because sputum is so easily obtainable in intubated patients, the organisms seen on Gram stain and grown on culture usually accurately reflect the identity of those in the lung tissue. The infecting bacteria are most commonly aerobic or facultative gram-negative bacilli, and the principles listed above apply in choosing an appropriate antimicrobial regimen.

EMPYEMA

The basic principles in treating empyema are to employ adequate antimicrobial therapy and to institute effective drainage of the pleural cavity. Often the pleural fluid obtained by thoracentesis will demonstrate the responsible organism on Gram stain, permitting a confident, immediate presumptive diagnosis; nearly always a properly cultured sample will grow the organisms. The clinician should expel any air present in the syringe following successful thoracentesis and then send the syringe directly to the laboratory for aerobic and anaerobic cultures, as well as tuberculous or fungal ones, if indicated. If the empyema originates from an underlying pneumonia, the responsible organism may already be known from results of sputum Gram stain or culture. The appropriate antimicrobial therapy can be determined from this information.

Although small empyemas due to an organism very susceptible to antimicrobial agents will occasionally subside with antibiotic treatment alone, nearly all empyemas require drainage of the infected pleural fluid. Sometimes repeated thoracenteses will suffice, but usually some surgical therapy is necessary. One approach, usually the initial technique in acute empyemas, is to insert one or more intercostal tubes percutaneously into the pleural space and connect the tubes to water seal. If this technique fails or if the empyema has been present long enough for the pleural surfaces to adhere, rib resection may be employed. This procedure involves removal of a portion of the rib overlying the empyema (often under local anesthesia) and insertion of a very large chest tube, which is left open to the atmosphere. Another surgical approach is to perform a thoracotomy and remove the infected pleural contents in the operating room. Empyemas following pneumonia can usually be managed with intercostal tube drainage; those occurring as complications of thoracic surgery often require another thoracotomy.[11] Management of the pleural space in empyema and other conditions is discussed more thoroughly in Chapter 92.

TUBERCULOSIS

The diagnosis of pulmonary tuberculosis usually requires growth of the organism from expectorated sputum. A positive sputum smear stained by the Ziehl-Neelsen or fluorochrome technique, however, allows a presumptive diagnosis until growth of the organism 2 to 6 weeks later definitively establishes the diagnosis.

Effective antituberculosis therapy, which involves at least two drugs, requires 6 to 9 months for most patients.[12] For patients infected with *Myobacterium tuberculosis* susceptible to isoniazid and rifampin, a 9-month course of daily therapy with these two drugs will provide a cure in almost all cases. An alternative approach is daily isoniazid and rifampin for 1 or 2 months followed by twice weekly therapy for the remainder of the 9-month course. A shorter course is possible when isoniazid, rifampin, and pyrazinamide are given daily for 2 months followed by 4 months of daily or twice weekly isoniazid and rifampin. The regimens are more complicated and protracted in patients infected with organisms resistant to one or more of these drugs. Such a situation should be suspected in patients who apparently acquired their infection from others known to have resistant organisms, in patients who have received sporadic and unreliable treatment in the past, or in patients from areas where drug resistance is common, such as Haiti, Southeast Asia, and some portions of Latin America. The basic principle underlying tuberculosis chemotherapy is to use at least two agents effective against the tubercle bacillus to prevent resistance from developing, for which the risk is considerable if only one active medication is used. In cases of suspected drug resistance, three or more agents are used until drug susceptibility testing is completed, to ensure that at least two of the agents are effective against the infecting organism.

References

1. Mandell GL, Douglas RG, Bennett JE (eds): Principles and Practice of Infectious Diseases. 3rd Ed. Churchill Livingstone, New York, 1990
2. Pennington JE (ed): Respiratory Infections: Diagnosis and Management. 2nd Ed. Raven Press, New York, 1989
3. DuPont HL (ed): Part VII. Infectious diseases. In Kelley WN (ed): Textbook of Internal Medicine. 2nd Ed. JB Lippincott, Philadelphia, 1992
4. Wilson JD, Braunwald E, Isselbacher KJ et al (eds): Harrison's Principles of Internal Medicine. Section 5: Infectious Diseases. 12th Ed. McGraw-Hill, New York, 1991, pp. 447–834
5. Kalin M, Lindberg AA, Tunevall G: Etiological diagnosis of bacterial pneumonia by Gram stain and quantitative culture of expectorates. Scand J Infect Dis 1983;53:153–160
6. Murphy TF, Fine BC: Bacteremic pneumococcal pneumonia in the elderly. Am J Med Sci 1984;288:114–118
7. Jay SJ, Johanson WG, Pierce AK: The radiographic resolution of *Streptococcus pneumoniae* pneumonia. N Engl J Med 1975;293:798–801
8. Van Metre TE: Pneumococcal pneumonia treated with antibiotics. N Engl J Med 1954;251:1048–1052
9. Pearlberg J, Haggar AM, Saravolatz L et al: *Hemophilus influenzae* pneumonia in the adult. Radiology 1984;151:23–26
10. Salata RA, Lederman MM, Shlaes DM et al: Diagnosis of nosocomial pneumonia in intubated, intensive care unit patients. Am Rev Respir Dis 1987;135:426–432
11. Lemmer JH, Botham MJ, Orringer MB: Modern management of the adult thoracic empyema. J Thorac Cardiovasc Surg 1985;90:849–855
12. Bass JB, Farer LS, Hopewell PC, Jacobs RF: Treatment of tuberculosis infection in adults and children. Am Rev Respir Dis 1986;134:355–363

Chapter 69

Clinical Approach to the Immunocompromised Patient

Jan V. Hirschmann

CHAPTER OUTLINE

The immune defense mechanisms that protect the normal host from serious infection are complex, interconnected systems. When defective, they render the individual susceptible to invasive disease from various pathogens, depending on the nature of the impairment. A clinically useful, although somewhat simplistic, classification is obtained by categorizing these disorders as affecting primarily neutrophil function,[1] humoral immunity (B-cell disorders),[2] and cell-mediated immunity (T-cell disorders).[2]

NEUTROPENIA

Although patients may have congenital or acquired disorders of neutrophil function, the most common clinical problem is an inadequate number of neutrophils.[1] Neutropenia is defined as a granulocyte count of less than 3000/mm^3, but infectious complications occur predominantly when the count drops below 1000/mm^3 and especially below 500/mm^3. Patients are at greatest risk when the number falls below 100/mm^3. The likelihood of infection also depends on the rapidity of the decline in granulocyte number and especially on the duration of the neutropenia. The most common causes of neutropenia are cytotoxic agents used to treat cancer and other diseases; invasion of the bone marrow by malignant cells, causing decreased production of normal white blood cells; aplastic anemia; and idiosyncratic drug reactions. The risk of infection with severe neutropenia is primarily from bacteria, especially aerobic and facultative gram-negative bacilli and *Staphylococcus aureus*. With prolonged granulocytopenia, especially when the patient has received lengthy courses of antibiotics, fungal infections, particularly from *Candida* and *Aspergillus* spp., may develop.

Most commonly, infections in patients with severe neutropenia cause fever, sometimes with bacteremia, but without a clear site of origin. Occasionally the anorectal area may be inflamed or cellulitis may develop on the skin, but most febrile episodes remain unexplained and perhaps are due to bacteria that enter the bloodstream from the bowel lumen.

When bacteremia occurs, it is usually from facultative or aerobic gram-negative bacilli, especially *Escherichia coli, Klebsiella* spp., and *Pseudomonas aeruginosa*, but other gram-negative bacilli or *S. aureus* may be responsible. When pneumonia from these organisms occurs, pulmonary symptoms such as cough or physical signs such as auscultatory crackles usually indicate a lung source. The radiographic appearance is typically a unilateral, patchy pneumonia. Since the patient has few neutrophils, sputum production is commonly absent or very scant, and, while cavitation may sometimes occur, empyema is rare.

The management of febrile neutropenic patients requires initiation of empiric antibacterial therapy promptly after obtaining blood cultures. Cultures of the oropharynx or expectorated saliva are unhelpful in establishing a diagnosis if a pneumonia is present, since the organisms isolated may not correspond to those infecting the lung. The antimicrobial combination chosen depends on many factors, including the susceptibility of bacteria found in that hospital, but a common approach is to give an aminoglycoside (e.g., gentamicin, tobramycin, or amikacin) plus an antipseudomonal penicillin (e.g., ticarcillin, mezlocillin, or azlocillin). Some clinicians use a third-generation cephalosporin (e.g., ceftazidime), alone or combined with an aminoglycoside. Antibiotics are commonly continued until the patient's granulocyte count exceeds 500 to $1000/mm^3$.

If the patient remains febrile for several days despite these agents, many clinicians add empiric amphotericin B because of the possibility of an unrecognized fungal infection. Fungal lung infections in this setting are primarily due to *Aspergillus spp.*, which can cause a progressive pneumonia, single or multiple pulmonary nodules, which may cavitate, or the abrupt onset of pleuritic chest pain and hemoptysis resulting from this organism's remarkable tendency to invade pulmonary blood vessels, producing thrombosis and pulmonary infarction. Occasionally mucormycosis, an infection by a type of fungus (*Absidia, Mucor, Rhizopus*) belonging to the family Mucorales, causes a similar clinical picture. Pulmonary aspergillosis and mucormycosis are usually fatal despite therapy with amphotericin B. Bacterial pneumonias in granulocytopenic hosts also have a significant mortality, survival depending mainly on whether bone marrow function recovers briskly to reverse the granulocytopenia.

Humoral Immunodeficiency

A marked decrease in immunoglobulins, primarily IgG, renders the host susceptible to infection, especially by encapsulated bacteria. *Streptococcus pneumoniae, Haemophilus influenzae*, and *Neisseria meningitidis* are the most common pathogens in congenital or acquired primary hypogammaglobulinemia. Diminished IgG also occurs with chronic lymphocytic leukemia and multiple myeloma. IgG-deficient patients also are frequently infected with *S. aureus*, and infections with *E. coli* and *Klebsiella* can occur, particularly with multiple myeloma. With congenital or acquired primary hypogammaglobulinemia, sinusitis, otitis media, and bronchiectasis are common respiratory infections, but these are rare in patients with chronic lymphocytic leukemia or multiple myeloma. When patients with humoral immunodeficiency develop pneumonia, sputum typically is produced, since the neutrophils are unaffected, and the diagnosis is usually evident on the sputum Gram stain and culture.

Cell-Mediated Immunodeficiency (other than AIDS)

Although congenital forms of cell-mediated immunodeficiency occur, a more common cause is the use of corticosteroids, cytotoxic agents, or other immunosuppressive agents such as cyclosporine to treat disease or to prevent rejection of cardiac, renal, or other organ grafts. The cell-mediated immunodeficiency from the human immunodeficiency virus (HIV) is discussed later in this chapter.

The infections to which these patients are most susceptible vary according to the underlying cause of the immunodeficiency, but in general the pathogens causing pulmonary infections are *Nocardia asteroides, Mycobacterium tuberculosis* or *avium-intracellulare, Cryptococcus neoformans*, cytomegalovirus, *Pneumocystis carinii*, herpes simplex, and herpes zoster. In the most severely immunocompromised hosts simultaneous infection with several of these agents may occur. In endemic areas severely immunocompromised patients are also susceptible to infections with *Histoplasma capsulatum* and *Coccidioides immitis*.

Pulmonary Nocardiosis

N. asteroides is a filamentous, branching, aerobic, gram-positive bacillus that resides in the soil.[3] Infection follows inhalation of the organism, with most patients having an insidious onset of cough, sputum production, anorexia, and weight loss. The organism may spread hematogenously to other sites, primarily the brain, where it causes a cerebral abscess, or the skin and subcutaneous tissues, where it causes nodules or abscesses. The sputum Gram stain may reveal gram-positive branching organisms, which are also visible on special acid-fast stains. The organism grows slowly on bacterial or fungal media, sometimes taking up to 4 weeks to be detectable. There are no useful serologic tests. The chest radiographic features are variable; commonly the appearance is that of a unilateral pneumonia involving one lobe, but single or multiple nodules, cavitation, and pleural involvement may occur. The optimal therapy for nocardiosis remains uncertain, but most commonly it involves sulfonamides alone or sulfamethoxazole-trimethoprim. For sulfonamide-allergic patients, minocycline or doxycycline have been used, but experience is limited. The duration of therapy is also unsettled; a minimum of 6 weeks is usual, but in immunocompromised hosts relapse is common, and many patients receive therapy for months or even indefinitely if the underlying immunosuppression persists.

Tuberculosis and Infection with *Mycobacterium avium-intracellulare*

Patients with cell-mediated immunodeficiency are at risk for tuberculosis. In developed countries, since the risk of acquiring tuberculosis is low, most cases are due to reactivation of organisms that were acquired years before and have since remained alive but dormant in the body. The risk is especially great for patients with AIDS who are from underdeveloped countries, but it may occur in lifelong citizens of developed countries, depending on their exposure to tuberculosis. A related organism, *M. avium-intracellulare* (MAI), also causes infection in compromised hosts.[4] This organism, found in soil, water, animals, birds, and foods, occurs worldwide, and infection develops from its inhalation or ingestion. It is not spread from person to person, and nearly all cases occur in patients with underlying lung disease or immunodeficiency. It often coexists with other pulmonary infections, especially with *P. carinii*. The organisms frequently spread via the bloodstream to cause infection in extrapulmonary sites, such as bone marrow and liver. This infection is difficult to treat, but successful therapy has sometimes occurred with combinations of several antituberculous drugs.

Cryptococcosis

C. neoformans is a fungus that exists as a yeast (single-cell organisms that reproduce by budding). It resides in the soil, predominantly in the droppings of pigeons, and it is widespread in nature in both urban and rural environments. It causes infection when inhaled into a susceptible host but is not spread from person to person. Once present in the lung, it has a remarkable tendency to travel via the bloodstream to distant sites, especially the meninges, but also to bone and skin. In many patients the pulmonary site of origin is not clinically evident, and they are symptomatic from the meningitis, which is usually a subacute or chronic disease with prominent headache, confusion, neck stiffness, nausea, and vomiting.[5] In others, the pulmonary source predominates, manifesting with fever, cough, sputum production, and chest radiographic abnormalities, which may include nodules, masses, unilateral infiltrates, or diffuse opacities.[6]

The diagnosis of cryptococcosis is established by growing the organism from blood, sputum, or cerebrospinal fluid. Cultures are usually positive within 10 days. The organism can be seen on India ink stains of the cerebrospinal fluid in 50 to 70 percent of patients with cryptococcal meningitis. A serologic test that detects cryptococcal antigen is positive in the cerebrospinal fluid in over 90 percent of patients with cryptococcal meningitis but is much less frequently positive in the serum of patients with only pulmonary involvement. The organism is also visible in tissue with use of special stains to detect fungi, including periodic acid-Schiff (PAS) and Gomori's methenamine silver (GMS). Treatment is with intravenous amphotericin B 0.3 mg/kg daily plus the oral agent flucytosine, 37.5 mg/kg q6h for 6 weeks. Intrathecal amphotericin B is usually unnecessary.

Pneumocystis carinii Pneumonia

P. carinii is an organism (probably a fungus) found worldwide but whose origin is unclear.[7] Since it is confined to the lungs in most patients, even those with severe immunocompromise, it is presumably inhaled from some unknown environmental source. It is probably not spread from person to person. As with so many organisms causing disease in immunosuppressed patients, most, if not all, normal hosts presumably have had contact with this agent, but disease occurs only when host defenses are severely compromised. Typically, the clinical features of *P. carinii* pneumonia (PCP) are fever (which may sometimes be present for several days or weeks before respiratory symptoms occur), dyspnea, and tachypnea. The chest radiograph usually reveals diffuse bilateral airspace pneumonia (Fig. 69-1), and patients are usually hypoxemic from the extent of their lung involvement. Sometimes, especially in the acquired immunodeficiency syndrome (AIDS), the chest film is normal but dyspnea and hypoxemia suggest the diagnosis. The organism is not rou-

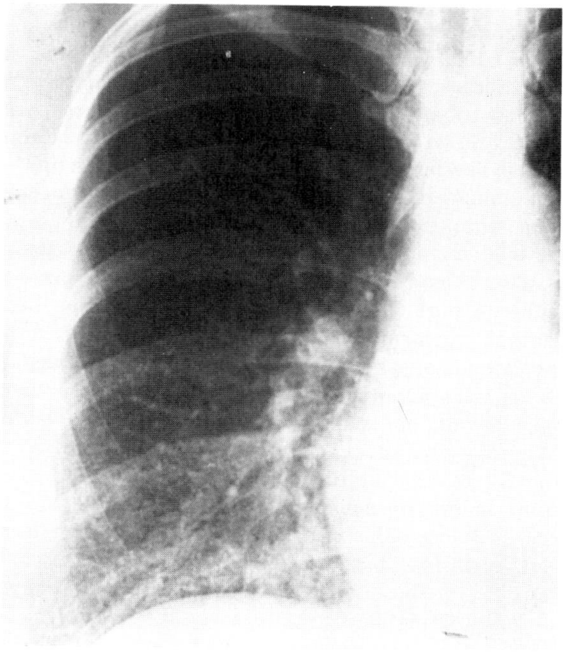

Figure 69-1. Typical chest radiographic appearance in *P. carinii* pneumonia, showing bilateral diffuse infiltrates more prominent at the bases (only the right lung is shown here). In this example the pattern is finely nodular; it may also be interstitial-alveolar and is occasionally less evenly spread throughout the lung. In many cases the abnormalities are much less prominent, and the chest radiograph can occasionally be normal early in the course of the illness. (From Blank,[19] with permission.)

tinely cultured; instead the diagnosis depends on demonstrating the typical cystic structures in tissue, bronchial brushings or washings, or sputum stained by the GMS or other technique. The disease is treated with intravenous pentamidine, parenteral or oral sulfamethoxazole-trimethoprim, or a combination of dapsone and pyrimethamine.

Cytomegalovirus Infection

Cytomegalovirus (CMV) is a herpes virus that infects most of the population without causing disease.[8] Its transmission is somewhat unclear, but in childhood it may travel from mother to infant in human milk or during childbirth through a contaminated uterine cervix. It may be transmitted from other infected children in newborn nurseries, daycare centers, schools, and family settings. Children can carry the organism in the respiratory tract or urine for prolonged periods. Normal adults, however, do not. The organism may be spread via sexual intercourse and blood transfusions.

When CMV disease occurs in immunocompromised hosts, it may develop from reactivation of latent infection acquired in the remote past, since the organism appears to remain alive but dormant in the body indefinitely after the initial, usually asymptomatic, infection. Alternatively, the immunosuppressed patient may acquire the organism for the first time through sexual intercourse, a blood transfusion, contact with an infected child, or receiving a transplanted organ that contains latent virus. This last mechanism has been well-documented with renal transplantation. Sometimes the manifestation of CMV infection in immunosuppressed patients is only fever, typically accompanied by elevation of hepatic enzymes. The infection may also cause a chorioretinitis, an eye infection that may decrease vision, as well as ulceration of the gastrointestinal tract. A serious complication is pneumonia, which is typically diffuse, with an "interstitial" pattern on the chest radiograph of widespread linear or nodular opacities in both lungs. Cytomegalovirus is often present with other organisms, and their individual contributions to the pneumonia may be difficult to assess. Usually the patient has fever, cough, and dyspnea combined with hypoxemia.

CMV pneumonia is often fatal, although ganciclovir, an antiviral, may be effective treatment in some patients. The diagnosis requires culture of the organism from blood, urine, sputum, or lung tissue. Growth usually takes several days to weeks. Because this virus may be found in asymptomatic patients or in lung tissue in which another agent is mainly responsible for the disease, histopathologic confirmation is helpful in determining its contribution to the clinical situation. Histologic analysis shows greatly enlarged bronchiolar and alveolar epithelial cells with nuclear and cytoplasmic inclusion bodies.

Varicella-Zoster Pneumonia

Two other herpes viruses occasionally cause pneumonia. Herpes varicella-zoster can cause pneumonia when the patient is exposed to the virus for the first time.[9] Typically, the skin lesions of varicella (chickenpox) appear, followed in a day or so by cough, dyspnea, and chest radiographic findings of a diffuse nodular pneumonia. In severely immunocompromised patients this pneumonia may be fatal. Immunocompromised patients with previous varicella infection are at risk for reactivation of the latent virus that persists indefinitely in the body following the initial infection. When reactivated it occurs as herpes zoster, the development of blisters unilaterally in a band along the distribution of a dermatome, the area of skin supplied by a single posterior spinal nerve root. These blisters usually begin on the face or trunk. In immunocompromised patients they tend to spread over several days to involve most of the patient's skin bilaterally. The blisters often become bloody and then necrotic. One complication of this spread of virus by the bloodstream is involvement of the lung, which causes diffuse nodular shadows on the chest radiograph, dyspnea, hypoxemia, and fever. This virus is susceptible to the antiviral agent acyclovir, which is recommended for the compromised host with varicella or herpes zoster. For immunocompromised hosts who have not had varicella but have been recently exposed, varicella-zoster immunoglobulin may prevent or lessen the severity of disease.

Herpes Simplex Pneumonia

Herpes simplex may cause a focal or diffuse pneumonia in immunocompromised patients, especially bone marrow transplant recipients.[10] Most patients have had concurrent or preceding mucocutaneous herpetic lesions, which are blisters that ulcerate or crust and occur on the lips, in the mouth, or on the genital area. Many cases of Herpes simplex pneumonia seem to occur from aspiration of oropharyngeal viruses into the tracheobronchial tree, causing focal or multifocal pulmonary infiltrates. A second mechanism may be hematogenous spread from an oral or genital site to cause diffuse pneumonia. The diagnosis can be made by culturing the virus from lower tracheobronchial secretions. The virus grows within a few days, but since it can be isolated from the upper airway in many patients without invasive disease, a positive culture from sputum or bronchoscopic specimens does not necessarily prove that it is causing the pneumonia. More convincing is isolation of the organism from lung tissue. Evidence that the organism is actually causing disease is buttressed by certain histologic changes, including intranuclear inclusion bodies in lung tissue cells, or by demonstrating the antigen in tissue by immunofluorescent staining. Very few cases have been diagnosed in life, but acyclovir therapy is presumably effective.

APPROACH TO PULMONARY INFECTIONS IN THE PATIENT WITH DEFECTIVE CELL-MEDIATED IMMUNITY

In evaluating a patient with cell-mediated immunodeficiency who has pulmonary infiltrates on chest radiography, it is useful to first divide the differential diagnostic possibilities into four groups: (1) the underlying disease or its known noninfectious complications, (2) complications of therapy, (3) infections, and (4) miscellaneous. Some immunocompromising diseases such as advanced Hodgkin's disease or non-Hodgkin's lymphoma may themselves involve the lung, occasionally causing an appearance that resembles that of an infectious process. Certain treatments such as radiation therapy or cytotoxic agents (e.g., methotrexate) may cause pulmonary processes characterized by dyspnea, fever, and opacities on chest radiographs. Finally, several miscellaneous problems such as intrapulmonary hemorrhage, pulmonary emboli, or congestive heart failure can mimic infections. The important clinical point is that clinicians should consider these possibilities rather than conclude immediately that every immunocompromised host with an abnormal chest radiograph has an infectious complication.

Second, it is wise to remember that if an infection is present, it may be due to common bacterial pathogens such as *S. pneumoniae* or *H. influenzae* rather than to nonbacterial causes. Blood cultures, sputum Gram stains, and cultures of sputum on conventional bacterial media should still be initial diagnostic measures in these patients. One clinical clue favoring a common bacterial pathogen is the sudden onset of an acute illness with a focal rather than a diffuse pattern on chest radiography.

If after consideration of noninfectious causes and common bacterial pathogens, a nonbacterial infection appears likely, some clinical clues may help direct the diagnostic approach. A bilateral diffuse process suggests a viral cause, especially cytomegalovirus, or *P. carinii*. Cavitation, hilar or mediastinal lymph node enlargement, unilateral involvement, or pleural effusion, however, indicates that the process is probably not due to viruses or *P. carinii*, at least not solely. In many cases, sputum should be stained for *P. carinii*, fungi, and mycobacteria by the GMS, Giemsa, and acid-fast techniques, since these may reveal the diagnosis. Fungal and mycobacterial cultures are often appropriate. If the diagnosis is still elusive, fiberoptic bronchoscopy with bronchoalveolar lavage and transbronchial biopsy is often the next step, and the specimens obtained should be sent for the stains and cultures indicated above. The yield of this approach varies considerably but is particularly low in bone marrow transplant recipients, in whom a nonspecific interstitial pneumonitis is common and difficult to diagnose with confidence from the small tissue specimens obtained by transbronchial biopsy. In these cases open lung biopsy may be preferable.

The possible etiologic agents causing pulmonary infections in patients with cell-mediated immunodeficiency are quite diverse, and the medications to treat them may have severe side effects. Accordingly, empiric treatment with several antimicrobial agents instead of an initial vigorous diagnostic approach poses several hazards. The regimen chosen may not cover the particular cause; the patient is usually exposed to at least one unnecessary agent; the duration of therapy needed is typically uncertain; and the appropriate response if adverse drug effects occur is often unclear, since discontinuing a critical medicine may be disastrous. Furthermore, many of these infections respond slowly rather than dramatically to treatment; when there is worsening or no substantial improvement after several days of empiric therapy, the clinician is uncertain whether the problem is inadequate antimicrobial coverage, an infection for which no therapy is effective, the expected slow response of an appropriately treated infection, or a noninfectious process. In seriously ill patients, however, these problems have to be weighed against the risks of invasive diagnostic procedures and the possibility that no definitive diagnosis will result from them. The choice between these two approaches requires careful, individualized clinical judgment.

HUMAN IMMUNODEFICIENCY VIRUS INFECTION AND AIDS

Human immunodeficiency virus type 1 (HIV-1) spreads from person to person by sexual contact, exposure to infected blood or blood products, and perinatal transmission from mother to child. In the United States the infection is most frequent in male homosexuals, intravenous drug abusers (because of needle sharing), recipients of blood products, and infants of infected mothers. Worldwide, however, over 60 percent of HIV infections have occurred from heterosexual transmission.[11]

When first infected, patients may have no symptoms or may develop an abrupt, mononucleosis-like illness consisting of fever, sweats, lethargy, muscle and joint pains, headache, sore throat, enlarged lymph nodes, and a rash on the trunk. The illness usually begins about 2 to 4 weeks after acquiring the virus and generally lasts 1 to 3 weeks. Some patients develop neurologic disorders, including aseptic meningitis and the Guillain-Barré syndrome, which are usually self-limited. Antibody against HIV typically becomes detectable 2 to 6 weeks after the illness begins. In patients without this illness, antibodies usually develop within 3 months of acquiring the virus.

Whether acute symptomatic illness occurs or not, patients have apparent good health for months to years, but eventually serious illness develops because the virus chronically infects several types of human cells, causing organ damage or defective immunity. HIV can infect brain cells, sometimes leading to neurologic damage, especially progressive dementia; gut epithelial cells, leading to a diarrhea-wasting syndrome; and bone marrow cells, producing hematologic abnormalities. Most importantly, HIV infects and destroys CD4+ lymphocytes, which regulate the normal immune response, leading to profoundly depressed cell-mediated immunity. This immunocompromise makes the patients susceptible to certain infections and malignancies, including Kaposi's sarcoma and central nervous system lymphoma. The average time from initial HIV infection to the profound immunocompromise and attendant complications that constitute AIDS is about 10 to 11 years, but probably all patients will eventually develop AIDS.

Among the most common complications of HIV infection are pulmonary problems,[12,13] whose differential diagnosis in-

Table 69-1. Pulmonary Complications of HIV Infection

Infections
Bacteria
S. pneumoniae
H. influenzae
Mycobacteria
M. tuberculosis
M. avium-intracellulare
Fungi
C. neoformans
H. capsulatum
C. immitis
Aspergillus spp.
Viruses
Cytomegalovirus
Herpes simplex
Herpes zoster
Malignancies
Kaposi's sarcoma
Non-Hodgkin's lymphoma
Other
Lymphocytic interstitial pneumonitis
Drug-induced disease

cludes a wide variety of infectious and noninfectious disorders (Table 69-1). Features helpful in distinguishing among these possibilities include the history of onset, the geographic area in which patients currently live or have resided in the past, extrapulmonary symptoms, and the radiographic patterns (Table 69-2). After a careful history and physical examination, the usual diagnostic approach is to obtain a chest radiograph and to examine a sample of expectorated sputum stained to detect bacteria (Gram stain), mycobacteria (acid-fast stain), and *P. carinii* (see below). If sputum is unavailable or unrevealing, most patients then undergo fiberoptic bronchoscopy with bronchoalveolar lavage, sometimes accompanied by transbronchial biopsies. These specimens are submitted for bacterial, mycobacterial, fungal, and viral cultures as indicated and for staining to detect the organisms mentioned above. These procedures usually yield a specific diagnosis. If no diagnosis is obtained, a second bronchoscopy may be warranted. Open-lung biopsies are somewhat hazardous and rarely disclose a treatable disease.[13]

Table 69-2. Radiographic Patterns of Infections in Patients with AIDS

Radiographic Pattern	Most Likely Infecting Agent
Diffuse reticulonodular infiltration	*P. carinii* *M. tuberculosis* *H. capsulatum* *C. immitis* Cytomegalovirus *C. neoformans*
Focal infiltrate	Bacterial infection *C. neoformans*
Lymph node enlargement	*M. tuberculosis* *M. avium-intracellulare*
Pleural effusion	*M. tuberculosis*
Normal	*P. carinii* *M. avium* complex *H. capsulatum*

(Data from Murray and Mills.[13])

PULMONARY INFECTIONS IN HIV-INFECTED PATIENTS

Bacterial Pneumonia

Community-acquired bacterial pneumonias, common in HIV-infected patients, are most commonly due to *S. pneumoniae* or *H. influenzae*. They are usually characterized by an acute onset of fever, dyspnea, pleuritic chest pain, and a productive cough of purulent sputum, which reveals the responsible organism on sputum Gram stain and culture. The chest radiograph generally discloses a focal airspace consolidation, although this may involve more than one lobe. Blood cultures are frequently positive.

Pneumocystis carinii Pneumonia

The most common pulmonary infection in HIV-positive patients in the United States is PCP, which is often their first serious complication. It usually occurs, however, when they are already profoundly immunocompromised, as evidenced by a CD4+ lymphocyte count less than 200/mm^3 (normal 800 to 1200) in over 90 percent. Patients typically develop fever and a nonproductive cough, with dyspnea worsening over a variable period of time. Many have symptoms for weeks before seeking medical attention; in others, the course is more fulminant. The physical examination of the lungs is usually normal, as is the white blood cell count. The chest radiograph, abnormal in more than 90 percent of cases, usually shows increased, diffuse interstitial and alveolar markings. Occasionally, patients develop cavities or pneumothoraces.

The diagnosis of PCP rests on detecting the organisms on special stains of sputum induced by inhalation of hypertonic saline, bronchoalveolar lavage fluid obtained at bronchoscopy, or tissue obtained by transbronchial biopsy (see Ch. 58). One or more of the samples are nearly always positive on GMS, modified Giemsa, or toluidine blue stains.

Drugs used to treat PCP include intravenous pentamidine, intravenous or oral sulfamethoxazole-trimethoprim (probably the drug of choice in those able to tolerate it), a combination of oral trimethoprim and dapsone, or inhaled pentamidine (8 mg/kg/d). Treatment is usually for 3 weeks. Systemic corticosteroids, when combined with one of these treatment protocols, reduce the incidence of respiratory failure and death when given within the first 72 hours of therapy to patients with moderate to severe infection, defined as a PaO_2 less than 70 mmHg when breathing room air or a $P(A\text{-}a)O_2$ greater than 35 mmHg. A common approach is oral prednisone 80 mg/d for 5 days, 40 mg/d for 5 days, and 20 mg/d for 11 days.[14]

After therapy of an episode of PCP, prophylactic medication is recommended to prevent a recurrence and is also suggested for all HIV-infected patients with CD4+ lymphocyte counts below 200 cells/mm^3, even without previous PCP. A common regimen is oral sulfamethoxazole-trimethoprim three times a week, dapsone daily, or aerosolized pentamidine 300 mg every 4 weeks—an effective but expensive program.[15]

Tuberculosis

Tuberculosis in HIV-positive patients usually occurs because latent infection, acquired years before, becomes reactivated. Those most at risk, therefore, are people with a high likelihood of previous exposure, including immigrants from foreign countries where tuberculosis is common and blacks and Hispanics living in impoverished urban areas. When the tuberculosis is primary rather than due to reactivation, concomitant HIV infection increases the likelihood of symptomatic progressive disease.[16] The incidence of tuberculosis in patients with AIDS is nearly 500 times that of the general population, and the chance of developing active disease in HIV-infected people with a positive tuberculin skin test (indicating past exposure and defined in this group as greater than 5 mm in diameter at 72 hours) is about 8 percent yearly. When tuberculosis develops in these patients, it is usually their first serious infection and typically occurs at a lesser level of immunocompromise than many other infections, presumably because *M. tuberculosis* is inherently more virulent than many other HIV-associated pathogens, such as *P. carinii*.

Tuberculosis in HIV-positive people differs from that in the general population by the frequency of both extrapulmonary involvement, especially in the lymph nodes, and bacteremia, with blood cultures positive for *M. tuberculosis* in about 25 to 40 percent of cases. Most patients have pulmonary involvement, with symptoms of fever, cough, and dyspnea. The chest radiographs, usually abnormal, commonly reveal hilar lymph node enlargement, predominantly upper lobe infiltrates, and pleural effusions. Cavities or a miliary pattern may occur, and occasionally bilateral interstitial infiltrates resembling those found in *P. carinii* infection develop. Acid-fast smears and cultures are often positive in expectorated sputum, but bronchoalveolar lavage or transbronchial biopsy is sometimes necessary to establish the diagnosis. Aspiration biopsy of involved peripheral lymph nodes is usually positive for acid-fast bacilli, but excision may be necessary for definitive diagnosis.

Treatment failures and relapses are uncommon with conventional antituberculous chemotherapy, although adverse reactions to the drugs, especially rifampin, are higher than in the general population. For drug-susceptible organisms, experts recommend a combination of isoniazid, rifampin, and pyrazinamide for 2 months, followed by rifampin and isoniazid for an additional 7 months or for 6 months after cultures become negative, whichever is longer.

All HIV-positive patients should have a tuberculin skin test. Those with induration greater than 5 mm in diameter at 72 hours should have a chest radiograph and a clinical evaluation to search for active tuberculosis. If none is present, they should receive prophylactive isoniazid for 12 months.

Infection with *Mycobacterium avium-intracellulare*

Patients with severe immunocompromise from HIV infection may develop disease caused by the organisms of the *M. avium* complex, which includes the closely related species, *M. avium* and *M. intracellulare* (commonly referred to as MAI).[17] These microbes, widespread in food, water, and soil, may be acquired by inhalation of aerosols or ingestion of contaminated material. Rarely pathogenic in normal hosts, they cause disseminated disease in about 15 to 25 percent of patients with severe HIV infection, usually those with CD4+ lymphocyte counts less than 100/mm^3. The typical clinical features are fever, weight loss, night sweats, diarrhea, anemia, and abdominal pain. Blood cultures grow the mycobacteria in most patients with disseminated disease. Although sputum cultures may be positive for the organism, respiratory symptoms are usually absent or related to another process, and the chest radiograph is typically normal, although lymph node enlargement is present in some. Although these mycobacteria cause systemic illness in HIV-positive patients, they rarely infect the lung parenchyma to cause clinical or radiographic abnormalities.

Fungal Infections

Infections with certain fungi can occur in patients with advanced HIV disease, and they have in common a tendency to disseminate widely to involve many organs, to resist therapy, to relapse, and to require lifelong suppression for control.[13]

The most frequent cause of fungal infection is *C. neoformans*, a yeast widespread in nature, predominantly residing in pigeon droppings. When inhaled, it causes lung infection and, especially in HIV-positive patients, commonly spreads via the bloodstream to involve distant areas, especially the meninges. In HIV disease meningoencephalitis is the most common clinical presentation, and the original pulmonary focus is often not clinically or radiographically evident. When pulmonary disease is present, cough and dyspnea are the prominent complaints, and chest radiographs usually demonstrate a focal pneumonia or nodules. Less common patterns are miliary disease, pleural effusion, cavitation, and lymph node enlargement. CD4+ lymphocyte counts are usually less than 100/mm^3. Treatment requires intravenous amphotericin B several times a week until the meningitis subsides and then lifelong regular suppressive medication, usually with oral fluconazole, because of the high frequency of relapse if antifungal therapy is completely stopped.

H. capsulatum resides in soil contaminated by bird or bat droppings, predominantly in the midwestern United States. Most immunocompetent hosts inhaling the organism have asymptomatic infection, but in patients with HIV infection, histoplasmosis is usually disseminated, causing symptoms of fever and weight loss.[13] Cough and dyspnea are frequent in those with lung involvement. Splenomegaly, hepatomegaly, and lymph node enlargement are common on physical examination. Chest radiographs, although often normal, most commonly demonstrate diffuse reticulonodular infiltrates. The organism is best isolated in cultures of blood, bone marrow, bronchoalveolar lavage fluid, or transbronchial biopsy specimens. Organisms are visible in tissue stained with special techniques to identify fungi with GMS or PAS. Treatment is with intravenous amphotericin B.

C. immitis lives in semiarid areas of the Western Hemisphere; in the United States it resides in the Southwest, especially Arizona and parts of southern California but also western Texas, Utah, New Mexico, and Nevada. When inhaled, it causes pulmonary infection but, in HIV-positive patients it commonly disseminates to involve many extrapulmonary sites,[13] causing fever, weight loss, cough, and fatigue in most. Chest radiographs usually demonstrate diffuse reticulonodular infiltrates. The diagnosis rests on finding the organism in lung secretions or tissue, blood cultures, or material from other infected sites. Treatment is intravenous amphotericin B.

Occasionally, usually in the terminal stages of HIV infection, *Aspergillus* spp. cause pulmonary infection.[18] CD4+ lymphocyte counts are generally less than 100/mm^3, and neutropenia is often present. Fever and an unproductive cough are the usual symptoms; dyspnea, pleuritic chest pain, and hemoptysis may also occur. The radiographic findings are diverse—unilateral or bilateral nodules, infiltrates, and cavities. The organism may be visible or may grow on culture from specimens obtained by bronchoalveolar lavage, transbronchial biopsy, or transthoracic needle aspiration. The infection is usually fatal, but some patients have responded to itraconazole.

Cytomegalovirus Pneumonia

Viral pneumonias are uncommon in HIV infection, although CMV frequently grows in bronchoalveolar lavage fluid or transbronchial biopsy specimens of patients with pulmonary disease. This virus is very common in the general population—about 50 percent have had prior infection—and is especially prevalent in sexually active homosexual men, affecting more than 90 percent. Reactivation of this infection is frequent in the later stages of HIV infection, with many patients shedding the organisms in their urine. When isolated from pulmonary secretions or tissue, CMV is not usually the cause of significant disease and is often present with another microbe that is the real pathogen, especially *P. carinii*. To qualify as a convincing etiology of a pulmonary process, the virus should be present on culture, present in lung cells (as demonstrated by inclusions in bronchoalveolar lavage cells or pulmonary tissue), and identified as the sole pathogen in a pneumonia that is progressing by clinical or radiographic criteria.[13] For the unusual case of convincing CMV pneumonia, intravenous ganciclovir may be effective treatment.

References

1. Hughes WT, Armstrong DA, Bodey GP et al: Guidelines for the use of antimicrobial agents in neutropenic patients with unexplained fever. J Infect Dis 1990;161:381–396
2. Rosenow EC, Wilson WR, Cockerill FR: Pulmonary disease in the immunocompromised host. Mayo Clin Proc 1985;60:473–487, 610–631
3. Wilson JP, Turner HR, Kirchner KA, Chapman SW: Nocardial infections in renal transplant recipients. Medicine (Baltimore) 1989;68:38–57
4. Horsburgh CR, Mason UG, Farhi DC, Iseman MD: Disseminated infection with *Mycobacterium avium-intracellulare*. Medicine (Baltimore) 1985;64:36–48
5. Perfect JR: Cryptococcosis. Infect Dis Clin North Am 1989;3:77–102
6. Feigin DS: Pulmonary cryptococcosis. AJR 1983;141:1263–1272
7. Peters SG, Prakash UBS: *Pneumocystis carinii* pneumonia: Review of 53 cases. Am J Med 1987;82:73–78
8. Schulman LL, Reison DS, Austin JHM, Rose EA: Cytomegalovirus pneumonitis after cardiac transplantation. Arch Intern Med 1991;151:1118–1124
9. Straus SE, Ostrove JM, Inchauspe G et al: Varicella-zoster virus infections. Biology, natural history, treatment, and prevention. Ann Intern Med 1988;108:221–237
10. Graham BS, Snell JD: *Herpes simplex* virus infection of the adult lower respiratory tract. Medicine (Baltimore) 1983;62:384–393
11. Green WC: The molecular biology of HIV-1 infection. N Engl J Med 1991;324:308–317
12. White DA, Matthay RA: Non infectious pulmonary complications of infection with the human immunodeficiency virus. Am Rev Respir Dis 1989;140:1763–1787
13. Murray JF, Mills J: Pulmonary infectious complications of human immunodeficiency virus infection. Am Rev Respir Dis 1990;141:1356–1372, 1582–1598
14. National Institutes of Health Consensus: Consensus statement on the use of corticosteroids as adjunctive therapy for *Pneumocystis carinii* pneumonia in AIDS. N Engl J Med 1990;323:1500–1504
15. Hughes WT: Prevention and treatment of *Pneumocystis carinii* pneumonia. Annu Rev Med 1991;42:287–295
16. Barnes PF, Bloch AB, Davidson PT, Snider DE: Tuberculosis in patients with human immunodeficiency virus infection. N Engl J Med 1991;324:1644–1650
17. Horsburgh CR: *Mycobacterium avium* complex infection in the acquired immunodeficiency syndrome. N Engl J Med 1991;324:1332–1338
18. Denning DW, Follansbee SE, Scolaro M et al: Pulmonary aspergillosis in the acquired immunodeficiency syndrome. N Engl J Med 1991;324:654–662
19. Blank N: Chest Radiographic Analysis. Churchill Livingstone, New York, 1989, pp. 215–293

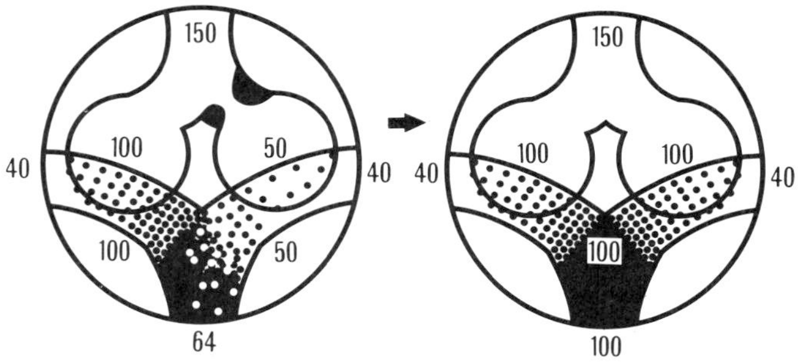

Section 5

Respiratory Care Practice

Chapter 70

Chest Physical Therapy

Colleen Kigin

CHAPTER OUTLINE

Breathing exercises and the techniques of positioning, percussion, vibration, and cough facilitation (commonly referred to as chest physiotherapy [CPT]) to remove excess secretions and maximize ventilation have been used since the late 1800s and early 1900s. The techniques employed have not changed dramatically through the years, but their efficacy has been more clearly established. The purpose of this chapter is to review the techniques and discuss indications and precautions for their use.

BREATHING EXERCISES TO REVERSE OR PREVENT ATELECTASIS

The term *breathing exercises* defines a series of maneuvers designed to modify the ventilatory pattern to enhance gas exchange and to maximize ventilatory muscle function. The focus can be divided into three distinct areas:

1. To reverse or prevent atelectasis
2. To optimize contraction of the diaphragm and other respiratory muscles
3. To train the respiratory muscles for increased strength or endurance

Atelectasis is the most common postoperative complication following major abdominal or thoracic surgery[1–3] but can occur in any patient ventilating at low lung volumes. As discussed in Chapter 41, the vital capacity of the postoperative upper abdominal surgery patient drops some 40 to 50 percent.[3,4] Breathing at these low lung volumes makes the gravity-dependent, peripheral areas of the lung most vulnerable to collapse, with these changes more striking in the obese or supine patient.[5]

Atelectasis may also occur as the level of surfactant in the lung drops.[6] Surfactant, produced by type II pneumocytes, decreases lung surface tension and thus the pressure gradient required for ventilation. The drop in surfactant and the consequent rise in surface tension occur very quickly postoperatively.[7] Collapse of the lung for 24 hours or longer is particularly difficult to reverse. It is also difficult to maintain expansion after reversal as time is required for the surfactant to reaccumulate. If atelectasis persists, a secondary infection often occurs, leading to the production of thick secretions and subsequently to airway obstruction.[8] Therefore prevention of atelectasis is the critical focus of treatment in the postoperative patient.

Stretch-Resistance Techniques

Striated muscles, including the diaphragm and intercostals, achieve maximal pressure or force by contracting from a lengthened rather than from a shortened or flattened position.[9] The patient who is splinting (or supporting) the thorax is rolled to the opposite side, and the clinician's hands are placed along the rib cage, palpating the decreased excursion (Fig. 70-1). The patient is instructed to exhale, with the clinician offering graded pressure to the rib cage. This should increase the stretch of the intercostals, facilitating contraction during inspiration. As the patient finishes exhalation, the clinician's hands offer graded resistance, after which the patient is instructed to breathe in maximally and to hold the inspiration for 2 to 3 seconds. This resistance, which is an "overload" on normal inspiratory muscle contraction, is provided in the hope of facilitating increased intercostal fiber firing and thereby facilitating thoracic excursion during inspiration. The activities of the clinician are paramount to the success of this procedure, and care must be taken to facilitate rather than inhibit thoracic expansion.

The patient is instructed to also palpate the rib cage and to concentrate on the normal action of the thorax as compared with that of the splinted area. Once this is achieved, the patient may be introduced to an incentive spirometer and instructed to pay attention to bilateral rib cage expansion during its use. However, use of the incentive spirometer does not replace careful attention to the patient's breathing pattern and the effects of splinting.

It has never been conclusively shown in the laboratory setting that expansion through proprioception can increase or facilitate airflow to an atelectatic area. However, when this technique is used clinically, breath sound changes and subsequent expectoration of mucus plugs lead one to assume that local muscle contraction and subsequent lung expansion have increased.[10] In fact, Thoren[11] in 1954 clinically demonstrated the benefit of inspiratory expansion through direct proprioception or stretch of the rib cage as compared with the normal stir-up technique.

It must also be remembered that airflow follows the path of least resistance. Consequently, when the patient splints the painful site, it seems logical that as long as the site is still splinted, a deep breath will not facilitate airflow to the atelectatic area. The stretch and resistance to the splinted

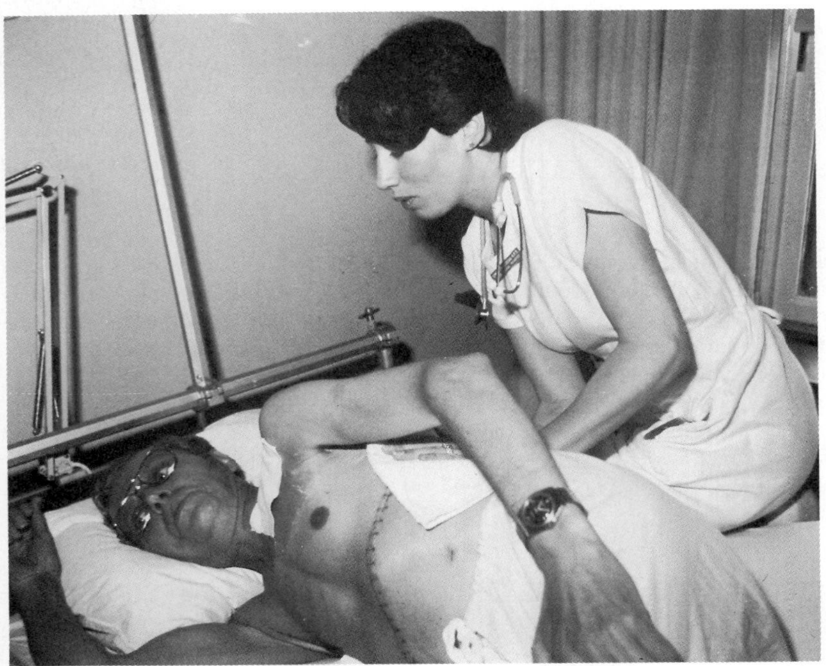

Figure 70-1. Patient with a thoracoabdominal incision receiving stretch immediately prior to inspiration and graded resistance during inspiration to promote maximal inspiratory volume. The resistance is provided below the incision site. Vibration (below the incision site) is provided during exhalation to promote clearance of secretions.

area promote normal contraction of intercostal muscles in the area and allows normal intercostal activity to resume, with subsequent motion or excursion of the rib cage on inspiration.

Sniff-Huff Technique

The patient who has undergone upper abdominal surgery often splints the diaphragm and abdominal area. The decrease in diaphragmatic contraction after upper abdominal surgery has been discussed since the 1950s.[11] Such a patient normally does not tolerate stretch or resistance to the abdominal area owing to the incision, and consequently different methods must be used to facilitate contraction.

The techniques I and my colleagues use to encourage diaphragmatic activity, maximal inspiratory volume, and effective expectoration of sputum are sniffing and huffing. Sniffing requires active contraction of the diaphragm, while huffing requires active contraction of the abdominal muscles. It seems to be easier for the patient to use these techniques in achieving maximum inspiratory volume and a forceful expectoration than to follow the more traditional instruction to breathe in deeply and cough. These techniques are also very effective in the intubated patient who is being weaned from mechanical ventilation.

Use of Adjunctive Devices

Frequently, clinicians have moved to adjunctive devices to assist in motivating a patient to take a deep breath. It must be remembered that use of an incentive spirometer without proper instruction may result in no changes in inspiratory volume or in reversal of atelectasis. The device should be used as an adjunct to the therapist's attention to the patient's breathing mechanics. The emphasis should be on breathing technique, with use of the spirometer for feedback regarding volume inspired (Fig. 70-2).

Postoperative pulmonary complications can be averted by frequent maximal inspiratory volumes. The process does not need to be complicated or expensive and may be accomplished with or without use of an adjunctive device. Maximal inspirations not only should be given attention while the patient is sitting upright but should also be incorporated with the use of other techniques, such as positioning and manual techniques (see later discussion).

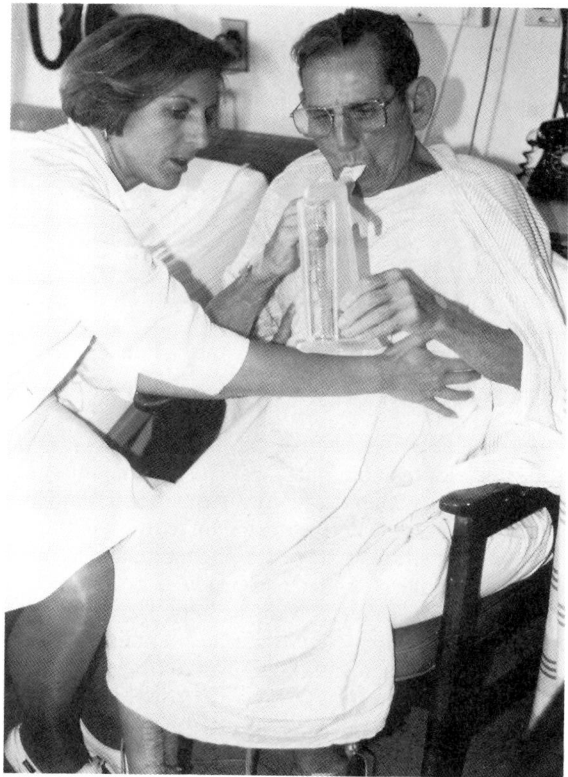

Figure 70-2. Patient using incentive spirometer as an adjunct to achieving maximal inspiratory volume. The therapist is monitoring the appropriate breathing pattern (bilateral expansion) as the patient is instructed in the use of the incentive spirometer.

BREATHING EXERCISES TO IMPROVE VENTILATORY MUSCLE FUNCTION

The postoperative patient generally needs stimulus or encouragement to perform maximal inspirations to resolve pulmonary complications. Other patient populations experiencing neuromuscular dysfunction or fatigue also require assistance to perform maximal inspirations. This section focuses on respiratory muscle fatigue and efficiency, both for the ventilator-supported patient who is attempting to wean and for the patient experiencing fatigue who potentially requires intubation and mechanical ventilation.

The Ventilatory Muscles

This discussion divides the ventilatory muscles into three groups: (1) the diaphragm; (2) the intercostal and accessory muscles; and (3) the abdominal muscles. Although this fact is commonly misunderstood, all three groups have both an inspiratory and expiratory function.[12]

Diaphragm

The diaphragm is the major inspiratory pump, particularly at low lung volumes.[13] It is well equipped for its constant work load, as it contains muscle fibers and mitochrondrial enzymes that favor aerobic metabolism.[14] About 75 percent of the diaphragm and intercostal muscle fibers are classified as slow- and fast-twitch high-oxidative fibers. These fibers have high endurance capability and are resistant to fatigue.[14]

For muscle contraction to be efficient and forceful, the length of the muscle prior to contraction must be optimized. The optimal resting length for maximal contraction of the diaphragm is just below functional residual capacity (FRC) in the normal individual. The contractile force is greatly reduced when the diaphragm contracts from a shortened position, as occurs with chronic obstructive pulmonary disease (COPD).[15] At any given load, hyperinflation of the lung caused by COPD also predisposes the inspiratory muscles to fatigue.[15]

Accessory Muscles

The accessory muscles include primarily the scalene and the sternocleidomastoid muscles. The scalene muscles, formerly thought to be inactive during quiet breathing, have in fact been found to be active during inspiration in the upright and supine position.[16] The sternocleidomastoid muscles, which are the muscles that can produce a ''pump handle'' action on the rib cage, are not usually active during quiet breathing but are very active during breathing at high lung volumes, which occurs in COPD or during high levels of ventilation, as in exercise.[16]

Abdominal Muscles

The abdominal muscles, traditionally considered to be only expiratory muscles, can be very important to the inspiratory phase of ventilation. As the abdominal muscles contract during active exhalation, the diaphragm is moved cephalad to a resting position of greater length or stretch. This more favorable resting length then permits a more efficient contraction, resulting in a larger inspiratory volume.[16]

Indicators of Ventilatory Muscle Fatigue

Fatigue generally occurs when energy demand exceeds energy supply. This could be due to many factors, including high resistive breathing, hypoxia, or low cardiac output.[16] Whatever the cause, the condition leads to alveolar hypoventilation and CO_2 retention. Clinical signs of inspiratory muscle fatigue include

1. Dyspnea (shortness of breath)
2. Increased respiratory rate
3. Asynchronous breathing pattern with abdominal and chest wall discoordination

Approaches to Therapy

The therapy to improve inspiratory muscle function can be divided into the following categories[17]:

1. Reducing the load on the inspiratory muscles and reducing the mechanical disadvantage
2. Improving the contractile characteristics, including strength and endurance
3. Resting the inspiratory muscles with mechanical ventilation if they are unable to maintain ventilatory function

Improvement in the above categories can be achieved by altering airway resistance and compliance and by decreasing the work of breathing by maximizing diaphragm resting length. Inhaled pharmacologic agents (Ch. 20) may markedly affect work of breathing by decreasing airway resistance. Drug therapy to promote bronchodilation and decrease airway resistance is discussed elsewhere in this text.

Maximizing the resting position of the diaphragm and intercostal muscles decreases the load on the ventilatory muscles and reduces the work of breathing. Barach[18] in the 1960s discussed the value of optimizing the resting position of the diaphragm. He believed he could decrease the work of breathing and reduce hyperinflation while maximizing the resting position of the diaphragm through use of the Barach belt. This elasticized belt allows patients to increase functional activity by simulating active abdominal contraction, moving the diaphragm to a more lengthened position prior to contraction. It also provides resistance against which the diaphragm can contract, thereby potentially increasing maximal inspiratory force.

Diaphragmatic breathing is often poorly taught. Instruc-

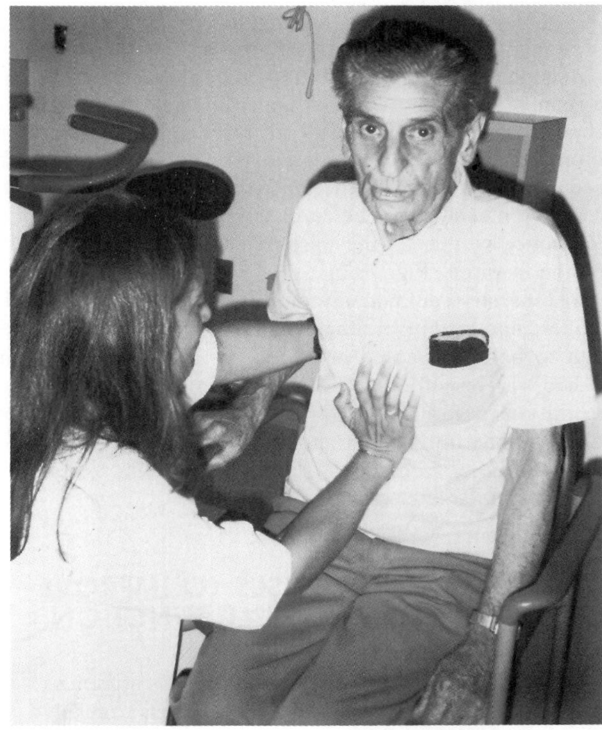

Figure 70-3. By pushing up and in during exhalation the therapist is optimizing the resting position of diaphragm in preparation for inspiration in a patient with COPD and a flattened or shortened diaphragm.

tions may be given such as "Place your hand on the patient's abdomen and have the patient make the abdomen protrude on inspiration." At the same time the therapist's hand is passive, simply indicating the place of expected movement.[19] Clinicians have noted that it is sometimes difficult for the patient to make the initial inspiratory movement. This is not surprising, since the shortened diaphragm is attempting to contract from an essentially dysfunctional position and is unable to increase its work load.

The techniques that we employ to maximize contraction are stretch and resistance to the diaphragm, with controlled abdominal contraction on exhalation. The patient is requested to exhale while the therapist's hand is placed below the rib cage over the diaphragm, pushing up and in during exhalation (Fig. 70-3). This ostensibly shifts the resting position of the diaphragm, as with the Barach belt. As the patient finishes exhalation, a "quick stretch" or slight increase in pressure immediately precedes the command for the patient to inhale. The therapist provides graded resistance or pressure on inhalation, increasing the fiber firing with some overload or resistance. Once inhalation is complete, the patient is instructed to exhale with slow, controlled contraction of the abdominal muscles. This action is, in fact, similar to that of the therapist's hand and is used with self-practice (Fig. 70-4).

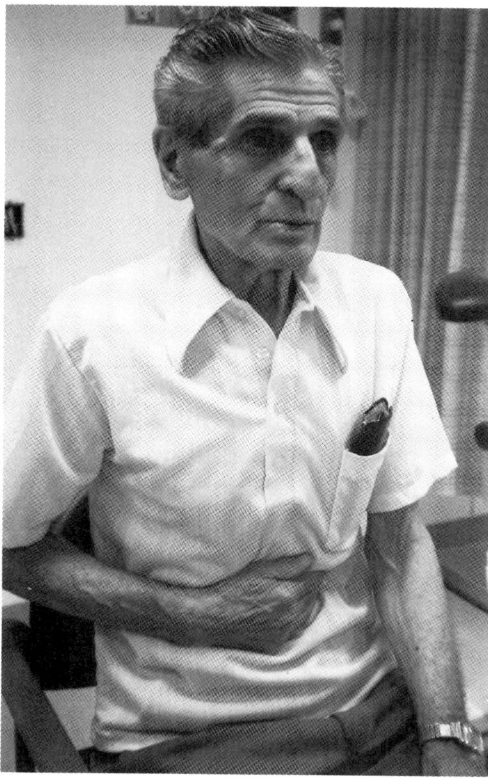

Figure 70-4. The patient is attempting to maximize the resting position of the diaphragm, moving it to a more lengthened position prior to inhalation, by performing a controlled, active *expiratory* maneuver.

These techniques have been used successfully in the nonintubated dyspneic patient in respiratory failure, as well as in the patient with diaphragmatic shortening and lung hyperinflation who is being weaned from mechanical ventilation.

Training for Strength versus Endurance

The definitions of strength, endurance, and fatigue for inspiratory and expiratory muscles are the same as those for skeletal muscle: strength is the maximal force that a muscle can develop; endurance is the length of time a muscle can contract against a given load; and fatigue is the inability to maintain a predetermined force during contraction.

The training concepts for ventilatory muscles, like those for other skeletal muscles, include overload, specificity, and reversibility.[20]

1. *Overload*: A muscle must experience a load greater than the stress it normally carries in order for training to take effect. The overload required to improve strength is of high intensity, with fast, short repetitions. The overload for endurance is of lower intensity and is sustained or repeated for long periods of time.
2. *Specificity*: Specificity reflects the concept that in order to train, for example, for endurance the load must be of lower intensity and must be sustained over a long period. The training must be similar to or the same as the activity one wishes to improve (i.e., directed toward the functional characteristics of the muscles to be trained).
3. *Reversibility*: Reversibility simply means that if the training or overload is stopped, the training effects will be lost and functional characteristics will return to baseline.

Strength and endurance capabilities are often both decreased in the patient with chronic respiratory failure or with respiratory failure due to neuromuscular or musculoskeletal defects. A training program may be designed to emphasize or to train for strength and/or endurance. Strength may be increased by contracting the muscles against high loads for short time periods; this can be accomplished by placing weights directly on the muscle,[21] by static maximal inspiratory efforts,[22] or by inspiratory resistive training.[23] Endurance may be increased by performing numerous contractions against lower resistance sustainable for long durations without a fatiguing load.

Direct Diaphragmatic Loading

Clinicians for years have advocated application of resistance directly to the diaphragmatic area to improve contractile force, which was often done by placing weights over the abdominal area. This approach was cumbersome and its efficacy was not documented. Today the technique receives little attention and has largely fallen into disuse except at isolated clinics. However, more recently it has been shown

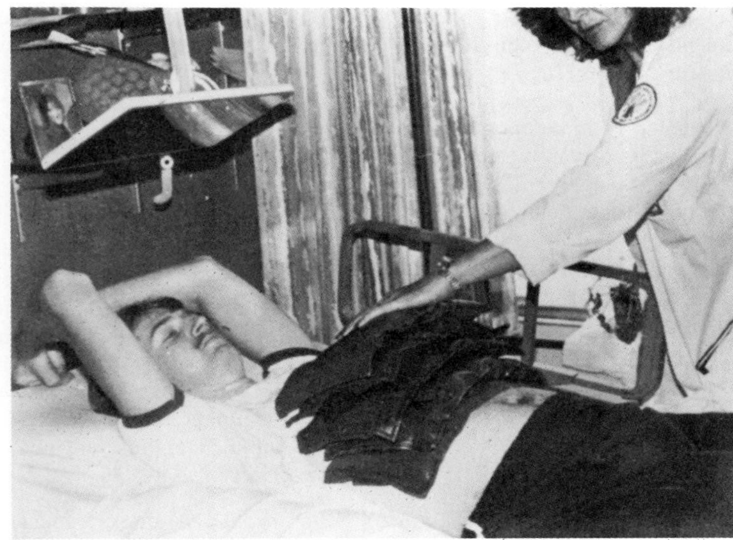

Figure 70-5. This patient, who is quadriplegic as a result of injury at the C5-C6 vertebral level, is undergoing respiratory muscle training by use of weights over the diaphragm. This individual is lifting 50 lb of weight 45 days after the injury. Vital capacity was 2.20 L initially and 3.63 L after training. (From O'Donohue,[1] with permission.)

to be successful in improving respiratory muscle strength in quadriplegic patients.[21] A weight program must be carefully initiated and evaluated but may result in a significant increase in vital capacity (Fig. 70-5).

Inspiratory Resistive Loading at the Mouth

The concept of training the ventilatory muscles for strength by resistance at the mouth has been generally applied to patients with COPD. The ventilatory muscles of the patient with COPD are in constant overload, which can easily lead to fatigue. The diaphragm is in an inefficient position, and the accessory muscles may be activated during quiet ventilation to assist the disadvantaged diaphragm. The goal of training is to enhance either the strength or endurance or *both* either by employing a resistance at the mouth or by having the patient breath rapidly.[24–26]

Resistance at the mouth can be applied through devices with variable apertures or openings, through which the patient breathes. Proper evaluation is essential for adjustment of the aperture so that the patient will be breathing against a resistance that can be sustained for 15 to 20 minutes without fatigue or a drop in arterial O_2 saturation (SaO_2).[27]

In my experience not all patients with chronic lung disease benefit from this form of therapy. If respiratory muscle fatigue or weakness is noted in a reliable, conscientious individual, the patient is evaluated and the appropriate aperture set to provide overload without accompanying O_2 desaturation. The patient is placed on a home care program with the resistance adjusted on subsequent clinical visits. This provides an endurance training program specific to the inspiratory muscles.

Hyperpnea

Hyperpnea is also used in respiratory muscle training.[28] This is accomplished by having the patient breathe as hard and fast as possible for short bursts of time. The loss of CO_2 is controlled by having the person breathe through a system that monitors CO_2 and provides a gas mixture to maintain baseline CO_2 levels during the training session. This approach is cumbersome, and a home care program is generally not possible.

POSITIONING

Rationale

Frequent position change is the hallmark of care for the immobilized bedridden patient. The rationale includes minimizing the prospect of pressure sores or skin breakdown and promoting ventilation and secretion removal. This section reviews the effects of position change on mucus clearance, ventilation (including inspiratory muscle excursion), ventilation/perfusion ($\dot{V}/\dot{Q}$) relationships, and oxygenation.

The normal individual has a mucociliary transport rate of 10 mm/min regardless of position, which decreases to about 6 mm/min with aging.[29] This transport rate also decreases significantly with smoking, pulmonary disease, or surgery. In addition, any patient in acute respiratory failure requiring mechanical ventilation will show a decrease from normal mucociliary transport.[29]

Excess or abnormal mucus in the presence of abnormal mucociliary transport moves caudally through the trachea or to the base of the lungs when a patient is upright and cranially or toward the trachea when the head is down.[29] Positioning takes advantage of gravity to help move retained secretions. The positions used to facilitate secretion flow are determined by placing the affected lung area as perpendicular as possible to the ground, thereby maximizing the effect of gravity on the secretions. If a position does not result in enhanced secretion flow, anatomic variations in the tracheobronchial tree should be considered. The thickness of the secretions and the need for adequate hydration, as well as potential obstruction of an airway due to bronchoconstriction or anatomic obstruction, should also be considered.

Bronchopulmonary Drainage Positions

The positions used for drainage of specific lobes are found in Figures 70-6 to 70-13. These positions are *optimal* for secretion clearance but may need modification according to the patient's clinical status. If a position results in cardiac arrhythmias, unacceptable changes in blood pressure, increased cranial pressure with head injury, or a drop in oxygenation as indirectly monitored by SaO_2, the position should be modified. It should be understood that contraindications to or inability to use the optimal drainage position does not contraindicate trying a modified position. The modified position may not allow the full effect of gravity, but secretions may still be mobilized with use of the manual techniques.

It is often suggested that drainage positions be maintained for 20 to 30 minutes.[30,31] However, if secretion transport mechanisms are abnormal, it is unrealistic to think that positioning alone will clear secretions in 20 minutes. Since 20 minutes or less (even as little as 5 minutes) may be the *maximum* amount of time that a person can tolerate a specific position, use of breathing/ventilatory assists such as deep breathing/huffing/coughing with the nonintubated patient and use of the manual techniques in conjunction with drainage are often necessary to clear secretions in an efficient, effective manner.

Positioning to Optimize Diaphragmatic Excursion

Specific positions may decrease the patient's sensation of dyspnea, and recognition of this can be very valuable in the treatment of the patient for whom mechanical ventilation is the last resort or for the patient who is being weaned from ventilatory support. Sharp et al.[32] reported that 7 of 17 nonintubated patients with COPD found relief of dyspnea in the

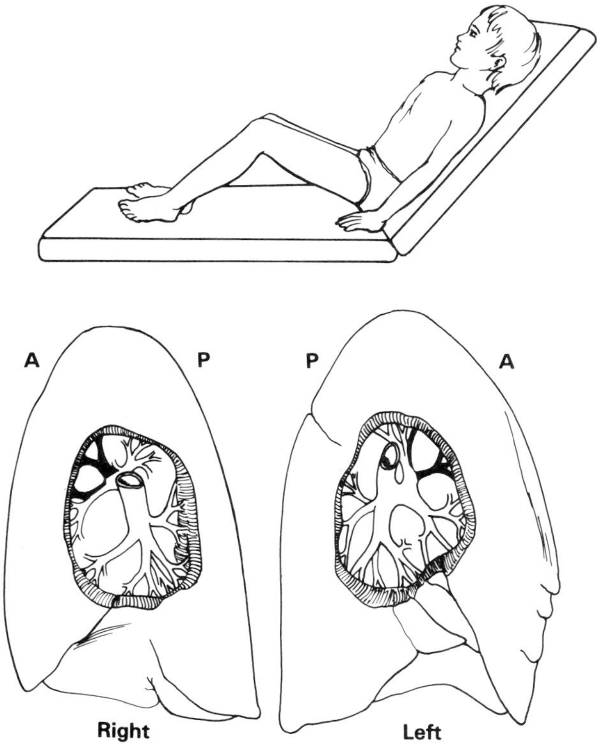

Figure 70-6. Position for drainage of anterior segments of right and left upper lobes. Note darkened insert on lung diaphragm for specific bronchioles drained. A, anterior; P, posterior.

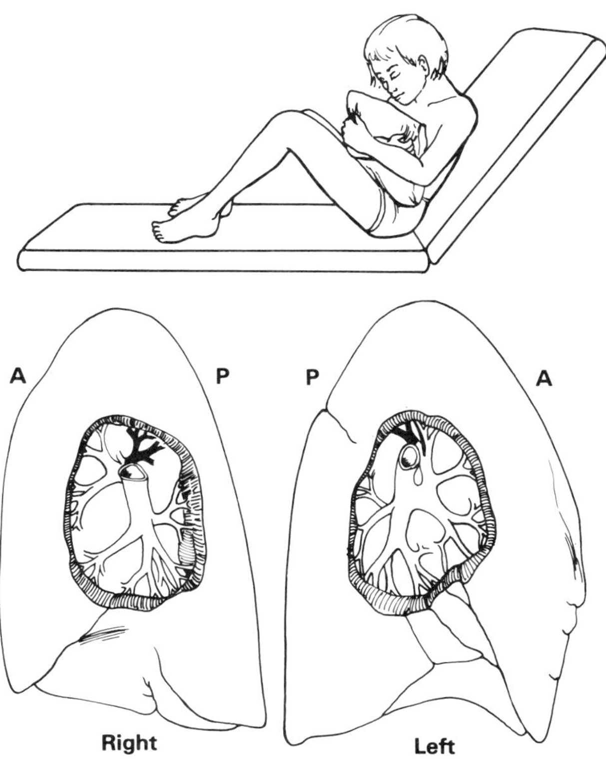

Figure 70-7. Position for drainage of posterior apices of upper lobes.

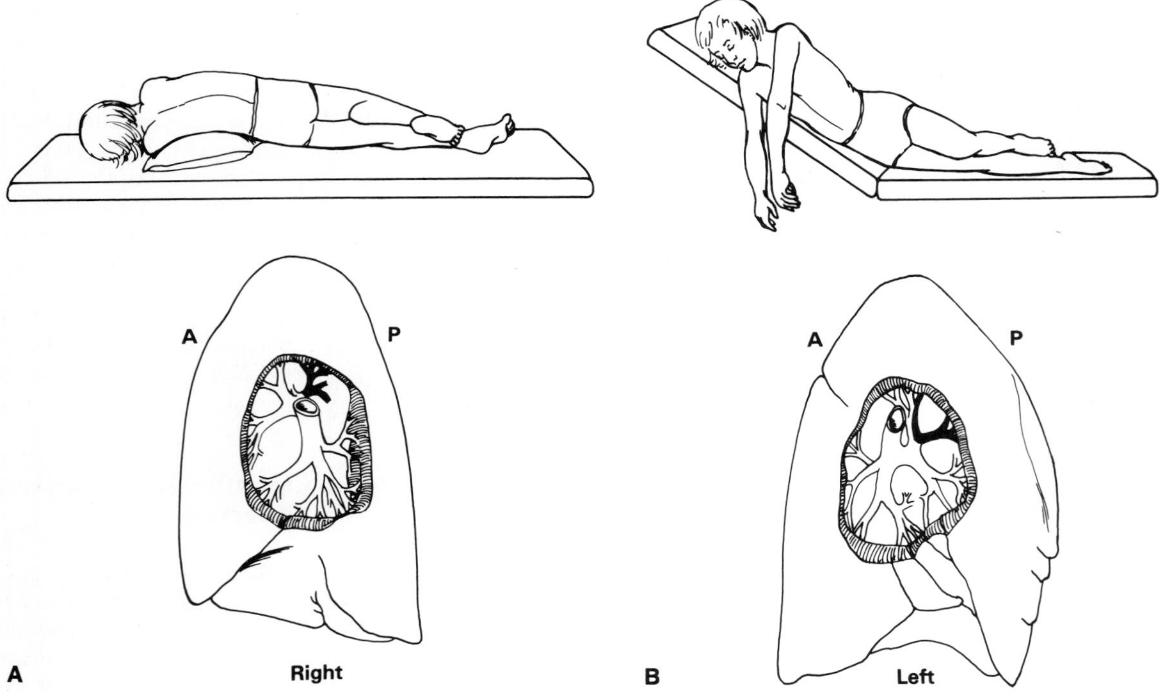

Figure 70-8. Alternate position for drainage of posterior apices of upper lobes. **(A)** Right upper lobe; **(B)** left upper lobe.

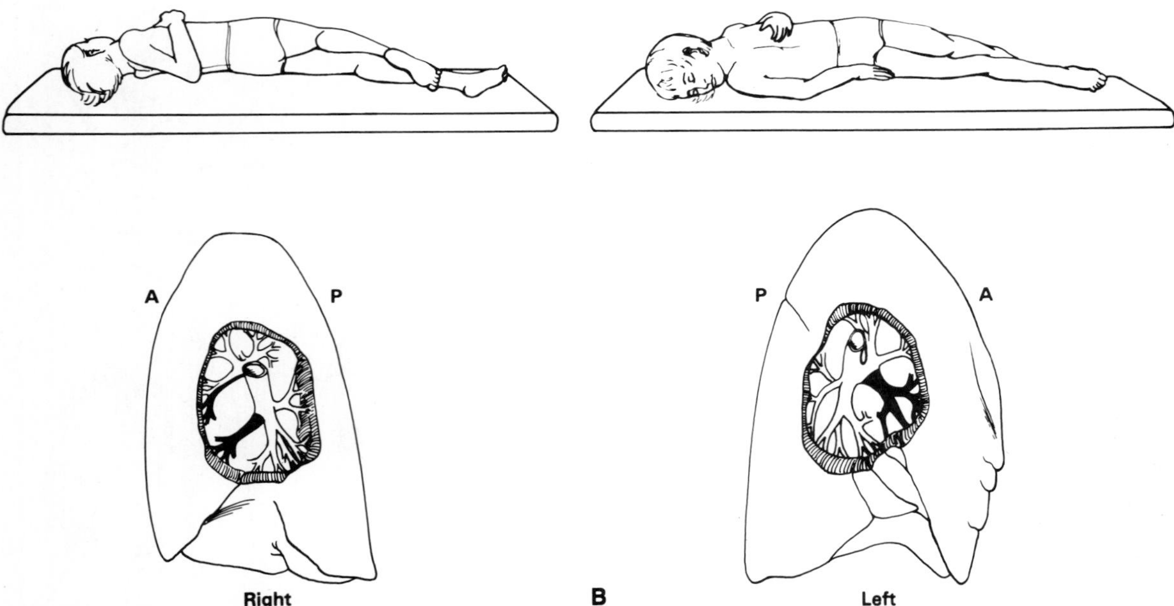

Figure 70-9. Position for drainage of the **(A)** right middle lobe or **(B)** lingular portion of the left upper lobe—one-fourth turn from prone.

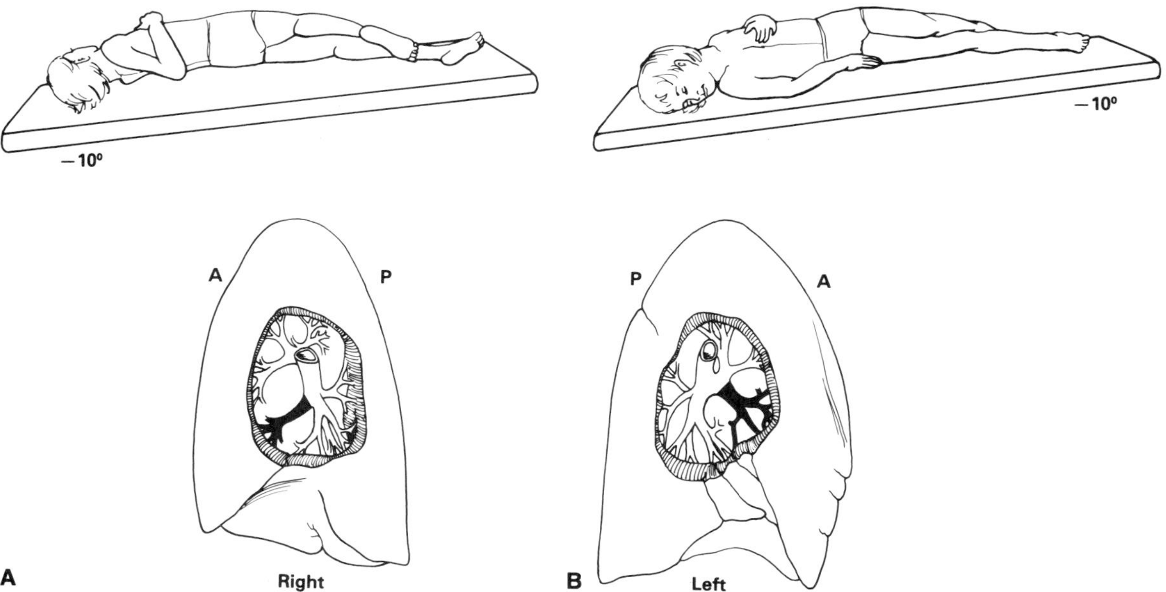

Figure 70-10. Alternate position for drainage of the (**A**) right middle lobe or (**B**) lingular portion of the left upper lobe—one-fourth turn from prone, head down 10 degrees.

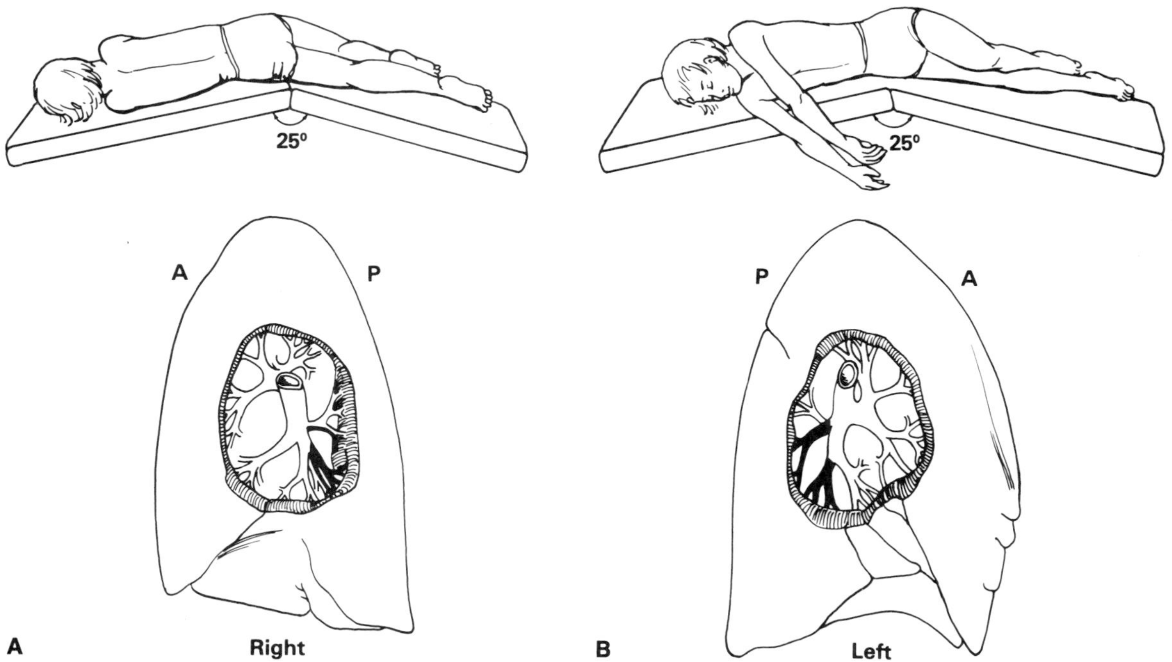

Figure 70-11. The right lower lobe (**A**) is ideally drained in the full prone position, with head tipped 10 to 25 degrees. However, in the acutely ill patient, this position is often modified to semiprone, as shown here. (**B**) The semiprone to full prone position is essential to draining the posterior aspect of the lower lobe.

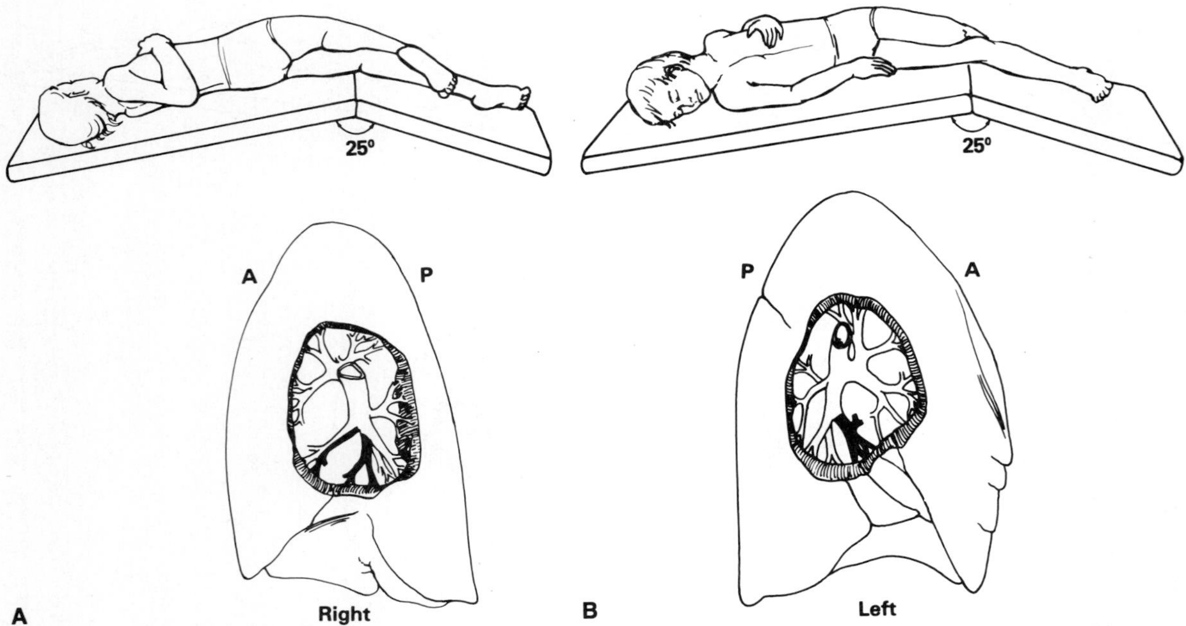

Figure 70-12. Position for drainage of the anterior bronchioles of the lower lobes—semisupine (partial roll to side), with head tipped 25 degrees. **(A)** right anterior lower lobe; **(B)** left anterior lower lobe.

forward-leaning position. These same seven patients had paradoxical breathing in the sitting or standing position. The authors attribute this relief of dyspnea to increased efficiency of diaphragmatic contraction in these positions.

These findings can be applied clinically with dramatic results. In my experience, optimum ventilatory function is achieved with the patient sitting forward, head flexed, and arms relaxed across lap (Fig. 70-14). The patient is instructed to exhale, while the therapist's hand follows the contour of the diaphragm, pushing up and in. This active assistance on exhalation may facilitate or assist in a diaphragmatic shift to a more efficient position. This can be useful when working

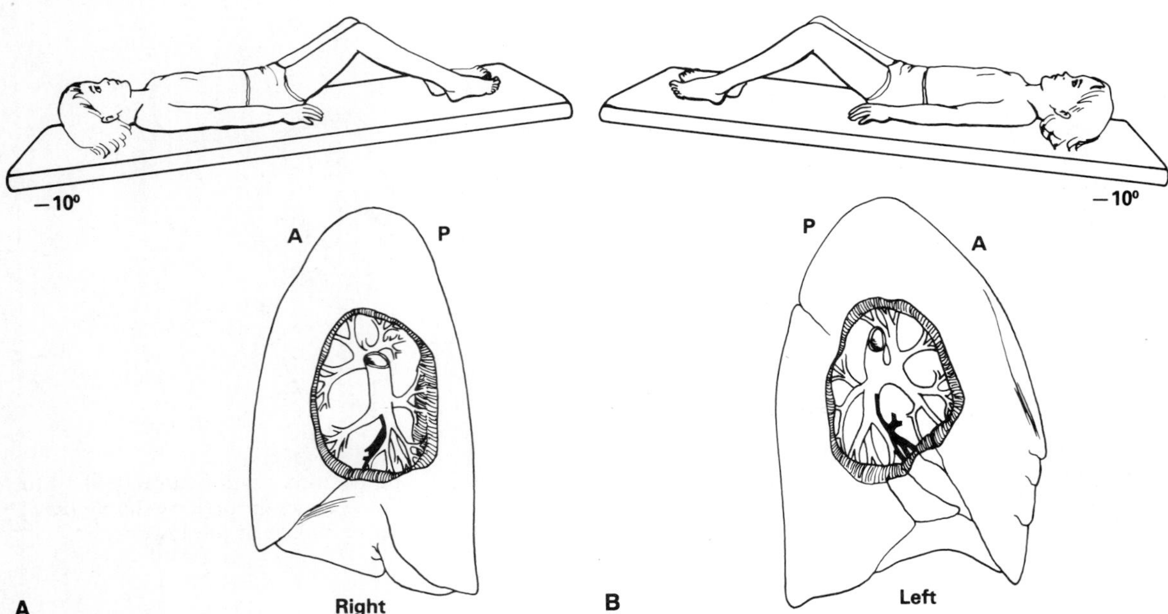

Figure 70-13. Alternate position for drainage of the **(A)** right and **(B)** left anterior bronchioles of the lower lobes—supine with head tipped 10 degrees.

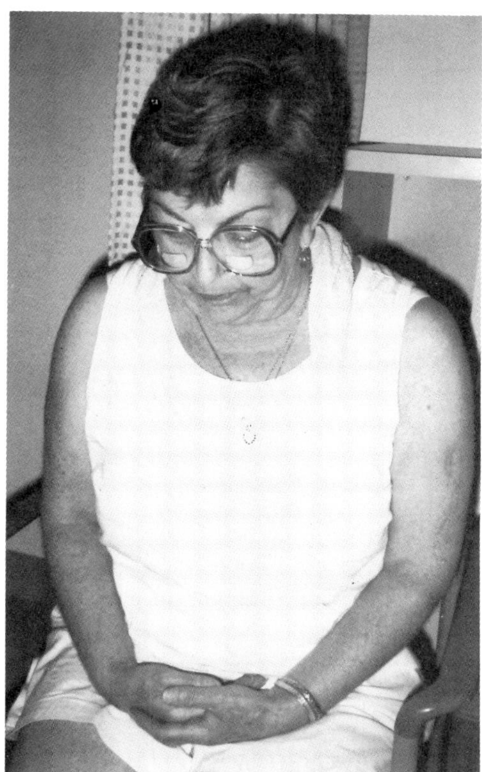

Figure 70-14. Positioning of a patient with head forward and upper extremities relaxed helps to optimize the resting position of the diaphragm prior to contraction.

with the COPD patient who is weaning from mechanical ventilation, as well as with the extubated patient who is dyspneic.

Lateral, supine, and prone positions can also affect diaphragmatic excursion. In the normal individual the dependent portion of the diaphragm has the greatest excursion.[33] In the supine position a greater force is exerted by the posterior or dorsal portion of the diaphragm; this is reversed when the person is prone.[34] However, if lung volume is low during either spontaneous or mechanical ventilation, airflow is more uniformly distributed—that is, greater proportions of the tidal volume move to the least gravity-dependent aspects of the lung. Consequently, atelectasis and secretion retention occur in the gravity-dependent zones.

Effects of Positioning on Oxygenation

Changes in oxygenation resulting from position change can be dramatic. An increase in oxygenation has been noted when persons with normal lungs as well as patients with chronic lung disease or post-thoracotomy patients are in the lateral rather than the supine position.[35,36] Increased oxygenation with the good lung down has also been observed with unifocal atelectasis, with pneumonia, and following lung resection.[37–39]

Treatment of patients with a unifocal process includes positioning with the good lung down in order to allow for maximal oxygenation as well as clearance of secretions from the affected lung (Fig. 70-15). Monitoring of SaO_2 and cardiopulmonary stress should occur throughout treatment. Post-treatment positioning emphasizes the lateral position, with the good or less affected lung dependent.

The patient with precarious ventilatory status, even with maximum ventilatory support, is often the patient with numerous tubes and lines in place. As a result, the patient's position is frequently supine or partially lateral. However, investigators have found that oxygenation can be increased by rolling these patients from supine to prone.[40] The prone position is believed to provide a means of counteracting the adverse ($\dot{V}/\dot{Q}$) ratio in the dependent portion of the lung, as well as to allow gravity to assist in secretion removal. Prone positioning requires numerous personnel and very careful

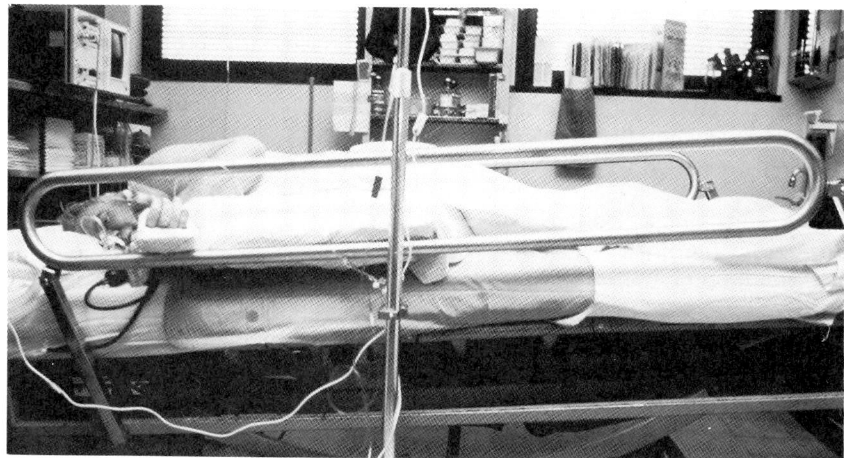

Figure 70-15. Patient with left lower lobe collapse is placed in a right lateral position. This position (with good lung down) should optimize oxygenation as well as promote secretion clearance of left lower lobe with gravity assistance. (From Kigin,[69] with permission.)

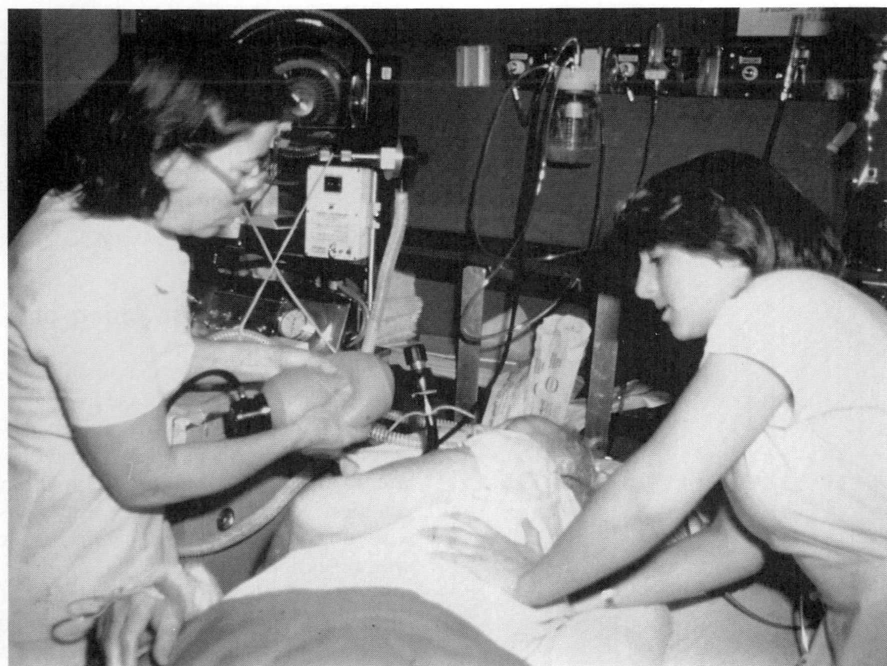

Figure 70-16. Patient in acute respiratory distress with *thick* secretions who was unable to adequately mobilize secretions in the modified lateral position. This patient tolerated the head-down, right lateral position while receiving vibration during manual ventilation with 100 percent O_2. (From Kigin,[69] with permission.)

monitoring. In my experience it is only attempted in the very acutely ill patients in whom mechanical ventilatory support is unable to provide adequate oxygenation.

Clinicians frequently hesitate to place patients with chronic or acute respiratory failure in the Trendelenburg or head-dependent position. However, it has been shown that the head-dependent position does not cause desaturation or a drop in FRC in stable chronic bronchitic patients[41] and can be safely used in patients with acute respiratory failure[42] who are not able to clear secretions in modified positions. In my experience the patient's needs should be carefully evaluated, and if retained secretions are the primary problem, use of optimum positioning to facilitate secretion clearance should be considered. Patients in acute failure should, however, be closely monitored during positioning. If the patient experiences increased dyspnea or a drop in SaO_2 a modified position should be attempted.

MANUAL TECHNIQUES FOR BRONCHOPULMONARY DRAINAGE

Rationale

Positioning alone may not be sufficient to promote secretion flow, and use of manual techniques in conjunction with positioning is frequently necessary[43] (Figs. 70-16 and 70-17).

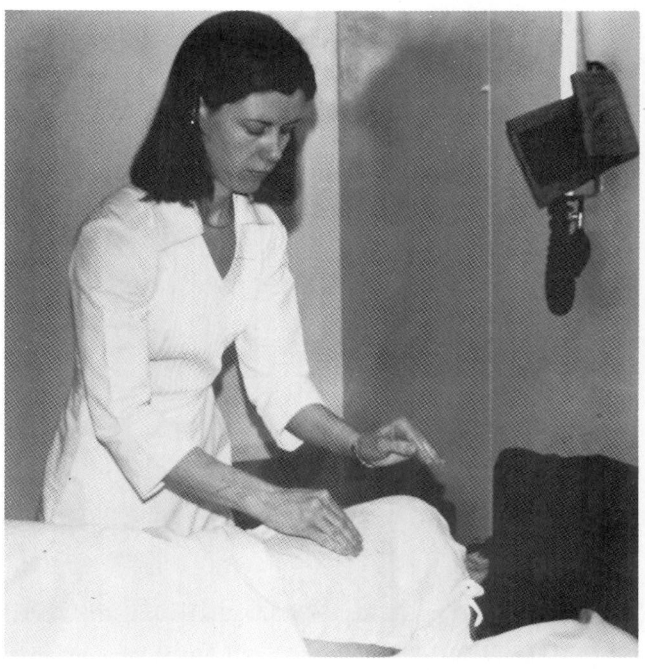

Figure 70-17. A patient with retention of left lingula/lower lobe secretions who is receiving percussion. Note cupped position of hands.

The manual techniques include percussion, vibration, and shaking (see boxed lists). These techniques have been used since the 1950s for patients in respiratory failure, including those requiring mechanical ventilation[44]; however, their success has been difficult to document. Investigators have either failed to define the treatment in terms of duration, force, or frequency of administration or have used clinical assessment techniques difficult to quantify (e.g., sputum production, radiographic changes).[45–48] Recent work has concentrated on establishing the optimum frequency of oscillation and vibration for secretion clearance. King et al.[49] found in dogs that the optimum frequency for secretion clearance was 13 Hz, with 5 to 17 Hz improving mucus flow, while Mellin[50] claims that a frequency of 5 to 6 Hz is optimum for secretion clearance. Other investigators, in attempting to control variables, have standardized the time or duration of the manual techniques. To attempt to standardize such a technique across a patient population with variable secretion retention and mucus clearance is similar to trying to standardize the dialysis time for patients with kidney failure and is a misuse of the techniques.

PERCUSSION

Definition

Percussion is a manual technique used to loosen secretions adherent to or lodged within the tracheobronchial tree. The procedure is used with postural drainage positions appropriate to affected areas. It is performed throughout inhalation and exhalation.

Indications

- Bronchial plugs
- Copious, tenacious secretions
- Lung abscess
- Bronchiectasis
- Segmental collapse
- Unoperative side of a thoracotomy (percussion is usually more comfortable than vibration to the patient resting on an incision site

Precautions/Conditions Necessitating Modification of Technique

- Rib fracture; sternal split
- Osteoporosis

Contraindications

- Recent pulmonary embolus prior to adequate anticoagulation
- Unstable flail chest

Method

Cup both hands, with the thumb aligned along the distal joint of the forefinger. The metacarpophalangeal joints are flexed 90 degrees, with the distal joints of the fingers extended and held together. The percussive surface of the hand is then made up of a "cup," with the borders consisting of the thenar and hypothenar eminences. With the hands well cupped, proceed with a relaxed swing of the forearm and wrist and clap over the posterior portion of the rib cage in an area bordered by (1) the spinal column, taking care not to clap directly over it; (2) the tenth rib, avoiding the floating ribs (eleventh and twelfth) and kidney area; and (3) the scapular region. The clap should sound hollow, with no slapping from excess pressure of the fingers or the heel of the hand. A light gown or towel over the chest often increases the patient's tolerance to the percussion procedure.

VIBRATION

Definition

Vibration is a manual technique used to loosen secretions lodged along the bronchial tree. This procedure, used in conjunction with postural drainage, is performed only during the exhalation phase of respiration. It is often an alternative treatment for patients who find percussion uncomfortable.

Indications

- Atelectasis
- Excessive, tenacious secretions
- Alternative to percussion
- Operative side of a thoracotomy (vibration is usually more comfortable than percussion around an incision site

Precautions/Conditions Necessitating Modification of Technique

- Osteoporosis
- Rib fractures; sternal split; flail chest

Contraindications

- Recent pulmonary embolus prior to adequate anticoagulation

Method

Place both hands firmly over the posterior and lateral thoracic rib cage of the affected area (one hand on top of the other). Stiffen the arms from the shoulder and with the elbows and wrists extended tensely, proceed with quick shakes, using short excursions of the oscillating hands. The magnitude of the vibrations may range from mere tension at the surface to slight springing of the rib cage. However, the treatment is not a shoving or heavy compression of the rib cage and these maneuvers should be avoided. The vibration is preceded by (1) hyperinflation of the intubated patient using an anesthesia bag or leaving the patient on the ventilator; or (2) basilar expansion with smooth, slow exhalation. The patient receives or takes a controlled deep breath and vibration is initiated on prolonged exhalation. The vibration is superficial and the rib cage should not be displaced, nor should the vibrations be uncomfortable to the patient. To be effective, however, the vibrations should not be so superficial as to move the patient's skin only; the hands must be placed on the chest firmly enough to transmit the vibrations through the chest wall.

Indications and Contraindications

The indication for use of the manual techniques is secretion retention—that is, inability to clear secretions by deep breathing and/or coughing activity. It should be remembered that decreased inspiratory volume postoperatively is corrected by maximal inspiratory volume. If secretion retention is also a problem, use of percussion or vibration in *conjunction* with maximal inspiratory volume is appropriate.

Contraindications for the use of percussion and vibration are relative. Depending on the patient's presentation and the clinician's evaluation, these techniques may be judiciously used even in patients with a flail chest. However, careful assessment and monitoring are required during therapy. Positioning is modified, as is the application of the manual techniques. For example, with an anterior chest wall fracture, a fine *vibration* would be used on the posterior rib cage even if the patient must remain supine. However, if there is any rib shift or other motion during treatment, treatment with these techniques is stopped.

Assessment of Efficacy

The effectiveness of CPT cannot be judged by the volume of secretions produced during therapy, although some clinicians believe secretion volume is the only indicator of success.[51] Improvements in expiratory flow,[52] vital capacity,[52] and specific airway conductance[53,54] have been associated with the volume of secretions produced.[55] However, Feldman et al.[56] demonstrated significant increases in expiratory flow at low lung volumes with as little as 5 mL of sputum production. As a result, especially in critically ill patients, sputum volume should not be used to evaluate treatment efficacy. Patients in acute respiratory failure may show dramatic improvement in oxygenation, chest radiographic findings, and lung compliance with as little as 2 mL of secretions removed.[57]

There are few objective data for comparing the efficacy of the manual techniques in sputum removal, although it is believed that percussion splatters or breaks up mucus plugs while vibration facilitates mucus flow. In an unpublished series studying the flow of an instilled bolus of propyliodone into the airways of dogs serving as their own controls, the movement of the bolus to the trachea was faster with the use of percussion or vibration than with positioning alone.

Bronchoscopy provides a mode of direct visualization of secretion movement and has been performed during vibration in our clinical setting. During lavage on a patient with alveolar proteinosis, clearance of secretions was subjectively less with saline alone than with saline and the manual techniques. In another institution, when a mechanical vibrator was compared with therapist-delivered percussion, the density of sputum removed during lavage was greater with percussion than with the mechanical device.[58] I and my colleagues favor use of the therapist's hands, which allows direct contact with the patient and evaluation and facilitation of thoracic motion and inspiratory volume during treatment, particularly when vibration is used.

BRONCHOPULMONARY DRAINAGE IN THE INTUBATED PATIENT

Effects on Oxygenation and Lung Compliance

Maintaining oxygenation during therapy in critically ill patients is possible but requires skilled application of CPT.[42] In my experience the acutely ill post-trauma or postoperative patient does not desaturate during CPT if ventilation is maintained with a manual ventilator and 100 percent O_2 (Fig. 70-16). Such patients frequently show dramatic increases in PaO_2, with the resolution of lobar collapse during treatment.

Increased total lung/thorax compliance following CPT has been documented in patients receiving mechanical ventilation.[59] This improvement has been attributed to clearance of secretions from the small airways. Dramatic resolution of atelectasis can occur with use of positioning, percussion, and vibration. Of note is a study by Marini et al.,[60] who compared the results of CPT and bronchoscopy in 31 patients with acute lobar atelectasis and found equal resolution (average 37 percent) of atelectasis with either treatment. The patients who received bronchoscopy subsequently received CPT and did not require further bronchoscopy. The authors compared these findings with other studies in which patients received bronchoscopy only and required repeated bronchoscopies to keep the lung reinflated.

Initial therapy for lung collapse is the use of positioning and the manual techniques. Such therapy is less invasive and less costly than other procedures and frequently results in resolution of the collapse. Should the collapse persist, bronchoscopy is then employed.

Cough, Huff, Forced Expiration, and Suction

Cough, the rapid expulsion of air from the lungs, can be either a voluntary effort or a reflex reaction. An effective cough requires a large inspiratory volume, followed by closure of the vocal cords and subsequent strong contraction of the abdominal muscles in conjunction with the elastic recoil of the lungs. This results in rapid expulsion of air through the suddenly opened vocal cords.[61]

A true cough cannot occur when an artificial airway is in place. In addition, the increased resistance of the airway reduces the maximum velocity of exhalation. However, during therapy the intubated patient should be asked to attempt to cough during suctioning, especially if the patient is ready for extubation. Ventilatory assistance (manual or mechanical) can greatly improve the efficacy of an attempted cough in the intubated patient. In addition, since the contractile ability of the diaphragm is decreased postoperatively,[62] the high pressures necessary for a cough may be better obtained in the sitting than in the supine position.[63] The force of the cough may be further enhanced by support or compression of the abdomen or thoracic area (post-thoracotomy)[64] during coughing.

Huffing, or forced expiration, is a maneuver that promotes the expulsion of air through an open glottis. The technique, when studied on stable patients with cystic fibrosis, asthma, or COPD, has been found to be an effective alternative to coughing or to the manual techniques for clearing secretions.[65] Clinically, I have found the technique to be of value in the acutely ill patient who is unable to cough effectively owing to pain or to highly reactive airways.

Detailed information regarding suctioning of artificial airways is discussed elsewhere in the text (Ch. 72). It should be noted, however, that the complications of mucosal damage and drop in PaO_2 can occur with the nonintubated as well as with the intubated patient. Adequate pre- and post-oxygenation can alleviate this drop in PaO_2, and the limitation of vacuum pressure can decrease the potential for mucosal damage.[66]

The use of "blind" nasotracheal suction in nonintubated patients is reserved for those with retained secretions and an ineffective cough. The irritation caused by the catheter may stimulate a cough that clears the secretions even without suction. Instillation of small amounts of saline (3 to 5 mL) through the catheter may also stimulate a cough. Vibration during the suctioning procedure may further facilitate secretion removal, particularly in the patient with a poor or ineffective cough reflex even with catheter insertion. Caution is necessary regarding possible laryngospasm during nasotracheal suctioning. Simulation of the larynx during suctioning may promote spasm. Manual ventilation with bag and mask must always be available when nasotracheal suctioning is performed.

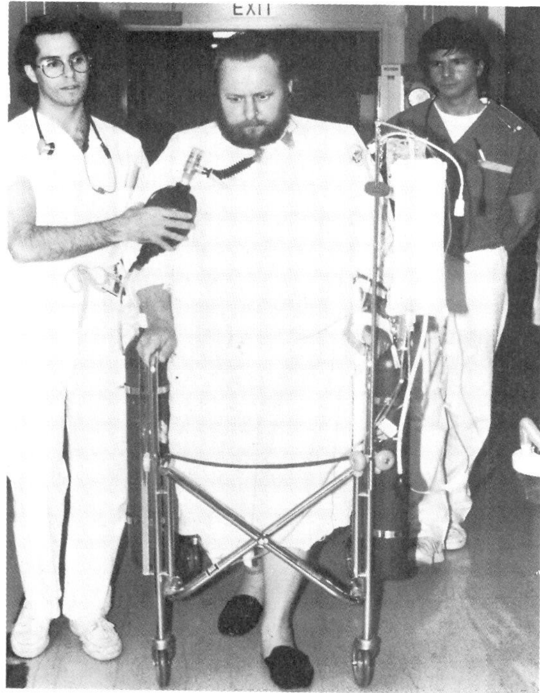

Figure 70-18. Ambulation of post-thorocotomy patient requiring continued mechanical ventilation. Ventilation and oxygenation are provided by manual ventilator. The patient, who is ventilator-dependent and is on an exercise program, has increased O_2 consumption whether exercising while sitting, standing, or during ambulation and requires adequate O_2 support during the exercise session. The patient's response to exercise is monitored by pulse oximetry, as well as heart rate, blood pressure, and respiratory rate.

MOBILIZATION AND EXERCISE

Early mobility and exercise are elements of therapy that are often overlooked in patients with pulmonary dysfunction. The postoperative patient extubated within 24 to 48 hours can usually ambulate easily, thereby minimizing the complications of prolonged bed rest, including venous thrombosis, pulmonary embolism, and increase in resting heart rate.[67,68] Prolonged supine positioning also causes demineralization of the long bones, with increased calcium excretion and potential osteoporosis.[67] Joint contracture and muscle atrophy contribute to potential prolonged debilitation.

The stabilized, alert, long-term ventilator-supported patient may be more easily weaned with a program of sitting, standing, and ambulating with ventilator support (Fig. 70-18). Patients requiring support should have their SaO_2 and heart rate monitored during ambulation. The focus should be on total rehabilitation of the long-term ventilator-supported patient, minimizing potential long-term musculoskeletal deficits that can occur with prolonged bed rest.

References

1. O'Donohue WJ (ed): Current Advances in Respiratory Care. Am College Chest Physicians, Park Ridge, IL, 1984
2. Palmer KNV, Sellick BA: The prevention of post-operative pulmonary atelectasis. Lancet 1953;1:164–168
3. Tisi GM: State of the art: Preoperative evaluation of pulmonary function. Am Rev Respir Dis 1979;119:293–299
4. Pontoppidan H: Mechanical aids to lung expansion in nonintubated patients. Am Rev Respir Dis 1980;(5, pt. 2)122:109–119
5. Ford GT, Whitelaw WA, Rosenal TW et al: Diaphragm function after upper abdominal surgery in humans. Am Rev Respir Dis 1983;127:431–437
6. Polgar G, Weng TR: The functional development of the respiratory systems. Am Rev Respir Dis 1979;120:625–632
7. Fraser RG, Pare JAP: Diagnosis of Disease of the Chest. WB Saunders, Philadelphia, 1977
8. Donnenfeld RS: Atelectasis: Preoperative and postoperative ventilatory care. Anesthesiol Clin 1971;9:103–127
9. Derenne J-P, Macklem PT, Roussos C: The respiratory muscles: Mechanics, control, and pathophysiology. Am Rev Respir Dis 1978;118:119–125
10. Bethune DD: Neurophysiological facilitation of respiration in the unconscious adult patient. Physiother C 1975;27:241–249
11. Thoren L: Postoperative pulmonary complications: Observations on their prevention by means of physiotherapy. Acta Chir Scand 1954;107:193–204
12. Luce JM, Culver BH: Respiratory muscle function in health and disease. Chest 1982;81:82–90
13. Loring SH, Mead J: Action of the diaphragm on the rib cage inferred from a force-balance analysis. J Appl Physiol 1982;53:756–764

14. Rochester DF, Aurora NS: Respiratory muscle failure. Med Clin North Am 1983;67:573–582
15. Rochester DF: Respiratory muscle function in health. Heart Lung 1984;13:349–360
16. Roussos C: Function and fatigue of respiratory muscles. Chest 1985;88:124S–132S
17. Sharp JT: Therapeutic considerations in respiratory muscle function. Chest 1985;88:1185–1192
18. Barach AL: Oxygen supported exercise and rehabilitation of patients with chronic obstructive lung disease. Ann Allergy 1966;24:51–59
19. Gaskell DV, Webber BA: The Brompton hospital guide to chest physiotherapy, Blackwell Scientific Publications, Oxford, 1973
20. Faulkner JA: New perspectives in training for maximum performance. JAMA 1968;205:741–748
21. Lane C: Inspiratory Muscle Weight Training and Its Effect on the Vital Capacity with Patients with Quadriplegia. Thesis, Northeastern University, Boston, 1982
22. Leith DE, Bradley M: Ventilatory muscle strength and endurance training. J Appl Physiol 1976;41:508–513
23. Gross D, Riley E, Grassino A et al: Influence of resistive training on respiratory muscle strength and endurance in quadriplegia. Am Rev Respir Dis 1978;117S:343
24. Belman MJ, Mittman C: Ventilatory muscle training improves exercise capacity in chronic obstructive pulmonary disease patients. Am Rev Respir Dis 1980;121:273–280
25. Pardy RL, Rivington RN, Despas PJ, Macklem PT: The effects of inspiratory muscle training on exercise performance in chronic airflow limitation. Am Rev Respir Dis 1981;123:426–431
26. Sonne LJ, Davis JA: Increased exercise performance in patients with severe COPD following inspiratory resistive training. Chest 1982;81:436–442
27. Jederlinic P, Muspratt JA, Miller MJ: Inspiratory muscle training in clinical practice: Physiologic conditioning or habituation to suffocation? Chest 1984;86:870–878
28. Belman MJ: Respiratory failure treated by ventilatory muscle training. Eur J Respir Dis 1981;62:391–398
29. Sackner MA: Pulmonary medicine: Tracheobronchial Toilet. Biomedia, Princeton, 1978
30. Cash JE (ed): Chest, Heart and Vascular Disorder for Physiotherapists. 5th Ed. Farber & Farber, London, 1976
31. Ingwersen U: Respiratory Physical Therapy and Pulmonary Care. Wiley Medical, New York, 1976
32. Sharp JT, Druz WS, Moisan T et al: Postural relief of dyspnea in severe chronic obstructive pulmonary disease. Am Rev Respir Dis 1980;122:201–209
33. Froese A, Bryan AC: Effects of anesthesia and paralysis on diaphragmatic mechanics in man. Anesthesiology 1974;41:242–250
34. Bryan C: Comments of a devil's advocate. Am Rev Respir Dis 1974;110:143S–144S
35. Clauss RH, Scalabrini BY, Ray JF, Reed GE: Effects of changing body position. Circulation, suppl. 2, 1968;37:214–221
36. Zack MB, Pontoppidan H, Kazemi H: The effect of lateral positions on gas exchange in pulmonary disease. Am Rev Respir Dis 1974;110:49–56
37. Prokocimer P, Garbino J, Wolff M, Regnier B: Influence of posture on gas exchange in artificially ventilated patients with focal lung disease. Intensive Care Med 1983;9:69–72
38. Remolina C, Khan AU, Santiago TV, Edelman NH: Positional hypoxemia in unilateral lung disease. N Engl J Med 1981;304:523–530
39. Seaton D, Lapp NL, Morgan WKC: Effect of body position on gas exchange after thoracotomy. Thorax 1979;34:518–526
40. Douglas WW, Rehder K, Beynen FM et al: Improved oxygenation in patients with acute respiratory failure: The prone position. Am Rev Respir Dis 1977;115:559–564
41. Marini JJ, Tyler LM, Hudson LD et al: Influence of head-dependent positions on lung volume and oxygen saturation in chronic airflow obstruction. Am Rev Respir Dis 1984;129:101–110
42. Mackenzie CF, Shin BB, McAslan TC: Chest physiotherapy: The effect on arterial oxygenation. Anesth Analg 1978;57:28–40
43. Frownfelter DL: Chest Physical Therapy and Pulmonary Rehabilitation. Year Book Medical Publishers, Chicago, 1978
44. Smith AC, Spalding JMK, Russell WR: Artificial respiration by intermittent positive pressure in poliomyelitis and other diseases. Lancet 1954;1:939–943
45. Gray L: Fatal pulmonary hemorrhage (letter). Phys Ther 1980;60:343–345
46. Flower KA, Eden RI, Lomax L et al: New mechanical aid to physiotherapy in cystic fibrosis. Br Med J 1979;2:630–631
47. Sutton PP, Pavia D, Bateman JRM, Clarke SW: Chest physiotherapy: A review. Eur J Respir Dis 1982;63:188–201
48. Maxwell M, Redmond A: Comparative trial of manual and mechanical percussion technique with gravity assisted bronchial drainage in patients with cystic fibrosis. Arch Dis Child 1979;54:542–550
49. King M, Phillips DM, Gross D et al: Enhanced tracheal mucus clearance with high frequency chest wall compression. Am Rev Respir Dis 1983;128:511–520
50. Mellins RB: Pulmonary physiotherapy in the pediatric age group. Am Rev Respir Dis 1974;110(6, pt. 2):137–142
51. Murray JF: The ketchup-bottle method. N Engl J Med 1979;300:1155–1160
52. Tecklin JS, Holsclaw DS: Evaluation of bronchial drainage in patients with cystic fibrosis. Phys Ther 1975;55:1081–1090
53. Cochrane GM, Webber BA, Clarke SW: Effects of sputum on pulmonary function. Br Med J 1977;2:1181–1186
54. Bateman JRM, Daunt KM, Newman SP et al: Regional lung clearance of excessive bronchial secretions during chest physiotherapy in patients with chronic airways obstruction. Lancet 1979;1:294–298
55. Mazzocco MC, Owens GR, Kirilloff LH, Rogers RM: Chest percussion and postural drainage in patients with bronchiectasis. Chest 1985;88:360–368
56. Feldman J, Traver GA, Taussig LM: Maximal expiratory flows after postural drainage. Am Rev Respir Dis 1979;119:239–246
57. Mackenzie CF, Ciesla N, Imle PC, Klemic N: Chest Physiotherapy in the Intensive Care Unit. Williams & Wilkins, Baltimore, 1981
58. Hammon WE, Martin RJ, Pennock B, Rogers RM: Percussion versus vibration for clearance of alveolar contents. Phys Ther 1980;60:589–596
59. Mackenzie CF, Shin B, Hadi F, Imle PC: Changes in total lung/thorax compliance following chest physiotherapy. Anesth Analg 1980;59:207–214
60. Marini JJ, Pierson DJ, Hudson LD: Acute lobar atelectasis: A prospective comparison of fiberoptic bronchoscopy and respiratory therapy. Am Rev Respir Dis 1979;119:971–981
61. Loudon RG: Cough: A symptom and a sign. Basics Respir Dis Spring, 1981
62. Byrd RB, Burns JR: Cough dynamics in post-thoracotomy state. Chest 1975;67:654–659
63. Curry LD, Van Eden C: The influence of posture on the effectiveness of cough. S Afr J Physiother 1977;33:8–16
64. Yamazaki S, Ogawa J, Shohzu A: Intra-pleural cough pressures in patients after thoracotomy. J Thorac Cardiovasc Surg 1980;80:600–610
65. Pryor JA, Webber BA, Hodson ME, Batten JC: Evaluation of the forced expiration technique as an adjunct to postural drainage in treatment of cystic fibrosis. Br Med J 1979;2:417–423
66. Adlkofer RM, Powaser MM: The effect of endotracheal suctioning on arterial blood gases in patients after cardiac surgery. Heart Lung 1978;7:1101–1109
67. Astrand PO, Rodahl K: Textbook of Work Physiology, McGraw-Hill, New York, 1977
68. Rose SD: Prophylaxis of thromboembolic disease. Med Clin North Am 1979;63:1205–1212
69. Kigin CM: Chest physical therapy for patients with acute respiratory failure. pp. 239–263. In Bone RC, George RB, Hudson LD (eds): Acute Respiratory Failure. Churchill Livingstone, New York, 1987

Chapter 71

Humidity and Aerosol Therapy

Robert M. Kacmarek

CHAPTER OUTLINE

Conditioning of the gas that we inspire is normally the role of the upper respiratory tract. As discussed in Chapter 4, the upper respiratory tract filters, humidifies, and warms inspired gases. Because provision of respiratory care frequently compromises the capability of the upper airway to perform these functions, the conditioning of inspired air must be considered during the performance of all respiratory care techniques.

Humidity therapy is best defined as the addition of water vapor, either heated or unheated, to inspired gas. Aerosol therapy, on the other hand, is the addition of both particulate and molecular water to inspired gas. Both humidity and aerosol therapy allow for variation in the inspired O_2 fraction (F_{IO_2}) delivered, and aerosol therapy is the method of choice for the delivery of drugs directly to the airways.

PHYSIOLOGIC CONSIDERATIONS

The amount of water vapor or molecular water that a given volume of air can hold is dependent on two factors, temperature and water availability. As discussed in detail in Chapter 1, the capacity of air for water (absolute humidity) is defined by temperature. At 37°C (body temperature) the maximum quantity of molecular water carried in air is 43.8 mg/L, with a water vapor pressure of 47 mmHg. Under normal physiologic conditions gas in the area of the carina is at 37°C and saturated with water vapor.[1,2] The exact location at which these conditions are reached may be as much as 5 cm beyond the carina and is referred to as the *isothermic saturation boundary*,[2] with its precise location primarily dependent on the condition of the inspired air. Nasal breathing is more efficient than oral breathing in conditioning inspired gas. As a result, the isothermic saturation boundary will be higher in the airway (closer to the trachea) during nasal breathing than during mouth breathing.

Normally, inspired gas is heated by convection within the respiratory tract, requiring 0.34 cal/L/°C.[3] Water vapor is added to inspired air by evaporation in the upper respiratory tract at an estimated rate of 250 mL/d.[4] That the respiratory tract must add water to inspired air defines the presence of a *humidity deficit* (Table 71-1), which is the amount of water added to inspired air to bring it to body temperature and pressure, saturated (BTPS). During health, systemic hydration provides the water necessary to meet the humidity deficit. However, during disease, when therapeutic gases are administered, the humidity deficit created may tax the body's ability to meet this deficit. As a result, secretions may be dried, leading to (1) impairment of ciliary activity; (2) impairment of mucus movement; (3) inflammatory change and necrosis of ciliated pulmonary epithelium; (4) retention of viscid, tenacious secretions with secondary incrustation; (5) bacterial infiltration; (6) atelectasis; and (7) pneumonia.[4,5]

INDICATIONS FOR HUMIDITY THERAPY

As defined in Table 71-2, humidity therapy is indicated in three settings[6]: (1) high flow therapeutic gas delivery to nonintubated patients; (2) conditioning of gas delivered via artificial airways; and (3) reduction of airway resistance in asthma. Historically, bubble-through humidifiers (see under Equipment Used for Humidity Therapy) have been used for the delivery of all therapeutic gases regardless of liter flow. This practice has spread because gases leaving cylinders or central gas piping systems are devoid of water vapor. Thus, humidifiers have been used to minimize the humidity deficit. As discussed later, unheated bubble-through humidifiers establish relative humidity at body temperatures in the range of 35 to 40 percent.[6–8] In fact, the most that can be expected is to establish a water vapor content in the therapeutic gas consistent with that of room air.

On theoretical grounds the need to humidify therapeutic gases delivered at low flow rates is questionable. At a 4 L/min flow from a nasal cannula, only about 66 to 166 mL of dry gas is inspired per breath (see Ch. 75), with the remaining tidal volume being room air. As a result, the National Consensus Conference on Oxygen Therapy of the American College of Chest Physicians[9] states "there is no evidence to indicate the need for routine humidification of therapeutic gas at flow rates of 1 to 4 L/min." Campbell et al.,[10] in a randomized study of the effects of low-flow humidified versus nonhumidified O_2 therapy, noted no difference in complications between the two groups (Table 71-3). As a result, my colleagues and I only recommend the routine use of unheated bubble-through humidifiers on simple O_2 masks, partial or nonrebreathing masks, high-flow systems, and nasal cannulas operated at more than 5 L/min, although there may be exceptions to this general rule based on the individual response of a given patient. In addition, these recommendations only apply to adults. All O_2 delivered to infants and children should be humidified.

Table 71-1. Calculation of Humidity Deficit

H_2O content necessary to prevent humidity deficit	= 43.8 mg/L
Minute ventilation	= 8.5 L
Actual H_2O content	= 20.0 mg/L
Deficit per liter 43.8 − 20.0	= 23.8 mg/L
Minute humidity deficit (23.8 mg/L) (8.5 L)	= 202.3 mg H_2O

Table 71-2. Indications for Humidity Therapy

Humidification of dry therapeutic gases
Liter flow >5 L/min
Delivery of heated humidified gas to artificial airways
During mechanical ventilation
During spontaneous breathing
Reduction of airway resistance during
Exercise-induced asthma
Nocturnal asthma

(Modified from Darin et al.,[6] with permission.)

In patients whose upper airway is bypassed by the presence of an endotracheal or tracheostomy tube, conditioning of inspired gas is required. Usually this is accomplished by the use of large-volume heated humidifiers or heated nebulizers (see under Equipment Used for Humidity Therapy and Equipment Used for Aerosol Therapy). Of concern is the delivery of gas at 100 percent relative humidity near body temperature (i.e., at or above 32°C). Since gas delivery to patients with artificial airways is via large-bore tubing, it is easy to monitor gas temperature near the patient's airway. Some of the units currently available (e.g., the Puritan-Bennett Cascade II and Concha humidifying systems) incorporate feedback from a temperature probe located near the airway to ensure that delivered gas is at the desired temperature. In patients with chronic tracheostomies, the respiratory system does adjust to the increased humidity deficit. Many of these patients may be able to adequately humidify their airways with the periodic use of heat and moisture exchangers (see Hygroscopic Condenser Humidifiers).

There is significant evidence that cooling and evaporative water loss increases airway resistance in specific groups of asthmatic patients.[11–13] The inhalation of cold unhumidified air by patients with exercise-induced asthma,[13] as well as by some who are not asthmatics,[14,15] results in increased airway resistance. Even in marathon runners, a 50 percent decrease in forced vital capacity (FVC) has been noted during exercise at −2 to −4°C.[15] This response is believed to occur via cholinergic mechanisms[16]; in fact, this response is blocked with ipratropium bromide in normal subjects and by cromolyn sodium along with ipratropium bromide in those with ex-

Table 71-3. Humidified versus Nonhumidified Low-Flow Oxygen Therapy

	Humidified O_2	Dry O_2
Number	99	86
Age ± SD	66.3 ± 13.6	65.9 ± 13.3
Men/women	66/35	56/30
Duration of O_2 therapy (days ± SD)	2.7 ± 2.5	2.8 ± 2.4
Range	1–20	1–20
Diagnoses		
Postoperative, coronary bypass	46	30
Postoperative other	16	15
Myocardial infarction	11	13
Malignancy	14	11
Other	12	17
Total	99	86

	Symptom Severity[a]									
	Humidified O_2					Dry O_2				
Symptom	1	2	3	4	5	1	2	3	4	5
Dry nose	22	52	39	7	20	1	48	40	3	13
Dry throat	0	36	53	11	26	0	23	40	10	31
Headache	2	4	9	4	8	0	13	18	1	6
Chest discomfort	1	2	16	5	14	0	8	10	0	9

[a] Data are number of patients rating symptoms at various degrees of severity at daily interviews. Severity scale ranged from 1 (minimal discomfort) to 5 (maximal discomfort).

(From Campbell et al.,[10] with permission.)

ercise-induced asthma.[16] It appears the combined effects of inspiring cool unhumidified gas and of the larger minute volumes associated with exercise moves the isothermal saturation boundary deeper into the lower airway, which results in a cholinergic response of the lower airways and increased resistance to gas flow. A similar mechanism is believed to account for nocturnal asthma.[17] However, the use of heated, humidified gas blocks this response. Although the data are preliminary, the use of heated humidification systems is recommended in chronic as well as acute management of exercise-induced and nocturnal asthma.

EQUIPMENT USED FOR HUMIDITY THERAPY

The following types of humidification systems are currently available:

- Bubble/diffusion/jet
- Large-volume bubble
- Large-volume wick
- Large-volume passover
- Large-volume temperature servo-controlled
- Spinning disc
- Heat and moisture exchanger

However, the efficiency of all types is based on the following specific factors:

1. Surface area of gas exposure to water
2. Duration of gas-water contact
3. Temperature of system

Ideally, humidifiers are designed to allow a large area of contact between therapeutic gas and water. This is accomplished differently by the various available systems, but in general, the larger the area of contact, the greater the relative humidity of the gas leaving the humidifier.

The duration of contact is critical for unheated humidifiers operating at high flows. To ensure maximum efficiency of any unit, it must be maintained near its maximum water fill level. Any reduction in water level, particularly for bubble-through humidifiers, results in decreased contact time and decreased relative humidity.

Temperature is by far the most important factor affecting the relative humidity of gas exiting a humidifier. As a result of the cooling produced by evaporation, gas exiting the humidifiers (unless heated) is cooler than room air. A drop of about 1°F occurs for every liter of gas passed through the humidifier. However, since with most unheated systems O_2 is delivered by 6 to 8 ft of small-bore tubing, gas temperature increases during delivery to the patient.

Bubble-Through Humidifiers

Figure 71-1 illustrates the operation of a bubble-through humidifier. Gas enters the unit via a flowmeter and tube extending into the water to the base of the unit. Depending on the model, a number of variations in design exist. In the

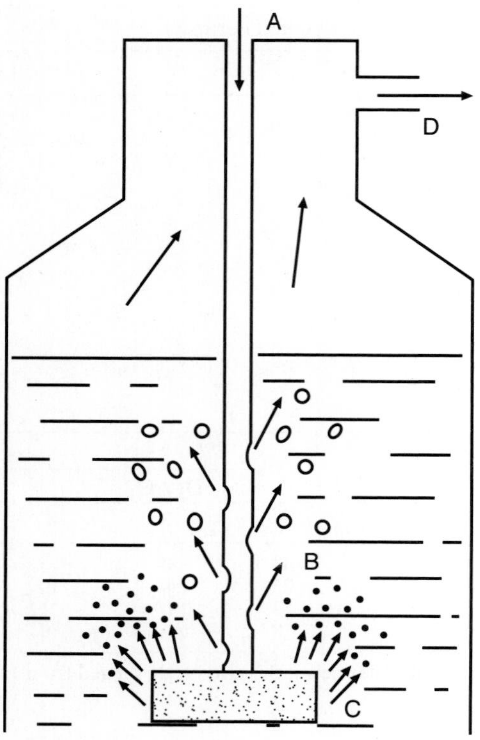

Figure 71-1. Bubble-diffusion humidifier. A, tube extending gas flow to the bottom of humidifier; B, holes in the side of the delivery tube, allowing bubbles of gas to exit; C, porous diffuser at base of unit; D, outflow port to patient (point where O_2 appliance is attached). (From Scanlon et al.,[22] with permission.)

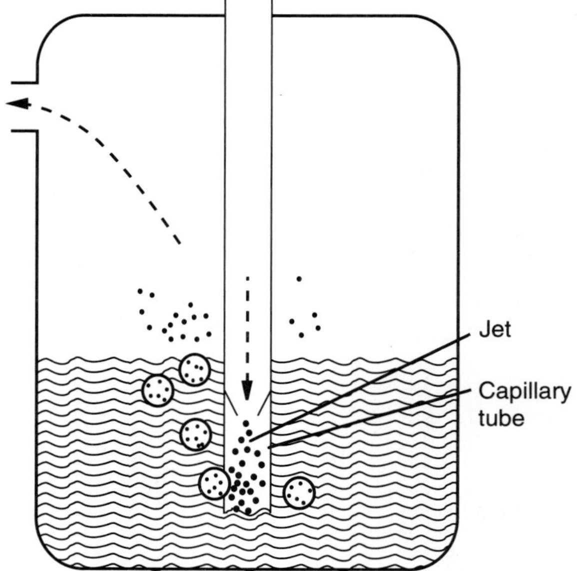

Figure 71-2. Bubble-jet humidifier: A small opening in the gas delivery tube under the surface of the water allows for entrainment of water into the gas delivery system. As water enters, an aerosol is created by the gas flow. The gas and aerosol exit the delivery tube at its tip. (From McPherson,[172] with permission.)

simplest, least efficient systems, gas is bubbled under water via holes in the sides and at the bottom of the delivery tube. Other units incorporate a porous stone-like diffusion head at the end of the tube, causing gas to exit the diffuser in small volume bubbles. Still others (Fig. 71-2) are listed as bubble-jet humidifiers because they include a venturi jet (see Ch. 1) in the gas delivery tube under the water level. This results in water being drawn into the delivery tube and water and gas exiting either via small holes in the delivery tube or from a diffuser. Use of the venturi jet increases the efficiency of the humidifier but may result in the delivery of particulate water to the patient, increasing the risk of contamination. This category of humidifiers is currently available in reusable or disposable units.

Large-Volume Bubble-Through Humidifiers

The Puritan-Bennett Cascade I humidifier (Fig. 71-3) is the prototype for large-volume bubble-through humidifiers. It is designed for use in ventilator circuits or high gas flow delivery systems. Gas entering the unit proceeds under water via a column inside the unit's tower reservoir, and gas exiting the column is forced through a grid-like diffuser. As a result of the high gas flow through the unit, a frothy interface between gas and air is created as gas moves up and out of the tower. This causes water to also cascade over the tower, increasing the time of gas-water contact. Gas then moves across the water surface before exiting the unit. A heating element with thermostat is submerged in the center of the unit. A shunt across the two aspects of this element ensures that it is turned off if the water level falls too far. This unit is highly efficient and is capable of delivering gas at BTPS at flows up to and exceeding 100 L/min.

Large-Volume Passover Heated Humidifiers

A typical large-volume passover heated humidifier is illustrated in Figure 71-4. These units are designed for use on ventilator or high-flow gas delivery systems. The water in the unit is separated from the gas flowing through the unit by a thin membrane permeable only to water vapor. Water resides in a thin layer between this membrane and a heating element. As the water is heated, it evaporates through the membrane into the unit's canister and is picked up by the gas flowing through the unit. These units are usually continuously fed via a reservoir, since only a small volume of water is actually present within the humidifier at any point in time. Like cascade-type units, these humidifiers are very efficient and capable of delivering high flows of gas at BTPS.

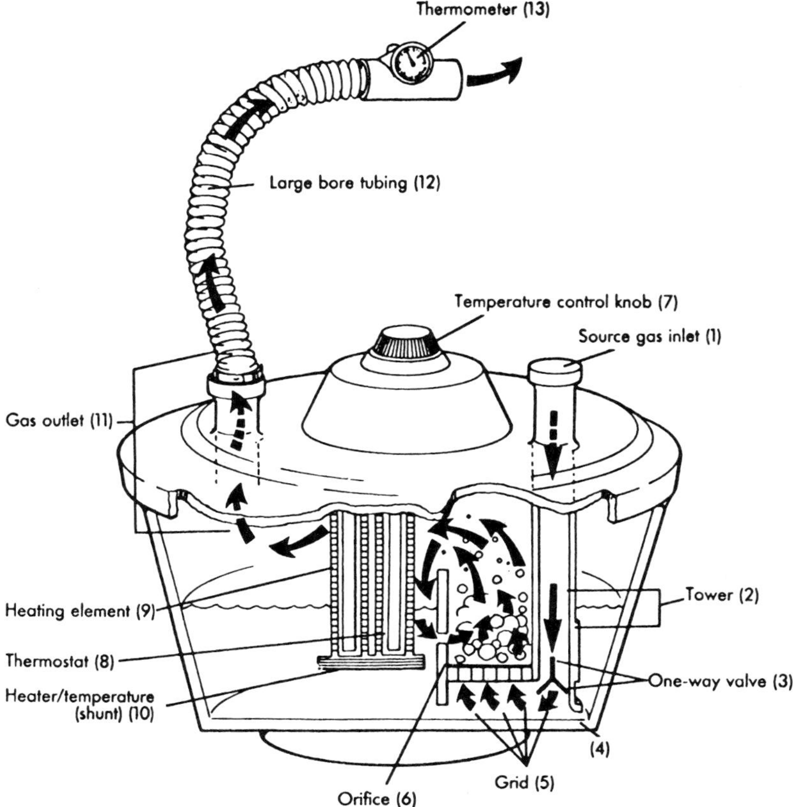

Figure 71-3. Puritan-Bennett Cascade I humidifier. See text for details. (From Scanlon et al.,[22] with permission.)

However, many lose efficiency at flows exceeding 100 L/min.

Wick-Type Humidifiers

The Bird model 3000 is the classic wick-type humidifier (Fig. 71-5). Like the heated passover units, wick systems are normally fed from a reservoir, and the actual volume of water in the unit is maintained at a minimum level. The wick, made of a porous hygroscopic material, is partially submerged in water but also extends into the humidifier body a considerable distance. As noted in Figure 71-5, the wick increases the surface area across which evaporation takes place. Wick humidifiers are also capable of delivering gas saturated with water vapor at body temperature, but like passover units they may lose efficiency at very high flows (above 100 L/min).

Servo-Controlled Humidifiers

Servo-controlled humidifiers use temperature probes placed at the Y of the ventilator circuit or near the airway in high-flow delivery systems to ensure that gas at the set temperature reaches the probe—that is, the temperature of the humidifier may need to be 45°C or higher to ensure that the temperature at the airway is near BPTS. Via electronic feedback these units ensure stability of airway temperature. Most include high- and low-temperature alarms and reservoir feed systems.

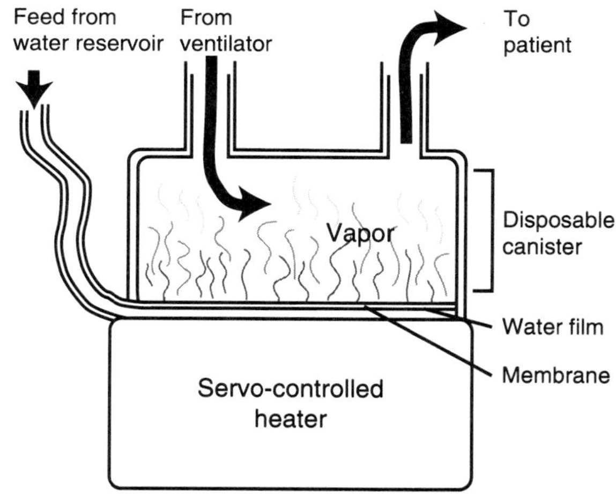

Figure 71-4. Schematic of a servo-controlled passover heated humidifier. (From Shapiro et al.,[4] with permission.)

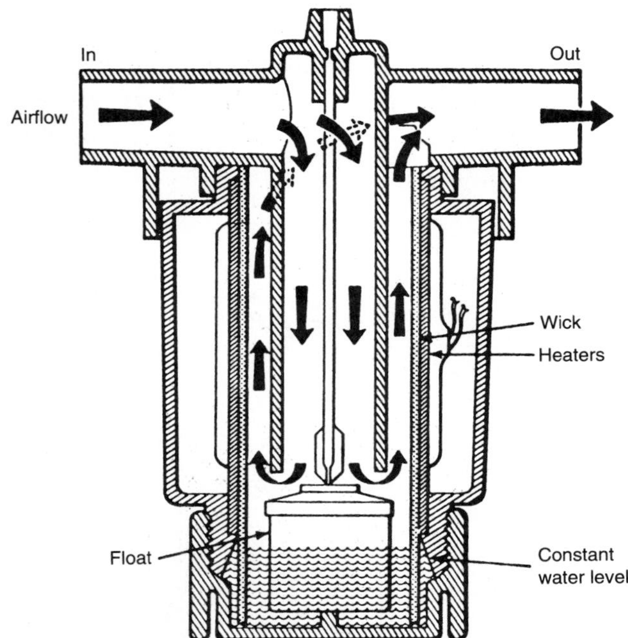

Figure 71-5. Bird model 3000 wick-type humidifier. (From McPherson,[173] with permission.)

Heated Wire Systems

Of major concern with all large-volume humidifier systems is the condensation of water in the large-bore tubing as temperature decreases between the humidifier and the patient. As much as a 14°C temperature drop can be noted over a 5-ft distance.[18] As a result, a number of manufacturers have introduced servo-controlled heated wire systems for use on mechanical ventilators. These systems prevent both temperature change from humidifier to patient and water condensation in the ventilator tubing, and as a result, concern regarding bacterial growth in ventilator circuits is also greatly reduced. My colleagues and I have demonstrated in neonatal/pediatric populations of ventilator-dependent patients that heated wire circuits can be used for up to 7 days without a circuit change.[19,20] To date, no data regarding the use of heated wire systems on adults are available. However, Dreyfuss et al.[21] have indicated no increase in nosocomial infection rate when adult ventilator circuits were left in place for the duration of a patient's ventilator course, as compared with the normal 48-hour change frequency.

Hygroscopic Condenser Humidifiers

Hygroscopic condenser humidifiers (HCHs) are also referred to as *heat and moisture exchangers* (HMEs). This type of humidifier functions as an artificial nose, and although normally used in ventilator circuits, it may be used on selected spontaneously breathing patients. Figure 71-6 illustrates the overall design of these units, all of which are small and designed to attach directly to the artificial airway. Each contains either a honeycomb or layers of hygroscopically treated material (cellulose, synthetic felt, or polypropylene).[22] As gas passes through the HCH, water vapor and heat are either added to or removed from the units. During exhalation, the HCH condenses water vapor and picks up heat from the exhaled gas, while during inspiration water vapor is evaporated into the inspired tidal volume and heat is transferred to the gas.

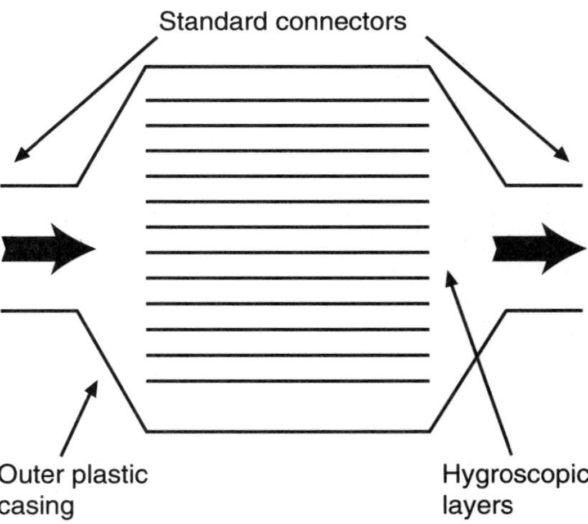

Figure 71-6. Hygroscopic condenser humidifier (heat and moisture exchanger). (From Scanlon et al.,[22] with permission.)

Table 71-4. Contraindications for the Use of Hygroscopic Condenser Humidifiers (Heat and Moisture Exchangers)

Type of Contraindication	Rationale for Contraindication
Neonatal and small pediatric patients	Mechanical dead space of the HCH or HME may be excessive relative to the patient's tidal volume
Patients who produce copious amounts of secretions	Secretions mobilized into HCH or HME compromise its humidification function and increase resistance
Patients who derive the majority of their minute ventilation via spontaneous breaths (IMV/SIMV/CPAP modes)	Mechanical dead space of the HCH or HME may be excessive relative to the patient's tidal volume
Patients whose tidal volume exceeds tidal volume specification listed by HCH or HME manufacturer	Finite capacity of HCH or HME for storage/delivery of water should not be exceeded
Patients who lose appreciable amounts of inhaled gas through a patent bronchopleural fistula	Volume of dry inspirate exceeds HCH or HME capacity to saturate it due to low recovery from expirate
Patients who lose appreciable amounts of inhaled gas by leakage around their intratracheal inflatable cuff	Volume of dry inspirate exceeds HCH or HME capacity to saturate it owing to low recovery from expirate

IMV, intermittent mandatory ventilation; SIMV, synchronized intermittent mandatory ventilation; CPAP, continuous positive airway pressure.

(Modified from Demers,[23] with permission.)

The efficiency of these devices depends on the design of the unit, as well as on atmospheric conditions and the size of the inspired tidal volume.[23] Branson and Seger[24] have demonstrated that adult HCHs can provide an absolute humidity of about 22 to 26 mg/L. However, because of the surface area of the particular HCH, this efficiency drops off as tidal volume increases, and therefore we do not recommend these units if tidal volume exceeds 1200 mL. In addition, the dead space volume and the resistance to gas flow through these units must be considered if they are used on spontaneously breathing patients. Dead space volumes of up to 90 mL are noted with some units,[23] while resistance to flow at normal peak inspiratory flow rates may necessitate pressure gradients of 2 to 4 cmH_2O[24] to maintain gas flow across the HCH. Care must also be exercised in the use of HCHs in patients with copious secretions, since if secretions enter the unit, resistance to gas flow may be markedly increased. Table 71-4 lists contraindications to the use of HCHs.

In spite of the problems with HCHs, they are useful for maintaining humidification during anesthesia and short-term mechanical ventilation (24 to 72 hours) and for periodic use in patients requiring long-term ventilatory support or those with chronic artificial airways. The units are particularly useful for short-term ventilatory support of postoperative patients.

Spinning Disc Humidifiers

Spinning disc humidifiers are commonly referred to as *room humidifiers* and function by creating a centrifugal force as a central disc with a siphon tube is spun at rapid rates. The centrifugal force created by the spinning causes water in a reservoir to rise up the siphon tube, to be thrown against baffles on the disc and the humidifier, and to be ejected from the unit by the air currents created by the centrifugal force (Fig. 71-7). These units would be more appropriately referred to as *room nebulizers* since aerosol particles are formed in large quantity and ejected into the room. Humidifiers of this type do help to increase the humidity of a small closed room in the winter, but they potentially contribute to the development of respiratory tract infections. Unless meticulous care is taken to clean the unit daily, bacterial growth within

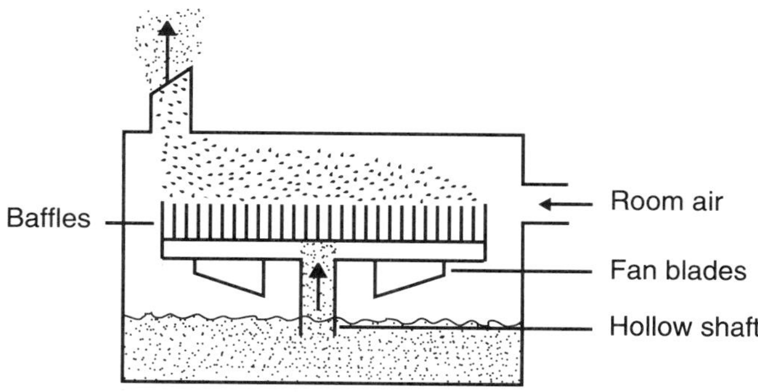

Figure 71-7. Spinning disk humidifier. (From Branson and Seger,[24] with permission.)

the unit will be excessive and since a mechanism for bacterial movement (aerosol particles) is present, airway contamination is probable. If used, the unit should be placed as far away from the patient as possible and its output directed away from the patient to increase the settling of aerosol particles prior to air currents reaching the patient.

PHYSICAL CHARACTERISTICS OF AEROSOLS

An *aerosol* is a suspension of liquid droplets or solid particles in a gaseous medium. The actual size of aerosol particles can vary considerably from 0.001 to 100 μ, although clinically useful particles are in the 1.0- to 10-μ range.[25,26] Therapeutic aerosols are normally produced by a technique referred to as *comminution*[27] (i.e., the shattering of a solid or liquid into minute particles), which requires input of energy to form the aerosol particles. Generally, three specific methods of comminution are used to produce therapeutic aerosols: (1) jet mixing; (2) the Babbington principle; and (3) ultrasonic nebulization. All three methods produce heterogeneous dispersion of aerosol particles, with jet mixing generally producing the greatest particle size variability.

Since aerosols are produced in variable size ranges, it is important to understand the relationship between particle size and mass. At a fixed density the volume of a particle varies with its mass. Specifically, the relation between the volume and the size of a sphere can be expressed as

$$\text{Volume} = 4/3\ \pi\ r^3 \qquad (1)$$

that is, the volume of a particle is directly proportional to the cube of its radius.[27] In other words, a small decrease in particle size dramatically lowers particle volume and thereby the available mass, while an increase in size increases the mass by the third power of the radius. A single 10-μ particle has the same mass as 1000 particles of 1-μ size and 1,000,000 particles of 0.1 μ size.[27]

Aerosol particle size distribution is usually characterized by the aerosol's mass median diameter (MMD) (i.e., 50 percent of the aerosol particles have a diameter larger and 50 percent have a diameter smaller than this value). Count median diameter is the particle size above and below which 50 percent of the aerosol by volume exists. These two values may differ considerably (Fig. 71-8), since most of the mass of the aerosol is found in the comparatively few large particles. Mode count refers to the most common particle size, or the particle size that occurs with highest relative frequency in the aerosol. If the logarithms of the diameters of aerosol particles are plotted, the familiar bell-shaped normal particle size distribution curve is obtained.[28] When the data are further graphed as a cumulative function on linear logarithmic paper, an elongated S-shaped sigmoidal curve results, from which the median diameter can be read directly at the 50 percent point.[28] This plot yields the geometric stan-

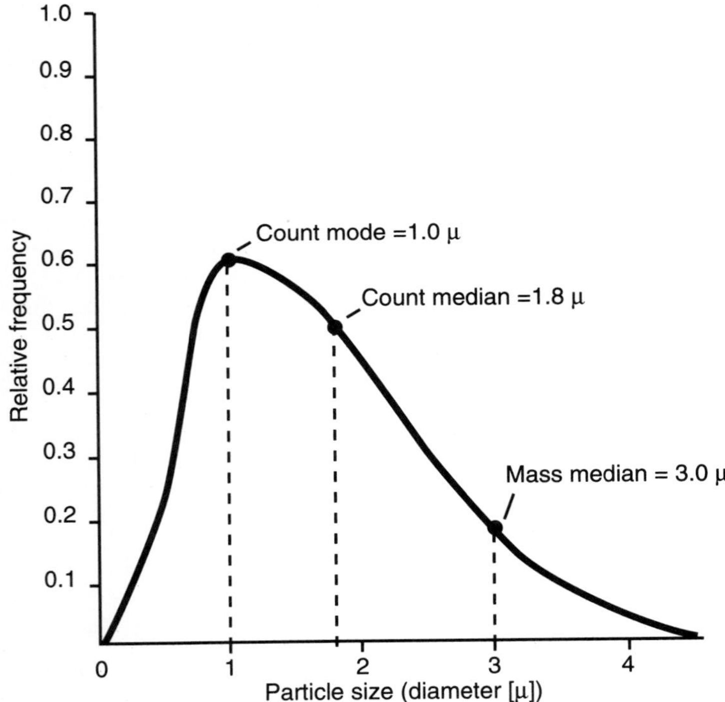

Figure 71-8. A hypothetical skewed distribution of aerosol particle sizes, illustrating the differences between the mode, the count, and the mass median diameter. (From Rau,[27] with permission.)

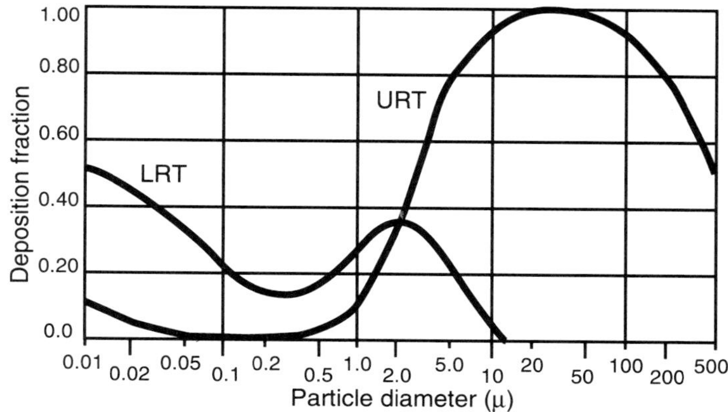

Figure 71-9. Particle size and respiratory tract deposition. The deposition probabilities of particles of different aerodynamic size are indicated for the upper respiratory tract (URT) and the lower respiratory tract (LRT), the demarcation of the two divisions being the epiglottis. These curves can be considered useful for associating the approximate deposition pattern and the amount deposited within the human respiratory system during spontaneous respiration. (From Morrow,[26] with permission.)

dard deviation, which is determined by the ratio of the median diameter to the diameter at 15.9 or 84.1 percent of the median diameter[28] and which is a measure of variability of particle diameter within the aerosol. As with all standard deviations, a large geometric standard deviation indicates a broad particle distribution.

As a result of the difficulty of measuring particle size and expressing aerosol size relationships, a simplified approach to identifying and comparing aerosols has been devised, which is based on the concept of an aerodynamic mass diameter. This value is a measure of a particle's terminal settling velocity. An aerodynamic scale is used to convert measurements of the particle being assessed into data for an equivalent water droplet (density 1 g/mL) of a diameter corresponding to the same settling velocity in still air.[28] The use of this standardized scale allows the behavior of different aerosols relative to the lung to be compared regardless of their density or structure. When estimating quantity of aerosol delivered to various aspects of the lung, the aerodynamic mass median diameter is normally used. This, like the MMD, is the diameter above and below which 50 percent of the mass of the aerosol resides.

In addition to particle size distribution, the concepts of penetration, deposition, retention, and clearance are used to describe the therapeutic efficiency of an aerosol.[29]

Penetration and Deposition

The term *penetration* defines the depth within the respiratory tract that particles of a given size are capable of reaching, whereas *deposition* refers to those mechanisms that enhance aerosol particle setting in the airway. In general, particles larger than 10 μ do not enter the lower respiratory tract (Fig. 71-9); however, the optimal size for maximum lower respiratory tract deposition is 1 to 5 μ. Particles smaller than 0.5 μ are stable in the delivery gas and do not deposit in the lower respiratory tract. Penetration to small airways requires particles of 3-μ or smaller size. In children, ribavirin aerosols require particle sizes of 1 to 2 μ for penetration to the bronchiolar level. Similar size distribution is desirable for the delivery of pentamidine, but beta-agonists primarily function in larger airways, where particle size in the 3- to 5-μ range is ideal.

Whether an aerosol particle that reaches a given level of the respiratory tract will deposit on that area is dependent on the following factors: inertia, sedimentation, brownian diffusion, interception, and electrostatic forces.[30] Of these, inertia, sedimentation, and brownian diffusion are the most important[30] (Table 71-5). Inertia is the tendency of a moving body to resist change in its direction and speed. Deposition occurs by inertial impacts as a result of the abrupt changes

Table 71-5. Mechanisms Important in Particle Deposition in the Lungs

	Inertia	Sedimentation	Diffusion
Particle size	Large particle diameter, ≥5 μ	Medium particle diameter, 1–6 μ	Smallest particle diameter, ≤1 μ
Anatomic site	Nose, pharynx, larger airways	Smaller airways	Terminal airways, alveolar ducts, alveoli
Aerodynamics	High airflow	Low airflow, breath-hold	Low to zero airflow, breath-hold
Geometric factors	Increased bifurcation angles	Horizontal airway surfaces	Small airspace dimensions, nearby surfaces

(From Brain and Valberg,[30] with permission.)

in airflow caused by branching of the airway. Sedimentation enhances deposition because gravity accelerates movement downward, and terminal settling velocity is reached when viscous resistive forces are equal and opposite in direction to gravity.[30] Aerosols undergo brownian motion as a result of collisions with molecules of gases; these collisions may force particles to strike the walls of the airway and therefore to deposit at that level.

Essentially, any factor that forces contact with the walls of the airway enhances deposition. Interception causes deposition, as a result of a fixed particle size entering a smaller and smaller airway. When the distance between the particle and the surface is less than the size of the particle, deposition occurs. If the aerosol is highly charged, electrostatic forces may enhance deposition as a result of attraction by opposite charges on the wall of the airway. However, normal therapeutic aerosols are not significantly charged. Other forces (magnetic or thermal) acting to enhance deposition of nontherapeutic aerosols are normally not significant within the respiratory tract.[30] The distance a particle travels before deposition due to either sedimentation or interception decreases in proportion as the square root of particle diameter increases.[28]

Retention and Clearance

Retention is defined as the amount of a substance present in the respiratory tract at a specific point in time. If aerosol delivery is continuous, the retention level, or equilibrium, is established when deposition rate equals clearance rate. Clearance is the removal of a deposited aerosol that is not soluble in the mucous membrane. The rate at which particles are cleared is dependent on the site of deposition. Retention in ciliated lung regions is much lower than in nonciliated regions because mucociliary transport and cough clear these areas. In nonciliated areas, clearance requires phagocytosis by alveolar macrophages then movement to ciliated areas, and finally removal by mucociliary transport and cough.

Factors Influencing Particle Deposition

In addition to the physical mechanism discussed above, a number of other factors influence the deposition of aerosol particles in the respiratory tract (Table 71-6). Alterations in the normal anatomy of airways can greatly influence deposition—the more tortuous the route that particles must take, the greater the likelihood of deposition in large airways.[31] Pathology of the respiratory tract affects deposition in a similar manner; local narrowing of airways or fibrotic parenchymal changes enhance distribution abnormalities and alter deposition.[32] Bypassing the upper airway with an artificial airway alters particle size distribution within the lower respiratory tract. Nasal breathing filters particles down to 5 μ in size,[33,34] whereas aerosol delivery via oral breathing may allow larger particles to enter the lower respiratory tract. The actual particle size distribution when an aerosol is generated may differ significantly from the particle size distribution that arrives at the lower respiratory tract because of evaporation or hygroscopicity of the aerosol. Volatile aerosols become smaller in particle size because of evaporation, while hygroscopic aerosols, particularly sodium chloride, may dramatically increase in size.[35] Finally, breathing can markedly affect the deposition site and the quantity of aerosol deposited. Rapid and shallow breathing decreases deposition overall but increases airway deposition, while slow and deep breathing increases the volume of aerosol deposited and the amount of deposition at the bronchial level.[36]

Table 71-6. Factors Affecting Deposition of Aerosol Particles

Factors
Particle size
Gravitational impaction
Sedimentation
Brownian diffusion
Interception
Electrostatic forces
Magnetic forces
Thermal forces
Anatomy of respiratory tract
Pulmonary pathology
Intact or bypassed upper airway
Evaporation
Hygroscopicity of aerosol
Breathing pattern

INDICATIONS AND GOALS FOR AEROSOL THERAPY

The overall goals of aerosol therapy are improvement in bronchial hygiene, conditioning of inspired gas, and delivery of medication[37] (Table 71-7). Essentially, any pathologic condition that adversely affects the respiratory system's ability to condition inspired gas or the function of the mucociliary escalator presents as an indication for aerosol therapy.

Improvement in Bronchial Hygiene

Desiccated retained secretions are hydrophilic (i.e., they absorb water). Since dried retained secretions are common

Table 71-7. Goals of Aerosol Therapy

- Improve bronchial hygiene
  - Hydrate dried retained secretions
  - Improve efficiency of cough
  - Restore and maintain normal function of the mucociliary escalator
- Sputum induction
- Humidify gases delivered to patients with artificial airways
- Deliver medication

in the presence of pulmonary pathophysiology and disrupt normal mucociliary movement as well as cough, hydration of these secretions is necessary to re-establish normal function. Systemic hydration is essential for mobilization of secretions; however, mobilization is enhanced if continuous aerosolized water is added to the airway, although it is important to remember that aerosols in general are irritants to the lung since they cause increased sputum production, giving rise to coughing and theoretically to increased clearance of secretions.[27] Bland aerosols stimulate irritant subepithelial receptors (cough receptors) in the trachea and bronchi, initiating vagally mediated reflex mucus production, cough, and to some extent increased airway resistance.[38] This seems to be a more realistic explanation for the effective use of short-term aerosol therapy to enhance sputum production in spontaneously breathing patients, since the inspiration of an aerosol for 10 to 20 minutes only results in a few milliliters of fluid being applied to the respiratory tract.

Upper Airway Inflammation

Children and adults with upper airway inflammation are primary candidates for the use of continuous cool aerosol therapy. Children with croup and all postextubation patients whether in the postoperative period or following long-term intubation, express subjective benefit from cool mist therapy. However, no systematic data are available to demonstrate objective benefit from this therapy. In spite of this, it is our clinical experience that cool aerosols are beneficial in these settings. In addition, any inflammatory injury of the upper airway may benefit from continuous cool aerosol therapy.

Humidification of Inspired Gases

As discussed earlier, administration of high-flow O_2 therapy may result in a humidity deficit, since O_2 is normally free of water vapor. This is particularly true in patients with artificial airways and acute pulmonary pathology. With these patients it is necessary to administer sufficient water vapor in the inspired gas to eliminate the humidity deficit; otherwise retained secretions develop and the potential for obstruction of the artificial airway exists.[4] In this setting either heated or cool aerosol therapy is used to condition the inspired gas. Presently, there are no data to determine which method of eliminating the humidity deficit is most effective. Cool aerosols may cause increased resistance to gas flow, especially in hyperreactive airways,[37] while heated systems may also increase resistance by deposition of larger amounts of fluid in the lung over prolonged periods and have been associated with an increased infection risk.[38] As a result, one can make a case for any one of three approaches: heated humidity, heated aerosol, or cool aerosol. In reality, whichever approach is best tolerated by the patient is considered by us to be the ideal for that patient.

Delivery of Aerosolized Medication

Many pharmacologic agents demonstrate maximum local effect when delivered by aerosol. These include beta-2-agonists, anticholinergics, steroids, and antiviral and antibacterial agents. The delivery of medication is by far the primary indication for the use of aerosol delivery systems. Generally, three broad groupings of medication delivery systems are currently in use: jet nebulizers (small-volume or large-volume), metered dose inhalers, and dry powder inhalers. Details of each of these systems is provided under Equipment Used for Aerosol Therapy, while information on the pharmacology of aerosolized drugs is presented in Chapter 20.

EQUIPMENT USED FOR AEROSOL THERAPY*

Equipment available for the delivery of aerosol therapy can be divided into two general categories; large-volume and small-volume aerosol generators. The large-volume group is normally used to provide continuous aerosol delivery or to deliver large volumes of physiologic saline for short periods, although ultrasonic nebulizers have also been used to deliver medication. On the other hand, the small-volume group is designed exclusively for the delivery of medications.

Large-Volume Aerosol Generators

Within the large-volume category are three types of generators, each operating by distinctly unique methods: ultrasonic nebulizers, hydrodynamic (Babbington) nebulizers, and jet nebulizers.

Ultrasonic Nebulizers

Figure 71-10 schematically depicts the general operating features of ultrasonic nebulizers. These units create an aerosol by applying electrical energy to a piezoelectric transducer, which converts the electrical energy to high-frequency sound waves. The sound waves are focused either directly or indirectly on the solution to be nebulized, forming a "geyser" in the solution. Continuous cavitation and disruption of the liquid surface of the nebulizing solution cause formation of an aerosol. The piezoelectric transducer is either a quartz crystal or a ceramic disc, which vibrates at a frequency of 1 to 2 MHz (normally about 1.30 to 1.40 MHz),[4,22] to form sound waves, which are transferred to the solution. The transducer is usually convex to allow focusing of the geyser produced.

As illustrated in Figure 71-10, the transducer sits in the bottom of the couplant compartment, which is filled with either physiologic saline or sterile distilled water (depending

---

* Significant portions of this section are from Kacmarek and Hess,[171] with permission.

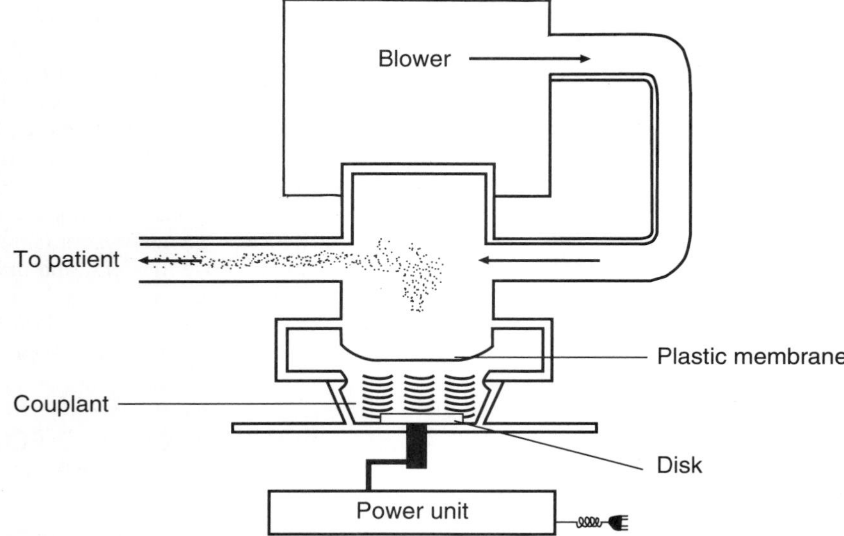

Figure 71-10. Schematic of an ultrasonic nebulizer. (From Shapiro et al.,[4] with permission.)

on the manufacturer). The solution to be nebulized is located in a container placed within the couplant compartment. At the base of the nebulizer container is a plastic membrane, which allows the energy from the couplant to be transferred to the nebulizer container. In some of the newer ultrasonic units the couplant compartment has been eliminated, and the solution to be nebulized is placed directly on the transducer. Most units come with an adjustable blower to deliver the solution from the nebulizer to the patient. In addition to a variable-speed blower, many units contain an amplitude control, which allows for variation in the intensity of the ultrasonic waves and thus in the volume of aerosol generated per unit time. It should be noted that the transfer of energy from the transducer to the couplant or nebulizing solution produces heat, increasing the temperature of the solution by about 3 to 10°C.[22] The transducer itself may become very hot.

Ultrasonic nebulizers are very efficient in their production of aerosols. Most (90 percent) of the particles produced are in the 1- to 10-μ range, with the MMD approximately 6 μ.[4] Depending on the amplitude setting, from 1 to 6 mL/min of nebulized solution is produced.[22]

Generally, ultrasonic nebulizers are used for short-term delivery of large volumes of physiologic saline (0.9 percent) or half normal (0.45 percent) saline solutions to facilitate expectoration of thick secretions. They are frequently used for sputum induction. Normally, these generators are not used for continuous aerosol delivery because of the large quantity of water potentially deposited on the airway and the finding in animals exposed to continuous ultrasonic therapy of microscopic pulmonary changes consistent with edema after 72 hours.[39,40] Also, ultrasonic nebulizers are generally not used for the delivery of aerosol medication because of concern that the vibratory energy of such high frequency waves would disrupt the chemical structure of the aerosolized drug.[41] In fact, it has been demonstrated that power outputs above 50 W/cm^2 can disrupt the chemical structure of nebulized medication.[42]

Overall, we believe that ultrasonic nebulizers play a very limited role in aerosol therapy. They are primarily used for the induction of sputum and for periodic treatment of retained secretions in patient refractory to other therapy.

Hydrodynamic Nebulizers

Hydrodynamic nebulizers, better known as Babbington nebulizers, create an aerosol by directing a high-pressure stream of gas perpendicular to a film of fluid coating a small sphere. The gas striking the film breaks it into aerosolized particles. A smaller sphere used as a baffle and located directly across from the high-pressure gas source removes the large particles from the aerosol.

A schematic of a Babbington nebulizer is presented in Figure 71-11. The solution to be nebulized is pumped by a small motor and dripped on the top of a small sphere. The solution moves over the surface of the sphere, passing a small orifice on one side, where gas exits under a pressure of about 10 psi. Solution not nebulized returns to a reservoir to be recycled over the sphere.

These nebulizers are available as single-sphere or double-sphere units and are as efficient as ultrasonic nebulizers, producing up to 6 mL/min of aerosol. The aerosol produced is also in the 1- to 10-μ range, with an MMD of 5 μ.[22] As a result of the energy lost when high-pressure gas expands, the aerosol produced by Babbington nebulizers is about 6 to 10°F below ambient temperature.[22]

The applications of Babbington nebulizers and restrictions on their use are similar to those of ultrasonic nebulizers. Babbington nebulizers are only recommended for intermittent use in selected patients and for sputum induction.

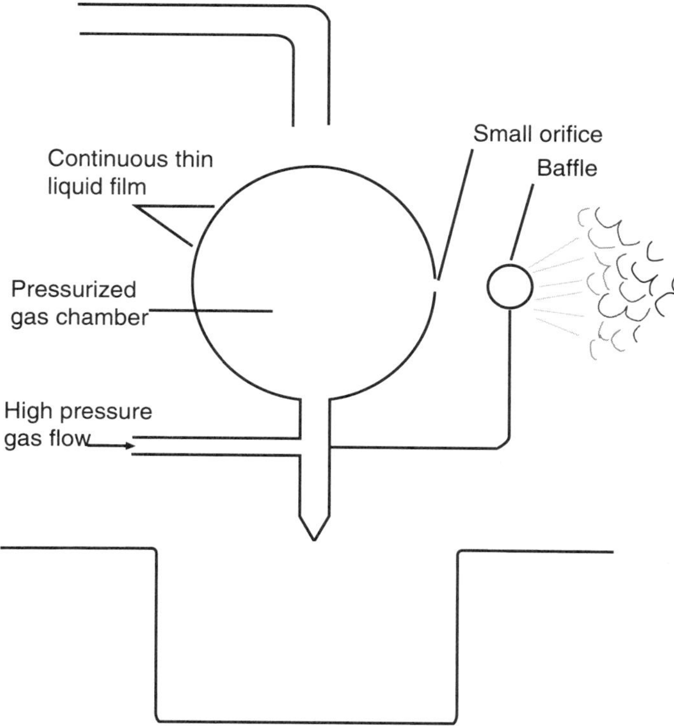

Figure 71-11. Schematic of a hydrodynamic (Babbington) nebulizer. (From Shapiro et al.,[4] with permission.)

Large-Volume Jet Nebulizers

The most commonly used large-volume nebulizer is the jet nebulizer (Fig. 71-12). These units function by jet mixing (see Ch. 1) as well as by the Bernoulli effect. As noted in Figure 71-13, a stream of high-pressure gas exits a small orifice located adjacent to a capillary tube sitting in the solution to be nebulized. The rapid flow of gas from the jet orifice creates a subatmospheric pressure in the capillary tube, allowing the solution to move up and out of the tube. As the solution exits the tube, the gas from the jet orifice strikes it, breaking it into an aerosol. The aerosol then strikes a fixed structure near the jet and the walls of the container, all of which function as baffles (i.e., structures that allow large aerosol particles to drop out of suspension or to fragment into smaller particles). Incidentally, perfume atomizers function in the same way as jet nebulizers, except that they do not contain baffles. All jet nebulizers, whether small- or large-volume and whether hand-, electrically, or pneumatically operated, create an aerosol by the same mechanism. The particle size range produced by jet nebulizers is very broad, although an appropriately baffled unit can produce microaerosols with an MMD of 0.5 μ. However, the typical large-volume jet nebulizer produces only about 55 percent of its particles in the 1- to 10-μ range.[4] Generally, these units only produce about 1 mL/min of aerosol.

Most large-volume jet nebulizers have a solution volume of 0.5 to 1.5 L. All are designed to function with a 50-psi gas source. However, even at this driving pressure, because of the small jet orifice size the flow exiting the jet is only about 12 to 15 L/min. Most units allow for air entrainment and various delivered F_{IO_2} levels (see Ch. 75). These units may also be heated or unheated. As discussed earlier, large-volume unheated humidifiers demonstrate up to a 12°F drop from ambient temperature within an hour of continuous use.[22] The same is true for large-volume nebulizers.

Jet nebulizers interfaced with ventilator circuits are generally referred to as sidestream or mainstream nebulizers. Mainstream nebulizers are usually of large volume, with the entire flow of therapeutic gas moving through the nebulizer (Fig. 71-13). Sidestream nebulizers are usually of small volume, are used to generate medicinal aerosols, and do not have the total volume of therapeutic gas moving through them.

Generally, large-volume nebulizers are the units of choice for continuous humidification of artificial airways and for delivery of O_2 therapy to postsurgical patients in the recovery room.

A special type of large-volume nebulizer is the small particle aerosol generator (SPAG) unit (Fig. 71-14), designed for the administration of ribavirin. This unit contains three jets and a drying chamber, in which a secondary flow of gas causes aerosol evaporation and stabilization of particle size. Of the particles produced by the SPAG unit, 95 percent are smaller than 5 μ, with an MMD of 1 μ (see Ch. 42 for details).

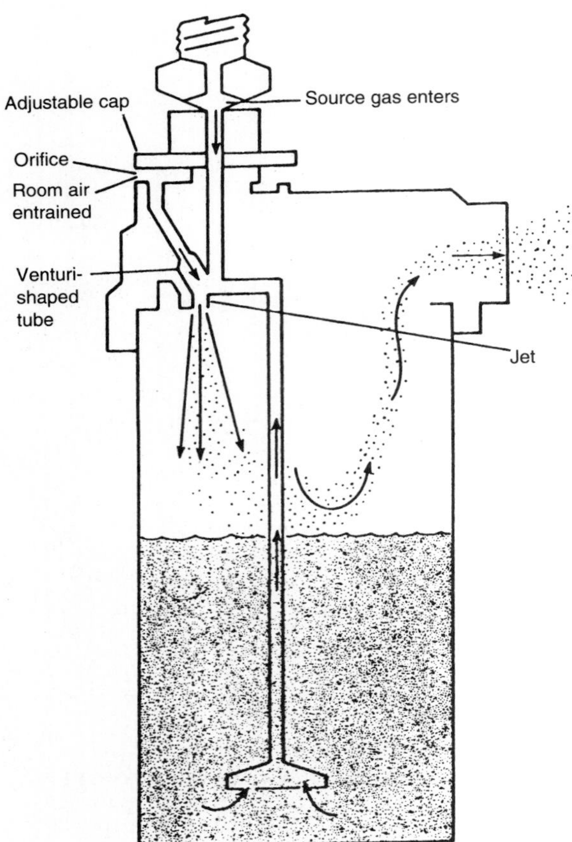

Figure 71-12. Schematic of a large-volume jet nebulizer. (From Branson and Seger,[24] with permission.)

Small-Volume Aerosol Generators

All small-volume aerosol generators are designed exclusively for administration of medication. Three specific types are represented: small-volume jet nebulizers (SVNs), metered dose inhalers (MDIs), and dry powder inhalers (DPIs). Both SVNs and MDIs use pressurized gas to create an aerosol, whereas DPIs use the patient's inspiratory efforts to create a dry powder aerosol.

Small-Volume Nebulizers

All SVNs, regardless of manufacturer, operate by the same mechanism that has been described for large-volume jet nebulizers but have a limited solution capacity of about 10 to 15 mL (Fig. 71-15). Since these units are used for delivery of medication, solution volumes in the range of 2 to 6 mL are normally used. Of concern is that each of these nebulizers, because of operational design, has a specific volume of solution (dead volume) that remains in the nebulizer after the unit ceases production of an aerosol. Depending on the manufacturer of the SVN selected, the dead volume varies from about 0.5 to 1.0 mL[43,44] and represents the solution that adheres to the walls, cap, and system connections (i.e., corrugated tubing, mouthpiece, and mask). During therapy, tapping the sides of the nebulizer causes droplets of solution adhering to the walls of the nebulizer to be renebulized, thus maintaining dead volume at a minimum. To ensure minimum dead volume and maximum aerosolization of the solution, nebulization with repetitive tapping of the nebulizer should continue until no aerosol is produced by the nebulizer or the nebulizer is "dry."

The quantity of the medication remaining in solution in the dead volume is dependent on the total volume of solution,[45–47] the nebulizer flow rate,[46,48,49] and the temperature and humidity of the solution, driving gas, and entrained gas.[50,51] Hess et al.[46] in a bench study demonstrated that the volume of drug aerosolized increased with increasing diluent volume and nebulizer flow rate, the maximum volume of drug being delivered at a total solution volume of about 4 mL and a nebulizer flow of 6 to 8 L/min. Clay et al.[48] demonstrated that the aerodynamic MMD of aerosol particles from four nebulizers decreased as flow rate increased from 4 to 8 L/min. As a result, we recommend that total solution volume be at least 4 mL and that nebulizers be operated at 6 to 8 L/min.

The temperature and humidity of the nebulized solution, as well as that of the driving and the entrained gas, affect the size of particles delivered by SVNs, as well as the concentration of the drug in the dead volume.[50,52] Evaporation of water and adiabatic expansion of the driving gas[53,54] reduce the temperature of aerosol solutions to about 8 to 12°F below the ambient temperature.[52] The evaporation of water also increases the concentration of the drug in the nebulizer solution. Since gas temperature increases as the aerosol is warmed to room temperature, the particle size of the aerosol is reduced. Therefore, although it is clinically impractical, nebulizer solutions should be maintained between ambient and body temperature and the gas entrained should be saturated with water vapor at room temperature to stabilize particle size. From a practical perspective, a mechanical compressor operating on room air is preferable to use of cylinder gas because of the water vapor content of room air, while temperature change in the solution can be minimized if the SVN is held firmly in a closed hand.

The aerosol produced by an SVN should be inhaled via the mouth in preference to the nose to minimize deposition of the drug in the nose and nasal pharynx[55] (Table 71-8). Deposition in the upper airway is enhanced with nasal breathing because of the tortuous route the aerosol must follow and the high nasal resistance to gas flow.[56] However, if patients with face masks are instructed to inspire through the mouth, no difference in response between mask and mouthpiece aerosol delivery has been demonstrated.[57,58] In fact, many patients prefer delivery via face mask, and the use of a face mask may improve compliance.

Intermittent activation of the SVN is preferred to continuous nebulization.[59,60] Both Kradjan and Lakshminarayan[60] and Hughes and Saez[59] found greater amounts of drug delivered to lung models with intermittent (inspiration only) activation of the SVN, since all the solution nebulized during

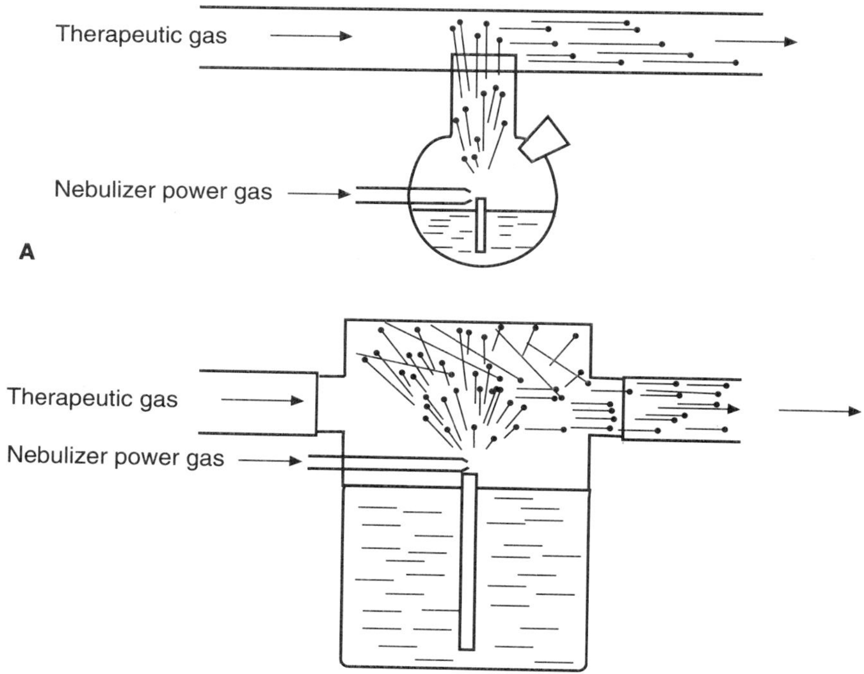

Figure 71-13. Schematic of (**A**) side-stream and (**B**) main-stream nebulizers. (From Scanlon et al.,[22] with permission.)

expiration is lost to the environment. Intermittent nebulization can be achieved by placement of a hand-operated Y or finger port in the driving gas line. This requires the patient to occlude the Y with a finger to direct gas to the nebulizer. However, intermittent nebulization greatly prolongs the treatment and affects compliance in the less than enthusiastic patient. As a result, even though intermittent nebulization is preferable from a deposition perspective, continuous aerosolization may be necessary from a practical perspective to ensure compliance. The actual protocol used must be individualized.

Ventilatory pattern does influence deposition of nebulized aerosols in the lower respiratory tract.[61–63] Although there is some controversy over the ideal ventilatory pattern, a slow

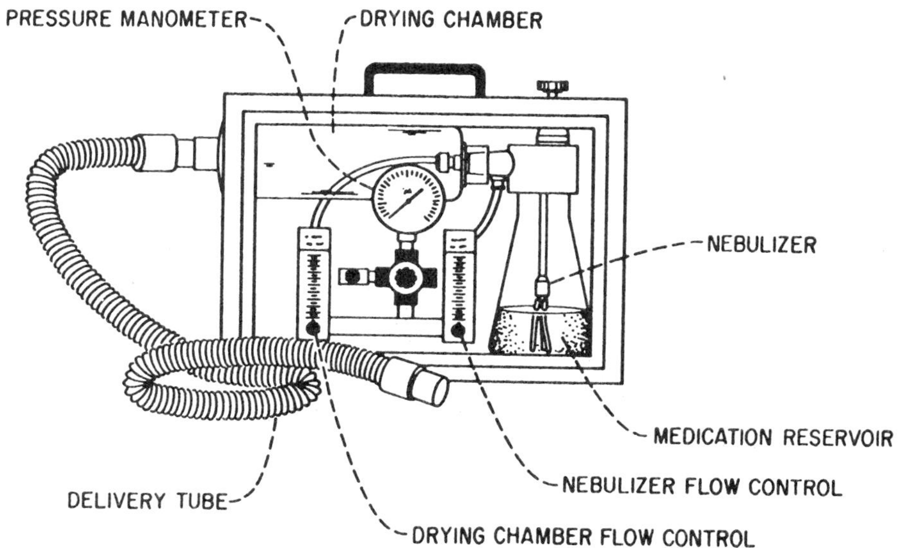

Figure 71-14. Schematic of the small particle aerosol generator (SPAG). (From Scanlon et al.,[22] with permission.)

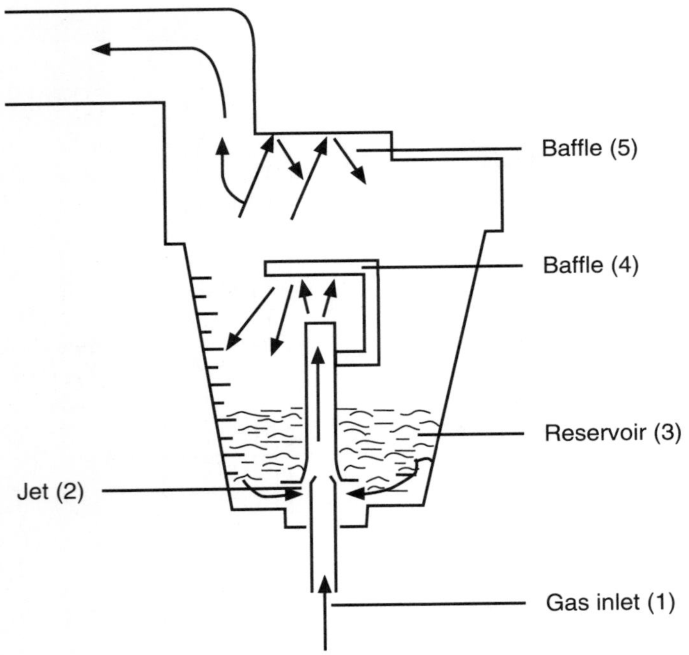

Baffle (5)
Baffle (4)
Reservoir (3)
Jet (2)
Gas inlet (1)

Figure 71-15. Schematic of small volume nebulizer. (From Eubanks and Bone,[173] with permission.)

Table 71-8. Technique for Use of a Small-Volume Nebulizer

1. Place drug in nebulizer.
2. Dilute with physiologic saline (0.9%) to 4 mL total volume.
3. Incorporate a finger port into the driving gas system to provide intermittent nebulization during inspiration only.
4. Set driving gas flow at 6–8 L/min.
5. Connect patient to nebulizer via a mouthpiece or mask (in some patients a nose clip may be necessary).
6. Instruct patient to inspire through open mouth if using a mask or to close lips around mouthpiece.
7. Grasp nebulizer chamber firmly in hand to maintain temperature during treatment.
8. Have patient inhale slowly (0.5 L/s) at normal tidal volume.
9. Have patient occasionally inspire to total lung capacity and incorporate (4–10 second) breath hold.
10. Tap sides of nebulizer to minimize dead volume.
11. Continue treatment until no aerosol is produced.
12. Monitor patient for presence of side effects (e.g., tachycardia or tremor) and beneficial effects (e.g., breath sounds, peak flow, & FEV_1)

FEV_1, forced expiratory volume in 1 second.
(From Kacmarek and Hess,[171] with permission.)

inspiratory flow (0.5 L/min)[61,62] at tidal volume, with an occasional inspiration to total lung capacity (TLC), and an inspiratory hold, is recommended[63] (see Table 71-8 for an outline of the technique for use of a SVN during spontaneous breathing).

Even when SVNs are administered ideally to the most cooperative, spontaneously breathing patients, only a small proportion (9 to 12 percent) of the drug placed in the nebulizer reaches the patient,[64,65] most of it being left in the apparatus itself or exhaled (Fig. 71-16). During mechanical ventilation the efficiency of aerosol deposition is decreased even further than during spontaneous breathing.[59,66–70] Numerous factors contribute to this inefficiency, including endotracheal tube size,[67] aerodynamic MMD,[67] continuous versus intermittent nebulization,[59,68,69] and placement of the nebulizer in the ventilator circuit.[59] MacIntyre et al.[66] reported that 2.9 ± 0.79 percent of a radioactively tagged aerosol was deposited in the lower respiratory tracts of seven stable adult patients receiving mechanical ventilatory support. Fraser et al.[70] using a lung model and SVN activation during inspiration, noted that only 4.8 percent of the initial dose was available for deposition in the large airways.

Evaluation of aerosol deposition in neonatal/pediatric lung models has demonstrated deposition even lower than that noted with adults.[68,71,72] Cameron et al.[68] noted a maximum of 1.52 percent of the generated aerosol deposited in a lung

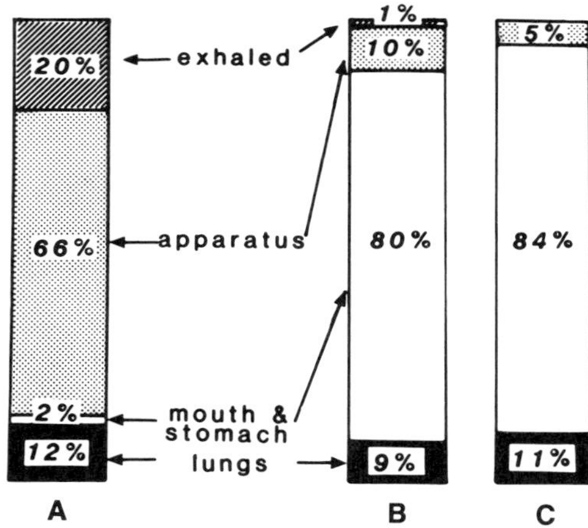

Figure 71-16. Fractional deposition of aerosol from (**A**) jet nebulizer compared with fractional deposition from (**B & C**) an MDI. Fig. B: Technetium 99m-labeled Teflon particles data from Newman et al.[106]; Fig. C: bromine 77-labeled ipratropium bromide data from Spiro et al.[105] (From Lewis and Fleming,[65] with permission.)

model used to evaluate the function of five SVNs in a neonatal ventilator circuit. Flavin et al.[71] reported similar findings in a rabbit model. A maximum of 1.96 ± 1.19 percent of the aerosol was deposited on the lower respiratory tract of the rabbits.

The effect of endotracheal tube size on percent deposition was demonstrated in a lung model by Ahrens et al.[67] Using 0.1 percent uranine as a tracer, they demonstrated a decrease in percent deposition as endotracheal tube size decreased from 9- to 6- to 3-mm ID. They also noted enhanced lung model deposition with decreasing aerodynamic MMD of the aerosol particles, observing maximum deposition past the 3-mm ID tube at particle diameter of 0.54 μ.

The volume of aerosol deposited in the lung can be enhanced by placement of the SVN at least 18 in. from the endotracheal tube.[59] Hughes and Saez[59] evaluated the amount of aerosol presented to the endotracheal tube of a lung model under four conditions: (1) continuous nebulization at the Y; (2) intermittent nebulization at the Y; (3) continuous nebulization at the ventilator circuit manifold; and (4) intermittent nebulization at the manifold. The highest percentage of aerosol (68.3 ± 1.2 percent) was presented to the endotracheal tube during intermittent nebulization at the manifold, while the lowest percentage (30 ± 2.0 percent) was presented during continuous nebulization at the circuit Y. Since 61.0 ± 1.5 percent of the aerosol was delivered during continuous nebulization at the manifold, nebulizer location would appear to be the most critical variable, with intermittent nebulization having a secondary effect.

As a result of the above-mentioned concerns, the efficacy of SVN therapy administered during mechanical ventilation has been questioned. Some authors have not been able to note a measurable response following SVN therapy[66] and others have noted only minimal changes in expiratory flows, peak airway pressure, or auto-PEEP (positive end-expiratory pressure) levels.[73,74] As a result, the dosage of the drug administered via SVN needs to be increased over standard recommended dosages to ensure that the same quantity of drug reaches the lower respiratory tract during mechanical ventilation as during spontaneous breathing. As an initial dose we use double the standard dose, that is, 1.0 mL of albuterol in 3 mL saline. Following the initial treatment, this dosage may need to be adjusted to elicit the desired response. Furthermore, inspiratory resistance, because of the presence of an artificial airway, may not be the ideal variable to monitor in order to establish response to therapy. Peak airway pressure, intrinsic PEEP (auto-PEEP) level, and expiratory flow and resistance would seem to provide a better evaluation of efficacy.

Administration Technique: Small-Volume Nebulizer via Mechanical Ventilators

Although little specific information regarding the optimal technique for the use of SVNs via ventilator circuits is available, the data from Hughes and Saez,[59] along with the information presented earlier on SVN technique during spontaneous breathing (Table 71-8), allow us to establish guidelines for the use of SVNs in ventilator circuits (Table 71-9).

Table 71-9. Technique for Use of Small-Volume Nebulizer during Mechanical Ventilation

1. Place drug in nebulizer.
2. Dilute with physiologic saline (0.9%) to 4 mL total volume.
3. Insert nebulizer into inspiratory limb of ventilator circuit ≥18 in. from Y.
4. Use intermittent nebulizer flow from ventilator, if available.
5. If continuous flow used, set at 6–8 L/min.
6. Ensure that mechanical ventilator rate is ≥4–8/min (unless contraindicated).
7. Ensure that V_T is ≥12 mL/kg (unless contraindicated).
8. If PSV rate drops, add back-up SIMV rate.
9. With children, adjust ventilator flow to ensure that total flow remains unchanged during pressure-limited ventilation.
10. With children (and some adults) readjust V_T during continuous flow nebulization to maintain constant V_T and peak airway pressure.
11. Tap sides of nebulizer to minimize dead space volume.
12. Continue prescribed procedure until no aerosol produced.
13. Remove equipment from ventilator circuit.
14. Return ventilator to pretreatment settings.
15. Monitor patient for side effects (e.g., tachycardia and tremor) and beneficial effects (e.g., improved breath sounds, peak flow, and FEV_1).

PSV, pressure support ventilation; SIMV, synchronized intermittent mandatory ventilation; V_T, tidal volume; FEV_1, forced expiratory volume in 1 second.

(From Kacmarek and Hess,[171] with permission.)

All SVNs should be placed at least 18 in. from the Y and powered intermittently through the ventilator (if possible). The volume of solution nebulized should be 4 mL, and if the unit is powered by a gas source external to the mechanical ventilator, a flow of 6 to 8 L/min should be used.

During use of an SVN for a spontaneously breathing patient, a periodic deep breath and a breath hold are recommended.[63] Although we realize that this may be impossible for the many mechanically assisted patients, it is encouraged. In order to maximize distribution and establish a more ideal ventilatory pattern during SVN treatments, we recommend the delivery of volume-limited mechanical breaths at a rate of 4 to 8 breaths per minute or higher, with tidal volumes set at 12 mL/kg or greater, unless contraindicated in a given patient. Patients on continuous positive airway pressure (CPAP) should be changed to synchronized intermittent mandatory ventilation (SIMV) or assist/control (A/C) during therapy, and patients receiving pressure support ventilation (PSV) with a SIMV back-up rate of less than 8 breaths per minute should have the PSV trigger rate carefully monitored. If PSV rate decreases, a back-up SIMV rate of 8 breaths per minute should be set. As noted by Beaty et al.,[75] the use of continuous nebulizer flow increases the pressure gradient that patients must overcome to trigger PSV. In those patients with marginal respiratory efforts, gross hypoventilation has been noted.

When continuous nebulization is used, the gas powering the nebulizer increases the mechanically delivered tidal volume and the peak airway pressure. This is normally not a concern in most adults but may create significant problems in children. With children and some adults, delivered tidal volume requires adjustment (decrease) to ensure consistency during aerosol therapy. During continuous flow pressure-limited ventilation in neonates and children, the flow from the ventilator must be reduced by a level equivalent to the added continuous nebulizer flow. If this adjustment is not made, peak airway pressure and delivered tidal volume may increase.

As with spontaneously breathing patients, dead volume should be minimized by tapping the sides of the SVN to allow nebulization of solution adhering to the SVN walls. Nebulization should be continued until no aerosol is produced.

Metered Dose Inhalers

Figure 71-17 illustrates the general design of an MDI. Each is a self-contained unit, consisting of a canister containing a propellant and the drug, along with a mouthpiece attachment. With each actuation a prescribed quantity of drug is delivered in a volume of inert gas between about 60 and 90 mL. The size of particles produced may be quite variable, with some particles as large as 40 μ.[76] However, most of the large particles are lost by baffling in the mouthpiece or the patient's mouth or are decreased in size by evaporation. Most of the particles produced are in the 2- to 5-μ range, but as with the SVN, only about 9 to 12 percent of the actuated drug actually deposits on the lower respiratory tract (Fig. 71-16). The propellants used are chlorofluorocarbons,

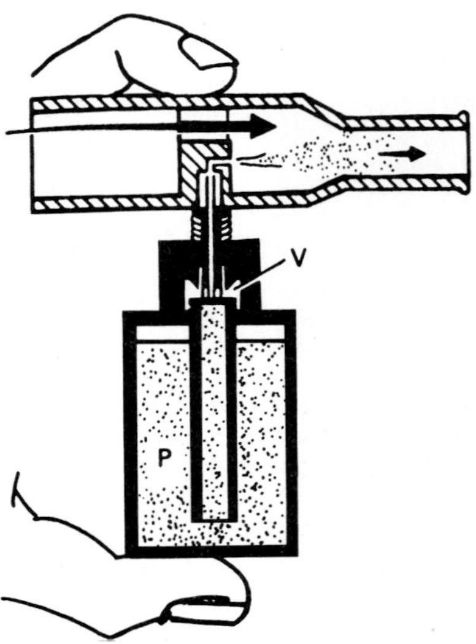

Figure 71-17. Diagram of an MDI. The material to be delivered is dissolved in fluid with a boiling point below room temperature, which is confined in a pressurized container (P). The valve (V) is designed to release a measured volume of fluid. Boiling liquid escapes and evaporates; particles of the active material continue in the airstream as a fine aerosol. (From Burton and Hodgkin,[174] with permission.)

which are generally considered inert but are blamed for depleting the ozone layer about the earth.[77] These propellants will be banned worldwide in the year 2000, and drug companies are presently attempting to develop suitable alternative propellants. A single MDI canister may contain hundreds of doses of drug.

There is much controversy over the technique that should be followed when an MDI is used. Differences of opinion exist over the lung volume at which the MDI should be actuated,[78–82] the position of the MDI in relation to the mouth during actuation,[82–84] the length of a postinhalation breath hold,[79,82–84] and the inspiratory flow rate.[78,79,82,85–87] Concern regarding the lung volume at which the MDI is actuated is based on peripheral distribution of the drug. Those favoring actuation at higher volumes believe that a more uniform peripheral distribution occurs at 80 percent of vital capacity (VC) than at 20 percent of VC, while proponents of early actuation believe that this enhances central airway deposition of the drug. Recent work by Dolovich et al.[82] and Newman et al.[79] suggests that the specific lung volume at which actuation takes place is unimportant provided that a slow maximal inspiration with a breath hold is performed. We agree with these authors, since it is difficult to instruct patients to precisely control the lung volume at which they actuate the MDI. As noted in Table 71-10, actuation should occur near the beginning of a complete slow inhalation from functional residual capacity (FRC).

Inspiratory flow during MDI use also contributes to the efficacy of therapy. Data from numerous authors[79,82,84–86] suggest that a slow inspiration maximizes the effect of the MDI (Fig. 71-18). The slow inspiratory flow encourages

Table 71-10. Technique for Use of Metered Dose Inhaler without Spacer

1. Warm MDI to body temperature.
2. Assemble apparatus.
3. Shake canister vigorously.
4. Hold canister upright.
5. Open mouth.
6. Place aerosol at mouth opening.
7. Begin to inspire slowly at inspiratory flows ≤0.5 L/min.
8. Actuate MDI.
9. Continue to inspire to TLC.
10. Hold breath for 4–10 seconds.
11. Wait 3–10 minutes between subsequent actuations.
12. Rinse mouth and pharynx if inhaling steroids.
13. Monitor patient for presence of side effects (e.g., tachycardia and tremor) and beneficial effects (e.g., improved breath sounds, peak flow, and FEV_1).

FEV_1, forced expiratory volume in 1 second.
(From Kacmarek and Hess,[171] with permission.)

laminar flow and deeper penetration of the aerosol before deposition.

After a complete inspiration, a breath hold of 4 to 10 seconds should be encouraged[79,82,84] (Fig. 71-19). Empirically, it would seem that the longer the breath hold, the greater the distribution and deposition of the inhaled drug. Although patients' ability to perform this maneuver must be considered, few patients with moderate to severe airflow obstruction are capable of a 10-second breath hold after a slow maximum inspiration.

The position of the MDI in relationship to the patient's mouth has been studied by several groups.[79,80,82–84] On the basis of the information currently available, it is difficult to draw conclusions about the proper placement of the MDI. Inspiration with the MDI placed 4 cm away from an open mouth may reduce potential side effects by decreasing oral deposition of large particles. However, it is difficult at best to consistently ensure that patients place the MDI in this position. In young and in elderly patients, this position frequently results in the aerosol missing the mouth. As a result, we recommend placement of the aerosol at the entrance of the open mouth rather than at 4 cm distance from the mouth. In patients having difficulty with this position, closure of the lips around the MDI mouthpiece is encouraged (Fig. 71-20).

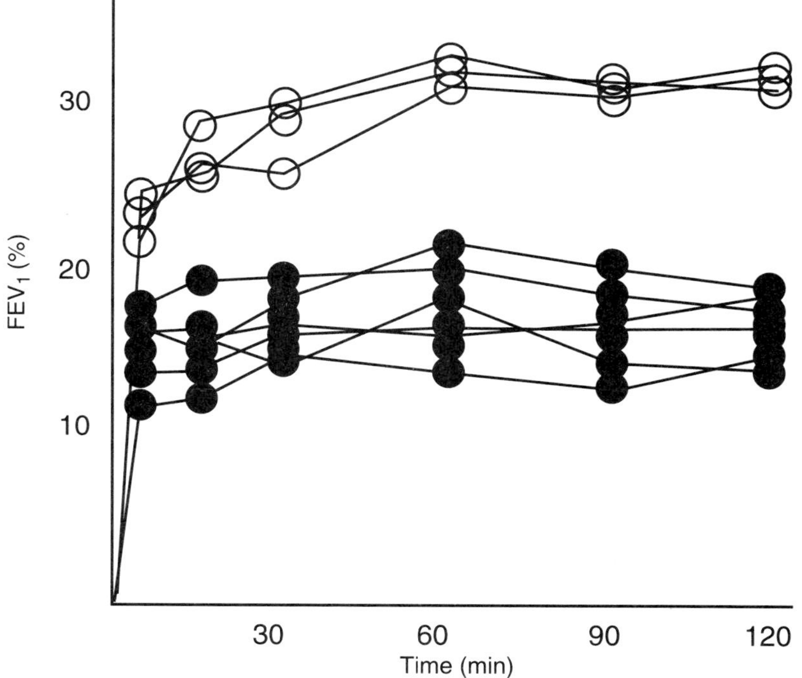

Figure 71-18. Percentage increases in forced expiratory volume in 1 second (FEV_1), plotted against time following controlled inhalation of 500 μg terbutaline at 25 L/min (open circles) and 80 L/min (solid circles) peak inspiratory flow. Each patient studied performed three studies at 25 L/min and six studies at 80 L/min involving various lung volumes and breath holding pauses. (From Newman et al.,[79] with permission.)

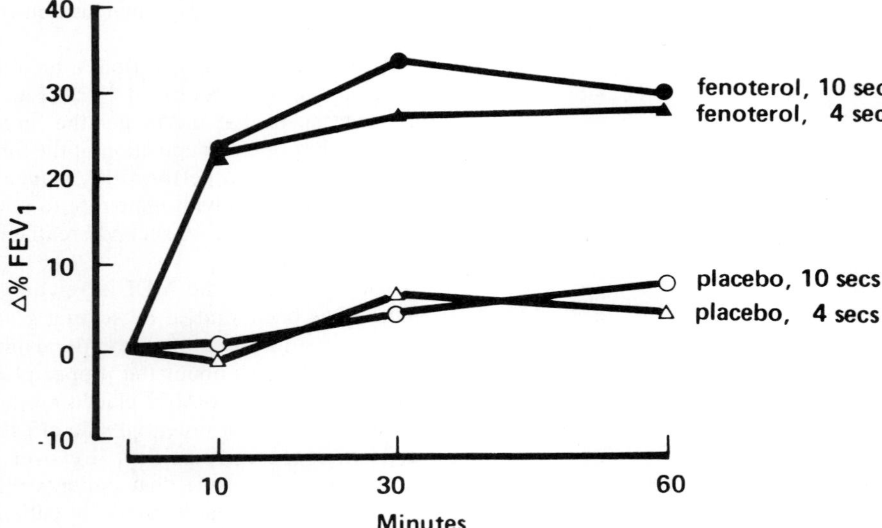

Figure 71-19. Mean percent change in FEV_1 at 10, 30, and 60 minutes after 400 μg fenoterol hydrobromide inhalation by MDI or placebo when breath-holding time was 4 or 10 seconds. Solid circle, 10 seconds fenoterol; solid triangle, 4 seconds fenoterol; open circle, 10 second placebo; open triangle, 4 second placebo. (From Lawford and McKenzie,[84] with permission.)

Temperature of the MDI prior to actuation also appears to affect percent deposition. Wilson et al.[87] in 1991 compared particle size produced and percentage of lower airway deposition in a lung model as the temperature of the MDI varied between 0°C and 42°C. Their data indicated greater deposition (17.4 percent at 4°C and 32.2 percent at 37°C) and smaller aerodynamic mass median diameter (3.65 μ at 0°C and 2.50 μ at 37°C) if MDI canisters were warmed to 37°C before actuation. Prewarming of the MDI, particularly in winter, should be encouraged. Patients should be instructed to carry the MDI close to the body to maintain temperature or to prewarm it by rolling the canister between their hands

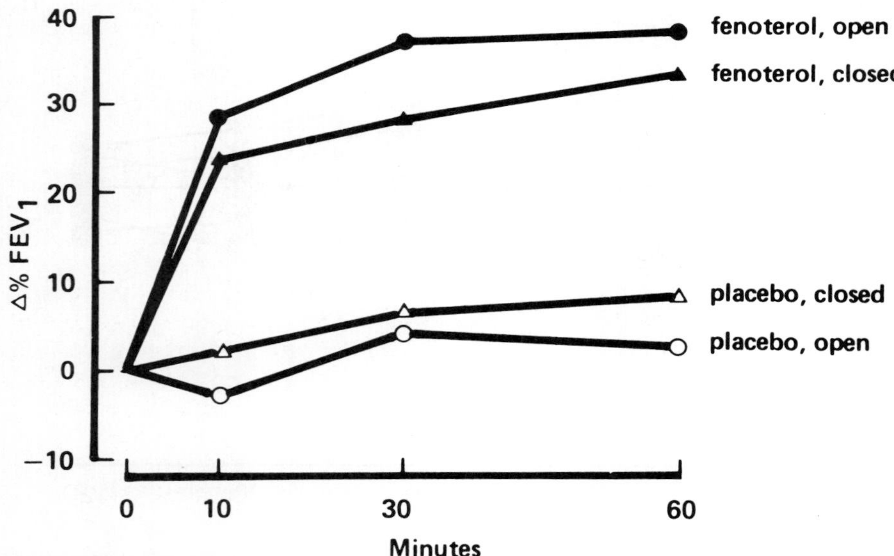

Figure 71-20. Mean percent change in FEV_1 at 10, 30, and 60 minutes after 400 μg fenoterol hydrobromide inhalation by MDI or placebo with closed or open mouth technique. Solid circle, open mouth fenoterol; solid triangle, closed mouth fenoterol; open triangle, closed mouth placebo; open circle, open mouth placebo. (From Lawford and McKenzie,[84] with permission.)

before actuation. Maintenance of the higher canister temperature increases vapor pressure in the canister and results in smaller aerosol particle size.[88]

Spacing of sequential actuations enhances the efficacy of the aerosol. Both Heimer et al.[89] and Pedersen[90] noted greater bronchodilator response when individual actuations were separated by a time interval; the enhancement of response resulted because the bronchodilating effect of the initial actuation improved the distribution of subsequent actuations. Ideally we recommend a 3- to 10-minute interval between actuations, but in many patients a more practical interval is 1 minute.

No difference in response between the MDI and the SVN has been demonstrated if the MDI is used properly.[91–97] When considering the detailed procedure (Table 71-10) required for proper administration of MDI, it is not surprising that a number of authors[98–101] have documented improper use of MDI. This, we believe, is the primary reason for the varied response to MDI noted by the medical community. The need for careful, detailed instruction to both patients and caregivers is essential if proper use of the MDI is to be ensured. The problems with technique are most pronounced with young children and the elderly, who required detailed, individualized performance-based education to ensure proper use. However, it should be emphasized that many patients may require a spacing device to obtain maximum benefit from an MDI.

Spacing Devices

Spacing devices (also called auxiliary or accessory devices) are extensions to the MDI (Fig. 71-21) designed (1) to eliminate the need for hand-breath coordination; and (2) to greatly reduce the deposition of large aerosol particles in the upper airway.[102–104]

These two effects of spacers eliminate the primary problems noted with the MDI as compared with the SVN. As already discussed, improper use of the MDI is common, as is deposition of a high percentage of the inhaled MDI aerosol in the oropharynx,[105,106] which enhances systemic absorption and local side effects (oral thrush and suppression of adrenocortical activity with steroids).[107] Numerous studies[108–114] have demonstrated reduced oropharyngeal deposition when spacers are used. This is accomplished by a two-stage process: (1) impingement of large particles on the walls of the spacer; and (2) evaporation, which reduces particle size during residence in the spacer.

MDIs with spacers perform at least as well as MDIs alone[82,115–124] or SVNs[126–135] and outperform MDIs that are used with incorrect technique. MDIs with spacers have also demonstrated equivalence to SVNs in the emergency department,[126,129,130] as well as during acute hospitalization.[126–128,132]

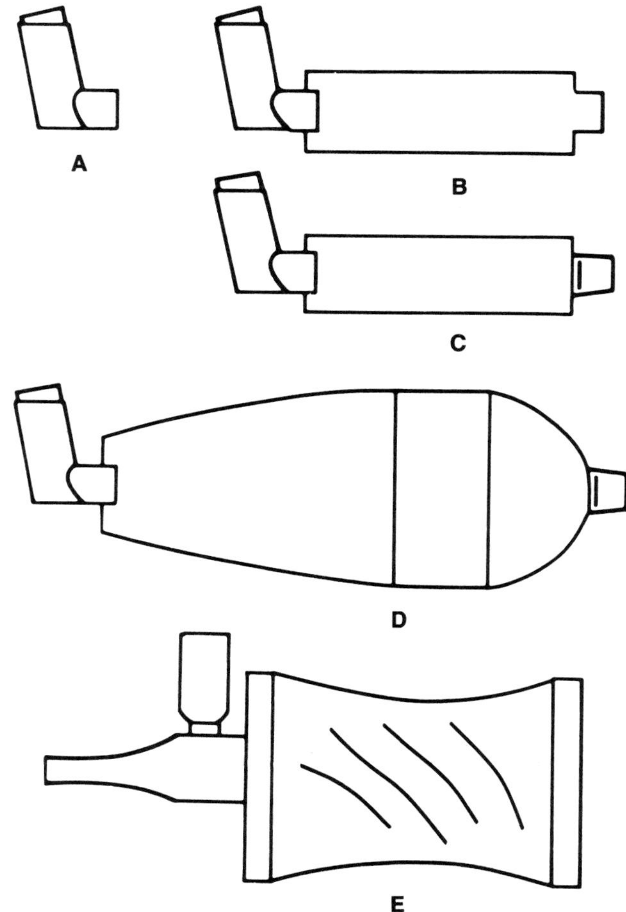

Figure 71-21. Schematics of MDI spacer systems: (**A**) actuator alone; (**B**) open-end straight tube; (**C**) Aerochamber; (**D**) Nebuhaler; and (**E**) InspirEase. (From Kim et al.,[175] with permission.)

Technique for Administration of Metered Dose Inhaler with Spacer

The technique for the use of an MDI with a spacer (Table 71-11) is essentially the same as with an MDI alone, with the following exceptions. (1) After warming, shaking, and assembling the apparatus and positioning it for use, the MDI is actuated, after which inspiration begins. (2) Since inspiration should continue to TLC and since spacer volume is relatively small (normally less than 800 mL), a tight lip seal about the spacer is relaxed as inspiration continues, allowing for inspiration of room air. As a result, a second inspiration from the spacer is recommended with some units (InspirEase) after an appropriate breath hold. This ensures that all of the aerosol from a single actuation is inspired. With other units (Aerochamber) this is not recommended. As with MDI alone, inspiration should be slow (at a rate of 0.5 L/s or less) and complete, beginning at FRC and continuing to TLC.

When to Use a Metered Dose Inhaler, Spacer, or Small-Volume Nebulizer

On the basis of efficacy, simplicity, and cost, it is difficult to argue against the use of MDIs in spontaneously breathing

Table 71-11. Technique for Use of Metered Dose Inhaler with Spacer

1. Warm MDI to body temperature.
2. Shake canister vigorously.
3. Assemble apparatus.
4. Hold canister upright.
5. Actuate MDI.
6. Place mouthpiece in mouth.
7. Close lips about mouthpiece.
8. Inspire slowly (≤0.5 L/s) from spacer.
9. Continue to inspire to TLC.
10. Hold breath for 4–10 seconds.
11. Repeat inspiration with breath hold if indicated by spacer manufacturer.
12. Wait 3–10 minutes between subsequent actuations.
13. Monitor patient for presence of side effects (e.g., tachycardia and tremor) and beneficial effects (e.g., improved breath sounds, peak flow, and FEV_1).

FEV_1, forced expiratory volume in 1 second.
(From Kacmarek and Hess,[171] with permission.)

patients. However, each patient's ability must be carefully analyzed before specific decisions on devices are made. Many patients do not properly use an MDI[98–101] in spite of detailed instruction and careful supervision. As a result, an MDI alone should only be used when the clinician is completely assured that proper technique will be followed. Since most hospitalized patients are anxious and experiencing some physiologic stress, unless they are experienced in the use of an MDI, we would recommend the use of a spacer. A spacer should always be used if steroids are being delivered.

The information presented above would lead one to question whether there ever is a role for SVNs in spontaneously breathing patients, particularly since masks can be adapted to spacers for use in infants, children, and uncooperative adults. However, before attempting to totally eliminate use of SVNs in this setting, the clinician should consider the ability of a distressed, uncooperative, or claustrophobic patients with asthma or chronic obstructive pulmonary disease (COPD) to follow the ideal breathing pattern outlined in Table 71-11 when an MDI with spacer and mask is held to the face. Because of the ventilatory pattern established by patients in these settings, optimal MDI therapy is impossible—slow inspiration from FRC to TLC with a 4- to 10-second end-inspiratory hold does not occur. We would thus not discard the SVN but use it (Table 71-12) in that group of patients unable to achieve a ventilatory pattern even remotely resembling the ideal during the use of an MDI with spacer.

Table 71-12. Patients for Whom SVN Is Preferred to MDI with Spacer or DPI

Confused, disoriented
Severely fatigued
Unable to master or tolerate MDI with spacer, even with face mask, or DPI
Experiencing severe acute asthma

(From Kacmarek and Hess,[171] with permission.)

Use of Metered Dose Inhaler during Mechanical Ventilation

As with the SVN, addition of an artificial airway decreases the quantity of MDI-delivered drug that deposits on the lower respiratory tract.[136–139] As noted earlier, about 9 to 11 percent[105,106] of the drug from an MDI is so deposited in spontaneously breathing patients. Most of the limited data available regarding deposition past the endotracheal tube indicate that at maximum, deposition is about 50 percent lower than during spontaneous breathing, with 4 to 6 percent of the actuated aerosol exiting the endotracheal tube.[136–139]

In a bench study on the effects of variation in ventilatory pattern and endotracheal tube size, Hess et al.[136] noted that an overall 3.3 ± 2.1 percent of the aerosol deposited in a filter beyond the endotracheal tube, an average of 89.2 ± 3.8 percent of the aerosol deposited on the endotracheal tube, and 7.4 ± 3.2 percent deposited on the MDI adapter. No differences in percent deposition were noted as flow rate (30 and 60 L/min), tidal volume (0.5 and 1.5 L), or endotracheal tube size (7.0 and 9.0 mm) changed. However, Crogan and Bishop,[137] again using a lung model, observed that a greater percentage of the aerosol exited the endotracheal tube as size increased (3.0 ± 1.9 percent for a 6.0-mm tube and 6.5 ± 4.4 percent for a 9.0-mm tube). They also noted that a greater quantity of aerosol exited the endotracheal tube if actuation occurred just after the start of a mechanical tidal volume delivery than if actuated before onset of the mechanical breath.

In a randomized comparison of SVN with MDI, Fuller et al.[138] demonstrated that 5.65 ± 1.09 percent of the aerosol delivered by MDI, as compared with 1.22 ± 0.35 percent of that delivered by SVN, is deposited in the lower respiratory tract. In this study four puffs of radiolabeled fenoterol were delivered, with successive actuations spaced 5 minutes apart. Fuller et al.[139] also noted no statistically significant differences in deposition from MDI between patients with endotracheal tubes (4.58 ± 3.03 percent) and those with tracheostomy tubes (6.69 ± 2.80 percent) in a series of patients receiving mechanical ventilation.

SVN versus MDI during Mechanical Ventilation

Few data[140–142] comparing the efficacy of SVNs and MDIs during mechanical ventilation are available. In 1991 Gay et al.[140] demonstrated no differences between MDI administration of 270 μg albuterol (three puffs) and 2.5 mg albuterol in a 3.5-mL solution volume given by SVN. Changes in passive expiratory flow at respiratory system recoil pressures of 6 to 10 cmH_2O were the same for both arms of this single-

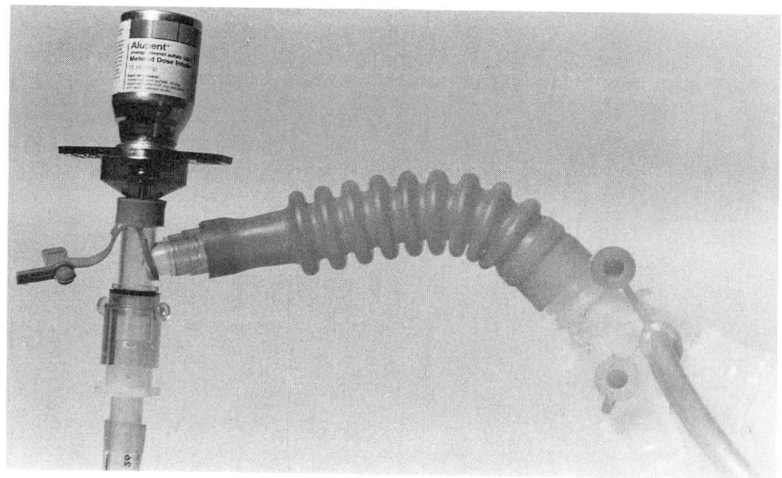

Figure 71-22. MDI and modified tracheal swivel adapter.

blind, randomized crossover comparison. Similar results have been provided by Hess et al.[141] and Gutierrez and Nelson[142] in patients receiving mechanical ventilation, while Fernandez et al.[143] noted no differences in effect between MDI-administered ipratropium bromide or salbutamol and IV aminophylline in a series of 20 ventilator-supported COPD patients. In spite of the limited data comparing these techniques in adults and older children receiving mechanical ventilation, we feel confident in concluding that SVN therapy and MDI therapy are equivalent in ventilator-supported patients, since extensive data establishing equivalence are available in spontaneously breathing individuals. At this time insufficient data are available to allow recommendations regarding MDI use in neonates, infants, and small children who are receiving mechanical ventilation.

Mechanical Ventilator MDI Adapters

Adapters designed to interface MDIs with the ventilator circuit can be classified as (1) modified tracheal swivel adapters (Fig. 71-22); (2) circuit inspiratory limb adapters (Fig. 71-23); and (3) circuit inspiratory limb spacers (Fig. 71-24). Specifics regarding available adapters have been recently reviewed by Hess.[147] However, few data are available to determine which of the adapters is most effective in depositing aerosol past the endotracheal tube and producing maximum patient response. Bishop et al.[144] demonstrated in a lung model that a larger volume of particles in the "respiratory range" (1 to 5 μ) was delivered beyond the endotracheal tube with the Monaghan AeroVent than with the Intermedical Intec 172275 and Instrumentation Industries RTC-22. More recently, catheters extending to the tip of the endotracheal tube have been used by Taylor and Lerman[145] as well as by Peterfreund et al.[146] to increase the delivery of metered dose drugs beyond the endotracheal tube. Taylor and Lerman[145] in a lung model demonstrated delivery of 97 percent of actuated salbutamol beyond the endotracheal tube when a 19-gauge catheter attached to the MDI was positioned at the tip of the tube. Peterfreund et al.[146] also using a lung model, demonstrated that attachment to the MDI of a 19-gauge, 12-

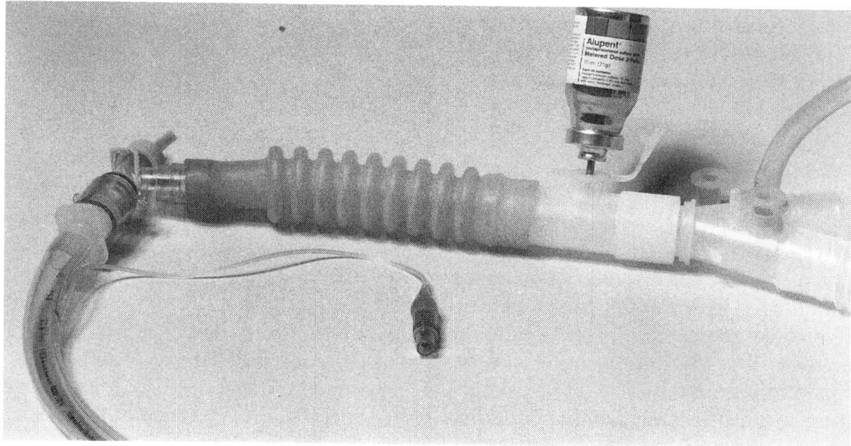

Figure 71-23. MDI and circuit inspiratory limb adapter.

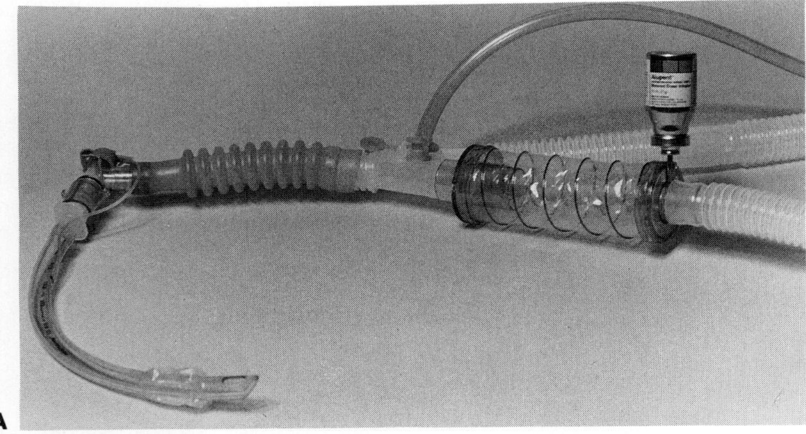

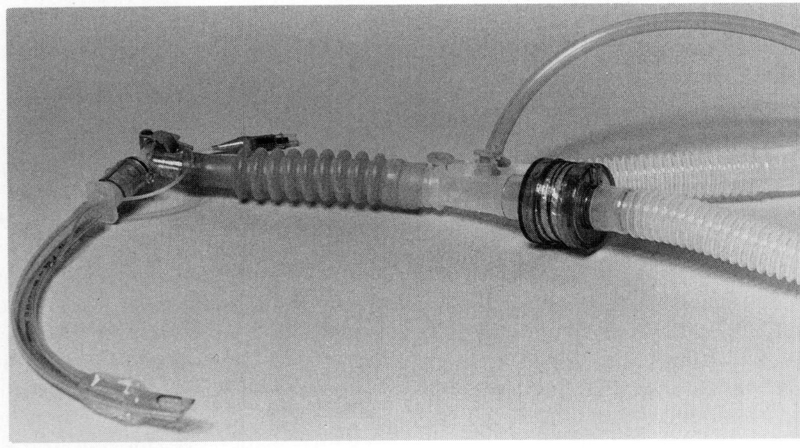

Figure 71-24. MDI and circuit inspiratory limb spacer (AeroVent). (**A**) Spacer with MDI ready for use. (**B**) Spacer closed, as in line when not in use.

in. intravenous catheter positioned in a tracheal swivel adapter resulted in delivery of 90 percent of the MDI-generated aerosol beyond the endotracheal tube. These preliminary data suggest an exciting alternative for MDI delivery in intubated patients but require additional research before application. Thus, currently available data on the placement of MDIs in ventilator circuits are too limited to permit a recommendation on best approach; additional studies are needed before guidelines in this area can be presented.

Technique for Use of MDI in Ventilator Circuits

Little information derived specifically from evaluations of MDI use during mechanical ventilation is available to assist in defining the ideal technique for MDI administration. However, it seems reasonable to extrapolate from the abundant information available on the use of MDI during spontaneous breathing. Gay et al.[140] administered the MDI to ventilator-supported patients during a large-volume manual inflation with a breath hold of several seconds, waiting 1 minute between actuations. Fernandez et al.[143] recommend slow delivery of a large tidal volume by manual ventilator, with a 10-second breath hold and a 5-minute wait between actuations. However, Hess et al.[136] noted no difference in drug deposition with MDI use based on tidal volume or on peak inspiratory flow, while Crogan and Bishop[137] found a flow of 60 L/min to be most efficient.

On the basis of this information, preliminary guidelines for MDI administration during mechanical ventilation are presented in Table 71-13. Ideally, a large tidal volume delivered at moderate flow rates of 30 to 60 L/min and held in the airway for at least 2 to 3 seconds is recommended. Whether this ventilatory pattern should be achieved by manual or mechanical ventilation has not been determined. As with spontaneously breathing, nonintubated patients, a pause between actuations is probably ideal, although this has not been extensively studied. Unless a true in-line spacer (AeroVent) is used, the MDI should be actuated immediately after the beginning of a mechanical breath. If the AeroVent is used, actuation should occur 1 to 2 seconds before the beginning of the mechanical breath or at the end of exhalation, depending on patient or mechanical ventilator rate.

Table 71-13. Technique for Use of MDI During Mechanical Ventilation

1. Place MDI adapter into circuit.
2. Adjust ventilator to deliver volume-limited breaths (rate ≥4/min, tidal volume 12–15 mL/kg) unless contraindicated, or use a manual ventilator.
3. Warm MDI to body temperature.
4. Shake MDI vigorously.
5. Place MDI in circuit.
6. Actuate MDI immediately after the beginning of a mechanical breath; if spacer used, actuate MDI 1–2 seconds before mechanical breath or near end-exhalation, depending on the rate.
7. Apply a 2–3 second inflation hold if not contraindicated.
8. Wait 1 minute between actuations.
9. Return ventilator to pretreatment settings.
10. Monitor patient for side effects (e.g., tachycardia and tremor) and beneficial effects (e.g., improved breath sounds, peak flow, and FEV_1).

FEV_1, forced expiratory volume in 1 second.
(From Kacmarek and Hess,[171] with permission.)

Dosing During Mechanical Ventilation Aerosol Therapy

As has been indicated, the relative amount of drug deposited beyond the endotracheal tube with either an MDI[136–140] or an SVN[59,66–70] is about 50 percent or less of that deposited during spontaneous breathing. As a result and as has been demonstrated in the studies reviewed here, a larger dose of bronchodilator should be administered during mechanical ventilation than during spontaneous breathing if deposition of an equivalent amount on the lower respiratory tract is desired. As a general rule, we would recommend doubling the standard dose used in spontaneously breathing patients; that is, four puffs from an MDI and approximately 0.6 to 1 mL of most aerosol drug solutions (dependent on specific drug) for use with an SVN. However, we caution that actual dosing should be further modified on the basis of patient response, and we find that many patients require and safely tolerate much higher doses than we have recommended as standards (see Ch. 20).

Dry Powder Inhalers

The use of DPIs for the delivery of aerosolized pharmacologic agents is less common in the United States than use of MDIs or SVNs, although it has become commonplace for the delivery of certain agents in Europe. The DPI most frequently used in the United States is the Spinhaler,[148] for administration of cromolyn sodium, although the availability of cromolyn sodium in liquid solution and of MDIs has limited the use of the powdered form. The Spinhaler[148] and the Rotahaler,[149] used for administration of albuterol and beclomethasone dipropionate, are single-dose devices. A multidose DPI, the Turbuhaler (Fig. 71-25), is presently available in Europe for administration of terbutaline sulfate.[150]

The principal advantages of DPIs are that (1) they are breath-activated and require less patient coordination to use properly; and (2) they do not require the use of Freon with its associated environmental problems as a propellant.[151] The principal disadvantage of the single-dose devices is that they must be loaded with a capsule prior to each use, which is considered cumbersome and difficult for some patients to coordinate during acute exacerbations. In addition, with the Rotahaler, care must be taken not to tilt the device after the capsule is loaded and opened in order to prevent loss of the drug.[152]

In contrast to SVNs or MDIs, inhalation from a DPI should be as rapid as possible,[152–154] since it is the inspiratory flow of the patient that creates the aerosol and moves the drug into the lung. However, efficacy has been demonstrated in patients unable to inspire rapidly.[150,155] Since the dry powder dissolves as it comes into contact with the mucosa, breath-holding is generally unnecessary,[152,155] although Auty et al.,[153] in a group of 6 normal volunteers and 20 patients, noted an increased effect from sodium cromoglycate when a 10-second breath hold was included in the administration protocol. As with the MDI, inhalation should be from FRC to TLC (Table 71-14). When these protocols are followed, the percentage of the inhaled drug that deposits on the respiratory tract is about 13 percent,[154] which is similar to the amount depositing with an MDI or SVN.

DPIs compare favorably with SVNs,[150,156,157] and MDIs.[155,158–166] In comparisons with asthmatic and COPD patients, essentially equivalent responses have been noted. Figure 71-26 depicts the results of the most detailed of these studies,[160] a randomized, double-blind, placebo-controlled evaluation of 231 patients with asthma and/or COPD receiving albuterol by either DPI or MDI. No differences in forced expiratory volume in 1 second (FEV_1), peak expiratory flow, or clinical efficacy were noted over a 12-week period.

From the data available it appears that the DPI is as effective as the MDI and SVN in most clinical settings and may be used interchangeably with them. The primary factor preventing more widespread use of DPI is availability. Only terbutaline, salbutamol, beclomethasone dipropionate, and cromolyn sodium are available in powder form. Moreover, all delivery devices except the Turbuhaler, incorporate single-use capsules for administration of terbutaline. This device (Fig. 71-25) contains 200 doses ready to inhale. In addition, the potential for side effects with steroids must be considered, since the required high inspiratory flows may enhance oropharyngeal deposition of large particles. The only situations in which we would not recommend a DPI are those in which we believe that an SVN is superior to either an MDI or a DPI because of lack of patient cooperation (Table 71-12). Table 71-15 contrasts the advantages and disadvantages of the SVN, MDI, and DPI. As a result of increasing worldwide concern over the use of Freon and the worldwide ban by the year 2000 on its use,[151] it seems reasonable to predict that the DPI will become more common and available for delivery of a greater variety of drugs, unless

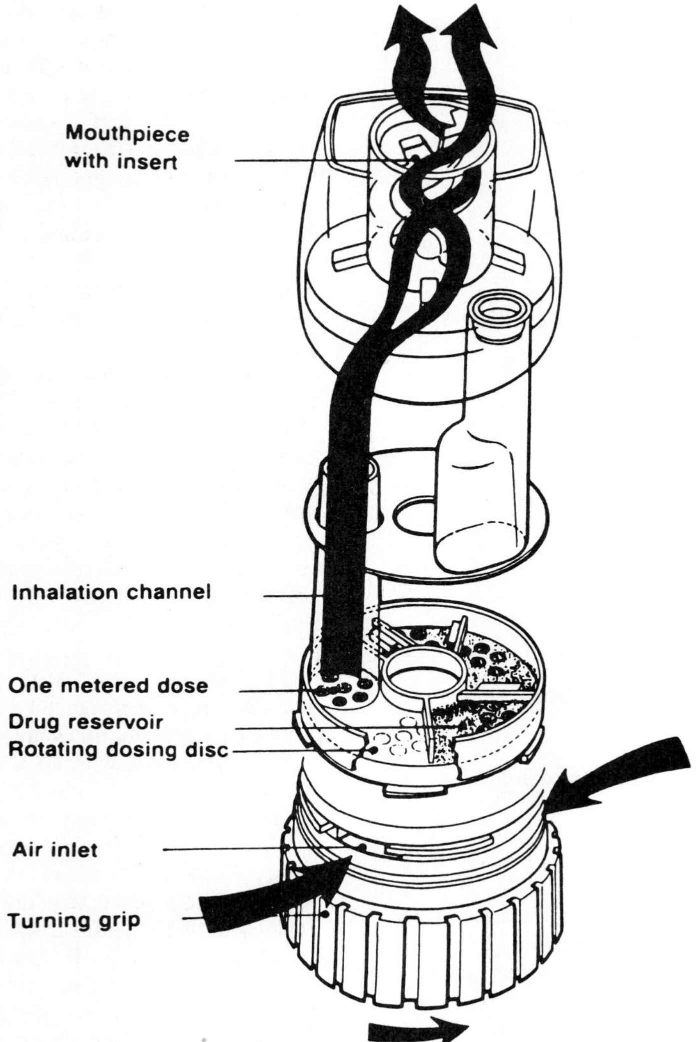

Figure 71-25. Turbuhaler for administration of terbutaline. This device contains 200 individual doses ready to inhale. (From Persson et al.,[161] with permission.)

suitable alternatives to Freon become readily available. Guidance on the selection of appropriate aerosol delivery devices during spontaneous breathing are provided in Table 71-16.

HAZARDS OF AEROSOL THERAPY

Although at initial assessment aerosol therapy appears to be without hazards, a number of concerns must be considered when it is applied. The specific hazards can be listed as (1) precipitation of bronchospasm; (2) swelling of dried retained secretions; (3) fluid overload; (4) drug-related side effects; and (5) infection.

Precipitation of Bronchospasm

As noted earlier, bland aerosol therapy is an irritant to the mucosal membrane. In some patients the irritation may be severe enough to elicit bronchospasm. A significant response is seen primarily during the use of ultrasonic or hydrodynamic nebulizers, in which potentially large volumes of fluid are deposited on the airway.[167] In patients showing an adverse response to these aerosols, use of bronchodilator therapy prior to bland aerosol therapy may significantly diminish the severity of the bronchospasm.

During all treatments with ultrasonic or hydrodynamic nebulizers, the patient's response should be carefully monitored. Periodic auscultation for adventitious breath sounds,

Table 71-14. Technique for Use of a Dry Powder Inhaler

1. Assemble apparatus.
2. Open capsule (specific techniques for use with each device).
3. Exhale normally to FRC.
4. Place inhaler in mouth.
5. Seal lips around mouthpiece.
6. Inhale rapidly (>60 L/min) through device (breath hold unnecessary).
7. Repeat process until capsule is empty.
8. Rinse mouth after inhalation of steroid.
9. Monitor patient for presence of side effects (e.g., tachycardia or tremor) and beneficial effects (e.g., improved breath sounds, peak flow, and FEV_1).

FEV_1, forced expiratory volume in 1 second.
(From Kacmarek and Hess,[171] with permission.)

as well as assessment of ventilatory pattern, should be carried out, and the patient's subjective response should be evaluated.[22]

Swelling of Dried Retained Secretions

Dry retained secretions occupy a small volume in the airway. Hydration of secretions can markedly increase secretion volume and have the potential to obstruct airways if the

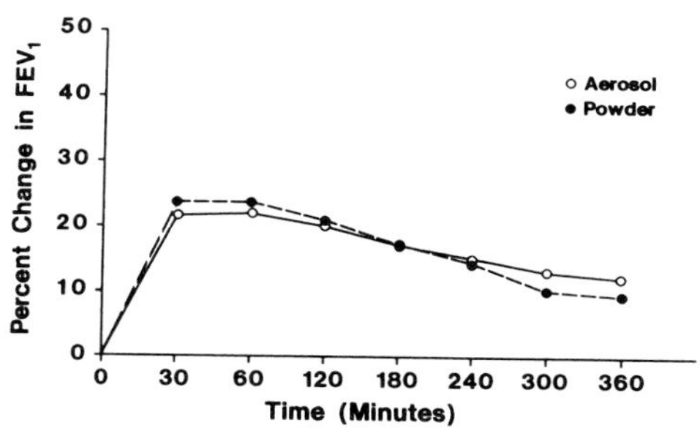

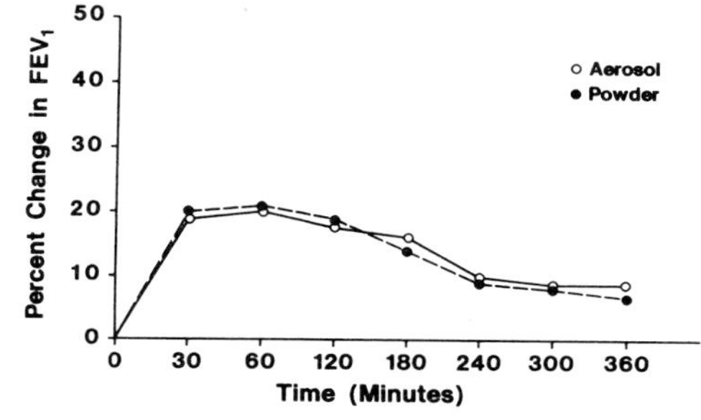

Figure 71-26. Comparison of effects of albuterol administered by MDI or by DPI. (**A**) Percentage of change from baseline in mean forced expiratory volume in 1 second (FEV_1) after treatment with albuterol by DPI (n = 115) or MDI (n = 116) at week 0. (**B**) Data are identical at week 12 to those obtained at week 0 after treatment with albuterol by DPI (n = 89) or MDI (n = 94). No differences were noted between the MDI and the DPI. (From Bronsky et al.,[160] with permission.)

Table 71-15. Advantages and Disadvantages of SVN, MDI, and DPI

Device	Advantages	Disadvantages
SVN	Less patient coordination required High (even continuous) doses possible No chlorofluorocarbon release	Expensive Wasteful Contamination occurs if not cleaned carefully Not all medications available Pressurized gas source required Time consuming
MDI	Convenient Inexpensive	Patient coordination required Patient activation required Results in pharyngeal deposition Has potential for abuse Difficult to deliver high doses Not all medications available Ozone-depleting chlorofluorocarbons released
MDI with auxiliary device	Less patient coordination required	More complex process for patient who can use MDI alone More expensive than MDI alone Less portable than MDI alone
DPI	Less patient coordination required Breath hold not required No chlorofluorocarbon release Breath-activated	Requires high inspiratory flow; most units are single-dose Can result in pharyngeal deposition Cannot be used with intubated patients Not all medications available Difficult to deliver high doses

(From Kacmarek and Hess,[171] with permission.)

Table 71-16. Considerations in Choosing a Specific Aerosol Delivery Device

Primary device of choice is MDI
If unable to use MDI properly, use MDI with spacer or DPI
If very high dose or continuous use is required or if patient is unable to tolerate MDI with spacer and mask, use SVN

(From Kacmarek and Hess,[171] with permission.)

patient is incapable of adequate cough and expectoration. Again, it is unlikely that this potential problem would arise except during ultrasonic or hydrodynamic therapy, in which the potential exists for deposition of large quantities of water on the airways.[4] During and after therapy with these nebulizers, patients should be carefully monitored for cardiopulmonary distress, and airway suctioning should be performed if secretion removal is inadequate.

Fluid Overload

Theoretically, fluid overload and its associated electrolyte imbalances can result from the prolonged use of ultrasonic or hydrodynamic nebulizers.[168] This is not a problem with jet nebulizers, since the output of jet nebulizers (1 mL/min) is much lower than with either ultrasonic or hydrodynamic nebulizers (up to 6 mL/min). The patients primarily at risk for fluid overload are infants and children. Therefore ultrasonic and hydrodynamic nebulizers are generally avoided in this group and are only used on a short-term, intermittent basis in adults.

Drug Reactions

Administration of aerosolized drugs can precipitate the same side effects noted during systemic administration of these agents, although because of localized administration, side effects with the newer aerosolized agents is minimal. Practitioners should be aware of the specific side effects of all agents administered in aerosolized form (see Ch. 20).

Infection

A potential for contamination of a patient's airway exists during administration of aerosol therapy. The wet, warm environment of aerosol generators provide an ideal medium for bacterial growth.[170,171] As a result, meticulous care should be exercised during the set-up and refilling of all aerosol generators, and appropriate infection control measures should be followed.

Infection Control

Careful adherence to equipment decontamination and equipment change schedules is imperative during aerosol therapy. All aerosol equipment used on patients should be sterile before set-up. In addition, all aerosol therapy equipment should be changed every 24 hours[22]; this includes small-volume as well as large-volume systems. Significant bacterial growth occurs on aerosol equipment after 24 hours of use. The same is not true for humidifiers, since they do not generate aerosol particles, no mechanism is available to transport bacteria from the water reservoir to the patient. In general, when nondisposable humidifiers are used for spontaneously breathing patients, weekly equipment change is adequate. This is not true, however, for large-volume heated humidifiers, in which large quantities of fluid condense in delivery tubing; these systems should be changed every 48 hours.

References

1. Darin J: The need for rational criteria for the use of unheated bubble humidifiers (editorial). Respir Care 1982;27:945–947
2. Dery R: The evolution of heat and moisture in the respiratory tract during anesthesia with a non-rebreathing system. Can J Anaesth 1973;20:296–309
3. Strauss RH: Influence of heat and humidity on the airway obstruction induced by exercise in asthma. J Clin Invest 1978;621:433–440
4. Shapiro BA, Kacmarek RM, Cane RD et al: Clinical Application of Respiratory Care. 4th Ed. Mosby-Year Book, St. Louis, 1991, pp. 57–73
5. Benson DM: Systemic and pulmonary changes with inhaled humid atmospheres. Anesthesiology 1969;30:199–206
6. Darin JD, Broadwell J, MacDonald R: An evaluation of water vapor output from four brands of unheated prefilled bubble humidifiers. Respir Care 1982;27:49–50
7. Dolan GK, Zawadski JJ: Performance characteristics of low-flow humidifiers. Respir Care 1976;21:393–403
8. Klein EF Jr, Shah DA, Shah NJ et al: Performance characteristics of conventional and prototype humidifiers and nebulizers. Chest 1973;64:690–696
9. American College of Chest Physicians, National Heart, Lung and Blood Institute: National conference on oxygen therapy. Respir Care 1984;29:922–935
10. Campbell EJ, Baker D, Crites-Silver P: Subjective effects of humidification of oxygen delivery by nasal cannula. A prospective study. Chest 1988;93:289–293
11. Chen WY, Horton DJ: Heat and water loss from the airways and exercise-induced asthma. Respiration 1977;34:305–313
12. Deal EC Jr, McFadden ER Jr, Ingram RH Jr et al: Role of respiratory heat exchange in production of exercise-induced asthma. J Appl Physiol 1979;46:467–475
13. Strauss RH, McFadden ER Jr, Ingram RH Jr et al: Influence of heat and humidity on the airway obstruction induced by exercise in asthma. J Clin Invest 1978;61:433–440
14. Mahler DA, Loke J: Lung function after marathon running at warm and cold ambient temperatures. Am Rev Respir Dis 1981;124:154–157
15. O'Cain CF, Dowlins NB, Slutsky AS et al: Airway effects of respiratory heat loss in normal subjects. J Appl Physiol 1980;49:875–880
16. Heaton RW, Henderson AF, Gray BJ, Costello JF: The bronchial response to cold air challenge: Evidence for different mechanisms in normals and asthmatic subjects. Thorax 1983;38:506–511
17. Chen WY, Chai H: Airway cooling and nocturnal asthma. Chest 1982;81:675–680
18. Wells RE, Perera RD, Kinney JM: Humidification of oxygen delivery during inhalation therapy. N Engl J Med 1963;268: 644–648
19. English PA, Kacmarek RM, Vallande N, Hopkins CC: Con-

tamination of heated neonatal ventilator circuits, abstracted. Respir Care 1990;35:1089
20. Kacmarek RM, Vallende N, English P, Hopkins CC: Extended use of heated neonatal-pediatric ventilator circuits, abstracted. Respir Care (in press)
21. Dreyfuss D, Djedaini K, Weber P et al: Prospective study of nosocomial pneumonia and of patient and circuit colonization during mechanical ventilation with circuit changes every 48 hours vs. no change. Am Rev Respir Dis 1991;143:738–743
22. Scanlon CL, Spearman CB, Sheldon RL: Egan's Fundamentals of Respiratory Care. 5th Ed. Mosby-Year Book, St. Louis, 1990, pp. 557–583
23. Demers B: Humidification system. pp. 19–23. In Kacmarek RM, Stoller J (eds): Current Respiratory Care. BC Decker, Toronto, 1988
24. Branson RD, Seger SM: Bland aerosol therapy. pp. In Kacmarek RM, Stoller JK (eds): Current Respiratory Care. BC Decker, Toronto, 1988
25. Lourenco RV, Cotromanes E: Clinical aerosols. I. Characterization of aerosols and their diagnostic uses. Arch Intern Med 1982;142:2163–2172
26. Morrow PE: Aerosol characterization and deposition. Am Rev Respir Dis 1974;110:88–99
27. Rau JL: Humidity and aerosol therapy. pp. 164–180. In Barnes T (ed): Respiratory Care Practice. Mosby-Year Book, St. Louis, 1988
28. Dolovich M: Clinical aspects of aerosol physics. Respir Care 1991;36:931–938
29. Morrow PE: Aerosol characterization and deposition. Am Rev Respir Dis 1974;710:88–99
30. Brain JD, Valberg PA: Deposition of aerosol in the respiratory tract. Am Rev Respir Dis 1979;120:1325–1333
31. Beeckmans JM: The deposition of aerosols in the respiratory tract: I. Mathematical analysis and comparison with experimental data. Can J Physiol Pharmacol 1965;43:157–164
32. Sweeney TD: Retention of inhaled particles in hamsters with pulmonary fibrosis. Am Rev Respir Dis 1983;128:138–145
33. Howmann RF, Black A, Walsh M: Deposition of aerosol particles in the nasopharyngeal region of the respiratory tract. Nature 1969;221:1254–1260
34. Lippmann M: Deposition and clearance of inhaled particles in the human nose. Ann Otol Rhinol Laryngol 1970;79:519–526
35. Cinkotai FF: The behavior of sodium chloride particles in moist air. J Aerosol Sci 1971;2:325–332
36. Valberg PA, Brain J: Breathing patterns influence aerosol deposition sites in excised dog lungs. J Appl Physiol 1982;53: 824–832
37. Gold WM: Vagally-mediated reflex bronchoconstriction in allergic asthma. Chest, suppl. 1973;63:11–15
38. Christopher KL, Saravolatz LD, Bush TL, Conway WA: The potential role of respiratory therapy equipment in cross infection. A study using a canine model for pneumonia. Am Rev Respir Dis 1983;128:271–275
39. Model JH: Effect of chronic exposure to ultrasonic aerosols on the lung. Anesthesiology 1967;28:680–685
40. Model JH: Effect of ultrasonic nebulized suspensions on pulmonary surfactant. Chest 1966;50:627–632
41. Allan D: Artificial humidification. Medical Sci 1966;17:41–47
42. Boucher RGM, Kreuter J: Fundamentals of the ultrasonic atomization of medicated solutions. Ann Allergy 1968;26: 591–598
43. Massey DG, Miyauchi D, Fournier-Massey G: Nebulizer function. Bull Eur Physiopathol Respir 1982;18:665–671
44. Arossa W, Quagliotti F, Sala N et al: Different performance of two commercial nebulizers. Respiration 1984;46:128–132
45. Clay MM, Pavia D, Newman SP et al: Assessment of jet nebulizers for lung aerosol therapy. Lancet 1982;2:592–594
46. Hess D, Horney D, Snyder T: Evaluation of hand-held nebulizer function. Respir Care 1989;34:717–723
47. Wood JA, Wilson RSE, Bray C: Changes in salbutamol concentration in the reservoir solution of a jet nebulizer. Respir Med 1986;80:164–169
48. Clay MM, Pavia D, Newman SP, Clarke SW: Factors influencing the size distribution of aerosols from jet nebulizers. Thorax 1983;38:755–759
49. Douglas JG, Leslie MJ, Brompton GK, Grant IWB: Is the flow rate used to drive a jet nebulizer clinically important? (Letter). 1985;290:92
50. Phipps PR, Gonda I: Droplets produced by medical nebulizers: Some factors affecting their size and solute concentration. Chest 1990;97:1327–1332
51. Porstendofer J, Gebhart J, Robig G: Effects of evaporation on the size distribution of nebulized aerosols. J Aerosol Sci 1977;8:371–380
52. Newman SP, Pellow PGD, Clarke SW: *In vitro* comparison of Devilbiss jet and ultrasonic nebulizers. Chest 1987;92:991–994
53. Davis SS: Physiochemical studies on aerosol solutions for drug delivery: I. Water-propylene glycol systems. Int J Pharmacol 1978;1:71–83
54. Mercer T: Production of therapeutic aerosols. J Aerosol Sci 1977;8:371–380
55. Heyder J: Mechanism of aerosol particle deposition. Chest 1981;80:820–823
56. Leiberman A, Ohki M, Forte V et al: Nose/mouth distribution of respiratory airflow in mouth breathing children. Acta Otolaryngol (Stockh) 1990;109:454–460
57. Stevenson RD, Wilson RA: Face mask or mouthpiece for delivery of nebulized bronchodilator aerosols? Respir Med 1981;75:88–90
58. Wood DO, Chandler D, Dugdale AE: Two methods of administering nebulized solbutamol, a controlled study. Aust Paediatr J 1978;14:150–155
59. Hughes JM, Saez J: Effects of nebulizer mode and position in a mechanical ventilator circuit on dose efficiency. Respir Care 1987;32:1131–1135
60. Kradjan WA, Lakshminarayan S: Efficiency of air compressor-driven nebulizers. Chest 1985;87:512–516
61. Pavia D, Thompson ML, Clarke SW, Shannon HS: Effect of lung function and mode of inhalation on penetration of aerosol in the human lung. Thorax 1977;32:194–197
62. Dolovitch M, Ryan G, Newhouse MT: Aerosol penetration into the lung. Influence on airway responses. Chest 1981;80: 834–836
63. Newman SP, Woodman G, Clarke SW: Deposition of carbenicillin aerosols in cystic fibrosis: Effects of nebulizer system and breathing pattern. Thorax 1988;43:318–322
64. Newman SP: Aerosol deposition considerations in inhalation therapy. Chest 1985;88:152S–160S
65. Lewis RA, Fleming JS: Fractional deposition from a jet nebulizer: How it differs from a metered dose inhaler. Respir Med 1985;79:361–367
66. MacIntyre NR, Silver RM, Miller CW et al: Aerosol delivery in intubated, mechanically ventilated patients. Crit Care Med 1985;13:81–85
67. Ahrens RC, Ries RA, Popendorf W, Wiese JA: The delivery of therapeutic aerosols through endotracheal tubes. Pediatr Pulmonol 1986;9:19–24
68. Cameron D, Clay M, Silverman M: Evaluation of nebulizers for use in neonatal ventilator circuits. Crit Care Med 1990;18:866–870
69. Henry WD, Chatburn RL: Effects of manual versus mechanical ventilation on aerosol dose efficiency, abstracted. Respir Care 1988;33:914
70. Fraser I, DuVall A, Dolovich M, Newhouse MT: Therapeutic aerosol delivery in ventilatory systems, abstracted. Am Rev Respir Dis 1981;123:107
71. Flavin M, MacDonald M, Dolovitch M et al: Aerosol delivery to the rabbit lung with an infant ventilator. Pediatr Pulmonol 1986;2:35–39
72. Cameron D, Arnot R, Clay M, Silverman M: Aerosol delivery in neonatal ventilator circuits: A rabbit lung model. Pediatr Pulmonol 1991;10:208–213
73. Gay PG, Rodarte JR, Tayyab H, Hubmayr RD: Evaluation of

bronchodilator responsiveness in mechanically ventilated patients. Am Rev Respir Dis 1987;136:880–885
74. Brudno D, Parker DH, Staton G: Responsiveness of pulmonary mechanics to terbutaline in patients with bronchopulmonary dysplasia. Am J Med Sci 1989;197:166–168
75. Beaty CD, Ritz RH, Benson MS: Continuous in-line nebulizers complicate pressure support ventilation. Chest 1989;96: 1360–1363
76. Newman SP: Aerosol deposition considerations in inhalation therapy. Chest, suppl. 1985;88:152S–156S
77. Balmes JR: Propellent gases in metered dose inhalers: Their impact on the global environment. Respir Care 1991;36: 1037–1044
78. Newman SP, Pavia D, Bateman RM, Clarke SW: Bronchodilator response after administration of pressurized aerosols at different lung volumes in patients with airway obstruction, abstracted. Clin Sci 1979;56:10P–11P
79. Newman SP, Pavia D, Clarke SW: Simple instructions for using pressurized aerosol bronchodilators. J R Soc Med 1980;73: 776–779
80. Riley DJ, Weitz BW, Edelman NH: The responses of asthmatic subjects to isoproterenol inhaled at differing lung volumes. Am Rev Respir Dis 1976;114:509–515
81. Riley DJ, Liu RT, Edelman NH: Enhanced responses to aerosolized bronchodilator therapy in asthma using respiratory maneuvers. Chest 1979;76:501–507
82. Dolovich M, Ruffin RE, Roberts R, Newhouse MT: Optimal delivery of aerosols from metered dose inhalers. Chest 1981;80:911S–915S
83. Williams TJ: The importance of aerosol technique: Does speed of inhalation matter? Respir Med 1982;76:223–228
84. Lawford P, McKenzie D: Pressurized bronchodilator aerosol technique: Influence of breath-holding time and relationship of inhaler to the mouth. Respir Med 1982;76:229–233
85. Grainger J: Correct use of aerosol inhalers. Can Med Assoc J 1977;116:584–585
86. Woolf CR: Correct use of pressurized aerosol inhalers. Can Med Assoc J 1979;121:710–711
87. Wilson AF, Mukai DS, Ahdout JJ: Effect of canister temperature on performance of metered dose inhalers. Am Rev Respir Dis 1991;143:1034–1037
88. Moren F: Drug deposition of pressurized inhalation aerosols: II. Influence of vapor pressure and metered volume. Int J Pharmacol 1985;1:213–218
89. Heimer D, Shim C, Williams H: The effect of sequential inhalations of metaproterenol aerosol in asthma. J Allergy Clin Immunol 1980;66:75–77
90. Pedersen S: The importance of a pause between the inhalation of two puffs of terbutaline from a pressurized aerosol with a tube spacer. J Allergy Clin Immunol 1986;77:505–509
91. Mestitz H, Copland JM, McDonald CF: Comparison of outpatient nebulized vs metered dose inhaler terbutaline in chronic airflow obstruction. Chest 1989;96:1237–1240
92. Jenkins SC, Heaton RW, Fulton TJ, Moxham J: Comparison of domiciliary nebulized salbutamol from a metered-dose inhaler in stable chronic airflow limitation. Chest 1987;91: 804–807
93. Cissik JH, Bode FR, Smith JA: Double-blind cross-over study of five bronchodilator medications and two delivery methods in stable asthma. Chest 1986;90:489–493
94. Gunawardena KA, Smith AP, Shankleman J: A comparison of metered dose inhalers with nebulizers for the delivery of ipratropium bromide in domiciliary practice. Respir Med 1986;80:170–178
95. Shim CS, Williams MH: Effect of bronchodilator therapy administered by canister versus jet nebulizer. J Allergy Clin Immunol 1984;73:387–390
96. Gomm SA, Keaney NP, Hunt LP et al: Dose-response comparison of ipratropium bromide from a metered-dose inhaler and by jet nebulization. Thorax 1983;38:197–201
97. Christensson P, Arborelius M, Lilja B: Salbutamol inhalation in chronic asthma bronchiale: Dose aerosol vs jet nebulizer. Chest 1981;79:416–419
98. Epstein SW, Manning CPR, Ashley MJ, Corey PN: Survey of the clinical use of pressurized aerosol inhalers. Can Med Assoc J 1979;120:813–816
99. Orehek J, Gayrard P, Grimand CH, Charpin J: Patient error in the use of bronchodilator metered aerosols. Br Med J 1976;1:76–77
100. Shin C, Williams MH: The adequacy of inhalation of aerosol from canister nebulizers. Am J Med 1980;69:891–896
101. Patterson IC, Crompton GK: Use of pressurized aerosols by asthmatic patients. Br Med J 1976;1:77–80
102. Dolovich OM, Ruffin R, Corr D, Newhouse MT: Clinical evaluation of a simple demand inhalation MDI aerosol delivery device. Chest 1983;84:36–41
103. Konig P: Spacer devices used with metered-dose inhalers. Breakthrough or gimmick? Chest 1985;88:276–284
104. Sackner MA, Kim CS: Auxiliary MDI aerosol delivery systems. Chest 1985;88:161S–170S
105. Spiro SG, Singh CA, Tolfree SEJ et al: Direct labeling of ipratropium bromide aerosol and its deposition pattern in normal subjects and patients with chronic bronchitis. Thorax 1984;39:432–435
106. Newman SP, Pavia D, Moren F et al: Deposition of pressurized aerosols in the human respiratory tract. Thorax 1981;36:52–55
107. Sackner MA, Kim CS: Recent advances in the management of obstructive lung disease: Auxiliary MDI aerosol delivery systems. Chest, suppl. 1985;88(2):161S–170S
108. Kim CS, Eldridge MA, Sackner MA: Oropharyngeal deposition and delivery aspects of metered-dose inhaler aerosols. Am Rev Respir Dis 1987;135:157–164
109. Corr D, Dolovich M, McCormack D et al: Design and characteristics of a portable breath actuated, particle size selective medical aerosol inhaler. J Aerosol Sci 1982;13:1–7
110. Newman SP, Moren F, Pavia D et al: Deposition of pressurized suspension aerosols inhaled through extension devices. Am Rev Respir Dis 1981;124:317–320
111. Newman SP, Woodman G, Clarke SW, Sackner MA: Effect of InspirEase on the deposition of metered-dose aerosols in the human respiratory tract. Chest 1986;89:551–556
112. Gleeson JGA, Price JF: Nebuhaler technique. Respir Med 1988;82:172–174
113. Niven RW, Haver K, Brain JD: An evaluation of the performance of several inhalation aerosol spacer devices using cascade impaction. J Aerosol Sci 1992 (in press)
114. Newman SP, Millar AB, Lennard-Jones TR et al: Improvement of pressurized aerosol deposition with Nebuhaler spacer device. Thorax 1984;39:935–941
115. Fairshter FD: Evaluation of a metered-dose aerosol delivery system using a partial flow-volume curve. Am Rev Respir Dis 1987;135:741–743
116. Crimi N, Palermo F, Cacopardo B et al: Bronchodilator effect of Aerochanger and InspirEase in comparison with metered dose inhaler. Eur J Respir Dis 1987;71:153–157
117. Lee H, Evans HE: Evaluation of inhalation aids of metered dose inhalers in asthmatic children. Chest 1987;91:366–369
118. O'Reilly JF, Gould G, Kendrick AH, Laszlo G: Domiciliary comparison of terbutaline treatment by metered dose inhaler with and without conical spacer in severe and moderately severe chronic asthma. Thorax 1986;41:766–770
119. Fuller HD: Comparison of two chamber devices in patients using a metered-dose inhaler with satisfactory technique. Can Med Assoc J 1986;135:625–629
120. Morris J, Milledge JS, Moszoro H, Higgins A: The efficacy of drug delivery by a pear-shaped spacer and metered dose inhaler. Respir Med 1984;78:383–387
121. Pauwels R, Lamont H, Hidinger K, Van der Straeten M: Influence of an extension tube on the bronchodilator efficacy of terbutaline delivered from a metered dose inhaler. Respiration 1984;45:61–66
122. Epstein SW, Parsons JE, Corey PN et al: A comparison of three

means of pressurized aerosol inhaler use. Am Rev Respir Dis 1983;128:253–255

123. Fuglsang G, Pedersen S: Cumulative dose response relationship of terbutaline delivered by three different inhalers. Allergy 1988;43:348–352
124. Tobin MJ, Jenoluri G, Danta J et al: Response to bronchodilator drug administration by a new reservoir aerosol delivery system and a review of other auxiliary delivery systems. Am Rev Respir Dis 1982;126:670–675
125. Newman SP, Millar AB, Lennard-Jones TR et al: Improvement of pressurized aerosol deposition with Nebuhaler spacer device. Thorax 1984;239:935–941
126. Salzman GA, Steele MT, Pribble JP et al: Aerosolized metaproterenol in the treatment of asthmatics with severe airflow obstruction. Chest 1989;95:1017–1020
127. Jasper AC, Mohsenifar Z, Kahan S et al: Cost-benefit comparison of aerosol bronchodilator delivery methods in hospitalized patients. Chest 1987;91:614–618
128. Summer W, Elston R, Tharpe L et al: Aerosol bronchodilator delivery methods. Relative impact on pulmonary function and cost of respiratory care. Arch Intern Med 1989;149:618–623
129. Berry RB, Shinto RA, Wong FH et al: Nebulizer vs spacer for bronchodilator delivery in patients hospitalized for acute exacerbations of COPD. Chest 1989;96:1241–1246
130. Turner JR, Corkery KJ, Eckman D et al: Equivalence of continuous flow nebulizer and metered-dose inhaler with reservoir bag for treatment of acute airflow obstruction. Chest 1988;93:476–481
131. Green AB, Jackson CL: Terbutaline metered-dose inhalation vs metaproterenol by hand-held nebulization. A comparison in black inner-city COPD patients. J Nat Med Assoc 1988;80: 393–396
132. Gervais A, Begin P: Bronchodilatation with a metered-dose inhaler plus an extension, using tidal breathing vs jet nebulization. Chest 1987;92:822–824
133. Berenberg MJ, Cupples LA, Baigelman W, Pearce L: Comparison of metered-dose inhaler attached to an aerochamber with an updraft nebulizer for the administration of metaproterenol in hospitalized patients. J Asthma 1985;22:87–92
134. Pedersen JZ, Bundgaard A: Comparative efficacy of different methods of nebulizing terbutaline. Eur J Clin Pharmacol 1983;25:739–742
135. Cushley MJ, Lewis RA, Tattersfield AE: Comparison of three techniques of inhalation on the airway response to terbutaline. Thorax 1983;38:908–913
136. Hess D, Beener C, Watson K: An evaluation of the effectiveness of metered dose inhaler (MDI) use with mechanical ventilation, abstracted. Respir Care 1988;33:910–911
137. Crogan SJ, Bishop MJ: Delivery efficiency of metered dose aerosols given via endotracheal tubes. Anesthesiology 1989;70:1008–1010
138. Fuller HD, Dolovich MB, Posmituck G et al: Pressurized aerosol versus jet aerosol delivery to mechanically ventilated patients. Am Rev Respir Dis 1990;141:440–444
139. Fuller HD, Dolovich MB, Turpie F et al: Aerosol deposition to the lungs by MDI in ventilated patients: ET tubes vs tracheostomy, abstracted. Chest 1990;98:27S
140. Gay PC, Patel HG, Nelson SB et al: Metered dose inhalers for bronchodilator delivery in intubated, mechanically ventilated patients. Chest 1991;99:66–71
141. Hess D, Fillman D, Daugherty A et al: Use of metered dose inhalers in intubated patients, abstracted. Respir Care 1989;34:1027
142. Gutierrez CJ, Nelson R: Short-term bronchodilation in mechanically ventilated patients receiving metaproterenol via SVN and MDI, abstracted. Respir Care 1988;33:910
143. Fernandez A, Lazaro A, Garcia A et al: Bronchodilators in patients with chronic obstructive pulmonary disease on mechanical ventilation. Am Rev Respir Dis 1990;141:164–168
144. Bishop MJ, Larson RP, Buschman DL: Metered dose inhaler aerosol characteristics are affected by the endotracheal tube actuator/adapter used. Anesthesiology 1990;73:1263–1265
145. Taylor RH, Lerman J: High efficiency delivery of salbutamol with a metered-dose inhaler in narrow tracheal tubes and catheters. Anesthesiology 1991;74:360–363
146. Peterfreund RA, Niven RW, Brain J: Improved delivery efficiency of the metered dose inhaler (MDI): Further laboratory evaluation of drug release from a nozzle extension, abstracted. Anesthesiology 1991;75:A396
147. Hess D: How should bronchodilators be administered to patients being mechanically ventilated? Respir Care 1991;36: 377–394
148. Nizami NP, Vakil DV, Lozynsky A, Nizami RM: Automatic piercing Spinhaler (Halermatic): A comparative study. Ann Allergy 1988;60:399–402
149. Crompton GK: Clinical use of dry powder systems. Eur J Respir Dis, suppl. 1982;122:96–99
150. Hansen NCG: Terbutaline as powder inhalation from Bricanyl Turbuhaler compared to terbutaline as nebulizer solution in severe chronic airways obstruction. Eur Respir J 1989;2: 716–720
151. Balmes JR: Propellent gases in metered dose inhalers: Their impact on the global environment. Respir Care 1991;36: 1037–1044
152. Pedersen S: How to use a Rotahaler. Arch Dis Child 1986;61:11–14
153. Auty RM, Brown K, Neale MG, Snashall PD: Respiratory tract deposition of sodium cromoglycate is highly dependent upon technique of inhalation using the Spinhaler. Respir Med 1987;81:371–380
154. Newman SP: Delivery of therapeutic aerosols. Probl Respir Care 1988;1:53–82
155. Tukiainen H, Terho EO: Comparison of inhaled salbutamol powder and aerosol in asthmatic patients with low peak expiratory flow level. Eur J Clin Pharmacol 1985;27:645–647
156. Assoufi BK, Hodson ME: High dose salbutamol in chronic airflow obstruction: Comparison of nebulizer with Rotacaps. Respir Med 1989;83:415–420
157. Grimwood K, Johnson-Barrett JJ, Taylor B: Salbutamol: Tablets, inhalational powder, or nebulizer? Br Med J 1981;282: 105–106
158. Johnsen CR, Weeke ER: Turbuhaler: A new device for dry powder terbutaline inhalation. Allergy 1988;43:392–395
159. Pover GM, Langdon CG, Jones SR, Fidler C: Evaluation of a breath-operated powder inhaler. J Int Med Res 1988;16: 201–203
160. Bronsky E, Bucholtz GA, Busse WW et al: Comparison of inhaled albuterol powder and aerosol in asthma. J Allergy Clin Immunol 1987;79:741–747
161. Persson G, Gruvstad E, Stahl E: A new multiple dose powder inhaler (Turbuhaler) compared with a pressurized inhaler in a study of terbutaline in asthmatics. Eur Respir J 1988;1:681–684
162. Swinburn PD, Sexton M: Inhaled bronchodilators: A comparison of different methods of inhaling. N Z Med J 1981;18:340–346
163. Sovijarvi ARA, Lahdensue A, Muittari A: Bronchodilating effect of salbutamol inhalation powder and salbutamol aerosol after metacholine-induced bronchoconstriction. Curr Ther Res 1982;32:566–573
164. Edmunds AT, McKenzie S, Tooley M, Godfrey S: A clinical comparison of beclomethasone dipropionate delivered by pressurized aerosol and as a powder from a Rotahaler. Arch Dis Child 1979;54:233–235
165. Muittari A, Ahonen A: Comparison of the bronchodilator effect of inhaled salbutamol powder and pressurized salbutamol aerosol. Curr Ther Res 1979;25:804–808
166. Smith JM, Gwynn CM: A clinical comparison of aerosol and powder administration of beclomethasone dipropionate in asthma. Clin Allergy 1978;8:479–481
167. Cheney FW, Butler J: The effects of ultrasonic nebulizers on airway resistance in man. Anesthesiology 1968;29:1099–1105

168. Lyons HA: Uses of therapeutic aerosols. Am J Cardiol 1969;12:462–468
169. Reinarz JA, Pierce AK, Mays BB: The potential role of inhalation therapy equipment in nosocomial pulmonary infections. J Clin Invest 1965;44:831–836
170. Pierce AK, Sanford JP: Bacterial contamination of aerosols. Arch Intern Med 1973;131:156–162
171. Kacmarek RM, Hess D: The interface between patient and aerosol generator. Respir Care 1991;36:952–976
172. McPherson SP: Respiratory Therapy Equipment. 2nd Ed. CV Mosby, St. Louis, 1981
173. Eubanks DH, Bone RC: Comprehensive Respiratory Care. 2nd Ed. Mosby-Year Book, St. Louis, 1990
174. Burton GG, Hodgkin JE (eds): Respiratory Care: A Guide to Clinical Practice. 2nd Ed. JB Lippincott, Philadelphia, 1984
175. Kim CS, Eldridge MA, Sackner MA: Oropharyngeal deposition and delivery aspects of metered dose inhaler aerosols. Am Rev Respir Dis 1987;135:157–164

Chapter 72

Airway Management

Michael J. Bishop
Ray H. Ritz

CHAPTER OUTLINE

Airway management is the provision of assistance to a patient in maintaining a patent airway. Clinicians place artificial airways in patients as dictated by four major indications:

1. *Maintaining the airway*: Unconscious patients or patients with facial, pharyngeal, or laryngeal trauma frequently obstruct their upper respiratory tract (see Ch. 42). The fixed wall of the artificial airway prevents such obstruction. The seal between the tube cuff and the trachea also provides protection from massive aspiration of secretions or gastric contents.
2. *Application of positive pressure to the airway*: Positive-pressure ventilation can be provided for short periods by using a mask, but long-term mechanical ventilation requires an intratracheal airway. Continuous positive airway pressure is also usually applied via a tracheal tube, although in some cooperative patients a tight mask seal may be adequate.
3. *Use of high O_2 concentrations*: Delivery of O_2 at high pressures is facilitated by a sealed system. While high inspired O_2 concentrations can be delivered by using high flow rates or a reservoir system with a mask, the rate of failure is

high owing to mask displacement and entrainment of room air.

4. *Facilitation of pulmonary toilet*: Frequent suctioning in the unintubated patient may be anatomically difficult to achieve or may result in substantial trauma to the oronasopharyngeal airway.

The skilled clinician can manage the airway for brief periods without a tracheal tube in place. In most patients, a tight seal can be achieved between a face mask and the patient's face, permitting positive-pressure ventilation. Proper mask technique is challenging to learn but is vital in many situations, including its use as an initial resuscitative measure, when the need for ventilation is very brief, or when it is impossible to intubate the trachea.

AIRWAY MANAGEMENT WITHOUT INTUBATION

While successful management of the airway in the unintubated patient is a skill learned primarily via experience, keeping in mind a few simple suggestions will help achieve success.

Mask Fit

Traditional black rubber anesthesia masks work well in many patients but do not provide a good seal in edentulous patients, patients with very large or small noses, or patients with beards. Masks with highly compliant, large, inflatable borders conform better to a wider variety of faces. Even so, in the edentulous patient a good fit may be difficult. Pulling the cheeks up on either side of the mask (Fig. 72-1) may provide a seal, but this requires a second person to squeeze the resuscitation bag. Other tricks include leaving dentures in place (but removing them prior to attempting intubation) or placing gauze pads between the alveolar ridge and the cheek.

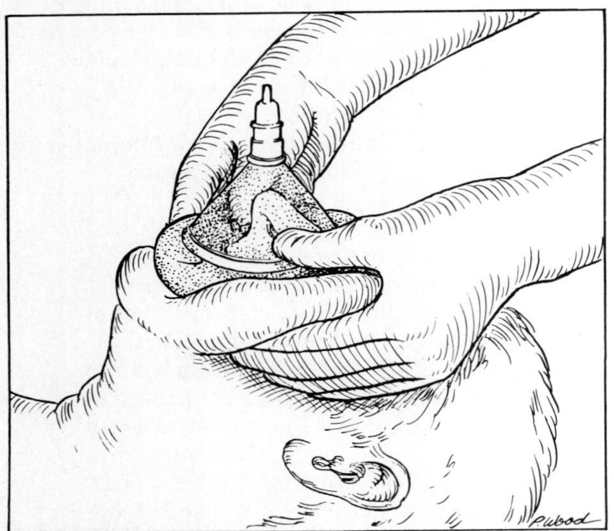

Figure 72-1. Pulling the cheeks to meet the rim of the mask helps to create a seal during positive pressure ventilation.

Head Position

Extension of the neck places traction on the hyoid and pulls the epiglottis and tongue away from the posterior pharynx. In some patients more traction may be required. This is best achieved by placing three fingers behind the posterior mandibular rami and providing firm force anteriorly while using the thumb and index finger to keep the mask tightly sealed to the face (Fig. 72-2).

Nasopharyngeal and Oropharyngeal Airways

In some patients airway obstruction persists even with anterior mandibular traction. This is especially common in obese patients but is by no means limited to them. In such cases maintaining a patent airway is greatly facilitated by insertion of a pharyngeal airway, which serves to separate the epiglottis and tongue from the posterior pharynx (Ch. 4).

ENDOTRACHEAL AND TRACHEOSTOMY TUBES

Tracheal Tubes

David Sheridan, one of the originators of the disposable tube quipped that the ideal tube was "all lumen and no wall." The heart of an endotracheal tube is the lumen. The materials surrounding that lumen provide additional features that are of benefit in specific circumstances but also are responsible for the complications associated with these devices.

Uncuffed Tubes

Uncuffed tubes for oral or nasal placement are now used primarily for pediatric patients. In children the subglottic region is the narrowest part of the airway. Since any damage to this area may eventually lead to laryngeal stenosis, every effort must be made to minimize pressure on the mucosa. Hence, inflatable cuffs are avoided, and uncuffed tubes are placed. The proper size tube will just fit through the subglottic opening and will provide a seal at pressures up to 30 cmH_2O. If the seal holds at higher pressures, the tube is likely to cause mucosal ischemia and possibly damage.

Many articles and formulas have been published suggesting the proper size for a child's tracheal tube. Ultimately, the proper fit must still depend on testing the seal and using the tube that provides an adequate seal to permit ventilation

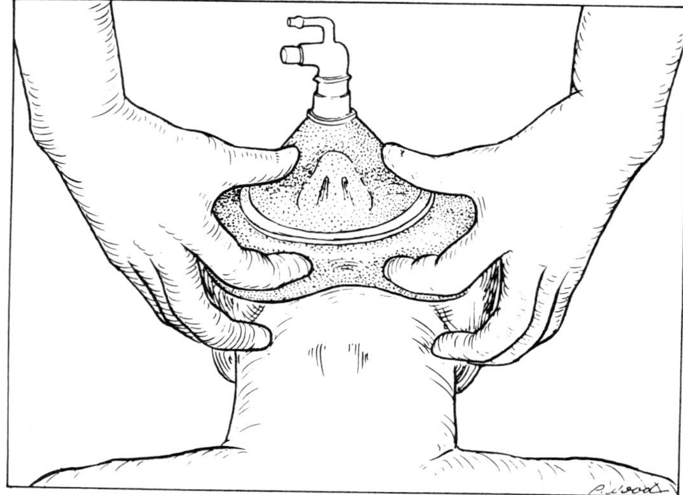

Figure 72-2. Traction underneath the mandible helps to pull the soft tissues of the anterior larynx and pharynx forward and thus to create an open airway.

but allows leakage at pressures above 30 cmH_2O. When intubating with an uncuffed tube, the clinician should have an assortment of sizes readily available. A good rule of thumb for the first tube to try is the formula ID = (age in years + 16)/4, where ID is internal diameter.

Cuffed Tubes

In 1928 Guedel and Waters provided a sensational demonstration of the value of adding a cuff to a tracheal tube. At the American Medical Association convention they intubated a dog named Airway and kept him anesthetized underwater for several hours without any obvious aspiration of water. The obvious utility of a cuff is twofold: it permits generation of positive pressure within the chest and it prevents massive aspiration.

Cuffed tubes have a second, small lumen, which serves to connect an inflation port with the cuff (Fig. 72-3). A small catheter fits into this lumen and has a valve at the inflation end. Each of these connections provides a site for potential failure, although system leaks most frequently occur at the valve owing to cracking or foreign material, with consequent malfunction.

Cuff sizes, shapes, and materials vary substantially among manufacturers, and a complete description of each is beyond the scope of this text.[1] However, it is useful to distinguish between high-volume, low-pressure and low-volume, high-pressure cuffs. Prior to the availability of modern plastic materials, cuffs were made of latex rubber, requiring pressures in excess of 100 cmH_2O to provide a seal. This high pressure led to ischemic necrosis of the tracheal wall.[2,3] Most tubes now used have a larger-volume, highly compliant cuff, which provides a much broader area of contact but seals at a substantially lower pressure. Low-volume, high-pressure cuffs are still used for short-term intubations in the operating room or in emergency situations because the cuffs are less obtru-

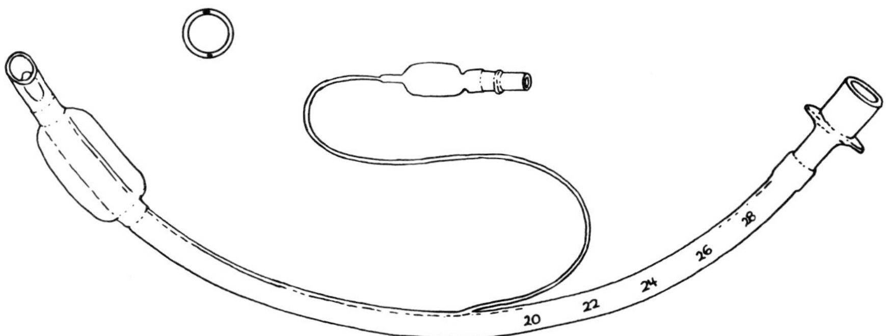

Figure 72-3. The various parts of a standard endotracheal tube are depicted. Notice the inflation lumen in the wall of the tube seen in cross section.

sive during intubation. Tubes with high-pressure cuffs should be removed from patients requiring long-term intubation.

In evaluating cuffed tubes, the clinician must consider several trade-offs. A thicker material, while more durable, forms folds, which may make intubation more difficult. A large cuff may wrinkle, allowing secretions to pass via the wrinkles into the trachea.[4]

Structural Considerations

Manufacturers construct tubes from a variety of materials. Latex rubber tubes, once the standard, have been largely replaced by synthetic materials, including polyvinylchloride (PVC) and silicone. Latex tubes are still used in some operating rooms, but their stiffness and the difficulty of passing suction catheters through them make them a poor choice for other than brief operations. In addition, they are generally manufactured with low-volume, high-pressure cuffs. PVC is inexpensive, stiff at room temperature and soft at body temperature, and nontoxic to tissue, which properties have made it the most widely used tube material for long-term intubation.

Although the cuff and the wall are the most obvious features of commonly used tubes, several other design features are noteworthy. The tip is beveled to facilitate visualization of the cords and to ease insertion. Edges are smooth to prevent trauma. The majority of tubes have a small fenestration near the tip called a *Murphy eye*, originally proposed as a safety device in case the tube tip became obstructed. Whether these tubes are in fact safer has not been studied. Most tubes also have a radiopaque line for radiographic visualization. Unfortunately, this line produces artifacts during computed tomography (CT). Tubes without such lines are available and can be used if the artifact interferes with a scan.

Specialized Tubes

In addition to the standard cuffed and uncuffed tubes, a wide variety of specialized tracheal tubes are manufactured.[5] Wire-reinforced tubes are made of soft material with a spiral wire to provide structural support. Their major advantage is their ability to withstand sharp bends without kinking. They are commonly used in situations in which the patient's head is in marked flexion or to intubate a tracheostomy stoma if a tracheostomy tube is not convenient. A major disadvantage of these tubes is difficulty in placement because of their lack of rigidity; a stylet is required. This lack of rigidity also results in easy displacement. Numerous complications have been reported with these tubes because of obstructions at the wire-rubber junction or because of bubbles in the tube wall related to the manufacturing process.[6–9]

Endobronchial Tubes

Endobronchial, or *double-lumen*, tubes are designed to isolate the lungs from each other. Most commonly, such isolation is desirable in the operating room to permit collapse of the operative lung while ventilation is maintained to the nonoperative side. In cases of unilateral infection, this also prevents drainage of purulent material into the dependent lung. Endobronchial tubes have also been used in several other situations, but their role in these is less well established. When hemoptysis is present, such a tube should prevent aspiration of blood into the contralateral lung. However, this remains more an ideal than a useful therapeutic intervention, since timely placement of such a tube is difficult in the face of massive hemoptysis. Double-lumen tubes have also been used for application of different levels of positive end-expiratory pressure (PEEP) to each lung and for differential lung ventilation.

Figure 72-4 depicts the basic design of available PVC disposable endobronchial tubes. The bronchial lumen has a

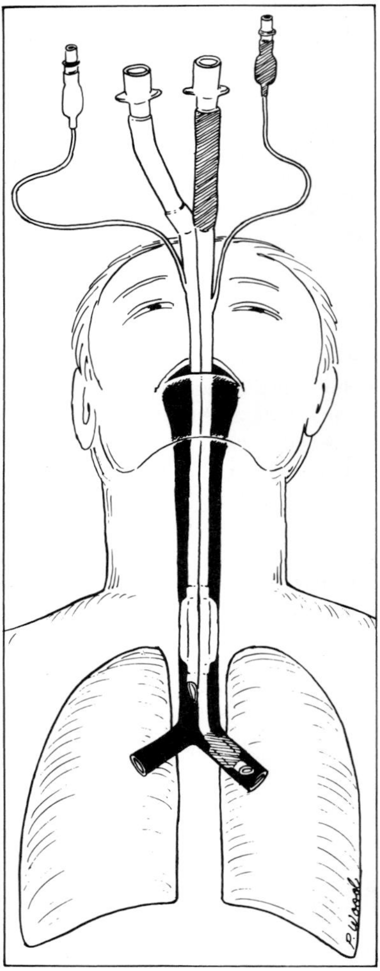

Figure 72-4. Schematic drawing of a double-lumen endotracheal tube. Positioning is critical, since if the tube is too far in, the bronchial lumen will occlude the upper lobe bronchus, and if the tube is not in far enough, both lungs will be ventilated.

small cuff, generally requiring no more than 3 mL of air. Overinflation can result in bronchial rupture.[10] A second, tracheal lumen has its outlet between the bronchial cuff and a tracheal cuff. Thus, gas flow to the unintubated bronchus actually comes via the tracheal lumen.

Prior to caring for a patient with an endobronchial tube in place, the clinician should review procedures for ensuring that the tube is properly situated,[11] using clinical signs of separate lung ventilation or fiberoptic bronchoscopy. Because of the need for precise localization, any significant patient movement may dislodge the tube and require re-establishment of proper positioning. Aside from the hazards of incorrect placement, endobronchial tubes also carry a high risk of obstruction because of their relatively narrow lumina.

Tracheostomy Tubes

Because they are shorter than endotracheal tubes, tracheostomy tubes create slightly less dead space. This is of little clinical significance. Their shorter length may result in slightly lower resistance than in an endotracheal tube of comparable diameter, but the right-angle bend creates significant turbulence, making the decrease in resistance less than might be expected.

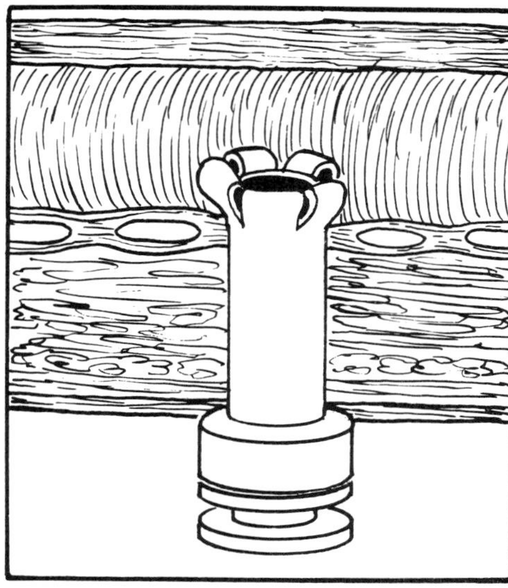

Figure 72-6. A tracheostomy button with the flange in the tracheal lumen.

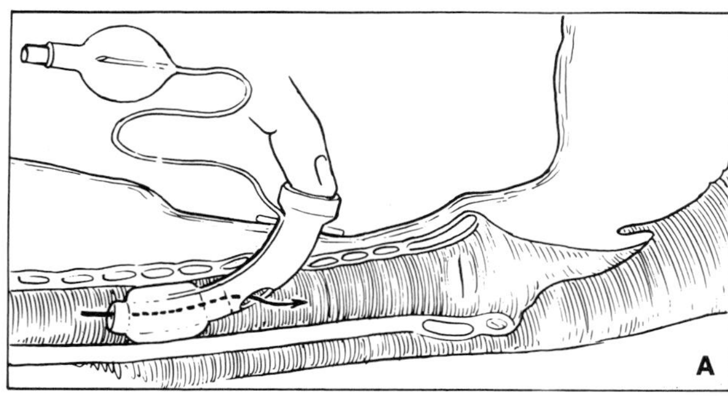

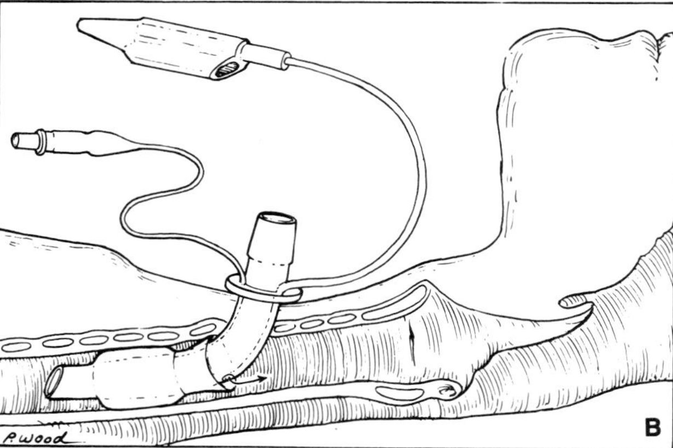

Figure 72-5. **(A)** Fenestrated tracheostomy tube. Occlusion of the lumen permits the patient to speak, but only when the patient does not require mechanical ventilatory support. **(B)** Speaking tracheostomy tube. The O_2 supply is connected to the extra lumen, and when the finger is placed over the hole, O_2 flows into the patient's trachea above the cuff and allows speech.

Uncuffed tracheostomy tubes may be used when positive-pressure ventilation is not required and there is no danger of aspiration of secretions from the pharynx. Fenestrated tracheotomy tubes may be useful when weaning patients from mechanical ventilation (Fig. 72-5A). These tubes permit gas flow either through the external orifice of the tube or via the upper airway. If the external orifice is plugged, flow to the lower respiratory tree is entirely through the patient's upper airway. This may be especially useful in promoting speech in the patient who can tolerate brief periods without mechanical ventilation, since plugging of the external orifice forces gas flow through the larynx.

An alternative for enabling tracheostomy patients to speak is a "speaking tube," which has a secondary lumen to provide gas flow above the main lumen[12] (Fig. 72-5B). The relatively low flows through such a lumen make normal speech impossible but may help in producing intelligible whispers.

Tracheostomy Buttons

Decannulation of a patient who has been mechanically ventilated for a prolonged period often produces anxiety as to whether the patient will require reintubation. A tracheostomy button (Fig. 72-6) is a small plastic device that plugs the tracheostomy but maintains stomal patency in case reinsertion of a tube is necessary.

RESPIRATORY PHYSIOLOGY IN THE INTUBATED PATIENT

Resistance

The normal upper airway provides about half of the resistance of the respiratory tree. Work to overcome that resistance constitutes approximately 10 percent of the normal work of breathing. Thus, a doubling or tripling of resistance results in a relatively small increase in the total work of breathing. The diameter of endotracheal tubes is constrained by the need to fit them through the larynx. For tracheostomy tubes, the constraint is the size of the incision, which is limited to prevent later tracheal scarring. The narrow lumen then produces an increase in resistance.

The resistance to gas flow follows Poiseuille's law, which states that resistance is directly proportional to length and inversely proportional to the fourth power of the radius. Thus, a tube that is 6 mm in diameter will have a resistance 3.2 times as high as an 8-mm diameter tube of comparable length, since $4^4/3^4 = 3.2$. The actual ratio may be even higher at high flow rates since turbulent flow alters the Poiseuille relationship.

Figure 72-7 provides a demonstration of the extra pressure a patient must develop to overcome tube resistance. Notice that the lines are curvilinear, rising sharply at high flows. At normal peak flows of 30 L/min most patients can breathe comfortably with tubes of an inner diameter as small as 6.5 mm. However, in patients with respiratory disease higher flow rates are often generated, and even large endotracheal tubes provide a significant impediment to ventilation.

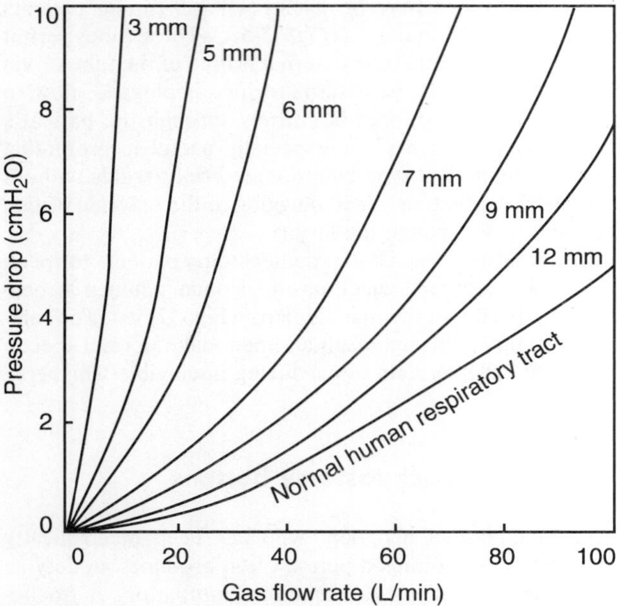

Figure 72-7. Pressure drop across endotracheal tubes of various size versus gas flow rate in liters per minute. (Adapted from Nunn,[48] with permission.)

Lower Airway Tone

In patients with reactive airways, insertion of an endotracheal tube often initiates or worsens wheezing. Even in apparently normal subjects, insertion of a tube may lead to increased resistance in the lower respiratory tree.[13] Because of this reflex, the clinician must recognize that intubation of a patient with reactive airways may result in deterioration in air flow.

Dead Space

Extrathoracic anatomic dead space in cadavers measures approximately 75 mL.[14] An endotracheal tube replaces this and obviously contains a smaller volume. Since the tube is a cylinder of known length and radius, its volume is easily calculated by the formula $V = \pi r^2 h$, where V is volume, r is radius, and h is height. An 8-mm (0.8-cm) diameter tube that is 25 cm in length will have a volume of $3.14 \times 0.4^2 \times 25$ or 12.6 cm^3. Tracheostomy tubes are generally a bit shorter and thus have slightly smaller volumes, although the difference as a proportion of tidal volume (V_T) is negligible. The decrease in anatomic dead space may be especially significant in patients with small V_T, since if V_T remains unchanged, alveolar ventilation should increase by 60 mL.

These calculations reflect the dead space of the tube only. Adding a Y piece adds several milliliters more and any connecting tubing between the tube and the Y piece adds still more volume. Again, by using the formula for the volume of a cylinder we can calculate that each centimeter of length of standard 22-mm (2.2-cm) tubing adds 3.8 mL of dead space.

Cough

An effective cough requires the ability to generate a high flow in the airways and the ability to collapse the airways so that the force of the flow is imparted to the sputum to be expectorated. Although intubated patients can generate adequate flow for a forceful cough,[15] the tube acts as a stint, holding the trachea open. Secretions often will accumulate below the tube, requiring suction to assist with their removal.

ENDOTRACHEAL INTUBATION

Intubation of the trachea is often a life-saving maneuver, but attempts to perform it by improperly trained individuals can result in great harm. The major danger arises from inability to support the airway once paralyzing drugs have been administered, inability to intubate the trachea, or lack of recognition that the esophagus has been inadvertently intubated. Because of these hazards, if the life of the patient is not in imminent danger, the procedure should be undertaken only by those schooled in alternative techniques for establishing and maintaining the patient's airway if the initial attempts at intubation fail.

Intubation

Intubation may be carried out under direct vision, by using fiberoptic endoscopy, or blindly. Whichever technique is used, a wide-bore rigid suction cannula with powerful vacuum and a face mask and bag for providing positive-pressure ventilation must both be available. These basic pieces of equipment may be life-saving in case of regurgitation or if the patient proves difficult to intubate.

Physiologic Response to Intubation

The rich innervation of the upper airway leads to a series of physiologic responses during intubation, including activation of both the sympathetic and parasympathetic nervous systems.[16] In children and occasionally in adults, vagal impulses lead to bradycardia. More commonly, intubation in adults produces tachycardia and hypertension. In the absence of a deep level of anesthesia, blood pressures may rise as high as 250/150 and the pulse may reach 180.

Patients with intracranial lesions carry a special risk because of the increase in intracranial pressure (ICP) that results from the rapid increase in blood flow.[17] If the patient already has high ICP from a tumor or hemorrhage, herniation of brain contents may occur. In patients in whom these physiologic responses are unacceptable, anesthetic drugs should be administered prior to intubation. Intravenous lidocaine also appears to be useful in attenuating hypertension, tachycardia, and increased ICP.[18,19]

Muscle Relaxant Drugs

Normal resting muscle tone in the muscles of the jaw is too great to permit intubation in all except the most feeble patients. A group of paralytic drugs termed *muscle relaxants* facilitate head positioning, mouth opening, and mandibular traction by abolishing the tone.

Muscle relaxants currently available are listed in Table 72-1. With the exception of succinylcholine, they act as competitive antagonists to acetylcholine and thus prevent muscle fiber depolarization and contraction. Succinylcholine acts by causing an initial depolarization and contraction followed by a prolonged refractory period (lasting several minutes) during which the muscles are unable to depolarize again. This property of succinylcholine is responsible for a major hazard associated with its use: in patients with recent burns or neurologic injury, massive potassium release may occur, with consequent cardiac arrest. Succinylcholine has the advantage of short duration of action. The nondepolarizing relaxants all require substantially longer time for their effect to wear off, and thus a mechanical ventilator must be available if they are used to intubate a patient.

Table 72-1. Doses of Muscle Relaxants Commonly Used for Intubation

Drug	Intubating Dose (mg/kg)
Succinylcholine	1.0
Succinylcholine after pretreatment with a nondepolarizer	1.5
Pancuronium	0.10–0.2
Metocurine	0.4–0.5
Atracurium	0.6–0.8
Vecuronium	0.07–0.15

Prevention of Aspiration during Intubation

Aspiration of gastric contents during intubation can lead to serious pulmonary compromise and is occasionally the ultimate cause of death. Unconscious patients cannot protect their airways. The likelihood of aspiration is increased if the stomach has been distended by mask ventilation or if the patient has recently eaten. If the patient is inadequately relaxed, insertion of the laryngoscope blade can result in vomiting. Aspiration results in either a chemical pneumonitis due to the acid in the stomach or an infectious process as particulate matter contaminates and obstructs the bronchial tree. In either case therapy is difficult, and hence prevention is critical.

In the emergency patient, the clinician should assume that the stomach is not empty. Keys to preventing aspiration are the avoidance of bag-and-mask ventilation, the application of pressure over the cricoid cartilage to occlude the esophagus, and the rapid completion of the intubation attempt. Complete preoxygenation of the patient by spontaneous ventilation with O_2 for 5 minutes will largely free the functional residual capacity (FRC) of nitrogen (N_2), permitting 5 to 7 minutes of complete apnea without desaturation. This eliminates the need for bag-and-mask ventilation after administration of relaxant. Following preoxygenation, a dose of succinylcholine is given and a period of 60 to 75 seconds allowed to ensure complete relaxation. During this time, an assistant should press firmly on the cricoid cartilage (Fig. 72-8), occluding the esophagus and preventing regurgitation of gastric contents. Intubation should be conducted by the most experienced individual available in the high-risk setting of a full stomach. The endotracheal tube should have a stylet in place to facilitate rapid placement. Finally, the assistant should release cricoid pressure only after placement of the tube in the trachea and inflation of the cuff have been confirmed.

Use of the Laryngoscope

A complete discussion of the many laryngoscope blades available is beyond the scope of this chapter. However, the blades fall into two basic categories, curved blades designed

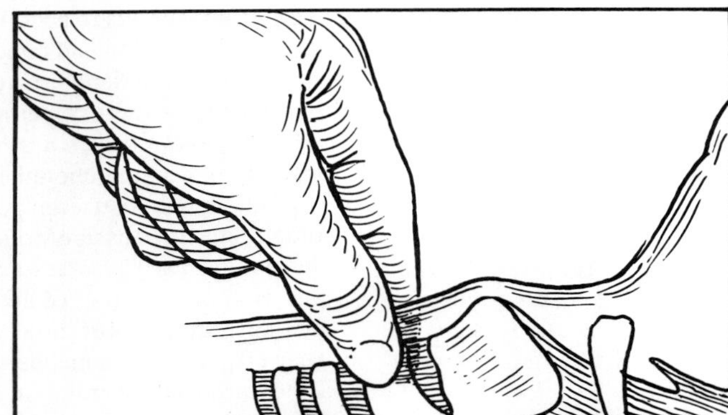

Figure 72-8. Proper technique for applying cricoid pressure during endotracheal intubation. Firm pressure needs to be applied to occlude the esophagus.

for placement in the vallecula (Fig. 72-9A) and straight blades designed to lift up the epiglottis (Fig. 72-9B). The curved blade is used to apply anterior traction on the tongue and the hyoid bone. This in turn pulls the epiglottis anteriorly since the traction is transmitted by the hyoepiglottic ligament. The curved blade provides ample room for the operator to insert an endotracheal tube between the vocal cords. The straight blades generally provide a clearer view of the glottis since they lift the epiglottis anterior to the cords. However, they generally provide much less room for insertion of the tube since they occupy space in the pharyngeal lumen. In some cases use of a straight blade means that a smaller tube must be inserted.

Nasal Intubation

Nasal intubation carries several advantages. The patient usually appears more comfortable with the mouth unencumbered, and nursing care is easier. In addition, "blind" nasal intubation can be accomplished without the need for muscle relaxants.

Nasal intubation can be performed under direct vision by passing the tube into the pharynx blindly and then guiding it into the larynx under direct laryngoscopy, but in most cases a Magill forceps (Fig. 72-10) is needed to maneuver the tube. In the spontaneously breathing patient, the tube can often be placed by using breath sounds as a guide. After

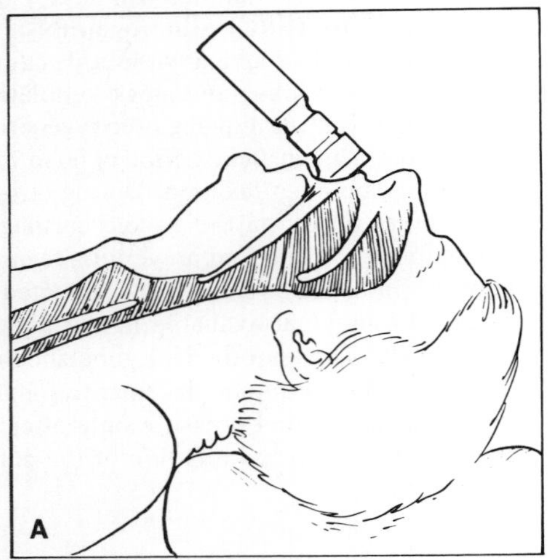

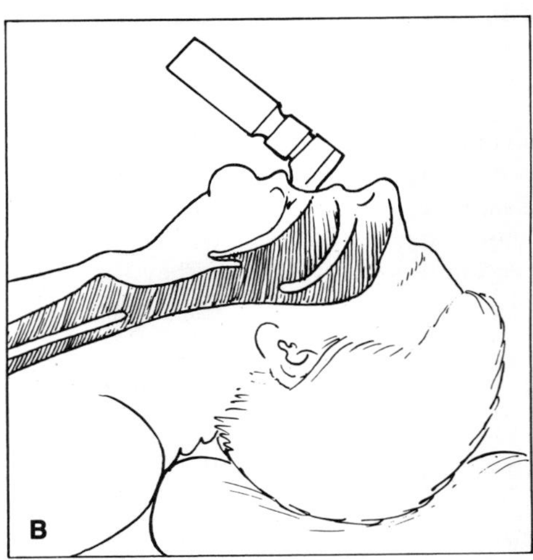

Figure 72-9. **(A)** A variety of straight blades are available. Straight blades are used to lift the epiglottis directly. While this often will provide a clear view of the cords, it leaves less room for the endotracheal tube to be inserted in the mouth and may actually prove more difficult to use. **(B)** The curved or Macintosh blade is used by placing the tip in the vallecula and pulling forward. The pull lifts the epiglottis out of the way because of the ligamentous attachments.

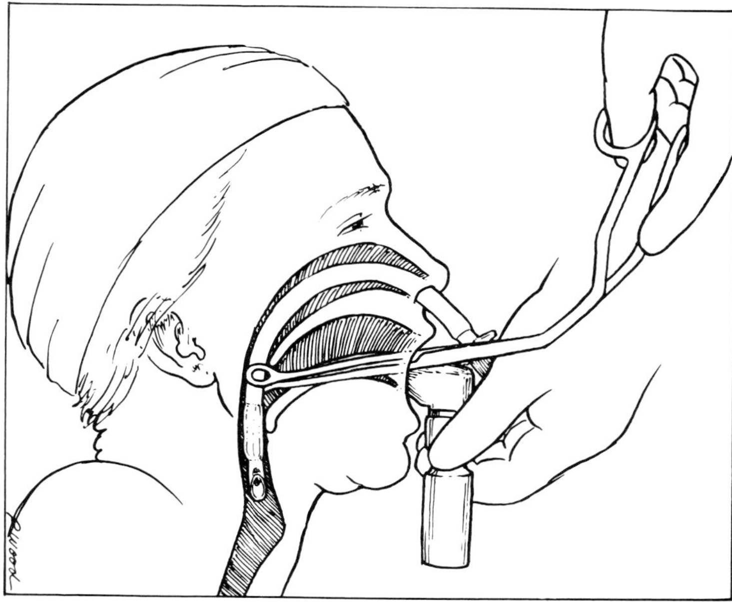

Figure 72-10. Use of Magill forceps to assist in the insertion of a tube through a larynx.

insertion into the pharynx, the tube is manipulated to maximize breath sounds and then advanced into the trachea. Vigorous coughing often but not always heralds entry into the trachea. Prior to attempting nasal passage, a topical vasoconstrictor should be applied to the mucosa to prevent nasal bleeding, which can be copious. Nasal intubation should not be performed if the patient has abnormal coagulation.

Fiberoptic Intubation

The fiberoptic bronchoscope can be used as a ''smart stylet'' for either nasal or oral intubation. Just as with direct laryngoscopy, proper use of the instrument requires training and practice under the guidance of an experienced operator. The fiberoptic bronchoscope is most useful in controlled situations in which a drying agent has been administered first and adequate topical anesthesia has been given. In emergency situations, secretions and/or blood make this method unsuitable.

AIRWAY CARE

Ascertaining Tube Placement

Perhaps the most disastrous complication of endotracheal intubation is the unrecognized placement of the tube in a main stem bronchus or in the esophagus. Severe hypoxia, with eventual brain damage or death, frequently results. Although such gross misplacement might seem simple to detect, even experienced clinicians can sometimes be fooled. Following a difficult intubation, clinical signs of correct placement are not always obvious.

Incorrect placement may also constitute a significant source of legal liability. Caplan et al.[20] reviewed a series of 1541 closed insurance claims from 20 insurance carriers involving anesthesia care and found that esophageal intubation or inadequate ventilation resulted in a median settlement of $200,000. In reviewing the cases they found that current standards of monitoring could have avoided a large proportion of these unfortunate events. The only cases they felt would not have benefited from proper monitoring were those in which the failure to intubate the trachea was recognized but all efforts to establish an airway failed.

Fatality from improper endotracheal tube placement can occur because of esophageal intubation, endobronchial intubation, or intubation of a false lumen. Although recognition of these events is crucial to the prevention of a disaster, many of the methods used to assess the position of the endotracheal tube after intubation are flawed. Tables 72-2 and 72-3, modified from a chapter by Birmingham and Cheney, illustrate the limitations of commonly used methods of evaluating tube placement.[21]

Recognition of Intratracheal Tube Placement

The traditional methods of recognizing proper tube placement, including observing chest rise, listening to bilateral breath sounds, and assessing V_T with respiratory effort, can all give misleading information following an esophageal intubation. Inflation of the stomach results in some movement

Table 72-2. Methods of Assessing Tracheal versus Esophageal Tube Position

Method	Documented Incidents of Failure	Comments
Direct visualization of vocal cords	None	Tube movement can occur before taping tube and with changes in head position
End-tidal CO_2	None	No CO_2 may be detected with severe bronchospasm or in the fully arrested patient with absent pulmonary blood flow; CO_2 may be exhaled from the stomach from prior mask ventilation
Breath sounds	Yes	Unreliable
Chest rise	Yes	Unreliable
Epigastric auscultation/observation	Yes	Unreliable
Reservoir bag compliance and refilling	Yes	Unreliable
Presence of tidal volumes with respiratory efforts	Yes	Unreliable
Quality of air leak around tube	Yes	Unreliable
Cuff palpation in trachea	Yes	Unreliable
Cuff volume necessary to occlude leak	None	Excessive cuff volume may indicate a tube above the cords or in the esophagus
Normal ventilator function	Yes	Unreliable
Chest radiography	Yes	Not fail-safe even when done
Tube condensation	None	Can be seen with esophageal tube
Fiberoptic bronchoscopy	None	Reliable but expensive, prone to breakage
Pulse oximetry	None	A late sign; may involve some alveolar gas exchange with esophageal ventilation and hence slow desaturation

(Modified from Birmingham and Cheney,[21] with permission.)

of the chest wall, creates some sounds of air movement, and results in some return of gas during the expiratory phase. Experimentally, Linko et al.[22] demonstrated that attempts to ventilate using a tube placed in the esophagus resulted in some gas exchange because of diaphragmatic movement.

Table 72-3. Methods for Prevention of Endobronchial Intubation

Method	Comments
Detection of equal breath sounds/chest rise	Unreliable
Tube position at incisors	Precut adult oral tubes to 25 cm; position tube 21 cm at incisors of normal-sized woman; position tube 23 cm at incisors of normal-sized man
Chest radiography	Tube tip at T2–T4 with head in neutral position (mandible overlying C5–C6)
Fiberoptic bronchoscopy	As reliable as radiography
Pulse oximetry	Desaturation does not necessarily occur
End-tidal CO_2	Has led to detection of endobronchial intubation

(Modified from Birmingham and Cheney,[21] with permission.)

This may be the explanation for cases in which a patient seems to survive for many minutes following an intubation that eventually proves to be esophageal. It may be especially difficult in the obese patient to ascertain from clinical signs whether the tube is in the esophagus or the trachea. Visualization of the vocal cords during intubation can guarantee accurate tube placement by an experienced intubator, but an inexperienced clinician may still confuse anatomy and place the tube incorrectly. There are numerous reported cases of esophageal intubation in which the clinicians stated the cords were seen. Also, visualization of the cords during intubation does not guarantee correct position after removal of an intubation stylet and tube taping.

While the experienced intubator uses multiple methods to confirm the proper positioning of the endotracheal tube, the "gold standard" now is to confirm the presence of expired CO_2. A quantitative end-tidal CO_2 monitor provides a characteristic wave form with endotracheal intubation and ventilation. If esophageal intubation follows mask ventilation, CO_2 may be detected initially because of exhaled gas that has entered the stomach[22–24]; however, the CO_2 levels will rapidly decrease to near zero as the gas becomes diluted, in contrast to the persistence of exhaled CO_2 following tracheal intubation. While in many areas capnometry has become the standard of care for ascertaining proper placement of endotracheal tubes in surgical patients, capnometers are not readily available in most emergency department or intensive care settings. An alternative to capnography is the use of colorimetric end-tidal CO_2 monitors, which indicate the presence of CO_2 by a color change from purple to yellow when the indicator (metacresol purple) is exposed to CO_2. In a study by Goldberg et al.,[25] colorimetric end-tidal CO_2 monitoring confirmed tracheal intubations and detected esophageal intubations 100 percent of the time as judged by capnography. Although capnography is highly reliable in most situations for the detection of proper placement, false negative results can occur during cardiac arrest, since no or very little CO_2 is delivered to the lungs in the absence of an adequate cardiac output.[26]

Preventing and Detecting Endobronchial Placement

Although unrecognized esophageal intubation usually results in rapid demise, the adverse effects of unrecognized intubation of a main stem bronchus may take longer to manifest themselves. Whether severe complications result will obviously depend on the severity of the underlying disease as well as the O_2 concentration being delivered.

A simple rule of thumb that results in correct positioning of the tube in nearly 100 percent of adults is to place the tube tip 23 cm from the teeth in men and 21 cm from the teeth in women.[27] This results in the cuff sitting well below the vocal cords with the tip above the carina and is valid except at the extremes of stature. Ideally, the tube should be situated with the tip at least 2 cm above the carina but with the cuff below the cricoid cartilage. Although most clinicians are aware of the need for the tip to be above the carina, the importance of the cuff being below the cricoid is not always appreciated. However, inflation of the cuff in the confines of the rigid cricoid cartilage can lead to mucosal or nerve damage and ultimately to subglottic stenosis or vocal cord paralysis. If the tube is within 2 cm of the carina, airflow distribution to the two lungs may not be equal. Furthermore, the tube can move several centimeters as the head is flexed and extended,[28] and a safety margin is needed to ensure that it does not move into the main stem bronchus during neck flexion.

Ultimately, tube position needs to be confirmed with a chest radiograph. If the carina is easily seen, tube position can be judged from that landmark. Occasionally the carina may not be visible, in which case vertebral bodies are valuable landmarks. The carina is generally within one vertebral body of T6 (T6 $\pm$ 0.6 vertebra),[29] and the tube tip should therefore be between T2 and T4.

Fixation of the Tube

Fixation of the tube serves to prevent either accidental extubation or migration of the tube further into the tracheobronchial tree with consequent endobronchial placement. The tube should be secured several centimeters above the carina, since during head movement the tube tip can move over a relatively broad range. The exact method of stabilization is usually determined by local preference in each hospital. The most common practice is to fix the tube with adhesive tape wrapped around it and along the lower part of the face. A key to maintaining stability is to place the tape high along the mandibular surface so that movement of the tube is relatively small when the jaw is moved.

Steps to ensure good fixation with minimal patient injury include (1) making sure that the surface is dry, which in some patients requires preliminary application of tincture of benzoin; and (2) if the patient is at risk for seizures or is likely to chew on the tube, placement of a bite block. If the patient is expected to be moving significantly, fixation should be placed around the back of the neck, with care used to place a backing along the hairline so that the tape does not stick to the hair.

When fixation is placed all the way around the head, care must be taken not to impede venous return. This is especially important in head-injured patients, since occlusion of venous return increases ICP and limits cerebral perfusion. Similarly, if significant facial swelling is present, the fixation must be inspected to ensure that flow is not occluded, since this increases the venous pressure and can worsen swelling. Pressure on areas of facial swelling can also result in eventual erosion of tissue. In patients in whom the endotracheal tube is in place for a prolonged period, the fixation may start to erode skin around the corner of the mouth. A protective covering, such as that used around intestinal stomas, provides added protection. Despite the clinician's best efforts, injury to the skin and loosening of the fixation are constant risks. Good practice includes reassessment of the fixation at least twice a day, with more frequent assessment if the patient has excessive secretions.

Once the taping is complete, tube position is verified as discussed above by a chest radiograph. If the tube is well positioned, the distance between the teeth and the end of the endotracheal tube should be measured. This can then be referred to during the routine checks of fixation to ensure that the tube has not migrated significantly from its initial position. An aid during these checks is to keep a tongue blade marked with the distance from the teeth to the end of the tube. Although useful, this technique is not absolutely fail-safe since in the occasional patient the movement of the tongue around the tube may cause curling of the tube in the back of the mouth, with migration of the tube up between the cords.

Since the mid-1980s a number of manufactured stabilization devices have become available. Harness devices work well but are expensive and can be cumbersome during routine care. Some of the less expensive devices, which do not pass around the back of the head, may not provide adequate stabilization.

Several categories of patients present special problems. In those with major facial injuries there may be little healthy tissue against which to fix the tube. With such patients, the tube can be wired to a tooth. A piece of surgical wire is inserted at the gum line between two incisors, and, one end is run behind the tooth and out on the other side of it. The wire is then twisted around the tooth, and the two ends are twisted around the tube. In patients with severe facial burns, the burn dressings often prevent the use of tape; in these cases a manufactured harness or umbilical tape around the back of the head provides the necessary fixation.

In children fixation is especially important because the short distance between the larynx and the carina means that even minimal movement can displace the tube from its proper position. To ensure that the tube remains in position, a good practice is always to have a second person assisting whenever the tube fixation is loosened in order to ensure that the tube has not moved following refixation.

Cuff Maintenance

The high incidence of tracheal stenosis that occurred in the era of high-pressure cuffs makes it imperative that the therapist conscientiously check cuff pressures. Even periods of a few hours at high cuff pressures can lead to mucosal necrosis and ultimately to tracheal stenosis. Animal research has indicated that the pressure should be maintained below 30 cmH_2O[30] in order to maintain adequate mucosal blood flow.

The pressure in the cuff should be checked a minimum of once a day. The more people who have the authority to put air into or remove air from the cuff, the more frequent the checks should be, since the pressure is more likely to have been altered. Intracuff pressure should also be checked if a leak develops around the cuff or if the apparent pressure or volume of the pilot balloon has changed. The major problem with frequent checks is that valves eventually may break, making replacement of the tube necessary. A wide variety of aneroid manometers is available for measuring pressure. If the cuff, a syringe, and the manometer are all connected via a stopcock, the pressure can be properly adjusted.

Another alternative for ensuring maintenance of appropriate pressure is the Pressure Easy device (Respironics, Inc.), which remains attached to the valve and provides continuous visual feedback of the pressure in the cuff, which should be in the range of 25 to 30 cmH_2O. It has the added capability of being continuously connected to the pilot valve and the breathing circuit which allows the cuff to receive additional inflation at peak inspiration. This technique can be useful in controlling difficult-to-abolish leaks around the cuff while still avoiding continuous high pressure.

In determining the appropriate minimum pressure for the cuff, the clinician should recognize that aspiration of secretions around the cuff is more likely to occur at lower pressures. Because of this, some clinicians have advocated trying to keep the pressure in the range of 25 to 30 cmH_2O at all times.[31]

Mouth Care

Maintenance of oral hygiene makes the patient feel better and is more aesthetically pleasing for visitors and staff. Tube fixation is removed, the patient's teeth are brushed, and the mouth is carefully suctioned. Because many patients in intensive care units are receiving broad-spectrum antibiotics, yeast overgrowth is common. In these cases the mouth may need to be swabbed with a topical fungicidal agent.

Suctioning

Even in the awake, alert patient, an artificial airway interferes with the cough mechanism. An integral part of an effective cough is the ability to collapse the airway so that high airflow rates and pressures impart significant momentum to the accumulated secretions.[15] The rigid nature of the tube prevents this and can limit the cough's effectiveness. In addition, many patients with tracheal tubes have weak coughs because of underlying illness, sedation, head injury, or pharmacologically induced paralysis. In order to facilitate secretion clearance, suctioning is an integral part of the care of the patient whose trachea is intubated.

In the intubated patient who is able to cough, secretions will move into the large airways and lower trachea rather effectively. In patients with weakened coughs, frequent turning and hyperinflation help to centralize the secretions. This is important, since the suctioning is really effective in removing secretions from the trachea and mainstem bronchi only.

The frequency of suctioning is dependent on the presence of secretions. Routine suctioning is warranted even in the absence of copious secretions to ensure that the tube remains fully patent. Adverse effects of suctioning are relatively minor but include physical damage to the airway, contamination of the airway, transient hypoxemia, and vagal stimulation.[32] In patients with head injuries, the increased ICP during suctioning may be a special hazard. This can be minimized by the administration of 1.5 mg/kg of lidocaine intravenously 1 to 3 minutes prior to suctioning.

Techniques available for suctioning include the traditional open system and the newer closed system. The open system uses a disposable single-use catheter, with the patient disconnected from the ventilator circuit. First the patient is ventilated with pure O_2 for a minimum of 1 minute, and a catheter is then gently inserted with use of sterile technique. Active suctioning is limited to 15 seconds to prevent significant hypoxemia. Irrigation with 3 to 10 mL of normal saline may be beneficial to help increase coughing and to loosen centrally located secretions. The catheter is actively twirled as it comes out to ensure that the surfaces are cleaned of secretions. While a larger-lumen suction catheter facilitates secretion removal, care must be taken not to create a system in which air cannot be drawn in between the catheter and the endotracheal tube, as this will result in complete collapse of the lungs.[33,34] The suction catheter should have a cross-sectional surface area equal to no more than half of the internal diameter of the endotracheal tube. As a rough approximation, this will be true if the suction catheter size in French units is twice the inner diameter of the tube in millimeters.[34]

Since about the early 1980s closed systems have been devised to allow suctioning without discontinuation of mechanical ventilation. These systems have the added benefit of avoiding opening the airway to contamination. Initial concerns about indwelling systems as a nidus for infection have not turned out to be warranted, as culturing of these catheters after 24 hours in place demonstrated no greater bacterial contamination than that seen on single-use disposable catheters.[35] Closed systems do appear to limit hypoxemia,[36] but preoxygenation with 100 percent O_2 still seems prudent. A final advantage of the closed system is limitation of contamination of the area around the patient by secretions.

Occasionally suctioning is performed for the specific purpose of obtaining a sputum specimen for culture. In this case use of bacteriostatic saline should be avoided so as not to limit bacterial growth of the culture. A suction trap can be placed in line to collect the specimen.

EMERGENCY SITUATIONS INVOLVING ARTIFICIAL AIRWAYS

Inability to Ventilate

A common yet frightening occurrence in critical care is the sudden inability to provide adequate ventilation to a patient. This is usually heralded by a machine alarm indicating either a delivered volume less than set volume or peak inspiratory pressures exceeding the set alarm value. The causes of such a sudden change can be divided according to the origin of the problem, namely, the machine, the artificial airway, or the patient. Causes intrinsic to the patient include tension pneumothorax, severe muscular rigidity, or severe bronchospasm. In all three of these cases there is still usually the ability to deliver some volume, and more often than not the cause is evident on a quick examination of the patient. Machine problems are relatively uncommon but may occur if a valve is inserted incorrectly into the circuit.

The most common cause of inability to ventilate is occlusion of the artificial airway. In patients with copious secretions and especially in children or patients with small tubes (Fig. 72-11), inspissation of secretions can lead to complete tube occlusion. A blood clot is a less common cause of obstruction but may occur if the patient has hemoptysis or a hemorrhagic tracheal erosion. Occasionally, the tube may develop an acute kink in the posterior pharynx. Often the patient can be ventilated very well initially, but as the tube heats to 37°C, it becomes more flexible and consequently kinks. Relatively uncommonly, overinflation of the cuff can result in tube occlusion.[37] Herniation of the cuff over the end of the tube has been reported in the literature, although neither of us has ever witnessed it over many years of respiratory care practice.

Every therapist needs to have firmly in mind the procedure for sudden inability to ventilate. Because the emergency is life-threatening, the steps must be moved through with rapidity. If the cause is not immediately obvious as being of patient origin, the circuit should be disconnected from the endotracheal tube and hand ventilation should be attempted. This will immediately rule out the machine as the source of the problem. If ventilation is still not possible, an attempt should be made to pass a suction catheter through the tube. In the event of a kink, occlusion by blood or secretions, or overinflation of the cuff, the catheter will not pass. If the catheter will not pass and a quick sweep of the finger into the back of the pharynx does not demonstrate occlusion and the cuff is not apparently overinflated, the tube should be removed immediately. At the same time help should be called for since the patient will need to be reintubated. Mask ventilation should be commenced while preparations are made to proceed with reintubation.

Leaking Tube

The construction of the endotracheal tube requires at least five junctions of component parts and thus produces multiple locations for failure in the cuff inflation system. Because of

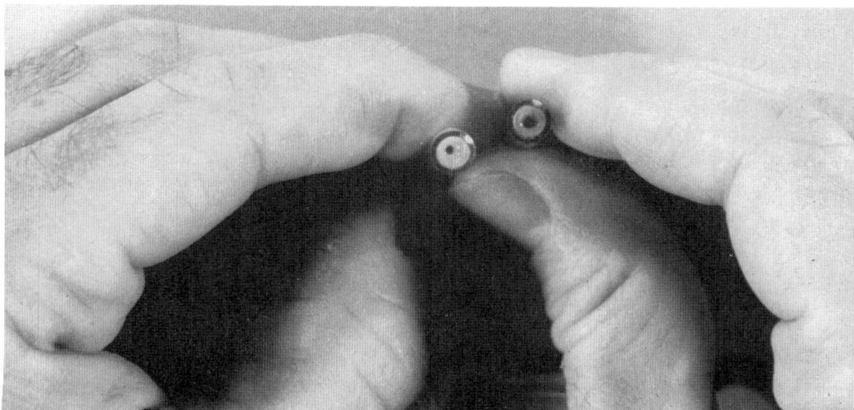

Figure 72-11. Endotracheal tube removed from a 6-month-old patient who developed sudden complete respiratory obstruction. The patient went from no difficulty with ventilation to complete obstruction in a matter of minutes. Note that secretions have virtually occluded the lumen.

this it is important to check the system prior to use of the tube by tube inspection and cuff inflation with syringe removal to test the pilot balloon valve as well as the cuff.

Failure of endotracheal tubes is surprisingly uncommon. The usual scenario is a call to the clinician that the patient has a leak around the tube, with a hole in the cuff suspected. While cuff leaks do occur, the most common cause of lost V_T is actually incorrect positioning of the tube. If the tube is positioned so that the cuff is between the cords, the seal will be inadequate. Further inflation of the balloon may seal the leak, but the leak gradually returns as the tube moves further out of the airway. Unfortunately, this often only serves to firmly convince the care team that the tube is defective and leaking. In view of the potential risks entailed in changing tubes in critically ill patients, the following protocol is useful to confirm the source of the problem:

1. The pharynx is suctioned, the cuff deflated, and the tube pushed further into the trachea. The cuff is reinflated and the amount of air required is noted. In most cases this solves the problem, since malposition is the cause of most ventilatory leaks. If this does solve the problem, care should be taken to ensure that the tube has not been passed to the other extreme and now rests in a main stem bronchus.
2. If step 1 does not resolve the problem, the cuff should be deflated, reinflated, and deflated again after 10 minutes. As much air should be retrieved as was put in. Failure to retrieve it suggests there really is a cuff leak (a relatively rare occurrence) and the tube needs to be changed. A further refinement to this technique is to inflate the cuff and then place a clamp—preferably one with padded ends to avoid damage—on the pilot tubing. This helps differentiate between the valve and the cuff as the site of a leak.
3. If step 2 does not reveal a cuff leak, then the likely culprit is the valve. This is the most common site of tube failure. Placing a blunt needle in the pilot tube and connecting it to a stopcock will provide a temporary solution to the problem.

Tube Replacement

In the critically ill patient replacement of the malfunctioning tube can be a life-endangering procedure. When the patient is receiving significant levels of PEEP, removing the tube results in an immediate drop in FRC, with hypoxemia often occurring within 10 or 15 seconds. The worse the underlying lung condition, the greater the risk. Reintubations are especially hazardous in patients who have been receiving mechanical ventilation with PEEP, since they often develop significant peripheral swelling, with swollen oral mucosa and lips.

When a tube is about to be replaced, all the same preparations need to be made as for any difficult intubation. A variety of laryngoscope blades and tubes need to be at hand, as well as suction and a bag and mask. The availability of an emergency airway kit (Table 72-4) also provides an additional measure of security.

Table 72-4. Contents of Emergency Airway Kit

High flow "jet" O_2 injector
Large-diameter needles for use with jet injector
Tube exchangers
Scalpel
Hemostats
Small endotracheal tubes (5–6 mm ID)

The patient should receive 100 percent O_2 for several minutes to provide an added margin of safety. If the patient is awake, the simplest method, which avoids the need for anesthesia, may be the use of a tube changer. These are flexible stylets, made by a variety of manufacturers and may be either plastic or woven. The stylet can be placed down the tube, the tube is then pulled out over the stylet, and a new tube is inserted. The operator should note the distance required and not place the tube changer further into the tracheobronchial tree than is needed, as pneumothoraces have occurred when the tube changers are pushed in too far. While generally successful, tube exchange using these devices does not always work satisfactorily. The replacement tube will sometimes become ensnared on the tongue or the larynx. When this occurs, pulling the jaw forward either manually or with a laryngoscope may be helpful.

In the heavily sedated patient or the patient who has received muscle relaxants, direct laryngoscopy is often the most efficient way to change the tube. The safest method is to place the laryngoscope alongside the existing tube and to then place the replacement tube near the opening of the larynx while an assistant pulls the old tube out as the new tube is advanced.

In the patient with severe facial swelling in whom the larynx cannot be visualized, a fiberoptic bronchoscope may be useful. The bronchoscope can be placed down the trachea alongside the existing cuff without loss of positive pressure in the chest. A new tube can then be slid along this and the old tube removed just at the last instant, leaving the patient without a protected airway for only a few seconds.

A special situation with extreme hazard is encountered in the patient with an unstable cervical spine who is in traction or an external fixation device. In such cases a tube exchanger may be useful. However, preparations should be made for surgical access to the airway via a cricothyroid puncture and/or a cricothyrotomy.

Accidental Extubation

Significant tube movement can occur during prolonged intubation from movements of the patient's head, from movement of the patient's tongue, or from traction when a tube is tethered to a ventilator. This can result in tube displacement, with consequent inadvertent extubation or main stem bronchial intubation. Premature extubation may also occur during routine tube care, while moving the patient, or as a result of self-extubation. In a recent prospective study, 12 self-extubations occurred in a group of 33 patients followed during prolonged tracheal intubation.[38] Although usually obvious, tube displacement may go undetected if the tube is in the pharynx, since some ventilation may still occur. Surprisingly, most patients who extubate themselves do not require reintubation.[39] Most likely, the patients who are able to do this are those in whom sedation has been minimized in anticipation of a weaning trial.

Accidental Decannulation of a Tracheostomy

In a patient with a mature tracheostomy, tube replacement is usually a simple, quick, and easy matter. However, this can occasionally be a life-threatening situation. In the first several days after tracheotomy the passages are not yet well formed, and attempts to replace the tube may result in its placement in mediastinal structures or subcutaneous fat. Rarely, in a mature stoma the tissue layers may separate and the tube be displaced into an extraluminal location. If it is not immediately obvious that there is a clear and direct opening into the trachea, it is usually best not to attempt to replace the tracheostomy tube. The most prudent approach is to place a translaryngeal tube via the oral route and to then reexplore the tracheostomy site. Alternatively, mask ventilation can be employed with manual occlusion of the stoma. This latter technique is definitely a second choice because it allows air to enter the peritracheal area and cause subcutaneous emphysema, which leads to eventual difficulty in identifying the structures.

Respiratory Complications from Nasogastric Tubes

Following the placement of a nasogastric tube, the patient may suddenly develop significant respiratory distress. The therapist should have in mind the differential diagnosis of respiratory complications of these tubes. If the nasogastric tube has accidentally been placed alongside the tracheal tube, it will no longer be possible to achieve a seal, and indeed if suction has been applied to the nasogastric tube, the lungs will rapidly deflate and hypoxemia will result. If the nasogastric tube has been placed far down into the lung, pneumothorax can occur.[40] Finally, if the tube is placed into the lung and the incorrect placement is not recognized, nasogastric feedings or antacids may inadvertently be allowed to enter the lung, resulting in aspiration pneumonitis.

COMPLICATIONS OF ARTIFICIAL AIRWAYS

Numerous case reports describe the complications that can beset an apparently simple procedure. Tubes have been swallowed and connectors have been aspirated. Enteral feedings have been administered into the cuff. The list goes on, and the reader is referred elsewhere for more details.[5,41] The ensuing sections describe some of the more common problems encountered.

Complications at the Time of Placement

The major complications occurring at the time of placement of an endotracheal tube result either from physical injury or from incorrect tube placement (Table 72-5). Tooth trauma is the most frequent intubation-related injury and is usually preventable with proper technique. The laryngoscope must never be used as a lever but should be pulled away from the body. Injury to the upper teeth results when they are used as a fulcrum. Should injury occur, immediate dental consultation must be instituted. The tooth can usually be saved by replacing it in the socket as soon as possible.

Port of Entry Complications

Artificial airways lead to complications at the site of entry into the body. Nasal tubes can cause nasal alar necrosis[42] and lead to accumulation of fluid in the sinuses because they obstruct sinus drainage.[43,44] Oral tubes can lead to stomatitis or tooth damage. Tracheostomy sites provide a locus for colonization by microorganisms. The artificial airway also provides a route of entry for contamination by the patient's own resident flora as well as by new flora introduced by nosocomial transmission. Colonization with microorganisms occurs rapidly in intubated patients.

Table 72-5. Acute/Early Complications of Tracheal Intubation

During intubation
- Traumatic-mechanical
  - Fracture-luxation of cervical spine with cord injury
  - Eye trauma
  - Epistaxis/hemorrhage
  - Trauma to teeth, lips, tongue, pharynx, larynx
  - Retropharyngeal dissection
  - Subcutaneous/mediastinal emphysema
  - Perforation of esophagus or pharynx, larynx, trachea
  - Aspiration (gastric contents, foreign bodies)
  - Esophageal intubation with gastric distension/hypoxemia
  - Arytenoid dislocation
  - Bronchial intubation
  - Pneumothorax

Reflex
- Vagal
  - Laryngeal spasm/apnea/bronchospasm/bradycardia/cardiac arrhythmias/hypotension
- Sympathetic
  - Arterial hypertension
- Spinal
  - Coughing, vomiting, bucking

Laryngeal Injury

Translaryngeal tubes left in place for more than 1 day result routinely in erosion of the laryngeal mucosa.[45] After several days, the pressure exerted by the tube results in formation of deep ulcers over the arytenoids, and ulceration will also often develop over the cricoid plate posteriorly.[46] However, in the vast majority of patients these ulcers will heal rapidly following extubation. In a small percentage of patients intubated for more than several days, permanent laryngeal damage occurs.

Tracheal Injury

Prior to the development of the high-volume low-pressure tracheal cuff, tracheal stenosis at the cuff site occurred in a high proportion of patients. This lesion is now relatively uncommon if cuff pressures are carefully monitored.

TRACHEOTOMY AS AN ALTERNATIVE TO PROLONGED INTUBATION

Tracheotomy offers many advantages over translaryngeal intubation when prolonged use of an artificial airway is anticipated. Nursing care is generally easier. Once the track from skin to trachea is formed, replacement of the tube is usually easy and requires little special skill or training. Patients appear more comfortable, and speech and eating are possible. Against these benefits should be weighed the risks and costs of the surgical procedure, including hemorrhage, infection, pneumothorax, and tracheo-innominate artery fistula.[47] In addition, some loss of airway diameter occurs routinely at the stomal level, although this is generally not functionally significant.

There are no absolute guidelines as to when tracheotomy should replace a translaryngeal tube. However, if intubation is clearly anticipated for more than 3 weeks, tracheotomy seems warranted. Conversely, for intubations under 10 days, a translaryngeal tube should suffice. For periods between these extremes, individual patient and hospital circumstances will dictate the choice.

References

1. Steen, JA: Impact of tube design and materials on complications of tracheal intubation. Probl Anesth 1988;2:211–224
2. Pearson FG, Goldberg M, DaSilva AJ: A prospective study of tracheal injury complicating tracheostomy with cuffed tube. Ann Otol Rhinol Laryngol 1968;77:867–872
3. Nordin U: The trachea and cuff-induced tracheal injury. Acta Otolaryngol, suppl (Stockh) 1977;345:1–85
4. Pavlin EG, Van Nimwegan D, Hornbein TF: Failure of a high compliance low pressure cuff to prevent aspiration. Anesthesiology 1975;42:216–219
5. Dorsch JA, Dorsch SE: Understanding Anesthesia Equipment: Construction, Care and Complications. Williams & Wilkins, Baltimore, 1984, pp. 353–400
6. Ohn K, Wu W: Another complication of armored endotracheal tubes. Anesth Analg 1980;59:215–216
7. Munson ES, Stevens DS, Redfern RE: Endotracheal tube obstruction by nitrous oxide. Anesthesiology 1980;52:275–276
8. Burns THS: Danger from flexometallic endotracheal tubes. Br Med J 1956;1:439–440
9. Kohli MS, Manku RS: Reinforced endotracheal tube-diversion of air from cuff balloon producing obstruction. Anesthesiology 1966;27:513–514
10. Burton NA, Fall SM, Graeber GM: Rupture of the left mainstem bronchus with a polyvinyl chloride double-lumen tube. Chest 1983;83:928–929
11. Brodsky JB: Complications of double-lumen tracheal tubes. Probl Anesth 1988;2:292–306
12. Heffner JE, Miller KS, Sahn SA: Tracheostomy in the intensive care unit. Part 1: Indications, techniques, management. Part 2: Complications. Chest 1986;90:269–274, 430–436
13. Gal TJ, Suratt PM: Resistance to breathing in healthy subjects following endotracheal intubation under topical anesthesia. Anesth Analg 1980;59:270–274
14. Nunn JF, Campbell EJM, Peckett BW: Anatomical subdivisions of the volume of respiratory dead space and effect of position of the jaw. J Appl Physiol 1959;14:174
15. Gal TJ: Effects of endotracheal intubation on normal cough performance. Anesthesiology 1980;52:324–329
16. Fox EJ, Sklar GS, Hill CH et al: Complications related to the pressor response to endotracheal intubation. Anesthesiology 1977;47:524–525
17. Shapiro HM, White SR, Harris AB et al: Acute intraoperative intracranial hypertension in neurosurgical patients: Mechanical and pharmacologic factors. Anesthesiology 1972;37:399–405
18. Abou-Madi MN, Keszler H, Yacoub JM: Cardiovascular reactions to laryngoscopy and tracheal intubation following small and large intravenous doses of lidocaine. Canu Anaesth 1977;24:12–19
19. Bedford RF, Persing JS, Probereskin L et al: Lidocaine or thiopental for rapid control of intracranial hypertension? Anesth Analg 1980;58:435–437
20. Caplan RA, Posner KL, Ward RJ et al: Adverse respiratory events in anesthesia: A closed claims analysis. Anesthesiology 1990;72:48–53
21. Birmingham PK, Cheney FW Jr: Incorrect tube placement: Prevention of a fatal complication. Probl Anesth 1988;2:278–291
22. Linko K, Paloheimo M, Tammisto T: Capnography for detection of accidental oesophageal intubation. Acta Anaesthesiol Scand 1983;27:199–202
23. Murry IP, Modell JH: Early detection of endotracheal tube accidents by monitoring cardon dioxide concentration in respiratory gas. Anesthesiology 1983;59:344–346
24. Ionescu T: Signs of endotracheal intubation. Anaesthesiology 1981;36:422
25. Goldberg JS, Rawle PR, Zehnder JL et al: Colorimetric end-tidal carbon dioxide monitoring for tracheal intubation. Anesth Analg 1990;70:191–194
26. Sanders AB, Kern KB, Otto CW et al: End-tidal carbon dioxide monitoring during cardiopulmonary resuscitation. JAMA 1989;262:1347–1351
27. Owen RL, Cheney FW: Endobronchial intubation: A preventable complication. Anesthesiology 1987;67:255–257
28. Conrardy PA, Goodman LR, Lainge F et al: Alteration of endotracheal tube position: Flexion and extension of the neck. Crit Care Med 1976;4:8–12
29. Goodman LR, Conrardy PA, Laing F et al: Radiographic evaluation of endotracheal tube position. AJR 1976;127:433–434
30. Nordin U, Lindholm CE, Wolgast M: Blood flow in the rabbit tracheal mucosa under normal conditions and under the influence of tracheal intubation. Acta Anaesthesiol Scand 1977;21:81–94
31. Bernhard WN, Cottrell JE, Sivakumaran C et al: Adjustment of intracuff pressure to prevent aspiration. Anesthesiology 1979;50:363–366
32. Brown SE, Stansbury DW, Merrill EJ, Linden GS, Light RW:

Prevention of suctioning-related arterial oxygen desaturation. Chest 1983;83:621–627
33. Fell T, Cheney FW: Prevention of hypoxia during endotracheal suction. Ann Surg 1971;174:24–28
34. Tiffin NH, Keim MR, Frewen TC: The effects of variations in flow through an insufflating catheter and endotracheal-tube and suction catheter size on test-lung pressures. Respir Care 1990;35:889–897
35. Ritz R, Scott LR, Coyle MB, Pierson DJ: Contamination of a multiple use suction catheter in a closed-circuit system compared to contamination of a disposable, single-use catheter. Respir Care 1986;31:1086–1091
36. Craig KC, Benson MS, Pierson DJ: Prevention of arterial oxygen desaturation during closed-airway endotracheal suction: Effect of ventilator mode. Respir Care 1984;29:1013–1018
37. Bishop MJ: Endotracheal tube lumen compromise from cuff overinflation. Chest 1981;80:100–101
38. Santos P, Afrassiabi A, Weymuller E: Prospective studies evaluating the standard endotracheal tube and a prototype endotracheal tube. Ann Otol Rhinol Laryngol 1989;98:935–940
39. Coppolo DP, May JJ: Self-extubations: A 12-month experience. Chest 1990;98:165–169
40. Roubenoff R, Ravich WJ: Pneumothorax due to nasogastric feeding tubes. Arch Intern Med 1984;149:184–188
41. Bishop MJ (ed): Physiology and Consequences of Tracheal Intubation. Probl Anesth 1988;2:163–306
42. Zwillich CW, Pierson DJ, Creagh CE et al: Complications of assisted ventilation: A prospective study of 354 consecutive episodes. Am J Med 1974;57:161–170
43. Deutschman CS, Wilton P, Sinow J et al: Paranasal sinusitis associated with nasotracheal intubation: A frequently unrecognized and treatable source of sepsis. Crit Care Med 1986;14:111–114
44. O'Reilly MJ, Reddick EJ, Black W et al: Sepsis from sinusitis in nasotracheally intubated patients: A diagnostic dilemma. Am J Surg 1984;147:601–604
45. Bishop MJ, Weymuller EA, Fink BR: Laryngeal effects of prolonged intubation. Anesth Analg 1984;63:335–342
46. Bishop MJ, Hibbard AJ, Fink BR et al: Laryngeal injury in a dog model of prolonged endotracheal intubation. Anesthesiology 1985;62:770–773
47. Stauffer JL, Olson DE, Petty TL: Complications and consequences of endotracheal intubation and tracheostomy. Am J Med 1981;70:65–76
48. Nunn JF: Applied Respiratory Physiology. 3rd Ed. Butterworth, London, 1987

Chapter 73

Lung Expansion Therapy

Robert L. Wilkins

CHAPTER OUTLINE

The major goal of lung expansion therapy is to prevent or correct significant atelectasis in the hospitalized patient. An important role in respiratory care is to identify those patients with or at high risk for atelectasis and to initiate a care plan that is effective and as inexpensive as possible. This challenge consumes a significant portion of the hospital-based clinician's time and therefore represents an important issue.

One of the most controversial questions in modern medicine is this approach to preventing and treating atelectasis. While the consequences of atelectasis can be serious, this concern should not motivate clinicians to routinely use costly measures. In many cases simple, inexpensive techniques are adequate, especially when only prophylactic measures are needed to prevent atelectasis. The key is the ability to determine when a modest approach is sufficient and when more extreme forms of therapy are needed. Thus, the goal of this chapter is not only to describe techniques for application of the various lung expansion modalities but also to provide guidelines that suggest when each modality should be applied.

VOLUNTARY DEEP BREATHING

Encouraging the patient to take sustained deep inspiratory efforts is one of the simplest yet most effective means of expanding the lung. The benefits of deep breathing appear to be enhanced by sustaining each breath for several seconds. The sustained inspiratory effort promotes collateral ventilation, which may help the inhaled gas to reach areas of atelectasis.[1]

Indications

Voluntary deep breathing should be a part of the care plan for any conscious patient at risk for atelectasis. This plan would include but not be limited to postoperative patients following abdominal or thoracic surgery or any patient who is bedridden for numerous days. This therapy would be contraindicated in patients with neuromuscular diseases such as myasthenia gravis, since spontaneous deep breathing is often not feasible and may exacerbate the patient's condition.

Technique

The key to utilization of deep breathing exercises is to motivate the patient. The patient must realize the importance of putting forth a sincere effort despite the apparent lack of respiratory problems and the discomfort produced. When motivation is poor, the use of incentive spirometry devices (see below) may be helpful. The patient should be instructed to sit as upright as possible and to take a minimum of 8 to 10 deep breaths every hour during the waking hours.[1] Instruction on technique should be given prior to surgery for optimal postoperative performance by the surgical patient, who may be less attentive after surgery owing to pain or to the effects of analgesics. In most cases the patient's sleep at night should not be interrupted for the performance of deep breathing maneuvers since sleep is important. If the patient awakens during the night, deep breathing exercises should be encouraged. As mentioned before, each deep breath should be held for several seconds to gain the most benefit. The patient should be cautioned to not perform the deep breathing exercises too quickly since this may lead to symptomatic hyperventilation.

As part of the care plan, coughing and changes in position provide excellent augmentation to the deep breathing exercises in the patient at risk for atelectasis.[2] Coughing is especially helpful when the patient has excessive airway secretions that have a tendency to be retained. Regular turning is very beneficial in preventing atelectasis in the bedridden patient. Since gravitational forces tend to promote atelectasis in the dependent lung regions, turning the bedridden patient frequently is advantageous as it will rotate the affected regions and thereby minimize the tendency for atelectasis.

Complications

Experience has shown that deep breathing exercises are not likely to lead to serious complications. This is not surprising, since deep breathing is a normal physiologic procedure. Hyperventilation that leads to syncope is possible but is easily avoided if the patient is advised to breath at a slow rate. It is possible for deep breathing exercises to result in barotrauma; however, the incidence of pneumothorax is very low.

INCENTIVE SPIROMETRY

Incentive spirometry (IS) represents a simple modification of the deep breathing exercises described above. With IS a device is used to provide the patient with immediate feedback regarding the quality of the inspiratory effort (Fig. 73-1). For many patients this feedback serves as motivation to reach a goal, such as a certain inspiratory volume, which may help to ensure that the patient's effort is meaningful. The desired level of performance by the patient with the IS device is usually determined by observation of the patient's initial effort.

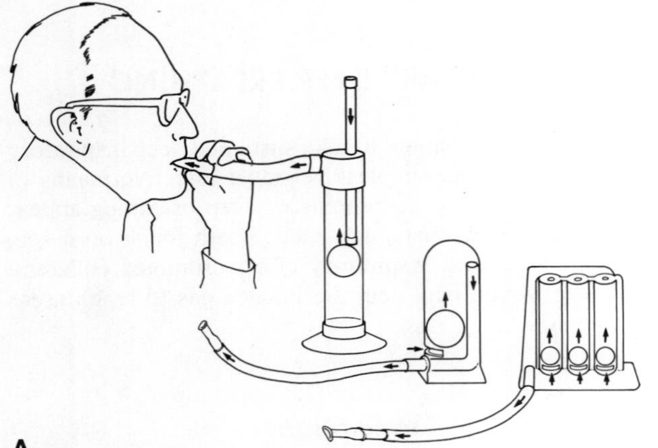

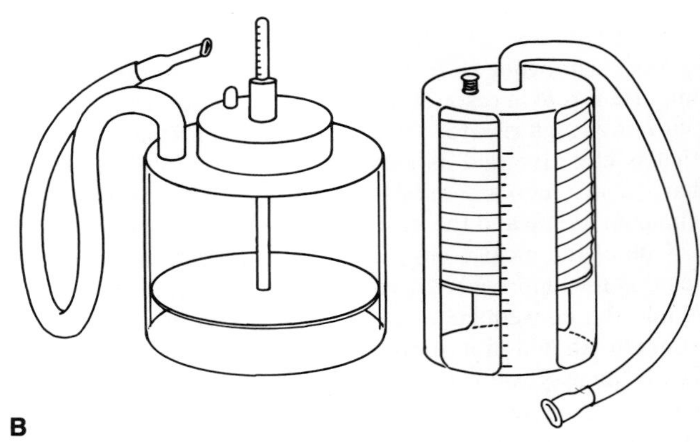

Figure 73-1. Incentive spirometry devices. **(A)** Flow-oriented incentive spirometers. Patients are instructed to inhale briskly to elevate the ball(s) and to keep them floating for as long as possible. The higher the ball is raised, the greater the flow (but not necessarily the volume) that the patient must generate. **(B)** Volume-oriented incentive spirometers. With these, unlike flow-oriented devices, the inhaled volume is known. Patients are instructed to inhale until the bellows or other volume indicator reaches a predetermined target level. (From Luce et al.,[25] with permission.)

Table 73-1. Evaluating Lung Infiltration Therapy

Modality	Goal	Criteria	Signs of Treatment Effectiveness
IS	Prevent atelectasis	Alert patient with adequate IC	Patient reaching goal; normal respiratory rate
IPPB	Correct atelectasis	Reduced IC; simpler measures not working	Improved breath sounds; reduced spontaneous respiratory rate; improved dyspnea; improved chest radiograph
	Reduce work of breathing	Severe dyspnea; reduced IC; no evidence of pneumothorax	Less dyspnea during and after treatment; reduced spontaneous respiratory rate; less breathing effort
CPAP	Correct atelectasis	Stable patient; other modalities not working	Improved breath sounds and chest radiograph; decreased work of breathing

IC, inspiratory capacity.

Indications

Many patients at risk for atelectasis can benefit from IS, especially cooperative postoperative patients with adequate vital capacity (VC), namely 10 to 15 mL/kg (Table 73-1). Since the additional cost of IS is minimal as compared with deep breathing exercises, it is reasonable to employ an IS device when motivation may be a problem or when the risk of atelectasis is especially high.

Technique

As with deep breathing exercises, the patient using IS should be encouraged to inhale slowly and sustain each inspiratory effort for several seconds. A brief rest of 30 seconds after each inspiratory effort can be helpful in obtaining maximal effort and avoiding hyperventilation. Instruction on the use of the IS device should be given to the surgical patient prior to surgery. For obvious reasons the IS device should be placed within reach of the patient at all times. In most cases the patient need not be observed using IS each hour; however, it is a good idea to scrutinize and coach the patient's technique once or twice each day. When the patient improves and is able to achieve the desired inspiratory goal with minimal effort, the expected level of achievement should be increased.

For patients with a poor inspiratory effort, the use of one-way valves that allow inhalation but not exhalation may be useful. This system has been shown to cause "breath stacking," which helps to achieve and sustain deep inspiration even in uncoached patients.[3]

Complications

The potential complications of IS are similar to those described above for deep breathing exercises. Respiratory alkalosis and syncope from hyperventilation represent the most common problems but are easily avoided with proper coaching in most cases.

INTERMITTENT POSITIVE-PRESSURE BREATHING

Intermittent positive-pressure breathing (IPPB) refers to the application of inspiratory positive pressure to the patient's airways, usually with an accompanying aerosol, for approximately 15 to 20 minutes as a treatment modality. This treatment is given to the spontaneously breathing patient through a mouthpiece or mask. It may be administered as frequently as every hour or less often (e.g., every 2 to 4 hours).

IPPB is a treatment modality that has suffered from lack of scientific study. It was originally introduced in 1947 by Motley and associates[4] and steadily gained in popularity over the next 25 years. Unfortunately this popularity resulted not from careful scientific investigations but rather from the strong desire to do something for patients suffering from respiratory problems. As a result, IPPB was overused and eventually sharply criticized. At a 1974 conference designed to study the scientific basis for respiratory therapy, the participants concluded that IPPB had little scientific basis.[5] While it continued to be popular for several years after the conference, the pendulum had begun to swing toward a decline in its use. Eventually, because of the widespread criticism that followed the 1974 conference, many clinicians totally avoided using IPPB. This attitude prevails today among many physicians and respiratory care clinicians.

In support of IPPB, numerous papers and editorials have been published pointing out that this therapy can be helpful in treating patients meeting specific criteria.[6–10] As a result of these publications and continued use in many centers, guidelines for the use of IPPB have been developed to promote its appropriate application. The reacceptance of IPPB by the medical community will depend on the use of these guidelines and the proper administration of IPPB treatment by trained personnel.

Indications

A possible use of IPPB is for the patient who has atelectasis despite the use of simple measures and is unable to maintain an adequate VC (10 to 15 mL/kg) (Table 73-1). For IPPB to be useful in this situation, the atelectasis cannot be the result of large airway obstruction. For many surgical patients VC may be adequate prior to surgery but will drop substantially in the postoperative period, as discussed in Chapter 41. This is most likely to occur in the patient undergoing upper abdominal or thoracic surgery.[11] The clinician must anticipate this drop in VC and consider IPPB as part of the treatment plan for these patients. IPPB treatments given to the postoperative patient not only expand the lung but also can improve the quality of the patient's cough and can thereby be instrumental in mobilizing secretions that, if retained, could lead to impaired gas exchange, atelectasis, and infection.

If given properly, IPPB can reduce the work of breathing.[9] This temporary respite may be appreciated by the patient with neuromuscular disease or chronic obstructive lung disease who cannot take deep breaths or cough effectively and is on the brink of respiratory failure. Although the long-term benefits of IPPB in such patients are difficult to document, the use of IPPB along with aggressive bronchial hygiene may avoid the need for intubation and mechanical ventilation.[12,13] IPPB treatments also can improve alveolar ventilation in this situation, which helps improve $PaCO_2$ and PaO_2.

Some investigators have claimed that IPPB with large tidal volumes can alter the lung mechanics of the patient with restrictive lung disease so that the work of breathing is decreased for hours after the treatment.[9] This potential benefit would be especially useful in treating the patient with neuromuscular disease or spinal cord injury or in weaning from mechanical ventilation. Whether any such effect occurs to a clinically important degree in most patients is unclear.

Contraindications

Although they are relatively few, there are some clinical situations in which IPPB should not be administered. The patient with an untreated pneumothorax should not receive IPPB treatments because of the risk of increasing the passage of air into the pleural space, with resultant tension pneumothorax. The patient who is hemodynamically unstable may deteriorate further when given an IPPB treatment, particularly in the presence of hypovolemia. The increase in intrathoracic pressure can worsen the condition of the hypotensive patient, especially when higher inflation pressures are used.

Technique

Before IPPB treatments are started, the specific goals of the therapy should be identified. The patient should be informed of the purpose, frequency, and expectations of the treatments. Just prior to the start of each IPPB treatment a baseline clinical assessment is essential to clarify the patient's clinical condition. This assessment should include vital signs, breath sounds, sensorium, symptoms, and simple spirometry results. During and after each treatment the patient should be re-evaluated and the results compared with the initial data.

For the patient with atelectasis, IPPB treatments must deliver large inspiratory volumes that exceed the patient's inspiratory capacity. Such treatments are referred to as volume-oriented IPPB treatments and require monitoring of the exhaled volume. A reasonable goal is that the tidal volume with IPPB should be at least 20 percent greater than the patient's measured inspiratory capacity. Since the patient with atelectasis typically has an abnormally low lung compliance, it will be necessary to use increased inspiratory pressures (higher than 20 cmH_2O) to achieve the optimal tidal volume in most cases.

Treatments should be given frequently during the waking hours (e.g., every 1 to 2 hours) for the best results when attempting to correct atelectasis. The clinician administering the treatment must make sure that the patient uses a very slow respiratory rate (4 to 8 breaths per minute) to diminish the possibility of hyperventilation. The patient should be seated in as upright a position as possible to encourage maximal lung inflation.

For the patient on the verge of respiratory failure who may benefit from a decrease in work of breathing, IPPB treatments need not be as volume-oriented as for the patient with atelectasis. In such cases the inspired volumes should be large enough, however, to provide appropriate expansion of the patient's lungs and increased CO_2 removal with each breath. Generally, a tidal volume of two to three times normal is appropriate.

When a pharmacologic aerosol such as a beta-adrenergic agonist is administered with the IPPB treatment, the patient should be encouraged to pause at the end of inhalation for 3 to 5 seconds before exhaling. This pause will allow better deposition of the aerosol in the airways. For the patient with moderate to severe dyspnea it is not reasonable to expect a pause with every breath or to expect the pauses to be lengthy.

After administration of an IPPB treatment, the clinician should chart all related information, including tidal volume, pressure, and duration of the treatment. Changes in vital signs, breath sounds, spirometry results (e.g., peak flow) and symptoms help document the response to treatment (Table 73-1). If the IPPB treatments are not accomplishing the desired goals, it is the responsibility of the clinician to communicate this information to the attending physician and suggest an alternative plan.

Complications

IPPB treatments can result in significant complications as outlined below. In most cases, however, the likelihood of serious complications is very low if the clinician administering the treatment is well trained. Clinicians must be aware of these potential complications and be able to recognize them when they occur. Close observation of the patient throughout the treatment is essential.

Decreased Cardiac Output

The application of positive pressure to the respiratory system can cause a decrease in cardiac output. While the exact mechanisms have been debated, most authors agree that elevation of intrathoracic pressure reduces venous return, which leads to decreased filling of the ventricles and diminished stroke volume.[14,15] This phenomenon is more common in hypovolemic patients.[16,17]

Small decreases in cardiac output can be difficult to identify but may be important in the patient with marginal cardiac function. A significant drop in perfusion may be recognized by deterioration of the patient's sensorium, peripheral cyanosis, tachycardia, cool extremities, and weak peripheral pulses. When these alterations are identified, the IPPB treatment should be discontinued and the patient monitored closely. Maintaining an appropriate inspiration/expiration ratio (i.e., 1:3 or 1:4) can be useful in minimizing the negative effect of positive pressure on cardiac output.

Hyperventilation

One of the most common problems associated with IPPB treatments is hyperventilation. The sudden drop in $PaCO_2$ will cause an immediate increase in blood pH. This acute respiratory alkalosis can have serious consequences, especially in the patient already experiencing metabolic alkalosis. Hyperventilation occurs when the patient is not properly coached and breathes too rapidly. Since the IPPB treatments typically increase the tidal volume to two to three times the normal value, the patient must breathe significantly more slowly during the treatments to avoid hyperventilation.

The patient experiencing hyperventilation may complain of being light-headed and of tingling or numbness in the extremities. If the patient begins complaining of these symptoms during the treatment, the procedure should be temporarily suspended for a few minutes to allow the patient to recover. The patient should be reminded to slow down by exhaling slowly and to pause at the end of exhalation for several seconds.

Barotrauma

The application of positive pressure to the airways can lead to rupture of lung tissue and result in air leaking into the pleural lining or other areas. As air leaks into the pleural lining, the pleural space fills with air (pneumothorax) and compresses the lung. Each subsequent positive pressure breath can cause more air to leak into the pleural space and produce progressive collapse of the lung. For this reason it is very important for the clinician to be able to use techniques that minimize the risk of barotrauma and to be able to recognize this problem if it occurs.

In patients with obstructive lung disease, air trapping may occur when the expiratory time is not sufficient to allow the entire inhaled volume to be exhaled. Air trapping leads to greater pressure in the distal lung and increases the chances of barotrauma in patients receiving positive pressure breaths. For this reason the patient must be instructed to exhale slowly and completely.

The patient who experiences pneumothorax may complain of chest pain and dyspnea. Examination typically reveals rapid pulse and breathing rates, as well as diminished breath sounds and increased resonance over the affected region.

Gastric Insufflation

As positive pressure is applied to the upper airways, the pressure may cause the esophagus to open and allow gas to enter the stomach. This problem is most likely to occur when high pressures (above 25 cmH_2O) are applied to the neurologically impaired patient, especially when a mask is used. A buildup of pressure in the stomach can lead to vomiting and aspiration as well as impair the function of the diaphragm. Swelling of the abdomen and belching are clues that gastric insufflation is occurring.

INTERMITTENT CONTINUOUS POSITIVE AIRWAY PRESSURE

Continuous positive airway pressure (CPAP) is a popular modality for the treatment of refractory hypoxemia due to acute restrictive lung diseases such as the adult respiratory distress syndrome. In this situation CPAP is applied on a continuous basis for days or weeks, depending on the course of recovery. *Intermittent* CPAP, however, is the periodic use of CPAP every 1 to 3 hours for the prevention and treatment of atelectasis. While this use of CPAP has not been popular, the results of some studies have been encouraging.[18–22] Before this modality of lung expansion therapy can be widely accepted, more study is needed to determine specific criteria for its use and the optimal technique.

Indications

The specific criteria for use of intermittent CPAP have not been determined. Hess has suggested that it may be most useful for uncooperative patients and those with excessive pain who cannot effectively cough or breathe deeply.[23] It seems reasonable to use intermittent CPAP for patients with atelectasis that persists despite use of conventional modalities such as IS and IPPB.

Intermittent CPAP is potentially hazardous in hemodynamically unstable patients and in those with untreated pneumothorax. For this reason, the patients with hypotension, acute myocardial infarction, shock, or recent chest trauma should probably not receive this therapy.

Technique

The optimal method for administering intermittent CPAP has not been determined by scientific study. Most studies have investigated its administration by way of a tight-fitting mask, and others have found that its application by use of a mouthpiece was effective.[18] The length and frequency of each treatment represent other key issues when intermittent CPAP is considered. In most studies CPAP was used every 1 to 2 hours while the patient was awake and applied for approximately 30 breaths and for up to as long as 15 minutes.

In most investigations 7.5 to 15 cmH_2O was an effective range for the level of CPAP. The best approach in applying intermittent CPAP may be to use a more conservative pressure initially while closely monitoring the patient's response. If the patient tolerates the therapy well and the atelectasis has not been resolved, increasing the CPAP level in 3- to 5-cmH_2O increments would seem reasonable.

Before CPAP is applied, the clinician should take time to explain the therapy to the patient. Emphasis on the importance of the tight-fitting mask and the typical sensations to be expected should be helpful.

During the treatment the patient must be closely monitored. Clinical signs of peripheral perfusion, such as sensorium, blood pressure, pulse rate, and temperature and color of extremities, should be closely observed, since CPAP has been known to decrease cardiac output. Because CPAP alone does not assist ventilation, the patient's ventilatory status must be assessed throughout the treatment. This is best accomplished through observation of respiratory rate and chest wall movement.

If the intermittent CPAP is effective, the patient's spontaneous respiratory rate should be slower and the level of dyspnea may be decreased after the treatment. Other indicators of treatment effectiveness would include improved breath sounds and a more normal chest radiograph (Table 73-1).

Complications

Like IPPB, intermittent CPAP can cause a variety of complications associated with increasing intrathoracic pressure. Since with CPAP the pressure is applied throughout the respiratory cycle, there may exist a greater chance of complications than with IPPB. Conversely, the pressure level with CPAP is not as great as the peak pressure typically used with IPPB or continuous mechanical ventilation. The hazards of barotrauma associated with positive pressure ventilation are discussed in the IPPB section earlier in this chapter and in Chapter 84.

Application of intermittent CPAP could lead to gastric insufflation. If pressure builds in the stomach, it could cause the patient to vomit, and since the patient is typically using a tight-fitting mask, the risk of aspiration is real. The patient should be coached to signal the clinician when any degree of nausea occurs during use of intermittent CPAP.

MISCELLANEOUS TECHNIQUES

Blow Bottles

In the past "blow bottles" (Fig. 73-2) have been used in an attempt to maintain optimal lung expansion in the postsurgical patient. The patient was instructed to blow forcefully into one water-filled bottle in an effort to move the water to another bottle. Today this approach is not popular since it places the emphasis on a forceful exhalation, which is of no benefit and may actually be harmful because of the attendant increase in intrathoracic pressure. If any benefit is derived from blow bottles, it probably lies in the deep inspiratory effort required prior to exhalation. However, the other techniques discussed in this chapter are both theoretically and practically preferable.

Carbon Dioxide Rebreathing

Rebreathing of CO_2 by means of rebreathing tubes and bags was popular in the late 1960s.[24] This technique was designed to cause patients to increase their breathing as the $PaCO_2$ level increased. While minute volume does increase with this therapy, this increase is primarily due to a faster respiratory rate rather than to an increase in the tidal volume. Rapid breathing at moderate volumes is of minimal or no value in the prevention or correction of atelectasis, and as a result rebreathing techniques are not effective or popular. In addition, this practice could induce dangerous acute respiratory acidosis in patients unable to augment total ventilation in response to the hypercapnic stimulus.

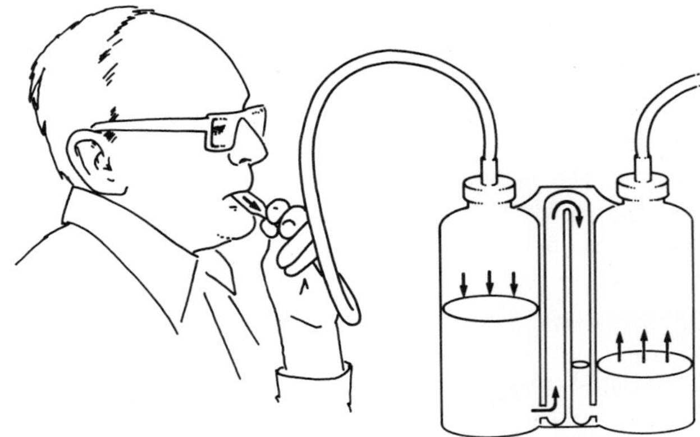

Figure 73-2. Blow bottles. The two containers are connected by a tube, and one is initially filled with water. With a series of slow, forced exhalations (each presumably preceded by a deep inspiration), the patient forces the water from the first chamber into the second. The other blow tube is then used to force water back into the first chamber, and the procedure is repeated. (From Luce et al.,[25] with permission.)

References

1. O'Donohue WJ: Perioperative measures for lung expansion. pp. 10–20. In O'Donohue WJ (ed): Current Advances in Respiratory Care. American College of Chest Physicians, Park Ridge, IL, 1984
2. Johnson NT, Pierson DJ: The spectrum of pulmonary atelectasis: Pathophysiology, diagnosis, and therapy. Respir Care 1986;31:1107–1120
3. Baker WL, Lamb VJ, Marini JJ: Breath-stacking increases the depth and duration of chest expansion by incentive spirometry. Am Rev Respir Dis 1990;141:343–346
4. Motley HL, Cournand A, Werko L et al: Intermittent positive pressure breathing: A means of administering artificial respiration in man. JAMA 1948;137:370–383
5. Pierce AK, Saltzman HA (chairmen): Conference on the scientific basis for respiratory therapy. Am Rev Respir Dis 1974;110:1
6. O'Donohue WJ: IPPB past and present, editorial. Respir Care 1982;27:588–590
7. Hughes RL: Improving postoperative tidal volumes. Respir Care 1981;26:985–986
8. American Association for Respiratory Care: The pros and cons of IPPB: AARC provides an assessment of its effectiveness. AARC Times 1986;10:48–50
9. Sinha R, Bergofsky EH: Prolonged alteration of lung mechanics in kyphoscoliosis by positive pressure hyperventilation. Am Rev Respir Dis 1972;106:47–51
10. O'Donohue WJ: Maximum volume IPPB for the management of pulmonary atelectasis. Chest 1979;76:683–687
11. Ali J, Weisel RD, Layug AB et al: Consequences of postoperative alteration in respiratory mechanics. Am J Surg 1974;128:376–382
12. Ziment I: Intermittent positive pressure breathing. pp. 529–555. In Burton GG, Hodgkin JE (eds): Respiratory Care: A Guide to Clinical Practice. 2nd ed. JB Lippincott, Philadelphia, 1984
13. Realy AM: Hyperinflation therapy. pp. 633–654. In Scanlon CL, Spearman CB, Sheldon RL (eds): Egan's Fundamentals of Respiratory Care. 5th Ed. CV Mosby, St. Louis, 1990
14. Cournand A, Motley HL, Werko L, Richards DW: Physiological studies of the effects of intermittent positive pressure breathing on cardiac output in man. Am J Physiol 1948;152:162–173
15. Luce JM: The cardiovascular effects of mechanical ventilation and positive end-expiratory pressure. JAMA 1984;252:807–811
16. Uzawa T, Ashbaugh DG: Continuous positive-pressure breathing in acute hemorrhagic pulmonary edema. J Appl Physiol 1969;26:427–432
17. Ashbaugh DG, Petty TL: Positive end-expiratory pressure. J Thorac Cardiovasc Surg 1973;65:165–170
18. Lindner KH, Lotz P, Ahnefeld FW: Continuous positive airway pressure effect on functional residual capacity, vital capacity and its subdivisions. Chest 1987;92:66–70
19. Anderson JB, Olesen KP, Eikard B et al: Periodic continuous positive airway pressure, CPAP, by mask in the treatment of atelectasis: A sequential analysis. Eur J Respir Dis 1980;61:20–25
20. Stock MC, Downs JB, Gauer PK et al. Prevention of postoperative pulmonary complications with CPAP, incentive spirometry, and conservative therapy. Chest 1985;87:151–157
21. Williamson DC, Modell JH: Intermittent continuous positive airway pressure by mask: Its use in the treatment of atelectasis. Arch Surg 1982;117:970–972
22. Ricksten SE, Bengtsson A, Soderberg C et al: Effects of periodic positive airway pressure by mask on postoperative pulmonary function. Chest 1986;89:774–781
23. Hess D: The use of PEEP in clinical settings other than acute lung injury. Respir Care 1988;33:581–597
24. Schwartz SI, Dale WA, Rahn H: Dead-space rebreathing tube for prevention of atelectasis. JAMA 1957;163:1248–1251
25. Luce JM, Tyler ML, Pierson DJ: Intensive respiratory care. WB Saunders, Philadelphia, 1984

Chapter 74

Assessment and Management of Acute Atelectasis

Robert L. Wilkins
David J. Pierson

CHAPTER OUTLINE

The term *atelectasis* refers to a collapsed or airless condition of the lung. Atelectasis is important in respiratory care because it is common and has the potential to severely impair lung function; in many cases, it can also be reversed by appropriate application of therapy.

Atelectasis can present as an acute or chronic problem in patients needing respiratory care. Chronic collapse of all or part of a lung is usually due to an obstructing neoplasm or other mechanical problem best approached by surgical or other specific intervention. This chapter limits discussion to that of acute atelectasis such as occurs in the postoperative setting. Specifically, this chapter addresses pathophysiology, assessment, and treatment of acute atelectasis. The techniques used in the prevention of atelectasis are described in Chapter 89, and the specific means of applying the lung expansion therapies mentioned in this chapter are discussed in Chapter 73.

PATHOPHYSIOLOGY OF ATELECTASIS

Atelectasis results when one or more of the following exists: (1) inadequate lung distending forces, (2) obstruction of the airways, or (3) insufficient surfactant. Although each mechanism is capable of causing atelectasis, in many cases a combination is present. Each mechanism is briefly described below.

Inadequate Lung Distending Forces

Typically, the primary distending force of the lung is provided by the negative pleural pressure, which is minimal during passive exhalation but increased (more negative) with contraction of the inspiratory muscles. Disorders that interfere with the generation and maintenance of the negative pleural pressure will encourage atelectasis.[1] A buildup of fluid, as in pleural effusion, or air, as in pneumothorax, and weakness of the inspiratory muscles are common problems that lead to atelectasis (Table 74-1).

Obstruction of the Airways

Although not all agree, some experts believe that the primary cause of postoperative atelectasis is occlusion of bron-

Table 74-1. Causes of Decreased Lung Distending Forces

Causes
Insufficient negative pleural pressure
Pleural space encroachment
By gas (e.g., pneumothorax)
By liquid (e.g., pleural effusion)
By solid (e.g., malignant mesothelioma)
Chest wall disorders (e.g., kyphoscoliosis, flail chest, cervical myelopathy or radiculopathy affecting intercostal nerves, myasthenia gravis)
Diaphragmatic disorders
Diaphragmatic apraxia (e.g., phrenic neuropathy, such as may occur following coronary bypass surgery, myopathy, or polyradiculopathy, such as that in Guillain-Barré syndrome)
Diaphragmatic loading (e.g., obesity, recumbency, ascites, increased intraperitoneal pressure from any cause)
Central nervous system dysfunction (e.g., coma, obtundation, or pain with resultant disinclination to breathe at normal tidal volumes or to sigh)

(Adapted from Johnson and Pierson,[1] with permission.)

chi by retained secretions.[2] Retention of secretions is common in the postoperative patient, especially when airway mucus transport is diminished by anesthetics and inadequate cough. Once the obstruction is present, absorption of the gases distal to the obstruction can lead to atelectasis. Absorption of the distal gas is enhanced when the patient is breathing an increased inspired O_2 fraction (F_{IO_2}) or readily absorbed anesthetic gases.[2–4] This phenomenon may be more crucial in children and infants since they do not have as much collateral ventilation as adults.

Insufficient Surfactant

The maintenance of lung expansion is assisted by the presence of surfactant, which lines the alveoli and bronchi and serves to reduce surface tension. This substance must be present in sufficient quantity and quality to be of optimal value in preventing atelectasis. Disorders such as respiratory distress syndrome, smoke inhalation, lung contusion, and pulmonary embolism have been shown to dramatically diminish surfactant function.[1,5,6] In addition, inhaled anesthetics, high inspired O_2 concentrations, and a lack of periodic deep breathing have been associated with inadequate surfactant.

ASSESSMENT OF THE PATIENT WITH ACUTE ATELECTASIS

Medical History

The first clue that may suggest that a patient should be closely examined for atelectasis is found in the medical history. If the patient was admitted for upper abdominal or thoracic surgery, the risk for atelectasis postoperatively is greater than with surgery at other anatomic sites.[7,8] A significant past medical history is also worth identifying. If the patient has a history of chronic bronchitis, asthma, cystic fibrosis, kyphoscoliosis, obesity, or other condition causing impaired pulmonary function, there is an increased risk for atelectasis in the postoperative period.[9,10] It is important to note that most of these factors also put patients at greater risk for atelectasis when they become bedridden because of illness or injury even if surgery has not been performed.

Once atelectasis develops, the patient may complain of dyspnea and chest pain. If the atelectasis involves a significant portion of the lung, dyspnea is more likely than if the involvement is minimal, since collapse of larger portions of the lung tends to increase the work of breathing. Severe dyspnea may be present when the patient develops acute atelectasis superimposed on a chronic lung disease or when the atelectasis is massive. In such cases effective therapy may require prompt intervention. Chest pain is likely if pneumothorax is present or if pleural inflammation exists.[1]

Physical Examination

How large a portion of the lung is involved in the atelectasis will determine the likelihood of significant physical findings. With minimal lung involvement the examination may be essentially normal; however, with more careful examination abnormalities are typically present when atelectasis exists.

Although often overlooked the physical examination findings are often capable of detecting the initial evidence of atelectasis in many cases. Typically, the patient will begin to breathe more rapidly as the lung starts to collapse.[11] Tachypnea is believed to occur in response to the decrease in compliance and subsequent drop in tidal volume that occurs with atelectasis. In addition to the tachypnea, tachycardia is also typically present if the atelectasis results in significant hypoxemia.

Although fever is commonly associated with atelectasis, scientific evidence for a causal relationship is scant.[1] Studies in dogs have not demonstrated fever following atelectasis induced by occlusion of the right middle lobe bronchus.[12] Fever that occurs with atelectasis is most likely related to infection of the retained secretions distal to an obstructed airway.[1,2] In this situation resolution of the obstruction and mobilization of retained secretions are vital to the patient's recovery.

Auscultation findings are varied but can be helpful in detecting the onset of atelectasis and the surrounding pathologic changes in the lung. While auscultating over the atelectatic section of the lung, late inspiratory crackles may be heard as the patient inhales deeply.[13,14] With subsequent deep breaths the crackles tend to decrease in number, and they may disappear entirely following several deep breaths. They usually occur in the dependent regions first, where the gravitational forces exert their greatest effect and promote atelectasis.

The breath sounds may be diminished, absent, or increased with atelectasis. If the major airway leading into the affected region is occluded, the breath sounds will be diminished or absent over the affected area. If the major airway is patent, a harsh or bronchial type of breath sounds will be heard over the affected region (see Ch. 44). The patient should be encouraged to breathe deeply during auscultation, since this will allow better assessment of the pathologic changes in the lung that occur with atelectasis.

With massive collapse of one lung, more obvious abnormalities will be present. In addition to tachycardia and tachypnea, signs of unilateral lung volume loss will be present. As one lung loses most of its volume, the trachea and cardiac impulse will shift toward the collapsed lung as detected by palpation. The diaphragm will tend to elevate on the affected side and can be identified by percussion.

Radiographic Findings

Acute atelectasis is most often initially detected because of abnormalities seen on the chest radiograph. This is probably related to routine use of chest radiographs and lack of clinical examination skills by many clinicians rather than to the sensitivity of the radiographic examination. There are situations, however, in which the atelectasis is not clinically apparent but is easily detected on the chest film. As a result, the chest radiograph has been and will continue to be a useful tool in the assessment of acute atelectasis.

When evaluating the chest film, the findings of opacification and volume loss suggest that atelectasis is present (see Ch. 57). The cause and extent of the atelectasis will dictate the abnormalities seen on the radiograph. If the atelectasis is caused by bronchial obstruction, as with airway tumor or mucus plugging, opacification of the corresponding lung distal to the obstruction will be present on the radiograph. If the airway obstruction involves a main stem or lobar bronchus, significant opacification and volume loss are seen (Fig. 74-1). With microatelectasis, as occurs postoperatively in the patient who does not breathe deeply, the chest film shows low lung volumes but may not demonstrate specific abnormalities unless the degree of lung involvement is substantial. In such cases the dependent regions typically show decreased radiolucency and volume loss.

The signs of volume loss associated with atelectasis include elevation of the hemidiaphragm, narrowing of the space between the ribs, and displacement of the hilum, airway(s), mediastinum, and fissures on the affected side (Fig. 74-1). Compensatory hyperinflation of the adjacent lung may be present.

When lobar atelectasis is present, the affected region on the radiograph should be closely inspected for the presence of an air bronchogram. The air bronchogram is seen by visualization of the lobar bronchus and its main branches as lucencies, in contrast to the water density of the surrounding lung tissue (Fig. 74-2). When present, this finding suggests that the atelectasis is not due to mucus impaction in the airways but rather to regional impairment of lung mechanics.[1] The presence or lack of an air bronchogram on the chest film of the patient with atelectasis therefore has therapeutic implications. This finding also predicts a slower rate of resolution of atelectasis, according to Marini and associates[15] (Fig. 74-3).

Arterial Blood Gas Findings

Ventilation/perfusion ($\dot{V}/\dot{Q}$) mismatching and an associated hypoxemia occur with atelectasis, as the ventilation of the affected area is severely compromised while perfusion is at least partially maintained. Complete collapse of an area of lung produces the ultimate $\dot{V}/\dot{Q}$ mismatch, right-to-left shunt, and the extent of the atelectasis will generally determine the degree of hypoxemia. With minimal atelectasis mild hypoxemia is commonly the only abnormality. If the hypoxemia is significant, it will stimulate the respiratory drive to increase ventilation and reduce $PaCO_2$. As a result, the common arterial blood gas findings associated with significant atelectasis are respiratory alkalosis with hypoxemia. If the patient has pre-existing pulmonary disease, the onset of acute atelectasis may severely compromise lung function. In this situation severe hypoxemia may result even when the atelectasis is minimal.

TREATMENT OF ACUTE ATELECTASIS

When it has been determined that the patient has atelectasis, generally on the basis of an abnormal chest radiograph, it is important to determine if it has caused physiologic compromise. If respiratory distress and significant hypoxemia are absent and the patient is expected to be ambulating soon, no treatment may be needed (Fig. 74-4). If the patient is not compromised but is not expected to be ambulating soon, lung expansion therapy should be given for 24 to 48 hours (see Ch. 73) to correct the atelectasis or at least to discourage its progression. When the patient is physiologically impaired by the atelectasis (e.g., has respiratory distress or significant hypoxemia), treatment must be initiated (Fig. 74-4).

With lobar atelectasis, treatment is aimed at removal of airway secretions and re-expansion of the affected region. Secretion removal is often best accomplished by encouraging the patient to generate an effective cough (Table 74-2). This usually requires effective pain relief in the surgical or trauma patient. In the unresponsive or uncooperative patient, stimulating a cough may be accomplished by administration of an irritating mist; although it is not recommended, some clinicians have also employed catherization of the trachea and periodic instillation of saline or sterile water to provoke cough in unresponsive patients. The administration of aerosol and chest physical therapy may be particularly useful when the retained secretions are thick and difficult to expectorate. Bronchodilators are useful when airway obstruction is present simultaneously with atelectasis, since they open airways and promote mucociliary escalator function.

In most cases the therapy just described is effective in promoting the removal of retained secretions. If this program proves inadequate, however, endotracheal suctioning or bronchoscopy may be needed. Bronchoscopy allows direct

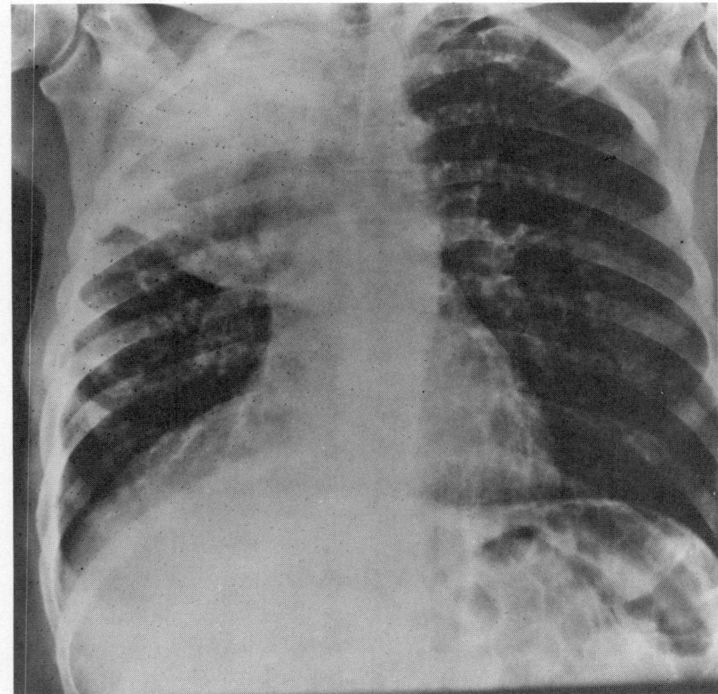

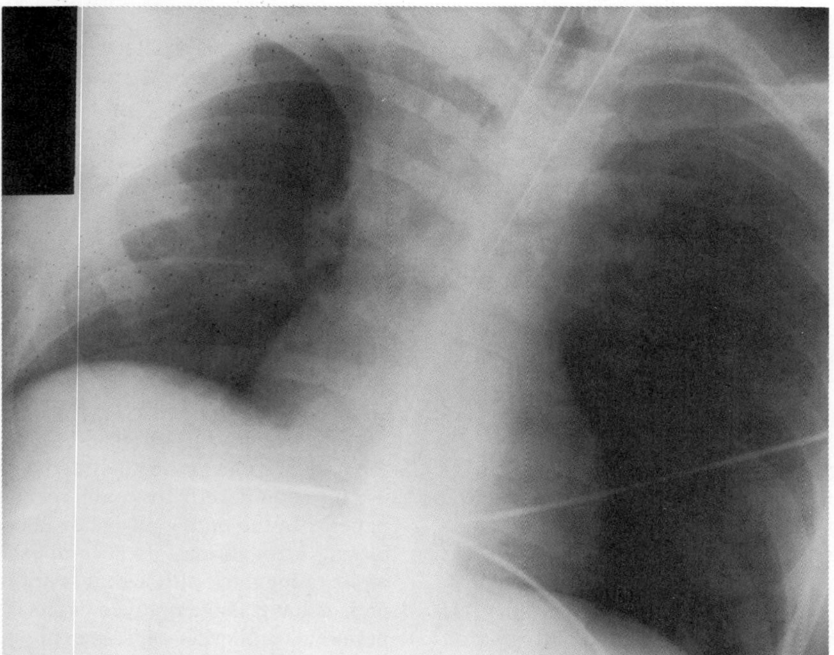

Figure 74-1. Right upper lobe atelectasis. **(A)** Chest radiograph demonstrating right upper lobe atelectasis because of a tumor obstructing the right upper lobe bronchus. Note the well-outlined horizontal fissure which is rotated upward and the elevation of the right hemidiaphragm. Although signs of atelectasis are present, right upper lobe volume loss is not marked, possibly because of partial filling of the lung by tumor tissue. (From Wilkins et al.,[22] with permission.) **(B)** Acute right upper lobe collapse in a critically ill, intubated patient, easily diagnosed despite the suboptimal patient positioning as commonly seen in the ICU. There is more volume loss than in Figure A.

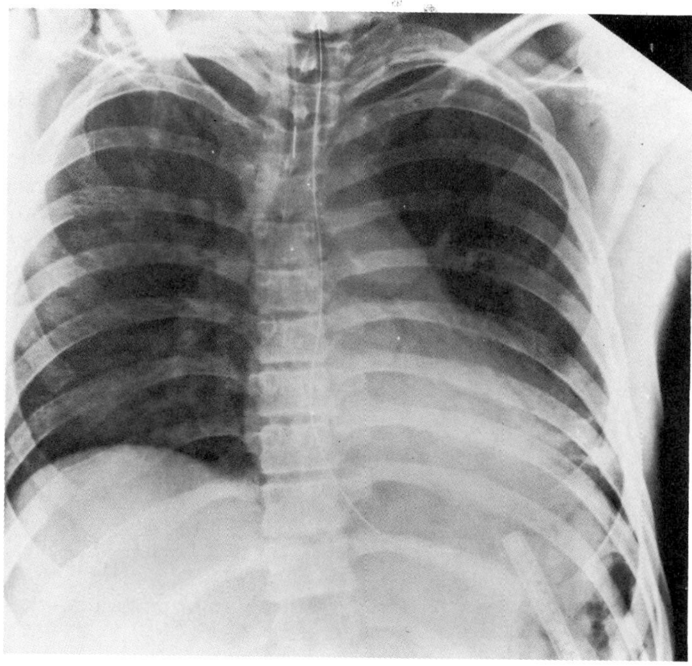

Figure 74-2. Acute atelectasis of the left lower lobe with prominent branching air bronchograms. (From Pierson,[23] with permission.)

Table 74-2. Methods Used to Prevent or Treat Atelectasis

- Reducing prolonged lobar dependence
  - Frequent position changes
  - Early ambulation
- Decreasing pleural pressure
  - Deep breathing exercises
  - Incentive spirometry
- Creating expiratory flow resistance or positive end-expiratory pressure (PEEP)
  - Blow bottles
  - CPAP by mask
  - PEEP
  - Positive expiratory pressure (PEP) mask
  - End-inspiratory breath hold/Valsalva maneuver
  - Positive end-inspiratory pressure
  - Voluntary coughing or tracheal catherization to induce cough
- Preventing or removing airway obstruction
  - Obstruction by mucus
    - Chest wall percussion or vibration; coughing; postural drainage; mucolytic drugs; blind catheter suction; bronchoscopic aspiration
  - Other obstruction
    - Percussion for foreign body removal; surgical extirpation; laser vaporization (e.g., carcinoma or benign airway lesions); bronchoscopic foreign body retrieval
- Increasing ventilatory drive
  - Respiratory stimulant drugs (e.g., doxapram)
  - CO_2 rebreathing
  - Minimizing sedation and narcotic analgesics/using local pain control
    - Electrical stimulation
    - Nerve blocks
    - Incisional anesthetic infiltration
  - Mechanical ventilation to obviate need for ventilatory drive (e.g., prolonged postoperative mechanical ventilation)
- Optimizing surfactant
  - Surfactant instillation (e.g., in neonatal respiratory distress syndrome)
  - Use of lowest possible F_IO_2 to reduce risk of O_2 toxicity and the rate of gas absorption from poorly ventilated alveoli
- Selectively insufflating atelectatic regions
  - Double-lumen endotracheal tube
  - Cuffed rigid bronchoscope
  - Cuffed flexible bronchoscope
  - Balloon catheter re-expansion
- Applying positive-pressure ventilation
  - Via mouthpiece or mask using intermittent positive-pressure breathing (IPPB)
  - Via endotrachael intubation

(From Johnson and Pierson,[1] with permission.)

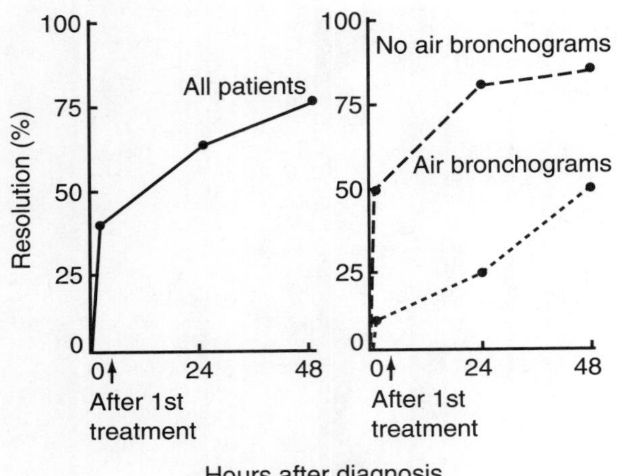

Figure 74-3. Resolution rate of acute lobar atelectasis with chest physical therapy showing delayed resolution in the presence of air bronchograms. (Redrawn from Marini et al.,[15] and reproduced from Johnson and Pierson,[1] with permission.)

instillation of mucolytics and lavage of the affected region. Bronchoscopy is likely to be ineffective if the chest radiograph has demonstrated the presence of an air bronchogram. As mentioned above, this finding suggests that mucus plugging is not the cause of the atelectasis, and bronchoscopy will be of minimal or no benefit.[16]

Expansion of the atelectatic region is best accomplished by encouraging the patient to breathe deeply. Spontaneous breathing promotes better distribution of the inhaled volume as compared with positive pressure breathing and is therefore more effective at reversing the atelectasis. Incentive spirometry offers an inexpensive and effective means of encouraging many patients who are alert and cooperative to breathe deeply.[2,17]

For patients who are weak and unable to generate significant inspiratory effort, intermittent positive-pressure breathing (IPPB) treatments may prove useful.[18] It is important that the IPPB treatments be given with tidal volumes larger than the patient's spontaneous vital capacity in order for the therapy to be of benefit (see Ch. 73). The application of IPPB to the patient with atelectasis from mucus plugging is likely to be futile until the retained secretions are mobilized.

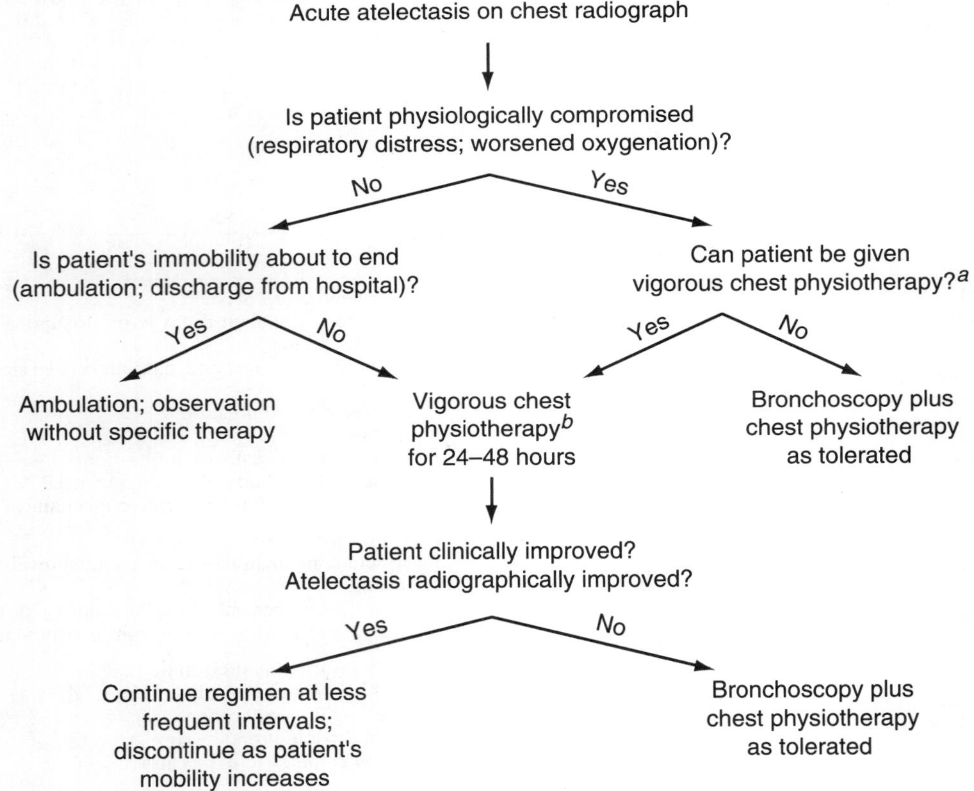

Figure 74-4. Algorithm for managing acute lobar atelectasis. [a]Patient not immobilized by traction or spinal injury; no intracranial hypertension or other contraindication to head-down position if required; no rib fractures or other injuries causing sufficient pain to prevent effective chest physiotherapy; sufficient personnel available to administer treatment. [b]Sample regimen: bronchodilator aerosol, followed by vigorous deep breathing and coughing, followed by postural drainage of affected lobe accompanied by chest percussion, repeated every 4 hours.

Continuous positive airway pressure (CPAP) has been shown to help maintain adequate lung expansion in postoperative patients.[19–21] This therapy can be applied through the use of a face mask, nasal mask, or endotracheal tube. During mechanical ventilation the use of sighs or inflation hold can be helpful in correcting atelectatic regions. Similar to IPPB, these positive pressure techniques are of little value when acute mucus plugging is present, and they may result in overinflation of nonatelectatic regions.

References

1. Johnson NT, Pierson DJ: The spectrum of pulmonary atelectasis: Pathophysiology, diagnosis, and therapy. Respir Care 1986;31:1107–1120
2. Marini JJ: Postoperative atelectasis: Pathophysiology, clinical importance, and principles of management. Respir Care 1984; 29:516–521
3. Dale WA, Rahn H: Rate of gas absorption during atelectasis. Am J Physiol 1952;170:606–615
4. Webb SJS, Nunn JF: A comparison between the effect of nitrous oxide and nitrogen on arterial PO_2. Anaesthesia 1967;22:69–75
5. Petty TL, Reiss OK, Paul GW et al: Characteristics of pulmonary surfactant in adult respiratory distress syndrome associated with trauma and shock. Am Rev Respir Dis 1977;115:531–536
6. D'Alonzo GE, Dantzker DR: Gas exchange alteration following pulmonary thromboembolism. Clin Chest Med 1984;5:411–419
7. Stein M, Cassara EL: Preoperative pulmonary evaluation and therapy for surgery patients. JAMA 1970;211:787–790
8. Latimer RG, Dickman M, Day WC et al: Ventilatory patterns and pulmonary complication after upper abdominal surgery determined by preoperative and postoperative computerized spirometry and blood gas analysis. Am J Surg 1971;122:622–632
9. Luce JM: Clinical risk factors for postoperative pulmonary complications. Respir Care 1984;29:484–495
10. Wightman JAK: A prospective survey of the incidence of postoperative pulmonary complication. Br J Surg 1968;55:85–91
11. Gravelyn TR, Weg JG: Respiratory rate as an indicator of acute respiratory dysfunction. JAMA 1980;244:1123–1128
12. Shields RT: Pathogenesis of postoperative pulmonary atelectasis. Arch Surg 1949;58:489–503
13. Forgacs P: The functional basis of pulmonary sounds. Chest 1978;73:399–409
14. Nath AR, Capel LH: Inspiratory crackles, early and late. Thorax 1974;29:223–228
15. Marini JJ, Pierson DJ, Hudson LD: Acute lobar atelectasis: A prospective comparison of fiberoptic bronchoscopy and respiratory therapy. Am Rev Respir Dis 1979;119:971–978
16. Fowler AA III, Scoggins WG, O'Donohue WJ Jr: Positive end-expiratory pressure in the management of lobar atelectasis. Chest 1978;74:497–500
17. Bartlett RH: Respiratory therapy to prevent pulmonary complications of surgery. Respir Care 1984;29:667–676
18. O'Donohue WJ Jr: IPPB past and present. Respir Care 1982;27:588–589
19. Duncan SR, Negrin RS, Mihm FG et al: Nasal continuous positive airway pressure in atelectasis. Chest 1987;92:621–624
20. Ricksten SE, Bengtsson A, Soderberg C et al: Effects of periodic positive airway pressure by mask on postoperative pulmonary function. Chest 1986;89:774–781
21. Lindner KH, Lotz P, Ahnefeld FW: Continuous positive airway pressure: Effect on functional residual capacity, vital capacity and its subdivisions. Chest 1987;91:66–70
22. Wilkins RL, Sheldon RL, Krider SJ et al (eds): Clinical Assessment in Respiratory Care. 2nd Ed. Mosby-Year Book, St. Louis, 1990
23. Pierson DJ: Acute respiratory failure. pp. 75–126. In Sahn SA (ed): Pulmonary Emergencies. Churchill Livingstone, New York, 1982

Chapter 75

Supplemental Oxygen and Other Medical Gas Therapy

Robert M. Kacmarek

CHAPTER OUTLINE

The foundation of respiratory care lies in the delivery of medical gases. Long before mechanical ventilator techniques became commonplace, O_2 was used as a therapeutic gas. Today, O_2 and other medical gases are commonly used within the hospital, as well as during home care. In this chapter the production, storage, and distribution of medical gases are discussed. In addition, indications, contraindications, and techniques used to administer medical gases are presented.

GASES IN THE ATMOSPHERE

O_2 is the second most abundant gas in the atmosphere, being exceeded in concentration only by N_2. These two gases comprise about 99 percent of the atmosphere. However, the final 1 percent is occupied primarily by eight other gases (Table 75-1). O_2 is also the third most abundant element in the universe behind hydrogen (H_2) (1st), and He (2nd), with carbon (C) (4th) and N_2 (5th) rounding out the top five. The quantity of O_2 in the environment remains relatively stable as a result of photosynthesis. This process, catalyzed by sunlight, produces a reaction of CO_2 with water in the presence of chlorophyll to form glucose and O_2. As a result of photosynthesis consuming CO_2 and producing O_2, and respiration producing CO_2 and consuming O_2, an atmospheric equilibrium is established that maintains the concentration of both CO_2 and O_2 essentially constant (Table 75-2).

PRODUCTION OF MEDICAL GASES

Many gases are produced commercially; however, only a small number (Table 75-3) are used medically, with O_2 being the most important. Medical gases are normally classified as

Table 75-1. Gaseous Composition of the Atmosphere

Gas	Composition (%)
N_2	78.08
O_2	20.95
Inert Gases	0.93[a]
CO_2	0.03
H_2	0.01

[a] Inert gases in the atmosphere include argon, neon, He, krypton, and xenon.

Table 75-3. Medical Gases

Nonflammable
- N_2
- CO_2
- He

Support combustion
- O_2
- Nitrous oxide (N_2O)
- Air
- O_2/N_2
- O_2/He
- O_2/CO_2

Flammable
- Cyclopropane [$(CH_2)_3$]
- Ethylene (C_2H_4)

nonflammable (will not burn), supporting combustion, and flammable (will burn readily) (Table 75-3). Flammable gases are used only in anesthesia.

The primary methods available for the production of O_2 are (1) electrolysis of water, (2) fractional distillation, and (3) physical separation. Of these, fractional distillation is the most important, producing the vast majority of O_2 used medically and also the process responsible for the production of most other gases present in the atmosphere. Historically, Joseph Priestly, in 1774, was the first individual to concentrate pure oxygen.[1] In his experiments he magnified sun rays to produce O_2 from mercuric oxide.

Electrolysis

If an electrical current is passed through a pool of water, the water decomposes into its component parts, one oxygen and two hydrogen atoms (Fig. 75-1). O_2 is accumulated at the anode, while H_2 is recovered from the cathode. Since water is a poor conductor of electricity, minerals are normally added to enhance conduction. Although O_2 is easily

Table 75-2. Physical Properties of Nonanesthetic Medical Gases

	O_2	Air	CO_2	He
Molecular weight	31.999	28.975	44.01	4.003
Percent by mole	20.946	—	0.0335	—
Partial pressure (ATPD)	158 mm Hg	—	0.25 mm Hg	0.000524
Density at 21°C and 1 atm viscosity	1.326 kg/m^3	1.2 kg/m^3	1.833 kg/m^3	0.1656 kg/m^3
Viscosity (poise)	201.8×10^{-6}	182.7×10^{-6}	148×10^{-6}	194.1×10^{-6}
Specific gravity at 21°C	1.1049	1	1.52	0.138
Boiling point at 1 atm	−297.3°F (−183°C)	−317.8°F (−194.3°C)	−29	−452.0°F (−268.9°C)
Freezing point at 1 atm	−361.1°F (−218.4°C)	−357.2 to −312.4°F (−216.2 to −191.3°C)	—	[a]
Critical temperature	−181.4°F (−118.6°C)	−221.2°F (−140.7°C)	87.9°F (31.1°C)	−450.2°F (−267.9°C)
Critical pressure	731.4 psia (5043 kPa, absolute)	547 psia (3770 kPa, absolute)	1070.6 psia (7382 kPa, absolute)	3 psia (227 kPa, absolute)
Triple point	−361.8°F (at 0.022 psia)	—	−69.9°F at 60 psig (416 kPa)	—
Sublimination temperature (1 atm)	—	—	−109.3°F (−78.5°C)	—
Solubility (v/v) H_2O at 0°C	0.0489	0.0292	0.90	0.0086
Color	Colorless	—	Colorless	Colorless
Odor	Odorless	—	Odorless	Odorless
Taste	Tasteless	—	Taste?	Tasteless
Flammability	Supports combustion	Nonflammable	Nonflammable	Nonflammable

ATPD, ambient temperature and pressure dry; psia, pounds per square inch absolute; psig, pounds per square inch gauge.
[a] Will not solidify at 1 atm −458°F (−272°C) and 25 atm, or 367.7 psi (2,335 kPa, absolute).
(From Ward,[1] as adapted from Gilbert,[42] with permission.)

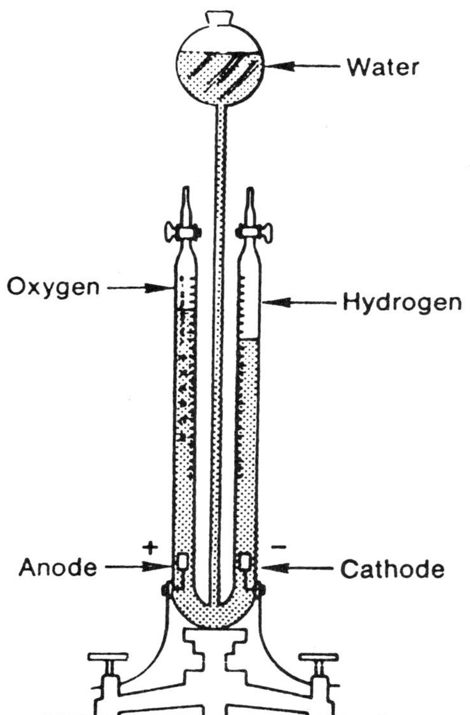

Figure 75-1. Apparatus used for the electrolysis of water. (From Webb et al.,[2] with permission.)

produced by this method, the cost is excessive because of the current that must be generated. As a result, electrolysis is not normally used for the production of O_2, but is still frequently used for the production of H_2.

Chemical Decomposition

Numerous chemical reactions result in the release of O_2. As Priestly demonstrated, the reaction of metallic oxides of Hg and silver (Ag_2) release O_2[1]:

$$2\ HgO \xrightarrow{Heat} 2\ Hg + O_2 \quad (1)$$

$$2\ Ag_2O \longrightarrow 4\ Ag + O_2 \quad (2)$$

The LeBrin process[2] has also been used to produce O_2. In this process, barium oxide (BaO) is heated to 500°C in air, which results in the production of barium peroxide. Continual heating of the barium peroxide to 800°C results in the release of O_2 and the original BaO.

The only chemical method used commercially to produce O_2 is controlled heating of solid sodium chlorate ($NaClO_3$), which produces O_2 and NaCl[3]:

$$2\ NaClO_3 \xrightarrow{Heat} 2\ NaCl + 3\ O_2 \quad (3)$$

This method can produce 4 to 5 L/min of O_2. The O_2 produced is 99.5 percent pure, with small quantities of CO_2, H_2O, and CO as by-products. This principle is used in some small, portable, emergency O_2 generators, referred to as solid-state O_2 generators (SSOG).

Fractional Distillation

The most common method of commercial production of O_2 is the fractional distillation of liquefied air, or the Joule-Kelvin method[1] (Fig. 75-2), which essentially proceeds in three phases[2]: (1) purification, (2) liquefaction, and (3) distillation of air. In the purification phase, air is passed through fine filters to remove pollutants, water, and CO_2. It is then compressed to 2000 psi. Waste liquid N_2 is used to remove some of the heat produced by this compression. The remaining generated heat is removed by water-cooled heat exchangers. As a result, the temperature of air is lowered below the freezing point of water, and most of the remaining water is removed. In the liquefaction phase, liquid ammonia is used to cool the purified air to about −40°C. This cooling removes the remainder of the water. The air is then decompressed to about 200 psi, which assists in cooling the gas to about −265°F; however, complete liquefaction requires a pressure of 530 psi at −265°F. With further decompression, the purified air is liquefied with its temperature below the boiling point of all gases. In the distillation phase, the liquid passes down vertically stacked distillation columns and various gases are boiled off.[4] All of the other gases in air boil at lower temperatures than O_2. As a result, O_2 at 99.5 to 99.9 percent purity is left after passing the columns. The Federal Drug Administration (FDA) requires that medical O_2 be 99 percent pure.

Physical Separation

The physical separation method of O_2 production uses filters to separate O_2 from the components of air. Essentially two distinct methods are used to produce O_2, primarily for use in home care (see Ch. 99). The first, the pressure swing absorbent or molecular sieve method (Fig. 75-3), draws room air by a vacuum pump into cylinders containing a silicate with ion exchange properties (crystal zeolite).[1] The air is then compressed to 200 to 300 psi and N_2 is absorbed by the zeolite. N_2 is released as an exhaust by the reversal of the compression. O_2 concentrations of between about 80 and 95 percent are possible, depending on O_2 liter flows. Flows up to 5 L/min can be provided.[5]

The second method uses a series of plastic polymer membranes to filter air (Fig. 75-4). Room air is drawn into the system by a pressure pump and forced across the membranes.[1] Both O_2 and water vapor move across the membranes. These units are much less efficient than molecular sieves. They produce concentrations ranging from 30 to 40 percent O_2, but the fraction of inspired O_2 ($F_{I}O_2$) is normally unaffected by alterations in delivered liter flows.[5]

Other Gases

Helium

He, although produced by fractional distillation of air, is produced in a quantity too small for large scale use. Most

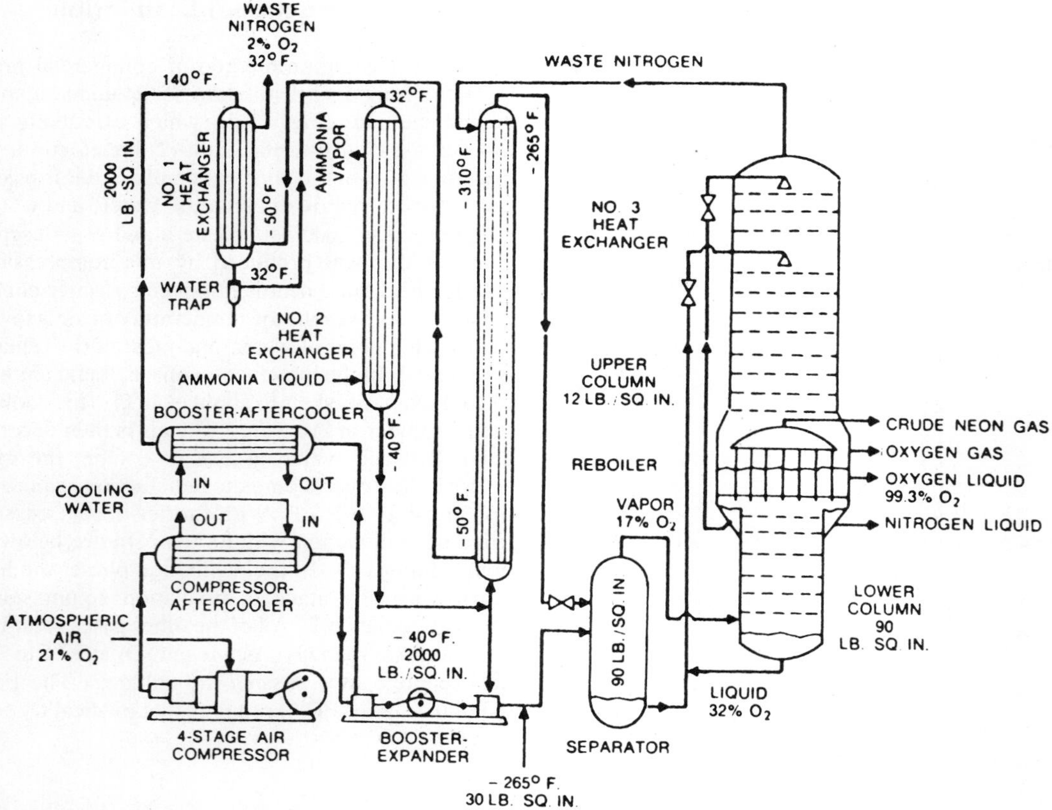

Figure 75-2. Air separation plant for the production of liquid oxygen. (From Webb et al.,[2] as borrowed from Union Carbide Corp., Linde Division, with permission.)

of the He used medically is collected and purified from natural gas fields around Amarillo, Texas; Saskatchewan, Canada; and the Black Sea.[1] Natural gas contains about 2 percent He.

Carbon Dioxide

As with He, CO_2 is a by-product of fractional distillation of air but, again, in quantities too small for large scale use. Most large scale production of CO_2 takes place in lime kilns.[2] The limestone is heated to a red glow in closed containers. Superheated steam is passed through the limestone, carrying with it the CO_2.

Compressed Air

Most of the compressed air used medically is produced in hospitals by filtering, drying, and compressing atmospheric gas. Commercial preparation of compressed air is performed in a similar manner.

Nitrogen

N_2 is produced as a by-product of the fractional distillation of air for the production of O_2.

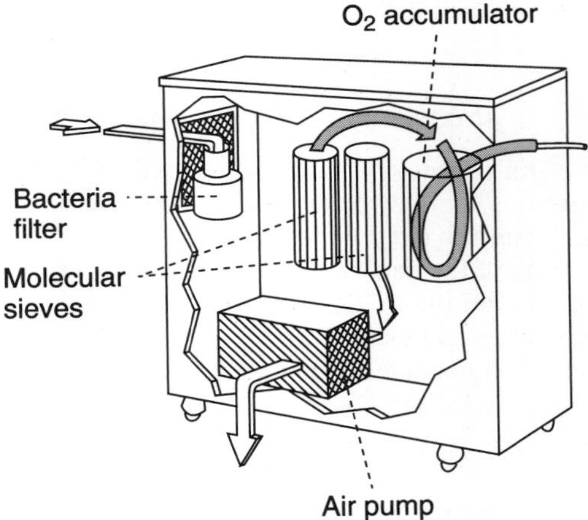

Figure 75-3. Molecular sieve oxygen concentrator. (From Webb et al.,[2] as borrowed from DeVilbis Company, Toledo, OH, with permission.)

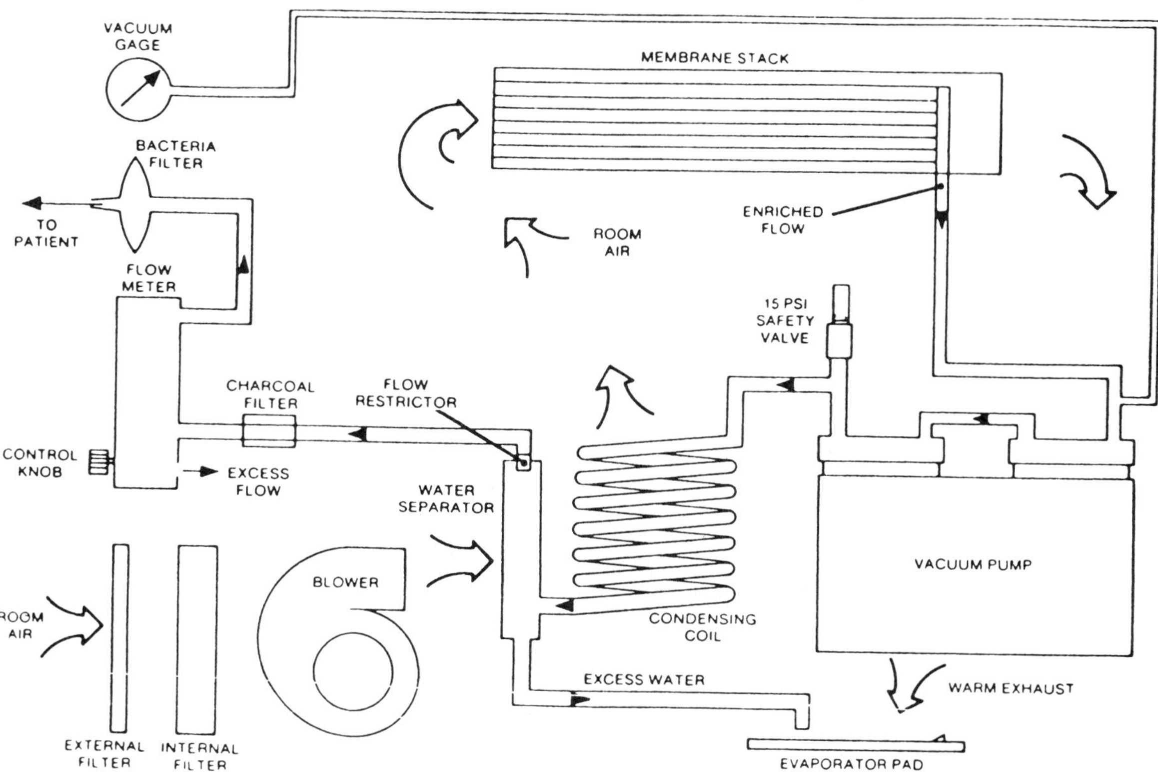

Figure 75-4. Membrane-type oxygen concentrator (enricher) flow diagram. (From Webb et al.,[2] as borrowed from Oxygen Enrichment Company, Schenectady, NY, with permission.)

REGULATION OF MEDICAL GASES

Numerous agencies, both governmental and nongovernmental, regulate the use of medical gases. These agencies (Table 75-4) promulgate regulations regarding compressed gas cylinders and bulk delivery systems, interstate as well as intrastate transport of gases, handling and storage of gases, purity, and educational standards.

Gas Storage Systems

Medical gases are generally available for use in one of three storage containers: portable cylinders, bulk (liquid cylinders), and fixed liquid systems. Of the three, the clinician comes into contact with fixed liquid systems most frequently, but interacts on a much more intimate basis with portable gas cylinder systems.

Portable Gas Cylinders

Regulations regarding the manufacture, testing, and transportation of all gas cylinders in the United States are established by the Department of Transportation (DOT), and were formerly established by the Interstate Commerce Commission. Generally, medical gas cylinders are produced by one of three construction methodologies.

The first is the steel billet, or single piece, construction. With this method, a tube of specific dimension is forced into a block of noncorrosive metal (high carbon steel, aluminum, heat-treated steel, manganese steel, or stainless steel), with a cylinder forming around it. Once formed, the bottom is shaped into a cup and the top is formed and treated.

The second approach uses two circular steel disks (two-piece construction). With this method the circular disks are formed into seamless cups, which are then heat-treated and welded into seamless shells. One of the disks forms the bottom of the cylinder with its cupped shape and the other disk is formed into the neck of the cylinder and threaded for attachment of the cylinder stem.

In the third method, the cylinder is formed from spun steel strands, which are spun around a mold of the actual cylinder. It is then heat-treated and the base and the neck are formed.

The DOT requires that high-pressure O_2 cylinders be made of seamless steel. Other cylinders may be formed from seamless, drawn, welded, or bronzed tubing.

Cylinder Markings

All cylinders have stamped markings on their shoulder, which are used to identify the process used to manufacture the cylinder, its maximum working pressure, serial number, owner, original hydrostatic test date, elastic expansion data, and retest date (Table 75-5). This information is provided to

Table 75-4. Governmental and Nongovernmental Agencies that Regulate or Determine Standards by Their Legal Authority

Agencies	Regulating Body	Activity/Responsibility
Governmental	Department of Transportation (DOT) inspection (prior to 1970, Interstate Commerce Commission [ICC])	Compressed gas cylinder specification & inspection
	Department of Health and Human Services (HHS) (formerly Department of Health, Education and Welfare), Food and Drug Administration	Purity levels of medical gases
	HHS, Bureau of Medical Devices	Classify, provide standards, and regulate medical devices
	Federal Department of Labor, OSHA	Occupational safety related to medical gases
Nongovernmental	Compressed Gas Association (CGA)	Specifications and recommendations in manufacture and safety systems
	National Fire Protection Association (NFPA)	Codes and safety recommendations for storage of flammable/oxidizing gases
	International Standards Organization (ISO)	Standards related to technical standards for manufacture
	American National Standards Institute (ANSI) and its Z-79 Committee	Coordination of standards for health devices (anesthesia, ventilatory equipment, adaptors, artificial airways, humidifiers, and nebulizers)
	Association for the Advancement of Medical Instrumentation (AAMI)	Education and standards related to a wide range of biomedical equipment
	American Society of Mechanical Engineers (ASME)	Standards for liquid gas bulk reservoir

(From Ward,[1] with permission.)

ensure both the user and the owner that a specific cylinder is safe and usable.

Hydrostatic Cylinder Testing

Cylinder testing for integrity is mandated by the DOT every 5 to 10 years, depending on the process used during manufacture.[6] Heat-treated cylinders require testing every 10 years, while non-heat-treated cylinders and the newer aluminum cylinders (much lighter) must be tested every 5 years. A star following cylinder markings (on shoulder of cylinder) indicates that testing is required every 10 years. Hydrostatic testing of cylinders is most commonly performed by the water-jacket volumetric expansion technique. The cylinder is suspended in a water bath and filled to five-thirds its normal working pressure. The quantity of water displaced at five-thirds filling pressure is the total expansion of the cylinder, while displacement by the empty cylinder is termed *permanent displacement*. The total expansion, minus the permanent displacement, is the elastic expansion, which is a measure of the average wall thickness of the cylinder at a given pressure. If the elastic expansion is outside the guidelines specific for the given cylinder, it is retired or used for storage of gases at lower working pressures.

The DOT also requires the owner to visually inspect the cylinder, both internally and externally, for surface defects such as arc burns, rust, dents, gouges, bulging, or corrosion. Finally, the dead ring or hammer test is performed. Striking the cylinder on its side should produce a clean ringing tone that lasts 2 to 3 seconds. Failing cylinders may have suffered fire damage or corrosion, or have been contaminated by oil or water, and are removed from circulation until the deficit is corrected.

Table 75-5. Cylinder Markings

Side 1	DOT.3AA.2015	Meets DOT regulations for type 3AA cylinders; maximum working pressure 2015 plus 10% for 3AA cylinders
	28300	Cylinder serial number
	PCGC	Owner symbol
	ABC	Manufacturers symbol
Side 2	8H52.EE 17.5	Original manufacturer hydrostatic test date; elastic expansion of 17.5 mL at ⅔ of maximum pressure
	Cr Mo Spun	Made from chrome molybdenum; spinning process used to manufacture
	3 X 58+	Retest date Inspectors mark Passed retest

Cylinder Handling and Storage

The DOT, Compressed Gas Association (CGA), and National Fire Protection Association (NFPA) have established guidelines regarding storage and handling of cylinders.[1,7,8] These include all of the following:

1. Storage areas must meet NFPA guidelines regarding construction materials, location, and actual structure; the area must be well ventilated, cool, and dry.
2. Only flame-resistant construction materials should be used in storage areas.
3. Full and empty cylinder areas must be separated to prevent confusion.
4. All cylinders should be restrained; usually chains are used for large cylinders and racks for small sized cylinders.
5. All storage areas should be locked.
6. No oil or petroleum-based lubricants should come into contact with valves, regulators, fittings, or gas hoses.
7. Soapy water should be used to detect system leaks.
8. Only regulators designed for a specific cylinder type and content should be used.
9. Valves on a cylinder should be cracked slowly before attachment of regulator to remove particulate matter from the valve and to dissipate heat of compression.
10. Damaged or unlabeled cylinders should not be used.
11. Cylinders should not be exposed to open flames or sparks, and should not be subjected to temperatures above 54.4°C.
12. Cylinder valves should be closed when not in use and cylinder caps (large cylinders) should be in place during storage and transport.
13. Cylinders should only be transported in suitable containers or carts.

A practice of some institutions that is not recommended because of the tremendous energy transfer and potential for contamination is the transfilling of small cylinders from large cylinders. If this process is performed, labeling and cylinder inspection must conform with DOT standards. In addition, the CGA recommends that the supply cylinder be isolated, that calibrated pressure gauges be used on the cylinder being filled, and that the filling rate be limited to 200 L/min.[9]

Gas Cylinder Sizes and Colors

As listed in Table 75-6, many sizes of gas cylinders are currently available. Of those listed, size D, E, and H, are the most commonly used for O_2 delivery. The other sizes are more commonly used for laboratory gas mixtures, or for emergency O_2 supply during travel. Color coding of E size cylinders in the United States is listed in Table 75-7. There is no standard for the color coding of cylinders; however, the compressed gas industry has adhered to the listed color scheme (Table 75-7) for over 30 years. This color coding may or may not be followed on cylinders of other sizes. It is important to note that the standard color code for O_2 in places other than the United States is white. As a result, it is imperative that the exact content of a cylinder be determined by the chemical name marked on the cylinder, and *not* by its color. Another method of identifying cylinder content is the "safety indexing system" (see Safety-Indexed Connection Systems) used to code cylinder valves to gas regulating devices.

Table 75-6. Dimensions and Capacities of Available Cylinders

Cylinder	Dimensions (in.)	Weight (lb)	Capacity[a]	
			cu ft	L
H	9 × 56	135	244	6907
G	8.50 × 55	100	187	5299
M	7 × 47	66	107	3028
E	4.25 × 29.75	15	22	625
D	4.25 × 20.25	10.25	13	359
B	3.50 × 16.50	5.75	5	151
A	3 × 10.75	2.50	2.5	75.7
DD	3.75 × 23.25	8.75	31	875
BB	2.75 × 19.75	4	1.3	379
AA	2.75 × 11	3	5	151

[a] Capacity varies for different types of gases; listed levels for H through A for O_2; DD, BB, and AA for $(CH_2)_3$.

Duration of Flow

Most gas cylinders are used for transport or emergency gas administration and, as noted in Table 75-6, contain limited quantities of gas; therefore, it is essential that clinicians precisely calculate the length of time a specific cylinder will last at a given liter flow. It is possible to calculate a cylinder flow conversion factor for any size gas cylinder and for each specific gas filling the cylinder. The conversion factor is dependent on the cylinder capacity and the pounds per square inch pressure level of a full cylinder.[10] Since cylinder size is

Table 75-7. Color Coding of E Cylinders in the United States

Gas	Color
O_2	Green[a]
Air	Yellow
He	Brown
$(CH_2)_3$	Red
CO_2	Gray
N_2O	Light blue
Cyclopropane	Orange
CO_2 and O_2	Gray and green
He and O_2	Brown and green

[a] The international color code for O_2 is white.

Table 75-8. Duration of Flow Conversion Factors

Gas	Cylinder Size D	E	G	H
O_2, O_2/N_2, air	0.16	0.28	2.41	3.14
O_2/CO_2	0.20	0.35	2.94	2.84
He/O_2	0.14	0.23	1.93	2.50

(From Chatburn and Lough,[10] with permission.)

normally listed in cubic feet of gas, one must use the factor 28.3 to convert cubic feet to liters.

$$\text{Conversion factor} = \frac{(\text{cu ft full cylinder})(28.3\ \text{L/cu ft})}{\text{psi of full cylinder}} \quad (4)$$

$$\text{Conversion factor} = \frac{(22\ \text{cu ft})(28.3\ \text{L/cu ft})}{2200\ \text{psi}} \quad (5)$$

$$= 0.28\ \text{L/psi (conversion factor for E-size cylinder of } O_2)$$

Because most cylinders are filled to 110 percent capacity, 2200 psi is used as cylinder capacity. The volume of gas in cylinders is also listed at the 110 percent capacity level. Liters per pounds per square inch conversion factors for commonly used cylinders are listed in Table 75-8.

To calculate the length of time a given cylinder will last at a specific liter flow, the number of pounds per square inch pressure in the cylinder is multiplied by the conversion factor for the cylinder and divided by the specific liter flow.

$$\text{Duration of flow (min)} = \frac{(\text{psi level})(\text{conversion factor})}{\text{flow (L/min)}} \quad (6)$$

For an H cylinder of O_2 with 1000 psi pressure, run at 5 L/min flow, the duration of flow is

$$\text{Duration of flow (min)} = \frac{(1000\ \text{psi})(3.14\ \text{L/psi})}{5\ \text{L/min}} = 628\ \text{min (10 h, 46 min)} \quad (7)$$

Generally, E size or smaller cylinders with 500 psi pressure or less should not be used since only limited time is available, even at 1 L/min flow. With these cylinders, calculating duration of flow by subtracting 500 from the gauge psi reading should prevent running out of gas in the middle of a transport.

Safety-Indexed Connection Systems

To prevent gas regulating devices designed for one gas or gas mixture from being used on another gas and to prevent the inadvertent use of a nontherapeutic gas, gas connection safety systems have been developed. Specifically, three systems have been designed for the delivery and regulation of medical gases: (1) The American Standard Compressed Gas Cylinder Outlet and Inlet Connections, or American Standard Safety System (ASSS), (2) The Pin-Index Safety System (PISS), and (3) the Diameter-Index Safety System (DISS).

American Standard Safety System

ASSS, adopted by both the United States and Canada, specifies attachment between high pressure (greater than 200 psi) gas cylinders of H, G, and M size and regulators or other attachments. Specifications are provided for mating nipple and hexagonal nuts with cylinder attachments (Fig. 75-5). In general, the threaded outlets of large cylinders are indexed in four basic divisions: internal or external, and left handed or right handed. Within each division, variation is established by altering the diameter and the pitch of the threads. Right-handed threads are used for medical gases, with most of the cylinder valve outlets having external threads and their corresponding nipples having internal threads. A total of 26 different connections are available for use with 62 gases. As a result, some gases have the same ASSS connection. The listing for O_2 is

CGA – 540 × 0.903 – 14 NGO – RH – Ext

indicating that the cylinder is listed by the CGA as connection No. 540, thread diameter of 0.903 in., and 14 threads per inch of the NGO type, and the threads are right-handed and external.

Large cylinders also incorporate a rupture (copper) disk within the valve stem designed to rupture at a cylinder pressure of 1.5 times maximum working pressure. This safety feature is included to prevent rupture of the cylinder itself. A fusible metal plug is also used on some large cylinder valves, although this safety device is more commonly seen on E size and smaller cylinders. It is composed of Woods

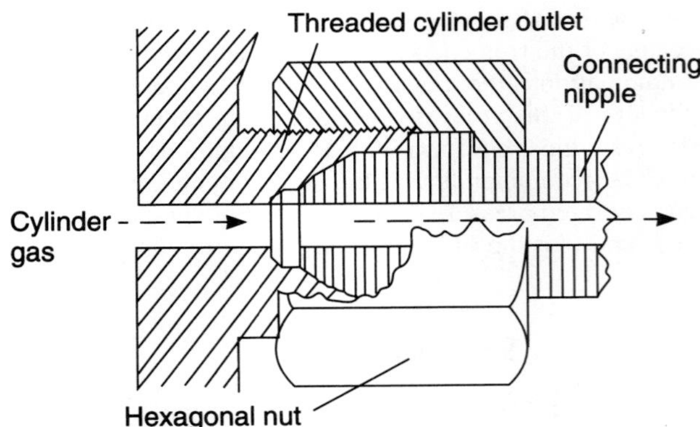

Figure 75-5. Diagram illustrating structure of a typical American standard connection, such as might be used to attach a reducing valve to a large high-pressure cylinder. The hexagonal nut is held onto the nipple of the reducing valve by a circular collar, seen as a cross-sectional projection on the nipple. As the hexagonal nut is tightened on the threaded cylinder outlet, the end of the nipple is snugly seated into the conical outlet. (From Thalken,[41] as modified from CGA Pamphlet V-1, Compressed Gas Association Inc., New York.)

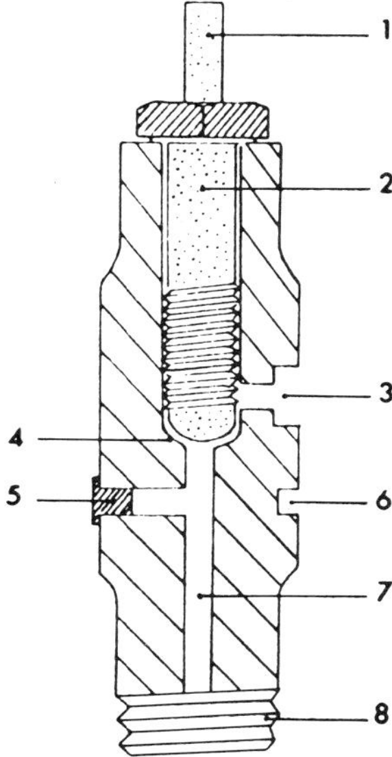

Figure 75-6. Cross-section of a small cylinder (E and smaller) valve: 1, valve stem; 2, threaded valve plunger; 3, cylinder outlet; 4, valve seat; 5, fusible plug pressure release valve; 6, PISS ports; 7, gas chamber; 8, threaded connection to body of cylinder. (From Thalken,[41] with permission.)

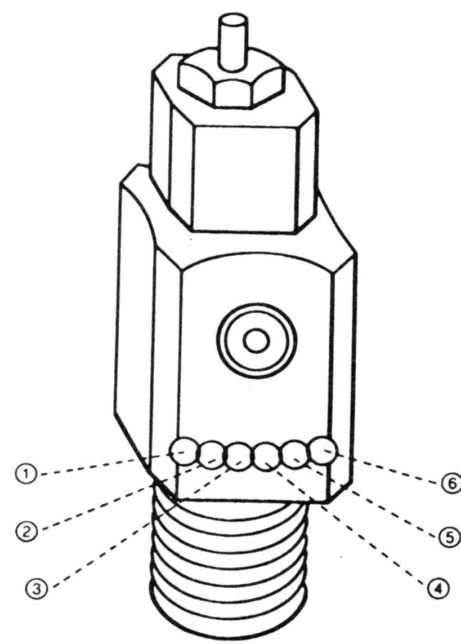

Figure 75-8. Yoke-type cylinder valve with identification of 6 possible holes for PISS. (From Ward,[1] with permission.)

metal, an alloy of bismuth, lead, cadmium, and tin, and melts at temperatures of 208°F to 220°F. A combination rupture disk and fusible plug is also used.

Pin-Index Safety System

The PISS is a subdivision of the ASSS for use on small (E size or smaller) cylinders with a maximum working pressure greater than 2000 psi. The actual stem of a small cylinder is illustrated in Figure 75-6. Two bore holes are placed in the stem valve assembly for positioning of pins located on the yoke type adapter used to attach regulators to these cylinders (Fig. 75-7). As with the ASSS system, the PISS is designed to prevent the wrong regulator from being attached to a given cylinder. The actual indexing consists of fitting the two pins on the yoke into the two holes on the valve stem. Since there are a total of 6 hole positions available on the stem (Fig. 75-8), a total of 10 specific two-pin combinations are available. All but one are currently in use (Table 75-9).

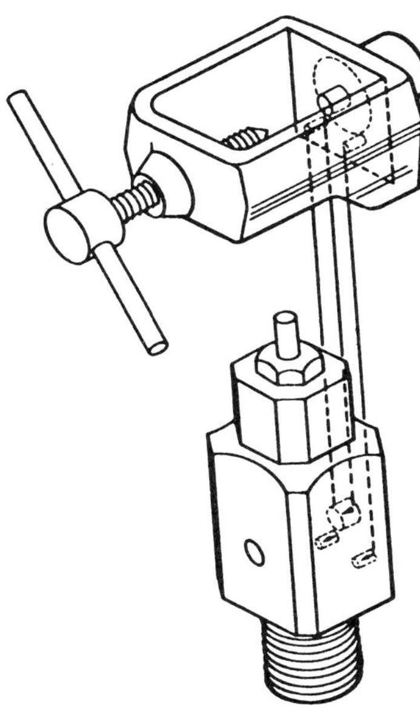

Figure 75-7. Yoke-type cylinder valve with yoke connector showing regulator inlet and pin placements. (From Ward,[1] with permission.)

Diameter-Index Safety System

For connections in which maximum gas pressure is 200 psi or less, the DISS regulates connections. It is designed to regulate connections between gas pressure reducing devices and gas delivery devices. DISS connections are used to connect O_2 humidifiers to flowmeters, or to connect 50 psi gas

Table 75-9. PISS Hole Positions of Indexed Gases

Gas	Indexed Holed Position
O_2	2–5
Air	1–5
C_2H_4	1–3
N_2O	3–5
$(CH_2)_3$	3–6
O_2/CO_2 ($CO_2 \leq 7\%$)	2–6
He/O_2 ($\leq 8\%$)	2–4
O_2/CO_2 ($CO_2 > 7\%$)	1–6
He/O_2 ($He > 8\%$)	4–6

C_2H_4, ethylene.

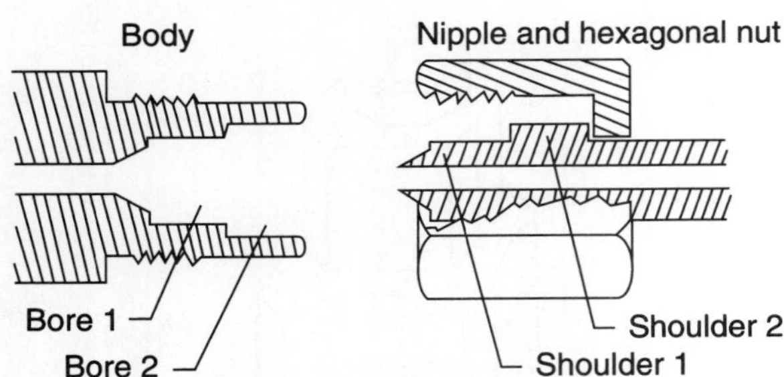

Figure 75-9. Schematic illustration of components of a representative DISS connection. The two shoulders of the nipple allow the nipple to unite only with a body that has corresponding borings. If the match is incorrect, the hexagonal nut will not engage the body threads. (From Thalken,[41] with permission as modified from CGA Pamphlet V-5, Compressed Gas Association Inc., New York.)

sources to ventilators (both O_2 and air). The DISS connection consists of three parts: body, nipple, and nut (Fig. 75-9). There are 11 indexed DISS connections, accommodating 11 gases or gas mixtures. The DISS connection number for O_2 is 1240; the connection is 0.5625 in diameter and has 18 threads per inch.

Quick-Connect Systems

Quick-connect systems (Fig. 75-10) represent a variation of the standard DISS connections and are specifically used to provide attachment of equipment to the wall outlets of gas piping systems (see Bulk Oxygen Delivery Systems). Each manufacturer has developed a unique set of wall attachments that are not interchangeable.

REGULATION OF GAS FLOW

Medical gas, whether exiting from a cylinder or a central piping system, must be regulated to the pressure and specific gas flow required by the patient or of equipment driven by that gas. Flowmeters are devices that regulate the specific flow of gas; regulators are devices that reduce system pressure to a working level, usually 50 psi.

Flowmeters

There are three commonly defined categories of flow-regulating devices: (1) Bourdon gauges, (2) back-pressure compensated flowmeters, and (3) non-back-pressure compensated flowmeters. In addition, regulation of flow can be accomplished by the use of a simple restriction using the law of flow:

$$\dot{V} = \frac{\Delta P}{R} \tag{8}$$

where $\dot{V}$ is flow of gas, ΔP is the pressure gradient across the restriction, and R is resistance to gas flow created by the restriction. As long as the pressure driving the gas through the restriction and the pressure downstream of the restriction are constant, a constant flow of gas is maintained. This type of flow regulator is referred to as a fixed-orifice, constant-pressure flowmeter.[1] Although the use of a restriction does establish a constant gas flow, the use of this device is limited to internal gas-flow regulation of equipment, since alteration in flow requires replacement of the restriction and the build-up of downstream pressure reduces flow delivery.

Bourdon Gauges

A Bourdon gauge is actually a low-pressure gas measuring device, normally operating between 0 and 50 psi system pressure (Fig. 75-11). Flow is not actually measured, but is based on the pressure measured by the gauge and the outflow orifice size (i.e., the gauge is calibrated in flow, based on specific pressure measurements and the actual measured flow leaving the device). For example, a measured pressure of 5 psi may equate to a flow of 1 L/min, or 10 psi may equate to a flow of 3 L/min. This device is referred to as a fixed-orifice, variable-pressure flowmeter.[1]

Bourdon gauges are usually used on adjustable high-pres-

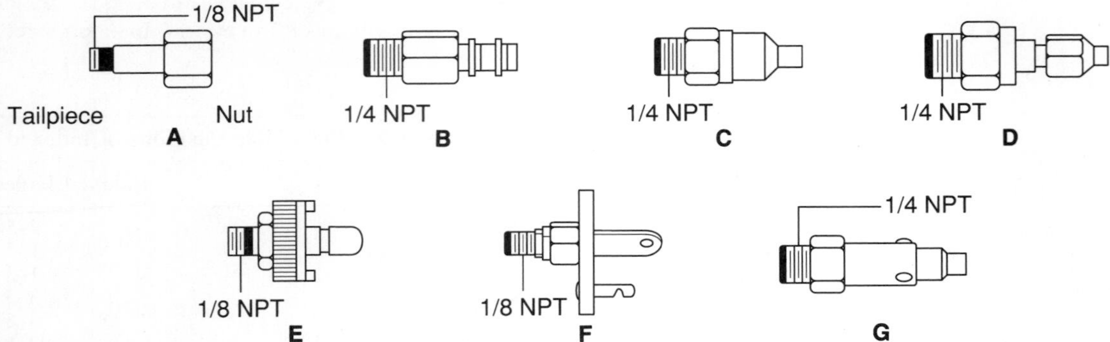

Figure 75-10. Common brands of quick connect systems. **(A)** Puritan DISS, **(B)** Puritan Q.C., **(C)** Hansen, **(D)** Schrader, **(E)** Ohio Diamond, **(F)** N.C.G., and **(G)** O.E.S. (From McPherson and Spearman,[11] with permission; courtesy of Puritan-Bennett Corp., Los Angeles.)

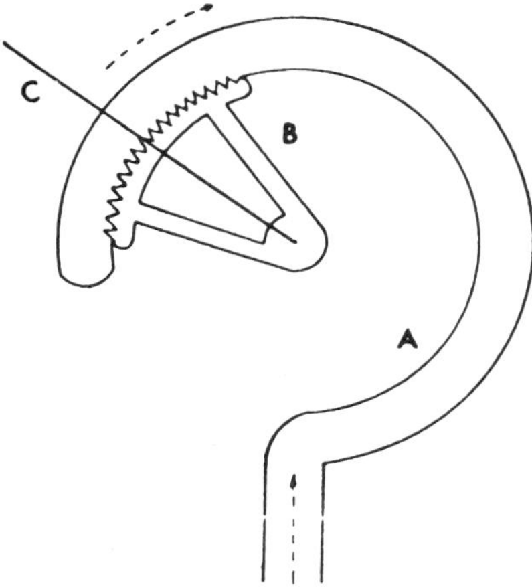

Figure 75-11. Internal function of a Bourdon gauge. A, curved, flexible, closed tube; B, gear mechanism; C, indicator needle, reflecting flow or pressure on face of valve. (From Thalken,[41] with permission.)

sure regulators. As noted in Figures 75-11 and 75-12, the gauge is actually a curved hollow copper tube connected to an indicator needle via a gearing mechanism. As pressure increases in the tube, the tube attempts to uncoil. This movement is transformed to the indicator dial by the gearing mechanism. The gauge reads accurately in any position and is commonly used on all size cylinders. Its primary limitation is that downstream (back) pressure results in a decreased pressure gradient establishing flow, and a decrease in flow of gas exiting the device. However, because the pressure sensed by the gauge is constant, its flow reading is unchanged (Fig. 75-12). As a result, total occlusion of the gas delivery orifice would still result in the gauge indicating that flow was delivered. Bourdon gauge flowmeters *always* indicate flow of gas *higher than delivered* in the face of back pressure.

Thorpe Tube Flowmeters

Thorpe tube flowmeters are the most common flow-regulating devices in use. In contrast to Bourdon gauges and fixed-orifice devices, Thorpe tubes actually measure flow of gas and are classified by Ward[1] as variable-orifice, constant-pressure, flowmeters. All Thorpe tubes are designed to operate from a low pressure gas source of 50 psi and are calibrated at atmospheric pressure for a specific gas. The diameter of the tube increases as the tube proceeds from base to top and within the tube is a float. As gas is allowed to enter the tube, the force of the gas under the float opposes the effect of gravity and moves the float up the tube. Since the diameter increases toward the top, more and more gas flow is required to raise the float. The position of the float stabilizes when the force below the float (P_1) equals the force above the float (P_2) (Fig. 75-13). As a result, Thorpe tubes must be upright when in use. If they are placed in anything but an absolute vertical position, they indicate flow inaccurately. Thus, their use during transport is limited. It should also be noted that since gas density determines the force

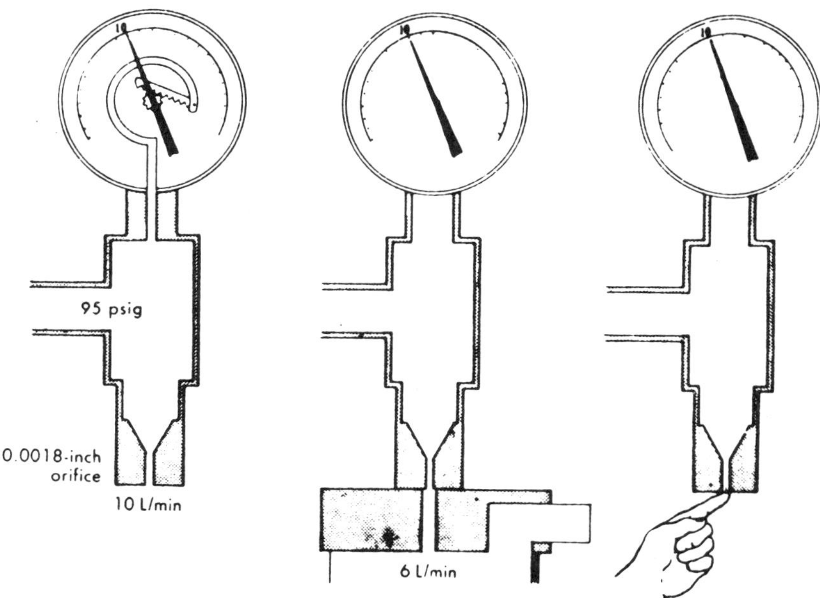

Figure 75-12. Bourdon regulator with resistance downstream. If resistance is placed on Bourdon regulator, postrestriction pressure is no longer constant; it will be somewhat higher than atmospheric pressure. Pressure gradient is then decreased and because only prerestriction pressure and not actual pressure gradient is monitored, the reading will be erroneously high. (From McPherson and Spearman,[11] with permission; courtesy of Puritan-Bennett Corp., Los Angeles.)

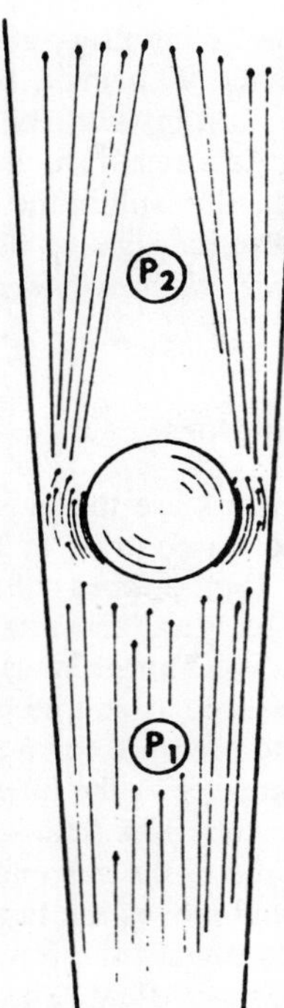

Figure 75-13. The position of the float in the Thorpe tube-type flowmeter is based on a balance between the force of gravity and the pressure difference ($P_1 - P_2$) across it, as determined by the variable-sized orifice created between the float and tube wall. (From Thalken,[41] with permission.)

applied to the float, Thorpe tubes are designed for use with specific gases. The use of an O_2 Thorpe tube flow meter on a gaseous system of He results in inaccurately low readings because of the low density of the He.

As indicated above, two types of Thorpe tubes, back-pressure compensated and non-back-pressure compensated, have been manufactured (Fig. 75-14). Today, only back-pressure compensated tubes are manufactured for clinical use. However, many non-back-pressure compensated units can be found in pulmonary function and physiology laboratories. The difference between the two types is a result of the location of the needle valve and its effect on the response of the unit to back pressure. Back-pressure compensated systems have the needle valve located downstream from the Thorpe tube. As a result, the pressure entering the Thorpe tube is always 50 psi. Thus, opening the needle valve drops the pressure downstream from the float but not upstream to the float; with a non-back-pressure compensated flowmeter, the needle valve is placed upstream from the Thorpe tube. Thus, the Thorpe tube is never directly affected by the 50 psi source pressure, unless the needle valve is wide open. The major difference in the operation of these two devices, as depicted in Figure 75-14, is the effect of downstream pressure. With both, downstream pressure decreases the flow exiting the meter. However, with the non-back-pressure compensated Thorpe tube, the *decrease* in *indicated flow* is *greater* than the *actual decrease* in *delivered flow*. Since the pressure across the float is rapidly equilibrated by downstream pressure, the float in non-back-pressure compensated systems drops more than the amount of gas flow that is moving past the float.

One can differentiate between back-pressure compensated and non-back-pressure compensated systems by closing the needle valve and then attaching the meter to a 50 psi pressure source. In a back-pressure compensated meter, the float will initially jump and then fall to its resting position. With non-back-pressure compensated systems, the float does not experience pressure unless the needle valve is opened. Most Thorpe tubes indicate whether they are back-pressure compensated.

Thorpe tube flowmeters are also referred to as rotometers, although some authors consider systems that use a ball as the float, Thorpe tubes, and those employing a bobbin, rotometers.[3] When flow settings are read on a Thorpe tube, the flow should be read at the middle of the ball, while with a rotometer it should be read at the top of the bobbin. Normally, Thorpe tubes are calibrated from 0 to 15 L/min. However, opening the needle valve to flush frequently establishes flows higher than 60 L/min. High-flow flowmeters are available that are calibrated to deliver up to 75 L/min. In addition, flowmeters calibrated to deliver less than 1 L/min are available.

The effect of various back pressures on Bourdon gauges, back-pressure compensated, and non-back-pressure compensated flowmeters is illustrated in Figure 75-15.

High-Pressure Regulators

As already indicated, gas within cylinders is maintained at up to 2200 psi, whereas gas flow regulatory devices are generally designed to operate from a source gas of 50 psi. High-pressure regulators are designed to reduce the pressure in cylinders and piping systems to a working pressure under which other equipment is designed to operate. They are also designed to modulate the variation in pressure noted as gas cylinders empty. There are three types of flow-regulating devices currently used: (1) preset regulators, (2) adjustable regulators, and (3) multistage regulators.

Preset Regulators

A preset regulator (Fig. 75-16) is designed to decrease cylinder working pressure to 50 psi and, as a result, gas flow is usually metered by a Thorpe tube. The regulator itself contains an ambient pressure chamber (D) and an actual working pressure chamber (C). The two are separated by a flexible diaphragm (E). Attached to the diaphragm in the ambient chamber is a spring (F) that maintains the valve stem (G) open unless the pressure in the working pressure chamber reaches 50 psi. Since the ambient chamber is open to atmosphere, no pressure builds up in it. A pressure pop-off valve (L) is included in the pressure chamber to prevent pressure from exceeding 200 psi, in the event that the valve stem is unable to be set at the gas entry valve (H). During operation, gas enters the regulator at the cylinder attachment

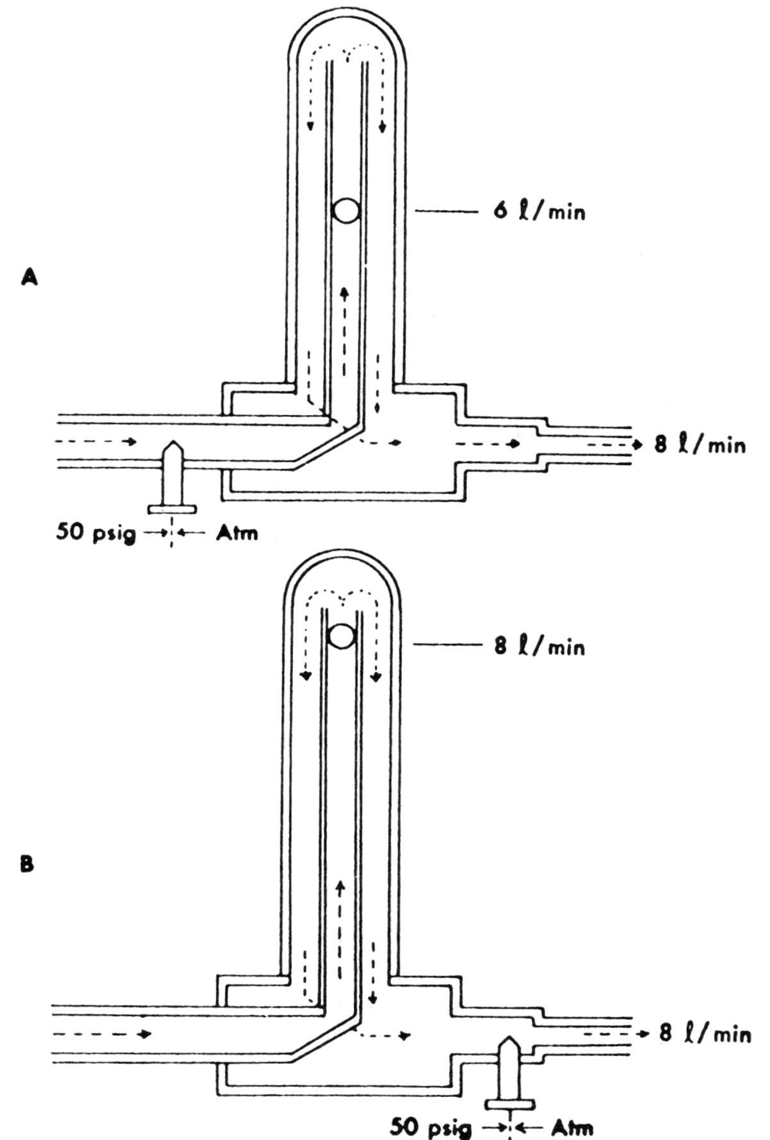

Figure 75-14. Comparison of (A) non-back-pressure compensated and (B) back-pressure compensated flowmeters. In the former, the flow-control valve is proximal to the meter and the gauge records less than the actual output. In the latter, location of the valve distal to the meter correlates the gauge reading with the output. (From Thalken,[41] with permission.)

(A), moves through the gas entry valve into the working chamber if the needle valve (K) is off; once pressure in the chamber reaches 50 psi, the diaphragm and spring are compressed, setting the valve stem, and thus preventing additional gas entry into chamber C. On opening the needle valve, the pressure in the chamber drops, opening the entry valve and allowing more gas to enter. In a short period, equilibrium between gas entering the working chamber and exiting the unit is established. Increasing the gas flow setting on the Thorpe tube increases the opening at the gas entry valve, while decreasing gas flow closes it.

Adjustable Regulators

An adjustable regulator functions in the same manner as a preset regulator, with one exception—the pressure necessary to set the valve stem (G) (Fig. 75-17) is variable. This is accomplished by varying the tension on the spring (F), by including a gas flow control at the needle valve. Thus, the pressure required to set the valve stem may vary from 0 psi on up, although it usually does not exceed 100 psi. With this type of regulator, a Bourdon gauge is used to indicate delivered flow.

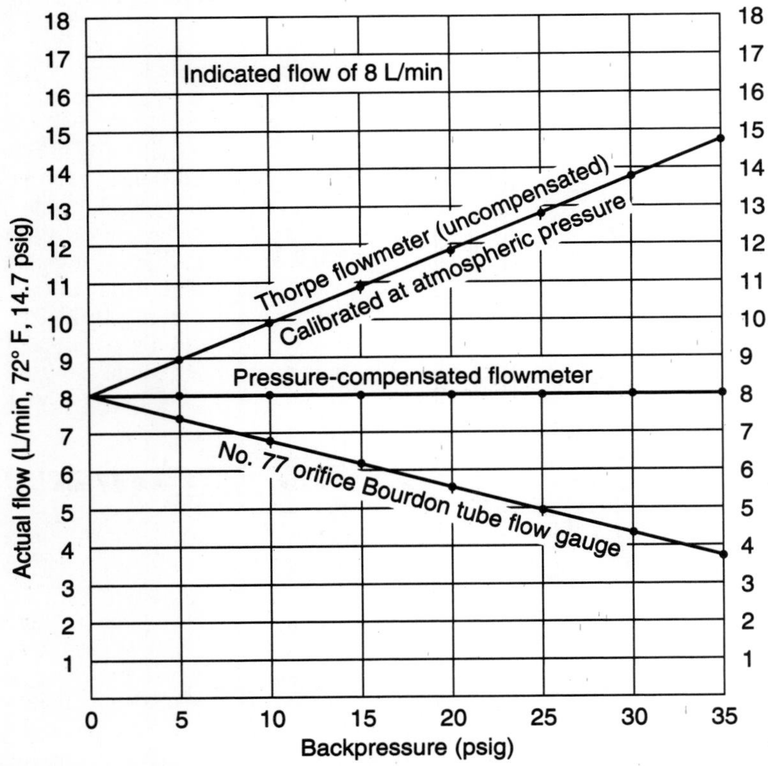

Figure 75-15. Comparative accuracy of flowmeters. (From McPherson and Spearman,[11] as modified from Puritan-Bennett Corp., Los Angeles.)

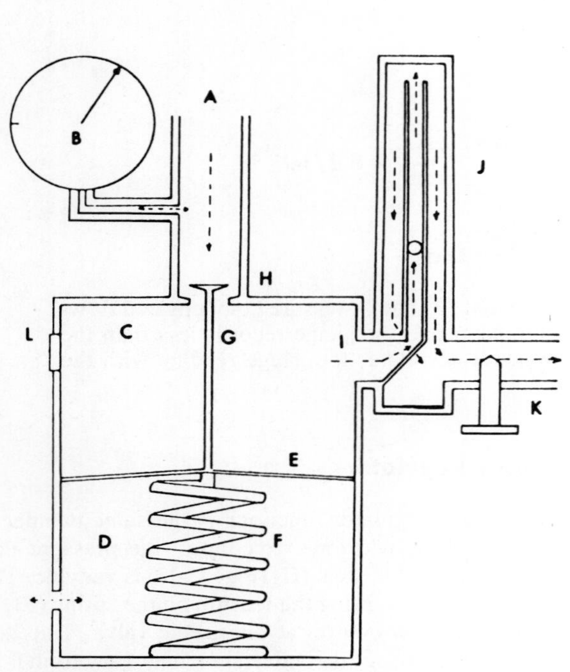

Figure 75-16. Diagram of preset, high-pressure gas regulator. A, attachment to cylinder; B, pressure gauge; C, pressure chamber; D, ambient pressure chamber; E, flexible diaphragm; F, spring; G, valve stem; H, gas entry valve; I, outflow port; J, Thorpe tube flowmeter; K, needle valve; L, pop-off valve. (From Thalken,[41] with permission.)

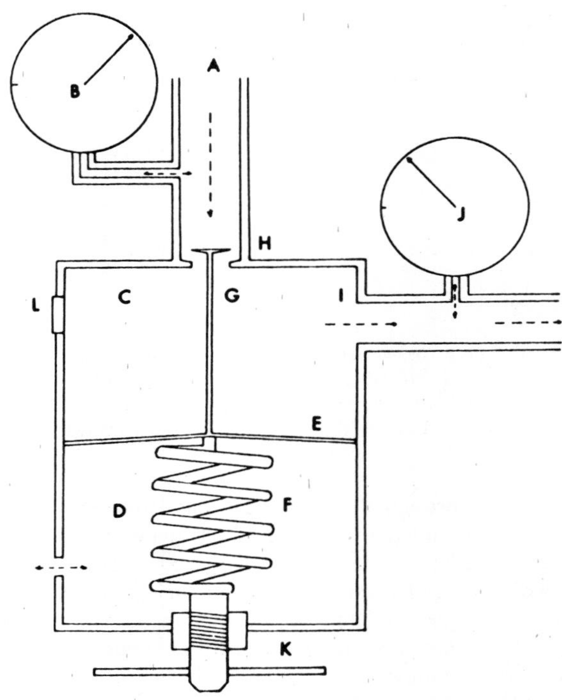

Figure 75-17. Diagram of an adjustable, high-pressure gas regulator. A, attachment to cylinder; B, pressure gauge; C, pressure chamber; D, ambient pressure chamber; E, flexible diaphragm; F, spring; G, valve stem; H, gas entry valve; I, outflow port; J, Bourdon flow gauge; K, threaded gas flow control; L, pop-off valve. (From Thalken,[41] with permission.)

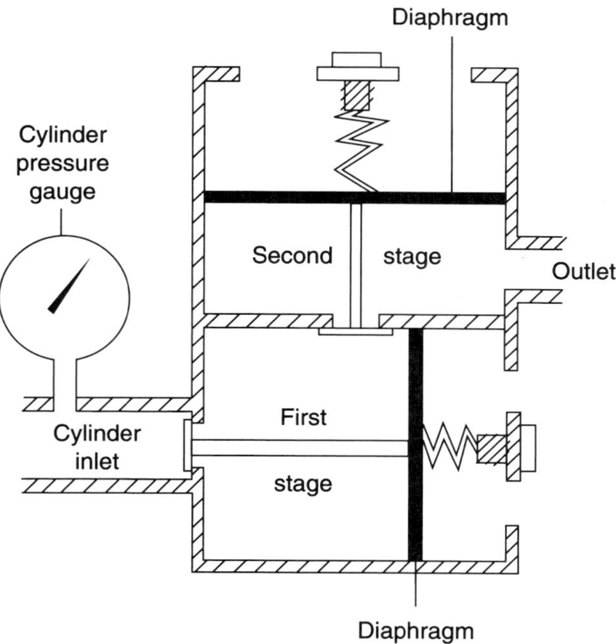

Figure 75-18. Multistage reducing valve. A double-stage reducing valve is two single-stage reducing valves working in series. Gas enters first stage (first reducing valve), and its pressure is lowered. Gas then enters second stage (second reducing valve), and pressure is lowered to desired working pressure (usually 50 psig). A three-stage reducing valve would have one more reducing valve in series. (From McPherson and Spearman,[11] with permission.)

Multistage Regulators

A multistage regulator (Fig. 75-18) is simply the combination of two preset or one preset and one adjustable regulator. Each of the stages function as described above. The first stage normally reduces cylinder pressure to between 200 and 700 psi, while the second stage further reduces it to the working pressure range. Each stage has its own safety pop-off valve. Multistage regulators are expensive and normally not used on a routine clinical basis. However, the reduction of pressure by multiple stages results in a precise gas flow, with minimal fluctuations in pressure. These devices are most frequently used in research activities.

BULK OXYGEN DELIVERY SYSTEMS

The average hospital uses enormous quantities of O_2 on a yearly basis, and therefore, the use of portable O_2 cylinders for the provision of continuous O_2 is not feasible. As a result, most institutions provide a bulk O_2 delivery system, or "piped-in O_2." These systems are referred to as low-pressure systems, because gas entering the hospital piping system is maintained at 50 psi (45 to 55 psi).

Bulk systems may use either gaseous or liquid O_2. However, regardless of the system used, the NFPA has guidelines that define system design. In general, a primary gas supply system and a secondary reserve system equal to usage for 1 day is established. The secondary system is designed for emergency use in the event that the primary system is depleted, or an accident disrupts the primary gas supply.

ntral piping systems (Fig. 75-19) are required to have

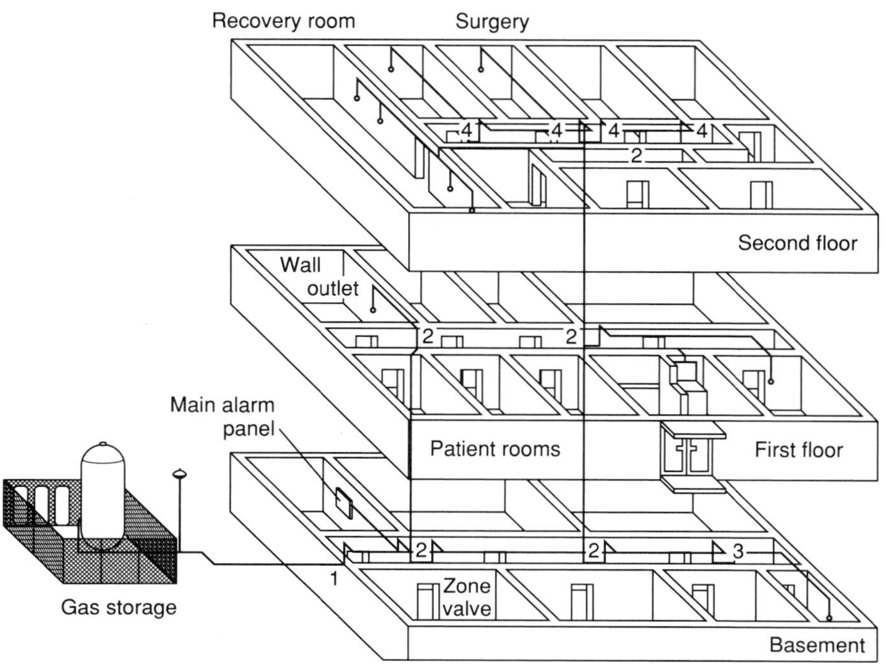

Figure 75-19. A hospital piping system. Numbers indicate zone, or area, values. (From McPherson and Spearman,[11] with permission; courtesy of Puritan-Bennett Corp., Los Angeles.)

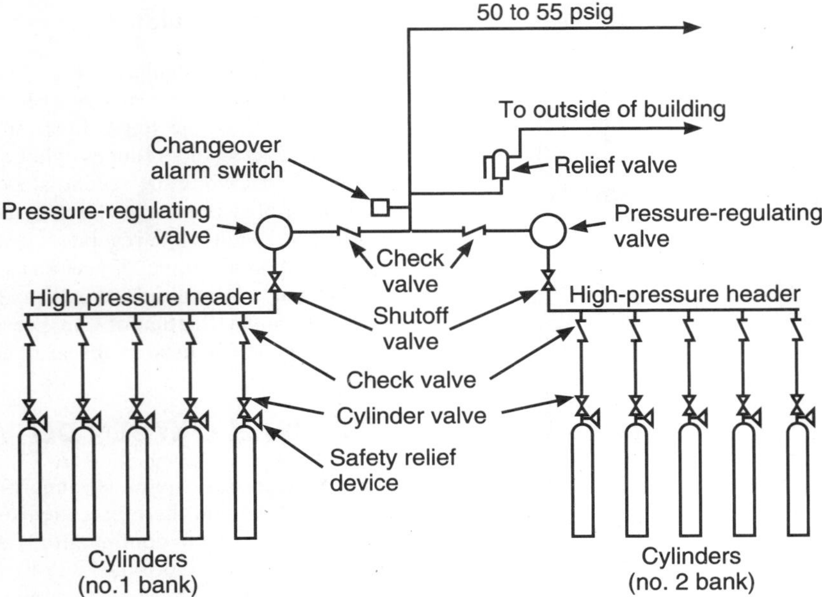

Figure 75-20. Alternating supply system is composed of primary and secondary supplies that alternate to charge the piping system. (From McPherson and Spearman,[11] with permission; © 1973 National Fire Protection Association, Boston.)

zone valves located in each patient care area, so that in the event of a leak or fire in that area the "zone" could be isolated. In addition, each zone, as well as the main gas feed line, is designed with system pressure alarms to ensure notification of a leak. Additional details regarding these systems are provided elsewhere.[10]

Gaseous Bulk Systems

There are three approaches used in a gaseous system. The first approach has a primary and secondary bank established by the side of the system in use at the time (Fig. 75-20). When gas pressure drops to a specific level, the bank switches to the secondary system. At the same time an alarm is activated and the primary bank is changed. The second approach is to use large fixed cylinders, also set up in a primary and secondary bank arrangement, which are filled on location from a liquid O_2 transport truck. The third system uses large trailer units, including up to 30 large cylinders, that are replaced in bulk. This system is frequently used as a back-up to a liquid system, or when system repairs are necessary.

Liquid Bulk Systems

Liquid O_2 systems (Fig. 75-21) are much more efficient than gaseous systems because 1 cu ft of liquid O_2 is equal to 860.6 cu ft of gaseous O_2, or 24,354.98 L of O_2. To store O_2 in liquid form it must be kept at a temperature below its critical temperature of −181.1°F and prevented from exerting a pressure greater than 250 psi (see Ch. 1). To accomplish this, large "thermos bottles" are used. The storage unit is composed of an inner and outer steel shell separated by an insulated vacuum to prevent transfer of heat to the liquid; the inner shell is coated with silver to aid in repelling heat. The unit is vented to allow vaporized O_2 to exit, maintaining internal pressure below 250 psi. Liquid O_2 leaving the storage unit is converted to gaseous O_2 by a vaporizer, after which its pressure is reduced to 50 psi for delivery into the central piping system. Both fixed stations with primary and secondary "tanks," as well as large, liquid-filled cylinders are currently available. As discussed in Chapters 99 and 100, liquid cylinders are commonly used in home care.

INDICATIONS FOR OXYGEN THERAPY*

As discussed in Chapter 11, O_2 is carried in blood and dissolved in plasma, as well as attached to hemoglobin, but to ensure O_2 availability to tissue, it must also be delivered to the tissue by the circulatory system. O_2 therapy can assist in preventing tissue hypoxia by reversing hypoxemia. In addition, O_2 therapy reduces the work of breathing, as well as the work of the myocardium.

---

* (Reproduced in part from Pierson,[43] with permission.)

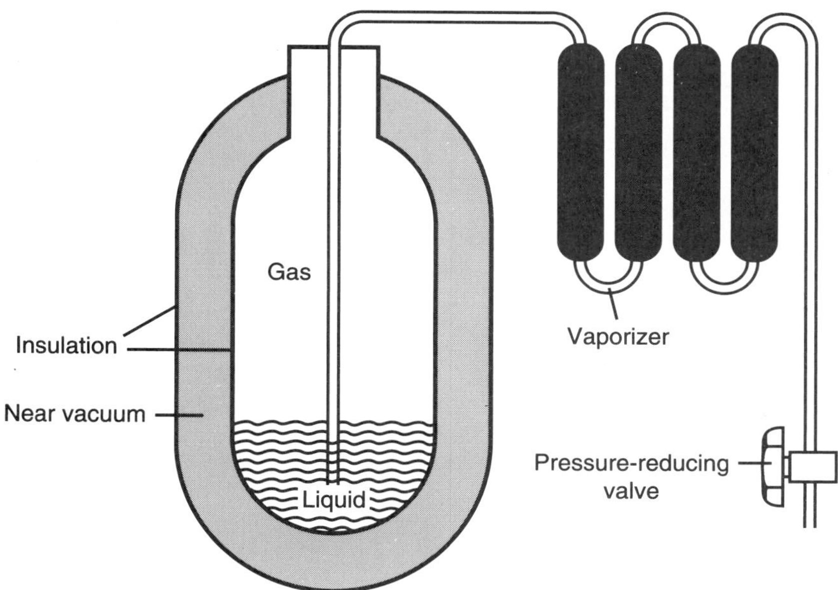

Figure 75-21. A liquid-O_2 system. (From McPherson and Spearman,[11] with permission.)

In general, O_2 therapy is only useful in reversing or preventing tissue hypoxia when the problem is hypoxemia. When diminished arterial O_2 content (CaO_2) is due to insufficient amounts of functioning hemoglobin, as in anemia, the administration of supplemental O_2 is of minimal benefit. When tissue hypoxia is caused by inadequate O_2 transport, the cause may be either failure to oxygenate the arterial blood, or failure to move it in sufficient quantity to the tissues. When the problem is a low cardiac output ($\dot{Q}_T$), further increases in PaO_2 will not correct the defect.

The classic example of failure of tissue O_2 utilization is cyanide poisoning, in which intracellular respiration is halted by the reaction of cyanide with cytochrome oxidase, which renders the cells incapable of using the O_2 presented to them. In cyanide poisoning, PaO_2, arterial O_2 saturation (SaO_2), CaO_2, and O_2 transport are all normal, but venous blood returns to the heart virtually unchanged because the tissues cannot use the O_2. Failure of tissue O_2 utilization can also be seen in septic shock, although the responsible mechanism is uncertain.

Causes of Hypoxemia

As shown in Table 75-10, there are four clinically important causes of hypoxemia.[3] Diffusion limitation is potentially a problem, but is not a cause of clinical hypoxemia, except perhaps during exercise at extreme altitude. Of the four, a reduced inspired O_2 tension is seldom a problem in clinical practice, although it is a possibility whenever patients become hypoxemic during supplemental O_2 therapy. For clinical purposes, the physiologic investigation of hypoxemia consists of distinguishing among alveolar hypoventilation, ventilation/perfusion ($\dot{V}/\dot{Q}$) mismatch, and right-to-left intrapulmonary shunt.

Alveolar hypoventilation causes hypoxemia because, as alveolar ventilation ($\dot{V}_A$) decreases, less and less O_2 is moved into the blood from each inspired breath. As this occurs, PaO_2 falls, concomitant with a rise in $PaCO_2$, which varies inversely with and can be considered a measure of $\dot{V}_A$. Because alveolar hypoventilation does not affect the alveolar-arterial oxygen tension difference [$P(A\text{-}a)O_2$], the fall in PaO_2 is of roughly the same magnitude as the rise in $PaCO_2$ (Fig. 75-22). This cause of clinical hypoxemia is thus easy to identify, as both $\dot{V}/\dot{Q}$ mismatch and right-to-left shunt increase the $P(A\text{-}a)O_2$, and in most clinical situations neither increases $PaCO_2$.

$\dot{V}/\dot{Q}$ mismatching and shunt can be distinguished clinically by their different responses to O_2 therapy.[12] This difference can be understood by examining how they cause hypoxemia (Fig. 75-23). As shown in Figure 75-23B, hypoxemia in $\dot{V}/\dot{Q}$ mismatch occurs because O_2 passes into the capillary blood faster than it can be replaced by $\dot{V}_A$ in the affected unit; therefore, the capillary blood leaves that unit incompletely saturated. Although ventilation to this region is reduced, it is still present to some degree, and correction of the hypoxemia can be achieved by raising the FIO_2, and hence the "driving pressure" of O_2 from the affected alveoli into the pulmonary capillaries, to the point at which the hemoglobin becomes fully saturated. Hypoxemia due to $\dot{V}/\dot{Q}$ mismatch is thus, in general, readily corrected by supplemental O_2 therapy. Hypoxemia due to this mechanism is typical in

Table 75-10. Effectiveness of Oxygen Therapy in Different Types of Tissue Hypoxia

Type of Defect	Mechanism of Tissue O_2 Deficiency	Clinical Examples	Supplemental O_2 Helpful?
Hypoxemia	Low inspired O_2 tension	High altitude, patient not receiving prescribed O_2	Yes
	Alveolar hypoventilation	Narcotic overdose, severe COPD, sleep apnea	Yes[a]
	$\dot{V}/\dot{Q}$ mismatch	COPD, asthma, diffuse lung disease	Yes
	Right-to-left shunt	Generalized cardiogenic pulmonary edema, ARDS Localized lobar pneumonia, acute atelectasis	Yes[b]
CaO_2	Hypoxemia, insufficient functional hemoglobin	See above; anemia, CO poisoning	No[c]
Decreased O_2 transport	Decreased CaO_2; decreased $\dot{Q}_T$	See above; cardiogenic shock, hemorrhagic shock, excessive PEEP	No
Decreased tissue O_2 use	Inadequate delivery of O_2 to hypoxic tissue bed	See above	
	Inability of tissues to use O_2	Cyanide poisoning	No

ARDS, adult respiratory distress syndrome; COPD, chronic obstructive pulmonary disease; PEEP, positive end-expiratory pressure; $\dot{V}/\dot{Q}$, ventilation/repufusion.

[a] Primary therapy is to increase alveolar ventilation.

[b] Improvement often minimal; other measures (PEEP, position changes, correction of primary problem) usually required.

[c] No clinically significant benefit from raising PaO_2 above 80–90 mmHg; if immediately available, hyperbaric O_2 therapy may temporarily reverse tissue hypoxia in selected circumstances.

(From Pierson,[43] with permission.)

chronic obstructive pulmonary disease (COPD), asthma, and diffuse lung diseases, such as interstitial pulmonary fibrosis.

Such is not the case with right-to-left shunt (Fig. 75-23C). Here, the affected alveoli are either collapsed or filled with edema, exudate, or blood, and hence they "see" no ventilation at all. Thus, raising the FIO_2, even to very high levels has virtually no effect on pure shunt, as hemoglobin in the normally ventilated units is already fully saturated with O_2, and hemoglobin in the shunt region still experiences no ventilation. Common clinical conditions in which hypoxemia shows these characteristics include generalized disorders, such as cardiogenic pulmonary edema and the adult respiratory distress syndrome (ARDS), and localized processes such as lobar pneumonia and acute lobar or whole-lung collapse. Improvement in severe hypoxemia due to right-to-left shunt generally requires measures in addition to supplemental O_2 administration, such as the use of positive end-expiratory pressure (PEEP) (see Ch. 76) in ARDS, and procedures to reinflate an acutely atelectatic lung (see Chs. 70, 73, and 74).

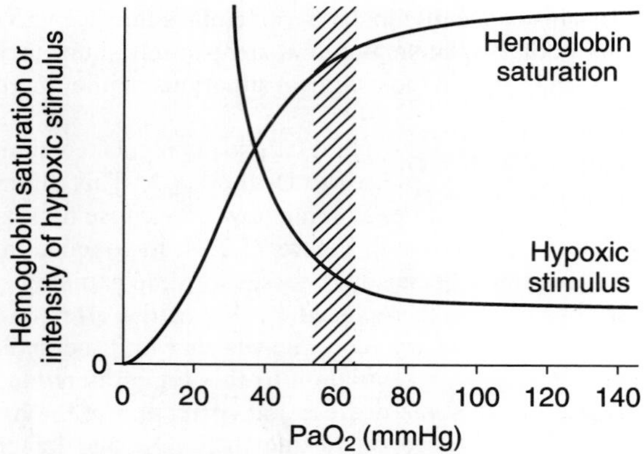

Figure 75-22. The approximately reciprocal relationship between $PaCO_2$ and PaO_2 when the $P(A\text{-}a)O_2$ does not change, as in hypoxemia due to alveolar hypoventilation. The PaO_2 falls about 1 mmHg for every 1 mmHg rise in $PaCO_2$; the opposite occurs when $\dot{V}_A$ is increased to correct the problem.

Distinguishing between V/Q mismatch and right-to-left shunt is important because it indicates the type and rigor of therapy that will likely be required to raise the PaO_2 out of the life-threatening range. Once severe hypoxemia is detected, O_2 therapy should be instituted promptly, and the PaO_2 response to this will identify which process is predominant. Table 75-11 provides hypothetical arterial blood gas results to illustrate how all three main causes of clinical hypoxemia—alveolar hypoventilation, $\dot{V}/\dot{Q}$ mismatch, and right-to-left shunt—respond to initial O_2 therapy.

Physiologic Basis for the Goals of Oxygen Therapy

In most patients with conditions for which O_2 therapy is physiologically appropriate, the goals of such therapy are derived directly from the shape of the oxyhemoglobin dis-

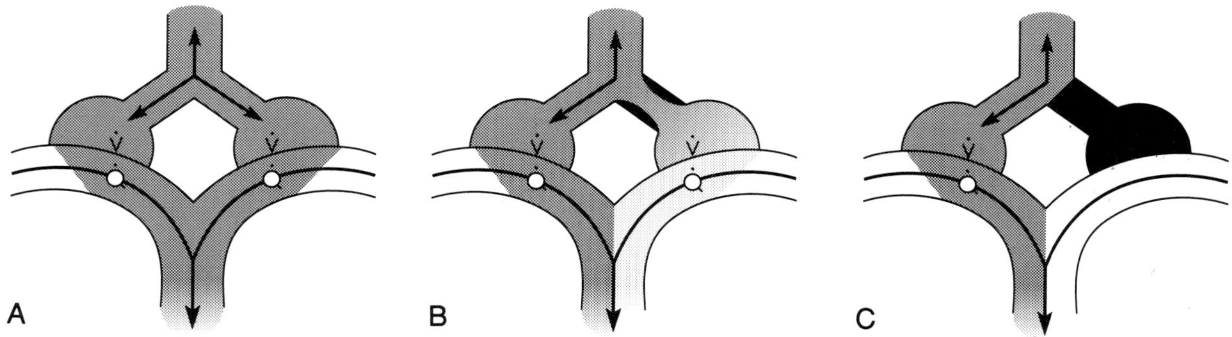

Figure 75-23. (A–C) Diagrammatic representation of $\dot{V}/\dot{Q}$ mismatch (Fig. B) and right-to-left shunt (Fig. C) as causes of hypoxemia, in relation to normal gas exchange (Fig. A). Whether the hypoxemia is readily correctable with supplemental O_2 depends on whether the abnormal lung units are ventilated, even to a relatively small degree. (See text for details.)

sociation curve. Enough O_2 should be given to saturate the available hemoglobin. With the exception of a few patients (see below), this means raising the PaO_2 to about 70 mmHg. Keeping the PaO_2 above around 100 mmHg produces no appreciable gain in blood oxygenation and runs the risk of exposing the patient to potentially toxic concentrations of O_2.

The exceptions just mentioned are patients who should be given less, not more, O_2 in the face of hypoxemia. These are generally certain individuals with severe COPD, who may develop life-threatening hypoventilation and respiratory acidosis in response to too much supplemental O_2.

Hypoxic drive is mediated by the peripheral chemoreceptors in the carotid bodies, which respond to PaO_2. At PaO_2 values above about 70 mmHg, there is little ventilatory drive from these receptors, and normally oxygenated persons are driven to breathe by $PaCO_2$ and other factors. As PaO_2 falls below about 60 to 65 mmHg, however, the hypoxic drive becomes more and more intense; in most individuals with PaO_2 values in the severely hypoxemia range (less than 50 mmHg), hypoxemia produces a strong stimulus to breathe. Some patients with COPD and certain other disorders have attenuated drives to hypercapnia, and are thus unusually dependent on their hypoxic drives to maintain adequate $\dot{V}_A$, especially during acute exacerbations. If such individuals are given enough supplemental O_2 to raise their PaO_2 to the point at which the hypoxic stimulus is removed, they may acutely hypoventilate.

As described below, it is therefore crucial that such individuals be administered O_2 with great caution, with care taken to preserve sufficient hypoxic drive to keep them breathing, while at the same time relieving life-threatening hypoxemia. It is, unfortunately, all too common for these patients to present to a medical care facility with acute respiratory distress, and be given too much O_2. This is followed quickly by somnolence and respiratory acidosis, which necessitates endotracheal intubation and mechanical ventilation, with all the attendant risks and disadvantages of these measures.[13]

Patients at Risk for Hyperoxic Respiratory Depression

As described above, certain patients with severe COPD, and occasionally other pulmonary diseases, should not be given O_2 as freely or in as large a dose as others. How can the clinician identify these patients in advance? Although there is no foolproof way, individuals most likely to develop hypoventilation in response to too much O_2 generally fit into the following categories:

1. Patients who have experienced this complication during previous acute episodes.
2. Patients with COPD and chronic hypoventilation (chronic CO_2 retention) who present with

Table 75-11. Response to Oxygen Therapy with Different Physiologic Mechanisms of Hypoxemia

Physiologic Mechanism	Clinical Example	$PaO_2/PaCO_2$	Treatment	$PaO_2/PaCO_2$
Alveolar hypoventilation	Narcotic drug overdose	50/70	Increase alveolar ventilation (no supplemental O_2)	80/40
$\dot{V}/\dot{Q}$ mismatch	Acute asthma attack	55/34	Nasal O_2, 2 L/min	80/38
Right-to-left shunt	Acute pulmonary edema	44/34	Nasal O_2, 2 L/min 100% O_2 by mask	46/34 52/35

(From Pierson,[43] with permission.)

acute respiratory decompensation and worsened hypoxemia.
3. Patients who fit the classic "blue bloater" stereotype, and who present with overt cor pulmonale (decompensated right-sided heart failure) and hypoxemia, but little or no dyspnea.
4. Patients with sleep apnea syndrome, especially those with daytime hypoventilation and hypersomnolence (pickwickian syndrome).
5. Other patients presenting with acute hypoxemia and hypersomnolence.

Patients are at risk for hyperoxic-induced hypoventilation during periods of acute decompensation, not when they are clinically stable. It is extremely rare for patients being started on long-term O_2 therapy, who are clinically stable, to experience clinically significant CO_2 retention when the O_2 is begun; the $PaCO_2$ may rise by 2 to 6 mmHg, but this is not enough to lower the arterial pH into a dangerous range.[14]

Although caution is warranted when administering O_2 to the patients described here, it is never justified to withhold O_2 therapy completely because of the risk of acute CO_2 retention. Severe hypoxemia (PaO_2 less than 50 mmHg in an acutely ill patient) is life-threatening, and should always be treated with O_2. If the patient is lethargic, uncooperative, or unresponsive, or becomes so during appropriate administration of O_2, endotracheal intubation may be required, but there is no safe alternative in such circumstances.

How can one give O_2 to such patients without suppressing their drive to breathe? The key is to work up to the target PaO_2 from below, rather than working down to it from above. This target level of oxygenation is a PaO_2 of at least 50, but less than 60 mmHg (Fig. 75-24). In Figure 75-24 the oxyhemoglobin dissociation curve is superimposed with the hypoxic ventilatory response curve, which shows how this PaO_2 range is related to the hypoxic drive to breathe. Although there is a certain amount of interindividual variability in hypoxic drive, keeping the PaO_2 in the mid-50s will avoid trouble in most cases.

In patients at risk for respiratory depression, O_2 should be started at 1 L/min by nasal prongs (a rare patient may even require 0.5 L/min), and the flow increased by increments of 0.5 L/min until the PaO_2 is at least 50 mmHg. A pediatric flowmeter is helpful at such times because it is calibrated in smaller gradations than the usual adult flowmeter, and it produces a more reliably constant O_2 flow. I prefer nasal cannulae to Venturi masks, because the latter inevitably prove difficult to keep on when the patient is dyspneic, and must be removed for eating, coughing, and such; nasal prongs guarantee a continuous flow of O_2, especially at such times, when the need for O_2 may be increased.

Patients should be monitored by arterial blood gas analysis during initial adjustments in O_2 therapy, rather than by pulse oximetry, because the changes in pH and $PaCO_2$ are as important as those in PaO_2. Once the required liter flow has been determined, pulse oximetry can be substituted as long as the patient is doing well clinically. Oxygenation should be assessed at least once daily during an acute illness requiring hospitalization, and blood gases should be measured

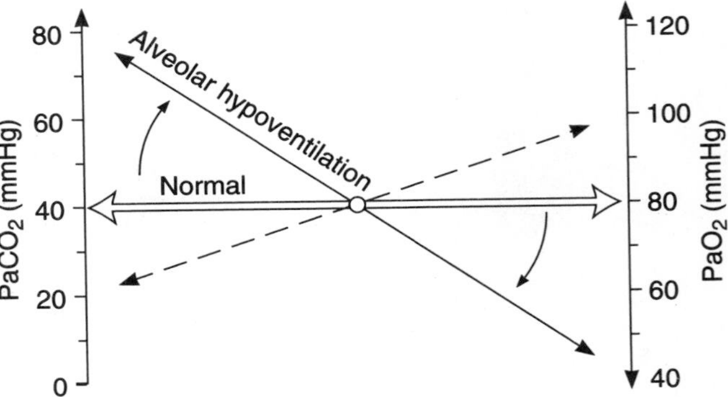

Figure 75-24. Conceptual superimposition of the oxyhemoglobin dissociation curve and the hypoxic ventilatory drive curve, showing the physiologic rationale for using an PaO_2 level of 50 to 60 mmHg as the "target" range for supplemental O_2 administration in patients at risk for acute CO_2 retention in response to too much O_2. A PaO_2 above 50 mmHg and not more than 60 mmHg will correct the immediate life-threatening aspect of acute hypoxemia, yet preserve enough hypoxic drive to prevent serious respiratory acidosis in most of these patients.

if unexplained tachycardia, tachypnea, or a change in mental status occurs.

In addition to O_2-induced hypoventilation, high concentrations of O_2 may be responsible for the development of nitrogen washout atelectasis (see Ch. 10), oxygen toxicity (see Ch. 35), or retinopathy of prematurity (see Ch. 88).

All Other Patients

Except in the case of the unusual individuals described above, the indications summarized in Table 75-11 apply to all hospitalized patients. A PaO_2 value below 50 mmHg, although admittedly arbitrary, has nonetheless been selected for sound physiologic reasons as an indication for supplemental O_2 in any patient. SaO_2, and hence CaO_2, drop off rapidly as PaO_2 falls progressively below 50 mmHg, which is at the top of the steep portion of the S-shaped oxyhemoglobin dissociation curve. The other components of O_2 transport should be recalled, and might dictate initiation of O_2 therapy at a higher PaO_2 value (e.g., in the presence of anemia or cardiac failure).

The indications for O_2 therapy in patients who are not hypoxemic are a bit less firm. As shown in Table 75-12, it seems prudent to supply an "O_2 reserve" when a patient is to undergo a procedure likely to induce hypoxemia. In certain conditions, such as acute asthma and sickle-cell crisis, there is theoretic justification for O_2 therapy, although studies directly demonstrating this benefit are lacking. In other situations, however, such as acute cerebrovascular accident, the postoperative period, and after trauma, it is even less clear whether the potential benefit from supplemental O_2 is worth its cost.

Table 75-12. Indications for Oxygen Therapy in Hospitalized Patients

Hypoxemia
PaO_2 <50 mmHg (SaO_2 <80%), while awake, in any patient
PaO_2 <55–60 mmHg (SaO_2 <85–89%) in any acutely ill patient
Substantial risk for developing hypoxemia
During endotracheal intubation
Bronchoscopy
Nasotracheal or endotracheal suctioning
Other procedures involving the airways, requiring positioning that impairs thoracic or abnormal excursion, or otherwise compromising respiration
Conditions in which supplemental O_2 is traditionally given, even in the absence of hypoxemia[a]
Acute asthma
Sickle-cell crisis
Acute myocardial infarction

[a] Benefits of O_2 therapy in these conditions are uncertain, and these indications are disputed by some clinicians.

(From Pierson,[43] with permission.)

A PaO_2 value in the range of 80 to 90 mmHg would seem ideal during O_2 therapy. For practical purposes it provides complete hemoglobin saturation, as well as a certain "safety margin" for patients whose oxygenation may fluctuate to a certain degree, as it does in those sufficiently ill to be in an intensive care unit (ICU).[15] However, for the physiologic reasons explained previously, there is little justification for maintaining the PaO_2 level of the patient above this range.

The oxygenation of patients should be checked once daily, and the therapy discontinued once it is no longer needed. A clinically stable and improving patient with a room air PaO_2 of 60 to 70 mmHg or higher (SaO_2 more than 90 percent) can safely have supplemental O_2 discontinued.

METHODS OF OXYGEN DELIVERY IN THE HOSPITAL*

> Oxygen makes up nearly 50 percent of the mass of this planet. It is a powerful therapeutic tool, yet it has been one of the most misused and abused remedies in medicine. Currently, its use still rarely conforms to the most elementary rational rules of therapeutics—that is, that a substance is given in a known dosage in a manner which produces a sustained optimal blood level.
> Julian M. Leigh, 1973[16]

In many respects this statement, presented to the Royal College of Surgeons, is still reflective of current medical practice regarding O_2 therapy. Even though O_2 is a drug widely used in the treatment of cardiopulmonary disease, provision of precise, consistent concentrations is rarely achieved. In fact, the methodology used to deliver O_2 to hospitalized adults has changed little over the last 20 years.

* (Reproduced in part from Kacmarek,[44] with permission.)

Classification of Delivery Systems

Equipment available to provide O_2 therapy to spontaneously breathing adults is normally classified into two groups: low-flow or variable performance equipment, and high-flow or fixed performance equipment.[1,17] Low-flow systems only provide a portion of the gas volume to be inspired, whereas high-flow systems provide the entire minute ventilation. With low-flow systems, the F_IO_2 provided is based on (1) the liter flow of O_2; (2) the size of the equipment reservoir (e.g., volume of a face mask); (3) the size of the anatomic reservoir (volume of nasal and oral pharynx); (4) the capability of filling the reservoir during the transition from exhalation to inspiration; and (5) the ventilatory pattern of the patient. Thus, the F_IO_2 varies, not only with alterations of liter flow for a given apparatus, but also with changes in ventilatory pattern. As a result, it is virtually impossible to specify the precise F_IO_2 a patient is receiving, nor is it possible to specify with any degree of accuracy the F_IO_2 a low-flow system delivers at a specific flow rate.

Shapiro et al.[17] have attempted to calculate the F_IO_2 level provided by various low-flow systems (Table 75-13) by assuming (1) a 50 mL volume of the anatomic reservoir; (2) the anatomic reservoir is filled with 100 percent O_2 during the transition between expiration and inspiration; and (3) a specific consistent ventilatory pattern (e.g., rate, 20 breaths per minute's tidal volume [V_T], 500 mL; inspiratory/expiratory [I/E] ratio, 1:2) is maintained. Application of these assumptions to the low-flow systems presented here forms the basis for the outlined F_IO_2 levels theoretically available at a given flow setting. However, it is imperative that clinicians realize that these F_IO_2 values are only gross guidelines, because increases or decreases in minute ventilation and alterations in ventilating pattern can markedly change *actual* delivered F_IO_2 (Table 75-13).

Conversely, high-flow systems provide a precise and consistent F_IO_2, independent of alterations in ventilatory pattern. To ensure a constant F_IO_2, system flow must exceed 3 to 4 times the measured minute volume, or, more importantly, peak inspiratory flow rates.[18] Because peak inspiratory flows during marked cardiopulmonary stress may exceed 80 to 100 L/min,[19] it is doubtful that even those systems classified as high flow are capable of meeting ventilatory demands of every patient under all circumstances. In most stable patients peak inspiratory flow averages approximately 30 to 40 L/min[19]; thus it is doubtful that any system providing less than 40 L/min functions as a high-flow system unless the system is closed (entrainment of room air impossible) and a sufficient reservoir is included.

Low-Flow Oxygen Systems

As previously defined, low-flow O_2 systems do not provide the entire inspired environment of the patient, but rely on reservoirs and volume of entrained room air to determine their delivered F_IO_2 levels. The four most commonly used low-flow systems are the nasal cannula, the simple mask

Table 75-13. Estimation of F_{IO_2} from Low-Flow Systems

Cannula	6 L/min	V_T	500 mL
Mechanical reservoir	None	I/E ratio	1:2
Anatomic reservoir	50 mL	Rate	20/min
100% O_2 provided per second	100 mL	Inspiratory time	1 sec

Volume inspired O_2[a]	
Anatomic reservoir	50 mL
Flow/s	100 mL
Inspired room air[a]	70 mL
O_2 inspired	220 mL

$$F_{IO_2} = \frac{220 \text{ mL } O_2}{500 \text{ mL } V_T} = 0.44$$

If V_T is decreased to 250 mL — Volume inspired O_2	
Anatomic reservoir	50 mL
Flow/s	100 mL
Inspired room air[b]	20 mL
O_2 inspired	170 mL

$$F_{IO_2} = \frac{170 \text{ mL } O_2}{250 \text{ mL } V_T} = 0.64$$

If V_T increased to 1000 mL — Volume inspired O_2	
Anatomic reservoir	50 mL
Flow/s	100 mL
Inspired room air[c]	170 mL
O_2 inspired	320 mL

$$F_{IO_2} = \frac{320 \text{ mL } O_2}{1000 \text{ mL } V_T} = 0.32$$

[a] Since 150 mL of 100% O_2 is inspired, the remainder of V_T is room air (350 mL), 20% of 350 mL = 70 mL—amount of O_2 in room air that is inspired.

[b] 20% of 250 − 150.

[c] 20% of 1000 − 150.

(From Kacmarek,[44] with permission.)

(without reservoir bag), the partial rebreathing mask and the so-called non-rebreathing mask (Table 75-14).

Nasal Cannula

The most commonly employed O_2 therapy delivery device is the O_2 cannula (Fig. 75-1). Because the nasal cannula is a low-flow device, the F_{IO_2} provided at a given flow rate may change dramatically from patient to patient, as well as from hour to hour in a given patient. Numerous authors have attempted to analyze the F_{IO_2} provided by a nasal cannula, and concentrations varying from 23 to 60 percent have been noted[20,21,22] at O_2 flows of 1 to 10 L/min. However, even wider ranges may be noted at extremes of ventilatory patterns. Shallow breathing, with small minute ventilations, may even increase delivered F_{IO_2} at moderate flow rates (5 L/min) to greater than 0.60.[17] A reasonable estimate of theoretic F_{IO_2} levels with nasal cannulae is provided in Table 75-15. The values listed are based on the assumptions outlined in Table 75-13. It must be remembered that these values are gross estimates and subject to vast changes, based on alterations in ventilatory patterns. Maximum efficiency of the nasal cannula does not require exclusive nasal breathing. Kory et al.[22] in 1962 demonstrated equivalent PaO_2 between nasal and oral breathing with constant O_2 flows. However, patency of the nasal pharynx must be ensured. The ability of the nasal cannula to increase F_{IO_2} levels peaks at about 6 L/min. This, coupled with increasing complaints of drying of the nasal mucosa and bleeding, have limited the maximum delivered flow from a nasal cannula to 6 L/min.

The nasal cannula is generally considered very comfortable by most patients; however, pressure sores at the crease between the ear and skull, across the maxilla, and on the nasal septum may develop.[1,17,18]

Table 75-14. Classification of Oxygen Delivery Systems

Low-flow systems	Cannula Simple mask Partial rebreathing mask Nonrebreathing mask[a]
High-flow systems[b]	Venturi masks Aerosol systems Large-volume aerosol systems

[a] The disposable nonrebreathing mask is not tight fitting and thus entrainment of room air normally occurs.

[b] For a system to be considered high-flow, it must provide ≥40 L/min flow.

(From Kacmarek,[44] with permission.)

Simple Mask

Of the various types of O_2 masks, the simple mask (Fig. 75-25) is the one most commonly used. Normally, only one size of mask is manufactured, which limits the efficiency of the mask on very large or very small faces. Generally, the poorer the mask fit, the greater the volume of air entrained between the mask and the patient's face. However, even with a well-fitting mask, F_{IO_2} levels vary greatly with ventilatory pattern, as noted with other low-flow systems. These masks are designed to be used with flows of at least 5 L/min. Flows at this level are necessary to clear exhaled gas from the mask and to prevent rebreathing of CO_2. With proper fit and a standard ventilatory pattern (Table 75-13),

Table 75-15. Theoretical F_{IO_2} Via Nasal Cannula[a]

L/min	F_{IO_2}
1	0.24
2	0.28
3	0.32
4	0.36
5	0.40
6	0.44

[a] These F_{IO_2} values are estimated, based on the assumptions listed in Table 75-13. Actual F_{IO_2} is greatly influenced by ventilatory patterns.

(From Kacmarek,[44] with permission.)

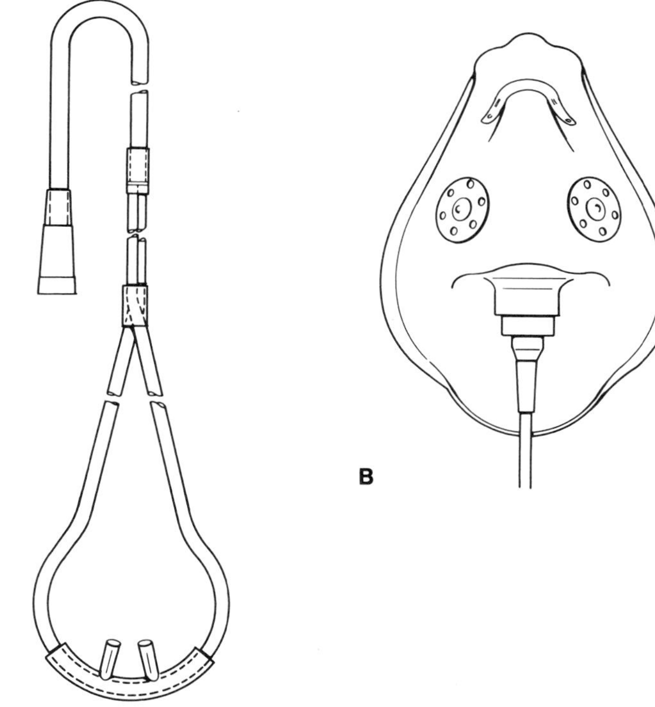

Figure 75-25. **(A)** Nasal cannula. **(B)** Simple O_2 mask. (From Kacmarek,[18] with permission.)

F_{IO_2} levels higher than those achieved with a nasal cannula are obtained (Table 75-16).

The maximum achievable F_{IO_2} level with a simple mask peaks at about 10 to 12 L/min because of the size of the mask reservoir. In addition, because peak inspiratory flow rates significantly exceed the liter flow capability to the mask, flows higher than about 12 L/min do not enhance F_{IO_2} levels.

Problems associated with simple masks are similar to those with nasal cannulae, pressure sores on the face and ear, but also include an increased potential for aspiration. Many patients complain that masks are hot and claustrophobic and, as a result, compliance may be low even during periods of marked hypoxemia. Finally, some patients complain of eye irritation, either as a result of the gas flow leaking at the bridge of the nose, or because the mask itself causes irritation.

Table 75-16. Theoretical F_{IO_2} Via Simple Mask, Partial Rebreathing Mask, and Non-Rebreathing Mask[a]

Mask	L/min	F_{IO_2}
Simple	≥5	0.40–0.60
Partial rebreathing	≥8	≥0.60
Nonrebreathing	≥10	≥0.80

[a] These F_{IO_2} values are estimated, based on the assumptions listed in Table 75-13. Actual F_{IO_2} is greatly influenced by ventilatory pattern.

(From Kacmarek,[44] with permission.)

Partial Rebreathing Mask

The partial rebreathing mask (Fig. 75-26) consists of a simple mask and, normally, a 1.0-L reservoir bag. It is classified as a partial rebreathing mask because there is no one-way valve between the mask and the reservoir bag, nor is there a one-way valve at the exhalation ports of the mask. During inspiration, O_2 is inspired from the mask, the reservoir bag, and the gas flow entering the system, while room air is entrained from the atmosphere. During exhalation, the first portion of the exhaled V_T enters the bag. Because this is dead space gas, no CO_2 enters the bag. The remainder of the exhaled volume exits the mask through the exhalation ports. If system flow is high enough to prevent the reservoir bag from deflating by more than half its volume during inhalation, no CO_2 accumulates during exhalation. However, accumulation of CO_2 in the reservoir bag and the mask can be expected if the bag deflates by more than half its capacity during inspiration. This mask provides greater than 60 percent O_2 if set up properly. A minimum of 8 L/min O_2 flow (Table 75-16) should enter the bag; however, in some patients, flows exceeding 15 L/min are required. Problems identified with the use of this mask are similar to those noted with simple masks.

Non-Rebreathing Mask

Ideally, a non-rebreathing mask should prevent entrainment of room air and deliver 100 percent O_2. This was pos-

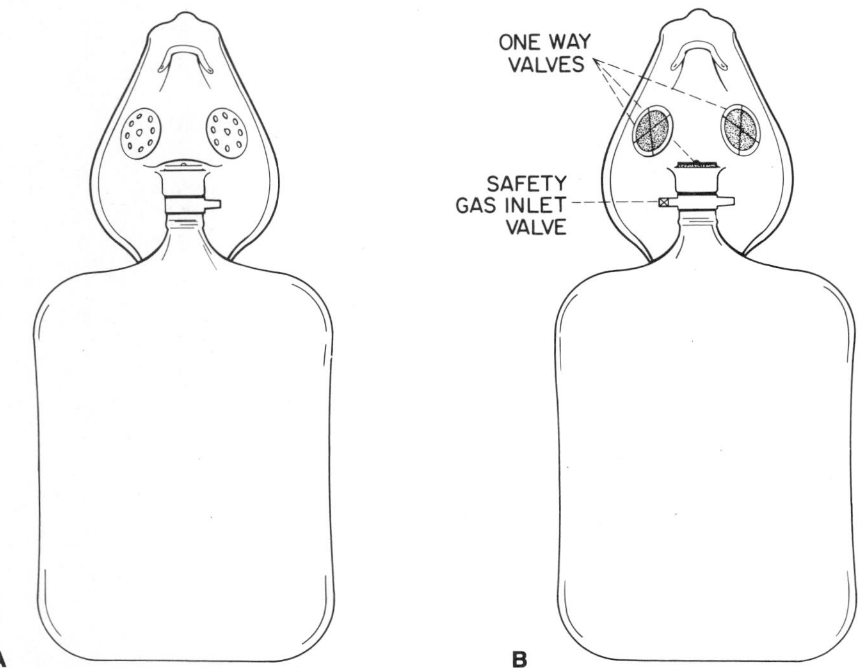

Figure 75-26. (**A**) Partial rebreathing mask and (**B**) nonbreathing mask. (From Kacmarek,[18] with permission.)

sible in certain patients with the old Boothby Lovelace Bulbulian (BLB) masks.[23] These were tight-fitting, non-disposable masks with spring-loaded exhalation valves capable of creating an expiratory retard. However, these masks were very hot and claustrophobic and greatly increased the risk of aspiration. As a result, they have given way to disposable non-rebreathing masks, which are usually capable of maintaining 80 percent or greater F_IO_2 levels.[24] Non-rebreathing masks have a one-way valve between the mask and the reservoir bag, as well as one-way valves at the exhalation ports of the mask (Fig. 75-26). In addition, a safety gas inlet valve is included at the attachment of the mask to the bag. With optimal operation, during the inspiratory phase the patient inspires gas from the mask, the bag, through the inlet valve, and from between the mask and the patient's face, if necessary. If available O_2 exceeds patient demand, only gas from the mask and bag are inspired. During the expiratory phase, all exhaled gas exits the mask. One-way valves and gas flow into the system should be great enough to ensure a flushing of the mask with 100 percent O_2 before the next inspiration. Proper operation normally requires a flow of at least 10 L/min, but usually requires flows in excess of 15 L/min. As a result of claustrophobia, compliance is good only for short periods, unless constant supervision is maintained. Problems associated with this mask are the same as those noted with the simple O_2 mask.

Humidifiers and Low-Flow Systems

Because O_2 from central gas delivery systems or tanks is dry, the addition of water vapor before delivery to the airway is normally provided. Bubble-diffusion humidifiers (Fig. 75-27) are normally used with low-flow O_2 systems. A relative humidity of about 60 to 100 percent at the exit port of the humidifier is normally achieved at a temperature 2 to 5°F below atmospheric temperature. This temperature differential is a result of heat loss from the heat of evaporation as O_2 bubbles through the humidifier. Three factors affect the efficiency of humidifiers: (1) the surface area of exposure between the gas and water; (2) the time the gas and water are in contact; and (3) the temperature of the system. Because gas leaves the humidifier at a temperature below atmosphere, when the gas is heated to body temperature, a relative humidity of about 35 to 40 percent is achieved. Thus, only a small volume of water vapor is added to the inspired gas by the standard bubble-diffusion humidifier. For this reason it can be argued that, at flow rates of 4 L/min or less with nasal cannulae, use of humidifiers can be eliminated.[25–28] Campbell et al.[26] have reported no difference in patients' subjective evaluation of comfort, with or without a humidifier, when O_2 is delivered at no more than 4 L/min using a nasal cannula. Specifically, no differences between the frequency of dry nose, dry throat, headache, chest discomfort, common cold symptoms, or sputum production alterations were noted. We therefore support the ACCP-NHLBI[28] recommendation that nasal O_2 at no more than 4 L/min need not be humidified. Because all other low-flow O_2 systems require flows of greater than 4 L/min, bubble-diffusion humidifiers should always be used with these appliances.

High-Flow Systems

High-flow O_2 delivery systems provide a patient's entire inspired minute volume. Generally, three apparatus are clas-

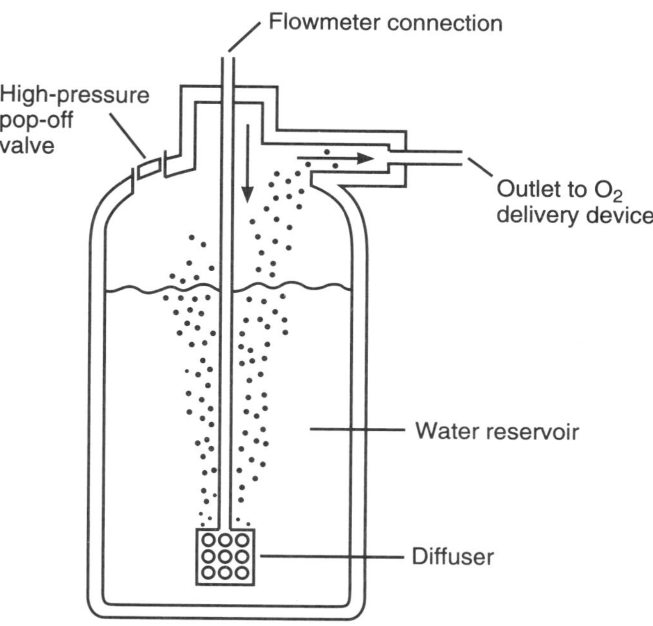

Figure 75-27. Bubble diffusion humidifier. (From Op't Hold,[45] with permission.)

sified as high-flow: (1) air entrainment masks; (2) large-volume aerosol systems; and (3) large-volume humidifier systems (Table 75-14).

Air Entrainment Masks

Also referred to as Venturi masks, air entrainment masks mix a specific volume of room air with every liter of O_2 flow through the mask (Fig. 75-28). O_2 under pressure is forced through a small nozzle on entering the mask. As a result, its velocity increases markedly, creating a jet drag or shearing effect, distal to the nozzle, which causes room air to be entrained into the mask (see Ch. 1).[25,26] The resulting F_{IO_2} is dependent on the size of the nozzle and the size of the entrainment ports. Thus, systems can be designed to provide very specific F_{IO_2} levels and deliver a specific gas volume to the patient's face (Fig. 75-29). With this system, the size of the entrainment port is constant, while the size of the nozzle is altered to ensure a specific entrainment ratio, a precise F_{IO_2}, and a delivery of a fixed gas volume. Aerosol entrainment collars are also available to allow entrainment of an aerosol instead of room air. However, because of the increased density of the aerosol, the F_{IO_2} provided by a specific nozzle tends to increase during aerosol entrainment. Entrainment mask systems are manufactured to deliver up to 50 percent F_{IO_2} (Table 75-17). It must be remembered that, for any of these systems to function as high-flow systems, at least 40 L/min must be delivered to the patient's face. Even this flow may be inadequate in patients with high ventilatory drives, for in critically ill patients, peak inspiratory rates may exceed 100 L/min.[29,30] The recommended minimal flows listed in Table 75-17 may be exceeded, and it is frequently necessary to deliver higher O_2 flows with the 28 to 40 percent systems to ensure adequate delivered total gas volume. As for systems delivering F_{IO_2} levels greater than 0.40, rarely do these systems operate as true high-flow systems because of their small entrainment ratios (1:1.7 or less). Finally, because these units are all mass-produced and disposable, the consistency of F_{IO_2} delivery between units may vary by up to 3 to 5 percent.[31,32]

Bubble-through humidifiers are normally not recommended for use with air entrainment masks because most gas flow (40 percent or less O_2 system) is room air and the patient's upper airway is intact. Problems associated with these systems include irritation of the face, ears, and eyes, an increased potential for aspiration, and poor compliance.

Large-Volume Aerosol Systems

Large-volume aerosol systems incorporate either disposable or nondisposable large-volume aerosol nebulizers and increased delivered gas volume, and vary F_{IO_2} by gas entrainment, as described in the previous section. Most nondisposable aerosol systems have fixed available F_{IO_2} levels (0.40, 0.60, and 1.0), whereas most disposable units provide a complete spectrum of available F_{IO_2} levels (0.21 to 1.0) by varying the size of the entrainment port. Each is designed with a fixed jet orifice. In addition to precise F_{IO_2} levels, these units can provide gas 100 percent humidified at body temperature, along with an aerosol. Figure 75-30 depicts the setup of these units as either single or tandem units. Tandem units are frequently used when high-flow and high F_{IO_2} levels are needed, because, as with air entrainment masks, a total flow of greater than 40 L/min is needed to ensure con-

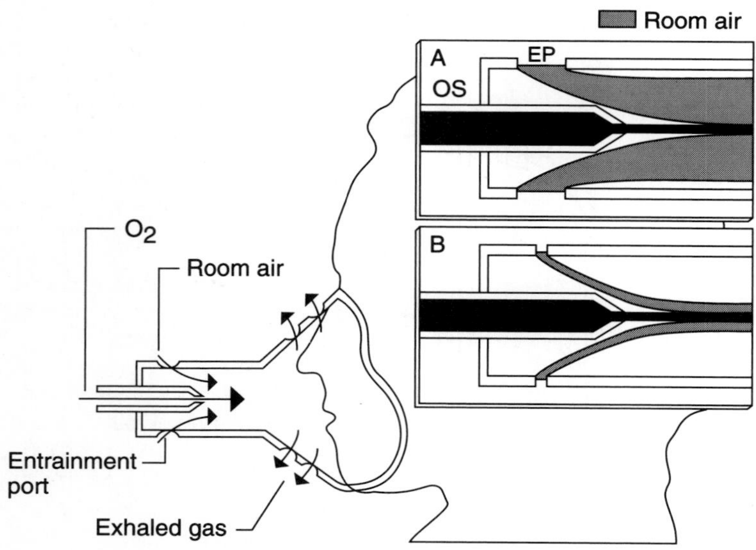

Figure 75-28. Principle of an air entrainment device. Pressurized O_2 is forced through a nozzle (constricted orifice); the increased gas velocity distal to the orifice creates a jet drag or shearing effect that causes room air to be entrained through the entrainment ports. The high flow of gas fills the mask (which has holes), allowing both exhaled and delivered gas to escape. **(A & B)** The size of the entrainment ports (EP) determines the amount of room air to be entrained; large ports, result in relatively higher F_IO_2 (Fig. A). For any size entrainment port, the F_IO_2 is stable; however, the total gas flow will vary with the pressurized O_2 flow. OS, O_2 source. (From Shapiro et al.,[17] with permission.)

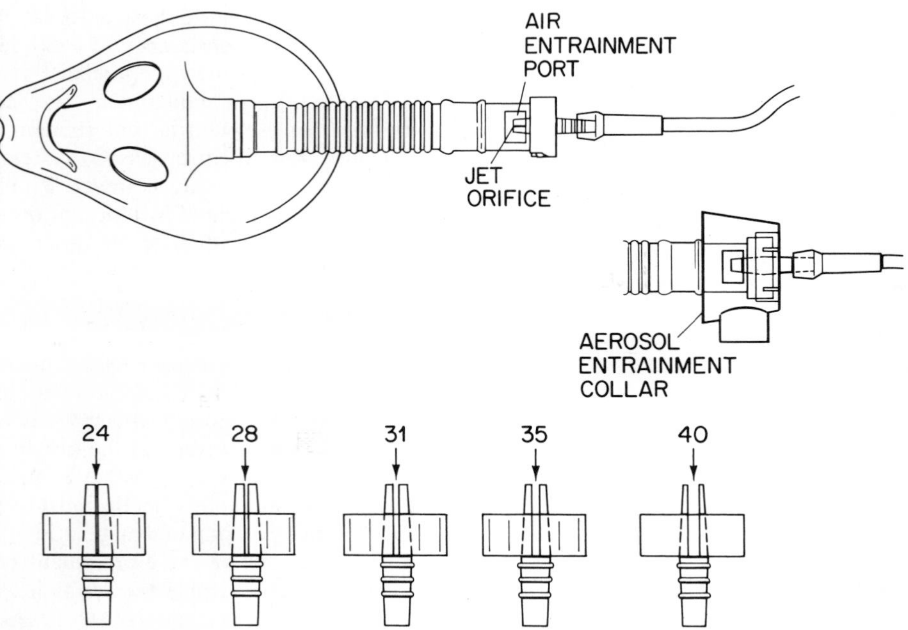

Figure 75-29. Depiction of an air entrainment mask, which operates the same as those in Fig. 75-28, except in this style the size of the entrainment port remains constant and various sized nozzles are available. Alteration of nozzle diameters alters the magnitude of the jet drag effect and entrainment ratio. (From Kacmarek,[18] with permission.)

Table 75-17. Entrainment Ratios and Outputs of Specific Air Entrainment Systems[a]

O_2/Air Entrainment Ratio	Minimal O_2 Flow	Total Flow[b]	FIO_2
1:25	4	104	0.24
1:10	4	44	0.28
1:7	6	48	0.31
1:5	8	48	0.35
1:3	8	32	0.40
1:1.7	12	32	0.50
1:1	12	24	0.60
1:0.6	12	19	0.70

[a] Variations in delivered FIO_2 may occur because systems are disposable.

[b] For the system to be classified high-flow, ≥40 L/min must be provided.

(From Kacmarek,[44] with permission.)

sistent and precise FIO_2 delivery. Normally, units are left unheated if they are delivered by face mask or head hood (Fig. 75-31). Most patients do not tolerate inspiring heated moist air through an intact upper airway; however, it is usually necessary to provide gas heated to near body temperature (33 to 37°C) when these systems are attached to artificial airways. Continuous monitoring of airway temperature should be maintained close to the attachment to the artificial airway. When precise FIO_2 levels must be maintained, a Briggs T-piece, with reservoir, is used. However, if small variations in FIO_2 can be tolerated and a tracheostomy tube is in place, a tracheostomy collar is preferred. The tracheostomy collar eliminates torque on the tracheostomy tube and decreases irritation of the trachea, but is easily displaced from the tracheostomy site. This system is limited by the flow capability of the nebulizer systems. A tandem setup is normally required if FIO_2 levels greater than 0.40 to 0.50 are needed. Problems with these systems are the same as those with all mask delivery systems.

Large-Volume Humidifier Systems

The most accurate and precise method of delivering O_2 outside of a ventilator or continuous positive airway pressure (CPAP) system is the use of a large-volume humidifier (Fig. 75-32). With these systems, blended gas at any FIO_2 (0.21 to 1.0) level is delivered at flow rates of up to 150 L/min through a large-volume humidifier (e.g., Puritan-Bennett-Cascade, Kansas City, KS). Gas then is transported by large-bore aerosol tubing to the patient. These systems can be heated or cooled and attached to an artificial airway or face mask. When attached to an artificial airway, a 10 to 15 in. reservoir tube is normally used to ensure room air is not entrained through the open port of the Briggs T-piece. The major drawback of these systems is the noise created as gas flows exceeding 80 to 100 L/min move through the system. Commonly, an O_2 analyzer and 3- to 5-L reservoir bag are added to the system.

Clinical Applications

When decisions are contemplated regarding O_2 delivery systems, the following questions should be addressed: (1)

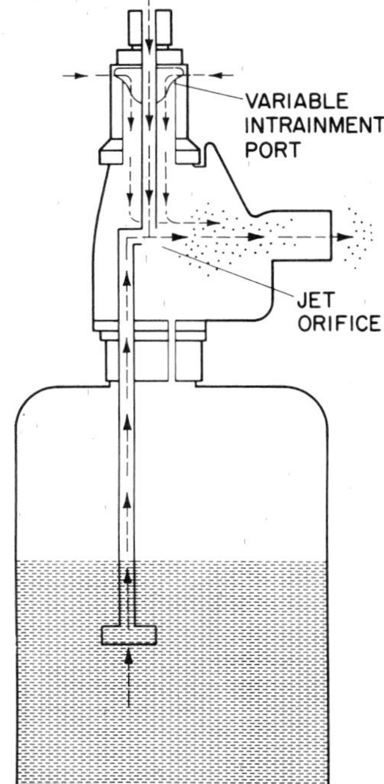

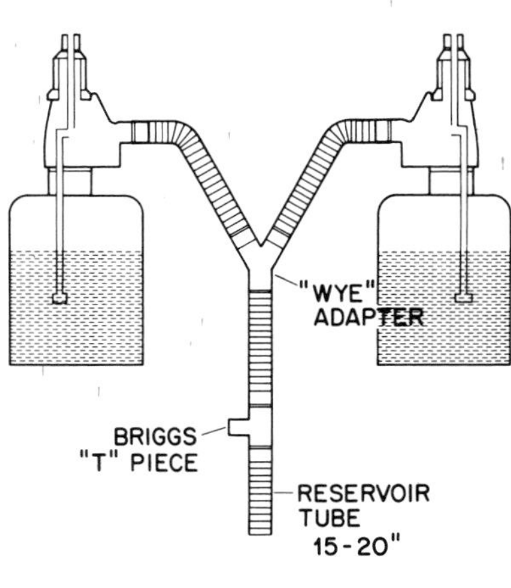

Figure 75-30. Mechanical aerosol delivery systems: single and tandem set-ups. (From Kacmarek,[18] with permission.)

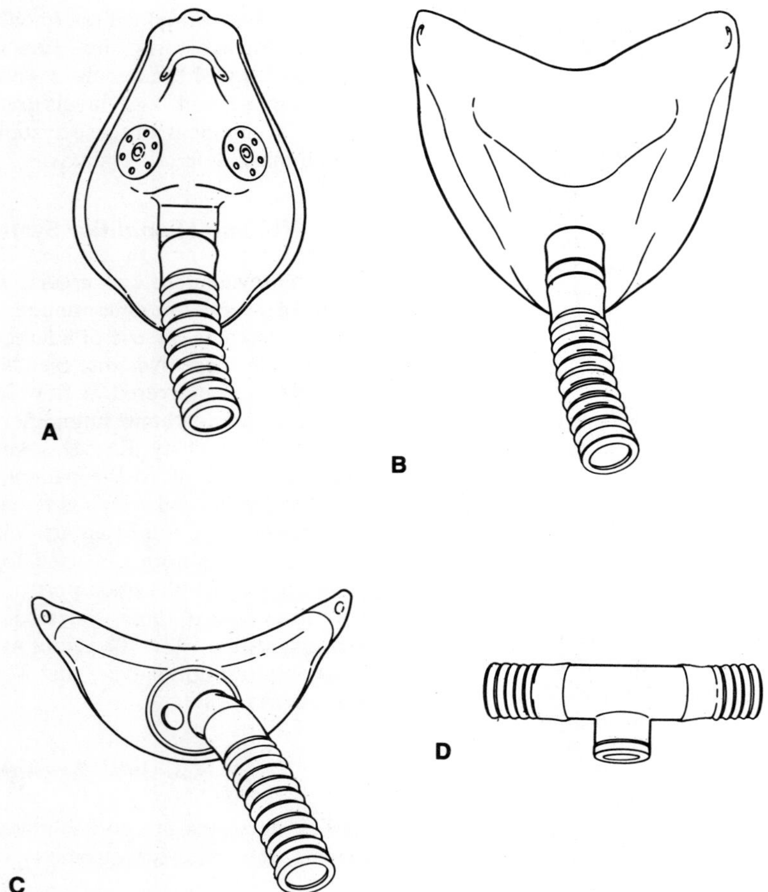

Figure 75-31. Aerosol delivery appliances. **(A)** Facemask; **(B)** head hood; **(C)** tracheostomy collar; and **(D)** Briggs T-piece. (From Kacmarek,[18] with permission.)

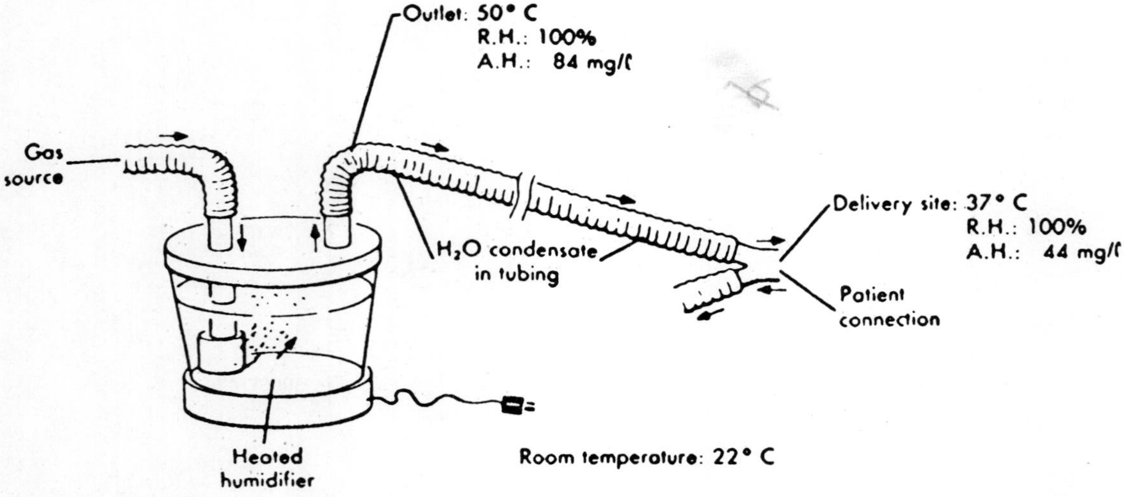

Figure 75-32. Large-volume humidifier system capable of providing heated or cool high-flow gas. (From Thalken,[41] with permission.)

What F_{IO_2} is needed? (2) Is consistency and accuracy of F_{IO_2} required? (3) Is there a need for high humidity? (4) Is an artificial airway present? and (5) Is tolerance and compliance a problem? Although the last question seems to deviate from concerns regarding the ideal approach, it may be the most critical question to answer, for regardless of how precise and accurate a delivery system is, it does not function optimally if not worn. For this reason, in patients without artificial airways, the O_2 cannula is the most frequently used apparatus. However, if compliance can be assured, the vital question becomes whether precise and accurate F_{IO_2} levels are needed.

Even though high-flow systems can be delivered to patients without artificial airways, we prefer to use low-flow systems. Patient tolerance and compliance with high-flow systems are normally low unless constantly monitored. As a result, the nasal cannula is the system we most commonly employ with this group. Even with patients with COPD, in whom the use of an air entrainment mask would seem ideal, we frequently use a nasal cannula. These patients are very claustrophobic, have a difficult time keeping the mask in place, and must take the mask off for eating, shaving, and oral hygiene. If patients tolerate an air entrainment mask, if they have frequent changes in their ventilatory pattern, and if small changes in F_{IO_2} affect their $PaCO_2$, we use the air entrainment mask. However, most non-intensive care, non-emergency patients are easily maintained on nasal cannula.

In the emergency department we use a simple O_2 mask or a partial rebreathing mask for immediate application of F_{IO_2} levels unobtainable with a cannula. Most of these patients requiring high F_{IO_2} levels are sent to the ICU; some are intubated. In the ICU we prefer the use of a high-flow system. Air entrainment masks or unheated mechanical aerosol systems are normally used if low F_{IO_2} levels are needed. In these cases, we base our decisions on the need for supplemental humidity. If high F_{IO_2} (greater than 0.40) is needed, we prefer high-flow humidifier systems.

In the recovery room, an unheated mechanical aerosol system with either a face mask or a face hood is ideal, depending on the need for O_2 and patient tolerance.

Only high-flow systems are adaptable to artificial airways. Compliance is normally not a concern with these patients, but comfort is important. If an endotracheal tube is in place, attachment to the system is always by way of a Briggs T-piece; however, with the tracheostomy tubes, a Briggs T-piece or tracheostomy mask can be used. If accurate and consistent F_{IO_2} is required, we always use a Briggs T-piece with reservoir. However, if heated humidified gas is the primary concern, with constant and accurate F_{IO_2} unnecessary, we use a tracheostomy collar to increase patient comfort. When 40 percent O_2 or less is needed, either an aerosol system or a high-flow humidifier system may be employed. We prefer the aerosol system because of ease of setup and maintenance and because of its ability to humidify the airway. When an F_{IO_2} above 0.40 is required, mechanical aerosol systems become impractical, even tandem setups. In this situation we use a high-flow humidifier system because of its accuracy, versatility, and flow capacity.

USE OF 100 PERCENT OXYGEN

Finally, when should we use 100 percent O_2? In spite of widespread concern regarding O_2-induced hypoventilation, absorption atelectasis, and the development of O_2 toxicity, 100 percent O_2 is indicated when marked concern regarding tissue hypoxia arises (i.e., 100 percent O_2 is indicated during cardiac arrest, transport, acute cardiopulmonary instability, and whenever carboxyhemoglobin levels are greater than 10 percent). However, once stabilization is achieved, the F_{IO_2} should be reduced to the lowest level that maintains an acceptable PO_2 for a given patient.

MONITORING OXYGEN THERAPY

One must be careful to evaluate the overall effect of O_2 therapy on the entire cardiopulmonary system when determining its efficacy. As noted in Table 75-18, profound changes in cardiopulmonary status may be noted, in spite of relatively minor changes in PO_2 or SaO_2. These changes indicate successful application of O_2 therapy, since O_2 is intended not just to improve hypoxemia but to also decrease the work of breathing and the work of the myocardium. In addition to arterial blood gas analysis and pulse oximetry, respiratory rate, ventilatory pattern, use of accessory muscles, heart rate, and blood pressure, as well as the patient's subjective assessment of wellbeing, should always be included in the assessment of O_2 therapy.

HELIUM THERAPY

The medical use of He can be traced to Barach in the 1930s.[33–36] He introduced mixtures of O_2 and He for the treatment of obstructive lesions of the larynx, trachea, and

Table 75-18. Response to Oxygen Therapy

Room Air Data	RR	35/min	PO_2	55 mmHg
	V_T	300/mL	PCO_2	32 mmHg
	Pulse	120/min	pH	7.28
	BP	160/110	SaO_2	88%
Patient A: 30% O_2 acceptable response	RR	18/min	PO_2	66 mmHg
	V_T	400/mL	PCO_2	39 mmHg
	Pulse	88/min	pH	7.41
	BP	138/96	SaO_2	92%
Patient B: 30% O_2 unacceptable response	RR	33/min	PO_2	66 mmHg
	V_T	300/mL	PCO_2	32 mmHg
	Pulse	118/min	pH	7.48
	BP	154/108	SaO_2	92%

BP, blood pressure.

In patient A, not only was PO_2 and SaO_2 increased, but ventilatory and cardiopulmonary stress were greatly reduced; whereas in patient B, ventilatory and cardiopulmonary stress persisted in spite of improvement in PO_2 and SaO_2. Patient B may require additional O_2 to meet demand.

Table 75-19. Physical Properties of Oxygen, Air, and Helium Mixtures

Gas	%	Density (g/L)	Viscosity (micropulse)
O_2	100	1.429	211.4
Air	—	1.293	188.5
He	100	0.179	201.75
He/O_2	20/80	1.178	209.5
He/O_2	40/60	0.678	207.5
He/O_2	80/20	0.428	203.6

(Modified from Gluck et al.,[37] with permission.)

airways. Helium use in management of airways obstruction is based on its inert nature and physical properties. As discussed in Chapter 1, the pressure gradient required to maintain turbulent flow [P = (RAW) ($\dot{V}^2$)] is much greater than that required to maintain laminar flow [P = (RAW) ($\dot{V}$)] (where P is pressure, RAW is airway resistance, and $\dot{V}^2$ is flow squared), and for any system the Reynold number determines whether flow will be laminar or turbulent. The key variables in the Reynold number that are related to gas composition are density and viscosity. The viscosity of He, air, and O_2 are similar (Table 75-19); however, the density of He is much lower than either O_2 or air. As a result, He is less likely to flow in a turbulent manner and thus requires less of a pressure gradient to move it past an airway obstruction. It is for this reason that He has been used in the management of certain patients. Recently, He/O_2 mixtures have been recommended in the management of asthma[37,38] and croup,[39] as well as tracheal stenosis.[40] However, no randomized study has been conducted to determine whether the benefit of using He outweighs its cost and technical difficulty over more conservative approaches to management. It is for this reason that, although He therapy appears theoretically beneficial, it is rarely used clinically.

From a practical perspective, He/O_2 mixtures must be administered with a tight-fitting mask, otherwise the low-density He rapidly diffuses into the room. In addition, a flowmeter calibrated for the precise He mixture administered should be used. If an O_2 flowmeter is used, it will read a lower flow than the actual, because of the lower density. Also, because of the low density of He, it is a poor vehicle for the transport of a pharmacologic aerosol, and the quality of a patient's cough is diminished during He therapy. Finally, the low density greatly distorts the voice—sound is high pitched and words are almost unintelligible. He/O_2 mixtures are commercially available as 80 percent He/20 percent O_2, or 70 percent He/30 percent O_2 mixtures.

CARBON DIOXIDE THERAPY

CO_2, also, has a long but unsupported history in the management of altered cerebral blood, hypoinflation, and singulation (hiccups).[41] At low concentrations (less than 10 percent), CO_2 is a respiratory stimulant; however higher concentrations result in respiratory depression and anesthesia. It is the stimulating effect of low concentrations of CO_2 that is expected to overcome hypoinflation and cause hyperinflation. However, most patients confronted with an increased inspired CO_2 concentration increase their respiratory rate in preference to their VT.

CO_2 has a dramatic effect on cerebral blood flow. Increased CO_2, mediated by changes in pH, dilates cerebral blood vessels, while decreased PCO_2 constricts blood vessels. However, many patients in need of increased cerebral blood flow respond to the increased F_ICO_2 by hyperventilation. In addition, sclerosis of cerebral blood vessels negates the effect of CO_2, although ophthalmologists do use CO_2 to dilate the blood vessels of the retina when thrombosis has impaired circulation.[41]

Singultation is one indication for increased F_ICO_2 that seems reasonable, although in our experience, it is of questionable efficacy. Singultation is a result of a spastic contraction of the diaphragm. Most approaches to reversing singultation, short of cutting the phrenic nerve, are based on increasing PCO_2 levels to increase phrenic nerve discharge and better coordinate diaphragm contraction. Inspiring 5 percent CO_2 mixtures with O_2 may stop singultation, although protracted singultation must be treated by addressing the cause of the problem.

Whenever CO_2 is administered, careful observation of the patient must be maintained and, normally, only 5 percent CO_2/95 percent O_2 mixtures are administered and only for periods of 10 to 15 minutes. Administration should be by tight-fitting mask, allowing the patient the option to remove the mask whenever necessary. Side effects include headache, palpitation, hypertension, dizziness, dyspnea, muscle tremor, paresthesia, and mental depression.[41]

References

1. Ward JJ: Equipment for mixed gas and oxygen therapy. pp. 285–355. In Barnes TA (ed): Respiratory Care Practice. Mosby-Year Book, St. Louis, 1988
2. Webb JM, Maguire J, Sych TE: Manufacture, storage, and transport of medical gases. pp. 289–317. In Burton G, Hodgkin T (eds): Respiratory Care. 3rd Ed. JB Lippincott, Philadelphia, 1991
3. Thalken FR: Production, storage, and delivery of medical gases. pp. 584–605. In Scanlan CI, Spearman CB, Sheldon RL (eds): Egan's Fundamentals of Respiratory Care. 5th Ed. Mosby-Year Book, St. Louis, 1990
4. Scott Aviation Products: Aviox Instruction Manual. A-T-O Corp., Lancaster, NY, 1980
5. Chusid EL: Oxygen concentrators. Int Anesthesiol Clin 1982; 20:235–247
6. Compressed Gas Association: Handbook of Compressed Gases. pp. 1–16. 2nd Ed. Van Nostrand, Reinhold, New York, 1981
7. Compressed Gas Association: Characteristics and safe handling of medical gases. Pamphlet P-1. pp. 1–35. Compressed Gas Association, Arlington, VA, 1965
8. National Fire Protection Association: Bulk Oxygen Systems. NFPA No. 50. pp. 1–50. National Fire Protection Association, Boston, MA, 1973
9. Compressed Gas Association: Transfilling of high pressure gas-

eous oxygen to be used for respiration. Pamphlet P-25. pp. 1–30. Compressed Gas Association, Arlington, VA, 1981
10. Chatburn R, Lough M: Handbook of Respiratory Care. 2nd Ed. Year Book Medical Publishers, Chicago, 1990
11. McPherson SP, Spearman CB: Respiratory Therapy Equipment. 3rd Ed. CV Mosby, St. Louis, 1985
12. Pierson DJ: Acute respiratory failure. pp. 75–126. In Sahn SA (ed): Pulmonary Emergencies. Churchill Livingstone, New York, 1982
13. Pierson DJ: Exacerbation of chronic bronchitis and emphysema: Ventilatory management. pp. 262–266. In Kacmarek RM, Stoller JK (eds): Current Respiratory Care. BC Decker, Toronto, 1988
14. Pierson DJ: The toxicity of low-flow oxygen therapy. Respir Care 1983;28:889–897
15. Thorson SH, Marini JJ, Pierson DJ et al: Variability of arterial blood gas values in stable patients in the ICU. Chest 1983;84:14–18
16. Leigh JM: Variation in performance of oxygen therapy devices. Ann Royal Coll Surg Engl 1973;52:234–253
17. Shapiro BA, Kacmarek RM, Cane RA et al: Application of Respiratory Care. pp. 123–150. 4th Ed. Mosby-Year Book, St. Louis, 1991
18. Kacmarek RM: In-hospital O_2 therapy. pp. 1–8. In Kacmarek RM, Stoller J (eds): Current Respiratory Care. BC Decker, Toronto, 1988
19. Nunn JF: Applied Respiratory Physiology. 2nd Ed. Butterworths, London, 1977
20. Schacter EN, Littner MR, Luddy P: Monitoring of oxygen delivery systems in clinical practice. Crit Care Med 1980;8:405–409
21. Miller WF: Oxygen therapy: Catheter, mask, hood, and tent. Anesthesiology 1962;23:445–451
22. Kory RC, Bergmann JC, Sweet RO et al: Comparative evaluation of oxygen therapy techniques. JAMA 1962;179:123–128
23. Leigh JM: The evolution of the oxygen therapy apparatus. Anaesthesia 1970;25:210–222
24. Hedley-Whyte J, Winter PM: Oxygen therapy. Clin Pharmacol Ther 1968;8:696–737
25. Lasky MS: Bubble humidifiers are useful—Fact or myth? [Letter.] Respir Care 1982;27:735–736
26. Campbell EJ, Baker D, Crites-Silver P: Subjective effects of humidification of oxygen for delivery by nasal cannula: A prospective study. Chest 1988;93:289–293
27. Estey W: Subjective effects of dry versus humidified low-flow oxygen. Respir Care 1980;25:1143–1144
28. Fulmer JD (chairman): ACCP-NHLBI National Conference on Oxygen Therapy. Chest 1984;86:234–247
29. Jones HA, Turner SL, Hughes BA: Performance of the large reservoir oxygen mask (Ventimask). Lancet 1984;1:1427–1431
30. Woolner DF, Larkin J: An analysis of the performance of a variable Venturi-type oxygen mask. Anaesth Intensive Care 1980;8:44–51
31. Canet J, Sanchis J: Performance of a low-flow O_2 Venturi mask diluting effects of the breathing pattern. Eur J Respir Dis 1984;65:68–73
32. Friedman SA, Weber B, Briscoe WA: Oxygen therapy: Evaluation of various air-entrainment masks. JAMA 1974;228:474–478
33. Barach AL: Use of helium as a new therapeutic gas. Proc Soc Exp Biol Med 1934;32:462–464
34. Barach AL: The use of helium in the treatment of asthma and obstructive lesions of the larynx and trachea. Ann Intern Med 1935;9:739–765
35. Barach AL: The therapeutic use of helium. JAMA 1936;107:1273–1275
36. Barach AL: The use of helium as a new therapeutic gas. Anaesthsia Analg 1935;14:210–215
37. Gluck EH, Onorato DJ, Castriotta R: Helium-oxygen mixtures in intubated patients with status asthmaticus and respiratory acidosis. Chest 1990;98:693–698
38. Shine ST, Gluck EH: The use of helium-oxygen mixtures in the support of patients with status asthmaticus and respiratory acidosis. J Asthma 1989;26:177–180
39. Nelson DS, McCellan L: Helium-oxygen mixtures an adjunctive support to refractory viral croup. Ohio Med J 1982;78:729–730
40. Sauder RA, Rafferty JF, Bilenki AL, Berkowitz ID: Helium-oxygen and conventinoal mechanical ventilation in the treatment of large airway obstruction and respiratory failure in an infant. South Med J 1991;84:646–648
41. Thalken FR: Medical gas therapy. pp. 606–630. In Scanlon CG, Spearman CB, Sheldon RL (eds): Egan's Fundamentals of Respiratory Care. 5th Ed. Mosby-Year Book, St. Louis, 1990
42. Gilbert DL: Cosmic and geophysical aspects of the respiratory gases. pp. 153–157. In Fenn WO, Rahn H (eds): Handbook of Physiology. Vol. 1. American Physiological Society, Washington, DC, 1964
43. Pierson DJ: Indications for oxygen therapy. Probl Respir Care 1990;3:549–561
44. Kacmarek RM: Methods of oxygen delivery in the hospital. Probs Respir Care 1990;3:563–574
45. Opt'Hold T: Humidity and aerosol therapy. pp. 356–405. In Barnes T (ed): Respiratory Care Practice, Year Book Medical Publishers, Chicago, 1988

Chapter 76

Positive End-Expiratory Pressure

Robert M. Kacmarek

CHAPTER OUTLINE

Although the use of positive end-expiratory pressure (PEEP) in the intensive care unit (ICU) was not popularized until after the description of Ashbaugh et al.[1] in 1967, the use of PEEP can be traced back to the late 1800s.[2] In fact, most of what we know regarding the physiologic effects of PEEP was addressed by Barach[3–7] and others[8–12] in the 1930s[3–10] and 1940s.[11,12] This technique to improve oxygenation has now become a cornerstone of therapy in the ICU. More than 10,000 articles have described and defined its use and physiologic effects.[13]

DEFINITIONS

A large number of acronyms (Table 76-1) have been used to describe the application of positive end-expiratory pressure, many of which are defined arbitrarily. PEEP is a term used both to refer generically to all techniques associated with the application of positive pressure at end-exhalation and to refer to specific applications of positive pressure at end-exhalation during mechanical ventilatory assistance[14] (Figs. 76-1 and 76-2). With the application of PEEP, the breaths patients take are mechanically assisted, with the baseline end-expiratory pressure elevated above that of the atmosphere. Continuous positive airway pressure (CPAP) is the application of PEEP to the spontaneously breathing individual. Here, the baseline pressure is again greater than atmospheric, but the patient inspires and expires spontaneously. An approach to the application of PEEP in spontaneously breathing individuals that is no longer recommended because of the marked increase in inspiratory work is expiratory positive airway pressure (EPAP). With EPAP, exhalation is at a pressure above atmosphere, but as a result of the use of a one-way valve, the patient must drop system

Table 76-1. Definition of Terms Referring to Positive End-Expiratory Pressure

Term	Definition
PEEP	Positive end-expiratory pressure: end-expiratory pressure applied during mechanical ventilation
CPAP	Continuous positive airway pressure: end-expiratory pressure applied during the entire spontaneous breathing cycle such that system pressures fluctuate minimally about the CPAP level
EPAP	Expiratory positive airway pressure: end-expiratory pressure applied only during the expiratory phase of a spontaneous breathing cycle such that system pressure must drop below atmospheric during inspiration
IMV + PEEP or IMV + CPAP	The use of end-expiratory pressure during intermittent mandatory ventilation (IMV)
SIMV + PEEP or SIMV + CPAP	The use of end-expiratory pressure during synchronized intermittent mandatory ventilation (SIMV)
IPS + PEEP or IPS + CPAP	The use of end-expiratory pressure during inspiratory pressure support (IPS)
CPPV	Continuous positive-pressure ventilation (or continuous positive-pressure breathing [CPPB]): the use of end-expiratory pressure during control mode or assist/control mode ventilation
Pressure control + PEEP	The use of end-expiratory pressure during pressure control ventilation

pressure below atmospheric in order to inspire. This large pressure drop greatly increases work of breathing.

Strict adherence to the above definitions has been lacking during the application of end-expiratory pressure in partial ventilatory support modes[15] (see Ch. 82). Here, the terms PEEP and CPAP have been mixed, especially in reference to intermittent mandatory ventilation (IMV), synchronized intermittent mandatory ventilation (SIMV), and inspiratory pressure support (IPS) ventilation. In these modes it is difficult to say if the patient is primarily receiving mechanical ventilation or breathing spontaneously. Either term, PEEP or CPAP, defines the technical approach used depending on the individual's frame of reference.

PHYSIOLOGIC EFFECTS

The elevation of end-expiratory pressure has profound effects on many bodily functions (Table 76-2). PEEP is normally applied to enhance the function of the lung; however, it also affects the cardiovascular system, the kidneys, and the central nervous system and it may also increase the probability of barotrauma.

Intrapulmonary and Intrapleural Pressures

Figure 76-3 illustrates the theoretical intrapulmonary and intrapleural pressure changes resulting from the application of PEEP. The effect that this pressure change has on intra-

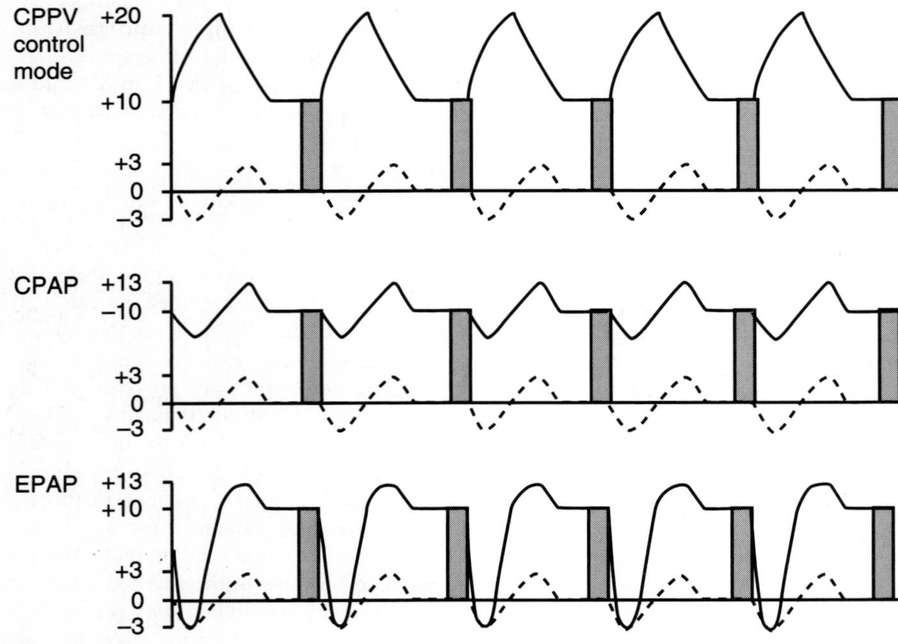

Figure 76-1. Airway pressure curves of various ventilatory modes during the application of PEEP/CPAP. Note that the only alteration in waveform is a change in baseline pressure except with EPAP, in which inspiration must still drop system pressure below atmosphere. (From Shapiro et al.,[59] with permission.)

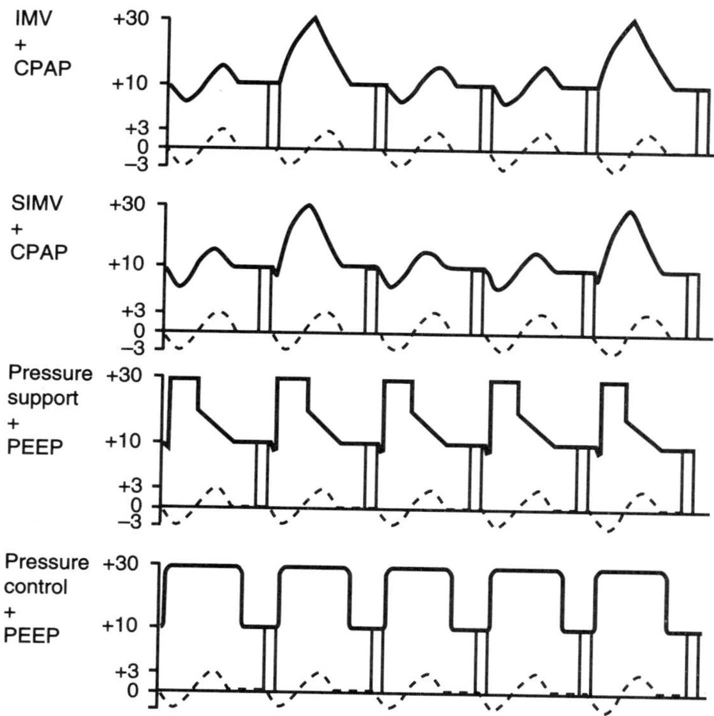

Figure 76-2. Airway pressure curves of various ventilatory modes during the application of PEEP/CPAP. Note that the only alteration in waveform is a change in baseline pressure. (From Shapiro et al.,[149] with permission.)

pleural pressure (Fig. 76-3) is dependent on the stiffness (compliance) of the lung-thorax system.[15] Generally, the more compliant the lung and the less compliant the chest wall, the greater the intrapleural (intrathoracic) and transpulmonary pressure change with any application of PEEP. Intrapleural pressure is least altered when lung compliance is low and chest wall compliance high; in other words, a stiff lung dampens the transmission of pressure to the intrapleural space. Although it is impossible to predict the precise intrathoracic pressure change in a given individual, regarding the application of PEEP it can be generally stated that in patients with normal lung and chest wall compliance who are passively exhaling, one-half of the applied PEEP is directly transmitted to the intrathoracic space. However, in patients with acute lung injury or adult respiratory distress syndrome (ARDS), only about one-fourth of the pressure is transmitted.[16] As noted later, this pressure transmission may have a profound effect on cardiovascular function.

Lung Volumes

With the application of PEEP, regardless of the status of the pulmonary system the functional residual capacity (FRC) increases.[17] This is a direct and primary result of three effects. First, since the lung and chest wall are elastic, any increase in baseline end-expiratory pressure must also increase lung volume[18] by an amount dependent on system compliance. Again, the stiffer the system, the smaller the volume change with a given application of PEEP. This volume change is a result of alveolar distension and is the primary mechanism for FRC enhancement up to about 10 cmH_2O PEEP. In addition, PEEP distends the conducting airways.[7,19] Barach and Swenson[7] showed a 1 to 2 mm increase in the diameter of small and moderate-sized airways with the application of 8 cmH_2O PEEP.

Second, PEEP levels above 10 cmH_2O increase FRC by recruitment of collapsed alveoli.[17,20] In general, the application of up to 10 cmH_2O PEEP distends alveoli to near their elastic limit, so that increasing PEEP beyond 10 cmH_2O has limited effect on alveolar distension. It is the recruitment of collapsed alveoli that generally results in the marked improvement in gas exchange noted in patients with ARDS as PEEP is applied above 10 cmH_2O.[21,22] Usually, in the patient in whom PEEP therapy is truly indicated (e.g., the ARDS patient) the lung volume change resulting from application of PEEP is directly related to the lung compliance change associated with its application.

Third, application of PEEP stabilizes alveoli, preventing their collapse during exhalation and thus maintaining lung volume.[21,23]

Lung Compliance

PEEP can markedly alter the compliance of the lung by the alveolar recruitment discussed above. Figure 76-4, taken

Table 76-2. Potential Physiologic Effects of Appropriately and Excessively Applied PEEP

	Appropriate Level	Excessive Level
Intrapulmonary pressure	Increased	Increased
Intrathoracic pressure	Increased	Increased
FRC	Increased	Increased
Lung compliance	Increased	Increased or decreased
Closing volume	Decreased	Decreased
PaO_2	Increased	Increased or decreased
$PaCO_2$	No change or decreased	Increased
$\dot{Q}_S/\dot{Q}_T$	Decreased	Decreased or increased
$P(A\text{-}a)O_2$	Decreased	Decreased or increased
$C(a\text{-}\bar{v})O_2$	Decreased	Decreased or increased
$P\bar{v}O_2$	Increased	Increased or decreased
$PaCO_2\text{-}P_{ET}CO_2$	Decreased	Increased
V_D/V_T	Decreased	Increased
Work of breathing	Decreased	Increased
Extravascular lung water	No change or increased	No change or increased
Pulmonary vascular resistance	Increased	Increased
Total pulmonary perfusion	No change or decreased	Decreased
Cardiac output	No change or decreased	Decreased
Pulmonary artery pressure	No change or increased or decreased	Decreased
Pulmonary capillary wedge pressure	No change or increased or decreased	Decreased
Central venous pressure	No change or increased or decreased	Decreased
Arterial pressure	No change or increased or decreased	Decreased
Intracranial pressure	No change or increased	Increased
Urinary output	No change or decreased	Decreased

FRC, functional residual capacity; $\dot{Q}_S/\dot{Q}_T$, shunt fraction; $P(A\text{-}a)O_2$, alveolar-arterial O_2 pressure difference; $C(a\text{-}\bar{v})O_2$, arterial-mixed venous O_2 content difference; $P\bar{v}O_2$, mixed venous O_2 pressure; $P_{ET}CO_2$, end-tidal CO_2 pressure; V_D/V_T, dead space/tidal volume ratio.

from the classic article by Suter et al.,[24] depicts the effect of PEEP on compliance. As noted, depending on the severity of lung disease during acute lung injury, lung compliance may be markedly altered. The greater the alveolar collapse and interstitial edema, the more the compliance curve shifts downward and to the right.[23] As PEEP is applied and alveoli recruited, the compliance curve shifts upward and to the left.[24] However, the application of excessive PEEP can overdistend alveoli, moving alveolar volume to the flat portion of the compliance curve, thus causing compliance to decrease.[24] Some authors have proposed the monitoring of compliance to assist in the establishment of the ideal PEEP level. Theoretically, as PEEP is applied, the premorbid FRC is re-established and the normal pressure volume relationship returned, but since lung disease, especially ARDS, is not homogeneous, this rarely occurs, although a conceptual goal of therapy is to re-establish normal FRC and compliance.

Closing Volume

The effect of PEEP on closing volume is controversial. It has been clearly established that the lung volume at which the most gravity-dependent airways close increases during anesthesia[25,26] and frequently rises above FRC.[27,28] This alteration favors the development of areas of low ventilation/perfusion ($\dot{V}/\dot{Q}$) ratio and shunting ($\dot{Q}_S/\dot{Q}_T$). This pattern can be altered by positional change[29] and the application of PEEP.[30] At least some authors[25,26,30] have indicated a decrease in closing volume below FRC with the application of 5 to 10 cmH_2O PEEP, along with improved $\dot{V}/\dot{Q}$ matching and oxygenation in obese[26] and postoperative[25,30] patients.

Gas Exchange

Improvement in gas exchange is the primary reason that PEEP is used in the treatment of generalized acute lung dis-

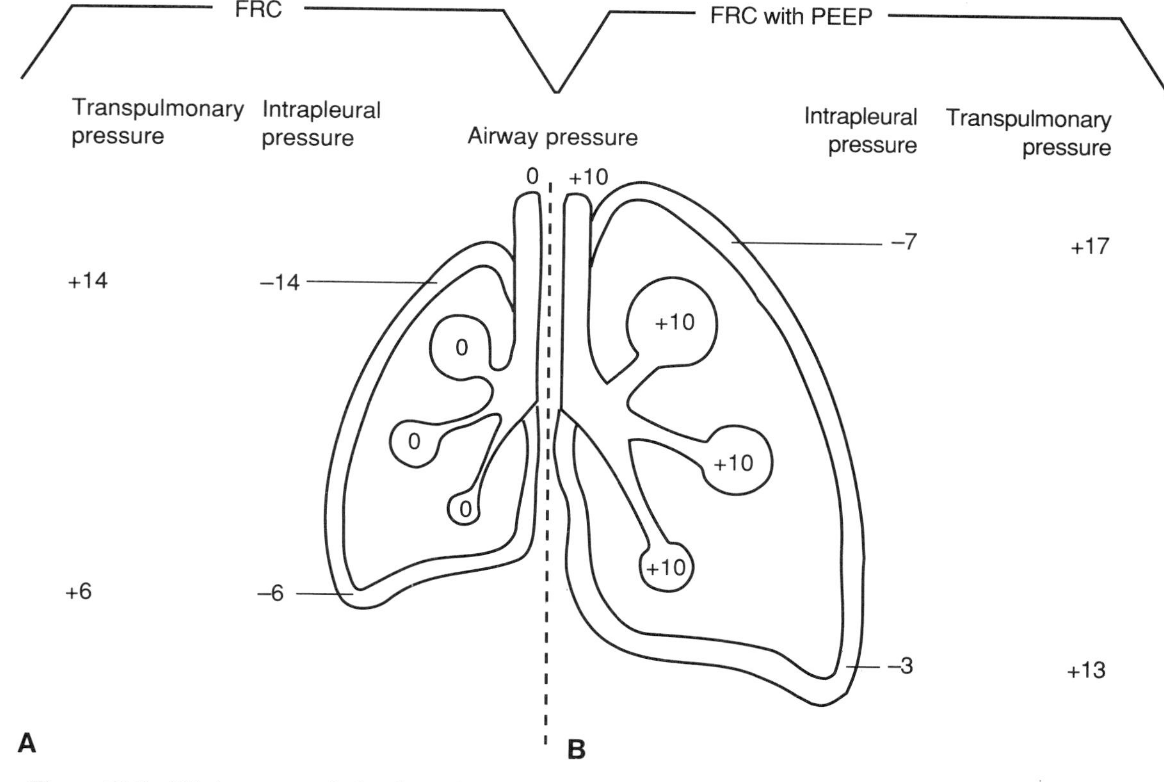

Figure 76-3. (**A**) Acute restrictive lung disease without PEEP results in greater than normal negative intrapleural pressures at functional residual capacity (FRC). (**B**) With 10 cmH_2O PEEP, more pressure is transmitted to the pleural space at the apex (7 cmH_2O transmitted) because of the normal apex-to-base variation in compliance than at the base (3 cmH_2O transmitted). Thus, transpulmonary pressure is increased by 7 cmH_2O at the base and only 3 cmH_2O at the apex. (From Shapiro et al.,[59] with permission.)

ease. Specifically, PEEP is expected to increase PaO_2 and decrease $\dot{Q}s/\dot{Q}_T$, alveolar-arterial O_2 pressure difference $[P(A\text{-}a)O_2]$, and arteriovenous O_2 content difference $[C(a\text{-}\bar{v})O_2]$ as it recruits lung volume. This effect of PEEP was first demonstrated in 1967 by Ashbaugh et al.[1] and has been shown by numerous others since.[31–34] The response in PaO_2 as a result of the application of PEEP is dependent primarily on the extent of alveolar recruitment.[34] As indicated above, initial application of PEEP results in distension of inflated alveoli, but this results in only modest increases in PaO_2 if alveolar recruitment is not established. However, once PEEP levels capable of recruitment are applied, large increases in PaO_2 are frequently seen. The time course of improved oxygenation varies considerably from patient to patient,[21–23] although frequently the initial increase in PaO_2 occurring after recruitment is followed by a more gradual increase in PaO_2 over the next hour.

PEEP has no direct effect on $PaCO_2$, but significant alterations in $PaCO_2$ may occur secondary to improved $\dot{V}/\dot{Q}$ matching resulting from recruitment or a deterioration in $\dot{V}/\dot{Q}$ relationships because of overdistension and decreased pulmonary perfusion.[35–38] Murray et al.[36] (Fig. 76-5) and Blanch et al.[38] have recommended the use of the gradient between $PaCO_2$ and end-tidal CO_2 pressure ($P_{ET}CO_2$) as an index of appropriate PEEP level. The $PaCO_2$-$P_{ET}CO_2$ gradient is normally about 3 to 5 mmHg. As PEEP is applied and $\dot{V}/\dot{Q}$ improved with a reduction in dead space/tidal volume ratio (V_D/V_T), the $PaCO_2$-$P_{ET}CO_2$ gradient should decrease and approach normal. However, if the application of PEEP decreases pulmonary perfusion and $\dot{V}/\dot{Q}$ deteriorates, the $PaCO_2$-$P_{ET}CO_2$ gradient increases because of increased V_D/V_T,[35,38] that is, $PaCO_2$ increases as $P_{ET}CO_2$ decreases. Although the change in $PaCO_2$-$P_{ET}CO_2$ can theoretically predict the appropriate level of PEEP, when evaluating a change in $PaCO_2$-$P_{ET}CO_2$ numerous other factors affecting pulmonary perfusion must be considered along with properly established PEEP levels.[35,38] As a result, the $PaCO_2$-$P_{ET}CO_2$ gradient is not a sufficiently reliable index of appropriate PEEP application for use without consideration of cardiac output and other functions.

Work of Breathing

Ideally, the application of PEEP/CPAP results in a decrease in the work of breathing by expanding collapsed alveoli and increasing compliance, by improving oxygenation and reducing ventilatory drive, or by minimizing the effects of auto-PEEP[39,40] (see under Auto-PEEP). However, if ov-

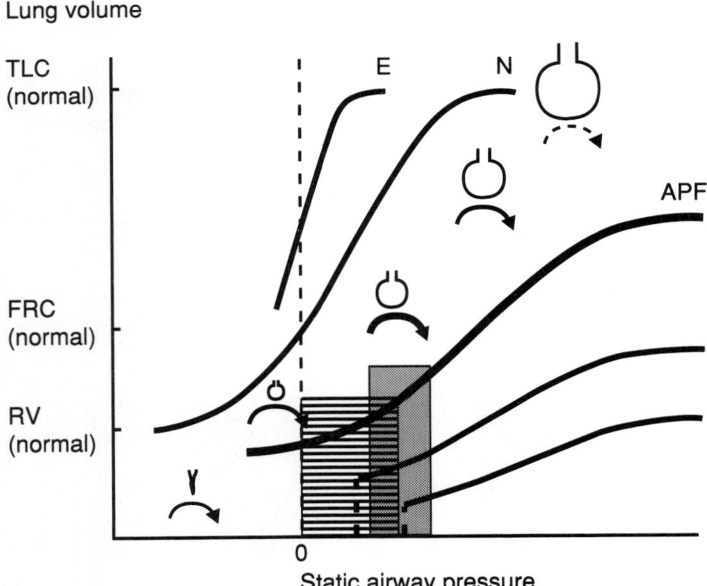

Figure 76-4. Family of regional pressure-volume curves of the respiratory system, in normal lungs (N) and in lungs of patients with emphysema (E) and acute pulmonary failure (APF). The whole lung APF curve is the sum of multiple regional compliance curves, some resembling normal and others very low compliance regions, two of which are shown in the diagram. Shaded areas show the pressure/volume relationship during the same tidal ventilation with and without PEEP. Broken vertical line denotes regional volume (RV) at which alveoli are unstable and readily "open" or "close." TLC, total lung capacity. (From Suter et al.,[24] with permission.)

erdistension occurs, reducing compliance, if EPAP is applied,[41] or if PEEP valves with high-flow resistance[42,43] are used, the work of breathing may be increased. Torres et al.,[44] in a post-thoracotomy sheep model noted increased gastric pressure and increased diaphragmatic electromyographic (EMG) activity when PEEP of 10 cmH_2O was applied (Fig. 76-6), while Hirsch et al.[43] found that the imposed work of breathing from ventilator systems markedly increased as CPAP levels were increased from 0 to 10 cmH_2O.

The potential for PEEP/CPAP to increase the work of breathing is greatest when PEEP is applied to the lung *without* recruitable volume and at levels equal to or greater than 10 cmH_2O. Under these conditions the diaphragm is disadvantaged while the lung is hyperinflated. Recruitment of abdominal muscles[44] during end-exhalation in an attempt to move the diaphragm to its normal resting position and decrease lung volume to the pre-PEEP level is an indication of increased work of breathing with PEEP/CPAP. As noted in Figure 76-6, addition of IPS is able to reduce the abdominal pressure and EMG activity to control levels. However it must be emphasized that when PEEP is applied appropriately in acute lung injury and properly titrated, the work of breathing is normally decreased.

Extravascular Lung Water

Much debate has occurred over the effect of PEEP on extravascular lung water (EVLW).[45–49] However, the consensus presently is that PEEP redistributes EVLW but maintains or actually increases its volume.[46–49] It is generally believed that PEEP moves fluid from the intra-alveolar to the perivascular interstitial space and that the application of PEEP may result in a greater transudation of fluid from the pulmonary vasculature into the peribronchial and hilar areas of the lung.[47–49]

Numerous series of blood vessels traverse the lung parenchyma, including alveolar vessels (across which gas exchange occurs), corner vessels (located in the peribronchial area), transitional vessels, and extra-alveolar vessels (see Ch. 10). In general the application of PEEP alters the transmural pressure across these vessels in relation to cardiac output.[49] If cardiac output is constant and vascular pressure is unchanged, PEEP increases the transmural pressure across the extra-alveolar and corner vessels, thereby increasing flux of fluid into the interstitial space (Fig. 76-7). However, if cardiac output and vascular pressures are decreased with the application of PEEP, EVLW remains con-

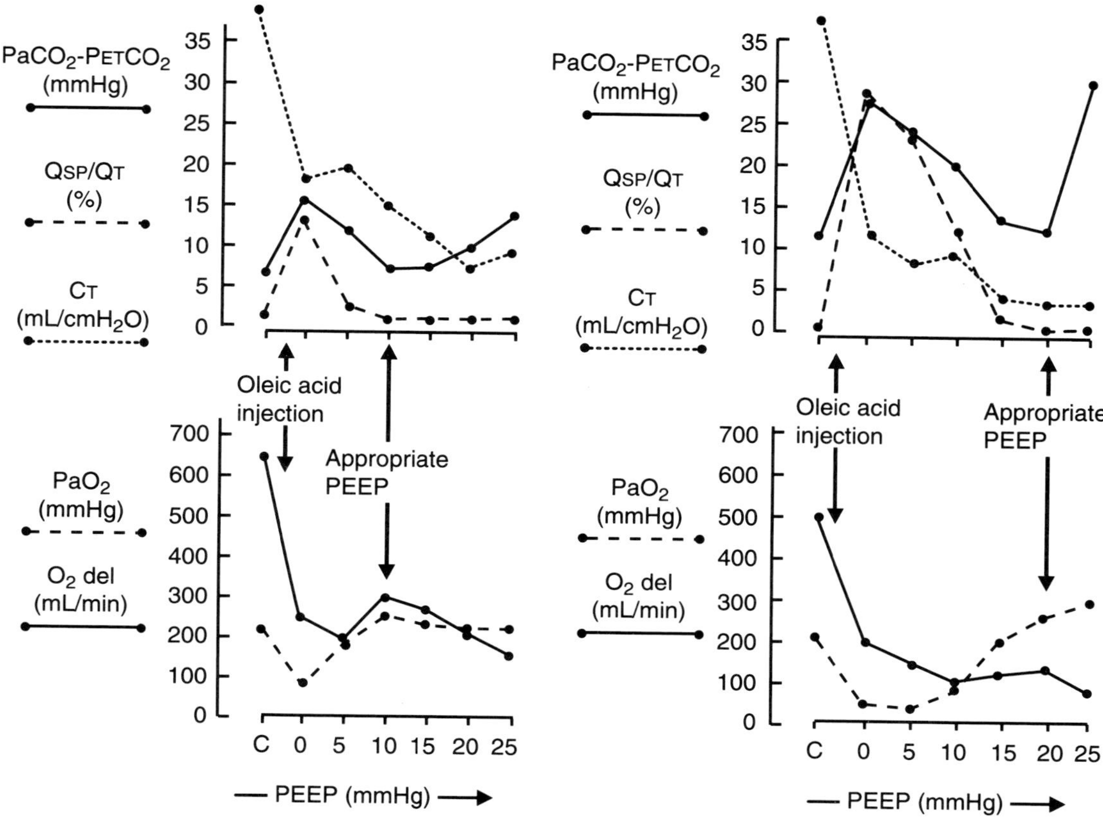

Figure 76-5. Data from two oleic acid-injured dogs during the application of PEEP. Total compliance (CT), PaO_2 and O_2 delivery (O_2 del) correlated with $PaCO_2$-$P_{ET}CO_2$; percent interpulmonary shunt ($\dot{Q}_{SP}/\dot{Q}_T$) did not. Minimal $PaCO_2$-$P_{ET}CO_2$ predicted appropriate PEEP level. (From Murray et al.,[36] with permission.)

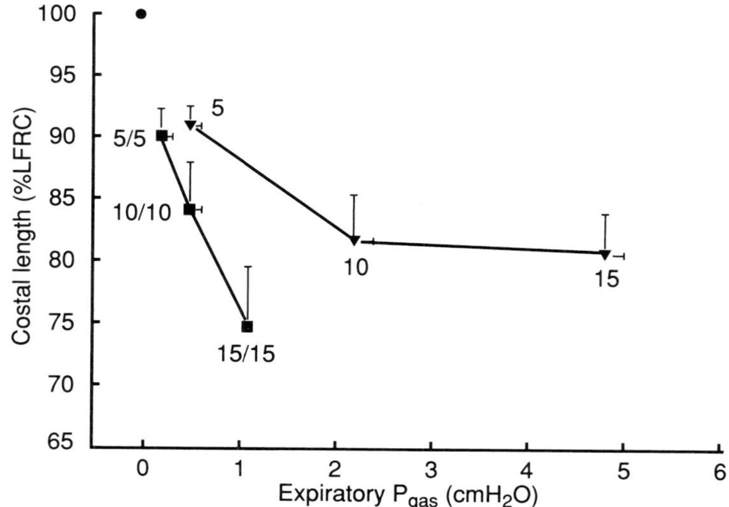

Figure 76-6. Effect of CPAP and IPS/CPAP on costal resting length and expiratory gastric pressure (P_{gas}) in sheep 24 hours post-thoracotomy. CPAP at 10 and 15 cm H_2O significantly increased P_{gas} by recruitment of abdominal muscle, thereby limiting the effect of CPAP on costal resting length. The addition of IPS to the CPAP significantly decreased P_{gas} and significantly decreased costal resting length ($P < 0.05$). (From Torres et al.,[44] with permission.)

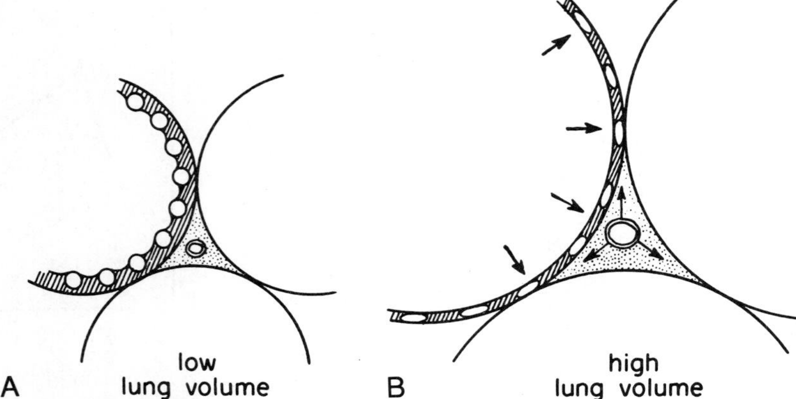

Figure 76-7. **(A & B)** As a result of PEEP increasing lung volume (Fig. B), the alveolar capillaries are stretched and compressed, potentially decreasing flow. However, the extra-alveolar and corner vessels between alveoli are expanded, which increases the flux of fluid into the interstitial space. At low lung volume (without PEEP) (Fig. A) these changes are reversed.

stant. In addition, the high intra-alveolar pressure with PEEP moves fluid from the alveoli into the interstitial space.[49] These effects can result in improved gas exchange in spite of constant or elevated EVLW levels.

Pulmonary Vascular Effects

PEEP increases pulmonary vascular resistance[50,51] and alters distribution of pulmonary blood flow[52] as well as bronchial venous drainage.[53] Increased vascular resistance is a direct result of vascular compression by alveolar distension.[50] PEEP also decreases total pulmonary blood flow, accentuating the normal gravity dependence of pulmonary perfusion and shifting blood flow to the perimeter of the lung as if the lung were exposed to centrifugal force.[52] Finally, PEEP decreases bronchial circulation to the conducting airways by compression of these vessels as the lung is distended.[53]

Cardiovascular Effects

The primary effect of PEEP on the cardiovascular system is a reduction in cardiac output as a result of impedance to systemic venous return because of increased intrathoracic pressure.[54] This increase in pressure surrounding the heart decreases cardiac transmural pressure, potentially decreasing the end-diastolic volume and stroke volume of both ventricles. Application of low levels of PEEP reduces right ventricular end-diastolic volume,[55] but right ventricular ejection fraction normally remains constant provided that no prior right ventricular dysfunction existed.[56] However, higher levels of PEEP cause marked increases in right ventricular afterload, increasing end-dias... volume and decreasing ejection fraction.[56] Increased right ventricular end-diastolic volume with high levels of PEEP causes right ventricular distension and a leftward shift of the interventricular septa.[57]

Left ventricular distensibility is reduced during PEEP as a result of interventricular septal shifting and decrease in pericardial pressure gradients due to the increased intrathoracic pressures.[58] These changes result in a decrease in left ventricular end-diastolic volume and stroke volume.

Actual changes in pulmonary hemodynamics following the application of PEEP depend on PEEP level, pulmonary and thoracic compliance, vascular volume to vascular space relationships, and myocardial contractility. In general, provided that pulmonary blood flow is not markedly reduced, application of PEEP results in an increase in the measured right ventricular preload (i.e., central venous pressure) and afterload (pulmonary artery pressure) and an increase in the measured left ventricular preload (pulmonary capillary wedge pressure [PCWP]). The higher the PEEP, the less the PCWP will reflect left atrial pressure.

The actual incremental effect of PEEP on intrathoracic pressure measurements is difficult at best to assess accurately. As indicated earlier, in normal lung with passive exhalation about 50 percent of the applied PEEP is transmitted to the intrathoracic space; however, in ARDS about 25 percent is transmitted.[16] When using these percentages to correct measured values it is imperative to ensure that the pulmonary artery catheter is placed in a zone 3 location (see Ch. 50) and the PEEP transmission estimate in centimeters of water is converted to millimeters of Hg (1 cmH_2O equals 0.7 mmHg).

Since cardiac output is usually decreased with PEEP, left ventricular afterload may also decrease as PEEP is applied. If pulmonary blood flow is markedly reduced by application of PEEP, the preload and afterload of both the left and right ventricles decrease, and as a result it is difficult to predict the precise effect that PEEP will have on hemodynamics. Any of the pressures commonly measured may increase, decrease, or stay the same, depending on the maintenance of pulmonary blood flow. However, it can be accurately surmised that a drop in pulmonary hemodynamic parameters with PEEP is a result of a marked decrease in pulmonary blood flow. In this case fluid or pharmacologic support is required if the PEEP level is to be maintained.

It is imperative that hemodynamic variables be assessed under conditions that best reflect a patient's ongoing status. As a result, measurement should be made during the application of PEEP and positive pressure ventilation, with data collected at end-expiration, because end-expiration represents the most consistent level of airway pressure therapy and the point of its least effect.[59]

Intracranial Pressure

Since PEEP increases right atrial pressure and decreases venous return, it also increases intracranial pressure and decreases cerebral blood flow.[60,61] However, since cerebral blood flow is controlled by a Starling resistor located between the sagittal sinus and the cerebral veins, cerebral blood flow is not markedly affected unless PEEP levels are high.[62] The effect of PEEP on the central nervous system (CNS) is greatest if cerebral autoregulation is impaired by closed head injury or other factors compromising CNS function.

Renal Function

Urinary output and sodium excretion are decreased by application of PEEP. Although the exact mechanisms for these physiologic responses have not been clarified, it is believed that the following factors contribute to the alteration in renal function: reduced renal blood flow,[63] redistribution of renal blood flow from cortical to medullary regions,[64] reduction in atrial natriuretic peptide levels,[65] and increase in antidiuretic hormone release.[66]

Barotrauma

For barotrauma to occur, three factors must be present: lung disease, overdistension, and pressure.[67] Since the primary indication for the use of PEEP is acute lung injury, disease is normally present when PEEP is applied. Thus, the amount of overdistension achieved at a given PEEP level essentially determines the probability of barotrauma. Because acute lung injury is patchy and heterogeneous,[68] overdistension of a given lung unit may be achieved at any PEEP level. As a result careful monitoring for the presence of barotrauma must be routinely performed, and PEEP must be maintained at the minimal level required to achieve the therapeutic end points of PEEP therapy. The pathogenesis, clinical features, and management of barotrauma are discussed further in Chapter 84.

INDICATIONS FOR USE

The primary indication for the use of PEEP is acute lung injury (noncardiogenic pulmonary edema or ARDS).[1,21,23]

Table 76-3. Clinical Settings in Which PEEP Is Commonly Used

Adult respiratory distress syndrome	Asthma
Chest trauma	Chronic obstructive pulmonary disease
Sleep apnea	Atelectasis
Neonatal apnea	Artificial airways
Tracheobronchomalacia	Cardiogenic pulmonary edema

Since the pathophysiology of ARDS results in decreased lung volumes and alveolar collapse, decreased compliance, and severe hypoxemia refractory to O_2 therapy, PEEP is ideal to support lung function and gas exchange. However, PEEP is used in many clinical settings other than ARDS (Table 76-3).

Adult Respiratory Distress Syndrome

The level of PEEP or CPAP required to support gas exchange during ARDS is dependent on the severity of the disease. Mild to moderate ARDS requires low levels of PEEP to support lung function. Since alveolar collapse is normally not as significant a problem in the early stages of ARDS, 5 to 15 cmH_2O PEEP is usually sufficient to return gas exchange to an acceptable level[34] (see section on titration and monitoring of PEEP). With severe ARDS, however, PEEP levels of 40 to 50 cmH_2O have been reported,[69,70] although we find that in these cases 15 to 20 cmH_2O is normally required to maintain gas exchange.

ARDS is the ideal indication for the application of PEEP; although ARDS is heterogenous, it presents in a more global homogenous pattern than other pulmonary disease. It also manifests itself pathophysiologically in a manner responsive to the application of PEEP. In the ICU, ARDS is by far the primary indicator for PEEP levels greater than 10 cmH_2O.

Chest Trauma

Traumatic chest injury, especially with pulmonary contusion, frequently progresses to ARDS,[11,12,71] and as a result, PEEP/CPAP is commonly used in this setting. PEEP/CPAP is also useful in stabilizing the chest wall and minimizing paradoxical chest wall movement. The use of PEEP on initial presentation may prevent the need for controlled mechanical ventilation by reducing the work of breathing and enhancing gas exchange as the chest wall is stabilized.[72,73]

Apnea

CPAP is used extensively in the treatment of apneas both in adults[74,75] and in neonates.[76,77] Nasal CPAP is the treatment of choice in obstructive sleep apnea.[74,78] The positive pressure applied to the oral and nasal pharynx "splints" the airway open during sleep, preventing obstruction and arterial

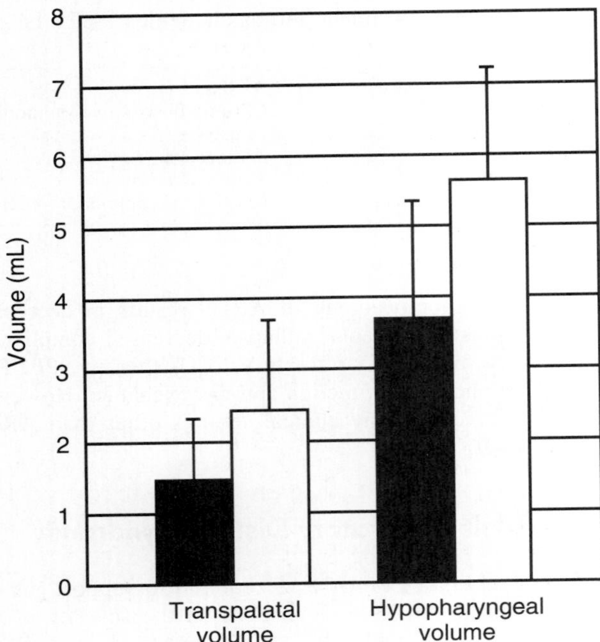

Figure 76-8. Calculated axial volume (on y axis) at two different sites in the airway, the transpalatal area and the hypopharyngeal area. The solid bars represent volumes calculated prior to the use of nasal CPAP and the open bars volumes calculated after nasal CPAP. Both sites showed a statistically significant increase in volume after application of nasal CPAP ($P < 0.05$). (From Abbey et al.,[150] with permission.)

desaturation (Fig. 76-8). A similar mechanism is believed to account for the effects of nasal CPAP in neonatal apnea. In adults 7 to 12 cmH_2O CPAP is normally used, while 2 to 4 cmH_2O is usually sufficient in children. CPAP has also been successfully used to treat tracheobronchomalacia in infants by splinting the unstable airways, preventing collapse.[79] Use of CPAP levels up to 30 cmH_2O for as long as 25 months has been reported.[80]

Asthma and Chronic Obstructive Pulmonary Disease

Historically, PEEP has been thought to be contraindicated in the treatment of asthma and chronic obstructive pulmonary disease (COPD) for fear of increased air trapping and barotrauma, although the successful use of PEEP in these clinical settings was described by Barach[3] and Barach and Swenson[7] in the 1930s. More recently, numerous authors have also shown beneficial effects of PEEP or CPAP during an acute asthmatic attack[81–84] or an acute exacerbation of COPD.[39,40,85–87] These beneficial effects seem to result from modification of the effects of auto-PEEP (see under Auto-PEEP) resulting from air trapping.[39,40] Martin et al.[81] demonstrated that during acute asthmatic attacks a decrease in airway resistance, less inspiratory pleural pressure drop, and decreased work of breathing can be achieved with the application of 12 cmH_2O CPAP. Similar findings have been reported by Qvist et al.[83] and Shivaram et al.[84] Explanations for the effects noted are controversial. We believe that these effects result from altering the level of equal intraluminal and extraluminal pressure (equal pressure point) and allowing for equilibration between alveolar and central airway pressure, thereby reducing the pressure gradient required to inspire.

In COPD dynamic airflow obstruction also results in air trapping and auto-PEEP. In the stable COPD patient this is modified by the patient's ventilatory pattern (long expiratory phase and pursed-lip breathing). However, the distress of an acute exacerbation or endotracheal intubation eliminates the patient's ability to modify the ventilatory pattern to compensate for air trapping. The use of CPAP or PEEP allows for equilibration of alveolar and central airway pressures, thus improving distribution of ventilation and reducing work of breathing in the presence of auto-PEEP[39,40] (see under Auto-PEEP).

Atelectasis

Postoperative atelectasis is a common complication of upper abdominal and thoracic surgery.[88] Numerous approaches to bronchial hygiene, including chest physical therapy, incentive spirometry, and intermittent positive-pressure breathing (IPPB), as well as coughing and deep breathing instruction, have been used in the postoperative period to prevent or reverse atelectasis. CPAP, either continuously or intermittently on a treatment basis, has been recommended for prophylaxis or treatment of atelectasis. It is believed that CPAP reverses atelectasis by increasing collateral airflow to collapsed lung regions, thereby assisting in reinflation and the removal of secretions.[89]

Andersen et al.[89] randomly compared CPAP with postural drainage and percussion in a group of postoperative patients with radiographic evidence of atelectasis and found that all patients receiving CPAP showed resolving atelectasis and increased PO_2 within less than 2 hours after the initiation of therapy. In addition, many of the patients nonresponsive to postural drainage and percussion subsequently also responded to CPAP. Stock et al.[90] noted a lower incidence of postoperative atelectasis with the use of CPAP as compared with deep breathing and coughing instruction as well as with incentive spirometry. Similar results have been noted by Williamson and Modell.[91] However, in separate studies Carlson et al.,[92] Stock et al.,[93] Linden et al.,[94] and Knodel et al.[95] could not demonstrate lower incidence or improved resolution of atelectasis with CPAP as compared with other forms of therapy.

For this indication CPAP has been used intermittently or continuously by mask. Although theoretically continuous CPAP would seem more advantageous, it is poorly tolerated and more likely to cause side effects than intermittent treatment (e.g., for 15 to 30 minutes every 2 to 6 hours). However, based on the conflicting data and the labor intensity of mask CPAP application, we normally recommend its intermittent use only in settings in which persistent atelectasis has been documented.

Artificial Airways

The placement of an artificial airway, whether an endotracheal or tracheostomy tube, eliminates the ability of the upper airway to modulate airflow and to exert back pressure during expiration. This leads to a reduction in the FRC as compared with the nonintubated state even in patients without acute or chronic lung disease.[96] In patients with chronic lung disease[97] and especially in infants,[98,99] a drop in PaO_2 is noted with the placement of an artificial airway (Fig. 76-9). The effect of bypassing the larynx can be reversed if low-level CPAP or PEEP (3 to 5 cmH_2O) is applied to the airway.[97–99] The use of CPAP has resulted in improved PO_2 and FRC in both children and adults during weaning from mechanical ventilation.[97–102] It is generally the rule in the neonatal or pediatric ICU to always apply low-level CPAP (3 to 5 cmH_2O) to artificial airways until extubation. We would extend this rule to the adult population and apply 5 cmH_2O CPAP to all airways placed acutely unless a compelling argument can be made against its use. We extubate adults from 5 cmH_2O CPAP without attempting to evaluate gas exchange while breathing at atmospheric pressure (O cmH_2O CPAP). This approach is particularly important in patients with chronic lung disease because of problems with air trapping and auto-PEEP (see under Auto-PEEP). This application of PEEP has been referred to as *physiologic PEEP*.

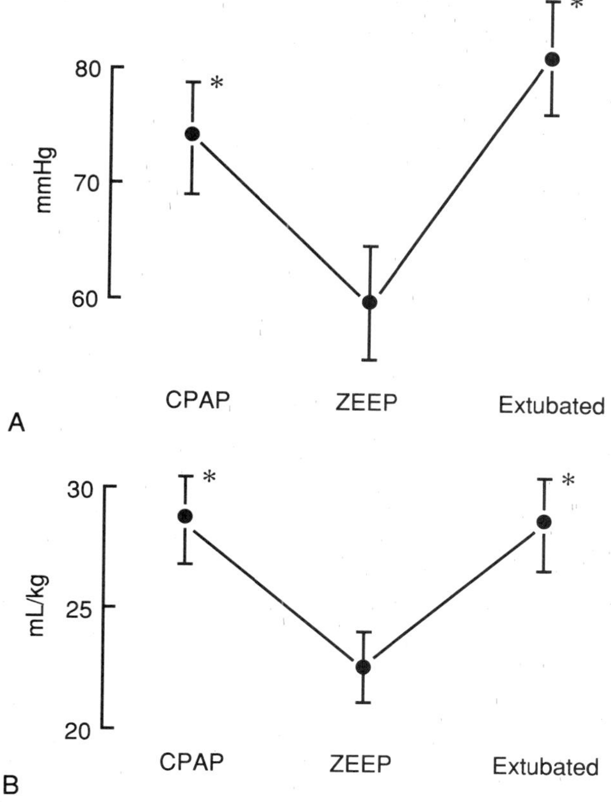

Figure 76-9. (**A**) PaO_2 during CPAP, with zero end-expiratory pressure (ZEEP), and following extubation. (**B**) FRC during CPAP, during ZEEP, and following extubation. Data on 16 infants recovering from acute respiratory distress (mean ± SD, *, $P < 0.01$ versus ZEEP). (From Gregory et al.,[151] with permission.)

Cardiogenic Pulmonary Edema

Pulmonary edema resulting from heart failure is a direct result of the increased preload of the left ventricle. In this setting the left ventricle is unable to increase its force of contraction and stroke volume as it is further distended. As discussed in other chapters, left ventricular failure is treated by pharmacologically improving contractility of the myocardium along with reducing preload and improving oxygenation. Use of CPAP or PEEP can have an indirect effect on left ventricular preload, particularly in the setting of a failing heart.[103,104] The increased mean intrathoracic pressure resulting from the application of CPAP or PEEP reduces venous return, thus decreasing preload, and as a result decreases fluid movement into the intrapulmonary space by altering the hydrostatic pressure relationships in the thorax. In addition, oxygenation improves[105,106] and work of breathing decreases.[107] Increased left-ventricular ejection fraction, decreased end-diastolic pressure, and improved cardiac output have also been demonstrated with the application of CPAP or PEEP.[108,109]

Frequently use of 10 cmH_2O CPAP sufficiently stabilizes the cardiopulmonary system to obviate the need for intubation[105] during initial management and to allow time for pharmacologic therapy to take effect. In the setting of acute cardiogenic pulmonary edema we would recommend a trial of mask CPAP. However, patient tolerance can be a significant problem in this setting.

AUTO-PEEP

Auto-PEEP,[85] also referred to as intrinsic PEEP,[110] unidentified PEEP, endogeneous PEEP, or occult PEEP, is a result of incomplete emptying of the lung at end-exhalation or air trapping.[111] The term *unidentified PEEP* is used because auto-PEEP is not identified on the pressure manometer of the ventilator unless an end-expiratory hold is imposed. Figure 76-10 illustrates this point. Figure 76-10A shows equal alveolar, central airway, and ventilator circuit pressures at end-exhalation as seen in most patients receiving mechanical ventilation. Figure 76-10B illustrates the presence of auto-PEEP as a result of dynamic airflow limitation or as a result of inadequate expiratory time. It should be noted that at end-exhalation alveolar pressure is above atmosphere but central airway pressure and ventilator manometer pressure are zero. As shown in Figure 76-10C, auto-PEEP can be quantified if an end-expiratory hold is applied.

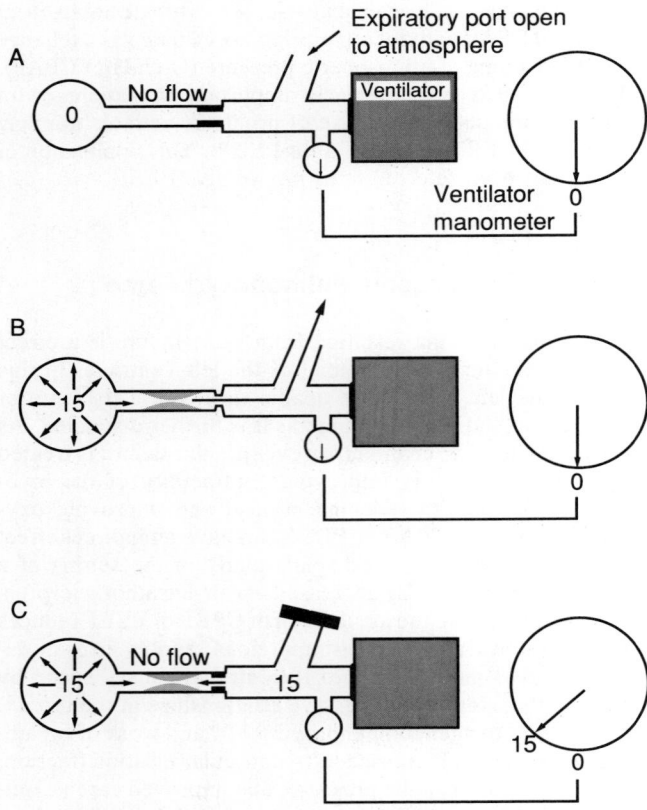

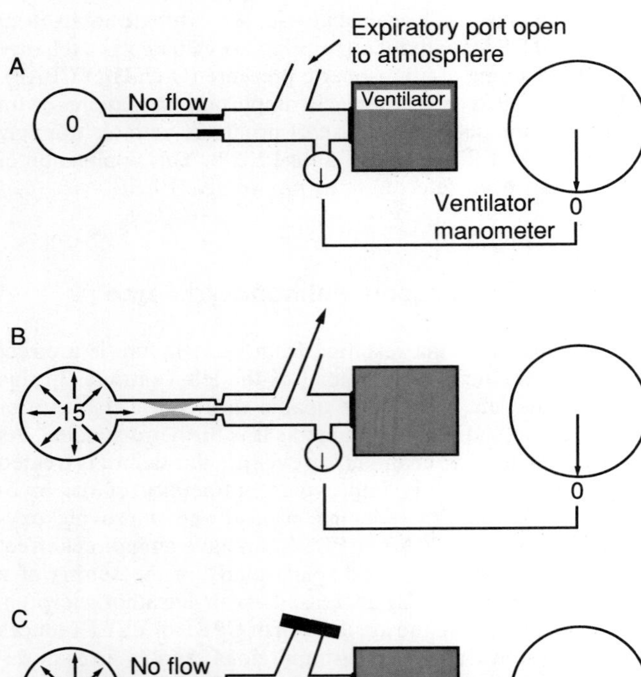

Figure 76-10. Relationship between alveolar, central airway, and ventilator circuit pressure under (**A**) normal conditions and in the presence of severe dynamic airway obstruction, (**B**) with expiratory port open, and (**C**) with expiratory port occluded. Auto-PEEP level is identified by creating an end-expiratory hold, allowing alveolar, central airway, and ventilator circuit pressure to equilibrate. Note that during equilibration auto-PEEP level can be read on the system manometer. (From Pepe and Marini,[85] with permission.)

This allows end-alveolar, central airway, and ventilator circuit pressure to equilibrate.

Generally, auto-PEEP occurs under two specific sets of circumstances: first, when insufficient expiratory time is available, even in the absence of lung disease, and second, in the presence of dynamic flow limitation.[112] In addition, auto-PEEP can develop without hyperinflation if exhalation is active.[112]

Complete passive exhalation requires at least three to four respiratory time constants (RCs) (Fig. 76-11). As noted in Chapter 1, the RC is dependent on the product of compliance (C) and resistance (R).

$$\text{RC} = (\text{C})\,(\text{R}) \qquad (1)$$

$$(\text{seconds}) = (\text{L/cmH}_2\text{O})(\text{cmH}_2\text{O/L/s})$$

When measured in the ICU, a global RC is determined. However, local RCs may differ markedly, some demonstrating large RCs (slow lung units) and others small RCs (fast lung units). The effect of inadequate expiratory time on air trapping in postoperative patients was illustrated by Bergman[111] in 1972 (Fig. 76-12). Air trapping in patients with normal lungs was noted at respiratory rates of 20 breaths per minute and in patients with COPD at rates of 12 per minute (inspiration/expiration [I/E] ratio 1:1). We have noted auto-PEEP and hyperinflation at rates as low as 6 per minute with an inspiratory time of 1 second in patients with acute exacerbation of COPD or asthma.

Auto-PEEP and air trapping in patients with dynamic airflow obstruction may occur at virtually any mechanical respiratory rate. All patients presenting with chronic or acute airflow limitation (Table 76-4) should be carefully monitored for auto-PEEP (see below). Brown and Pierson[113] in a consecutive series of 62 patients receiving controlled mechanical ventilation, identified auto-PEEP at levels up to 16 cmH_2O in 24 patients (Fig. 76-13). They noted that the likelihood as well as the level of auto-PEEP increased with age, the presence of chronic lung disease, and the need for minute ventilations greater than 10 L/min. Similar data have been published by Wright and Gong.[114] In our medical ICU, it is common to identify auto-PEEP levels of 3 cmH_2O or higher when ventilatory rates reach 10 per minute.

Physiologic Effects

The effects of auto-PEEP are similar to those defined earlier for applied PEEP. However, since auto-PEEP most commonly develops in patients with increased or normal compliance, the effects on pulmonary hemodynamics and cardiac output are frequently greater than those seen when PEEP is applied to the patient with acute lung injury. If auto-PEEP is unrecognized, inappropriate management of cardiovascular status may result.

Auto-PEEP may have a dramatic effect on PCO_2 if it markedly affects the distribution of pulmonary blood flow. Large increases in dead space may occur in the patient with asthma or severe COPD if high levels of auto-PEEP develop. We have noted PCO_2 increases of 10 to 20 mmHg simply as a result of auto-PEEP development. Auto-PEEP during manual ventilation is frequently an unidentified problem. Clinicians tend to apply manual ventilation at a much higher rate than they would use with mechanical ventilation. As a result, ineffective ventilation (high PCO_2) may be a result of too rapid a ventilatory rate. Decreasing the ventilatory rate (minute ventilation) in any of the above settings normally results in a decrease in PCO_2.

As noted in Chapter 84, barotrauma occurs when the diseased lung is overinflated by high distending pressure. The localized development of auto-PEEP in the COPD or asthmatic patient greatly increases the likelihood of barotrauma.[67]

As discussed in Chapter 1, both applied PEEP and auto-PEEP affect the determination of compliance. When compliance is determined, *total* end-expiratory pressure (applied PEEP plus auto-PEEP) must be subtracted from the plateau pressure to determine the actual pressure required for static lung inflation.[115] If auto-PEEP is not considered in this cal-

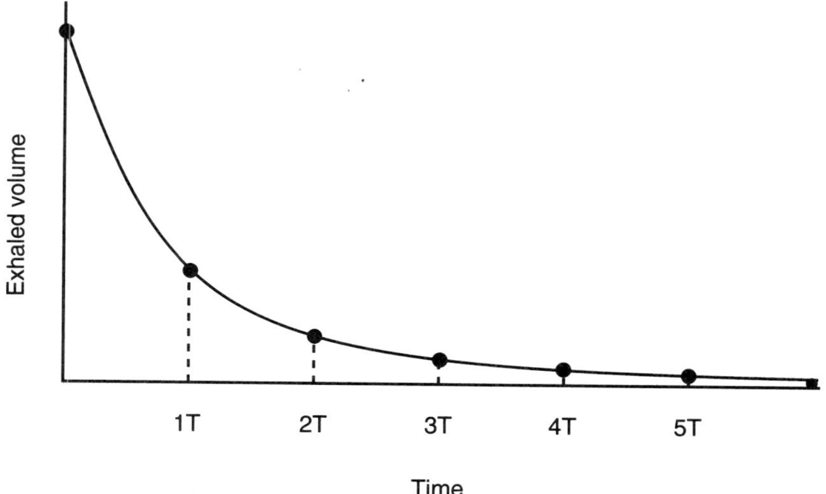

Figure 76-11. Relationship between volume passively exhaled and number of elapsed time constants (RCs): 63, 86.5, 95, 98.2, and 99.3 percent of VT is exhaled in one, two, three, four, and five RC, respectively.

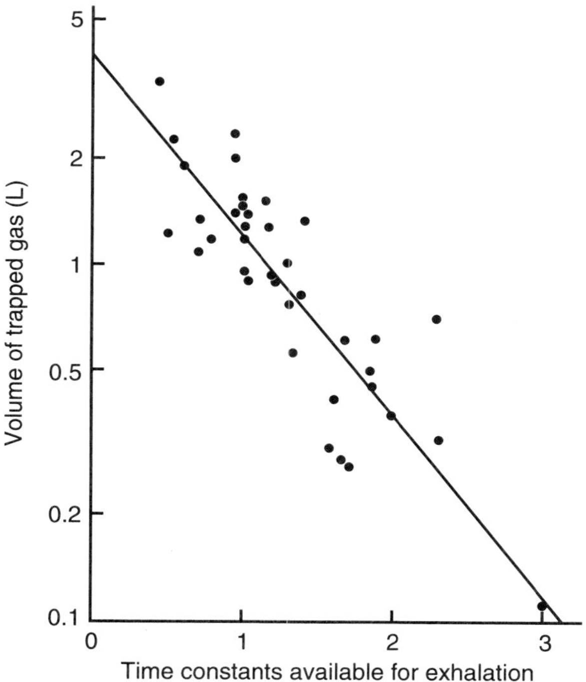

Figure 76-12. Volume of trapped gas as a function of the number of time constants available for exhalation for inspired VT of 1000 mL. The volume of trapped gas increased logarithmically as the number of time constants available for exhalation decreased. The regression line for these data, calculated by the method of least squares, was, volume of trapped gas = $3873e^{-1.156T}$, where T is the number of time constants available for exhalation. By using this equation, it can be shown that for breaths of 1000 mL, 95 percent completion of passive exhalation required 3.7 time constants in subjects of this study. Similar results could be demonstrated for breaths of 500 mL. (From Bergman,[111] with permission.)

culation, an erroneously low compliance valve is obtained.[116,117]

In spontaneously breathing patients the presence of auto-PEEP greatly increases the work of breathing. A normal esophageal pressure-volume loop of a spontaneously breathing individual without auto-PEEP is illustrated in Figure 76-14. If auto-PEEP develops, work of breathing increases as a result of the patient's need to create a pressure gradient to overcome the auto-PEEP before gas can enter the airway. Both Smith and Marini[39] and Petrof et al.[40] have documented the marked increase in work of breathing in the presence of auto-PEEP (Tables 76-5 and 76-6). Data from Smith and Marini[39] (Table 76-5) come from a series of COPD patients requiring assisted ventilation, while the information provided by Petrof et al.[40] is from patients capable of breathing spontaneously on CPAP. These studies illustrate increased work of breathing during ventilatory assistance because the artificial airway prevents normal function of the glottis and pursed-lip breathing. (The effect of applied PEEP or CPAP on auto-PEEP is discussed later.) Frequently, spontaneously breathing patients with auto-PEEP (in the presence of an artificial airway) perform less work and demonstrate less

Table 76-4. Clinical Settings in Which Auto-PEEP Is Most Likely to Develop

Chronic bronchitis Secretions Mucosal edema	Pulmonary burns Mucosal edema Secretions
Emphysema Airway destruction	Rapid respiratory rates
Asthma Mucosal edema Bronchoconstriction Secretions	Large tidal volume

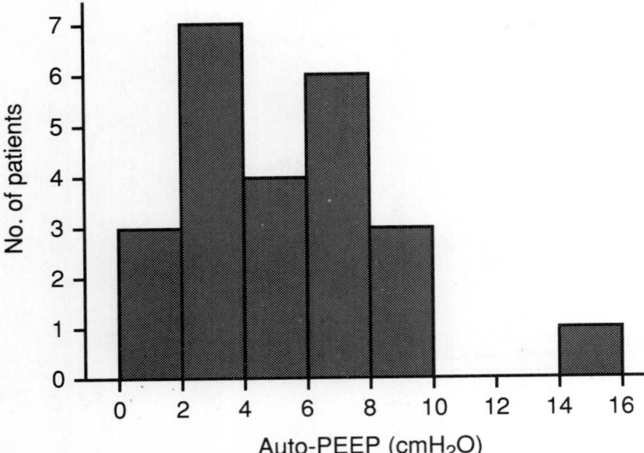

Figure 76-13. Magnitude of auto-PEEP in 24 patients receiving controlled mechanical ventilation detected during routine ventilator checks out of a total of 62 patients receiving mechanical ventilation. (From Brown and Pierson,[113] with permission.)

auto-PEEP once they have been extubated. However, it should be remembered that the spontaneously breathing patient *without* an artificial airway also may develop auto-PEEP in an acute exacerbation of asthma or COPD.

My colleagues and I have found that the inability of patients to trigger assisted ventilation with every inspiratory effort is most commonly a result of auto-PEEP. In other words, when the patient's spontaneous ventilatory rate exceeds that of the mechanical ventilator, either the sensitivity of the ventilator is set inappropriately or the increased work of breathing associated with auto-PEEP prevents the patient from decompressing the auto-PEEP and triggering the ventilator on every spontaneous breath. When this occurs, steps to modify the level of auto-PEEP should be taken (see discussion on management of auto-PEEP).

Detection and Quantitation

Unfortunately, identifying the presence of and quantifying the level of auto-PEEP is no easy task (Table 76-7). The presence of ronchi or wheezing is normally associated with auto-PEEP, as is an end-expiratory flow rate above zero.[117] From observation of the plot of expiratory gas flow during ventilation (Fig. 76-15), the presence but not the magnitude of auto-PEEP can be identified. A change in peak airway pressure when respiratory rate is decreased but delivery of tidal volume is unaltered also identifies the presence but not the precise magnitude of auto-PEEP, since both compliance and resistance may have been affected by the decrease in auto-PEEP associated with the decrease in rate.

During controlled mechanical ventilation the easiest method of identifying auto-PEEP is the application of an end-expiratory hold (Fig. 76-16). The Servo 900C, the Hamilton Veolar, the Ohmeda Advent, and the Liquid Air Cesar have incorporated an end-expiratory hold feature. With these units the auto-PEEP level is identified by viewing either the digital readout of auto-PEEP or the end-expiratory pressure on the ventilatory manometer during the end-expiratory pause. Figure 76-17 illustrates the use of the Braschi valve for determination of auto-PEEP.[118] This valve consists of a Briggs adapter with a one-way valve on its proximal opening to allow gas flow only toward the patient. It can be used on any ventilator in which closure of the exhalation valve is independent of the development of pressure in the inspiratory limb of the circuit. A pressure manometer must be added at the Y of the circuit if the ventilator senses pressure on the inspiration side of the circuit; otherwise the auto-PEEP level is indicated on the ventilator manometer. To use this valve, the port allowing gas to exit the circuit is opened once the patient begins exhalation. When the next controlled mechanical breath is delivered, the exhalation valve closes, the delivered volume exits the Braschi valve, and an end-expiratory hold is developed for the length of the inspiratory phase. This valve functions well provided the patient's mechanical respiratory rate is not excessive (greater than 25

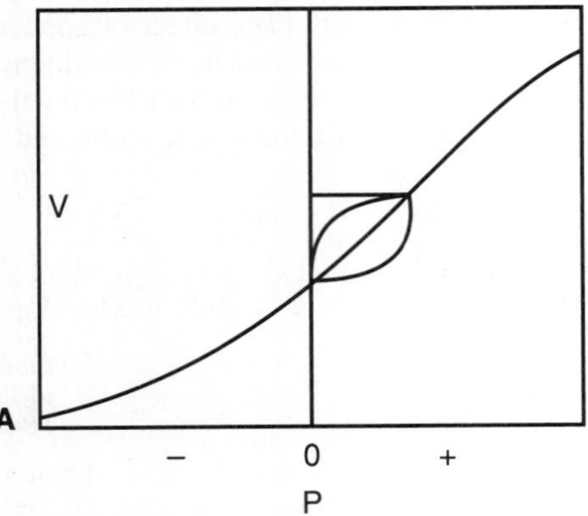

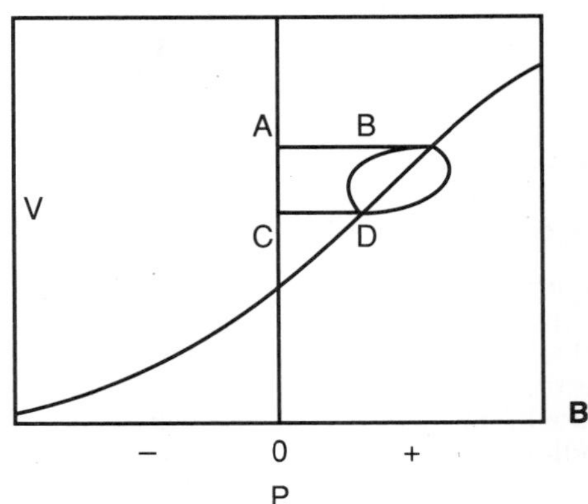

Figure 76-14. **(A)** Normal spontaneously breathing esophageal pressure-volume (P-V) loop. **(B)** Effect of auto-PEEP on area of P-V loop, reflecting marked increase in work of breathing as a result of the need to decompress the auto-PEEP prior to changing lung volume. (From Otis,[152] with permission.)

Table 76-5. Effects of PEEP on Work of Breathing during Mechanical Ventilation in the Presence of Auto-PEEP, as a Result of Dynamic Airflow Obstruction[a]

	PEEP (cmH_2O)		
	0	5	10
Inspiratory $\dot{W}b_I$ (J/L)	0.83 ± 0.53	0.67 ± 0.39	0.39 ± 0.23[b]
Synchronous	0.75 ± 0.46	0.61 ± 0.34	0.36 ± 0.19
Asynchronous	0.09 ± 0.12	0.06 ± 0.09	0.03 ± 0.04
Expiratory $\dot{W}b_E$ (J/L)	0.33 ± 0.37	0.25 ± 0.24	0.15 ± 0.17
Synchronous	0.21 ± 0.17	0.15 ± 0.13	0.11 ± 0.13
Asynchronous	0.12 ± 0.24	0.09 ± 0.14	0.04 ± 0.06
Total $\dot{W}b$ (J/L)	1.16 ± 0.48	0.91 ± 0.38[b]	0.54 ± 0.28[c]
$\dot{W}b_{min}$ = total $\dot{W}b \times \dot{V}_E$ (J/min)	10.58 ± 5.89	8.42 ± 4.56	4.77 ± 3.21[c]

$\dot{W}b_I$, inspiratory work of breathing; $\dot{W}b_E$, expiratory work of breathing; $\dot{W}b$, work of breathing; $\dot{W}b_{min}$, work of breathing over 1 min; $\dot{V}_E$, minute ventilation.

[a] Values are means ± SD; $n = 10$.

[b] $P \leq 0.05$ compared with 0 PEEP.

[c] $P \leq 0.01$ compared with 0 PEEP.

(From Smith and Marini,[39] with permission.)

breaths per minute) and the patient is not breathing spontaneously.

Hoffman et al.[119] demonstrated that respiratory inductive plethysmography (Fig. 76-18) could also be used to identify the level of auto-PEEP. With this method, applied PEEP is slowly added until the baseline sum display begins to increase. The lowest level of applied PEEP not causing an increase in the baseline valve approximates the auto-PEEP level.

Determination of auto-PEEP during spontaneous breathing, whether or not ventilatory assistance is provided, requires insertion of an esophageal balloon and simultaneous measurement of esophageal pressure and airway opening pressure or flow at airway opening.[39] Normally there is only a minor nonmeasurable delay between the change in esophageal pressure and airway opening pressure or flow. However, if auto-PEEP is present, esophageal pressure may decrease significantly from baseline before flow or pressure change at the airway opening occurs. The difference between baseline esophageal pressure and the esophageal pressure required to alter flow or pressure at the airway is equal to the auto-PEEP level. Figure 76-19 depicts the determination of auto-PEEP by this method.

Table 76-6. Effects of CPAP on Work of Breathing during Weaning in the Presence of Auto-PEEP, as a Result of Dynamic Airflow Obstruction[a]

	$\dot{W}_I$ (J/min)	$\dot{W}_I/\dot{V}_E$ (J/L)	$\dot{W}_{Iel}/\dot{V}_E$ (J/L)	$\dot{W}_{Ires}/\dot{V}_E$ (J/L)
Control	17.37 (1.92)	1.61 (0.12)	0.89 (0.08)	0.76 (0.12)
CPAP 5	14.47 (1.34)	1.31 (0.11)	0.63 (0.06)	0.71 (0.09)
P value[b]	<0.05	<0.01	<0.005	NS
Control	17.47 (1.91)	1.61 (0.11)	0.86 (0.05)	0.72 (0.08)
CPAP 10	12.28 (1.19)	1.16 (0.07)	0.55 (0.05)	0.68 (0.07)
P value	<0.01	<0.005	<0.005	NS
Control	19.94 (2.78)	1.70 (0.15)	0.94 (0.08)	0.70 (0.07)
CPAP 15	10.81 (1.78)	1.02 (0.11)	0.46 (0.06)	0.65 (0.08)
P value	<0.005	<0.005	<0.005	NS

$\dot{W}_I$, total inspiratory work; $\dot{W}_{Iel}$, elastic component of inspiratory work; $\dot{W}_{Ires}$, resistive component of inspiratory work; $\dot{V}_E$, minute ventilation; NS, not statistically significant ($P > 0.05$).

[a] Values are mean ± (SE) for all patients.

[b] *P* values refer to CPAP versus control (paired *t* test).

(From Petrof et al.,[40] with permission.)

Management

The primary approach to managing auto-PEEP, if it is a result of dynamic airflow obstruction, is to treat the obstruction (Table 76-8) by appropriate bronchial hygiene techniques and aerosolized as well as systemic drug therapy. Auto-PEEP level can also be reduced if the approach used to ventilate is modified[117]; specifically, by lengthening expiratory time by decreasing rate and increasing tidal volume or by decreasing inspiratory time by increasing peak inspiratory flow and decreasing compressible volume loss with the use of low compressible volume circuits.[120] The use of a large (9-mm ID) endotracheal tube,[121] particularly in patients with large minute volume requirements, as well as the avoidance of I/E ratio inversion, may also reduce auto-PEEP.

Maintaining a normal pH by administration of $NaHCO_3$ in the presence of a metabolic acidosis, instead of maintaining alveolar hyperventilation, normally reduces auto-PEEP.[117] In addition to the above, the use of a low IMV rate supplemented with spontaneous ventilation may reduce the auto-PEEP level in patients receiving assisted ventilation.[39]

Under certain conditions the application of PEEP or CPAP may reduce the work of breathing as a result of auto-PEEP

Table 76-7. Methods Used to Quantify Auto-PEEP

End-expiratory hold	Use of Braschi valve
Servo 900C	Respiratory inductive plethysmography
Hamilton Veolar	Servo 940 mechanics calculator
Ohmeda Advent	Esophageal pressure monitoring

in spontaneously breathing patients. Figure 76-20, from Smith and Marini,[39] depicts the three settings in which auto-PEEP may develop: (1) inadequate expiratory time without dynamic airflow obstruction; (2) generalized dynamic airflow obstruction; and (3) localized dynamic airflow obstruction.

When auto-PEEP is a result of inadequate expiratory time without concomitant dynamic airflow obstruction, the applied PEEP and the auto-PEEP are additive. This additive effect occurs because there is no alteration in dynamic airflow limitation as external PEEP is applied. On the other hand, if auto-PEEP is purely a result of dynamic airflow obstruction, the applied PEEP may reduce the auto-PEEP level by improving gas distribution and minimizing the transpulmonary pressure differential during exhalation.[39,40] Smith and Marini[39] demonstrated a reduction in overall auto-PEEP level, an increase in peak expiratory flow, a decrease in end-expiratory flow, a reduction in expiratory resistance, and a reduction in RC as PEEP was applied to a series of ICU patients maintained on partial ventilatory support. Similar findings were demonstrated by Petrof et al.[40] in a group of COPD patients being weaned from ventilatory support to whom varying levels of CPAP were applied (Tables 76-5 and 76-6).

The third situation, and probably the one most commonly encountered clinically, is localized dynamic airflow obstruction (i.e., the development of auto-PEEP in specific lung units). This may result in overdistension of affected lung units and compression of nearby normal lung units. The application of PEEP in this setting may or may not improve overall gas distribution. Theoretically, the applied PEEP would decrease expiratory resistance in units with dynamic airflow obstruction and as a result would decrease end-expiratory volume in these units while increasing the end-expiratory volume in normal lung units. However, care must be exercised in this setting not to cause generalized overdistension.

The application of PEEP/CPAP to minimize the effects of auto-PEEP must be carried out very cautiously. If applied PEEP is positively affecting auto-PEEP, peak airway pressure should only increase a minimal amount as PEEP is applied. The same should occur with plateau pressure unless significant overdistension occurs. In the study by Petrof et al.,[40] a mean increase in FRC of only 450 mL occurred as 15 cmH_2O CPAP was applied. If peak airway pressure and plateau pressure increase sufficiently to equal or exceed the level of PEEP applied, the applied PEEP is simply adding to the auto-PEEP and should be removed. In patients failing to trigger the mechanical ventilator on every spontaneous effort because of auto-PEEP, slowly increasing the applied PEEP by 1- or 2-cmH_2O increments allows end-expiratory and ventilator circuit pressure to equilibrate. The proper level of applied PEEP is determined by the lack of dyssynchrony between the patient and the ventilator.

Applied PEEP should only be used to modify the effects of auto-PEEP after the other approaches outlined above have been tried. My colleagues and I routinely use 5 cmH_2O PEEP in patients dependent on mechanical ventilation and in patients being weaned who have dynamic airflow limitation, and have used higher levels in the management of acute auto-PEEP in the patient with asthma or COPD. Qvist

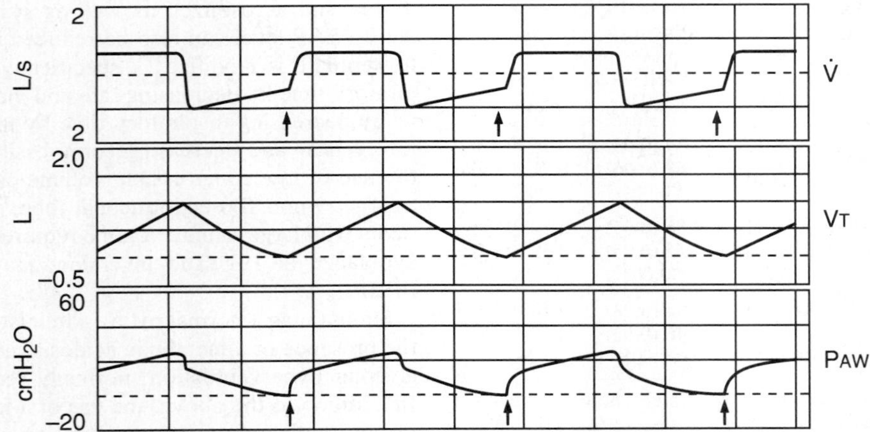

Figure 76-15. Airway pressure (PAW) and flow waveforms during volume-limited controlled ventilation in the presence of auto-PEEP. The initial airway pressure demonstrates a rapid initial increase (arrow), approximating the auto-PEEP level and then gradually increasing to peak airway pressure. Expiratory gas flow does not return to zero (arrow) in the presence of auto-PEEP.

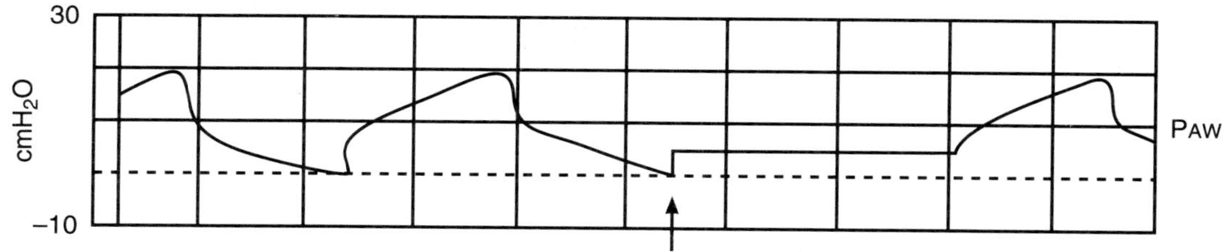

Figure 76-16. Measurement of auto-PEEP (arrow) using an end-expiratory hold on the Servo 900C ventilator. Note that peak airway pressure is not affected on the inspiration following measurement since auto-PEEP is present even though unnoticed on every breath.

et al.[83] have used up to 20 cmH_2O applied PEEP to manage the patient with acute asthma.

INADVERTENT PEEP

The term *inadvertent PEEP* refers to the PEEP developed in the ventilator system as a result of the ventilator operation. As noted later, under Technical Application of PEEP, ventilator exhalation valves and PEEP valves can inadvertently develop PEEP in the circuit in spite of the PEEP level being set at zero. This is particularly true of continuous gas flow systems because of the flow-resistant properties of all PEEP devices. Inadvertent PEEP is real PEEP. Regardless of the reason for its presence, PEEP is being applied, and its effects should be monitored if it cannot be eliminated by technical alterations of the mechanical ventilator system.

CLINICAL USE IN ARDS

Goals

Overall, the goal of ventilatory support is to maintain tissue oxygenation. This, of course, is the primary goal of PEEP, but more specifically, the goals of PEEP include (1) reversal of hypoxemia, (2) decreased work of the myocardium, and (3) decreased work of breathing, all accomplished without adversely affecting cardiac output.[34] Since the severity of illness in ARDS is frequently marked, it is necessary to define specific end points of PEEP therapy. In general, because of the adverse physiologic effects of PEEP discussed earlier, our focus during application of PEEP is to apply the least PEEP necessary to maintain a PO_2 of about 55 mmHg with an inspired O_2 fraction (FIO_2) of 0.60 to 0.80 or less (Table 76-9). A PO_2 of 55 mmHg may be questioned

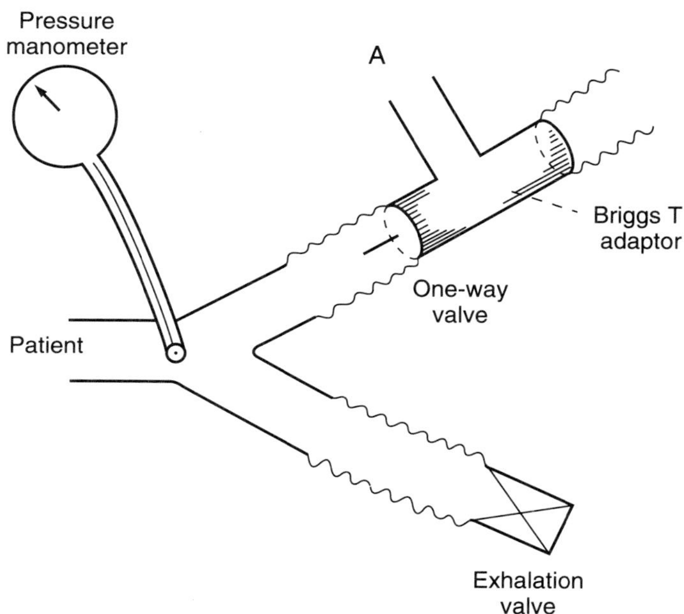

Figure 76-17. Placement of the Braschi valve (Briggs adapter with one-way valve) in the inspiratory limb of the ventilator circuit. A, occlusion port to atmosphere. See text for details on use to determine auto-PEEP.

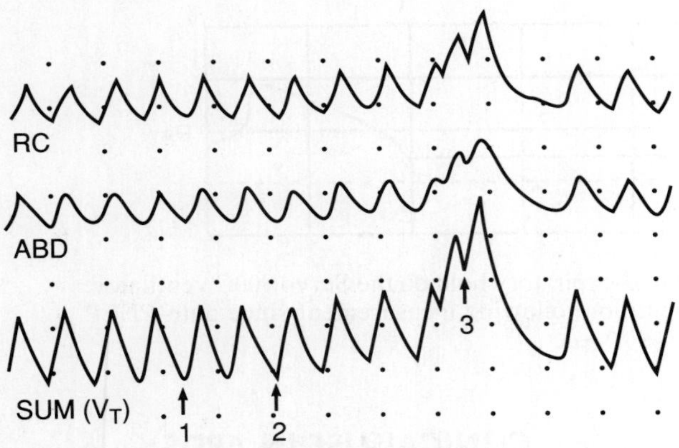

Figure 76-18. Auto-PEEP as measured by respiratory inductive plethysmography. External PEEP was applied at arrow 1 (4 cmH_2O), at arrow 2 (6 cmH_2O), and at arrow 3 (8 cmH_2O). The level of auto-PEEP is equal to the highest applied PEEP value without an increase in external thoracic/abdominal gas volume (6 cmH_2O), RC, rib cage; ABD, abdomen; Sum (V_T), total rib cage plus abdomen. (From Hoffman et al.,[119] with permission.)

Table 76-8. Approaches Used to Modify the Level of Auto-PEEP

Decrease dynamic airflow obstruction
- Aggressive bronchodilation
- Chest physical therapy
- Airway suctioning
- Large-size endotracheal tube

Normalize pH
- Administer $NaHCO_3$ during metabolic acidosis
- Avoid purposeful hyperventilation

Allow PCO_2 to rise into the 50–60 mmHg range by decreasing rate and normalizing pH

Modify ventilatory pattern
- Increase expiratory time
  - Decrease rate
  - Increase V_T
- Decrease inspiratory time
  - Increase peak inspiratory flow
  - Use low compressible volume circuit
- Use low rate SIMV

Apply PEEP/CPAP

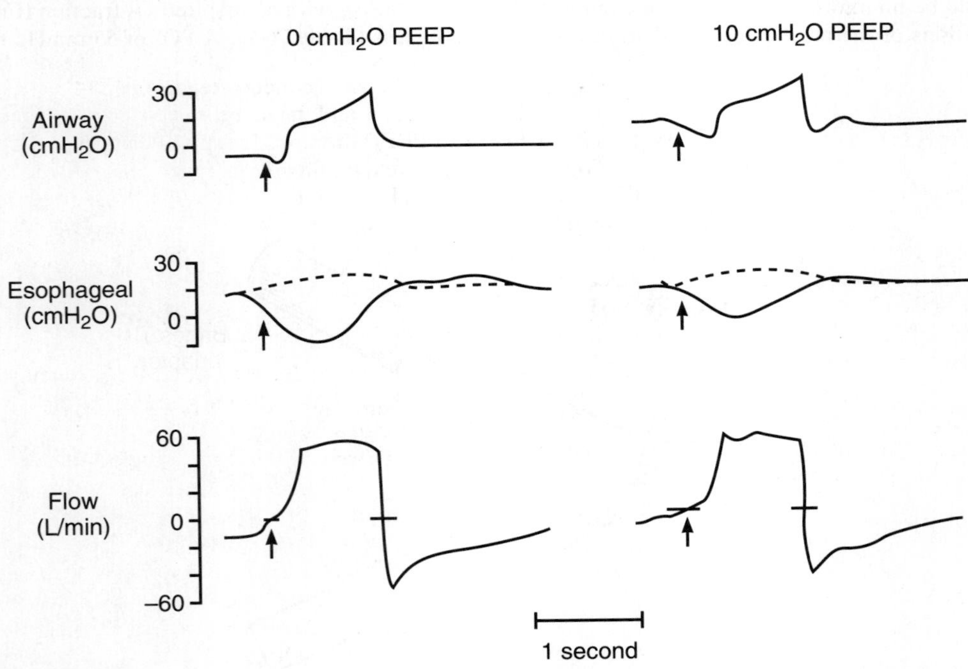

Figure 76-19. Assessment of the level of auto-PEEP in spontaneously breathing patients by evaluation of esophageal pressure change relative to either airway opening pressure or flow at airway opening. Arrows indicate pressure and flow change at airway opening. The change in esophageal pressure between baseline and the level that allows change in airway opening pressure or in flow is equal to the auto-PEEP level. Note effect of 10 cmH_2O applied PEEP on the level of auto-PEEP (left side). (From Smith and Marini,[39] with permission.)

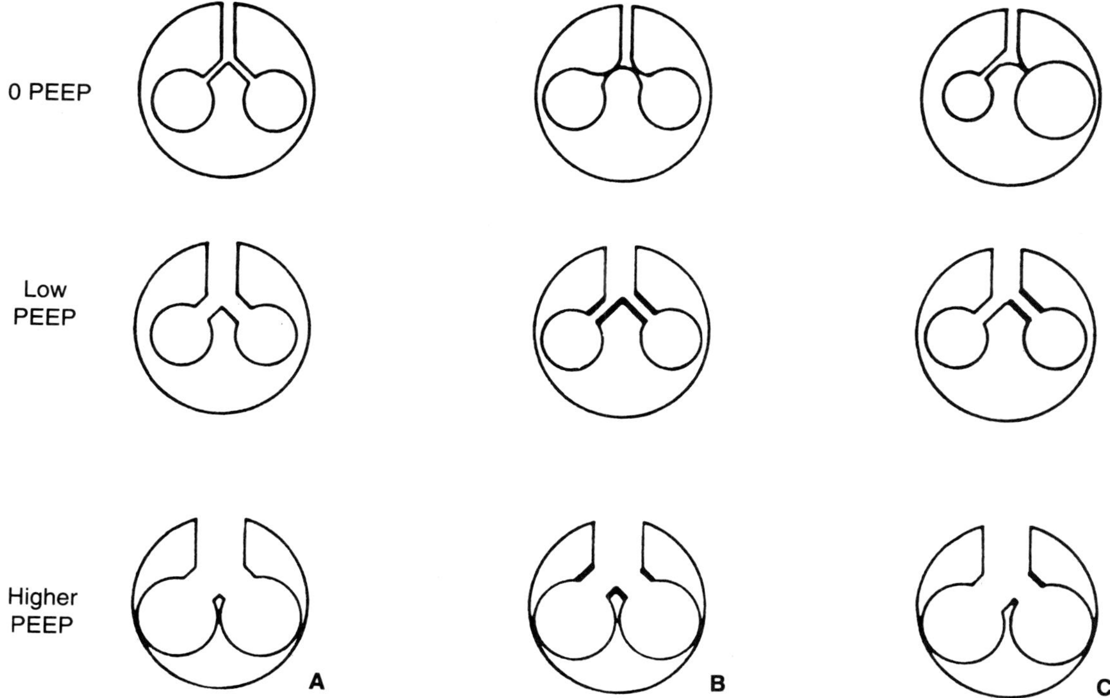

Figure 76-20. Theoretical model of airflow obstruction causing auto-PEEP, as proposed by Smith and Marini. **(A)** Auto-PEEP caused by insufficient expiratory time, not dynamic airflow limitation. **(B)** Generalized dynamic airflow limitation. **(C)** Localized dynamic airflow limitation. Also illustrated is the effect of applied PEEP in each setting. See text for discussion. (From Smith and Marini,[39] with permission.)

as inadequate by some; however, the critically ill ARDS patient is normally paralyzed and sedated with a reduced O_2 consumption provided body temperature is normal. As long as hemoglobin content (above 10 g) and cardiac output are acceptable and acid-base status is normal, a PO_2 of 55 mmHg provides about 88 percent saturation of the hemoglobin and an O_2 content of about 12 Vol%. It should be remembered that home O_2 therapy is not considered to be indicated unless PO_2 levels are less than 55 mmHg.[116] Chapter 65 discusses O_2 toxicity and raises concern about the use of high F_IO_2 levels. However, because of the lack of convincing evidence documenting the adverse effect of high F_IO_2 in the presence of severe ARDS, we have begun to accept higher F_IO_2 levels when high PEEP levels (above 15 cmH_2O) are required to maintain PO_2 in the 50 to 60 mmHg range.

Table 76-9. Goals of PEEP Therapy in Severe ARDS

PO_2 of about 50–60 mmHg
Hb content >10 g
Normal body temperature
$F_IO_2 \leq 0.60$–0.80
Normal cardiac output
Cardiac index 2.5–4.0 L/min/m^2

Finally, concern regarding cardiac output almost always exists and must be factored into discussions on goals of PEEP therapy. Ideally, we attempt to maintain the cardiac index within normal range (2.5 to 4.0 L/min/m^2) and use fluid and beta-agonists when necessary to maintain the cardiac index.

Monitoring

Since PEEP has a potentially significant effect on the entire cardiopulmonary system, as many of the variables potentially affected by PEEP as can be monitored should be monitored. Essentially, these include all those variables listed in Table 76-2. Realistically, gas exchanges, pulmonary mechanics, and hemodynamics must be monitored during the use of PEEP. The PO_2, along with hemoglobin content and saturation, are the most direct measurements of ability to oxygenate blood. Hemoglobin saturation is useful provided it is directly measured. Pulse oximetry data, although lacking accuracy, are ideal for monitoring changes in oxygenation state as PEEP is applied. Pulse oximetry also provides immediate notification of an alteration in oxygenation state if a patient's clinical status changes. We would recommend the use of pulse oximetry in any patient requiring the therapeutic application of PEEP in ARDS.

Monitoring of peak, mean, and plateau airway pressures,

as well as calculation of static lung compliance, helps to define pulmonary mechanics at a given PEEP level.[123] Some believe that mean airway pressure plays an important role in determining the appropriate PEEP level.[124] We have found that it is not unusual for a mean airway pressure of about 20 cmH_2O to be necessary to maintain oxygenation in severe ARDS. Monitoring of alteration in peak and plateau airway pressure can help evaluate the effect of PEEP application on overdistension. If overdistension has occurred, a small increase in PEEP, 2 to 3 cmH_2O, may result in a marked increase (5 to 10 cmH_2O) in peak and plateau pressure. Normally, peak and plateau pressures should stay the same or decrease if lung has been recruited with the application of PEEP. At worst, peak and plateau pressure should only increase by an amount equivalent to the amount of PEEP added.

Since PEEP has the capability of decreasing cardiac output and intrathoracic vascular pressures, careful monitoring of hemodynamics is essential during its application. Ideally, pressures measured within the thoracic cavity should remain the same or increase as PEEP is applied. If they decrease, the increase in mean intrathoracic pressure as PEEP is applied has decreased flow. This may necessitate an adjustment of PEEP level or administration of fluid or beta-agonists. Whether a pulmonary artery catheter is necessary for appropriate management of PEEP is questionable. We believe a pulmonary artery catheter is advisable for more detailed assessment of pulmonary hemodynamics whenever PEEP levels reach 15 cmH_2O.

Clinical Approach

Numerous approaches to the application of PEEP (Table 76-10) have been described. These include "optimal,"[24] "best,"[125] and "super-PEEP,"[69,70] each with its defined end points evolving about specific variables (e.g., compliance, $P\bar{v}O_2$, shunt fraction). We would use the term *least PEEP* to define the most appropriate level of PEEP for a given patient. As defined above, our end points include a PO_2 of about 55 mmHg and an F_IO_2 less than or equal to 0.60 to 0.80 while maintaining cardiovascular status. During the initial application and daily adjustment of PEEP, we recommend the performance of a PEEP trial (Table 76-11), in which varying levels of PEEP are carefully applied in successive increments until the least PEEP level achieving the goals of therapy is identified. Ideally, the highest PEEP level still on the steep aspect of the compliance is preferred. Comparisons of airway pressure, gas exchange, and hemodynamics are correlated with compliance to determine the appropriate setting. Once PEEP level is established, the F_IO_2 is decreased to that level while maintaining the PO_2 in the 50- to 60-mmHg range. In unstable patients, adjustments in PEEP and F_IO_2 are normally made in small increments of 2 to 3 cmH_2O or 0.05 F_IO_2, and the effect of these changes completely assessed, as outlined, to avoid the marked decrease in oxygenation occasionally seen as therapy is withdrawn.

Table 76-10. Approaches Used to Achieve the Most Appropriate PEEP Level

Investigators	Date	End Points	Terminology
Suter et al.[24]	1975	Maximum lung-thorax compliance	Optimal PEEP
Kirby et al.[69]	1975	Reduction of shunt to 0.15	Super-PEEP
Douglas & Downs[70]	1977	Reduction of shunt to 0.12	Super-PEEP
Walkinshaw & Shoemaker[126]	1980	Maximal $\dot{V}O_2$	Preferred PEEP
Murray et al.[36]	1984	Minimal $PaCO_2$-$P_{ET}CO_2$	—
Demers et al.[125]	1977	Highest $P\bar{v}O_2$	Best PEEP

PEEP Withdrawal

PEEP withdrawal should not require an abrupt change from a very high level of PEEP. If PEEP trials are performed on a daily basis, the need to make large changes in PEEP should rarely exist. In fact, abrupt changes in PEEP may lead to hemodynamic instability if fluid had been administered during the application of PEEP or if a marked change in oxygenation status has occurred, requiring time for recovery.[127] This is particularly true in patients with compromised left ventricular function.[128] The level of PEEP applied may be maintaining a delicate pulmonary vascular fluid balance in association with a compromised left ventricular function. PEEP reduction in this setting can cause marked alteration in left ventricular function, with pulmonary hypertension and subsequent cardiopulmonary failure.

In general, PEEP is reduced in 2- to 5-cmH_2O increments, with careful assessment 10 to 15 minutes after the decrease. The criteria used by Hudson et al.[127] during PEEP withdrawal (Table 76-12) can be applied in most clinical settings.

PEEP during Manual Ventilation

As a result of the potential alterations in pulmonary mechanics, gas exchange, and hemodynamics when PEEP is abruptly discontinued, a level of PEEP equivalent to that applied by the mechanical ventilator should be applied to all manual ventilators whenever mechanical ventilation is momentarily discontinued. All the manual ventilation equipment currently on the market allows for the application of PEEP (see below for details).

TECHNICAL APPLICATION

Regardless of whether PEEP is being applied to a spontaneously breathing patient or one supported by mechanical

Table 76-11. Representative PEEP Trials for Determining the Level of PEEP Used in Initial Management of Patients with ARDS

	PEEP (cmH_2O)	PaO_2 (mmHg)	BP (mmHg)	CO (L/min)	C (mL/cmH_2O)
Example 1 (FIO_2 = 0.60)[a]					
0 min	0	54	120/80		28
15 min	5	72	120/80		32
30 min	10	128	120/80		36
Example 2 (FIO_2 = 1.00)[b]					
0 min	0	52		6.0	20
15 min	5	55		6.0	20
40 min	10	67		6.0	22
60 min	15	96		5.8	25
80 min	20	124		4.5	26
Example 3 (FIO_2 = 1.00)[c]					
0 min	0	46		5.5	22
20 min	5	50		5.5	22
40 min	10	66		5.7	28
60 min	15	97		5.3	30
80 min	20	128		5.3	25

BP, blood pressure; CO, cardiac output; C, patient/system compliance.

[a] Example 1 is a trial to a PEEP of 10 cmH_2O in a patient with uncomplicated ARDS whose mental status, BP, and urine output are normal and stable. Although acceptable arterial oxygenation is achieved at a PEEP of 5 cmH_2O, continuing on to 10 cmH_2O produces a large enough increase in PaO_2 to permit lowering FIO_2 to 0.5 or below. Pulmonary artery catheterization and measurement of cardiac output are unnecessary.

[b] Example 2 is an initial trial in a severely hypoxemic, hemodynamically unstable patient with underlying cardiac disease and unclear central volume status. In such patients the time intervals may have to be longer because of the number and complexity of measurements and other care procedures required, but should be less than 30 minutes if possible. Cardiac output measurements are necessary because a PEEP of 15 cmH_2O and higher is used, the patient has cardiac disease, rendering hemodynamic responses unpredictable, and hypovolemia is a possibility. The most appropriate PEEP in our opinion is at 15 cmH_2O; arterial O_2 content (CaO_2) is not significantly improved at 20 cmH_2O, and O_2 transport ($CaO_2 \times CO$) falls by approximately 25% despite an increase in PaO_2.

[c] Example 3 is a clinical setting similar to that in Example 2. Cardiac output measurement is needed for the same reasons as above, to monitor for adverse cardiac effects of PEEP. Although PaO_2, CaO_2, and O_2 transport continue to increase up to a PEEP of 15 cmH_2O and PaO_2 is raised further at 20 cmH_2O without a drop in cardiac output, we believe that the drop in C at 20 cmH_2O signifies an increased likelihood of alveolar rupture and pneumothorax and therefore would use 15 cmH_2O as the best PEEP level. Decreasing V_T may permit the use of 20 cmH_2O by diminishing the peak distending volume and the risk of barotrauma.

(From Bolin and Pierson.[148])

ventilation, a mechanism must be incorporated into the gas delivery system to allow for the application of PEEP. Generally, devices capable of generating PEEP are defined as either flow resistors or threshold resistors.

Flow Resistors

A flow resistor is a device that establishes a fixed resistance at the expiratory limb of a ventilator or continuous positive airway pressure circuit. The PEEP level established is dependent on the flow of gas ($\dot{V}$) through the system and the physical characteristics (resistance [R]) of the device that affects gas flow; that is, PEEP level is governed by the law of flow (analogous to Ohm's law)

$$P \approx (R)(\dot{V}) \tag{2}$$

where P is the expiratory pressure established. The level of PEEP in this system can be altered by altering either R or $\dot{V}$. If $\dot{V}$ is a constant (K), alterations in R directly affect PEEP level:

$$K \approx \frac{R}{P} \tag{3}$$

For a given R, PEEP increases linearly with an increase in total flow through the valve.

Banner and associates[129] have argued that the pressure exerted during exhalation is more appropriately represented by

$$\text{Expiratory pressure} \approx R(\dot{V}_{exh} + \dot{V}_{sys}) \tag{4}$$

Table 76-12. Criteria Used for Initiation of PEEP Reduction

Hemodynamic stability
Sepsis under control
FIO_2 reduced to 0.5
PaO_2 ≥70 mmHg
Monitor effect after 5–15 min
Use pulse oximeter to maintain SaO_2 ≥90%
Decrease PEEP in increments of 2–5 cmH_2O
If ARDS of short duration, decrease PEEP q6h
If ARDS of prolonged duration, decrease PEEP q6–12h

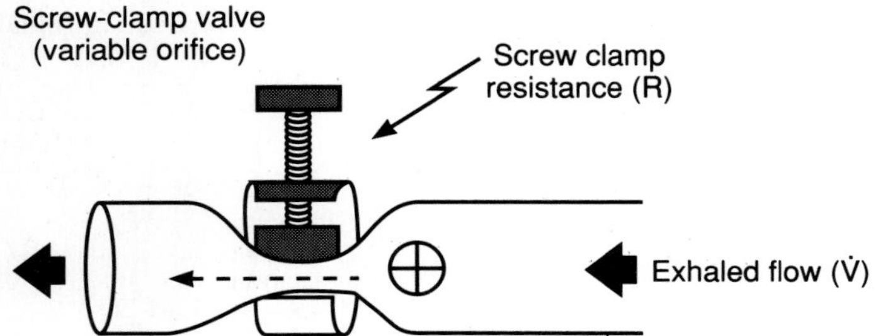

Figure 76-21. Variable-orifice flow resistor PEEP device. Restriction of gas flow is controlled by alteration of the screw clamp setting. (From Banner et al.,[129] with permission.)

where $\dot{V}_{exh}$ is the patient's exhaled flow rate and $\dot{V}_{sys}$ is the set system flow rate. Increased total system flow occurs throughout exhalation, and it is this flow that determines the pressure established. Therefore, patients must maintain system pressure above that created by the flow resistor prior to exhalation in order for exhalation to occur. The general operation of a flow resistor is illustrated in Figure 76-21.

Threshold Resistors

Threshold resistors generate a pressure (P) by exerting a force (F) over a discrete surface area (SA).

$$P \approx F/SA \quad (5)$$

Theoretically threshold resistors, in contrast to flow resistors, generate pressure without causing flow resistance. However, in reality most devices classified as threshold resistors actually function as partial flow resistors.[42,124] Their function, as described by Banner,[130] is best characterized by the following equation:

$$P \approx F/SA + R(\dot{V}_{exh} + \dot{V}_{sys}) \quad (6)$$

That is, the PEEP level is established both by the design of the valve and the gas flow through it. The greater the dependence on flow to establish PEEP in any exhalation-PEEP valve, the greater the work of breathing imposed by the valve. As inspiration occurs, the diversion of system flow from the exhalation valve to the patient lowers system end-expiratory pressure; this requires the patient to generate a greater pressure to maintain diversion of flow, and results in greater work of breathing.[43] The flow-resistive properties of threshold resistors operating as exhalation-PEEP valves have been demonstrated by many.[129,131–133]

Threshold resistors can be classified as either gravity-dependent or non-gravity-dependent.[134] Gravity-dependent resistors include the original PEEP device, the underwater seal (Fig. 76-22), the Emerson water column, and the Boehringer weighted ball valve. Most non-gravity-dependent resistors are spring-loaded valves (Fig. 76-23) or magnetic valves (Fig. 76-24). Mechanical ventilators normally use a mushroom or diaphragm-type (Fig. 76-25) exhalation valve to exert PEEP. These valves usually possess significant flow resistive properties.[135] On the other hand, some of the newest ventilators have sophisticated exhalation valves designed with virtually no flow resistance.[129,131] One such system is the Hamilton exhalation valve (Fig. 76-26). Because it is mechanically opened by an electromagnetic system, it has virtually no flow resistance effects, nor does it impose significant work of

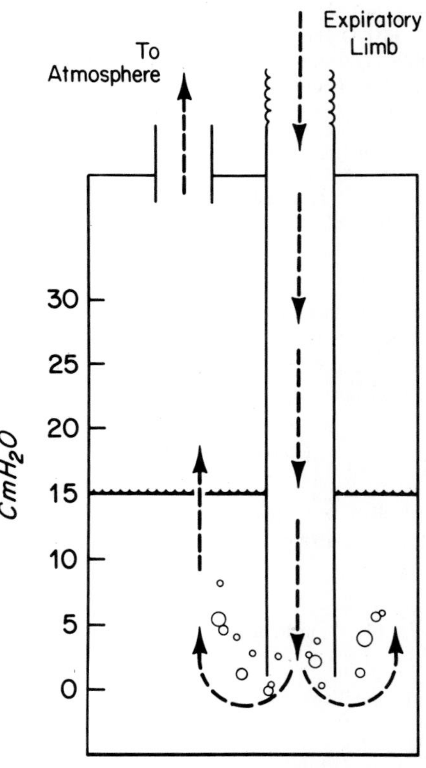

Figure 76-22. Underwater-seal threshold resistor PEEP device. PEEP level is determined by the depth of submersion of the expiratory limb. (From Kacmarek and Goulet,[42] with permission.)

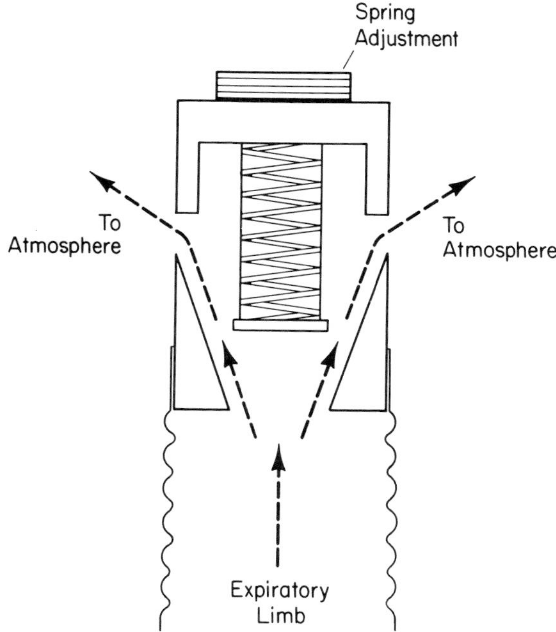

Figure 76-23. Spring-loaded threshold resistor PEEP device. Expired gas must exert sufficient force to lift the spring-loaded valve off its seat to allow gas to exit from the system. (From Kacmarek and Goulet,[42] with permission.)

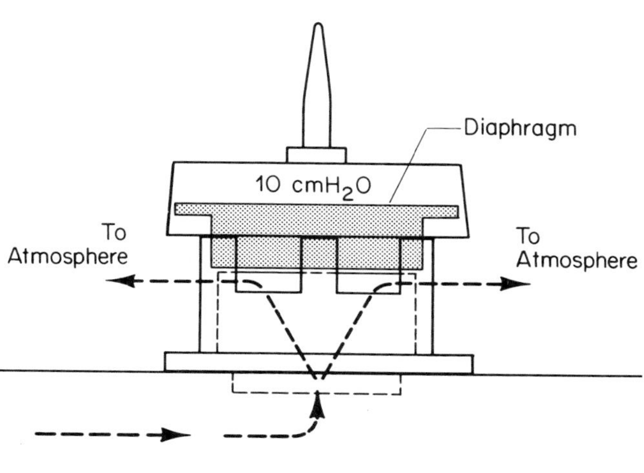

Figure 76-25. Diaphragm-type exhalation valve PEEP device. Sufficient force must be exerted during expiration to overcome the end-expiratory pressure maintained over the diaphragm during exhalation. Surface area of the valve seat and outlet ports may increase resistance to gas flow. (From Kacmarek and Goulet,[42] with permission.)

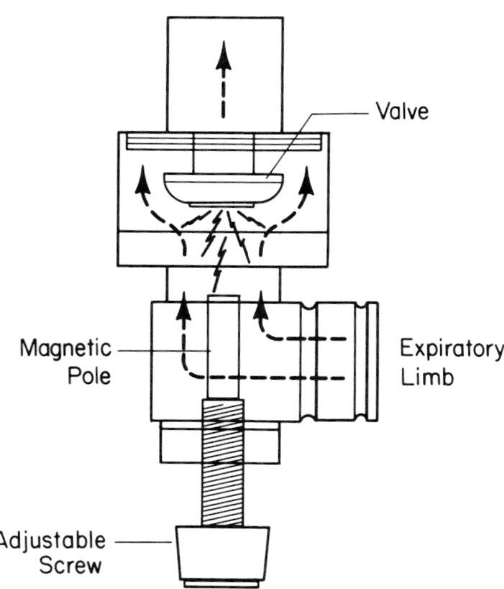

Figure 76-24. Magnetic-valve threshold resistor PEEP device. The force exerted by the exhaled gas must be sufficient to overcome the magnetic attraction between the magnetic pole and the metallic disc. (From Kacmarek and Goulet,[42] with permission.)

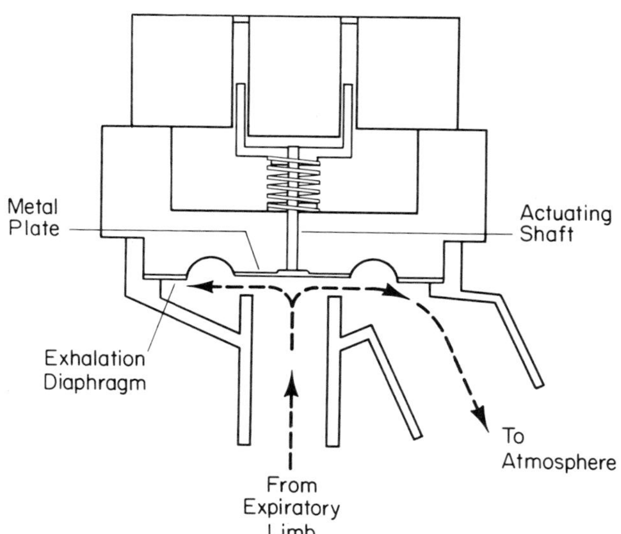

Figure 76-26. Hamilton ventilator exhalation valve PEEP device. The exhalation diaphragm is electromagnetically positioned by the actuating shaft. During exhalation sufficient force must be exerted to overcome the end-expiratory pressure maintained by the actuating shaft on the diaphragm. (From Kacmarek and Goulet,[42] with permission.)

Table 76-13. Classification of PEEP Devices

Type	Manufacturer	Part No.	Method of Operation	Gravity Dependence	Range (cmH_2O)	Flow Resistance
Underwater seal	—	—	Hydrostatic force	Dependent	Unlimited	Low
Water column	Emerson	KS PEEP bottle	Hydrostatic force	Dependent	0–25 0–50	Moderate
Ball valve	Boehringer	2715-2719	Weighted ball	Dependent	2.5, 5, 10, 15	Moderate to high
Spring-loaded	Vital Signs	9003-9022	Flexion of multiple springs	Nondependent	2.5, 5, 7.5, 10, 12.5, 15, 20	Low
	Ambu, Inc.	194-001-000	Compression of spring	Nondependent	0–20	High
	Anesthesia PEEP-20 PEEP-10	 177000 137-002-000	 Compression of spring Compression of spring	 Nondependent Nondependent	 0–20 0–10	 High Moderate
	Boehringer (Maxi-PEEP)	4830	Compression of spring	Nondependent	0–30	High
	Life Design Systems	LDS-8870	Compression of spring	Nondependent	0.20	Moderate
	Lifeguard	11346	Compression of spring	Nondependent	0.16	Moderate
	Intertech	PL-2958	Compression of spring	Nondependent	0.20	Moderate
Magnetic valve	Instrumentation Industries	BE 171	Magnetic attraction	Nondependent	2.5, 5, 7.5, 10, 12.5, 15	Low to moderate
		BE 142	Magnetic attraction	Nondependent	0–20	Low to moderate
Mushroom valve	Puritan-Bennett	MA-1, MA-2, 7200	Inflatable balloon	Nondependent	Limit of ventilator	Moderate to high
	Intermed	Bear 1, 2, 3, 5	Inflatable balloon	Nondependent	Limit of ventilator	Moderate
	Newport	E 100i, Breeze Wave	Inflatable balloon	Nondependent	Limit of ventilator	Moderate
Scissor valve	Siemens	900, 900B, 900C	Variable orifice	Nondependent	Limit of ventilator	High
Diaphragm	Hamilton	Alveolar, Amadaeus	Magnetic attraction	Nondependent	Limit of ventilator	Low
	Ohmeda	CPU-1, Advent	Magnetic attraction	Nondependent	Limit of ventilator	Low
	Disposable		Gaseous compression	Nondependent	Limit of ventilator	High
Mushroom valve	Disposable		Inflatable balloon	Nondependent	Limit of ventilator	High

breathing.[129] More detailed reviews of the function of PEEP devices are available elsewhere.[98,134] Table 76-13 lists the general characteristics of currently available PEEP devices.

CPAP Systems

Many approaches are available to deliver PEEP to the spontaneously breathing patient. However, CPAP systems may be grouped into two general categories, demand systems and continuous flow systems. Each approach has its merits, but the clinician must be aware of concerns with each.

Demand Systems

All the mechanical ventilators manufactured today allow for administration of CPAP, with spontaneous gas flow provided by a demand system. These systems are designed to provide rapid flow of gas into the ventilator circuit to meet the patient's inspiratory needs and to maintain the system at baseline pressure. In most of these systems PEEP is maintained by a mushroom or diaphragm exhalation valve. As already discussed, these valves, because of individual design, are highly resistant to gas flow. However, because a continuous flow is not provided, increased system pressure during patient exhalation is normally a clinical problem only in patients forcefully exhaling[132]; passive exhalation rarely results in significant alterations in PEEP level.[134] Care must be taken when patients do actively expire or "buck" against the system during attempts to cough.

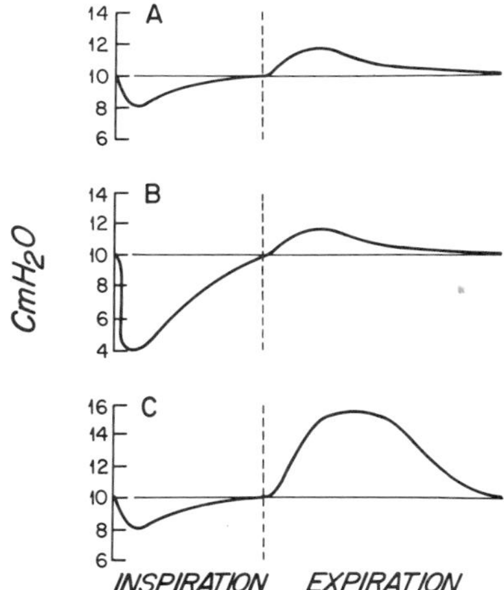

Figure 76-27. Airway pressure curves with the application of CPAP. Curve A represents an ideal curve; maximum pressure deviation from baseline is ± 2 cmH_2O. Curve B represents excessive pressure drop during inspiration, normally a result of insensitive demand systems or insufficient flow with continuous flow systems. Curve C represents excessive expiratory resistance resulting from the use of a high flow resistance PEEP device. (From Kacmarek and Goulet,[42] with permission.)

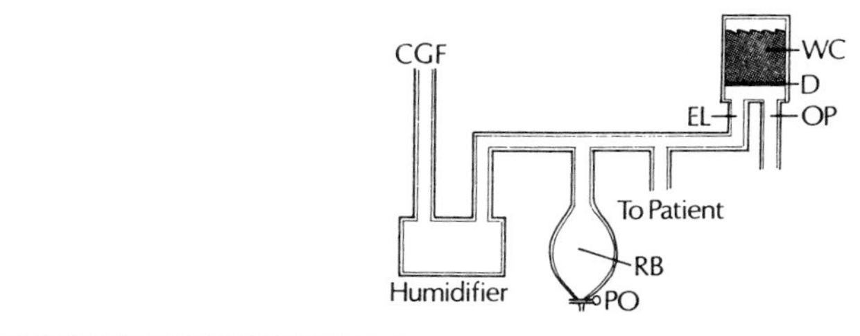

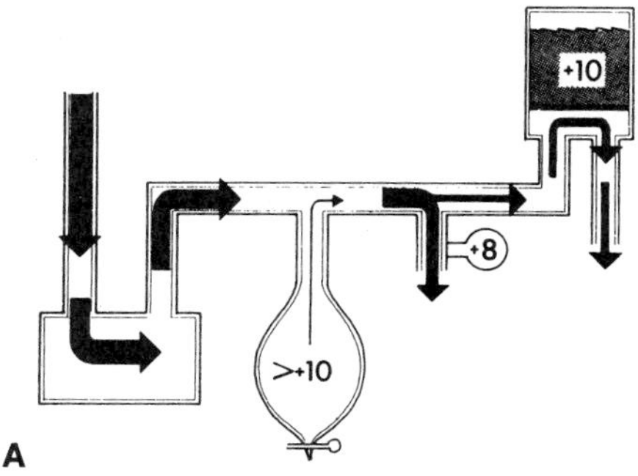

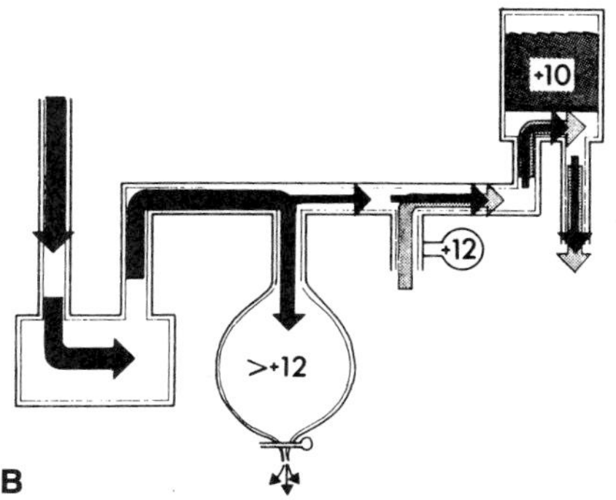

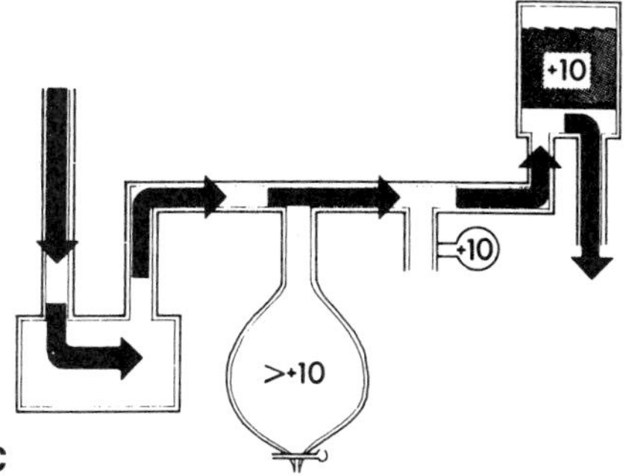

Figure 76-28. Schematic representation of a continuous flow CPAP system. (**A**) During inspiration the patient must create a pressure differential in order to inhale. However, system pressure should decrease by no more than 2 cmH_2O, and continuous gas flow out of the system should be measurable, even during peak inspiration. (**B & C**) During expiration a pressure differential must also be created; however, an ideal PEEP device should not cause pressures to increase over the end-expiratory level by more than 2 cmH_2O. CGF, continuous gas flow; PO, pop-off valve; RB, reservoir bag; EL, expiratory limb; D, diaphragm; WC, water column; OP, output port. (From Shapiro et al.,[59] with permission.)

Figure 76-27 depicts a series of airway pressure curves when CPAP is applied. Curve A represents the ideal curve on which little alteration in baseline pressure is noted. Generally, a ± 2 cmH_2O variation in baseline pressure is the accepted limit.[135–137] Curve C illustrates the effect of resistance to gas flow through the system during a forced exhalation; a significant rise of baseline pressure and an increase in patient expiratory work of breathing are noted.[42] The most common problem with the use of demand CPAP systems, however, is depicted in curve B, namely, a significant drop in system pressure because of an inability of the demand system to meet the patient's inspiratory needs.

The lack of responsiveness and the inability of demand systems to meet patients' inspiratory needs are well documented[137–140] and represent the primary concern with the use of demand CPAP systems. These systems can impose a significant amount of work and result in failure of a patient to tolerate the administration of CPAP. However, recent data indicate that provided the demand system is operating properly, the appropriate humidifier is used, and the sensitivity is appropriately set, demand systems function as well as or better than continuous flow systems which are dependent on the PEEP device used in such systems.[42,141,142] As discussed in detail in Chapter 87, to ensure that imposed work of breathing is not a factor, 5 to 10 cmH_2O inspiratory pressure support should be used during demand CPAP administration.[42]

Continuous Flow CPAP

Numerous variations in the design of continuous flow CPAP systems have been described in the literature.[143–146] In each of these systems the circuit is designed to minimize the imposed work of breathing. As depicted in Figure 76-28, one must be concerned with changes in pressure during inspiration that reflect inspiratory work imposed on the patient[42,43] and changes in system pressure during expiration that reflect imposed expiratory work.[132] Pressure changes during expiration are dependent on the PEEP device selected, while inspiratory pressure changes are affected by the system's capability of providing sufficient gas volume to satisfy continuous patient inspiratory demands,[134,135] as well as by the PEEP device itself.

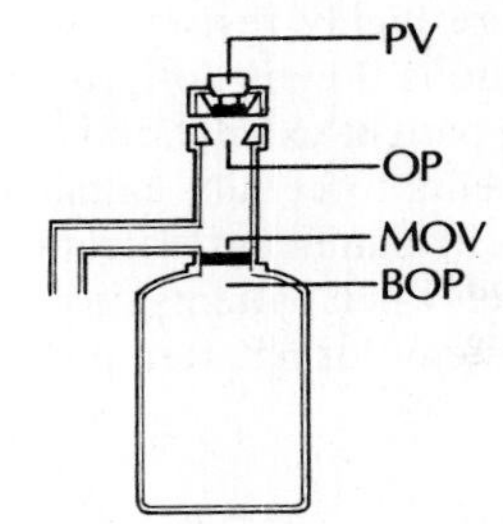

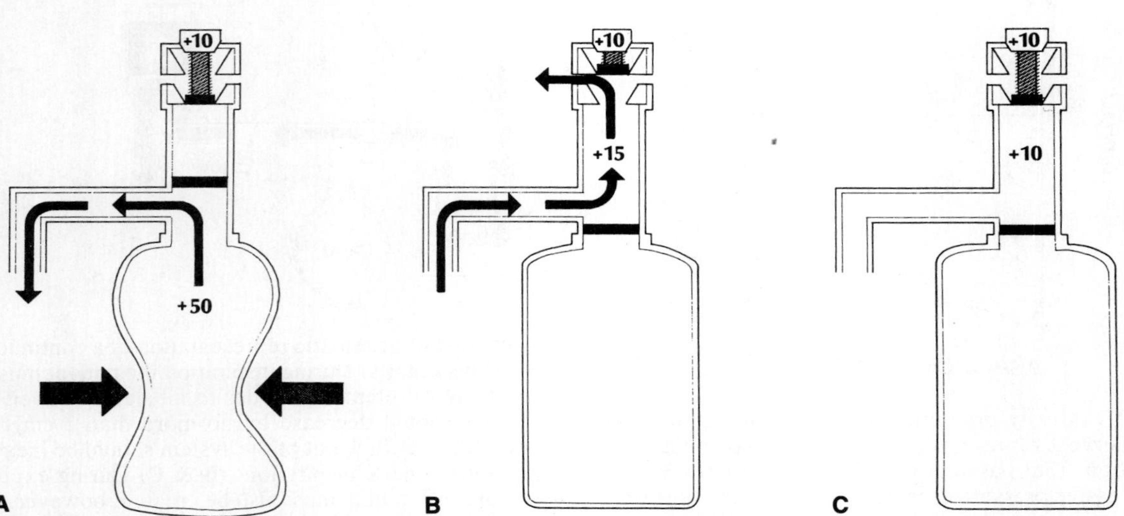

Figure 76-29. Schematic representation of a spring-loaded PEEP valve attached to a manual ventilator with a single gas-collecting head. **(A)** positive pressure ventilation (PPV); **(B)** exhalation; **(C)** end exhalation. PV, spring-loaded valve; OP, outlet port; MOV, movable occluding valve of manual ventilator; BOP, outlet port of manual ventilator. (From Shapiro et al.,[59] with permission.)

A typical CPAP continuous flow system is illustrated in Figure 76-28. This system includes a medium-volume high-compliance reservoir bag (3 to 5 L) and maintains system flow in excess of patient peak inspiratory flow demands. Characteristically, system continuous flows are maintained at 60 to 90 L/min, the adequacy of continuous flow being evaluated by gas exiting the system. Gas exiting the system during peak inspiratory flow periods should be measurable. For the agitated patient with high inspiratory flow requirements, it is advisable to use a high-capacity (10-L) reservoir or to employ two smaller-volume (5-L) bags in series. Figure 76-28 depicts the use of a water column PEEP device; however, any low flow resistance device may be employed. In addition to the device illustrated, a system pressure manometer and, ideally, an O_2 analyzer should be continuously included in all CPAP circuits. The analyzer should be located before the humidifying device and the pressure manometer attached at or near the patient's airway.

With all circuits some fluctuations in system pressure are noted. However, these fluctuations must be kept to a minimum, the acceptable range being within about ± 2 cmH_2O.[134,135] Fluctuations of greater magnitude during inspiration may be corrected by increasing system flow or increasing the size of the circuit reservoir. Changes in baseline pressure during exhalation are primarily affected by the flow resistance properties of the PEEP device employed.

Finally, a pressure pop-off valve is included in all systems. In the circuit illustrated it is located at the tail of the reservoir bag. A relief valve is included to prevent excessive pressure from building up in the system (as when a patient coughs with high flow resistance PEEP device or system obstruction).

PEEP with Mechanical Ventilation

Concerns and cautions when PEEP is applied in conjunction with mechanical ventilation are essentially the same as those discussed for CPAP systems. In all ventilator applications, concerns about the design of the exhalation valve must be raised; as always, the least flow-resistant exhalation valve should be used. Of major concern is the use of disposable exhalation valve systems, since some of those currently available exhibit high flow resistance.[132] Continuous flow IMV systems require the same consideration given to continuous flow CPAP systems.

PEEP with Manual Ventilation

PEEP can be applied to any manual ventilator,[42,134] but it is best accomplished when the manual ventilator has a single gas-collecting head (Fig. 76-29) that allows for the attachment of a spring-loaded or magnetic PEEP valve.[147] Any patient requiring more than 5 cmH_2O PEEP while receiving mechanical ventilation should always have PEEP applied via the manual ventilator. This will prevent the changes in lung mechanics and gas exchange that are otherwise noted when the PEEP level is periodically decreased.[127]

References

1. Ashbaugh DG, Bigelow DB, Petty TL, Levine BE: Acute respiratory distress in adults. Lancet 1967;2:319–323
2. Oertel MJ: In Yeo JB (transl): Von Ziemssen's Handbook of Therapeutics. Vol 3. William Wood, New York, 1885, p. 448
3. Barach AL: The use of helium in the treatment of asthma and obstructive lesions in the larynx and trachea. Ann Intern Med 1935;9:739–765
4. Barach AL: The effects of inhalation of helium mixed with oxygen on the mechanics of respiration. J Clin Invest 1936;15:47–61
5. Barach AL: Recent advances in inhalation therapy in the treatment of cardiac and respiratory disease. NY State J Med 1937;37:1095–1110
6. Barach AL, Martin J, Eckman M: Positive pressure respiration and its application in the treatment of acute pulmonary edema. Ann Intern Med 1938;12:754–795
7. Barach AL, Swenson P: Effect of breathing gases under positive pressure on lumens of small and medium-sized bronchi. Arch Intern Med 1939;63:946–948
8. Poulton EP, Oxon DM: Left-sided heart failure with pulmonary edema. Lancet 1936;2:981–983
9. Lovelace WR: Oxygen for therapy and aviation: An apparatus for the administration of oxygen or oxygen and helium by inhalation. Mayo Clin Proc 1938;13:646–654
10. Eckman M, Barach AL: Inhalation therapy equipment. Mod Hosp 1939;52:78–84
11. Burford TH, Burbank B: Traumatic wet lung: Observations on certain physiologic fundamentals of thoracic trauma. J Thorac Surg 1945;14:415–424
12. Brewer LA, Burbank B, Samson PC: The "wet lung" in war casualties. Ann Surg 1946;123:343–362
13. Kacmarek RM: History of PEEP in acute lung injury. Respir Care 1988;33:422–433
14. Spearman CB: Positive end expiratory pressure: Terminology and technical aspects of PEEP devices and systems. Respir Care 1988;33:434–443
15. Hurford WE, Teboul JL: Cardiovascular function during acute respiratory failure. pp. 253–284. In Zapol WM, Lemaire F (eds): Adult Respiratory Distress Syndrome. Marcel Dekker, New York, 1991
16. Marini JJ, Wheeler AP: Critical Care Medicine: The Essentials. Williams & Wilkins, Baltimore, 1989, pp. 20–21
17. Stoller JK: Respiratory effects of positive end-expiratory pressure. Respir Care 1988;33:454–463
18. Daly BDT, Edmonds CH, Norman JC: *In vivo* alveolar morphometrics with positive end-expiratory pressure. Surg Forum 1973;24:217–219
19. Dueck R, Wagner PD, West JB: Effects of positive end-expiratory pressure on gas exchange in dogs with normal and edematous lungs. Anesthesiology 1977;47:359–366
20. Cane RD, Shapiro BA: Ventilator discontinuance and weaning. Anesthesiol Clin North Am 1987;5:749–761
21. Kumar A, Falke KJ, Geffin B et al: Continuous positive-pressure ventilation in acute respiratory failure. N Engl J Med 1970;273:1430–1436
22. McIntyre RW, Laws AK, Ramachandraw PR: Positive expiratory pressure plateau: Improved gas exchange during mechanical ventilation. Can J Anaesth 1969;16:477–486
23. Katz JA, Ozanne GM, Zinn SE, Fairley HB: Time course and mechanisms of lung-volume increase with PEEP in acute pulmonary failure. Anesthesiology 1981;54:9–16
24. Suter PM, Fairley HB, Isenberg MD: Optimum end-expiratory airway pressure in patients with acute pulmonary failure. N Engl J Med 1975;292:284–289
25. Gilmour I, Burnham M, Craig DB: Closing capacity measurements during general anesthesia. Anesthesiology 1976;45:477–481
26. Hedenstierna G, Santesson J, Norlander O: Airway closure and distribution of inspired gas in the extremely obese, breathing

spontaneously and during anesthesia with IPPV. Acta Anaesthesiol Scand 1976;20:334–340
27. Weenig CS, Pietak S, Hickey RF et al: Relationship of preoperative CV to FRC and alveolar-arterial oxygen differences during anesthesia with controlled ventilation. Anesthesiology 1974;41:3–9
28. Wyche MD, Teichner RL, Kallos T et al: Effects of continuous positive-pressure breathing on functional residual capacity and arterial oxygenation during intra-abdominal operations. Anesthesiology 1973;38:68–76
29. Craig DB, Wahba WM, Dow HR: Closing volume and its relationship to gas exchange in seated and supine positions. J Appl Physiol 1971;31:717–723
30. Alexander JI, Spence AA, Rarikh RK: The role of airway closure in postoperative hypoxemia. Br J Anaesth 1973;45:34–39
31. Downs JB, Klein EF, Modell JH: The effect of incremental PEEP on PaO_2 in patients with respiratory failure. Anesth Analg 1973;52:210–215
32. Kirby RR, Perry JC, Calderwood HW et al: Cardiorespiratory effects of positive end-expiratory pressure. Anesthesiology 1975;43:533–539
33. Weisman IM, Rinaldo JE, Rogers RM: Current concepts: Positive end-expiratory pressure in adult respiratory failure. N Engl J Med 1982;307:1381–1384
34. Shapiro BA, Cane RD, Harrison RA: Positive end-expiratory pressure therapy in adults, with special reference to acute lung injury: A review of the literature and suggested clinical correlations. Crit Care Med 1984;12:127–141
35. Zinn SE, Ozanne GM, Fairley HB: Mixed expired gas transients as a non-invasive index of the effects of PEEP. Anesthesiology 1980;52:261–264
36. Murray IP, Modell JH, Gallagher TJ, Banner MJ: Titration of PEEP by the arterial minus end-tidal CO_2 gradient. Chest 1984;85:100–104
37. Jardin F, Genvray B, Pazin M, Margairaz A: Inability to titrate PEEP in patients with acute respiratory failure using end-tidal carbon dioxide measurement. Anesthesiology 1985;62:530–533
38. Blanch L, Fernandez R, Benito S et al: Effect of PEEP on the arterial minus end-tidal carbon dioxide gradient. Chest 1987;92:451–454
39. Smith TC, Marini JJ: Impact of PEEP on lung mechanics and work of breathing in severe airflow obstruction. J Appl Physiol 1988;65:1488–1499
40. Petrof BJ, Legare M, Goldberg P et al: Continuous positive airway pressure reduces work of breathing and dyspnea during weaning from mechanical ventilation in severe COPD. Am Rev Respir Dis 1990;141:281–289
41. Douglas ME, Downs JB: Response to cardiopulmonary effects of PEEP and CPAP (letter). Anesth Analg 1978;57:346–350
42. Kacmarek RM, Goulet RL: PEEP devices. Anesthesiol Clin North Am 1987;5:757–776
43. Hirsch CA, Kacmarek RM, Stanek K: Work of breathing during CPAP and PSV imposed by the new generation mechanical ventilators: A lung model study. Respir Care 1991;36:815–828
44. Torres T, Kacmarek RM, Kimball WR et al: Regional diaphragmatic length and EMG activity during inspiratory pressure support and CPAP in awake sheep. J Appl Physiol (in press)
45. Russell JA, Hoeffel J, Murray JF: Effect of different levels of positive end-expiratory pressure on lung water content. J Appl Physiol 1982;53:9–15
46. Hopewell PC, Murray JF: Effects of continuous positive pressure ventilation in experimental pulmonary edema. J Appl Physiol 1976;40:568–574
47. Slutsky RA: Reduction in pulmonary blood volume during positive end-expiratory pressure. J Surg Res 1983;35:181–187
48. Pare PD, Warriner B, Baile EM, Hogg JC: Redistribution of pulmonary extra-vascular water with positive end-expiratory pressure in canine pulmonary edema. Am Rev Respir Dis 1983;127:590–593
49. Hopewell PC: Failure of positive end-expiratory pressure to decrease lung water content in alloxan-induced pulmonary edema. Am Rev Respir Dis 1979;120:813–819
50. Hobelmann CF, Smith DE, Virgilio RW et al: Hemodynamic alterations with positive end-expiratory pressure: The contribution of the pulmonary vasculature. J Trauma 1975;15:951–959
51. Baile EM, Albert RK, Kirk W et al: Positive end-expiratory pressure decreases bronchial blood flow in the dog. J Appl Physiol 1984;56:1289–1293
52. Hedenstierna G, White FC, Wagner PD: Spatial distribution of pulmonary blood flow in the dog with PEEP ventilation. J Appl Physiol 1979;47:938–946
53. Cassidy SS, Haynes MS: The effects of ventilation with positive end-expiratory pressure on the bronchial circulation. Respir Physiol 1986;66:269–278
54. Qvist J, Pontoppidan H, Wilson RS et al: Hemodynamic responses to mechanical ventilation with PEEP. Anesthesiology 1975;42:45–49
55. Fewell JE, Abendschein DR, Carlson CJ: Mechanism of decreased right and left ventricular end-diastolic volumes during continuous positive-pressure ventilation in dogs. Circ Res 1980;47:467–473
56. Lenfant C, Howell BJ: Cardiovascular adjustment in dogs during continuous positive pressure breathing. J Appl Physiol 1960;15:425–432
57. Robotham JL, Lixfield W, Holland L et al: The effects of positive end-expiratory pressure on right and left ventricular performance. Am Rev Respir Dis 1980;121:677–684
58. Dorinsky PM, Whitcomb ME: The effects of PEEP on cardiac output. Chest 1983;84:210–218
59. Shapiro BA, Kacmarek RM, Cane RA et al: Clinical Application of Respiratory Care. 4th Ed. Mosby–Year Book, St. Louis, 1990
60. Doblar DD, Santiago TV, Kah AAV et al: The effect of positive end-expiratory pressure ventilation (PEEP) on cerebral blood flow and cerebrospinal fluid pressure in goats. Anesthesiology 1981;55:244–250
61. Huseby JS, Pavlin EG, Butler J: Effect of positive end-expiratory pressure on intracranial pressure in dogs. J Appl Physiol 1978;44:25–32
62. Luce JM, Huseby JS, Kirk W, Butler J: A Starling resistor regulates cerebral venous outflow in dogs. J Appl Physiol 1982;53:1496–1503
63. Gabriele G, Rosenfeld CR, Fixler DE et al: Continuous airway pressure breathing with the head-box in the newborn lamb; effects on regional blood flows. Pediatrics 1977;59:858–865
64. Manny J, Justice R, Hechtman HB: Abnormalities in organ blood flow and its distribution during positive end-expiratory pressure. Surgery 1979;85:425–432
65. Leithner C, Frass M, Pacher R et al: Mechanical ventilation with positive end-expiratory pressure decreases release of alpha-atrial natriuretic peptide. Crit Care Med 1987;15:484–488
66. Venus B, Mathru M, Smith R et al: Renal function during application of positive end-expiratory pressure in swine. Effect of hydration. Anesthesiology 1985;62:765–769
67. Pierson DJ: Alveolar rupture during mechanical ventilation: Role of PEEP, airway pressure and distending pressure. Respir Care 1988;33:472–486
68. Maunder RJ, Shuman WP, McHugh JW et al: Preservation of normal lung regions in the adult respiratory distress syndrome. JAMA 1986;255:2463–2465
69. Kirby RR, Downs JB, Civetta JM et al: High level positive end-expiratory pressure (PEEP) in acute respiratory insufficiency. Chest 1975;67:156–163
70. Douglas ME, Downs JB: Pulmonary function following severe acute respiratory failure and high levels of positive end-expiratory pressure. Chest 1977;71:18–23
71. Jensen NK: Recovery of pulmonary function after crushing injury to the chest. Chest 1952;22:319–346
72. Hurst JM, DeHaven CB, Branson RD: Sole use of mask CPAP in respiratory insufficiency. J Trauma 1985;25:1065–1068

73. Branson RD, Hurst JM, DeHaven CB: Mask CPAP: State of the art. Respir Care 1985;30:846–857
74. Frith RW, Cant BR: Severe obstructive sleep apnea treated with long-term nasal continuous positive airway pressure. Thorax 1985;40:45–50
75. Strohl KP, Redline S: Nasal CPAP therapy, upper airway muscle activation, and obstructive sleep apnea. Am Rev Respir Dis 1986;134:555–558
76. Miller MJ, Carlo WA, Martin RJ: Continuous positive airway pressure selectively reduces obstructive apnea in preterm infants. J Pediatr 1985;106:91–94
77. Kattwinkel J, Nearman HS, Fanaroff AA et al: Apnea of prematurity: Comparative therapeutic effects of cutaneous stimulation and nasal continuous positive airway pressure. J Pediatr 1975;86:588–592
78. Issa FG, Sullivan CE: Reversal of central sleep apnea using nasal CPAP. Chest 1986;90:165–171
79. Kanter RK, Pollack MM, Wright WW, Grundfast KM: Treatment of tracheobronchomalacia with continuous positive airway pressure. Anesthesiology 1982;57:54–56
80. Pizer BL, Freeland AP, Wilkinson AR: Prolonged positive airway pressure for severe neonatal tracheobronchomalacia. Arch Dis Child 1986;61:908–909
81. Martin JG, Shore S, Engel LA: Effect of continuous positive airway pressure on respiratory mechanics and pattern of breathing in induced asthma. Am Rev Respir Dis 1982;126:812–817
82. Wilson BA, Jackson PJ, Evans J: Effects of positive end-expiratory pressure breathing on exercise-induced asthma. Int J Sports Med 1981;2:27–30
83. Qvist J, Pemberton M, Bennike K: High-level PEEP in severe asthma (letter). N Engl J Med 1982;307:1347–1348
84. Shivaram U, Donath J, Khan F et al: Continuous positive airway pressure (CPAP) in the treatment of acute bronchial asthma: Clinical study of 20 patients, abstracted. Am Rev Respir Dis 1984;129:A41
85. Pepe PE, Marini JJ: Occult positive end-expiratory pressure in mechanically ventilated patients with airflow obstruction: The auto-PEEP effect. Am Rev Respir Dis 1982;126:166–170
86. Barat G, Asuero MS: Positive end-expiratory pressure: Effect on arterial oxygenation during respiratory failure in chronic obstructive airway disease. Anaesthesia 1975;30:183–189
87. Barach AL, Bickerman HA, Rodgers J: Continuous positive pressure breathing in chronic obstructive lung disease: Effect on minute ventilation and blood gases. Ann Allergy 1973;31:72–78
88. Ford GI, Guenter CA: Toward prevention of postoperative pulmonary complications. Am Rev Respir Dis 1984;130:4–8
89. Andersen JB, Olesen KP, Eikard B et al: Periodic continuous positive airway pressure, CPAP, by mask in the treatment of atelectasis. A sequential analysis. Eur J Respir Dis 1980;61:20–25
90. Stock MC, Downs JB, Gauer PK, Cooper RB: Prevention of atelectasis after upper abdominal operations. Crit Care Med 1983;11:220–224
91. Williamson DC, Modell JH: Intermittent CPAP by mask. Arch Surg 1982;117:970–972
92. Carlson C, Sonden B, Tyhlen U: Can postoperative continuous positive airway pressure prevent pulmonary complications after abdominal surgery? Intensive Care Med 1981;7:225–229
93. Stock MC, Downs JB, Gauer PK et al: Prevention of postoperative pulmonary complications with CPAP, incentive spirometry and conservative therapy. Chest 1985;87:151–157
94. Lindner KH, Lotz P, Ahnefeld FW: Continuous positive airway pressure effect on functional residual capacity, vital capacity and subdivisions. Chest 1987;92:66–70
95. Knodel AR, Covelli HD, O'Reilly M: The role of mask CPAP in preventing postoperative atelectasis, abstracted. Am Rev Respir Dis 1984;126:A110
96. Venus B, Copiozo GB, Jacobs K: Continuous positive airway pressure: The use of low levels in adult patients with artificial airways. Arch Surg 1980;115:824–828
97. Feeley TW, Saumarez R, Klick JM et al: Positive end-expiratory pressure in weaning patients from controlled ventilation: A prospective randomized trial. Lancet 1975;2:725–728
98. Berman LS, Fox WW, Raphaely RC, Downes JJ: Optimum levels of CPAP for tracheal extubation of newborn infants. J Pediatr 1976;89:109–112
99. Fox WW, Berman LS, Dinwiddie R, Shaffer TH: Tracheal extubation of the neonate at 2 to 3 cmH_2O continuous positive airway pressure. Pediatrics 1977;59:257–261
100. Annest SJ, Gottlieb M, Paloski WH et al: Detrimental effects of removing end-expiratory pressure prior to endotracheal extubation. Ann Surg 1980;191:539–545
101. Quan SF, Falltrick RT, Schlobohm RM: Extubation from ambient or expiratory positive airway pressure in adults. Anesthesiology 1981;55:53–56
102. Katz JA, Marks JD: Inspiratory work with and without continuous positive airway pressure in patients with acute respiratory failure. Anesthesiology 1985;63:598–607
103. Calvin JE, Drieder AA, Sibbald WJ: Positive end-expiratory pressure (PEEP) does not depress left ventricular function in patients with pulmonary edema. Am Rev Respir Dis 1981;124:121–128
104. Grace MP, Greenbaum DM: Cardiac performance in response to PEEP in patients with cardiac dysfunction. Crit Care Med 1982;10:358–360
105. Rasanen J, Heikkila J, Downs J et al: Continuous positive airway pressure by face mask in acute cardiogenic pulmonary edema. Am J Cardiol 1985;55:296–300
106. Rasanen J, Vaisanen IT, Heikkila J, Nikki P: Acute myocardial infarction complicated by left ventricular dysfunction and respiratory failure: The effects of continuous positive airway pressure. Chest 1985;87:158–162
107. Vaisanen IT, Rasanen J: Continuous positive airway pressure and supplemental oxygen in the treatment of cardiogenic pulmonary edema. Chest 1987;92:481–485
108. Perel A, Williamson DC, Modell JH: Effectiveness of CPAP by mask for pulmonary edema associated with hypercarbia. Intensive Care Med 1983;9:17–19
109. Mathru M, Venus B, Smith RA: All positive airway pressures are not created equal! (editorial). Chest 1985;87:137–138
110. Rossi A, Gottfried SB, Zocchi L et al: Measurement of static compliance of the total respiratory system in patients with acute respiratory failure during mechanical ventilation: The effect of intrinsic positive end-expiratory pressure. Am Rev Respir Dis 1985;131:672–677
111. Bergman NA: Intrapulmonary gas trapping during mechanical ventilation at rapid frequencies. Anesthesiology 1972;37:626–633
112. Marini JJ: Should PEEP be used in airflow obstruction? (editorial). Am Rev Respir Dis 1989;140:1–3
113. Brown DG, Pierson DJ: Auto-PEEP is common in mechanically ventilated patients: A study of incidence, severity, and detection. Respir Care 1986;31:1069–1074
114. Wright J, Gong H: Auto-PEEP: Incidence, magnitude, and contributing factors. Heart Lung 1990;19:352–357
115. Fernandez R, Mancebo J, Blanch LI et al: Intrinsic PEEP on static pressure-volume curves. Intensive Care Med 1990;16:233–236
116. Rossi A, Gottfried SB, Zocchi L et al: Measurement of static compliance of the total respiratory system in patients with respiratory failure during mechanical ventilation. Am Rev Respir Dis 1985;131:672–677
117. Benson MS, Pierson DJ: Auto-PEEP during mechanical ventilation of adults. Respir Care 1988;33:557–568
118. Iotti G, Braschi A: Respiratory mechanics in chronic obstructive pulmonary disease. pp. 223–232. In Vincent JL (ed): Critical Care Update 1990. Springer-Verlag, Berlin, 1990
119. Hoffman RA, Ershowsky P, Krieger BP: Determination of auto-PEEP during spontaneous and controlled ventilation by

monitoring changes in end-expiratory thoracic gas volume. Chest 1989;96:613–616
120. Scott LR, Benson MS, Bishop MJ: Relationship of endotracheal tube size to auto-PEEP at high minute ventilation. Respir Care 1986;31:1080–1082
121. Scott LR, Benson MS, Pierson DJ: Effect of inspiratory flowrate and circuit compressible volume on auto-PEEP during mechanical ventilation. Respir Care 1986;31:1075–1079
122. Nocturnal Oxygen Therapy Trial Group: Continuous or nocturnal oxygen therapy in hypoxemic chronic obstructive lung disease: A clinical trial. Ann Intern Med 1980;93:391–398
123. Beydon L, Lemaire F, Jonson B: Lung mechanics in ARDS: Compliance and pressure-volume curves. pp. 139–162. In Zapol WM, Lemaire F (eds): Adult Respiratory Distress Syndrome. Marcel Dekker, New York, 1991
124. Pesenti A, Marcolin R, Prato P et al: Mean airway pressure vs. positive end-expiratory pressure during mechanical ventilation. Crit Care Med 1985;13:34–37
125. Demers RR, Irwin RS, Bramen SS: Criteria for optimum PEEP. Respir Care 1977;22:596–601
126. Walkinshaw M, Shoemaker WC: Use of volume loading to obtain preferred levels of PEEP. Crit Care Med 1980;8:81–86
127. Hudson LD, Weaver LJ, Haisch CE, Carrico CJ: Positive end-expiratory pressure: Reduction and withdrawal. Respir Care 1988;33:613–619
128. Hurfod WF, Lynch KE, Strauss HW et al: Myocardial perfusion as assessed by thallium-201 scintigraphy during the discontinuation of mechanical ventilation in ventilator-dependent patients. Anesthesiology 1991;74:1007–1016
129. Banner MJ, Lampotang S, Boysen PG: Flow resistance of expiratory positive pressure valve systems. Chest 1986;90:212–217
130. Banner MJ: Expiratory positive-pressure valves: Flow resistance and work of breathing. Respir Care 1987;32:431–439
131. Banner MJ, Lampotang S, Boysen PG et al: Resistance characteristics of expiratory pressure valves. Anesthesiology 1986;65:A80
132. Marini JJ, Culver BH, Kirk W: Flow resistance of exhalation valves and positive end-expiratory pressure devices used in mechanical ventilation. Am Rev Respir Dis 1985;131:850–854
133. Hall JR, Rendleman DC, Downs JB: PEEP devices: Flow-dependent increases in airway pressure. Crit Care Med 1978;6:100
134. Kacmarek RM, Dimas S, Reynolds J, Shapiro BA: Technical aspects of positive end-expiratory pressure (PEEP). Parts I, II, and III. Respir Care 27:1982;1478–1519
135. Kacmarek RM, Wilson RS: IMV systems, do they make a difference? (editorial). Chest 1985;87:557
136. Gherini S, Peters RM, Virgilio RW: Mechanical work on the lungs and work of breathing with positive end-expiratory pressure and continuous positive airway pressure. Chest 1979;76:251–256
137. Kirby RR: Positive airway pressure: System design and clinical application. pp. G1–G52. In Shoemaker WC (ed): Critical Care: State-of-the-Art. Society of Critical Care Medicine, Fullerton, CA, 1985
138. Gibney RTN, Wilson RS, Pontoppidan H: Comparison of work of breathing on high gas flow and demand valve continuous positive airway pressure systems. Chest 1982;82:692–694
139. Lemaire F, Rleut P, Rauss A et al: A clinical comparison of the work of breathing (WOB) through demand-valve systems. Am Rev Respir Dis 133:A121, 1986
140. Viale JB, Annat G, Bertrand D et al: Additional inspiratory work in intubated patients breathing with continuous positive airway pressure systems. Anesthesiology 1985;63:536–639
141. Katz JA, Kraemer RW, Gjerde GE: Inspiratory work and airway pressure with continuous positive airway pressure delivery system. Chest 1985;88:519–526
142. Samodelov LF, Falke KJ: Total inspiratory work with modern demand valve devices compared to continuous flow CPAP. Intensive Care Med 1988;14:632–639
143. Civetta JM, Brons R, Gel JC: A simple and effective method of employing spontaneous positive pressure ventilation. J Thorac Cardiovasc Surg 1972;63:312–317
144. Henry WC, West GA, Wilson RS: A comparison of the oxygen cost of breathing between a continuous flow CPAP system and a demand-flow CPAP system. Respir Care 1983;28:1273–1281
145. Braschi A, Lotti G, Locatelli A et al: Functional evaluation of a CPAP circuit with a high compliance reservoir bag. Intensive Care Med 1985;11:85–89
146. Hillman K, Friedlos J, Davey A: A comparison of intermittent mandatory ventilation systems. Crit Care Med 1986;14:499–502
147. Greenbaum DM, Schwartz JO, Goldblatt MB: More on PMR modification for PEEP (letter). Respir Care 1978;23:1137–1140
148. Bolin RW, Pierson DJ: Ventilatory management in acute lung injury. Crit Care Clin 1986;2:585–599
149. Shapiro BA, Harrison RA, Kacmarek RM, Cane RD: Clinical Applications of Respiratory Care. 3rd Ed. Year Book Medical Publishers, Chicago, 1985
150. Abbey NC, Black AJ, Green D et al: Measurement of pharyngeal volume by digitized magnetic resonance imaging: Effect of nasal continuous positive airway pressure. Am Rev Respir Dis 1989;140:717–723
151. Gregory GA, Kitterman JA, Phibbs RH et al: Treatment of the idiopathic respiratory distress syndrome with continuous positive airway pressure. N Engl J Med 1971;284:1333–1340
152. Otis AB: Work of breathing. pp. 463–467. In Fenn WU, Rahn H (eds): Handbook of Physiology: The Respiratory System. Vol. 1. American Physiological Society, Washington, DC, 1964

Chapter 77

Preservation and Augmentation of Cardiac Output

David J. Pierson

CHAPTER OUTLINE

The pathogenesis, manifestations, and treatment of acute respiratory failure and other pulmonary disorders seen in the intensive care unit (ICU) cannot be understood without consideration of the heart as well as the lungs. Although a thorough discussion of cardiac function and its changes in response to disease and therapy is beyond the scope of this book, the clinician must nevertheless have a general, conceptual knowledge of these things. This chapter reviews the determinants of cardiac output, describes the most common clinical situations in which reduced cardiac function is encountered in ICU patients, and gives an overview of approaches to therapy of this aspect of these patients' illness. Because such a synopsis cannot hope to provide complete information for clinical management, the therapies are presented conceptually only, and no drug doses or other specifics are mentioned. For more comprehensive information the reader should consult recent authoritative texts[1–8] and reviews.[9–11] The practical aspects of assessing and monitoring cardiac function in the ICU are discussed in Chapter 50.

DETERMINANTS OF CARDIAC OUTPUT

Cardiac output (CO or $\dot{Q}_T$) is the volume of blood pumped by the heart in liters per minute. Both the right and the left side of the heart pump this quantity of blood. *Stroke volume* (SV) is the output of blood from the heart per beat (i.e., $\dot{Q}_T$ divided by heart rate [HR]). The SV reflects the difference between the end-diastolic volume (EDV) and end-systolic volume (ESV) of the ventricle, and when expressed as a percentage of EDV it is called the *ejection fraction* (EF). In order to "normalize" $\dot{Q}_T$ (i.e., to compare results from different patients of varying body sizes), it is commonly divided by body surface area and expressed as the *cardiac index*, in liters per minute per square meter.

The heart's function as a pump is determined by three factors, as described in Chapter 8, namely, preload, afterload, and contractility.[4,12] *Preload* is the length of the heart muscle at the start of contraction (i.e., the stretch on the muscle at EDV). *Afterload* is the tension that the muscle is called on to develop when it contracts. The heart muscle's *contractility* (also called its *inotropic state*) is the velocity of fiber shortening for any given preload and/or afterload (i.e., effectiveness of cardiac squeeze given the work load placed on the ventricle and its state of distension at that moment).

Preload and the Frank-Starling Relationship

The observation that the force of contraction of a heart muscle fiber is related to the initial length of that fiber was made in 1895 by Frank based on studies of the hearts of frogs. Starling in 1914 extended Frank's findings with the statement that the mechanical energy released on passage from the resting to the contracted state depends on the available chemically active surfaces on the muscle fibers. These concepts became known as the "law of the heart." More recently, Sarnoff and Mitchell modified the Frank-Starling law to specify that the above relationship holds for any given state of responsiveness (e.g., contractility) of the cardiac muscle and showed that there is a family of function curves (Starling curves) for each ventricle depending on the conditions under which the ventricle is contracting at that moment.[12] Examples of such curves are shown in Figure 77-1.

Figure 77-1 shows that SV, and thus to a large extent $\dot{Q}_T$, depends on the EDV of the ventricle (e.g., its preload), although this relationship is different for different states of contractility. Because EDV is difficult to measure at the bedside, pulmonary capillary wedge pressure (PCWP), which is determined by using a pulmonary artery (Swan-Ganz) catheter (see Ch. 50), is used instead. As long as there is no obstruction (as in cases of mitral stenosis) between the left ventricle and the pulmonary artery containing the catheter, PCWP is clinically equivalent to left atrial pressure; left atrial pressure is in turn equivalent to left ventricular end-diastolic pressure (EDP), which may be considered to reflect left ventricular EDV. In general, the greater the preload the greater the $\dot{Q}_T$, but the curves are not linear, and a point is eventually reached beyond which further increases in preload do not produce further gain in $\dot{Q}_T$.

Figure 77-2 shows the relationships between EDV (preload) and EDP,[12] which would be assessed as PCWP, in two different conditions of *ventricular compliance*. The compliance of the left ventricle is analogous to that of the respiratory system as measured during mechanical ventilation. Curve A in Figure 77-2 (normally compliant ventricle) shows that EDV can increase substantially before EDP begins to rise; curve B (decreased compliance, as with a healing myocardial infarction) demonstrates a much greater increase in EDP for a smaller increase in EDV. In other words, a less compliant (stiffer) ventricle generates a higher pressure (reflected in PCWP) for any given increase in volume (EDV).

Figures 77-1 and 77-2 demonstrate that either an increase in EDV or a decrease in ventricular compliance can cause PCWP to rise. Because the delicate alveolar-capillary membrane (see Fig. 7-12) and the requirements for effective pulmonary gas exchange demand that the pressure in the pulmonary capillaries and venules remain low, an increase in EDP (i.e., PCWP) may quickly lead to hydrostatic (cardiogenic) pulmonary edema.

Preload is affected both by the total intravascular blood volume and by its distribution. Thus, severe blood loss, as

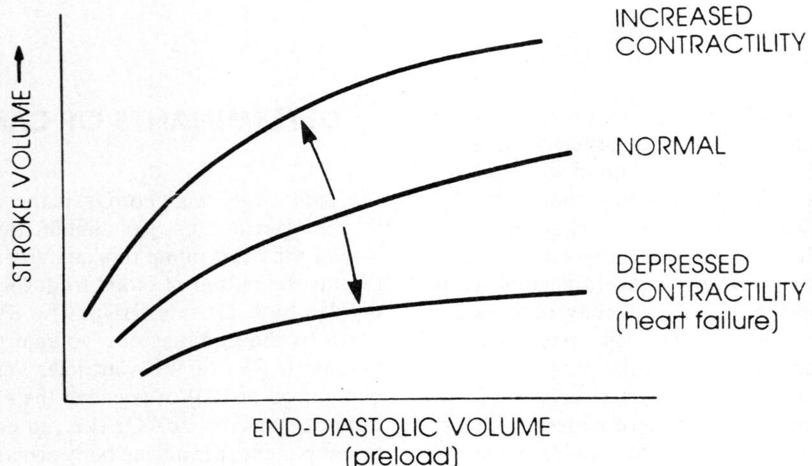

Figure 77-1. A family of ventricular function (Starling) curves, plotting SV against EDV. SV is essentially the same here as $\dot{Q}_T$; EDV may be taken to represent preload and is clinically equivalent to pulmonary capillary wedge pressure (PCWP) assuming there is no structural abnormality between the left ventricle and the pulmonary capillary. The normal curve demonstrates that for any given EDV there is a corresponding subsequent SV (and $\dot{Q}_T$). An increase in EDV (or PCWP) results in a corresponding increase in SV, until the curve reaches a plateau. The curves showing increased or decreased contractility relate a shift in the direction of SV to EDV under these different circumstances. (From Gilbert and Hew,[12] with permission.)

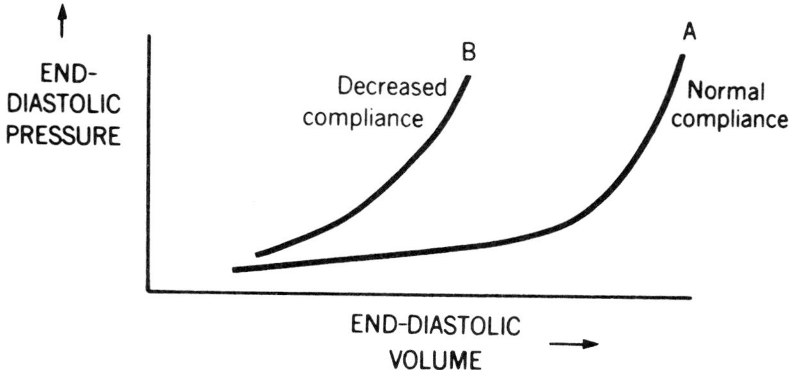

Figure 77-2. Relationship between ventricular EDV and end-diastolic pressure (EDP). Curve A depicts this normal relationship: relatively large increases in EDV are accompanied by relatively small increases in EDP until higher volumes are reached. Curve B demonstrates a much greater increase in EDP for a relatively smaller increase in EDV, as seen in healing myocardial infarction. (From Gilbert and Hew,[12] with permission.)

in trauma or surgery, decreases preload, and so does a fall in venous return to the right side of the heart because of increased intrathoracic pressure (e.g., coughing, tension pneumothorax, or positive-pressure ventilation). The effectiveness of atrial contraction also influences preload, especially in the presence of ventricular hypertrophy or decreased left ventricular compliance.[12]

Afterload

Afterload can be thought of as the stresses against which the ventricle must work in generating $\dot{Q}_T$. Another term for afterload is *outflow resistance*, often clinically measured as systemic vascular resistance (SVR). The ability of the ventricle to generate $\dot{Q}_T$ is related to the amount of resistance against which it must work.

Figure 77-3 shows the relationship between outflow resistance (*impedance*, the peripheral component of afterload) and SV (i.e., $\dot{Q}_T$), in the presence of three different states of ventricular function.[12] If ventricular function is normal, increasing outflow resistance leads to little change in SV. With increasing ventricular dysfunction, however, the higher the outflow resistance, the greater the reduction in SV and hence the lower the $\dot{Q}_T$. In such situations (e.g., decompensated congestive heart failure) the use of peripheral vasodilating drugs such as sodium nitroprusside can improve heart failure by decreasing impedance and increasing SV.

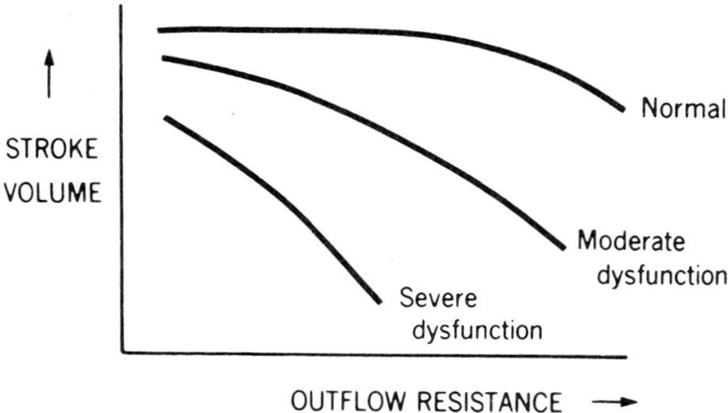

Figure 77-3. Relationship between resistance to ventricular ejection and the subsequent SV in different states of ventricular contractility. The normal curve demonstrates that increase in outflow resistance (e.g., increase in systemic vascular resistance) is associated with little change in SV. However, the curves indicating moderate and severe ventricular dysfunction demonstrate that a marked fall in SV may occur in these abnormal states. (From Gilbert and Hew,[12] as adapted from Cohn and Franciosa,[16] with permission.)

Contractility

The third major determinant of $\dot{Q}_T$, *contractility*, influences ventricular function independently of preload and afterload.[1,2,4] According to the force-velocity relationship for both skeletal and cardiac muscle, the greater the force, tension, or load against which a muscle is called on to work, the lower the velocity of shortening; the reverse of this relationship also holds. Variations in myocardial contractile function can be described through the use of force-velocity curves constructed by plotting the instantaneous velocity of fiber shortening against the force or afterload that individual fibers develop[4] (Fig. 77-4).

Although the concepts depicted in Figure 77-4 are complicated, they help to understand the behavior of the heart under different clinical conditions. If Figure 77-4 is compared with Figure 77-1, it is apparent that an increase in contractility is associated with an increase in SV in the absence of a change in preload. A decrease in contractility has the opposite effect. Heart failure is usually accompanied by a decrease in contractility and a drop in $\dot{Q}_T$; increasing contractility in this setting may also improve $\dot{Q}_T$.

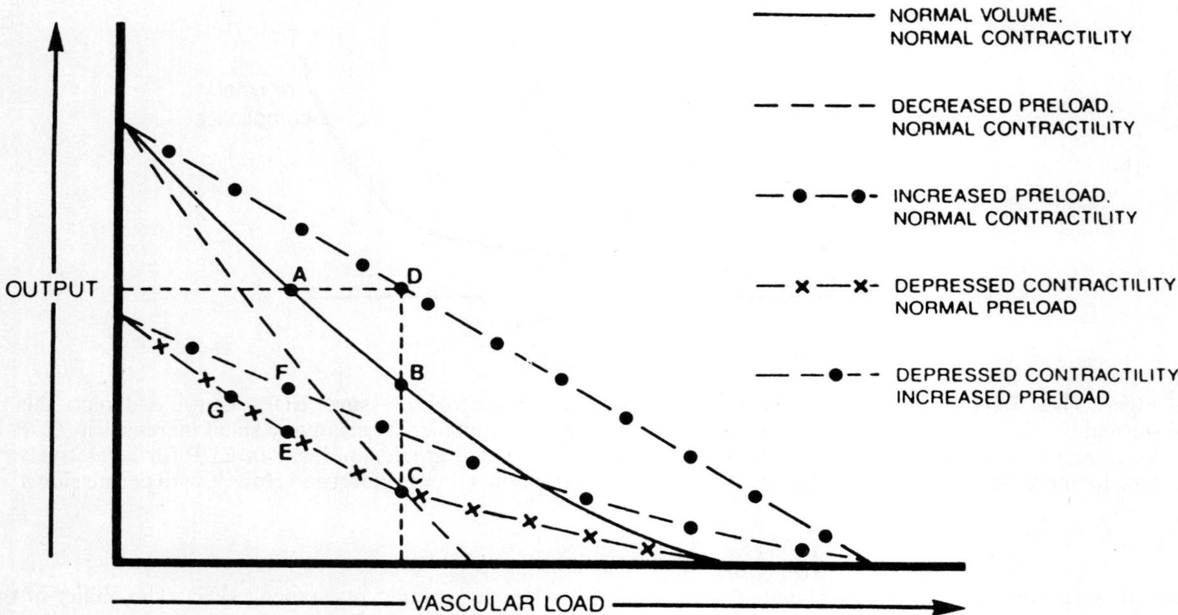

Figure 77-4. The relationship between cardiac output and vascular load (which can be thought of here as outflow resistance, systemic vascular resistance, or afterload) under differing conditions of contractility and preload is shown as a family of five curves. A normal individual functions at point A ("normal volume, normal contractility"). An isolated increase in vascular load causes this patient to function at point B of the same curve, with a resultant decrease in $\dot{Q}_T$, which can be compensated for by an increase in preload (point D ["increased preload, normal contractility"]). Depressed contractility also results in decreased output for a given vascular load (point C ["depressed contractility, normal preload"]). This can be compensated for by increasing preload (point F ["depressed contractility, increased preload"]). By diminishing vascular load (afterload or SVR), one can also increase $\dot{Q}_T$ independently of the state of contractility or preload (e.g., shifting from point C to point E or G or from point B to point A). (From Calvin and Sibbald,[4] with permission.)

CLINICAL SETTINGS AND APPROACH TO THE PATIENT

Table 77-1 outlines the possible mechanisms for decreased cardiac output as encountered in the ICU, along with their manifestations, usual clinical presentations, and potential therapy.

Preload

Decreased

Decreased preload essentially means volume depletion with respect to what the heart "sees." This may be systemic volume depletion (e.g., as in massive bleeding) or regional volume depletion. The latter is especially important in respiratory care in that ventilator management is a frequent cause (see Ch. 84 and Fig. 84-1). With positive-pressure ventilation, especially when positive end-expiratory pressure (PEEP) is used, mean intrathoracic pressure is increased and venous return from the rest of the body to the right side of the heart is thereby impeded. This problem becomes especially important in patients who are marginally hypovolemic systemically.

Decreased preload is manifested at the bedside by hypotension and tachycardia; if a pulmonary artery (Swan-Ganz) catheter is in place, PCWP will be found to be low. Therapy essentially consists of repleting intravascular volume. If decreased preload becomes a clinical problem at the initiation of mechanical ventilation or application of increased PEEP, the settings should be adjusted so that mean airway pressure and PEEP are minimized, as with the use of pressure support ventilation or low-rate intermittent mandatory ventilation; volume challenge should be attempted if hypotension persists once these adjustments have been made.

Increased

Manifestations of increased preload commonly occur in the presence of impaired myocardial contractility and are dominated by (hydrostatic) pulmonary edema. The PCWP will be elevated. In the presence of increased pulmonary capillary permeability, as in the adult respiratory distress syndrome (ARDS), pulmonary edema due to increased preload occurs at lower hydrostatic pressures than in the normal individual. Thus, "cardiogenic" pulmonary edema can develop at "normal" PCWP in patients with ARDS.

Therapy for increased preload consists essentially of decreasing the vascular volume "seen" by the heart. This can

Table 77-1. Conceptual Overview of Mechanisms and Potential Therapies for Improving Cardiac Output

Problem	Manifestations	Usual Clinical Settings	Therapy
Decreased preload	↓ BP; ↑ HR; ↓ PCWP	Intravascular volume depletion (e.g., hemorrhage; sepsis) Positive-pressure ventilation, especially with PEEP	Volume (treat underlying cause)
Increased preload	↑ PCWP; pulmonary edema	Volume overload; cardiogenic pulmonary edema (seen with ↓ contractility)	Decrease overall vascular volume (diuresis, ultrafiltration) Redistribute vascular volume away from the heart (arterial vasodilators [nitrates, nitroprusside, ACE inhibitors]; venous vasodilators [TNG, morphine])
Decreased afterload	↓ SVR	Septic shock	Treat underlying disorder Volume; vasoconstrictor drugs (neosynephrine; high-dose dopamine; norepinephrine)
Increased afterload	↑ SVR	Decompensated congestive heart failure Hypertensive crisis	Arterial vasodilators (nitrates)
Decreased contractility	↓ BP; ↑ HR; ↑ PCWP; pulmonary edema	Acute MI; acute myocardial ischemia; cardiomyopathy	Treat primary disorder Increased O_2 supply to heart (supplemental O_2; RBC transfusion) Inotropic drugs (dopamine, dobutamine, amrinone) Afterload reduction (e.g., with sodium nitroprusside)

ACE, angiotensin-converting enzyme; BP, blood pressure; MI, myocardial infarction; PEEP, positive end-expiratory pressure; RBC, erythrocyte; TNG, nitroglycerin

take the form of overall volume reduction, as with diuretics, or of volume redistribution within the circulatory system, as with drugs that pool blood in the periphery.

Afterload

Decreased

Decreased afterload is seen typically in sepsis (septic shock), and manifested by a low SVR. Therapy focuses on treating the primary cause while providing increased volume, with or without infusion of sympathomimetic amines in an attempt to increase peripheral vascular tone. Table 77-2 lists the most commonly used sympathomimetic amines, along with their effects on various aspects of cardiovascular function.[13,14]

Increased

Increased afterload, indicated by an increase in SVR, occurs in hypertensive crisis and as the result of decompen-

Table 77-2. Hemodynamic Effects of Sympathomimetic Amines Used to Support Circulatory Function in the ICU[a]

Drug	Effects				
	Cardiac Output	Venous Return (Preload)	Contractility	Heart Rate	Systemic Vascular Resistance (Afterload)
Norepinephrine	Variable	↑↑↑	↑	Variable	↑↑↑
Epinephrine	↑↑	↑	↑↑	↑↑	↑
Low-dose ("renal") dopamine	↑	↑	↑	NC	NC or ↓
Mid-dose dopamine	↑↑	↑	↑↑	↑↑	↑↑
High-dose dopamine	Variable	↑↑↑	↑	Variable	↑↑↑
Dobutamine	↑↑	↓	↑↑	NC or ↑	↓
Isoproterenol	↑	↓	↑↑↑	↑↑↑	↓↓

NC, no change.
[a] When given as intravenous infusion, listed in order of decreasing alpha- and increasing beta-adrenergic effects.

sated congestive heart failure. Like increased preload, it is generally encountered in patients with impaired myocardial contractility. Therapy focuses on lowering afterload with arterial vasodilators such as sodium nitroprusside, hydralazine, or angiotensin-converting enzyme inhibitors.[3,9,15]

Contractility

Decreased

Decreased contractility is seen in acute myocardial infarction and ischemia, and also in cardiomyopathies of a variety of etiologies. It is typically manifested by pulmonary edema, hypotension, and tachycardia; the PCWP is elevated. Improvement in the primary disorder producing the decreased contractility is the primary concern in management. Administration of supplemental O_2 is important when hypoxemia is present, and transfusion should be considered in the presence of reduced blood O_2-carrying capacity (e.g., in anemia), even in the absence of hypoxemia. In patients who are hypotensive, inotropic drugs such as norepinephrine, dobutamine, and dopamine are used (Table 77-2). Afterload reduction with agents such as sodium nitroprusside is another important aspect of the management approach.

References

1. Braunwald E (ed): Heart Disease. 3rd Ed. WB Saunders, Philadelphia, 1988
2. Braunwald E: Normal and abnormal myocardial function. pp. 880–890. In Wilson JD, Braunwald E, Isselbacher KJ et al (eds): Harrison's Principles of Internal Medicine. 12th Ed. McGraw-Hill, New York, 1991
3. Braunwald E: Heart failure. pp. 890–900. In Wilson JD, Braunwald E, Isselbacher KJ et al (eds): Harrison's Principles of Internal Medicine. 12th Ed. McGraw-Hill, New York, 1991
4. Calvin JE, Sibbald WJ: Applied cardiovascular physiology in the criticallly ill with special reference to diastole and ventricular interaction. pp. 312–326. In Shoemaker WC, Ayres S, Grenvik A et al (eds): Textbook of Critical Care. 2nd Ed. WB Saunders, Philadelphia, 1989
5. Cohn JN: Approach to the patient with heart failure. pp. 340–347. In Kelley WN (ed): Textbook of Internal Medicine. 2nd Ed. JB Lippincott, Philadelphia, 1992
6. Zelis R, Sinoway LI: Pathophysiology of congestive heart failure. pp. 104–112. In Kelley WN (ed): Textbook of Internal Medicine. 2nd Ed. JB Lippincott, Philadelphia, 1992
7. Leier CV: Approach to the patient with hypotension and shock. pp. 353–361. In Kelley WN (ed): Textbook of Internal Medicine. 2nd Ed. JB Lippincott, Philadelphia, 1992
8. Francis GS, Donat WE, Weiner BH: Syndromes of left ventricular failure. pp. 391–406. In Rippe JM, Irwin RS, Alpert JS, Fink MP (eds): Intensive Care Medicine. Little Brown, Boston, 1991
9. Parmley WM: Pathophysiology and current therapy of congestive heart failure. J Am Coll Cardiol 1989;13:771–785
10. Passmore JM, Goldstein RA: Acute recognition and management of congestive heart failure. Crit Care Clin 1989;5:497–532
11. Katz AM: Changing strategies in the management of heart failure. J Am Coll Cardiol 1989;13:513–523
12. Gilbert BW, Hew EM: Physiologic significance of hemodynamic measurements. pp. 12–24. In Armstrong PW, Baigrie RS (eds): Hemodynamic Monitoring in the Critically Ill. Harper & Row, Philadelphia, 1980
13. Brater DC: Clinical pharmacology of cardiovascular drugs. pp. 315–335. In Kelley WN (ed): Textbook of Internal Medicine. 2nd Ed. JB Lippincott, Philadelphia, 1992
14. Lawson NW, Wallfisch HK: Cardiovascular pharmacology: A new look at the "pressors." p. 195. In Stoelting RK, Barash PG, Gallagher TJ (eds): Advances in Anesthesia. Year Book Medical Publishers, Chicago, 1986
15. Abrams J: Vasodilator therapy for chronic congestive heart failure. JAMA 1985;254:3070–3074
16. Cohn JN, Franciosa JA: Vasodilator therapy of cardiac failure. N Engl J Med 1977;297:27–31

Chapter 78

Extracorporeal Membrane Oxygenation and Carbon Dioxide Removal

David H. Ingbar

CHAPTER OUTLINE

In severe respiratory failure, conventional mechanical ventilation occasionally is unable to oxygenate the blood adequately or to remove CO_2. These limits of ventilation may be the result of very large amounts of physiologic dead space (massive pulmonary embolus), intrapulmonary right-to-left shunt (adult respiratory distress syndrome [ARDS]), severe ventilation/perfusion mismatch (severe asthma), loss of ventilating gas (bronchopleural fistula), and/or rapid rates of CO_2 production and O_2 consumption (sepsis). Clinically this situation is most frequently encountered in patients with severe ARDS in the acute phase. Under these difficult circumstances, the mechanical ventilation itself also may contribute to the primary cause of lung damage. In animal models high alveolar pressures may overstretch compliant alveoli and cause pulmonary edema with protein leak and hemorrhage. In turn, atelectasis is believed to result from deficient surfactant function in these regions. Since the early 1970s extracorporeal gas exchange of several different types has been used at selected centers to "rest" the lung and provide adequate gas exchange for a temporary period while the lung is healing.

Extracorporeal gas exchange to replace alveolar ventilation by gaseous diffusion across membranes was first introduced in the 1950s. However, early models were limited by membranes that provided poor diffusion of O_2. With the realization that silicone supported O_2 diffusion well, in the late 1960s extracorporeal membrane oxygenation (ECMO) was first used for adults with severe respiratory failure. After use in selected patients in a nonrandomized fashion, the National Institutes of Health (NIH) sponsored a large randomized study of ECMO treatment for severe acute respiratory failure at nine centers across the United States.[1] When this study showed no survival benefit, ECMO for adult respiratory failure was virtually abandoned in the United States. Subsequently, a different method, extracorporeal CO_2 removal with low-frequency positive-pressure ventilation ($ECCO_2R$-LFPPV), has been reported in Europe to have strikingly beneficial effects on lung function and survival in similar patients.[2,3] This method now is undergoing a randomized trial in the United States.[4] ECMO is thought to be beneficial for many newborns with severe respiratory failure of several different causes.[5] The discrepancies in reported results highlight the importance of critical assessment of these expensive, invasive techniques and of understanding the different methods of extracorporeal support currently in use.

TYPES OF EXTRACORPOREAL BYPASS SYSTEMS

The components of extracorporeal support include (1) blood drainage and return systems, (2) pumps, (3) membrane filter, (4) humidified gas supply, (5) in-line vascular filters, and (6) monitoring and alarm systems. Typically all patients are systemically heparinized and paralyzed or heavily sedated during these procedures. Priming of the system with heparinized solutions is required.

There are four potential modes of extracorporeal circulation: arteriovenous (AV), venoarterial (VA), venovenous (VV), and mixed combinations. Of these, the VA system has received the most attention and was used in the original NIH ECMO study.[1] Venous blood is removed and is pumped through a membrane lung, where it is oxygenated and CO_2 is removed. The blood is returned to the arterial circulation for distribution to systemic vascular beds. In this type of ECMO circuit, pulmonary blood flow is diminished by the rate of flow through the bypass circuit. This could have either positive or negative effects. Fewer inflammatory mediators may be brought to the lung endothelium, and theoretically, blood cells such as neutrophils might be less likely to travel into the lung and amplify the injury state.

With VA ECMO, the right ventricle (RV) does not respond positively to pulmonary hypertension or to increases in filling volume, and this technique reduces the preload on the RV. On the other hand, the lung endothelium is the site of metabolism and inactivation of many vasoactive mediators that may exacerbate ARDS. In addition, since pulmonary blood flow is reduced, there could be ischemic necrosis of portions of the lung, especially in regions that are overdistended or are being ventilated at very high alveolar pressures.

The decreased blood flow in VA ECMO may cause in situ thrombosis and sludging within pulmonary vessels. There also is the possibility of reperfusion injury when the blood flow returns. The filtering function of the lung is lost, so that any particulates formed within the ECMO circuit have direct access to systemic vascular beds, such as the cerebral circulation. Finally, the oxygenated blood must be returned high in the aortic arch so as to mix well with the poorly oxygenated blood that has passed through the lungs and left heart; otherwise the coronary and carotid arteries may be perfused with relatively deoxygenated blood. Typically, an arterial catheter must be advanced in retrograde fashion from the femoral artery up to a position high in the aortic arch.

The advantages of VV bypass are that the lung receives the full systemic cardiac output and the problems of mixing and systemic embolism are eliminated. It is possible to alter peripheral blood flow patterns if there is high flow through the bypass circuit. The other methods have been used only rarely.

COSTS AND COMPLICATIONS

The potential benefits of these techniques must be weighed carefully against the costs and potential complications. Clearly, even when the technique is used successfully, the cost is very high. This is due to the technology itself, the need for at least one full-time nurse per patient, and the blood components used. Most ECMO patients have required 1 L of blood product replacement per day. In addition, this multidisciplinary technique must be performed frequently by a staff that works together well and often. Patients must be heparinized and paralyzed for extracorporeal support. Usually the catheters are inserted in the operating room, but recently catheters that can be placed percutaneously have been reported.

Technical problems with the circuits have been rare in the experience of most investigators.[6–9] However, if use were more widespread and the operators were less experienced, such problems would likely arise. Intravascular pressures across the circuit must be monitored to detect clotting and increased circuit resistance. For multiple days of VA bypass (standard ECMO), the efficacy of oxygenation also is followed, so that the membrane can be changed if it becomes less effective.

Bleeding has been the most common serious complication. Some investigators have been able to use relatively low doses of heparin, but virtually all patients develop platelet counts below 100,000/μL. Bleeding tendencies particularly are manifest during surgical procedures, but these very ill patients usually tolerate surgery as well as their non-ECMO peers. In neonates, intracranial hemorrhage is a major concern, occurring in up to 30 percent of premature infants.[5] Heparin-bonded tubing systems that limit systemic heparin delivery and avoid systemic anticoagulation now are being tested.

Infection and sepsis have been the other major feared complications. Sepsis occurs frequently, but again it is not clear that ECMO increases the sepsis rate in these very ill patients.

Other complications have included: deep venous thrombosis and pseudoaneurysm formation at the site of cannulation; renal failure; central nervous system emboli; seizures in neonates; and, very rarely, hemolysis. Since neonatal ECMO often has involved ligation of the right carotid artery, some infants manifest changes in left-sided muscle tone and right-sided auditory evoked potentials.

CLINICAL UTILITY IN ADULT RESPIRATORY FAILURE

The major usage in adult patients has been for severe acute respiratory failure, most commonly due to ARDS.[3,4,6,8] The results to date of the three major investigations of these techniques for treatment of ARDS are inconsistent and are summarized below.

NIH-Sponsored Randomized Trial

The randomized trial sponsored by the NIH included patients with many causes of respiratory failure.[1] For example, 57 percent of the patients had respiratory failure due to pneumonia. Although the arterial blood gas criteria required for entry represented the most severe end of the spectrum of ARDS, many of these patients may have been missing features of ARDS such as diffuse bilateral infiltrates. Patients were entered under "fast" or "slow" criteria, as summarized in Table 78-1. There was no common protocol for management, and different centers used different membrane oxygenators, mechanical ventilator management, and ancillary therapy. The patients had received ventilation for a mean of 9 days prior to entry.

A total of 90 patients were randomly assigned to either conventional mechanical ventilation or ECMO. For the ECMO patients ventilation was provided at lower inspired O_2 fraction (F_{IO_2}), tidal volume (V_T), and respiratory rate than for the conventional patients. These patients also had lower platelet and white blood cell counts. Pulmonary blood flow was reduced by ECMO from 3.5 L/m^2/min in the conventional group to 2.4 L/m^2/min in the ECMO group. Although there was a suggestion of early stabilization by ECMO, the survival rates in both groups were very poor and showed no significant difference (9.5 percent survival of ECMO and 8.3 percent of conventional patients).[1] Five patients who were failing conventional therapy were transferred to ECMO, but all of them died. There was slightly better survival of patients who had been intubated for shorter periods prior to entry in the study. Requirements for blood and plasma were greater in the ECMO than in the conventional patients (2.5 versus 1.0 L/d), but there was no difference in the occurrence of sepsis or pneumothorax.

Table 78-1. NIH ECMO Trial—Entry and Exclusion Criteria

Entry criteria
Fast entry
PaO_2 <50 mmHg for >2 hours on F_{IO_2} = 1.0 and PEEP >4 cmH_2O
Slow entry
PaO_2 <50 mmHg for >12 hours on F_{IO_2} > 0.59 and PEEP >4 cmH_2O with true shunt fraction >30%
Exclusion criteria
Age <12 or >65 years
Pulmonary insult of >21 days duration
Pulmonary capillary wedge pressure >25 mmHg
Chronic systemic disease
Lack of consent from patient or physician

F_{IO_2}, inspired oxygen fraction; PEEP, positive end-expiratory pressure.

Italian $ECCO_2R$-LFPPV Trials

The Italian group of Gattinoni and colleagues have pioneered the use of a combination of VV bypass to remove CO_2 with low-frequency pressure control ventilation for treatment of severe respiratory failure.[2,3] Studies with this system began in the late 1970s and still continue. Their membrane bypass system can remove large quantities of CO_2, even at very low blood flow rates. It uses a 9-m^2 surface area membrane ventilated with 15 L/min of humidified, O_2-enriched gas (Fig. 78-1).

Venovenous bypass was selected to avoid potential ischemic necrosis of the lung caused by decreases in pulmonary blood flow. To complement this, their ventilatory method lessened airway pressure. Patients received pressure control ventilation at rates of 3 to 5 breaths per minute with positive end-expiratory pressure (PEEP). The initial PEEP level used was selected to keep mean airway pressure constant and then was adjusted to achieve the optimal measured static compliance for the individual patient's lungs. PEEP levels in most patients ranged from 15 to 25 cmH_2O. There also was a small-bore catheter supplying a continuous flow of 1 to 2 L/min of 100 percent O_2 just above the main carina. Consequently, the true alveolar F_{IO_2} was 0.10 to 0.15 above the F_{IO_2} set on the ventilator.

In Gattinoni and co-workers' protocol,[2,3] patients with respiratory failure and stiff lungs initially were treated with pressure control ventilation. Patients who responded were gradually switched to continuous positive airway pressure (CPAP) for weaning. Nonresponders were placed on the $ECCO_2R$-LFPPV system. Treatment was continued until the patients' arterial blood gas values were adequate on CPAP, with an F_{IO_2} of 0.4 and PEEP of 10 to 15 cmH_2O.

Of the patients treated with $ECCO_2R$-LFPPV in this study,[3] the great majority (38 of 43) entered by the "slow" criteria. In contrast to the NIH ECMO trial,[1] the survival rate was 49 percent. The best survival was in patients with pulmonary and fat emboli or other miscellaneous causes of respiratory failure (shock, sepsis, near drowning). Mortality was greatest in patients with post-traumatic respiratory failure. These results are somewhat surprising, since most studies of ARDS outcome have found that survival is better in surgical patients. Lung function improved in 73 percent of all patients during bypass, usually beginning within 48 hours. Although bleeding was common and often a significant clinical problem, the lack of an increase in sepsis compared with the pre-bypass period was surprising.

There are several potential reasons for the greatly improved survival in Gattinoni's patients as compared with those in the NIH trial. First, the Italian study was nonrandomized and lacked a control group. Patient selection may have biased the results favorably. Second, their system may have caused less ischemic and pressure necrosis of the lung. Third, the lower airway pressures may have decreased the amplification of epithelial injury. Fourth, the paralysis and heparinization may have been beneficial. Finally, the patients may have received unusually attentive care because of the study.

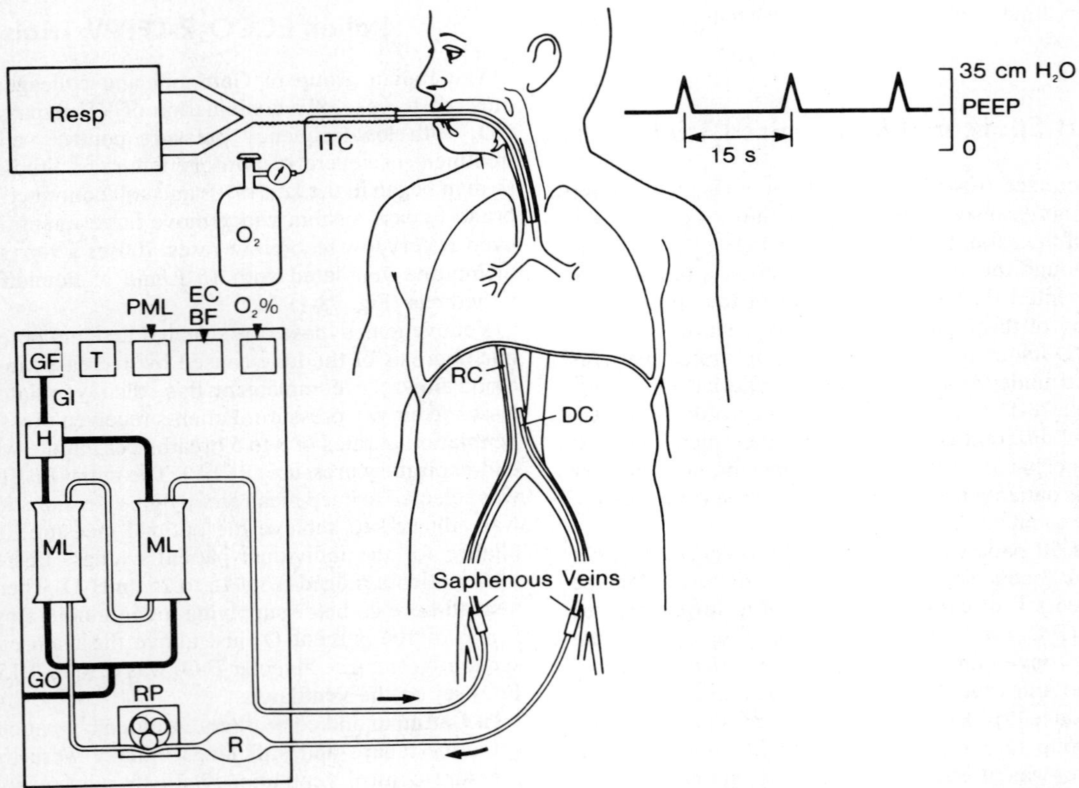

Figure 78-1. Configuration of system for patient support with extracorporeal CO_2 removal and low-frequency positive-pressure ventilation (ECCO$_2$R-LFPPV), as popularized by Gattinoni and colleagues in Milan. DC, drainage catheter; RC, return catheter; ITC, intratracheal catheter for O_2 flow; ML, membrane lung; RP, roller pump; R, venous reservoir; H, humidifier; GI, gas inlet; GO, gas outlet; GF, gas flow monitor; PEEP, positive end-expiratory pressure; Resp, positive-pressure ventilator; PML, pressure across lung; ECBF, extracorporeal blood flow; T, temperature. (From Gattinoni et al.,[3] with permission.)

University of Utah ECCO$_2$R-LFPPV Randomized Trial

In view of the conflicting results of these two large studies, a randomized, controlled trial of ECCO$_2$R-LFPPV was initiated at the University of Utah by Morris and colleagues.[4] This trial employed bypass and ventilator systems identical to those of Gattinoni and used the same entry criteria. The study design eliminated many of the concerns about patient selection and comparison with historical controls. To further eliminate bias by physicians in patient management, protocols for patient care and decision making were developed for both the ECCO$_2$R-LFPPV and conventional ventilation groups. These management protocols were developed through the consensus of 15 multidisciplinary critical care specialists.[4] The algorithms were embedded in bedside computers so that they were almost continuously available.

This study is still underway, but since it is not double-blind, interim results are available. The preliminary results indicate that ECCO$_2$R-LFPPV does not markedly improve survival. Both groups have had survival rates somewhat better than those reported by Gattinoni and those of historical control ARDS patients at the University of Utah. It is not clear whether the improvement is due to general improvements in the care of these critically ill patients or whether it is due specifically to the patient management algorithms used with all patients.

OTHER MISCELLANEOUS USES IN ADULTS

ECMO has been used rarely for the transient support of patients with severe gas exchange defects, such as massive pulmonary emboli. It also has proved beneficial when undertaking large-volume bilateral bronchoalveolar lavage, as in treating pulmonary alveolar proteinosis.

CLINICAL USES IN NEONATES

ECMO has been used much more widely in the treatment of severe respiratory failure in the newborn.[5] Some of the common indications are listed in Table 78-2. In neonates believed to be extremely likely to die, the survival rate with

Table 78-2. Possible Uses of Extracorporeal Support

In adults
Brief support for
Bilateral alveolar lavage for pulmonary alveolar proteinosis
After lung transplant respiratory failure
Massive pulmonary embolus
Intermediate-term support for
??Acute respiratory failure & ARDS
CO_2 removal without intubation
In neonates
Meconium aspiration
Infant respiratory distress syndrome
Persistent pulmonary hypertension of the newborn
Congenital diaphragmatic hernia
?Newborn sepsis

VA ECMO was as high as 80 percent in a large series from the national neonatal ECMO registry.[5] Controlled studies have been considered to be unethical because of these results. A major problem specific to neonates is the use of the right carotid artery for access with subsequent ligation. This can cause central nervous system damage in a significant number of infants. ECMO also may increase the likelihood of cerebral hemorrhage.

SUMMARY OF CLINICAL STATUS

At present ECMO therapy of respiratory failure in adults remains experimental, and its use should be restricted to clinical protocols at centers with appropriately experienced and committed personnel teams. Clinical benefit has not yet been convincingly demonstrated for any particular subgroup of patients with respiratory failure. The relative benefits of $EECO_2R$-LFPPV in comparison with VA bypass ECMO are not yet clear but the difference in survival suggests that iatrogenic barotrauma due to positive pressure ventilation may be decreased with the former method. In comparison with ECMO, greater benefit probably results from the development of consistent, well conceived management algorithms for these complex critical ailments. Extremely rarely, ECMO offers life-sustaining support for short periods of time to patients with severe respiratory failure due to loss of alveolar ventilation or capillary blood flow. Consequently, this modality should not be forgotten altogether while awaiting further results from randomized trials.

References

1. Zapol WM, Snider MT, Hill JD et al: Extra-corporeal membrane oxygenation for severe acute respiratory failure: A randomized prospective study. JAMA 1979;242:2193–2196
2. Gattinoni L, Pesenti A, Rossi GP et al: Treatment of acute respiratory failure with low-frequency positive-pressure ventilation and extracorporeal removal of CO_2. Lancet 1980;2:292–294
3. Gattinoni L, Pesenti A, Mascheroni D et al: Low-frequency positive-pressure ventilation with extracorporeal CO_2 removal in severe acute respiratory failure. JAMA 1986;256:881–886
4. Morris AH, Wallace CJ, Clemmer TP et al: Extracorporeal CO_2 removal therapy for adult respiratory distress syndrome patients. Respir Care 1990;35:224–231
5. Toomasian JM, Snedecor SM, Cornell RG et al: National experience with extracorporeal membrane oxygenation for newborn respiratory failure. ASAIO Trans 1988;34:140–147
6. Hickling KG: Extracorporeal CO_2 removal in severe adult respiratory distress syndrome. Anaesth Intensive Care 1986;14:46–53
7. Hirschi RB, Bartlett RH: Extracorporeal membrane oxygenation support in cardiorespiratory failure. Adv Surg 1987;21:189–212
8. Kolobow T: An update on adult extracorporeal membrane oxygenation–extracorporeal CO_2 removal. ASAIO Trans 1988; 34:1004–1005
9. Ryckman FC: Extracorporeal membrane oxygenation in the management of respiratory and cardiac failure. Probl Respir Care 1989;2:98–110

Chapter 79

Hemoglobin and Synthetic Oxygen Carriers

David H. Ingbar

CHAPTER OUTLINE

The potential usefulness of artificial blood substitutes has tantalized investigators for many years. In addition to substituting for red blood cell (RBC) transfusion, they also could be useful for organ preservation for transplantation, treatment of organ ischemia, sensitization of tumor cells for chemotherapy or radiation therapy, or treatment of anaerobic infections. Avoiding the use of RBCs obviously is advantageous in situations in which blood is difficult to cross-match, cross-matched blood is unavailable, or the patient (e.g., a Jehovah's Witness) refuses RBC transfusion. In addition, it may decrease complications, including transfusion reactions; transmission of infectious diseases such as hepatitis, acquired immunodeficiency syndrome (AIDS), and cytomegalovirus (CMV) infection; and volume overload.

The four major functions of RBCs are (1) loading O_2 in the pulmonary capillaries and releasing it in the systemic capillaries; (2) picking up CO_2 from the capillaries of peripheral tissues and releasing it in the lungs; (3) buffering acid present in the blood; and (4) maintaining intravascular volume. The ideal blood substitute would have a number of similar properties: it would take up large volumes of O_2 at the normal pulmonary capillary PO_2 and release CO_2 in the lungs; in the capillary it would release large volumes of O_2 while binding large volumes of CO_2; and it also would support circulatory dynamics and buffer tissue acidosis. It should be nontoxic and stable for long periods and over a wide range of temperatures, and cross-matching should be unnecessary. Finally, the blood substitute should survive for a reasonably long half-life without auto-oxidation. Not surprisingly, none of the currently available blood substitutes meet these criteria.

Three major groups of synthetic blood substitutes have been studied and are reviewed here briefly.[1] Perfluorocarbons (PFCs) have been investigated the most extensively.[2] Since about 1980 interest also has focused on stroma-free hemoglobin (SFH) solutions and repackaging of hemoglobin (Hb) within small microspheres of different types.

PERFLUOROCHEMICAL EMULSIONS

The intrinsic solubility of O_2 in PFCs is high, presumably owing to the high density of adjacent fluorine atoms. Most of the PFCs are fluorinated 8- to 10-carbon organic compounds, which are chemically inert and of fairly high density. Since they are immiscible with water, they would occlude capillaries if they were not emulsified by dispersion prior to

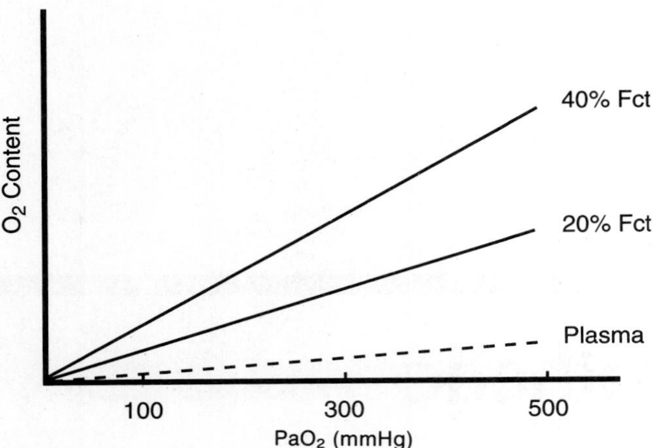

Figure 79-1. O_2 content versus PaO_2 with 20 and 40 percent concentrations of perfluorocarbon emulsion as compared with plasma alone. Compare with normal oxyhemoglobin dissociation curve (see Fig. 11-1). Fct, fluorocrit.

use. Unfortunately, this requirement limits the PFC concentration that can be achieved within the bloodstream. The low vapor pressure of PFCs prevents their rapid excretion from the lungs. Emulsification results in very small droplets, 0.1 to 0.2 μm in diameter, which therefore have a very high surface area with a very low viscosity.

Both O_2 and CO_2 are 20 times as soluble in PFCs as in water or plasma. As with plasma, the amount of O_2 dissolved in PFCs is directly proportional to the PO_2 (Fig. 79-1). This differs markedly from the normal Hb-O_2 dissociation curve (see Ch. 11, Fig. 11-1). The volume percent of PFC that can be obtained in the blood after dispersion and infusion, the fluorocrit (Fct), is a major limitation on the total dissolved content of O_2. In most animal studies the Fct does not exceed 5 to 10 percent. A second major problem is that a very high PaO_2 must be achieved to dissolve significant amounts of O_2. At a PaO_2 of 400 mmHg, 1 percent Fct corresponds to half the O_2 content of 1 percent hematocrit (Hct). At lower PaO_2, the PFCs are even less effective.

Excretion of PFCs occurs primarily through the lungs. The intravascular half-life in humans is dose-dependent but usually is between 6 and 24 hours. Some PFCs accumulate in the reticuloendothelial system and can still be found in the liver months after a single dose. Small amounts are excreted in urine and stool.

Early Studies

In 1966 Clark and Gollan[3] demonstrated that mice immersed in preoxygenated PFCs could survive for hours. Subsequently, Geyer demonstrated that rats could survive a complete transfusion and continue to eat, drink, and grow for as long as 7 days.[4] The only commercially available PFC emulsion, Fluosol-DA 20 percent (FDA-20), was first used in the 1970s. It consists of the O_2 carrier perfluorodecalin, the stabilizer perfluorotripropylamine, the nonionic surfactant Pluronic F-68, yolk phospholipids as emulsifiers, glycerol as a preservative, hydroxyethyl starch as an oncotic agent, glucose, and salts. Overall there is 20 g of PFC in every 100 mL of solution. FDA-20 was first given to human volunteers in 1978. In Japan it has been used for patients with a variety of conditions in addition to hemorrhagic shock.[5] Clinical trials in the United States, begun at the same time, have been restricted to Jehovah's Witnesses with severe anemia who refuse transfusion therapy.

Treatment of Anemia

There is considerable controversy about the clinical utility of FDA-20 for treatment of anemia. Table 79-1 gives the results in five series of patients receiving FDA-20 for severe anemia. An ideal blood substitute should increase tissue O_2 delivery, tissue O_2 consumption, and mixed venous PO_2 ($P\bar{v}O_2$). In addition, cardiac output might drop, since this compensation for tissue hypoxia might no longer be necessary. The effects of FDA-20 transfusion varied significantly in the different studies. For example, Tremper et al.[6] showed beneficial effects on O_2 consumption and $P\bar{v}O_2$ with an Fct of 2.9 percent and an F_IO_2 of 84 percent. By contrast, Gould

Table 79-1. Clinical Effects of Perfluorocarbon Blood Substitute (FDA-20) Infusion in Five Reported Series

Authors	Year	Patients No.	Patients Type	mL/kg	Cardiac Output	DO_2	$\dot{V}O_2$	$P\bar{v}O_2$
Mitsuno and Ohyanagi[5]	1985	225	Mixed	≥20	?Increase	Increase	?Stable	Stable
Tremper et al.[6]	1982	7	Anemia	20	Stable	Increase	Increase	Increase
Waxman et al.[7]	1984	6	Anemia (Hb <7)	20	Stable	Increase	Increase	Increase
Stefaniszyn et al.[8]	1985	3	Anemia prior to surgery	10–20	Varied	Increase	Varied	Increase
Gould et al.[9]	1986	8	Anemia	20	Stable	Stable	Stable	Increase

DO_2, systemic O_2 delivery; $\dot{V}O_2$, O_2 consumption.

and colleagues[9] achieved a mean maximal Fct of 5 percent, a mean PaO_2 of 430 mmHg and an FIO_2 of 100 percent. Although $P\bar{v}O_2$ was increased, there was no change in cardiac index, O_2 transport, or O_2 delivery. Patients in the Gould et al.[9] study had more severe anemia (Hb below 3.5 g/dL) than those in the Tremper et al.[6] study (mean Hb 5.4 g/dL).

The clinical utility of FDA-20 in these situations is limited by the maximum achievable PaO_2 and the potential for O_2 toxicity during prolonged use of very high FIO_2. In addition, repeated dosing or continuous infusion is needed to maintain a reasonable Fct. Finally, significant volume expansion and hemodilution occur and may adversely affect the patient.

Other Uses

PFCs may carry O_2 to sites distal to partial vascular obstruction or regions of microvascular damage. FDA-20 has decreased experimental myocardial infarct size in dogs, and in humans it has prevented the drop in ejection fraction that occurs during balloon inflation in percutaneous transluminal coronary angioplasty. There is controversy about the effects on cerebrovascular ischemia. Another microvascular problem in which FDA-20 may be useful is sickle cell crisis.

Another major potential use is to better preserve organs for transplantation. Experimentally, cardiac muscle damage and oxidant production are decreased with FDA-20 and O_2.

PFCs may sensitize tumor cells to radiation and chemotherapy. Hypoxia protects cells against radiation cytotoxicity. By selectively increasing the O_2 content of tumor cells but not normal cells, PFCs make the former more susceptible to injury. In ongoing clinical trails, FDA-20 and hyperbaric O_2 are being used to treat central nervous system gliomas, head and neck carcinomas, and lung cancer. They also are synergistic with a variety of alkylating agents for retarding growth of experimental tumors.

Complications

Early reactions to FDA-20 include rapid onset of chest pressure and shortness of breath, possibly related to complement activation by Pluronic F-68. Patients also may become hypotensive or have a normotensive bradycardia. Several days after treatment it is not uncommon for patients to develop abnormal chest x-ray findings, fever, elevated white blood cell count, and worsening oxygenation.[10] However, the mechanism of this problem may be heterogeneous and is not well defined. PFCs also may diminish host defenses by decreasing neutrophil migration, adherence, and activation. The combination of chemotherapy with hyperoxia and PFC exposure may increase lung inflammation and theoretically might cause increased lung damage. However, normal rats tolerated exchange transfusion and exposure to 85 percent O_2 for 5 days with no morphologic alteration in the lungs other than PFC accumulation in alveolar and interstitial macrophages.

Current Usefulness

The current usefulness of PFCs is limited by their short half-life, the inability to achieve a high Fct, the requirement for very high PaO_2 and FIO_2, and their relatively low O_2-carrying capacity as compared with RBCs. PFCs are not of great value for severe anemia but may be more useful in treating microvascular problems. Particularly exciting are their potential uses in myocardial ischemia or sickle cell crisis and as sensitizers for radiation therapy and chemotherapy of tumors.

STROMA-FREE HEMOGLOBINS

Attempts to replace the blood with infusion of purified Hb have a long history. Sellards and Minot first gave very small volumes of Hb intravenously to 33 patients in 1916. Three patients had chills, fever, and headache. Rare use of Hb infusion in the 1930s and 1940s resulted in significant complications, including renal injury and hypertension. In 1934 Mulder[11] transfused cats with Hb solutions and showed that they were physiologically intact by their ability to land upright after being dropped out of high windows.

The use of SFH offers several advantages over the use of PFCs.[12,13] First, the need to use a very high FIO_2 is eliminated. Second, SFH can be easily stored, shipped, and handled. Third, the O_2-carrying capacity of SFH is potentially much greater than that of PFCs, and the Hb-O_2 dissociation curve retains its normal shape. It is believed that eliminating the stromal component avoids most of the toxic effect, particularly renal damage, seen when intravascular RBC lysis occurs.

SFH typically is prepared by hemolysis of washed, outdated RBCs, which have been further purified by multiple crystallizations and then lyophilized. In this process 2,3-diphosphoglycerate (2,3-DPG) is lost, and there is potential for oxidation to methemoglobin. The O_2 affinity of SFH is significantly increased because of loss of the 2,3-DPG, dissociation of Hb tetramer, and the change in pH from the normal value of RBCs. The P_{50} shifts to the left, from its usual value of 26 to 27 mmHg to 12 to 16 mmHg.

Experimental Trials

In 1976 complete exchange transfusion with SFH was performed in baboons. Their O_2 consumption was maintained, but their $P\bar{v}O_2$ diminished markedly, which suggests that release of O_2 to the tissues might be a problem in ill humans. Consequently the SFH was converted to its pyridoxylated form (P-SFH) to normalize P_{50}; this led to higher whole blood P_{50} and somewhat higher $P\bar{v}O_2$ levels in baboons after exchange transfusion. The efficacy of P-SFH was diminished by the use of relatively low Hb concentrations to avoid major increases in oncotic pressure. In addition, SFH and P-SFH were rapidly cleared from the blood, which caused both an osmotic diuresis and the need for frequent SFH infusions.

Because of this, methods of polymerizing Hb have been developed. For example, copolymerization of P-SFH with glutaraldehyde creates large complexes, which are not filtered in the kidney. Studies in rats and baboons indicate that the half-life of polymerized as compared with nonpolymerized P-SFH is markedly prolonged (38 versus 4 hours). Other methods of cross-linking hemoglobin that result in even lower O_2 affinity are being explored.[14]

In comparison with PFCs, Hb solutions have much greater O_2-carrying capacity at normal PaO_2 levels. One comparative study of SFH and FDA-20 in ventilated baboons showed that both blood substitutes could maintain O_2 consumption; however, P-SFH contributed more to O_2 delivery and achieved this in animals breathing room air.[15]

The major complication of concern with SFH is nephrotoxicity. One clinical safety trial of SFH in normal volunteers in 1977 showed early onset of reversible decrease in urine volume and creatinine clearance. Other complications have included mild hypertension, transient bradycardia, and occasionally fevers, chills, or shortness of breath. Further human toxicity studies using polymerized forms of P-SFH are currently awaited, following which efficacy studies can proceed more rapidly.

ENCAPSULATED HEMOGLOBINS

The use of encapsulated Hbs has recently attracted attention. Patients with chronic anemia have been treated with resealed RBCs loaded with Hb modified by inositol hexaphosphate (IHP). The IHP improves O_2 unloading by shifting the Hb-O_2 dissociation curve to the right. These resealed RBCs are quite large and their ability to enter distorted microvasculature is lower than that of SFH and PFCs.

Hb also has been encapsulated within small liposomes of 0.7 μm diameter.[16] The liposomes contain large quantities of hemoglobin (15 g/dL) with a P_{50} of 24 mmHg. Rats survive 50 percent and near complete exchange transfusions with these "neohemocytes" without kidney or liver damage and with maintenance of O_2 consumption at an Hct of 3 percent. The half-life of the liposomes is approximately 6 hours.

Liposomal size and lipid composition must be optimized in order to prolong their half-life and minimize toxicity. Given their significant O_2-carrying capacity, liposome-encapsulated Hbs have potential application to humans provided their toxicity is sufficiently low.

SUMMARY OF CLINICAL STATUS

PFCs have been tested more extensively than other blood substitutes, but results in treating patients with severe anemia have been disappointing. Instead, they may be most useful in situations of abnormal microcirculation with ischemia and as sensitizers for chemotherapy and radiation therapy. At present their use is limited by the need for a very high FiO_2 for prolonged periods, the need for repeated dosing to achieve a high Fct, and their significant toxicities. New PFCs are being developed that may alleviate some of these limitations.

Polymerized P-SFH and encapsulated Hb solutions are of greater potential usefulness for increasing tissue O_2 delivery. However, at present relatively few human studies and few toxicity data are available. These uses of outdated Hb may permit treatment of patients with severe anemia in outlying locations where RBCs are not available.

Finally, studies on all these substances have focused predominantly on O_2 carrying and delivery. Other properties of RBCs such as CO_2 transport and acid buffering need investigation. The ultimate test of efficacy of new blood substitutes will occur when they are used in the critically ill patient with multiple stresses on the O_2 transport system.

References

1. Ingbar DH: The quest for a red blood cell substitute. Respir Care 1990; 35:260–272
2. Tremper KK, Anderson ST: Perfluorochemical emulsion oxygen transport fluids: A clinical review. Annu Rev Med 1985;309–313
3. Clark LC, Gollan F: Survival of mammals breathing organic liquids equilibrated with oxygen at atmospheric pressure. Science 1966;152:1755–1756
4. Geyer RP: Fluorocarbon-polyol artificial blood substitutes. N Engl J Med 1973;289:1077–1082
5. Mitsuno T, Ohyanagi H: Present status of clinical studies of Fluosol-DA (20%) in Japan. Int Anesthesiol Clin 1985;23:169–184
6. Tremper KK, Friedman AE, Levine EM et al: The preoperative treatment of severely anemic patients with a perfluorochemical oxygen-transport fluid, Fluosol-DA. N Engl J Med 1982;307:277–283
7. Waxman K, Tremper KK, Cullen BF et al: Perfluorocarbon infusion in bleeding patients refusing blood transfusions. Arch Surg 1984;119:721–724
8. Stefaniszyn HJ, Wynands JE, Salerno TA: Initial Canadian experience with artificial blood (Fluosol-DA-20%) in severely anemic patients. J Cardiovasc Surg 1985;26:337–342
9. Gould SA, Rosen AL, Sehgal LR et al: Fluosol-DA as a red-cell substitute in acute anemia. N Engl J Med 1986;314:1653–1656
10. Police AM, Waxman K, Tominaga G: Pulmonary complications after fluosol administration to patients with life-threatening blood loss. Crit Care Med 1985;13:96–98
11. Mulder AG, Amberson WR, Steggerda FR et al: Oxygen consumption with hemoglobin-Ringer. J Cell Comp Physiol 1934;5:383–397
12. Moss GS, Gould SA, Sehgal LR et al: Hemoglobin solution—from tetramer to polymer. Surgery 1984;95:249–255
13. Gould SA, Sehgal LR, Rosen AL et al: Red cell substitutes: An update. Ann Emerg Med 1985;14:796–803
14. Winslow RM: Blood substitutes—current status. Transfusion 1989;29:753–773
15. Gould SA, Rosen AL, Sehgal LR et al: Red cell substitutes: Hemoglobin solution or fluorocarbon? J Trauma 1982;22:736–740
16. Hunt CA, Burnette RR, MacGregor RD et al: Synthesis and evaluation of a prototypal artificial red cell. Science 1985;230:1165–1168

Chapter 80

Hyperbaric Oxygen Therapy

Richard L. Sheldon

CHAPTER OUTLINE

The term *hyperbaric oxygen* (HBO) refers to the exposure of patients to air and/or O_2 at pressures greater than one atmosphere (1 atm). The earliest historical reference to hyperbaric medicine was in the seventeenth century, when use of air under pressure to treat decompression sickness was described by Sir Robert Boyle.[1] Since that time the therapeutic use of HBO has an interesting history not unlike the historical progression of many other medical treatment modalities. Currently many centers throughout the world use hyperbaric chambers to treat multiple medical problems. Over the years many applications have proved to be at best fads, and at worst blatant absurdities. It would be correct to say that as with most medical treatment modalities, there is controversy over which applications of HBO are useful.[2] Presently, applications of HBO that are of absolutely proven benefit are few.

BASIC HYPERBARIC PHYSIOLOGY

The physiologic effects of HBO can be divided into two categories, those due to the increased pressure exerted by the chamber and those due to inhalation of O_2 at high concentrations in a hyperbaric environment.

Physiologic Effects Due to Pressure

At sea level and at standard temperature and pressure, the pressure is said to be 1 atmosphere absolute. However, a common gauge would say 0 atm, 14.7 psi, or 760 mmHg. Some confusion may come when the term *atmospheres absolute* (ATA) is used. The term is meant to simplify the concept of *atmospheric pressure* and to point out that at sea level there is "absolutely" 1 atm of pressure. Most hyperbaric chambers use two to three times atmospheric pressure, or 2 to 3 ATA, which is equivalent to the pressure at a depth of 33 to 66 ft in the ocean. As shown in Table 80-1, as the pressure increases, the volume of a given amount of gas decreases progressively. This physical fact makes possible the treatment of gas-related injuries such as air embolism and the "bends" of decompression sickness.

Physiologic Effects Due to Oxygen

The effects of increased PO_2 can be categorized into four types.[3] First, blood flow is reduced because high O_2 concentrations in the precapillary and capillary bed result in vasoconstriction and consequently in less edema. Second, high O_2 concentrations can detoxify certain bacterial toxins produced during the normal metabolism of the particular

Table 80-1. Pressure Effects of Hyperbaric Oxygen Therapy as Related to an Easily Visualized Activity in Nature—Submersion in Water[a]

Depth (ft under H_2O)	Indicated Gauge Pressure (atm)	Absolute Pressure (ATA)	Relative Gas Volume of Bubble (Fraction)	Relative Diameter of Bubble (%)
0	0	1	1	100
33	1	2	$\frac{1}{2}$	79.3
66	2	3	$\frac{1}{3}$	69.3
99	3	4	$\frac{1}{4}$	63
132	4	5	$\frac{1}{5}$	58.5
165	5	6	$\frac{1}{6}$	55

[a] Gauge readings and changes in bubble size with increasing depth are shown.

bacteria. Third, the restoration of normal or greater than normal PO_2 to traumatized tissue or dead and devitalized tissue can stimulate growth and differentiation of fibroblasts, osteoblasts, osteoclasts, and granulocytes, thereby accelerating wound healing. Restoration of microcirculation (angioneogenesis) is improved in hyperbaric states. Finally, HBO can exert antibacterial effects on certain anaerobic and aerobic bacteria,[3] probably via improvement of the immune system due to "switching on" of the neutrophils, made possible by more O_2 substrate. Oxygen radicals produced by activated neutrophils are very toxic to bacteria.[4]

TYPES OF HYPERBARIC CHAMBERS

Multiplace Chambers

Early hyperbaric chambers were referred to as *decompression chambers* and could take the form of entire operating rooms and the necessary equipment and staff to run them or of walk-in chambers in which the patient or group of patients plus attending personnel could all be present. Multiplace hyperbaric chambers[4] (Fig. 80-1) are still in use in large centers and are maintained at considerable expense. A multiplace chamber consists of an inner and an outer chamber with appropriate locking systems so that equipment, supplies, and staff can be moved from the outer to the inner chamber in which the patients are being treated without losing pressure. These chambers are brought to pressures as high as 6 ATA with air. Masks inside the chamber are then used to supply 100 percent O_2 or other gases such as He/O_2 mixtures to the patient. Compression times and pressures are carefully controlled in accordance with the U.S. Navy Diving Tables.[3]

Monoplace Chambers

The recent proliferation of HBO treatments has been due largely to the development and marketing of monoplace hyperbaric chambers[4] (Fig. 80-2). These chambers are somewhat portable, low-maintenance, relatively low cost devices, which can be purchased by anyone, installed easily, and operated after short training periods. They can be transported in a trailer or van to different facilities, so that a single chamber can be made available to many hospitals or clinics.

Monoplace chambers are pressurized with 100 percent O_2 to 2 to 3 ATA, and usually one patient is treated at a time. On occasions, during emergencies, two patients can be in the chamber at once. For the most part these chambers can accomplish everything that the larger, multiplace chambers can do. If a complication occurs during treatment, the decompression can be accomplished in a matter of seconds and the patient removed from the chamber for care. Multiplace and monoplace HBO chambers are compared in Table 80-2.

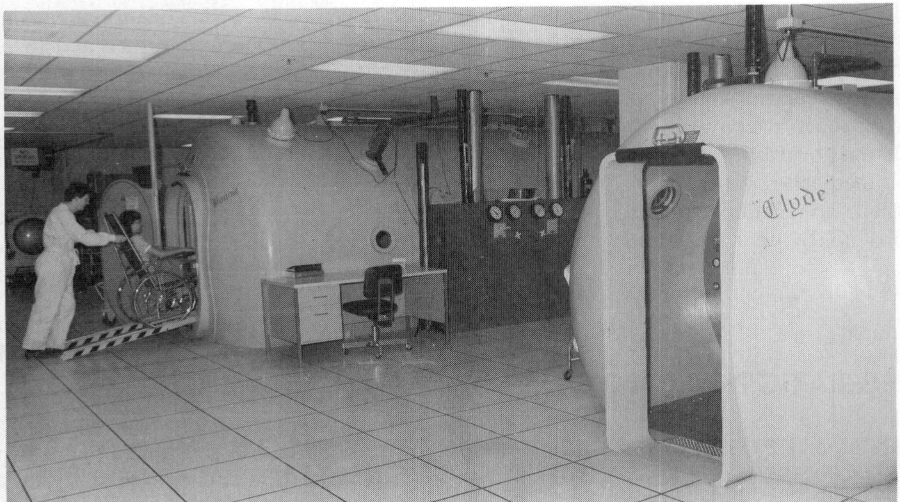

Figure 80-1. Multiplace hyperbaric chambers. (From Grim et al.[4]; reproduced courtesy of St. Lukes Medical Center, Milwaukee.)

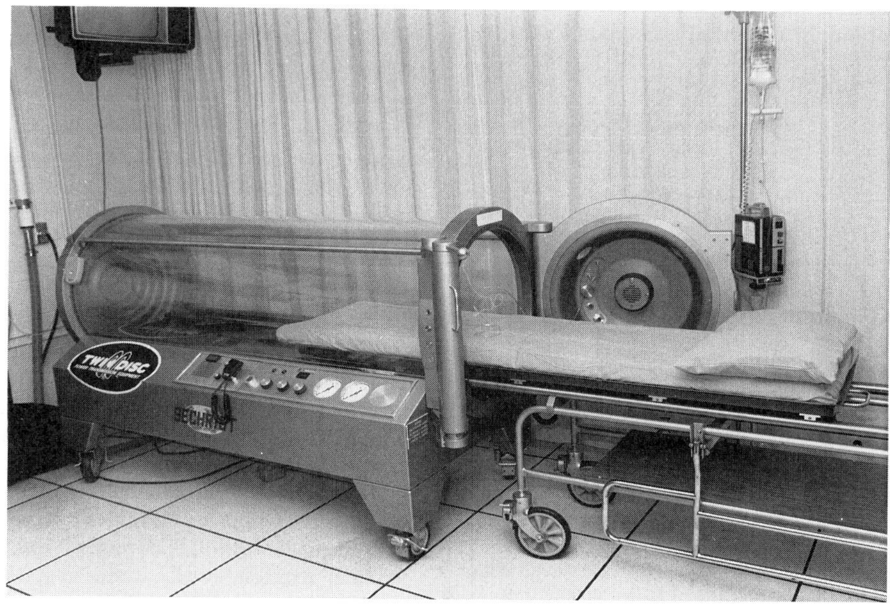

Figure 80-2. A monoplace hyperbaric chamber. (From Grim et al.[4]; reproduced courtesy of David Teplica, MD.)

CLINICAL SITUATIONS IN WHICH HYPERBARIC OXYGEN IS USED

The Undersea and Hyperbaric Medical Society, Inc. (UHMS) makes the following statement about the clinical use of HBO[3]:

> Hyperbaric oxygen treatment, in which a patient breathes 100% oxygen intermittently while the pressure of the treatment chamber is increased to a point higher than sea level pressure [i.e. >1 atmosphere absolute (ATA)], can be viewed as the new application of an old, established technology to help resolve certain recalcitrant, expensive, or otherwise hopeless medical problems.

The UHMS has become the recognized "clearing house" for HBO information and is generally accepted by third party payers in American medicine as an authority in evaluating new and old applications of HBO. Each application is the subject of a position paper describing in detail the new indication and all applicable research; this position is then reviewed and critiqued and submitted to committee for discussion and vote.[3] Table 80-3 lists the UHMS's currently approved applications of HBO.

Air or Gas Embolism

When gas bubbles embolize to an organ, serious compromise of the organ system can occur since the bubble can effectively block blood flow distal to where it comes to rest.

Table 80-2. Comparison of Multiplace and Monoplace Hyperbaric Oxygen Chambers

Chamber	Advantages	Disadvantages	Special Considerations
Multiplace	Can treat several patients at once Can go to higher pressures Can use several combinations of gases Attendant can handle emergency inside chamber	Very expensive Fixed High maintenance Higher staffing needs Hard to install	Good for research Can handle wide range of problems Training of operators is extensive and ongoing
Monoplace	Less expensive Portable Low maintenance Minimal staffing required Easily installed	Only one patient treated at a time Limited low range of pressures Uses only 100% O_2 Must decompress if emergency occurs	Handles all "approved" applications of HBO Operator training time is short

Table 80-3. Applications of Hyperbaric Oxygen Therapy Currently Approved by the Undersea and Hyperbaric Medical Society

Condition	Presumed Mechanism of Action of HBO
Air or gas embolism	Increase in pressure decreases bubble size
CO poisoning and smoke inhalation	Forces CO off hemoglobin
CO poisoning complicated by cyanide poisoning	
Clostridial myonecrosis (gas gangrene)	Inactivates the toxin
Crush injury, compartment syndrome, and other acute traumatic ischemias	Decreases edema
Decompression sickness	Increase in pressure decreases bubble size
Enhanced healing of selected problem wounds	Enhances fibroelastic activity and collagen production
Exceptional blood loss (anemia)	Dissolves enough O_2 in serum
Necrotizing soft tissue damage	Accelerates healing and reduces infection rate
Osteomyelitis (refractory)	Accelerates healing of new bone
Radiation tissue damage (osteoradionecrosis)	Stimulates formation of new microcirculation
Compromised skin grafts and flaps	Stimulates formation of new microcirculation
Thermal burns	Reduction of edema and infection Accelerates wound healing

This results in ischemia, which is most noticeable when the brain is involved. Modern medicine with its varied procedures has made exposure to air embolism more common. The following is a brief and incomplete list of documented situations in which air embolism has occurred: placement of burr holes in the skull, removal of large tumors, neurosurgery while the patient is in the sitting position, surgery on opened arteries and veins, cardiopulmonary bypass, angioplasty, total hip replacement, bronchoscopy with biopsy, liver transplantation, use of intra-aortic balloon pumps, pulmonary artery catheterization, kidney dialysis, abortions using air in the uterus, gunshot to head or chest, autotransfusion during surgery, and breath holding by scuba divers during ascent.[3]

Hyperbaric chambers can reduce the volume of an intravascular gas bubble and increase the diffusion gradient of embolized gas (Table 80-1). As with all treatment modalities, the sooner HBO is initiated, the better the result in cases of air embolism.[3] The improvement seen usually occurs promptly.

Carbon Monoxide Poisoning

CO binds to hemoglobin with an affinity more than 200 times that of O_2[1]; thus O_2 is displaced and not allowed to bind because the binding sites are filled with CO.[5] Tissue hypoxia results. The classic blood gas finding is that of a normal PaO_2 with a reduced measured O_2 saturation. CO bound to hemoglobin can be measured directly as carboxyhemoglobin. The organ systems most commonly affected in CO poisoning are the central nervous system and the heart.[5]

Indications for treatment are currently under review. It is accepted that increasing levels of carboxyhemoglobin correlate with worsening symptoms.[5] Central nervous system symptoms of CO poisoning range all the way from headache to coma and death. Carboxyhemoglobin levels above 50 percent are usually considered severe intoxication. However, occasionally only mild symptoms are seen despite levels of 50 percent or higher. Treatment for severe CO intoxication includes high-flow O_2 (100 percent) by tight-fitting mask, mechanical artificial ventilation, and HBO.[5,6] Some reports show a 30 percent mortality if HBO is delayed for over 6 hours but a decrease in mortality to 13.5 percent if HBO is started within 6 hours of discovery of the poisoning.[5]

Also of concern is the incidence of delayed central nervous system complications of poisoning. These delayed symptoms usually occur within 1 month after exposure and have been known to last for many months. The incidence of these delayed neurologic problems has been reported to drop from approximately 12 percent to near zero if HBO is used.[5]

Gas Gangrene

Gas gangrene (clostridial myonecrosis) is caused by anaerobic, spore-forming, gram-positive, encapsulated bacilli, the most common of which is *Clostridium perfringens*. Clostridia produce many toxins, of which the most important is a tissue-necrotizing and cell-lethal phospholipase C (lecithinase C).[3] The high O_2 tensions in HBO are both bacteriostatic and bactericidal to Clostridia; HBO is also able to stop the production and toxic effects of clostridial toxin.[3] The treatment schedules used to treat documented cases of gas gangrene with HBO vary from center to center, but it is usually agreed that three or four treatments of 100 percent O_2 at 2 to 3 ATA are all that is required to at least stop the advancing tissue destruction caused by the toxin.

Traumatic Ischemia

Crush injury can result in damage to both large and microscopic blood vessels,[7] which frequently compromises blood flow. If swelling occurs secondary to crush in a compartmentalized area such as the hand, ischemia may result owing to compression of the microcirculation. When perfusion in an area falls to the point at which tissue O_2 tensions are less than 30 mmHg, several important defense mechanisms are damaged.[7] Killing of microorganisms by white blood cells is reduced, as is the secretion of collagen by fibroblasts, which is essential to wound healing. Another important effect of HBO in crush injuries is the lessening of edema in the involved area by an estimated 20 percent.[3]

The UHMS guidelines recommend three 90-minute treatments per day during the first 48 hours, followed by two 90-minute treatments each day for 2 days and finally one 90-minute treatment each day for 2 days, as a complete standard treatment course.[3] Early application of HBO (4 to 6 hours after injury) is essential for this form of therapy to be useful in traumatic ischemia.

Decompression Sickness

When decompression (ascent) occurs at a rate faster than nitrogen (N_2) can be removed from tissue by simple diffusion, bubbles are formed. When the bubbles enter the bloodstream and are large enough, obstruction can occur, resulting in potentially life-threatening organ dysfunction.[1,7a] The most common circumstance in which this occurs is the case of an underwater diver who rises from depth to the surface too rapidly to allow the N_2 to leave the body. Signs and symptoms of decompression sickness include fatigue, joint and muscle pain (the "bends"), brain dysfunction, and in severe enough cases, shock and death.[1]

Immediate recompression in a hyperbaric chamber remains the treatment of choice.[4,7a] Delays of over 6 hours in treatment can result in serious injury; however, positive results have been reported even after such long delays.[3] The choice of which recompression schedule is used depends on several factors. Essentially, all treatment facilities have available the U.S. Navy Diving Tables, which take into account all these factors and clearly spell out which recompression schedule will give the best results.[3] The patient should be treated until all symptoms are resolved.

Wound Healing

The physiology of wound healing is remarkably complex.[3] A degree of hypoxia is required in order for healing to occur. Wounds are not only usually underperfused but also infected. In order for healing to proceed, fibroblastic activity, which is O_2-dependent, must be supported and collagen production must be enhanced.[4] High O_2 tensions in the tissues stimulate the production of capillaries.[3]

Venous stasis ulcers and decubitus ulcers are usually dealt with by a combination of surgical techniques or conservative measures such as good nursing care. When these measures fail, HBO may be of use. It is usually called on when the situation is so severe that loss of a limb is feared.[3] Wounds associated with arterial insufficiency are rarely helped by HBO, but HBO is useful in this setting when vascular surgery has re-established blood flow to the area and skin grafting is anticipated. HBO will then prepare a well granulated base that is ready to accept the skin graft.[3] Diabetic ulcers may respond when treated with HBO before they reach an advanced stage. HBO can help with both the polymicrobial infected state and the hypoxic condition represented in the usual diabetic ulcer.

Other Clinical Situations

Exceptional Blood Loss (Anemia)

If blood loss and impairment of O_2 content become so severe that cellular respiration is impaired, exceptional blood loss is said to have occurred. If blood replacement is not possible for medical or religious reasons, repetitive "dives" via hyperbaric chamber have sometimes been employed. Enough O_2 can be dissolved in plasma to sustain life even if no hemoglobin-containing red blood cells are present[8] (Fig. 80-3). Since the O_2 stored in the plasma is rapidly consumed and HBO cannot be used continuously, its clinical utility in this setting is questionable.

Necrotizing Soft Tissue Infections

When traumatic or surgical wounds are compromised by underlying disorders affecting the microcirculation, such as diabetes mellitus or atherosclerotic vascular disease, mixed aerobic and anaerobic bacteria can establish terrible and life-threatening infections. Usually surgical debridement and antibiotics are adequate, but if mortality and morbidity are expected to be high, HBO is sometimes added as supporting therapy.[3]

Refractory Osteomyelitis

Osteomyelitis can usually be treated adequately with antibiotics and surgical debridement, but occasionally the infection will resist standard treatment for months or years. In this setting HBO has been useful as adjunctive therapy. Animal studies show that HBO promotes osteoclast formation, thus helping to accelerate the tissue repair.[9]

Radiation Tissue Damage (Osteoradionecrosis)

Protection of irradiated tissues should be directed to two tissue types: bone and soft tissues. In the clinical setting of compromised vascularity in the area to be irradiated, severe tissue sloughs can be seen. It has been shown that a schedule of presurgical and preirradiation HBO, followed by post-surgery and intrairradiation HBO, can significantly improve the results of therapy.[10] The mechanisms are believed to be related to HBO's ability to stimulate the rapid development of microcirculation (angioneogenesis).[3]

Compromised Skin Grafts and Flaps

It is sometimes, although infrequently, necessary to place a skin graft or rotate a flap of skin onto an area of denuded

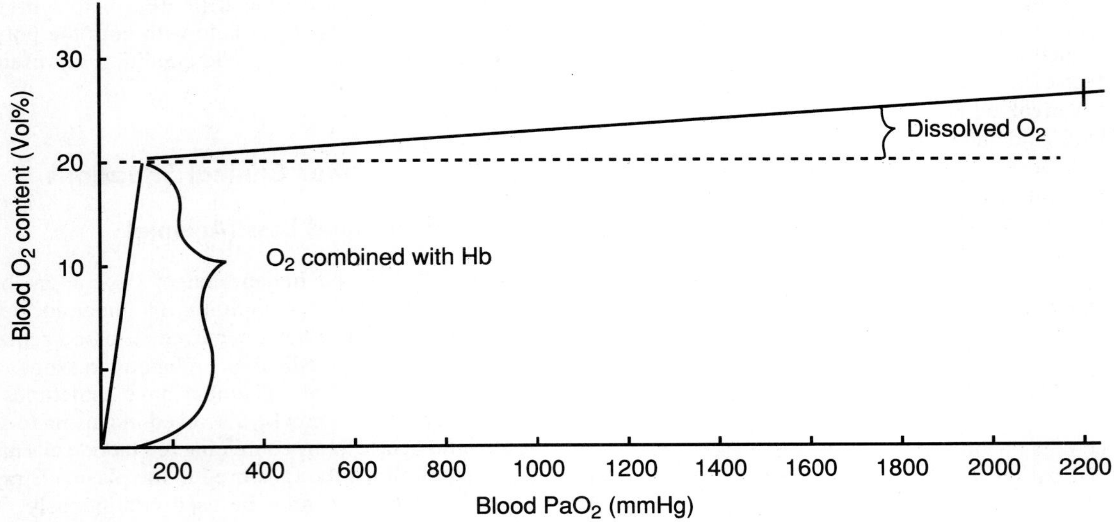

Figure 80-3. Extrapolation of oxyhemoglobin dissociation curve (Fig. 11-1) into ranges of PaO_2 and blood O_2 content encountered in hyperbaric O_2 therapy. Increment in dissolved O_2 with increasing PaO_2 equals 0.003 mL O_2/100 mL blood/mmHg, or 2.3 mL O_2/100 mL blood/ATA. By using HBO it is possible to dissolve enough O_2 in plasma to sustain life even in the complete absence of Hb.

tissue that is poorly perfused. Preoperative and postoperative application of HBO have been associated with improvement in survival of grafts and flaps managed in this manner.[3]

Thermal Burns

The prompt application of HBO to the management of thermal burns in animals has been associated with reduction in edema formation, reduction of local infection, preservation of partially burned tissues at the margins, and improved wound healing.[3] There are some burn centers in the United States in which hyperbaric chambers are a prominent aspect of routine care. Good randomized prospective studies need to be made by these centers in order to clarify the efficacy of HBO in burns.

Table 80-4. Major Complications of Hyperbaric Oxygen Therapy

Barotrauma (complications due to pressure)
Ear or sinus trauma
Tympanic membrane rupture
Pneumothorax
Air embolism
O_2 toxicity
Central nervous system toxic reactions
Pulmonary toxic reactions
Other complications
Fire
Reversible visual changes
Claustrophobia

(From Grim et al.,[4] with permission.)

COMPLICATIONS

Although numerous potentially serious complications of HBO exist[4] (Table 80-4), this therapy is remarkably safe when properly applied. Complications can generally be grouped into two categories: those due to pressure and those due to O_2 toxicity.[3,11] The most common injury from pressure is to the tympanic membrane (''ear squeeze''). Other injuries include pneumothorax and serous otitis. Injuries associated with the high O_2 concentrations include convulsions, eye changes, and extremely rare pulmonary damage.

Perhaps one of the most vexing ''complications'' is claustrophobia. This problem not infrequently limits the patient's willingness to return to the chamber to complete a course of therapy. Anxiolytic drugs can help some patients control their fear.

References

1. Strauss RH: Diving Medicine. Grune & Stratton, Orlando, FL, 1976
2. Gabb G, Robin ED: Hyperbaric oxygen. A therapy in search of diseases. Chest 1987;92:1074–1082

3. Hyperbaric Oxygen Therapy: A Committee Report. Undersea and Hyperbaric Medical Society, Bethesda, MD, 1989
4. Grim PS, Gottlieb LJ, Boddie A, Batson E: Hyperbaric oxygen therapy. JAMA 1990;263:2216–2220
5. Kiem LW: Oxygen, hyperbaric oxygen therapy, and carbon monoxide intoxication. Cardiopulmonary News and Interviews (American College of Chest Physicians) 1988;3:19–21
6. Ilano AL, Raffin TA: Management of carbon monoxide poisoning. Chest 1990;97:165–169
7. Skyhar MJ, Hargens AR, Strauss MB et al: Hyperbaric oxygen reduces edema and necrosis of skeletal muscle in compartment syndromes associated with hemorrhagic hypotension. J Bone Joint Surg [Am] 1986;68:1218–1224
7a. Melamed Y, Shupak A, Bitterman H: Medical problems associated with underwater diving. N Engl J Med 1992;326:30–35
8. Boerema I, Meyne NG, Brummelkamp WK et al: Life without blood: A study of the influence of high atmospheric pressure and hypothermia on dilution of the blood. J Cardiovasc Surg 1960;1:133–146
9. Esterhai JL, Pisarello J, Brighton CT et al: Adjunctive hyperbaric oxygen therapy in the treatment of chronic refractory osteomyelitis. J Trauma 1987;27:763–768
10. Fattore L, Strauss RA: Hyperbaric oxygen in the treatment of osteoradionecrosis: A review of its use and efficacy. Oral Surg Oral Med Oral Pathol 1987;63:280–286
11. Thom SR: Hyperbaric oxygen therapy. J Intensive Care Med 1989;4:58–74

Chapter 81

Determining the Need for Mechanical Ventilation

James K. Stoller

CHAPTER OUTLINE

Assessing patients with respiratory failure and determining the need for mechanical ventilation are common challenges for the clinician working in respiratory care. The decision to initiate mechanical ventilation begins with consideration of the two major purposes that mechanical ventilation can serve:

1. To support the patient during an episode of acute respiratory failure or
2. To reverse chronic ventilatory failure in the hope of providing a more durable ventilatory improvement

In this chapter, the spectrum of acute respiratory failure and the pathophysiology of respiratory failure are first briefly reviewed, and the indications for initiating mechanical ventilation are then discussed for the specific settings of acute oxygenation failure, acute ventilatory failure, and chronic ventilatory failure.

Respiratory failure occurs when either of the two major gas exchange functions of the lung—oxygenation and ventilation—deteriorates.[1,2] In approaching potential candidates for mechanical ventilation, a clear understanding of the type of respiratory failure at hand and its pathophysiology will help focus the expected benefits of mechanical ventilation and initial ventilatory strategies in such a way as to maximize benefits.

FAILURE OF OXYGENATION

As listed in Table 81-1 and discussed more fully in Chapters 29 and 31, impaired oxygenation of the arterial blood is generally ascribed to one of five pathophysiologic mechanisms, of which ventilation/perfusion mismatching, anatomic (right-to-left) shunting, and alveolar hypoventilation are the most common. Diffusion impairment rarely causes significant hypoxemia at sea level, and so-called diffusion-perfusion impairment, which may be considered a variant of diffusion limitation, is also an uncommon cause of hypoxemia and is usually associated with the specific clinical circumstance of intrapulmonary capillary dilation, which may accompany chronic liver disease.[3] Inspiration of gas of decreased O_2 pressure is readily identified and also occurs only in specific, known settings (e.g., controlled laboratory circumstances or hypobaric chambers).

In the acute setting, calculation of $P(A\text{-}a)O_2$, also called the A-a gradient, may help to differentiate alveolar hypo-

Table 81-1. Physiologic Mechanisms of Hypoxemia

Alveolar hypoventilation (see Table 81-2)
Ventilation-perfusion mismatch
Anatomic (right-to-left) shunt
Intracardiac (e.g., interatrial shunt)
Intrapulmonary (e.g., pulmonary arteriovenous malformation)
Diffusion impairment[a]
Reduced inspired O_2 pressure (P_IO_2)
Inhaling gas with inspired O_2 fraction (F_IO_2) <0.21
Exposure to lower than normal barometric pressure

[a] Includes a variant, diffusion-perfusion impairment (e.g., pulmonary capillary dilation associated with liver disease).

ventilation from other causes of hypoxemia. As discussed in Chapter 19, normal values of $P(A\text{-}a)O_2$ while breathing room air rise with advancing age[1] from nadir values of approximately 10 mmHg in young individuals to zenith values of 25 mmHg in octogenarians (Fig. 81-1). Age-related mean values for room air $P(A\text{-}a)O_2$ are predicted from the following equation:

$$P(A\text{-}a)O_2 = 2.5 \pm (0.21)(\text{age in years}) \quad (1)$$

$P(A\text{-}a)O_2$ is the difference between the calculated P_AO_2 and the measured PaO_2[1] (i.e., $P(A\text{-}a)O_2 = P_AO_2 - PaO_2$), where P_AO_2 is calculated from a variant of the alveolar air equation (see Ch. 10), as follows:

$$P_AO_2 = P_IO_2 - (PaCO_2)\left(F_IO_2 + \frac{1 - F_IO_2}{R}\right) \quad (2)$$

where R is the respiratory exchange ratio, P_IO_2 is the inspired O_2 pressure, and F_IO_2 is the inspired O_2 fraction,

$$P_IO_2 = (F_IO_2)(P_b - PH_2O) \quad (3)$$

Assuming that the subject breathes room air (F_IO_2, 0.21), that the barometric pressure (P_b) is 760 mmHg, and that water vapor pressure (PH_2O) at 37°C is 47 mmHg, Equation 2 becomes

$$P_AO_2 = 149 - (PaCO_2)(1.25) \quad (4)$$

and $P(A\text{-}a)O_2$ is given by

$$P(A\text{-}a)O_2 = 149 - [(PaCO_2)(1.25) + PaO_2] \quad (5)$$

As noted above, hypoxemia in the face of a normal $P(A\text{-}a)O_2$ value identifies alveolar hypoventilation as the cause of hypoxemia and should lead the clinician to examine causes of hypoventilation. The response to breathing pure O_2 can also help to identify the mechanism of hypoxemia in an individual patient. Specifically, in anatomic (right-to-left) shunt—whether intracardiac (i.e., interatrial) or intrapulmonary (i.e., due to a pulmonary arteriovenous malformation)—hypoxemia occurs because desaturated venous blood mixes directly with arterial blood without first being exposed to alveolar O_2, which would cause it to become oxygenated. With true anatomic shunt, therefore, breathing pure O_2 generally will not relieve hypoxemia. By contrast, breathing pure O_2 does improve oxygenation when the cause of hypoxemia is ventilation/perfusion mismatch, diffusion impairment, or, to a lesser extent, diffusion-perfusion impairment.[3]

FAILURE OF VENTILATION

Ventilatory failure is the second type of respiratory dysfunction for which treatment by mechanical ventilation may be indicated.[4] As with hypoxemia, knowledge of the pathophysiology of hypercapnia and its acuity will help clarify the need for ventilatory support in an individual patient.

Hypercapnia exists when $PaCO_2$ exceeds the normal range (e.g., 44 mmHg at sea level). As summarized in Equation 6 below, $PaCO_2$ will rise when CO_2 production increases (without a commensurate increase in alveolar ventilation) or when alveolar ventilation falls:

$$PaCO_2 = (0.863\ \text{mmHg}) \left[\frac{CO_2\ \text{production rate (mL/min, STPD)}}{\text{alveolar ventilation (L/min, BTPS)}}\right] \quad (6)$$

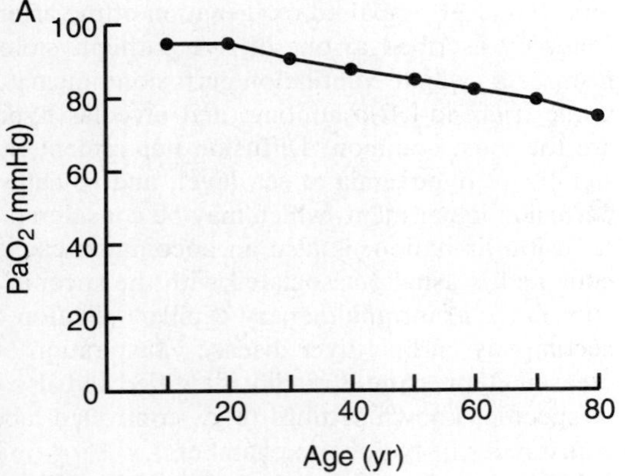

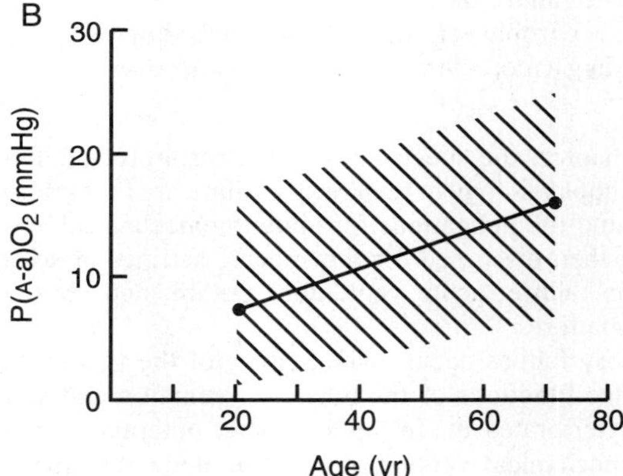

Figure 81-1. **(A)** Variation of PaO_2 with age. **(B)** Variation of $P(A\text{-}a)O_2$ with age, given by $[P(A\text{-}a)O_2] = 2.5 \pm (0.21)$ (age); bold line indicates mean values, shaded area ± 2 SD. $P(A\text{-}a)O_2 \leq 25$ mmHg at *all* ages. (From Tisi,[1] with permission.)

where STPD is standard temperature and pressure, dry and BTPS is body temperature and pressure, saturated.

Under clinical circumstances, increased CO_2 production usually accompanies increased metabolic rates (e.g., as reflected in fever or protracted muscular contraction) or increases in the respiratory quotient (RQ), most commonly seen when patients receive high concentrations of glucose instead of lipid during total parenteral nutrition. Specifically, fever increases CO_2 production by 13 percent for every 1°C elevation above normal.[4] As discussed in Chapter 51, the RQ varies with the caloric source, such that the RQ is 0.7 for fat oxidation and rises to values of 0.8 and 1.0, respectively, during protein and glucose oxidation.[5,6] Under normal circumstances, rising CO_2 production is accompanied by increased alveolar ventilation and $PaCO_2$ is maintained, but $PaCO_2$ will rise with increasing CO_2 production when alveolar ventilation is fixed (e.g., when the patient is paralyzed on a mechanical ventilator or when airflow obstruction is severe). As suggested by Equation 6, $PaCO_2$ may also rise when alveolar ventilation decreases.

Alveolar ventilation is the component of total minute ventilation that participates in CO_2 elimination by reaching perfused alveoli. Under normal circumstances, the ratio of dead space to tidal volume (V_D/V_T) is approximately 0.3, but any process that augments wasted ventilation (e.g., bullous emphysema with increased ventilation to poorly perfused lung) can increase V_D/V_T. Unless accompanied by an increased ventilatory rate, rising V_D/V_T will cause alveolar ventilation to fall. Extreme degrees of wasted ventilation can outstrip even these compensatory benefits of increased ventilatory rate.

Other causes of alveolar hypoventilation include decreased ventilatory rate, such as that which may accompany decreased respiratory drive, and dysfunction of the respiratory bellows, which may accompany phrenic nerve dysfunction or respiratory muscle dysfunction associated with metabolic derangement (e.g., hypophosphatemia or hypokalemia), with neuromuscular diseases (e.g., Duchenne muscular dystrophy, Guillain-Barré syndrome, or acid maltase deficiency), or with structural derangement of the chest wall (e.g., kyphoscoliosis). A classification scheme for causes of hypercapnia and alveolar hypoventilation is presented in Table 81-2.

Because the diaphragm generates the major component of inspiratory force under normal circumstances, diaphragmatic fatigue is the common pathway by which acute ventilatory failure frequently develops.[7,8] As shown by Cohen et al.[9] in a study of seven patients who developed ventilatory failure after discontinuing mechanical ventilation, the failing inspiratory muscles demonstrate a consistent physiologic sequence, beginning with a fall in the high/low power spectrum ratio of the diaphragmatic electromyogram (EMG), progressing to an increasing respiratory rate, respiratory alternans (in which abdominal breathing by diaphragmatic descent alternates with rib breathing in which the diaphragm passively ascends during inspiration), and respiratory paradox (in which the diaphragm passively ascends with each inspiratory effort). As shown in Figure 81-2, respiratory paradox heralds the development of hypercapnia.[9]

Table 81-2. Causes of Hypercapnia

Alveolar hypoventilation
- Decreased ventilatory drive (i.e., patient won't breathe)
  - Pharmacologic suppression of ventilatory drive (e.g., narcotics, benzodiazepines, barbiturates)
  - Pathologic suppression of ventilatory drive (e.g., brain stem stroke, obesity-hypoventilation syndrome, Ondine's curse, hypothyroidism)
- Decreased respiratory bellows activity or response (i.e., patient can't breathe)
  - Bilateral phrenic nerve dysfunction
  - Bilateral diaphragmatic dysfunction (unilateral diaphragmatic dysfunction usually does not cause hypoventilation)
    - Metabolic causes (e.g., hypophosphatemia, shock, diaphragmatic fatigue)
    - Associated with systemic neuromuscular diseases (e.g., Duchenne muscular dystrophy, Guillain-Barré syndrome, acid maltase deficiency, amyotrophic lateral sclerosis)

Increased dead space ventilation
- Lung vascular or parenchymal dysfunction (markedly increased dead space ventilation)
  - Pulmonary vascular occlusion (without compensatory hyperventilation) (e.g., pulmonary embolism in a paralyzed, mechanically ventilated patient)
  - Parenchymal lung dysfunction (e.g., severe bullous emphysema)

Increased CO_2 production
- Endogenous causes (e.g., fever)
- Exogenous causes (e.g., increased RQ associated with carbohydrate feedings)

In addition to acute insults, such as hypophosphatemia[10–12] and shock, which can weaken the force of diaphragmatic contraction, prolonged loaded inspiratory effort can also cause diaphragmatic fatigue. Key determinants of diaphragmatic fatigue are the fraction of the maximal transdiaphragmatic pressure ($P_{di}max$) expended with each breath ($P_{di}/P_{di}max$) (Fig. 81-3) and the fraction of the total breathing cycle devoted to inspiration (T_I/T_{TOT}), also called the *duty cycle*.[7] For example, with a duty cycle of approximately 0.5, breathing that requires inspiratory pressures equal to or higher than 40 percent of $P_{di}max$ will eventually cause diaphragmatic fatigue (Fig. 81-2). Over a broad range of inspiratory patterns, the offsetting effects of increasing $P_{di}/P_{di}max$ and decreasing duty cycle are such that diaphragmatic fatigue is predictable when the product of $P_{di}/P_{di}max$ by the duty cycle (called the tension-time index [TT_{di}]) exceeds 0.15 (Fig. 81-4).

ACUITY OF RESPIRATORY FAILURE

After recognizing and characterizing the type of respiratory failure in a patient, assessing the need for mechanical ventilation poses three additional questions to the clinician:

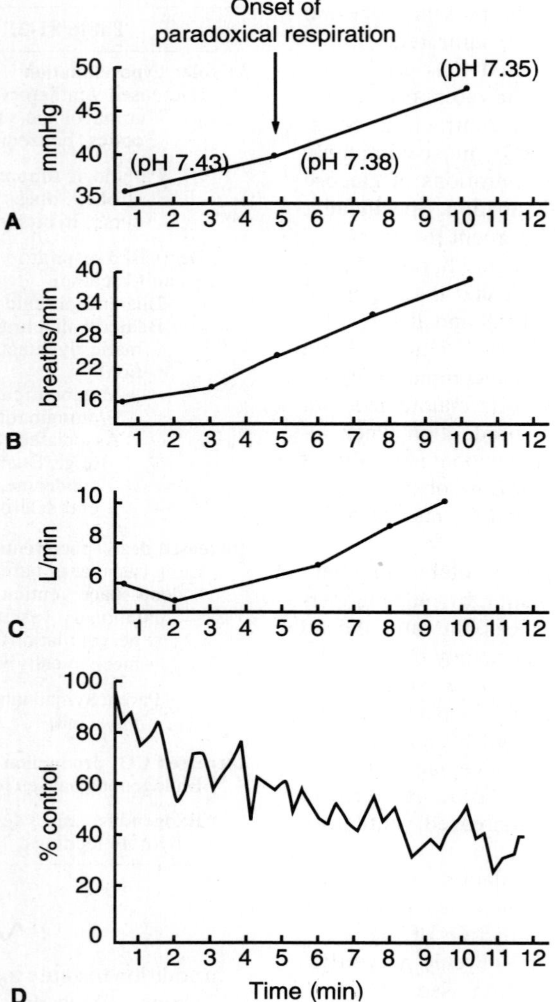

Figure 81-2. Sequence of changes in **(A)** $PaCO_2$, **(B)** respiratory rate, **(C)** minute ventilation, and **(D)** high/low (H/L) EMG ratio of the diaphragm in a patient during a 20-minute attempt at discontinuation. The initial change was a fall in H/L ratio, which was followed by a progressive increase in respiratory rate. The $PaCO_2$ initially fell, and the patient became alkalemic. Paradoxical abdominal displacements were not noted until after there had been a substantial increase in respiratory rate and minute ventilation. Hypercapnia and respiratory acidosis did not develop until after abdominal paradox and alteration between rib cage and abdominal breaths had been noted. Just before artificial ventilation was reinstituted, there was a sharp fall in respiratory frequency and minute ventilation. (From Cohen et al.,[9] with permission.)

1. Is the respiratory failure acute or chronic?
2. If the respiratory failure is acute, is the patient unstable or compromised, and if not, at what rate is such compromise developing?
3. If the need for mechanical ventilation is not immediate, what maneuvers can avert this need?

To assess the acuity of respiratory failure, current data should be compared with baseline arterial blood gas levels to clarify the acuity and magnitude of change of current hypoxemia or hypercapnia. If baseline arterial blood gas values are unavailable, reviewing the patient's past hemoglobin values (looking for past evidence of erythrocytosis, which may accompany chronic hypoxemia) and serum HCO_3^- values (looking for evidence of antecedent metabolic alkalosis, which may accompany chronic respiratory acidosis) may help to clarify the acuity of respiratory failure.

Regardless of whether old data are available, the patient's current clinical status is the preeminent determinant of the need for initiating mechanical ventilation. Signs of upper airway compromise (e.g., stridor, intercostal retractions) or unfavorable trends in gas exchange following an insult that is

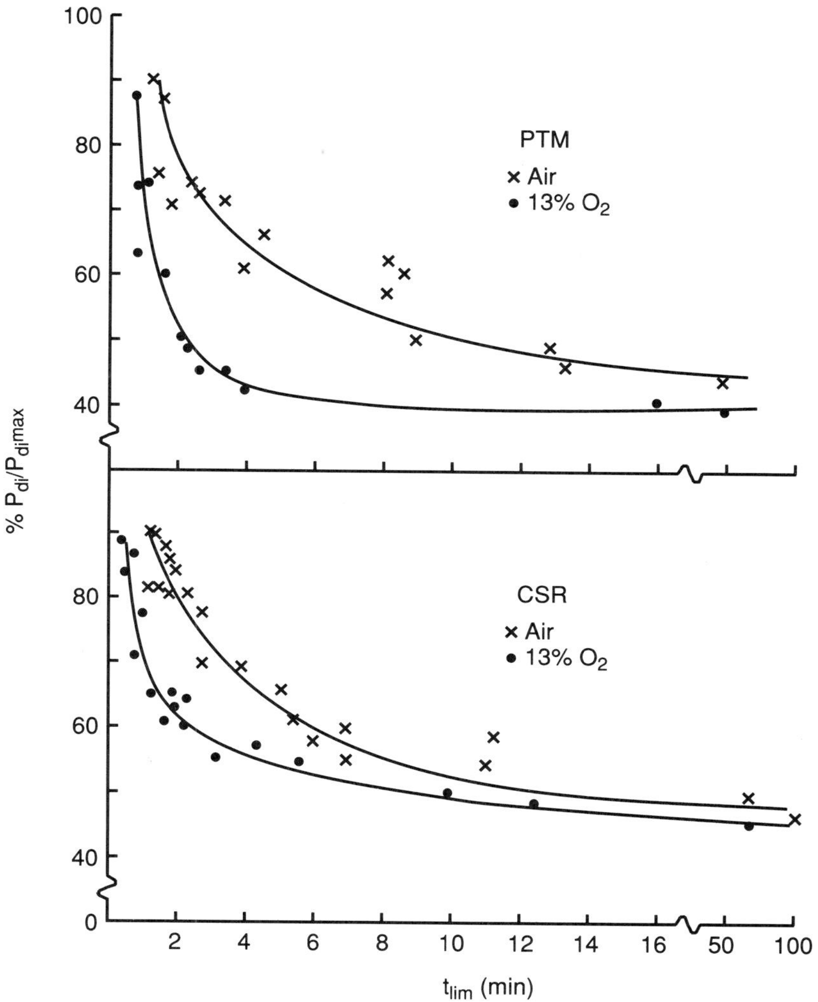

Figure 81-3. Relationship between transdiaphragmatic pressure (P_{di}), expressed as a percentage of maximum inspiratory P_{di} (P_{di}max) and endurance time (T_{lim}). Each point represents an individual run from a given subject. (From Roussos and Macklem,[8] with permission.)

likely to progress (e.g., early hypoxemia following sepsis or other precipitants of acute lung injury) should prompt consideration of intubation and mechanical ventilation.

Specific indications for initiating ventilatory support in acute respiratory failure can be stated in several ways. Based on empirical observation, numerous attempts have been made in the past to identify specific measures of ventilatory mechanics, gas exchange, and other aspects of respiratory function that would indicate the need for mechanical ventilation (Table 81-3). These measures can be grouped according to categories of physiologic dysfunction for easier conceptualization (Table 81-4). Finally, Table 81-5 offers a practical breakdown of indications for ventilatory support, based on the key distinction between acute failure of ventilation (Chs. 30 and 64) and failure of oxygenation (Chs. 31–34 and 65).

As discussed in Chapters 82 and 83, initial ventilatory strategies should be individualized according to the indications for mechanical ventilation in each patient; to preserve the patency of the upper airway in an otherwise awake and stable patient, intubation without positive pressure ventilation may suffice. On the other hand, in the case of impending hypoxemia following sepsis, use of positive end-expiratory pressure (PEEP) to enhance oxygenation would be more appropriate.

When unfavorable gas exchange trends are evolving slowly and the patient remains stable, identifying and treating remediable causes of respiratory failure may avert the need for intubation and/or mechanical ventilation. For example, repletion of serum phosphate levels in severely hypophosphatemic patients has been shown to increase diaphragmatic contractility.[10] Other drugs capable of enhancing

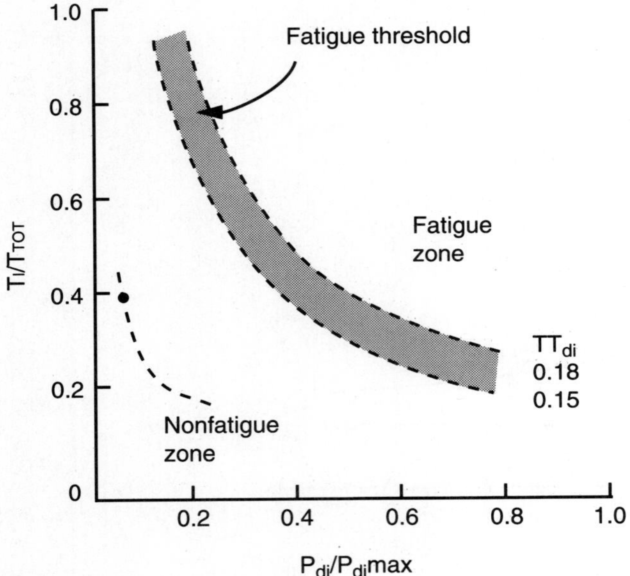

Figure 81-4. T_I/T_{TOT}, relationship between inspiratory time and cycle duration; P_{di}/P_{di}max, mean transdiaphragmatic pressure expressed as percentage of maximal P_{di}; solid circle, pattern of breathing during resting breathing; fatigue threshold; breathing patterns falling in this zone can be sustained for 45 minutes or longer; TT_{di}, product of P_{di}/P_{di}max by T_I/T_{TOT}; fatiguing patterns, breathing sustained with any pattern falling in this area will result in respiratory muscle failure in less than 1 hour. (From Grassino and Macklem,[7] with permission.)

Table 81-4. Indications for Mechanical Ventilation in Acute Respiratory Failure, Classified by Physiologic Mechanism

Mechanism	Best Available Indicator[a]
Inadequate alveolar ventilation	$PaCO_2$ and pH
Inadequate lung expansion	V_T; VC; f
Inadequate respiratory muscle strength	MIF; MVV; VC
Excessive work of breathing	$\dot{V}_E$ required to keep PCO_2 normal; V_D/V_T; f
Unstable ventilatory drive	Breathing pattern, clinical setting
Severe hypoxemia	$P(A\text{-}a)O_2$. PaO_2/P_AO_2; PaO_2/F_IO_2; $\dot{Q}_S/\dot{Q}_T$

[a] Definitions of abbreviations and symbols are given in Table 81-2.
(From Pierson,[20] with permission.)

Table 81-3. Some Measurements Used for Determining the Need for Mechanical Ventilation

Measurement	Values: Normal	Values: Mechanical Ventilation Indicated[a]
Tidal volume (V_T), mL/kg	5–8	<5
Vital capacity (VC), mL/kg	65–75	<10; <15
Forced expiratory volume in 1 second (FEV_1), mL/kg	50–60	<10
Functional residual capacity (FRC), % of predicted value	80–100	<50
Respiratory rate (f), breaths/min	12–20	>35
Maximum inspiratory force (MIF), cmH_2O	80–100	<20; <25; <30
Minute ventilation ($\dot{V}_E$), L/min	5–6	>10
Maximum voluntary ventilation (MVV), L/min	120–180	<20; <(2 × $\dot{V}_E$)
Dead space fraction (V_D/V_T), %	0.25–0.40	>0.60
$PaCO_2$, mmHg	36–44	>50; >55
PaO_2, mmHg	75–100 (breathing air)	<50 (air); <70 (mask O_2)
Alveolar-to-arterial PO_2 gradient [$P(A\text{-}a)O_2$], breathing 100% O_2, mmHg	25–65	>350; >450
Arterial/alveolar PO_2 ratio (PaO_2/P_AO_2)	0.75	<0.15
Arterial Po_2/inspired O_2 fraction ratio (PaO_2/F_IO_2), mmHg	350–450	<200
Intrapulmonary right-to-left shunt fraction ($\dot{Q}_S/\dot{Q}_T$), %	≤5	>20; >25; >30

[a] Multiple cutoff values indicate different recommendations by different sources.
(From Pierson,[20] with permission.)

Table 81-5. Indications for Initiating Mechanical Ventilation in the Two Basic Forms of Acute Respiratory Failure

Development of acute ventilatory failure
- $PaCO_2$ above baseline (i.e., $PaCO_2$ increased by ≥5 mmHg without easily correctable cause, such as excess narcotic or hypophosphatemia)
- Signs of impending ventilatory failure (e.g., abdominal paradox, respiratory alternans)
- Signs of upper airway compromise (e.g., stridor, intercostal retractions)

Development of progressive hypoxemia
- PaO_2 <65 mmHg despite high inspired O_2 concentration (e.g., FIO_2 ≥0.50)
- Less severe hypoxemia but in a setting in which progressive deterioration is expected (e.g., acute lung injury, massive aspiration)

diaphragmatic contractility are dopamine,[13] aminophylline,[14] and digoxin,[15] but patients who receive these agents in attempts to "tide them over" must be watched closely for failure to respond. Continuous positive airway pressure (CPAP) by mask is another maneuver that is sometimes used to avert the need for intubation and mechanical ventilation. However, as suggested by Suter and Kobel,[16] this maneuver is most appealing when the underlying cause of respiratory failure is self-limited and reversible over the short term (e.g., short-lived congestive heart failure).

INITIATING MECHANICAL VENTILATION FOR CHRONIC RESPIRATORY FAILURE

In addition to its use in acute respiratory failure, mechanical ventilation has recently been advocated for treating chronic ventilatory failure accompanying stable, hypercapnic chronic obstructive pulmonary disease (COPD). Based on the notion that chronic ventilatory failure reflects inspiratory muscle fatigue, the goal of mechanical ventilation in this setting is to rest the inspiratory muscles, thereby improving ventilation during spontaneous breathing. Studies to date have used both negative pressure ventilation[17–19] (e.g., cuirass or tank ventilators) and positive pressure ventilation without intubation (e.g., intermittent positive pressure ventilation with a nasal CPAP mask).

Several available studies demonstrate the benefits of intermittent negative pressure ventilation for respiratory muscle function and gas exchange in patients with hypercapnic COPD. Cropp and DiMarco[17] performed a randomized, controlled study in which eight hypercapnic COPD patients underwent negative pressure ventilation for 3 to 6 hours daily over 3 consecutive days, while control patients (who were comparable at baseline for forced expiratory volume in 1 second [FEV_1] and arterial blood gas values) did not receive mechanical ventilation. Unlike the control group, recipients of intermittent negative pressure ventilation experienced improved maximal inspiratory and expiratory pressures, prolonged time over which isocapnic hyperventilation could be sustained, and improved $PaCO_2$, which decreased from 60 mmHg before therapy to 52 mmHg measured 2 to 3 hours after discontinuing mechanical ventilation.

In a subsequent study by Gutierrez and colleagues,[18] five patients with stable hypercapnic COPD (mean baseline $PaCO_2$, 58.6 mmHg) were treated by weekly 8-hour daytime sessions with a cuirass-type negative pressure ventilator over a minimum of 4 months. As in the prior study by Cropp and DiMarco,[17] $PaCO_2$ after negative pressure ventilation decreased to a nadir value of 51.9 mmHg by the second month of the therapy and remained stable over the duration of weekly ventilation sessions. This decline in resting $PaCO_2$ was accompanied by an increase in the maximal inspiratory mouth pressure, V_T, 12-minute walk distance, and functional status as measured by increased Karnovsky scores. Cessation of weekly negative pressure ventilation was associated with a gradual increase in $PaCO_2$ toward baseline hypercapnia.

More recently, another randomized, controlled trial has failed to support the efficacy of external negative pressure ventilation for patients with severe COPD.[19] Control patients underwent a 3-week inpatient pulmonary rehabilitation program without ventilatory muscle training. In addition to participating in the same pulmonary rehabilitation program, patients in the treatment group used a PulmoWrap for a mean of 4.5 h/d, adjusting the PulmoWrap to allow restful inspiration without dyspnea or evidence of accessory muscle contraction. Outcome measures were reassessed after 3 weeks of treatment, and while both patient groups experienced improvements in leg cycling endurance, transdiaphragmatic pressures, and tension-time indices, no differences in the magnitude of improvement between treated and control patients were seen. Mean resting $PaCO_2$ decreased from 46 ± 8 to 42 ± 1 mmHg in the PulmoWrap group, although a single patient experienced a more substantial decline from 56 to 46 mmHg following treatment.

Overall, the mixed conclusions from the currently available literature leave the question of the efficacy of intermittent mechanical ventilation for patients with stable severe COPD unresolved. The data from Celli et al.[19] can be reconciled with earlier studies if the benefits associated with intermittent negative pressure ventilation in the earlier studies are also conferred by an aggressive pulmonary rehabil-

Table 81-6. Indications for Initiating Intermittent Negative Pressure Ventilation or Mask Positive Pressure Ventilation in Chronic Ventilatory Failure

Chronic ventilatory failure (i.e., $PaCO_2$ >45 mmHg) and
Resultant functional impairment in the setting of
- Chronic neuromuscular disease (e.g., amyotrophic lateral sclerosis, Guillain-Barré, acid maltase deficiency, refractory myasthenia gravis)
- Chest wall deformity (e.g., kyphoscoliosis)
- Obesity hypoventilation syndrome
- Chronic obstructive pulmonary disease (?)

itation program. Overall, available studies do not permit endorsement of intermittent mechanical ventilation for patients with stable hypercapnic COPD, but suggestive evidence will continue to foster interest in this possibility. Results of intermittent negative pressure ventilation and mask positive pressure ventilation for patients with chronic hypercapnia due to neuromuscular diseases and/or kyphoscoliosis have been generally more promising (Table 81-6).

References

1. Tisi GM: Arterial blood gases and pH. pp. 75–92. In Pulmonary Physiology in Clinical Medicine. Williams & Wilkins, Baltimore, 1980
2. Stoller JK: Respiratory effects of positive end-expiratory pressure. Respir Care 1988;33:454–463
3. Krowka MJ, Cortese DA: Hepato-pulmonary syndrome: An evolving perspective in the era of liver transplantation. Hepatology 1990;11:138–142
4. Weinberger SE, Schwartzstein RM, Weiss JW: Hypercapnia. N Engl J Med 1989;321:1223–1231
5. Edems NK, Gil KM, Elwyn DH: The effects of varying energy and nitrogen intake on nitrogen balance, body composition, and metabolic rate. Clin Chest Med 1986;7:3–17
6. Kemper MS, Askanazi J: Nutritional considerations in respiratory failure. pp. 201–206. In Kacmarek RM, Stoller JK (eds): Current Respiratory Care. BC Decker, Toronto, 1988
7. Grassino A, Macklem PT: Respiratory muscle fatigue and ventilatory failure. Annu Rev Med 1984;35:625–647
8. Roussos C, Macklem PT: Diaphragmatic fatigue in man. J Appl Physiol 1977;43:189–197
9. Cohen CA, Zagelbaum G, Gross D et al: Clinical manifestations of inspiratory muscle fatigue. Am J Med 1982;73:308–316
10. Aubier M, Murciano D, Lecocguic Y et al: Effect of hypophosphatemia on diaphragmatic contractility in patients with acute respiratory faiulre. N Engl J Med 1985;313:420–424
11. Agusti AG, Torres A, Estopa R, Agustividal A: Hypophosphatemia as a cause of failed weaning: The importance of metabolic factors. Crit Care Med 1984;12:142–143
12. Laaban JP, Grateau G, Psychoyos I et al: Hypophosphatemia induced by mechanical ventilation in patients with chronic obstructive pulmonary disease. Crit Care Med 1989;17:1115–1119
13. Aubier M, Murciano D, Menu Y et al: Dopamine effects on diaphragmatic strength during acute respiratory failure in chronic obstructive pulmonary disease. Ann Intern Med 1989; 110:17–23
14. Aubier M, DeTroyer A, Sampson M et al: Aminophylline improves diaphragmatic contractility. N Engl J Med 1981;305:249–252
15. Aubier M, Murciano D, Viires N et al: Effects of digoxin on diaphragmatic strength generation in patients with chronic obstructive pulmonary disease during acute respiratory failure. Am Rev Respir Dis 1987;135:544–548
16. Suter PM, Kobel N: Treatment of acute pulmonary failure by CPAP via face mask: When can intubation be avoided? Klin Wochenschr 1981;59:613–616
17. Cropp A, DiMarco AF: Effects of intermittent negative pressure ventilation on respiratory muscle function in patients with severe chronic obstructive pulmonary disease. Am Rev Respir Dis 1987;135:1056–1061
18. Gutierrez M, Beroiza T, Contreras G et al: Weekly cuirass ventilation improves blood gases and inspiratory muscle strength in patients with chronic air-flow limitation and hypercarbia. Am Rev Respir Dis 1988;138:617–623
19. Celli B, Lee H, Criner G et al: Controlled trial of external negative pressure ventilation in patients with severe chronic airflow obstruction. Am Rev Respir Dis 1989;140:1251–1256
20. Pierson DJ: Indications for mechanical ventilation in acute respiratory failure. Respir Care 1983;28:570–577

Chapter 82

Methods of Providing Mechanical Ventilatory Support

Robert M. Kacmarek

CHAPTER OUTLINE

Regardless of the approach used, provision of mechanical ventilatory support requires the development of a transpulmonary pressure (P_{TP}) gradient. As discussed in Chapter 5,

$$P_{TP} = P_{pul} - P_{pl} \quad (1)$$

where P_{pul} is intrapulmonary or alveolar pressure and P_{pl} is pleural pressure. The most common approach to providing ventilatory support is positive pressure ventilation, which increases P_{TP} by increasing P_{pul} with application of pressure above atmospheric. Negative pressure ventilation provides ventilatory support by creating a negative extrathoracic pressure, thus creating a more negative P_{pl}. As a result, the P_{TP} is increased because of the more negative P_{pl}. Even the rocking bed and pneumobelt enhance gas exchange by altering P_{TP} (see Ch. 94).

Within this chapter, the basic concepts of positive pressure ventilation are discussed. Emphasis is on definitions of modes, waveforms, and the other variables that are set during ventilatory support. Management strategies are presented in Chapter 83; mechanical ventilators are discussed in Chapter 85.

POSITIVE PRESSURE VENTILATION

During the delivery of mechanically assisted breaths, four variables must be coordinated: pressure, flow, volume, and time. This is true regardless of the specific approach used. Figure 82-1 depicts typical airway pressure, flow, and volume delivery waveforms per unit time during volume-limited mechanical ventilation. Generally, inspiration is begun either by the patient beginning to inspire, which activates the gas delivery system of the ventilator, or when a specific time interval has elapsed. The end of the inspiratory phase occurs when the cycling mechanism variable has reached its defined limit. Specifically, a given volume of gas has been delivered, a given period of inspiratory time has expired, a pressure limit has been met, or a minimal flow has been delivered. During positive pressure ventilation, the clinician generally defines the limits of pressure, flow, volume, and time, although if patients are breathing spontaneously, they can modify the limits set on many programmed variables (see Ch. 85).

Since positive pressure mechanical ventilation greatly in-

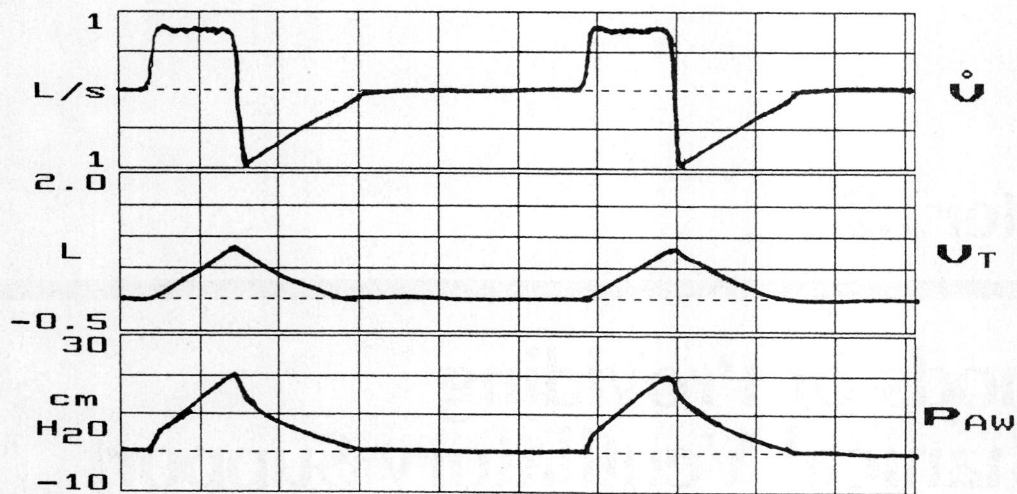

Figure 82-1. Pressure, volume, and flow waveforms during volume control positive pressure ventilation. (Waveforms recorded with a Bicore CP-100 monitor.)

creases P_{TP} gradients above those that occur during normal spontaneous breathing, and results in the development of a positive, instead of a negative intrathoracic pressure, a number of physiologic systems can be adversely affected. The potential adverse effects of positive pressure are as follows:

- Increased mean intrathoracic pressure
- Decreased venous return
- Increased ventilation/perfusion ($\dot{V}/\dot{Q}$) ratio
- Decreased cardiac output ($\dot{Q}_T$)
- Increased intracranial pressure
- Decreased renal blood flow
- Airtrapping and auto-PEEP (intrinsic positive end-expiratory pressure) (Ch. 76)
- Barotrauma (see Ch. 84)
- Nocosomial pneumonia (see Ch. 97)
- Respiratory alkalosis
- Agitation and increased respiratory distress
- Increased work of breathing

It is important to emphasize the potential for positive pressure to adversely affect the relationship between ventilation and perfusion (see Ch. 10). Since positive pressure ventilation increases mean intrathoracic pressure and distorts the normal movement of the diaphragm (Fig. 82-2), the normal matching of ventilation and perfusion may be markedly altered.[1] In general, perfusion to well-ventilated areas is decreased with positive pressure ventilation and, as a result, dead space ventilation is increased. In the normally healthy individual, dead space/tidal volume (V_D/V_T) ratios may increase to about 50 percent from their normal 20 to 40 percent level. Thus, a larger minute ventilation usually must be delivered during positive pressure ventilation than during normal breathing. However, the clinician should not continually increase the level of ventilation in the presence of a continually rising PCO_2. Most commonly, marked increases in PCO_2 during mechanical ventilation are a result of a system malfunction (e.g., change in set rate or V_T or system leak), or a decrease in $\dot{Q}_T$ and pulmonary perfusion. If altered perfusion is the cause, increasing minute ventilation may only enhance CO_2 increase because of the adverse effect of increased P_{TP} on pulmonary circulation (see Ch. 83).

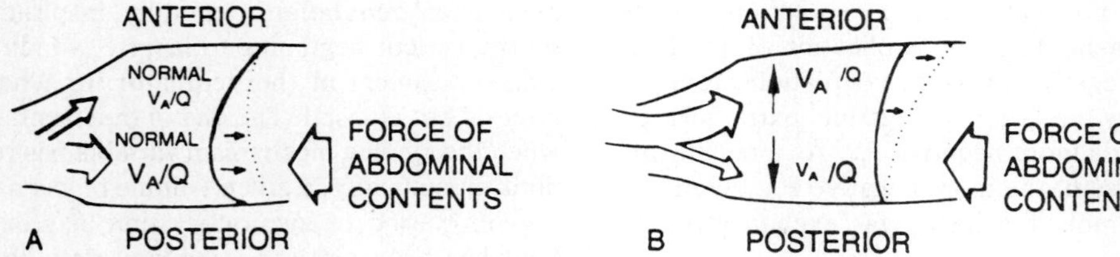

Figure 82-2. **(A)** Spontaneous breathing in the supine position is associated with greater posterior diaphragmatic and lung movement. Accordingly, $\dot{V}/\dot{Q}$ relationships here are more closely matched. Less ventilation and perfusion are present anteriorly. **(B)** When the diaphragm does not contract and the patient is mechanically ventilated, most ventilation is anterior (high $\dot{V}/\dot{Q}$), while most perfusion remains posterior (low $\dot{V}/\dot{Q}$). The result is a potentially significant alteration in normal overall $\dot{V}/\dot{Q}$. (From Rasanen and Downs,[1] with permission.)

MODES OF POSITIVE PRESSURE VENTILATION

Modes of positive pressure ventilation (PPV) can be divided into two major groups, volume targeted and pressure targeted, each of which can be applied to either the spontanously breathing patient or the sedated patient. In addition, volume-targeted and pressure-targeted modes can be integrated so that a percentage of breaths in the spontaneously breathing patient are volume targeted, while others are pressure targeted. Finally, patients can breathe spontaneously through the ventilator circuit without any ventilatory support, while maintaining all of the alarm capabilities of the ventilator. This is accomplished in the CPAP (continuous positive airway pressure) setting, as discussed in Chapter 76. In this setting, baseline pressure is maintained at or above atmospheric, with all ventilatory effort provided by the patient. This approach is used frequently during weaning from ventilatory support (Ch. 86). However, with most ventilators in use today, this approach increases the imposed work of breathing[2] (see Ch. 87).

Volume-Targeted versus Pressure-Targeted Ventilation

The differences between the volume- and pressure-targeted approaches to ventilatory support are outlined in Table 82-1. The key difference is the assurance of VT delivery, or the assurance of a peak inspiratory pressure plateau limit. With volume-targeted ventilation, a specific VT is delivered without variation, although the peak airway pressure may vary. In pressure-targeted ventilation, a peak inspiratory pressure plateau (Fig. 82-3) is established for the duration of inspiration, but the VT may vary, depending on changes in the resistance and compliance of the patient–ventilator system. In addition, with pressure targeted, a decelerating flow pattern is always established. As noted in Figure 82-3, a very high peak flow is delivered to establish the plateau pressure rapidly, after which the flow rapidly decreases, while the pressure is maintained throughout the timed inspiratory period. In volume targeted, any of a series of flow waveforms and peak flows may be set by the clinician and gas delivery does not vary from that programmed. Little data are available to determine which (volume or pressure targeted) is more efficacious.[3–10] Many uncontrolled, non-randomized studies have indicated that pressure targeted is more beneficial in adult respiratory distress syndrome (ARDS)[3–6]; however, the controlled studies, to date, have produced conflicting results.[7,8] In theory, because of the rapid rise to plateau pressure and the maintenance of this pressure during inspiration, gas exchange should be enhanced wherever $\dot{V}/\dot{Q}$ mismatch is great.[11] The limiting of peak airway pressure in pressure-targeted ventilation does not, in our opinion,

Table 82-1. Volume-Targeted versus Pressure-Targeted Ventilation

	Volume Control	Pressure Control
Rate	Set or variable	Set or variable
VT	Set	Variable
Peak pressure	Variable	Set
Peak flow	Set	Variable
Flow wave	Set but variable	Set
A/C	Yes	Yes
Control	Yes	Yes
Inspiratory time	Variable	Variable
I/E ratio	Variable	Variable

A/C, assist/control; I/E, inspiration/expiration.

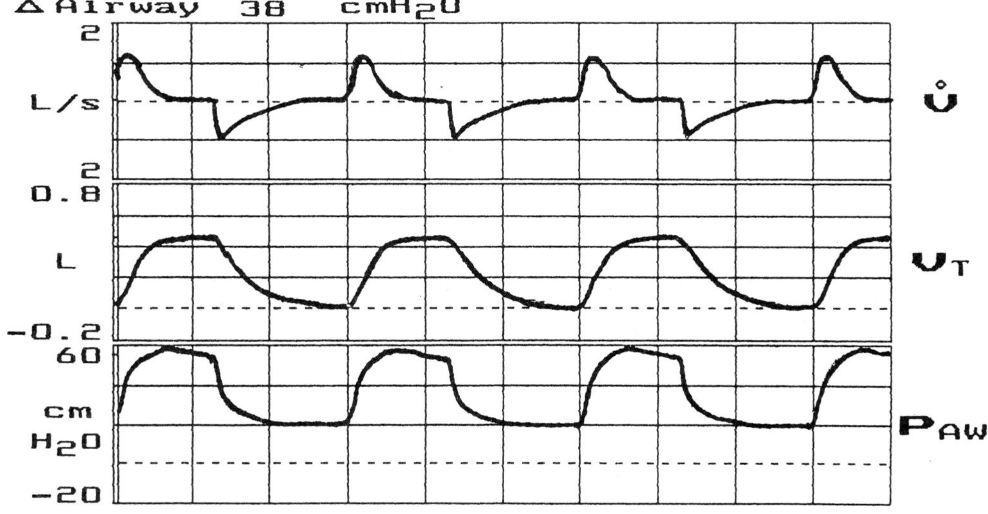

Figure 82-3. Pressure, volume, and flow waveform during pressure control positive pressure ventilation. (Waveforms recorded with a Bicore CP-100 monitor.)

constitute a significant benefit because it is alveolar pressure, not peak ventilator circuit pressure, that contributes to barotrauma (see Ch. 84). As a result, we believe no conclusive data exist that would lead one to favor pressure targeted over volume targeted. If one is most concerned about maintaining consistent volume delivery, then volume-targeted ventilation modes are most appropriate; however, if concern centers on limiting peak airway pressure, then pressure-targeted modes are most appropriate.

Volume-Targeted Modes

The various methods of delivering volume-targeted ventilation are volume control, volume assist/control (A/C), volume assisted, intermittent mandatory ventilation (IMV), synchronized IMV (SIMV), and mandatory minute ventilation (MMV) (Table 82-3); pressure waveforms for each approach are illustrated in Figures 82-4 and 82-5. As discussed below, volume-targeted ventilation can be provided under total ventilator control, total patient control, or a combination of the two.

Volume Control

During volume control, the ventilator delivers a fixed ventilatory pattern regardless of the patient's breathing pattern. As a result, volume control requires either sedation, sedation and paralysis, or hyperventilation beyond the apneic threshold to prevent active patient interaction with and active opposition to (fighting) the ventilator. If sedation and/or paralysis wears off or the ventilatory drive of the patient changes, the patient will begin to breathe spontaneously and will fight the ventilator. This will normally affect gas exchange and hemodynamics adversely. As a result, we recommend against the use of volume-control ventilation. The goals of complete ventilatory control can be achieved with volume A/C or SIMV, without preventing spontaneous interaction with the ventilator should the patient's ventilatory drive change.

Volume Assist/Control

With volume A/C (assisted mechanical ventilation [AMV]), as with volume control, the clinician programs the

Table 82-2. Volume-Targeted Modes

Mode	Description	Advantages	Disadvantages
Volume control	Complete control of ventilation; patients unable to interphase with machine; V_T constant, peak pressure variable; FVS only	Control over minute volume and method of delivery	Patient unable to interact with machine; requires sedation, sedation/paralysis, or hyperventilation; spontaneously breathing patient fights ventilator; peak airway pressure variable
Volume A/C	Volume control, however, spontaneous breathing can increase rate; V_T constant, peak pressure variable; FVS only	Patients may determine rate over set level; control over minimum minute volume and delivery methodology can provide volume control with sedation, sedation/paralysis, or hyperventilation	May cause respiratory alkalosis, air trapping, auto-PEEP, cardiovascular compromise with high rates; peak airway pressure variable
IMV	Volume control with continuous flow in between control breaths allowing spontaneous breathing; PVS to FVS	Able to provide any level of ventilatory support; at low levels patient able to breath spontaneously; air trapping, auto-PEEP, and patient-induced respiratory alkalosis less likely than in volume A/C; can provide volume control with sedation, sedation/ paralysis, or hyperventilation; less cardiovascular compromise than volume control or A/C	Stacking of mechanical breaths on spontaneous breaths; increased work of breathing at low IMV mandatory rate; may cause respiratory alkolosis, air trapping, auto-PEEP at rapid spontaneous respiratory rates; peak airway pressure variable
SIMV	Volume A/C with demand spontaneous breathing in between A/C breaths; PVS to FVS	No stacking of mechanical breaths on spontaneous breaths; same as IMV	Same as IMV
MMV	Ventilator maintains minimum minute volume, may provide volume control, total spontaneous breathing, or anything in between dependent on patient's spontaneous minute ventilation; PVS to FVS	Allows some patients to wean themselves	Rapid shallow breathing when setting of MMV is low may prevent mandatory volume A/C breaths; increased WOB at low mandatory rate; requires clinician to decrease MMV if weaning is to continue; peak airway pressure variable

WOB, work of breathing.

Mode	Description	Advantages	Disadvantages
Pressure control	Complete control of ventilation; peak airway pressure constant, VT variable; FVS only	Control over method of delivery except VT, which may vary from breath to breath	Generally requires sedation, sedation/paralysis, or hyperventilation; spontaneously breathing patient may fight gas delivery
Pressure A/C	Pressure control; however, patient may increase rate of ventilation; pressure constant, VT variable; FVS only	Patient may determine rate over set level; peak pressure constant; pressure control available with sedation, sedation/paralysis, or hyperventilation	May cause respiratory alkalosis, air trapping, auto-PEEP, cardiovascular compromise with high rates; VT variable
Pressure support	Peak pressure set, otherwise all aspects of ventilation controlled by patient; PVS to FVS	Patient has control over process of ventilation; machine responds to patient demands; gas is delivered in response to patient desires; peak airway pressure set	VT variable; no backup rate, continuous nebulizer therapy may cause hypoventilation; air trapping, auto-PEEP possible if rate high
Airway pressure release ventilation	Delivery of two levels of CPAP using continuous flow system; normally I/E ratio inversed; spontaneous breathing at each CPAP level possible; designed for use via artificial airway; PVS to FVS	Simple set up; airway pressure controlled; spontaneous breathing	VT variable; increased WOB at inspiratory CPAP level, no alarms, no patient monitors
BiPAP	Delivery of two levels of CPAP (IPAP and EPAP) commercially available, designed for use via nasal mask; normal I/E ratio, patient can control rate, length of inspiration; PVS to FVS	Commercially available; airway pressure controlled; patient controls all aspects of ventilation except pressure level; designed for noninvasive use	VT variable; no alarms, no patient monitors
MMV pressure limited	Ventilator maintains minimum minute volume by varying PSV level in response to patient's ability to maintain MMV level; PVS to FVS	Allows some patients to wean themselves; peak airway pressure maintained within specified range	Rapid shallow breathing can defeat goal of MMV; requires clinician to decrease MMV level if weaning is to continue; VT variable

Table 82-3. Pressure-Targeted Modes

WOB, work of breathing; IPAP, inspiratory positive airway pressure; EPAP, expiratory positive airway pressure.

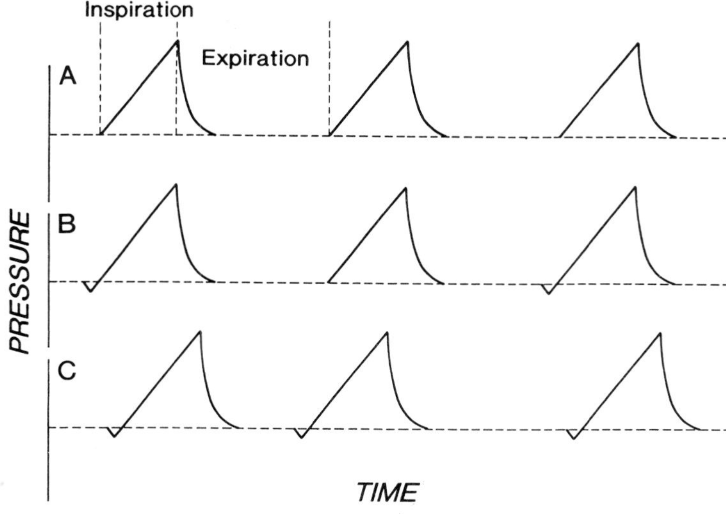

Figure 82-4. Pressure versus time waveform during **(A)** volume control, **(B)** volume A/C, and **(C)** volume-assisted positive pressure ventilation. Note no patient triggering occurs with volume control, all breaths are patient triggered with volume assist (Fig. C), and only some breaths are patient triggered with volume A/C. Defections below baseline indicate patient triggering.

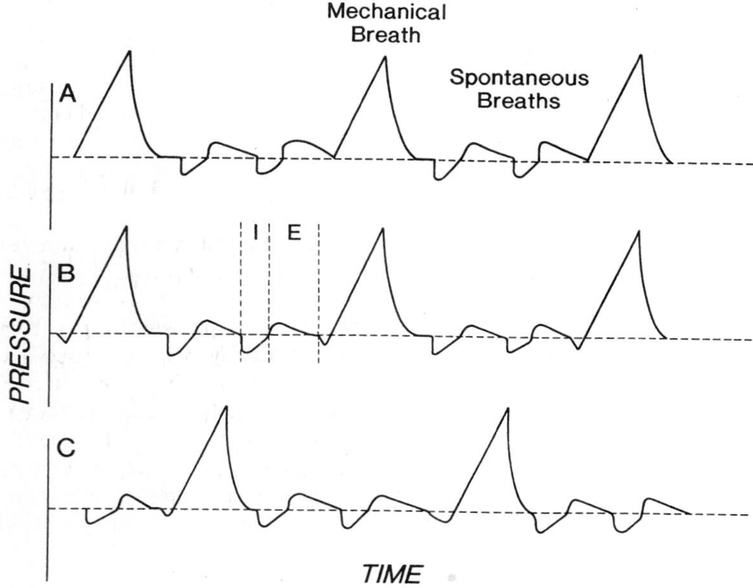

Figure 82-5. Pressure versus time waveforms during **(A)** IMV, **(B)** SIMV, and **(C)** volume-controlled MMV positive pressure ventilation. Note each spontaneous breath occurs between volume-targeted breaths. With IMV, mandatory volume breaths are controlled, while with SIMV, they are patient triggered. MMV pressure waveforms are exactly the same as SIMV. Defections below baseline are created by patient inspiratory efforts. I, spontaneous inspiration; E, spontaneous expiration.

ventilator to provide a volume-targeted ventilatory pattern. However, the major difference between volume control and volume A/C is the patient's ability to trigger the ventilator at a rate more rapid than that programmed. During normal set-up, the ventilatory rate is programmed at the level that would provide adequate baseline ventilation. Alterations in the patient's drive to breathe will establish a more rapid ventilatory rate with volume A/C. To establish controlled ventilation, sedation, sedation and paralysis, or hyperventilation beyond the apneic threshold (higher set rate) is necessary. The disadvantage is that volume A/C allows the patient to increase minute ventilation by altering breath rate. This may promote hyperventilation and alkalosis, air trapping, and auto-PEEP, as well as hemodynamic compromise.[12,13]

Volume Assisted

With volume-assisted ventilation, the clinician programs V_T, peak flow, flow waveform, fraction of inspired O_2 (F_{IO_2}), and PEEP, but does not program rate. Rate determination is left entirely up to the patient. As a result, gross hypoventilation and respiratory arrest may occur if the patient does not have an intact ventilatory drive. Some of the newer generations of mechanical ventilators incorporate back-up or apneic ventilation modes as safeguards against profound hypoventilation. However, we recommend against the use of volume-assisted ventilation. Again, the goals of ventilatory assistance can be achieved with the use of volume A/C ventilation.

Intermittent Mandatory Ventilation

The historic development of mechanical ventilatory assistance has progressed from complete ventilatory support, with no patient involvement, to attempts to allow greater and greater patient–ventilator interaction. IMV potentially allows significant patient interaction with the ventilator. It was first described by Downs et al. in 1973 as a mode to assist in weaning patients from ventilatory support.[14] Since then, IMV has been established as a mode of mechanical ventilation for use during all indications for ventilatory support. IMV is best defined as volume-control ventilation that allows spontaneous breathing by a continuous gas flow in between volume-control breaths. As with volume A/C, total ventilatory control can be established with the proper mandatory control rate and sedation, sedation and paralysis, or hyperventilation beyond the apneic threshold. If the patient's ventilatory drive becomes active, the patient can breathe spontaneously in between the IMV rate (volume-control breaths). The volume-limited breath is volume controlled; thus, concern that spontaneous patient effort will interfere with the volume-control rate exists. However, Hasten et al.[14] could not document adverse effects from stacking of mechanical breaths on spontaneous breaths.

At lower IMV mandatory volume-control rates, the patient assumes a greater and greater percentage of ventilatory support (PVS). During attempts to wean patients with IMV (actually SIMV), Marini et al.[15] demonstrated that patient work per breath increases during both mandatory and spontaneous breaths, as the percentage of ventilatory support provided by the mandatory volume-targeted breath rate decreases (see Ch. 87). As a result, clinicians must be acutely aware of those factors that may adversely affect patient workload during low mandatory rates with IMV (or SIMV). In general, we do not recommend maintaining patients at low mandatory volume-control rates (≤4 breaths per minute) unless approaches to unload work during the spontaneous breathing phase are included. (see Pressure Support Ventilation).

Synchronized Intermittent Mandatory Ventilation

SIMV is essentially the same as IMV, with the following exceptions. Instead of the mandatory breaths being volume controlled, they are volume assist/controlled. In addition, during the spontaneous breathing phase, gas is provided from a patient-triggered demand flow system. In general, most mechanical ventilators offering SIMV function by allowing the patient's effort to trigger either mandatory or spontaneous breathing, depending on programmed time intervals. In other words, all patient effort results in activation of a demand system, unless during the window of time that results in triggering of an assisted breath. Generally, these (A/C) time windows last 1 to 2 seconds. If triggering does not occur within this time interval, a volume-control breath is delivered. The clinical applications and potential problems of SIMV are the same as those listed for IMV, except that breath stacking does not normally occur.

Mandatory Minute Ventilation

MMV is the first approach to ventilatory support that incorporates computer control of ventilation. It was introduced on the Engstrom Erica ventilator in the mid-1980s.[16] Essentially, MMV is SIMV, with the ventilator deciding how many mandatory breaths to be delivered. The clinician programs a typical SIMV mandatory breath delivery, setting V_T, flow rate, waveform, rate, F_{IO_2}, and PEEP. In addition, a minimum MMV rate is set. If the patient is apneic, the ventilator delivers the MMV as programmed. If the patient is breathing spontaneously and is capable of maintaining minute volume at or above the minimum level, no mandatory breaths are delivered. If spontaneous minute volume falls below that set, it is supplemented by mandatory volume A/C breaths at a rate sufficient to meet the programmed minute ventilation. Although this seems ideal for weaning patients from ventilatory support, the initial volume control-based systems could be easily defeated by an ineffective ventilatory pattern in spite of meeting the established minute ventilation. That is, rapid, shallow breathing, although ineffective, would not activate a mandatory breath unless minute volume was below the set level. In addition, it is our experience that patients "settle in" to a combination of spontaneous and mandatory breaths that they consider "comfortable." As a result, the mandatory minute volume has to be continuously decreased to force the patient to provide a greater percentage of total minute volume. This is essentially no different from that noted with IMV or SIMV. However, modifications (see below) using either pressure-targeted approaches or combined pressure- and volume-targeted approaches seem, at least theoretically, more advantageous.

Pressure-Targeted Modes

As with volume-targeted modes, pressure-targeted (pressure-limited) approaches to ventilation can be classified as control, A/C, or assisted. In addition, variations on the application of pressure-targeted ventilation have been developed: airway pressure release ventilation (APRV) and bilevel positive airway pressure (BiPAP), as well as MMV modes based on pressure targeting. Regardless of the specific description, all of these modes have the limitation of peak airway pressure in common. The advantages and disadvantages of pressure-targeted modes are listed in Table 82-3; pressure waveforms are illustrated in Figures 82-6, 82-7, and 82-8.

Pressure Control

Pressure-control ventilation is the same as volume control in that the patient is not involved in the process of ventilation. In true pressure-control ventilation, the patient is unable to control the rate of ventilation. However, *theoretically* the patient can inspire spontaneously during the pressure plateau inspiratory phase. During the inspiratory phase, the demand system of the machine provides sufficient flow to maintain system pressure; however gas flow may be zero before end inspiration (Fig. 82-3). If the patient chooses to inspire spontaneously during machine inspiration, demand flow would be provided to the system to maintain the plateau pressure. If the inspiratory time is sufficiently long, the patient could attempt to exhale at the plateau level before the machine cycles to exhalation. However, in actuality, patients receiving pressure-control ventilation must be sedated, sedated and paralyzed, or hyperventilated beyond their apneic threshold or they tend to fight gas delivery. As with volume control, we do not recommend pressure control because of the tendency of patients to fight the ventilator when their ventilatory drive increases.

Pressure Assist/Control

Gas delivery for pressure A/C is the same as for pressure control, except that a minimum rate is set. The machine sensitivity is also set to allow patient triggering at a rate higher than set, if so desired. Otherwise, the two modes (pressure control and pressure A/C) are identical. As with volume A/C, patients may breathe rapidly, which may result in respiratory alkalosis, air trapping, and auto-PEEP, as well as cardiovascular compromise.[15] With volume A/C, if the patient fights the ventilator and peak pressure exceeds the high pressure limit/alarm setting, inspiration is terminated; in pressure A/C, no such mechanism exists. A patient fighting the de-

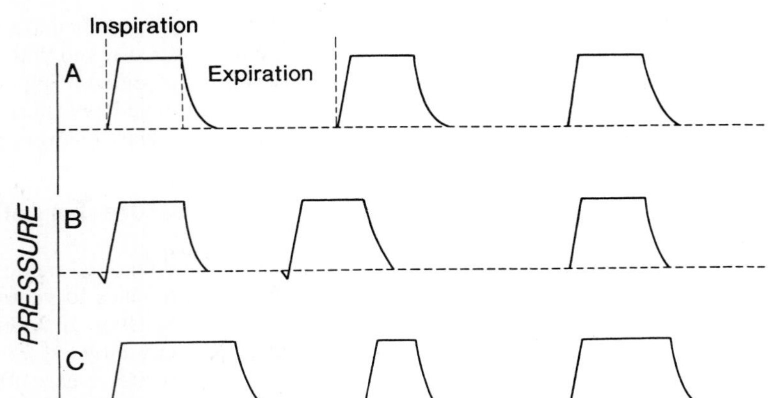

Figure 82-6. Pressure versus time waveforms during **(A)** pressure control, **(B)** pressure A/C, and **(C)** PSV. Note, in pressure control all aspects of gas delivery are programmed. With pressure A/C, the patient may exceed the set rate; however, all other aspects of gas delivery are programmed. In PSV (pressure assist) the only programmed variable is pressure plateau level; the patient selects rate, VT, and inspiratory time.

livered breath may receive a decreased VT, but no change in inspiratory time occurs.

Pressure Support

The mode of ventilation analogous to volume assist is pressure support ventilation (PSV) or pressure assist ventilation. This is a true pressure assist mode of ventilation because no back-up rate is set. However, as described earlier, many new mechanical ventilators have back-up modes or apneic modes that activate in the event of apnea or hypoventilation. Of all the modes of ventilation currently in general use, this mode is the approach most capable of responding on a breath-to-breath basis to a patient's ventilatory demand.[17] The only variable set by the clinician is the pressure support plateau level. The inspiratory time, peak inspiratory flow, VT, and rate are all determined by the patient's ventilatory demands, as well as by the impedance of the patient–ventilator system. Table 82-4 contrasts PSV with pressure A/C and volume A/C ventilation. Numerous authors[2,17–21] have demonstrated the ability of PSV to relieve the patient of the imposed work of breathing that results from endotracheal tubes and ventilator demand systems, as well as from the impedance to gas flow that is associated with pulmonary pathophysiology. We have also found PSV useful in the management of patients with acute ventilatory failure once they have passed the acute phase of their disease. MacIntyre,[20] in 1986, demonstrated that PSV was equivalent to SIMV in providing ventilatory support in a series of acutely ill patients. However, PSV is primarily used as a mode of weaning from ventilatory support (see Ch. 86). Because of the level of patient involvement during PSV, and the ability of titrating patients' work of breathing by varying the level of PSV, which improves gas exchange and minimizes transdiaphragmatic pressure changes (Table 82-5), PSV has established itself as an extremely useful ventilatory assist mode during PVS (see under Full and Partial Ventilatory Support). Of particular interest is the use of PSV during SIMV (Figure 82-7). As noted by Hurst et al.[21] (Table 82-6), the addition of low levels of PSV to SIMV spontaneous breaths can greatly improve gas exchange and, at least in this uncontrolled study, facilitate weaning.

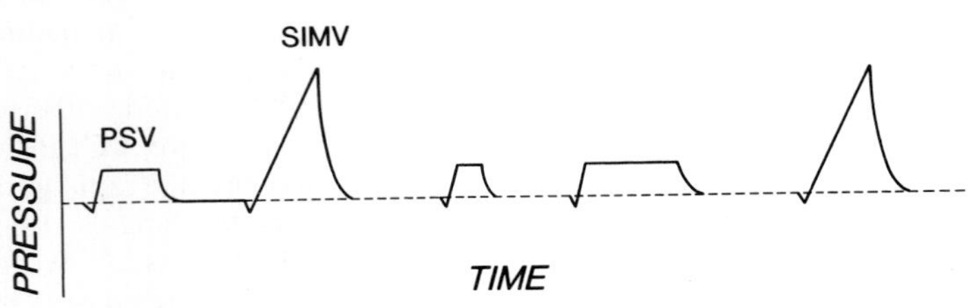

Figure 82-7. Pressure versus time waveform during SIMV with PSV. Note both SIMV and PSV function independently. All spontaneous breaths are supported with PSV.

Table 82-4. Comparison of PSV, Volume Control, and Pressure Control

	PSV	Volume Control	Pressure Control
Rate	Variable	Set/variable	Set/variable
V_T	Variable	Set	Variable
Peak pressure	Set	Variable	Set
Peak flow	Variable	Set	Variable
Flow wave	Set	Variable	Set
Ability to assist	Yes	Yes	Yes
Control ventilation available	No	Yes	Yes
Inspiratory time	Variable	Set	Set
I/E ratio	Variable	Set	Set

Airway Pressure Release Ventilation/Bilevel Positive Airway Pressure

In our opinion, APRV and BiPAP define essentially the same mode of ventilation, and are a variation of pressure control or pressure A/C ventilation. Idealized airway pressure waveforms versus time waveforms during APRV and BiPAP are illustrated in Figure 82-8. One of the major differences between APRV/BiPAP and pressure control is that APRV/BiPAP maintains a continuous flow of gas past the patient's airway, while, with pressure control, gas is deliv-

Table 82-6. Effects of SIMV with PSV in Surgical Patients

Value	IMV	IMV ± PSV[a]
PaO_2 (mmHg)	87 ± 10	99 ± 16
$PaCO_2$ (mmHg)	50 ± 4	43 ± 5[b]
RR (spontaneous breaths per minute)	36 ± 5	16 ± 3[c]
$\dot{V}_E$ (L/min)	13.5 ± 2	8.9 ± 1.5[b]
$\dot{V}O_2$ (mL/min)	299 ± 59	278 ± 68
$\dot{V}CO_2$ (mL/min)	270 ± 23	245 ± 27
REE (kJ/d)	8316 ± 714	7843 ± 743
P_{AW} (cmH_2O)	12 ± 4	16 ± 5
V_D/V_T (%)	0.68 ± 0.1	0.42 ± 0.05[b]
MAP (mmHg)	84 ± 7	82 + 9
SP (mmHg)	139 ± 15	130 + 16

RR, respiratory rate; $\dot{V}_E$, expired volume; $\dot{V}O_2$, O_2 consumption; $\dot{V}CO_2$, CO_2 consumption; REE, energy expenditure; P_{AW}, mean airway pressure; MAP, mean arterial pressure; SP, systolic pressure.

[a] A mean level of 9 cmH_2O PSV provided.

[b] $P < .05$

[c] $P < .01$.

(From Hurst et al.,[21] with permission.)

Table 82-5. Changes in Ventilatory Parameters, Gas Exchange, and Transdiaphragmatic Pressure with Increasing Levels of Pressure Support[a]

	Pressure Support Levels (cmH_2O)			
	0	10	15	20
V_T (mL)	377 ± 80	459 ± 63[c]	491 ± 82[e]	533 ± 131[f]
RR (min^{-1})	31 ± 8	29 ± 8	26 ± 8[f]	24 ± 7[f]
$\dot{V}_E$ (L/min)	11.2 ± 2.2	13.0 ± 2.9[d]	13.1 ± 2.9[d]	12.3 ± 2.3
P_{di} (cmH_2O)	21 ± 12	14 ± 11[f]	10 ± 8[f]	9 ± 8[f]
$PEEP_i$ (cmH_2O)[b]	2.7 ± 1.7	1.5 ± 1.2[d]	0.9 ± 1.2[d]	0.7 ± 0.7[d]
PaO_2 (mmHg)	76 ± 18	79 ± 19	79 ± 16	83 ± 19
$PaCO_2$ (mmHg)	45 ± 8	40 ± 6[d]	39 ± 5[e]	36 ± 6[f]
$\dot{V}O_2$ (mL/min)	288 ± 49	241 ± 55[e]	235 ± 48[e]	213 ± 54[f]
$\dot{W}$ (J/min)	19.5 ± 19.7	13.8 ± 13.6	10.9 ± 10.9[d]	5.0 ± 2.6[e]
W/V (J/L)	15.8 ± 1.15	0.95 ± 0.76[d]	0.74 ± 0.63[e]	0.39 ± 0.14[f]

RR, respiratory rate; $\dot{V}_E$, minute ventilation; P_{di}, difference between peak inspiratory and peak expiratory transdiaphragmatic pressure; $PEEP_i$, intrinsic positive end-expiratory pressure; $\dot{V}O_2$, O_2 consumption; $\dot{W}$, work of breathing per unit of time; W/V, work of breathing per liter of ventilation.

[a] All data are expressed as mean ± SD; statistical analysis compares the value with pressure support zero value.

[b] The mean value for the six patients in whom it was present.

[c] $P < 0.06$.

[d] $P < 0.05$.

[e] $P < 0.01$.

[f] $P < 0.001$.

(From Brochard et al.,[19] with permission.)

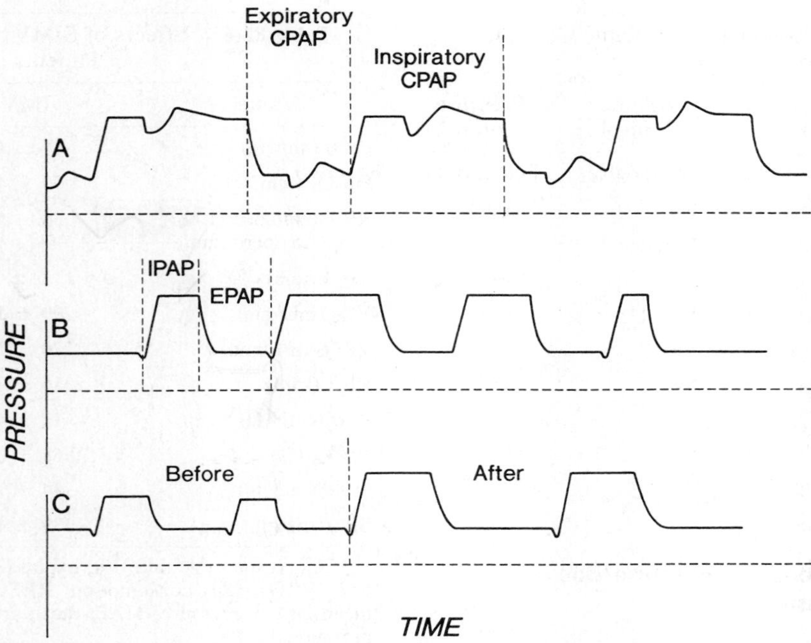

Figure 82-8. Pressure versus time waveforms during **(A)** airway pressure release ventilation (APRV), **(B)** bilevel positive airway pressure (BiPAP), and **(C)** pressure limited MMV. By design, APRV is usually adjusted with the inspiratory time longer than expiratory time and it is expected that patients will superimpose a spontaneous breath at both the inspiratory and expiratory CPAP levels. With BiPAP, normal application is via the timed/spontaneous mode (A/C), in which the patient is allowed to control all aspects of gas delivery except the IPAP (inspiratory positive airway pressure) level (EPAP, expiratory positive airway pressure). In pressure limited MMV, the PSV level is periodically adjusted to ensure MMV. PSV levels are depicted before and after adjustment.

ered by a demand system. As a result, it is easier for patients to inspire spontaneously at baseline pressure or plateau pressure with APRV/BiPAP than with pressure control. Generally, all of the approaches discussed maintain a baseline pressure above atmospheric. With APRV/BiPAP, this is generally required by design, while with pressure control it is a result of the clinician's approach to patient management. APRV is provided by a "homemade" continuous gas flow system[22] (Fig. 82-9). This system includes two PEEP valves, each set for a different CPAP level. A solenoid valve changes the direction of gas flow from one valve to the other, and thus alternates from baseline pressure to plateau pressure, based on the timing of the solenoid valve. BiPAP is provided by a stand-alone commercial unit that provides alternating levels of continuous gas flow to establish two levels of "CPAP."[23] In addition, the BiPAP unit (available from Respironics Inc.) incorporates three specific "mode" settings: timed (control), timed/spontaneous (A/C), and spontaneous (assist).[23]

The uses of APRV and BiPAP diverge along grossly different routes. Proponents of APRV believe it is best used in intubated patients with mild to moderate acute ventilatory failure. By contrast, BiPAP has been designed for noninvasive ventilatory support through a nasal mask.[23,26,27] Its primary use is in patients with chronic ventilatory failure, who require nocturnal ventilatory muscle rest. However, we have also used BiPAP to reverse acute ventilatory failure in patients with chronic ventilatory insufficiency, and as a transition from invasive mechanical ventilation, again in those patients with chronic ventilatory failure.

Mandatory Minute Ventilation

Pressure-targeted approaches to MMV are essentially the same as those with volume-limited approaches. A minimum minute volume is programmed, with the level of ventilatory support provided dependent on the level of minute ventilation provided by the patient. The Hamilton Veolar ventilator provides pure pressure-targeted MMV.[16] It accomplishes this by varying the level of PSV to ensure the MMV level. Although this appears to overcome some of the problems of rapid, shallow breathing, patients are still able to defeat the basic operational premise of MMV by breathing rapidly. East et al.[28] have demonstrated in a dog model that combining volume-targeted MMV with pressure-support ventilation prevents hypoventilation during pharmacologic depression (Fig. 82-10). Since PSV is a pure assist form of ventilation, its combination with volume-targeted MMV would defeat the problems associated with PSV and ventilatory depression.

The Bear 5 ventilator has the most unique method of applying MMV. In this unit SIMV and PSV are combined. The

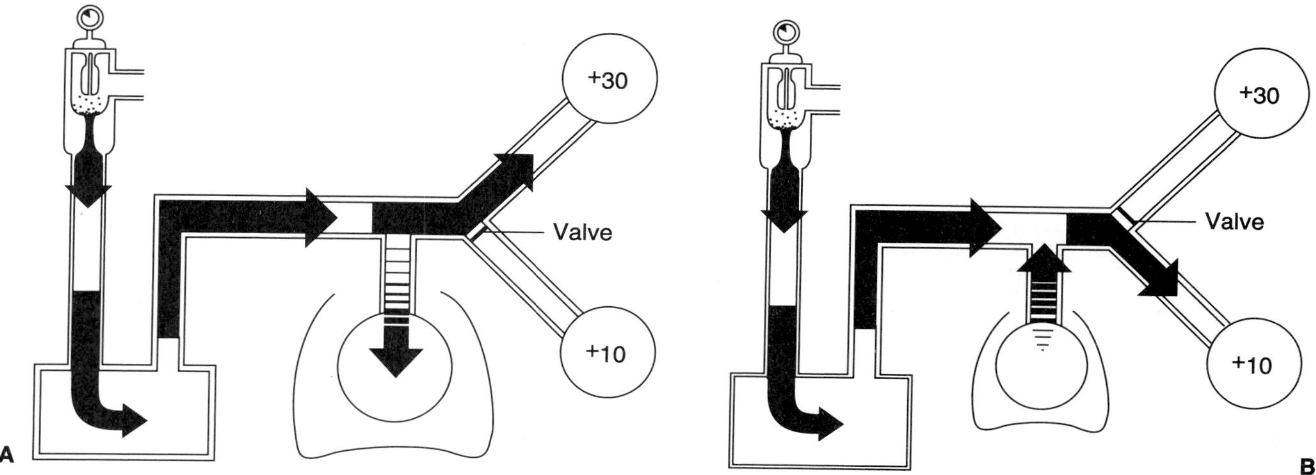

Figure 82-9. Schematic presentation of APRV set with $P_{inflation}$ at 30 cmH_2O and $P_{release}$ at 10 cmH_2O. **(A)** $P_{inflation}$ generated by continuous-flow system with threshold resistor set at 30 cmH_2O. Flow into lungs is determined by $P_{inflation}$ and forces impeding flow (resistance and compliance). Inspiratory lung volume is determined by $P_{inflation}$ and pulmonary compliance. **(B)** Release valve positioned to allow flow through threshold resistor, which is set at 10 cmH_2O. This drops airway pressure to release the pressure level, and gas exits lung. (From Cane et al.,[22] with permission.)

clinician can set an SIMV mandatory rate that is provided, regardless of the patient's ventilatory pattern; in addition, PSV can be added. Thus, a reasonable level of ventilation with appropriate VT is assured. MMV is operative about these settings.

Full and Partial Ventilatory Support

Controversy has long existed regarding the optimal mode of ventilation to employ during various phases of acute ventilatory failure. However, regardless of the mode selected, ventilatory support can be categorized into two general approaches: full ventilatory support (FVS) and partial ventilatory support. During FVS, the mechanical ventilator provides all, or nearly all the effort required to maintain gas exchange. As noted below, many of the commonly available modes of ventilation can provide FSV, provided they are appropriately set and the patient properly sedated. This is true even if patients are triggering the ventilator, as long as the adjustment of gas delivery is consistent with patient demands.

Most patients requiring ventilatory support for acute respiratory failure present with hypercarbia, hypoxemia, acidosis, and either ventilatory muscle dysfunction or failure, and are commonly exhausted. For these reasons we normally employ FVS techniques during the first 24 to 72 hours of ventilatory support.

During partial ventilatory support, the patient provides a significant percentage of the effort required to maintain gas exchange. Partial ventilatory support can be provided by IMV, SIMV, PSV, APRV, BIPAP, or MMV. Each of these approaches allows the clinician to titrate the level of support provided by the ventilator. With IMV, SIMV, or MMV, the frequency of the predetermined volume-limited breath can vary, allowing the patient to breathe spontaneously between the mandatory breaths. By contrast, inspiratory pressure support (IPS or PSV), APRV, and BIPAP allows the clinician to select the level of ventilatory effort required of the patient for each breath by varying the pressure limit selected. Each of these modes (IMV, SIMV, PSV, MMV, APRV, and BIPAP) allows various levels of patient–ventilator interaction from almost completely spontaneous ventilation to FVS. PSV has the advantage of contouring the delivered flow of gas to meet the patient's demand to a greater extent than any of the other modes.

Partial ventilatory support is a more physiologic approach to mechanical ventilation and a generally recommended approach to managing patients once they are past the acute phase of respiratory failure.[1,29,31] Allowing patients to play a more significant role in the process of ventilation normally improves $\dot{V}/\dot{Q}$ matching,[31] decreases hemodynamic compromise,[1,30,32] and may prevent further deterioration of diaphragmatic function. The key to appropriate application of PVS techniques is to titrate the level of patient–machine interaction so that active patient involvement is present but sufficient support is provided to prevent deterioration of ventilatory muscle function and overall cardiopulmonary status. Because of the delicate balance required, FVS is generally easier to employ appropriately than PVS, with clinical judgment being the key to the optimal titration of PVS.

Proportional Assist Ventilation

The newest approach to PVS is proportional assist ventilation (PAV). Although its application is entirely experimental and currently only used at a limited number of in-

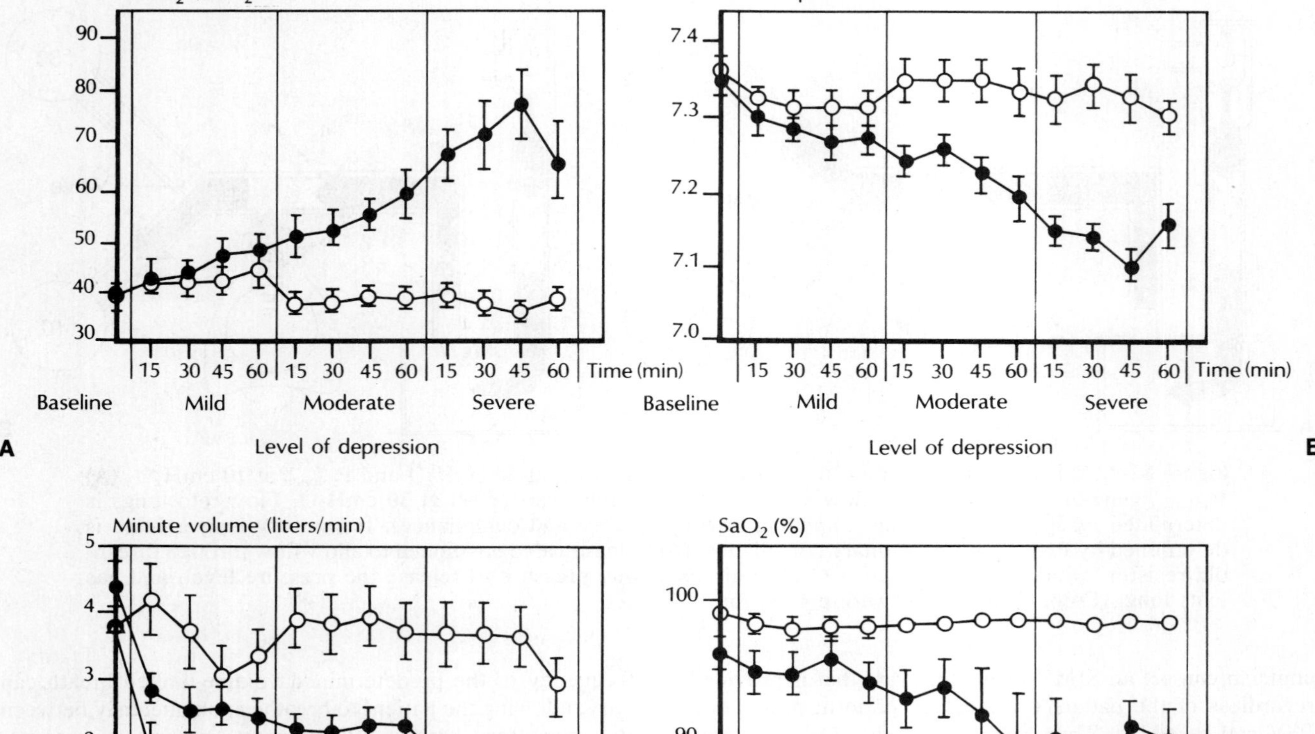

Figure 82-10. Ventilatory variables **(A)** $PaCO_2$, **(B)** arterial pH, **(C)** minute volume, and **(D)** SaO_2 during the use of PSV and PSV plus MMV measured over four respiratory depression levels. PSV only, solid squares; PSV + MMV, open circles; level of spontaneous ventilation during PSV + MMV, solid triangles; and spontaneous minute ventilation, open triangles. (From East et al.,[22] with permission.)

stitutions, it is at least theoretically the ultimate approach to PVS. With PAV, the ventilator responds to each patient effort in an independent manner, dependent on actual patient effort as well as the compliance and resistance of the system.[33] In effect, PAV amplifies patient effort, thus normalizing the relationship between patient effort and level of ventilation achieved, while leaving the patient entirely in control of all aspects of breathing. Thus, for a given breath pressure, volume, time, and flow may differ from previous and subsequent breaths, although the level of amplification of patient effort would be the same with each breath. Recently PAV has been shown effective in supporting a group of five ventilator-dependent patients, without compromise of gas exchange, with lower peak airway pressure for a period of 3 to 4 hours.[34]

RESPIRATORY RATE AND TIDAL VOLUME

Numerous factors play a role in establishing the spontaneous ventilatory pattern of an individual: height, weight, sex, total lung thoracic compliance (CT), airway resistance (RAW) and cardiopulmonary stress. During mechanical ventilation similar factors play a role in determining the VT selected. VT levels delivered by a mechanical ventilator are frequently 50 percent larger than those normally inspired spontaneously. The two primary factors mandating these large volumes are circuit compressible volume and physiologic dead space, although a number of other factors should be considered,[35] including

Patient's dyspnea
Circuit compressible volume
Physiologic dead space
Oxygenation
Ventilation
Cardiovascular stability
Barotrauma
Respiratory time constants

Dead Space

Since ventilator circuits contain large-volume humidifiers and large-bore corrugated tubing up to 10 ft in length or longer, a considerable percentage of the volume delivered by the ventilator never reaches the patient. Most systems have compressible volume loss factors of 3 to 5 mL/cm-H_2O[16]; if the peak airway pressure minus total system PEEP level is 50 cmH_2O, 150 to 250 mL of the delivered V_T is lost in compressible volume. None of the ventilators currently on the market, with the exception of the Puritan-Bennett 7200, allows for compressible volume factors. With the 7200, a compressible volume factor is calculated and gas delivery is monitored so that set V_T is the volume that enters the patient's airway.[16] With other units, the set V_T minus the compressible volume is the volume that actually enters the patient airway.[35]

The physiologic V_D is equal to both alveolar and anatomic V_D. In normal, healthy individuals the physiologic V_D is primarily anatomic and equals approximately 2.2 mL/kg body weight. At a normally inspired V_T, the V_D/V_T ratio varies from 0.20 to about 0.40. The V_D/V_T ratio is important in mechanical ventilation because it determines the efficiency of ventilation[35]:

$$\text{Efficiency of ventilation} = 1 - V_D/V_T \qquad (2)$$

(i.e., the lower the V_D/V_T, the greater the efficiency of ventilation and, thus, the greater the fraction of minute ventilation providing minute alveolar ventilation).

Mechanical ventilation dilates the airways and usually decreases venous return and $\dot{Q}_T$ thus altering the distribution of intrapulmonary $\dot{V}/\dot{Q}$. These changes also tend to increase the physiologic dead space.[36,37] However, the effect of mechanical ventilation on V_D/V_T is not clearly defined. Hedley-Whyte et al.[38] reported that V_D/V_T remained constant as V_T was increased from 7 mL/kg, with the ventilatory rate constant at 20 breaths per minute (control mode). Hedenstierna[39] noted similar results if the rate was kept constant, but also reported that V_D/V_T decreased with increasing V_T, if the minute ventilation was kept constant by adjusting the ventilatory rate. V_D/V_T remained unchanged when Marshall and Grange[40] doubled the V_T with a constant ventilation rate in a group of anesthetized patients. However, Visick et al.[41] noted a decreased V_D/V_T at a V_T of 15 mL/kg, as compared to 5 mL/kg in anesthetized adults.

These seemingly conflicting data can be explained by analyzing the relationship between physiologic V_D and V_T at various levels of delivered V_T. When delivered V_T is extremely small, V_D (primarily anatomic) represents a large percentage of V_T. As the mechanical V_T increases, the V_D/V_T decreases until it reaches a level at which positive pressure significantly distends the conducting airways. At this level there is a proportional increase in V_D and V_T; thus, V_D/V_T remains constant. As mechanical V_T is increased further, the movement of V_T onto the plateau segment of the patient's compliance curve (Fig. 82-11) results in a disproportionate increase of alveolar dead space because venous return and $\dot{Q}_T$ are reduced. From this point, V_D/V_T increases with increasing V_T.

Oxygenation and Ventilation

Both oxygenation and ventilation tend to improve as larger V_T levels with slow rates are applied, in distinction to rapid rates and small volumes in patients with normal lung thoracic mechanics.[35] This is a result of reversal of atelectasis and intrapulmonary shunting that tends to occur with small mechanical V_T.[42,43,44] In addition, patients with acute pulmonary pathology normally experience acute dyspnea that may persist in spite of the correction of hypercarbia and hypoxemia. Such patients, particularly those with a neurologic or neuromuscular disease, may experience a lessening of dyspnea when V_T levels larger than normal are administered mechanically.[45] From these data it would appear that a mechanical V_T of approximately 10 to 15 mL/kg results in the average patient maintaining the V_D/V_T ratio at its lowest level.

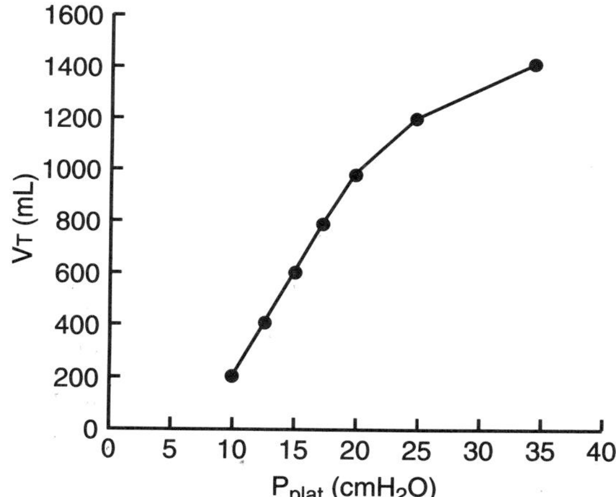

Figure 82-11. Total lung-thorax compliance curve developed by increasing the exhaled V_T in 200-mL increments. The ideal maximum V_T in this example, located on the steep aspect of the compliance curve, is about 1000 mL. V_T over this level markedly increases static and dynamic pressures. (From Kacmarek,[68] with permission.)

Respiratory Time Constants

When determinations of mechanical VT and rate are made at the bedside, the time required to allow the lung and thorax to return to its resting end-expiratory level must be considered. In 1969, Bergman[46] analyzed the exhalation of anesthetized subjects and developed an equation that described the time course of passive exhalation:

$$V_{(t)} = V_O\, e^{-} \left(\frac{1}{RC}\right) t \tag{3}$$

where $V_{(t)}$ is the volume of gas remaining in the thorax at any time after the start of exhalation; V_O is the gas volume above resting FRC at the beginning of exhalation; log e is the base of the natural logarithm; R is total resistance; C is total compliance, and t is time. RC is thus defined as the time constant of the respiratory system:

$$(\text{resistance})\ (\text{compliance}) = \text{time} \tag{4}$$

$$(\text{cmH}_2\text{O/L/s})\ (\text{L/cmH}_2\text{O}) = \text{s} \tag{5}$$

If it is assumed that airway resistance and compliance are independent of volume, a finite time interval is necessary for complete passive exhalation. In one time constant, 37 percent of VT is exhaled. It requires about 4 time constants (98 percent of VT) for passive exhalation to be complete. If less time is available, air trapping and auto-PEEP develop (see Ch. 76), a common problem of mechanically ventilated patients with chronic obstructive pulmonary disease (COPD).[47] In general, patients with normal lungs begin to develop air trapping and auto-PEEP at a rate of 20 breaths per minute or greater. However, patients with chronic pulmonary disease may experience air trapping at rates of 8 breaths per minute or more.

These data provide crude guidelines for determining optimal mechanical ventilatory rates. In patients with a large RC (pulmonary obstruction), rapid ventilatory rates will result in air trapping even if exhalation is active, while in patients with small RC values (pulmonary restriction), rapid rates may be employed without fear of air trapping.

Barotrauma

Of primary concern to many clinicians when selecting respiratory rate and VT is barotrauma. This concern has caused many clinicians to deliver small VT levels in an attempt to reduce peak inspiratory pressure (PIP). Although reduction of PIP is desirable, the combination of lung disease, overdistension and high alveolar pressure must be present to cause barotrauma.[48,49,50] Bone[49] has reported a major reduction in the incidence of barotrauma by basing mechanical VT on total compliance (CT).

We recommend using pressure-volume curves to establish the appropriate VT. In Figure 82-11, 200 mL changes in VT are plotted against plateau pressure. Note that a VT of 1000 mL is the largest VT still remaining on the steep aspect of the compliance curve. Volumes greater than this may stretch the lung beyond its elastic limit and increase the probability of barotrauma. Although this approach provides a rough approximation of the appropriate VT for a large portion of adults, one should be aware that the actual compliance of the lungs can vary daily with acute disease and the selected VT will require adjustments as the clinical course progresses.

The discussions of compression volume, dead space, time constants, and barotrauma suggest the use of large VT levels and slow mechanical rates. This ventilatory pattern has also been shown to be effective in decreasing the patient's sense of dyspnea,[45] improving oxygenation,[42] and maintaining adequate ventilation,[43,44] when compared with approaches employing smaller VT levels and higher ventilatory rates.

Guidelines

In general, an initial mechanical VT of 12 to 15 mL/kg[1,30,35,51] at rates of 8 to 12 breaths per minute is recommended. Variations from this level may be necessary in patients with severe chronic lung disease or ARDS (Table 82-7). Volume selection is based on ideal, not actual body weight; however, obese patients normally require a VT of at least 15 mL/kg for effective ventilation, while cachectic patients may require 12 mL/kg or less. The initial machine rate is set to meet the metabolic requirements for CO_2 elimination. Adjustment of settings is subsequently based on the results of arterial blood gas (ABG) analysis.

In patients with severe acute lung injury, large VT and slow rates may not maintain adequate gas exchange without generating dangerously high peak and mean alveolar pressures. Markedly altered pulmonary mechanics (i.e., severely decreased compliance) is an indication for the use of higher rates (greater than 12 to 20 breaths per minute) with smaller VT (less than 10 mL/kg). In these patients, effective distribution of ventilation is compromised by inhomogeneous regional pulmonary compliance. Overall, RC is small, but significant local variations occur. With slow ventilatory rates, lung regions with large RC values receive most of the ventilation, and localized areas of overdistension may develop. At rapid ventilatory rates, the distribution of gas is less affected by CT, and RAW becomes the more prominent factor affecting inspired gas distribution. As a result, overdistension of regions with a normal RC value is decreased.

The presence of chronic pulmonary restriction results in

Table 82-7. Initial Settings for Rate and VT for Mechanically Ventilated Patients with Differing Pathophysiology

Patient Type	Rate (breaths/min)	VT[a] (mL/kg)
Normal lungs	8–12	12–15
COPD (lengthened expiratory time)	≤8–10	12–15
Chronic pulmonary restriction	>12–20	<10
Severe, acute lung injury	>12–20	<10

[a] Based on ideal body weight.

severe alterations of C_T, which markedly decreases the size of the mechanical V_T that remains on the steep aspect of the compliance curve. Thus, when ventilating this type of patient, a much smaller V_T (<10 mL/kg) than those used in patients with relatively normal lungs is indicated. In these patients, RC is usually small, and faster ventilatory rates can be used without hyperinflation to maintain effective gas exchange at the smaller V_T. Ventilatory frequencies over 12 to 20 breaths per minute should be selected.

Slower rates are generally advantageous in patients with severe COPD because of the increased C_T, increased R_{AW}, increased RC value, the possibility of air trapping (auto-PEEP) and the need to maintain $PaCO_2$ near the patient's normal level (usually above 45 to 50 mmHg). Initially, low ventilatory rates of 8 to 10 breaths per minute are recommended. Because the primary pathophysiology affecting gas distribution is an increased R_{AW}, slow rates generally optimize ventilatory gas distribution. V_T is adjusted to maintain appropriate CO_2 elimination and usually ranges from 12 to 15 mL/kg.

INSPIRATORY FLOW WAVEFORMS AND PEAK FLOW

Mechanical ventilators provide up to four inspiratory flow waveforms: square, sine, accelerating, and decelerating (Fig. 82-12). Data evaluating when each should be employed are minimal. Little difference has been noted from either a gas exchange or cardiovascular function perspective with square and sine waves[52,53,54] and generally their use is equivocal. Decelerating inspiratory gas flows enhance the distribution of ventilation if the peak inspiratory flow is low and inspiratory time long.[52,53] No data supporting the use of accelerating gas flows are available.[53,54] We commonly employ either square or sine wave patterns in spontaneously breathing patients and use decelerating patterns in patients receiving controlled ventilation, especially if abnormalities of ventilation distribution exist, which result in oxygenation difficulties. It is our opinion that the decelerating waveform is beneficial in improving oxygenation in the patient with ARDS.

Patient synchrony with an assisted positive-pressure breath depends on the ability of the ventilator to meet the patient's inspiratory demands.[55,56,57] Two technical factors primarily affect this: trigger sensitivity[55,56] and peak inspiratory flow.[57] The greater the force necessary to trigger the ventilator, and the lower the peak flow rate, the greater the patient dyssynchrony. Marini et al.[57] have demonstrated that the patient's work of breathing during volume-assisted ventilation may equal that during spontaneous breathing if inspiratory flows are inadequate (see Ch. 87). This phenomenon is demonstrated in Figure 82-13. Figure 82-13A represents the work performed by the ventilator during a controlled breath and an ideal assisted breath, whereas Figure 82-13B shows an actual pressure-volume curve during an assisted breath. The difference in the area between the two curves (Fig. 82-13B) is the work performed by the patient during the volume-assisted breath. To minimize this problem, peak inspiratory flow in most spontaneously breathing adults should be set at 60 to 90 L/min. In those ventilators without peak flow controls, inspiratory times of 0.8 to 1.2 seconds are usually appropriate (Table 82-8). In addition, the combination of demand flow with volume-limited ventilation, as recently described by Bonasset et al.[58] and Amato et al.[59] and currently available on the new Servo 300 ventilator,[60] appears to be capable of providing the variation in flow delivery necessary to meet patients' spontaneous breathing requirements, while maintaining a constant V_T. Most of the pressure-limited approaches are capable of meeting patients' inspiratory demands, as noted by the rapid ini-

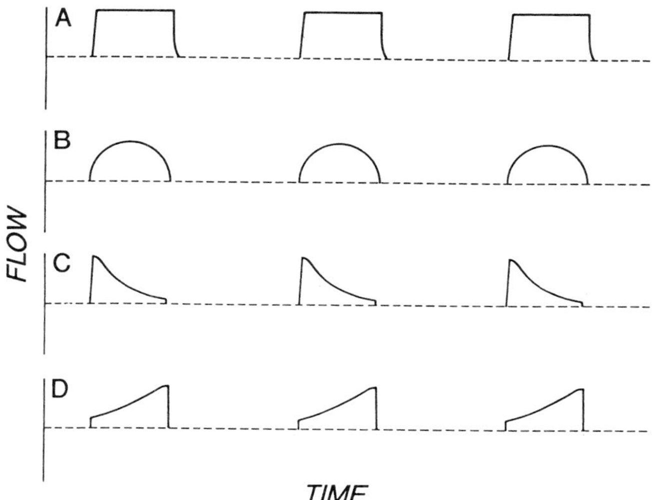

Figure 82-12. Inspiratory flow waveforms available on today's mechanical ventilators. **(A)** Square wave, **(B)** sine wave, **(C)** decelerating wave, and **(D)** accelerating wave.

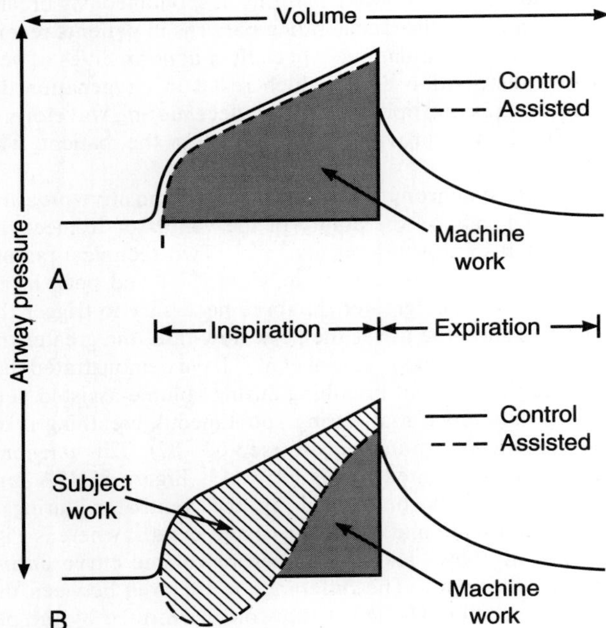

Figure 82-13. Estimation of patient work of breathing during assisted, volume-limited (square wave flow) ventilation. **(A)** Actual total work of breathing during controlled ventilation and ideal assisted ventilation. **(B)** Controlled ventilation compared to actual assisted ventilation. The hatched area represents work performed by a patient during assisted ventilation. (From Marini et al.,[69] with permission.)

tial flows delivered to establish peak airway pressure early in the inspiratory phase.

It should be remembered that the above discussions concern spontaneously breathing patients. In patients who are sedated and receiving controlled ventilation, manipulation of inspiratory time and/or peak flows is based on effective distribution of gas and hemodynamic compromise, not on work of breathing.

Table 82-8. Ranges for Setting of Variables Affecting Inspiratory Time during Spontaneous and Controlled Ventilation

	Spontaneous Breathing	Controlled Ventilation
Peak flow	60–90 L/min	Whatever accomplishes the goals of ventilation/oxygenation
Inspiratory time	0.8–1.2 s	0.8–3.0 s
I/E ratio	≥1:3	≥1:3–1.5:1
Flow waveform	Square/sine, decelerating	Square/sine, decelerating

INSPIRATORY TO EXPIRATORY RATIOS

Most healthy adults ventilate spontaneously with an inspiratory/expiratory (I/E) ratio of 1:1.5 to 1:2 (i.e., expiration is about 50 to 100 percent longer than inspiration). This is necessary to avoid use of the accessory muscles of exhalation and air trapping. Generally the same standard should be applied to mechanical ventilation. However, since mechanical rates are generally slow in most patients, I/E ratios are normally less than 1:3, with actual inspiratory time being of most importance. In patients with COPD or asthma, because of air trapping and auto-PEEP, even smaller ratios (longer expiratory times), are normally employed.

Much recent interest has been given to prolonging, to the point of inversal, the I/E ratio in the management of ARDS.[3–7,9–11] Since gas distribution and loss of lung volume are the primary pathophysiologic changes that lead to decreased compliance and hypoxemia, many authors believe prolongation of the I/E ratio improves oxygenation.[3–6] While much anecdotal data[3–6] exist in this area, little if any information supporting inversal of the I/E ratio to the levels used by some authors (4:1) exist.[3–6] The major concern with marked inversal of the I/E ratio is the development of auto-PEEP, which, as outlined in Chapter 76, is difficult to assess and may cause localized hyperinflation and increase the probability of barotrauma. For these reasons, we recommend a conservative approach when lengthening the I/E ratio to increase mean airway pressure and improve oxygenation.[9] We frequently use a 1:1 ratio, but normally do not exceed a 1.5:1 ratio. (See Chapter 83 for discussions regarding the management of patients requiring prolonged inspiratory times.)

Inflation Hold

One method of increasing inspiratory time and I/E ratio is the use of an inflation hold. This maneuver stops active delivery of gas into the lung but maintains the exhalation valve closed for the hold period. On many ventilators inflation holds can be programmed from a minimum of 0.1 seconds to a maximum of 3 seconds. In addition to allowing better equilibration of gas in the lungs and lengthening inspiratory time, the inflation hold is used periodically to establish a plateau pressure for the determination of lung-ventilator system compliance (see Ch. 83).

PEEP AND F_{IO_2}

Maintaining adequate oxygenation is a major challenge during acute respiratory failure, especially for patients with acute lung injury. Assuming hemoglobin levels, ventilation, and $\dot{Q}_T$ are optimized, PEEP (or CPAP) and O_2 therapy are the major methods available to improve oxygenation status. O_2 therapy is normally the first and most immediate therapy. However, regional reduction in lung volume due to airway closure, atelectasis, $\dot{V}/\dot{Q}$ inequality, and increased shunting are common pulmonary complications in hospitalized patients with acute lung injury. Restoration of functional residual capacity toward normal values can be achieved with PEEP or CPAP. Therapy is usually directed toward improving arterial oxygenation. The improvement in functional residual capacity is directly related to the level of PEEP and total respiratory system compliance. Although there is a linear increase in PaO_2 with an increase in FRC, increasing levels of PEEP are associated with other less favorable changes, including increases of mean intrathoracic pressure and pulmonary vascular resistance and the risk of pulmonary barotrauma. The use of PEEP must balance both benefits and complications of therapy; thus no agreement on what level of PEEP is optimal in any given clinical setting exists.

During the tritration of PEEP, monitoring the composite effect of PEEP on PaO_2, lung compliance, $\dot{Q}_T$, pulmonary hemodynamics and O_2 delivery can assist in determining the most appropriate level for any patient. Since the overall goal of PEEP is to provide tissue oxygenation at the minimal end-expiratory pressure and FIO_2 setting (usually a PaO_2 of 60 to 70 mmHg at an $FIO_2 \leq 0.60$ to 0.70), while maintaining a normal cardiac index, these may be considered the desired endpoints when adjusting PEEP and FIO_2. (See Ch. 76 for a detailed discussion of PEEP and FIO_2 settings.)

SIGH BREATHS

During normal, quiet spontaneous breathing an individual normally inspires deeply a number of times per hour. These sign breaths help to reestablish lung volume that has diminished as a result of shallow breathing and to reverse microatelectasis. Historically, patients with normal lungs who were mechanically ventilated with small V_T were "sighed" periodically by the ventilator. However, since most ventilators use large V_T to ventilate patients with normal or increased compliance, sighs are normally not administered. In fact, few ventilators now incorporate the sigh option.

If a sigh is to be delivered, it is usually programmed for 1.5 times the set V_T and administered anywhere from 6 to 20 times per hour. Situations for which we believe sighs are indicated are as follows:

- Before and after suctioning
- During chest physical therapy
- After and during bronchoscopy
- Before and during extubation
- If small V_T are used with normal or increased compliance during controlled ventilation
- During re-expansion of lung collapse

However, we would also recommend that they be administered with a manual ventilator and an inspiratory hold. This usually allows the clinician to determine whether an appropriate change in compliance has occurred and to assist in secretion removal, as described in Chapter 72. We do not recommend use of the sigh as it is programmed on some mechanical ventilators.

Table 82-9. High-Frequency Ventilation

	HFPPV	HFJV	HFO
Rate	60–150/min	60–1600/min	60–3600/min
V_T	3–5 mL/kg	2–5 mL/kg	1–3 mL/kg
I/E ratio	1:3–1:2	1:3–1:2	1:3–1:2
Technical application	Conventional ventilator	Special ventilator	Special ventilator
FIO_2	21–100	21–100	21–100
PEEP	0–40	0–40	0–40
Exhalation	Passive	Passive	Active
Gas movement	Convection	Convection	Diffusion

HIGH FREQUENCY VENTILATION

High frequency ventilation (HFV) techniques (Table 82-9) are based on using ventilatory rates of greater than 60 breaths per minute. Initially HFV approaches were believed to improve gas exchange over conventional approaches at lower PEEP, peak airway, and mean airway pressures, with a lower risk of barotrauma.[61–63] Initial studies indicated this was, in fact, true in patients with normal lungs; however, these techniques have at best only demonstrated equivalence to conventional mechanical ventilation in patients with ARDS.[64–67]

Three different techniques are presently available: high-frequency positive-pressure ventilation (HFPPV), high-frequency jet ventilation (HFJV), and high-frequency oscillation (HFO). HFPPV is available on conventional ventilators. Some of the neonatal units currently available allow rates up to the 150 breaths per minute. Both HFJV and HFO require ventilators specifically designed for the purpose of HFV. Across these three approaches rates from 60 (1 Hz) to 3600 (60 Hz) per minute are available.

HFJV is the only one of the three techniques that has been subjected to randomized trials. Four studies[64–67] in ARDS patients have been conducted to date. None have demonstrated superiority to conventional ventilation techniques. As a result, at least in adults, HFV has not found a place in the average intensive care unit. It is still considered experimental and is beyond the scope of this text.

References

1. Rasanen J, Downs JB: Modes of mechanical ventilatory support. pp. 180–203. In Kirby RR, Banner JM, Downs JB (eds): Clinical Application of Ventilatory Support. 2nd Ed. Churchill Livingstone, New York, 1990

2. Hursh C, Kacmarek RM, Stanek K: Work of breathing during CPAP and PSV imposed by the new generation mechanical ventilators: A lung model study. Respir Care 1991;36:815–828
3. Gurevitch MJ, VanDyke J, Young ES, Jackson K: Improved oxygenation and lower peak airway pressure in severe adult respiratory distress syndrome: Treatment with inverse ratio ventilation. Chest 1986;89:211–213
4. Tharratt RS, Allen RP, Albertson TE: Pressure controlled inverse ratio ventilation in severe adult respiratory failure. Chest 1988;94:755–762
5. Lain DC, DeBenedetto R, Morris SL, et al: Pressure control inverse ratio ventilation as a method to reduce peak inspiratory pressure and provide adequate ventilation and oxygenation. Chest 1989;95:1081–1088
6. Abraham E, Yoshihara G: Cardiorespiratory effects of pressure controlled inverse ratio ventilation in severe respiratory failure. Chest 1989;96:1356–1359
7. Cole AGH, Weller SF, Sykes MK: Inverse ratio ventilation compared with PEEP in adult respiratory failure. Intensive Care Med 1984;10:337–339
8. Abraham E, Yoshihara G: Cardiorespiratory effects of pressure controlled ventilation in severe respiratory failure. Chest 1990; 98:1445–1449
9. Kacmarek RM, Hess D: Pressure-controlled, inverse-ratio ventilation: Panacea or auto-PEEP? (editorial). Respir Care 1990; 35:945–948
10. Duncan SR, Rizk NW, Raffin TA: Inverse ratio ventilation. PEEP in disguise? (editorial). Chest 1987;92:390–391
11. Marini JJ, Crooke PS, Truwit JD: Determinants and limits of pressure-preset ventilation: A mathematical model of pressure control. J Appl Physiol 1989;67:1081–1092
12. Benson MS, Pierson DJ: Auto-PEEP during mechanical ventilation in adults. Respir Care 1988;33:557–568
13. Smith TC, Marini JJ: Impact of PEEP on lung mechanics and work of breathing in severe airflow obstruction. J Appl Physiol 1988;65:1488–1499
14. Hasten RW, Downs JB, Heenen TJ: A comparison of synchronized and non-synchronized intermittent mandatory ventilation. Respir Care 1980;25:554–561
15. Marini JJ, Smith TC, Lamb VJ: External work output and force generation during synchronized intermittent mechanical ventilation: Effect of machine assistance on breathing effort. Am Rev Respir Dis 1988;138:1169–1179
16. McPherson SP: Mechanical ventilators. pp. 391–492. In Respiratory Therapy Equipment. 3rd Ed. Mosby-Year Book, St. Louis, 1990
17. Kacmarek RM: The role of pressure support ventilation in reducing the work of breathing. Respir Care 1988;33:99–120
18. Brochard L, Rua F, Lorino H et al: The extra work of breathing due to endotracheal tube is abolished during inspiratory pressure support breathing. Am Rev Respir Dis 1987;137:64–73
19. Brochard L, Harf A, Lorino H, Lemaire F: Inspiratory pressure support prevents diaphragmatic fatigue during weaning from mechanical ventilation. Am Rev Respir Dis 1989;139:513–521
20. MacIntyre NR: Respiratory function during pressure support ventilation. Chest 1986;89:677–683
21. Hurst JM, Branson RD, Davis K, Barrette RR: Cardiopulmonary effects of pressure support ventilation. Arch Surg 1989; 124:1067–1070
22. Cane RD, Peruzzi WT, Shapiro BA: Airway pressure release ventilation in severe respiratory failure. Chest 1991;200:460–463
23. Strumpf DA, Carlisle CC, Millman RP et al: An evaluation of the Respironics BiPAP bi-level CPAP device for delivery of assisted ventilation. Respir Care 1990;35:415–422
24. Downs JB, Stock MC: Airway pressure release ventilation: A new concept in ventilatory support. Crit Care Med 1987;15:459–465
25. Garner W, Downs JB, Stock MC: Airway pressure release ventilation (APRV). Chest 1988;94:779–785
26. Goldstein RS, Avendano MA: Long-term mechanical ventilation as elective therapy: Clinical status and future prospects. Respir Care 1991;36:297–304
27. Goldstein RS, DeRosie JA, Avendano MA, Dolmage M: Influence of non-invasive positive pressure ventilation on inspiratory muscles. Chest 1991;99:408–415
28. East TD, Elkhuizen HM, Pace NL: Pressure support with mandatory minute ventilation supplied by the Ohmeda CPU-1 prevents hypoventilation due to respiratory depression in a canine model. Respir Care 1989;34:795–800
29. Wilson RS, Kacmarek RM: Airway management and mechanical ventilation during acute respiratory failure. pp. 407–422. In Tinker J, Zapol WM (eds): Care of the Critically Ill Patient. 2nd Ed. Springer-Verlag, London, 1991
30. Shapiro BA, Kacmarek RM, Cane RD et al: Positive pressure ventilation. pp. 281–302. Clinical Application of Respriatory Care. 4th Ed. Mosby-Year Book, St. Louis, 1991
31. Shah DM, Newell JC, Dutton RE: Continuous positive airway pressure versus positive end-expiratory pressure in respiratory distress syndrome. J Thorac Cardiovasc Surg 1977;74:557–564
32. Venus B, Jacobs HK, Mathru M: Hemodynamic responses to different modes of mechanical ventilation in dogs with normal and acid aspirated lungs. Crit Care Med 1980;8:620–625
33. Younes M: Proportional assist ventilation, a new approach to ventilatory support: Theory. Am Rev Respir Dis 1992;145:114–120
34. Younes M, Puddy A, Roberts D et al: Proportional assist ventilation: Results of an initial clinical trial. Am Rev Respir Dis 1992;145:121–129
35. Kacmarek RM, Venegas J: Mechanical ventilatory rates and tidal volumes. Respir Care 1987;32:466–478
36. Cooper EA: Physiological dead space in passive ventilation: Relationship with tidal volume, frequency, age, and minor upsets of respiratory health. Anaesthesia 1967;22:199–208
37. Hedenstierna G, McCarthy G: Mechanics of breathing, gas distribution and functional residual capacity at different frequencies of respiration during spontaneous and artificial ventilation. Br J Anaesth 1975;47:706–711
38. Hedley-Whyte J, Pontoppidan H, Morris MJ: The response of patients with respriatory failure and cardiopulmonary disease to different levels of constant volume ventilation. J Clin Invest 1966;45:1543–1554
39. Hedenstierna G: The anatomical and alveolar deadspace during respiratory treatment. Br J Anaesth 1975;47:993–999
40. Marshall BE, Grange RA: Changes in respiratory physiology during ether/air anesthesia. Br J Anaesth 1966;38:329–338
41. Visick WD, Fairley HB, Hickey RF: The effects of tidal volume and end-expiratory pressure on pulmonary gas exchange during anesthesia. Anesthesiology 1973;39:285–290
42. Hedenstierna G, Johansson H: Ventilation of a lung model with the Engstrom repsirator: The effect of different settings on gas distribution. Acta Anaesthesiol Scand 1972;16:206–215
43. Bendixen HH, Hedley-Whyte J, Chir B, Laver MB: Impaired oxygenation in surgical patients during general anesthesia with controlled ventilation: A concept of atelectasis. N Engl J Med 1963;269:991–996
44. Bendixen HH, Bullwinkel B, Hedley-Whyte J: Atelectasis and shunting during spontaneous ventilation in anesthetized patients. Anesthesiology 1964;25:297–301
45. Hotchkiss RS, Wilson RS: Mechanical ventilatory support. Surg Clin North Am 1983;63:417–438
46. Bergman NA: Properties of passive exhalation in anesthetized subjects. Anesthesiology 1969;30:378–387
47. Brown DG, Pierson DJ: Auto-PEEP is common in mechanically ventilated patients: A study of incidence, severity and detection. Respir Care 1986;31:1069–1073
48. Pierson DJ: Alveolar rupture during mechanical ventilation: Role of PEEP, peak airway pressure and distending volume. Respir Care 1988;33:472–486
49. Bone RC: Pulmonary barotrauma complicating mechanical ventilation (abstracted). Am Rev Respir Dis 1976;113:118
50. Bone RC, Francis PB, Pierce AK: Pulmonary barotrauma complicating positive end-expiratory pressure (abstracted). Am Rev Respir Dis 1975;111:921
51. Williams-Colon S, Thalken FR: Management and monitoring of

the patient in respiratory failure. pp. 780–826. In Scanlon C, Spearman CB, Sheldon RL (eds): Egan's Fundamentals of Respiratory Therapy. 5th Ed. CV Mosby, St. Louis, 1990

52. Al-Saady N, Bennett ED: Decelerating flow waveform improves lung mechanics and gas exchange in patients on intermittent positive pressure ventilation. Intensive Care Med 1985;11:68–75
53. Baker AB, Babington PCB, Colliss, Cowie RW: Effects of varying inspiratory flow waveform and time in intermittent positive pressure ventilation. Br J Aneaesth 1977;49:1221–1233
54. Baker AB, Restall R, Clark BW: Effects of varying inspiratory flow waveform and time in intermittent positive pressure ventilation emphysema. Br J Anaesth 1982;54:547–554
55. Christopher KL, Neff TA, Bowman JL: Demand and continuous flow intermittent mandatory ventilation systems. Respir Care 1984;33:625–630
56. Marini JJ, Capps JS, Culver BH: The inspiratory work of breathing during assisted ventilation. Chest 1985;87:612–618
57. Marini JJ, Smith TC, Lamb VJ: External work output and force generation during synchronized intermittent mandatory ventilation. Am Rev Respir Dis 1988;138:1169–1179
58. Bonassa J, Marcelo BP, Amato MD et al: Volume-assisted pressure supported ventilation (abstracted). Respir Care 1990; 35:1113
59. Marcelo A, Bonassa J, Carmen SV et al: Volume-assisted-pressure supported ventilation: Clinical study (abstracted). Respir Care 1990;35:1113
60. Servo Ventilator 300. Product literature. WS 06915. Siemens Life Support Systems, Sweden, 1991
61. Slutsky AS, Drazen JM, Ingram RH Jr: Effective pulmonary ventilation with small-volume oscillations at high frequency. Science 1980;209:609–611
62. Klain M, Smith RB: High frequency percutaneous transtracheal jet ventilation. Crit Care Med 1977;5:280–287
63. Rossing TH, Slutsky AS, Lehr JL: Tidal volume and frequency dependence of carbon dioxide elimination by high-frequency ventilation. N Engl J Med 1981;305:1375–1379
64. Carlon GC, Howland WS, Groeger JS et al: Role of high-frequency jet ventilation in the management of respiratory failure. Crit Care Med 1984;12:777–779
65. Holzapfel L, Robert D, Perrin F et al: Comparison of high-frequency jet ventilation to conventional ventilation in adults with repsiratory distress syndrome. Intensive Care Med 1987;13:100–104
66. MacIntyre NR, Follett JV, Dietz JL et al: Jet ventilation at 100 breaths per minute in adult respiratory failure. Am Rev Respir Dis 1986;134:897–901
67. Schuster DP, Klain M, Snyder JV: Comparison of high frequency jet ventilation to conventional ventilation during severe acute respiratory failure in humans. Crit Care Med 1982;10:625–630
68. Kacmarek RM: Noninvasive monitoring techniques in the ventilated patient. pp. 182–187. In Kacmarek RM, Stoller J (eds): Current Respiratory Care, Marcel Dekker, New York, 1988
69. Marini JJ, Rodriguez M, Lamb V: The inspiratory workload of patient-initiated mechanical ventilation. Am Rev Respir Dis 1986;134:902–909

Chapter 83

Management of the Patient–Mechanical Ventilator System

Robert M. Kacmarek

CHAPTER OUTLINE

Management of the patient–mechanical ventilator system is one of the most important and demanding tasks of the respiratory care clinician. Under this broad umbrella is the assessment of patient response to ventilatory assistance, subsequent modification of methodology used during assistance, and assurance of proper ventilator function. To ensure that the goals of ventilatory assistance are accomplished, the clinician must carefully evaluate the patient–ventilator system on a regular basis. It is important that the clinician does not forget that a patient is attached to the end of the ventilator tubing. As a result of the sophisticated technology used today, it is easy to be conditioned into managing numbers and machines and not patients.

This chapter presents in a systematic manner many of the overall processes involved in bedside assessment and management of the patient–ventilator system. Because the patient is the primary concern, we begin with the patient, followed by assessment of the ventilator system. Options for management decisions during specific settings are also presented.

PHYSICAL ASSESSMENT

As stressed by MacIntyre[1] there is specific information regarding patient clinical status that can only be gathered with our senses (Table 83-1). Direct assessment of the patient should always precede assessment of the ventilator system. Patients requiring ventilatory support should *appear comfortable*; they should not be at the same level of physiologic distress noted before initiation of ventilation. Reasons for physiologic distress (Table 83-2) should be identified and corrected immediately. For example, patients on full ventilatory support should not be breathing out of phase with the ven-

Table 83-1. Information Based on Physical Assessment

Ventilatory pattern	Sputum
Paradoxical breathing	Volume
Respiratory alternans	Color
Asymmetric movement	Consistency
Rate, depth	Dyspnea
Effort	General appearance
Breath sounds	Relaxed
Wheezing	Sedated
Consolidation	Anxious
Percussion note	

tilator—the patient should not be inspiring as the ventilator is expiring. A uniform, bilateral rise of the chest, and descent of the diaphragm should be observable. If the chest is rising unevenly, or one side is lagging behind the other, pneumothorax or obstruction of a large airway may be present, requiring chest tube insertion or bronchial hygiene therapy.

Tension Pneumothorax

The recognition, diagnosis, and treatment of a pneumothorax during positive pressure ventilation is a critical skill required of all respiratory care clinicians. If a pneumothorax develops during positive pressure ventilation, it always results in a tension pneumothorax, which requires immediate treatment. The specific signs associated with the development of a tension pneumothorax are listed in Table 82-3. Generally, a marked precipitous decline in the patient's status is noted. Progressive hemodynamic instability is present. As a result of a decrease in lung/chest wall compliance, peak airway pressure rises (volume-targeted ventilation), and potentially can increase with each breath. High pressure alarms are activated and tidal volume (V_T) delivery decreased (both volume- and pressure-targeted ventilation). Breath sounds on the affected side are diminished or absent, and the chest becomes more hyperinflated, without showing the normal rhythmic change in chest wall dimensions. The affected chest wall is tympanic to diagnostic percussion, and in severe cases the trachea is deviated away from the affected side. If a tension pneumothorax is suspected, 100 percent O_2 via a manual ventilator is delivered. A rapid rate with small V_T should be established, being careful not to exert excessive pressure that would extend the pneumothorax. Definitive diagnosis is made by radiograph, although rapid decompression of the chest before the radiograph is obtained may be necessary in those cases in which the extent of the pneumothorax is increased on a breath-by-breath basis and cardiovascular collapse is imminent. Rapid decompression is accomplished by insertion of a 19-gauge needle into the second or third intercostal space anteriorly at the nipple line.[2] To avoid blood vessels perfusing the intercostals, the needle is inserted over the lower rib.

Table 83-2. Signs of Distress during Ventilatory Support

Out of phase with ventilator	General agitation
Tachypnea	Use of accessory muscles
Tachycardia/bradycardia	Paradoxical breathing
Hypotension/hypertension	Respiratory alternans

Table 83-3. Signs Associated with Tension Pneumothorax during Mechanical Ventilation

Decreased chest wall compliance
- Increased peak airway pressure (volume targeted)
- High-pressure alarm sounding (volume targeted)
- Decreased delivered V_T (both volume and pressure targeted)
- Low V_T or minute volume alarm sounding (both volume and pressure targeted)

Increased intrathoracic pressure
- Hypertension very early
- Hypotension as tension progresses
- Tachycardia initial response
- Bradycardia as cardiovascular collapse develops

Physical assessment
- Breath sounds diminished on affected side
- Chest hyperinflated on affected side
- No expiratory chest movement on affected side
- Tympanic diagnostic percussion note
- Trachea shifted to unaffected side in very severe cases

Assisted Ventilation

In patients breathing spontaneously the following should be evaluated: (1) respiratory rate, (2) V_T, (3) abdominal-chest wall coordination, (4) use of accessory muscles, (5) presence of retractions, (6) respiratory alternans, and (7) paradoxical breathing.[3] Patients exhibiting rapid, shallow breathing and discoordinate ventilatory patterns are exerting significant effort to breathe and work loads may be fatiguing.[4] Adjustments to enhance a more appropriate ventilatory pattern are normally necessary (e.g., increasing synchronized intermittent mandatory ventilation [SIMV] rate, increase pressure support ventilation [PSV] level, discontinue continuous positive pressure airway pressure [CPAP]/T-piece trial) (see Ch. 87).

Chest Assessment

Auscultation and palpation of the chest wall provide invaluable information regarding the patient's pulmonary status. Chest wall and diaphragm movement can be evaluated by palpation; distribution of gas flow and presence of secretions and bronchospasm, as well as the likelihood of air trapping can be evaluated by auscultation. It is particularly important to auscultate the chest before and after bronchial hygiene, aerosol therapy, and suctioning, to evaluate the efficacy of therapy.

Finally, touching the patient can help identify the presence of fever, poor peripheral perfusion, and diaphoresis. (See Ch. 44 for more details on clinical assessment.)

MONITORING OF GAS EXCHANGE

Mechanical ventilatory support is normally instituted because of inadequate gas exchange, and as a result, monitoring of gas exchange is a key element in the management of the patient–ventilator system. Normally, arterial blood gas levels are assessed when clinical signs of alterations in gas exchange are noted, or when changes are made in settings of the ventilator. However, continuous monitoring of arterial blood gases by indwelling arterial probes is rapidly becoming a reality[5] and is expected to become an integral part of the intensive care unit (ICU) in the future.

Pulse oximetry is useful during mechanical ventilation of those patients in whom oxygenation is a major problem. Patients with adult respiratory distress syndrome (ARDS) or requiring high inspired O_2 fraction (F_{IO_2}) (0.50 or more) and positive end-expiratory pressure (PEEP) (more than 5 cmH_2O) should be monitored continuously with pulse oximetry, although in today's ICU is it unlikely that pulse oximetry would not be available for any patient requiring ventilatory support. As noted in Chapter 47, we do not recommend the use of capnometry in the critically ill patient, since there is a high probability that end-tidal PCO_2 ($P_{ET}CO_2$) and $PaCO_2$ will change in opposite directions because of alterations in ventilation/perfusion ($\dot{V}/\dot{Q}$) relationships.[6] (See Ch. 47 for more details on assessment of gas exchange.)

MONITORING PULMONARY MECHANICS

The term *pulmonary mechanics* has been used to encompass the assessment of the resistance, both elastic and nonelastic, of the patient–ventilator system, as well as of the patient's ability to spontaneously ventilate (respiratory rate and V_T), and of the patient's ventilatory reserve or ventilatory muscle capability (vital capacity [VC] and maximum inspiratory pressure). All of these variables provide direct data on the status of the pulmonary system. If monitored regularly, they help in defining the ongoing status of the pulmonary system and also in determining when ventilatory support can be decreased or discontinued.

Patients receiving partial ventilatory support require evaluation and documentation of spontaneous V_T and rate whenever the patient–ventilator system is evaluated. Increased spontaneous V_T may be the first indication that the patient is capable of assuming a greater role in the maintenance of ventilation. Decreases in V_T, with increases in respiratory rate, usually indicate decreased ventilatory capability and increased effort required to maintain gas exchange. This should alert the clinician to the possible need for increased ventilatory support. Decreased respiratory rate in the intermittent mandatory ventilation (IMV)/SIMV mode occurs when patients sleep or are sedated but, if associated with an increased V_T, may also be an indication of greater spontaneous ventilatory capability.

V_T and rate do provide data on a patient's spontaneous breathing capabilities; however, the best indicator of ventilatory reserve is the patient's ability to breathe deeply.[7] Thus, careful monitoring of VC and maximum inspiratory pressure (see Chs. 52 and 86) provides a useful index of ventilatory reserve. Increases in these values are associated with an increase in ventilatory reserve and a greater probability of sustained spontaneous ventilation.[2] If ventilatory reserve is improving, a decrease in ventilatory support may be indicated (e.g., decreasing IMV/SIMV rate, decreasing PSV level, switching from assist/control [A/C] to IMV/SIMV or PSV, or beginning weaning).[8]

Compliance and Resistance

Estimations of system compliance and inspiratory resistance provide quantitative data on the progression of pulmonary pathology.[9] They reflect the stiffness of the system and gas flow resistance, although inspiratory resistance only provides a gross evaluation of system resistance and is greatly affected by the artificial airway. As noted later in this section, expiratory resistance provides more useful and sensitive information regarding resistance to gas flow and response to therapeutic interventions. Compliance and resistance should be periodically evaluated in all mechanically ventilated patients. Values determined in this setting are not consistent with those obtained in the pulmonary function laboratory; however, when measurements are consistently determined, changes over time reflect changes in elastic or nonelastic resistance to ventilation.

An inspiratory positive pressure curve with a 1.5-second inflation hold (Fig. 83-1) provides a gross estimate of

1. The amount of pressure required to overcome total patient–ventilator system impedance to ventilation (peak inspiratory pressure [PIP])

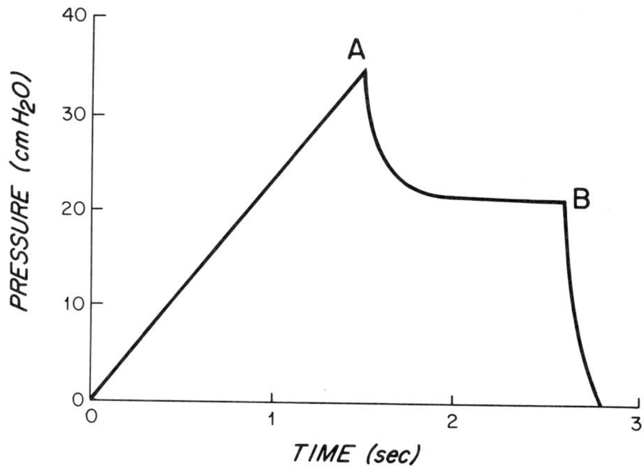

Figure 83-1. An inspiratory positive pressure waveform with a 1.5-second inflation hold. As noted in the text, the plateau pressure is a reflection of the peak alveolar pressure (point A, peak airway pressure; point B, plateau pressure).

2. Total system elastic resistance (compliance) to ventilation (plateau pressure [P_{plat}])
3. Total system nonelastic inspiratory resistance to ventilation (PIP minus P_{plat})

It must be remembered that these pressures are reflective of the total patient–ventilator system, and thus may markedly differ from true patient values. It is also essential that these data be determined during a passive inflation and with a square wave flow pattern. If the flow pattern is other than square wave, estimation of inspiratory resistance is erroneous.

Compliance

Effective static compliance (CES) is determined by dividing the measured exhaled-, or corrected expired-mechanical VT (VET) by the P_{plat}, minus the total PEEP level. (It should be remembered that the P_{plat} is equal to the peak alveolar pressure.) A measured exhaled mechanical VT is used because it is a more accurate estimation of the volume received on the previous breath than the machine volume setting. In addition, the exhaled volume, if measured other than at the patient endotracheal tube, must be corrected for compressible volume loss (i.e., the volume compressed in the ventilator circuit per delivered pressure [in centimeters of water] [P_{plat} − total PEEP]). Compressible volume factors (CF) equal about 2 to 5 mL/cmH_2O for most ventilator circuits. Total PEEP is subtracted from the P_{plat} to reflect the true static pressure maintaining gas in the airway. Total PEEP is equal to the applied PEEP ($PEEP_A$) plus any auto-PEEP ($PEEP_I$) measured above the applied PEEP.

Assuming that VET is 1000 mL, P_{plat} is 50 cmH_2O, $PEEP_A$ is 10 cmH_2O, $PEEP_I$ is 5 cmH_2O, and CF is 2 mL/cmH_2O, then

$$C_{ES} = \frac{V_{ET} - [(P_{plat} - PEEP_A - PEEP_I)(CF)]}{P_{plat} - PEEP_A - PEEP_I}$$

$$= \frac{1000 - [(50 - 10 - 5)(2\ mL)]}{50 - 10 - 5\ cmH_2O}$$

$$= \frac{930\ mL}{35\ cmH_2O}$$

$$= 26.6\ mL/cmH_2O$$

Many clinicians exclude the use of the CF because consistent ventilator set-ups are used, and as a result, a consistent error is associated with each calculation. This is acceptable because compliance calculations during ventilatory support are only gross estimates of system compliance. The key factor is assurance that all calculations are performed in a consistent manner. We have used the term *effective static compliance* in this calculation, because the value determined is an estimate of total system static compliance. Total PEEP level is subtracted from the P_{plat} because the PEEP applied is not reflective of the amount of pressure required to maintain the static VT in the system. Including PEEP in the determination of compliance increases the error in the calculation. If this error were constant, it could be tolerable; however, because PEEP levels change or are eliminated, the magnitude of the error also changes. Figure 83-2 illustrates the effect of calculating CES without PEEP correction, with applied PEEP correction only, and with applied auto-PEEP correction. Table 83-4 lists the common causes of alteration in CES and RAW (airway resistance).

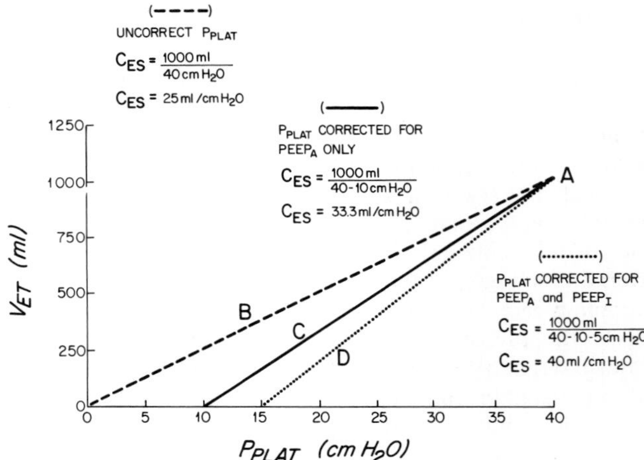

Figure 83-2. Effects of applied PEEP ($PEEP_A$) and auto-PEEP ($PEEP_I$) on determination of CES. A, P_{PLAT}; B, atmospheric pressure; C, $PEEP_A$ level; and D, $PEEP_I$. BA, compliance curve without correlation for $PEEP_A$ or $PEEP_I$; CA, compliance curve with correction for $PEEP_A$ only; DA, compliance curve for corrections for $PEEP_A$ and $PEEP_I$. (From Kacmarek,[56] with permission.)

Dynamic compliance (C_{dyn}) is an estimate of total patient–ventilator system resistance to ventilation or impedance to

Table 83-4. Causes of Static Compliance and Airway Resistance Changes

- CES decreased
  - System stiffer
    - Atelectasis
    - Consolidation
    - Pneumothorax
    - ARDS
    - Endobronchial intubation
    - Total airway obstruction
- CES increased
  - System more elastic
    - Resolution of above problems
- RAW (inspiration) increased
  - Lumen of airway decreased
    - Bronchospasm
    - Mucosal edema
    - Secretions
    - Compression of airway (tumors)
- RAW (inspiration) decreased
  - Lumen of airway increased
    - Resolution of above problems

gas movement. It is based on peak airway pressure instead of P_{plat}, and is ideally determined when gas is delivered in a square waveform.

Assuming that V_{ET} is 1000 mL, PIP is 70 cmH_2O, $PEEP_A$ is 5 cmH_2O, $PEEP_I$ is 5 cmH_2O, and CF is 2 mL/cmH_2O, then

$$C_{dyn} = \frac{V_{ET} - [PIP - PEEP_A - PEEP_I)(CF)]}{PIP - PEEP_A - PEEP_I}$$

$$= \frac{1000 - [(70 - 5 - 5)(2\ mL)]}{70 - 5 - 5\ cmH_2O}$$

$$= \frac{880\ mL}{60\ cmH_2O}$$

$$= 14.7\ mL/cmH_2O$$

C_{dyn} is less useful than C_{ES} because it does not differentiate between alterations in values that are a result of changes in elastic from those that are a result of nonelastic system resistance to ventilation. For this reason the determination of C_{ES}, along with an estimate of system resistance, is recommended.

A decrease in C_{ES} indicates the system is stiffer. Decreased C_{ES} occurs with endotracheal intubation, total airway obstruction, atelectasis, consolidation, pneumothorax, or ARDS.[10] Basically, any change that limits the expandability of the system decreases C_{ES}. An increase in C_{ES} signals an improvement of pulmonary pathology, expansion of an atelectatic area, the resolution of a consolidation, decompression of a pneumothorax, or the resolution of ARDS. Increased C_{ES} may signal the need to evaluate the level of ventilatory support provided, whereas a decrease in C_{ES} may indicate the need for greater ventilatory support, increased PEEP levels, or bronchial hygiene.

It is important to note that single values for C_{ES} have limited usefulness, although markedly decreased values do indicate a stiffer system. More appropriately, the trend in C_{ES} should be followed. If the C_{ES} is decreasing, the cause should be determined and appropriate action taken. When C_{ES} increases, appropriate steps to decrease therapy or level of support should be taken. Determination of C_{ES} at different levels of PEEP or delivered V_T is useful in determining the proper settings for these variables (see Ch. 82).

Resistance

Nonelastic resistance to ventilation, or system resistance (R_{AW}), can be estimated by dividing the difference between PIP and P_{plat} by the peak flow rate, provided the flow rate is delivered in a square wave pattern. With a sine wave pattern, peak flow occurs at mid-inspiration and with a decelerating pattern, peak flow occurs at the beginning of inspiration; thus the pressure differential (PIP − P_{plat}) may grossly underestimate the pressure necessary to overcome system resistance if a square waveform is not provided.

Assuming that PIP is 70 cmH_2O, P_{plat} is 50 cmH_2O, and peak flow is 60 L/min, then patient/ventilatory system resistance (R_{AW}) is calculated as follows:

$$R_{AW} = \frac{(PIP - P_{plat})}{\text{peak flow}}$$

$$= \frac{70 - 50\ cmH_2O}{60\ L/min}$$

$$= 0.33\ cmH_2O/L/min$$

This calculation is a very gross estimate of system resistance, because the flow rate delivered by ventilators is inconsistent. Even if a ventilator is designed to provide a square waveflow, an end-inspiratory flow taper is common with many systems. For this reason, many practitioners simply record PIP and P_{plat}, but do not actually calculate R_{AW}.

Increases in R_{AW} are caused by pathophysiologic changes that decrease airway lumen: edema, partial airway obstruction, or bronchospasm. Thus, bronchial hygiene therapy or aerosolized sympathomimetics may be indicated when estimates of R_{AW} increase. In addition, the pressure necessary to overcome R_{AW} can be decreased by one of two alterations in gas delivery. First, inspiratory flow rate can be decreased. Since the magnitude of PIP is dependent on flow, decreased flow lowers PIP. However, a decrease in peak flow increases inspiratory time.

Thus, if V_T is 1000 mL (1.0 L), peak flow ($\dot{V}$) is 60 L/min (1.0 L/s), then inspiratory time (t_I) can be calculated as follows:

$$\dot{V} = \frac{V_T}{t_I}$$

$$t_I = \frac{V_T}{\dot{V}}$$

$$= \frac{1.0\ L}{1.0\ L/s}$$

$$= 1.0\ s$$

However, if the peak flow is decreased to 30 L/min, and V_T is 1000 mL (1.0 L) and $\dot{V}$ is 30 L/min (0.5 L/s), then

$$\dot{V} = \frac{V_T}{t_I}$$

$$t_I = \frac{V_T}{\dot{V}}$$

$$= \frac{1.0\ L}{0.5\ L/s}$$

$$= 2.0\ s$$

The change in flow rate may have markedly decreased peak airway pressure, but because of the increased inspiratory time, the mean airway pressure and mean intrathoracic pressure may have increased. Caution must be exercised whenever a change such as this is performed. Second, the peak airway pressure can also be decreased by decreasing the V_T and increasing the rate, but maintaining a consistent minute volume. Again, if this maneuver is performed, care must be taken to evaluate the effect on gas exchange and cardiovascular status. In general, the source of the increased RAW should be treated with only minor alterations in the relationship between flow rate, VT, and rate attempted. As with CES, RAW measurements that are evaluated over time are a more valuable index of change in the system than is a single value.

It has become increasingly more apparent that the endotracheal tube is the primary resistor in the patient–ventilatory system[11,12] and that evaluation of inspiratory resistance to gas flow varies little with pharmacologic treatment, unless significant bronchospasm is present.[13,14] Also, airways narrow during exhalation and expiratory flow through an endotracheal tube results in greater resistance to flow than does inspiratory flow because of turbulence at the point of entry (trachea) into the endotracheal tube.[15] All of the above (taken together) have led clinicians to evaluate expiratory resistance in addition to inspiratory resistance. The evaluation of expiratory resistance is more complex than inspiratory resistance and requires the measurement of expiratory flow.

The Siemens Servo mechanics package uses the following equation to calculate expiratory resistance from the expiratory gas flow, provided a short inspiratory hold is incorporated in the gas delivery system (Fig. 83-3):

$$\text{Expiratory resistance} = \frac{\text{pause pressure} - \text{early expiratory pressure}}{\text{early expiratory flow}}$$

As noted, expiratory resistance is more difficult to determine than inspiratory resistance. However, expiratory resistance is very useful in determining the response to bronchodilators or the probability of a given patient developing air trapping and auto-PEEP.

MONITORING OF AUTO-PEEP

Detailed discussions on pathophysiology, measurement, and management of auto-PEEP are provided in Chapter 76. Suffice it to say that the monitoring of auto-PEEP is critical in the management of any patient with airflow obstruction, rapid ventilatory rates, or short expiratory times and should be a part of the routine evaluation of all patients. We particularly note the presence of auto-PEEP in the medical ICU when rates are 8 breaths per minute or more. The frequency of auto-PEEP development has been reported to be 40 percent of all patients ventilated.[16,17]

PRESSURE, FLOW, AND VOLUME WAVEFORMS

The ability to monitor pressure, flow, and volume waveforms has become a reality on most mechanical ventilators. In addition, free-standing monitoring systems designed to display waveforms, as well as to produce other derived variables are being manufactured. Of all the data we are able to accumulate at the bedside of the ventilator-dependent patient, the single variable most reflective of the patient's interaction with the mechanical ventilator is the airway pressure waveform. It is available on any patient who is mechanically ventilated, provided a pressure transducer and display screen are available. In most ICUs pressure waveforms can be displayed on the cardiac monitor screen, provided a pressure measuring port is available. If the waveform cannot be displayed continuously, it can at least be displayed during periods of patient evaluation.

The question, where is the ideal location to measure pres-

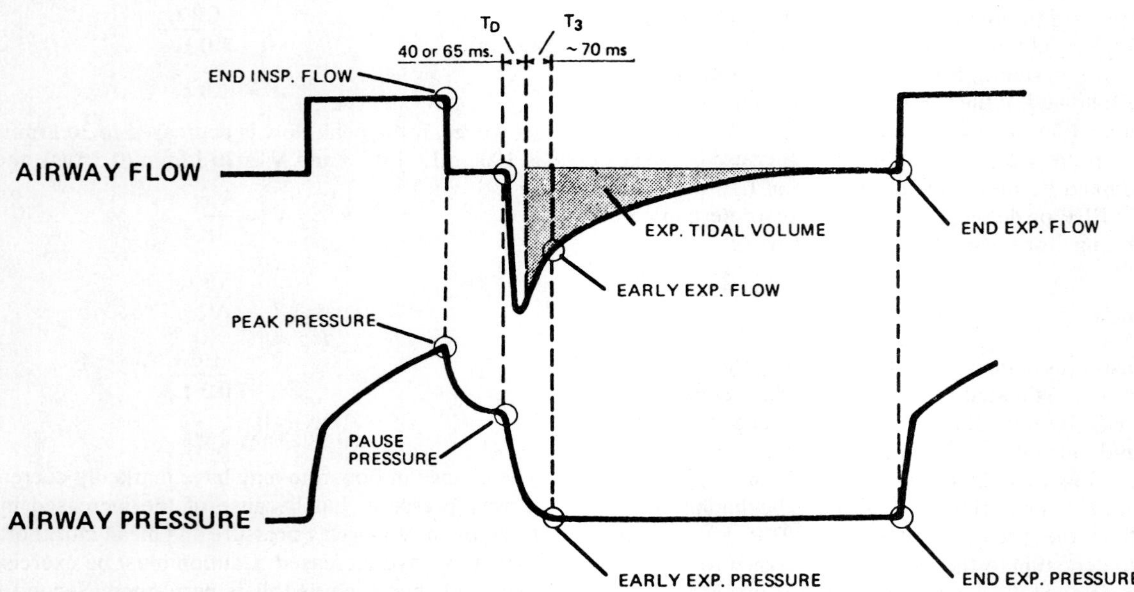

Figure 83-3. Airway pressure and flow waveforms with an inflation hold, depicting the methodology used by the Siemens mechanics calculator for the determination of expiratory resistance. The pressure differential used is pause pressure minus early expiratory pressure with expiratory flow measured at the same time early expiratory pressure is recorded. (From Siemens,[57] with permission.)

Table 83-5. Information Provided by Pressure, Flow, and Volume Waveforms

Pressure waveform
Trigger sensitivity
Inadequate inspiratory peak flow
Patient dyssynchrony
Auto-PEEP
Compliance
Resistance
Flow waveform
Auto-PEEP
Patient dyssynchrony
Response to bronchodilator
Volume waveform
Quantification of system leak

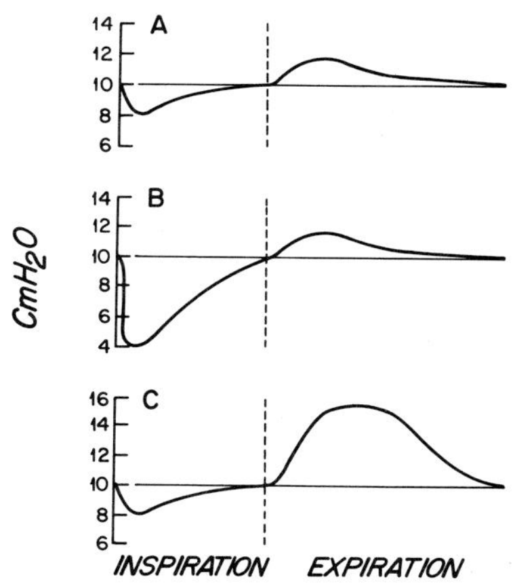

Figure 83-4. Airway pressure waveforms during continuous flow CPAP. (**A**) Normal pressure deflections ±2 cmH_2O during unstressed breathing. (**B**) Excessive inspiratory effort. (**C**) Excessive expiratory effort. (From Kacmarek and Goulet,[19] with permission.)

sure waveform, has been debated.[18] In our opinion, the closer to the source of pressure generation, the greater the reflection of patient effort and actual pressure affecting the lung itself. Most mechanical ventilators measure pressure and flow internal to the ventilator itself. As a result, higher than actual pressures are displayed during inspiration and lower than actual pressures are displayed during expiration; during spontaneous breathing, pressure measured internal to the ventilator may grossly underestimate the pressure within the patient's airway. Ideally, pressure should be monitored at the tip of the endotracheal tube, so that the effect of the endotracheal tube on patient effort or pressure dampening can be assessed. However, the technology to allow this on a routine basis is not currently available. As a result, we recommend routine monitoring of pressure and flow at the Y of the ventilator circuit (Table 83-5).

Pressure Waveform

As noted above and in Chapter 76, the airway pressure waveform is useful for determination of compliance, resistance, and auto-PEEP; however, its primary value is in the identification of patient effort and patient–ventilator synchrony.[19] Figure 83-4 depicts airway pressure curves during CPAP, measured at the Y of the ventilator circuit. Figure 83-4A depicts the normal inspiratory and expiratory pressure changes during continuous flow CPAP; Figure 83-4B illus-

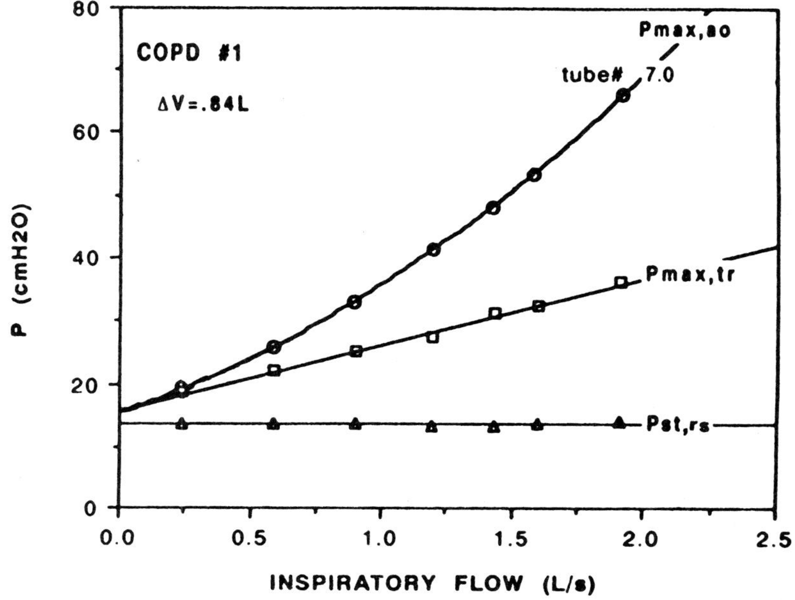

Figure 83-5. Plots of peak airway pressure (Pmax), peak tracheal pressure (Pmax,tr), and static (plateau) airway pressure (Pst,rs) at varying peak inspiratory flows in a COPD patient intubated with a no. 7 endotracheal tube. Note the marked increase and difference between Pmax and Pmax,tr as peak flow increases. However, Pst,rs remains constant because actual volume delivered was unchanged. Remember Pst,rs is equal to peak alveolar pressure. (From Milic-Emili et al.,[20] with permission.)

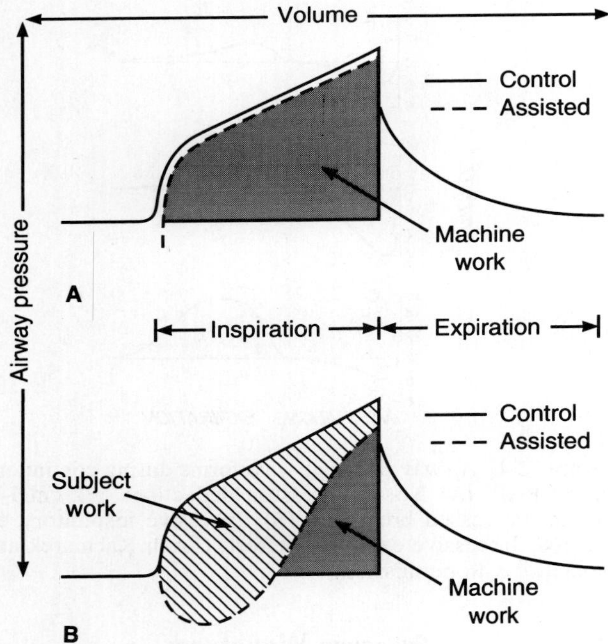

Figure 83-6. **(A)** Plot of an ideal pressure-time waveform during volume targeted ventilation. **(B)** Plot of actual pressure-time curve (dotted line) superimposed on the ideal curve. Note the scooped-out actual pressure waveform. The hatched area reflects the work performed by the patient during assisted volume-targeted ventilation. This type of actual pressure waveform is indicative of inadequate peak inspiratory flow or too lengthy an inspiratory time. (From Marini et al.,[21] with permission.)

trates increased effort during inspiration; and Figure 83-4C illustrates increased effort during expiration. Although these are not precisely the same curves noted during demand-flow CPAP, the initial pressure deflections are the same. When evaluating airway pressure waveforms during spontaneous breathing, one must remember that the pressure deflections only represent the work imposed by the mechanical ventilator system. To determine the work imposed by the endotracheal tube and the ventilator, the waveform measured at the carina must be evaluated. As noted in Figure 83-5, the pressure difference across the endotracheal tube is dependent on tube size and peak inspiratory flow.[20] However, it is fair to say that during spontaneous breathing, if airway pressures are decreasing 3 to 5 cmH_2O, then carinal pressures are decreasing about 10 to 15 cmH_2O and pleural pressures are decreasing about 15 to 20 cmH_2O. Thus, in spite of the dampened pressure curve at the Y, reasonable assumptions regarding effort can be made from these data.

Similar information is available for airway pressure curves during ventilatory assistance.[21] Figure 83-6 is an airway pressure-time curve during volume-limited ventilation. The top curve depicts the ideal waveform during controlled ventilation; the bottom curve shows the ideal superimposed on an actual curve during assisted ventilation. Note the scooped-out actual pressure curve. This waveform always indicates patient effort is exceeding the ventilator's ability to provide flow. Figures 83-7 to 83-9 also depict situations in which patients are dyssynchronous with the mechanical ventilator, or for whom triggering effort is excessive.

Calculation of total work of breathing can also be determined from the airway pressure-time trace during constant-flow ventilation if passive inflation is ensured.[22] This estimate is determined by multiplying the average inflation pressure (P_{avg}) by the V_T (Fig. 83-10). Under the above conditions, P_{avg} is a reflection of total system impedance to gas movement and is equal to work of breathing, divided by V_T. P_{avg} is calculated from the pressure-time curve by the following equation:

$$P_{avg} = \frac{PIP - (P_{plat} - PEEP_{total})}{2}$$

where $PEEP_{total}$ is equal to applied PEEP plus auto-PEEP.

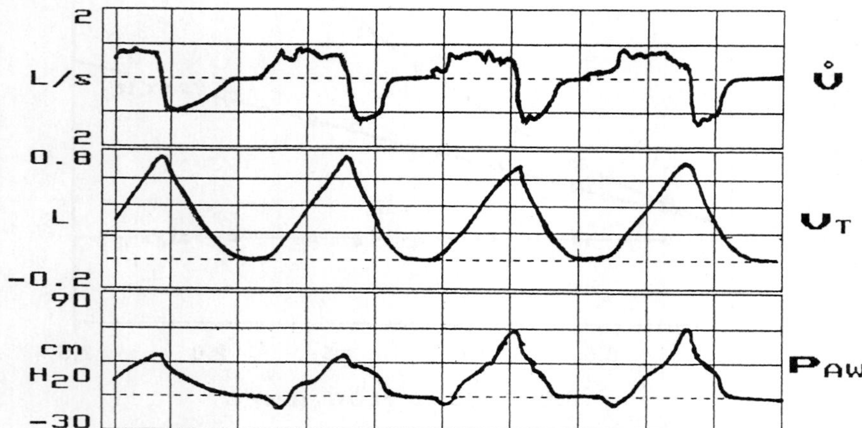

Figure 83-7. Airway pressure (PAW), flow (V̇) and volume (VT) waveforms during volume-targeted ventilation. Note the marked alterations in the airway pressure trace indicative of patient dyssynchrony. This patient's dyssynchrony is also reflected in the inability of the ventilator to maintain a constant flow pattern. (Waveforms recorded with a Bicore CP-100 monitor.)

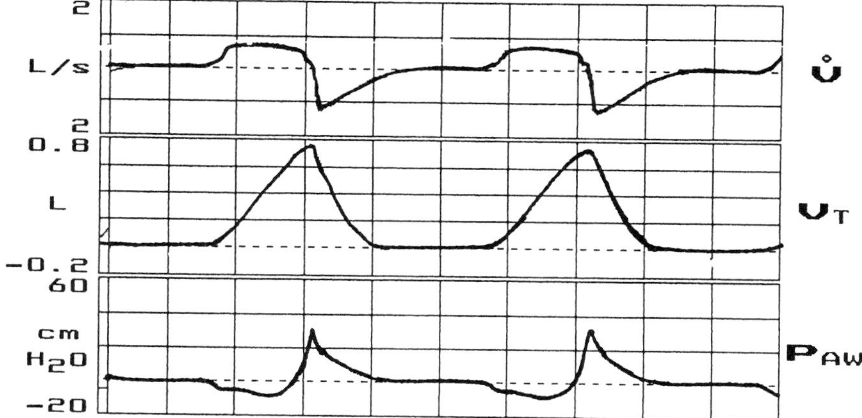

Figure 83-8. Airway pressure (PAW), flow (V̇), and volume (VT) waveforms during volume-targeted ventilation. The PAW illustrates grossly inadequate peak inspiratory flow. This patient's work of breathing is excessive, in spite of ventilatory assistance. (Waveforms recorded with a Bicore CP-100 monitor.)

Flow Waveform

As discussed above, expiratory resistance can be determined from the expiratory flow waveform. In addition, as described in Chapter 76 and illustrated in Figure 83-11, the presence, but not the level of auto-PEEP can be identified from the flow-time curve. The effectiveness of bronchodilator therapy can also be evaluated from the expiratory flow-time curve (Fig. 83-12), by evaluating the shape of the curve, the peak expiratory flow, and the length of time it takes for expiratory flow to return to zero. Effective bronchodilator therapy should increase peak expiratory flow and decrease the time for expiratory flow to return to zero.

For pressure-control ventilation to be most effective, inspiratory flow should fall to zero before the end of inspiration, and in cases with lengthy inspiratory times, an infla-

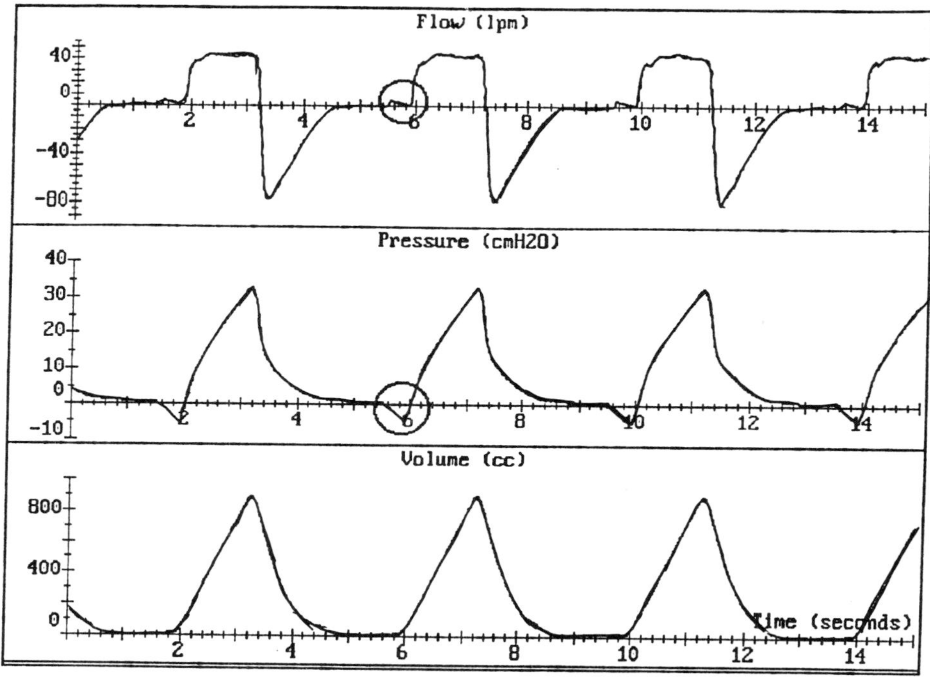

Figure 83-9. Flow, pressure, and volume waveforms in a patient for whom the trigger sensitivity is inappropriately set. A 5- to 6-cmH_2O pressure change is necessary to trigger the ventilator (circled area, pressure curve). Flow is measurable at the airway (circled area, flow curve) but the volume-targeted breath is not activated. (Waveforms recorded with a Ventrak monitor.)

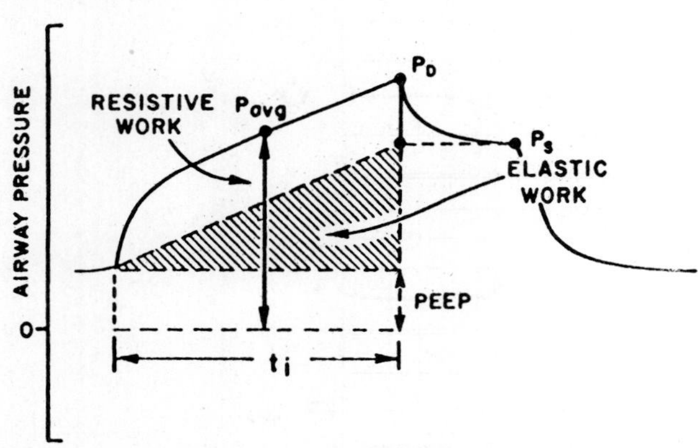

Figure 83-10. Airway pressure-time trace during passive inflation with the ventilator delivering a volume-targeted breath in a square waveform. The average airway pressure (P_{avg} in this setting is equal to the work necessary to overcome the total impedance of the patient–ventilator system. P_D, peak inspiratory pressure; P_S, plateau pressure. (From Truwit and Marini,[22] with permission.)

tion hold should be established. Figure 83-13 illustrates two pressure control delivery settings: one in which inspiratory flow returns to zero before end-inspiration, and the second, in which it does not. Finally, a flow-time curve allows for verification of the actual flow waveform being delivered (square, decelerating, or sine).

Volume Waveform

The volume waveform displayed by most monitoring systems is simply the integration of the flow-time curve, and as a result, provides little additional data. The one exception to this is the quantification of airleak (Fig. 83-14). As noted, the volume-time trace very nicely allows for the determination of the difference between inspiratory and expiratory volume. The amount of gas lost via bronchopleural fistulas is easily quantified with volume-time curves.

Esophageal Pressure Waveform

Although rarely used clinically because of the difficulty in placing the catheter and performing measurements, esophageal catheters capable of measuring the esophageal pressure waveform are commonly used for research purposes. However, the use of esophageal pressure monitoring is becoming more commonplace due to newer instrumentation.[23,24] Normally, esophageal pressure changes in direct relationship to airway pressure. However, during spontaneous breathing the esophageal pressure change is much greater than the airway pressure change, and during controlled mechanical ventilation it may be considerably dampened. Monitoring of esophageal pressure is most useful in two distinct clinical settings: (1) management of ARDS and (2) during the management of the difficult-to-wean patient. In ARDS esophageal pressure monitoring allows for the direct estimate of the

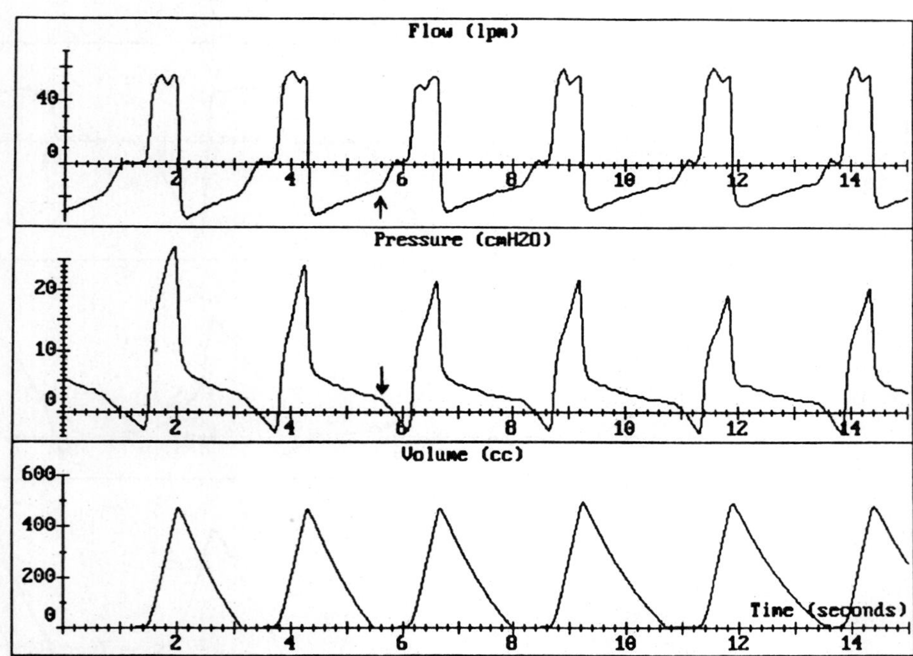

Figure 83-11. Flow, pressure, and volume waveforms in a patient dyssychronous with the mechanical ventilator (variable airway pressure curves) and with auto-PEEP present. Arrow on pressure and flow curves indicates end of exhalation. Note the considerable expiratory flow at this transition. Whenever expiratory flow does not return to zero, air trapping and auto-PEEP are present. (Waveforms recorded with a Ventrak monitor.)

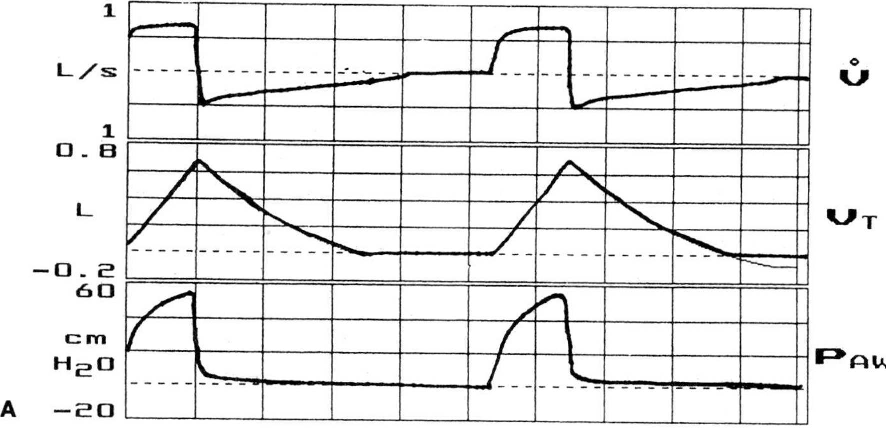

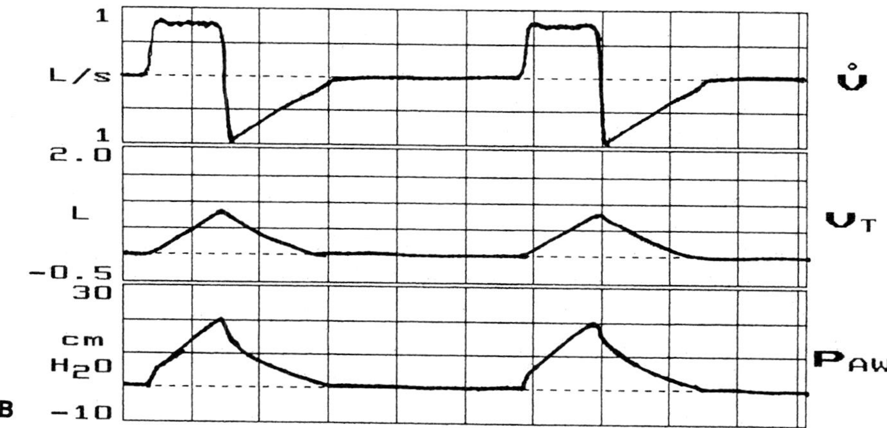

Figure 83-12. **(A)** Airway pressure (PAW), flow (V̇), and volume (VT) waveforms, before bronchodilator therapy, during volume-control ventilation. Note the peak expiratory flow is 0.5 L/s and the length of expiration is 3 seconds. **(B)** After bronchodilator therapy, peak expiratory flow increased to 1.0 L/s and expiratory time decreased to 1.5 seconds. In addition, peak airway pressure dropped considerably, while peak inspiratory flow remained constant at 0.75 L/s. (Waveforms recorded with a Bicore CP-100 monitor.)

pressure transmitted across the lung, which affects intrathoracic hemodynamics. However, the most important use of esophageal pressure is in the management of the difficult-to-wean patient, in whom auto-PEEP and increased work of breathing are common problems.

In spontaneously breathing patients the only reliable method for evaluating auto-PEEP is simultaneous evaluation of esophageal pressure and airway opening pressure or flow (see Ch. 76). The change from baseline end-expiratory esophageal pressure to the esophageal pressure that causes flow or pressure change at the airway opening equals the auto-PEEP level. To measure lung effort plus imposed work, esophageal pressure change is essential (see Pressure-Volume Loops and Chs. 26 and 52 for details on determination of work of breathing). This measurement can be invaluable in titrating partial ventilatory support levels and determining the effectiveness of various approaches to weaning, although no specific level predictive of weaning has been defined. Fiastro et al.[25] found that work loads of greater than 12 J/min were associated with failure of weaning trials.

PRESSURE-VOLUME LOOPS

A typical airway pressure-volume (P-V) loop is shown in Figure 83-15. From this loop, work, as well as compliance, are easily determined (Table 83-6). Loops shifted to the right (Fig. 83-16) always represent a decrease in total patient–ventilator system compliance. Overdistension of the lung/thorax is also easily noted from a P-V loop. In Figure 83-17,

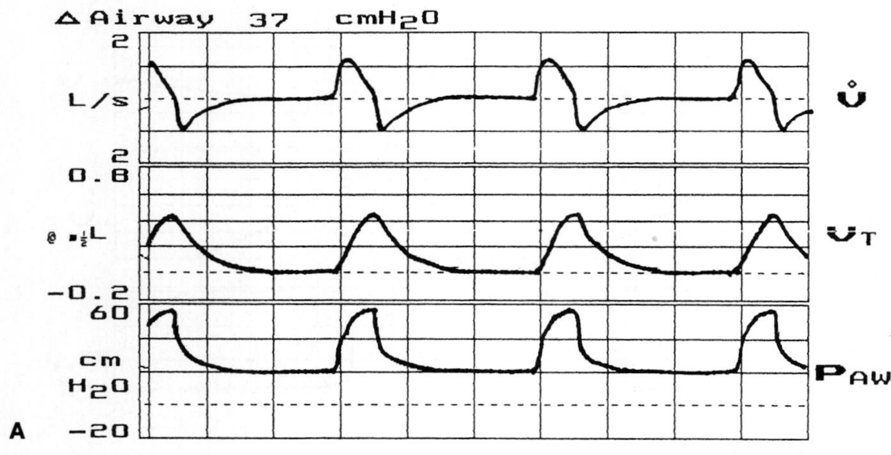

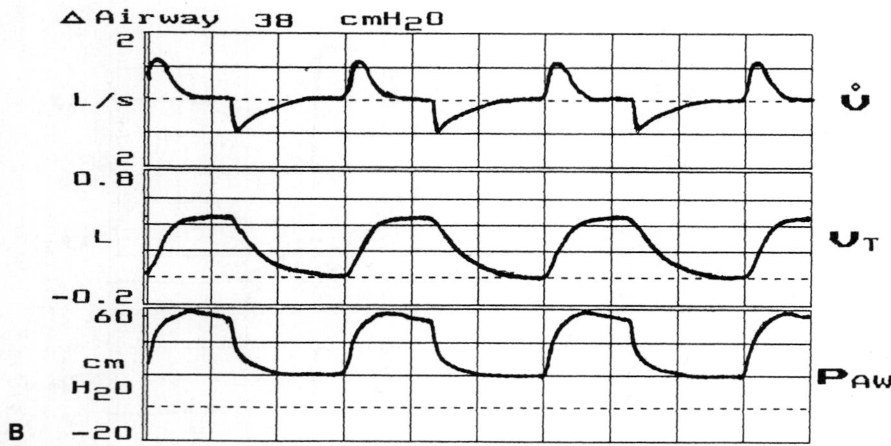

Figure 83-13. **(A)** Airway pressure (PAW), flow ($\dot{V}$), and volume (VT) waveforms during pressure-control ventilation. Note, inspiratory time is inadequate; flow rate has not returned to zero, nor is an inflation hold (zero flow period) observed. **(B)** Results of increasing inspiratory time. Now flow returns to zero about midway through the inspiratory time period. The remaining inspiratory time illustrates an end-inspiratory hold. (Waveforms recorded with a Bicore CP-100 monitor.)

note that at the top end of the loop a very small volume change occurs for a large pressure change. In this case, VT is excessive and should be decreased to ensure the VT delivery remains on the steepest aspect of the P-V curve.

The P-V loop can also be used to titrate pressure support levels. Figure 83-18A depicts spontaneous breathing in demand CPAP, Figure 83-18B shows the effect of 5 cmH_2O PSV, and Figure 83-18C, the effect of 15 cmH_2O PSV. Note the change in the contour of the loop from 0 to 15 cmH_2O PSV. Even though this is airway pressure, not esophageal pressure, the P-V loop does assist in the titration of PSV to ensure unloading imposed work of breathing. Adequacy of trigger sensitivity can be identified from a pressure-time trace; however, the effort associated with triggering is even more dramatically illustrated from an airway P-V loop (Fig. 83-19).

The esophageal P-V loop provides the same information as the airway pressure loop, only more precisely (i.e., precise titration of patient work load can be accurately per-

Table 83-6. Information Provided by Pressure-Volume and Flow-Volume Loops

Pressure-Volume Loops	Flow-Volume Loops
Compliance	Airway resistance
Trigger sensitivity	Expiratory flows
Overdistension	Response to bronchodilator
Work of breathing	

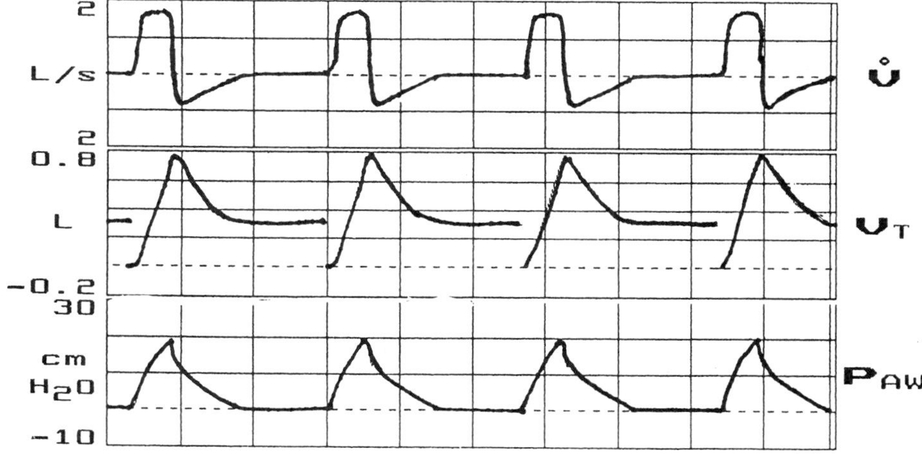

Figure 83-14. Airway pressure (PAW), flow ($\dot{V}$), and volume (V_T) in the presence of a large airleak. Note the pressure and flow waveforms provide little help in quantifying the airleak. However, one look at the volume waveform identifies a 300-mL airleak. The gap between end expiration and the next inspiration is a result of the pneumotachograph zeroing itself as inspiration begins. (Waveforms recorded with a Bicore CP-100 monitor.)

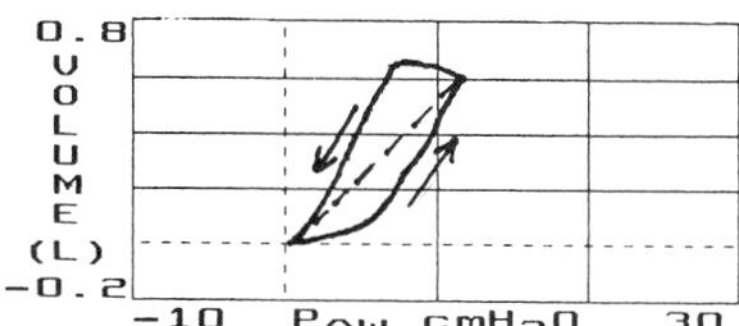

Figure 83-15. Illustration of a normal airway pressure-volume loop with actual work performed by the ventilator during volume controlled ventilation. Arrow extending upward indicates inspiration; arrow extending downward indicates expiration; dotted line connecting the points of zero flow is the compliance curve. (Loop recorded with a Bicore CP-100 monitor.)

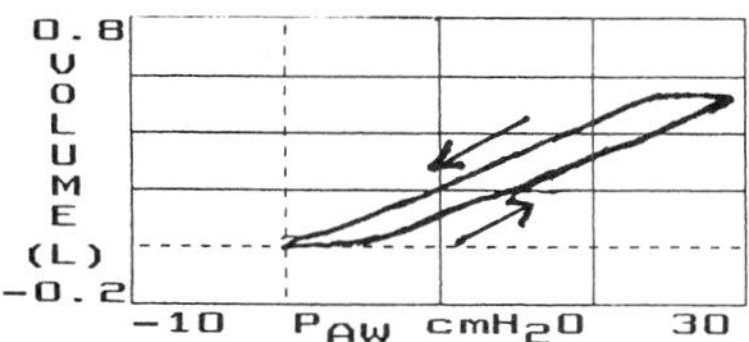

Figure 83-16. Airway pressure-volume loop during controlled volume-targeted ventilation, with compliance reduced. Note the loop is shifted downward to the right. At a slightly lower V_T than in Figure 83-15, more than twice the work is required to overcome the patient–ventilator impedance. (Loop recorded with a Bicore CP-100 monitor.)

formed only with an esophageal P-V loop. The airway P-V loop only reflects the work of breathing imposed by the ventilator system; whereas the esophageal P-V loop reflects the lung work, as well as the work to overcome the endotracheal tube and the ventilator circuit. As a result, the esophageal P-V is the ideal loop to monitor.

FLOW-VOLUME LOOPS

The flow-volume loop is useful in quantifying the effect of bronchodilator therapy. As illustrated in Figure 83-20, a dramatic change in the contour of the loop can be noted in responsive patients after bronchodilator therapy. Peak expiratory flow should increase, expiratory time should decrease, and expiratory flow at various points on the expiratory curve should increase.

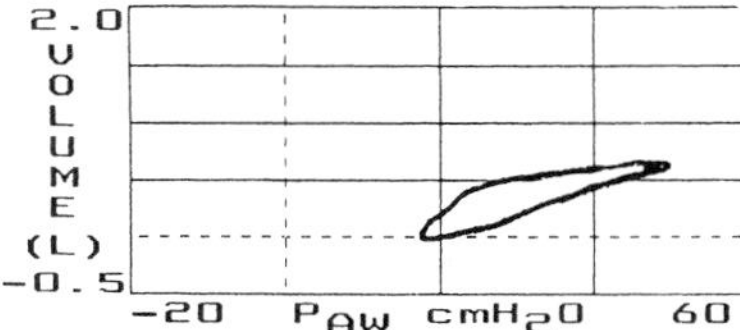

Figure 83-17. Airway pressure-volume loop in a patient with severe ARDS who is receiving volume-targeted ventilation. At the time this loop was measured V_T was 600 mL, rate was 19 breaths per minute, and peak inspiratory flow was 50 L/min. Notice the top end of the loop: very little volume change occurs during the last 10 to 15 cmH_2O pressure increase. This type of loop is illustrative of overdistension, which requires a decrease in V_T to about 500 mL. (Loop recorded with a Bicore CP-100 monitor.)

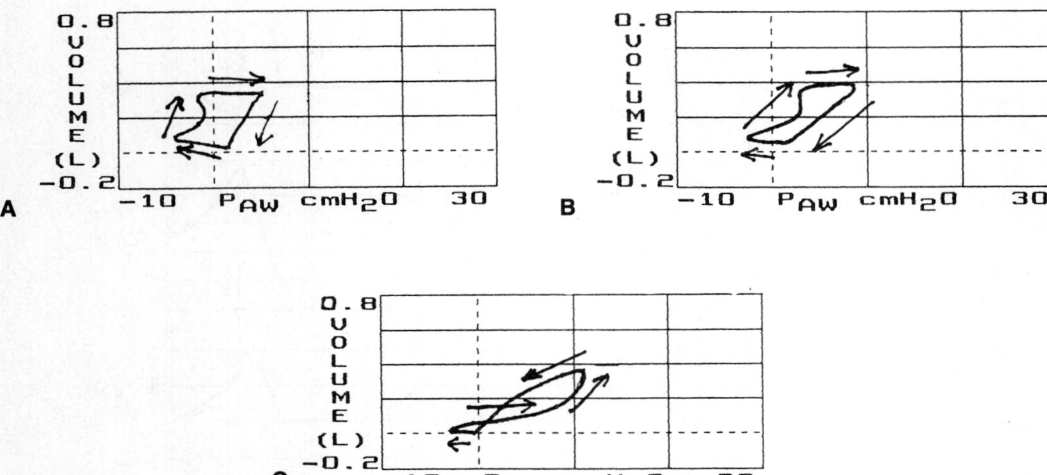

Figure 83-18. **(A)** An airway pressure-volume loop during demand CPAP. The area to the left of the vertical line indicates work imposed by the ventilator system. Although this is not lung work, the greater the area to the left of the vertical zero pressure line the greater the lung work. **(B)** Effect of 5 cmH_2O PSV on imposed work; **(C)** effect of 15 cmH_2O PSV. Ideal PSV in this setting is somewhere between 5 to 15 cmH_2O. (Loops recorded with a Bicore CP-100 monitor.)

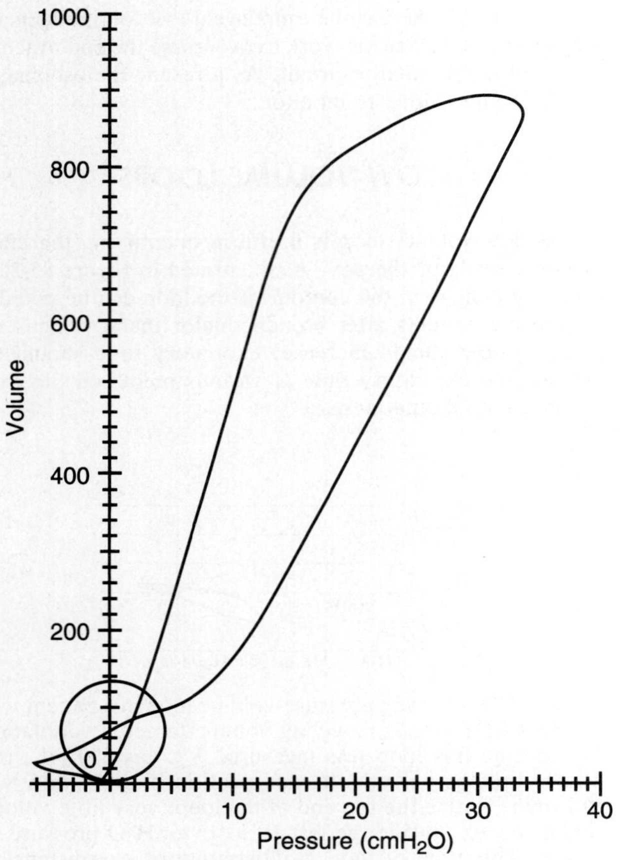

Figure 83-19. Pressure-volume loop indicating excessive effort (6 cmH_2O pressure) required to trigger ventilator. Sensitivity of ventilator requires adjustment. (Loop recorded with a Ventrak monitor.)

EVALUATION OF THE PATIENT–VENTILATOR SYSTEM

Today's mechanical ventilators are highly sophisticated computerized systems capable of being programmed to provide a spectrum of approaches to ventilatory support. However, because of their sophistication and ability to evaluate their own function, they provide a false sense of security.[26] It is all too frequently assumed that ventilators always function as programmed. Miscalibration, inadvertent alterations of settings, and technical problems or limitations all can result in the ventilator functioning differently than initially programmed.

To ensure proper function of the patient–ventilator system, one must perform independent periodic evaluations of the system. The frequency of system evaluation is dependent on the clinical status of the patient and the frequency of ventilator adjustments. In acutely ill, unstable patients, constant evaluation of the patient–ventilator system may be necessary, whereas in chronic ventilator-assisted patients, one check per shift may be adequate. In general, evaluations are performed every 4 hours.

Protocol

It is important to realize that whenever a system evaluation is made, the patient's cardiopulmonary status (as discussed above) should be evaluated. Alterations in a patient's clinical status (e.g., pneumothorax, hypotension, airway obstruction) have a profound effect on the ventilator system, as well as on the patient.

The ventilator flow sheet used by the Massachusetts Gen-

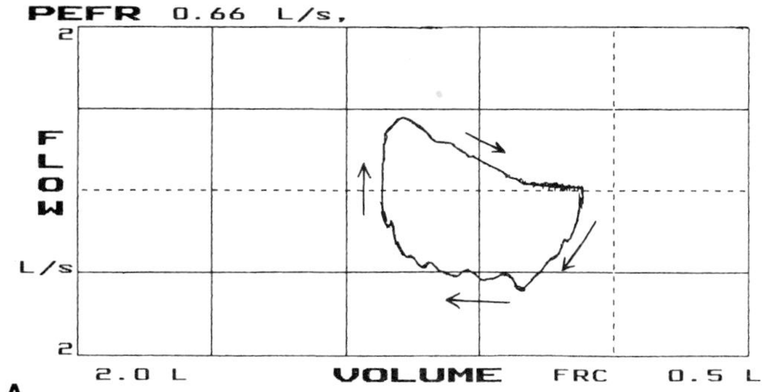

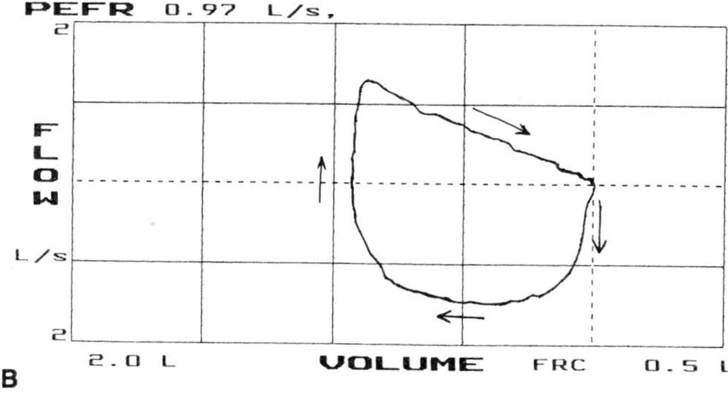

Figure 83-20. (**A**) Flow-volume loop recorded on an asthmatic patient before bronchodilator therapy. Portion of curve above dotted line represents exhalation; portion below, inspiration. Note peak expiratory flow rate (PEFR) (0.66 L/s) and scooped-out contour of expiratory curve. (**B**) Flow-volume loop measured on same patient 30 minutes after bronchodilator therapy and 100 mL V_T increase. PEFR has increased to 0.97 L/s and scooped-out contour of expiratory curve has been eliminated, indicating appropriate response to bronchodilator. (Loops recorded with a Bicore CP-100 monitor.)

eral Hospital Respiratory Care Department is shown in Figure 83-21. In addition to ventilator parameters, information concerning the type and size of the artificial airway used; the volume of gas and the gas pressure in the cuff of the artificial airway; arterial blood gas data; and the patient's spontaneous V_T, respiratory rate, VC, and maximum inspiratory pressure are included.

Whenever a ventilator check is performed, the clinician should first verify that all variables on the ventilator are set as ordered.[26] When this check is finished, it is important to review the previous clinician's notes to identify machine calibration problems. For example, the machine rate is set at 11 breaths per minute, but the machine at this setting delivers only 10 breaths per minute; or the V_T is set at 900 mL, but the machine is delivering 1000 mL. Ideally, the machine should deliver what is indicated on the control panel; however, many ventilators do not always function as designed. Any machine that is significantly out of calibration should be removed from the clinical area and scheduled for maintenance (Table 83-7).

The second step is the evaluation of what the patient is actually receiving.[26] A discrepancy between findings in step 1 and step 2 identifies variables that are out of calibration and possible machine malfunctions. Machine rate is counted, and exhaled V_T is measured with an independent spirometer. (It must be remembered that, because of compressible volume loss, the V_T setting on the machine, and the actual delivered V_T will differ.) F_IO_2 is measured with a calibrated O_2 analyzer.

Table 83-7. Protocol for Patient–Ventilator System Evaluation

Verify that all variables are set as ordered
Determine what the patient is actually receiving
Verify the alarm setting
Check system temperature and function of humidifier
Evaluate pulmonary mechanics

With continuous-flow IMV systems, the system flow is evaluated. Under all circumstances, at least four times the patient's measured spontaneous minute volume should be assured.[27] However, in most patients, 60 to 90 L/min of continuous flow is needed.[27] Adequacy of flow in meeting patients' inspiratory demands is also evaluated by observing the machine pressure manometer and airway pressure waveform and by measuring flow exiting the system via the exhalation valve. If adequate flow is being provided to meet the patient's peak inspiratory demand, the system pressure during spontaneous ventilation should only fluctuate ± 2 cmH_2O.[28] Greater fluctuations indicate increased patient effort and insufficient continuous flow. Second, continuous flow exiting the exhalation valve should be measurable during peak spontaneous inspiration.[28] If flows are inadequate, the continuous gas flow rate should be increased, being careful not to create a significant expiratory retard.

When demand valves or demand system ventilators are used to provide spontaneous inspiratory gas flow during SIMV, fluctuation of greater than ± 2 cmH_2O also indicates increased patient spontaneous inspiratory effort.[19,28] If increased effort is noted, the sensitivity setting should be evaluated or the level of mechanical ventilation increased, the patient sedated, or PSV added to unload the work during spontaneous breathing.

The pressure-time trace during mechanical breaths should be evaluated to ensure the patient is in synchrony with the ventilator. If dyssynchrony is present, evaluation of adequacy of peak flow, inspiratory time, sensitivity setting, need for bronchial hygiene (aerosol therapy, suctioning, or chest physiotherapy), or improved oxygenation and ventilation is necessary. Again, sedation may be required if the patient is out of phase with the ventilator after the above adjustments have been made.

The third step is the evaluation of alarm settings (see under Alarm Systems).[26] All patient–ventilator systems have a minimum of two alarms: ventilator disconnect and high airway pressure. In addition, continuous use of an in-line O_2 analyzer is highly recommended, as is a loss of pressure alarm when PEEP is employed.

SHEET #

MASSACHUSETTS GENERAL HOSPITAL
RESPIRATORY CARE DEPARTMENT

VENTILATOR RECORD

DATE: ____________ to 7 AM ____________

DIAGNOSIS	PERTINENT HISTORY

CURRENT PERTINENT PROBLEMS	TODAY'S THERAPEUTIC OBJECTIVES	VENT TYPE	
1.	1.	NUMBER	
2.	2.	TODAY'S WEANING SCHEDULE	
3.	3.		
4.	4.	AIRWAY TYPE @	LIP NARE
		DATE OF PLACEMENT	CUFF VOLUME

TIME	PROGRESS NOTES	SIGNATURE

FORM NO. 10173 (9/89)

Figure 83-21. Ventilator flow sheet used by the Respiratory Care Department of the Massachusetts General Hospital. (Courtesy of Massachusetts General Hospital, Boston, MA.)

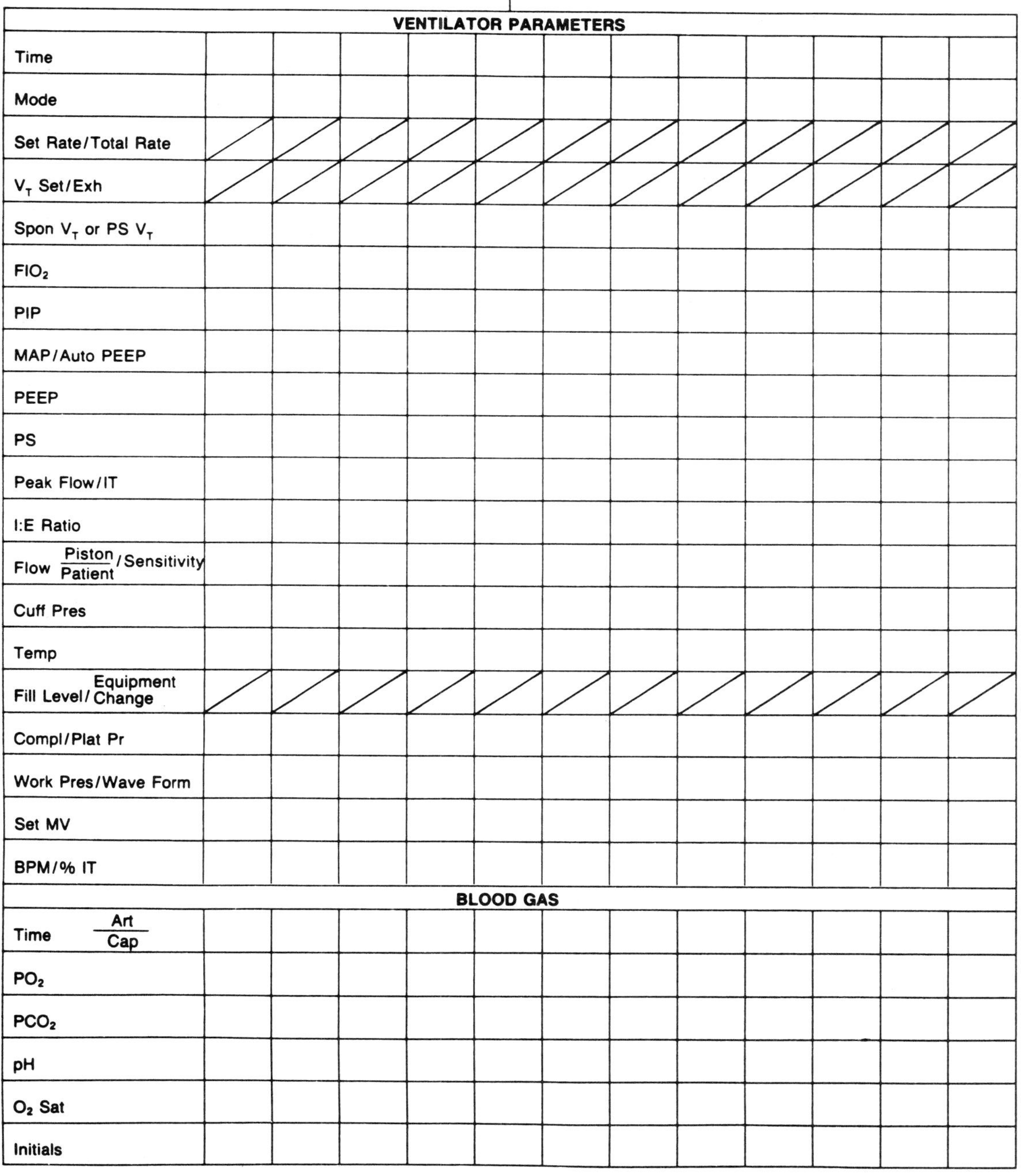

VENTILATOR RECORD

PAGE 2

VENTILATOR PARAMETERS												
Time												
Mode												
Set Rate/Total Rate												
V_T Set/Exh												
Spon V_T or PS V_T												
FIO_2												
PIP												
MAP/Auto PEEP												
PEEP												
PS												
Peak Flow/IT												
I:E Ratio												
Flow $\frac{\text{Piston}}{\text{Patient}}$/Sensitivity												
Cuff Pres												
Temp												
Fill Level/Equipment Change												
Compl/Plat Pr												
Work Pres/Wave Form												
Set MV												
BPM/% IT												
BLOOD GAS												
Time $\frac{\text{Art}}{\text{Cap}}$												
PO_2												
PCO_2												
pH												
O_2 Sat												
Initials												

Figure 83-21. (*Continued*).

VENTILATOR RECORD

Page 3

ALARMS												
Time												
O_2 High/Low												
O_2 Cal												
O_2 Sat High/Low												
HIP/POP												
LIP/Delay												
Low PEEP/CPAP												
Low V_T/Delay												
BUR/HRR												
Apnea Delay												
V_E High/Low												
Temp Alarm												
Initials												
SPONTANEOUS VENTILATION AND WEANING												
Time												
RR												
HR												
Sp V_T												
VC												
IF												
PS V_T												
% Sat												
Wean Time/Daily Total												
NON-VENTILATOR DEVICES												
Time												
FIO_2												
CPAP												
Flow O_2/Air												
Temp												
Fill Level												
Cuff Pres												
Device												
Initials												

Figure 83-21. (*Continued*).

Step 4 is the assurance of proper function of the system's humidification device.[26] Accumulation of water in system tubing can affect peak airway pressure and delivered V_T. Circuits should include water traps or have condensated water drained frequently. Fluid should always be drained away from the patient to prevent contamination. In addition, system temperature and humidifier water level should be checked. System temperature is normally maintained at 32°C to 35°C to assure the delivery of gas at 100 percent relative humidity near body temperature.

Step 5 is the assessment of the patient's pulmonary mechanics.[26] The specific variables assessed may vary with each patient. However, in all patients, PIP, spontaneous respiratory rate, and V_T, as well as P_{plat}, can easily be evaluated. Compliance and resistance, as well as VC and maximum inspiratory force are normally determined on a daily basis, or more frequently, as dictated by patient management.

TROUBLESHOOTING A MALFUNCTIONING VENTILATOR*

Any aspect of the operation of a mechanical ventilator can malfunction. However, certain problems are more common than others; specifically, system leaks, controls out of calibration, and alarm system failures. When troubleshooting a malfunctioning ventilator, the patient's status should never be compromised. Once a malfunction is noted, the patient should be disconnected from the mechanical ventilator and manually ventilated. If the malfunction cannot be readily identified and rectified, a different ventilator should be used and the malfunctioning unit sent for repair.

Method of Finding Leaks

During initial set-up and calibration, many ventilators perform a self-test that ensures a competent system, without significant leaks. In older units, where this is not provided, an independent evaluation of the circuit integrity must be performed (Table 83-8). In spite of assurance of system integrity at the onset of ventilatory support, system leaks can develop anytime during continuous ventilatory support. The most common source of leaks is the humidifier, particularly if the humidifier is periodically opened for refilling. The second most common source is worn-out diaphragms on exhalation valves. Third, small holes in both disposable and permanent large-bore tubing is common. If the presence of a leak is established and the source cannot be identified, the complete circuit should be changed. If this change does not correct the problem, the leak may be internal, and the machine should be removed from the patient area to be serviced (Table 83-9).

Table 83-8. Test for System Leaks[a]

1. Set high-pressure alarm at maximum
2. Set V_T at 1.0 L
3. Occlude patient Y and prevent exhalation
4. Deliver V_T

[a] Pressures to 80 cmH_2O should be held for 2 to 4 seconds; if not, leak exists.

Table 83-9. Primary Causes of Ventilator System Leaks

Humidifier
Exhalation valve diaphragm
Connections and tubing
Internal machine leak

(From Kacmarek,[26] with permission.)

Machine Calibration

Theoretically, if a ventilator is to deliver 10 breaths per minute, an independent assessment should verify that 10 breaths per minute are delivered. However, each manufacturer lists a tolerance range for all variables on mechanical ventilators. Thus, the rate setting may have a ±10 percent error or the V_T setting may have a ±5 percent error. Whenever the difference between a set and delivered variable exceeds the manufacturer's tolerance ranges, the ventilator should be removed from patient care and sent for servicing.

Alarm Systems

Patient–ventilator alarm systems are designed to notify clinicians of system malfunctions or changes in a patient's clinical status. Ideally, these alarms should notify the clinician of an ongoing problem, not a single event.[29] Unfortunately, few ventilator manufacturers have included "smart" alarms on their ventilators. As a result, mechanical ventilators contribute greatly to the noise pollution in the ICU and program clinicians to disregard all alarms.[29,30] Thus, alarms must be appropriately set and carefully monitored to avoid their simply becoming a nuisance.[30]

Generally, all ventilators have nonadjustable alarms that identify machine function, presence of electrical power, and pressurized gases. The clinician, however, must set the alarms associated with gas delivery (Table 83-10).

System pressure alarms are generally one of three types: (1) high pressure, (2) low pressure, and (3) loss of PEEP. High-pressure alarms are designed to identify an acute increase in system pressure and should be set about 10 cmH_2O above the average peak airway pressure. The actual level above peak airway pressure is dependent on the patient's clinical status. In patients tolerating ventilation well, with fairly stable peak airway pressure, setting the alarm less than 10 cmH_2O above peak airway pressure may be appropriate.

* Adapted from Kacmarek,[26] with permission.

Table 83-10. Setting of Ventilator Alarms

Alarm	Setting
High minute ventilation	10–15% > set or target minute volume
Low minute ventilation	10–15% < set or target minute volume
High V_T	10–15% > set or target V_T
Low V_T	10–15% < set or target V_T
High-system pressure	About 10 cmH_2O > average peak airway pressure
Low-system pressure	5–10 cmH_2O < average peak airway pressure
Loss of PEEP	3–5 cmH_2O < PEEP level
O_2 analyzer	0.05 > F_IO_2 0.05 < F_IO_2

However, in the agitated patient whose peak airway pressure fluctuates considerably, the high-pressure alarm may have to be set 10 cmH_2O above peak airway pressure or greater, to prevent periodic alarming simply because of agitation. In most ventilators, the high-pressure alarm, venting of additional pressure and volume, and the termination of inspiration coincide. However, in a few ventilators these variables may not apply. If machines with independent controls for the high-pressure alarm and pressure release are used, they should be set with the alarm 2 or 3 cmH_2O lower than the pressure that results in pressure release. If the high-pressure pop-off is set at a level lower than the high-pressure alarm, clinicians may not be alerted to the presence of increased peak airway pressures. This increase may result in a significant decrease in ventilation if most of the V_T is vented. This scenario is particularly serious if a pneumothorax or endobronchial intubation should occur.

The low-pressure alarm is designed to identify system leaks that result in a decrease in peak airway pressure. This alarm should be set 5 to 10 cmH_2O below average peak airway pressure.

The loss of PEEP alarm is used to identify minor leaks in the system, which cause PEEP levels to decrease, or to identify circumstances in which increased patient spontaneous inspiratory effort causes PEEP level to fall significantly. Generally, the loss of PEEP alarm is set 3 to 5 cmH_2O below PEEP level. The actual setting is dependent on patient spontaneous inspiratory effort. The greater the fluctuation in PEEP level during inspiration, the lower the setting.

Continuous monitoring of F_IO_2 with an independent O_2 analyzer is highly recommended. This alarm should be able to recognize increased or decreased F_IO_2. Generally, the alarm is set to sound if F_IO_2 increases or decreases by 0.05.

During pressure-limited and spontaneous breathing modes the setting of V_T and minute ventilation alarms is critical. Generally in pressure-limited ventilation, both the V_T and minute ventilation alarms are set about 10 to 15 percent above and below the set or targeted volumes. As with pressure alarms, these ranges may vary, depending on patient status. During CPAP, similar ranges are set; however, frequently, greater variation exists than during mechanical ventilation.

The function of all alarms should be evaluated with each ventilator check. This evaluation is accomplished by creating the circumstance under which the alarm should sound (e.g., causing the system pressure to increase, creating system leaks, and exposing the O_2 analyzer to increased and decreased F_IO_2).

As a final note, even the most sophisticated alarm will function only when activated. Thus, as a general rule, patient–ventilator system alarms should *never* be turned off. When patients are disconnected from the ventilator for short periods (e.g., for suctioning) time delays only should be activated.

SYSTEMATIC ALTERATION IN LEVEL OF OXYGENATION*

Tissue oxygenation is based on a number of variables, but can be simplified for general discussion to two primary factors: O_2 delivery and O_2 content. O_2 delivery is based primarily on cardiac output ($\dot{Q}_T$), acid-base status, blood volume, and tissue perfusion. If we assume that acid-base balance is normalized, the major nonventilatory concern regarding O_2 delivery is $\dot{Q}_T$. For this reason, alterations in level of ventilation should always be made with their impact on $\dot{Q}_T$ considered. Thus, alterations in V_T, rate, minute ventilation, inspiration/expiration (I/E) ratios, inspiratory times, inspiratory pauses, and PEEP level should be made only after consideration of their effect on cardiovascular stability.

O_2 content is based on hemoglobin content, oxyhemoglobin saturation, and PaO_2. Of these variables, PaO_2 is the only one directly affected by manipulation of respiratory care equipment, although oxyhemoglobin percent saturation is indirectly affected by changes in $PaCO_2$ and/or pH. PaO_2 is affected essentially by the adjustment of two variables, F_IO_2 and PEEP, although increasing inspiratory time and mean airway pressure have a direct effect on PaO_2 in some settings. Improvement in venous return does reduce to some extent the hypoxemic effects of shunting and venous admixtures; however, F_IO_2 and PEEP are the primary variables normally manipulated (see Chs. 75 and 76).

Increasing a Decreased PaO_2

In general, in most critically ill patients, a decreased PaO_2 is one below 60 to 70 mmHg.[31] If we assume that venous return and $\dot{Q}_T$ are adequate, two alterations to increase PaO_2 are possible: increasing F_IO_2 or increasing PEEP. If the F_IO_2 is 0.40 or less and the pulmonary problem is not a result of a generalized disease process causing increased intrapulmonary shunting, the F_IO_2 is normally the first variable to

* Adapted from Kacmarek,[26] with permission.

Table 83-11. Increasing a Decreased PaO_2[a]

FiO_2 <0.40
Localized or generalized disease
1. Increase FiO_2
2. Add or increase PEEP
FiO_2 >0.40
Localized disease
1. Increase FiO_2
2. Add or increase PEEP
Generalized disease
1. Add or increase PEEP
2. Increase FiO_2
3. Increase inspiratory time

[a] An adequately functioning cardiovascular system and appropriate sedation are assumed.

(Modified from Kacmarek,[26] with permission.)

be increased. However, if the FiO_2 is greater than 0.40 and the disease process has caused generalized intrapulmonary shunting, applying PEEP or increasing its level should be considered. Whenever FiO_2 is above 0.40 and the problem is localized, or is a result of venous admixture, increasing the FiO_2 is normally considered first, because the addition of PEEP in this circumstance may foster $\dot{V}/\dot{Q}$ inequalities.[32,33] The use of PEEP is indicated primarily when a generalized disease process is present.[34,35] However, PEEP may be useful with localized problems that are not responsive to increases in FiO_2 (Table 83-11).

In general PEEP levels are increased in increments of 2 to 5 cmH_2O, followed by careful assessment of the impact of the change on the cardiovascular system. FiO_2 changes are normally 0.05 to 0.10. However, FiO_2 is increased more rapidly in the face of severe hypoxemia. The long-term use of FiO_2, at or near 1.0, should always be discouraged because it increases intrapulmonary shunt and has potentially toxic effects on lung parenchyma,[36,37] although we are willing to accept FiO_2 levels of 0.7 to 0.8 in patients with severe ARDS.

In severe ARDS mean airway pressure, along with PEEP level, appear to be the primary factors that determine PO_2 levels at a given FiO_2.[38–40] In addition to adding PEEP, lengthening the inspiratory time and using pressure control ventilation have been cited as important approaches to improving oxygenation status.[41] Longer inspiratory times normally translate into higher mean airway pressures, regardless of whether volume- or pressure-control ventilation is employed. However, we do not recommend inversing the I/E ratio to the level that auto-PEEP is created (see Ch. 76). Generally this limits the I/E ratio to 1.5:1.0, depending on the ventilatory rate. Pressure control ventilation is more effective in establishing a lengthy inspiratory time and increasing mean airway pressure than volume control. However, as depicted in Figure 83-22, if a decelerating waveform, along with an inflation hold are applied, volume control should be as effective as pressure control.

Decreasing an Increased PaO_2

Whether to decrease the FiO_2 or the PEEP level when PaO_2 is elevated is dependent on the actual FiO_2 and PEEP level. If the FiO_2 is 0.80 or more, the primary concern is decreasing the FiO_2 because of the potential toxic effects of O_2 at high concentrations.[36,37] Once the FiO_2 is below 0.75, the PEEP level can be slowly decreased, alternating with further decreases in the FiO_2. PEEP is decreased in 2 to 5

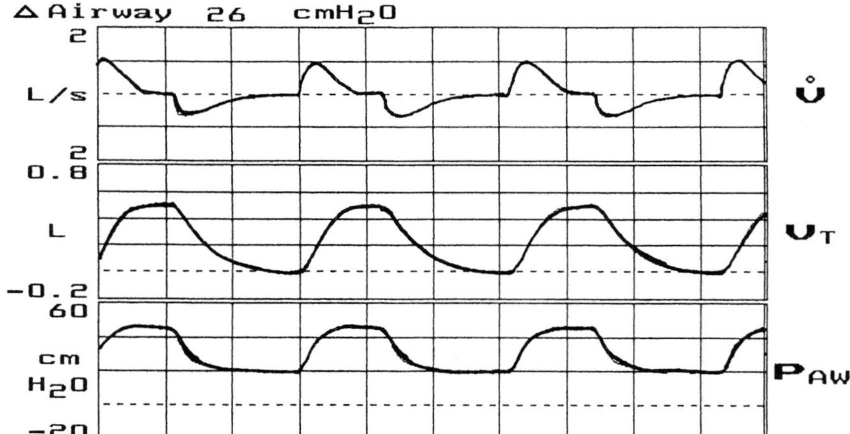

Figure 83-22. Airway pressure (PAW), flow ($\dot{V}$), and volume (VT) waveforms during volume-targeted ventilation of a patient with severe ARDS. The ventilator was set to deliver gas in a decelerating waveform, with a 0.6-second inflation hold resulting in an I/E ratio of about 1:1 at a rate of 19 breaths per minute. Note, expiratory flow rate returned to zero long before the end of expiration. As a result, inspiratory time could be lengthened without causing air trapping. Note the pressure waveform is similar to pressure control. VT was set at about 500 mL and peak flow at 75 L/min. (Waveforms recorded with a Bicore CP-100 monitor.)

Table 83-12. Decreasing an Increased PaO_2

$FIO_2 \geq 0.80$
1. Decrease FIO_2
2. Decrease PEEP

$FIO_2 < 0.80$
1. Decrease PEEP
2. Decrease FIO_2

$FIO_2 = 0.50$
Normalize inspiratory time

cmH_2O increments, whereas FIO_2 may be decreased by 0.05 to 0.10 or more at each alteration. Decreasing the PEEP level may result in increased venous return; therefore, careful monitoring of the cardiovascular system should be performed whenever PEEP is decreased or increased. After changes in either FIO_2 or PEEP, the patient's cardiopulmonary status should be evaluated (Table 83-12).

If lengthy inspiratory times are employed, the protocol above can still be followed. However, as PEEP levels fall below 10 cmH_2O and FIO_2 reaches 0.50, inspiratory times and I/E ratios should be normalized.

SYSTEMATIC ALTERATION IN LEVEL OF VENTILATION*

Alterations in level of ventilation should be made only after consideration of the cardiovascular effects of each alternative. In general, changes that least affect cardiovascular status (increase mean intrathoracic pressure) should be considered first, followed by those with a more profound effect on the cardiovascular system.

Increasing a Decreased $PaCO_2$

Before adjusting the ventilator of a patient with a respiratory alkalosis, one must determine the cause of the alkalosis. In the A/C, IMV, or SIMV modes patients hyperventilate because of pain, anxiety, fear, hypoxemia, metabolic acidosis, and/or central nervous system trauma. If one of these problems is noted to be the cause of the hyperventilation, correction of the primary problem should eliminate the hyperventilation. If true mechanical hyperventilation exists, regardless of mode, hyperventilation may be corrected by decreasing the ventilatory rate, which is normally the first choice in all but the A/C mode. V_T is usually not decreased unless volumes greater than 12 to 15 mL/kg ideal body weight are used, or the V_T is on the flat portion of the compliance curve. It should be remembered that decreasing the rate helps most to decrease the mean intrathoracic pressure. In the A/C mode, alterations in rate and V_T do little to correct mechanical hyperventilation. If the V_T is excessive, it can be decreased. However, in most circumstances, patients in A/C ventilation require sedation to eliminate mechanical hyperventilation because it is the patient who is selecting the higher mechanical rate, not the machine (Table 83-13).

* Adapted from Kacmarek,[26] with permission.

Table 83-13. Increasing a Decreased $PaCO_2$

Determine cause

Correct primary problem
- Sedate for anxiety, pain, fear
- Increase FIO_2 or PEEP if hypoxemic
- Treat metabolic acidosis
- If central nervous system problem, manage appropriately

If simply mechanical hyperventilation
- IMV/SIMV or control mode
  1. Decrease rate
  2. Decrease V_T
- A/C mode
  - Decrease V_T if excessive
  - Normally, sedation is required

Decreasing an Increased $PaCO_2$

An increased $PaCO_2$ in patients mechanically ventilated is normally caused by mechanical hypoventilation. However, in patients with chronic obstructive pulmonary disease (COPD) or asthma, air trapping and auto-PEEP may be the cause, and in patients with cardiovascular instability, high mean airway pressure may be the cause. In both of these situations, marked $\dot{V}/\dot{Q}$ mismatch may result in an elevated PCO_2. If the hypercarbia is a result of mechanical hypoventilation, it is essentially corrected by increasing the level of ventilation. This is accomplished either by increasing the mechanical rate or the V_T. The decision of which to increase depends on the actual rate and V_T. Adjustment of the variable that has the least effect on mean intrathoracic pressure should always be attempted first (Table 83-14).

As a general guideline, 12 to 15 mL/kg ideal body weight is the V_T required by most patients mechanically ventilated.[2,42,43] This level, however, may be modified for each patient. For example, obese patients may require a much larger V_T, whereas patients with chronic restrictive pulmonary disease may require a much smaller one. In patients who are mechanically hypoventilated, with a mechanical rate of 8 breaths per minute or greater, the clinician should first ensure that the V_T is appropriate. If the V_T is low, it should be increased before changes in mechanical rate are

Table 83-14. Decreasing an Increased $PaCO_2$[a]

Rate ≥ 8 breaths/min	Rate <8 breaths/min
1. Increase V_T	1. Increase rate
2. Increase rate	2. Increase V_T

[a] It is assumed that V_T is not excessive; optimally, about 12 to 15 mL/kg.
(From Kacmarek,[26] with permission.)

made. If the V_T is set appropriately, the rate should be increased.

V_T is usually increased before rate because a change of 100 mL normally does not cause as great an increase in mean intrathoracic pressure as a 1 to 2 breath per minute increase in rate.[2] This observation is true only if the V_T delivered is on the steep aspect of the patient's compliance curve. Once the V_T extends into the flat part of the compliance curve, increases in V_T markedly increase mean and peak airway pressure.

It is always difficult to apply any hard and fast rules to altering ventilator parameters. However, the following always applies: Whenever any change in the level of ventilation is made, concern for its cardiovascular effects must be foremost, and a careful evaluation of the cardiovascular system before and after making the change is essential.

In the patient with COPD and asthma, *decreasing the ventilatory rate* frequently results in a decrease in the PCO_2. This may not appear logical, but if significant auto-PEEP, along with an elevated mean airway pressure are present, perfusion to well-ventilated areas may be dramatically reduced. As a result, a marked increase in dead space occurs. With a decrease in the mechanical rate, the mean airway pressure is decreased and the auto-PEEP level is decreased because of longer expiratory time. As a result, $\dot{V}/\dot{Q}$ matching improves and dead space ventilation decreases, which ensures more effective ventilation and a decrease in the PCO_2. The same general argument can be made for the cardiovascularly unstable patient, except the probability of auto-PEEP is less. A concern regarding excessive mean airway pressure should always be raised whenever increases in mechanical minute ventilation result in no change, or minimal change, in the PCO_2. It is not unusual to see minute ventilation increased 20 to 30 percent by overly aggressive clinicians, without a change in the PCO_2 but accompanied by cardiovascular instability. Frequently, decreasing the ventilator rate in these situations improves the PCO_2 level.

USE OF PRESSURE SUPPORT VENTILATION

Of all the modes of ventilation currently available, PSV has received the most scientific investigation. As discussed in Chapter 82, PSV is capable of unloading the ventilatory muscles,[44] normalizing the ventilatory pattern[44–46] and cardiovascular status of patients,[45] as well as functioning as a mode of ventilation.[46,47] In general, we recommend the use of PSV at low levels (5 to 15 cmH_2O) in any patient who is breathing spontaneously (CPAP), with or without a back-up SIMV rate. PSV is particularly indicated in the presence of a small endotracheal tube (less than 8.0 mm in males and less than 7.5 mm in females) and in those patients with a high ventilatory drive (minute ventilation greater than 12 L/min).[45] We also find PSV useful as a mode of ventilation in the recovering ARDS patient. In many of these patients, PSV has been the only mode that did not require significant sedation to ensure patient–ventilator synchrony.

FULL VERSUS PARTIAL VENTILATORY SUPPORT

As discussed in Chapter 82, great debate exists over selection of the appropriate mode of ventilation for a given setting. As a result, we will not try to add to this debate, but discuss the use of full (FVS) versus partial (PVS) ventilatory support. During initial management (12 to 72 hours) of all patients requiring ventilatory support, we recommend the use of FVS. This is to ensure control over the process of ventilation and to establish appropriate gas exchange, rest ventilatory muscles, and minimize cardiovascular swings from hypo- to hypertension because of anxiety, hypoxemia, hypercarbia, or pain during the early phases of ventilatory support. Beyond this period, the decision to continue with FVS or to change to PVS depends on patient presentation. In those patients whose disease process is getting worse, or in whom the pathophysiology requiring ventilatory support has not begun to resolve, we continue with FVS. However, once the most acute phase of the disease process is over, or when decisions are made to begin weaning, PVS is begun. However, in the vast majority of patients, we use FVS during the night to ensure maximum ventilatory muscle rest, which we believe, along with a good night's sleep, benefits all patients.

TARGETS

The severe ARDS patient, more so than any other patient we mechanically ventilate, taxes our ability to provide effective ventilation. As a result, we must frequently accept end points of therapy considered unacceptable in other settings. In severe ARDS, lung function is affected in a nonhomogeneous manner.[41,49] Some lung units are nonaerated due to edema or atelectasis, while others may have normal compliance and $\dot{V}/\dot{Q}$ ratio. As a result, the functioning lung in ARDS is not so much stiff as it is small.[41,49] Thus, as indicated in Chapter 82 and by Hickling et al.,[50] V_T delivery in ARDS needs to be much smaller (10 mL/kg or less) than during ventilation of the average patient. This is not to infer that respiratory rates need to be significantly high. The goal, as defined by Marcy and Marini,[41] is to prevent excessive peak alveolar pressures (assessed by monitoring end-inspiratory plateau pressure). They consider pressures greater than 35 to 40 cmH_2O at the alveolar level excessive. In addition, the goal is to maintain mean airway pressure at the lowest level necessary to ensure "adequate" oxygenation by a combination of PEEP, inspiratory time, and V_T using minimal PEEP levels (15 cmH_2O or less). To accomplish these goals, in addition to accepting a low V_T and higher FIO_2, lower PO_2 and higher PCO_2 levels must be expected.[50,51]

No data derived in patients with severe ARDS indicate that high FIO_2 levels in this setting cause toxicity. All data implicating FIO_2 to O_2 toxicity have been determined in previously healthy animals[52–54] and there are data to suggest that prior lung injury guards against the development of tox-

Table 83-15. Ventilatory Gas Exchange Targets in Severe ARDS

$PO_2 \geq 55$ mmHg Hct 30–35% $\dot{Q}_T$ normal
$PCO_2 > 60$ mmHg Allow gradual increase Buffer acid if pH <7.25
PEEP ≥10 but ≤15
Peak alveolar pressure <35–40 cmH_2O
V_T <10 ml/kg
I/E ratio Lengthen inspiratory time to 1:1 If no auto-PEEP is noted, may increase I/E to 1.5:1
$F_IO_2 \leq 0.80$
Mean airway pressure minimum needed to maintain oxygenation

Hct, hematocrit.

icity.[53,54] As a result, we are willing to accept an F_IO_2 up to 0.75 to 0.80 to avoid the excessive use of PEEP (greater than 15 cmH_2O) and high mean airway pressures with their potential for barotrauma (see Chs. 76 and 84). In light of the difficulty in oxygenating the ARDS patient, we accept a PO_2 of 55 mmHg or more. In doing this we are assuming a normal $\dot{Q}_T$ and an acceptable hematocrit of 30 to 35 percent or more.

Permissive hypercapnia is a term used by Hickling et al.[50] to define the decision to allow the PCO_2 to rise to levels well above 60 mmHg during the most acute phase of ARDS, provided the pH is normalized (7.30 or more).[51,55] In fact, we have managed a number of patients with PCO_2 levels in the range of 90 to 100 mmHg for several days until their disease process improved, allowing better ventilation at a given mechanical minute volume. If the decision to allow PCO_2 to rise is made early in the patient's course, its rise is usually slow, with renal mechanisms allowing for normalization of the pH. However, if the decision is made later in the course of the disease, HCO_3^-, or other buffers must be administered to normalize the pH. Although this approach to therapy is contrary to normal logic, there is no direct physiologic insult associated with an elevated PCO_2, provided the pH is normal (Table 83-15).

This strategy is intended to minimize the effects of lung overdistension and consequent damage to alveolar tissue by high alveolar pressures. Although defined here for the ARDS patient, limiting alveolar pressures and accepting lower PO_2 levels and higher PCO_2 levels is an approach to ventilator management that we have also applied to patients with asthma, COPD, and large air leaks.

References

1. MacIntyre NR: Respiratory monitoring without machinery. Respir Care 1990;35:546–556
2. Shapiro BA, Kacmarek RM, Cane RD et al: Clinical Application of Respiratory Care. 4th Ed. Mosby-Year Book, 1991
3. Yang KL, Tobin MJ: A prospective study of indexes predicting the outcome of trials of weaning from mechanical ventilation. N Engl J Med 1991;324:1445–1450
4. Cohen CA, Zagelbaum G, Gross D et al: Clinical manifestations of inspiratory muscle fatigue. Am J Med 1982;73:308–316
5. Shapiro BA, Cane RD, Chomka CM et al: Preliminary evaluation of an intra-arterial blood gas probe in dogs and humans. Crit Care Med 1989;17:455–460
6. Hess D, Schlottag A, Levin B et al: An evaluation of the usefulness of end-tidal PCO_2 to aid weaning from mechanical ventilation following cardiac surgery. Respir Care 1991;36:837–843
7. Bendixen H, Egbert LD: Respiratory Care. CV Mosby, St. Louis, 1965
8. Millbern SM, Downs JB, Junper LC et al: Evaluation of criteria for discontinuing mechanical ventilatory support. Arch Surg 1978;113:1441–1443
9. Bone R: Monitoring ventilatory mechanics in acute respiratory failure. Respir Care 1983;28:597–603
10. Kacmarek RM, Mack CM, Dimas S: The Essentials of Respiratory Care, 3rd Ed. Year Book Medical Publishers, Chicago, 1990
11. Shapiro M, Wilson RK, Casar G et al: Work of breathing through different sized endotracheal tubes. Crit Care Med 1986;14:1028–1031
12. Wright PE, Marini JJ, Bernard GR: In vitro versus in vivo comparison of endotracheal tube airflow resistance. Am Rev Respir Dis 1989;140:10–16
13. MacIntyre NR, Silver RM, Miller CW et al: Aerosol delivery in intubated mechanically ventilated patients. Crit Care Med 1985; 13:81–85
14. Fuller HD, Dolovich MB, Posmituck G et al: Pressurized aerosol versus jet aerosol delivery to mechanically ventilated patients. Am Rev Respir Dis 1990;141:440–444
15. Mathews J, Ingenito E, Davison B et al: Airflow resistance characteristics of endotracheal tubes, abstracted. Anesthesiology (submitted)
16. Brown DG, Pierson DJ: Auto-PEEP is common in mechanically ventilated patients: A study of incidence, severity and detection. Respir Care 1986;31:1069–1074
17. Wright J, Gong H: Auto-PEEP: Incidence, magnitude and contributing factors. Heart Lung 1990;19:352–357
18. Kacmarek RM, Shimada Y, Ohmura A et al: The second Nayoga conference: Triggering and optimizing mechanical ventilatory assist. Respir Care 1991;36:45–52
19. Kacmarek RM, Goulet RL: PEEP devices. Anesth Clin North Am 1987;5:757–770
20. Milic-Emili J, Tantucci C, Chasse M, Corbeil C: Introduction with special reference to ventilator-associated barotrauma. pp. 1–8. In Benito S, Net A (eds): Pulmonary Function in Mechanically Ventilated Patients. Springer-Verlag, Berlin, 1991
21. Marini JJ, Rodriguez RM, Lamb V: The inspiratory workload of patient-initiated mechanical ventilation. Am Rev Respir Dis 1986;134:902–909
22. Truwit JD, Marini JJ: Evaluation of thoracic mechanics in the ventilated patient. Part II. Applied Mechanics. J Crit Care 1988; 3:199–213
23. Bicore: Bicore CP-100 pulmonary monitor. Product literature. Bicore, Irvine, CA, 1991
24. Med-Science Inc: VenTrak respiratory monitor. Product literature. Med-Science Inc., Jacksonville, FL, 1992
25. Fiastro JF, Habib MP, Shon BY, Campbell SC: Comparison of standard weaning parameters and the mechanical work of breathing in mechanically ventilated patients. Chest 1988; 94:232–238
26. Kacmarek RM: Systematic modification of mechanical ventilation. pp. 516–534. In Barnes T (ed): Respiratory Care Practice. Year Book Medical Publishers, Chicago, 1988
27. Kacmarek RM, Wilson RS: IMV systems: Do they make a difference? (editorial). Chest 1985;87:557–558
28. Kacmarek RM, Dimas S, Reynolds J, Shapiro BA: Technical aspects of positive end-expiratory pressure: II. PEEP with positive pressure ventilation. Respir Care 1982;27:1490–1504

29. Kacmarek RM: Noninvasive monitoring in respiratory care: Conference summary. Respir Care 1990;35:740–746
30. Hess D: Noninvasive monitoring in respiratory care—present, past and future: An overview. Respir Care 1990;35:482–499
31. Shapiro BA, Cane RD, Harrison RA: Positive end-expiratory pressure in acute lung injury. Chest 1983;83:558–563
32. Hobelmann CF, Smith DE, Virgilio RW et al: Mechanics of ventilation with positive end-expiratory pressure. Ann Thorac Surg 1977;24:68–74
33. Douglas ME, Downs JB: Cardiopulmonary effects of PEEP and CPAP. Anesth Analg 1978;57:347–350
34. Suter PM, Fairly HB, Isenberg MD: Optimal end-expiratory airway pressure and patients with acute pulmonary failure. N Engl J Med 1975;292:284–290
35. Gallagher TJ, Civetta JM: Goal-directed therapy of acute respiratory failure. Anesth Analg 1980;59:831–836
36. Block ER: Recovery from hyperoxic depression of pulmonary 5-hydroxytryptamine clearance—effect of inspired PO_2 tension. Lung 1978;155:131–140
37. Frank L, Massaro D: The lung and oxygen toxicity. Arch Intern Med 1979;139:347–350
38. Mang H, Kacmarek RM, Ritz R et al: Cardiopulmonary effects of volume and pressure controlled CPPV at various I:E ratios in an acute lung injury model, abstracted. Am Rev Respir Dis (in press)
39. Presenti A, Marolin R, Prato P et al: Mean airway pressure vs positive end-expiratory pressure during mechanical ventilation. Crit Care Med 1985;13:34–37
40. Gattinoni L, Marcolin R, Caspanic ML et al: Constant mean airway pressure with different patterns of positive pressure breathing during the adult respiratory distress syndrome. Bull Eur Physiopathol Respir 1985;21:275–279
41. Marcy TW, Marini JJ: Inverse ratio ventilation in ARDS: Rationale and implementation. Chest 1991;100:495–504
42. Hotchkiss RS, Wilson RS: Mechanical ventilatory support. Surg Clin North Am 1983;63:417–437
43. Kacmarek RM, Venegas J: Mechanical ventilator rates and tidal volumes. Respir Care 1987;32:466–480
44. Brochard L, Harf A, Lorino H, Lemaire F: Inspiratory pressure support prevents diaphragmatic fatigue during weaning from mechanical ventilation. Am Rev Respir Dis 1989;139:513–521
45. Kacmarek RM: The role of pressure support ventilation in reducing work of breathing. Respir Care 1988;33:99–120
46. Brochard L, Pluskwa F, Lemaire F: Improved efficiency of spontaneous breathing with inspiratory pressure support. Am Rev Respir Dis 1987;136:411–415
47. McIntyre NR: Respiratory function during pressure support ventilation. Chest 1986;89:677–683
48. Tokioka H, Saito S, Kosaka F: Comparison of pressure support ventilation and assist control ventilation in patients with acute respiratory failure. Intensive Care Med 1989;15:364–367
49. Gattinoni L, Pesenti A, Bambino M et al: Relationships between lung computed tomographic density, gas exchange and PEEP in acute respiratory failure. Anesthesiology 1988;69:824–832
50. Hickling KG, Henderson SJ, Jackson R: Low mortality associated with low volume pressure limited ventilation with permissive hypercapnia in severe adult respiratory distress syndrome. Intensive Care Med 1990;16:372–377
51. Pesenti A: Target blood gases during ARDS ventilatory management. Intensive Care Med 1990;16:349–351
52. Frank L, Massaro D: Oxygen toxicity. Am J Med 1980;69:117–126
53. Deneke SM, Fanburg BL: Normobaric oxygen toxicity of the lung. N Engl J Med 1980;303:76–86
54. Frank L, Massaro D: The lung and oxygen toxicity. Arch Internal Med 1979;139:347–350
55. Stoller JK, Kacmarek RM: Ventilatory strategies in the management of the adult respiratory distress syndrome. Clin Chest Med 1990;11:755–772
56. Kacmarek RM: Noninvasive monitoring techniques in the ventilated patient. pp. 182–187. In Kacmarek RM, Stoller JK (eds): Current Respiratory Care. BC Decker, Toronto, 1988
57. Seimens: Seimens Lung Mechanics Calculator 940. Product literature No. 6928782E313E. Seimens, Solna, Sweden, 1980

Chapter 84

Complications of Mechanical Ventilation

David J. Pierson

CHAPTER OUTLINE

Mechanical ventilation is often life-saving, but as with other interventions in medicine it is also associated with a constellation of adverse occurrences, which may themselves be life-threatening. Some of these, such as machine malfunction, are obviously due to mechanical ventilation. In other cases, however, such as pneumothorax and nosocomial pneumonia, the role of the ventilator per se in something that happens to a critically ill patient is less certain. This distinction should be kept in mind, and a better title for this chapter might be "Adverse Clinical Events *Associated with* Mechanical Ventilation."

Table 84-1 lists the general categories of ventilator-related complications. Those shown in boldface are discussed here, while the others are covered in the other chapters indicated. For more comprehensive discussions of the general topic of ventilator complications, the reader is referred to three recent reviews.[1–3]

ADVERSE PHYSIOLOGIC EFFECTS OF MECHANICAL VENTILATION

Impaired Cardiac Function

The effects of positive-pressure ventilation on cardiac function were first reported in 1948 by Cournand et al.[4] and have been reviewed more recently by several authors.[5,6] These effects are much more likely to occur with application of positive end-expiratory pressure (PEEP), and most research has focused on this setting.[6–8] Cardiac output may fall precipitously on initiation of mechanical ventilation or addition of PEEP. Although various mechanisms have been postulated, the two effects diagrammed in Figure 84-1 are mainly responsible.[9]

The likelihood of cardiac impairment depends on the pa-

Table 84-1. Complications of Mechanical Ventilation[a]

Adverse physiologic effects
Unintended air trapping and auto-PEEP
Extra-alveolar air (barotrauma)
  Pneumomediastinum
  Subcutaneous emphysema
  Pneumothorax
  Bronchopleural fistula (see Ch. 92)
Ventilator malfunction
Nosocomial pneumonia (also see Chs. 68 and 97)
Agitation and respiratory distress during mechanical ventilation
Worsening oxygenation during mechanical ventilation
Adverse effects of inappropriate ventilator management (see Ch. 83)
Complications of intubation, endotracheal tubes, and tracheostomy (see Ch. 72)
O_2 toxicity (see Ch. 75)
Psychosocial complications (see Ch. 104)
Ethical problems associated with mechanical ventilation (see Ch. 103)

[a] Complications shown in bold type are discussed in this chapter.

tient's baseline cardiac function and fluid status and the extent to which the mean intrathoracic pressure is increased: patients who have underlying cardiac disease, who are relatively hypovolemic, or who are treated with levels of PEEP exceeding 10 cmH_2O should be monitored closely for this complication. For any given state of hydration and cardiac function, cardiac impairment is more likely to occur with volume-limited than with pressure-limited modes, and with intermittent mandatory ventilation (IMV) it is more likely at high than at low rates. Its likelihood is increased whenever PEEP or continuous positive airway pressure (CPAP) is employed.

Increased Intracranial Pressure

Positive-pressure ventilation in the presence of head injury or other cause of increased intracranial pressure may impair cerebral blood flow, especially when PEEP is used.[10–12] Mechanical ventilation and PEEP can raise jugular venous pressure, which in turn can impede venous return from the brain and raise intracranial pressure. Fortunately, conditions that require PEEP to support oxygenation such as adult respiratory distress syndrome (ARDS) also reduce lung compliance, so that less pressure is transmitted to the jugular venous system.

Gastric Distension

Gastric distension (also termed *meteorism*) can be massive[13] and can even rupture the stomach.[14] It commonly occurs during bag-mask manual ventilation when mouth pressure is raised above lower esophageal sphincter pressure. Even with an inflated endotracheal tube cuff, gastric distension may occur when tracheal pressure becomes higher than both cuff pressure and lower esophageal sphincter pressure in the presence of a closed or occluded mouth. This complication, most commonly seen with nasotracheal intubation and in patients with low lung-thorax compliance, can be prevented or relieved by passage of a small-caliber nasogastric tube.

Respiratory Alkalosis

Unintended hyperventilation is common when patients are first placed on mechanical ventilation, particularly when they have underlying chronic obstructive pulmonary disease

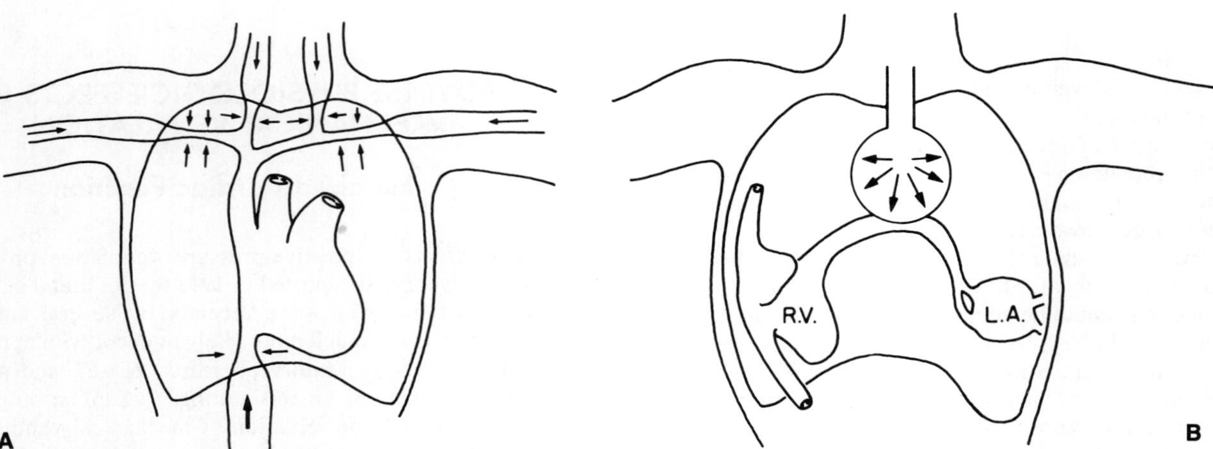

Figure 84-1. The two main effects of positive-pressure ventilation on cardiac function. **(A)** Increased intrathoracic pressure impedes venous return to the right side of the heart. **(B)** Increased lung volume stretches pulmonary vessels, raising pulmonary vascular resistance. Both effects are accentuated by the application of positive end-expiratory pressure. (From Harken et al.,[9] with permission.)

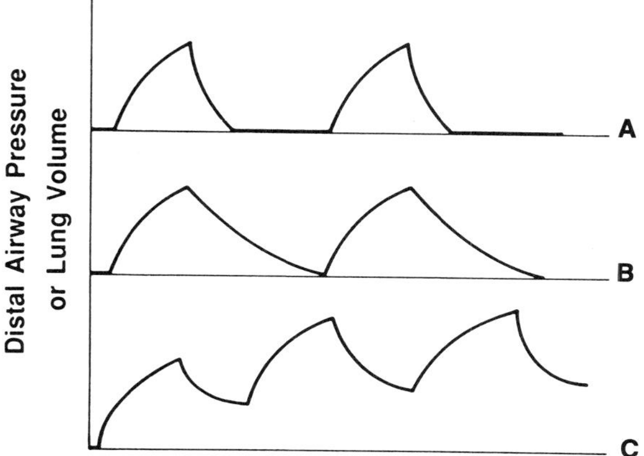

Figure 84-2. Development of air trapping and auto-PEEP during mechanical ventilation. **(A)** With adequate exhalation time and no expiratory airflow obstruction, distal airway pressure returns to zero and lung volume returns to baseline (functional residual capacity) between ventilator breaths. **(B)** As in Figure A but with less expiratory time or with airflow obstruction, so that exhalation is just completed when each successive ventilator breath is delivered. **(C)** As cycling rate increases or airflow obstruction worsens, incomplete exhalation prior to the next breath results in air trapping and auto-PEEP. (From Benson and Pierson,[18] with permission.)

(COPD) with chronic CO_2 retention and compensatory metabolic alkalosis.[1,15] The most frequent consequence of this hyperventilation is inability to wean the patient from the ventilator, but it can also be life-threatening: development of arterial pH above 7.55 during mechanical ventilation may precipitate seizures or cardiac arrhythmias and may increase the overall mortality of acute respiratory failure.[13] Respiratory alkalosis can be avoided or corrected if arterial pH (pHa), rather than $PaCO_2$, is used to guide ventilator adjustment (see Ch. 83).

Other Effects

Renal and hepatic dysfunction occur frequently among patients who require mechanical ventilation. Most investigators believe that reduced blood flow resulting from the effects of positive-pressure ventilation on cardiac output is the most likely mechanism, although hormonal and other changes have also been postulated.[1,3] Many patients who require ventilatory support during critical illness have other conditions that are potential causes of fluid retention and liver dysfunction, and any direct effects of mechanical ventilation remain largely conjectural.

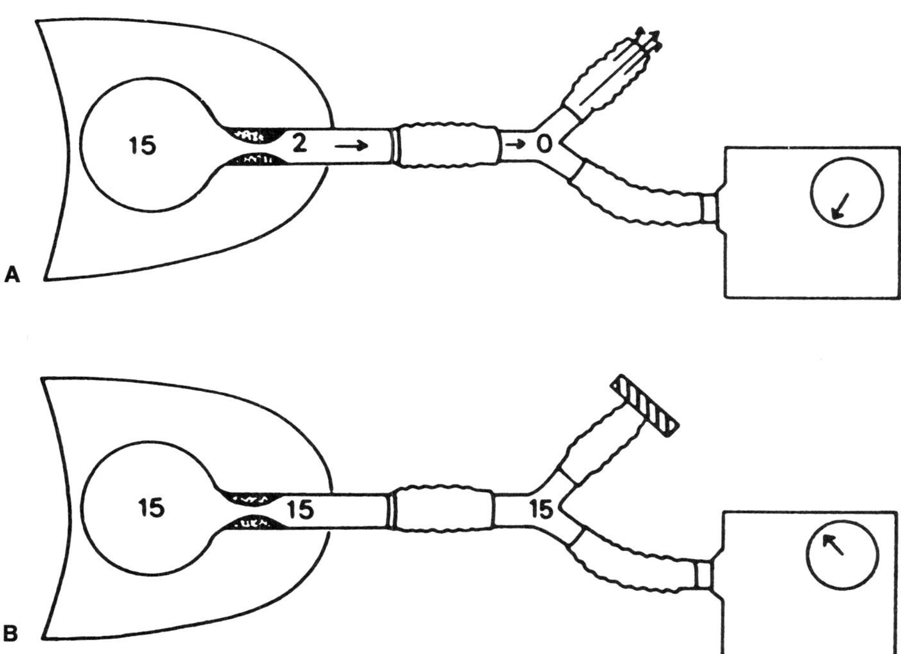

Figure 84-3. Detection of auto-PEEP during mechanical ventilation. **(A)** Auto-PEEP is present (15 cmH_2O at alveoli) but not detected at ventilator manometer because exhalation circuit is open to the atmosphere. **(B)** Occlusion of exhalation port just as next ventilator breath would normally be delivered permits pressure to equilibrate throughout the system and auto-PEEP to be detected and quantitated on pressure manometer. (From O'Quin and Marini,[19] with permission.)

Table 84-2. Techniques for Minimizing Auto-PEEP and Its Physiologic Effects

Eliminate unnecessary ventilation
- Correct overventilation and respiratory alkalosis
- If auto-PEEP severely impairs cardiac function, allow $PaCO_2$ to rise above normal, keeping arterial pH >7.30

Decrease expiratory airflow obstruction
- Treat bronchospasm aggressively with aerosolized bronchodilators and other therapy as indicated
- Keep airways free of secretions
- Replace small-diameter endotracheal tube with larger one

Maximize expiratory portion of ventilatory cycle
- Increase inspiratory flow rate to 80–100 L/min
- Replace standard, corrugated ventilator circuit with low-compressible-volume tubing[a]

Decease patient's work of breathing by adding external PEEP[b]

[a] This will decrease the total tidal volume the ventilator must deliver for each breath, enabling more rapid delivery and thus increasing the time for exhalation.

[b] Amount of external PEEP added should be at or below level of measured auto-PEEP and should be reduced promptly as auto-PEEP decreases; this applies only to auto-PEEP in the setting of obstructive airway disease and not to auto-PEEP occurring with very high minute ventilation, as in ARDS.

UNINTENDED AIR TRAPPING AND AUTO-PEEP

If a delivered breath is incompletely exhaled prior to the onset of the next inspiration, air will be trapped in the chest, lung volume will increase, and end-expiratory alveolar pressure will be raised, which creates intrinsic or auto-PEEP[16–18] (Fig. 84-2). Unlike externally applied PEEP, auto-PEEP cannot be detected unless it is deliberately sought[19,20] (Fig. 84-3).

Auto-PEEP is more common than originally believed.[20] Patients especially at risk for this potentially life-threatening complication of mechanical ventilation are those with obstructive airway disease (e.g., COPD or asthma) and those with ARDS, burns, or other conditions in which the required ventilation exceeds 15 to 20 L/min, especially with a small-diameter endotracheal tube.[18]

The technique for measuring auto-PEEP varies according to the ventilator and mode used. Once detected, auto-PEEP and its physiologic consequences can be eliminated or at least reduced by following the steps listed in Table 84-2.

EXTRA-ALVEOLAR AIR (BAROTRAUMA)

Pneumothorax, pneumomediastinum, subcutaneous emphysema, and other forms of extra-alveolar air detected during mechanical ventilation are collectively termed *barotrauma*. Although this term implies that excessive pressure is the cause, it is more likely that alveolar disruption, whether during mechanical ventilation or spontaneous breathing, results from overdistension (i.e., excessive peak inflating *volume*) rather than from high pressure per se.[21,22] Figure 84-4 illustrates this mechanism.[23,24] Extra-alveolar air that first becomes evident during ventilatory support may also be unrelated to this therapy (Table 84-3).

Figure 84-5 shows schematically how alveolar rupture can be followed by several kinds of clinical manifestation depending on how much air enters the pulmonary interstitium and where the path of least resistance takes it. The radiographic signs of the various forms of extra-alveolar air are discussed in Chapter 57. Pneumomediastinum, pneumoperitoneum, and subcutaneous emphysema are rarely of physiologic significance and do not require specific treatment. However, pneumothorax is different in that the air collects in a space (the pleural cavity) from which it cannot naturally

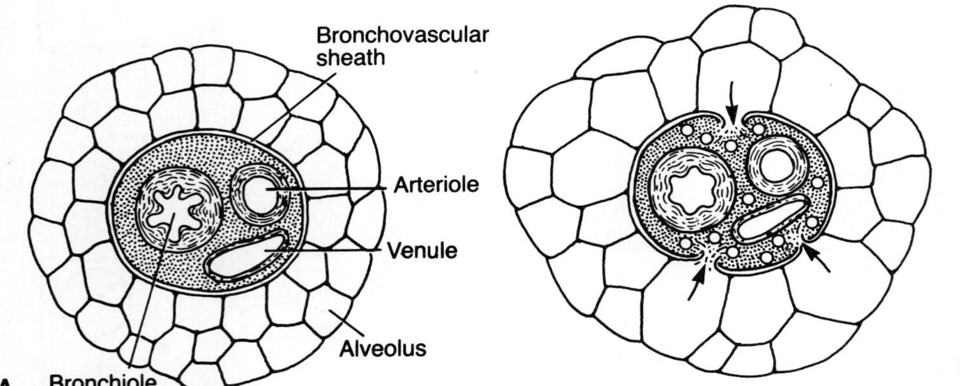

Figure 84-4. Mechanism of alveolar rupture, **(A)** showing normally distended structures and **(B)** overdistended alveoli, such as are found at peak lung inflation during mechanical ventilation. Pressures between adjacent alveoli equilibrate rapidly, even when the alveoli are unequally distended. However, pressure in the adjacent bronchovascular sheath remains somewhat lower than in the alveoli, so that when these are overdistended, a transient pressure gradient is created and the delicate alveolar membranes may rupture. (From Maunder et al.,[22] with permission.)

Table 84-3. Possible Sources of Extra-alveolar Air in Mechanically Ventilated Patients

- Alveolar rupture or airway disruption prior to initiation of mechanical ventilation
  - Penetrating or blunt chest trauma
  - Mouth-to-mouth or manual ventilation
  - Attempted placement of subclavian or internal jugular lines
  - Inadvertent perforation of diaphragm or pleura during surgery or biopsy
- Direct laceration of visceral pleura or airway during mechanical ventilation
  - Attempted central venous line placement
  - Transbronchial biopsy; bronchial brushing
- Spontaneous alveolar rupture during mechanical ventilation
  - As a manifestation of patient's underlying disease
    - Primary disease process (e.g., ARDS, pneumonia)
    - Complicating conditions (e.g., nosocomial infection, malnutrition)
    - Defective or uneven healing (e.g., late in ARDS course)
  - Caused by mechanical ventilation, with or without PEEP
    - Primarily due to high peak distending lung volume
    - (?) Primarily due to high peak airway pressure
    - (?) Other mechanisms

Table 84-4. Techniques for Reducing the Likelihood of Alveolar Rupture during Mechanical Ventilation

- Use small tidal volumes in patients with obstructive lung disease or other cause for pulmonary hyperinflation
- Decrease tidal volume as PEEP is increased
- Use PEEP cautiously in patients at increased risk due to
  - Unilateral, patchy, or cavitary lung disease
  - Nosocomial pneumonia or sepsis syndrome
  - ARDS late in clinical course (i.e., after 1–2 weeks)
  - COPD or asthma
- Monitor lung-thorax compliance during PEEP trials as a predictor of increased risk for alveolar rupture
- Avoid or promptly correct right main stem bronchus intubation
- Avoid end-inspiratory pause
- Keep inspiration/expiration ratio low (short inspiration, long expiration)
- Avoid intermittent "sigh" breaths of increased tidal volume, especially when PEEP is in use
- Monitor patient for auto-PEEP; follow steps in Table 84-2 to reduce it if present

(Modified from Pierson,[21] with permission.)

escape as pressure increases. Pneumothorax in a patient receiving positive-pressure ventilation can quickly progress to tension pneumothorax, which may rapidly cause cardiovascular collapse and death; for this reason it should always be relieved promptly if ventilatory support cannot immediately be discontinued (see Ch. 92).

Table 84-4 outlines steps to minimize the risk of alveolar rupture and barotrauma during mechanical ventilation. These steps are especially important in high-risk patients, such as those with obstructive or unevenly distributed lung disease, pulmonary infection, and late-phase ARDS (i.e., beyond 1 to 2 weeks).[21]

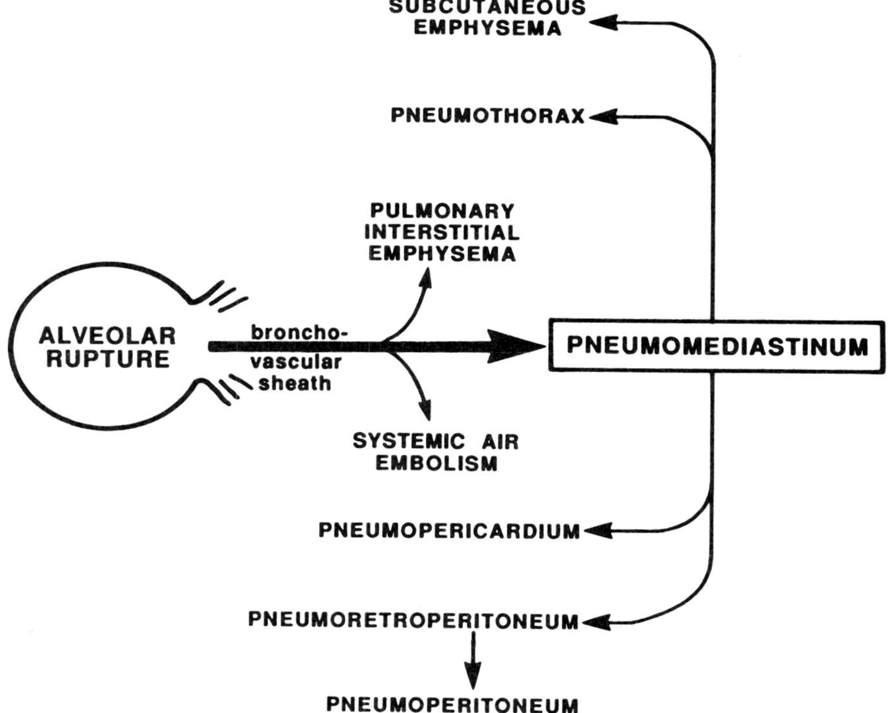

Figure 84-5. Pathogenesis of the different clinical manifestations of extra-alveolar air once alveolar disruption has occurred. (From Pierson,[24] with permission.)

CONSEQUENCES OF VENTILATOR MALFUNCTION

Ventilator malfunctions of clinical importance include failure to cycle or to deliver the desired inspired O_2 fraction, tidal volume, inspiratory flow, pressure waveform, humidification, or temperature. The possibility of these and other problems cannot be eliminated, but their incidence can be minimized if proper maintenance, alarms, quality assurance, and routine ventilator checks are used.

Today's high-capacity, microprocessor-based critical care ventilators have pressure, flow, and minute volume capabilities far exceeding those of the early 1970s.[25–27] One would like to think that they are also safer, although few actual clinical data are available to substantiate this; published experience with ventilator malfunction deals with older-generation equipment.[13,28,29]

NOSOCOMIAL PNEUMONIA

Hospital-acquired pneumonia has a high mortality rate and is common in patients who require mechanical ventilation. One study of medical and surgical patients in intensive care showed that 21 percent of those who were mechanically ventilated for more than 48 hours developed nosocomial pneumonia.[30] Although impaired host resistance in those ill enough to require ventilatory assistance is a key factor,[3,31,32] it is important to understand the role of ventilators and other respiratory care equipment in the development of this complication.[33–38] The pathogenesis of nosocomial pneumonia is considered in more detail in Chapter 36. Table 84-5 summarizes current concepts in the prevention of pneumonia in mechanically ventilated patients.[31]

Table 84-5. Prevention of Nosocomial Pneumonia during Mechanical Ventilation

General principles
- Treatment of underlying disease and complications
  - Appropriate use of antibiotics
  - Aggressive treatment of hypotension
- Extubation and removal of nasogastric tube as clinically indicated
- Provision of stress ulcer prophylaxis
  - Assessment of risk-benefit
  - Maintenance of natural gastric acid barrier
- Maintenance of patient in upright position to reduce reflux and aspiration of gastric bacteria
- Assessment of nutritional state and need for tube feeding
- Possible selective decontamination of oropharynx and stomach with antibiotics in certain subsets of patients

Infection control (see Ch. 97)
- Surveillance in the intensive care unit
- Awareness programs
- Review of techniques for airway suctioning
- Hand washing and appropriate use of gloves
- Appropriate methods of disinfection

Respiratory care equipment
- 48-hour circuit changes for ventilators with humidifiers
- Awareness and proper handling of condensate
- No transfer of equipment between patients
- Care of in-line medication nebulizers
- Proper disinfection of tubing, bags, spirometers, etc.
- Careful use of heat and moisture exchangers
- Consideration of expiratory-phase gas-outflow traps or filters

(Adapted from Craven and Steger,[31] with permission.)

Table 84-6. Protocol for Assessment of Agitation and Respiratory Distress That Develop during Mechanical Ventilation

- Remove patient from ventilator
- Ventilate patient manually with 100% O_2
- Perform rapid physical examination, emphasizing cardiopulmonary aspects
- Note results of physiologic parameters being monitored
  - Absolute values
  - Trends over last several hours
- Assess airway patency and suction airway
- If death appears imminent, treat likely causes of deterioration
  - Airway obstruction
  - Tension pneumothorax
- Once patient is adequately supported, perform more time-consuming diagnostic and therapeutic maneuvers as indicated by clinical status

(Adapted from Hudson,[39] with permission.)

AGITATION AND RESPIRATORY DISTRESS THAT DEVELOP DURING MECHANICAL VENTILATION

Although not usually included under complications of mechanical ventilation, the new onset of agitation and respiratory distress in a patient who previously tolerated ventilatory support is a distinct entity to which the clinician needs to have a prompt, well organized approach.[39,40] Distress may simply reflect failure to match ventilator settings to the patient's needs or may indicate the wearing off of sedating drugs, but it may also be a sign that a new, life-threatening complication has developed. Those of immediate concern include failure of the ventilator to cycle or to deliver an adequate tidal volume, obstruction of the airway, and tension pneumothorax.

The protocol given in Table 84-6 emphasizes immediate disconnection of the patient from the ventilator and institution of manual ventilation; if the problem is in the ventilator, the patient's distress should abruptly resolve.[39] If not, the sequence listed in the table should be rapidly followed, first to detect immediately life-threatening problems and then to investigate less serious possibilities.

WORSENING OXYGENATION DURING MECHANICAL VENTILATION

Although not a complication in the usual sense, the new onset of hypoxemia or worsening oxygenation is a common occurrence in ventilated patients and has recently been re-

Table 84-7. Possible Causes of Worsening Oxygenation during Mechanical Ventilation

Ventilator-related problems
Endotracheal or tracheostomy tubes
Ventilator circuit
Function of ventilator itself
Inappropriate ventilator settings
Progression of underlying disease process
ARDS
Cardiogenic pulmonary edema
Pneumonia; sepsis
Acute exacerbation of asthma or COPD
Onset of new medical problem
Pneumothorax
Atelectasis (lobar collapse; diffuse microatelectasis)
Aspiration of gastric or oropharyngeal contents
Nosocomial pneumonia; sepsis
Pulmonary thromboembolism
Fluid overload
Bronchospasm
Retained secretions
Shock; any process causing a fall in cardiac output in the presence of a right-to-left intrapulmonary shunt
Effects of interventions and procedures
Endotracheal suctioning
Changes in body position
Chest physical therapy
Bronchoscopy
Thoracentesis
Peritoneal dialysis
Hemodialysis
Medications
Bronchodilators
Vasodilators
Beta blockers

(Adapted from Glauser et al.,[41] with permission.)

viewed in depth by Glauser et al.[41] Table 84-7 lists possible causes that should be considered when this situation arises. These include problems with the ventilator or other apparatus, evolution of the patient's primary disease or condition, onset of a new medical problem, and the effects of various therapeutic agents and maneuvers that can worsen oxygenation.

References

1. Pierson DJ: Complications of mechanical ventilation. pp. 19–46. In Simmons DH (ed): Current Pulmonology. Vol. 11. Mosby-Year Book, St. Louis, 1990
2. Pingleton SK: Complications of acute respiratory failure (state of the art). Am Rev Respir Dis 1988;137:1463–1493
3. Strieter RM, Lynch JP III: Complications in the ventilated patient. Clin Chest Med 1988;9:127–139
4. Cournand A, Motley HL, Werko L et al: Physiological studies of the effects of intermittent positive pressure breathing on cardiac output in man. Am J Physiol 1948;152:162–174
5. Biondi JW, Schulman DS, Matthay RA: Effects of mechanical ventilation on right and left ventricular function. Clin Chest Med 1988;9:55–72
6. Hudson LD: Cardiovascular complications in acute respiratory failure. Respir Care 1983;28:627–631
7. Craig KC, Pierson DJ, Carrico CJ: The clinical application of positive end-expiratory pressure (PEEP) in the adult respiratory distress syndrome (ARDS). Respir Care 1985;30:184–201
8. Schulman DS, Biondi JW, Matthay RA et al: Effect of positive end-expiratory pressure on right ventricular performance. Am J Med 1988;84:57–67
9. Harken AH, Brennan MF, Smith B et al: The hemodynamic response to positive end-expiratory pressure ventilation in hypovolemic patients. Surgery 1974;76:786–793
10. Shapiro HM, Marshall LF: Intracranial pressure responses to PEEP in head-injured patients. J Trauma 1978;18:254–260
11. Sherman CB, Dacey RG, Pierson DJ et al: The use of hyperventilation in head injury. Respir Care 1986;31:1121–1127
12. Luce JM: Cerebral resuscitation. pp. 403–418. In Bone RC (ed): Critical Care: A Comprehensive Approach. American College of Chest Physicians, Park Ridge, IL, 1984
13. Zwillich CW, Pierson DJ, Creagh CE et al: Complications of assisted ventilation: A prospective study of 354 consecutive episodes. Am J Med 1974;57:161–170
14. Barker SJ, Karagianes T: Gastric barotrauma: A case report and theoretical considerations. Anesth Analg 1985;64:1026–1028
15. Pierson DJ: Exacerbation of chronic bronchitis and emphysema: Ventilatory management. pp. 267–272. In Kacmarek RM, Stoller JK (eds): Current Respiratory Care. BC Decker, Philadelphia, 1988
16. Pepe PE, Marini JJ: Occult positive end-expiratory pressure in mechanically ventilated patients with airflow obstruction: The auto-PEEP effect. Am Rev Respir Dis 1982;126:166–170
17. Wright J, Gong H Jr: "Auto-PEEP": Incidence, magnitude, and contributing factors. Heart Lung 1990;19:352–357
18. Benson MS, Pierson DJ: Auto-PEEP during mechanical ventilation of adults. Respir Care 1988;33:557–565
19. O'Quin R, Marini JJ: Pulmonary artery occlusion pressure: Clinical physiology, measurement, and interpretation. Am Rev Respir Dis 1983;128:319–326
20. Brown DG, Pierson DJ: Auto-PEEP is common in mechanically ventilated patients: A study of incidence, severity, and detection. Respir Care 1986;31:1069–1074
21. Pierson DJ: Alveolar rupture during mechanical ventilation: Role of PEEP, peak airway pressure, and distending volume. Respir Care 1988;33:472–484
22. Maunder RJ, Pierson DJ, Hudson LD: Subcutaneous and mediastinal emphysema: Pathophysiology, diagnosis, and management. Arch Intern Med 1984;144:1447–1453
23. Macklin MT, Macklin CC: Malignant interstitial emphysema of the lungs and mediastinum as an important occult complication in many respiratory diseases and other conditions: An interpretation of the clinical literature in the light of laboratory experiment. Medicine (Baltimore) 1944;23:281–352
24. Pierson DJ: Pneumomediastinum. pp. 1782–1808. In Murray JF, Nadel JA (eds): Textbook of Respiratory Medicine. WB Saunders, Philadelphia, 1988
25. Pierson DJ, Capps JS, Hudson JD: Maximum ventilatory capabilities of four current-generation mechanical ventilators. Respir Care 1986;31:1054–1058
26. Spearman CB, Sanders HG Jr: The new generation of mechanical ventilators. Respir Care 1987;32:403–414
27. Evaluation: Microprocessor-controlled third-generation critical care ventilators. Health Devices 1989;18:59–83
28. Abramson NS, Wald KS, Grenvik A et al: Adverse occurrences in intensive care units. JAMA 1980;244:1582–1584
29. Feeley TW, Bancroft ML: Problems with mechanical ventilators. Int Anesthesiol Clin 1982;20:83–93
30. Craven DE, Make B, McCabe WR et al: Risk factors for pneumonia in patients receiving continuous mechanical ventilation. Am Rev Respir Dis 1986;133:792–795
31. Craven DE, Steger KA: Pathogenesis and prevention of nosocomial pneumonia in the mechanically ventilated patient. Respir Care 1989;34:85–97
32. Summer WR, Nelson S: Nosocomial pneumonia: Characteristics of the patient-pathogen interaction. Respir Care 1989; 34:116–124

33. Cross AS, Roup B: Role of respiratory assistance devices in endemic nosocomial pneumonia. Am J Med 1981;70:681–685
34. Reinarz JA, Pierce AK, Mays BB et al: The potential role of inhalation-therapy equipment in nosocomial pulmonary infection. J Clin Invest 1965;44:831–839
35. Pierce AK, Sanford JP, Thomas GD et al: Long-term evaluation of decontamination of inhalation-therapy equipment and the occurrence of necrotizing pneumonia. N Engl J Med 1970;282:528–531
36. Craven DE, Lichtenberg DA, Goularte TA et al: Contaminated medication nebulizers in mechanical ventilator circuits: Source of bacterial aerosols. Am J Med 1984;77:834–838
37. Craven DE, Goularte TA, Make BJ: Contaminated condensate in mechanical ventilator circuits: A risk factor for nosocomial pneumonia? Am Rev Respir Dis 1984;129:625–628
38. Chatburn RL: Decontamination of respiratory care equipment: What can be done, what should be done. Respir Care 1989; 34:98–110
39. Hudson LD: Diagnosis and management of acute respiratory distress in patients on mechanical ventilators. pp. 201–213. In Moser KM, Spragg RG (eds): Respiratory Emergencies. 2nd Ed. CV Mosby, St. Louis, 1982
40. Tobin MJ: What should the clinician do when a patient "fights the ventilator"? Respir Care 1991;36:395–406
41. Glauser FL, Polatty RC, Sessler CN: Worsening oxygenation in the mechanically ventilated patient: Causes, mechanisms, and early detection. Am Rev Respir Dis 1988;138:458–465

Chapter 85

Critical Care Ventilators

Robert M. Kacmarek

CHAPTER OUTLINE

The mechanical ventilators used in today's intensive care units (ICUs) are a product of decades of research and engineering refinement. The operational capabilities of these units dwarf those of the original positive pressure ventilators introduced in the 1940s through the 1960s.[1] Most of the newest generation of mechanical ventilators are highly sophisticated microprocessor-controlled instruments, many incorporating several interdependent microprocessors. The following is a listing of most of the units that would be classified as the "newest generation of mechanical ventilators":

Siemens, Servo 900C
Siemens, Servo 900E
Siemens, Servo 300
Puritan-Bennett, 7200spe
Puritan-Bennett, 7200e
Puritan-Bennett, 7200ae
Ohmeda, Advent
Infrasonics, Adult Star
Newport, Wave
Hamilton, Veolar
Hamilton, Amadeus
Bird, 6400 ST
Bird, 8400 ST
Intermed, Bear 5
Drager (Biomedical Systems), IRISA
Sechrist, 2000
Engstrom, ERICA
Liquid Air, CESAR

Although I believe this list is complete, I am also confident that it will be obsolete by the time this text is published, because newer units seem to be introduced almost monthly.

This chapter provides an overview of the general functional characteristics of the newest generation of mechanical ventilators. It does not systematically review the capabilities of each unit. A detailed discussion of individual units is provided by the specific manufacturer and in a number of other texts.[2–5] This chapter begins with a presentation of the ventilator classification system recently introduced by Chatburn.[6]

CLASSIFICATION OF MECHANICAL VENTILATORS*

The classification of mechanical ventilators into a specific, well-defined system is intended to enhance communication between clinicians. For example, if the mechanism designed to terminate inspiration is referred to by a number of different terms, it is difficult to determine whether a series of individuals or manufacturers are referring to the same mechanism. In this sense, a mechanical ventilator classification system is a language purely designed to enhance communication.

In general, a ventilator is simply a machine, a system of related elements designed to alter, transmit, and direct applied energy in a predetermined manner to perform useful work.[7] We input energy into mechanical ventilators in the form of electricity or compressed gas. The ventilator translates, or transforms, the energy in a predetermined manner to augment or replace the patient's muscles in the performance of the work of breathing. Thus, the mechanical ventilator can be described by four basic but global functions: (1) power input, (2) power transmission or conversion, (3) control, and (4) output. In addition, alarms can be considered. It is imperative that a good classification scheme describe how a given ventilator works in general terms, but have enough detail to allow one ventilator to be distinguished from another.

Input Variable

Two forms of input energy are used to operate mechanical ventilators:

- Pneumatic
- Electric
  - Alternating current (ac)
  - Direct current (dc, battery)
- Pneumatic/electric

Most mechanical ventilators only require input from one of these energy forms for the unit to function, although it is feasible that both input forms of energy would be necessary for a given unit to operate properly.

Power Conversion and Transmission

Power conversion and transmission refer to the exact mechanism or mechanisms used to drive the machine (i.e., providing gas delivery). As noted in Table 85-1, this usually takes the form of a compressor and/or motor linkage or proportional valving system, both potentially controlled by feedback from the actual output variables. Thus, a closed loop, computer-controlled feedback loop may be established to enhance performance of the driving mechanism (Fig. 85-1). Details on driving mechanisms are provided elsewhere.[2,3,7]

Table 85-1. Power Conversion and Transmission

External compressor
Internal compressor
Motor and linkage
Compressed gas, direct
Electric motor, rotating crank and piston rod
Electric motor, rack and pinion
Electric motor, direct
Output Control Valves
Pneumatic diaphragm
Pneumatic poppit valve
Electromagnetic poppit valve
Electromagnetic proportional valve

(From Chatburn,[6] with permission.)

Control

During the process of normal breathing or mechanical ventilatory assistance, four independent but interrelated variables must be coordinated: volume, pressure, flow, and time. In general, if any of these variables is programmed to operate in a specified manner, the others must respond, based on the variable or variables controlled. Therefore, if a ventilator is programmed to deliver a specific volume of gas in a precise flow waveform, airway pressure and time of delivery are dependent on the volume and flow waveform chosen, as well as on the impedance of the patient–ventilator system. Table 85-2 lists those factors considered under the area of control.

To establish control over pressure, flow, volume, and time, a control circuit must be incorporated into the ventilator's design. The control circuit is the subsystem respon-

Table 85-2. Mechanical Ventilator Control

Control circuit
Mechanical
Pneumatic
Fluidic
Electric
Electronic
Control variables and waveforms
Pressure
Volume
Flow
Time
Phase variables
Trigger
Limit
Cycle
Baseline
Conditional variables

(From Chatburn,[6] with permission.)

* Adapted from Chatburn,[6] with permission.

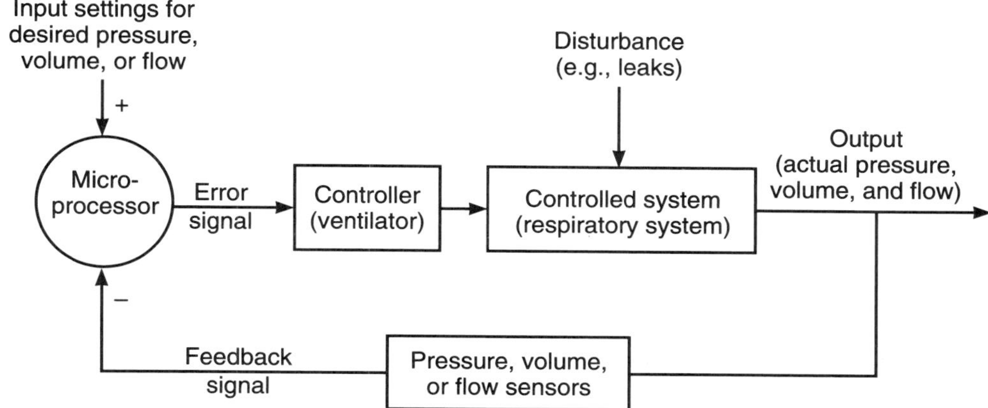

Figure 85-1. Energy flows from input to output via the unit's driving mechanism under the control of a microprocessor. Feedback from the output variable is provided, allowing closed-loop or servo control of output variables. (From Chatburn,[6] with permission.)

sible for controlling the driving mechanism and/or the output valve. A given ventilator may incorporate more than one type of control circuit (Table 85-2). For details, refer to McPherson,[2] Dupuis,[3] Chatburn,[6] and Spearman and Sanders.[7]

If the control variable for a given approach is ventilatory pressure, the ventilator controls airway pressure in a definite manner, causing it to rise above end-expiratory pressure in a predetermined pressure waveform. Generally, when this type of control is established, volume and flow are variable. A ventilator is classified as a volume controller if it measures and controls the volume it delivers. Delivered volume can be measured directly by the volume change of the ventilator's compressor, such as the displacement of a piston or bellows.[8] If the volume change remains consistent when compliance or resistance changes, and if volume change is not directly measured, the ventilator is classified as a flow controller. Most ventilators currently believed to be volume controllers (7200, 900C, Veolar) are actually flow controllers. If both pressure and volume are affected substantially by changes in lung mechanics, then the only form of control is time. Figure 85-2 defines the criteria used to determine the type of controller.

Phase Variables

Once the control variables and the associated waveforms are identified, more detail can be obtained by examining the events that take place during a ventilatory cycle (i.e., the period of time between the beginning of one breath and the beginning of the next). Mushin et al.[9] divided this time span

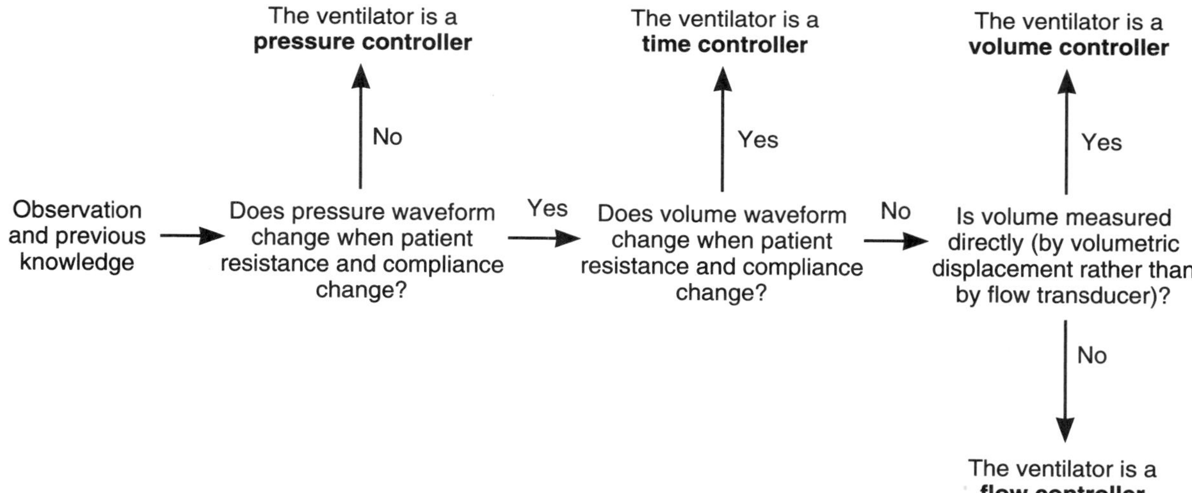

Figure 85-2. Criteria for determining the control variable during a ventilator-supported inspiration. Beginning with observations and previous knowledge of this ventilator, decisions are based on the effect of load on ventilator output. (From Chatburn,[6] with permission.)

into four phases: (1) the change from expiration to inspiration, (2) inspiration, (3) the change form inspiration to expiration, (4) and expiration. This convention is useful for examining how a ventilator starts, sustains, and stops an inspiration, and what it does between inspirations. In each phase a particular variable is measured and used to start, sustain, and end the phase. In this context, pressure, volume, flow, and time are referred to as phase variables[10] (Fig. 85-3).

Trigger

The phase variable that *initiates inspiration* is referred to as the trigger variable. In general, ventilators are triggered to inspiration by time or pressure. However, some of the newest ventilators have incorporated flow triggering (Siemens 300, Puritan-Bennett 7200) and, at least theoretically, volume could be used as a trigger.

Limit

Inspiratory time is defined as the time interval between the start of inspiratory flow and the start of expiratory flow. During inspiration pressure, volume, and flow increase above their end-expiratory values. If one (or more) of these variables rises no higher than some preset value, the variable is called a limit variable; but it must be distinguished from the variable used to end inspiration (called a cycle variable). Therefore, we impose the additional criteria that inspiration is not terminated because a variable has met its preset limit value. Thus, a variable is limited if it increases to a preset value before inspiration ends.

Cycle

Inspiration always ends (i.e., is cycled off) because some variable has reached a preset value. The variable that is measured and used to terminate inspiration is called the cycle variable. The criteria for determining cycle variables are given in Figure 85-3.

Baseline

The significant characteristic of expiration is how the ventilator affects the way the control variables return to their baseline values. The variable controlled during the expiratory time is the baseline variable. The ability of a ventilator to control the baseline variable means, for practical pur-

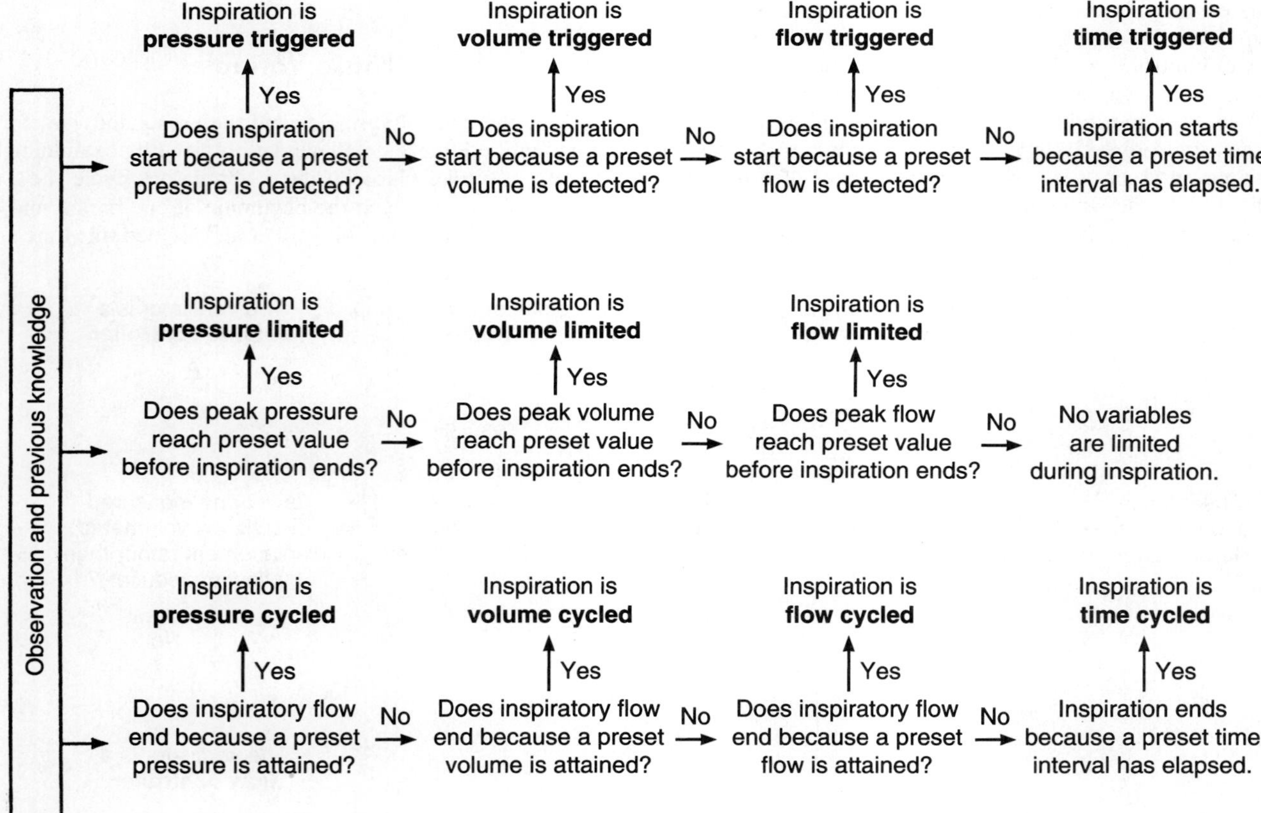

Figure 85-3. Criteria for determining the phase variables during a ventilator-supported breath. (From Chatburn,[6] with permission.)

poses, the ability to control expiratory pressure (i.e., positive end-expiratory pressure [PEEP], continuous positive airway pressure [CPAP]).

Conditional Variables

For each breath provided by the mechanical ventilator, there is a specific pattern of control and phase variables. The ventilator may either keep this pattern constant for each breath, or it may introduce other patterns (e.g., one for mandatory and one for spontaneous breaths). Some ventilators are capable of complex patterns, such as two types of mandatory breaths (one normal, one sigh) and two types of spontaneous breaths (e.g., two different pressure limits). In essence, the ventilator must decide which pattern of control and phase variables to implement before each breath, depending on the value of some preset conditions. The specific conditions under which variable patterns of ventilation are delivered are referred to as *conditional variables*.

Output

Just as the study of cardiovascular physiology involves the study of electrocardiograms and blood pressure waveforms, the study of ventilator operation requires the examination of output waveforms. The waveforms of interest are the pressure, volume, and flow waveforms (Table 85-3).

No ventilator is an ideal controller, and ventilators are designed only to approximate a particular waveform. Idealized or standard waveforms are nevertheless helpful because they characterize a ventilator's capabilities. However, the ideal waveforms, as depicted in Figure 85-4, differ considerably from actual waveforms (see Chs. 82 and 83).

Table 85-3. Mechanical Ventilator Output

Pressure waveforms
Rectangular
Exponential
Sinusoidal
Oscillating
Volume waveforms
Ramp
Sinusoidal
Flow waveforms
Rectangular
Ascending ramp
Descending ramp
Sinusoidal
Effects of the patient circuit

(From Chatburn,[6] with permission.)

Pressure Waveforms

Rectangular

A rectangular waveform is referred to mathematically as a step or instantaneous change in transrespiratory pressure from one constant value to another. In response, volume rises exponentially from zero to a steady-state value equal to compliance times the change in airway pressure, or peak inspiratory pressure (PIP) minus PEEP (i.e., PIP − PEEP). Inspiratory flow falls exponentially from a peak value (at the start of inspiration) equal to (PIP − PEEP)/resistance.

Exponential

Exponential pressure waveforms are commonly used during neonatal ventilation. Ventilators such as the Bear Cub are designed to deliver a modified rectangular waveform that typically results in a gradual, rather than instantaneous change in pressure at the start of inspiration. Thus, depending on the specific ventilator settings (e.g., short inspiratory time, low flow rate, and high PIP), the pressure waveform may never attain a constant value and resembles an exponential curve instead. In response, the volume and flow waveforms are also exponential, but their peak values are less than with a rectangular pressure waveform.

Sinusoidal

A sinusoidal pressure waveform can be created by attaching a piston either to a rotating crank or to a linear-drive motor driven by an oscillating signal generator. In response, the volume and flow waveforms are also sinusoidal, but they attain their peak values at different times.

Volume Waveforms

Ramp

Volume controllers that produce an ascending-ramp waveform produce a linear rise in volume from zero at the start of inspiration to the peak value (i.e., the set tidal volume [V_T]) at end-inspiration. In response, the flow waveform is rectangular in shape. The pressure waveform rises instantaneously from zero to a value equal to resistance times flow at the start of inspiration, from which it rises linearly to its peak value (i.e., PIP) equal to

$$\text{PIP} = \frac{V_T}{\text{compliance}} + [(\text{flow})(\text{resistance})] + \text{PEEP}$$

Sinusoidal

The sinusoidal waveform is most often produced by ventilators driven by a piston attached to a rotating crank. The output waveform of this type of ventilator is approximated by the first half of a cosine curve (in this case, sometimes referred to as a sigmoidal curve). Because the volume is sinusoidal during inspiration, pressure and flow are also sinusoidal.

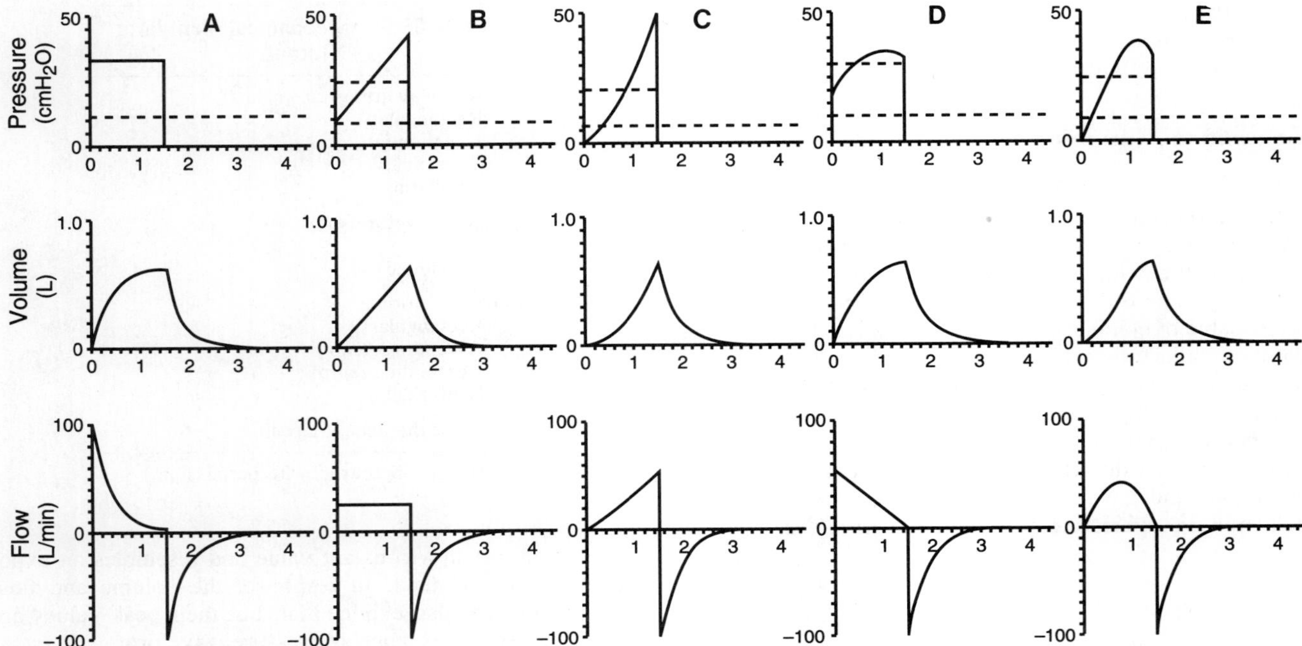

Figure 85-4. Theoretical output waveforms for **(A)** pressure-controlled inspiration with rectangular pressure waveform, identical to flow-controlled inspiration with an exponential-decay flow waveform; **(B)** flow-controlled inspiration with rectangular flow waveform, identical to volume-controlled inspiration with an ascending-ramp volume waveform; **(C)** flow-controlled inspiration with an ascending-ramp flow waveform; **(D)** flow-controlled inspiration with a descending-ramp flow waveform; and **(E)** flow-controlled inspiration with a sinusoidal flow waveform. Dashed lines that stop at the vertical line represent mean inspiratory pressure while the longer dashed lines denote mean airway pressure (assuming zero end-expiratory pressure). For the rectangular pressure waveform (Fig. A), the mean inspiratory pressure is the same as the peak inspiratory pressure. These output waveforms were created by (1) defining the control waveform (e.g., an ascending-ramp flow waveform is specified as flow = constant × time) and specifying that V_T equals 644 mL (about 9 mL/kg for a normal adult); (2) specifying the desired values for resistance and compliance (compliance, 20 mL/cmH_2O; resistance, 20 cmH_2O × s × L^{-1}, according to ANSI recommendations[11]); (3) substituting the above information into the equation of motion; and (4) using a computer to solve the equation for pressure, volume, and flow and plotting the results against time. (From Chatburn,[6] with permission.)

Flow Waveforms

Rectangular

A rectangular flow waveform is perhaps the most common output. When the flow waveform is rectangular, volume has a ramp waveform, and pressure is a step followed by a ramp, as described for the ramp volume waveform.

Ascending Ramp

A true ascending-ramp waveform starts at zero and increases linearly to the peak value. Ventilator flow waveforms are usually truncated; inspiration starts with an initial instantaneous flow (e.g., the Bear 5 starts inspiration at 50 percent of the set peak flow). Flow then increases linearly to the set peak flow rate. In response to an ascending-ramp flow waveform, the pressure and volume waveforms are exponential, with an upward concave shape.

Descending Ramp

A true descending-ramp (decelerating) waveform starts at the peak value and decreases linearly to zero. Ventilator flow waveforms are usually truncated; inspiratory flow rate decreases linearly from the set peak flow until it reaches some arbitrary threshold at which flow drops immediately to zero (e.g., the Bennett 7200a ends inspiration when the flow rate drops to 5 L/min). In response to a descending-ramp flow waveform, the pressure and volume waveforms are exponential, with a concave downward shape.

Sinusoidal

Some ventilators offer a mode in which the inspiratory flow waveform approximates the shape of the first half of a sine wave. As with the ramp waveform, ventilators often truncate the sine waveform by starting and ending flow at some percentage of the set peak flow, rather than starting and ending at zero flow. In response to a sinusoidal flow waveform, the pressure and volume waveforms are sinusoidal but out of phase with each other.

Effects of the Patient Circuit

So far in this discussion, it has been implied that what comes out of the ventilator is the same as what goes into the patient. However, the pressure, volume, and flow measured inside the ventilator are never the same as the pressure, volume, and flow measured at the patient's airway opening. The reason is that the patient's circuit has its own compliance (actually, the compliance of the tubing material, plus the compressibility of the inspired gas) and resistance. Therefore, the pressure measured inside the ventilator on the inspiratory side is always higher than the pressure at the airway opening, because of the elastic and flow-resistive pressure drops created by the patient circuit. Volume and flow coming out of the ventilator are always higher than the volume and flow delivered to the patient because of the effect of compliance of the patient circuit. This compliance effect absorbs both volume and flow. In addition, it must be remembered that, in general, the set values for pressure, volume, and flow differ from the output (ventilator) values because of calibration errors and from the input (patient) values because of the effects of the patient circuit. Thus, there are two general sources of error that cause discrepancies between the desired and actual patient values.

Alarm Systems

Ventilator alarms have also increased in number and complexity. Day and MacIntyre[12] have stressed that the goal of ventilator alarms is to warn of *events*. They define an event as any condition or occurrence that requires clinician awareness or action. Technical events are those involving an inadvertent change in the ventilator's performance; patient events are those involving a change in the patient's clinical status.[12] A ventilator may be equipped with any conceivable vital sign monitor, so the appropriate scope of surveillance needs to be defined. The most logical scope would include the ventilator's mechanical-electronic operation and those variables associated with the mechanics of breathing (i.e., pressure, volume, flow, time) (Table 85-4).

Alarms may be audible, visual, or both, depending on the seriousness of the alarm condition. Visual alarms may be as simple as colored lights or as complex as alphanumeric messages indicating the exact nature of the fault condition. Specifications for an alarm event should include

1. Conditions that trigger the alarm
2. The alarm response in the form of audible and/or visual messages
3. Any associated ventilator response, such as termination of inspiration or failure to operate
4. Whether the alarm must be manually reset or resets itself when the alarm condition is rectified

Table 85-5 outlines the various levels of alarm priority along with characteristics and appropriate categories. Alarm categories are based on the ventilator classification scheme.

Input Power Alarms

Loss of Electrical Power

Most ventilators have some sort of battery backup in case of electrical power failure. Ventilators typically have alarms that are activated if the electrical power is cut off while the machine is still switched on (e.g., if the power cord is accidentally pulled out of the wall socket). If the ventilator is designed to operate on battery power (e.g., transport ventilators), an alarm usually warns of a low-battery condition.

Loss of Pneumatic Power

Ventilators that use pneumatic power have alarms that are activated if either the O_2 or air supply is cut off or reduced below some specified driving pressure. In some cases the

Table 85-4. Mechanical Ventilator Alarm Systems

Input power alarms
- Loss of electrical power
- Loss of pneumatic power

Control circuit alarms
- General systems failure (ventilator inoperative)
- Incompatible ventilator settings
- Inverse I/E ratio

Output alarms
- Pressure
  - High and low peak airway pressure
  - High and low mean airway pressure
  - High and low baseline pressure (PEEP or CPAP)
  - Failure of airway pressure to return to baseline within a specified period
- Volume
- Flow
- Time
  - High or low ventilatory frequency
  - High or low inspiratory time
  - Long or short expiratory time (long expiratory time = apnea)
- Inspired gas
  - High or low inspired gas temperature
  - High or low F_{IO_2}

F_{IO_2}, inspired O_2 fraction.
(From Chatburn,[6] with permission.)

Table 85-5. A Four-Level Classification of Ventilator Alarms[a]

	Level 1	Level 2	Level 3	Level 4
Alarm characteristics				
Mandatory?	Yes	Yes	No	Yes
Redundant?	Yes	No	No	No
Noncancelling?	Yes	No	No	Yes
Audible?	Yes	Yes	Yes	No
Visual?	Yes	Yes	Yes	Yes
Automatic backup response?	Yes	No		No
Automatic reset			No	
Audible?	Yes	Yes	Yes	Yes
Visual?	No	Yes	Yes	Yes
Applicable alarm categories				
Input				
Electric power?	Yes	No	No	No
Pneumatic power?	Yes	No	No	No
Control circuit				
Inverse I/E?	No	Yes	No	Yes
Incompatible settings?	No	No	No	Yes
Mechanical/electronic fault?	Yes	No	No	No
Output				
Pressure?[b]	Yes	Yes	Yes	Yes
Volume?[c]	Yes	Yes	Yes	Yes
Flow?[d]	Yes	Yes	Yes	Yes
Minute ventilation?	Yes	Yes	Yes	Yes
Time?[e]	Yes	Yes	Yes	Yes
Inspired gas (F_{IO_2}, temperature)?	Yes	Yes	No	Yes

[a] Level 1, critical ventilator malfunction; level 2, noncritical ventilator malfunction (not immediately life-threatening); level 3, patient status change; level 4, operator alert (inappropriate control setting or alarm threshold).
[b] Pressure alarms: high and low peak, mean, and baseline.
[c] High and low inhaled and exhaled V_T; may include alarm for leak.
[d] Alarm triggered if expiratory flow does not fall below set threshold (gas trapping).
[e] Inspiratory or expiratory times too long or too short.
(From Chatburn,[6] with permission.)

alarm is activated by an electronic pressure switch (e.g., Bennett 7200); however, in others the alarm is pneumatically operated as a part of the blender (e.g., Siemens Servo 900C).

Control Circuit Alarms

Control circuit alarms are those that either warn the operator that the set control variables are incompatible (e.g., inverse inspiration/expiration [I/E] ratio) or that some aspect of a ventilator self-test has failed. In the latter case, there may be something wrong with the ventilator control circuitry itself, (e.g., a microprocessor failure) and the ventilator generally responds with a generic message such as "ventilator inoperative."

Output Alarms

Output alarms are those triggered by an unacceptable state of the ventilator's output. More specifically, an output alarm is activated when the value of a control variable (pressure, volume, flow, or time) falls outside an expected range. Some possibilities include

1. **Pressure**
   High and low peak airway pressure—indicating a possible endotracheal tube obstruction or leak in the patient circuit, respectively
   High and low mean airway pressure—indicating a possible leak in the patient circuit or a change in ventilatory pattern that might lead to a change in the patient's oxygenation status (i.e., within reasonable limits, oxygenation is roughly proportional to mean airway pressure)
   High and low baseline pressure (PEEP or CPAP)—indicating a possible patient-circuit or exhalation-manifold obstruction (or inadvertent PEEP), and disconnection of the patient from the patient circuit, respectively
   Failure of airway pressure to return to baseline within a specified period—indicating a possible patient-circuit obstruction or exhalation-manifold malfunction
2. **Volume**
   High and low exhaled V_T—indicating changes in respiratory system-time constant during pressure-controlled ventilation or possible

disconnection of the patient from the patient circuit

3. **Flow**
   High and low exhaled minute ventilation—indicating hypertension (or possible machine self-triggering) and possible apnea or disconnection of the patient from the patient circuit, respectively
4. **Time**
   High or low ventilatory frequency—indicating hyperventilation (or possible machine self-triggering) and possible apnea, respectively
   Inspiratory time too long or too short—too long indicates a possible patient-circuit obstruction or exhalation-manifold malfunction; too short indicates that adequate VT may not have been delivered (in a pressure-control mode) or that gas distribution in the lungs may not be optimal
   Expiratory time too long or too short—too long indicates apnea; too short indicates warning of alveolar gas trapping (i.e., expiratory time should be three to four time constants or more of the respiratory system)
5. **Inspired gas**
   High/low inspired gas temperature
   High/low inspired O_2 fraction (F_IO_2)

NEW GENERATION MECHANICAL VENTILATORS*

The primary factor distinguishing the newest generation of mechanical ventilators from previous generations is microprocessor control. Microprocessors have expanded the function and enhanced the performance of mechanical ventilators, which has resulted, at least theoretically, in the following advantages[1,13]:

1. Flexibility and variability in gas delivery pattern
2. Back-up/apnea ventilation availability in all modes (assist/control [A/C], synchronized intermittent mandatory ventilation [SIMV], pressure support ventilation [PSV], and CPAP)
3. Ability to evaluate/monitor overall function
4. Need for fewer moving parts
5. Extensive patient–ventilator system monitoring capabilities
6. Ease of repair
7. Ease of updating systems
8. Improved spontaneous breathing capabilities
9. RS 232 outputs
10. The capability of interfacing with computer systems

* Adapted from Kacmarek and Meklaus,[1,5] with permission.

Gas Delivery System

The internal gas delivery circuitry of a microprocessor ventilator is generally much simpler than its earlier counterparts. Figure 85-5, a schematic of the Hamilton Veolar ventilator, illustrates the overall simplicity of the pneumatic systems of microprocessor ventilators. Air and O_2 at 50 psi enter the ventilator at independent connections and immediately pass through check valves (A) and by pressure switches (B) to regulators (C) that reduce pressure to 20 psi before proceeding to a mixing chamber (D) to establish the concentration of inspired gas. From here, gas enters a reservoir tank (E), which maintains pressure at 3 to 5 psi. The reservoir ensures sufficient gas is available to meet peak inspiratory demands. During inspiration, gas proceeds to the unit's flow control valve (F), where gas movement across the valve is controlled by a linear potentiometer and differential pressure transducer (G). After exiting the flow control valve, gas on the way to the patient's inspiratory circuit passes an ambient antisuffocation valve (H), a high pressure relief valve (I), and a proximal flow meter (J).[13,14] Although at first inspection this may seem complex, it is a large improvement over the yards of small-bore tubing directing gas flow in earlier generations of ventilators.

The flow control mechanism is the heart of the gas delivery system in all of these ventilators. It controls flow during spontaneous, as well as mechanical ventilation, and allows for variability in inspiratory waveform. These valves, whether they are proportional solenoids or variable orifice flow controllers, are all regulated by servo feedback mechanisms, most via microprocessors. As a result, consistency in gas delivery, as well as variability in waveform production, is enhanced over earlier generations of mechanical ventilators. Figure 85-6 is a schematic of the Hamilton flow control valve, which consists of an electrodynamically-controlled plunger valve with a triangular opening. During inspiration, as the valve opens, a differential pressure transducer measures pressure across the valve, providing feedback to the microprocessor, which controls the opening via a linear potentiometer.[14] As a result, inspiratory gas flow wave patterns can be contoured to provide all possible inspiratory waveforms.

A second enhancement resulting from the use of sophisticated flow control mechanisms has been a marked decrease in the work of breathing imposed by this generation of ventilators over that of previous generations.[15,16] The development of more responsive flow control valves and the addition of microprocessor control has resulted in a 10-fold reduction in imposed work.[17,18] All of these units also allow "spontaneous" ventilation to be assisted by inspiratory pressure support.

Versatility in operation of these units goes beyond the gas flow mechanism. Because moving parts are few in all of these ventilators, and those present are under microprocessor control, the introduction of new modes or gas delivery patterns can usually be accomplished without significant changes in the gas delivery system. For example, the incorporation of airway pressure release ventilation[19] is, at least theoretically, feasible on every microprocessor ventilator marketed, with-

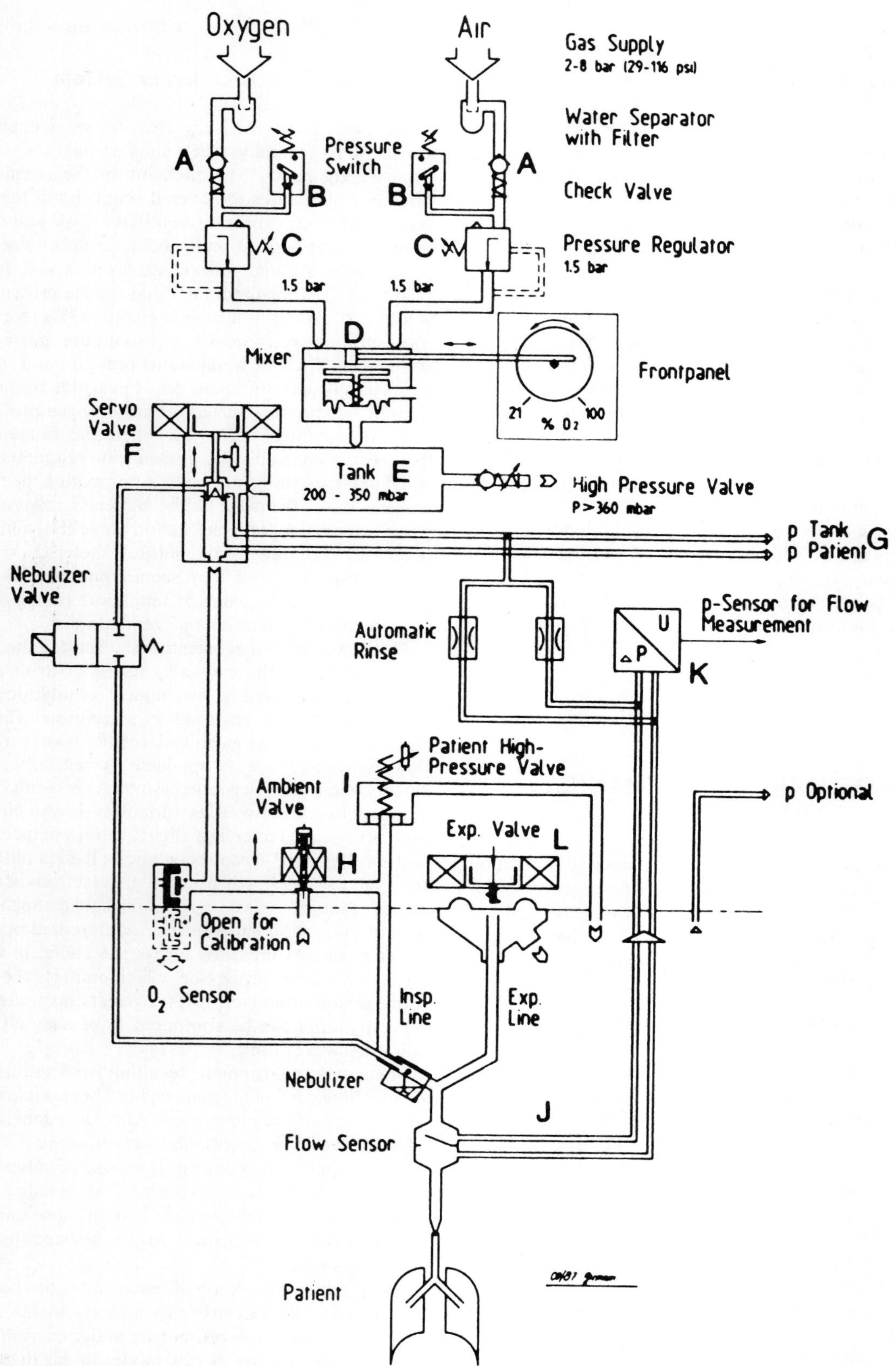

Figure 85-5. Internal schematic of the Hamilton Veolar ventilator. A, Check valve; B, pressure switch; C, internal pressure regulators; D, mixing valve; E, reservoir tank; F, plunger valve; G, pressure sensors; H, ambient valve; I, patient high-pressure valve; J, low compliance tubing; K, differential pressure transducer; L, exhalation valve. (From Hamilton Medical,[13] with permission.)

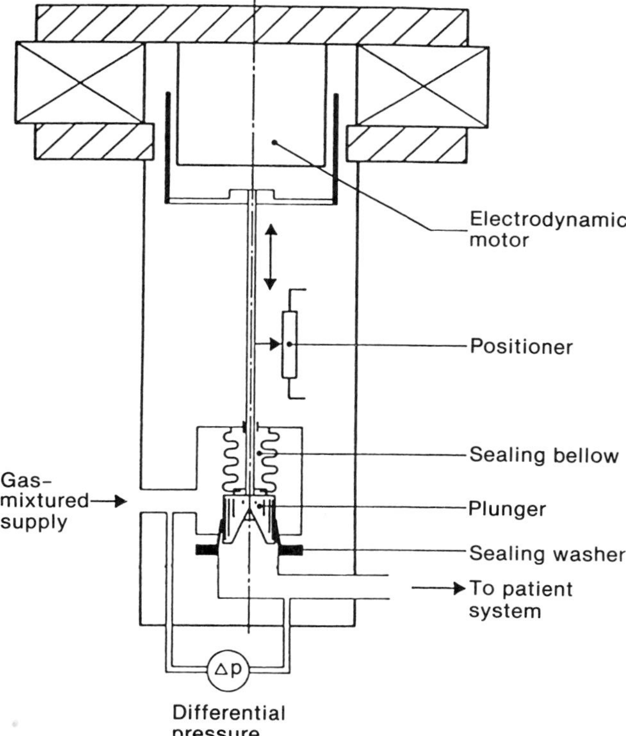

Figure 85-6. Schematic of Hamilton Veolar and Amadeus flow control valve. (From Hamilton Medical,[13] with permission.)

out significant alteration in internal hardware. Although the reprogramming of a given unit may be extensive, once the algorithm is completed it may only require the changing of circuit boards and the addition of panel controls to incorporate it. A primary example of this flexibility is the Puritan-Bennett 7200 ventilator. Since its introduction in 1983, at least eight updates have occurred without significant hardware alterations.

Back-Up/Apnea Ventilation

Microprocessors have enabled back-up/apnea ventilation to be expanded beyond the A/C mode. Most of these units have added this feature during SIMV, PSV, and CPAP. This has greatly increased the safety of applying any of the spontaneous breathing modes.

Patient–Ventilator System Monitoring

All of the microprocessor-based units perform a detailed systems check before they become functional. If specific systems fail this evaluation, the unit may be rendered inoperable, although with some units noncritical problems can be overridden. In addition, during use the unit continues to evaluate its function and notifies the operator of its inability to perform as programmed. The diagnostic capabilities of these machines have greatly increased the ease with which they can be repaired. Normally error codes identify malfunctioning systems for repair personnel. If problems are related to electrical components, simple replacement of a circuit board usually rectifies the problem. Because relatively few moving parts are included, hardware problems are rare.

Patient monitoring capabilities are greatly expanded in this generation of ventilators. Essentially, every aspect of the patient's ventilatory pattern can be assessed, monitored, and displayed. Additionally, each monitored patient variable, as well as machine functions, can have alarms. Some of these units monitor up to 17 variables, all of which have alarms (Bear 5).

Graphic displays of inspiratory pressure and gas flow waveforms are available on the Bear 5, IRISA, and Infrasonics ventilators, as well as being optional on the Ohmeda monitoring system, the Hamilton "Leonardo," the 7200a display screen, and the Servo computer-assisted ventilation model. These displays assist in the evaluation of patient effort during both spontaneous breathing and positive pressure ventilation and improve the clinician's ability to contour gas delivery to ventilatory demand (see Ch. 83 for detailed discussion). In addition, most of these units have an RS 232 output available, which allows the interface of the ventilator with a computer for data storage or more extensive trending of monitored variables, as well as documentation of alarm conditions and alterations in machine parameter settings.

Disadvantages of Microprocessor Ventilators

Overall, the function of microprocessor ventilators is enhanced over that of previous generations of mechanical ventilators because they are capable of a greater scope of performance. However, they are relatively expensive. The top-of-the-line units of most manufacturers, with options, list between $25,000 and $35,000. In addition, many of these units are highly complex and difficult to operate, requiring extensive training and retraining to ensure a complete understanding of all their nuances. For example, the Hamilton Veolar and the Drager IRISA each incorporate controls with dual functions. The Veolar uses single dials to adjust somewhat related but different variables (e.g., PEEP and pressure support, as well as inspiratory and expiratory pause percentage and I/E ratio). On the other hand, selected controls on the IRISA have entirely different functions in various modes (e.g., speed with which peak flow is obtained in the pressure support mode, and sensitivity, as well as intermittent PEEP and pressure support level). Even the 7200 and the Bear 5, which appear initially to have their control panel laid out logically, frequently are perceived as difficult to operate, because multiple entries are required to set parameters and special functions are hidden by a single key (+ + key on the 7200). Additionally, with most of these units it is impossible for the clinician to view the control panel and understand how the patient is being mechanically ventilated without detailed knowledge of the machine's operation.

Many of these machines are capable of providing every documented approach to ventilation available, but as a result, their capabilities far exceed the need of 70 to 80 percent of patients requiring mechanical ventilation. Exceptions to this are the step-down units recently introduced by Puritan-Bennett (7200e), Siemens (900E) and Hamilton (Amadeus), as well as the Bird 6400 ST. Although each of these units is microprocessor-based, their mode capabilities (control, A/C, SIMV, and PSV), monitoring functions, and alarm functions are downgraded from those incorporated in top-of-the-line models. These units, it appears, better occupy the niche where 70 to 80 percent of patients' needs lie.

References

1. Kacmarek RM, Meklaus GL: The new generation of mechanical ventilators. Crit Care Clin 1990;6:551–578
2. McPherson SP: Respiratory Therapy Equipment. 3rd Ed. CV Mosby, St. Louis, 1990
3. Dupuis YG: Ventilators—Theory and Clinical Application. CV Mosby, St. Louis, 1986
4. Banner MJ, Blanch P, Desautels DA: Mechanical ventilators. pp. 401–503. In Kirby RR, Banner MJ, Downs JB (eds): Clinical Applications of Ventilatory Support. Churchill Livingstone, New York, 1990
5. Kacmarek RM, Meklaus GL: Microprocessor controlled mechanical ventilators. Probl Crit Care 1990;4:161–183
6. Chatburn RL: A new system for understanding mechanical ventilators. Respir Care 1991;36:1123–1155
7. Spearman CB, Sanders HG Jr: Physical principles and functional designs of ventilators. pp. 63–104. In Kirby RR, Banner MJ, Downs JB (eds): Clinical Applications of Ventilatory Support. Churchill Livingstone, New York, 1990
8. Miller WF, Scacci R, Gast LR: Laboratory Evaluation of Pulmonary Function. JB Lippincott, Philadelphia, 1987, pp. 39–44
9. Mushin WW, Rendell-Baker L, Thompson PW, Mapleson WW: Automatic Ventilation of the Lungs. 3rd Ed. Vol. 225. Blackwell Scientific Publications, Oxford, 1980
10. Desautels DA: Ventilator performance evaluation. pp. 121–144. In Kirby RR, Banner MJ, Downs JB (eds): Clinical Applications of Ventilatory Support. Churchill Livingstone, New York, 1990
11. Chatburn RL, Primiano FP Jr: Mathematical models of respiratory mechanics. pp. 59–100. In Chatburn RL, Craig KC (eds): Fundamentals of Respiratory Care Research. Appleton & Lange, East Norwalk, CT, 1988
12. Spearman CB, Sanders HG: The new generation of mechanical ventilators. Respir Care 1987;32:403–418
13. Hamilton Medical: Hamilton Veolar Ventilator Operator's Manual. Part number 610131. Hamilton Medical, Reno, NV, 1985
14. Vandine JD: Mechanical ventilators. pp. 438–466. In Barnes TA (ed): Respiratory Care Practice. Year Book Medical Publishers, Chicago, 1988
15. Gibney TRN, Wilson RS, Pontoppidan H: Comparison of work of breathing on high gas flow and demand valve continuous positive airway pressure systems. Chest 1982;82:692–695
16. Katz JA, Kraemer RW, Gjerde GE: Inspiratory work and airway pressure with continuous positive pressure delivery systems. Chest 1985;88:519–526
17. Hirsch CA, Kacmarek RM, Stanek K: Work of breathing during CPAP and PSV imposed by the new generation mechanical ventilators: A lung model study. Respir Care 1991;36:815–828
18. Samodelov LF, Falke KJ: Total inspiratory work with modern demand valve devices compared to continuous flow CPAP. Intensive Care Med 1988;14:632–639
19. Downs JB, Stock MC: Airway pressure release ventilation: A new concept in ventilatory support. Crit Care Med 1987;15:459–461

Chapter 86

Discontinuing Ventilatory Support

Thomas L. Higgins
James K. Stoller

CHAPTER OUTLINE

Weaning a patient from mechanical ventilation is a common challenge for the respiratory care clinician. Deciding when and how to wean a patient encompasses both art and science, since no single indicator or group of parameters predicts either weaning success or failure with 100 percent accuracy. For the purposes of this chapter, weaning is defined as the staged withdrawal of support by mechanical ventilation. Weaning is not synonymous with extubation, since there is a subset of patients, primarily those with upper airway edema or compression or those with glottic dysfunction with aspiration, who may no longer require mechanical ventilation but cannot be extubated because airway patency is threatened or because the airway cannot be protected against aspiration. This chapter considers the purpose of weaning and extubation, the rationale and clinical utility of predictive indices in weaning, application of weaning parameters in general and in specific patient subsets, specific impediments to weaning, practical details (or "how to") of the weaning process, and ancillary issues related to withdrawal of ventilatory support.

Gradual withdrawal of mechanical support is not always necessary. Patients undergoing short-term intubation and ventilation for surgical procedures under general anesthesia are usually managed by simply discontinuing ventilation when they have sufficient neurologic function and muscular strength to breathe on their own. While these patients occasionally require some assisted ventilation (and rarely, reintubation with resumption of mechanical ventilation), most do well since the cause of their ventilator dependence is only the presence of anesthetic agents, which can be rapidly reversed, eliminated, or metabolized. Weaning, or gradual withdrawal from mechanical ventilation, becomes more important in the patient whose reason for needing mechanical ventilation is only slowly resolving, particularly after systemic sepsis and multisystem organ failure. Recovery from surgical procedures in patients with pre-existing compromise of the respiratory system may also be associated with a long weaning period.

Intubation and prolonged mechanical ventilation are associated with considerable morbidity.[1–4] In one study vocal cord granulomas and ulceration of the true cords were seen in almost two-thirds of patients intubated for more than 24 hours.[1] Early tracheal lesions were seen in one-third of these patients and progressed to circumferential fibrous stenosis in 10 percent. Another study has reported significant tracheal lesions in 20 percent of intensive care unit (ICU) survivors and 95 percent of those dying while intubated.[2] Use of a compliant, deformable endotracheal cuff and continuous monitoring and adjustment of cuff pressure, preferably to less than 30 mmHg, may minimize these complications.[3] Functional concerns also favor removing the endotracheal tube as soon as possible, since tracheal intubation causes epithelial damage, loss of cilia, and impairment of tracheal mucus clearance, particularly with cuffed tubes.[5,6] Intubation impairs cough efficiency by limiting the velocity of expiratory airflow that can be achieved.[7] Instrumentation of the airway is a risk factor for nosocomial pneumonia,[8] although other factors (severity of illness, smoking history, prolonged operative procedure) are also contributory.[9] Proper decontamination of respiratory equipment,[10] measures to reduce tracheal colonization from the stomach,[11,12] and use of selective digestive tract decontamination[13,14] all reduce but do not eliminate the risk of nosocomial pneumonia. Intubation practically precludes oral feeding, mandating the use of either enteral feedings or parenteral nutrition. Iatrogenic malnutrition was identified in 23 of 26 patients on ventilators in one study[15]; this is of critical importance, since inadequate nutrition impairs skeletal and respiratory muscle function.[16] The adverse consequences of prolonged ventilator support underscore the importance of weaning at an optimal time to minimize the occurrence or severity of these complications.

RESPIRATORY PARAMETERS

Guidelines for weaning are desirable, since they may prevent premature weaning trials and avoid unnecessarily prolonged ventilatory support. A number of respiratory parameters have been proposed as guidelines for weaning patients from mechanical ventilation, but no single indicator or score performs flawlessly. Because no parameters have yet proved infallible in predicting successful extubation or inevitable failure of extubation, most experienced clinicians regard these parameters as guidelines rather than rigid rules. Nevertheless, measuring parameters remains important as a training device, to reduce dependence on the skills of an individual physician, and as a guide to management. Critical examination of the various weaning parameters can help the clinician to understand the reasons for ventilator dependency in a given patient and can often redirect management approaches when weaning fails.

The major determinants of ability to wean can be classified into three categories (Table 86-1): oxygenation, ventilatory pump function (i.e., the ability to eliminate CO_2), and neuropsychiatric status. Failure in each of these categories may have multiple causes. For example, hypoxemia as the result of hypoventilation may occur owing to suppression of respiratory drive or respiratory bellows dysfunction. Hypox-

Table 86-1. Determinants of Ability to Wean

Oxygenation
- Criteria of Adequacy
  - PaO_2 >60 mmHg on FIO_2 <0.35 at minimal PEEP, PaO_2/FIO_2 >200; $P(A\text{-}a)O_2$ <350 mmHg
- Selected causes of failure
  - Hypoventilation due to neurologic injury or drugs
  - Ventilation/perfusion mismatch (e.g., airspace disease, congestive heart failure)
  - Anatomic (right-to-left) shunt (e.g., intracardiac shunt, pulmonary arteriovenous malformation), decreased venous O_2 content/excessive O_2 extraction due to low cardiac output or hypermetabolism

Ventilation
- Criterion of Adequacy
  - $PaCO_2$ <50 mmHg or within 8 mmHg of baseline
- Selected causes of failure
  - Decreased respiratory drive (e.g., sedation, obesity/hypoventilation syndrome)
  - Decreased respiratory bellows function; diaphragmatic weakness; neuromuscular disease (e.g., Duchenne muscular dystrophy)
  - Increased CO_2 production without compensatory increase in alveolar ventilation (fever, hypermetabolism, carbohydrate overfeeding)
  - Increased dead space ventilation without compensatory increase in alveolar ventilation (e.g., pulmonary embolus, bullous emphysema)

Neuropsychiatric integrity
- Criteria of adequacy
  - Awake, alert, cooperative, with intact gag and swallowing
- Selected causes of failure
  - Cerebrovascular accident
  - Sleep deprivation/ICU psychosis
  - Drug therapy
  - Depression
  - Psychological dependency on ventilator

emia may also occur because of ventilation/perfusion inequalities (e.g., parenchymal disease, airflow obstruction) or anatomic shunt (e.g., decreased venous O_2 content as the result of inadequate cardiac output or increased peripheral O_2 uptake, intracardiac shunt, or pulmonary arteriovenous malformation). Impaired CO_2 elimination may be caused by suppression of the respiratory rate, impaired respiratory bellows function, increased dead space ventilation, or increased CO_2 production without compensatory hyperventilation. While outside the scope of this discussion, lack of airway patency can also cause hypoventilation, with resultant hypoxemia and hypercarbia. A variety of lesions, including vocal cord paralysis, tracheal mucosal edema, or compression of the airway by foreign bodies, aneurysms, or tumor can occur and must be considered in the patient who fails extubation despite normal mechanics and blood gases while intubated. Neuropsychiatric impediments to weaning include difficulties with mentation and cooperation as the result of cerebrovascular accident, medications, sleep deprivation, "ICU psychosis" or depression, and psychologic dependency on the ventilator.[17]

The assessment of weaning proceeds in two phases (Table 86-2): phase 1 is to ensure that certain basic criteria regarding the initial reason for mechanical ventilation are satisfied; and phase 2 is to determine whether weaning is likely to succeed on the basis of specified criteria. In phase 1 of the decision to wean, the condition for which mechanical ventilation was initiated must be resolved or resolving. The presence of ongoing sepsis is a contraindication to weaning because of increased metabolic requirements and the propensity for hemodynamic compromise. The presence of positive blood cultures predicts the need for reintubation in medical patients.[18]

Table 86-2. Two Phases of Decision Making for Weaning

Phase 1: general criteria to be satisfied
- Resolution of the process for which mechanical ventilation was initiated
- Absence of septicemia
- Hemodynamic stability
- Management secretions

Phase 2: satisfaction of specific weaning criteria
- Oxygenation/O_2 transport
  - PaO_2 >60 mmHg with FIO_2 <0.35 on low-level PEEP
  - $P(A\text{-}a)O_2$ <350 mmHg
  - Cardiac index >2.1 L/min/m^2
  - No lactic acidosis
- Mechanical function of the respiratory system
  - VC >10 mL/kg ideal body weight
  - $\dot{V}_E$ (rest) <10 L/min
  - MVV at least twice resting $\dot{V}_E$
  - TT_{di} <0.15
  - Tracheal occlusion pressure ($P_{0.1}$) <6 cmH_2O
  - Patient/ventilator system compliance >25 mL/cmH_2O
  - MIP >30 cmH_2O
  - F/V_T ≤105

FIO_2, inspired O_2 fraction; $P(A\text{-}a)O_2$, alveolar-arterial gradient; VC, vital capacity; $\dot{V}_E$, minute ventilationj; MVV, maximal voluntary ventilation; TT_{di}, tension-time index of the diaphragm; MIP, maximum inspiratory pressure; F/V_T, respiratory rate divided by tidal volume.

Similarly, an active infectious pulmonary process or tracheobronchitis may be an indication for continued mechanical ventilation if secretions are thick or copious, especially in the presence of diminished pulmonary reserve. Next, hemodynamic stability must be ensured. The transition from intermittent mandatory ventilation (IMV) at a rate of 10 to 12 breaths per minute to continuous positive airway pressure (CPAP) is associated in postoperative patients with a 10 percent increase in both O_2 consumption and CO_2 production.[19] Rapid weaning in patients with obstructive lung disease results in marked increases in transmural pulmonary artery pressure,[20] which suggests that acute left ventricular dysfunction may occur during the transition from supported to spontaneous ventilation, particularly when chronic obstructive pulmonary disease (COPD) and heart disease coexist. Finally, in phase 1 the patient's general strength must be restored. Prolonged bed rest causes muscle atrophy, partly from disuse and partly from protein catabolism during illness.[16] Proper nutritional support is essential in allowing recovery from acute lung injury and successful weaning from mechanical ventilation.[16,21] Electrolyte abnormalities, particularly hypocalcemia[22] and hypophosphatemia,[23] should be addressed. In general, the longer the need for mechanical ventilation, the longer the weaning process will take. Successful weaning, however, has been reported even after 5 years of mechanical ventilation.[24]

Once these general considerations have been satisfied in phase 1 of the weaning process, attention may turn to the measurable ventilatory parameters: oxygenation, ventilation, and quantification of endurance. Most parameters of oxygenation and O_2 transport have been derived empirically, seldom with prospective validation of the chosen threshold values. Oxygenation is deemed adequate when PaO_2 is above 60 mmHg at an inspired O_2 fraction (FIO_2) below 0.35 percent on low levels (i.e., not more than 5 cmH_2O) of positive end-expiratory pressure (PEEP), or if the alveolar-arterial gradient [$P(A\text{-}a)O_2$] is below 350 mmHg. Conventional criteria of adequate O_2 transport include mixed venous PO_2 ($P\bar{v}O_2$) above 35 mmHg, cardiac index greater than 2.1 L/min/m^2, and absence of lactic acidosis.

A number of measurements are used to evaluate the mechanical function of the respiratory system, including vital capacity (VC), tidal volume (V_T), minute ventilation ($\dot{V}_E$), maximal voluntary ventilation (MVV), and maximal inspiratory pressure (MIP). Among the earliest proposed weaning criteria were a VC of at least 10 mL/kg (ideal) body weight,[25] a VC of at least 1 L in an average-sized adult,[26] and a resting $\dot{V}_E$ less than 10 L/min with the ability to double the resting rate.[27] Table 86-3 summarizes prospective evaluations of the more common weaning parameters, beginning in 1973 with those of Sahn and Lakshminarayan.[28] In the sections that follow, each of the commonly proposed criteria is discussed.

Maximal Inspiratory Pressure

MIP is widely used as an index for evaluating ventilatory reserve, although it is not always measured in a standardized manner.[29] Multiple alternative terms and abbreviations are

Table 86-3. Literature Evaluation of Conventional Weaning Parameters

Author and Type of Patients	Parameters Evaluated						Best Predictors
	VC	V_T	$\dot{V}_E$	MVV/$\dot{V}_E$	MIP	V_D/V_T	
Sahn and Lakshminarayan[28] 100, mostly surgical	−	−	+	+	+	−	MIP < −30 cm H_2O
Tahvanainen et al.[18] 47 long-term medical	+	+	+	+	+	+	Urine output, RQ, positive blood culture, temperature
Morganroth et al.[49] 10 long-term medical/surgical	+	+	+	−	+	−	Score consisting of multiple ventilator and adverse factors
Fiastro et al.[34] 17 mixed-term medical/ surgical	+	+	+	−	+	−	Mechanics for short-term; WOB for long-term
Menzies et al.[88] 55 long-term COPD	+	+	−	−	+	−	Premorbid level of activity, FEV_1, albumin level, MIP, and respiratory rate during T-piece trial
DeHaven et al.[35] 48 postoperative/trauma	+	+	+	−	+	−	Gas exchange more useful than relying on mechanics (which may prolong support)
Millbern et al.[36] 38 short-term postoperative	+	−	−	−	+	−	pH >7.35 while decreasing IMV rate

−, not examined; +, included; WOB, work of breathing; RQ, respiratory quotient; FEV_1, forced expiratory volume in 1 second; IMV, intermittent mandatory ventilation; V_T, tidal volume; V_D/V_T, dead space/tidal volume ratio.

used to describe this characteristic, including inspiratory force (IF), negative inspiratory force (NIF), negative inspiratory pressure (NIP), maximum inspiratory force (MIF), peak negative pressure (PNP), and maximal static inspiratory pressure.[30] Recent studies have concluded that technical considerations influence the outcome of the MIP procedure and that proper technique requires airway occlusion for up to 20 seconds and use of a one-way valve that allows the patient to exhale after attempting inspiration[29,31] (Fig. 86-1). MIP will be reflected as a negative value on the pressure manometer but should be expressed in its absolute value to avoid confusion when using the terms *greater than* or *less than*. Normal values of MIP exceed 100 cmH_2O in men and are approximately 25 percent lower in women.[32] The technique of performing the MIP maneuver varies at different institutions but should be standardized. Ideally, it should be performed at complete expiration when lung volume approaches residual volume (RV), with use of a one-way valve and with 20 seconds of occlusion, while watching for any distress that occurs during the procedure.[29–31] Simple occlusion without the use of a one-way valve[29] or the use of manometers built into ventilators such as the Puritan Bennett 7200A[33] may underestimate the true MIP.

Because the method used will affect the results obtained, much of the literature supporting the use of MIP requires careful interpretation. An early critical examination of MIP in 1973 by Sahn and Lakshminarayan,[28] found that a MIP below 20 cmH_2O predicted weaning failure while a MIP above 30 cmH_2O guaranteed weaning success. Most of the patients in that study were postsurgical and had brief du-

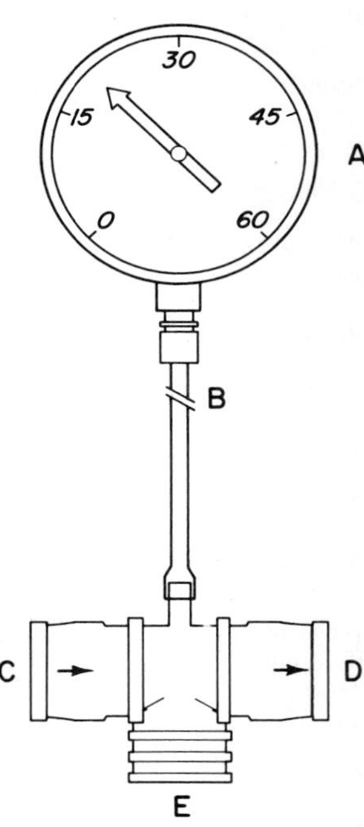

Figure 86-1. Apparatus used to determine MIP in patients with artificial airways. (**A**) manometer; (**B**) connecting tubing; (**C**) inspiratory one-way valve with port for thumb occlusion; (**D**) expiratory one-way valve with port; (**E**) 22-mm ID port for attachment to artificial airway. (From Kacmarek et al.,[29] with permission.)

rations of mechanical ventilation (mean duration 37 hours, maximal duration 168 hours). Thus, these results may not be generalizable to patients on long-term ventilatory support, as suggested by other studies in which the predictive utility of MIP was less favorable.[18,34–36] Prospective examination of MIP by Tahvanainen et al.,[18] who used similar criteria but a different patient group, resulted in a 26 percent false-positive rate and a 100 percent false-negative rate for weaning prediction. Major problems with using MIP are that the compliance of the patient's respiratory system is not considered and that it depends on the patient's cooperation. Serial use of MIP during T-piece trials may be helpful in detecting fatigue,[30] but MIP is a measure of strength rather than endurance. Therefore, in our view MIP is best employed for serial evaluation of patients receiving short-term ventilation rather than as a sole criterion for extubating the patient on long-term ventilation. Also, it is important to remember that an MIP that reflects adequate mechanical strength may still be insufficient to ensure airway protection.[37]

Vital Capacity

VC is defined as the volume of gas exhaled after maximum inspiration and has a normal value of approximately 70 mL/kg. Traditionally, a VC greater than 10 to 15 mL/kg has been considered sufficient reason for discontinuing mechanical ventilation.[25] Prospective evaluation of VC by Tahvanainen and colleagues[18] found no significant difference in VC between the successful and unsuccessful weaning groups (Table 86-3). Even when applied to short-term postoperative patients, VC was found to be a less reliable predictor for extubation than the ability to maintain pH above 7.35 while decreasing the IMV rate.[36] Like MIP, VC is a measure of strength, not endurance, and is highly dependent on patient cooperation.

Minute Ventilation and Maximal Voluntary Ventilation

Two objective measures of ventilation that have been extensively studied are the resting $\dot{V}_E$ and the ability to double the resting $\dot{V}_E$ during MVV. Sahn and Lakshminarayan[28] found that all patients with $\dot{V}_E$ less than 10 L and MVV twice $\dot{V}_E$ were successfully weaned. Failure to satisfy both criteria predicted weaning failure in 17 of 24 (70.8 percent) patients. Despite these early data, the usefulness of both $\dot{V}_E$ and MVV has been debated. Tahvanainen and colleagues[18] showed that a $\dot{V}_E$ of 10 L/min or lower falsely predicted weanability in 11 percent of patients and falsely underestimated weanability in 75 percent. (Table 86-3). In this same study the criterion of doubling voluntary $\dot{V}_E$ falsely predicted both success and failure in 76 percent of patients, which has led to reluctance to accept these parameters as sole criteria for extubation.

Both the patient's spontaneous $\dot{V}_E$ and the $\dot{V}_E$ provided during mechanical ventilation should be considered. If a $\dot{V}_E$ greater than approximately 10 L/min is necessary to maintain a $PaCO_2$ of 40 mmHg, the demand placed on the patient's ventilatory apparatus may be excessive, precluding successful weaning. Such an elevated $\dot{V}_E$ requirement indicates that one or more of three possible mechanisms is present: hyperventilation, increased CO_2 production, and/or increased dead space ventilation (V_D/V_T).

Endurance Measurements

Fatigue, or lack of endurance, is perhaps the most common precipitant of reintubation. Short of allowing fatigue to develop, it is difficult to predict an individual patient's endurance. Criteria regarding the diaphragmatic response to phrenic nerve stimulation and the power spectrum of the diaphragmatic electromyogram (EMG) have been developed. Cohen and colleagues[38] examined diaphragmatic EMGs in 12 patients during weaning attempts, 7 of whom developed EMG evidence of fatigue (i.e., appearance of a power spectral shift); in 6 of the 7 this was associated with an abnormal breathing pattern characterized by paradoxical abdominal motion with inspiration (see Fig. 52-4). The study is important because it characterizes the clinical sequence of respiratory muscle fatigue (Table 86-4) and suggests that the onset of chest wall and abdominal paradox is an early indicator, followed by the development of hypercarbia. The amount of dyssynchrony between the rib cage and abdominal musculature can be measured as an indicator of fatigue. Normally, rib cage and abdominal movements are synchronous; the ribs expanding as the abdomen protrudes with inspiration. With inspiratory muscle fatigue, dyssynchrony between rib and abdominal movement develops.[39] Inspiratory paradox does not distinguish between successful and unsuccessful weaning, although measurement of the maximal amplitude of diaphragm excursion divided by V_T, and the relationship between rib cage excursion and V_T have been found to be nonspecific but sensitive indicators of respiratory muscle fatigue.[39]

Evaluation of Breathing Pattern

The pattern of breathing is particularly important, since rapid shallow breathing and abdominal paradox are associ-

Table 86-4. Clinical Sequence of Inspiratory Muscle Fatigue

Shift of EMG power spectrum
Tachypnea
Respiratory alternans
Paradoxical abdominal motion
Fall in respiratory rate and minute ventilation
Elevation of $PaCO_2$
Arterial acidemia

EMG, diphragmatic and intercostal electromyogram.
(Adapted from Cohen et al., with permission.)

ated with ventilatory failure. Unlike MIP, VC, and MVV, the breathing pattern is not highly dependent on patient cooperation. Rapid shallow breathing can be quantified by dividing the respiratory rate by the V_T (in liters) to produce a rapid shallow breathing index (frequency/tidal volume [F/V_T] ratio).[40] A value of F/V_T equal to or greater than 105 breaths/min/L indicates rapid shallow breathing and in one recent study represented the most accurate predictor of failure in weaning patients from mechanical ventilation.[40]

Bellemare and Grassino[41] have shown that the tension-time index of the diaphragm (TT_{di}) can predict the ability to sustain spontaneous respiration. This index is the product of the fraction of maximal transdiaphragmatic pressure (P_{di}) expended with each breath ($P_{di}/P_{di}max$) and the fraction of the breathing cycle time spent in inspiration. TT_{di} values below 0.15 (T_I/T_{TOT}, or duty cycle) predict ability to sustain respiration for longer than 45 minutes. Values of TT_{di} above 0.15 indicate a decrease in the maximum time ventilation can be sustained and predict eventual ventilatory failure, possibly because of limitation of diaphragmatic blood flow[41] (Fig. 86-2). This method is currently practical only as an investigational tool; neither transdiaphragmatic pressure nor inspiratory time is routinely measured clinically.

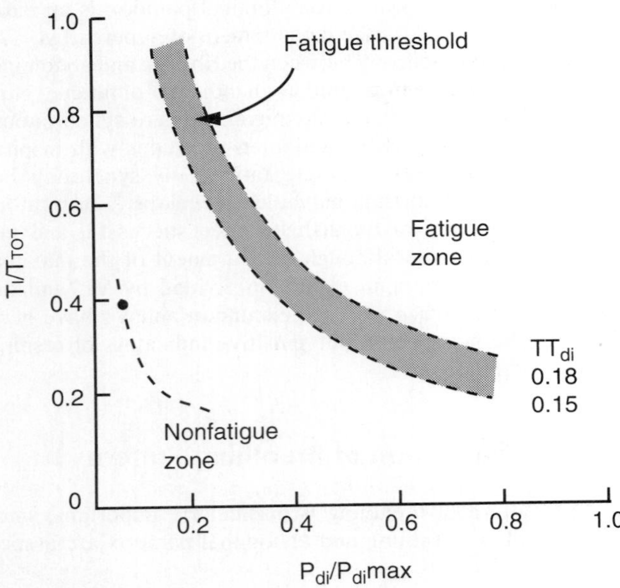

Figure 86-2. Tension-time index for the human diaphragm (TT_{di}). The inspiratory time total ventilatory cycle time (T_I/T_{TOT}) ratio is plotted against transdiaphragmatic pressure during normal breathing/maximum P_{di} possible ($P_{di}/P_{di}max$) ratio. The fatigue threshold represents a TT_{di} that can be sustained for 1 hour or longer and has a value of 0.15 to 0.18 in the normal human diaphragm. The TT_{di} threshold can be achieved with a large variety of P_{di} and T_I/T_{TOT} values. Patterns in the fatigue zone result in fatigue in less than 1 hour, whereas patterns in the nonfatigue zone can be sustained indefinitely. The circle represents the TT_{di} during resting breathing in normal subjects. (From Grassino et al.,[118] with permission.)

Patient/Ventilator System Compliance

The patient/ventilator system compliance (measured in units of milliliters per centimeter of H_2O, is the ratio between the volume of gas delivered and the difference between plateau pressure (P_{pl}) and positive end-expiratory pressure (i.e., V_T/P_{pl} − PEEP). Normal values are 60 to 100 mL/cmH_2O. Weaning failure is likely when patient/ventilator system compliance is less than 25 mL/cmH_2O. Unfortunately, measured compliance for patients on or off the ventilator does not discriminate sufficiently to use this as a sole predictor of weaning.[42]

Work of Breathing

Since the O_2 cost of breathing relates to the ability to sustain respiration,[43,44] work of breathing must be considered as a determinant of weaning. It may be expressed as either work per minute or work per liter of ventilation.[34] Work per minute is defined as the amount of work done per breath multiplied by the respiratory rate and reflects ventilatory requirements. Work per liter is the work per minute divided by $\dot{V}_E$ and is a better measure of efficiency of breathing. Fiastro and colleagues[34] found that in patients requiring prolonged ventilation, work of breathing was a better indicator of successful weaning than standard bedside weaning criteria. Work calculations, either work per minute or total work per liter, give better discrimination than compliance.[42] Further data suggest that work per liter of ventilation significantly correlates with lung mechanics and that while work per minute and work per liter of ventilation are both increased with acute exacerbations of COPD, only the latter relates to the severity of pulmonary mechanical impairment.[45]

Work of breathing can also be assessed by comparing O_2 consumption during complete inspiratory muscle rest (i.e., controlled mechanical ventilation) and O_2 consumption during spontaneous ventilation to determine the O_2 cost of breathing,[43] which can predict time to weaning and extubation in patients recovering from respiratory failure[44] and can identify patients unable to sustain spontaneous ventilation because of excessive ventilatory work.[43] In one study patients who were unable to be weaned demonstrated a 25 percent change in O_2 consumption with weaning.[43] Because O_2 utilization measurements require indirect calorimetry with a metabolic cart, clinical applicability may be limited.

Tracheal Occlusion Pressure

Respiratory center drive is particularly important in patients with COPD and is assessed by measuring the airway pressure generated during the first tenth of a second of occluded inspiratory effort. This measurement is called *tracheal occlusion pressure* ($P_{0.1}$). Elevated $P_{0.1}$ (above 6 cmH_2O) has been reported to predict weaning failure.[46] In Murciano et al.'s study[47] $P_{0.1}$ was followed in patients be-

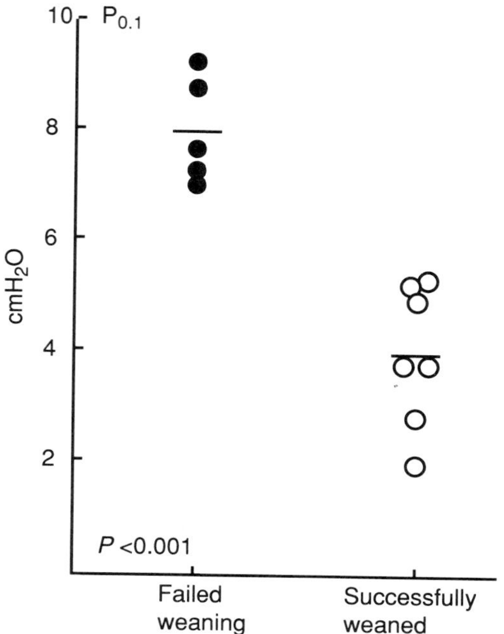

Figure 86-3. Airway occlusion pressure ($P_{0.1}$) during the immediate weaning period without assisted ventilation in patients who failed to wean and in those who were successfully weaned. (From Sassoon et al.,[46] with permission.)

ginning with the first day of acute respiratory failure and was found to decrease before extubation in successfully extubated patients. In patients in whom $P_{0.1}$ did not change significantly from the value measured at the onset of respiratory failure, diaphragmatic fatigue eventually developed, and reintubation was necessary within 2 to 6 days[47] (Fig. 86-3). These investigators concluded that measurement of $P_{0.1}$ provides a simple and valid index to assess the likelihood of respiratory muscle fatigue.[47] A modification of this test incorporating CO_2 stimulation has been reported to augment sensitivity and specificity.[48]

SCORING SYSTEMS AND OTHER CRITICAL FACTORS

A number of studies have examined alternative measures of weaning readiness and have combined previously identified variables into new indices to improve predictive ability. Renal function, the presence of sepsis, and arterial pH have been identified as important cofactors. Among the scoring systems that have been proposed are the Ventilator Dependency and Adverse Factor Scores of Morganroth and colleagues[49] and the Integrative Index of Yang and Tobin.[40]

Morganroth and colleagues developed a scoring system with six ventilator items (F_{IO_2}, level of PEEP, static and dynamic compliance, delivered ventilator $\dot{V}_E$, and triggered respiratory rate) plus 21 "adverse factors," which were based on retrospective analysis of 10 patients undergoing 11 weaning attempts after prolonged (30 days or longer) mechanical ventilation.[49] The weaning protocol called for progression from assist control to T-piece. Of the 11 patients, 9 were successfully weaned in this study, and standard criteria did not distinguish between successful and unsuccessful weaning attempts. An adverse factor score of 55 was found to best separate weaning success from failure, and scores were useful in informing treatment in the original study group. However, the scoring system is cumbersome, and the study must be viewed as an hypothesis-generating study that requires independent confirmation before the criteria can be endorsed. In a preliminary prospective study of thoracic and open heart surgical patients receiving ventilation for 72 hours or longer, the Morganroth score inadequately predicted weaning, and other factors such as renal failure were found to be more important than the items included in the score.[50]

Studying medical ICU patients, Yang and Tobin[40] examined traditional predictors of weaning and two new indices: the rapid shallow breathing index, discussed earlier, and "CROP," which integrates compliance (C), rate (R), oxygenation (O), and pressure (P) measurements. The CROP index is defined as the product of dynamic compliance, MIP, and the ratio of PaO_2 to P_AO_2 divided by the respiratory rate. Threshold values developed from data on 36 patients were prospectively applied to 64 additional patients. The rapid shallow breathing index (with V_T expressed in liters) was found to be the best predictor of successful weaning[40] (Fig. 86-4). Specifically, among patients requiring an extended duration of mechanical ventilation (i.e., longer than 8 days), 64 percent of those with F/V_T values of 105 or lower were successfully weaned, the highest positive predictive value of any of the other parameters examined (including $\dot{V}_E$ of 15 L/min or less, respiratory frequency of 38/min or less, V_T of 0.325 L or more, V_T/weight of 4 or more, MIP of -15 cmH_2O or less, dynamic compliance of 22 mL/cmH_2O or less, static compliance of 33 mL/cmH_2O or higher, PaO_2/P_AO_2 ratio of 0.35 or higher, and CROP index of 13 mL/breath/min or higher). The negative predictive value of F/V_T higher than 105 in such longer-term patients was 0.89, only slightly lower than that for respiratory frequency and MIP (both 1.00), which suggests that the F/V_T ratio is useful in predicting both weaning success and failure. Even better predictive performance for the F/V_T parameter was observed in patients requiring shorter durations (i.e., less than 8 days) of mechanical ventilation (positive and negative predictive values of 0.82 and 1.00 respectively).

A study by Millbern and colleagues examining 33 short-term postoperative patients without pulmonary disease concluded that the intubated patient's ability to maintain a pH above 7.35 while breathing spontaneously was a better predictor of the ability to sustain spontaneous respiration than was MIP or VC.[36] Just like the results of Sahn and Lakshminarayan,[28] these results may not be generalizable to long-term ventilator patients because the study was conducted with healthy patients who received ventilation for short periods. Importantly, these investigators do point out that when pH is used as a criterion for weaning decisions, weaning occurred more rapidly than when standard criteria were

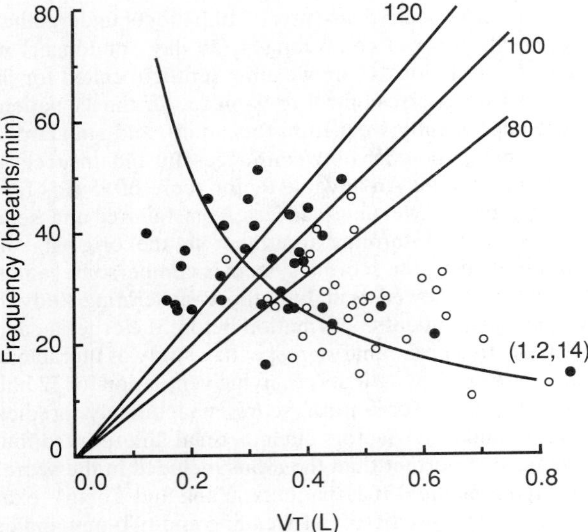

Figure 86-4. Isopleths for the breathing frequency/V_T (F/V_T) ratio representing different degrees of rapid shallow breathing. For the patients indicated by the points to the left of the isopleth, representing 100 breaths/min/L, the likelihood that a weaning trial would fail was 95 percent, whereas for the patients indicated by the points to the right of this isopleth, the likelihood of a successful weaning outcome was 80 percent. The hyperbola represents a minute ventilation of 10 L/min, a criterion commonly used to predict weaning outcome; apparently, this criterion was of little value in discriminating between successfully weaned patients (open circles) and the patients in whom weaning failed (solid circles). Values for one patient (V_T 1.2 L and respiratory frequency of 14 breaths per minute) lay outside the graph. (From Yang and Tobin,[40] with permission.)

used to make the jump from IMV to T-piece trial. Like Tahvanainen et al.,[18] they also observed that Sahn and Lakshminarayan's criteria[28] lacked predictive utility because some patients not meeting these criteria were successfully extubated and another (1 of 33) meeting the criteria required reinstitution of mechanical ventilation.[36] In Tahvanainen et al.'s study of 47 medical patients, traditional weaning criteria and blood gas data did not distinguish successful from unsuccessful weaning attempts, but patients requiring reintubation were distinguished by lower urine volume, lower respiratory quotient values, and a higher incidence of positive blood cultures.[18]

A valuable resource sometimes overlooked is the nurses' overall assessment of the patient. In one intriguing study,[51] a number of physiologic parameters (including negative inspiratory force, $P_{0.1}$, forced vital capacity [FVC], and abdominal paradox), were compared with the nurses' global predictions of weaning success, arbitrarily assigned a score ranging from 1 to 4. In this series of 30 patients, ultimate weaning success was predicted better by this "nurse wean index"[51] than by any other criterion or combination of criteria.

Overall, we suspect that the nonuniform performance of the various indices across studies reflects differences in the type of patients, length of ventilatory support, lack of standardization in making measurements, choice of threshold value, nonuniform or vague definition of end points, and failure to include the true determinants of weaning outcome.

NONRESPIRATORY FACTORS AND OTHER IMPEDIMENTS TO SUCCESSFUL WEANING

Despite extensive investigation of pulmonary function parameters (e.g., gas exchange and mechanical function) as indicators of weaning, little attention has been given to other, nonrespiratory features that may prove equally important. Indeed, failure to consider such factors as nutritional status and nonpulmonary organ dysfunction may contribute to the nonuniformity of results obtained in studies of traditional (pulmonary function) weaning parameters.[18,49,50,52] Factors that determine weaning, in addition to pre-existing respiratory status and the reason for mechanical ventilation, include baseline function of other organ systems, complications developing while on the ventilator, duration of critical illness, and duration of mechanical ventilation. Nonrespiratory factors of particular importance include nutritional status, fluid balance, metabolic and acid-base derangements, cardiac and renal function, pharmacologic therapy, and neuropsychiatric factors (Table 86-5).

Nutritional Status

Patients with acute respiratory failure are often malnourished either on admission or during hospitalization as a result of increased metabolic demands with inadequate nutritional support.[53] Malnutrition has adverse effects on the respiratory system, including decreased respiratory muscle strength and function, decreased diaphragmatic mass (both area and thickness) and contractility, and decreased endurance.[16]

Malnutrition, particularly amino acid deficiency, decreases the ventilatory response to hypoxemia.[57] The immune system responds to malnutrition with decreased cell-mediated immunity, altered IgG turnover, and impaired

Table 86-5. Nonrespiratory Parameters Affecting Ability to Wean

Nutritional status
Fluid balance
Metabolic and acid-base derangements
Cardiac function
Renal function
Pharmacologic therapy
Neuropsychiatric factors

macrophage function.[53] Malnutrition develops or worsens in most patients undergoing mechanical ventilation.[15] In a retrospective review of 47 patients who received mechanical ventilation for 3 days or more, 93 percent of those with adequate nutritional support could be weaned; however, only half of those with inadequate nutritional support could be weaned.[54] Among 14 "unweanable" medical patients, all those who responded with increases in albumin and transferrin during parenteral nutrition were all weaned eventually, whereas those who had no biochemical response to nutrition remained unweanable.[21] Weight gain after nutritional repletion of malnourished emphysema patients is accompanied by significant improvements in ventilatory and muscle strength.[55]

While undernutrition is obviously an impediment to weaning, overnutrition or the wrong kind of nutrition can also frustrate weaning efforts. High minute ventilation, a common cause of inability to wean, may be produced by excessive carbohydrate loading,[56] resulting in increased CO_2 production and increased work of breathing to eliminate this CO_2. Other causes of increased CO_2 production include fever, sepsis, shivering, seizures, and agitation. Hyperventilation may also be caused by increased central drive, dyspnea, pain, agitation, or inappropriate ventilator settings. Increased CO_2 production may also be caused by inefficient ventilation due to increased dead space; this occurs in the setting of pulmonary embolism without compensatory hyperventilation, in obstructive lung disease, late in the course of the adult respiratory distress syndrome (ARDS), and with acute hyperinflation due to a rapid cycling rate, extrinsic PEEP or auto-PEEP.

Amino acids are an essential part of parenteral nutrition, and have been shown to restore ventilatory drive and improve both minute ventilation and respiratory rate when these have been disrupted as the result of prolonged glucose infusion.[57]

Metabolic Abnormalities

Metabolic causes of weaning failure are legion and include hypophosphatemia, hypocalcemia, and hypothyroidism. Hypophosphatemic patients demonstrate increased P_{di} after repletion to normal levels of phosphate.[23] Hypocalcemia decreases diaphragmatic strength, without relation to diaphragmatic blood flow.[22] Hypothyroidism can affect weaning, as the hypoxic ventilatory response is markedly blunted with low thyroid activity.[58]

Acid-Base Disturbances

Acid-base abnormalities are important considerations in weaning. The most common problem is seen with patients who develop acute ventilatory failure in the face of chronic CO_2 retention. As the baseline $PaCO_2$ is frequently unknown, these patients may be ventilator-supported during their acute illness to a presumed normal baseline $PaCO_2$ of 40 mmHg, resulting in acute alkalemia; 3 to 4 days later, a new compensatory state develops as the kidneys dump the excess HCO_3^-, but the patient is now unable to be weaned from the ventilator in this new steady state. Allowing the $PaCO_2$ to gradually normalize over several days may allow weaning to resume. Other acid-base problems that can develop during weaning include respiratory alkalosis, metabolic alkalosis (commonly due to nasogastric drainage and diuretic therapy), and metabolic acidosis as with renal disease or diabetic ketoacidosis. Complex disorders involving partial compensation and failure of two or more systems frequently confound the issue (see Ch. 28).

Perception of Breathing

In patients with obstructive lung disease, the pulmonary stretch receptors may be activated because the mechanically delivered volumes are much larger than those that can be attained during spontaneous breathing. Because V_T changes are accurately sensed under different load conditions,[59] failure to recreate these volumes during weaning can lead to agitation. One approach to this problem is to decrease the V_T during periods of mechanical ventilation and then to increase the rate as necessary to maintain alveolar ventilation. During weaning periods, narcotics can be added judiciously to manage undue agitation.

Endotracheal Tube Caliber

Airway resistance increases as endotracheal tube size decreases.[60] To the extent that smaller-caliber tubes (e.g., for nasal intubation) can greatly increase the imposed work of breathing, they impair weaning. The minimum caliber tube for women should be 7 mm ID, and for men 8 mm ID if weaning appears compromised. Recent guidelines developed by the American College of Chest Physicians[61] suggest that a tracheotomy should be considered when weaning will likely extend beyond 14 days. Tracheotomy appears to help patients who are having trouble clearing secretions and may also improve patient comfort. It is not always necessary, however, and there is a trend toward leaving endotracheal tubes in place for longer periods of time as long as the cuff pressure is minimized and appropriate care is taken to prevent airway infection.

Sleep Deprivation and Psychological Issues

The role of sleep deprivation as an impediment to weaning has not been well studied. The ICU is frequently noisy, the lights are always on, and there is a constant level of activity that makes it difficult for patients to establish a daily routine. The result may be a level of twilight awareness in which patients are neither fully awake nor asleep, frequently nap throughout the day, or completely shift their day-night cycle.

Any of these insults can impair successful weaning. One common approach is to give patients sedative-hypnotic drugs at bedtime to promote a good night's sleep and to restore a normal daily cycle. Because depression is commonly a problem in the long-term ICU patient, a tricyclic antidepressant at bedtime may be useful both for sedative effect and to forestall depression, it should be realized that the fully antidepressant effect of tricyclics may not be apparent for 2 to 3 weeks after their initiation.[62]

The attitude of the patient, although important, is often difficult to assess or change. Patients who are well informed about what is expected and who strive to meet daily goals seem to progress more rapidly than those who are uninvolved in the process or who are depressed. Weaning goals set by the clinical team should be attainable, should avoid precipitating fatigue or undue discomfort, and should cause each session of weaning to end in success rather than failure. From the practical viewpoint a daily weaning strategy should be developed early in the day and can be canceled if the day is otherwise occupied with laboratory tests or if the patient has a medical setback that makes it impossible to successfully wean that day. Some patients with psychological dependency will hyperventilate at the onset of weaning trials without relation to physiologic need and may have to be weaned surreptitiously. Formal biofeedback can also facilitate weaning by allowing the patient to visualize different breathing patterns.[63] Potential solutions to the problem of dysfunctional breathing patterns include adequate sedation with narcotics[64,65] and very slow changes in the level of pressure support or IMV rate to prevent anxiety induced by sudden changes in the response of the lung stretch receptors during the active weaning process.

Other Factors

Anemia, by virtue of decreasing O_2-carrying capacity, may interfere with weaning by forcing increases in minute ventilation or cardiac output. Interference with the weaning process may also be caused by multiple medications, including narcotics, tranquilizers, sedative hypnotics, paralytic agents and aminoglycoside antibiotics, which can cause myasthenia-like muscle weakness.

WEANING IN SPECIFIC PATIENT SETTINGS

The Postoperative Patient

The uncomplicated surgical patient is generally easy to wean, although if extubation criteria based on conventional respiratory mechanics are used, extubation will be delayed in nearly half.[35] Blood gas values on CPAP constitute the preferred criterion for extubation.[35,36] Special considerations apply when the abdomen or the chest has been opened. Abdominal muscle activity after laparotomy results in changes in intra-abdominal pressure, which may be mistaken for diaphragmatic impairment.[66] Median sternotomy for open heart [illegible] produces decreases in a number of pulmonary parameters, including VC, total lung capacity (TLC), inspiratory capacity, and functional residual capacity (FRC), both immediately and as late as 7 days postoperatively.[67] Sternotomy and internal mammary artery (IMA) harvesting may adversely affect postoperative respiratory function by disrupting chest wall stability and affecting intercostal muscle blood supply. Sternotomy has been shown to decrease postoperative pulmonary function tests, and when the IMA is harvested, there is greater impairment than when saphenous vein grafts alone are used.[68] Some of the immediately observed changes may be due to discomfort from mediastinal and pleural chest tubes; pulmonary mechanics generally improve and pain scores decrease after removal of chest tubes on the first postoperative day.[69]

The decision to extubate after open heart surgery must take into account not only hemodynamic stability and the amount of mediastinal bleeding but also the patient's temperature and ability to metabolize narcotics and neuromuscular blockers, which are typically not reversed at the end of cardiac surgery. The high-dose narcotic technique commonly used for open heart surgery may result in pulmonary or gastric sequestration of fentanyl with subsequent reabsorption and renarcosis, and this must also be taken in account when early extubation is planned.[70] One study of patients undergoing uncomplicated open heart surgery concluded that early extubation (within 3 hours of ICU arrival) was possible if spontaneous ventilation rate did not exceed 26 breaths per minute, expired V_T was at least 10 mL/kg body weight, and end-tidal CO_2 was less than 6.5 percent.[71] Another study by Michel et al.,[72] which examined 44 post-open heart surgery patients who met criteria of mental alertness, recovery of muscle strength, hemodynamic stability, and adequacy of pulmonary gas exchange, demonstrated that it is not necessary to satisfy criteria of VC at least 15 mL/kg or MIP at least 28 cmH_2O and that adherence to these guidelines would have led to unduly long intubation. These authors also point out that patients undergoing mitral valve replacement are at high risk for pulmonary complications and are more likely than coronary bypass patients to require delayed extubation.[72] As compared with patients undergoing isolated coronary artery bypass grafting, those undergoing reoperation, emergency operation, or valve surgery are more likely to be ventilator-supported for more than 24 hours, to require reintubation, and to have late complications such as CO_2 retention, bronchospasm, pleural effusion, and pneumonia.[73]

The Hemodynamically Unstable Patient

Weaning the ventilator-dependent patient requires particular attention to hemodynamics, particularly following open heart surgery or myocardial infarction. Beach and colleagues noted that postcardiotomy patients ready for weaning by the usual criteria sometimes responded to discontinuing mechanical ventilation with a sudden reduction in cardiac output associated with reduced O_2 availability and increased pulmonary vascular resistance.[74] The relationship between left ventricular function and ventilation is complex, and the hemodynamic response to changes in ventilatory patterns depends on left ventricular function. Negative intrathoracic pressure can increase left ventricular afterload by increasing left ventricular transmural pressures.[75] In coronary bypass patients with normal left ventricular function, significant increases in cardiac index and stroke volume index occur on switching from controlled ventilation to IMV.[76] By contrast, patients with impaired left ventricular function (ejection fraction less than 60 percent) respond to changing from controlled ventilation to IMV with increased right atrial and pulmonary artery occlusion pressures and significantly decreased mean arterial pressure, cardiac index, and stroke index[76] (Fig. 86-5). Gated blood pool imaging of patients undergoing unsuccessful weaning from mechanical ventilation demonstrates increases in the left ventricular end diastolic volume index with changes from controlled to spontaneous ventilation.

The Patient with Renal Impairment or Volume Overload

Volume overload can be an impediment to successful weaning. Application of PEEP can be used to treat pulmonary edema, since increased intrathoracic pressure discourages venous return. Lemaire and colleagues noted that prolonged (10-day) diuretic therapy with reduction of body weight by an average of 5 kg was necessary to achieve weaning in patients with left ventricular dysfunction.[20] In our experience weaning the long-term cardiac patient is highly dependent on normal renal function, perhaps because of the fluid overload that may occur with renal insufficiency. Extravascular lung water is increased in patients undergoing coronary artery bypass surgery, but if left ventricular function is normal, it decreases by 24 hours postoperatively.[77] Animal studies have suggested that ultrafiltration is beneficial in reducing extravascular lung water, although diuretics may achieve the same effect.[78] Application of slow continuous ultrafiltration or continuous arteriovenous hemofiltration (CAVH) to reduce fluid overload in patients after coronary artery bypass surgery may facilitate their weaning from mechanical ventilation.[79] CAVH has also been proposed to eliminate a myocardial depressant factor, thus allowing catecholamine support to be reduced after cardiac surgery.[79]

The Patient with Diaphragmatic Dysfunction

Phrenic nerve injury is surprisingly common after coronary artery bypass grafting, causing diaphragmatic dysfunction in approximately 1 percent of patients.[80] Injury to the left phrenic nerve is more common and is thought to occur as a result of cold injury to the nerve during surgery,[81] although recent studies suggest that phrenic nerve dysfunction following internal mammary dissections may be caused by

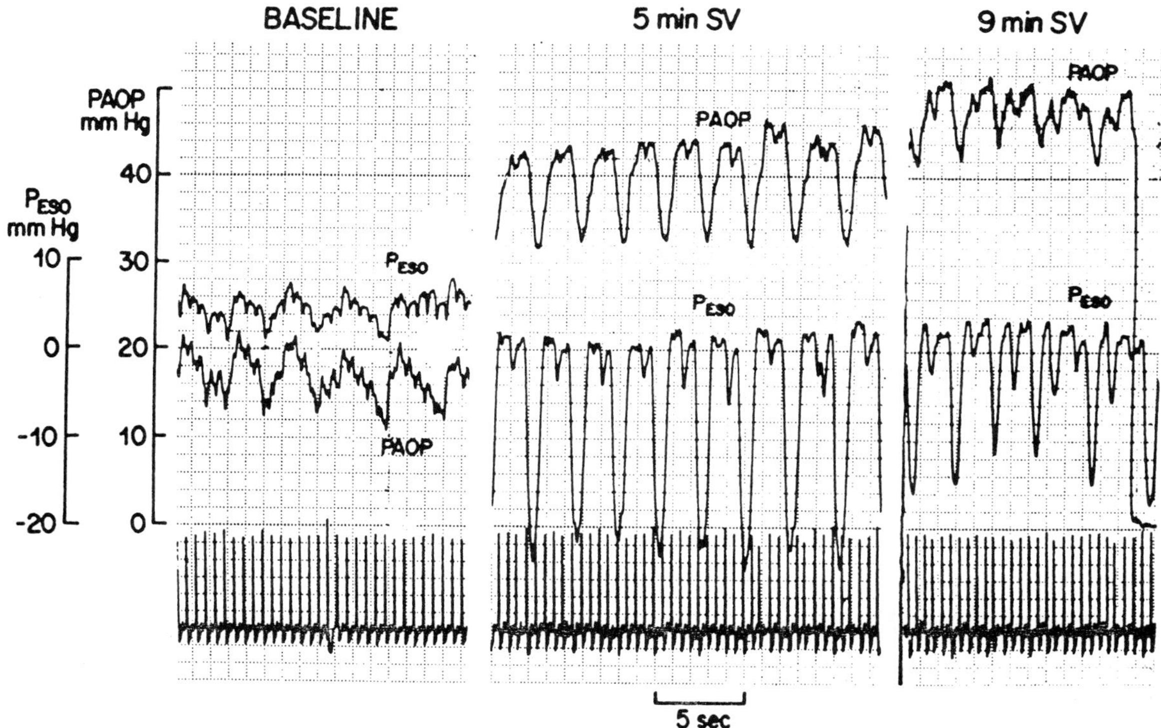

Figure 86-5. Weaning of a patient from a mechanical ventilation (baseline) to spontaneous ventilation (SV). There is a progressive increase of pulmonary artery occlusion pressure (PAOP) from 14 mmHg (baseline) to 50 mmHg (9 min SV). The esophageal pressure (P_{R50}) is reduced during SV with marked negative inspiratory excursions. (From Lemaire et al.,[20] with permission.)

ischemia to the phrenic nerve.[80] Less often, a phrenic nerve may be transected during dissection of the internal mammary artery or injured during manipulation of the heart for valve replacement. Bilateral diaphragmatic dysfunction should be considered in the differential diagnosis of orthopnea after extubation and is confirmed if the decrement in VC exceeds 20 percent on moving from an upright to a supine posture. Atelectasis following coronary artery bypass surgery is another marker of phrenic nerve dysfunction.[82] More severe atelectasis may occur when a larger number of grafts are used, when operative and bypass times are longer, when the pleural space is entered, when a cardiac insulating pad is not used to protect from local cooling, and when body temperatures are low for surgery.[80–82] Phrenic nerve recovery after injury may require up to 27 months.[80] When bilateral phrenic nerve dysfunction precludes weaning, long-term management with rocking beds[80] or nighttime positive-pressure ventilation[83] is required until respiratory muscle strength and endurance improve.

The Patient with Thoracic Cage Dysfunction

Disorders of the thoracic cage include abnormalities due to scoliosis, thoracoplasty, obesity, and neuromuscular impairments. General principles of managing these patients include minimizing the degree of hypoxemia due to reversible ventilation/perfusion imbalance, precisely titrating O_2 to avoid CO_2 retention related to blunted hypoxic drive, treating cor pulmonale with careful attention to acid-base status, and occasionally using respiratory stimulants such as doxapram.[84–86] In the specific instance of difficult-to-wean patients with neuromuscular weakness, Aldrich et al.[87] in 1989 suggested in an uncontrolled trial that inspiratory muscle training can facilitate weaning.

The Patient with Chronic Obstructive Pulmonary Disease

Patients with COPD pose a special weaning challenge. As suggested by Menzies et al.[88] rates of failure to wean in such patients may be as high as 24 percent, with most patients (up to 58 percent) requiring up to 2 weeks of mechanical ventilation before weaning could be achieved. Morganroth et al.[49] have observed that standard weaning parameters of mechanical function apply poorly to patients with COPD after prolonged ventilatory support, and that the adverse factor score, although cumbersome, may be better suited to predicting weaning in this group.

In ventilating and weaning COPD patients, special consideration must be given to the phenomenon of auto-PEEP, also known as intrinsic PEEP.[89,90] Auto-PEEP occurs when end-expiratory pressure persists in the alveoli without being registered at the airway manometer and must be distinguished from the PEEP that is purposefully applied and recorded at the proximal airway. Though undetectable without the special maneuver of occluding the expiratory port of the ventilator at end expiration (and with any continuous flow interrupted), auto-PEEP may have the same hemodynamic consequences as routine PEEP (i.e., decreased venous return, hypotension) and occurs commonly in COPD patients on mechanical ventilation (see Chs. 76 and 84).

Auto-PEEP is increased when airflow resistance is increased and when exhalation time is decreased, both of which effects impair alveolar emptying prior to the next ventilator breath. Maneuvers to decrease auto-PEEP therefore include treating bronchospasm and secretions, slowing the respiratory rate, maximizing the time for expiration, and using low-compliance ventilator tubing to permit rapid gas delivery and to maximize exhalation time. Auto-PEEP may frustrate weaning by increasing the work of breathing associated with having to overcome residual alveolar pressure before inhalation can begin, and some investigators have proposed adding conventional PEEP in COPD patients to offset this adverse effect of auto-PEEP.[91] (See Ch. 76 for more details on managing auto-PEEP.)

The Elderly Patient

Like patients with COPD, elderly patients pose special challenges in weaning. In general, the elderly are more prone to multisystem failure and have less functional reserve than younger patients.[92,93] For example, in one study octogenarians had a threefold increase in the incidence of respiratory failure and a fourfold increase in the need for tracheotomy after open heart surgery as compared with younger patients.[44] As with COPD patients, conventional criteria for predicting successful weaning have shown little diagnostic accuracy when applied to elderly patients (over 70 years old).[75] Weaning prediction in such patients must be individualized, and close attention must be given to trends in parameters rather than to single-state cutoff values.

PRACTICAL ISSUES IN WEANING

Discussion of weaning methods provokes controversy. There are several accepted methods of weaning, each of which has advantages and disadvantages, and the well-versed clinician should be familiar with all methods so that alternative strategies can be employed when others fail. A survey of methods used by American physicians for weaning from mechanical ventilation found that IMV to T-piece weaning was used by 64 percent of respondents, IMV to CPAP weaning by 26 percent, assist-control ventilation to T-piece by 8 percent, and controlled ventilation to assist ventilation to T-tube by 2 percent.[96] Pressure support strategies for weaning became popular after this survey was completed. Our practice is to use IMV for routine, short-term weaning and CPAP with pressure support, alternating with periods of rest on assist-control, when confronted with failure of IMV weaning. A practical approach is presented in Figure 86-6.

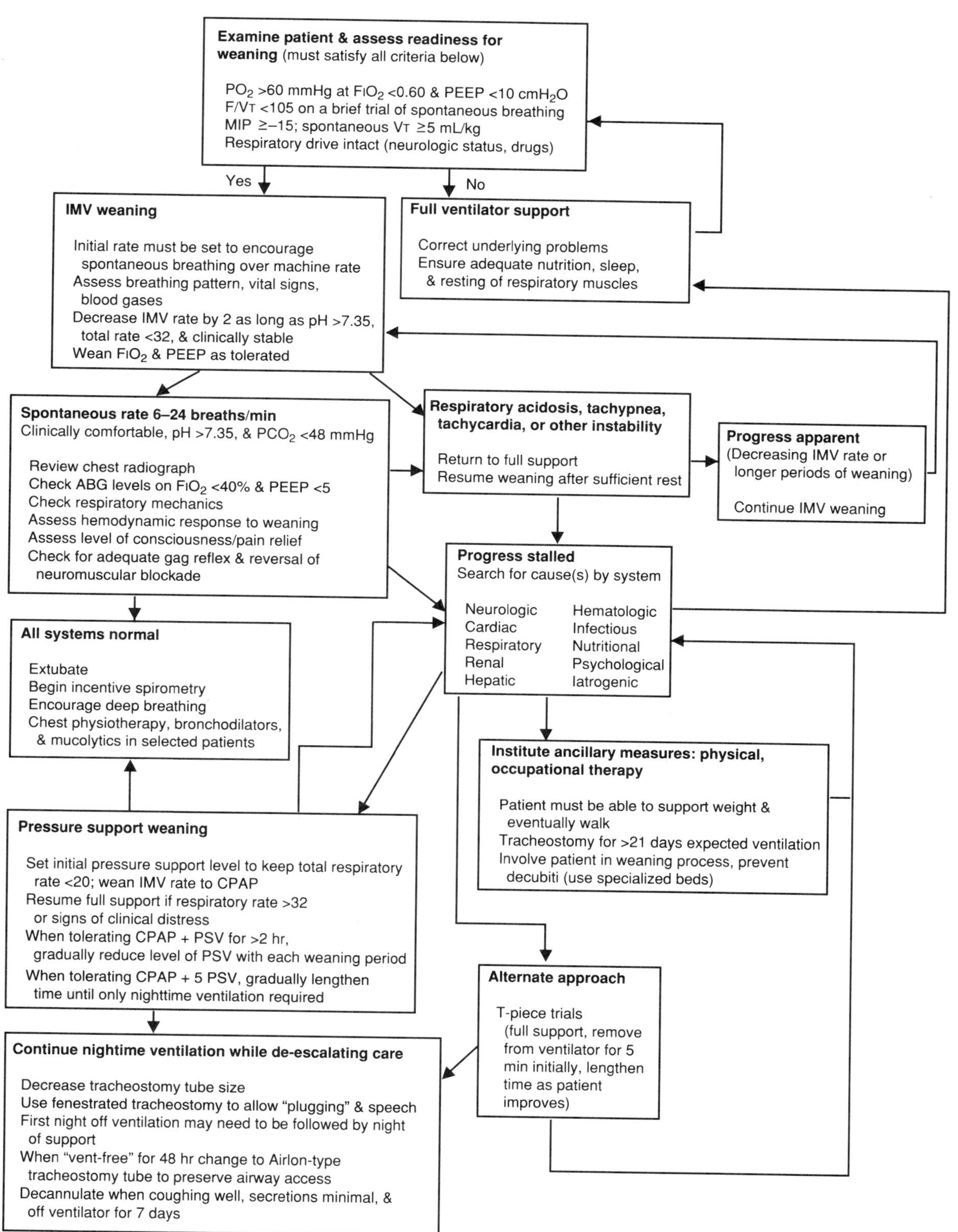

Examine patient & assess readiness for weaning (must satisfy all criteria below)
PO2 >60 mmHg at FIO2 <0.60 & PEEP <10 cmH2O
F/VT <105 on a brief trial of spontaneous breathing
MIP ≥–15; spontaneous VT ≥5 mL/kg
Respiratory drive intact (neurologic status, drugs)
Yes
No
IMV weaning
Initial rate must be set to encourage spontaneous breathing over machine rate
Assess breathing pattern, vital signs, blood gases
Decrease IMV rate by 2 as long as pH >7.35, total rate <32, & clinically stable
Wean FIO2 & PEEP as tolerated
Full ventilator support
Correct underlying problems
Ensure adequate nutrition, sleep, & resting of respiratory muscles
Spontaneous rate 6–24 breaths/min
Clinically comfortable, pH >7.35, & PCO2 <48 mmHg
Review chest radiograph
Check ABG levels on FIO2 <40% & PEEP <5
Check respiratory mechanics
Assess hemodynamic response to weaning
Assess level of consciousness/pain relief
Check for adequate gag reflex & reversal of neuromuscular blockade
Respiratory acidosis, tachypnea, tachycardia, or other instability
Return to full support
Resume weaning after sufficient rest
Progress apparent
(Decreasing IMV rate or longer periods of weaning)
Continue IMV weaning
All systems normal
Extubate
Begin incentive spirometry
Encourage deep breathing
Chest physiotherapy, bronchodilators, & mucolytics in selected patients
Progress stalled
Search for cause(s) by system
Neurologic
Cardiac
Respiratory
Renal
Hepatic
Hematologic
Infectious
Nutritional
Psychological
Iatrogenic
Institute ancillary measures: physical, occupational therapy
Patient must be able to support weight & eventually walk
Tracheostomy for >21 days expected ventilation
Involve patient in weaning process, prevent decubiti (use specialized beds)
Pressure support weaning
Set initial pressure support level to keep total respiratory rate <20; wean IMV rate to CPAP
Resume full support if respiratory rate >32 or signs of clinical distress
When tolerating CPAP + PSV for >2 hr, gradually reduce level of PSV with each weaning period
When tolerating CPAP + 5 PSV, gradually lengthen time until only nighttime ventilation required
Alternate approach
T-piece trials
(full support, remove from ventilator for 5 min initially, lengthen time as patient improves)
Continue nightime ventilation while de-escalating care
Decrease tracheostomy tube size
Use fenestrated tracheostomy to allow "plugging" & speech
First night off ventilation may need to be followed by night of support
When "vent-free" for 48 hr change to Airlon-type tracheostomy tube to preserve airway access
Decannulate when coughing well, secretions minimal, & off ventilator for 7 days

Figure 86-6. An approach to weaning.

T-Piece Weaning

The traditional method of weaning is to disconnect the patient from the ventilator for a specific period of time and allow the patient to breathe on T-piece or CPAP. This is a time-honored but labor-intensive method, since the patient must be monitored continuously for distress or fatigue. Beginning intervals may be as brief as 2 minutes each hour and be progressively lengthened by 2 min/h or more as endurance develops. A reasonable starting point is 5 minutes of T-piece followed by 60 minutes of rest. If this first trial is successful, the trial can be increased in 5-minute intervals, allowing at least 1 hour of rest between attempts. Signs of T-piece weaning failure include respiratory rate above 35 to 40; heart rate above 110 to 120; and increased blood pressure, diaphoresis, air hunger, and signs of respiratory muscle fatigue. Elevated end-tidal CO_2 is a very late sign of decompensation.[38] Optimally, the weaning should be stopped just prior to signs of distress to avoid inducing "weaning anxiety." Between weaning periods full support should be provided with use of assist-control at a rate sufficient to blunt the patient's own respiratory drive.

Intermittent Mandatory Ventilation Weaning

IMV is a mode of mechanical ventilation in which the patient may breathe spontaneously from a reservoir or demand system between ventilator breaths while the ventilator provides positive pressure breaths of adjustable size and frequency. IMV weaning is the method most commonly used in the United States at present.[96]

Is IMV superior to conventional weaning (T-piece trials)? Early studies suggested that IMV was preferable to controlled mechanical ventilation, resulting in less alkalosis, less time on the ventilator, and less increase in O_2 consumption.[97] Unfortunately, initial claims that IMV was a preferred weaning mode because it could shorten weaning time have not been validated by later studies.[98] More recent controlled trials comparing time to weaning using this mode versus progressive T-piece weaning have also failed to show any difference in weaning time between the two modes.[99] In our view, IMV weaning remains an attractive initial weaning strategy, especially with a continuous flow circuit but the versatile clinician must be prepared to try alternate strategies (e.g., T-piece trials, pressure support) when the IMV approach fails.

Pressure Support Weaning

Microprocessor-controlled ventilators now incorporate a pressure support function, which allows the patient to breathe spontaneously while receiving mechanical assistance with each breath. Specifically, inspiratory pressure is servocontrolled to maintain a preset pressure until inspiratory flow falls below a specified threshold (usually 25 percent or less of peak inspiratory flow). During pressure support weaning, the level of inspiratory pressure support is slowly decreased, and the patient gradually assumes more of the inspiratory work. While evidence recommending pressure support for weaning is sparse, its demonstrated advantages include increased patient comfort, ability to offset increased work of breathing imposed by the ventilator or the endotracheal tube, and increased efficiency for the clinician overseeing its use.[100,101] We use pressure support combined with CPAP as the preferred method of weaning long-term patients. The initial pressure level is set at approximately half the peak inspiratory pressure, and CPAP is set for optimal PEEP (generally 5 to 10 cmH_2O). The level of pressure support is then adjusted up or down to maintain a respiratory rate between 12 and 24. This allows the patient to perform some respiratory muscle training while minimizing tachypnea and its associated stress. Weaning using inspiratory pressure support can often be continued for 1 hour or more; the patient is placed back on full support when the respiratory rate exceeds 32 breaths per minute or clinical signs of distress develop.

Assist-Control

The assist-control mode is not a mode of weaning but a ventilatory mode in which a backup rate is provided over which the patient can breathe by triggering machine breaths with inspiratory effort. Unlike the situation with IMV, spontaneous tidal breathing is not possible. Each breath the patient takes results in delivery of a full assisted breath; thus, assist-control is best used for support between weaning trials rather than for weaning.

Positive End-Expiratory Pressure

The advisability of extubating patients from small amounts of PEEP has been the subject of some debate. Relatively little literature is available, but in one study by Feeley and colleagues[102] of 25 patients with acute respiratory failure who were otherwise ready to be weaned, patients extubated from 5 cmH_2O CPAP experienced less increase in $P(A\text{-}a)O_2$ after extubation than patients extubated without PEEP. To the extent that no difference was observed between the two compared groups with respect to rise in the $PaCO_2$ or in the duration of the weaning effort, the use of 5 cmH_2O PEEP is not believed to contraindicate an extubation effort.

In summary, no evidence supports the superiority of any one weaning method. The available literature suggests that each mode may occasionally succeed when the other has failed, although these crossover successes may reflect improvement in the patient's clinical status. The clinician should be able to employ all available approaches: T-piece trials, IMV, and pressure support.

ANCILLARY ISSUES IN WEANING

Tracheotomy

Tracheotomy is indicated for relief of upper airway obstruction, for access for pulmonary hygiene, and for control of the airway for long-term positive pressure ventilation.[103] During long-term weaning the presence of a tracheostomy permits bronchial hygiene, improves patient comfort, and allows use of a fenestrated tracheostomy tube, which may be occluded to allow the patient to speak during periods when mechanical ventilation is not required. Relative contraindications to tracheotomy include recent sternotomy and the presence of burned tissue or infection in the area of the tracheotomy. Complications include pneumothorax, pneumomediastinum, subcutaneous emphysema, incisional hemorrhage, aerophagia, aspiration, and tube displacement.[104] Late complications also include tracheal stenosis, tracheoinnominate and tracheoesophageal fistulae, tube obstruction, aspiration, swallowing dysfunction, and stomal infections.[104]

Controversies regarding tracheotomy are well summarized in recent reviews.[61,103,104] In the absence of definitive studies regarding the timing of tracheotomy, we suggest the following indications for tracheotomy during the weaning process:

1. Anticipation of a prolonged (i.e., more than 1 month) need for intubation and mechanical ventilation
2. Absence of a contraindication to tracheotomy (e.g., upper airway burn, mediastinitis)
3. Expectation of copious or tenacious secretions requiring direct access to the airway for suctioning
4. Chronic aspiration requiring long-standing airway protection in the absence of other strategies to minimize aspiration (e.g., gastrostomy tubes, jejunostomy tubes, nasogastric feeding)

Pharmacologic Aids to Weaning

Beta-adrenergic agents, aminophylline, and anticholinergics are frequently helpful in the patient with reactive airway disease. Aminophylline has also been shown to improve diaphragmatic contractility[105] and to partially reverse reduced diaphragmatic activity seen after abdominal surgery.[106] Dopamine improves diaphragmatic strength and blood flow in patients with COPD and acute respiratory failure: on average, an infusion of 10 μg/kg/min increases heart rate by 17 percent, cardiac output by 40 percent, and both diaphragmatic blood flow and transdiaphragmatic strength by 30 percent.[107] Opioids, particularly dihydrocodeine, have been shown to decrease breathlessness and improve exercise tolerance in patients with COPD and may have a role in improving patient comfort during weaning.[108] Respiratory stimulants such as doxapram have been successfully employed in patients with primary alveolar hypoventilation[84] but are not generally recommended in weaning.

Weaning Failure

Despite the best efforts to prepare the patient for weaning and ultimately for extubation, some patients will inevitably fail to sustain respiration on their own and require resumption of mechanical ventilation. The rate of extubation failure in general surgical patients averaging 65 years of age is approximately 5 percent.[109] Patients failing extubation, however, have a disproportionate increase in mortality and morbidity, particularly pulmonary edema and pneumonia. In patients with head injury, approximately 5 percent require reintubation, primarily for airway protection.[109] Patients undergoing open heart surgery have an overall reintubation rate of approximately 5 percent, with patients undergoing reoperation, emergency surgery, and valve surgery having a much higher rate of reintubation than those undergoing isolated coronary artery bypass surgery.[73] Patients recovering from smoke inhalation and burns have a 13 percent incidence of extubation failure, primarily because of the need to protect the airway.[109] The wide variation in reintubation rates in various populations of ventilator-assisted patients point out the importance of careful assessment of the reason for extubation failure and correction of the underlying problem.

Outcome

Prognosis after successful weaning from mechanical ventilation also varies widely, depending on the age of the patient, the underlying disease process, and the presence of other complicating factors. Diseases such as ARDS are associated with high hospital mortality (e.g., up to 65 percent), but similar survivals at hospital discharge, 1 year, and 3 years suggest that long-term results are excellent in those who survive the acute illness.[110] In a study of 100 patients receiving mechanically assisted ventilation in a community hospital, all patients under the age of 50 years who survived the ICU stay survived to leave the hospital and were alive at 1 year.[111] In the subset of patients age 70 years and older, however, hospital survival was only 49 percent and 1 year survival was only 27 percent, which suggests that successful extubation in elderly patients is not necessarily indicative of a good prognosis.[111] A number of other studies also emphasize that prognosis after mechanically assisted ventilation is far worse than many clinicians realize, particularly in the elderly population, and in those with COPD.[112–116] Important ethical, legal, and economic questions are being raised regarding prolonged ventilation, and more detailed studies will clearly be welcomed to assist the clinician to make responsible decisions. Preliminary results indicate that scoring systems such as APACHE may be useful in making early estimates of hospital mortality[117] but predictive models still have severe limitations when applied to individual patients.[88]

References

1. Kastanos N, Miro RE, Perez AM et al: Laryngotracheal injury due to endotracheal intubation: Incidence, evolution, and predisposing factors. A prospective long-term study. Crit Care Med 1983;11:362–367
2. Stauffer JL, Olson DE, Petty TL: Complications and consequences of endotracheal intubation and tracheotomy. A prospective study of 150 critically ill adult patients. Am J Med 1981;70:65–76
3. Lewis FR Jr, Schlobohm RM, Thomas AN: Prevention of complications from prolonged tracheal intubation. Am J Surg 1978;135:452–457
4. Colice GL, Stukel TA, Dain B: Laryngeal complications of prolonged intubation. Chest 1989;96:877–884
5. Sackner MA, Hirsch J, Epstein S: Effect of cuffed endotracheal tubes on tracheal mucus velocity. Chest 1975;68:774–777
6. Alexopoulos C, Jansson B, Lindholm C-E: Mucus transport and surface damage after endotracheal intubation and tracheostomy. An experimental study in pigs. Acta Anaesthesiol Scand 1984;28:68–76
7. Gal TJ: Effects of endotracheal intubation on normal cough performance. Anesthesiology 1980;52:324–329
8. LaForce FM: Hospital-acquired gram-negative rod pneumonias: An overview. Am J Med 1981;70:664–669
9. Garibaldi RA, Britt MR, Coleman ML et al: Risk factors for postoperative pneumonia. Am J Med 1981;70:677–680
10. Pierce AK, Sanford JP, Thomas GD, Leonard JS: Long-term evaluation of decontamination of inhalation-therapy equipment and the occurrence of necrotizing pneumonia. N Engl J Med 1970;282:528–531
11. Pingleton SK, Hinthorn DR, Liu C: Enteral nutrition in patients receiving mechanical ventilation. Multiple sources of tracheal colonization include the stomach. Am J Med 1986;80:827–832
12. Driks MR, Craven DE, Celli BR et al: Nosocomial pneumonia in intubated patients given sucralfate as compared with antacids or histamine type 2 blockers. The role of gastric colonization. N Engl J Med 1987;317:1376–1382
13. Kerver AJH, Rommes JH, Mevissen-Verhage EAE et al: Prevention of colonization and infection in critically ill patients: A prospective randomized study. Crit Care Med 1988;16:1087–1093
14. Van Uffelen R, Rommes JH, Van Saene HKF: Preventing lower airway colonization and infection in mechanically ventilated patients. Crit Care Med 1987;15:99–102
15. Driver AG, LeBrun M: Iatrogenic malnutrition in patients receiving ventilatory support. JAMA 1980;244:2195–2196
16. Wilson DO, Rogers RM: The role of nutrition in weaning from mechanical ventilation. J Intensive Care 1989;4:124–133
17. Cassem NH, Hackett TP: The setting of intensive care. pp. 319–341. In Hackett TP, Cassem NH (eds): Massachusetts General Hospital Handbook of General Hospital Psychiatry. CV Mosby, St. Louis, 1978
18. Tahvanainen J, Salmenpera M, Nikki P: Extubation criteria after weaning from intermittent mandatory ventilation and continuous positive airway pressure. Crit Care Med 1983;11:702–707
19. Kemper M, Weissman C, Askanazi J et al: Metabolic and respiratory changes during weaning from mechanical ventilation. Chest 1987;92:979–983
20. Lemaire F, Teboul J-L, Cinotti L et al: Acute left ventricular dysfunction during unsuccessful weaning from mechanical ventilation. Anesthesiology 1988;69:171–179
21. Larca L, Greenbaum DM: Effectiveness of intensive nutritional regimes in patients who fail to wean from mechanical ventilation. Crit Care Med 1982;10:297–300
22. Aubier M, Viires N, Piquet J et al: Effects of hypocalcemia on diaphragmatic strength generation. J Appl Physiol 1985;58:2054–2061
23. Aubier M, Murciano D, Lecocguic Y et al: Effect of hypophosphatemia on diaphragmatic contractility in patients with acute respiratory failure. N Engl J Med 1985;313:420–424
24. Downs JB, Perkins HM, Sutton WW: Successful weaning after five years of mechanical ventilation. Anesthesiology 1974;40:602–603
25. Bendixen HH, Egbert LD, Hedley-White J et al: Management of patients undergoing prolonged artificial ventilation. Respir Care, 1965;10:149–153
26. Safar, Kinkel HG: Prolonged artificial ventilation. p. 126. In Safar P (ed): Respiratory Therapy. FA Davis, Philadelphia, 1965
27. Stetson JB: Introductory essay in prolonged tracheal intubation. Int Anesthesiol Clin 1970;8:774–775
28. Sahn SA, Lakshminarayan S: Bedside criteria for discontinuation of mechanical ventilation. Chest 1973;63:1002–1005
29. Kacmarek RM, Cycyk-Chapman MC, Young-Palazzo PJ, Romagnoli DM: Determination of maximal inspiratory pressure: A clinical study and literature review. Respir Care 1989;34:868–878
30. Hess D: Measurement of maximal inspiratory pressure: A call for standardization. Respir Care 1989;34:857–859
31. Marini JJ, Smith TC, Lamb V: Estimation of inspiratory muscle strength in mechanically ventilated patients: The measurement of maximal inspiratory pressure. J Crit Care 1986;1:32–38
32. Black LF, Hyatt RE: Maximal respiratory pressures: Normal values and relationship to age and sex. Am Rev Respir Dis 1969;99:696–702
33. Branson RD, Hurst JM, Davis K Jr, Campbell R: Measurement of maximal inspiratory pressure: A comparison of three methods. Respir Care 1989;34:789–794
34. Fiastro JF, Habib MP, Shon BY, Campbell SC: Comparison of standard weaning parameters and the mechanical work of breathing in mechanically ventilated patients. Chest 1988;94:232–238
35. DeHaven CB Jr, Hurst JM, Branson RD: Evaluation of two different extubation criteria: Attributes contributing to success. Crit Care Med 1986;14:92–94
36. Millbern SM, Downs JB, Jumper LC, Modell JH: Evaluation of criteria for discontinuing mechanical ventilatory support. Arch Surg 1978;113:1441–1443
37. Pavlin EG, Holle RH, Schoene RB: Recovery of airway protection compared with ventilation in humans after paralysis with curare. Anesthesiology 1989;70:381–385
38. Cohen CA, Zagelbaum G, Gross D et al: Clinical manifestations of inspiratory muscle fatigue. Am J Med 1982;73:308–316
39. Tobin MJ, Guenther SM, Perez W et al: Konno-Mead analysis of ribcase-abdominal motion during successful and unsuccessful trials of weaning from mechanical ventilation. Am Rev Respir Dis 1987;135:1320–1328
40. Yang KL, Tobin MJ: A prospective study of indexes predicting the outcome of trials of weaning from mechanical ventilation. N Engl J Med 1991;324:1445–1450
41. Bellemare F, Grassino A: Effect of pressure and timing of contraction on human diaphragm fatigue. J Appl Physiol 1982;53:1190–1195
42. Peters RM, Hilberman M, Hogan JS, Crawford DA: Objective indications for respirator therapy in post-trauma and postoperative patients. Am J Surg 1972;124:262–269
43. Lewis WD, Chwals W, Benotti PN et al: Bedside assessment of the work of breathing. Crit Care Med 1988;16:117–122
44. Harpin RP, Baker JP, Downer JP et al: Correlation of the oxygen cost of breathing and length of weaning from mechanical ventilation. Crit Care Med 1987;15:807–812
45. Fleury B, Murciano D, Talamo C et al: Work of breathing in patients with chronic obstructive pulmonary disease in acute respiratory failure. Am Rev Respir Dis 1985;131:822–827
46. Sassoon CSH, Te TT, Mahutte CK, Light RW: Airway occlusion pressure. An important indicator for successful weaning in patients with chronic obstructive pulmonary disease. Am Rev Respir Dis 1987;135:107–113
47. Murciano D, Boczkowski J, Lecocguic Y et al: Tracheal occlusion pressure: A simple index to monitor respiratory muscle

fatigue during acute respiratory failure in patients with chronic obstructive pulmonary disease. Ann Intern Med 1988;108:800–805

48. Montgomery AB, Holle RHO, Neagley SR et al: Prediction of successful ventilator weaning using airway occlusion pressure and hypercapnic challenge. Chest 1987;91:496–499
49. Morganroth ML, Morganroth JL, Nett LM, Petty TL: Criteria for weaning from prolonged mechanical ventilation. Arch Intern Med 1984;144:1012–1016
50. Higgins TL, Kraenzler EJ, Blum JM: Evaluation of criteria for discontinuing mechanical ventilation following open heart surgery. Chest 1988;94:40S
51. Muir JF, Defouilloy C, Pawlicki JP et al: Acute respiratory failure (ARF) in COPD patients: IMV vs non IMV (NIMV) weaning. Am Rev Respir Dis 1985;131:A13
52. Hilberman M, Kamm B, Lamy M et al: An analysis of potential physiological predictors of respiratory adequacy following cardiac surgery. J Thorac Cardiovasc Surg 1976;71:711–720
53. Pingleton SK, Harmon GS: Nutritional management in acute respiratory failure. JAMA 1987;257:3094–3099
54. Bassili HR, Deitel M: Effect of nutritional support on weaning patients off mechanical ventilators. JPEN J Parenter Enteral Nutr 1981;5:161–163
55. Wilson DO, Rogers RM, Sanders MH et al: Nutritional intervention in malnourished patients with emphysema. Am Rev Respir Dis 1986;134:672–677
56. Covelli HD, Black JW, Olsen MS, Beekman JF: Respiratory failure precipitated by high carbohydrate loads. Ann Intern Med 1981;95:579–581
57. Weissman C, Askanazi J, Rosenbaum S et al: Amino acids and respiration. Ann Intern Med 1983;98:41–44
58. Zwillich CW, Pierson DJ, Hofeldt FD et al: Ventilatory control in myxedema and hypothyroidism N Engl J Med 1975;292:662–665
59. Wolkove N, Altose MD, Kelsen SG et al: Perception of changes in breathing in normal human subjects. J Appl Physiol 1981;50:78–83
60. Habib MP: Physiologic implications of artificial airways. Chest 1989;96:180–184
61. Plummer AL, Gracey DR: Consensus conference on artificial airways in patients receiving mechanical ventilation. Chest 1989;96:178–180
62. Tesar GE, Stern TA: Evaluation and treatment of agitation in the intensive care unit. J Intensive Care 1986;1:137–148
63. Holliday JF, Hyers TM: The reduction of weaning time from mechanical ventilation using tidal volume and relaxation biofeedback. Am Rev Respir Dis 1990;141:1214–1220
64. Higgins TL: Anesthetic and paralytic techniques in the intensive care unit. pp. 207–213. In Kacmarek RM, Stoller JK (eds): Current Respiratory Care. BC Decker, Toronto, 1988
65. Santiago TV, Edleman NH: Opioids in breathing. J Appl Physiol 1985;59:1675–1685
66. Duggan JE, Drummond GB: Abdominal muscle activity and intraabdominal pressure after upper abdominal surgery. Anesth Analg 1989;69:598–603
67. Braun SR, Bimbaum ML, Chopra PS: Pre- and postoperative pulmonary function abnormalities in coronary artery revascularization surgery. Chest 1978;73:316–320
68. Berrizbeitia LD, Tessler S, Jacobowitz IJ et al: Effect of sternotomy and coronary bypass surgery on postoperative pulmonary mechanics. Comparison of internal mammary and saphenous vein bypass grafts. Chest 1989;96:873–876
69. Higgins TL, Barrett C, Riden DJ et al: Influence of pleural and mediastinal chest tubes on respiration following coronary artery bypass grafting (CABG). Chest 1989;96:237S
70. Caspi J, Klausner JM, Safadi T et al: Delayed respiratory depression following fentanyl anesthesia for cardiac surgery. Crit Care Med 1988;16:238–240
71. Prakash O, Meij S, Van der Borden B, Saxena PR: Cardiorespiratory monitoring during open heart surgery. Crit Care Med 1981;9:530–535
72. Michel L, McMichan JC, Marsh HM, Rehder K: Measurement of ventilatory reserve as an indicator for early extubation after cardiac operation. J Thorac Cardiovasc Surg 1979;78:761–764
73. Higgins TL: Postoperative care of the cardiac surgery patient. Probl Anesth 1989;3:211–227
74. Beach T, Millen E, Grenvik A: Hemodynamic response to discontinuance of mechanical ventilation. Crit Care Med 1973;1:85–90
75. Buda AJ, Pinsky MR, Ingels NB et al: Effect of intrathoracic pressure on left ventricular performance. N Engl J Med 1979;301:453–459
76. Mathru M, Tadikonda LK, Rao TLK et al: Hemodynamic response to changes in ventilatory patterns in patients with normal and poor left ventricular reserve. Crit Care Med 1982;10:423–426
77. Sivak ED, Starr NJ, Graves JW et al: Extravascular lung water values in patients undergoing coronary artery bypass surgery. Crit Care Med 1982;10:593–599
78. Sivak ED, Tita J, Meden G et al: Effects of furosemide versus isolated ultrafiltration on extravascular lung water in oleic acid-induced pulmonary edema. Crit Care Med 1986;14:48–51
79. Coraim FJ, Coraim HP, Ebermann R, Stellwag FM: Acute respiratory failure after cardiac surgery: Clinical experience with the application of continuous arteriovenous hemofiltration. Crit Care Med 1986;14:714–718
80. Abd AG, Braun NMT, Baskin MI et al: Diaphragmatic dysfunction after open heart surgery: Treatment with a rocking bed. Ann Intern Med 1989;111:881–886
81. Wheeler WE, Rubis LJ, Jones CW et al: Etiology and prevention of topical cardiac hypothermia-induced phrenic nerve injury and left lower lobe atelectasis during cardiac surgery. Chest 1985;88:680–683
82. Wilcox P, Baile EM, Hards J et al: Phrenic nerve function and its relationship to atelectasis after coronary artery bypass surgery. Chest 1988;93:693–698
83. Sivak ED, Razavi M, Groves LK, Loop FD: Long-term management of diaphragmatic paralysis complicating prosthetic valve replacement. Crit Care Med 1983;11:438–440
84. Lugliani R, Whipp BJ, Wasserman K: Doxapram hydrochloride: A respiratory stimulant for patients with primary alveolar hypoventilation. Chest 1979;76:414–419
85. Bergofsky EH: State of the art. Respiratory failure in disorders of the thoracic cage. Am Rev Respir Dis 1979;119:643–669
86. Sivak ED: Prolonged mechanical ventilation. An approach to weaning. Cleve Clin J Med 1980;47:89–96
87. Aldrich TK, Karpel JP, Uhrlass RM et al: Weaning from mechanical ventilation. Adjunctive use of inspiratory muscle resistive training. Crit Care Med 1989;17:143–147
88. Menzies R, Gibbons W, Goldberg P: Determinants of weaning and survival among patients with COPD who require mechanical ventilation for acute respiratory failure. Chest 1989;95:398–405
89. Pepe PE, Marini JJ: Occult positive end-expiratory pressure in mechanically ventilated patients with airflow obstruction. Am Rev Respir Dis 1982;126:166–170
90. Rossi A, Gottfried SB, Zocchi L et al: Measurement of static compliance of the total respiratory system in patients with acute respiratory failure during mechanical ventilation. The effect of intrinsic positive end-expiratory pressure. Am Rev Respir Dis 1985;131:672–677
91. Smith TC, Marini JJ: Impact of PEEP on lung mechanics and work of breathing in severe airflow obstruction. J Appl Physiol 1988;65:1488–1499
92. Lakatta EG, Mitchell JH, Pomerance A, Rowe GG: Human aging: Changes in structure and function. J Am Coll Cardiol 1987;10:42A–47A
93. Wahba WM: Influence of aging on lung function: Clinical significance of changes from age twenty. Anesth Analg 1983;62:764–776
94. Higgins TL, Starr NJ, Loop FD, Estafanous FG: Perioperative course of octogenarians undergoing open heart surgery, ab-

stracted. Society of Cardiovascular Anesthesiologists 11th Annual Meeting, April 1989. Society of Cardiovascular Anesthesiologists, Seattle, 1989
95. Krieger BP, Ershowsky PF, Becker DA, Gazeroglu HB: Evaluation of conventional criteria for predicting successful weaning from mechanical ventilatory support in elderly patients. Crit Care Med 1989;17:858–861
96. Venus B, Smith RA, Mathru M: National survey of methods and criteria used for weaning from mechanical ventilation. Crit Care Med 1987;15:530–533
97. Downs JB, Perkins HM, Modell JH: Intermittent mandatory ventilation. Arch Surg 1974;109:519–523
98. Schachter EN, Tucker D, Beck GJ: Does intermittent mandatory ventilation accelerate weaning? JAMA 1981;246:1210–1214
99. Tomlinson JR, Miller KS, Lorch DG et al: A prospective comparison of IMV and T-piece weaning from mechanical ventilation. Chest 1989;96:348–352
100. Kacmarek RM: The role of pressure support ventilation in reducing work of breathing. Respir Care 1988;33:99–120
101. MacIntyre NR: Weaning from mechanical ventilatory support. Volume-assisting intermittent breaths versus pressure-assisting every breath. Respir Care 1988;33:121–125
102. Feeley TW, Klick JM, Saumarez R, McNabb TG: Positive end-expiratory pressure in weaning patients from controlled ventilation. A prospective randomized trial. Lancet 1975;2:725–728
103. Heffner JE, Scott Miller K, Sahn SA: Tracheostomy in the intensive care unit. Part 1: Indications, technique, management. Chest 1986;90:269–274
104. Heffner JE, Scott Miller K, Sahn SA: Tracheostomy in the intensive care unit. Part 2: Complications. Chest 1986;90:430–436
105. Aubier M, De Troyer A, Sampson M et al: Aminophylline improves diaphragmatic contractility. N Engl J Med 1981;305:249–252
106. Dureuil B, Desmonts JM, Mankikian B, Prokocimer P: Effects of aminophylline on diaphragmatic dysfunction after upper abdominal surgery. Anesthesiology 1985;62:242–246
107. Aubier M, Murciano D, Menu Y et al: Dopamine effects on diaphragmatic strength during acute respiratory failure in chronic obstructive pulmonary disease. Ann Intern Med 1989;110:17–23
108. Woodcock AA, Gross ER, Gellert A et al: Effects of dihydrocodeine, alcohol, and caffeine on breathlessness and exercise tolerance in patients with chronic obstructive lung disease and normal blood gases. N Engl J Med 1981;305:1611–1616
109. Demling RH, Read T, Lind LJ, Flanagan HL: Incidence and morbidity of extubation failure in surgical intensive care patients. Crit Care Med 1988;16:573–577
110. Schmidt CD, Elliott CG, Carmelli D et al: Prolonged mechanical ventilation for respiratory failure: A cost-benefit analysis. Crit Care Med 1983;11:407–411
111. Witek TJ, Schachter EN, Dean NL, Beck GJ: Mechanically assisted ventilation in a community hospital. Arch Intern Med 1985;145:235–239
112. Nunn JF, Milledge JS, Singaraya J: Survival of patients ventilated in an intensive therapy unit. Br Med J 1979;1:1525–1527
113. Spicher JE, White DP: Outcome and function following prolonged mechanical ventilation. Arch Intern Med 1987;147:421–425
114. Davis H II, Lefrak SS, Miller D, Malt S: Prolonged mechanically assisted ventilation. An analysis of outcome and charges. JAMA 1980;243:43–45
115. Martin TR, Lewis SW, Albert RK: The prognosis of patients with chronic obstructive pulmonary disease after hospitalization for acute respiratory failure. Chest 1982;82:310–314
116. Elpern EH, Larson R, Douglass P et al: Long-term outcomes for elderly survivors of prolonged ventilator assistance. Chest 1989;96:1120–1124
117. Knaus WA: Prognosis with mechanical ventilation: The influence of disease, severity of disease, age, and chronic health status on survival from an acute illness. Am Rev Respir Dis 1989;140:S8–13
118. Grassino A, Bellemare F, Laporta D: Diaphragm fatigue and the strategy of breathing in COPD. Chest 1984;85:51S

Chapter 87

Optimizing Ventilatory Muscle Function during Mechanical Ventilation

Robert M. Kacmarek

CHAPTER OUTLINE

Mechanical ventilation is begun for a number of reasons, as outlined in Chapter 81. High on the list is ventilatory failure as a result of ventilatory muscle dysfunction. It is generally assumed that once mechanical ventilation is instituted, the ventilator does all the work of breathing. This assumption is generally true during full ventilatory support if patients are appropriately sedated; however, whenever the patient must interact with the ventilator during either full or partial ventilatory support (Ch. 82), the potential exists for the patient to perform the majority of the work of breathing and thereby delay the recovery of dysfunctional ventilatory muscles.[1]

In addition to manipulation of the mechanical ventilatory system, work of breathing can also be decreased by reducing ventilatory demand, improving respiratory impedance, and improving efficiency of ventilation. Ventilatory demand can be reduced by decreasing CO_2 production and ventilatory drive by treating fever, correcting metabolic acidosis, reducing psychogenic stress, and using appropriate sedation. Impedance of gas flow can be improved by appropriate bronchial hygiene techniques, chest physical therapy, and use of aerosolized drugs, as well as by control of systemic and pulmonary vascular volume. Ventilatory efficiency is also improved by proper positioning to favor more normal lung tissue and the elimination of intrinsic positive end-expiratory pressure (auto-PEEP). These techniques, discussed elsewhere in this text, should always be considered as other manipulations are made to improve the patient-ventilator interface.

The remainder of this chapter focuses on manipulations of the patient–mechanical ventilator interface that enhance synchrony between patient and machine and decrease the work of breathing imposed by the ventilator system (Table 87-1).

PEAK INSPIRATORY FLOW

During all volume-limited, assisted breaths in synchronized intermittent mandatory ventilation (SIMV) or assist/control, the practitioner must adjust the peak inspiratory flow rate either directly or indirectly. However, few machines allow an accurate assessment of the patient's spontaneous peak inspiratory flow. As a result, a difference be-

Table 87-1. Primary Factors Affecting Ventilatory Muscle Function and Work of Breathing during Ventilatory Assistance

Peak inspiratory flow	Presence of heat and moisture exchanges
Sensitivity setting	Auto-PEEP
Humidification system	Level of ventilatory support
Demand valve function	
Continuous flow system function	

tween the peak inspiratory flow desired by the patient and that delivered by the ventilator can exist. Patients' peak inspiratory flows during stress may exceed 100 to 150 L/min, while most mechanical ventilators are capable of providing peak flows only up to 100 to 120 L/min during volume-limited breaths.[2]

Marini and co-workers[3,4] have clearly demonstrated that patients may perform as much work during volume-assisted breaths as during spontaneous breathing if peak inspiratory flow is inadequate. Figure 87-1A shows an airway pressure-volume curve during controlled mechanical ventilation (solid line), which defines the total work of breathing. If the ventilator were to provide the total work of breathing during assisted ventilation under the same clinical circumstances, the same curve (dotted line) should be established. That is, the curve during controlled ventilation and assisted ventilation should be identical. The airway pressure-volume curve of Figure 87-1B depicts an actual pressure-volume curve during assisted ventilation (dotted line) superimposed on a patient's ideal curve (solid line). It should be noted that the machine work is greatly diminished; thus, the large hatched area completing the ideal curve and falling below baseline represents patient work during the assisted breath. Any time a difference exists between the peak inspiratory flow or inspiratory time of the machine and the patient, the potential exists for the patient to perform a high percentage of the work during volume-assisted ventilation.[5]

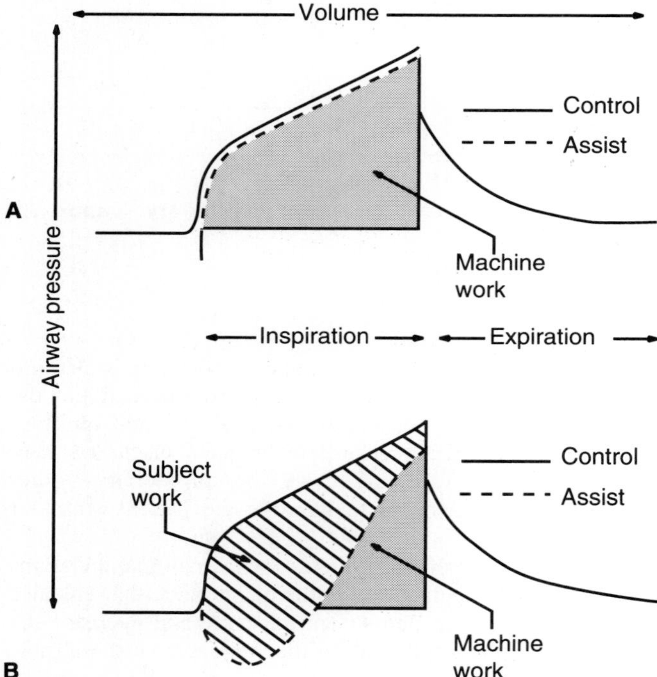

Figure 87-1. **(A)** Theoretical relationship between actual and ideal airway pressure curve during assisted mechanical breaths (assist/control or SIMV). No difference should exist between control breath and assisted breath. **(B)** Actual airway pressure curve differences. The hatched area represents work performed by the patient during an assisted volume-limited breath. If inspiratory flows and inspiratory times are inappropriate, the patient's work of breathing during assisted breathing may equal that during spontaneous breathing. (From Marini et al.,[4] with permission.)

During all volume-assisted breaths, care must be taken to ensure that patients are in synchrony with the ventilator. Frequently, this requires peak inspiratory flow settings of 80 to 100 L/min or inspiratory times set at 0.8 to 1.0 second. One way of ensuring that volume-limited breaths are delivered in the appropriate manner is to determine spontaneous inspiratory time and then to adjust the peak inspiratory flow of the ventilator or inspiratory time to match inspiratory time during spontaneous breathing.

It should be remembered that this concern over peak inspiratory flow only exists during assisted breaths. During controlled mechanical ventilation, inspiratory time or peak inspiratory flow may be set to achieve other goals of mechanical ventilation, such as mean airway pressure, inspiration/expiration (I/E) ratio, and hemodynamic stabilization (see Ch. 83).

SENSITIVITY SETTING

During any mechanically assisted breath or continuous positive airway pressure (CPAP), patients must trigger the mechanical breath or open a demand valve.[2] This requires the patient to generate a negative intrathoracic pressure and perform some work.[6–8] The more negative the sensitivity is set in relation to baseline pressure, the greater the effort the patient must exert to trigger the ventilator. Ideally, the sensitivity should be set at -0.5 to -1.0 cmH_2O.[5] Some ventilators (Drager IRISA) have fixed sensitivity settings in this range (-0.7 cmH_2O); others allow large variation in sensitivity settings.[9]

The accumulation of water in the ventilator tubing and its oscillation can trigger the ventilator.[10] As a result, ventilator sensitivity is frequently set at -2 or -2.5 cmH_2O. These settings impose work on ventilatory muscles and delay the delivery of gas into the ventilator circuit.[10–12] Gurevitch and Gelmont[12] have demonstrated this effect in a case study, using multiple ventilators on a single patient (Fig. 87-2). They noted that the less sensitive the ventilator, the greater the delay in gas delivery, which always reflects increased ventilatory muscle effort. In this case study the Bear 5 ventilator stopped triggering once the sensitivity was decreased below -2.0 cmH_2O. There is a twofold explanation for this finding:

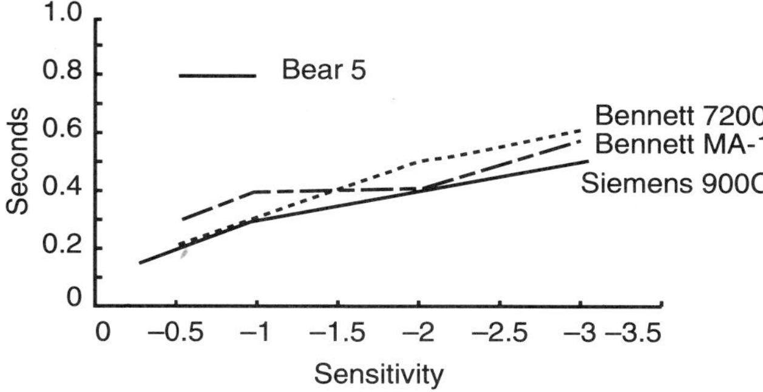

Figure 87-2. Ventilator response delay at various trigger sensitivities with the Bear 5, Bennett 7200, Bennett MA-1, and Siemens 900C ventilators in one patient. As trigger sensitivity became more negative, the time from onset of inspiratory effort to ventilator response increased. (From Gurevitch and Gelmont,[12] with permission.)

(1) the patient studied had a very weak inspiratory drive; and (2) this ventilator maintains a 5 L/min bias flow to ensure calibration of monitoring systems.[2,9] The addition of a bias flow increases the patient effort required for triggering regardless of sensitivity setting.

On certain ventilators (e.g., the Hamilton Veolar and Amadeus, Ohmeda CPU-1 and Advent) inspiratory effort is sensed internally on the inspiratory side.[2,10] In such ventilators the use of a bubble-through humidifier markedly increases the patient effort required for triggering[13] because patient effort must be sensed either through a column of fluid or through a small hole in the humidifier system. With any ventilator that senses patient effort internally on the inspiratory side, a pass-over humidifier should always be used.

DEMAND SYSTEMS

During spontaneous, non-mechanically supported breaths via ventilator systems, work of breathing is imposed.[6–13] The magnitude of the imposed work is related to the humidifier[9,10] used and the sensitivity setting[12] (see above), but also to the basic design of the ventilator.[6–8,10,11] As noted by Gurevitch and Gelmont,[12] there is a delay between the patient's initiation of inspiratory effort and the ventilator's initiation of flow into the system. This delay can be marked during spontaneous breaths (CPAP), particularly with older-generation ventilators.[6–8] Most of the newest generation of mechanical ventilators have minimized this imposed work of breathing by adding 1 to 4 cmH_2O of inspiratory pressure support during demand breathing when the pressure support control is set at zero.[10,14]

With all available units, the addition of CPAP to demand flow increases the imposed work of breathing.[10] This appears to be a result of the flow-resistive function of exhalation and PEEP valves in common use.[15] As a result of the effects of demand systems and the use of artificial airways (see below), most recommend the use of low levels of inspiratory pressure support to overcome the imposed work of breathing (see Ch. 83 for details) and return patient total work to a level at or below that during premorbid spontaneous breathing.[16]

The Puritan-Bennett 7200a ventilator modified the effect of demand systems by including a flow-triggering option (flow-by).[9] With this triggering mechanism, demand flow is initiated when a bias flow (5 to 20 L/min) is decreased by 1 to 8 L/min (sensitivity setting). The major difference between pressure triggering and flow triggering of this type is that in the former the unit attempts to maintain the baseline pressure minus the sensitivity setting, but with flow-by, maintenance of actual baseline pressure is attempted. The use of flow-by has improved the basic demand function of the 7200a and reduces the imposed work of breathing.[10,17]

CONTINUOUS FLOW SYSTEMS

Although continuous flow systems normally impose less work of breathing than demand systems, few ventilators include continuous-flow options. In order to ensure minimum imposed work of breathing, continuous flow systems must meet patient peak inspiratory flow demands. This requires the use of a large gas reservoir (3 to 5 L) and the maintenance of continuous flow at or above patient peak inspiratory flow, which means at about 60 to 90 L/min.[15] Flows less than this may result in marked increases in patient work (see Ch. 76 for details on continuous flow systems).

Some new ventilators include continuous low flow systems (Bear 5) or combine continuous flow with demand flow (Puritan-Bennett 7200a, flow-by). These systems only work efficiently if they are designed to meet patient peak flow demands, as is the case with the 7200a flow-by system, but the Bear 5, because of a limited available flow (40 L/min), is usually incapable of meeting most patients' demands.[10]

ARTIFICIAL AIRWAYS

The single most significant factor affecting ventilatory muscle function and work of breathing during ventilatory assistance is the artificial airway.[16] Regardless of type, the artificial airway provides the greatest resistance to gas flow into the patient.[18] This effect is more prominent with endotracheal tubes than with tracheostomy tubes because endotracheal tubes are longer and more likely to be compressed as they pass through the upper airway.[5]

The effect of decreasing endotracheal tube size on work load and resistance to gas flow is depicted in Figure 87-3, from which it may be seen that the smaller the endotracheal tube and the greater the minute ventilation, the greater the work load.[19] Generally, artificial airways of less than 7.5 mm internal diameter in women and 8.0 mm internal diameter in men result in marked additional work loads.[5] This increase is most devastating in patients with pre-existing ventilatory muscle dysfunction but may also precipitate fatigue in previously healthy individuals if minute ventilation is high.

Most of the studies evaluating resistance to gas flow

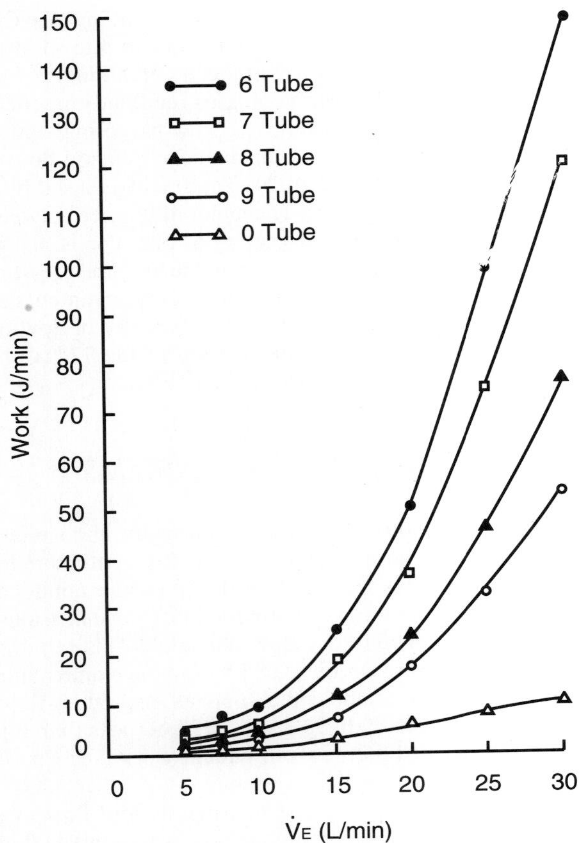

Figure 87-3. Relationship between work of breathing and increasing minute ventilation through endotracheal tubes of different size. Fatiguing work loads occurred at minute ventilations greater than 25 L/min with tubes of 6 and 7 mm internal diameter. (From Shapiro et al.,[19] with permission.)

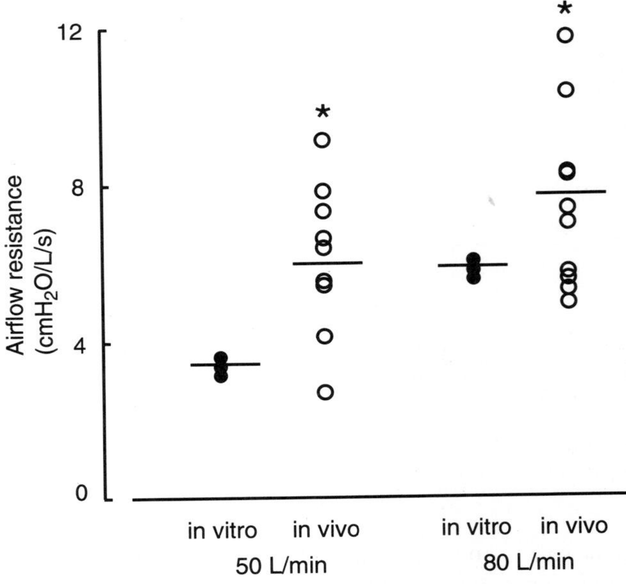

Figure 87-4. Comparison of the calculated endotracheal tube (for a #8.0 tube) airflow resistance in vitro (an average of inspiratory and expiratory flow) with measurements made in vivo. Flow resistance was higher when measured in vivo at both flow rates. In vitro, N equals 5; in vivo, N equals 10. (From Wright et al.,[20] with permission.)

through endotracheal tubes have been performed in lung models[18] or individuals breathing through tubes[19] but not actually intubated. This has resulted in an underestimation of the effect of tubes, as noted by Wright et al.[20] (Fig. 87-4). Gas flow resistance is greater in vivo than in vitro primarily because the contour of the tube is changed as it is warmed by the body and passes through the airway. In addition, the adhesion of secretions to the walls of the tube increases gas flow resistance.

The airway resulting in the greatest increased work load is the nasotracheal tube.[5] Since these tubes must pass through the nose and nasopharynx, their shape can be markedly altered, and frequently they are kinked as they pass from the nasal into the oral pharynx. This is not sufficient to stop gas flow but is enough to decrease the lumen of a tube from 8.0 to 7.5 mm. The point of kinking also provides an ideal location at which secretions can adhere.

From the perspective of ventilatory muscle function, the largest oral endotracheal tube should always be used. However, other factors may affect the actual selection of a specific airway (see Ch. 72). Patients with compromised ventilatory muscle function should not be forced to breathe through any endotracheal tube for prolonged periods. Inspiratory pressure support can be used to offset the work imposed by the ventilator and the artificial airway (see Ch. 82), particularly in the presence of a small nasotracheal tube.[16]

HEAT AND MOISTURE EXCHANGERS

Heat and moisture exchangers have become commonplace in operating rooms and during short-term ventilatory support. Although these units are capable of providing adequate humidification to select patient populations, they also increase resistance to ventilation[21] and ventilatory muscle work (see Ch. 71). As a result, they are not recommended for routine use in patients on CPAP, T pieces, or low levels of SIMV. This is particularly true if small nasal endotracheal tubes are in place.

AUTO-PEEP

Of all those factors that may adversely affect ventilatory muscle function and work of breathing, auto-PEEP is the most difficult to evaluate (see Ch. 76). In the spontaneously breathing patient the presence of an esophageal balloon is normally necessary to accurately measure auto-PEEP,[22] although some clinicians have attempted to assess auto-PEEP level by determining a reproducible end-expiratory plateau for three or four consecutive breaths.[23]

Auto-PEEP established as a result of dynamic airflow restriction has a significant effect on work of breathing because it increases the transpulmonary pressure gradient necessary to establish flow.[24] As shown in Figure 87-5, the end alveolar pressure and the central airway pressure differ in the presence of auto-PEEP. Thus, the patient must reduce the alveolar pressure before the central airway pressure and the ventilator circuit pressure can decrease. This results in a marked increase in work of breathing. As noted in Chapter 76 and Table 87-2, numerous approaches are available to decrease the level of auto-PEEP. The most effective in the spontaneously breathing patient is to apply PEEP[24] or CPAP,[23] thereby allowing an equilibration between central

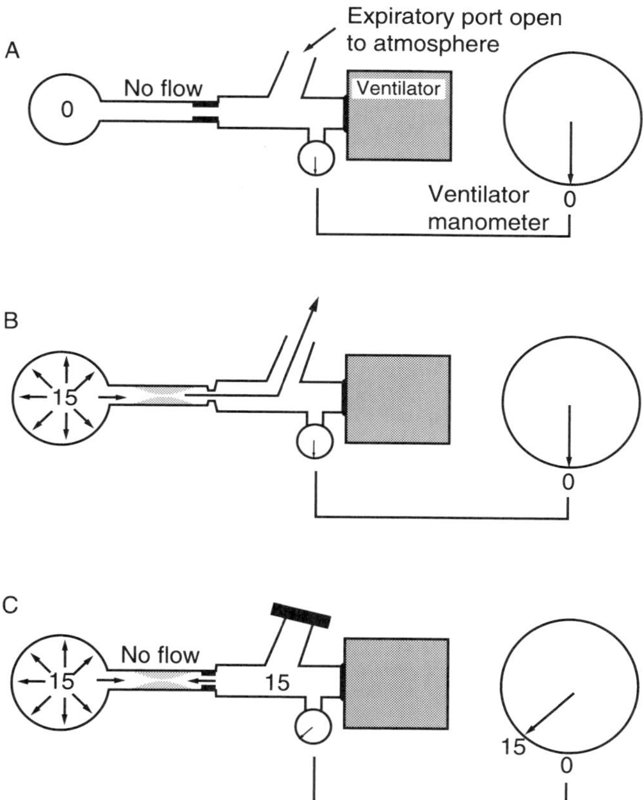

Figure 87-5. Measurement of auto-PEEP by expiratory port occlusion. **(A)** Normally alveolar pressure is atmospheric at the end of passive exhalation. **(B)** With severe airflow obstruction (and the expiratory port open), alveolar pressure remains elevated and slow flow continues even at the end of the set exhalation period. The ventilator manometer senses negligible pressure because it is open to the atmosphere through large-bore tubing and downstream from the site of flow limitation. **(C)** With the gas flow stopped by occlusion of the expiratory port at the end of the set exhalation period, pressure equilibrates throughout the lung ventilator system and is displayed on the ventilator manometer. (From Pepe and Marini,[22] with permission.)

Table 87-2. Approaches Used to Modify the Level of Auto-PEEP

Decrease dynamic airflow obstruction
- Aggressive bronchodilation
- Chest physical therapy
- Airway suctioning
- Large sized enotracheal tube

Normalize pH
- Administer $NaHCO_3$ during metabolic acidosis
- Avoid purposeful hyperventilation

Allow PCO_2 to rise into the 50s and 60s by decreasing rate and normalizing pH

Modify ventilatory pattern: increase expiratory time
- Decrease rate/increase V_T
- Decrease inspiratory time
  - Increase peak inspiratory flow
  - Use low compressible volume circuit
- Use low rate SIMV

Apply PEEP/CPAP

airway pressure and end alveolar pressure (auto-PEEP). As a result, the transpulmonary pressure gradient required to trigger the ventilator decreases and is normalized if applied PEEP is equal to the initial auto-PEEP[23,24] (Fig. 87-6).

Since auto-PEEP is difficult to determine in spontaneously breathing patients, the primary clue to its presence may be an inability to trigger an assisted breath or demand flow with

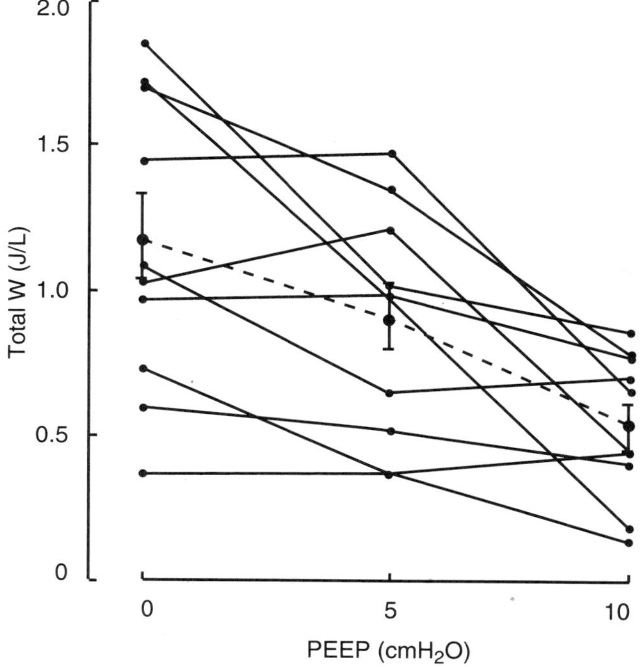

Figure 87-6. The effect of applied PEEP on total work of breathing in the presence of auto-PEEP. Total work ($\dot{w}$) decreased as applied PEEP increased to 5 and then 10 cmH_2O. (From Smith and Marini,[24] with permission.)

every inspiratory effort (assuming sensitivity is properly set). When the patient's ventilatory rate exceeds the machine rate, only one of two problems exists, either an insensitive or malfunctioning trigger mechanism or the pressure of auto-PEEP. After careful evaluation of the machine, PEEP can be applied in 1 to 2 cmH_2O increments until the patient is able to trigger the ventilator with every breath.[5] At this time the applied PEEP has eliminated the effect of auto-PEEP on work of breathing. Since auto-PEEP is very common when the glottic mechanism is bypassed by an artificial airway, I recommend the use either of 5 cmH_2O CPAP or of PEEP on a routine basis and have used up to 12 cmH_2O of CPAP or PEEP because of recognized auto-PEEP.

LEVEL OF VENTILATORY SUPPORT

SIMV, although advantageous, may result in excessive patient work loads if improperly adjusted.[25] This mode incorporates spontaneous breathing and volume-limited mechanical ventilation at variable percentages of total minute ventilation, depending on machine rate setting and patient ventilatory drive. Many clinicians maintain the lowest level of machine SIMV rate that produces normal CO_2 elimination regardless of the patient's spontaneous breathing rate. This practice must be questioned in the light of data provided by Marini et al.[25] (Fig. 87-7). In a series of critically ill patients, they compared the work of breathing during volume-limited and spontaneous breaths at various levels of SIMV corresponding to percent provision of total minute ventilation. As noted (Fig. 87-7), the work of breathing increased during both the mechanical and the spontaneous breaths as percent SIMV rate decreased.

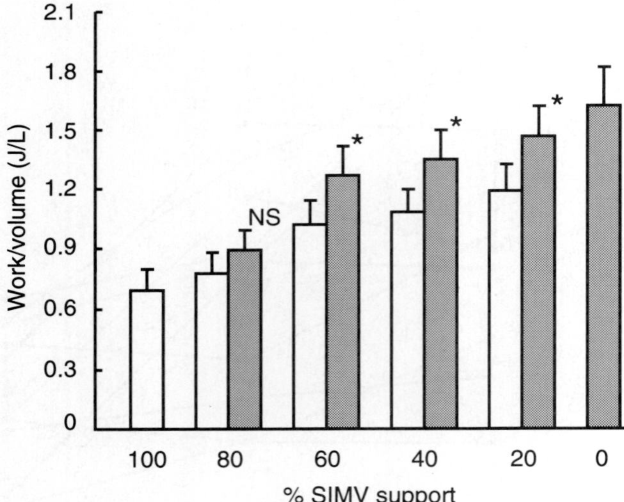

Figure 87-7. Inspiratory work per unit volume (in joules per liter) done by a patient during SIMV breaths (open squares) and spontaneous breaths (darkened squares). Work increased with decreasing SIMV percentage for both types of breath. Normal work of breathing for spontaneous breaths tended to exceed that for SIMV breaths. Asterisks indicate a significant difference between spontaneous and assisted breaths. NS, not significant. (From Marini et al.,[25] with permission.)

This is a particular concern in the long-term, ventilator-dependent patient, where SIMV or intermittent mandatory ventilation (IMV) is used as a weaning mode. Maintaining patients at low SIMV rates for prolonged periods may result in ventilatory muscle dysfunction. Problems with SIMV can be avoided if careful assessment of patients' spontaneous ventilatory patterns are made and machine rate is adjusted to ensure a normal spontaneous breathing pattern and a relatively slow (less than 20 breaths per minute) spontaneous rate. In addition, the use of inspiratory pressure support[16,26] along with SIMV is very useful in normalizing spontaneous ventilatory patterns and minimizing work of breathing.

References

1. Marini JJ: Minimizing breathing effort during mechanical ventilation. In Zapol W, Lemaine F (ed): Acute Respiratory Failure. Marcel Dekker, New York, 1990
2. McPherson S: Respiratory Therapy Equipment 3rd Ed. Mosby-Year Book, St. Louis, 1990
3. Marini JJ, Capps JS, Culver BH: The inspiratory work of breathing during assisted mechanical ventilation. Chest 1985;87:612–618
4. Marini JJ, Rodriguez RM, Lamb V: The inspiratory work load of patient-initiated mechanical ventilation. Am Rev Respir Dis 1986;134:902–909
5. Kacmarek RM: Interactions between patients and mechanical ventilators. Curr Opinion Anesthesiol 1990;3:228–234
6. Gibney RTN, Wilson RS, Pontuppidan H: Comparison of work of breathing on high gas flow and demand valve continuous positive airway pressure systems. Chest 1982;82:692–695
7. Katz JA, Kraemer RW, Gjerde GE: Inspiratory work and airway pressure with continuous positive airway pressure delivery system. Chest 1985;88:519–526
8. Viale JP, Annat G, Bertrand O: Additional inspiratory work in intubated patients breathing with continuous positive pressure systems. Anesthesiology 1985;63:536–539
9. Kacmarek RM, McKlaus G: The new generation mechanical ventilators. Crit Care Clin 1990;6:551–578
10. Hirsch C, Kacmarek RM, Stanek K: Work of breathing during CPAP and IPS imposed by the new generation mechanical ventilators. Respir Care 1991;36:815–828
11. Beydon L, Chasse M, Harf A, Lemaire F: Inspiratory work of breathing during spontaneous ventilation using demand valve and continuous flow systems. Am Rev Respir Dis 1988;138:300–304
12. Gurevitch MJ, Gelmont D: Importance of trigger sensitivity to ventilator response delay in advanced chronic obstructive pulmonary disease with respiratory failure. Crit Care Med 1989; 17:354–359
13. Kacmarek RM, Stanek K, McMahon K: Imposed work of breathing during synchronized intermittent mandatory ventilation using home care ventilators. Respir Care 1990;35:405–414
14. Samodelov LF, Falke F: Total inspiratory work with modern demand valve devices compared to continuous flow CPAP. Intensive Care Med 1988;14:632–639
15. Kacmarek RM, Goulet RL: PEEP devices. Anesthesiol Clin North Am 1987;5:757–776
16. Kacmarek RM: The role of pressure support in reducing the work of breathing. Respir Care 1988;33:99–120
17. Sassoon CSH, Giron AE, Ely EA, Light RW: Inspiratory work

of breathing on flow-by and demand flow continuous positive airway pressure. Crit Care Med 1989;17:1108–1114
18. Bolder PM, Healy TEJ, Bolder AR et al: The extra work of breathing through endotracheal tubes. Anesth Analg 1986; 65:853–859
19. Shapiro W, Wilson RK, Casar G et al: Work of breathing through different sized endotracheal tubes. Crit Care Med 1986;14:1028–1031
20. Wright PE, Marini JJ, Bernard GR: In vitro versus in vivo comparison of endotracheal tube airflow resistance. Am Rev Respir Dis 1989;140:10–16
21. Ploysongsang Y, Branson RD, Rashkin MC, Hurst JM: Effect of flow rate and duration of use on the pressure drop across six artificial noses. Respir Care 1989;34:902–907
22. Pepe PE, Marini JJ: Occult positive and end-expiratory pressure in mechanically ventilated patients with airflow obstruction. Am Rev Respir Dis 1982;126:166–170
23. Petrof BJ, Legare M, Goldberg P et al: Continuous positive airway pressure reduces work of breathing and dyspnea during weaning from mechanical ventilation in severe chronic obstructive pulmonary disease. Am Rev Respir Dis 1990;141:281–289
24. Smith TC, Marini JJ: Impact of PEEP on lung mechanics and work of breathing in severe airflow obstruction. J Appl Physiol 1988;65:1488–1499
25. Marini JJ, Smith TC, Lamb VJ: External work output and force generation during synchronized intermittent mandatory ventilation. Am Rev Respir Dis 1988;138:1169–1170
26. Hurst JM, Branson RD, Davis K, Barrette RR: Cardiopulmonary effects of pressure support ventilation. Arch Surg 1989; 124:1067–1070

Chapter 88

Intensive Respiratory Care of Children

Eve Medvidofsky
Patricia B. Koff
Joan Balik

CHAPTER OUTLINE

Respiratory care provided to infants and children is guided by essentially the same criteria that guide therapy in adults. However, because of the size and varied pulmonary physiology seen, especially in infants, modification of some basic approaches to care must be considered. The intention of this chapter is not to provide a detailed description of the management of critically ill children but to review specific aspects of respiratory care that require modification when applied to children. Accordingly, information is presented regarding O_2 and aerosol therapy and chest physiotherapy, as well as airway care and positive-pressure ventilation.

OXYGEN THERAPY

Equipment decisions regarding delivery of O_2 therapy to children differ somewhat from those made for adult patients. Not only the efficiency of the system but also patient comfort and the likelihood of continuous use must be considered. Generally, O_2 cannulas, tents, and hoods are tolerated best, while mask therapy such as that used with adults (by means of venturi, simple O_2, or aerosol mask) is poorly tolerated by young pediatric patients.

The biggest difference between low-flow O_2 therapy in adult and pediatric patients is that higher O_2 concentrations are achieved at lower flow rates in children. This occurs because of the effect on entrained room air of children's smaller tidal volumes and minute volumes (see Ch. 75). Concentrations also may vary from patient to patient as with adults, since minute volumes vary considerably. Oxygenation should be monitored by pulse oximeter, transcutaneous PO_2, or arterial blood gas measurements.

Nasal Cannulas

Nasal cannulas are made in infant, pediatric, and adult sizes (Fig. 88-1B). Flow rates with adults generally vary from

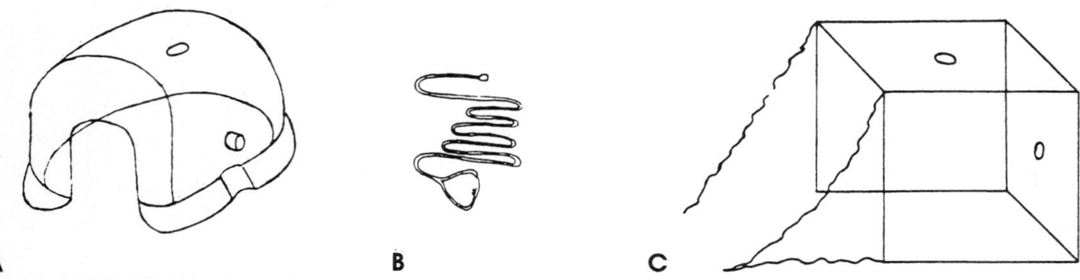

Figure 88-1. O_2 delivery for pediatric patients. **(A)** O_2 hood, **(B)** nasal cannula, and **(C)** tot-hut.

0.5 to 6 L/min; however, with pediatric patients it is rare to need a rate higher than 4 L/min. With infants flow rates as low as 0.125 L/min have been used and blended gas has sometimes been delivered to the cannula.

The prongs on the cannula may not be tolerated by some patients. To relieve the irritation, some practitioners trim the prongs, leaving wide holes in the tubing. From our experience it is better to find the best fitting cannula and thus avoid modification. Cannulas without prongs do not remain in place under the nares, and the holes may face outward or become obstructed with the tape used for securing nasogastric tubes.

Oxygen Hoods

Hoods are used for small infants 0 to 6 months of age who are minimally active (Fig. 88-1A). Hoods can provide up to about 50 percent O_2 on a consistent basis and should be humidified. Since the delivery of a cool gas in an enclosed environment to a small infant results in heat loss and stress, a heated humidifier or heated nebulizer is frequently used to deliver O_2 in these cases. More active infants and older infants may use a "tot-hut" (Fig. 88-1C), which is larger than a hood but smaller than an O_2 tent. Adequate flow through either device must be provided to maintain a constant O_2 concentration and to flush expired gases. The necessary flow depends on the size of the hood used and the desired O_2 concentration. Inspired O_2 fraction (F_{IO_2}) should be monitored continuously or at frequent intervals, and the O_2 analyzer probe should be placed near the infant's face since O_2 gradients do occur within the hood.[1] Supplemental O_2 via cannula or mask is normally provided if it is necessary to remove the patient from the hood.

Oxygen (Mist) Tents

Mist tents are used for children with acute or chronic respiratory disease associated with increased sputum production (Fig. 88-2). Mist tents provide cool aerosols, which assist in reducing the edema that often accompanies pediatric airway diseases such as croup or bronchiolitis. The tent also can furnish an O_2-enriched environment up to approximately 40 percent. At least 10 L/min of O_2 should be provided to avoid CO_2 buildup. The F_{IO_2} should be analyzed continuously or at frequent intervals to ensure O_2 delivery. When the child is removed from the tent, an additional source of O_2 is used. As with adult O_2 delivery systems, no smoking should be permitted in the room, and in addition, the child should not be given spark-producing toys in an O_2-enriched enclosure.

AEROSOL THERAPY

In addition to the use of cool aerosols with hoods or tents, aerosolized medications are frequently delivered to pediatric patients with respiratory problems such as asthma, bronchiolitis, or cystic fibrosis. The use of gas-powered or jet nebulizers is common in the neonatal unit as well as with older children. Infant and pediatric pulmonary function evaluation systems developed in the late 1980s have begun to provide objective data on the effectiveness of this type of therapy, as well as information to determine the appropriate dosages for individual patients. However, widespread variation in doses currently exists, as discussed by Post and Lambert[2] (e.g., albuterol doses vary between institutions from 0.005 to 1.3 mg/kg).

Various devices are available for the delivery of aerosolized medications.[3] Commonly, infant masks are attached to jet nebulizers, or a large-bore corrugated tube is attached to the nebulizer and the mist is directed to the patient's face.

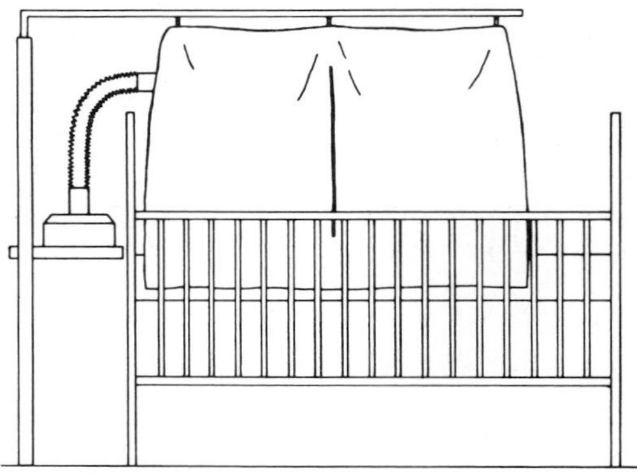

Figure 88-2. O_2 mist tent.

Some centers advocate the use of manual resuscitator bags for delivery of aerosolized drugs to both spontaneously breathing infants and those receiving mechanical ventilation. In-line nebulizer therapy is also commonly used in pediatric ventilator-supported patients. Since nebulizers are commonly run at 6 to 8 L/min, careful adjustment of the ventilator-delivered tidal volume or continuous gas flow system is necessary during therapy to avoid marked increases in tidal volume and airway pressure. Again, the effectiveness of this therapy, as well as the influence of the gas powering the nebulizer on the patient's respiratory mechanics, is just beginning to be documented.

Metered dose inhalers (MDIs) are frequently used in older children. Their ease of use, portability, and effectiveness make them attractive in this population. With the development of spacer devices, MDI use has even been possible with toddlers, who generally do not have the coordination required for the breathing and squeezing sequences[4] (see Ch. 71).

CHEST PHYSIOTHERAPY

The goals of chest physiotherapy (CPT) in pediatric patients are similar to those in adults. Pediatric patients who benefit most from CPT are those at risk for retained secretions, atelectasis, and pneumonia, as well as postoperative thoracoabdominal surgery patients, and comatose patients with neuromuscular or pre-existing chronic lung disease (bronchopulmonary dysplasia or cystic fibrosis).

Possible complications from percussion, vibration, and postural drainage in pediatric patients include

1. Increased intracranial pressure with certain postural drainage positions
2. Transient PaO_2 decreases and dyspnea
3. Rib fractures in small infants or patients predisposed to skeletal disease
4 Infection of the contralateral lung[5]

There are special considerations in the pediatric patient that need to be noted. The endotracheal tube is not as stable as in the adult. When repositioning the ventilator patient, one should remove the patient from the circuit, turn the patient quickly, and then reattach the ventilator. Emptying the water from the ventilator circuits prior to positioning is essential to avoid accidental lavage. Treatments should be carried out before eating or at least 1 to 2 hours after eating; oral or nasogastric feeding systems must be turned off at least 30 minutes prior to treatment. A child who appears upset should be held during treatment. Children with status asthmaticus or acute congestive heart failure may be adversely affected by the Trendelenberg position.[6]

There is some controversy over using percussion as a prophylactic treatment in the care of postoperative cardiac patients.[7] These patients, at minimum, should be treated by position changes, mobility, and deep breathing and coughing exercises. Percussion should be performed on patients with excessive secretions or mucus plugging and those at risk for pulmonary complications. Percussion may be performed with cupped hands, or with commercially available devices, or cups created from resuscitation masks, bulb syringes, and other such items. Percussion should not be performed below the posterior or anterior ribs. Use of a towel or light blanket to cover a patient who is not gowned is recommended. Identifying the border of the ribs before starting therapy is also helpful. Vibrators are available and are sometimes better tolerated by smaller infants than the therapist's hand. In our experience, postoperative cardiac patients also may tolerate mechanical vibrators better than manual methods. Postural drainage along with percussion may be carried out with the smaller patient in the therapist's lap to reduce anxiety and increase comfort (Fig. 88-3). See Chapter 70 for details on chest physiotherapy.

THE PEDIATRIC AIRWAY

The airway of a child is different from that of an adult. It is more flexible, and the tongue can occlude the airway easily because of its large size in proportion to the oral cavity. The infant's epiglottis is short and narrow and angles away from the trachea. It is more difficult to pass an endotracheal tube through a pediatric patient's airway because the narrowest area of the airway is the cricoid cartilage, below the glottic opening,[8] whereas the narrowest portion of the adult airway is the glottic opening (Table 88-1).

Intubation

In children up to the age of 5, the airway is most easily visualized with a straight blade (e.g., the Miller blade).[9] The blade should be long enough to reach the epiglottis to enable lifting and visualization of the vocal cords. To ensure that the length of the blade is adequate, the blade should be placed next to the child's face; it should reach from the mouth to the larynx.[10] An infant should be placed with the head in the neutral position while an older child should be placed in the sniffing position during intubation.[5] Hyperextension of the neck, particularly in infants, must be avoided during intubation in order to prevent obstruction of the airway.

Pediatric patients may be orally or nasally intubated. Orotracheal tubes are chosen for short-term intubation because a larger tube, which is easier to suction and less resistant to gas flow, can be used. The oral route also provides easier access than the nose. On the other hand, to ensure tube stabilization and to decrease the chance of accidental extubation, the nasal tube is the best choice. The nasal tube enhances communication and sucking and appears to provide greater patient comfort.[9]

Tube selection is of utmost importance. The most common error in pediatric intubation is to use a tube that is too small.[9] According to Poiseuille's law, resistance to airflow varies

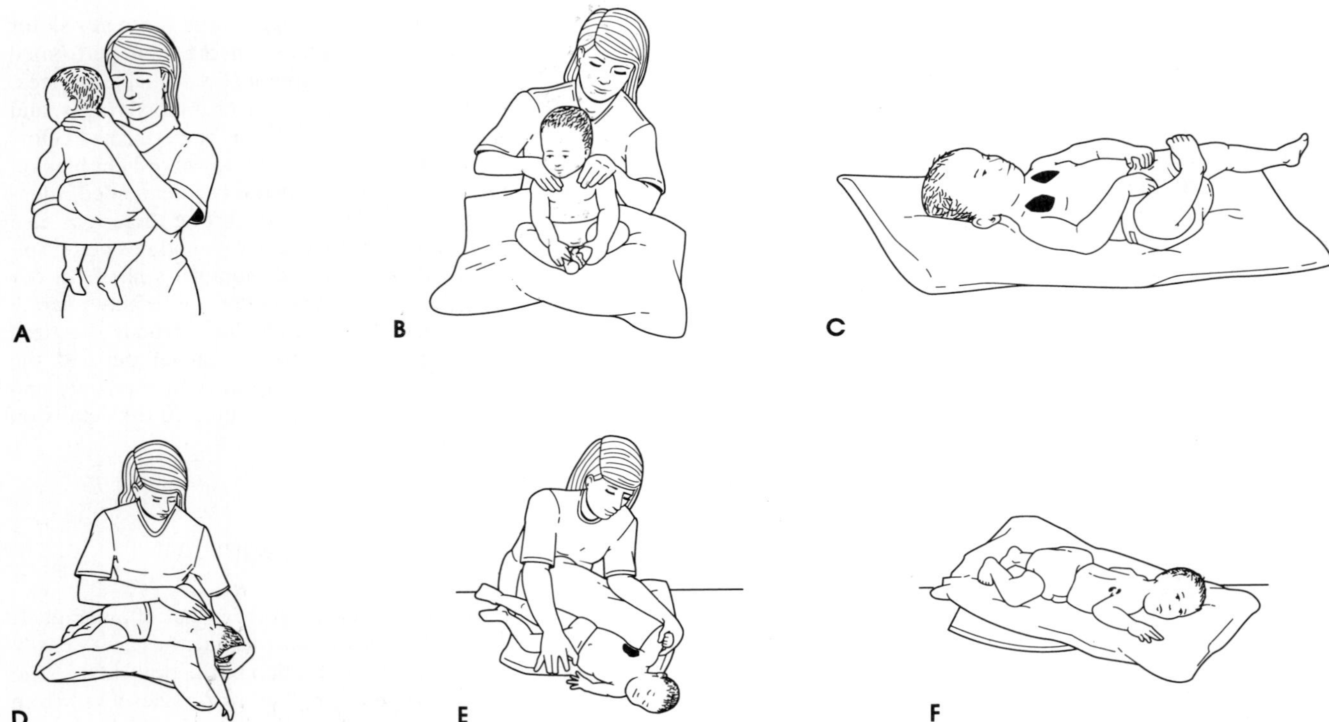

Figure 88-3. Postural drainage and percussion positions for infant and child. **(A)** Posterior segments of right and left upper lobes are drained with patient in upright position at 30-degree angle forward. Percussion should be over upper posterior thorax. **(B)** Apical segments of right and left upper lobes are drained with patient in upright position, leaning forward 30 degrees. Percussion should be over area between clavicle and top of scapula on each side. **(C)** Anterior segments of right and left upper lobes are drained with patient in flat, supine position. Percussion should be over anterior side of chest directly under clavicles to around nipple area (shaded). Avoid direct pressure on sternum. **(D)** Right and left lateral basal segments of lower lobes are drained at 30 degrees Trendelenburg position. Patient lies on appropriate side, rotated 30 degrees forward. Percussion should be over uppermost portions of lower ribs. **(E)** Right and left anterior basal segments of lower lobes are drained at 30 degrees Trendelenburg position. Patient lies on appropriate side with 30-degree turn backwards. Percussion should be above anterior lower margin of ribs. **(F)** Right and left superior segments of lower lobes are drained at 15 degrees Trendelenburg position, with patient in prone position. Percussion should be below scapula in midback area. (From Badgett and Casselberry,[14] with permission.)

inversely with the fourth power of the tube radius. Therefore, choosing the largest tube possible minimizes the effect of tube resistance. A tube that is too small makes suctioning difficult and does not provide a tight enough fit to protect against aspiration and air leaks. It must be noted, however, that some risk is involved in choosing too large a tube since perfusion to the wall of the airway may be decreased by tube pressure, causing necrosis or stenosis of the airway.

Table 88-1. Pediatric versus Adult Airway

	Infant	Adult
Larynx	C3–C4	C4–C5
Epiglottis	Short, narrow	Flat
Trachea	Narrowest at cricoid ring	Narrowest at rima glottidis
Cords	Slant anteriorly	Straight

(Adapted from Mastropietro,[8] with permission.)

The ideal endotracheal tube size varies with the age and size of the child. Since the narrowest portion of the child's airway is the cricoid cartilage below the vocal cords, endotracheal tubes with inflatable cuffs are not used with young children. However, a child above the age of 8 may need a cuffed tube. Sometimes all that is needed is the presence of the cuff, with the cuff left deflated. Cuffed tubes are about 0.5 mm larger in external diameter than uncuffed tubes.[9]

The use of a pediatric intubation tray enhances the efficiency of intubation. This tray should include a chart with the approximate relationship between endotracheal tube size and child's age (see Ch. 42). One can estimate the appropriate tube size for a child by using the tube that most closely approximates the diameter of the child's little finger.[11] In addition, two formulas are available to estimate tube size:

$$\text{Age} + 16 \div 4 = \text{tube ID}$$

or

$$\text{Height (cm)} \div 20 = \text{tube ID}$$

Appropriate tube placement above the carina can be estimated by multiplying the ID by 3. For example, 4 (ID) $\times$ 3 equals 12 cm.

Securing Endotracheal Tubes

Taping endotracheal tubes is a precarious procedure in the pediatric patient. Slight movement may pull the tube out or push it in too far. Before proceeding to tape or retape an endotracheal tube, the clinician should listen to breath sounds and note the marking on the tube at the gum line or nares.

Taping the pediatric patient's tube is a two-person procedure, requiring one person to hold the tube in place and restrain the patient from movement and the other person to perform the actual taping (Fig. 88-4). If an oral tube is used, the tube should be moved frequently from one side of the mouth to the other side to minimize damage to developing dentition.[12] After the first layer of tape is applied, chest auscultation should be performed to ensure equal breath sounds and proper tube placement. Tube placement should be checked periodically to ensure proper positioning. Excessive secretions may loosen the adhesive and allow the tube to move.

Extubation

Postextubation stridor, caused by edema or stenosis, is a more common complication in the pediatric than in the adult setting. A nebulizer should be ready for use with 0.25 to 0.5 mL racemic epinephrine (Vanponefrin) and 3.5 mL normal saline if stridor is present. If the patient has had either numerous intubations or a traumatic intubation and airway swelling is therefore suspected, systemic steroids should be administered 24 hours prior to extubation.

Preparation for extubation is the first step in removing an endotracheal tube. The intubation tray should be at the bedside, along with a resuscitation bag and suction equipment. The steps for removing the tube are similar to those in an adult extubation. The airway and the oropharynx should be suctioned to prevent aspiration of the oral contents. Hyperinflation and hyperoxygenation should be provided and the endotracheal tube removed during inspiration while positive pressure is applied with a manual ventilator. Immediately following extubation, the neck should be auscultated for stridor. The patient should then be placed in a hood, or cool mist should be provided by mask with an F_{IO_2} about 0.10 higher than that of the mixture administered via the

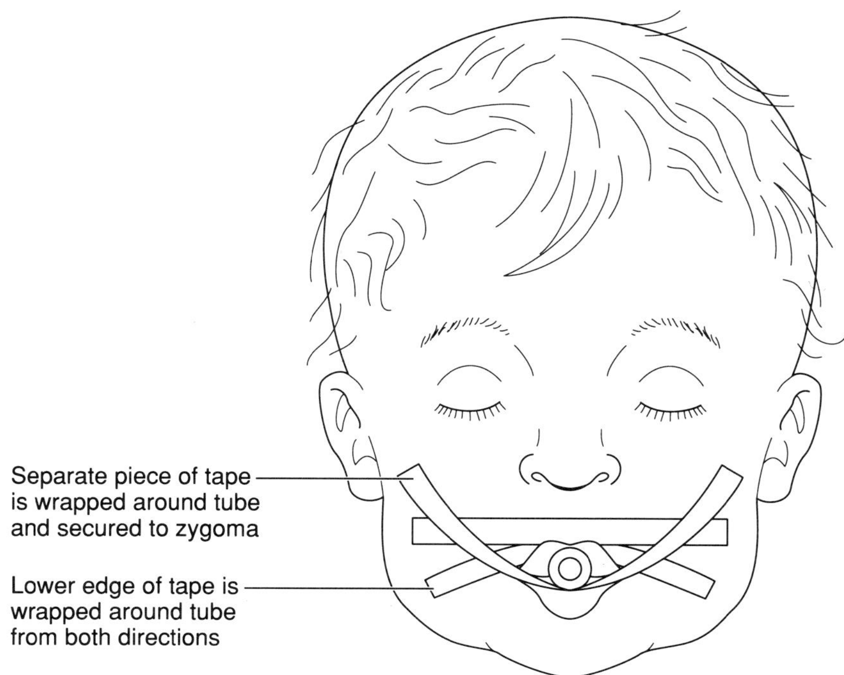
Separate piece of tape is wrapped around tube and secured to zygoma
Lower edge of tape is wrapped around tube from both directions

Figure 88-4. Endotracheal tube taping method described by Brown,[13] which uses benzoin on child's face, elastic tape cut into an H configuration, and pink Hy-tape (Hy-tape Surgical Products Corp., New York) wrapped once around elastic tape and tube.

endotracheal tube. Arterial blood gas levels and/or pulse oximetry should be used to monitor postextubation O_2 status, and the patient should be frequently assessed clinically for respiratory distress.

Accidental extubations may occur in the pediatric setting during suctioning, turning the patient, or retaping the tube.[13] If the patient displays signs of increased respiratory distress, decreased O_2 saturations that do not respond to bagging with an increased F_{IO_2} mixture, crying around the tube, or decreased tidal volumes during mechanical ventilation, an accidental extubation may have occurred. The clinician should listen for breath sounds and, if these are questionable, remove the endotracheal tube, bag/mask, ventilate, and reintubate.

Suctioning

Normally it is recommended that the outer diameter of the suction catheter be no more than half the inner diameter of the endotracheal tube. In our experience it is difficult to suction thick secretions with small suction catheters. We believe it is more efficient to use a larger catheter but one that easily passes through the endotracheal tube.[14] Frequent suctioning is required with small endotracheal tubes to ensure patency; we routinely suction our pediatric patients approximately every 2 hours. Close monitoring during suctioning is required, as these patients are susceptible to hypoxia and bradycardia during the suctioning process (see Ch. 72).

Suctioning the pediatric patient requires the same techniques used with adults; however, the suction pressure is usually set at 80 to 100 mmHg (60 to 80 mmHg for neonates). Hyperoxygenation via manual ventilation should be provided before suctioning. If secretions are difficult to mobilize, the patient may be lavaged with normal saline: in the infant and small child a few drops of saline will suffice, and in the older patient 1 to 3 mL may be used. The actual suctioning procedure is to insert the catheter until an obstruction is felt and then to withdraw the catheter 0.5 cm and start suctioning while rotating and removing the catheter. Total suction time should not exceed 10 seconds. In infants we recommend turning the head during suctioning to allow the catheter to enter the right or left bronchus. Turning the head to the left allows the catheter to enter the right main stem bronchus, and turning it to the right may allow the left main stem to be suctioned.

The clinician should monitor the patient's heart rate, blood pressure, and O_2 saturation for signs of respiratory distress during suctioning. With the pediatric patient who is receiving mechanical ventilation, routine suctioning is preferred to suctioning on an as-required basis to ensure a patent airway. Given the small inner diameter of pediatric endotracheal tubes, occlusion or partial obstruction by secretions may easily occur. Risks and complications of endotracheal suction include bronchial stenosis, formation of granulation tissue, mucosal damage, and hypoxia, leading to bradycardia, dysrhythmias, or hypotension.

Tracheostomy

Pediatric tracheostomy management requires special care and expertise since younger patients have a greater complication rate and a higher mortality rate than adults.[15] Tracheotomies are performed to relieve upper airway obstructions, to facilitate secretion removal, to ensure airway protection, and to allow prolonged mechanical ventilation or because of severe laryngotracheobronchitis.[16] A tracheostomy tube allows more movement by the patient and easier application of varied techniques of ventilatory support and weaning. Some authors believe that tracheotomies may allow the patient an earlier discharge from the intensive care unit (ICU), as well as shortening their hospitalization.[17]

The infant and smaller pediatric tracheostomy tubes are not cuffed. The neonatal tube is shorter than the pediatric tube although it may have the same diameter. In our experience some pediatric patients require tube lengths to be specially cut. This may be done by checking the chest film and measuring where the tip of the tube lies relative to its desired location above the carina.

To ensure proper tracheostomy tube placement, a chest radiograph should be obtained immediately post-tracheotomy. The radiograph can also rule out pneumothorax or subcutaneous emphysema. Other problems that arise early with children less than 5 years of age include bleeding, airway obstruction, dysplasia, tracheoesophageal fistula, accidental decannulation, and apnea.[18] The use of adequate humidification cannot be overemphasized to prevent plugging. Obstruction of the tracheostomy tube may be due to secretions or the distal end of the tube having become lodged against the posterior wall of the trachea (which is noted by an expiratory wheeze).[18]

Decannulation must take place under close observation, preferably in the pediatric ICU setting. Prior to decannulation, bronchoscopy should be performed to rule out subglottic stenosis and to verify adequate vocal cord mobility.[19] Children may develop respiratory distress even after they have been assessed as having an adequate airway. This distress may be a result of increased airway resistance, tracheal collapse (due to weakening of the cartilage in the region of the tracheostomy), or reduced laryngeal abductor activity.[20]

Decannulation can begin once the conditions for which the tracheostomy was performed have been resolved. The first step in the decannulation process involves gradually substituting tubes of smaller and smaller diameter. There are several reasons for gradually reducing the size of the tube before its actual removal: reduced anxiety, improved tolerance, and gradual return of reflex laryngeal abductor activity.[20] Gradual weaning involves replacing the tracheostomy tube with one of the next smaller diameter every 24 hours. The tube is not plugged because the child's airway is so small that even the smallest tubes may obstruct the airway. Once the smallest size tube has been tolerated successfully, that tube is removed and the stoma is covered with sterile gauze.

If the patient has had a bronchoscopy that indicates a healthy airway and a noticeable leak is present around the tracheostomy tube, the tube can often be removed without the previously mentioned steps. (The patient's airway may have increased in diameter with normal growth and development and the tracheostomy tube may have become "smaller" relative to this growth.) The patient should be NPO before removing the tracheostomy tube, and extra tubes should be at the bedside. Following decannulation, the patient should be monitored for signs of distress such as decreased O_2 saturation, increased work of breathing, and stridor due to airway obstruction. We recommend aggressive pulmonary hygiene postdecannulation.

RESUSCITATION BAGS

The most common cause of cardiac arrest in pediatric patients is respiratory in origin; therefore, efficient use of a resuscitation bag is essential to pediatric care. Two types of bags are available for use in the pediatric setting: self-inflating, which are similar to those used in adult resuscitation, and anesthesia bags, which are flow-inflating (Fig. 88-5).

Self-inflating resuscitator bags are more easily operated by the clinician in the emergency situation than are the flow-inflating bags.[21] These bags have some restrictions, including variations in F_IO_2 from 0.5 to 0.9, even when reservoirs are attached. In fact, studies have shown that F_IO_2 decreases when the 40 cmH_2O relief value is activated. The F_IO_2 can be increased by occluding the pressure relief valve or by increasing the flow to the bag.[22] We do not recommend using self-inflating bags when 100 percent O_2 is required. The pop-off valve is normally set at 30 to 40 cmH_2O, and one must exclude the relief valve to receive the higher pressures that may be required during resuscitation or with a noncompliant lung.[21] Barotrauma resulting from the generation of high airway pressures is a concern. To closely monitor the pressures being delivered, a pressure manometer may be placed in line with self-inflating bags.

Flow-inflating bags when used properly have advantages over self-inflating bags.[21] The relief valve on these bags allows the clinician to adjust both positive end-expiratory pressure (PEEP) and peak airway pressures. The practitioner is able to monitor the pressures delivered with the use of an in-line manometer. F_IO_2 is set at 100 percent, or an O_2 blender may be used to obtain other appropriate O_2 concentrations. When using a mask with the flow-inflating bag, the clinician is assured of a tight seal when the bag inflates at flow rates of 8 to 10 L/min.[23] Care should be taken to check PEEP and peak airway pressures before using flow-inflating bags which are best used by clinicians experienced in this operation.

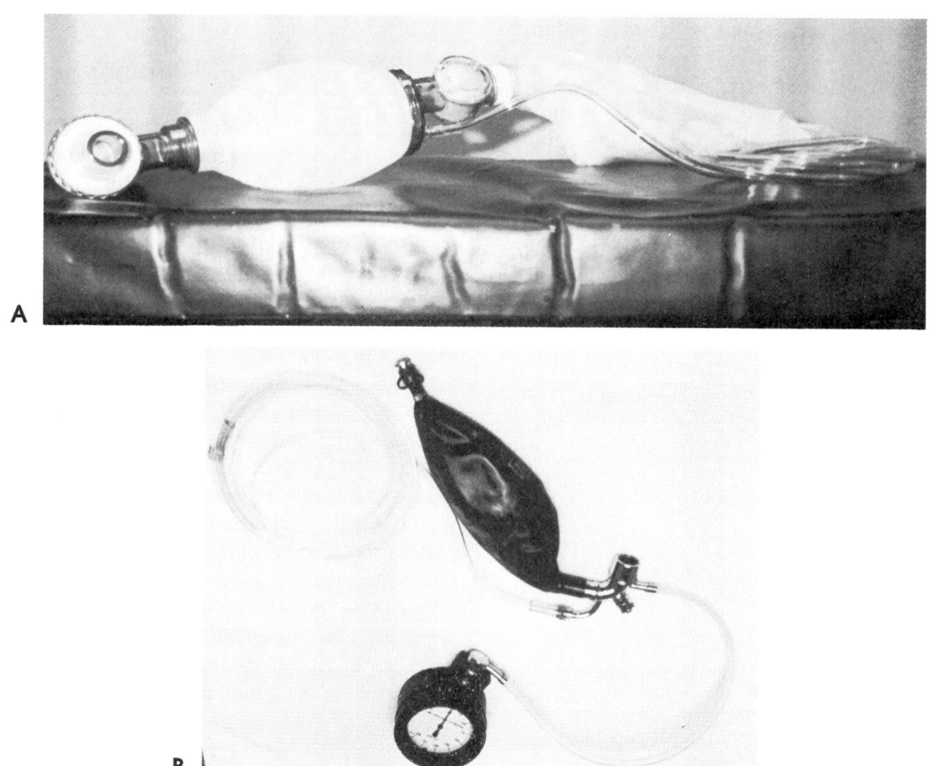

Figure 88-5. Resuscitator bags used in pediatrics. **(A)** Laerdal self-inflating bag with reservoir. **(B)** Anesthesia Associates flow-inflating bag with pressure manometer.

POSITIVE-PRESSURE VENTILATION

Pediatric patients are frequently placed on mechanical ventilators that differ considerably from those used for adults. Pressure-limited, time-cycled ventilators are normally used in infants weighing less than 15 kg, patients without frequent changes in compliance or resistance, and infants at risk for barotrauma. Volume-cycled ventilators are best used for patients with severe pulmonary disease or with rapidly changing compliance or resistance, postoperative cardiac patients, or patients heavier than 15 kg (Table 88-2).

Compressible Volume

Tubing compliance in adult ventilatory support presents minimal problems, whereas in the pediatric patient the volume lost in compressible tubing may be a considerable portion of the tidal volume. It is possible to calculate the compressible volume in all volume-cycled ventilator circuits. Variables in determining the compressible volume factor include the tubing size, ventilator, and type of humidifier used.[5] To calculate an approximation of the compressible volume factor, a tidal volume of 200 mL, a flow rate of 40 L/min, a rate of 5 breaths per minute, and a maximum pressure limit should be set. The patient's Y-piece should be occluded, and after the ventilator cycles, the peak pressure reached should be noted and the exhaled volume measured. The compressible volume factor is equal to the tidal volume divided by the peak pressure (e.g., a tidal volume of 200 mL divided by a peak pressure of 80 cmH_2O equals a compressible volume factor of 2.5 mL/cmH_2O). This factor is multiplied by the peak pressures generated by the patient, minus PEEP, and the result is subtracted from the tidal volume returned during normal ventilation in order to estimate the actual delivered tidal volume (e.g., a peak pressure 35 cmH_2O less 5 cmH_2O PEEP multiplied by 2.5 mL/cmH_2O, equals 75 mL, which is the volume lost in the tubing; subtraction of this volume from the returned tidal volume of 200 mL gives the patient's actual tidal volume of 125 mL).[24] The compressible volume may be decreased by using smaller-diameter circuits with rigid walls, limiting the length of the inspiratory side of the circuit, placing the exhalation valve near the airway opening, using smaller-volume humidifiers, and maintaining fluid levels in humidifiers.[5]

Table 88-2. Pediatric Ventilator Selection

Pressure-limited, time-cycled
Neonatal population
Infants weighing 15 kg
Infrequent changes in compliance and resistance
Barotrauma concerns
Inspiratory flow requirements versus ventilator capability
Volume-cycled
Pediatric population
Infants weighing >15 kg
Changing compliance and resistance
Inspiratory flow requirements

When setting up a pressure-limited, time-cycled ventilator, one should select the smallest amount of pressure necessary to visualize good bilateral chest expansion. If the patient initially receives manual ventilation with a pressure manometer in line, the same ventilator pressures needed during manual ventilation should be set. The inspiratory time should be set according to the patient's respiratory rate to achieve an inspiration/expiration ratio of approximately 1:2. PEEP is set at 3 to 5 cmH_2O to elevate the resting lung volume, and F_{IO_2} is set at 0.8 to 1.0. An F_{IO_2} of 0.8 is preferred because it reduces the possibility of atelectasis after denitrogenation in areas of the lung with low ventilation.[25] The parameters are then adjusted on the basis of arterial blood gas and noninvasive monitoring data.

With a volume-cycled ventilator, the tidal volume is calculated by multiplying the patient's weight in kilograms by a factor of 12 to 15 and adding the tubing compliance volume to the result (e.g., a weight of 6 kg × 12 equals 72 mL, which yields a tidal volume of 132 mL after adding a tubing compressible volume of 60 mL [calculated from the tubing compressible volume factor and the estimated peak airway pressures]). Chest excursion, breath sounds, and arterial blood gas levels need to be assessed, and the volume may need to be adjusted accordingly. The remainder of the ventilator parameters are set at the same values as during pressure ventilation.

Weaning

Intermittent mandatory ventilation (IMV) "has emerged as the standard technique for weaning infants and children."[5] Once a child's underlying reason for mechanical ventilation has been stabilized or reversed, weaning should be considered. The infant and young child are usually weaned to an IMV rate of 4 breaths per minute in increments of 2 to 4 breaths per minute and the PEEP is decreased to 3 to 4 cmH_2O and the F_{IO_2} to 0.4 on the basis of arterial blood gas levels and clinical signs. A patient who has an active cough with arterial blood gas parameters within normal limits and clinical signs stable may be ready for extubation. Older children may be placed on a continuous positive airway pressure (CPAP) trial and their spontaneous parameters (similar to those used with adult patients, including vital capacity and maximum inspiratory pressure) evaluated; extubation is then performed if the assessed parameters are adequate. Rarely is an infant or young child placed on a CPAP trial in view of the increased airway resistance associated with small endotracheal tubes.[26] Specific criteria predictive of successful extubation in infants are lacking. One study has demonstrated a positive correlation with a crying vital capacity greater than 15 mL/kg and a maximum inspiratory pressure greater than 45 cmH_2O.[27]

The use of pressure support as a weaning technique is growing in popularity. It appears to be most useful in pediatric patients who have failed to wean by conventional methods.[28] Typically, these patients may have required extended periods of mechanical ventilation and/or have had depressed respiratory muscle function (see Chs. 82 and 83).

Intermittent Mandatory Ventilation Systems

Volume-cycled ventilators may be adapted with external continuous-flow IMV systems. These systems have been added to ventilators used in the ICU setting to decrease the work of breathing imposed on the infant,[29] which is otherwise increased in small infants by the ventilator demand valves. These IMV bags provide an easy and readily available alternative. Additionally, supplemental IMV systems may be used with home mechanical ventilators (Fig. 88-6).

There are several points one should remember when using a supplemental IMV system: (1) the F_{IO_2} supplying the IMV system should match that provided by the ventilator; (2) the sensitivity setting on the ventilator should be adjusted so that the patient inspires from the external IMV system, not the ventilator; (3) the IMV bag must receive sufficient flow to meet the demand of the patient; (4) the IMV supplemental flow should be turned off when measuring tidal volumes delivered from the ventilator; and (5) the ventilator alarm settings may need to be reset (or a separate disconnect alarm added), in view of the additional flow.

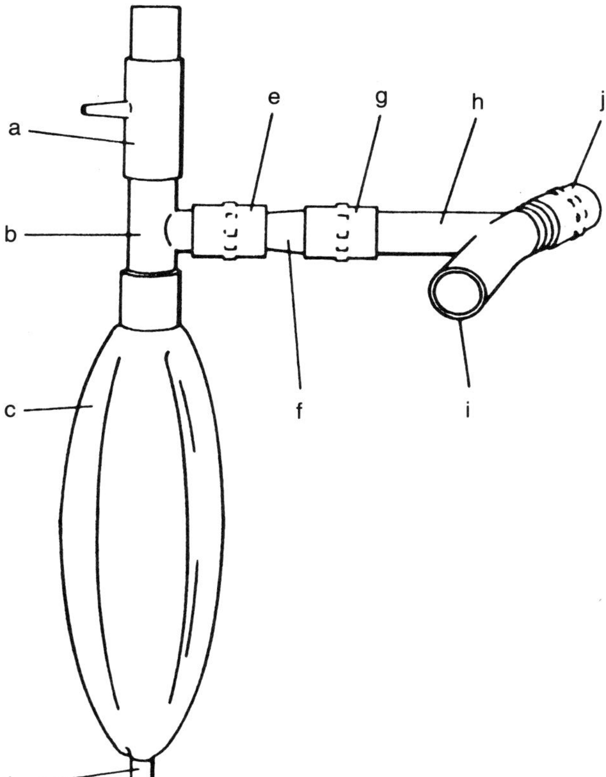

Figure 88-6. Supplemental IMV attachment used with pediatric critical care or home care ventilators: **(A)** Hudson one-way valve with bleed-in port for blended gas; **(B)** Hudson #1077 T-adapter; **(C)** Anesthesia Associates nondisposable anesthesia bag; **(D)** Anesthesia Associates bag tail pop-off; **(E)** Intec 22-mm cuff connector #172222; **(F)** Inspiron #1671 one-way adapter; **(G)** Intec 22-mm cuff connector; **(H)** Hudson #1630 Y connector; **(I)** inlet for gas coming from ventilator; **(J)** Intec 22-mm cuff connector for connection to humidifier.

Monitoring

Monitoring the pediatric mechanical ventilator-dependent patient involves routine ventilator checks, airway assessment, and assessment of oxygenation, ventilation, and acid-base balance.

Ventilator checks vary depending on the type of ventilator being used. Figure 88-7 shows a respiratory care flow sheet, which has separate sections for "volume" and "pressure" ventilators. Regardless of ventilator type, ongoing attention must be paid to F_{IO_2}, the volume and/or pressure being delivered, and the patient's spontaneous respiratory rate, as well as to the machine rate. As with all ventilators, alarms must also be frequently checked. The temperature of the gas and the efficient delivery of humidity is also essential, given the ease with which thick secretions can obstruct the small airway.

Airway assessment should routinely include tube position relative to a fixed point (e.g., gum line, teeth), tube stability, type of secretions present, and the position of the tube determined radiographically. Any question regarding tube stability or position should be immediately addressed, as accidental extubations can be life-threatening to the pediatric patient.

Arterial blood gas determinations remain the "gold standard" for assessment of oxygenation, ventilation, and acid-base balance in the pediatric ventilator patient. Arterial lines are generally placed if frequent arterial blood gas values are needed, since arterial punctures are difficult procedures in pediatric patients. Occasionally, capillary blood gases may be used for management. Capillary blood provides useful information regarding PCO_2 and pH but is of little value in assessing PO_2.

Transcutaneous PO_2 and PCO_2 measurements are frequently used for trending in the newborn period and may also be used with infants and pediatric patients. The American Academy of Pediatrics has issued a consensus statement on the use of transcutaneous monitors.[30] Caution is advised in using such monitors as predictors of actual PaO_2 as they may underestimate high PaO_2 values (above 100 mmHg).

Pulse oximetry is commonly used for both ventilator-supported and spontaneously breathing pediatric patients. While it can be most helpful as a trending tool, care must be exercised to avoid relying on it to the exclusion of arterial blood gas measurements.

Intensive respiratory care of children can be an extremely challenging and rewarding aspect of health care. Clinicians must constantly balance the care they are providing with its

UNIVERSITY HOSPITAL
Respiratory Care
NICU Ventilator Flowsheet

Circuit Changed	
Date	Initials

Please include in comment section:
—Suction info
—Treatments
—Patient Position
—Pt alertness and cooperation
—NIF, Spirometry

ET TUBE OR TRACH SIZE	POSITION

Pt. Wgt ________ ICU Day # ________

		VOLUME VENTILATOR TYPE ________						ALARM SETTINGS			PRESSURE VENTILATOR TYPE ________					ABGs				ALARMS
DATE / TIME	MODE / WAVE	ACT $\dot{V}$ / $\dot{V}$ SET	Vt exh / Vt set	ACT f / SET f	PRES SUP / Pause	Peak / Static	Static C / PEEP CPAP	IX / MAP	FIO2 / TEMP	Flow Rate	PEAK PRES / PEEP CPAP	ACT f / SET f	I time / I:E	MAP / Pop Off	TcPO2 / TcCO2	TIME / SITE	pH / pCO2	PO2 / HCO3	O2 Sat / ETCO2	
Therapist																				
Therapist																				
Therapist																				
Therapist																				
Therapist																				
Therapist																				

Figure 88-7. Neonatal ICU ventilator flow sheet. (Courtesy of Respiratory Care Department, University Hospital, Denver, CO.)

effect on the child's long-term welfare. Little margin for error is possible with these patients.

References

1. McPherson SP: Respiratory Therapy Equipment. 2nd Ed. CV Mosby, St. Louis, 1981
2. Post DJ, Lambert GH: Inhaled bronchodilator use in infants: A national survey. Respir Care 1989;34:1024–1032
3. Koff PB: Pharmacology. pp. 212–224. In Koff PB, Eitzman DV, Neu J (eds): Neonatal and Pediatric Respiratory Care. CV Mosby, St. Louis, 1988
4. Levison H, Reilly PA, Worsly GH: Spacing devices and metered dose inhalers in childhood asthma. J Pediatr 1985;107:662–670
5. Gioia FR, Stephenson RL, Alterwitz SA: Principles of respiratory support and mechanical ventilation. pp. 113–169. In Rogers MA (ed): Textbook of Pediatric Intensive Care. Vol. 1. Williams & Wilkins, Baltimore, 1987
6. Lough MD, Williams TJ, Rawson JE: Pediatric Respiratory Therapy. 3rd Ed. Year Book Medical Publishers, Chicago, 1985
7. Reines D, Sade RM, Bradford BF, Marshall J: Chest physiotherapy fails to prevent postoperative atelectasis in children after cardiac surgery. Ann Surg 1982;195:451–458
8. Mastropietro C: The potentially difficult airway. J Am Assoc Nurse Anesth 1988;56:25–32
9. Rosen P, Barkin R: Respiratory distress in the child. J Emerg Med 1985;3:157–164
10. McClarty RS: Pediatric Advanced Life Support. Children's Orthopedic Hospital, Seattle, 1985
11. Hochbaum SR: Emergency airway management. Emerg Med Clin North Am 1986;4:411–418
12. Loochtan AM, Loochtan RM: Damage to neonatal oral structures: Effects of laryngoscopy and intubation. Respir Care 1989;34:879–886
13. Brown MS: Prevention of accidental extubation in newborns. Am J Dis Child 1988;142:1240–1247
14. Badgett D, Casselberry C: Chest Physiotherapy. pp. 557–561. In Levin DL, Morriss FC, Moore G (eds): A Practical Guide to Pediatric Intensive Care. 2nd Ed. CV Mosby, St. Louis, 1984
15. Newlands WJ, McKerrow JS: Paediatric tracheostomy: Fifty-seven operations on fifty-three children. J Laryngol Otol 1987;101:929–935
16. Swift AC, Rogers JH: The changing indications for tracheostomy in children. J Laryngol Otol 1987;101:1258–1264
17. Stock MC, Woodward CG, Shapiro BA et al: Perioperative complications of elective tracheostomy in critically ill patients. Crit Care Med 1986;14:110–117
18. Kirchner JA: Avoiding problems in tracheostomy. Laryngoscope 1986;96:55–62
19. Myer C, Willis R, Miller R, Cotton RT: Tracheostomy decannulation in the pediatric patient. Laryngoscope 1987;97:764–769
20. Black RJ, Baldwin DL, Johns AN: Tracheostomy decannulation panic in children: Fact or Fiction? J Laryngo Otol 1984;98:297–304
21. Kanter RK: Evaluation of mask-bag ventilation in resuscitation of infants. Am J Dis Child 1987;141:761–769
22. Hirschman A, Kravath RE: Venting versus ventilating. Chest 1982;3:369–374
23. Finer NN, Barrington KJ, Al-Fadley F, Peters KL: Limitation of self-inflating resuscitators. Pediatrics 1986;77:417–425
24. Demers RR, Pratter MR, Irwin RS: Use of the concept of ventilator compliance in the determination of static total compliance. Respir Care 1981;26:644–652
25. Kanter RK: Initial mechanical ventilator settings for pediatric patients. Am J Emerg Med 1987;5:113–118
26. Wall MA: Infant endotracheal tube resistance: Effects of changing length, diameter, and gas density. Crit Care Med 1980;8:38–46
27. Shimada Y, Yoshiya I, Tanaka K et al: Crying vital capacity and maximal inspiratory pressure as clinical indicators of readiness for weaning of infants less than a year of age. Anesthesiology 1979;51:456–462
28. Betit P, Thompson JE: Mechanical ventilation. pp. 282–295. In Koff PB, Eitzman DV, Neu J: Neonatal and Pediatric Respiratory Care. CV Mosby, St Louis, 1988
29. Bingham RM, Hatch DJ, Helms PJ: Assisted ventilation and the servo ventilator in infants. Anaesthesia 1986;41:168–174
30. Task Force on Transcutaneous Oxygen Monitors: Report of consensus meeting, Dec. 5–6, 1986. Pediatrics 1989;83:122–133

Chapter 89

Perioperative Respiratory Care

Richard D. Branson

CHAPTER OUTLINE

Perioperative respiratory care encompasses treatment and/or patient education prior to, during, and after completion of a surgical procedure. As previous chapters have described the usefulness of perioperative evaluation and the untoward effects of surgery on respiratory function, these topics are not considered here. Instead, this chapter describes methods available to prevent and treat postoperative pulmonary complications through intervention during the preoperative, intraoperative, and postoperative periods.

PREOPERATIVE CONSIDERATIONS

Preoperative interventions rely heavily on the prediction of patients at risk for developing complications in the postoperative period. High-risk patients include the elderly, the obese, those with a smoking history, those with poor nutritional status, and those with pre-existing chronic pulmonary disease (COPD).[1] Additionally, patients without preoperative risk may incur high risk owing to intraoperative complications or risk factors, including unrecognized esophageal intubation, aspiration of gastric contents, prolonged operative procedures, and upper abdominal and thoracic incisions. Potential preoperative therapies for each group are discussed below.

Patients with pre-existing respiratory impairment represent the group most likely to receive and benefit from preoperative therapy. Tisi[2,3] and others[4,5] have found the incidence of postoperative pulmonary complications in patients with abnormal preoperative spirometry and/or arterial blood gases to be 40 to 60 percent, as compared with 0 to 10 percent in normal patients. Preoperative interventions in this group include education, secretion mobilization, hydration, bronchodilator therapy, smoking cessation, O_2 therapy, nutritional supplementation, and administration of miscellaneous medications.

Patient Education

Perhaps the most important preoperative intervention is education of the patient in the importance and proper use of planned postoperative therapy. Common sense dictates that a patient can learn the use of incentive spirometry (IS), intermittent positive-pressure breathing (IPPB), or any other therapy more effectively preoperatively than postoperatively, when sedation and pain limit understanding and compliance. Those patients with chronic sputum production may benefit from a variety of techniques designed to mobilize retained secretions, including deep breathing, coughing, IS, postural drainage, and chest percussion and vibration. When appropriately applied for several days preoperatively, postural drainage, coughing, and deep breathing appear to be effective in reducing postoperative complications.[6,7]

Fluid Resuscitation

Fluid resuscitation toward normovolemia improves hemodynamic stability intraoperatively and thus may reduce postoperative morbidity.[8] This may require placement of a pulmonary artery catheter preoperatively to guide fluid replacement therapy.

Nutrition

Malnutrition is a systemic disease with specific pulmonary effects, including blunting of ventilatory drive, decreased respiratory muscle mass and strength, and impaired pulmonary defense mechanisms.[9–11] The literature is replete with contradictory evidence concerning the effect of preoperative nutritional support on postoperative morbidity and mortality. There is some evidence that patients with protein energy malnutrition who receive 3 to 6 weeks of nutritional repletion have a reduced incidence of septic complications and a reduced hospital stay.[12] However, aside from intuition, which says a properly nourished patient will tolerate the stress of surgery better than a malnourished one, no clinical studies have been made in this area with respect to pulmonary complications. However if time permits, preoperative nutritional supplementation should be considered for the malnourished patient even though any benefit is speculative.[12–15]

Smoking Cessation

Cessation of cigarette smoking prior to surgery is also frequently recommended. Abstinence for even a short period (48 hours) results in improved ciliary function, eliminates the hemodynamic effects of nicotine, and reduces carboxyhemoglobin levels by as much as 15 percent.[16] Longer periods of abstinence provide further benefits—sputum production can be reduced in 2 weeks and respiratory function improved in 6 weeks.[16] Smoking cessation in and of itself will not reduce postoperative morbidity, but it is an important facet of a multifactorial treatment plan.

Oxygen Therapy

Preoperative O_2 therapy in patients with chronic hypoxemia (PaO_2 below 60 mmHg when breathing room air) may prove beneficial.[17] If time allows, several weeks of continuous home O_2 therapy can help reduce polycythemia, improve cardiovascular function by decreasing pulmonary hypertension, and enhance the patient's intellectual capabilities.[18] Like nutritional support, the benefits of O_2 therapy would seem intuitively obvious. However, no clinical trials have demonstrated reduced postoperative morbidity and mortality following preoperative O_2 therapy.

Pharmacologic Agents

Patients with pre-existing pulmonary disease frequently receive a myriad of pharmacologic agents aimed at reducing bronchospasm, enhancing secretion removal, improving cardiac function, and preventing infection. Prior to surgery strict adherence to the current medical regimen should be ensured. Preoperative optimization of theophylline levels is recommended, as both low and high levels are associated with complications.[19] In patients not currently receiving theophylline preparations, bronchodilation with beta-2-agonists is recommended because the combination of theophylline and surgically induced catecholamine discharge may result in ventricular ectopy. Preoperative drugs that may be beneficial in the patient with pulmonary disease are listed in Table 89-1. For a more comprehensive discussion of the use of these and other respiratory drugs, see Chapter 20.

Obesity

Pulmonary disorders are also common in obese patients because of an increase in the work of breathing, greater minute ventilation requirements to meet the metabolic needs of the increased body mass, and small airway closure resulting in ventilation/perfusion ($\dot{V}/\dot{Q}$) mismatching and hypoxemia.[20–25] Pulmonary compliance is reduced in obesity, which results in abnormally low vital capacity, total lung capacity, and functional residual capacity (FRC), with FRC in some instances falling below closing capacity during normal breathing. When this occurs, alveoli that continue to be perfused are not ventilated, and venous admixture increases. This problem is exacerbated by positioning (Fig. 89-1).

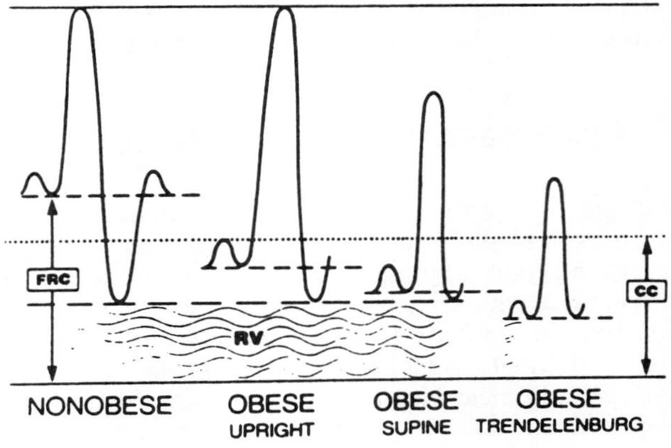

Figure 89-1. Effect of position change on lung volume in obese subjects. Further decline in FRC worsens the relationship between FRC and closing capacity. (From Vaughan,[47] with permission.)

Table 89-1. Pharmacologic Agents for Bronchospasm

Drug	Acuity	Comments
Methylxanthines (e.g., aminophylline)	Chronic asthma and COPD Acute bronchospasm	Serum levels 10–20 μg/mL Levels may vary widely Adjunct to beta-2-agonists May cause tachycardia Interact with halothane to cause ventricular ectopy
Beta-2-agonists (e.g., albuterol)	Acute or chronic bronchospasm	Sole treatment in many cases Education necessary for proper inhalation technique Frequent doses needed to reach distal airways Potential for tachycardia
Anticholinergics (e.g., ipratropium)	Acute or chronic bronchospasm	Better for COPD than for asthma Slower onset than beta-2-agonists Preventive action Effective against reflex or irritant bronchospasm
Corticosteroids (e.g., prednisone)	Chronic or acute asthma or COPD	Anti-inflammatory Not bronchodilators; reduce hyperreactivity Multiple systemic side effects Take hours to work
Topical anesthetics (e.g., lidocaine)	Acute bronchospasm	May be given via endotracheal tube for reflex bronchoconstriction Serum levels 1.5–5 μg/mL

Preoperatively the obese patient should be instructed in the use of whatever method of lung inflation therapy will be used postoperatively. Avoiding premedications that cause respiratory depression is advisable. Weight loss prior to surgery may improve cardiovascular and pulmonary function but may require an inordinate amount of time to achieve.

INTRAOPERATIVE CONSIDERATIONS

Regardless of preoperative status, intraoperative management should include adequate control of the airway, prevention of gastric aspiration, selection of an appropriate anesthetic agent, and maintenance of adequate ventilation and oxygenation. Current standards dictate that capnography and pulse oximetry be used during all operations performed under general anesthesia. When combined, these monitoring techniques help to warn of esophageal intubation and of worsening gas exchange. In many cases placement of an arterial line for frequent blood gas monitoring and blood pressure measurement is warranted.[26]

Aspiration

Aspiration of gastric contents is a potentially life-threatening complication. Proper airway maintenance, including frequent checking of the endotracheal tube cuff, positive pressure ventilation, and preoperative management (antacids, keeping the patient NPO) are keys to prevention.

Anesthesia

Selection of the proper type of anesthesia and specific anesthetic agent can also reduce postoperative complications. While regional anesthesia is often believed to be more favorable than general anesthesia in patients with lung disease,

Table 89-2. Advantages and Disadvantages of General and Regional Anesthesia

	Advantages	Disadvantages
General anesthesia	Complete control of the airway Alleviates anxiety and apprehension Provides for a "cooperative" patient Allows for easy removal (suctioning) of secretions	Airway instrumentation, which may cause reflex bronchospasm Need for muscle relaxants Respiratory depression
Regional anesthesia	Instrumentation of the airway not required Muscle relaxants not required No respiratory depression	Airway is not controlled Sedation may be required Secretion removal is hampered Uncooperative patient may cause disaster

no clinical studies have borne this out. Table 89-2 lists the potential advantages and disadvantages of the two anesthetic techniques. No one anesthetic method is foolproof, and these advantages and disadvantages should be considered on an individual basis. Intraoperative position and length of the surgical procedure also affect postoperative pulmonary morbidity and mortality.

Obesity

The obese patient also represents a significant intraoperative challenge. Airway management is frequently complicated and complex. The combination of reduced lung compliance, excess soft tissue mass, and altered anatomy make the risk of aspiration of gastric contents extremely high in this population.[27] Rapid sequence induction or awake intubation are recommended for the morbidly obese. The intraoperative use of positive end-expiratory pressure (PEEP) to restore FRC and improve PaO_2 is controversial. Santesson[28] found that progressive increases in PEEP improved PaO_2 (Fig. 89-2) but at the expense of O_2 delivery (reduced cardiac output), and Salem et al.[29] demonstrated that intraoperative PEEP improved PaO_2 and that PEEP withdrawal resulted in worsening oxygenation. Current practice dictates that large tidal volumes and high inspired O_2 concentrations should be used during anesthesia for obese patients and that if PEEP is to be used, its effect on O_2 delivery should be considered. Wyner et al.[30] in 1981 recommended mechanical suspension of the abdominal panniculus as a method of improving intraoperative pulmonary status. This is accomplished by suspending the panniculus from the ceiling via special surgical clips and heavy rope. Wyner et al.[30] have shown that this method results in marked improvement in arterial oxygenation.

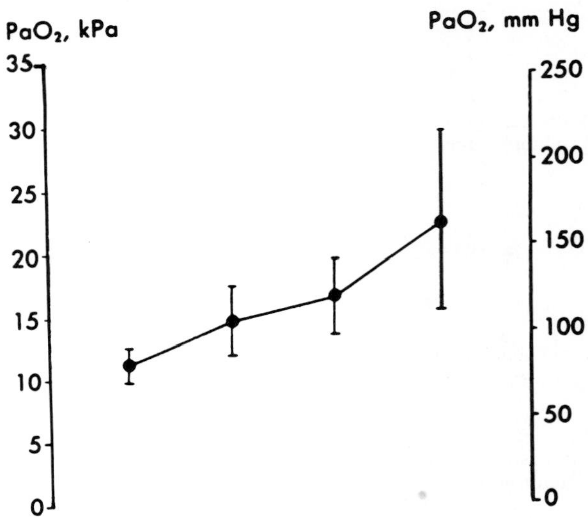

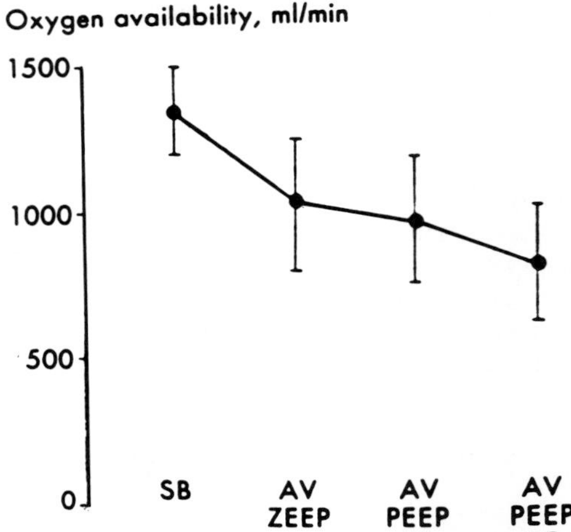

Figure 89-2. PaO_2 and O_2 availability during spontaneous breathing (SB) and artificial ventilation with zero end-expiratory pressure and with PEEP of 10 and 15 cmH_2O. (From Santesson,[28] with permission.)

POSTOPERATIVE TREATMENT

Following the operative procedure, the focus of care turns toward prevention of complications in most patients and treatment of complications in those already affected. Regardless of preoperative etiology, postoperative measures are aimed at restoring lung volume through passive or active lung inflation techniques.

Lung Inflation Techniques

The most frequently used lung inflation techniques include coughing and deep breathing (CDB), chest percussion and postural drainage (CPPD), IS, IPPB, and continuous positive airway pressure (CPAP).[31] Each technique uses a different method to achieve the goal of lung inflation, and each is based on sound physiologic principles. As stated earlier, use of these techniques is indicated in patients with preoperative risk, specifically those who have undergone upper abdominal or thoracic procedures. Use of any of these methods following lower abdominal procedures or extremity surgery is unnecessary and expensive.

Numerous studies have compared several or all of these techniques with one another, with or without use of an untreated control group. The most significant are considered here. In a study of 48 patients, Stein and Cassara[5] compared patients treated by CDB with untreated control subjects and found that the incidence of postoperative pulmonary complications (PPCs) was nearly three times as great in the untreated group (60 versus 22 percent). Craven et al.[32] compared the use of IS with no treatment in 70 patients following upper abdominal operations and demonstrated a significant decrease in the incidence of PPCs in the IS group (46 versus 71 percent). Celli and colleagues[33] compared patients given CDB, IS, or IPPB with untreated control patients and found that all three lung inflation techniques were better than no treatment and roughly equivalent to each other. Among the 81 patients studied, the control group had a PPC rate of 88 percent, the CDB group 33 percent, the IS group 30 percent, and the IPPB group 32 percent. The conclusion from this study was that some lung expansion technique is needed and its application should be based on availability and cost. Schwieger et al.[34] found no difference between untreated control subjects and those receiving IS in a "low-risk" group of patients; this further strengthens the argument for use of respiratory care services only in those patients at risk for PPCs. In 1988 Roukema and colleagues[35] compared a CDB group with a control group in a total patient population of 153 and confirmed the findings of Stein and Cassara. In this study control patients had a PPC rate of 60 percent, versus 19 percent for those receiving CDB therapy.

Several studies have used CDB patients as the control group and compared the PPC incidence among them with that in patient groups treated with other modalities.[36–39] Bartlett et al.[36] treated 150 patients and found the PPC incidence to be 25 percent in the CDB group and 19 percent in the IS group. Lyager et al.,[37] following up the study of Bartlett et al., showed that CDB was superior to IS in preventing PPC. In their study of 94 patients Lyager et al.[37] demonstrated a complication rate of 51 percent in the IS group but only 33 percent in the CDB group. Stock and colleagues[38] compared PPCs in three groups—CDB, IS, and CPAP by mask—on days 1 and 3 following cardiac surgery. They found that CPAP was superior to IS and CDB on both days (CDB, 33 and 41 percent; IS, 50 and 41 percent; and CPAP, 23 and 11 percent incidence of PPCs). Rickstein et al.[39] carried out a study similar to that of Stock and found that CPAP was better than CDB on both days 1 and 3 following upper abdominal operations (CDB, 33 and 40 percent; CPAP, 11 and 4 percent incidence of PPCs). In comparative studies (no control group), Van De Water et al.[40] found IS to be superior to IPPB and Jung et al.[41] found IPPB superior to IS.

Choice of treatment for PPCs often starts off a heated debate as to the superiority of one method over another. However, as with most therapy, no cookbook answer is suitable for all patients. CDB is least expensive and appears to be of value. This technique relies on patient cooperation and motivation, something that cannot always be counted on. IS adds cost by virtue of the mechanical device but may lend itself to more frequent use by the patient. However, patient motivation remains imperative for its successful application. IPPB requires more expensive treatment and more clinician time, with little gain in most patients. IPPB should be considered in cases in which the patient is unable to take a deep breath (e.g., in neuromuscular disease) and CDB and IS are ineffective. Intermittent application of CPAP by mask clearly improves FRC and has the advantage of passive operation. The passive inflation of the lungs may reduce pain and improve compliance in some patients.

Many criticisms of the studies mentioned can be levied. These include diagnosis of PPCs, randomization, and in some cases lack of a control group. The main points to be remembered are (1) the incidence of PPCs in untreated patients is approximately 70 percent in high-risk groups; (2) lung inflation techniques applied judiciously can reduce the incidence of PPCs; (3) therapy should be chosen on the basis of the patient's tolerance and ability to use the therapy; and (4) despite treatment approximately 25 percent of high-risk patients will develop PPCs.

Pain Control

Another postoperative therapy to prevent PPCs is proper pain control. Narcotics may relieve pain but suppress respiration, leading to hypoventilation and atelectasis. Epidural analgesia appears to be more effective than systemic analgesics, with fewer side effects. Studies show that epidural analgesia improves forced vital capacity, forced expiratory volume in 1 second, and peak expiratory flow rate. These improvements in pulmonary function allow the patient to cough more effectively with less pain and to cooperate with lung inflation therapies, thus helping to reduce the incidence of PPCs.[42–46]

The combined effect of epidural analgesia and a lung inflation technique on reducing PPCs is greater than either therapy alone.

References

1. Garibaldi RA, Britt MR, Coleman ML et al: Risk factors for postoperative pneumonia. Am J Med 1981;70:677–680
2. Tisi GM: Preoperative evaluation of pulmonary function: Validity, indications and benefits. Am Rev Respir Dis 1979;119:293–310
3. Tisi GM: Preoperative identification and evaluation of the patient with lung disease. Med Clin North Am 1987;71:399–412
4. Latimer RG, Dickman M, Day WC et al: Ventilatory patterns and pulmonary complications after upper abdominal surgery determined by preoperative and postoperative computerized spirometry and blood gas analysis. Am J Surg 1971;122:622–632
5. Stein M, Cassara EL: Preoperative pulmonary function and therapy for surgery patients. JAMA 1970;211:787–790
6. Torrington KG, Henderson CJ: Perioperative respiratory therapy (PORT): Program of preoperative risk assessment and individualized postoperative care. Chest 1988;93:946–951
7. Ford GT, Guenter CA: Toward prevention of postoperative pulmonary complications. Am Rev Respir Dis 1984;130:4–5
8. Thomas A, Valabhji P: Arrhythmia and tachycardia in pulmonary heart disease. Br Heart J 1969;31:491–495
9. Rochester DF, Esau SA: Malnutrition and the respiratory system. Chest 1984;85:411–415
10. Arora NS, Rochester DF: Effect of body weight and muscularity on human diaphragm muscle mass, thickness and area. J Appl Physiol 1982;52:64–70
11. Arora NS, Rochester DF: Respiratory muscle strength and maximal voluntary ventilation in undernourished patients. Am Rev Respir Dis 1982;126:5–8
12. Buzby GP, Mullen JL, Matthews DL et al: Prognostic nutritional index in gastrointestinal surgery. Am J Surg 1980;139:160–162
13. Buzby GP, Knox LS, Crosby LO et al: Study protocol: A randomized clinical trial of total parenteral nutrition in malnourished surgical patients. Am J Clin Nutr, suppl. 1988;47:366–381
14. Cerra FB: Hypermetabolism, organ failure and metabolic support. Surgery 1987;101:1–14
15. Fleck A: The acute phase response: Implications for nutrition and recovery. Nutrition 1988;4:109–117
16. Pearce AC, Jones RM: Smoking and anesthesia: Preoperative

abstinence and perioperative morbidity. Anesthesiology 1984;61:576–584

17. Fletcher EC, Levin DC: Cardiopulmonary hemodynamics during sleep in subjects with chronic obstructive pulmonary disease. Chest 1984;85:6–14
18. Nocturnal Oxygen Therapy Trial Group: Continuous or nocturnal oxygen therapy in hypoxemic chronic obstructive pulmonary disease. Ann Intern Med 1980;93:391–398
19. Murciano D: Effects of theophylline on diaphragmatic strength and fatigue in patients with chronic obstructive pulmonary disease. N Engl J Med 1984;311:349–353
20. Craig DB, Wahba WM, Don HF et al: "Closing volume" and its relationship to gas exchange in seated and supine positions. J Appl Physiol 1971;31:717–721
21. Don HF, Wahba WM, Craig DB: Airway closure, gas trapping, and the functional residual capacity during anesthesia. Anesthesiology 1972;36:533–539
22. Don HF, Wahba M, Cuadrado L et al: The effects of anesthesia and 100 per cent oxygen on the functional residual capacity of the lungs. Anesthesiology 1970;32:521–529
23. Don HF, Craig DB, Wahba WM et al: The measurement of gas trapped in the lungs at functional residual capacity and the effects of posture. Anesthesiology 1971;35:582–590
24. Drenick EJ: Definition and health consequences of morbid obesity. Surg Clin North Am 1979;59:963–976
25. Vaughan RW, Conahan TJ: Cardiopulmonary consequences of morbid obesity. Life Sci 1980;26:2119–2127
26. Gardner R, Schwartz R, Wong HC et al: Percutaneous indwelling radial artery catheters for monitoring cardiovascular function. N Engl J Med 1974;290:1227–1231
27. Fisher A, Waterhouse TD, Adams AP: Obesity: Its relation to anaesthesia. Anaesthesia 1975;30:633–647
28. Santesson J: Oxygen transport and venous admixture in the extremely obese. Influence of anaesthesia and artificial ventilation with and without positive end-expiratory pressure. Acta Anaesthesiol Scand 1976;20:387–394
29. Salem MR, Dalal FY, Zygmunt MP et al: Does PEEP improve intraoperative arterial oxygenation in grossly obese patients? Anesthesiology 1978;48:280–281
30. Wyner J, Brodsky JB, Merrell RC: Massive obesity and arterial oxygenation. Anesth Analg 1981;60:691–693
31. Kigin CM: Advances in physical therapy. pp. 37–71. In O'Donohue WJ (ed): Current Advances in Respiratory Care. American College of Chest Physicians, Park Ridge IL, 1984
32. Craven JL, Evans GA, Davenport PJ et al: The evaluation of the incentive spirometer in the management of postoperative pulmonary complications. Br J Surg 1974;61:793–797
33. Celli BR, Rodriguez KS, Snider GL: A controlled trial of intermittent positive pressure breathing, incentive spirometry, and deep breathing exercises in preventing pulmonary complications after abdominal surgery. Am Rev Respir Dis 1984;130:12–15
34. Schwieger I, Gamulin A, Forster A et al: Absence of benefit of incentive spirometry in low-risk patients undergoing elective cholecystectomy. Chest 1988;89:652–656
35. Roukema JA, Carol EJ, Prins JG: The prevention of pulmonary complications after upper abdominal surgery in patients with noncompromised pulmonary status. Arch Surg 1988;123:30–34
36. Bartlett RH, Brennan MD, Gazzaniga AB et al: Studies on the pathogenesis and prevention of postoperative pulmonary complications. Surg Gynecol Obstet 1973;137:926–933
37. Lyager S, Nielsen L, Nielsen HC et al: Can postoperative pulmonary complications be improved by treatment with the Bartlett-Edwards incentive spirometer after upper abdominal surgery? Acta Anaesthesiol Scand 1979;23:312–319
38. Stock MC, Downs JB, Cooper RB et al: Comparison of continuous positive airway pressure, incentive spirometry, and conservative therapy after cardiac operations. Crit Care Med 1984;12:969–972
39. Rickstein S, Bengtsson A, Sodomerberg C et al: Effects of periodic airway pressure by mask on postoperative pulmonary function. Chest 1986;89:774–781
40. Van De Water JM, Watring WG, Linton LA et al: Prevention of postoperative pulmonary complications. Surg Gynecol Obstet 1972;135:229–233
41. Jung R, Wight J, Nusser R et al: Comparison of three methods of respiratory care following upper abdominal surgery. Chest 1980;78:31–35
42. Bromage PR, Camporesi E, Chestnut D: Epidural narcotics for postoperative analgesia. Anesth Analg 1980;59:473–480
43. Jayr C, Mollie A, Bourgain TL et al: Postoperative pulmonary complications: General anesthesia with postoperative parenteral morphine compared with epidural analgesia. Surgery 1988;104:57–63
44. Rawal N, Sjostrand UH, Dahlstrom B et al: Epidural morphine for postoperative pain relief: A comparative study with intramuscular narcotic and intercostal nerve block. Anesth Analg 1982;61;93–98
45. Shuman M, Sandler AN, Bradley JW et al: Postthoracotomy pain and pulmonary function following epidural and systemic morphine. Anesthesiology 1984;61:569–575
46. Simonneau G, Vivien A, Sartene R et al: Diaphragm dysfunction induced by upper abdominal surgery: Role of postoperative pain. Am Rev Respir Dis 1983;128:899–903
47. Vaughan RW: Pulmonary and cardiovascular derangements in the obese patient. pp. 115–131. In Brown BR (ed): Anesthesia and the Obese Patient. FA Davis, Philadelphia, 1982

Chapter 90

Respiratory Care of the Patient Who Is Unresponsive, Immobilized, or Paralyzed

David J. Pierson
Dean R. Hess

CHAPTER OUTLINE

Although lying motionless during daily rest and sleep is normal, spending too much time in bed can impair normal physiologic processes and have adverse effects on health[1] (Table 90-1). When patients are unresponsive and do not move spontaneously, when they are rendered immobile because of injury or therapy, or when they are unable to move spontaneously owing to disease or the effects of drugs, a set of special needs and problems is created quite apart from the underlying illness itself. Among these special needs and problems, those pertaining to the respiratory system are particularly important because they are common, may develop very soon after a patient is rendered immobile, and are often potentially life-threatening.[2,3]

Maintenance of airway protection, secretion clearance and adequate lung inflation dominate the special needs of immobilized patients; acute atelectasis, pneumonia, and pulmonary embolism constitute the most serious potential problems. Assessment of these needs and prevention, recognition, and management of these problems are important "core material" for everyone involved in respiratory care.

Common clinical settings in which immobility occurs are listed in Table 90-2. Although these represent a spectrum of medical conditions whose causes and expected duration vary markedly, all of them have in common the needs and problems just identified. This chapter provides an overview of the circumstances in which the clinician may encounter immobility, discusses in detail the respiratory consequences of high cervical spinal cord injury, and offers a review of the methods currently used to prevent and treat complications. The topics covered integrate material addressed in several other chapters, to which the reader should refer for more detail. These include the series of chapters dealing with ventilatory muscle function (Chs. 5, 26, 52, and 87), those discussing the airway and secretion clearance (Chs. 53, 70, and

Table 90-1. Adverse Effects of Bed Rest

Structure/System	Adverse Effects
Joints	Contractures; loss of normal range of motion
Muscles	Disuse atrophy; 15% loss per week of inactivity
Bone	Osteoporosis; pathologic fractures
Urinary tract	Infection; kidney stones
Heart	Deconditioning: decreased cardiac reserve; decreased stroke volume; tachycardia at rest and following exercise
Circulation	Orthostatic hypotension; thrombophlebitis
Lung	Pulmonary embolism; atelectasis; pneumonia
Gastrointestinal tract	Anorexia; hospital-acquired malnutrition; constipation; impaction
Skin	Decubitus ulcers
Psyche	Anxiety; depression; disorientation

(Modified from Corcoran,[1] with permission.)

72), and those that focus on ensuring adequate lung inflation (Chs. 73, 74, and 76).

THE UNRESPONSIVE PATIENT

Patients who do not respond normally to external stimulation may be comatose, stuporous, or in a vegetative state.[4–6] *Coma* is a pathologic state in which neither arousal nor awareness is present. Comatose patients maintain a sleep-like unresponsiveness, from which they cannot be aroused. Such patients do not open their eyes in response to stimuli, produce comprehensible speech, or move their extremities on command or in an appropriate response to noxious stimuli.[4,5] Comatose patients may move spontaneously, showing either decorticate (reflexive flexor movement) or decerebrate (extensor posturing movement) patterns. *Stupor* may be considered a less profound version of coma in which patients remain capable of arousal if strong enough external stimulation is produced.

Patients who have suffered anoxic brain injury or severe head trauma may retain brain stem function despite severe damage to the cerebral hemispheres. Such patients may appear to awaken after an initial period of coma, but evidence of purposeful behavior or awareness of their surroundings is absent. This condition of functional decortication is referred to as the *vegetative state*.[4]

The differential diagnosis of stupor and coma is extensive,[4,6] and only the main entities encountered in respiratory care are listed in Table 90-2. Two clinical settings familiar to clinicians are drug overdose and postresuscitation anoxic encephalopathy. The overdose patient is often comatose on presentation, subsequently progressing through stupor to normal mental status over a period of hours to days. During this time neurologic status may fluctuate, as may the patient's state of immobility. Along with provision of adequate alveolar ventilation in cases of frank ventilatory failure, airway protection is a main concern. Extubation in such patients must be deferred until consistent, complete alertness has returned; in the meantime, care must be taken that self-extubation does not occur, as this increases the likelihood of aspiration of pharyngeal contents as well as of laryngeal injury.

Anoxic encephalopathy, commonly following incomplete cerebral resuscitation in the setting of cardiac arrest, is another common condition requiring care of the comatose patient. Ethical issues such as the appropriateness of continued vigorous supportive measures come to the forefront in such patients, particularly as days pass since the event. The goals of respiratory care in such settings are to prevent complications and to continue support until the patient's prognosis is certain and agreement can be reached between the care-

Table 90-2. Clinical Settings Characterized by Unresponsiveness or Inability to Move

The unresponsive (comatose) patient
- Central nervous system depression by drugs
  - Self-induced: intentional overdose; accidental overdose
  - Iatrogenic, intentional: anesthesia and surgery; treatment of status epilepticus; sedation for agitation, combativeness, or alcohol withdrawal; to reduce O_2 consumption in severe refractory hypoxemia
  - Iatrogenic, unintentional: inadvertent oversedation; adverse reaction to lidocaine, cimetidine, or other drugs
- Poisoning; ingestion of toxic substances
- Anoxic encephalopathy (e.g., following cardiac arrest)
- Head injury
- Primary central nervous system disease
  - Space-occupying lesion: tumor; subdural hematoma; hydrocephalus; brain abscess
  - Cerebrovascular accident: thrombosis; hemorrhage
  - Infection: meningitis; encephalitis
  - Epilepsy
- Metabolic abnormalities (e.g., hyponatremia; hypercalcemia; myxedema; hepatic encephalopathy)

The immobilized patient
- Fractures and other skeletal injuries: spine; pelvis; femur; humerus
- Skin grafting; other specialized surgical procedures requiring immobility
- Burns; severe exfoliative dermatitis
- Extensive casting or bracing: pelvis, cervical spine, etc.
- Restraints: delirium tremens; manic states; uncontrollable agitation

The paralyzed patient
- High cervical spinal cord injury: acute; chronic
- Primary neuromuscular disease: Guillain-Barré syndrome; botulism; severe myasthenia gravis; postpoliomyelitis; amyotrophic lateral sclerosis
- Use of muscle relaxants (e.g., pancuronium bromide; doxacurium chloride): anesthesia and surgery; to decrease O_2 consumption during severe refractory hypoxemia; uncontrollable agitation during mechanical ventilation

givers and the patient's family as to what further measures are in the patient's best interests.

THE IMMOBILIZED PATIENT

Patients who are capable of moving may be immobilized deliberately because of the requirements of management. In the presence of conditions such as those listed in Table 90-2, immobilization may be the result of skeletal traction devices, casts, bandages, or measures to restrain agitated or violent patients. The patient with a cervical spinal injury, with or without accompanying neurologic deficit, is a familiar example. Another is the individual who develops severe alcohol withdrawal syndrome after hospitalization for trauma or some other reason and must be restrained for the protection of the patient and others.

Delirium tremens may complicate the management of pneumonia, trauma, or another condition to which the patient's alcoholism was predisposing and which may have initially brought about admission to the hospital. The most extreme form of alcohol withdrawal, delirium tremens, is a life-threatening condition characterized by disorientation, hallucinations, tremulousness, agitation, and markedly increased autonomic nervous system activity, manifested by tachycardia, fever, and diaphoresis. It usually appears 2 to 4 days after cessation of sustained heavy alcohol ingestion but may develop after as much as 1 week of abstinence; the clinical syndrome typically lasts 4 to 7 days, but recovery may occasionally take 2 weeks or longer. Full-blown delirium tremens is a difficult disorder to manage and may be associated with mortality rates of 10 to 20 percent or even higher. Mortality results primarily from the sequelae of inadvertent oversedation, failure of airway protection, and aspiration of gastric contents. Careful attention must be given to airway management and secretion clearance, and conscious efforts must be made not to administer more sedation than necessary to control violent agitation.

THE PARALYZED PATIENT

Paralysis refers to the physical inability to move, apart from any motivation to do so. Complete or partial paralysis may occur in a wide variety of disorders[3] (Table 90-3). In respiratory care this state is most often encountered in two settings: weakness of the muscles themselves and mechanical interruption of the nerves supplying those muscles.

Muscle Weakness

In the management of critically ill patients the most common circumstance for muscle weakness is the deliberate use of muscle relaxant drugs such as pancuronium bromide. Such therapeutic paralysis may be necessary to control agitated or combative patients when sedation is ineffective and is also occasionally employed to reduce excessive O_2 consumption associated with muscle activity in the presence of refractory hypoxemia in severe adult respiratory distress syndrome (ARDS). Paralysis is also required during the use of some modes of ventilatory support, such as pressure control with inverse inspiration/expiration ratio and low-frequency positive-pressure ventilation with extracorporeal CO_2 removal, which without paralysis and heavy sedation would be intolerable for patients.

Severe muscle weakness leading to the complications of immobility is also encountered in several diseases, including the Guillain-Barré syndrome,[7] myasthenia gravis,[8] and the other conditions listed in Table 90-2. In such cases the weakness may affect mainly the peripheral musculature, with sufficient preservation of ventilatory muscle function that adequate ventilation and secretion clearance can be maintained, but severe cases generally involve paralysis of these muscles as well, requiring establishment of an artificial airway and institution of ventilatory support.[2,3,9]

The most effective means for assessing and monitoring the adequacy of ventilatory muscle function in patients with muscle weakness is the repeated measurement of maximum inspiratory force (MIF) and vital capacity (VC). As discussed in Chapter 64, the clinician should not wait for the development of acute respiratory acidosis but should be prepared to institute mechanical ventilation when serial measurements of MIF and VC show progressive deterioration to the range of -20 to -25 cmH_2O and 10 to 15 mL/kg, respectively. Figure 90-1 illustrates the clinical use of these monitors and also the prolonged nature of the (eventually reversible) ventilatory paralysis that can occur.[10]

Cervical Spinal Cord Injury

Patients with acute cervical spinal cord injury, such as may occur from motor vehicle accidents, diving accidents, and gunshot wounds, constitute an important subset of the intensive care unit (ICU) population with unique clinical problems and needs.[11–14] Such patients often continue to need respiratory care following the acute phase of their illness and may be encountered by the clinician months or years after the original injury.

The impact of cervical spinal cord injury on respiratory function is determined primarily by the anatomic level of the injury (Fig. 90-2[11]; Table 90-4[2]). Injury below C7 causes impairment mainly of expiratory muscles and so interferes with effective cough and secretion clearance. Above this level, muscle function is markedly affected by how high the injury is (Table 90-5). The phrenic nerves, originating at spinal cord level C3–C5, remain intact in lower cervical injuries, although some impairment of inspiratory capacity occurs and forced expiratory function is lost.

With midcervical injuries (C3–C5) there is partial to complete diaphragmatic paralysis as well as loss of the intercostal and scalene muscle function. Patients with this functional level cannot cough and are prone to atelectasis from loss of resting thoracic muscle tone and inability to fully expand the lungs; most are ventilator-dependent initially, although many can eventually breathe without assistance. Individuals

Table 90-3. Disorders of Ventilatory Neuromuscular Function

Level	Examples	Associated Clinical Characteristics	Nerve Conduction	Electromyographic Findings
Upper motor neuron	Hemiplegia Quadriplegia Extrapyramidal disorders	Weakness Hyperreflexia Increased muscle tone May have sensory and autonomic changes	Normal	Normal
Lower motor neuron	Paralytic poliomyelitis Amyotrophic lateral sclerosis Werdnig-Hoffmann disease Spinal muscular atrophies Postpolio syndrome	Weakness Atrophy Flaccidity Hyperreflexia Fasiculations Bulbar involvement No sensory changes	Normal	Denervation potentials Giant motor units
Peripheral neurons	Guillain-Barré syndrome Acute intermittent porphyria Diphtheria Lyme disease Toxins (lead, thallium triorthocresyl phosphate) Saxitoxin Polyneuropathies associated with lupus or polyarteritis Critical illness polyneuropathy	Weakness Flaccidity Hyporeflexia Bulbar involvement Sensory and autonomic changes	Reduced	Denervation potentials in axonal neuropathies
Myoneural junction	Myasthenia gravis Botulism Eaton-Lambert syndrome Organophosphate poisoning Tick paralysis Black widow spider bite	Fluctuating weakness Fatigability Ocular and bulbar involvement Normal reflexes No sensory changes	Normal	Changes in the amplitude of the muscle response to repetitive nerve stimulation
Muscle	Muscular dystrophies Polymyositis Acid maltase deficiency Carnitine palmityl transferase deficiency	Weakness, usually proximal Normal reflexes No sensory or autonomic changes Often have pain	Normal	Small motor units

(From Kelly and Luce,[3] with permission.)

who sustain high cervical spinal cord injury (C1–C2) have paralysis of all the major ventilatory muscles and retain potential activity only in the sternomastoids, trapezii, platysma, mylohyoids, and sternohyoids (Table 90-5). Only a few such patients eventually attain substantial ventilator independence.[15]

The acute phase of cervical spinal cord injury[12,13,16] typically lasts several weeks and is characterized by instability in several body systems (Table 90-6). The initial neurologic deficit may either improve or worsen in the hours to days following injury. During the phase of *spinal shock*, related primarily to acute sympathetic denervation, patients are hypotensive, bradycardic, and susceptible to hypothermia. In this setting they are also prone to development of cardiac arrhythmias, particularly severe bradycardia and asystole, on stimulation of the main airways during suctioning. This potentially life-threatening problem tends to be particularly severe in patients receiving positive end-expiratory pressure (PEEP); this is probably related to the airway pressure changes that occur during disconnection from the ventilator circuit for suctioning. In such settings the use of an in-line multiple-use suction catheter,[17,18] such as that shown in Figure 90-3, can reduce the frequency and severity of suctioning-related bradyarrhythmias.

Also common in the acute postinjury period is segmental, lobar, or even whole lung atelectasis. The atelectasis tends to recur, often on the opposite side (so-called ping-pong atelectasis). Although in postoperative and other patients acute lobar collapse usually does not cause severe hypoxemia and is not a medical emergency, such is not the case in the acute

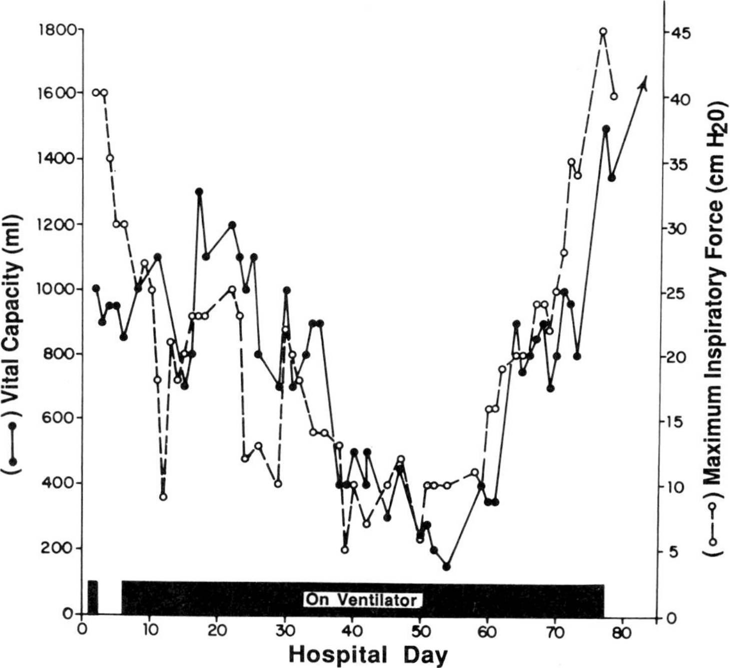

Figure 90-1. Clinical course of ventilatory muscle weakness in a patient with neuromuscular paralysis due to postdiphtheritic neuropathy. The first 80 days of this patient's 142-day hospital course to full recovery are shown, including 72 days of mechanical ventilation. The progression and persistence of the ventilatory muscle weakness, as well as the patient's eventual recovery, were effectively monitored by repeated measurements of VC (solid line) and MIF (dashed line). (From Pierson and Brown,[10] with permission.)

quadriplegic, who frequently develops profound hypoxemia and cardiovascular instability. As discussed further in Chapter 74, immediate bronchoscopy is often required in this setting. Aggressive measures to maintain lung expansion (see Ch. 73) should be begun early in the patient with acute cervical spinal cord injury so that development of major atelectasis can be prevented.

After the period of physiologic instability has passed and patients with cervical spinal cord injury have recovered from the acute phase of their injury, those whose injuries are at the midcervical and lower levels tend to display characteristic patterns of pulmonary and ventilatory muscle function,[2] as summarized in Table 90-7. They typically have a mild restrictive ventilatory defect as gauged by total lung capacity, but proportionally greater reduction in VC and especially expiratory reserve volume.[2] Maximum inspiratory pressure tends to be preserved more than maximum expiratory pressure.

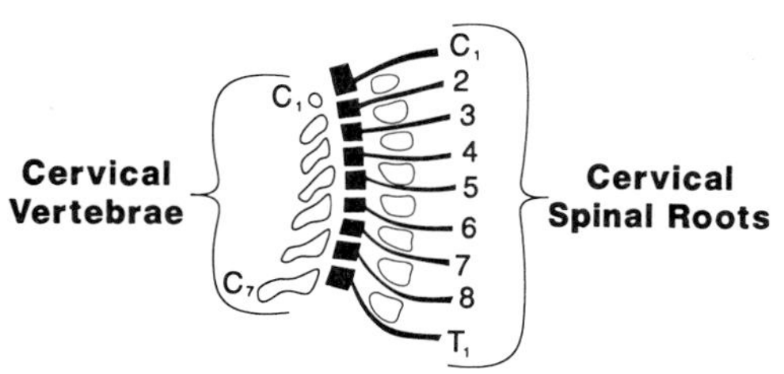

Figure 90-2. Relationship of cervical vertebrae to cervical spinal nerve roots. (From Mansel and Norman,[11] with permission.)

Table 90-4. Innervation of the Ventilatory Muscles

Muscle Group	Spinal Cord Level	Nerve(s)
Inspiratory muscles		
Diaphragm	C3–C5	Phrenic
Parasternal intercostals	T1–T7	Intercostal
Lateral external intercostals	T1–T12	Intercostal
Scalenes	C4–C8	
Sternomastoid	XI	Cranial nerve, C1, C2
Expiratory muscles		
Lateral internal intercostals	T1–T12	Intercostal
Rectus abdominis	T7–L1	Lumbar
External and internal obliques	T7–L1	Lumbar
Transversus abdominis	T7–L1	Lumbar

(From Rochester and Findley,[2] with permission.)

Table 90-5. Effects of Spinal Cord Level on Pulmonary Function in Quadriplegia

Cord Level	Ventilatory Muscles Affected	Clinical Effects
High cervical (C1, C2)	Paralysis of diaphragm (C3–C5), intercostals, and abdominals Inspiratory electromyographic (EMG) activity in sternomastoids, trapezii, platysma, mylohyoids, and sternohyoids	Virtually total ventilatory muscle paralysis Initial ventilator dependence in all patients Eventual partial independence in a few, via glossopharyngeal respiration, etc.
Midcervical (C3–C5)	Partial to complete phrenic nerve paralysis with bilateral hemidiaphragm weakness Paralysis of intercostals and abdominals	Variable inspiratory capacity Severe restrictive defect No expiratory muscle activity Inability to cough Eventual ventilator independence in half or more of patients
Lower cervical (C5–C7)	Intact phrenic nerves (diaphragm function intact) Paralysis of intercostals and abdominals	Mild to moderate reduction in inspiratory capacity Moderate restrictive defect Ventilator-independent Inability to cough; problems clearing secretions
Below C7	Diaphragm intact Other inspiratory muscles paralyzed Expiratory muscles paralyzed	Inspiratory capacity mildly reduced to normal Forced exhalation and cough impaired in proportion to number of thoracic and abdominal segments affected Atelectasis uncommon; variable difficulty in clearing secretions

KINETIC BED THERAPY FOR IMMOBILIZED PATIENTS

The complications of prolonged immobility are well known.[19] These include atelectasis and pneumonia, venous thrombosis and pulmonary embolism, skin breakdown and decubitus ulcer formation, and urinary stasis with urinary tract infection. It has also been long appreciated that turning the patient can decrease the frequency of these complications, and side-to-side turning at 2-hour intervals is considered standard nursing care of immobilized patients. Since normal persons during sleep make one gross postural change every 11.6 minutes, it has been suggested that this is the minimal physiologic mobility requirement for patients supported on a soft surface.[20] Because frequent turning is labor-

Table 90-6. Complications of Acute Cervical Spinal Cord Injury

Flaccid paralysis below level of injury

Spinal shock syndrome
- Hypotension (increased venous capacitance; loss of sympathetic tone)
- Bradycardia (can progress to heart block)
- Poikilothermia (usually hypothermia)

Propensity to cardiac dysrhythmias (especially bradycardia and asystole) on stimulation of airways (e.g., by suction catheter)

Ventilatory muscle paralysis or weakness depending upon level of injury (see Table 90-4)

Hypoxemia (from ventilation-perfusion mismatching and right-to-left intrapulmonary shunting due to inadequate lung expansion, with or without alveolar hypoventilation)

Loss of ability to cough

Gastric atony (risk for aspiration, gastric distension, gastric rupture, and further compromise of diaphragm function)

Paralytic ileus (leading to abdominal distension and further compromise of diaphragm function)

Denervation of urinary bladder (overdistension; urinary tract colonization and infection associated with catheterization)

Catabolic state (hypoalbuminemia; hypocalcemia; increased risk for malnutrition)

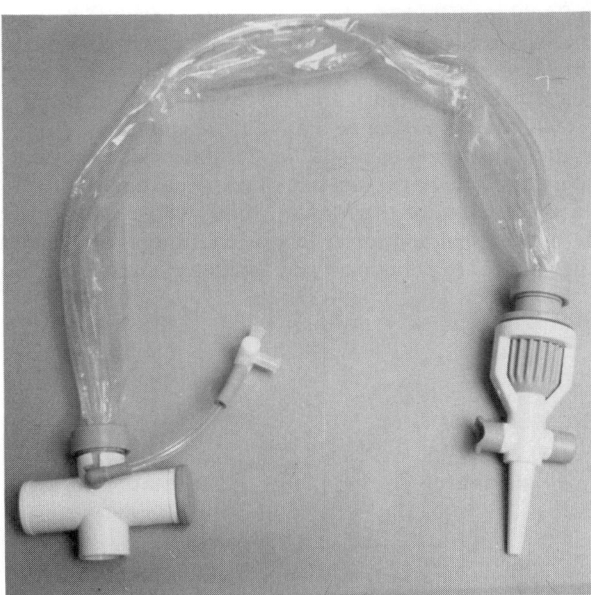

Figure 90-3. Multiple-use, closed-system suction catheter system (TrachCare, Ballard Medical Products, Midvale, UT), permitting endotracheal suctioning without disconnection from ventilator circuit and sudden loss of PEEP.

Table 90-7. Pulmonary and Ventilatory Muscle Function in Quadriplegic Patients with C4–C7 Spinal Cord Injury

Variable	Mean ± SD
VC (% predicted)	52 ± 11
FEV_1/FVC (%)	85 ± 3
Inspiratory capacity (% predicted)	71 ± 16
Expiratory reserve volume (% predicted)	21 ± 12
Total lung capacity (% predicted)	70 ± 4
Functional residual capacity (% predicted)	86 ± 14
Residual volume (% predicted)	141 ± 20
Maximum voluntary ventilation (% predicted)	49 ± 10
Maximum inspiratory pressure (cmH_2O)	64 ± 12
Maximum expiratory pressure (cmH_2O)	41 ± 22

FEV_1/FVC, ratio of forced expiratory volume in 1 second to forced vital capacity.

(Adapted from Rochester and Findley,[2] with permission.)

intensive, there has been increasing interest in recent years in the use of beds that automatically turn the patient. *Kinetic therapy* is the use of a bed that automatically and continuously turns a patient from side to side.

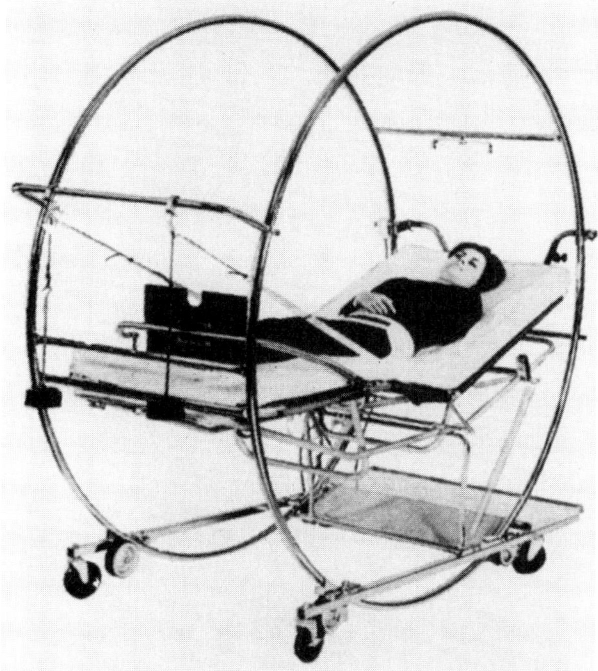

Figure 90-5. Stryker Circ-O-Lectric bed (Stryker Medical, Kalamazoo, MI).

Technical Aspects

The Stryker Wedge Turning Frame and Stryker Circ-O-Lectric bed (Stryker Medical, Kalamazoo, MI) are designed to allow spinal cord-injured patients to be turned from supine to prone position (Figs. 90-4 and 90-5). Although these beds have become less commonly used since the early 1980s, when kinetic beds became more popular, they continue to be used in some spinal cord injury centers. These beds do not represent true kinetic therapy because they do not automatically and continuously turn the patient. Although the currently available Stryker beds are easier to use than previous models, they do require considerable nursing staff time to position the patient. Care must be taken to avoid injury when positioning patients on the Wedge Turning Frame and Circ-O-Lectric bed, as complications and death have been associated with these beds.[21–23]

The Roto-Rest bed (Kinetic Concepts, Inc., San Antonio, TX) (Figs. 90-6 and 90-7) rotates continuously on its long

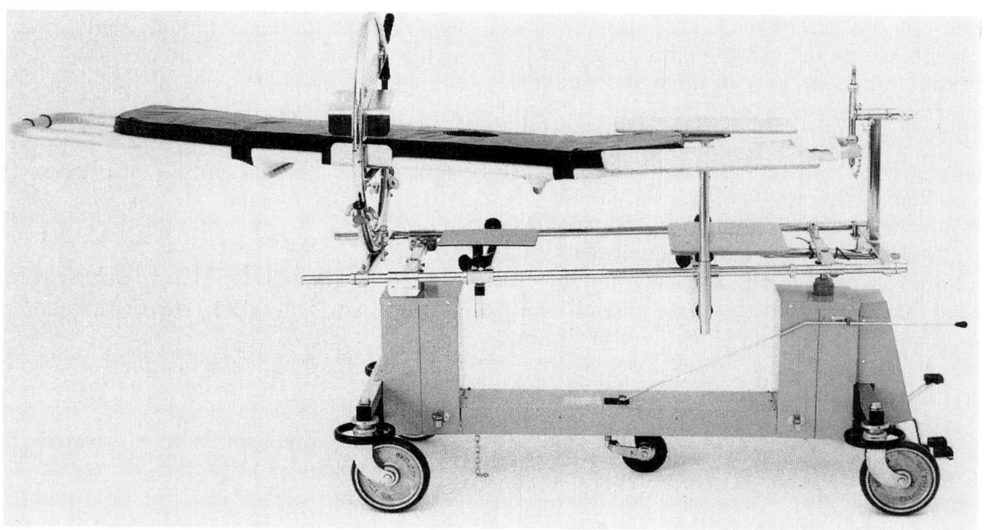

Figure 90-4. Stryker Wedge Turning Frame (Stryker Medical, Kalamazoo, MI).

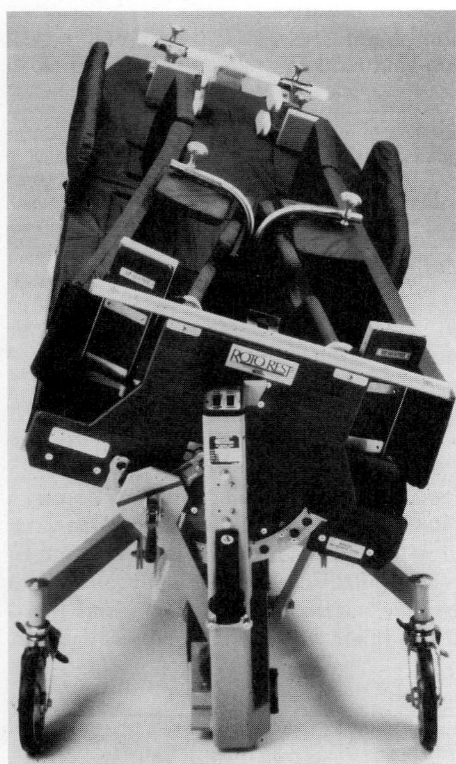

Figure 90-6. Roto-Rest bed (Kinetic Concepts Inc., San Antonio, TX).

axis through an arc of 124 degrees (62 degrees from a level plane) approximately every 3.5 minutes (1 degree every 1.7 seconds). Trendelenburg's and reverse Trendelenburg's positions (maximal 13 degrees in either direction) can be used. Patient position can be locked at a variety of positions along the arc of rotation of the bed. Hatches in the occipital, thoracic, rectal, and extremity areas allow for patient care and evaluation. For chest physiotherapy the patient is positioned and the thoracic hatch can be opened to provide chest percussion. Variable rotation allows precise unilateral rotation for patients with unilateral lung disease. The Roto-Rest bed can be used for patients with spinal cord injury and those in skeletal traction.

Another form of kinetic therapy involves the use of air suspension (fluid air, air loss) beds. These are intended to reduce skin breakdown by providing an air support surface, and they also provide continuous side-to-side rotation (up to 45 degrees). These include air-filled beds (e.g., BioDyne, Kinetic Concepts, San Antonio, TX) (Fig. 90-8) and beds filled with fluidized silicone-coated microspheres (e.g., FluidAir, Kinetic Concepts, San Antonio, TX). Unlike the Roto-Rest bed, these beds should not be used for patients with an unstable spine or those in spinal traction. Virtually nothing has been reported about these beds in the scientific literature.

Anecdotal reports,[24–27] retrospective studies,[28,29] prospective controlled clinical trials,[30–36] and a literature review[37] of kinetic therapy (in each case, the Roto-Rest bed) have been published. The studies in the literature use a variety of research methodologies of varying scientific rigor, are generally short-term, and usually include a small number of patients. Kinetic therapy has been evaluated in stroke patients, medical patients, and multiple trauma patients. Use of kinetic bed therapy has been reported to prevent deep venous thrombosis, atelectasis, and pneumonia. Although the cost of a kinetic bed is greater than that of a conventional bed, kinetic bed therapy may reduce the length of stay in the ICU, so that the total patient cost for a kinetic bed or a conventional bed may be similar (when the kinetic bed is indicated).[35,36]

Indications

Indications for kinetic bed therapy are listed below:

Immobilized patients (coma, spinal injury, stroke)

Obese patients who cannot be easily turned and are at risk for complications of immobility

Patients with unilateral lung disease who cannot be easily placed on one side

Generally, kinetic bed therapy should only be considered in patients who are immobile and are expected to remain immobile for a prolonged period. Kinetic bed therapy may also be considered for patients with limited mobility (e.g., obese patients) who require turning for therapeutic procedures (e.g., chest physiotherapy). Kinetic therapy may also be useful in some patients with unilateral lung disease, who may show a postural improvement in pulmonary shunt (the kinetic bed can be programmed to favor positioning to one side). Because of the cost associated with kinetic therapy, the decision to use it should be carefully considered and individualized for the specific patient; kinetic therapy should *never* be considered routine for any group of patients.

Although kinetic therapy is designed to provide continuous rotation, this often does not occur in critically ill patients, in whom bed rotation is often interrupted for therapeutic and diagnostic procedures. It is ironic that the amount of rotation time is most limited when the patient is most ill, which may be the time at which continuous rotation is most beneficial. At this time there has been no scientific evaluation of the minimal amount of rotation time needed each day to provide benefit.

Hazards, Complications, and Contraindications

The hazards and complications of kinetic therapy[37,38] are as follows:

Ventilator disconnection, inadvertent extubation, accidental aspiration of ventilator circuit condensate

Disconnection of intravenous, intra-arterial, or urinary catheters

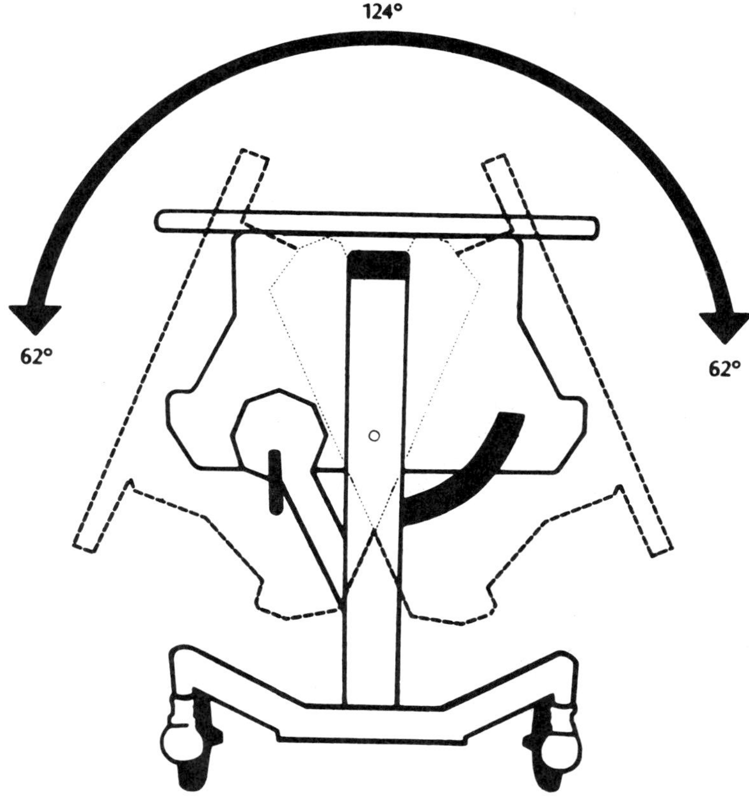

Figure 90-7. Schematic drawing illustrating the continuous rotation of the Roto-Rest bed along its rotational axis. (From Kelly et al.,[31] with permission.)

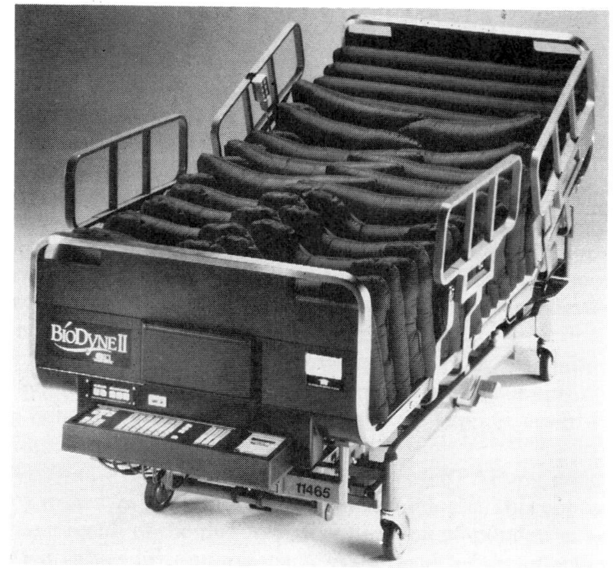

Figure 90-8. Biodyne air-filled bed (Kinetic Concepts Inc., San Antonio, TX).

Arrhythmias
Patient intolerance (agitated, combative patients)
Increased intracranial pressure
Worsening dyspnea and hypoxemia
Difficult examination of the posterior
Chest x-ray artifact
Cost

Some of these are potentially life-threatening (e.g., ventilator disconnection or intra-arterial catheter disconnection). The complication rate associated with the use of kinetic beds is unknown and probably under-reported. For example, frequent ventilator disconnections that are promptly recognized and corrected are likely not to be reported but nonetheless are frustrating and time-consuming for those caring for the patient. In the case of ventilator tubing and vascular lines, it is important that these be of sufficient length to allow patient rotation, and this must be determined before rotation is begun.

Kinetic therapy interferes with patient assessment in several ways. First, physical assessment of the patient's posterior is limited, particularly if an air suspension bed is used. Second, the quality of the chest radiograph is diminished (Fig. 90-9). Although the Roto-Rest bed has a radiolucent

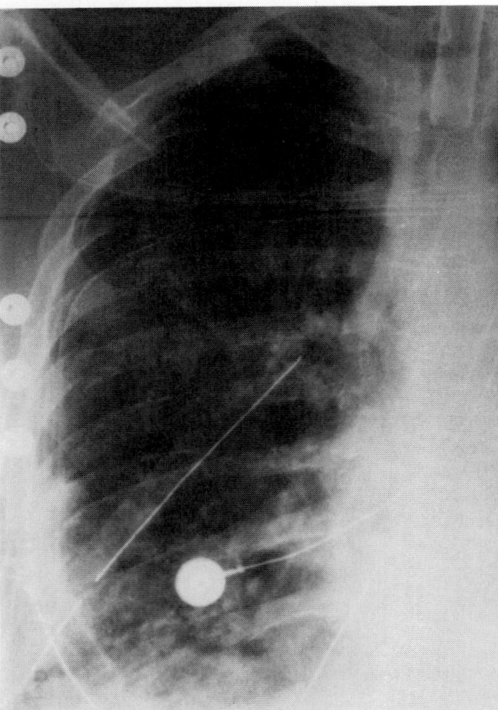

Figure 90-9. Chest x-ray of a patient on a Roto-Rest bed. A small pneumothorax is present on the right side, which is nearly obscured by the artifact from the bed.

surface, artifacts (lines and shadows) appear on the chest x-ray, which can make interpretation difficult. Also, the chest x-ray taken on a Roto-Rest bed places the heart further from the x-ray film, resulting in magnification (Fig. 90-10).

Positioning has been shown to result in intracranial pressure changes in head-injured patients.[39] This is of concern relative to kinetic therapy because these beds are commonly used for head-injured acute trauma patients. However, in one study it was found that kinetic therapy did not adversely affect intracranial pressure in comatose neurosurgical patients.[40]

Table 90-8 lists contraindications to kinetic therapy.[37] The only absolute contraindications are unstable spinal cord injuries and traction of the arm abductors.

Criteria for Discontinuation

Criteria for discontinuation of kinetic therapy are listed below:

- Occurrence of a complication associated with rotation (arrhythmia, increased intracranial pressure, hemodynamic instability, etc.)
- Increased spontaneous mobility

The principal reason for discontinuation of kinetic therapy is the ability of the patient to mobilize spontaneously. Kinetic therapy should also be discontinued if the patient has an adverse response.

A

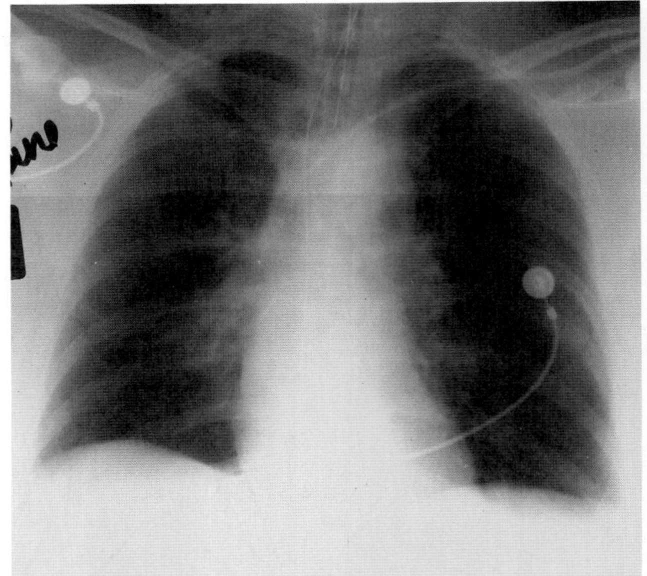

B

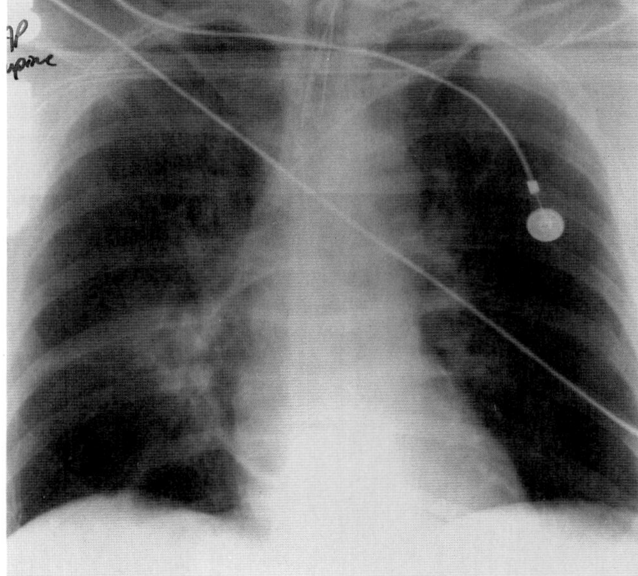

Figure 90-10. Anteroposterior 48-in. portable supine chest radiographs taken on the same patient **(A)** before and **(B)** after she was placed on a Roto-Rest bed. In Figure B the heart appears to have enlarged because it is now farther away from the film cassette, and part of the bed appears as an artifact overlying the clavicles.

BREATHING ASSISTANCE AND COUGHING FOR QUADRIPLEGIC PATIENTS

The degree of respiratory dysfunction following injury to the spinal cord depends on the level of injury.[3,11] If the injury occurs above the level of C3, there is paralysis of the diaphragm, intercostal muscles, and abdominal muscles; this is

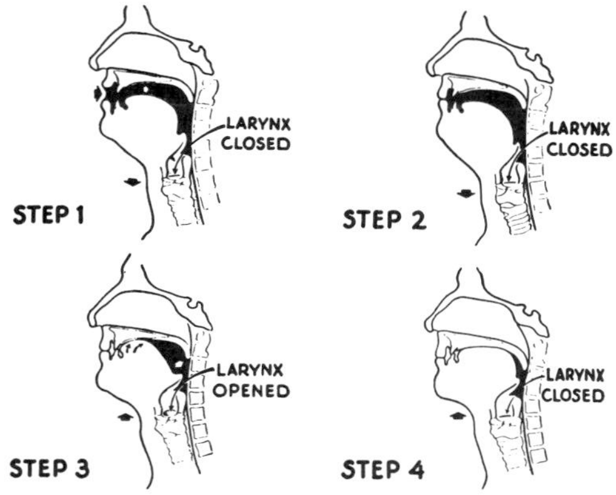

Figure 90-11. Glossopharyngeal breathing. Step 1: The mouth and pharynx are filled with air, with depression of the tongue, jaw, and larynx to achieve maximum volume. Step 2: The lips are closed and the soft palate is raised to trap the air. Step 3: The jaw, floor of the mouth, and larynx are raised; this, with progressive motion of the tongue, forces air through the opened larynx. Step 4: After as much air as possible is forced through the larynx, it is closed and the air is retained in the lungs until the cycle is reinitiated. (From Dail et al.,[41] with permission.)

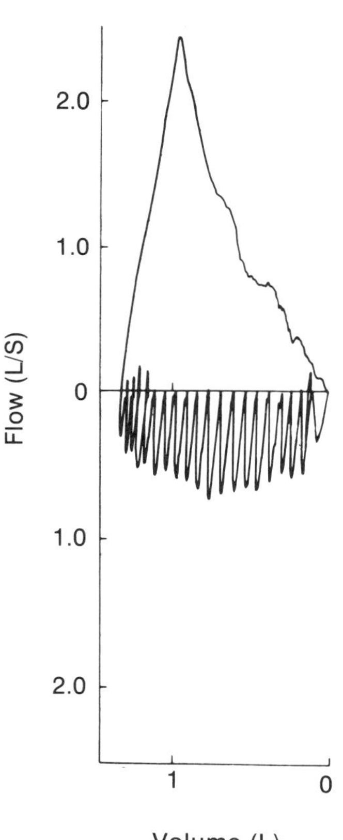

Figure 90-12. The flow-volume loop obtained from a patient performing glossopharyngeal breathing. Inspiration (below horizontal axis) was achieved by 20 consecutive inspiratory maneuvers. (From James et al.,[43] with permission.)

Table 90-8. Contraindications to Kinetic Therapy

Absolute
Unstable spinal injuries
Traction of the arm abductors
Relative
Marked agitation
Severe diarrhea
Rise in intracranial pressure
Greater than 10% decrease in blood pressure
Worsening dyspnea and hypoxia
Cardiac arrhythmias

(From Sahn,[37] with permission.)

not compatible with life unless mechanical ventilation is provided. If the injury is below C5, the function of the diaphragm is not impaired. With low cervical or high thoracic spinal injury, however, expiratory muscle function is severely limited. Such patients may be able to breathe without ventilatory support but are at considerable risk for retained secretions, atelectasis, and pneumonia because of their impaired ability to cough (see Table 90-5).

Glossopharyngeal Breathing

Glossopharyngeal breathing, sometimes called "gulping" or "frog breathing," is a technique for ventilating the lungs that does not require use of the respiratory muscles.[41–44] In patients with high cervical spinal injury this technique can be used to provide breathing for short periods (and longer periods in some patients) without mechanical assistance. In patients with lower cervical injury this breathing technique can be used to increase the inspiratory capacity and to facilitate coughing.

Glossopharyngeal breathing uses the muscles of the mouth and pharynx to force air into the lungs under positive pressure. About 50 to 80 mL of air is trapped in the pharynx when the mouth and nasopharynx are closed (Fig. 90-11). The air is then forced into the trachea by constricting the pharyngeal muscles and displacing the tongue upward. The trapped air is held in the lower respiratory tract by closing the glottis until the next volume of air is forced into the trachea. It typically takes about 20 such maneuvers and about 15 seconds to force 1000 mL of air into the lungs. The larynx is then opened, and exhalation occurs as the result of the passive elastic recoil of the lungs. Although this technique requires several weeks for patients to learn, it results in a significant increase in inspiratory capacity and expiratory flow (Fig. 90-12).

Quad Coughing

Owing to loss of abdominal muscle function, the cough of quadriplegic patients is very ineffective.[45] Cough effectiveness in these patients can be improved by use of a manual cough technique, commonly called *quad coughing*.[46] The pa-

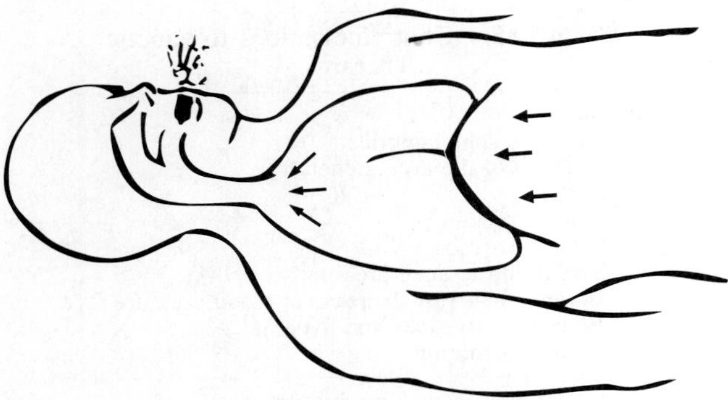

Figure 90-13. To produce quad coughing, external abdominal pressure is applied under the diaphragm during exhalation following maximal inspiration, resulting in an increased expiratory flow and secretion removal.

tient is instructed to take a deep breath and hold the air in the lungs by closing the glottis. The patient is then asked to exhale as a caregiver presses inward and upward on the upper abdominal and epigastric area (Fig. 90-13). The abdominal pressure should be directed toward the diaphragm; it should be applied during exhalation only and must be coordinated with the efforts of the patient. Compression on the lateral aspect of the chest can also be effective. Because of the discomfort that this technique can produce in patients with a functioning afferent nervous system, quad coughing should only be used with quadriplegic patients.

Positioning and Abdominal Binders

Quadriplegic patients often have a postural dependence of the VC.[47] In normal persons VC decreases when changing from an upright to a supine position, but in quadriplegic patients VC paradoxically increases in the supine position as a result of a decrease in residual volume due to the effect of gravity on the abdominal contents. This effect is also related to the relatively high compliance of the abdomen and low compliance of the lungs in these patients. In the erect posture, the abdominal contents fall, which flattens the diaphragm and makes it less effective. This can result in less efficient ventilation and dyspnea in the sitting position (platypnea).

The postural dependence of VC can be inhibited by use of an abdominal binder (Fig. 90-14), which prevents the movement of abdominal contents when the patient is moved from the supine to Fowler's position.[47,48] To facilitate breathing in quadriplegic patients, they should not be placed into a sitting position unless the abdomen is supported with a binder.

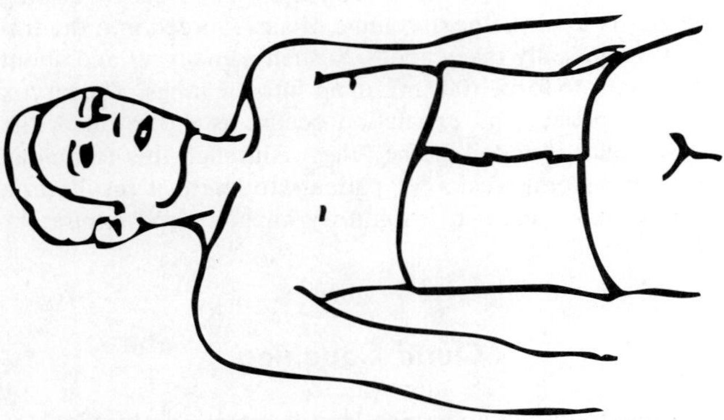

Figure 90-14. Schematic illustration indicating position of abdominal binder in quadriplegic patient.

Respiratory Muscle Training

Although quadriplegic patients have compromised expiratory muscle function, it has been shown that many have a measurable expiratory reserve volume. This has been shown to result from the contraction of the clavicular portion of the pectoralis major muscle,[49,50] which has a motor innervation arising from C5–C7. Contraction of the pectoralis major muscle in quadriplegic patients results in constriction of the upper rib cage, with a subsequent decrease in lung volume (Fig. 90-15). It has been shown that isometric contractions can be used to train the pectoralis muscle for strength[51] (Fig. 90-16). Over a 3-week training period, the quadriplegic subjects in that study developed a 55 percent

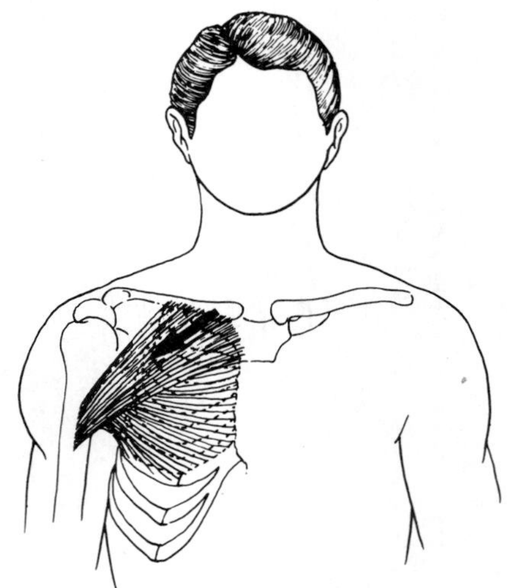

Figure 90-15. Diagram illustrating the expiratory action of the clavicular portion of the pectoralis major in quadriplegic patients. The muscle fibers run caudally and laterally from the medial half of the clavicle to the humerus. If the arms are fixed, these fibers (arrow) on both sides of the chest displace the clavicles and the manubrium of the sternum in a caudal direction. As a result, the upper part of the rib cage, which is closely attached to the sternum, moves caudally as well and contracts. (From Estenne et al.,[51] with permission.)

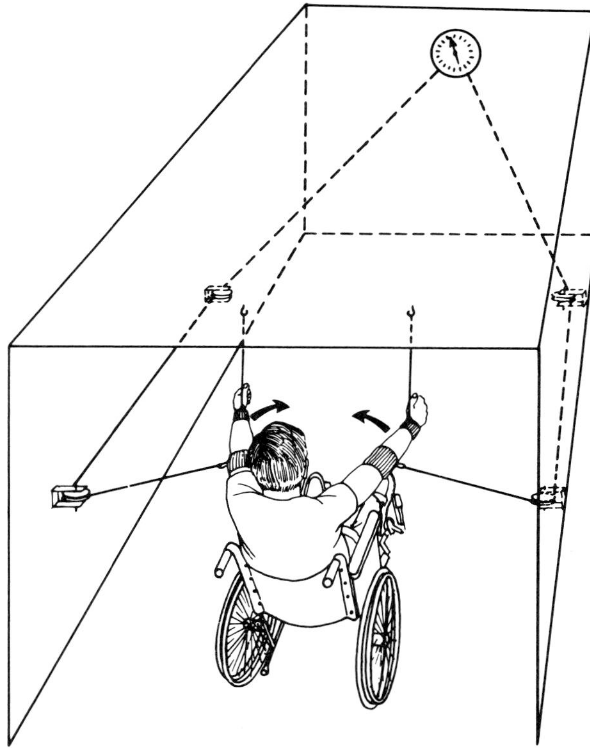

Figure 90-16. Apparatus used for measuring the strength of the pectoralis major muscle and for training it. The subject sits in a wheelchair, and straps are positioned around each wrist and elbow. Ropes are then used to attach the wrists to the ceiling in such a manner that the arms are maintained horizontal and abducted 30 to 40 degrees. Additional ropes and pulleys connect the elbows to a dynamometer placed in front of the subject. When the subject performs a horizontal adduction of the arms (arrows), the contraction of the pectoralis muscles is virtually isometric. (From Estenne et al.,[51] with permission.)

increase in pectoralis muscle strength and a 47 percent increase in expiratory reserve volume.

Inspiratory muscle training has also been reported in quadriplegic patients. In one study[52] there was a 40 percent increase in diaphragmatic strength following regular breathing against inspiratory resistances for 16 weeks. Thus, inspiratory muscle training in quadriplegic patients may be useful for protecting against fatigue, and expiratory muscle training may be useful for improving expiratory flow and cough effectiveness.

Tracheostomy and Suctioning

Prolonged (or permanent) tracheostomy is required in some quadriplegic patients.[53] Such patients include those who require frequent suctioning for secretion removal, those with swallowing difficulty who are likely to aspirate, and those who cannot be entirely weaned from ventilator support (e.g., those who require nocturnal ventilation). For patients who require a tracheostomy only for suctioning, an uncuffed fenestrated tube or tracheostomy button may be used. Except for the periods of suctioning, these tubes can be plugged, allowing the patient to breathe through the upper airway (and to speak) (see Chapter 53).

Other Therapy

Quadriplegic patients benefit from deep breathing. In those who can voluntarily breathe deeply, incentive spirometry can be used. In those quadriplegic patients who have difficulty deep breathing, a trial of intermittent positive-pressure breathing (IPPB) is reasonable.[54] However, IPPB should only be used if it results in a deeper breath than the patient can produce voluntarily, if it is tolerated by the patient, and if it is not associated with side effects such as gastric insufflation. A trial of aerosolized bronchodilator therapy is also reasonable in these patients to decrease airway smooth muscle tone and facilitate secretion removal.[53,54] In those patients who have problems with secretion removal, a trial of chest physiotherapy is also reasonable.

References

1. Corcoran PJ: Use it or lose it—the hazards of bed rest and inactivity. West J Med 1991;154:536–538
2. Rochester DF, Findley LJ: The lungs and neuromuscular and chest wall diseases. pp. 1942–1971. In Murray JF, Nadel JA (eds): Textbook of Respiratory Medicine. WB Saunders, Philadelphia, 1988
3. Kelly BJ, Luce JM: The diagnosis and management of neuromuscular diseases causing respiratory failure. Chest 1991; 99:1485–1494
4. Caronna JJ: Approach to the patient with impairment of consciousness. pp. 2302–2308. In Kelley WN (ed): Textbook of Internal Medicine. 2nd Ed. JB Lippincott, Philadelphia, 1992
5. Ropper AH, Martin JB: Coma and other disorders of consciousness. pp. 193–203. In Wilson JD, Braunwald E, Isselbacher KJ et al. (eds): Harrison's Principles of Internal Medicine. 12th Ed. McGraw-Hill, New York, 1991
6. Felice KJ, Schwartz WJ, Drachman DA: Evaluating the patient with altered consciousness in the intensive care unit. pp. 1546–1553. In Rippe JM, Irwin RS, Alpert JS, Fink MP (eds): Intensive Care Medicine. 2nd Ed. Little Brown, Boston, 1991
7. Chad DA: The Guillain-Barré syndrome. pp. 1591–1595. In Rippe JM, Irwin RS, Alpert JS, Fink MP (eds): Intensive Care Medicine. 2nd Ed. Little Brown, Boston, 1991
8. Long RR: Myasthenia gravis in the intensive care unit. pp. 1596–1601. In Rippe JM, Irwin RS, Alpert JS, Fink MP (eds): Intensive Care Medicine. 2nd Ed. Little Brown, Boston, 1991
9. Growdon JH, Fink JS: Paralysis and movement disorders. In Wilson JD, Braunwald E, Isselbacher KJ et al. (eds): Harrison's Principles of Internal Medicine. 12th Ed. McGraw-Hill, New York, 1991
10. Pierson DJ, Brown GF: Prolonged respiratory paralysis following cutaneous diphtheria. Respir Care 1986;31:1102–1106
11. Mansel JK, Norman JR: Respiratory complications and management of spinal cord injuries. Chest 1990;97:1446–1452
12. Luce JM: Medical management of spinal cord injury. Crit Care Med 1985;13:126–131

13. Albin MS, Gilbert TJ: Acute spinal cord trauma. pp. 1277–1285. In Shoemaker WC, Ayres S, Grenvik A et al. (eds): Textbook of Critical Care. 2nd Ed. WB Saunders, Philadelphia, 1989
14. Weeks EJ, Fiandaca MS: Spinal cord injury. pp. 1478–1489. In Rippe JM, Irwin RS, Alpert JS, Fink MP (eds): Intensive Care Medicine. 2nd Ed. Little Brown, Boston, 1991
15. Bach JR, Alba AS: Noninvasive options for ventilatory support of the traumatic high level quadriplegic patient. Chest 1990; 98:613–619
16. Bouchard C: Acute spinal-cord injury. N Engl J Med 1991; 324:1885–1886
17. Brown SE, Stansbury DW, Merrill EJ et al: Prevention of suctioning-related arterial oxygen desaturation: Comparison of off-ventilator and on-ventilator suctioning. Chest 1983;83:621–627
18. Craig KC, Benson MS, Pierson DJ: Prevention of arterial oxygen desaturation during closed-airway endotracheal suction: Effect of ventilator mode. Respir Care 1984;29:1013–1018
19. Harper CM, Lyles YM: Physiology and complications of bed rest. J Am Geriatr Soc 1988;36:1047–1054
20. Keane FX: The minimum physiological mobility requirement for man supported on a soft surface. Paraplegia 1978–1979;16:383–389
21. Slabaugh PB, Nickel VL: Complications with use of the Stryker frame. J Bone Joint Surg [Am] 1978;60:1111–1112
22. Coppola AR: Stryker frame death. Va Med 1977;104:477–478
23. Smith TK, Whitaker J, Stauffer ES: Complications associated with the use of the circular electrical turning frame. J Bone Joint Surg [Am] 1975;57:711–713
24. Keane FX: Roto-Rest. Br Med J 1967;3:731–732
25. Keane F: Roto-Rest. Paraplegia 1970;7:254–258
26. Schimmel L, Civetta JM, Kirby RR: A new mechanical method to influence pulmonary perfusion in critically ill patients. Crit Care Med 1977;5:277–279
27. Green BA, Green KL, Klose KJ: Kinetic nursing for acute spinal cord injury patients. Paraplegia 1980;18:181–186
28. Brackett TO, Condon N: Comparison of the wedge turning frame and kinetic treatment table in the acute care of spinal cord injury patients. Surg Neurol 1984;22:53–56
29. Reines HD, Harris RC: Pulmonary complications of acute spinal cord injuries. Neurosurgery 1987;21:193–196
30. Becker DM, Gonzalez M, Gentili A et al: Prevention of deep venous thrombosis in patients with acute spinal cord injuries: Use of rotating treatment tables. Neurosurgery 1987;20:675–677
31. Kelly RE, Vibulsresth S, Bell L, Duncan RC: Evaluation of kinetic therapy in the prevention of complications of prolonged bed rest secondary to stroke. Stroke 1987;18:638–642
32. Gentilello L, Thompson DA, Tonnesen AS et al: Effect of a rotating bed on the incidence of pulmonary complications in critically ill patients. Crit Care Med 1988;16:783–786
33. Demarest GB, Schmidt-Nowara WW, Vance LW, Altman AR: Use of the kinetic treatment table to prevent the pulmonary complications of multiple trauma. West J Med 1989;150:35–38
34. Summer WR, Curry P, Haponik EF et al: Continuous mechanical turning of intensive care unit patients shortens length of stay in some diagnostic-related groups. J Crit Care 1989;4:45–53
35. Kelly RE, Bell LK, Mason RL: Cost analysis of kinetic therapy in the prevention of complications of stroke. South Med J 1990; 83:433–434
36. Fink MP, Helsmoortel CM, Stein KL et al: The efficacy of an oscillating bed in the prevention of lower respiratory tract infection in critically ill victims of blunt trauma. Chest 1990; 97:132–137
37. Sahn SA: Continuous lateral rotational therapy and nosocomial pneumonia. Chest 1991;99:1263–1267
38. Kollef MH, Witte MC: Pacing wire-induced recurrent ventricular tachycardia secondary to kinetic therapy bed motion (letter). Crit Care Med 1988;16:651–652
39. Lee S: Intracranial pressure changes during positioning of patients with severe head injury. Heart Lung 1989;18:411–414
40. Gonzalez SM, Goldberg ML, Baumgartner R et al: Analysis of the effect of kinetic therapy on intracranial pressure in comatose neurosurgical patients. Neurosurgery 1983;13:654–656
41. Dail CW, Affeldt JE, Collier CR: Clinical aspects of glossopharyngeal breathing. JAMA 1955;158:445–449
42. Feigelson CI, Dickinson DG, Talner NS, Wilson JL: Glossopharyngeal breathing as an aid to the coughing mechanism in the patient with chronic poliomyelitis in a respirator. N Engl J Med 1956;254:611–613
43. James WS, Minh V, Minteer MA, Moser KM: Cervical accessory respiratory muscle function in a patient with a high cervical cord lesion. Chest 1977;71:59–64
44. Montero JC, Feldman DJ, Montero D: Effects of glossopharyngeal breathing on respiratory function after cervical cord transection. Arch Phys Med Rehabil 1967;48:650–653
45. Siebens AA, Kirby NA, Poulos DA: Cough following transection of spinal cord at C-6. Arch Phys Med Rehabil 1964;45:1–8
46. Kirby NA, Barnerias MJ, Siebens AA: An evaluation of assisted cough in quadriplegic patients. Arch Phys Med Rehabil 1966; 47:705–710
47. Estenne M, DeTroyer A: Mechanism of the postural dependence of vital capacity in tetraplegic subjects. Am Rev Respir Dis 1987; 135:367–371
48. Goldman JM, Rose LS, Williams SJ et al: Effect of abdominal binders on breathing in tetraplegic patients. Thorax 1986; 41:940–945
49. Estenne M, DeTroyer A: Cough in tetraplegic subjects: An active process. Ann Intern Med 1990;112:22–28
50. DeTroyer A, Estenne M, Heilporn A: Mechanism of active expiration in tetraplegic subjects. N Engl J Med 1986;314:740–744
51. Estenne M, Knoop C, Vanvaerenbergh J et al: The effect of pectoralis muscle training in tetraplegic subjects. Am Rev Respir Dis 1989;139:1218–1222
52. Gross D, Ladd HW, Riley EJ et al: The effect of training on strength and endurance of the diaphragm in quadriplegia. Am J Med 1980;68:27–35
53. Wicks AB, Menter RR: Long-term outlook in quadriplegic patients with initial ventilator dependency. Chest 1986;90:406–410
54. McMichan JC, Michel L, Westbrook PR: Pulmonary dysfunction following traumatic quadriplegia. Recognition, prevention, and treatment. JAMA 1980;243:528–531

Chapter 91

Management of the Patient with Chest Trauma

Ray H. Ritz
David J. Pierson

CHAPTER OUTLINE

The human thorax is commonly the unfortunate target for traumatic injury. More than 25 percent of the fatalities associated with automobile accidents result from chest injuries.[1] At the same time, the chest can absorb surprising amounts of trauma without serious injury to the patient. The bony yet flexible rib cage can fend off potentially penetrating objects and diffuse significant blunt shock. Early attention to the maintenance of ventilation and cardiovascular function can help reduce the mortality associated with chest trauma. One study suggested that almost one-third of more than 600 traumatic deaths could have been prevented if a more organized approach had been used in caring for the injured.[2]

Chest trauma occurs in two forms; blunt chest trauma and penetrating injuries. Either type of injury can be categorized either as immediately life-threatening or as potentially life-threatening. This chapter reviews briefly the different forms of traumatic chest injury encountered by the clinician and outlines current approaches to stabilization and management. For more comprehensive information the reader is referred to several recent texts[3–7] and reviews[8–10] on thoracic trauma.

Trauma to the chest may be thought of as involving four general anatomic regions or types of structure: the thoracic cage, the conducting airways, the lung parenchyma, and the pleural space. A fifth category, diaphragmatic injury, although uncommon, is nonetheless clinically important when it does occur. Within several of these regions or categories there are important clinical subgroupings, as outlined in Table 91-1.

RIB FRACTURES AND FLAIL CHEST

Although the rib cage affords significant protection to underlying thoracic organs, blunt or penetrating trauma can damage this bony system. Ribs 4 to 10 are those most likely to be fractured during blunt chest trauma. The shoulder girdle and scapula provide protection to ribs 1 to 3 and ribs 11

Table 91-1. Chest Trauma: Types of Injury, Clinical Presentations, and Approaches to Management

Injury	Clinical Presentation	Assessment and Management
Rib fractures	Chest wall pain (may not correlate with number of fractures) Splinting Dyspnea Hypoxemia (especially if associated contusion)	Suspect hemothorax/pneumothorax Suspect major vessel or tracheobronchial injury with fracture of ribs 1 and/or 2 Pain control; consider intercostal or epidural analgesics Supplemental O_2
Flail chest	Paradoxical chest wall motion with breathing; palpable fractures and/or flail Severe respiratory distress Acute oxygenation and/or ventilation failure	Suspect contusion, hemothorax, pneumothorax Pain management; consider epidural catheter Supplemental O_2 Lung expansion therapy Consider mechanical ventilation and/or positive end-expiratory pressure (PEEP)
Tracheobronchial injury	Pneumothorax Bronchopleural air leak Failure of lung to re-expand with chest tube suction Massive subcutaneous emphysema Hemoptysis	Suspect in presence of rib 1 and/or 2 or scapular fractures Suspect associated great vessel injury Bronchoscopy to confirm diagnosis Surgical repair
Pulmonary laceration	Pneumothorax Bronchopleural air leak Hemoptysis Hemothorax	Chest tube Bronchoscopy to rule out large airway injury Surgical exploration if air leak unmanageable or continued massive bleeding
Pulmonary contusion	Focal infiltrate on chest radiograph in same area as blunt trauma Hypoxemia (risk for developing adult respiratory distress syndrome [ARDS]) Hemoptysis	Supplemental O_2 PEEP therapy if required to support oxygenation Mechanical ventilation if severe or associated injuries
Pneumothorax	Pleuritic chest pain Dyspnea; tachypnea Evidence of other forms of extra-alveolar air Increased resonance and decreased breath sounds on ipsilateral side, if large (inconsistent, unreliable)	Chest tube drainage[a] Supplemental O_2
Tension pneumothorax	Expansion and hyperresonance of affected side Tracheal deviation Severe respiratory distress Cardiovascular collapse	Immediate decompression with chest tube or (if not immediately available) large-gauge needle
Pneumomediastinum	Air in mediastinum and/or neck on chest radiograph Chest pain Crunching sound with cardiac cycle on auscultation	Suspect airway injury Be prepared to treat pneumothorax (no specific therapy needed)
Subcutaneous emphysema	Crepitus over anterior neck and/or chest, spreading widely over body Subcutaneous/intermuscular air on chest radiograph	Suspect airway injury Suspect pneumothorax (no specific therapy needed)
Air embolism	Focal neurologic symptoms or signs without evidence for head injury Cardiovascular collapse	Positioning Hyperbaric O_2 therapy
Hemothorax	Dyspnea Dullness to percussion and diminished breath sounds over affected side Radiographic signs of pleural fluid (nonspecific on supine film)	Suspect in penetrating chest trauma Chest tube Thoracotomy if massive or continued bleeding
Diaphragmatic injury	Bowel air in hemithorax on initial radiograph Presence may only be detected during surgery	Surgical exploration and repair

[a] Some have advocated simple aspiration of small uncomplicated traumatic pneumothorax; all cases should be followed closely.

and 12 are flexible and small so that fractures of these two groups are rare.[11] Fractures of ribs 1 and 2 are frequently accompanied by severe head, neck, and thoracic organ injuries; and the mortality rate can approach 50 percent.[12]

The fracture of one or two ribs, albeit painful, may be of little consequence. Without significant injury to the underlying lung, effective pain management outside the hospital may be all that is required. On the other hand, the same injury may cause laceration of the lung beneath the rib or be accompanied by a serious contusion to the parenchyma.

In patients with advanced chronic lung disease, inadequate pain control alone may compromise pulmonary mechanics, leading to atelectasis or pneumonia.

No specific treatment is generally required to repair rib fractures (Table 91-1). In any patient whose pain is so severe as to limit normal breathing, intercostal nerve blocks can be useful in providing adequate relief while avoiding the respiratory depression that accompanies systemic analgesia. Once the pain is controlled, effective lung inflation and pulmonary hygiene techniques (incentive spirometry, deep breathing, and coughing) can be employed with much more success.

As the number of rib fractures increases, so does the incidence of thoracic and abdominal organ injury. When multiple ribs are fractured in more than one place, the chest wall may become unstable and a *flail chest* may develop[13] (Fig. 91-1). With this condition, during inspiration the affected portion of the chest wall moves inward owing to the more negative pleural pressure and then moves outward during exhalation. The actual paradoxical movement may not appear immediately after injury because of the splinting provided by the intercostal muscles. As the patient fatigues or relaxes in response to sedation or as lung compliance decreases with fluid resuscitation or progression of consolidation from contusion or aspiration, the flail may then develop.

Until recently there has been controversy over the need for stabilization of the chest wall via mechanical ventilation. However, it is now established that patients with flail chest should not be managed differently from others with blunt chest trauma.[13–16] With only minor complicating injuries, appropriate supplemental O_2 and analgesia, along with aggressive pulmonary hygiene, may suffice. In the face of poor gas exchange, increased work of breathing, or significant other injuries, mechanical ventilation is indicated. Development of impaired gas exchange and increased work of breathing, while associated with an unstable chest wall, are in reality related to underlying pulmonary contusion and other injury.

TRACHEOBRONCHIAL INJURY

Tracheobronchial injuries are uncommon but may occur after major chest injury.[17–19] Because the trachea is free to move from the neck down to the carinal bifurcation and the bronchi are tethered to the lung parenchyma beyond the lobar level, shear forces during deceleration injury are greatest within 5 cm of the main carina, and the great majority of tracheobronchial injuries occur here. These injuries range from barely visible mucosal tears to through-and-through transection of the trachea or a main bronchus. These injuries usually produce large air leaks, often with failure of the collapsed lung to re-expand under chest tube suction[17] (Fig. 91-2), and there is often bleeding into the airway. Early diagnosis and repair are essential, even with smaller tears, as these can lead to the later formation of strictures, with post-obstructive pneumonias and eventual bronchiectasis.

INJURY TO THE LUNG PARENCHYMA

Pulmonary Laceration

Pulmonary lacerations can accompany rib fractures, penetrating injuries (from knives, bullets, etc), or rapid deceleration injuries.[20–22] They can involve pneumothorax, hemothorax, or airway injuries and surgical repair may be necessary (Table 91-1). If the injury involves a major bronchus, extensive airway bleeding may occur. Pulmonary lacerations

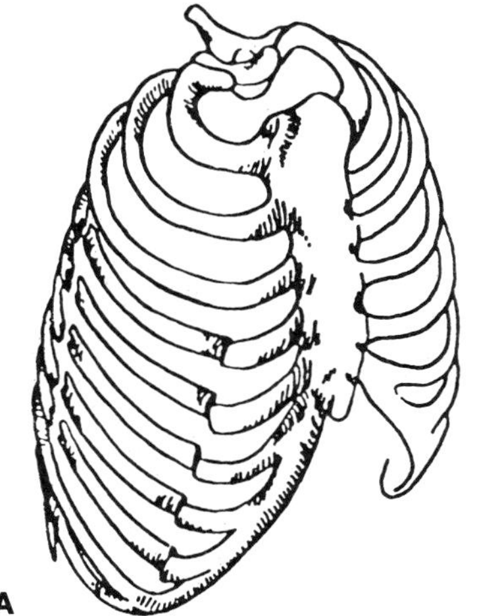

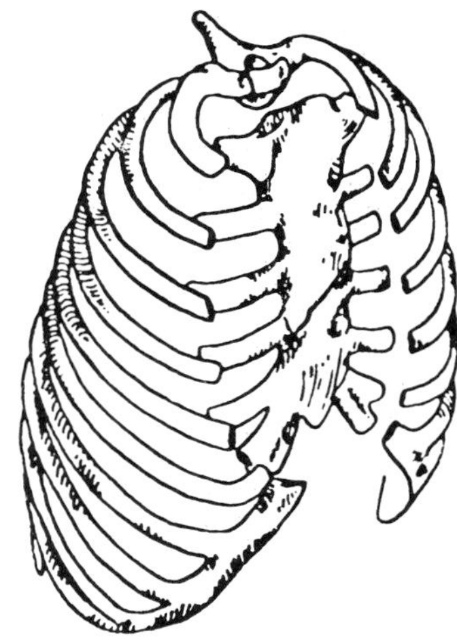

Figure 91-1. Flail chest. The fracture of three or more ribs in two places seriously affects the integrity of the chest wall, which can allow the injured portion to become free-floating. (**A**) A lateral injury and (**B**) an anterior injury resulting from trauma to the sternum are shown. Paradoxical movement may occur as the patient fatigues or as narcotics or sedatives are administered. The accompanying impairment of gas exchange is generally related to the underlying lung contusion. (From Moore,[5] with permission.)

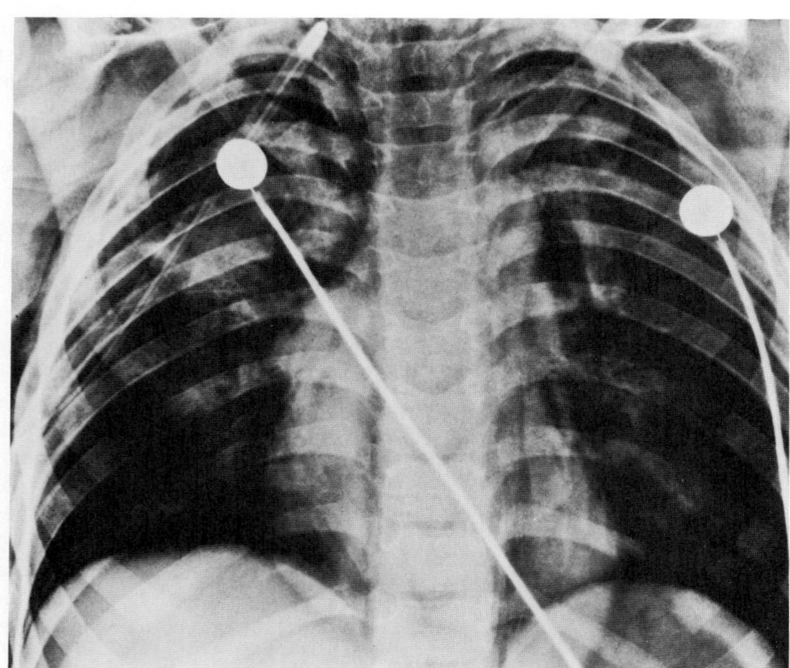

Figure 91-2. Chest radiograph of a patient with traumatic right upper lobe bronchial rupture. There is a large persistent pneumothorax despite the presence of a chest tube, and the right upper lobe has fallen away from the hilum. (From Groskin et al.,[52] with permission.)

often lead to localized hematomas in the lung, and these may subsequently cavitate. Localized collections of extra-alveolar air in an area of lung contusion should suggest the presence of pulmonary laceration (Fig. 91-3).

If the injury is unilateral and massive, selectively ventilating the unaffected lung may be useful. Selective intubation of a main-stem bronchus can be difficult to accomplish and requires a skilled physician. Once intubation is achieved, the patient must be quickly transported to the operating room for repair.

If mechanical ventilation is required once the bronchus is repaired, excessive airway pressures should be avoided. Pressure-limited ventilation offers the advantage of controlling airway pressures, but tidal volumes and minute ventilation may vary depending on the patient's synchrony with the ventilator. Volume-controlled ventilation provides constant minute ventilation but can allow unacceptable pressures to develop unless tidal volumes are limited to those on the steep portion of the compliance curve. However, either mode of ventilation can be used if carefully applied.

Pulmonary Contusion

As traumatic force is transmitted through the chest wall to the lung parenchyma, the result may be a focal injury characterized by interstitial and intra-alveolar hemorrhage and edema.[22] This disruption of the alveolar-capillary interface is accompanied by increased intrapulmonary shunting, decreased functional residual capacity, and impaired oxygenation. The appearance of these physiologic events can be delayed by as much as 8 to 24 hours, although a focal radiographic abnormality is generally present on admission to the emergency department (Fig. 91-4). As the process progresses, compliance decreases and work of breathing increases. Atelectasis and pneumonia can often accompany the injury.

Treatment of pulmonary contusion includes the use of supplemental O_2 to reverse any hypoxemia and diligent pulmonary hygiene (Table 91-1). If significant impairment to gas exchange or increased work of breathing occurs, the application of continuous positive airway pressure (CPAP) or positive end-expiratory pressure (PEEP) and mechanical ventilation is warranted. Without complications, a pulmonary contusion will gradually resolve within 7 days. Pulmonary contusions may progress into severe adult respiratory distress syndrome (ARDS) and be associated with high mortality.

EXTRA-ALVEOLAR AIR (BAROTRAUMA)

Pneumothorax

Pneumothorax and tension pneumothorax may present either at the time of injury or during the recuperative period. The initial thoracic assessment should include investigation for the presence of free air in the pleural space.

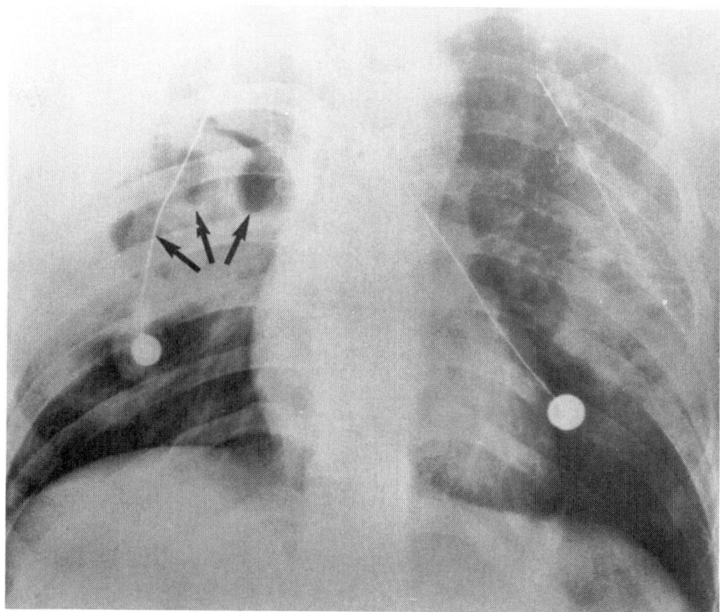

Figure 91-3. Chest radiograph of a patient with bilateral lung contusions and right-sided pulmonary lacerations, leading to extra-alveolar air collections within the contused lung (arrows). The contused areas are seen as focal areas of airspace density. A chest tube is present on the left side. (From Shulman and Samuels,[17] with permission.)

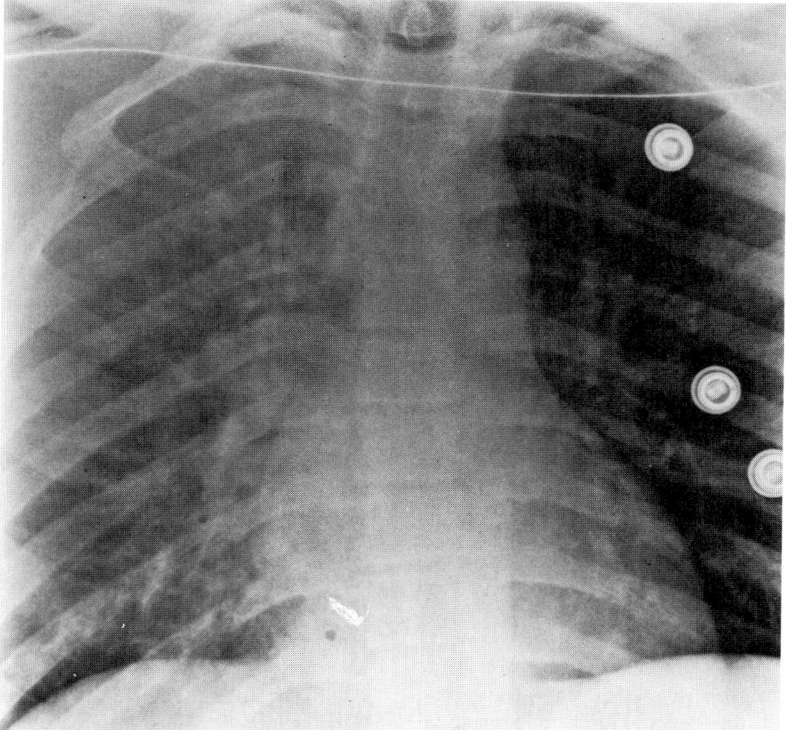

Figure 91-4. A more diffuse lung contusion is seen on this chest radiograph obtained on arrival in the emergency department following blunt trauma. The entire upper right lung is denser than the left, although not yet so densely consolidated as the contused areas in Figure 91-3. (From Groskin et al.,[52] with permission.)

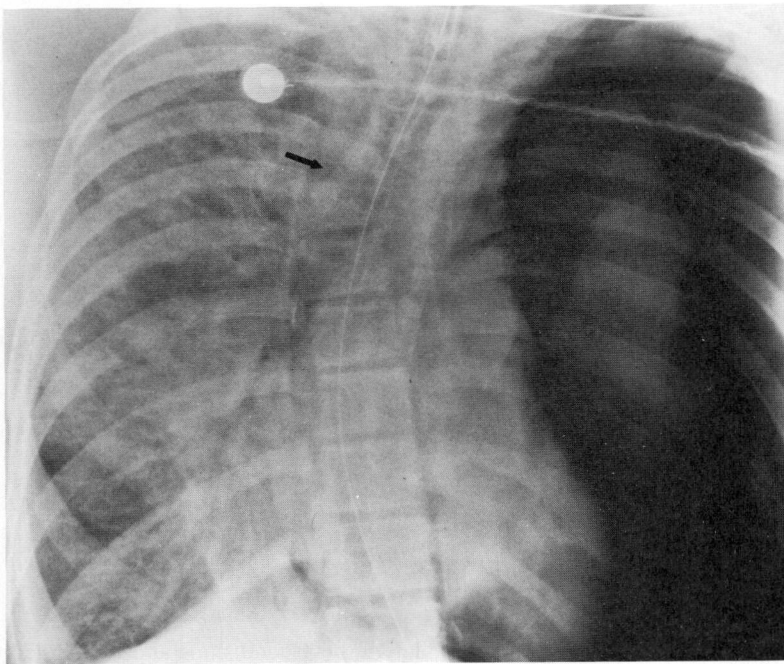

Figure 91-5. Left-sided tension pneumothorax, with contralateral whole lung atelectasis, following blunt chest trauma. The mediastinum is shifted dramatically away from the pneumothorax, and the atelectatic left lung is seen as a contracted mass about the hilum. The arrow points to a T5–T6 vertebral fracture dislocation. (From Groskin et al.,[52] with permission.)

The presence of one or more of the physical findings listed in Table 91-1 should trigger a further assessment with a posteroanterior chest film rather than the usual anteroposterior bedside radiograph. Small pneumothoraces may be overlooked by a physical examination, and a pneumothorax of less than 10 percent may even be difficult to determine radiographically. The presence of rib fractures should prompt a careful examination for pneumothoraces, since the jagged ends of broken ribs can easily injure the underlying parenchyma; however, the absence of rib fractures in blunt trauma does not eliminate the risk of pneumothorax. It has been demonstrated that deceleration injuries can produce barotrauma without injury to the rib cage.[23]

The presence of tracheal deviation and hyperinflation of a hemithorax are indications of a medical emergency due to a tension pneumothorax (Fig. 91-5). Immediate placement of a chest tube is essential. If this is not immediately possible, a large-bore needle may be inserted into the second intercostal space at the midclavicular line.

Chest trauma patients who are supported by mechanical ventilation can develop pneumothoraces as a result of air trapping or parenchymal defect.[24] In this setting, the event is generally accompanied by a sudden reduction in arterial O_2 saturation (SaO_2), alteration in blood pressure, tachycardia or bradycardia, and increased ventilating pressures. Placement of an anterior chest tube into the affected area is the definitive therapy.

Pneumomediastinum

Pneumomediastinum (Fig. 91-6) can occur both with chest injury and with facial trauma.[24,25] In patients with pneumomediastinum the possibility of tears of the esophagus and the tracheobronchial tree should be considered. The development of a pneumothorax is also possible, and the capability for emergent pleural decompression should be readily at hand. Treatment of the underlying cause of the pneumomediastinum generally results in resolution of the complication, and no specific therapy is needed[25,26] (Table 91-1).

Subcutaneous Emphysema

Subcutaneous emphysema often presents as free air in the neck and chest wall and may develop by several mechanisms. It may dissect into the tissue planes from wounds in the skin or may move up the mediastinum and into the subcutaneous tissues from the root of the lung after alveolar laceration or rupture. Although subcutaneous emphysema itself is of little concern, it may indicate the presence of other barotrauma. It also complicates the assessment of chest radiographs by obscuring many features. No specific treatment is required[25,26] (Table 91-1). The condition generally presents

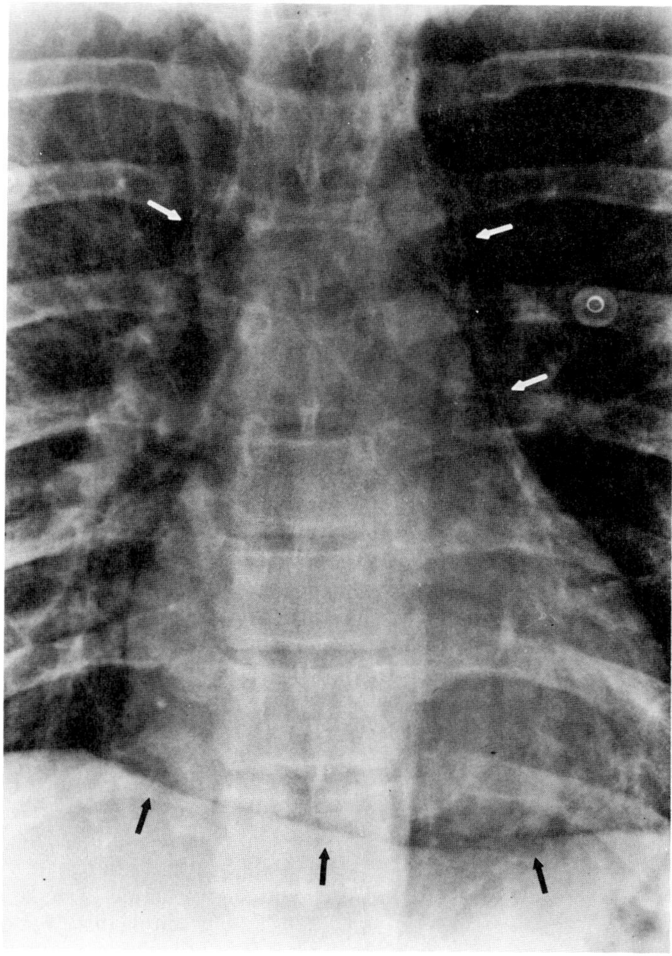

Figure 91-6. Pneumomediastinum, seen on a frontal chest radiograph taken following blunt chest trauma. There is lateral displacement of the mediastinal (parietal) pleura (white arrows), clear definition of the aortic knob, and the "continuous diaphragm sign" (black arrows) characteristic of pneumomediastinum. (From Groskin et al.,[52] with permission.)

no significant discomfort for the patient and will resolve as the air is reabsorbed.

Air Embolism

Air embolism is a rare complication associated with chest trauma and surgical procedures.[27–29] It may occur with pulmonary lacerations, as a result of accidental entry through central intravenous lines, or during cardiopulmonary bypass. Diagnosis of air embolism is difficult. Patients with focal neurologic symptoms and no evidence of head injury or with sudden cardiovascular collapse in the presence of the above risk factors should be evaluated for this devastating complication.

HEMOTHORAX

Hemothorax can range in severity from asymptomatic to the cause of profound shock. Studies have reported over 70 percent of patients with blunt chest trauma have accompanying hemothorax of some degree.[20,30] The source of bleeding for small hemothoraces is often pulmonary contusions or lacerations. Massive hemothorax (greater than 2000 mL) generally results from the rupture of a major pulmonary artery or vein and may also be the result of an injury to one of the great systemic vessels of the thorax.

Hemothorax is treated by insertion of a posterolateral chest tube and adequate fluid resuscitation as needed (Table 91-1). If substantial bleeding continues (e.g., at a rate exceeding 200 mL/h) after the chest tube is placed, surgical intervention is required. Undrained hemothoraces may result in the development of empyema or eventual scarring and calcification of the pleura, producing a restrictive ventilatory defect.

INJURY TO THE DIAPHRAGM

Diaphragmatic injury has been reported in association with both blunt and penetrating chest trauma.[31–34] It is more common with the latter, particularly with gunshot and knife injuries. If the injury is significant, abdominal contents can spill into the thorax and compress the adjacent lung (Fig. 91-7). The invading gastrointestinal tissue is also at risk for ischemia. Unless abdominal contents spill into the chest, diaphragmatic injuries may go undetected[35]; many are discovered only while exploring the abdomen for other injuries. Even small diaphragmatic tears must be surgically repaired, but the injury, if small, may present no immediate risk since the use of accessory muscles can provide adequate ventilation (Table 91-1).

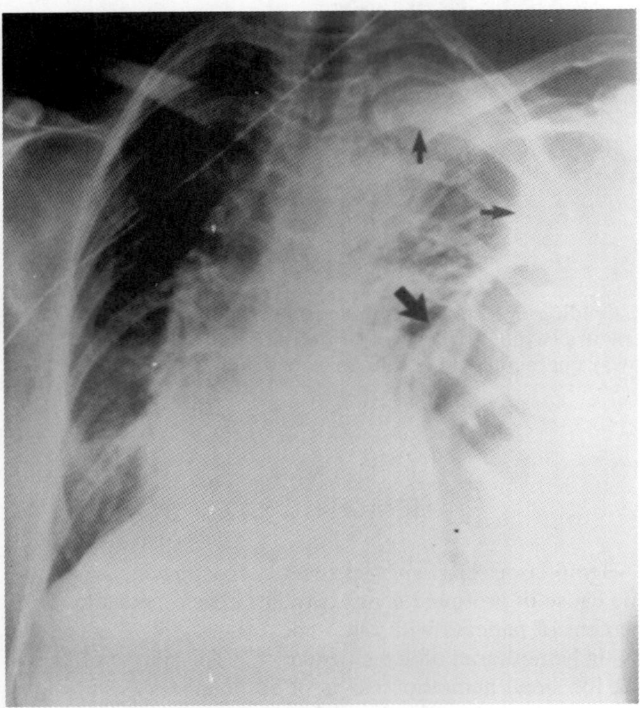

Figure 91-7. Chest radiograph of a patient with a ruptured left hemidiaphragm secondary to blunt thoracoabdominal trauma. The stomach has herniated into the left chest (large arrow), and there is a large hemothorax (small arrows). The splenic flexure of the colon has also herniated into the chest and can be seen through the stomach bubble. The mediastinum has shifted to the right. At laparotomy the spleen was also found to be ruptured. (From Shulman and Samuels,[17] with permission.)

APPROACHES TO MANAGEMENT

Initial Stabilization

The fundamental considerations that apply to cardiopulmonary resuscitation (CPR) (see Ch. 95) also apply to patients with chest trauma.[8,9,36] The first priority is to ensure that there is a patent airway.[37–39] The appearance of spontaneous ventilation is a favorable sign but represents no guarantee that the patient possesses a fully patent airway or that ventilation is adequate. The quality of the airway and the patient's overall work of breathing should be quickly assessed, since evidence of increased work of breathing can be an indication of any number of injuries. If spontaneous ventilation is absent or significantly compromised or if there is evidence of injury to the airway itself, the prompt placement of an artificial airway is indicated. Supra- and substernal retractions, nasal flaring, intercostal retractions, inspiratory stridor, and agonal respirations all require ruling out injury to the upper airway. If intubation is indicated, placement of an oral endotracheal tube is generally the procedure of choice. This procedure is complicated in trauma patients, since cervical injury should be assumed until definitively ruled out. In a review of over 10,000 automobile accident victims, 1 in 300 sustained severe neck injuries.[40]

Once patency of the airway is achieved, adequate oxygenation and ventilation must be ensured. Application of O_2 at an inspired O_2 fraction (F_{IO_2}) of 1.0 until the patient's status is determined is rarely contraindicated. Manual ventilation with a self-inflating resuscitator is the quickest method to achieve adequate ventilation. During manual ventilation, it is simple to make a gross assessment of the patient's lung compliance. Patients for whom it is difficult to provide ventilation should be immediately examined for the presence of a pneumothorax. Auscultation of the chest is simple to perform and its findings, combined with other symptoms such as tracheal deviation away from the silent lung and hyperresonance of the affected side, make the presence of free air in the pleural space probable. Decompression of the thorax is essential.

A rapid assessment of cardiovascular status should be made simultaneously with the stabilization of ventilation. Blood pressure should be normalized by administration of appropriate fluid, improvement of cardiac performance, and closed chest compressions if necessary. Once the patient is hemodynamically stable, attention can be directed to other systems and injuries. It is critical that the initial assessment be made and initial treatment instituted as rapidly as possible.

Bronchopulmonary Hygiene

The more severe the trauma to the chest, the more attentive one must be to issues of pulmonary hygiene. Patients must be encouraged to vigorously cough and breathe deeply with regular frequency. Splinting the chest wall with pillows may help promote adequate effort. An incentive spirometry device is often useful for quantifying for both patient and clinician the appropriateness of inspired volumes. The patient should be coached to inspire slowly to maximal lung volume on each maneuver. Lung inflation adjuncts such as intermittent positive-pressure breathing (IPPB) should be used only when there is evidence of their effectiveness. Patients should demonstrate an improvement in inspiratory capacity during IPPB of more than 25 percent over their spontaneous effort.[41]

Frequent position changes are of great benefit. Turning from side to side is important for patients unable to get out of bed. Individuals who are able to walk unassisted may need little assistance in their pulmonary hygiene.

Chest percussion and postural drainage are useful when the cough mechanism is poor and secretion production is high. For treating acute lobar collapse, it has been shown that vigorous chest physiotherapy can be as effective as bronchoscopy in re-expanding the atelectatic area.[42] This is less true in the radiographic presence of air bronchograms, since the collapse in that case is a result of tissue edema and not of excessive secretions and therefore therapies directed at clearing secretions are less effective.

Chest percussion and postural drainage are not without complications. Decreases in PaO_2 and SaO_2 have been noted, as well as increases in intracranial pressure.[43] Recent pulmonary hemorrhage and rib fractures are considered relative contraindications to these therapies. Patients experiencing cardiovascular instability, arrhythmias, or significant hypoxemia may not tolerate chest percussion and drainage and must be closely monitored if treated.[44] This should include continuous monitoring of cardiac rhythm, blood pressure, and SaO_2.

Aggressive pulmonary hygiene is essential in mechanical ventilator-supported chest trauma patients with pneumonia, pulmonary contusions, or underlying chronic lung disease. Regular nasotracheal or endotracheal suctioning is important if secretion clearance is compromised. Manual hyperinflation at regular intervals will help avoid atelectasis and low lung volumes. The frequency of hyperinflation and suctioning should be directly related to the severity of illness. Suctioning should be performed when the patient shows signs of increased work of breathing such as increased respiratory rate, shallow tidal volumes, or retractions or when breath sounds indicate the presence of secretions.

Pain Control

Effective pain control is essential in managing patients with chest injuries. Without it, pulmonary hygiene is significantly complicated, as is the ability to maintain adequate lung volumes. The use of intravenous narcotics is useful as long as the patient is not oversedated. If the patient is receiving full ventilation, this may not be a concern—indeed it may be preferable. Oversedation can blunt respiratory drive, however, and reduce the patient's participation in secretion clearance.

Two techniques that are useful are patient-controlled analgesia (PCA) and epidural narcotics. Microprocessor-controlled systems used with PCA allow the patient to self-administer programmed amounts of narcotics at designated intervals. Over-medication can be avoided by programming the system to limit the amount and frequency of administration. Epidural narcotic analgesics are administered through a catheter placed in the epidural space of the spinal column. When the catheter is correctly placed, this technique avoids the respiratory depression associated with narcotics while effectively eliminating chest wall pain.

Patients being managed with epidural narcotics must be closely monitored after the catheter is placed. Improper catheter placement can result in respiratory depression by failing to contain the narcotic inside the epidural space. Some have advocated that patients receiving epidural narcotics be monitored with capnographs to detect periods of hypoventilation or apnea, but this is seldom necessary—regular observation by nurses or respiratory care clinicians is generally adequate. With the pain controlled, the patient may feel comfortable and not motivated to regularly cough and breathe deeply. Atelectasis can occur in spite of the patient's apparent sense of well-being.

Mechanical Ventilation

Mechanical ventilation is indicated in chest trauma patients when gas exchange is impaired, work of breathing is excessive, or the patient's overall physiology is unstable. The variety of modes of ventilation available today allows great flexibility in supporting ventilation.

Blunt chest trauma with accompanying pulmonary contusion generally requires support of oxygenation. Conservatively, this can be accomplished with supplemental O_2 or CPAP. CPAP can be used successfully when treating the hypoxemia accompanying mild to moderate pulmonary contusions or to assist in stabilizing a flail chest. It also is useful in reducing the work of breathing in patients who develop air trapping from early airway closure.[45]

If the patient's $PaCO_2$ rises to unacceptable levels or fatigue is eminent owing to excessive work of breathing, the use of intermittent mandatory ventilation (IMV) is common. As the patient's need for ventilation increases, the base rate should be increased to keep the imposed work at an acceptable limit. When the goal is to minimize work of breathing, the IMV rate should be increased to a level that provides the patient's total minute ventilation needs. To completely eliminate patient work, sedation or paralysis may be necessary.

An alternative to IMV is pressure-support ventilation (PSV). This mode is completely patient-triggered and supports spontaneous ventilation by providing preset levels of pressure during inspiration. As discussed further in Chapter 83, PSV can be used to overcome the resistance of the endotracheal tube or to reduce the patient's overall work. PSV can be used in conjunction with IMV or as a stand-alone mode.

PEEP is often used to increase lung volumes,[46] to improve oxygenation, to avoid high F_{IO_2} values,[47] or to reduce work of breathing in patients with chest trauma.[48] It can be applied in conjunction with either IMV or PSV. However, it carries the risk of impaired cardiac output[49] and barotrauma.[24] PEEP is applied by mechanical ventilators and CPAP devices by controlling the amount of gas exhaled from the system (see Ch. 76).

PEEP can also develop inadvertently as a result of incomplete exhalation.[50] This effect, termed *auto-PEEP*, is not evident on pressure-sensing devices positioned in the external breathing circuit. The risk factors for auto-PEEP include obstructive lung disease, advanced age, high minute ventilations and respiratory rates, bronchospasm, and small endotracheal tubes.[51] The clinical responses are directed at increasing expiratory time, allowing increased spontaneous ventilation, and reducing the resistance to expiratory flows (see Chs. 76 and 84).

Chapter 92 deals in detail with management of persistent bronchopleural air leaks. Severe chest trauma can include injuries that allow significant amounts of delivered tidal volumes to leak out of chest tubes. Increasing the delivered tidal volume to compensate for this is not generally recommended.

References

1. Blair E, Topuzlu C, Deane RS: Major blunt chest trauma. Curr Probl Surg 1969;17:1–64
2. Van Wagoner FH: Died in the hospital: A three year study of deaths following trauma. J Trauma 1961;1:401–408
3. Moore EE, Mattox KL, Feliciano DV (eds): Trauma. 2nd Ed. Appleton & Lange, East Norwalk, CT, 1991
4. Trunkey DD, Lewis FR Jr, (eds): Current Therapy of Trauma. BC Decker, Philadelphia, 1991
5. Moore EE (ed): Early Care of the Trauma Patient. BC Decker, Philadelphia, 1990
6. McMurtry RY, McLellan BA (eds): Management of Blunt Trauma. Williams & Wilkins, Baltimore, 1990
7. Zuidema GD, Rutherford RB, Ballinger WF II (eds): The Management of Trauma. 4th Ed. WB Saunders, Philadelphia, 1985
8. Trunkey D: Initial treatment of patients with extensive trauma. N Engl J Med 1991;324:1259–1263
9. Brunko MW, Rosen P: Blunt and penetrating chest trauma. pp. 98–104. In Callaham ML (ed): Current Practice of Emergency Medicine. 2nd Ed. BC Decker, Philadelphia, 1991
10. Clemmer TP, Fairfax WR: Critical care management of chest injury. Crit Care Clin 1986;2:759–773
11. Bertelson S, Bugge-Asperheim B, Geiran O et al: Thoracic injuries. Ann Chir Gynaecol 1981;70:237–250
12. Wilson JM, Thomas AN, Goodman PC et al: Severe chest trauma: Morbidity implication of first and second rib fractures in 120 patients. Arch Surg 1978;113:846–849
13. Moore FA, Haenel JB, Moore EE: Flail chest/pulmonary contusion: A surgical critical care challenge. Curr Pulmonol 1991;12:223–259
14. Trinkle JK, Richardson JD, Franz JL et al: Management of flail chest without mechanical ventilation. Ann Thorac Surg 1975;19:355–363
15. Sladen A, Aldredge CF, Albarran R: PEEP vs ZEEP in the treatment of flail chest injuries. Crit Care Med 1973;1:187–191
16. Shackford SR, Virgilio RW, Peters RM: Selective use of ventilator therapy in flail chest injury. J Thorac Cardiovasc Surg 1981;81:194–201
17. Shulman HS, Samuels TH: The radiology of blunt chest trauma. Can Assoc Radiol J 1983;34:204–217
18. Wiot JF: Tracheobronchial trauma. Semin Roentgenol 1983;18:15–22
19. Mulder DS, Barkum JS: Injury to the trachea, bronchus, and esophagus. pp. 343–356. In Moore EE, Mattox KL, Feliciano DV (eds): Trauma. 2nd Ed. Appleton & Lange, East Norwalk, CT, 1991
20. Gray AR, Harrison WH, Coures CM et al: Penetrating injuries to the chest. Am J Surg 1960;100:709–714
21. Beall AC, Bricker DL: Considerations in the management of penetrating thoracic trauma. J Trauma 1968;8:408–417
22. Eddy AC, Carrico CJ, Rusch VR: Injury to the lung and pleura. pp. 357–372. In Moore EE, Mattox KL, Feliciano DV (eds): Trauma. 2nd Ed. Appleton & Lange, East Norwalk, CT, 1991
23. Robertson HT, Lakshminarayan S, Hudson LD: Lung injury following a 50 meter fall into water. Thorax 1978;33:175–180
24. Pierson DJ: Alveolar rupture during mechanical ventilation: Role of PEEP, peak airway pressure, and distending volume. Respir Care 1988;33:472–486
25. Cianchetti JA, Carroll GF: Traumatic pneumomediastinum resulting from facial trauma. Ann Emerg Med 1980;9:218–221
26. Maunder RJ, Pierson DJ, Hudson LD: Subcutaneous and mediastinal emphysema: Pathophysiology, diagnosis, and management. Arch Intern Med 1984;144:1447–1453
27. Von Bahr V: Gas embolism originating in the pulmonary veins. Ups Lakareforenings Fordandlingar 1944;49:259–265
28. Macho JR: Air embolism. pp. 226–227. In Trunkey DD, Lewis FR Jr (eds): Current Therapy of Trauma. BC Decker, Philadelphia, 1991
29. Yee ES, Verrier ED, Thomas AN: Management of air embolism in blunt and penetrating trauma. J Thorac Cardiovasc Surg 1983;85:661–668
30. Harrison WH, Gray AR, Coures CM et al: Severe nonpenetrating injuries to the chest: Clinical results in the management of 216 patients. Am J Surg 1960;100:715–722
31. Drews JA, Mercer EC, Benfield JR: Acute diaphragmatic injuries. Ann Thorac Surg 1973;16:67–78
32. Horn JK: Diaphragm injuries. pp. 240–243. In Trunkey DD, Lewis FR Fr (eds): Current Therapy of Trauma. BC Decker, Philadelphia, 1991
33. Taylor GA: Traumatic rupture of the diaphragm. pp. 199–205. In McMurtry RY, McLellan BA (eds): Management of Blunt Trauma. Williams & Wilkins, Baltimore, 1990
34. Root HD: Injury to the diaphragm. pp. 427–440. In Moore EE, Mattox KL, Feliciano DV (eds): Trauma. 2nd Ed. Appleton & Lange, East Norwalk, CT, 1991
35. Blair E: Delayed or missed diagnosis in blunt chest trauma. J Trauma 1971;11:129–145
36. Collicott PE: Initial assessment of the trauma patient. pp. 109–126. In Moore EE, Mattox KL, Feliciano DV (eds): Trauma. 2nd Ed. Appleton & Lange, East Norwalk, CT, 1991
37. Grande CM, Stene JK, Bernhard WN: Airway management: Considerations in the trauma patient. Crit Care Clin 1990;6:37–59
38. Phillips TF: Airway management. pp. 127–146. In Moore EE, Mattox KL, Feliciano DV (eds): Trauma. 2nd Ed. Appleton & Lange, East Norwalk, CT, 1991
39. Stewart RD: Airway management in trauma resuscitation. pp. 37–64. In McMurtry RY, McLellan BA (eds): Management of Blunt Trauma. Williams & Wilkins, Baltimore, 1990
40. Huelke DF, O'Day J, Mendelsohn RA: Cervical injuries suffered in automobile crashes. J Neurosurg 1981;54:316–322
41. American Thoracic Society Respiratory Care Committee. Guidelines for the use of intermittent positive pressure breathing (IPPB). Respir Care 1980;25:365–370
42. Marini JJ, Pierson DJ, Hudson LD: Acute lobar atelectasis: A prospective comparison of fiberoptic bronchoscopy and respiratory therapy. Am Rev Respir Dis 1979;119:971–978

43. Tyler ML: Complications of positioning and chest physiotherapy. Respir Care 1982;27:458–466
44. Luce JM, Tyler ML, Pierson DJ: Intensive Respiratory Care. 2nd Ed. WB Saunders, Philadelphia, 1992
45. Stock CM, Downs JB, Gauer PK: Prevention of pulmonary complications with CPAP, incentive spirometry, and conservative therapy. Chest 1985;87:151–157
46. Daley BD, Edmonds CH, Norman JC: In vivo morphometrics with positive end-expiratory pressure. Surg Forum 1973;24:217–219
47. Pepe PE, Hudson LD, Carrico CJ: Early application of positive end-expiratory pressure in patients at risk for the adult respiratory distress syndrome. N Engl J Med 1984;311:281–286
48. Smith TC, Marini JJ: Impact of PEEP on lung mechanics and work of breathing in severe airflow obstruction. J Appl Physiol 1988;65:1488–1499
49. Harken AH, Brennan MF, Smith B et al: The hemodynamic effect of positive end-expiratory ventilation in hypovolemic patients. Surgery 1974;76:786–793
50. Pepe PE, Marini JJ: Occult positive end-expiratory pressure in mechanically ventilated patients with airflow obstruction. Am Rev Respir Dis 1982;126:166–170
51. Benson MS, Pierson DJ: Auto-PEEP during mechanical ventilation of adults. Respir Care 1988;33:557–565
52. Groskin S, Maresca M, Heitzman ER: Thoracic trauma. pp. 75–127. In McCort JJ (ed): Trauma Radiology. Churchill Livingstone, New York, 1990

Chapter 92

Management of Pneumothorax, Bronchopleural Fistula, and Pleural Effusion

David J. Pierson

CHAPTER OUTLINE

Disorders of the pleural space are encountered in many clinical settings, and a conceptual understanding of the principles of their management is important for effective therapy and patient safety. This chapter presents the basic approaches to therapy for the three categories of pleural disease most often dealt with in respiratory care. Background information on the disorders covered here can be found in Chapters 6 and 84 and also in several general references to the management of pleural disease.[1–4]

PNEUMOTHORAX

Therapy for pneumothorax[4,5] depends in part on its cause and clinical setting but in general requires evacuation of the pleural air (Table 92-1). The only exceptions are primary (simple) spontaneous pneumothorax (a specific disorder most commonly seen in slender young men without other pulmonary disease) and iatrogenic pneumothorax (as may occur following bronchoscopic lung biopsy or central intravenous line placement), and even then only when the air collection is small. In certain settings simple aspiration of the pneumothorax is sufficient, but in all seriously ill patients and in those with underlying lung disease, insertion of a chest (thoracostomy) tube is necessary. The lung will usually re-expand spontaneously, although it is common practice to initially connect the chest tube to suction. Once the lung has re-expanded and no air has leaked through the chest tube for 24 hours, the tube is connected to water seal for another day; if the lung remains expanded, the tube is then removed.

Care must be used in rapidly evacuating a large pneumothorax, particularly when the lung is completely collapsed and the pneumothorax has been present for several days or longer. Hypotension[6] and life-threatening re-expansion pulmonary edema[7] may occur in this setting, but their likelihood can be reduced by re-expanding the lung in several stages rather than all at once.

If a pneumothorax recurs, acutely or after an interval of months or years, chemical pleurodesis (inflammatory adhesion of the visceral and parietal pleurae) is usually attempted. This procedure (see under Chemical Pleurodesis) consists of instilling a sclerosing agent into the pleural space via a chest tube; tetracycline is most often used in the United States,[8] although talc may be less painful for the patient and at least as effective in preventing recurrent pneumothorax.[9] If chem-

Table 92-1. Management of Pneumothorax (PTX)

Clinical Setting	Appropriate Treatment
Primary spontaneous (simple) PTX	
Patient not dyspneic and PTX small (<10–20%)	Observation[a]
PTX >10–20% or patient dyspneic on exertion	Simple aspiration[b] or minitube with Heimlich valve
Recurrence	Chest tube
Secondary spontaneous (complicated) PTX[c]	Chest tube
Iatrogenic PTX	
Small (<10–20%) and patient not dyspneic	Observation[a]
Larger (>10–20%) or patient dyspneic	Simple aspiration[b] or minitube with Heimlich valve
Traumatic PTX	Chest tube
Bilateral PTX	Chest tubes
Complete lung collapse (total PTX)	Chest tube
Failure of lung to re-expand with aspiration or minitube	Chest tube
Persistent air leak or bronchopleural fistula	Chest tube
Hydropneumothorax or hemopneumothorax	Chest tube
Pleurodesis planned	Chest tube
Tension PTX	Chest tube[d]

[a] Chest radiograph repeated at least daily until no further increase, then less often as indicated.
[b] Chest radiograph obtained immediately to confirm re-expansion; appropriate repeat films to check for recurrence.
[c] Spontaneous PTX in a patient with underlying lung disease.
[d] Emergency needle decompression if chest tube cannot be placed immediately.

ical pleurodesis fails, surgical escarification or obliteration of the pleural space may be required.

Tension pneumothorax is a true medical emergency that can cause death within minutes. The pressure can be relieved temporarily by percutaneous insertion of a large-bore needle through the upper anterior chest wall if a chest tube cannot be inserted immediately.

Pneumothorax developing during positive-pressure ventilation is always a life-threatening complication and must be treated promptly by insertion of a chest tube. It is often preceded by pneumomediastinum, but the latter also commonly occurs without progression to pneumothorax. For this reason "prophylactic" chest tube placement when air is detected subcutaneously or in the mediastinum during mechanical ventilation poses unnecessary risks for the patient and is not recommended. However, a chest tube and insertion tray should be kept at the bedside for immediate insertion if signs of tension pneumothorax appear.

Intermittent positive pressure breathing (IPPB) treatments, blow bottles, and other maneuvers that increase airway pressure are dangerous in patients with untreated pneumothorax. Similarly, transportation of such patients by air and hyperbaric O_2 therapy pose unacceptable risks, as discussed in Chapters 96 and 80, respectively. When indicated, these maneuvers may be carried out once the pneumothorax has been evacuated and a properly functioning chest tube is in place.

BRONCHOPLEURAL FISTULA

Air commonly continues to leak into the pleural space after placement of a chest tube for pneumothorax, but these leaks usually stop spontaneously in hours to a few days as the injury heals. When they do not, a persistent bronchopleural air leak, or bronchopleural fistula (BPF), is present. Spontaneous communication between the airways and the pleural space can also occur in tuberculosis, suppurative lung infections, and malignancy and when a bronchial stump breaks down after lung resection. However, BPF is most often encountered in respiratory care in the setting of alveolar disruption during mechanical ventilation for severe respiratory failure (Fig. 92-1; see also Figs. 84-4 and 84-5).

Although bronchopleural air leak during mechanical ventilation most often produces only a few bubbles through the water seal of the collection apparatus during inspiration, leaks of several hundred milliliters per breath are sometimes encountered. The leaked volume can be estimated by subtracting the expired from the inspired tidal volume as long as the leak exceeds 100 to 200 mL per breath and the measurements are made at the same point in the ventilator circuit to avoid error due to air compression in the inspiratory circuit. For smaller leaks or if more precision is desired, two accurate methods of quantitation are available. The "gold standard" is the 120-L Tissot-type water-seal spirometer, which can easily be adapted to collect the leaked gas under the same suction as is being applied to the chest tube.[10] A heated pneumotachometer of appropriate diameter also

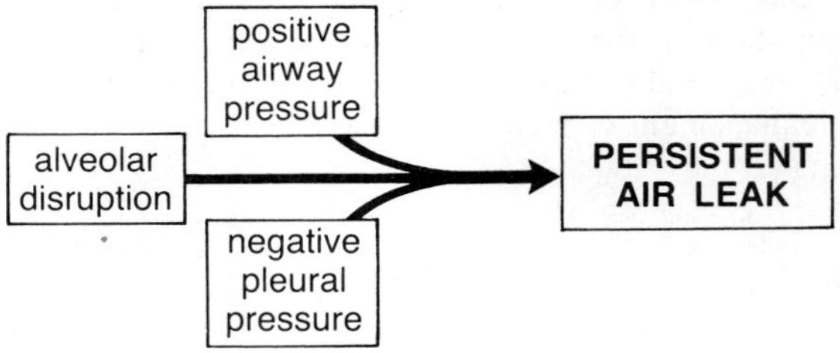

Figure 92-1. Pathogenesis of persistent bronchopleural air leak (bronchopleural fistula) during mechanical ventilation. The extent of alveolar disruption, particularly if infection is present, and the additive effects of airway pressure and chest tube suction determine the magnitude of the leak. Management should attempt to reduce the contribution of each of the factors shown. (From Pierson,[12] with permission.)

gives accurate results at all leak volumes and flow rates, but portable hand-held spirometers of the spinning-vane type and electronic spirometers are too inaccurate under certain conditions of flow to be satisfactory for this purpose.[11]

Potential adverse effects of BPF in the patient receiving mechanical ventilation include incomplete expansion of the affected lung, inability to maintain positive end-expiratory pressure (PEEP), and acute respiratory acidosis.[4,12] although the last of these is fortunately rare.[13] Appearance of a BPF during the later stages of the adult respiratory distress syndrome (ARDS) indicates a particularly poor prognosis,[13] although this probably reflects the severity of the underlying pulmonary disease rather than an effect of the BPF itself. Studies of ARDS patients with BPF have demonstrated that the component of each tidal volume "lost" via the chest tube does in fact participate in gas exchange, sometimes even having a higher PCO_2 than the gas exiting the endotracheal tube.[14] Hypercapnia and respiratory acidosis in such patients thus reflect severe mismatching of ventilation and perfusion rather than an effect of the fistula per se. Even in the 5 percent of such patients with refractory respiratory acidosis unresponsive to conventional ventilator adjustments,[13] the CO_2 retention probably reflects parenchymal lung dysfunction rather than the BPF.

It follows, then, that the management of patients with BPF complicating severe respiratory failure should be essentially the same as if the BPF were not there, provided that a functioning chest tube and pleural drainage system are in place. Several commonsense measures should be taken, as shown in Table 92-2. However, despite the large number of anecdotal reports touting various measures, such as high-frequency jet ventilation (HFJV), independent lung ventilation via double-lumen endotracheal tube, and application of PEEP to the chest tube(s),[12,15] none of these has been evaluated systematically for effectiveness and safety in comparison with conventional management. In the case of HFJV, in fact, gas exchange in patients with BPF complicating ARDS may actually be worsened rather than improved.[16]

Table 92-2. Management of Bronchopleural Fistula during Mechanical Ventilation

Use lowest number of mechanical breaths that permits adequate alveolar ventilation
- Spontaneous ventilation with pressure support
- Intermittent mandatory ventilation (MV) at lowest mandatory rate that maintains normal $PaCO_2$ and keeps spontaneous rate <30 breaths per minute, with use of pressure support if necessary

Avoid or correct respiratory alkalosis to minimize inspiratory minute ventilation

Reduce effective (returned) tidal volume to ≤10 mL/kg

Minimize inspiratory time
- Low inspiration/expiration ratio
- High inspiratory flow rate (e.g., 70–100 L/min)
- No inflation hold (end-inspiratory pause)

Avoid or minimize PEEP, both dialed-in and intrinsic (auto-PEEP)

Use least amount of suction on chest tube(s) that maintains lung inflation

Explore positional differences, avoiding positions that substantially increase leak

Sedate patient and paralyze if necessary if spontaneous movements increase leak

Treat bronchospasm and other causes of expiratory airflow obstruction

Consider HFJV, independent lung ventilation, and other experimental techniques only if above measures fail to maintain complete lung inflation and control $PaCO_2$ to keep arterial pH consistently >7.30

Treat underlying cause of respiratory failure, maintaining nutritional and other support, in order to discontinue mechanical ventilation as soon as possible

PLEURAL EFFUSION

Accumulation of excess fluid in the pleural space is a sign of serious disease,[1,3] and its cause should almost always be investigated by thoracentesis, as described in Chapter 58. The only instances in which a pleural effusion should not be tapped for diagnosis are those in which the cause is clinically obvious (e.g., clear-cut congestive heart failure), with no unusual or atypical features. An effusion in a patient with pneumonia must be tapped promptly[17] or if small, followed with serial chest radiographs until it is certain that it is not enlarging. Ultrasound or computed tomography (CT) can help to localize small or loculated effusions, although these procedures tend to be overused and must not delay the making of a diagnosis.

Management of most pleural effusions is directed at the primary disease process rather than at the pleural fluid per se.[18–23] A therapeutic thoracentesis (removal of fluid for treatment rather than to assist in diagnosis) is indicated when the presence of the pleural fluid itself causes marked dyspnea or other symptoms and the patient's underlying illness cannot be readily treated.

Pleural fluid must be drained promptly with a chest tube in two specific instances, traumatic hemothorax and thoracic empyema. Bleeding into the pleural space cannot be assessed accurately without drainage, and the rate of blood loss after blunt or penetrating chest trauma is a primary determinant of the need for operation; in addition, undrained blood, fibrin, and clot may eventually lead to fibrothorax, producing significant restrictive pulmonary impairment. An empyema needs to be drained immediately with a chest tube, both because "pus in an enclosed space" cannot be cured unless physically removed and because loculations of the fluid can form quickly, making a more extensive surgical procedure necessary to achieve adequate drainage.[17,21] When an empyema cannot be completely evacuated with a chest tube, early surgical drainage instead of multiple chest tubes and repositionings can reduce morbidity and shorten the patient's hospital stay.[22]

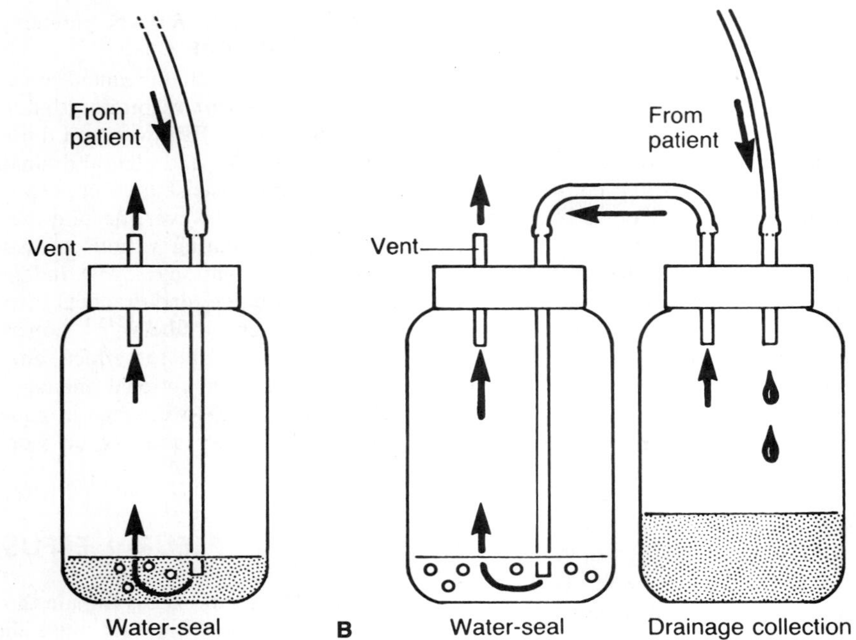

Figure 92-2. **(A)** One-bottle pleural drainage system. **(B)** Two-bottle pleural drainage system. Proximal (right-hand) bottle permits accumulation of drainage fluid without increasing the pressure necessary to vent the pleural space. (From Luce et al.,[2] with permission.)

CHEST TUBES AND PLEURAL DRAINAGE SYSTEMS

The size, positioning, and handling of chest tubes vary with the clinical indication. A smaller-diameter tube is required to drain air and it should be seated high in the pleural cavity. Larger tubes are needed to drain fluid, particularly hemothoraces, empyemas, and inflammatory effusions; these tubes should be placed posteriorly and directed downward into the pleural gutter. Proper, sterile insertion technique[24,25] should be used to position the tube so that its most proximal drainage hole is at least 2 cm inside the pleural cavity.

Several kinds of pleural drainage systems are available. Their purposes are to permit air and fluid to be evacuated from the pleural space while preventing air from entering and maintaining a closed, sterile system. All are variations of a few basic types,[25,26] notably the one-, two-, three-, and four-bottle systems illustrated schematically in Figures 92-2 and 92-3. Present commercial units have different appearances, but most can be understood by reference to these diagrams. While most are effective for fluid drainage and small air leaks, the currently available models vary considerably in their ability to handle larger air leaks.[27] An Emerson suction pump connected to an old-fashioned bottle system is the setup most capable of maintaining adequate suction in the presence of a large bronchopleural air leak.[27]

The simplest pleural drainage system is the Heimlich valve,[28] a short length of collapsible tubing, like a Penrose drain, enclosed in a protective sheath, which vents air from the pleural space to the atmosphere but collapses when there is no air leak. It is helpful in draining uncomplicated pneumothoraces but is not appropriate when pleural fluid is present.

An "underwater seal," or single-bottle system (Fig. 92-2A), prevents air from entering the pleural space by means of a 2-cm water seal. When fluid as well as air drains from the chest, however, fluid accumulates in the bottle and increases the intrapleural pressure required to break the water seal and vent the chest; fluid could also run back into the pleural space if the bottle were raised during patient transport. These problems are circumvented by a two-bottle system (Fig. 92-2B), which provides separate vessels for fluid drainage and water seal. For one- and two-bottle systems, a regulated suction system such as an Emerson suction pump must be used rather than wall suction. Wall suction can be used with a three-bottle system (Fig. 92-3A), in which the pressure gradient between collection system and pleural space is determined by the depth of the water in the far left-hand bottle, minus the 2 cm of the water seal in the middle bottle. A four-bottle system (Fig. 92-3B) incorporates a second water seal.

When the suction is momentarily turned off, the level of the water seal fluctuates with the respiratory cycle if the tube is patent. If the tube becomes occluded by clot or exudate, gentle milking or stripping may open it. Manually stripping a chest tube can generate a negative pressure of up to 400

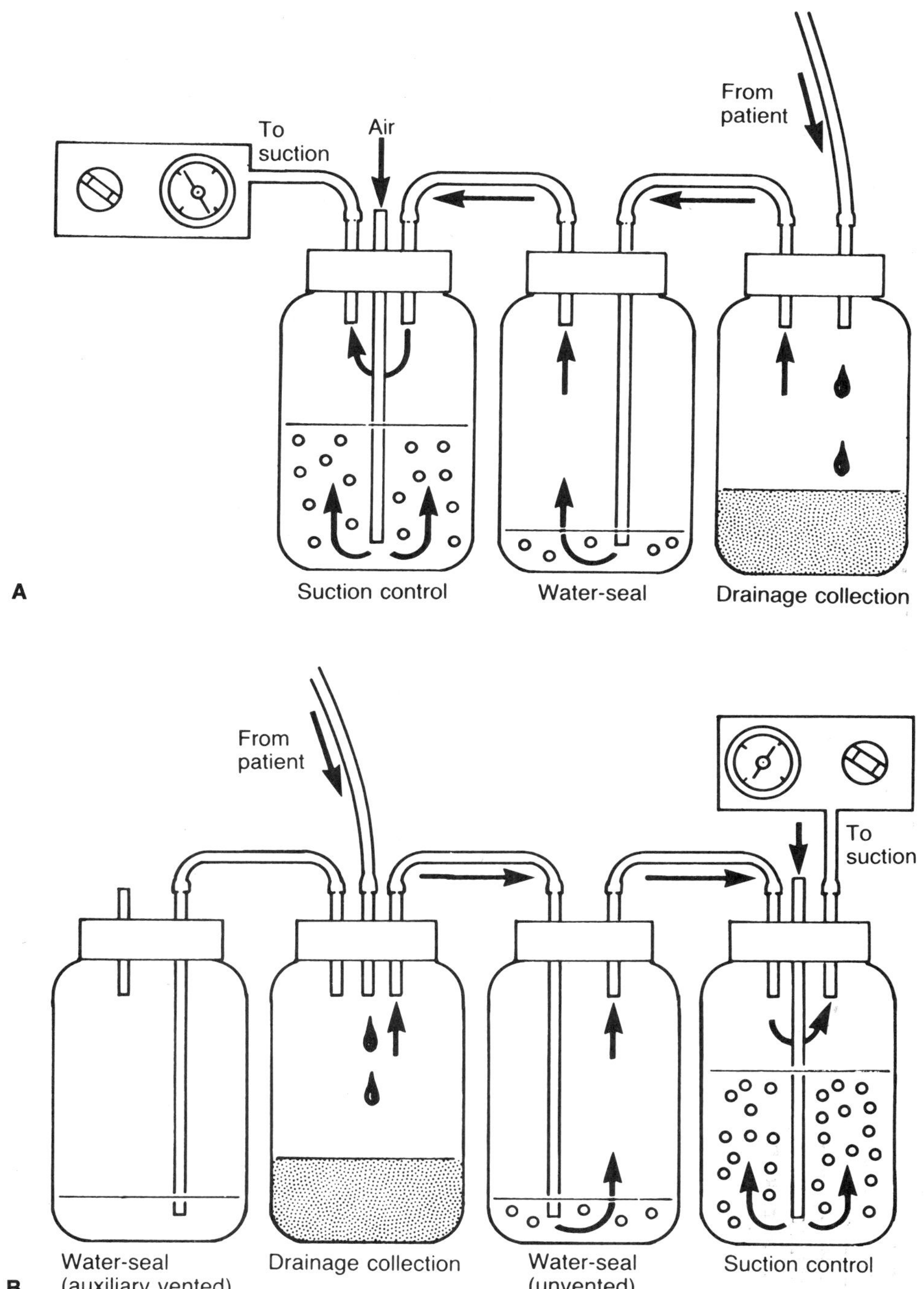

Figure 92-3. **(A)** Three-bottle pleural drainage system, which permits use of wall suction to increase the pressure gradient between the pleural space and the collection bottle. (**B**) Four-bottle pleural drainage system, which has the features of the system shown in Figure A plus a second water seal. Commercial systems such as the Pleur-Evac and others are variants of these basic systems, some incorporating a self-contained air vent to prevent pressure build-up within the system. (From Luce et al.,[2] with permission.)

mmHg inside the tube,[29] however, so that this procedure should be carried out gingerly; routine stripping of chest tubes has been shown to be unnecessary.[30]

A nonfunctioning chest tube is dangerous and should be removed. Not only can it not vent the chest in case a tension pneumothorax develops, but it also permits buildup of pleural fluid and may serve as a conduit for the introduction of bacteria.

CHEMICAL PLEURODESIS

Chemical pleurodesis is most commonly used for malignant effusions,[19] but it can also be helpful in refractory benign inflammatory effusions[18] and in some cases of recurrent pneumothorax.[5,8] The procedure is painful, and both systemic and local analgesia should be used. For pleurodesis to be most effective, the lung must be completely expanded and the pleural space completely drained of fluid. The sclerosing agent, commonly tetracycline 20 mg/kg in 50 mL saline, is instilled through the chest tube, often along with a topical anesthetic, and the tube is clamped for 2 hours while the patient is moved through several positions to facilitate spread of the agent throughout the pleural cavity. The tube is then unclamped, and suction is applied until the drainage is less than 100 to 150 mL/d.

References

1. Light RW: Pleural Diseases. 2nd Ed. Lea & Febiger, Philadelphia, 1990
2. Luce JM, Tyler ML, Pierson DJ: Intensive Respiratory Care. WB Saunders, Philadelphia, 1984
3. Sahn SA: State of the art: The pleura. Am Rev Respir Dis 1988; 138:184–234
4. Luce JM, Pierson DJ: Critical Care Medicine. WB Saunders, Philadelphia, 1988
5. Light RW: Pneumothorax. pp. 1745–1759. In Murray JF, Nadel JA (eds): Textbook of Respiratory Medicine. WB Saunders, Philadelphia, 1988
6. Pavlin DJ, Raghu G, Rogers TR, Cheney FW: Re-expansion hypotension: A complication of rapid evacuation of prolonged pneumothorax. Chest 1986;89:70–74
7. Mahfood S, Hix WR, Aaron BL et al: Reexpansion pulmonary edema. Ann Thorac Surg 1988;45:340–345
8. Stephenson LW: Treatment of pneumothorax with intrapleural tetracycline, editorial. Chest 1985;88:803–804
9. Almind M, Lange P, Viskum K: Spontaneous pneumothorax: Comparison of simple drainage, talc pleurodesis, and tetracycline pleurodesis. Thorax 1989;44:627–630
10. Ritz R, Benson M, Bishop MJ: Measuring gas leakage from bronchopleural fistulas during high-frequency jet ventilation. Crit Care Med 1984;12:836–837
11. Larson RP, Capps JS, Pierson DJ: A comparison of three devices used for quantitating bronchopleural air leaks. Respir Care 1986;31:1065–1068
12. Pierson DJ: Persistent bronchopleural air leak during mechanical ventilation: A review. Respir Care 1982;27:408–416
13. Pierson DJ, Horton CA, Bates PW: Persistent bronchopleural air leak during mechanical ventilation: A review of 39 cases. Chest 1986;90:321–323
14. Bishop MJ, Benson MS, Pierson DJ: Carbon dioxide excretion via bronchopleural fistulas in patients with adult respiratory distress syndrome. Chest 1987;91:400–402
15. Powner DJ, Grenvik A: Ventilatory management of life-threatening bronchopleural fistulae: A summary. Crit Care Med 1981; 9:54–58
16. Bishop MJ, Benson MS, Sato P, Pierson DJ: Comparison of high-frequency jet ventilation with conventional mechanical ventilation for bronchopleural fistula. Anesth Analg 1987; 66:833–838
17. Sahn SA, Light RW: The sun should never set on a parapneumonic effusion, editorial. Chest 1989;95:945–947
18. Chetty KG: Transudative pleural effusions. Clin Chest Med 1985;6:49–54
19. Winterbauer RH: Nonneoplastic pleural effusions. pp. 2139–2157. In Fishman AP (ed): Pulmonary Diseases and Disorders. 2nd Ed. McGraw-Hill, New York, 1988
20. Ruckdeschel JC: Management of malignant pleural effusion: An overview. Semin Oncol, suppl. 1988;15:24–28
21. Light RW: Parapneumonic effusions and empyema. Clin Chest Med 1985;6:55–62
22. Ashbaugh DG: Empyema thoracis. Factors influencing morbidity and mortality. Chest 1991;99:1162–1165
23. Pierson DJ: Disorders of the pleura, mediastinum, and diaphragm. pp. 1111–1116. In Wilson JD, Braunwald E, Isselbacher KJ et al. (eds): Harrison's Principles of Internal Medicine. 12th Ed. McGraw-Hill, New York, 1990
24. Miller KS, Sahn SA: Chest tubes: Indications, technique, management and complications. Chest 1987;91:258–264
25. Symbas PN: Chest drainage tubes. Surg Clin North Am 1989; 69:41–46
26. Kersten L: Chest tube drainage system—indications and principles of operation. Heart Lung 1974;3:97–101
27. Rusch VW, Capps JS, Tyler ML, Pierson DJ: The performance of four pleural drainage systems in an animal model of bronchopleural fistula. Chest 1988;93:859–863
28. Heimlich HJ: Valve drainage of the pleural cavity. Chest 1968; 53:282–287
29. Duncan C, Erickson R: Pressures associated with chest tube stripping. Heart Lung 1982;11:166–171
30. Lim-Levy F, Babler SA, deGroot-Kosolcharoen J et al: Is milking and stripping chest tubes really necessary? Ann Thorac Surg 1986;42:77–80

Chapter 93

Management of the Patient with Head Trauma

John M. Luce

CHAPTER OUTLINE

Head trauma is the most common cause of disability and death among trauma patients, particularly those under 50 years of age.[1] Head trauma also imposes a large social burden, accounting for over 5 million days of hospitalization and over 30 million days of work lost annually in the United States.[2] Although most of the morbidity and mortality of patients with head trauma is due to their initial insult, further preventable damage may occur during the resuscitative period. Such resuscitation takes place in the intensive care unit (ICU) for the most part and frequently involves measures designed to reduce intracranial hypertension. This chapter discusses the pathophysiology and management of head trauma and intracranial hypertension from a critical care rather than a neurosurgical point of view.

PATHOPHYSIOLOGY OF HEAD TRAUMA

Diffuse or focal injury may result from head trauma.[3] Despite the common occurrence of *diffuse brain damage* due to head trauma, its exact mechanism is unknown. Ommaya and Gennarelli[4] believe that the basic phenomenon is cerebral concussion, in which rotational shear forces following abrupt acceleration or deceleration disrupt axons and myelin sheaths. The shear forces are maximal at the brain surface, minimal at its center, and intensified where the brain is exposed to bony or dural protrusions such as those at the frontal or temporal tips. The forces therefore cause a centripetal pattern of nerve fiber injury which affects subcortical structures only after the cortex is involved. The end result is diffuse injury that can cause transient and varying degrees of coma and death with or without intracranial hypertension.[5]

Focal brain injuries may occur alone or in concert with concussion. Such injuries include cerebral contusion, which is characterized by subpial and intracerebral extravasation of blood, and cerebral laceration in which the pia mater is torn. Contusion and laceration usually occur under areas of extreme impact and most often involve the frontal and temporal lobes. Other focal injuries are called *mass lesions* because they involve the collection of blood in specific areas. Epidural hematomas, for example, most often arise from lacerations of the posterior branch of the middle meningeal artery, frequently in association with temporal skull fractures. By contrast, subdural bleeding usually emanates from small cerebral veins bridging the cortex and the superior sagittal sinus, especially in the frontal region. Such hematomas may result from penetrating injuries or other conditions in which great force is applied to a small area of the brain.[2]

Cerebral swelling often accompanies or follows diffuse and focal brain injury and has two causes, one of which is an increase in cerebral blood flow (CBF). Although this increase may not be observed clinically, Brown and Brown[6] demonstrated in monkeys that head blows cause a transient decrease in mean arterial pressure (MAP) and CBF that is followed within 30 seconds by a marked increase in both variables. The increase in MAP, which is similar to that originally observed by Cushing[7] in patients with brain stem ischemia, presumably results from a catecholamine release, which causes profound peripheral vasoconstriction and redistribution of blood into the central circulation. MAP and CBF usually fall in adults within minutes to hours following head trauma, and the fall in CBF generally is paralleled by a reduction in cerebral O_2 consumption ($CMRO_2$).[7] However, children and adolescents characteristically manifest a sustained increase in CBF.[8,9]

The second cause of cerebral swelling, and the most common cause in adults, is vasogenic edema.[10] Such edema accumulates gradually after head injury, usually reaching a peak after several days. It requires an increase in permeability of the cerebral microvasculature, which could be caused by the initial surge of blood to the brain. In support of this hypothesis, punctate superficial hemorrhages were observed by Brown and Brown[6] in the brains of animals following concussive trauma. Cerebral edema may result from either diffuse or focal brain damage. It injures the brain largely by causing intracranial hypertension, just as do mass lesions.

PATHOPHYSIOLOGY OF INTRACRANIAL HYPERTENSION

Intracranial hypertension is diagnosed if the intracranial pressure (ICP), which is the same as the pressure in the cerebrospinal fluid (CSF) of the subarachnoid space, is elevated above the normal level of 10 mmHg. ICP exceeds this level in more than 80 percent of patients with severe head injury requiring hospital admission and is almost invariably elevated in those with rapidly expanding mass lesions.[11] Lundberg et al.,[12] who introduced the concept of continuous ICP monitoring in neurosurgical patients, observed that ICP rose as high as 115 mmHg in some individuals. Pitts and Martin[2] noted that ICP generally reaches its zenith some 2 to 3 days after head trauma in patients with diffuse brain injury, a point at which cerebral swelling is most pronounced.

The pathophysiology of intracranial hypertension can best be understood by examining the contents of the cranium, (Fig. 93-1), which include brain solids, brain water, brain blood, and the CSF. Because these components are enclosed in the normally solid skull, an increase in the volume of any one of them must be balanced by a decrease in the volume of another, or the ICP will rise; this in the Monroe-Kellie principle.[3] When the volume of brain solids, water, or blood increases, CSF is displaced into the subarachnoid space surrounding the spinal cord. CSF production then decreases

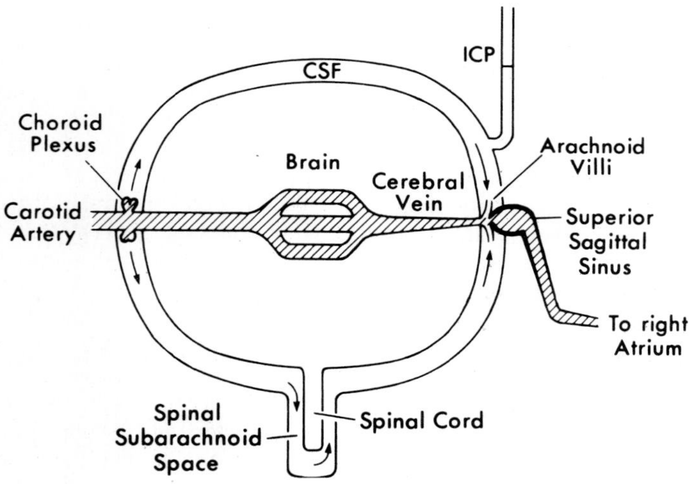

Figure 93-1. Schematic representation of intracranial anatomy. Arterial inflow is represented by the carotid artery; venous outflow occurs through the cerebral veins that enter the superior sagittal sinus. ICP impinges on the cerebral veins and causes their pressure to rise, acting like a Starling resistor. Indeed, ICP and cerebral venous pressure are so similar that ICP is used as the effective venous outflow pressure. It is measured in the CSF space around the brain, which is continuous in health with the space around the spinal cord. CSF is made in the choroid plexus and resorbed by the arachnoid villi.

after this displacement has become maximal, thereby preventing or limiting the rise in ICP. Nevertheless, ICP eventually rises as the volume of one or more intracranial components increases or, in the case of hydrocephalus, as CSF continues to accumulate. The rate at which the ICP rises depends on the total volume of the brain contents; if this volume is low, a large further increase in volume will be required for the pressure to increase. However, the pressure will increase rapidly if the volume of the brain contents is abnormally high to begin with and only a small volume is added (Fig. 93-2).

Intracranial hypertension may damage the brain by compressing or displacing tissue. The latter effect is seen most dramatically during transtentorial herniation, when the ICP rises on the cephalad side of the tentorial notch between the temporal lobe and the cerebellum and forces brain structures caudad because pressure is lower on that side (Fig. 93-3). During the descent, compression of the brain stem and the third nerve by the temporal lobe is responsible for a combination of (1) ipsilateral oculomotor nerve paresis, which results in dilatation of the pupil on that side; (2) contralateral hemiparesis, progressing to decerebrate rigidity in which the arm and leg are flexed; and (3) altered level of consciousness. Respiratory irregularities that culminate in apnea result from increased pressure in the posterior fossa with ischemia of the brain stem, as does the hypertensive (Cushing) response.

A less dramatic but equally important consequence of intracranial hypertension is a global reduction in CBF, which may damage the entire brain. As may be seen from Figure 93-4, CBF normally is determined by four factors: (1) the cerebral metabolic rate, which is reflected in the $CMRO_2$; (2) the $PaCO_2$, which indicates the availability of CO_2 to cross the blood-brain barrier, increase the H^+ concentration of the brain's extracellular fluid and cause cerebral vasodilatation; (3) the PaO_2, which will cause cerebral vasodilatation if it falls below approximately 60 mmHg; and (4) the cerebral perfusion pressure (CPP), which is the difference between MAP and ICP, as will be discussed. Cerebral blood flow normally is directly proportional to CPP and inversely proportional to cerebral vascular resistance (CVR). In health CBF remains constant over wide variations in CPP because CVR changes accordingly; this is the principle of *cerebral autoregulation*. However, autoregulation usually is impaired after head trauma and other brain insults, so that CVR becomes fixed and as a result, CBF is entirely dependent on CPP.

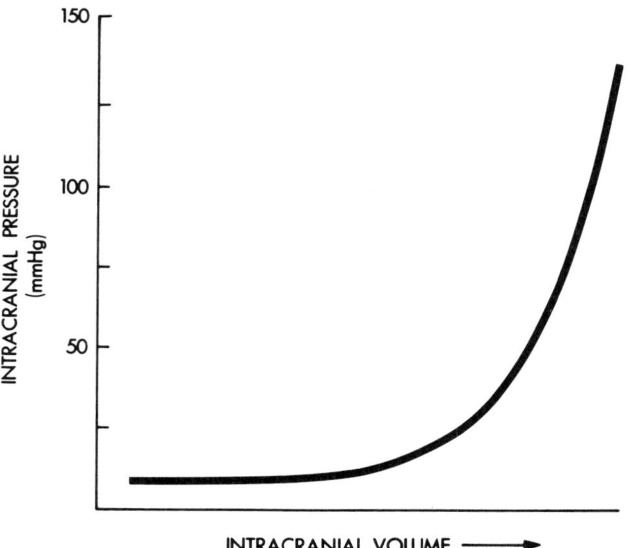

Figure 93-2. Relationship between ICP and volume of brain contents. Small increases in volume yield large increases in pressure as the curve becomes steeper.

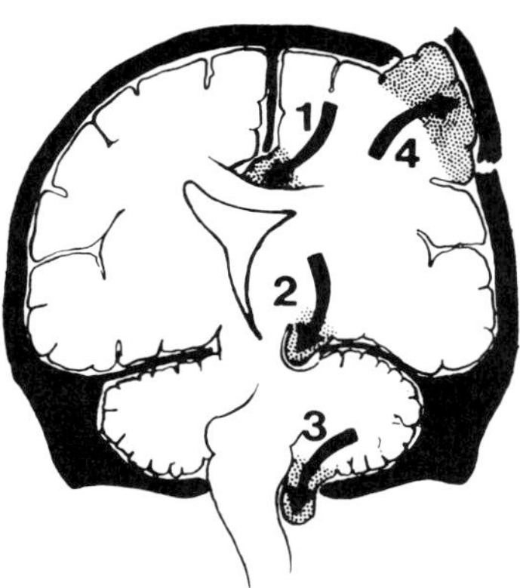

Figure 93-3. Translocation of brain tissue can occur if the pressure on one side of a structure exceeds that on the other side in patients with intracranial hypertension. For example, tissue may move across the falx cerebri (1), the tentorium cerebelli (2), or the foramen magnum (3) or through a bony defect in the skull (4). (From Fishman,[10] with permission.)

The perfusion pressure of any organ is the difference between the arterial inflow and the venous outflow pressures. The MAP represents the cerebral arterial inflow pressure, and pressure in the delicate cerebral veins represents the outflow pressure. However, this venous pressure cannot be easily measured, and pressures in the sagittal sinus, the jugular veins, and the right atrium, which drain the cranial vault, may differ somewhat from cerebral venous pressure. Several investigators, including Luce et al.,[13] have demonstrated that ICP more closely resembles cerebral venous pressure and actually helps determine venous pressure by impinging on the veins where they enter the sagittal sinus (Fig. 93-1). Because of this relationship, ICP can be used as the effective outflow pressure of the brain, and CPP may be defined as MAP minus ICP. Kety and co-workers[14] and Greenfield and Tindall[15] have demonstrated that CBF decreases significantly when ICP exceeds 40 mmHg under experimental circumstances; assuming a normal MAP of 90 mmHg, this ICP rise would produce a CPP of 50 mmHg. Recent evidence has correlated a poor outcome after head injury with a CPP of 60 mmHg or less.[16]

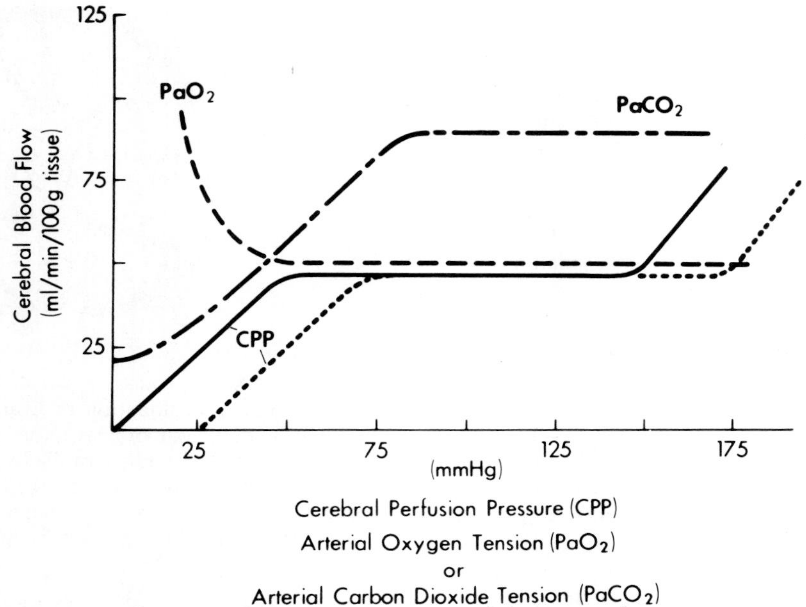

Figure 93-4. Three determinants of cerebral blood flow are $PaCO_2$, PaO_2, and CPP, which is the difference between MAP and ICP. When autoregulation is present, large changes in CPP do not alter CBF. The CPP curve is shifted to the right in chronically hypertensive patients. Autoregulation usually is lost following severe head trauma, so that blood flow varies directly with CPP.

It is important to stress that a CPP of 50 to 60 mmHg or less can be reached by decreasing MAP as readily as by increasing ICP. Hypotension generally is uncommon among patients with head injury unless there is failure of the medulla oblongata, the lower portion of the brain stem, in which the cardiovascular as well as the respiratory control centers are located. However, hypotension may be seen with concurrent spinal cord trauma or other insults. In fact, hypotension due to multiple injuries was observed in 13 of 100 consecutive head injury patients transferred to a major trauma center.[17] The MAP of such patients deserves as much attention as their ICP.

CARDIOVASCULAR COMPLICATIONS

As noted above, hypotension is rare following head trauma in the absence of severe brain stem damage or concurrent injuries. Indeed, most head-injured patients show little cardiovascular compromise, in marked contrast with patients with cervical spinal cord injury, who frequently manifest spinal shock. Perhaps the most common cardiovascular problems in head injury patients are dysrhythmias ranging from tachycardia to impaired atrioventricular conduction and electrocardiographic changes such as T-wave inversion or ST segment depression. Like the centrally mediated hypotension discussed earlier, these abnormalities presumably result from injury of the cardiovascular control center in the brain stem.

RESPIRATORY COMPLICATIONS

The effects of head trauma on the regulation of ventilation have been evaluated by Plum and Posner,[18] who described six respiratory patterns resulting from lesions in the central nervous system: (1) eupneic or normal respiration, which may occur even in the presence of small lesions; (2) Cheyne-Stokes or periodic respiration, which is associated with bilateral hemispheric disease; (3) central neurogenic hyperventilation, which may be due to lesions at the pontine level; (4) apneustic respiration, which also may reflect damage to the pons; (5) ataxic respiration related to injury in the medulla; and (6) apnea caused by overwhelming damage to the medullary respiratory control center. However, North and Jennett[19] were unable to predict such a precise localization of lesions based on respiratory pattern. Therefore, it must be stressed that any of these six patterns may be observed immediately after head trauma or may develop later, especially if transtentorial herniation occurs.

Although many respiratory patterns are possible, hyperventilation or eucapnic respiration with a normal $PaCO_2$ is usually seen in patients with severe head injury. In fact, the most common arterial blood gas abnormality in these individuals is hypoxemia, with a decreased PaO_2. Frequently hypoxemia can be explained by bacterial pneumonia, gastric aspiration, lobar atelectasis, pulmonary edema, or other processes that alter the lungs on radiographic examination, however, the radiograph also may appear normal.[20]

Several explanations have been offered for the hypoxemia

of head-injured patients with normal chest radiographs. One is that the patients have microatelectasis related to a reduction in their functional residual capacity (FRC). Although FRC was normal in the head-injured patients studied by Schumacker and associates,[21] Cooper and Boswell[22] in 1983 described 24 persons who manifested an increase in venous admixture associated with a significant reduction in FRC following head trauma. In an editorial accompanying Cooper and Boswell's article, deTroyer and Martin[23] speculated that head injury might depress involuntary activity in the intercostals and other respiratory muscles and thereby reduce FRC by relaxation of the chest wall.

Another possible explanation for both the hypoxemia and the decreased FRC of head-injured patients is that extravascular water accumulates in their lungs. The patients therefore might be thought to manifest clinical or subclinical neurogenic pulmonary edema (NPE). Frost and associates[24] concluded that neurologic factors accounted for hypoxemia in over two-thirds of head-injured patients, many of whom had normal chest radiographs. MacKensie et al.[25] demonstrated increased extravascular lung water in 9 of 18 patients with severe head trauma or spontaneous subarachnoid hemorrhage. None of the patients had evidence of pulmonary contusion, pneumonia, gastric aspiration, or cardiac failure. Although several of the patients did not exhibit intracranial hypertension, overall there was a significant correlation between increases in extravascular lung water and ICP.

Theodore and Robin[26] have argued that NPE results from the hypertensive response that is provoked by intracranial hypertension and brain stem ischemia. The simultaneous increase in systemic and pulmonary microvascular pressure seen in this response causes water to leak from the blood vessels into the lung interstitium. The vessels then leak proteins as well as water because they have been injured in the hydrostatic phase. Whatever the underlying mechanism, NPE should be suspected in patients who manifest hypoxemia with or without chest radiographic abnormalities immediately following head injury. Nevertheless, NPE usually should be considered a diagnosis of exclusion, and other causes of hypoxemia such as drug-induced pulmonary edema, gastric aspiration, and overly vigorous fluid resuscitation should be ruled out after injury.

The most common lingering respiratory effect of head trauma is depression of respiratory defense mechanisms, which may occur in several ways. The best known alteration is depression of the gag reflex, a reflex that ordinarily limits bacterial contamination of the lower airways. Profound coma also may depress the cough reflex and cause upper airway obstruction through relaxation of the tongue musculature. Impairment in mucociliary clearance has not been evaluated in head-injured patients but remains a theoretical possibility, as do abnormalities in surfactant metabolism in areas of microatelectasis and alteration in alveolar macrophage function in the presence of pulmonary edema fluid.[27]

Presumably these changes in host defenses, coupled with iatrogenic insults such as endotracheal intubation and residence in the ICU, are responsible for respiratory complications during the resuscitation phase. Bacterial pneumonia is the most common of these complications, occurring in over 50 percent of head-injured patients intubated for longer than 5 days at San Francisco General Hospital. Lobar atelectasis also may occur after injury, along with pulmonary edema caused by fluid overload, sepsis, and other conditions. If the chest radiograph appears normal but hypoxemia exists, bronchospasm and pulmonary embolism should be considered.

MEDICAL MANAGEMENT

The initial evaluation of head-injured patients is essential in determining the extent of damage to the brain and other vital organs, directing treatment, and estimating prognosis. However, thorough history-taking and physical examination should not be performed until the cervical spine is immobilized, the airway is protected, bleeding is controlled, seizures are treated, arterial blood gases are drawn, a nasogastric tube and bladder catheter are passed, and ventilation is supported if necessary. Conscious patients or onlookers then may be questioned about the type and circumstances of injury, if and when the patients lost consciousness, and whether they have concurrent medical or surgical problems.

Bruce et al.[3] stress that the examination of head-injured patients should focus on level of consciousness, pupillary size and reaction to light, corneal reflexes, oculomotor function (usually determined by oculovestibular rather than oculocephalic testing because of the possibility of spinal cord damage), retinal vessels, gag reflex, cough reflex, rectal tone, and pattern of ventilation. In addition to noting these variables, it may be helpful to categorize patients by means of the Glascow Coma Scale (GCS),[28,29] which is based on their best level of eye opening and verbal and motor response (Table 93-1).

Table 93-1. Glasgow Coma Scale

Eye opening	
Spontaneous	4
To speech	3
To pain	2
Nil	1
Motor response	
Obeys commands	6
Localizes	5
Withdraws	4
Abnormal flexion	3
Abnormal extension	2
Nil	1
Verbal response[a]	
Oriented	5
Confused conversation	4
Inappropriate words	3
Incomprehensible sounds	2
Nil	1

[a] If the patient is intubated, the letter T is substituted for the verbal response, and the highest possible score is 10T.

Patients with signs of tentorial herniation may be candidates for exploratory burr holes at this stage in their evaluation. However, if time permits and proper facilities are available, diagnostic radiographic studies should be performed, which usually should include cervical spinal views and chest x-ray. Plain skull radiographs once were taken routinely in trauma patients, but computed tomography (CT) can visualize brain structures in addition to the skull.[30] Angiography may be used if CT is not available or if additional information is required.

The medical management of head injury is intended to ensure systemic and cerebral homeostasis. From a cardiovascular standpoint this means that MAP should be maintained in the normal range so that CPP does not fall near the critical level of 50 to 60 mmHg or rise to such an extent that CBF level is greatly increased. Fluids or vasopressors may be used to support CPP if necessary. Alternatively, MAP may be lowered by vasodilator therapy in the occasional hypertensive patient; this should be done with extreme caution, however, because an elevated MAP may reflect chronic hypertension or the hypertensive response to brain stem ischemia.

From a respiratory standpoint, airway protection is the first priority. Mechanical ventilation also should be instituted in hypercapnic patients because the elevated $PaCO_2$ may dilate cerebral vessels and increase CBF. Hypoxemia should be corrected by supplemental O_2 therapy with the addition of positive end-expiratory pressure (PEEP) if necessary to avoid O_2 toxicity, despite the fact that PEEP may compromise venous return. The ideal PaO_2 level is uncertain in head-injured patients, but generally it should exceed 100 mmHg to avoid cerebral tissue hypoxia during hyperventilation therapy.[31]

Measures to ensure cerebral homeostasis include administration of metabolic substrates and the normalization or reduction of cerebral metabolic needs. All patients in coma should receive treatment with 100 mg of thiamine and 0.4 mg of naloxone as soon as possible; dextrose should be added if hypoglycemia is demonstrated.[2] Adequate nutrition is essential thereafter; caloric intake should be greater than the basal needs of 25 cal/kg/d to offset the stress of injury. Cerebral metabolic needs can be normalized by therapeutic or prophylactic administration of phenytoin to abolish seizures, administration of antipyretics and appropriate antibiotic therapy to treat fever, and administration of sedatives and muscle relaxants to reduce agitation.

MONITORING

Following initial management, severely head injured patients customarily are monitored by means of serial physical examinations and GCS evaluation. Furthermore, because responsiveness, pupillary reflexes, and other variables frequently are altered by drugs and other therapeutic interventions, additional monitoring may be required. This requirement is met most commonly by continuous recording of CPP with an indwelling systemic arterial catheter to measure MAP (and facilitate arterial blood gas analysis) and an epidural,[32] subdural,[33] or intraventricular[34] catheter to measure ICP. The advantages and disadvantages of these devices are given in Table 93-2.

Table 93-2. Intracranial Pressure Monitoring Devices

Device	Limitations	Accuracy	Infection (%)
Ventriculostomy catheter	Cannot be inserted into small ventricles	Excellent	2–5
Subdural screw	Cannot be used to drain CSF	Good	1–2
Epidural transducer	Cannot be used to drain CSF	Fair	<1

Given the poor correlation among CPP, CBF, and $CMRO_2$ in many head-injured patients,[8] clinicians have long sought a way of directly measuring the last two variables. CBF can be quantitated by observing the washout curves of radionuclides introduced into the brain via carotid artery injection[35] or inhalation.[36] However, these techniques are either invasive or cumbersome and cannot easily be repeated in serial fashion. Some attention therefore has focused on position emission tomography (PET)[37] and single-photon emission computed tomography (SPECT).[38] As yet experimental, PET and SPECT are potentially portable and noninvasive. Although these techniques are complicated and expensive, they may be able to provide clinical information about both CBF and $CMRO_2$.

Another potential monitoring tool in head-injured patients is determination of multimodality-evoked potentials (MEPS). This technique involves the recording of brain activity following auditory, visual, or peripheral stimulation and can be performed easily at the bedside. Greenberg et al.[39,40] have demonstrated the usefulness of MEPS in determining the location and extent of traumatic central nervous system lesions.

Other ICU monitoring techniques may be applicable in certain head-injured patients. One of these is on-line measurement of end-tidal CO_2 tensions ($P_{ET}CO_2$), which correlate well with $PaCO_2$ level unless large increases in physiologic dead space limit CO_2 excretion by the lungs. A second frequently used technique is estimation of right and left ventricular end-diastolic filling pressure (and, by inference, volume) with catheters in the superior vena cava or pulmonary artery. The latter are particularly helpful in patients who are receiving therapy with barbiturates, diuretics, and other agents that reduce effective intravascular volume and in patients with co-existing respiratory or cardiovascular disease.

TREATMENT OF INTRACRANIAL HYPERTENSION

Intracranial hypertension may occur if cerebral blood volume increases as a result of decreased venous drainage. Because this may be caused by kinking of the jugular veins[41] and lowering the brain below the level of the heart, the patient's head and neck should be kept near the midline position and elevated 30 degrees. These simple measures often serve to blunt the diminution in venous drainage that is caused by coughing, straining, and other activities that increase intrathoracic pressure. If they do not, sedatives and muscle relaxants may be given to limit muscle activity.

Positive pressure ventilation with or without PEEP also may increase ICP by decreasing cerebral venous return.[42] Cotev et al.[43] and Burchiel et al.[44] have demonstrated in dogs and humans, respectively, that PEEP is more likely to increase ICP if intracranial compliance is low or if respiratory system compliance is high because PEEP-induced increases in intrathoracic pressure are applied more profoundly to intrathoracic vessels in the latter circumstance. Because PEEP is indicated primarily to treat pulmonary edema, which decreases respiratory system compliance, it should not adversely affect ICP in most circumstances. Nevertheless, both MAP and ICP levels should be followed closely in head-injured patients receiving this therapy.

Hyperventilation may be expected to decrease CBF by causing cerebral vasoconstriction via an increase in the pH level of brain extracellular fluid.[3] The CBF reduction probably is maximal at a $PaCO_2$ of 20 mmHg because the vasoconstriction is offset by the vasodilatory effect of cerebral tissue hypoxia. Although Harper[45] has shown that the cerebrovascular responsiveness to hyperventilation varies even in health, most head-injured patients manifest at least some reactivity to changes in $PaCO_2$.[46] However, after 8 hours or more of hyperventilation, the H^+ concentration of brain extracellular fluid is restored to normal by active transport processes.[47] The $PaCO_2$ level, therefore, should be normalized as soon as possible provided that ICP does not increase.

Hyperosmolar agents reduce ICP (1) by decreasing brain water through the creation of an osmolar gradient between the bloodstream and brain cells and (2) through a reduction in total body water.[48] Most clinicians administer treatment with a 20 percent mannitol solution either in high intermittent doses (0.25 to 0.5 g/kg every 1 to 2 hours) or by continuous infusion (0.05 to 0.1 g/kg). A serum osmolality of approximately 325 mOsm should not be exceeded because excessive hyperosmolality may injure neurons. Mannitol depletes the body of sodium and potassium as well as water and must be used cautiously. It also should be given cautiously to head-injured children because it may transiently increase intravascular volume, CBF, and ICP.[3]

Diuretics are given to decrease ICP by reducing intravascular volume. Furosemide in doses of 40 to 80 mg most commonly is employed for this purpose; it has the additional advantage of reducing CSF production by unknown mechanisms.[49] Acetazolamide is a carbonic anhydrase inhibitor that limits ion exchange across the choroid plexus. This agent is used to reduce CSF production in head-injured patients, particularly those with communicating hydrocephalus. The usual therapeutic dose of acetazolamide is 250 mg, two to four times a day. Although acetazolamide therapy may be helpful in reducing CSF, drainage via a ventriculostomy usually is more effective.

Corticosteroids have been assumed to prevent vasogenic brain edema through their stabilizing effects on vascular membranes. This assumption is supported by studies such as that of Rovit and Hagan,[50] who reported a reduction in the size of experimental lesions in animals pretreated with dexamethasone. Nevertheless, neither low-dose (16 mg/d) nor high-dose (96 mg/d) dexamethasone therapy sufficiently affected ICP or outcome in severely head-injured patients studied by Cooper et al.[51] Corticosteroid therapy is not routinely used in patients with head trauma at San Francisco General Hospital.

Treatment with barbiturates may reduce CBF and ICP by decreasing $CMRO_2$ or by lowering the effective circulating intravascular volume through peripheral venodilation and mild depression of the cardiac output.[52] Marshall et al.[53] reported that high-dose pentobarbital therapy (3 to 5 mg/kg) normalized ICP and reduced daily mannitol requirements in a majority of severely head-injured patients, although subsequent controlled trials failed to demonstrate any benefit from barbiturate therapy.[54,55] A 1980 study suggested that lidocaine was as effective as thiopental for rapid reduction of ICP and caused less cardiovascular depression.[56]

Other therapies to reduce ICP include hypothermia,[57] which reduces CBF as barbiturates do but is logistically difficult to administer; and hyperbaric oxygenation,[58] which causes cerebral vasoconstriction similar to that achieved by hyperventilation but is much more expensive and cumbersome. Dimethyl sulfoxide (DMSO) treatment also reduces ICP in some patients but has not been shown to improve outcome.[59]

PROGNOSIS

Two important questions relate to the issue of outcome from head trauma: (1) How can outcome be predicted? and (2) Is it altered by medical intervention? Regarding the first question, Overgaard and associates[60] have demonstrated that the initial clinical evaluation focusing on level of consciousness, motor behavior, and pupillary reflexes is most predictive of recovery from blunt head trauma. Jennett and Teasdale[28,29] introduced the GCS in part to facilitate prognostication on the basis of early physical examination, and their approach has been validated by Braakman et al.[61] Indeed, Narayan and co-workers[62] have since demonstrated that GCS was accurate in 80 percent of predictions, and that CT data and ICP level were less useful prognostic indicators.

After initial evaluation, age is the most important determinant of outcome. Bruce et al.[63] in 1978 reported that children and adolescents frequently recover from severe head injury despite pronounced intracranial hypertension and the presence of potentially ominous physical findings such as decerebrate rigidity. This good outcome may relate to the facts that young people manifest cerebral hyperemia after head trauma and have fewer mass lesions than adults. Berger et al.[64] determined that the death rate from head injury in an unselected pediatric population should be as low as 33 percent or less. This figure contrasts markedly with the death rate in older adults, which often is twice as high.

That initial clinical evaluation and age are highly predictive of outcome following head trauma suggests that morbidity and mortality cannot be greatly influenced by therapy. This conclusion is supported by the uniform death rate of 50 percent among 700 severely head-injured patients, most of them adults, in three countries with different care systems and management techniques.[65] In marked contrast, Becker and colleagues[66] have claimed that aggressive head injury management has lowered mortality to 30 percent. Studies such as these have engendered attitudes ranging from therapeutic pessimism to enthusiastic optimism among various clinicians and have not settled the issue of whether therapy is beneficial.

An intermediate viewpoint is that clinical outcome depends on both the degree of initial damage and the recognition and management of treatable injuries. The value of CPP measurement and manipulation has been questioned[67] but this approach has not been subjected to a prospective, randomized trial. Nevertheless, these therapies have been shown to be helpful in detecting deterioration in patients with mass lesions,[68] and their use is supported by extensive clinical experience.[69] Furthermore, early identification and intervention have greatly influenced the outcome from intracerebral and subdural hematoma.[70] Future improvements in outcome after traumatic brain insults will require innovative new therapies. Until these treatments are available, the medical management of head injury should involve the skillful use of the techniques described in this chapter.

References

1. Sevitt S: Fatal road accidents: Injuries, complications, and causes of death in 250 subjects. Br J Surg 1968;55:481–505
2. Pitts LH, Martin N: Head injuries. Surg Clin North Am 1982; 62:47–60
3. Bruce DA, Gennarelli TA, Langfitt TW: Resuscitation from coma due to head injury. Crit Care Med 1978;6:254–269
4. Ommaya AK, Gennarelli TA: Cerebral concussion and traumatic unconsciousness: Correlation of experimental and clinical observations on blunt head injuries. Brain 1974;97:633–654
5. Strich SJ: Shearing of nerve fibres as a cause of brain damage due to head injury: A pathological study of twenty cases. Lancet 1961;2:443–448
6. Brown GW, Brown ML: Cardiovascular responses to experimental cerebral concussion in the rhesus monkey. Arch Neurol Psych 1954;71:707–713
7. Cushing H: Concerning a definite regulatory mechanism of the vaso-motor centre which controls blood pressure during cerebral compression. Bull Johns Hopkins Hosp 1901;12:290–291
8. Bruce DA, Langfitt TW, Miller JD et al: Regional blood flow, intracranial pressure, and brain metabolism in comatose patients. J Neurosurg 1973;38:131–145
9. Bruce DA, Alavi A, Bilaniuk L et al: Diffuse cerebral swelling following head injuries in children: The syndrome of "malignant brain edema." J Neurosurg 1981;54:170–178
10. Fishman RA: Brain edema. N Engl J Med 1975;293:706–711
11. Miller JD, Becker DP, Ward JD et al: Significance of intracranial hypertension in severe head injury. J Neurosurg 1977;47:503–516
12. Lundberg N, Troupp H, Lorin H: Continuous recording of the ventricular-fluid pressure in patients with severe acute traumatic brain injury: A preliminary report. J Neurosurg 1965;22:581–590
13. Luce JM, Huseby JS, Kirk W, Butler J: A Starling resistor regulates cerebral venous outflow in dogs. J Appl Physiol 1982; 53:1496–1503
14. Kety SS, Shenkin HA, Schmidt CF: The effects of increased intracranial pressure on cerebral circulatory functions in man. J Clin Invest 1948;27:493–499
15. Greenfield JC, Tindall GT: Effect of acute increase in intracranial pressure on blood flow in the internal carotid artery of man. J Clin Invest 1965;44:1343–1351
16. Shields CB, McGraw CP: ICP and CPP as predictors of outcome following closed head injury. Presented at 6th International Symposium on Intracranial Pressure, Glasgow, June 9–13, 1985
17. Miller JD, Sweet RC, Narayan R, Becker DP: Early insults to the injured brain. JAMA 1978;240:439–442
18. Plum F, Posner JB: The Diagnosis of Stupor and Coma. 2nd Ed. FA Davis, Philadelphia, 1972
19. North JB, Jennett S: Abnormal breathing patterns associated with acute brain damage. Arch Neurol 1974;31:338–344
20. Frost EAM: The physiopathology of respiration in neurosurgical patients. J Neurosurg 1979;50:699–714
21. Schumacker PT, Rhodes GR, Newell JC et al: Ventilation-perfusion imbalance after head trauma. Am Rev Respir Dis 1979; 119:33–43
22. Cooper KR, Boswell PA: Reduced functional residual capacity and abnormal oxygenation in patients with severe head injury. Chest 1983;84:29–35
23. De Troyer A, Martin JG: Respiratory muscle tone and the control of functional residual capacity, editorial. Chest 1983;84: 3–4
24. Frost EAM, Arancibia CU, Shulman K: Pulmonary shunt as a prognostic indicator in head injury. J Neurosurg 1979;50:768–772
25. Mackensie RC, Christensen JM, Pitts LH, Lewis FR: Pulmonary extravascular fluid accumulation following intracranial injury. J Trauma 1983;23:968–975
26. Theodore J, Robin ED: Pathogenesis of neurogenic pulmonary oedema. Lancet 1975;1:749–751
27. La Force FM, Mullane JF, Boehme RF et al: The effect of pulmonary edema on antibacterial defenses of the lung. J Lab Clin Med 1973;82:631–648
28. Teasdale G, Jennett B: Assessment of coma and impaired consciousness. Lancet 1974;1:81–84
29. Jennett B, Teasdale G: Aspects of coma after severe head injury. Lancet 1977;1:878–881
30. Naidich TP, Moran CJ, Pudlowski RM, Hanaway J: Advances in diagnosis: Cranial and spinal computed tomography. Med Clin North Am 1979;63:849–895
31. Kennealy JA, McLennan ME, Loudon RG, McLaurin RL: Hyperventilation-induced cerebral hypoxia. Am Rev Respir Dis 1980;122:407–412
32. Jacobson SA, Rothballer AB: Prolonged measurement of experimental intracranial pressure using a subminiature absolute pressure transducer. J Neurosurg 1967;26:603–608
33. Vries JK, Becker DP, Young HF: A subarachnoid screw for monitoring intracranial pressure. J Neurosurg 1973;39:416–419
34. Luce JM: Neurologic monitoring. Respir Care 1985;30:471–480
35. Lassen NA, Hoedt-Rasmussen K, Sorensen SC et al: Regional

cerebral blood flow in man determined by krypton. Neurology 1963;9:719–727

36. Obrist WD, Thompson HK, King CH, Wang HS: Determination of regional cerebral blood flow by inhalation of 133-xenon. Circ Res 1967;20:124–135
37. Mazziotta JC, Phelps ME, Miller J, Kuhl DE: Tomographic mapping of human cerebral metabolism: Normal unstimulated state. Neurology 1981;31:503–516
38. Kuhl DE, Barrio JR, Huang S-C et al: Quantifying local cerebral blood flow by N-isopropyl-p-[^{123}I] iodoamphetamine (IMP) tomography. J Nucl Med 1982;23:196–203
39. Greenberg RP, Mayer DJ, Becker DP, Miller JD: Evaluation of brain function in severe human head trauma with multimodality evoked potentials. Part 1: Evoked brain-injury potentials, methods, and analysis. J Neurosurg 1977;47:150–162
40. Greenberg RP, Becker DP, Miller JD, Mayer DJ: Evaluation of brain function in severe human head trauma with multimodality evoked potentials. Part 2: Localization of brain dysfunction and correlation with posttraumatic neurological conditions. J Neurosurg 1977;47:163–177
41. Toole JF, Tucker SH: Influence of head position upon cerebral circulation: Studies on blood flow in cadavers. Arch Neurol 1960;2:616–623
42. Luce JM, Huseby JS, Kirk W, Butler J: Mechanism by which positive end-expiratory pressure increases cerebrospinal fluid pressure in dogs. J Appl Physiol 1982;52:231–235
43. Cotev S, Paul WL, Ruiz BC et al: Positive end-expiratory pressure (PEEP) and cerebrospinal fluid pressure during normal and elevated intracranial pressure in dogs. Intensive Care Med 1981; 7:187–191
44. Burchiel KJ, Steege TD, Wyler AR: Intracranial pressure changes in brain-injured patients requiring positive end-expiratory pressure ventilation. Neurosurgery 1981;8:443–449
45. Harper AM: The inter-relationship between $aPCO_2$ and blood pressure in the regulation of blood flow through the cerebral cortex. Acta Neurol Scand 1965;14:94–163
46. Paul RL, Polanco O, Turney SZ et al: Intracranial pressure responses to alterations in arterial carbon dioxide pressure in patients with head injuries. J Neurosurg 1972;36:714–720
47. Severinghaus JW: Role of cerebrospinal fluid pH in normalization of cerebral blood flow in chronic hypocapnia. Acta Neurol Scand 1965;14:116–120
48. Wise BL: Effects of infusion of hypertonic mannitol on electrolyte balance and on osmolarity of serum and cerebrospinal fluid. J Neurosurg 1963;20:691–697
49. McCarthy KD, Reed DJ: The effect of acetazolamide and furosemide on cerebrospinal fluid production and choroid plexus carbonic anhydrase activity. J Pharmacol Exp Ther 1974; 189:194–201
50. Rovit RL, Hagan R: Steroids and cerebral edema: The effects of glucocorticoids on abnormal capillary permeability following cerebral injury in cats. J Neuropathol Exp Neurol 1968;27:277–299
51. Cooper PR, Moody S, Clark WK et al: Dexamethasone and severe head injury. J Neurosurg 1979;51:307–316
52. Traeger SM, Henning RJ, Dobkin W et al: Hemodynamic effects of pentobarbital therapy for intracranial hypertension. Crit Care Med 1983;11:697–701
53. Marshall LF, Smith RW, Shapiro HM: The outcome with aggressive treatment in severe head injuries. J Neurosurg 1979; 50:26–30
54. Schwartz ML, Tator CH, Rowed DW et al: The University of Toronto head injury treatment study: A prospective, randomized comparison of pentobarbital and mannitol. Can J Neurol Sci 1984;11:434–440
55. Ward JD, Becker DP, Miller JD et al: Failure of prophylactic barbiturate coma in the treatment of severe head injury. J Neurosurg 1985;62:383–388
56. Bedford RF, Persing JA, Pobereskin L, Butler A: Lidocaine or thiopental for rapid control of intracranial hypertension? Anesth Analg 1980;59:435–437
57. Rosomoff HL, Shulman K, Raynor R, Grainger W: Experimental brain injury and delayed hypothermia. Surg Gynecol Obstet 1960;109:27–32
58. Miller JD, Ledingham IM: Reduction of increased intracranial pressure. Arch Neurol 1971;24:210–216
59. Pitts LH, Lovely MP, Bartowski HM: The effect of dimethylsulfoxide (DMSO) on intracranial pressure and outcome after severe head injury. Presented at 6th International Conference on Intracranial Pressure, Glasgow, June 9–13, 1985
60. Overgaard J, Hvid-Hansen O, Land AM et al: Prognosis after head injury based on early clinical examination. Lancet 1973; 2:631–635
61. Braakman R, Gelpke GJ, Habbema JDF et al: Systematic selection of prognostic features in patients with severe head injury. Neurosurgery 1980;6:362–369
62. Narayan RK, Greenberg RP, Miller JD et al: Improved confidence of outcome prediction in severe head injury. J Neurosurg 1981;54:751–762
63. Bruce DA, Schut L, Bruno LA et al: Outcome following severe head injuries in children. J Neurosurg 1978;48:679–688
64. Berger MS, Pitts LH, Lovely M et al: Outcome from severe head injury in children and adolescents. J Neurosurg 1985; 62:194–199
65. Jennett B, Teasdale G, Galbraith S et al: Severe head injuries in three countries. J Neurol Neurosurg Psychiatry 1977;40:291–298
66. Becker DP, Miller JP, Ward JD et al: The outcome from severe head injury with early diagnosis and intensive management. J Neurosurg 1977;47:491–502
67. Fleischer AS, Payne NS, Tindall GT: Continuous monitoring of intracranial pressure in severe closed head injury without mass lesions. Surg Neurol 1976;6:31–34
68. Seelig JM, Greenberg RP, Becker DP et al: Reversible brainstem dysfunction following acute traumatic subdural hematoma. J Neurosurg 1981;55:516–523
69. Miller JD, Butterworth JF, Gudeman SK et al: Further experience in the management of severe head injury. J Neurosurg 1981;54:289–299
70. Seelig JM, Becker DP, Miller JD et al: Traumatic acute subdural hematoma: Major mortality reduction in comatose patients treated within four hours. N Engl J Med 1981;304:1151–1157

Chapter 94

Respiratory Care of the Patient with Burns or Smoke Inhalation

Ray H. Ritz

CHAPTER OUTLINE

Between 2 million and 2.5 million individuals are treated for burn injuries each year in the United States, of whom approximately 70,000 are admitted to intensive care units.[1,2] Burn-related fatalities number 10,000 to 12,000 annually.[3,4] Advances in burn care have improved the chances of surviving major thermal injuries, but the mortality rate for healthy young adults who suffer a 60 to 75 percent total body surface area (TBSA) burn still hovers around 50 percent.[5] The direct cause of death in hospitalized burn patients is most commonly severe infection and/or cardiopulmonary failure. Those patients who suffer injuries in addition to their cutaneous burn injury have significantly higher mortality rates.[6]

Patients with burn injuries present a series of unique complications to their management. Initial care of the burn patient is centered around support of basic pulmonary and cardiovascular systems. Those who survive the initial injury are at risk for a variety of respiratory complications during the course of their hospitalization, including CO poisoning, airway obstruction, pulmonary edema, pneumonia, and pulmonary thromboembolism[7] (Fig. 94-1). These patients may pose some of the most difficult clinical management problems encountered in respiratory care. The following pages address the fundamental clinical principles that are unique to thermal and inhalation injuries, while other chapters of this text describe in detail the full spectrum of complications and issues that apply to all critically ill patients.

AIRWAY MANAGEMENT

The initial decision to intubate a patient is based on the degree of thermal and/or toxic inhalation injury (Table 94-1). When airway edema develops following inhalation injury, this generally occurs within 24 hours of the initial injury, and prophylactic intubation may be indicated to avoid the difficulties associated with tube placement in an edematous airway. Also, if the degree of cutaneous injury is significant, early intubation and application of mechanical ventilation and positive end-expiratory pressure (PEEP) may be useful.[8] A quick estimation of the TBSA affected can be made by applying the "rule of nines," which allocates a set percentage of surface area to each geographic portion of the body (Fig. 94-2). Intubation may be appropriate if the thermal injury exceeds 30 to 40 percent of TBSA, if there are indications of inhalation injury (burns of the oral pharynx, singed nasal hair, soot in upper or lower airway), or if there is loss of consciousness or evidence of shock.

When intubation is indicated, the largest-caliber endotra-

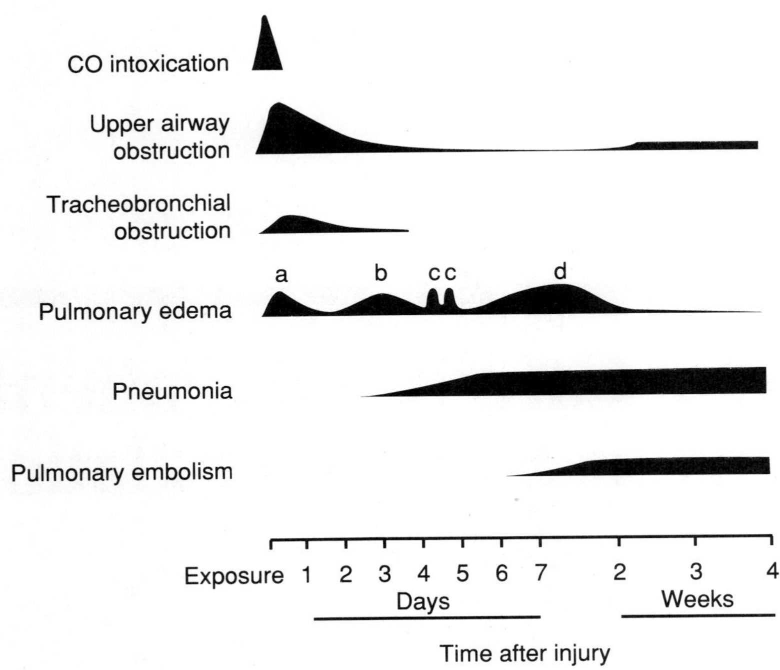

Figure 94-1. Pulmonary complications present at various times in patients with burn and toxic inhalation injuries. The most common complications are shown against time on the horizontal axis. The development of pulmonary edema may have numerous etiologies. The sequence represented here includes such causes as a, hypervolemia secondary to initial fluid resuscitation; b, hypervolemia secondary to fluid shifts as edema dissipates; c, iatrogenic hypervolemia during surgery; and d, general sepsis. (Adapted from Haponik and Summer[17] with permission.)

Table 94-1. Clinical Predictors of Inhalation Injuries

Exposure characteristics
Closed space setting, entrapment
Unconsciousness
Known inhaled toxin
Facial, cervical burns
Carbonaceous sputum
Respiratory symptoms
Hoarseness
Sore throat
Cough
Dyspnea
Chest pain
Hemoptysis
Respiratory signs
Pharyngeal burns/inflammation
Stridor
Tachypnea
Cyanosis
Wheezes, rhonchi, crackles

(From Haponik and Summer,[7] with permission.)

cheal tube possible should be used in order to accommodate possible future bronchoscopies and to simplify pulmonary hygiene. Oral endotracheal tubes are generally preferred initially owing to their ease of placement. Nasal tubes carry the associated risk of infections of the sinuses and middle ear. Once intubation is accomplished, it may not be possible to change the airway for weeks. Elective reintubation with a nasal tube may be acceptable in the stable patient if long-term mechanical ventilation is anticipated. This may provide a greater degree of comfort to the patient as well as being simpler to stabilize, but in a patient with facial burns, erosion of the nares is common. Early tracheotomy should be avoided in burn patients because of their inherent increased risk of infection.[10] Tracheotomy may be considered if long-term ventilatory support is required and aggressive surgery or healing has reduced the percent of open wound.

Maintenance of an oral or nasal endotracheal tube in burn patients is complicated by the rapid and extreme shifts in extravascular fluid during the initial phases of the injury. Uncut tubes should be placed and cut conservatively, so that if facial swelling occurs, an adequate length of tube is externally available to allow for effective stabilization. The method of securing the tube should facilitate simple loos-

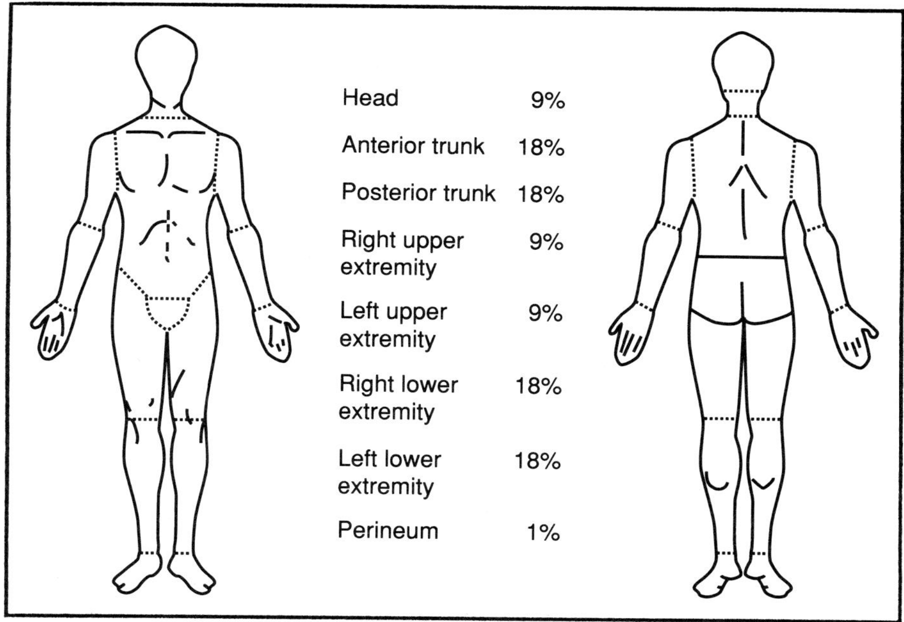

Figure 94-2. The rule of nines. Although not accurate in children, this rule allows a quick estimate of the percent surface area burned. The body is divided into regions and each is allocated 9 or 18 percent of the TBSA. (Adapted from Deitch,[9] with permission.)

ening or tightening as needed. When facial burns are present, adhesive-backed tape is seldom useful. Cloth ties or commercially available harnesses can secure tubes adequately but are often difficult to apply. Frequent assessment of tube stability is necessary. The stabilizing system should also be checked to ensure that it is not too tight as a result of swelling.

Extubation should be approached cautiously. It should be clear that the patient possesses adequate reserve to maintain ventilation. If an inhalation injury was present or if intubation was long-term (longer than 3 to 4 weeks), removal of an artificial airway should be performed carefully. With the cuff down, airflow through the upper airway should be audible at pressures of 30 cmH_2O or less. The absence of a leak may mean the presence of edema or the development of stenosis or webbing of the vocal cords. If the patient has a tracheostomy tube, a conservative approach may include changing the airway to a fenestrated tube, which allows the use of the upper airway during monitored periods. In this fashion, the adequacy of the cough can be assessed as well as patients' ability to protect themselves from aspiration.

TOXIC INHALATION

Even without thermal injury to the airway, inhalation of the toxic products of incomplete combustion presents considerable risks to victims. The presence of inhalation injuries substantially increases the mortality rate associated with cutaneous burns[11] (Fig. 94-3). In two well-studied catastrophic fires, the 1942 Coconut Grove fire in Boston and the 1981 MGM Grand Hotel fire in Las Vegas, a significant number of victims died without cutaneous burns.[12,13] Inhaled agents can be classified as either asphyxiants or irritants (Table 94-2).

Tissue hypoxia is common with smoke inhalation, and prompt administration of high concentrations of O_2 is essential. CO, the most common asphyxiant, is rapidly absorbed into the blood and interferes with O_2 delivery by binding with hemoglobin. Although this process is reversible, the superior affinity of hemoglobin for CO (230 to 270 times as great as for O_2)[14] means that exposure to low levels of CO can have serious consequences. This is clearly demonstrated by the effect of breathing automobile exhaust, which contains approximately 9 percent CO.[15]

One interesting clinical finding of CO poisoning is the absence of cyanosis in the presence of potentially profound tissue hypoxia. The presence of carboxyhemoglobin can actually result in a "cherry red" appearance of the lips.[16] Co-oximetry (automated differential spectrophotometry) is the most common method of determining carboxyhemoglobin levels and may be performed on either venous or arterial blood. The physiologic effects of CO poisoning are directly proportional to the levels present in the blood (Table 94-3).

Treatment of CO poisoning is directed toward improving tissue oxygenation and breaking the carboxyhemoglobin bond to allow transport of O_2. Under ambient conditions (an inspired O_2 fraction [F_IO_2] of 0.21 at 1 atm), half of the ab-

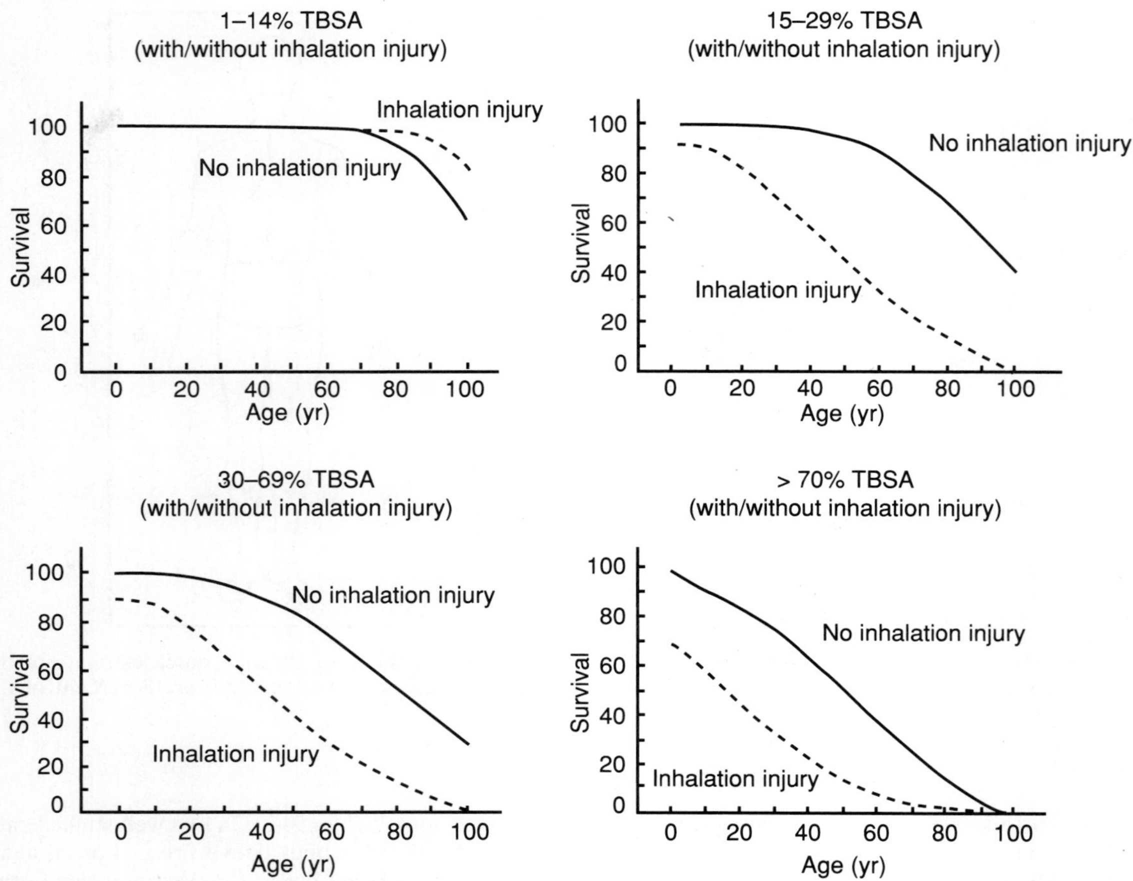

Figure 94-3. The impact of superimposing an inhalation injury onto cutaneous burns is dramatically illustrated in these graphs, based on a retrospective study of the medical records of 1705 patients over a 10-year period. As the percent TBSA burned increases, so does the mortality. Inclusion of age only serves to magnify the seriousness of the injury. (Adapted from Tredget et al.,[11] with permission.)

sorbed CO (half-life [t1/2]) is eliminated by the lungs every 5.3 hours. If 100 percent O_2 is provided, t1/2 is reduced to approximately 1.5 hours. The application of O_2 at 3 atm in a hyperbaric chamber will reduce t1/2 to 23 minutes[17,18] (Fig. 94-4). An F_{IO_2} of 1.0 should be provided as soon as possible and maintained until the patient's condition is assessed. Although any threshold level is arbitrary in view of the available data, patients with carboxyhemoglobin levels of 40 percent or greater should probably be treated with hyperbaric O_2 therapy if it is available.[18,19] The F_{IO_2} may generally be reduced when the CO level is less than 10 percent as long as the patient's arterial O_2 saturation (SaO_2) is 90 percent or greater.

Table 94-2. Inhaled Toxic Agents

Irritants
Hydrogen chloride
Nitrogen oxide
Sulfur dioxide
Isocyanates
Phosgene
Chlorine
Ammonia
Acrolein
Asphyxiants
Carbon monoxide
Cyanide

Inhalation of irritants may occur in conjunction with CO poisoning or as the primary injury. Such inhalation results in a variety of injuries, including inflammation of the airways and parenchymal damage, which in turn result in pulmonary edema, laryngospasm, bronchospasm, increased work of breathing, loss of surfactant, and hypoxemia. Intubation and mechanical ventilation are indicated if the injury is severe. Upon physical examination individuals may present with soot in the oral airway, burns around the nose or mouth, or other indications of inhalation injuries. The decision to intubate the patient must be based on overall condition, but

Table 94-3. Effects of Carbon Monoxide Poisoning

F_ICO	COHb (%)	Response in Healthy Adult
0	0.3–0.7	No effect
0.003	1–5	Selective increase in blood flow to vital organs to compensate for reduced O_2-carrying capacity
0.007	5–10	Visual light threshold increased, dyspnea on vigorous exercise, dilation of cutaneous blood vessels
0.012	10–20	Abnormal vision evoked response, dyspnea on mild exertion, throbbing headache
0.022	20–30	Marked headache, irritability, easy fatiguability, poor judgment, diminished vision and fine manual dexterity, nausea/vomiting
0.035–0.052	30–40	Severe headache, nausea/vomiting, confusion, syncope on exertion
0.082–0.122	50–60	Intermittent convulsions, respiratory failure, coma, death if prolonged exposure
0.199	70–80	Coma, rapidly fatal

(From Waffle,[32] with permission.)

if an airway injury is present, this procedure only becomes more difficult as the effects of the injury become more pronounced.

Bronchospasm should be treated by administration of aerosolized bronchodilators, although "mechanical wheezing" that results from airway edema may not respond to such therapy. Bronchospastic patients being mechanically ventilated who are refractory to bronchodilator therapy should be regularly assessed for the presence of auto-PEEP.[20] The use of steroids in smoke inhalation injuries is generally contraindicated owing to the increased risk of infection.[2,21] Airway edema and pulmonary edema may be a result of cell wall injury to the bronchial or alveolar structures or may be a function of fluid resuscitation and massive cutaneous burns.

VOLUME RESUSCITATION

Thermal injuries can cause a significant and rapid accumulation of edema in both burned and unburned tissue. This shift of intravascular fluid into the extravascular regions may result in profound hypotension and shock if not treated by appropriate fluid resuscitation. The magnitude of the burn injury will dictate how aggressively the volume replacement is administered. Fluid management is a critical component of burn care, and scrupulous attention must be paid to fluid balance to avoid either underhydration or overhydration.

A common approach to fluid management is the Parkland formula.[3,22] Using this approach, in the first 24 hours after the initial injury the patient is given 4 mL/kg/% burn of lactated Ringer's solution. The fluid is infused at a rate of 50 percent of the total calculated volume in the first 8 hours and the balance in the following 16 hours. Individual variation from patient to patient requires careful monitoring of urinary output, blood pressure, heart and respiratory rate, and mental status. Titration of infusion rates should be based on obtaining acceptable values of those variables. Fluid administration may need to be increased by as much as 50 percent if significant inhalation injury accompanies the surface burn injury.[23]

Excessive administration of fluids can increase the amount of edema and may contribute to impaired tissue oxygenation. Urinary output in excess of 2 mL/kg/h may be an indication of over-resuscitation, but it may also be a result of hyperglycemic osmotic diuresis. This distinction should be made, and if diuresis is a result of overhydration, fluid administration should be reduced by 25 percent every 2 to 4 hours until urine output is within the acceptable range.

Patients with compromised cardiac function may be intolerant of adequate fluid replacement unless medications such as dobutamine and dopamine are administered. In this population it may be appropriate to administer the above drugs prophylactically to prevent cardiac failure.[24,25] If fluid management is complicated, the placement of a pulmonary artery catheter may be necessary, but it should be used conservatively since the risk of infection is high.

After 24 hours the lactated Ringer's solution should be changed to 5 percent dextrose in water with additional plasma or albumin, since vascular permeability to proteins will have returned to near normal. After 72 hours postinjury, the tissue edema will begin to subside, with a resulting significant increase in urinary output. Fluid administration must be titrated to maintain a stable output. Significant amounts of potassium may be lost, so serum levels should be monitored to prevent serious complications of hypokalemia such as cardiac arrhythmias. During hospitalization patients should also be monitored for hypernatremia as well as for adequate serum albumin and hemoglobin levels.

NUTRITIONAL CONSIDERATIONS

No other major injury elicits as great a hypermetabolic response as does a burn injury.[26] Aggressive nutritional support is necessary to control the massive weight and nitrogen loss that results from the catabolic process accompanying this excessive hypermetabolism. Since rapid fluid shifts occur in addition to alterations in serum albumin and nitrogen levels due to the thermal injury, assessing the nutritional status of burn patients is difficult. Even with today's automated bedside metabolic carts, there is some controversy concerning the best approach to providing nutritional support.

The best conventional wisdom dictates that 50 to 60 percent of the total caloric intake consist of carbohydrates. This

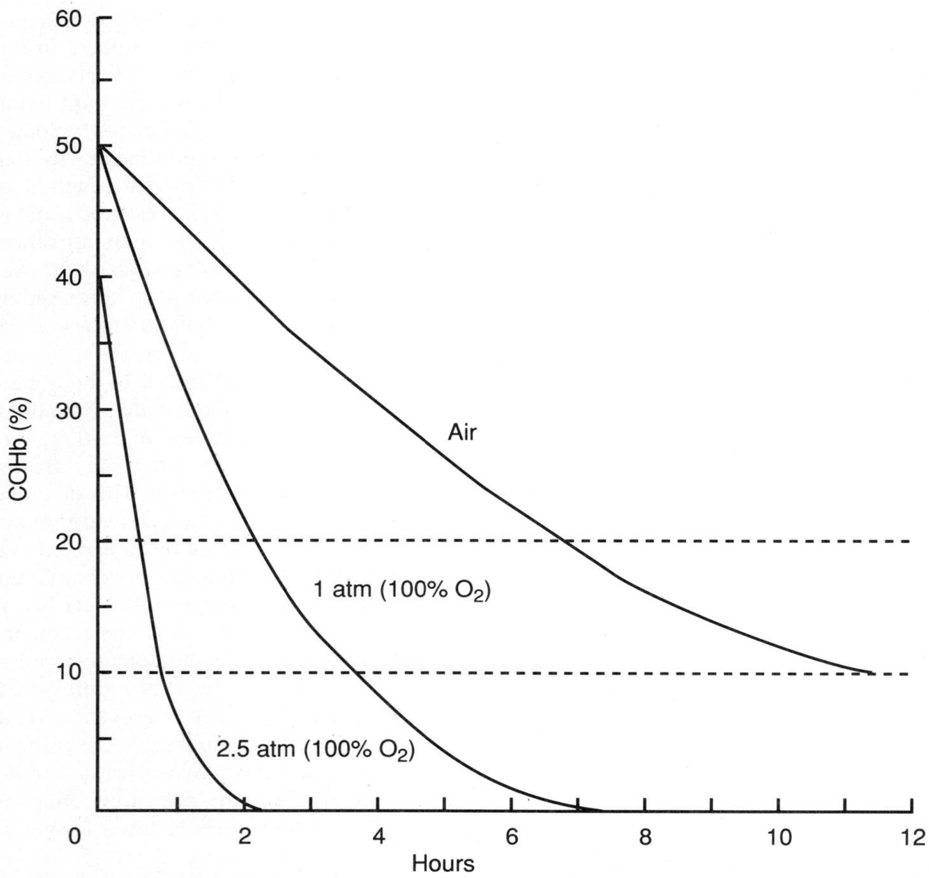

Figure 94-4. The effect of supplemental O_2 at an F_IO_2 of 1.0 at ambient pressure and at 2.5 atm on CO elimination is compared with the elimination rate on room air. (Adapted from Winter,[15] with permission.)

is owing to the high consumption of glucose secondary to the burn injury. Survival among patients receiving a high-protein diet may be greater than among those receiving a more standard diet, particularly if nutritional support can be provided enterally.[27]

Enteral feeding has some advantages over the parenteral route since it carries a lower risk of infection than does the invasive method. It also maintains gut function. Unfortunately, the high metabolic demands of the major burn patient are often not satisfied by this method. The ability to rapidly adjust parenteral support and to give large amounts of nutritional substrate make this form of administration common. As gastrointestinal function returns, conversion to the enteral route of support is appropriate.

Overfeeding can complicate the management of burn patients as well. If excessive carbohydrate (glucose) is administered, glucose intolerance, polyuria, and increased CO_2 production may occur. The latter requires increased minute ventilation in order to maintain CO_2 elimination and acid-base balance. Large minute ventilation values can result in the development of auto-PEEP.[20] Reduction of the amount of administered carbohydrate may allow reduction of the minute ventilation requirement. The only other alternative is to reduce the minute ventilation and allow the patient's $PaCO_2$ to rise and to adjust the pH with $NaHCO_3$.

INFECTIONS

Infection presents a grave risk to the burn patient. Although stringent measures are used to avoid contamination, infections are virtually unavoidable. Wounds should be covered with sterile dressings immediately upon admission to the hospital. Isolation practices vary, but generally include strict gowning and gloving prior to each contact with the patient.

A major cause of wound sepsis in thermal injuries is *Pseudomonas aeruginosa*.[28] This organism reproduces rapidly on necrotic tissue and spreads quickly to adjacent unburned areas. Topically applied antimicrobial agents such as sulfadiazine cream or silver nitrate are effective at treating initial colonization, but they do not penetrate eschar. Heavy colonization requires an agent that does penetrate the scar tissue, such as mafenide acetate cream. Frequent debridement of necrotic tissue is essential. As sepsis becomes more pronounced, the use of systemic antibiotics is indicated. The need for surgical excision of necrotic tissue may require transporting the patient to the operating room. Given the amount of ventilatory support required by some burn patients, this can be an extremely complicated process.

MECHANICAL VENTILATION

Although the basic concepts of mechanical ventilation generally apply to the management of burn patients, there are some complications unique to major thermal injuries.

Patients with full thickness circumferential burns around the thorax may develop a severe restriction of the chest wall, which limits their ability to ventilate and which may be so severe that the ability to mechanically ventilate is impaired. This usually presents immediately after the injury and is evident by extremely high ventilating pressures. Once other potential causes (pneumothorax, airway obstruction, etc.) have been ruled out, the traditional approach to relieving the chest wall restriction is to make a set of midaxillary incisions, one on either side running perpendicular to the ribs, and one incision horizontally just below the rib cage. This eliminates the mechanical restriction and allows ventilation at a lower pressure.

Since the early 1980s increasing evidence has accumulated to support the concept that early surgical excision of the burn reduces mortality[29,30] and shortens hospital stays.[31] As this new approach to burn care becomes more widely adopted, early pulmonary restriction in burned patients and the need for escharotomies will be eliminated.

Bronchospasm is another common complication, particularly if an inhalation injury is present. Aggressive treatment with bronchodilators as frequently as once every hour may be necessary. Inhalation injuries may trigger excessive secretion production requiring frequent suctioning. The airway may also become irritated and hypersensitive, which results in spasmodic coughing, and this may become so severe as to limit the ability to ventilate. Administration of narcotics may be necessary to stabilize ventilation.

The high metabolic demand and the profound degree of sepsis may necessitate extremely high levels of minute ventilation, which may exceed the ability of some ventilators owing to the high pressures or flows required. As indicated previously, a common complication of high minute ventilation is the development of auto-PEEP. Patients should be monitored regularly for this, and maneuvers to minimize auto-PEEP should be used, including intermittent mandatory ventilation (IMV), shortened inspiratory times, and reduced respiratory rates and minute ventilations. When auto-PEEP is minimized, addition of applied PEEP (that provided intentionally with the ventilator) should be considered, at a level equal or close to that of the auto-PEEP, in order to minimize work of breathing. However, when balancing the applied PEEP to the auto-PEEP, frequent assessments of the auto-PEEP (i.e., total PEEP) should be made to ensure that the latter is not increased by this process (see Ch. 76).

Caution should be used in increasing minute ventilation in order to maintain normal blood gases. Accepting a PaO_2 of 60 mmHg and allowing the $PaCO_2$ to rise to 60 mmHg or higher may be preferable to the complications associated with high minute ventilations and airway pressures. The patient's pH can be adjusted with $NaHCO_3$ infusion if necessary, and an SaO_2 of 90 percent will generally provide adequate tissue oxygenation.

Weaning from mechanical ventilation can be difficult in burn patients. This may be particularly true when burns have been extensive and long-term ventilation has been employed. While major portions of the burned surface remain open, taking over the preponderance of the ventilatory work allows more energy to be devoted to other systems. As long as minute ventilation remains high and lung compliance is low, the overall work of breathing may be great enough to obviate weaning. As these parameters improve and infections are brought under control, a larger portion of ventilatory work may be done by the patient. Reductions in IMV rates or low levels of pressure support are approaches to weaning that may be useful in this setting.

Although advances in technology have improved the morbidity and mortality of burn injuries, burn patients can be the most labor-intensive and complicated patients found in today's intensive care unit. Such individuals require meticulous attention to the details of care as well as some of the most sophisticated monitoring used in medicine. The emotional toll on those caring for them is great, and yet the satisfaction derived from meeting the challenges they present can be substantial.

References

1. Demling RH: Burns. N Engl J Med 1985;313:1389–1398
2. Markley K: Burn care: Infection and smoke inhalation. Ann Intern Med 1979;90:269–270
3. Deitch EA: The management of burns. N Engl J Med 1990;323:1249–1253
4. Cahalane M, Demling RH: Early respiratory abnormalities from smoke inhalation. JAMA 1984;251:771–773
5. Herndon DN, Curreri PW, Abston S et al: Treatment of burns: An overview of clinical aspects of burn care. Curr Probl Surg 1987;24:341–397
6. Shairani KZ, Pruitt BA, Mason AD: The influence of inhalation injury and pneumonia on burn mortality. Ann Surg 1987;205:82–87
7. Haponik EF, Summer WR: Respiratory complications in burn patients: Diagnosis and management of inhalation injury. J Crit Care 1987;2:121–141
8. Venus B, Matsuda T, Copiozo JB et al: Prophylactic intubation and continuous positive airway pressure in the management of inhalation injury in burn victims. Crit Care Med 1981;9:519–523
9. Deitch EA: Keys to the early care of burn patients. J Crit Illness 1990;5:1213–1222
10. Epstein BS, Rudman HL, Hardy DL, et al: Comparison of orotracheal intubation with tracheostomy for anesthesia in patients with face and neck burns. Anesth Analg 1966;45:352–359
11. Tredget EE, Shankowsky HA, Taerum TV et al: The role of inhalation injury in burn trauma: A Canadian experience. Ann Surg 1990;212:720–727
12. Finland M, Davidson CS, Levenson SM: Clinical and therapeutic aspects of the conflagration injuries to the respiratory tract sustained by victims of the Coconut Grove disaster. Medicine (Baltimore) 1946;25:215–283

13. Crapo RO: Smoke inhalation injuries. JAMA 1981;246:1694
14. Aronow WS: Effect of cigarette smoking and carbon monoxide on coronary heart disease. Chest 1976;70:514–518
15. Winter PM: Carbon monoxide poisoning. JAMA 1976;236:1502–1504
16. Smith JS, Brandon S: Acute carbon monoxide poisoning: 3 year experience in a defined population. Postgrad Med J 1970;46:65–70
17. Norkool DM, Kirkpatrick JN: Treatment of acute carbon monoxide poisoning with hyperbaric oxygen: A review of 115 cases. Ann Emerg Med 1985;14:1168–1171
18. Thom SR, Keim LW: Hyperbaric oxygen therapy. Probl Respir Care 1990;3:575–590
19. Kindwall EP: Carbon monoxide and cyanide poisoning. pp. 177–190. In Davis JC, Hunt TK (eds): Hyperbaric Oxygen Therapy. Undersea Medical Society, Bethesda, MD, 1977
20. Pepe PE, Marini JJ: Occult positive end-expiratory pressure in mechanically ventilated patients with airflow obstruction: The auto-PEEP effect. Am Rev Respir Dis 1982;126:166–170
21. Herndon DN, Thompson PB, Traber DL: Pulmonary injury in the burned patient. Crit Care Clin 1985;1:79–96
22. Baxter CR, Shires GT: Physiological response to crystalloid resuscitation of severe burns. Ann NY Acad Sci 1968;150:874–893
23. Navar PD, Saffle JR, Warden GD: Effect of inhalation injury on fluid resuscitation requirements after thermal injury. Am J Surg 1985;150:716–720
24. Pruitt BA Jr: Advances in fluid therapy and the early care of the burn patient. World J Surg 1978;2:139–150
25. Aikawa N, Ishkari K, Naito C et al: Individualized fluid resuscitation based on hemodynamic monitoring in the management of extensive burns. Burns Incl Therm Inj 1982;8:249–255
26. Wilmore DW, Aulick LH: Metabolic changes in burned patients. Surg Clin North Am 1978;58:1173–1187
27. Alexander JW, MacMillan BG, Sinnett JD et al: Beneficial effects of aggressive protein feeding in severely burned children. Ann Surg 1980;192:505–517
28. Pruitt BA, Lindberg RB, McManus WF et al: Current approach to prevention and treatment of *Pseudomonas aeruginosa* infections in burn patients. Rev Infect Dis 1983;5:S889
29. Engrav LH, Heimbach DM, Reus JL et al: Early excision and grafting vs nonoperative treatment of burns of indeterminant depth: A randomized prospective study. J Trauma 1983;23:1001–1004
30. Herndon DH, Barrow RE, Rutan RL et al: A comparison of conservative versus early excision therapies in severely burned patients. Ann Surg 1989;209:547–553
31. Gray DT, Pine RW, Harnar TJ et al: Early surgical excision versus conventional therapy in patients with 20 to 40 percent burns: A comparative study. Am J Surg 1982;144:76–80
32. Waffle CM: Carbon monoxide poisoning. pp. 259–271. In Brenner BE (ed): Comprehensive Management of Respiratory Emergencies. Aspen Publication, Rockville, MD, 1985

Chapter 95

Cardiopulmonary and Cerebral Resuscitation

John M. Luce

CHAPTER OUTLINE

The term *cardiopulmonary resuscitation* (CPR) refers to the restoration of heartbeat and breathing after these functions have been temporarily lost. CPR is the treatment for cardiopulmonary arrest, a condition in which the heart no longer pumps oxygenated blood to the tissues of the body. Cardiopulmonary arrest may result from obstruction of the airway due to an aspirated food bolus, depression of breathing during a sedative or narcotic drug overdose, or flooding of the lungs in a drowning accident. More commonly, however, it is caused by disturbances in the heart's normally rhythmic beating. These rhythm disturbances, or dysrhythmias, include ventricular tachycardia, in which the cardiac ventricles that pump blood beat independently of the atria that supply them; ventricular fibrillation, in which all four cardiac chambers quiver chaotically; and asystole, in which there is no heartbeat. Although these dysrhythmias may occur in the context of a myocardial infarction, commonly known as a heart attack, they also may develop spontaneously in patients with underlying electrical instability of the heart.

Most people lose consciousness if their brains are deprived of oxygenated blood for more than 5 or 10 seconds, and permanent neurologic damage, if not complete brain death, is likely if cerebral blood flow is compromised for 4 minutes or longer. The heart itself cannot regain rhythmic electrical activity if its blood flow is diminished for much longer than 10 minutes, because tissues in the cardiac conduction system that normally generate and propagate electrical impulses die for lack of O_2. Even those organs, such as the kidney, that can function longer without O_2 ultimately fail owing to the effects of *ischemia* (a diminution in blood flow) and *hypoxia* (a reduction in O_2). Therefore, CPR must be performed expeditiously and effectively if it is to restore life.

Although prompt restoration of heart beat and breathing should aid the brain along with other organs, the effects of ischemia and hypoxia on the central nervous system also may be prevented or anticipated by measures specifically designed to improve neurologic function. Most of these measures had been used in patients with head trauma and other neurosurgical catastrophes before they were applied to patients with cardiopulmonary arrest and became known collectively as *cerebral resuscitation*. Because cardiopulmonary and cerebral resuscitation are inseparable in patients with cardiopulmonary arrest, Safar[1] and others have suggested that the terms be combined as cardiopulmonary-cerebral resuscitation. This chapter follows the more traditional approach of describing the technique of cardiopulmonary and cerebral resuscitation separately. However, these descriptions are preceded by a discussion of the history of CPR and the possible mechanisms of blood flow during closed chest compression because CPR is an evolving science and art that can best be appreciated if its ongoing development is known.

HISTORY OF CARDIOPULMONARY RESUSCITATION

Although the need for speed in CPR was not unknown to earlier practitioners, their efforts were handicapped by their misunderstanding of the causes of cardiopulmonary arrest. Most of these efforts were aimed at problems in breathing, not heart beat, with their greatest emphasis on restoring the breath of life. The first recorded example of CPR comes from the Bible,[2] in which Elisha is reported to have revived a child by lying on his body and breathing into his mouth. In eighteenth century Europe unconscious persons were slung over the backs of trotting horses or rolled over barrels in an attempt to move air into and out of their chests. The Schafer prone pressure method of artificial respiration involved squeezing the lower back to force the abdominal contents against the diaphragm, and empty the lungs. This technique persisted until 1954, when Elam et al.[3] demonstrated that mouth-to-mouth and mouth-to-nose resuscitation were simpler and much more effective.

Attention was first given to the heart's role in cardiopulmonary arrest in the operating room, where surgeons and anesthesiologists occasionally were confronted with patients whose hearts had stopped or were beating irregularly. Asystole in these instances was due most often to anesthetic agents, whereas ventricular tachycardia or fibrillation most often resulted from metabolic abnormalities. Because external electrocardiographic (ECG) monitoring was not available, cardiac dysrhythmias could be diagnosed only by opening the chest. Treatment consisted of manually squeezing the cardiac ventricles, that is, performing open chest or internal cardiac massage, until the heart could be defibrillated by the direct application of a strong electrical current. Although associated with serious complications, including occasional laceration of the heart and lungs as the chest was hastily penetrated as well as eventual infection of the open thorax, internal cardiac massage was successful in many instances—so successful, in fact, that scalpels were made available throughout hospitals to open the chests of patients who suffered cardiopulmonary arrest outside the operating room.

The Cardiac Pump Model

Open chest cardiac massage remained the standard in-hospital CPR until it became unnecessary for diagnostic and therapeutic purposes. The diagnostic breakthrough was the development in the 1950s of external ECG monitoring, which allowed detection of dysrhythmias using electrodes placed on the chest wall. Then in 1960 Kouwenhoven et al.[4] reported that the circulation could be supported easily and with few complications through the rhythmic application of firm pressure to the lower sternum. In their initial study these investigators demonstrated that *closed-chest cardiac massage*, as they called their new technique, provided palpable pulses and an adequate blood pressure in dogs in ventricular fibrillation. They subsequently reported that external compression, combined with artificial respiration, restored cardiac and neurologic function in patients before electrical defibrillation could be accomplished with paddles applied to the chest.

Kouwenhoven and co-workers[4] attributed the success of their new technique to the position of the heart in the thorax. They noted that the heart fills most of the space between the sternum and the thoracic spine and is restricted in lateral movement by the lungs and the pericardium. Because of this anatomic relationship, they reasoned, pressure applied to the anterior sternum should squeeze the right and left ventricles, raising ventricular pressures above those in the pulmonary artery and aorta and creating a pressure gradient that should force blood through these vessels. Release of the pressure should allow the chest to recoil to its original position, causing a negative intrathoracic pressure, which would enhance blood return to the heart. Although pressure would be exerted also on the venous system with each cardiac compression, Kouwenhoven et al.[4] argued that blood flows primarily in a forward direction because of the one-way arrangement of the heart valves (Fig. 95-1).

The reports of Kouwenhoven and associates[4] were well received by some physicians, but others were quick to challenge noninvasive CPR. For example, Weale and Rothwell-Jackson[5] noted that external cardiac massage could lead to rib fractures and liver laceration and also pointed out that the presence of palpable pulses was not proof of organ perfusion, since an artery can pulsate at its site of ligation. Furthermore, they maintained, closed-chest compression was based on erroneous physiologic assumptions. Their argument was as follows: Many patients, including those with emphysema, have deep chests in which the heart falls away from the sternum, and in most instances the propagation of pressure pulses during external cardiac massage is not due to the heart being squeezed between the sternum and vertebral column. Instead, closed-chest compression causes a generalized increase in intrathoracic pressure that is transmitted equally to the heart and vessels in the chest and then to extrathoracic arteries and veins because the heart valves are rendered incompetent. Forward flow cannot occur because the generalized increase in pressure precludes the development of a gradient necessary to force blood from the heart into the aorta and pulmonary artery; blood also cannot cross peripheral arteriovenous circuits because pressures are equal in the arteries and the veins. As a result of these several factors, during closed-chest compression the heart cannot act as a unidirectional pump, as occurs with internal cardiac massage.

Confronted with these conflicting viewpoints, Mackenzie and co-workers[6] measured vascular pressures and cardiac outputs in three patients who sustained cardiopulmonary arrest that was treated with external massage. They demon-

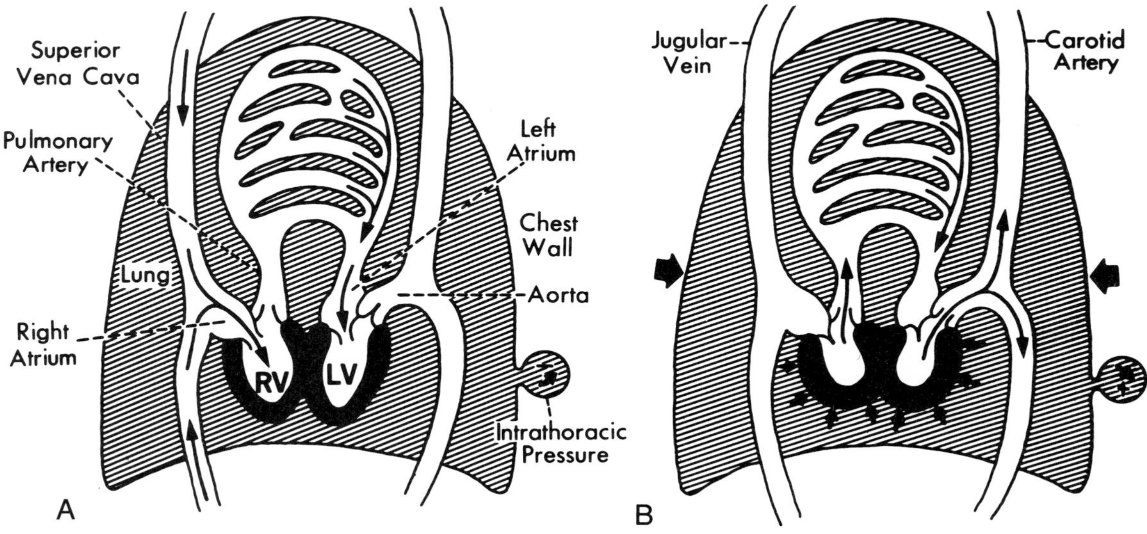

Figure 95-1. Traditional cardiac pump model of cardiopulmonary resuscitation: (**A**) relaxation, (**B**) compression. During relaxation or mechanical "diastole," negative pressure in the chest enhances blood return to the heart. Blood is preferentially stored in the right (RV) and left ventricle (LV). During closed-chest compression or mechanical "systole," the heart is squeezed between sternum and spine, a pressure gradient is developed between the two ventricles and the pulmonary artery and aorta, and antegrade flow occurs through the large vessels owing to the one-way arrangement of heart valves. (Adapted from Luce et al.,[2] with permission.)

strated that pressures in the cardiac chambers and large vessels in the chest were elevated equally, supporting Weale and Rothwell-Jackson's claim that closed-chest compression causes a generalized increase in intrathoracic pressure. The investigators also showed that external massage produces peripheral arterial and venous pressure pulses of equal magnitude and inferred, as Weale and Rothwell-Jackson had, that those pressures might damage the normally low-pressure cerebral circulation. Yet they did not describe cerebral vascular damage in their patients, and they reported that closed-chest compression could provide a cardiac output that, although significantly less than that achieved during normal heart rhythm, was enough to suggest that the heart acted as a pump during external massage. These findings led them and other physicians to recommend closed-chest compression without resolving the issue of its physiology. In 1974 the American Heart Association (AHA) published its standards for Cardiopulmonary Resuscitation and Emergency Cardiac Care,[7] which called for CPR at 60 chest compressions per minute, with each compression lasting 50 percent of the cardiac cycle, and a lung inflation following every 5 chest compressions. These recommendations were so well accepted by professionals and lay persons alike that until recently they constituted conventional CPR.

The Thoracic Pump Model

Despite this acceptance, certain investigators have continued to question how CPR works and how it might be improved. Among them have been Criley et al.,[8] who believed that rhythmic coughing, which previously had been recommended to clear contrast material from the coronary arteries during angiography, might also cause an increase in intrathoracic pressure that could maintain cerebral blood flow. The unexpected chance to study this occurred when three patients developed ventricular fibrillation at the time of angiography. Since external cardiac massage could not be initiated immediately, Criley et al. urged their patients to cough while a defibrillator was brought into position. The patients did so, restoring their blood pressures and remaining conscious for longer than would be possible without adequate flow to the cerebral circulation. Although Criley and co-workers had experience with only a few patients, they noted that cough CPR has several advantages. It is patient-initiated and less hazardous than other forms of CPR because external force is not applied to the chest. In addition, since each cough is preceded by a negative pressure inspiration, cough CPR enhances venous return to the heart and might thereby be expected to improve cardiac output.

Werner and colleagues[9] were among the first to study what actually happens to the heart during CPR. Their insights were gained with a technique called *echocardiography*, in which sound waves are bounced off the intrathoracic structures to provide a two-dimensional picture of cardiac activity. These investigators performed echocardiography on patients with severe hypoxic brain damage who were undergoing CPR for ventricular fibrillation. They found that the valves of the fibrillating hearts were indeed incompetent during the application of closed-chest compression, as Weale and Rothwell-Jackson had predicted. At the same time, they noted that the cardiac ventricles did not change in size during closed-chest compression, as would be expected if the heart were alternately being filled with and then emptied of blood.

From this finding, Werner et al. inferred that the heart does not act as a pump during CPR but instead serves as a conduit for blood that is being pumped by the entire chest, with most of its volume located in the largest intrathoracic vascular reservoir, the lungs.

How blood might be pumped by the entire chest rather than the heart itself was explored by Rudikoff et al.[10] using a portable CPR device that employs a pneumatic piston to deliver uniform chest compressions and ventilations at a preset airway pressure; compression rate, duration, and ventilations can be set by a built-in computer. Resuscitating dogs in ventricular fibrillation with this device, the investigators demonstrated that pressures in the atria, ventricles, pulmonary artery, and aorta were identical during external cardiac massage. Antegrade flow occurred in the carotid artery to the brain during the compression phase, and there was little pressure differential between the intrathoracic aorta and the extrathoracic carotid artery; at the same time, retrograde flow in the jugular vein was negligible despite a large gradient between the right atrium, which normally receives jugular venous blood before it passes into the right ventricle, and the extrathoracic jugular vein. These findings again confirmed Weale and Rothwell-Jackson's claim that external cardiac massage causes a generalized increase in intrathoracic pressure but for the first time refuted their assumption that it is transmitted equally to all extrathoracic vessels. In place of the latter hypothesis, Rudikoff et al.[10] and then Yin et al.[11] postulated that this pressure gradient necessary for cerebral perfusion exists outside the chest between the carotid artery and the jugular veins. This gradient occurs because the thick-walled carotid artery remains open as long as intrathoracic pressure is not raised so high that the vessel collapses at the thoracic outlet, whereas the thin-walled jugular vein is squeezed shut by the high pressure at the point where it enters the chest.

Although differences in wall strength between the carotid artery and jugular vein are important, cerebral blood flow during CPR may also be made possible by the presence of valves in the veins. These valves, which are located at the thoracic inlet of the jugular vein, were identified by sixteenth century anatomists but still are unknown to many physicians. However, Fisher and co-workers[12] demonstrated that the valves prevent retrograde flow up the jugular circulation during coughing and other maneuvers that increase intrathoracic pressure and speculated that the valves help to establish the extrathoracic arteriovenous pressure gradient during CPR. Niemann et al.,[13] performing angiography with oily contrast material in dogs that were fibrillated and then resuscitated with the pneumatic device described earlier, similarly demonstrated that closure of the jugular venous valves during CPR was responsible for the development of a pressure gradient across the cerebral circulation that would allow antegrade blood flow. These investigators also showed that the left ventricle has a small and relatively fixed volume during closed-chest compression, further demonstrating that the heart serves as a conduit for blood pumped by the thorax during CPR (Fig. 95-2).

THE "NEW" CARDIOPULMONARY RESUSCITATION

Elucidation of the thoracic pump model of CPR has been paralleled by new clinical approaches based on the belief that

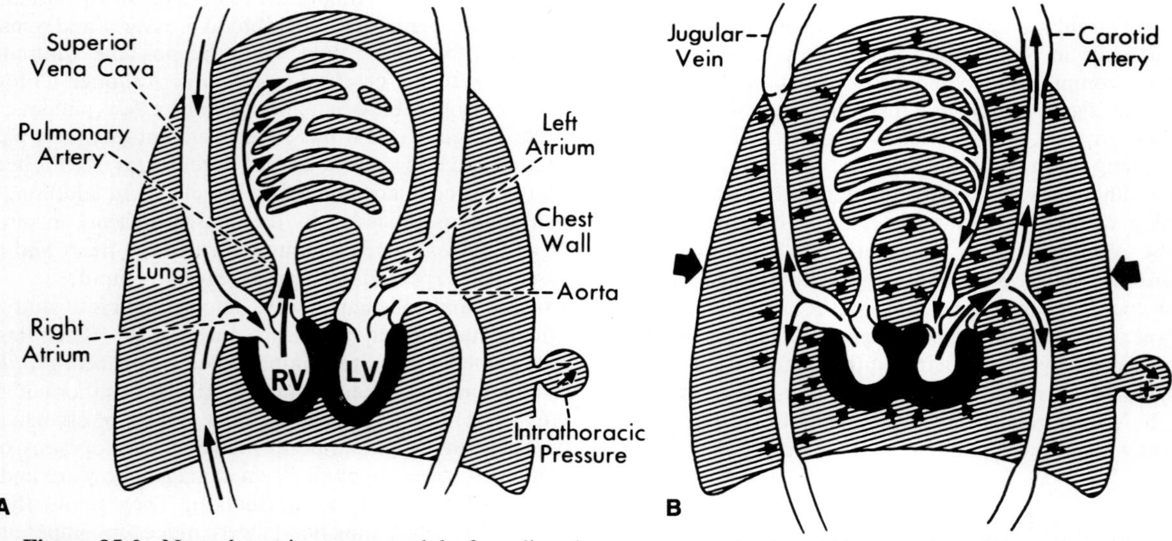

Figure 95-2. New thoracic pump model of cardiopulmonary resuscitation: (**A**) relaxation, (**B**) compression. Closed-chest compression ("systole") causes a generalized increase in intrathoracic pressure that squeezes all structures in the chest, including the pulmonary blood vessels, which have been filled during relaxation ("diastole") phase. The cardiac valves are incompetent. A pressure gradient between intrathoracic and extrathoracic vessels is developed, and blood flows into head because the thick-walled carotid artery remains patent while the thin-walled jugular vein is squeezed shut and also because valves are present in the vein. (Adapted from Luce et al.,[2] with permission.)

cerebral blood flow might be enhanced during resuscitation by measures that increase intrathoracic pressure and its duration. Taylor et al.[14] were the first to determine whether alterations in the rate or duration of closed-chest compression might affect cerebral blood flow. In one study, eight patients were given mechanical CPR by means of the pneumatic device at compression rates of 40, 60, and 80 per minute and compression durations of 30 percent, 40 percent, 50 percent, and 60 percent of the cardiac cycle. The investigators gained a rough idea of carotid blood flow by noninvasive Doppler flow technology. They found that a compression duration of 60 percent increased antegrade carotid flow over that attained with shorter durations, whereas changing the compression rate at a duration of 60 percent had no substantial effect. This finding supported the thoracic pump model because cardiac output should be rate-dependent if the heart itself is pumping blood. It led Taylor et al.[14] to suggest that undue emphasis was generally being placed on compression rate rather than duration of chest compression in CPR.

Chandra and co-workers[15] sought to determine whether the timing of chest compressions and artificial ventilation was important. In their study they initially adhered to the sequence of five chest compressions followed by one ventilation, as recommended by the AHA; the ventilation was delivered at a low airway pressure of around 40 cmH_2O. However, because they believed that external massage causes a generalized increase in intrathoracic pressure, these investigators wondered whether the pressures that could be achieved by simultaneous compression and ventilation at high airway pressures might not augment cerebral blood flow during CPR. They therefore modified their pneumatic device to deliver chest compressions with a variable rate and a 60 percent duration simultaneously with ventilation aimed at providing airway pressures of 100 cmH_2O. They found that this approach, which they called the new CPR, generated almost twice the carotid flow of conventional CPR at a compression duration of 50 percent in fibrillating dogs.

Chandra and colleagues[16] next extended the new CPR to humans who had not recovered from cardiopulmonary arrest despite prolonged resuscitation. Using the pneumatic device, these investigators gave the patients brief periods of conventional CPR at a compression rate of 60 per minute and a duration of 60 percent alternating with the new CPR at a rate of 40 per minute and a duration of 60 percent. The new CPR increased mean arterial pressure and carotid flow over the levels observed with conventional CPR in this study. Lowering airway pressure during chest compression decreased arterial pressure and flow, which suggests that the elevation in intrathoracic pressure was largely responsible for the beneficial effects of CPR.

PERFUSING THE HEART AS WELL AS THE HEAD

Although studies such as these demonstrated that the new CPR based on the thoracic pump model could improve cerebral blood flow, they did not examine its effects on other organs. However, in 1983 Luce et al.[17] studied blood flow to the heart, kidneys, and brain using radiolabeled microspheres in dogs during normal cardiac rhythm and ventricular fibrillation. These microspheres are 15-μm polystyrene beads labeled with isotopes such as radioactive cobalt or indium. After being injected as a bolus into the left ventricle, the spheres are distributed with the rest of the cardiac output to the tissues of the body, where they lodge in capillaries because of their size. By counting the radioactivity in the organs of experimental animals after autopsy, investigators can measure regional blood flow.

In this study[17] microspheres were injected into dogs during either normal cardiac rhythm or ventricular fibrillation. The fibrillation was treated either with nonsimultaneous compressions and ventilations at a low airway pressure or with simultaneous compressions and ventilations at a high airway pressure delivered either with a pneumatic device or a rapidly inflatable vest surrounding the chest and upper abdomen. A compression duration of 60 percent was used. Blood flow to the brain was better during simultaneous compression and ventilation CPR than during nonsimultaneous compression and ventilation CPR and depended on the intrathoracic pressure achieved with both mechanical devices, in keeping with the findings of Chandra and associates. However, perfusion of the heart and kidneys was poor during all types of CPR.

The limited blood flow to the heart during CPR can be understood by examining normal cardiac physiology. Although the heart pumps blood to other organs during its contraction, or systolic phase, its own circulation is perfused for the most part with blood from the aortic root when the heart muscle relaxes during diastole. Closed-chest compression during ventricular fibrillation is a form of mechanical "systole," which might be expected to produce antegrade blood flow outside the chest regardless of whether the cardiac pump or thoracic pump mechanism is operative. However, blood flow through the coronary arteries, especially those supplying the left ventricle of the heart, is a diastolic phenomenon, which occurs during the relaxation phase of closed-chest compression. When the heart is beating normally, enough pressure remains in the aortic root during diastole to perfuse the coronary circulation. However, as Bellamy et al.[18] demonstrated in fibrillating swine, this pressure falls during cardiopulmonary arrest regardless of the rise in intrathoracic and aortic root pressure caused by closed-chest compression.

The importance of diastolic aortic pressure actually was pointed out as early as 1965 by Pearson and Redding.[19] Using an asphyxiated dog model of cardiopulmonary arrest, these investigators demonstrated that return of circulation during and survival after CPR were directly dependent on maximal artificial diastolic pressure. They also showed that the highest mean diastolic pressures, averaging 35 to 45 mmHg, were achieved in animals infused with drugs possessing alpha-adrenergic properties, which caused the constriction of peripheral blood vessels and a redistribution of blood volume into the central circulation. Among these vasoconstrictor drugs were methoxamine, metaraminol, phenylephrine, and epinephrine. The vasodilating beta-adrenergic drug isoproterenol was of no value in this study.

Using radiolabeled microspheres to document blood flow, Holmes et al.[20] recently confirmed the findings of Pearson and Redding that alpha-adrenergic agents such as epinephrine improve vital organ perfusion during CPR and that isoproterenol and other beta-adrenergic agents worsen it. In addition, Michael et al.[21] combined saline or epinephrine infusion with either nonsimultaneous or simultaneous compression and ventilation CPR to see which combination was superior. They found that the use of epinephrine plus simultaneous compression and ventilation CPR maintained cerebral blood flow at 73 percent of control values and left ventricular blood flow at 28 percent of control values in fibrillating dogs. The improved blood flows correlated with increased electroencephalographic activity and the restoration of spontaneous circulation. This study, like that of Pearson and Redding, supports the use of alpha-adrenergic agents during CPR.

CURRENT GUIDELINES FOR CARDIOPULMONARY RESUSCITATION

The 1986 Standards and Guidelines for Cardiopulmonary Resuscitation and Emergency Cardiac Care of the AHA[7] are divided into two parts: basic life support (BLS) and advanced cardiac life support (ACLS). Basic life support is intended either to prevent cardiopulmonary arrest or insufficiency through speedy recognition and intervention or to support the ventilation and circulation of patients following cardiopulmonary arrest. Its well known sequence involves patient assessment and attention to the "ABCs" of airway, breathing, and circulation. Because BLS usually precedes ACLS and may determine the overall success of resuscitation, it is discussed here in some detail.

Basic Life Support

A clinician who arrives at the scene of cardiopulmonary arrest without assistance should first determine unresponsiveness by shouting at and gently shaking the patient. Care should be taken not to distort the neck if trauma has occurred to the cervical spine. The clinician then should call for help and position the patient supine on a firm, flat surface. By kneeling at the level of the patient's shoulders, the clinician can perform artificial ventilation and chest compression with relative ease. After this position is assumed, the clinician should open the patient's airway by placing one hand on the patient's forehead and tilting it backwards, while simultaneously lifting the chin upward with the other hand. This head tilt–chin lift maneuver should create an air passage by moving the tongue forward and out of the throat (Fig. 95-3).

The clinician's ear should next be placed over the patient's nose and mouth to assess the presence or absence of spontaneous breathing. The clinician should look for the chest to rise and fall, listen for airflow, and feel the flow of air. If the patient is not breathing, the airway should be kept open with the head tilt–chin lift maneuver, the nose gently pinched shut, the clinician's lips sealed around those of the patient, and two breaths given of a volume sufficient to make the patient's chest rise. Mouth-to-nose or mouth-to-stoma breathing also may be employed. If none of these techniques provides ventilation, the patient's head should be repositioned. If this is unsuccessful, subdraphragmatic abdominal thrusts (also called the Heimlich maneuver), followed by a finger sweep of the patient's mouth, should be performed.

Once ventilation is supported, the patient's circulatory adequacy should be assessed by palpating the large carotid arteries in the neck. If no pulse is palpated within 5 to 15 seconds, the Emergency Medical System should be activated (by calling 911 in most areas) and closed-chest compressions should be begun. The clinician's hands should first be positioned, with the fingers locked, over the patient's lower sternum. The clinician's elbows should be locked, the arms straightened, and the shoulders oriented directly over the hands so that the upper body moves up and down like a piston. The adult patient's sternum should be depressed 4 to 5 cm with each chest compression.

The closed-chest compression rate for adults is now set at 80 to 100 per minute in place of the 60 per minute rate recommended in previous AHA guidelines. This change is in keeping with both the cardiac pump and the thoracic pump theories outlined earlier in this chapter. If external massage of the heart actually occurs during closed-chest compression, a faster rate should increase cardiac output. At the same time, if an increase in intrathoracic pressure is the true mechanism of blood flow, a compression duration of 50 percent, which is easier to achieve with a rapid rate, should improve perfusion of the brain and the heart.

In one-person CPR, the clinician is now expected to perform 15 closed chest compressions followed by two artificial ventilations. This requires less shifting of position than the previous practice of delivering five compressions followed by one ventilation. Two-person CPR, which usually is available in the hospital or when an ambulance arrives in the field, still uses the five compressions and one ventilation sequence long recommended by the AHA. The chest compressions should be performed by one clinician kneeling by the patient's side; the second clinician remains at the head to maintain an open airway, monitor the carotid pulse for the adequacy of chest compressions, and breathe for the patient.

It will be noted that simultaneous compression and ventilation CPR is not recommended in the new AHA guidelines. This is not to say that the AHA is unfamiliar with ongoing research regarding mechanisms and improvement of blood flow during CPR; indeed, much of that research is described in the new guidelines. Nevertheless, despite its success in laboratory animals and a few patients, simultaneous compression and ventilation CPR cannot be widely recommended in humans until it has been subjected to large clinical trials. Furthermore, despite all the experimental evidence supporting the thoracic pump model of CPR, it should not replace the cardiac pump model until more research is performed. Besides, both mechanisms may play a role during closed chest compression.

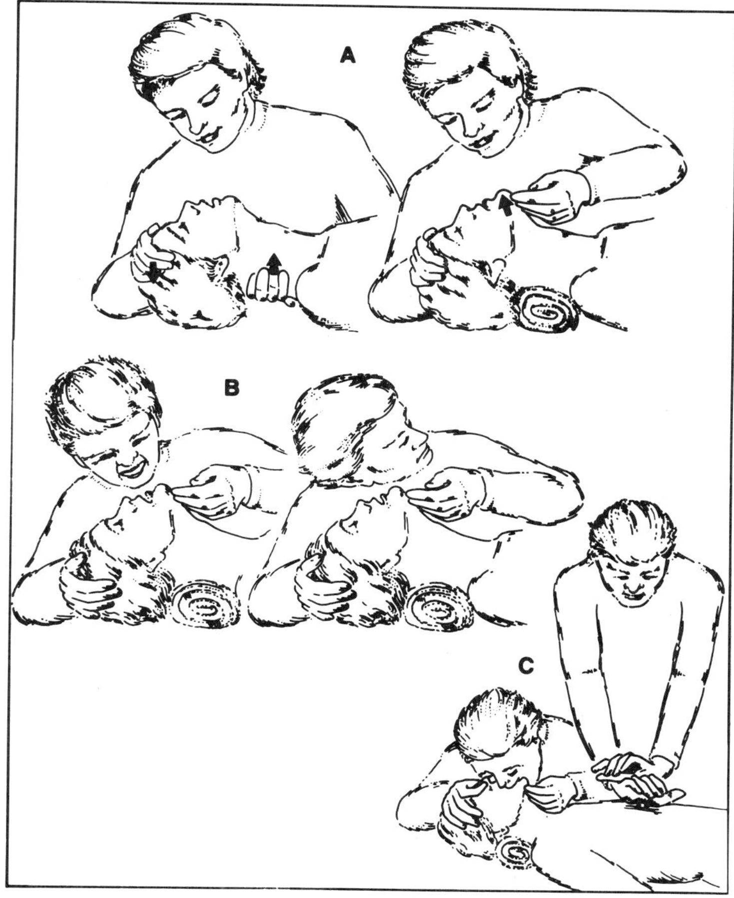

Figure 95-3. (**A**) Chin lift technique to open the upper airway, followed by (**B**) examination for airflow and (**C**) administration of artificial ventilations and closed chest compressions. (From Luce et al.,[29] with permission.)

Advanced Cardiac Life Support

ACLS includes: (1) BLS; (2) the use of adjunctive equipment for establishing effective ventilation and circulation; (3) ECG monitoring and dysrhythmia detection; (4) establishment and maintenance of intravenous access; (5) employment of electrical and drug therapies; and (6) treatment of patients with known or suspected myocardial infarction. The key aspects of ACLS are covered in this chapter; readers are referred to the 1986 AHA guidelines[7] for further information.

One of the most important features of ACLS is the use of adjuncts for oxygenation, ventilation, and airway protection as soon as possible in CPR. Such adjuncts include supplemental O_2, which should be delivered to practically every patient with cardiopulmonary arrest; close-fitting face masks to aid artificial ventilation, whether it involves mouth-to-mask breathing or insufflation of the lungs with an anesthesia bag; and artificial airways, which facilitate oxygenation and ventilation. Although devices such as oropharyngeal, nasopharyngeal, and esophageal obturator airways may be helpful in some patients, endotracheal intubation by either the oral or the nasal route is the preferred method to control the airway. Endotracheal intubation is not without potential complications, of course, and it should be attempted only by experienced clinicians.

ECG monitoring should be established as soon as possible following cardiopulmonary arrest. Augmented by a 12-lead ECG, such monitoring can help make the diagnosis of myocardial infarction and is particularly helpful in detecting dysrhythmias that either follow infarction or are responsible for cardiopulmonary arrest in the first place. Once such dysrhythmias are diagnosed, they should be treated immediately if they are judged to be responsible for hemodynamic compromise. This is true with brady- and tachydysrhythmias of either supraventricular or ventricular origin; it is particularly

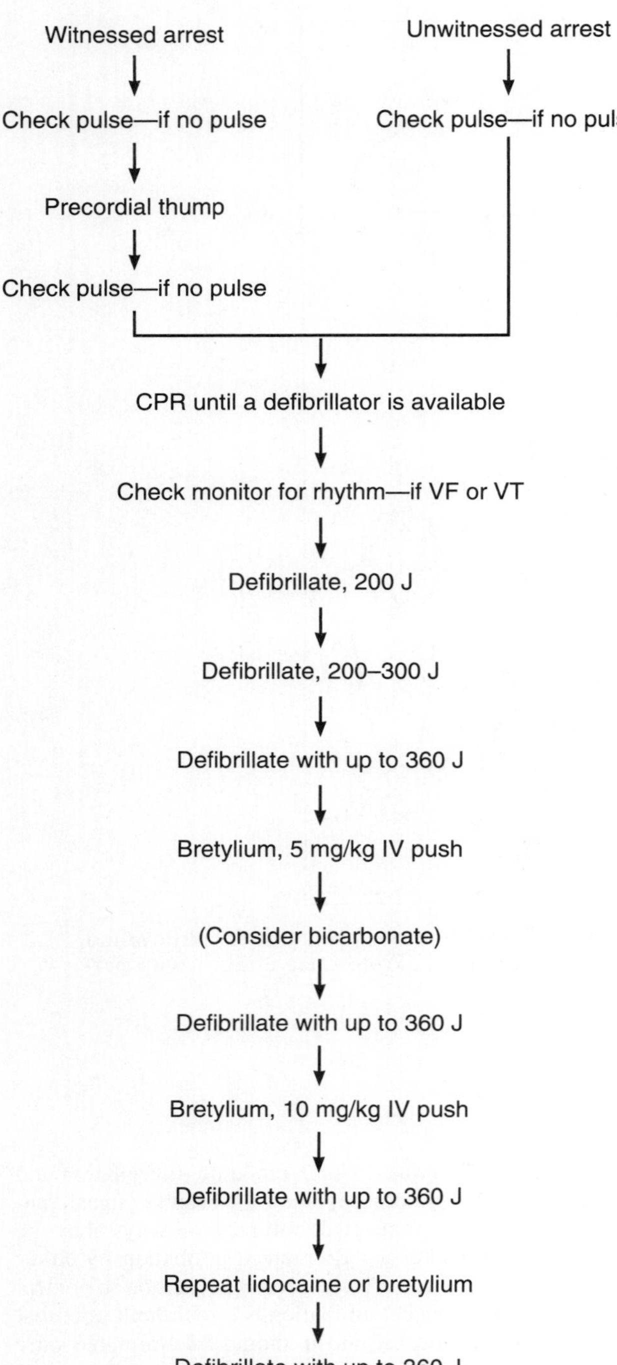

Figure 95-4. American Heart Association algorithm for treatment of pulseless ventricular tachycardia (VT) and ventricular fibrillation (VF). Pulse and rhythm should be checked after each shock, and epinephrine should be repeated every 5 minutes. Sodium bicarbonate is not recommended routinely. (Adapted from American Heart Association,[7] with permission.)

true of pulseless ventricular tachycardia and ventricular fibrillation because the rapidity of reversal of these latter two dysrhythmias is the major determinant of survival. Indeed, the current AHA guidelines[7] for the treatment of pulseless ventricular tachycardia and ventricular fibrillation call for three sequential attempts at defibrillation, with increasingly high levels of electrical energy as soon as these conditions are diagnosed and a defibrillator is available. Electrical defibrillation may be preceded by a precordial thump if cardiopulmonary arrest due to pulseless ventricular tachycardia or ventricular fibrillation is confirmed by the ECG.

When defibrillation (or cardioversion, in the case of significant supraventricular dysrhythmias) is not successful, or when a pulse is present and the patient is stable, an intravenous route should be established for the administration of drugs and fluids. Cannulation of either a peripheral or central vein is preferable to intracardiac injection during CPR, but central access through either the subclavian or the internal jugular veins should be sought wherever possible. A 1984 study[22] demonstrated a long delay in the arrival of drugs to the heart when peripheral intravenous sites are used for injection during CPR, even when effective chest compressions are performed. If an endotracheal tube is in place and central venous access is delayed, epinephrine, lidocaine, and atropine can be administered via the endotracheal tube.

Of all the drugs used during CPR, the AHA has affirmed that epinephrine is the most important. Previous guidelines had recommended the liberal administration of sodium bicarbonate, calcium, and isoproterenol in many forms of cardiopulmonary arrest. Now sodium bicarbonate, which is of little benefit in making the body less acidic and indeed probably causes the venous pH to fall, is to be used sparingly, if at all.[23] Calcium also is contraindicated owing to its possible role in causing intracellular injury, and isoproterenol is limited to patients with intolerable bradycardia. Epinephrine in repeated doses is now recommended for pulseless ventricular tachycardia, ventricular fibrillation, and asystole. Research in progress suggests that even higher doses of epinephrine may be appropriate; if verified, this finding undoubtedly will find its way into future AHA guidelines.

Several other drugs that are useful in controlling heart rhythm and rate deserve mention here. They include lidocaine, which decreases electrical conduction through the heart and is the drug of choice for the management of ventricular tachycardia and fibrillation; procainamide hydrochloride, which prolongs the myocardial refractory period and is recommended when lidocaine is contraindicated or has failed to suppress ventricular ectopy; bretylium tosylate, which exerts a postganglionic adrenergic blocking action and is useful in the treatment of resistant ventricular tachycardia and fibrillation; and atropine sulfate, a parasympatholytic drug, which enhances cardiac conduction and is used to treat bradycardia associated with hemodynamic compromise. Figures 95-4 to 95-6 present the current AHA algorithms for the use of these agents along with epinephrine and defibrillation in the therapy of ventricular fibrillation and ventricular tachycardia with or without pulse, as well as asystole.

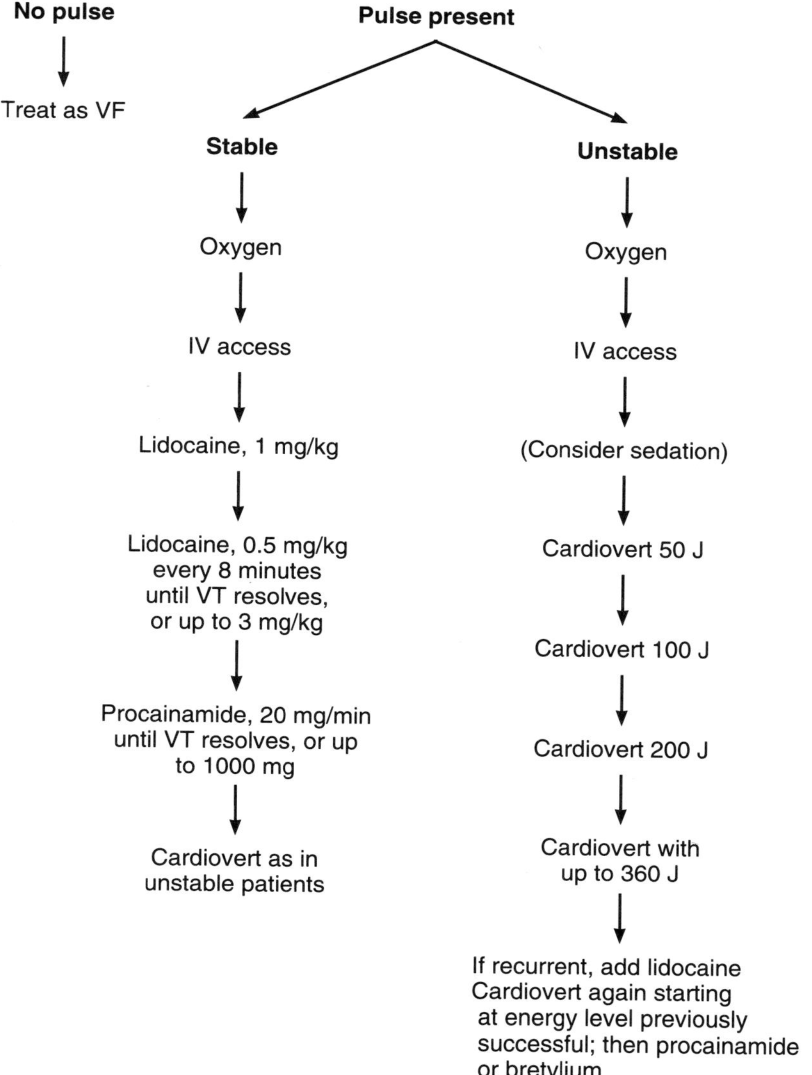

Figure 95-5. American Heart Association algorithm for treatment of sustained ventricular tachycardia with pulse. Patients without pulse and treated as shown in Figure 95-4; those with a pulse who become unstable move to the "unstable" arm of the algorithm. If hypotension, pulmonary edema, or loss of consciousness occurs, unsynchronized cardioversion (i.e., defibrillation) should be used. A precordial thump may be employed prior to cardioversion. (Adapted from American Heart Association,[7] with permission.)

TECHNIQUES OF CEREBRAL RESUSCITATION

As mentioned earlier, the term *cerebral resuscitation* is used to describe certain measures designed to improve neurologic outcome following a variety of insults to the central nervous system. Many of these measures were developed to reduce intracranial pressure by decreasing cerebral blood flow or by diminishing cerebral edema in patients with neurosurgical disease. Such resuscitative techniques include sustained hyperventilation to a $PaCO_2$ in the range of 20 to 25 mmHg, which causes cerebral vasoconstriction and thereby reduces cerebral blood flow; the administration of hyperosmolar agents such as mannitol and diuretics such as furosemide to dehydrate the brain; and the use of corticosteroids such as dexamethasone to enhance microvascular integrity and reduce cerebral edema.

Although these and other therapies may be appropriate in patients with documented intracranial hypertension due to, say, head trauma (see Ch. 93), their efficacy has not been demonstrated in patients with global ischemia and hypoxia secondary to cardiopulmonary arrest. These patients certainly do not have intracranial hypertension during either the time of arrest, when cerebral perfusion is absent, or during CPR, when cerebral perfusion is poor. Furthermore, they

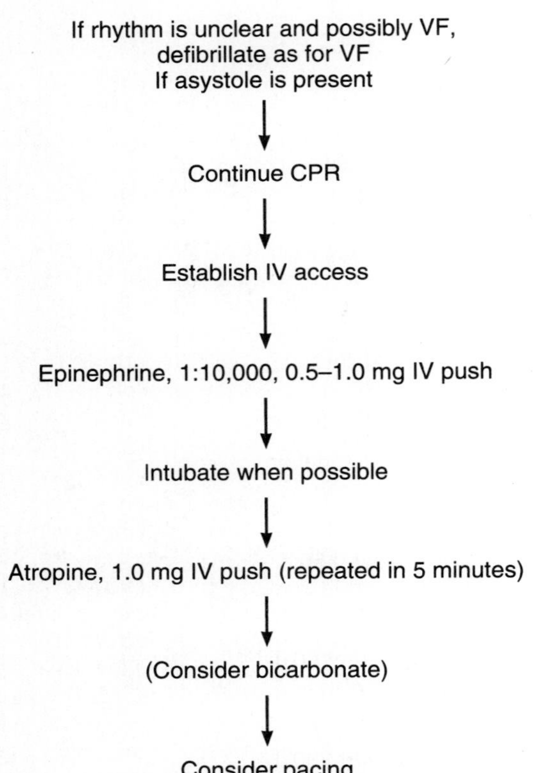
If rhythm is unclear and possibly VF, defibrillate as for VF
If asystole is present
Continue CPR
Establish IV access
Epinephrine, 1:10,000, 0.5–1.0 mg IV push
Intubate when possible
Atropine, 1.0 mg IV push (repeated in 5 minutes)
(Consider bicarbonate)
Consider pacing

Figure 95-6. American Heart Association algorithm for treatment of asystole. Defibrillation for possible or presumed ventricular fibrillation (VF) may be used. Epinephrine should be given every 5 minutes. Sodium bicarbonate is not recommended routinely. (Adapted from American Heart Association,[7] with permission.)

are unlikely to have a markedly elevated intracranial pressure after resuscitation. Therefore, patients with cardiopulmonary arrest do not appear to be logical candidates for this type of therapy.

One cerebral resuscitation approach that may be useful after cardiopulmonary arrest involves decreasing cerebral metabolic needs to balance the patient's decrease in brain blood supply. Hypothermia, which is employed in some neurosurgical patients, would be a possibility here but it is logistically too difficult to establish as part of ACLS. Another logistically feasible possibility is intravenous administration of rapidly acting barbiturates such as thiopental, which put the brain to rest and also reduce cerebral edema. Thiopental loading has been demonstrated to improve neurologic outcome in primates subjected to occlusion of the cerebral circulation. Unfortunately, however, thiopental administration shortly after cardiopulmonary arrest was not beneficial to patients in a recent international trial.[24]

Another group of drugs that may be useful in cerebral resuscitation are the calcium antagonists or calcium channel blockers. These agents have vasodilating properties and also limit the flux of calcium into cells, thereby potentially ameliorating ischemic cellular injury. To date, calcium antagonists such as flunarazine and lidoflazine have been shown to increase cerebral blood flow and to improve neurologic outcome in experimental models of cardiopulmonary arrest.[25] Although generally they cannot be recommended until they are studied in clinical circumstances, these drugs someday may prove to be protective of the brain.

ETHICAL ISSUES IN CARDIOPULMONARY RESUSCITATION

Cardiopulmonary resuscitation was originally developed to restore the heartbeat and breathing of otherwise healthy people whose cardiac rhythm and spontaneous ventilation had failed following surgery, near drowning, and other treatable problems. Because of its success in such persons, CPR soon came to be regarded as one of the most dramatic and promising medical technologies. Unlike other technologies, however, CPR was and is of potentially universal application because cardiopulmonary arrest occurs at some time in the death of every individual. Furthermore, CPR must be initiated promptly and sustained fully to be effective, so that decisions about CPR must be made in advance or foregone in favor of a policy of resuscitation in all circumstances. Finally, the conjectural aspects of advance deliberations about whether to provide CPR are difficult for patients, families, and health professionals to deal with. Because of all these factors, CPR was declared obligatory for physicians functioning in their official capacity, and it was considered appropriate for all people in cardiopulmonary arrest by the President's Commission on Deciding to Forego Life-Sustaining Treatment.[26]

As the universal appropriateness of CPR became accepted, the AHA and other groups stepped up their efforts to educate health professionals and lay people alike about this therapy. BLS involving the technique of closed-chest compression and ventilation was taught to all physicians, and proof of current knowledge of BLS became mandatory for medical licensing in many states. ACLS, which also includes the administration of drugs and defibrillation, was learned by many hospital physicians as well as by paramedics manning ambulances on the streets, and annual certification in ACLS also became available. Meanwhile, a significant proportion of the adult nonmedical population of the United States became trained in the techniques of CPR. Although statistics on the number of knowledgeable adults are hard to come by, the AHA reports that more than one-third of all adults are trained in CPR in some areas.

Although many Americans are now familiar with CPR, the application of this therapy to chronically sick patients as well as to persons who were healthy except for their temporary cardiac rhythm and breathing problem has prompted health professionals and lay people alike to question the wisdom of a universal resuscitation policy. One argument against CPR is that this mode of therapy often was unsuccessful in seriously ill individuals and could cause morbidity and mortality. Second, the blanket application of CPR runs counter to the wishes of some patients and thereby violates their right of self-determination, a right that is increasingly respected in our society. Third, CPR often is not always medically indicated in that it cannot benefit patients who are brain dead or dying from terminal illness. Finally, when initiated in persons who are near death, CPR interferes with their dying with dignity.

Because of these and other objectives, CPR has come to be regarded as a technology that can be withheld in certain situations. For example, CPR is not medically indicated in patients who are brain dead, although determining neurologic function may be difficult in an emergency. CPR also may be withheld from competent patients who refuse such treatment. And finally, in the words of the recent AHA guidelines, CPR is not indicated in patients with terminal irreversible illnesses whose death is imminent. The term *imminent* here means not only that death is near (some have suggested a time frame of 2 weeks) but that it is threatening, and that resuscitation from death would leave a life filled with pain.

The principle of withholding CPR from brain-dead or near dead patients and competent persons who refuse resuscitation is now well accepted by the medical and legal professions. Furthermore, the American public seems relieved by the thought that semicomatose cancer patients, among others, will not suffer unnecessarily through the mandatory administration of CPR. However, consensus has not been reached on the withholding of support from patients who are neither brain dead nor terminally ill, especially when their wishes are not known. Some of these patients may have survived successful CPR and now be in a persistently vegetative state. Others have chronic conditions, such as Alzheimer's disease, that preclude rational decision making and diminish the quality of life but are not imminently fatal. Patients of both these types are present in large numbers in United States nursing homes. Often their families cannot or will not deal with the issue of resuscitation, and their physicians are uncertain about the propriety of withholding care.

A third group of individuals who pose ethical problems in resuscitation are those with inevitably lethal illnesses whose deaths are nevertheless not imminent and who develop potentially treatable problems. In this group are patients with the acquired immunodeficiency syndrome (AIDS) who develop *Pneumocystis carinii* pneumonia (PCP). Wachter et al.[27] have demonstrated that short-term survival in patients with AIDS who require intubation and mechanical ventilation for respiratory failure due to PCP approximates 40 percent, and that patients who are knowledgeable about this poor prognosis frequently choose not to receive intensive care or be resuscitated. Nevertheless, difficulties arise as to the appropriate time to raise these subjects with the patients. Should it be done when AIDS is first diagnosed and the patients are most lucid—and when death seems far away? Should it be done when PCP develops, with recognition that this complication may be the initial manifestation of immune deficiency? Or should discussions be held when respiratory failure is close at hand, a time when informed consent may be impossible owing to the progressive decline in neurologic status often associated with AIDS?

Although responses to these questions differ among physicians and patients, the general approach to the issue of resuscitation and intensive care of patients with AIDS described by Wachter et al.[27] may be helpful. The policy of these investigators is to raise issues of CPR and other life support as early as possible, and certainly when PCP is diagnosed, so that patients with AIDS can decide for themselves whether they want intensive care and resuscitation. If AIDS has just been diagnosed and respiratory failure seems as yet a remote possibility, Wachter et al. encourage patients to make a living will or appoint another person, usually a relative or trusted friend, to make decisions about medical care if the patient becomes incapable of making such decisions. This latter act is called the designation of a *durable power of attorney for health care*.

Raising the issue of resuscitation early in the course of illness has done much to affirm the right of self-determination of competent AIDS patients. But what of a final group of persons whose illness could not be anticipated and who have a marginal ability to give formal consent, if at all? This group includes patients hospitalized in intensive care units for acute processes such as trauma who then develop bacterial infections of their bloodstream and other complications. Although these people started with reversible problems, their long-term survival becomes highly unlikely owing to the complications, and caring for them may strain medical resources. Yet the patients and their families usually were unprepared for these complications, and because the patients can be kept alive almost indefinitely by mechanical ventilators and other devices, their deaths are only as imminent as their physicians allow. In such patients, the withholding of CPR is less a decision in itself than the last step in withdrawing other forms of supportive but not curative technology.

Although intensive care unit patients pose unique ethical problems, the same basic principles of resuscitation should apply to them as to other individuals. Whenever possible, the wishes of these patients should be respected, and support should be continued until patients and physicians alike agree that it is no longer medically indicated. When patients cannot make decisions for themselves and a living will or durable power of attorney for health care has not been previously arranged, which is usually the case, family and friends should be asked to communicate what they believe the patients' wishes regarding prolonged intensive care and resuscitation would be. Unfortunately, these wishes rarely are clear in a proxy situation. As a result, the physicians must decide whether the patients have an irreversible illness that would cause imminent death if technological support were not available. After all, the patients would die without such support. And, as Jonsen et al.[28] counsel, "It should not be forgotten that the patient who suffers cardiac arrest is, at least in one sense, dead. Cardiopulmonary resuscitation, then, brings back to life by restoring heartbeat. Thus, if the patient is imminently dying of a lethal process, bringing back to life would be the ultimate in futility."

References

1. Safar P: Cardiopulmonary-Cerebral Resuscitation. WB Saunders, Philadelphia, 1981

2. Luce JM, Cary JM, Ross BK et al: New developments in cardiopulmonary resuscitation. JAMA 1980;244:1366–1370
3. Elam JO, Brown ES, Elder ED: Artificial resuscitation by mouth-to-mask method. N Engl J Med 1954;250:749–754
4. Kouwenhoven WB, Jude JR, Knickerbocker GG: Closed-chest cardiac massage. JAMA 1960;173:1064–1067
5. Weale FE, Rothwell-Jackson RL: The efficiency of cardiac massage. Lancet 1982;1:990–992
6. MacKenzie GJ, Taylor JH, McDonald AH et al: Hemodynamic effects of external cardiac compression. Lancet 1964;1:1342–1345
7. American Heart Association: Standards and guidelines for cardiopulmonary resuscitation (CPR) and emergency cardiac care (ECC). JAMA 1986;255:1366–1370
8. Criley JM, Blaufuss AH, Kissel GL: Cough-induced cardiac compression: Self-administered form of cardiopulmonary resuscitation. JAMA 1976;236:1246–1250
9. Werner JA, Green HL, Janko LL et al: Visualization of cardiac valve motion during external chest compression using two-dimensional echocardiography: Implications regarding the mechanism of blood flow. Circulation 1980;63:1417–1421
10. Rudikoff MT, Maughan WL, Effron M et al: Mechanisms of blood flow during cardiopulmonary resuscitation. Circulation 1980;61:345–352
11. Yin FCP, Cohen JM, Tsitlik J et al: Role of carotid artery resistance to collapse during high-intrathoracic-pressure CPR. Am J Physiol, Heart Circ Physiol 12, 1982;243:H259–H267
12. Fisher J, Vaghaiwalla BS, Tsitlik J et al: Determinants and clinical significance of jugular venous valve competence. Circulation 1982;65:188–196
13. Niemann JT, Rosborough JP, Hausknecht M et al: Pressure-synchronized cineangiography during experimental cardiopulmonary resuscitation. Circulation 1981;64:985–991
14. Taylor GJ, Tucker WH, Greene HL et al: Importance of prolonged compression during cardiopulmonary resuscitation in man. N Engl J Med 1977;296:1515–1517
15. Chandra N, Weisfeldt ML, Tsitlik J et al: Augmentation of carotid flow during cardiopulmonary resuscitation by ventilation at high airway pressure simultaneous with chest compression. Am J Cardiol 1981;48:1053–1063
16. Chandra N, Rudikoff M, Weisfeldt ML: Simultaneous chest compression and ventilation at high airway pressure during cardiopulmonary resuscitation. Lancet 1980;1:175–178
17. Luce JM, Ross BK, O'Quin RJ et al: Regional blood flow during cardiopulmonary resuscitation in dogs using simultaneous and nonsimultaneous compression and ventilation. Circulation 1983;67:258–265
18. Bellamy RF, DeGuzman LR, Pedersen DC: Coronary blood flow during cardiopulmonary resuscitation in swine. Circulation 1984;69:174–180
19. Pearson JW, Redding JS: Influence of peripheral vascular tone on cardiac resuscitation. Anesth Analg 1965;44:746–752
20. Holmes HR, Babbs CF, Voorhees WD et al: Influence of adrenergic drugs upon vital organ perfusion during CPR. Crit Care Med 1980;8:137–140
21. Michael JR, Guerci AD, Koehler RC et al: Mechanisms by which epinephrine augments cerebral and myocardial perfusion during cardiopulmonary resuscitation in dogs. Circulation 1984;69:822–835
22. Hedges JR, Barsan WB, Doan LA: Central versus peripheral intravenous rates in cardiopulmonary resuscitation. Am J Emerg Med 1984;2:285–293
23. Graf H, Leach W, Arieff AL: Evidence for a detrimental effect of bicarbonate therapy in hypoxic lactic acidosis. Science 1984;227:754–757
24. Brain Resuscitation Clinical Trial I Study Group: Randomized clinical study of thiopental loading in comatose survivors of cardiac arrest. N Engl J Med 1986;314:397–403
25. Vaagenes P, Cantadove R: Amelioration of brain damage by lidoflazine after prolonged ventricular fibrillation in dogs. Crit Care Med 1984;12:846–853
26. President's Commission on Deciding to Forego Life-Sustaining Treatment: A Report on Ethical, Medical and Legal Issues in Treatment Decisions. U.S. Government Printing Office, Washington, D.C., 1983, pp. 231–235
27. Wachter RM, Russi MB, Bloch DA et al: *Pneumocystis carinii* pneumonia and respiratory failure in AIDS: Improved outcomes and increased use of intensive care units. Am Rev Respir Dis 1991;143:251–256
28. Jonsen AR, Siegler M, Winslade W: Clinical Ethics. Macmillan, New York, 1982
29. Luce JM, Tyler ML, Pierson DJ: Intensive Respiratory Care. WB Saunders, Philadelphia, 1984

Chapter 96

Intrahospital Transport of the Critically Ill Patient

Ray H. Ritz

CHAPTER OUTLINE

Intensive care medicine today depends on an ever-widening array of diagnostic and therapeutic services as part of the accepted community standards of practice. These specialized services often require use of large, sophisticated devices, which are neither available nor practical to use in an intensive care unit (ICU). Additionally, facilities such as emergency departments, patient wards, and outpatient clinics need access to these same diagnostic services, which makes their centralized location important. Hospitals that have added new services to older buildings may not have been able to place them in the patient care areas that need them the most.

This situation requires that patients be transported from their rooms to departments such as radiology, angiography, to operating rooms, and so forth much more frequently than ever before. The more severe a patient's illness, the greater the risk associated with transporting that patient outside of the home unit. Patients once considered too ill to be moved from an ICU are now frequent candidates for intrahospital transport. Maintaining physiologic support during transport of some patients can be extremely complicated, and the clinician's skills play an important role in the success and safety of this process.

ASSOCIATED RISKS

Critically ill patients being transported can experience significant cardiovascular changes and frequently require treatment.[1,2] Perhaps those most at risk are postoperative patients being transported from the operating room, but the risk for ICU patients increases with the severity of their illness and the level of physiologic support provided. Patients receiving mechanical ventilation have developed life-threatening alterations in gas exchange and hemodynamic status during intrahospital transport.[3,4]

Erratic manual ventilation during the course of a transport can result in either hypercarbia or hypocarbia, with a corresponding shift in pH. Respiratory alkalosis is associated with reduced blood flow to the heart and brain and creates a left shift of the oxyhemoglobin dissociation curve. The increased affinity of hemoglobin for O_2 can further limit O_2 delivery to vital organs already compromised. Hyperventilation may cause coronary vasospasm, which in turn can lead to ischemia of the myocardium. Another complication of manual hyperventilation is the possibility of thoracic gas trapping or auto-PEEP (positive end-expiratory pressure).

The effect of auto-PEEP is well known,[5] yet monitoring for it during transport is extremely difficult at best.

Inadvertent hypoventilation during transport may cause respiratory acidosis, leading to increased myocardial irritability and arrhythmias. Insufficient tidal volume (V_T) can also contribute to lower overall lung volume, leading to decreased PaO_2 levels.

Increased pain and/or anxiety during transport can cause patients to alter their breathing patterns, which can have the same adverse effects as alterations imposed by the transport team. The goal during all patient transports should be to maintain consistent physiologic support as similar as possible to that provided in the ICU.

TRANSPORT OF THE NON-VENTILATOR-SUPPORTED PATIENT

Stable, nonintubated ventilator-supported patients can safely be transported outside of the ICU with little difficulty. Maintaining a semirecumbent position and ensuring frequent deep breathing can help prevent hypoxemia in low-risk patients.[6] Supplemental O_2 therapy often can be maintained during transport with the same equipment used in the ICU, the only alteration needed being a portable O_2 source. The most common type of portable O_2 device is the E cylinder, which contains approximately 615 L of O_2 when pressurized at 2200 psi (pounds per square inch). The cylinder's contents must be adequate to provide the appropriate flow for a time that exceeds the anticipated transport time. Table 96-1 lists the estimated life for an E cylinder at various pressurization levels and liter flows. Pressure gauges used on transport cylinders are exposed to frequent abuse, which can affect their accuracy, and unanticipated obstacles may slow down the transport. Consequently, no patient requiring O_2 should be transported with a cylinder containing less than 1000 psi of O_2.

Intubated, spontaneously breathing patients can also be simply and safely transported. Again, O_2 therapy can be provided with a variety of standard devices. However, bypassing of the upper airway requires that the patient not be deprived of warmed, humidified inspiratory gas for extended periods. It is not clear how long an intubated patient can be maintained without humidification.

Table 96-1. Variation in E Cylinder Life[a] at Different Content Levels and O_2 Use Rates

Flow Rate (L/min)	Cylinder Contents (psi)			
	500	1000	1500	2200
2	70	140	210	308
4	35	70	105	154
6	23	47	70	103
8	18	35	53	77
10	14	28	42	62
12	12	23	35	51
14	10	20	30	44
16	9	18	26	39

[a] Gas supply duration in minutes.

Humidification provided by continuous aerosol generators or pass-over humidifiers is generally not practical during transport. However, heat and moisture exchangers (HMEs) can provide adequate conditioning of inspiratory gas over the range of most normal minute ventilations. They are simple to use and reasonably priced, but they have some limitations. HMEs become less efficient as the patient's V_T and respiratory rate increase. They can also become clogged by secretions, which will increase their resistance and necessitate changing them.[7] Dead space is also increased by the addition of an HME to the breathing circuit although the amount will vary with the specific device used.[8] Since most patients spend less than 2 hours outside the ICU (except for operative procedures) the use of HMEs seems to provide a satisfactory solution to most humidification needs during extended transports. Short transports of 30 minutes or less may be safely made without addition of an HME.

In patients with artificial airways, care must be taken to avoid applying tension on the airway. Devices attached to the airway must be well stabilized, and tubing connecting the O_2 supply to the patient should be managed in such a way that it does not drag on the floor or catch on doorknobs or other obstacles. The centimeter markings on oral or nasal endotracheal tubes and their relationship to the lip or nostril should be noted prior to moving the patient. A self-inflating resuscitator and a resuscitation mask should be taken along during transport in case of an emergency.

In the two groups described above, standard monitoring of cardiac rhythm and rate are generally sufficient. Pulse oximetry would only be indicated in patients having periods of hypoxemia or other evidence of instability. If hypoxemia is an issue, an inspired O_2 fraction (F_IO_2) of 1.0 should be used during transport. In most instances respiratory care personnel would not be needed to accompany the patient unless the O_2 therapy is unique or the patient unstable.

TRANSPORT OF THE PATIENT RECEIVING MECHANICAL VENTILATION

Maintaining ventilatory support equal to that provided in an ICU during transport is complex. As minute ventilation ($\dot{V}_E$), F_IO_2, and PEEP requirements increase, more sophisticated systems must be used to ensure adequate support. There are several methods of providing ventilation during transports.

Manually Operated Devices

Mapleson Systems

Anesthesiologists employ a variety of manual ventilation devices which may be suitable for use during intrahospital transport of patients receiving mechanical ventilation. These systems were classified by Mapleson[9,10] (hence their name) into six basic configurations, A through F (Fig. 96-1). Five of these are suitable for use in the transportation of patients receiving mechanical ventilation (system E lacks a reservoir bag, which limits its application). These systems employ, in various arrangements, some or all of the following components: a fresh gas inlet, a length of corrugated tubing, a pressure relief valve, and a non-self-inflating reservoir bag.

The Mapleson A circuit provides fresh gas flow from the rear of the assembly and allows an acceptable amount of rebreathing as long as adequate flow is provided. Decompression of the circuit is accomplished by allowing excess gas to vent from the pressure relief valve proximal to the patient. This also serves to regulate the delivered V_T. The Mapleson B circuit is similar to the A system except that the fresh gas inlet is moved in front of the reservoir bag and rebreathing is slightly reduced. The Mapleson C circuit jomits the corrugated tubing, which further reduces rebreathing but decreases the mobility of the operator. The Mapleson D system places the fresh gas inlet proximal to the patient and moves the pressure relief valve close to the operator. This allows easy adjustment of the valve and keeps rebreathing at a minimum. Model F is similar to model D except that it omits the pressure relief valve and allows decompression of the circuit by venting excess gas from the base of the reservoir bag, which has been cut off. This system requires the operator to pinch the open end of the reservoir bag shut during inspiration and to release it during exhalation.

In addition to those pictured in Figure 96-1, numerous other modifications have been used effectively. To keep rebreathing at an acceptable level, Mapleson systems require a flow of fresh gas at a rate that is two to three times the patient's $\dot{V}_E$ requirement.[11]

Patients with modest $\dot{V}_E$ requirements (6 to 12 L/min) who are clinically stable can be safely and easily managed with these devices. Many anesthesiologists prefer this method of manual ventilation because sudden changes in compliance or resistance can easily be detected and the rhythmic refilling of the bag with exhaled gas provides a sense of confidence in the adequacy of ventilation. Also, these devices provide F_IO_2 in excess of 0.90.

The Mapleson systems have several drawbacks when employed during transport. If the patient's $\dot{V}_E$ is too high, rebreathing of CO_2 can occur. The gas consumption of this system is high and the reservoir bag is not self-inflating, so that a loss of compressed gas supply results in inability to provide ventilation even with room air. Also, PEEP is not maintained by a preset valve but is applied by controlling the leak from the system manually while observing a pressure manometer connected to the breathing circuit. Despite these limitations, manual ventilation with Mapleson systems can be safely accomplished during transport as long as patients are carefully selected and adequate compressed O_2 is available.

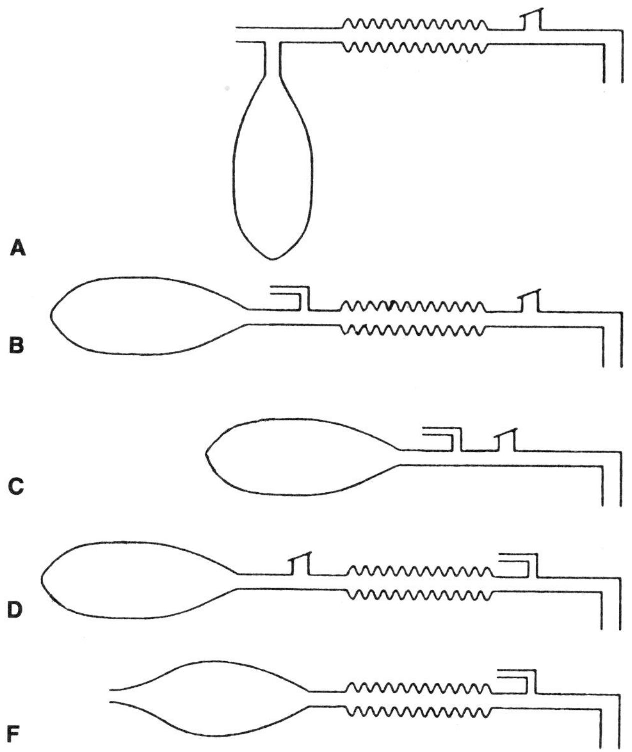

Figure 96-1. Mapleson circuits acceptable for manual ventilation during transport: models A, B, C, D, and F offer various combinations of (1) fresh gas inlet, (2) corrugated tubing, (3) pressure relief valve, (4) non-self-inflating reservoir bag, and (5) patient connection (on right), which can be used to manually provide ventilation to intubated patients during intrahospital transport. Model E was omitted owing to its lack of a reservoir bag. (Redrawn from Mapleson,[9] with permission.)

Self-Inflating Resuscitators

Most manual ventilation provided to ICU patients is supplied by self-inflating resuscitators. These come in a variety of models, both disposable and reusable (Fig. 96-2). Comparisons of various models have revealed varying degrees of performance, although most models meet basic standards. Most investigators have focused on the adherence of these devices to American National Standards Institute (ANSI) standards, which define acceptable levels of valve performance, durability, maintenance of adequate $F_{I}O_2$ at modest $\dot{V}_E$ levels, average stroke volumes, and maximum available rates.

In clinical use self-inflating resuscitators can meet most ventilation needs if used properly. The patient's $F_{I}O_2$ can be maintained or exceeded if an O_2 reservoir is attached to the device's entrainment port. Even with the reservoir, significant gas consumption may be necessary. PEEP can be applied from either a built-in or an add-on valve attached to the exhaled gas port of the resuscitator. The PEEP level may be limited by the type of valve used. Any PEEP valve used during intrahospital transport should provide a stable PEEP level regardless of its position. A V_T of 1.0 L or more and rates above 30 breaths per minute can be achieved by many self-inflating resuscitators, although not always at the same time.[12] These devices also provide the assurance of being able to maintain ventilation with room air if the compressed gas source fails.

Rebreathing Circuits

A closed-circuit system using a CO_2 absorber offers a unique option for providing manual ventilation during transport[13] (Fig. 96-3). This device uses a non-self-inflating reservoir bag placed between two unidirectional valves to drive inspiratory gas into the patient's lungs. Exhaled gas is returned into the bag via the expiratory limb of the circuit. CO_2 is scrubbed from the inspiratory gas by placing a CO_2 absorber in the inspiratory limb of the circuit between the reservoir bag and the patient. A PEEP valve can be placed in the expiratory limb of the circuit if required.

This system offers the advantage that only the O_2 consumed by the patient, generally less than 1 L/min, needs to be replaced. This dramatically lowers the gas consumption during transport and extends the amount of time for which the portable gas source can be used. A length of tubing inserted between the reservoir bag and the unidirectional valve gives the operator additional mobility while in transit. An $F_{I}O_2$ of 1.0 can be easily maintained.

Several precautions must be taken when using a rebreathing system. The patient must receive adequate preoxygenation at an $F_{I}O_2$ of 1.0 prior to being connected to the device. If this is not done, the patient will wash out N_2 into the closed system and lower the $F_{I}O_2$ delivered by the closed system. Also, given the significant total internal volume of the reservoir bag, absorber, and tubing, care should be taken to ensure that an adequate V_T is delivered to the patient at

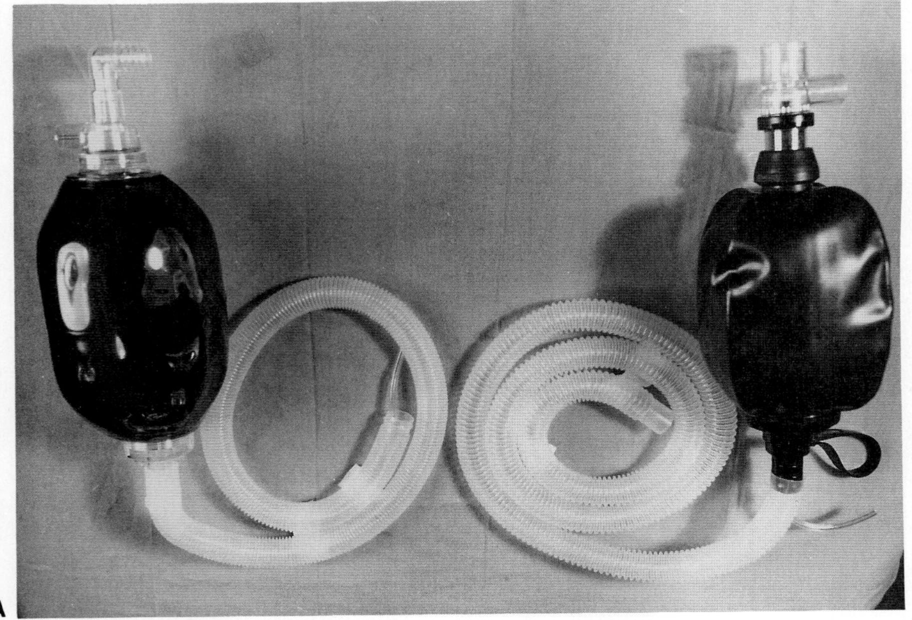

Figure 96-2. Self-inflating resuscitators are available from numerous manufacturers in both **(A)** nondisposable, and **(B)** disposable models. Minor performance variations occur between different models, but most models meet or exceed ANSI standards for operation. Reservoirs are necessary on all models in order to ensure maintenance of adequate $F_{I}O_2$.

Rebreathing Circuit for Transport

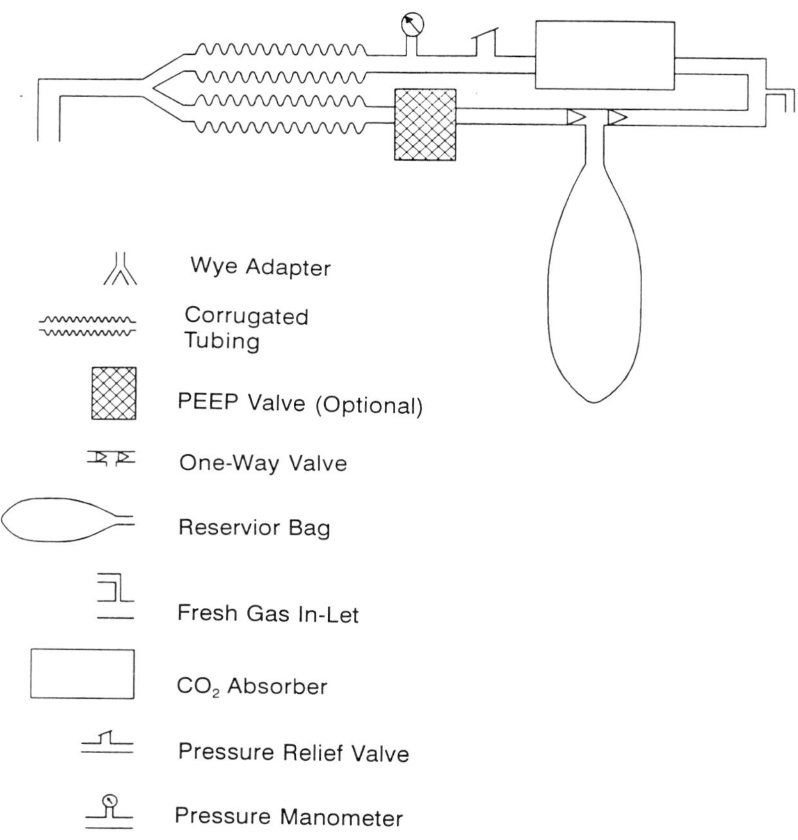

Figure 96-3. The closed-circuit breathing system pictured above offers the ability to maintain a wide variety of V_T and respiratory rate combinations while minimizing the consumption of compressed O_2 during transport. The one-way valves provide unidirectional gas flow, and the CO_2 absorber scrubs the inspiratory gas free of CO_2. An optional non-position-dependent PEEP valve placed in the circuit allows the application of end-expiratory pressure in addition to an F_{IO_2} of 1.0.

high ventilating pressure. This device may seem to be somewhat complicated, but for patients who require high F_{IO_2} and $\dot{V}_E$ levels or who may be in transport for extended periods and for whom compressed gas conservation is therefore critical, it offers some distinct advantages over other manual systems.

Variability of Manual Ventilation

Numerous investigators have evaluated factors that affect the quality of ventilation provided by self-inflating resuscitators. In a study in which clinicians ventilated a test lung, V_T increased by approximately 0.25 L with the use of two-handed versus one-handed ventilation. This study also demonstrated that increasing airway resistance or decreasing lung compliance both significantly decrease V_T.[14] Another bench study, which measured the effect on V_T of hand size and the type of self-inflating resuscitator used, showed that V_T varied from 0.49 L with one small hand to 0.98 L with two large hands.[15]

Measurements made during patient transport demonstrate that V_T decreases and respiratory rate, $\dot{V}_E$, and pH increase in response to the subsequent hyperventilation.[16] Another study demonstrated a deterioration of $\dot{V}_E$ and rate over time, apparently in response to operator fatigue.[17] Since the average actual time spent in transport ranges from 15 to 25 minutes,[18] the previously listed physiologic alterations can exist for a like amount of time. This makes the addition of portable spirometers and/or pressure manometers essential if a precise $\dot{V}_E$ or PEEP level is required.

Portable Mechanical Ventilators

An alternative to manual ventilation during intrahospital transport is use of a portable ventilator. These ventilators are of various configurations and include models specifically designed for transport application, home care ventilators, and portable ICU ventilators (Tables 96-2 and 96-3).

Small portable emergency ventilators have been used for field transport by the military and by paramedics, but these devices may vary in their ability to provide consistent $\dot{V}_E$ levels.[19–21] Also, they can limit the range and combinations of V_T levels and rates available,[22] and they usually provide an F_{IO_2} that is a direct reflection of the source gas powering the device. Devices of this type often use pneumatically powered logic circuits and consume compressed gas in addition to that used for the patient. PEEP can generally be applied with an external valve. The design of ventilators of this type continues to improve rapidly as the technology they employ changes. As new devices become available, each must be studied to determine its usefulness during intrahospital transport.

Home care ventilators are conveniently sized and have the ability to provide consistent ventilatory parameters while being powered by built-in batteries. These systems were traditionally designed to provide ventilation with room air only, but many have been adapted to allow administration of some amount of supplemental O_2. This is generally accomplished either by addition of an O_2 accumulator/reservoir from which the inspiratory gas is drawn from or else by the bleeding-in of O_2 into the inspiratory gas. With either system it may be difficult to maintain adequate F_{IO_2} levels if the requirement is significant. The mechanical limitations on home care ventilator flow rates and peak pressures may render these devices inadequate for patients who require extreme levels of ventilatory support. Nevertheless, studies have shown that fewer incidents of deterioration in gas exchange occur with the use of these devices during transport.[3] The purchase cost may limit making a transport ventilator available for all transports.

Some ICU ventilators are designed with internal battery packs and when portable compressed gas sources are added, will maintain the same ventilation as in the ICU. The addition of external batteries to ICU ventilators that lack internal power sources has been described as a modification for transport application.[23] The drawback of this alternative is the size of the ventilator and attachments. The standard 96-in. by 63-in. hospital elevator is crowded enough by the patient, bed, accompanying staff, and other required devices (e.g., intravenous lines, monitors), and a full-sized ventilator simply may not fit.

Table 96-2. Comparison of Pulmonary Variables in Common Portable Mechanical Ventilators[a]

Ventilator	Tidal Volume (L)	Rate (breaths/min)	F_{IO_2}[b]	PIP_{max} (cmH_2O)	PEEP (cmH_2O)	Flow Rate (L/min)	Logic Gas Consumption
Bio-Med IC-2A	0.000–3.0	1.33–66	100% source	0–120	0–25	0–75	12.0
Ohmeda Logic 7	0.100–2.0	10.00–40	0.50 or 1.0	40–80	Add-on	0–65	2.0
Omni-Vent D/MRI	0.030–3.0	1.00–50	100% source	20–140	0–20	0–98	0.40–2.0
LSP Autovent 2000	0.200–0.6	8.00–20	100% source	0–55	N/S	N/S	5.0
LSP Autovent 3000	0.200–1.2	8.00–30	100% source	0–55	N/S	N/S	1.0
Newport e100i	0.005–+	1.00–120	0.21 to 1.0	0–100	0–25	3–100	4.0–9.0
Aequitron LP6	0.100–2.2	1.00–38	via bleed-in	0–100	Add-on	N/S	0.0
Aequitron LP10	0.100–2.2	1.00–38	0.21–1.0	15–100	Add-on	20–100	0.0
Lifecare PLV-100	0.050–3.0	2.00–40	via bleed-in	5–89	Add-on	10–120	0.0
Lifecare PLV-102	0.050–3.0	10.00–120	0.21–0.90	5–95	Add-on	10–120	0.0
PB Companion 2801	0.050–2.8	1.00–69	via bleed-in	10–100	Add-on	20–120	0.0
Bear 33	0.100–2.2	2.00–40	via bleed-in	0–80	Add-on	20–120	0.0
Hamilton Max	0.050–1.5	2.00–30	100% source	0–90	Add-on	0–90	0.0
Bird Mini-TPX	0.050–2.5	4.00–15	0.45–0.60	N/S	Add-on	0–120	0.0
Impact Uni-Vent 750	0.010–3.0	1.00–150	100% source	N/S	Add-on	0–100	0.0
Pneupac Model 2-R	0.340–1.4	11.00–21	0.45 or 1.0	N/S	Add-on	0–40	0.5
Stein-Gates	0.030–3.0	1.00–150	100% source	N/S	Add-on	0–45	0.0

N/S, data not supplied; PIP_{max}, highest peak inspiratory pressure.
[a] Data based on manufacturer's specifications.
[b] Devices noted as using O_2 bleed-in valves may also use reservoirs.

Table 96-3. Comparison of Other Variables in Common Portable Mechanical Ventilators[a]

Ventilator	Dimensions H × W × D (in.)	Weight (lb)	Internal Battery	Battery Duration (hr)	SIMV/IMV Available[c]
Bio-Med IC-2A	10.25 × 8.17 × 3.17	9.0	Pneumatically powered		Yes (internal)
Ohmeda Logic 7	7.16 × 8.27 × 4.96	11.0	Pneumatically powered		No
Omni-Vent D/MRI	7.00 × 4.00 × 5.00	4.5	Pneumatically powered		Yes (external)
LSP Autovent 2000	5.75 × 3.50 × 1.75	2.5	Pneumatically powered		Yes (internal)
LSP Autovent 3000	5.75 × 3.50 × 1.75	2.5	Pneumatically powered		Yes (internal)
Newport e100i	10.50 × 9.50 × 6.50	13.0	Yes (external)	2.2	Yes (internal)
Aequitron LP6	9.25 × 13.5 × 12.5	32.0	Yes (internal)	1.0	Yes (internal)
Aequitron LP10	9.75 × 14.5 × 13.25	34.0	Yes (internal)	1.0	Yes (internal)
Lifecare PLV-100	9.00 × 12.3 × 12.3	28.3	Yes (internal)	1.0	Yes (internal)
Lifecare PLV-102	9.00 × 12.3 × 12.3	28.9	Yes (internal)	1.0	Yes (internal)
PB Companion 2801	19.00 × 20.5 × 20.5	35.5	Yes (internal)	1.0	Yes (internal)
Bear 33	7.50 × 14.0 × 12.8	29.0	Yes (internal)	1.0	Yes (internal)
Hamilton Max	3.40 × 11.8 × 6.50	11.0	Yes (internal)	8.0	Yes (internal)
Bird Mini-TPX	2.40 × 2.75 × 3.30	2.6	Pneumatically powered		No
Impact Uni-Vent 750	11.40 × 8.66 × 4.33	10.0	Yes (internal)	9.0	Yes (internal)
Pneupac Model 2-R	3.54 × 7.09 × 2.36	2.9	Pneumatically powered		No
Stein-Gates	5.12 × 3.94 × 5.91	5.5	Pneumatically powered		No

N/S, data not supplied.
[a] Data based on manufacturer's specifications.
[b] Devices noted as using O_2 bleed-in valves may also use reservoirs.
[c] Specific SIMV/IMV design may not function in the same fashion as nonportable ventilators.

CHEST TUBE MANAGEMENT DURING TRANSPORT

Patients with chest tubes can present an additional challenge for transport. If the drainage system is being managed by water seal (or other passive method of preventing ambient air from entering the pleural space), no special precautions are required as long as the water seal is maintained (with the bottle below the patient's chest) at all times. If active suction is required to prevent accumulation of a pneumothorax, transport may not be feasible unless suction is provided.

Portable suction devices are available, which operate with varying degrees of effectiveness. Battery-powered systems can maintain adequate levels of suction as long as their power source functions. Rechargeable batteries unfortunately can develop memories, recharge incompletely, and fail abruptly. Pneumatically powered systems, which use a venturi valve to develop negative pressure, can consume significant amounts of compressed gas.

Any portable system must be tested to ensure that it will remove an adequate volume of gas per minute to prevent an inadvertent pneumothorax. If the air leak is small, switching to a water seal for the duration of the transport may be acceptable. This may be determined by running a trial for the anticipated transport time while still in the ICU. The same trial can be made with a portable suction system to ensure its adequacy. Monitoring the patient's arterial O_2 saturation (SaO_2) by pulse oximetry during this type of trial will often help to quickly determine their tolerance of any alteration in the drainage system.

RISKS, COSTS, AND BENEFITS

Although some would advocate inclusion of numerous monitors during transports,[24] reducing the complexity of this difficult activity is just as desirable. The average transport takes the patient out of the ICU for an average of 76 minutes.[25] This period requires the undivided attention of a team of nurses, respiratory therapists, and physicians. One hospital's patient cost averaged $424 per transport, and the overall cost to the hospital was $26,712 for 63 transports.[25] Many ICU directors are concerned about patient safety during transport, but written policies often do not exist.[26] Transports are expensive and dangerous. Given the high risks and the cost to the institution, the benefit of the study or treatment for which the transport is made should be carefully considered and policies developed that ensure a safe and effective process.

References

1. Insel J, Weissman C, Kemper M et al: Cardiovascular changes during transport of critically ill and postoperative patients. Crit Care Med 1986;14:539–542
2. Ehrenwerth J, Sorbo S, Hackel A: Transport of critically ill adults. Crit Care Med 1986;14:543–547
3. Weg JG, Haas CF: Safe intrahospital transport of critically ill ventilator-dependent patients. Chest 1989;96:631–635
4. Braman SS, Dunn SM, Amico CA, Millman RP: Complications of intrahospital transport in critically ill patients. Ann Intern Med 1987;107:469–473
5. Pepe PE, Marini JJ: Occult positive end expiratory pressure in mechanically ventilated patients with airflow obstruction: The auto-PEEP effect. Am Rev Respir Dis 1982;166–170
6. Biddle CJ, Holland MS, Schreiber TR, Mathewson HS: Prevention of hypoxemia in good-risk patients during postoperative transport by positioning and deep breathing. Respir Care 1987; 32:24–28
7. Reynolds FB: Humidification and humidifiers. Problems in the performance of anesthetic and respiratory equipment. Int Anesthesiol Clin 1974;12:79–91
8. Heat and moisture exchangers. Health Devices 1983;12:155–167
9. Mapleson WW: The elimination of rebreathing in various semiclosed anesthetic systems. Br J Anaesth 1954;26:323–332
10. Willis BA, Pender JWM, Mapleson WW: Rebreathing in a T-piece: Volunteer and theoretical studies of the Jackson-Rees modification of Ayer's T-piece during spontaneous respiration. Br J Anaesth 1975;47:1239–1246
11. Greene NM: Flow rates into anesthetic circuits. 9th Annual Anesthesiology Symposium, Naval Regional Medical Center, Portsmouth, VA, Aug. 31–Sept. 2, 1978
12. Maynard HR, Madsen R: Evaluation of three disposable adult manual resuscitators, abstracted. Respir Care 1986;31:934
13. Viegas OJ, Cummins DF, Shumacker CA: Portable ventilation system for transport of critically ill patients. Anesth Analg 1981; 60:760–761
14. Hess D, Goff G: The effects of two-handed versus one-hand ventilation on volumes delivered during bag-valve ventilation at various resistances and compliances. Respir Care 1987;32:1025–1028
15. Hess D, Goff G, Johnson K: The effect of hand size, resuscitator brand, and the use of two hands on volumes delivered during adult bag-valve ventilation. Respir Care 1989;34:805–810
16. Adams KS, Branson RD, Hurst JM: Variabilities in delivered tidal volume and rate during manual ventilation, abstracted. Respir Care 1986;31:950
17. Law GD: Effects of hand size on $\dot{V}_E$, V_T, and F_{IO_2} during manual resuscitation, abstracted. Respir Care 1982;27:1236–1237
18. Gervias HW, Eberle B, Konietzke D et al: Comparison of blood gases of ventilated patients during transport. Crit Care Med 1987;15:761–763
19. Johanningman JA, Branson RD, Campbell R, Hurst JM: Laboratory and clinical evaluation of the MAX transport ventilator. Respir Care 1990;35:952–959
20. Heinrichs W, Mertzluff F, Dick W: Accuracy of delivered versus preset minute ventilation of portable emergency ventilators. Crit Care Med 1989;17:682–685
21. Branson RD, Hurst JM, Adams KS et al: A new transport ventilator: Laboratory and clinical evaluation, abstracted. Respir Care 1985;30:874
22. Morash C, Potash RJ, Kacmarek RM: Performance evaluation of the Ohmeda Logic 07 transport ventilator, abstracted. Respir Care 1986;31:938
23. Gildersleeve JA, Snider MT, Tantun KR, Shore M: Mechanical ventilation of patients requiring high-level PEEP during in-hospital transport, abstracted. Respir Care 1982;27:1263
24. Moore FA, Haenel JB, Moore EE et al: Safe intrahospital transport of ventilated patients—the value of transcutaneous monitoring, abstracted. Crit Care Med 1988;16:433
25. Indeck M, Peterson S, Brotman S: Risk, cost, and benefit of transporting patients from the ICU for special studies, abstracted. Crit Care Med 1987;15:350
26. Smith IU, Flemming S, Bekes CE: Written policy and patient transport from the intensive care unit (letter). Crit Care Med 1987;15:1162

Chapter 97

Infection Control and Isolation Procedures in Respiratory Care

Jan V. Hirschmann

CHAPTER OUTLINE

Primarily because of the current epidemic of the acquired immunodeficiency syndrome (AIDS), infections and infection control are more in the minds of clinicians than at any time in recent memory.[1–6] Hospital infection control and an understanding of how infections are and are not spread in the health care setting are no longer topics solely for epidemiologists and hospital policy makers but are at the very heart of everyday practice and pertinent to every interaction between health care provider and patient.

This chapter summarizes current recommendations for infection control and isolation procedures in respiratory care. It first discusses principles and procedures for controlling disease transmission from patients to hospital personnel. Next, measures to control the transmission of disease from hospital personnel to patients are covered. Information is then presented on controlling disease transmission via respiratory equipment and respiratory care procedures. The chapter concludes with a brief discussion of several additional aspects of the prevention of hospital-acquired (nosocomial) pneumonia.

CONTROLLING DISEASE TRANSMISSION FROM PATIENTS TO HOSPITAL PERSONNEL

"Universal Precautions" and Body Substance Isolation

Although infections in hospitalized patients are common, most are not transmissible to other patients or hospital personnel. Because of the risk of transmission of hepatitis B virus and the human immunodeficiency virus (HIV) especially, the Centers for Disease Control (CDC) recommended "universal precautions,"[7] an approach that requires health care workers to wear gloves and other protective barriers to reduce the risk of parenteral, mucous membrane, and nonintact skin exposures to blood and body fluids known to transmit bloodborne infections. The underlying principle is to assume that *all* patients, regardless of their clinical condition, are potentially infective. The CDC specified as potential sources of infection blood, semen, vaginal secretions, tissues, cerebrospinal fluid, synovial fluid, pleural fluid, pericardial fluid, amniotic fluid, bloody saliva in dental settings, breast milk in special circumstances, and any other fluid containing visible blood. Some hospitals adopted this guideline, while others believed it simpler to state that all body fluids require careful handling, including saliva, feces, nasal secretions, sputum, sweat, tears, and urine.

One widely practiced approach that adopts the latter view is body substance isolation (BSI), which specifies the following precautions, all of which involve placing a barrier, (e.g., gloves, gown, etc) between the health care worker and patients' moist body substances: (1) when direct contact with these substances (e.g., pus, urine, sputum, feces, blood) is anticipated, caregivers wear gloves; (2) when soilage of the clothes of the hospital personnel is expected, they wear gowns; (3) when spattering of these substances into the mouth, nose, or eyes is possible, health care workers wear gowns and eye protection (eyeglasses or goggles). If unexpected contact with these substances occurs, the health care worker should promptly wash the affected area. Other elements of BSI include care in handling all patients' laboratory specimens. Soiled trash and linen are bagged and managed identically for all patients. Syringes, needles, and other sharp objects are discarded into rigid, puncture-resistant containers and needles are not recapped in order to avoid the risk of needle stick punctures. When health care personnel, such as respiratory care clinicians or nurses, perform suction on patients or otherwise come into contact with their sputum, they should use gloves (and gowns if soilage of clothes is likely) and should wash their hands after contact. When dealing with open skin lesions, pustules, boils, wounds, or wound infections, they likewise should use gloves when any contact takes place and gowns when soilage of clothing is likely and should wash their hands after contact. The same recommendations apply for contact with urine. After all physical interactions with patients or their body substances, hospital personnel should wash their hands.

A few serious infections transmitted by the respiratory route are sufficiently contagious that patient isolation is warranted, either in a private room or sometimes with roommates who are similarly infected or immune to the disease (Table 97-1). These infections include measles, mumps, varicella-zoster, rubella, tuberculosis, diphtheria, pertussis (whooping cough), meningococcal meningitis (until treated for 24 hours), and plague. Ideally, hospital personnel caring for these patients are immune to the disease because of vaccination or previous infection (possible for measles, mumps, varicella-zoster, diphtheria, and pertussis). Otherwise, masks, although not proven to protect personnel from airborne agents, are recommended. A more detailed discussion of some important contagious infections is given below.

Table 97-1. Infections Requiring Respiratory Isolation[a]

Measles	Diphtheria
Mumps	Pertussis (whooping cough)
Varicella-zoster	Meningococcal meningitis[b]
Rubella	Plague
Tuberculosis	

[a] For rationale and details see text.
[b] Until treated for 24 hours.

Tuberculosis

Patients with active pulmonary tuberculosis can transmit the infection by aerosolizing organisms when coughing or sneezing. The droplets evaporate, and the tubercle bacilli can remain suspended in the air for prolonged periods of time. Acquisition of infection requires inhalation of the bacilli into the *alveoli* of a susceptible host, because the upper airway and tracheobronchial tree are resistant to the organisms. Infection by other routes such as ingestion of bacilli or contact with clothing, dishes, or other material (including respiratory equipment) that the patient has touched or coughed on does not occur. Accordingly, the major preventive measures are to put infected patients into rooms in which special ventilation prevents spread of aerosolized organisms to other areas of the hospital and to instruct patients to cover their mouths and noses with a tissue when coughing or sneezing. If the patients cannot comply, medical personnel should wear masks when entering the room. Clinicians collecting expectorated sputum specimens from infected patients should wear masks and gloves. Gowns are unnecessary unless soilage of clothing is likely.

Usually, patients transmit infection only when the concentration of tubercle bacilli in the sputum is sufficiently great (about 10^4/mL) for organisms to be visible on the special stains used to detect them. Those with negative sputum smears but positive cultures represent a low risk for spreading infection. Patients with suspected tuberculosis who have three negative sputum smears can therefore be removed from respiratory isolation. Although the precise time when contagiousness ceases is unknown, patients who have received appropriate antituberculous therapy for at least 2 weeks are generally no longer capable of transmitting infection, even if their smears and cultures are markedly positive, and also can be removed from isolation.

Viral Infections

The major risk to hospital personnel comes from viruses. Viral respiratory infections are most likely to occur during the winter months in community outbreaks. Most of these, such as the common cold or pharyngitis, are mild, and no measures can reliably prevent their spread among medical personnel. Influenza, however, can be quite debilitating, and vaccination is recommended for health care workers to prevent infection from seriously depleting the hospital staff during epidemics. Since the virus undergoes regular antigenic changes, annual immunization is necessary to ensure protection against the current strain. Vaccination is especially desirable for medical personnel who themselves have cardiac or pulmonary disorders (see Ch. 62), for they are at highest risk for serious complications from influenza. In epidemics from influenza A, the most common type, unvaccinated personnel can receive prophylaxis with amantidine, an agent that is 70 to 90 percent effective in preventing illness.

Hospitalized patients with varicella or herpes zoster infection can transmit the virus to those who have not previously had varicella. Women of childbearing age without a previous history of varicella should be especially careful because varicella during the first trimester of pregnancy can occasionally cause fetal malformations. Varicella is also a very serious infection for women about the time of delivery. People with a prior history of varicella are not at risk of developing infection following contact with patients who have either varicella or herpes zoster.

Hospital personnel can acquire mucocutaneous infection from contact with skin lesions or respiratory secretions of patients with herpes simplex, who may harbor the virus in the upper airway without having any mucosal abnormalities.[8] When inadvertently introduced onto the lips, skin, or mucous membranes, the virus may cause vesicles and erosions, which may recur. Inoculation of the virus into a finger may cause a herpetic whitlow, characterized by swelling, redness, and pain in the digit accompanied by vesicles or pustules. Painful, swollen lymph nodes may develop in the axilla, and fever is common. Herpetic whitlows may periodically recur after resolution, as do other mucocutaneous infections with this virus. The possibility of developing this problem is one of the many reasons that hospital personnel should wear gloves when they touch the mucous membranes, respiratory secretions, or broken skin of patients.

Hepatitis B

Hepatitis B is a viral infection that can cause serious liver damage. It is transmitted by three routes: sexual contact, parenteral exposure to contaminated blood or blood products, and perinatal transmission from mother to offspring. It is not communicable by casual contact, contaminated food or water, or airborne or fecal-oral routes. The risk for health care personnel in the workplace is from contact with blood or with sharp objects, such as needles, contaminated with blood. These risks are the same as for infection with HIV, which causes AIDS. Precautions to prevent infections with these viruses are discussed in the next section. Hospital personnel exposed to blood or material contaminated with blood should receive immunization against hepatitis B. The vaccine is very effective and safe. Immunization against HIV is currently unavailable.

Acquired Immunodeficiency Syndrome

AIDS is caused by HIV, a virus that is transmitted by sexual contact, parenteral exposure to contaminated blood or blood products, or perinatal transmission from mother to offspring.[9] The virus has been isolated from blood, semen, saliva, tears, breast milk, and urine, but studies of those who have lived with AIDS patients but have not had sexual contact with them indicate that spread of infection by casual contact with saliva or tears does not occur. As with hepatitis B, the risk of transmission of HIV to health personnel in the workplace is by parenteral exposure to blood by a contaminated needle or other sharp instrument, although the risk is very small. While the likelihood of acquiring hepatitis B infection following puncture with a needle contaminated with hepatitis B positive blood is 6 to 30 percent, the risk of HIV infection following puncture with a needle contaminated with HIV is about 0.3 percent, and such cases have often involved a large inoculation of blood. HIV transmission from skin or mucous membrane contact with blood, although reported, has been very rare. No body fluid other than blood has been implicated as a source of occupational acquisition of HIV.[9]

Precautions to prevent these exposures include disposal of contaminated sharp items into puncture-resistant containers. Needles should not be recapped, purposely bent, or otherwise manipulated by hand. When the possibility of exposure to blood or other body fluids exists, gloves should be worn. Health personnel should wear gowns, masks, and eye coverings when extensive contact with blood or potentially infective body fluids is expected, as during endoscopic procedures or postmortem examination. If the hands become contaminated with blood, they should be washed thoroughly immediately.

No transmission of HIV during mouth-to-mouth resuscitation has been documented, but it is theoretically possible. Resuscitation equipment and devices suspected to be contaminated with blood or body fluids should be discarded or thoroughly cleaned and disinfected. Effective disinfectants include germicides approved as hospital disinfectants that kill mycobacteria, a characteristic that ensures adequate potency against viruses as well. Another effective substance is a freshly prepared solution of sodium hypochlorite (household bleach) in dilutions of 1:10 to 1:100.

Since airborne infection with HIV has not been documented, respiratory isolation of patients with AIDS is unwarranted. Furthermore, most of the respiratory infections that they have are not contagious, the major exception being tuberculosis. With reasonable precautions, the chance that medical personnel will develop HIV infection from caring for patients with AIDS is exceedingly low.

CONTROLLING DISEASE TRANSMISSION TO PATIENTS VIA HOSPITAL PERSONNEL

Occasionally medical personnel can transmit disease directly to patients. Health care workers with apparent viral respiratory infections should not care for high-risk patients such as neonates, young infants, patients with chronic obstructive pulmonary disease (COPD), and those with severe immunocompromise. Hospital personnel who are obviously contagious with some serious infection should refrain from all patient contact until contagiousness ceases. Examples include active pulmonary tuberculosis and varicella infection.

More frequently, however, hospital personnel indirectly

transmit disease by transporting hospital flora to ill patients, whose skin, respiratory tract, or alimentary canal becomes colonized with these organisms. Infection may occur if these microbes gain access to normally sterile sites, such as the lung, urinary tract, or subcutaneous tissue, because of impaired host defenses, trauma, surgery, or other forms of instrumentation such as bladder catheterization. The main route by which health care workers convey these organisms to patients from the hospital environment or from other patients is via the hands, and the major way to avoid this contamination of patients is by washing the hands before and after contact with all patients. Hand washing is especially important in the intensive care unit (ICU), for serious pathogens abound there, and ICU patients are the most ill and thus the most susceptible to infection with these organisms. The object of hand washing is not to sterilize the hands, an unattainable goal, but to reduce the number of these transient hospital organisms and prevent their colonization. Hand washing is especially important after contact with respiratory secretions, regardless of whether gloves have been worn, and after any contact with patients who are intubated or have had recent tracheotomies.

CONTROLLING DISEASE TRANSMISSION VIA RESPIRATORY EQUIPMENT AND THERAPY

Most outbreaks of infections traced to respiratory equipment have been from contaminated reservoir nebulizers. Humidifiers are rarely responsible, because they bubble a gas through water without producing an aerosol. Nebulizers, however, create aerosols containing particles of water of a size that can reach the distal areas of the respiratory tract. If these droplets are contaminated with organisms, typically gram-negative bacilli, pneumonia may result. To prevent this problem, reservoirs should be completely emptied and refilled with sterile solutions at least every 24 hours. Only sterile fluid dispensed aseptically should be put into a nebulizer or humidifier, and the unused fluid from the original container should be discarded after 24 hours.

In contrast to nebulizers, most equipment used for mechanical ventilation has humidifying cascades that do not generate aerosols, and the risk of infection is therefore much lower. The humidifying cascade should be changed every 24 hours, but the ventilator circuit (disposable tubing, temperature sensor, swivel adapter) need not be changed more often than every 48 hours.[10] A 1991 study by Dreyfuss et al.[11] suggests that even routinely changing ventilator circuits every 48 hours may be unnecessary. Unless special problems occur, microbiologic sampling of respiratory equipment while in use by a patient is not recommended, and unless there is a high rate of hospital-acquired pneumonias implicating respiratory equipment, the disinfection process need not be monitored by cultures. Because the internal machinery of mechanical ventilators is not an important source of bacterial contamination of inhaled air, it should not be routinely sterilized or disinfected between patients.

When a respiratory therapy machine is used for several patients, the breathing circuit should be replaced by a sterile or disinfected one between patients. Respiratory equipment that touches patients' mucous membranes should be sterilized or disinfected before use in other patients. Respirometers or other equipment that monitor several patients consecutively should not directly touch parts of the breathing circuit but should be attached by extension pieces or be sterilized or disinfected between patients. Hand-powered resuscitation (e.g., Ambu) bags should be sterilized or disinfected before use on other patients.

Contamination and excessive trauma may occur during suctioning of the respiratory tract. Suctioning should not be done routinely but only when secretions cause easily audible gurgling sounds or impaired ventilation. A sterile catheter should be used each time and fresh (but not necessarily sterile) gloves worn on both hands. If flushing of the catheter is required, sterile solutions should be used and then discarded.

OTHER MEASURES TO CONTROL HOSPITAL-ACQUIRED PNEUMONIAS

A very high percentage of nosocomial pneumonias follow surgical procedures, especially on the thorax and abdomen. These operations may impair important defense mechanisms, such as coughing and mucociliary transport, and they may cause diminished consciousness and altered swallowing, which predispose to aspiration. Other risk factors for postoperative pneumonias include obesity, cigarette smoking, COPD, and age older than 70 (see Chs. 54 and 68). Preoperative measures that may help prevent pneumonias in these patients include treatment of any respiratory infections, discontinuance of smoking, optimal bronchodilator management for those with COPD, and instruction in postoperative methods to prevent pneumonia, as discussed in Chapter 89. These methods include frequent coughing, deep breathing, turning in bed, early ambulation, and use of an incentive spirometer. Control of pain with analgesics and appropriate wound support help to allow coughing and deep breathing. Measures that may be helpful for patients with profuse respiratory secretions include suctioning, postural drainage, and percussion.

Also at high risk for pneumonia are patients who aspirate frequently. These patients usually have altered consciousness, a swallowing disorder, or an indwelling nasogastric tube. Pneumonia may be difficult to prevent, but correcting the impairment of consciousness, removing nasogastric tubes promptly when indicated, and avoiding oral feeding of patients with abnormal swallowing or impaired consciousness are obviously reasonable measures. Positioning these patients on their sides rather than on their backs and suctioning their airways when airway secretions accumulate may also be effective. One source of organisms causing aspiration pneumonia is the stomach. The stomach is ordinarily sterile or possesses a sparse flora because the acid environment is hostile to organisms and because gastric motility sweeps the stomach contents, including swallowed organisms, downstream. When motility is impaired or stomach pH raised, organisms, especially gram-negative bacilli, thrive. A common cause of reduced acidity in ICU patients is H-2 blockers or antacids, given in an attempt to prevent gastric bleeding. These agents, by encouraging bacterial growth in the stomachs of patients who may aspirate gastric contents, increase the risk of nosocomial pneumonia. Studies suggest that sucralfate, an agent that coats the gastric mucosa, is as effective in preventing gastric hemorrhage as H-2 blockers or antacids without changing the gastric acidity or encouraging bacterial proliferation.[12] Agents that markedly change stomach pH, such as antacids, H-2 blockers, or omeprazole, therefore should be avoided in these patients.

In patients receiving mechanical ventilation the main preventive measures are to observe infection control techniques when caring for them and to extubate them promptly when clinical circumstances warrant. Administration of systemic antibiotics in the absence of infection does not reduce the frequency of infection but tends to encourage colonization, and often subsequent infection, with organisms resistant to the agent used. Indeed, prudent use of systemic antibiotics and selection of those with the narrowest spectrum of activity that will treat an established infection probably help to decrease the incidence of serious infections. Prophylactic antibiotics administered in aerosol or solution form down tracheal tubes do reduce colonization by some bacteria but do not prevent fatal pneumonias. Prolonged or widespread use in ICUs promotes the emergence of resistant bacteria, and this method of attempting to control nosocomial pneumonia is not recommended.[12] Whether systematic decontamination of the gastrointestinal tract with topically administered, poorly absorbed antibiotics applied to the oropharynx decreases the incidence of nosocomial pneumonia or reduces ICU stays is unsettled, although several studies from Europe suggest that this may prove to be the case.[13,14]

References

1. Pierson DJ: Infection and infection control in respiratory care: An introduction to the 1988 Schering Symposium papers. Respir Care 1989;34:80
2. Schaberg DR: How infections spread in the hospital. Respir Care 1989;34:81–84
3. Craven DE, Steger KA: Pathogenesis and prevention of nosocomial pneumonia in the mechanically ventilated patient. Respir Care 1989;34:85–97
4. Chatburn RL: Decontamination of respiratory care equipment: What can be done, what should be done. Respir Care 1989;34:98–110
5. Hooton TM: Protecting ourselves and our patients from nosocomial infections. Respir Care 1989;34:111–115
6. Summer WR, Nelson S: Nosocomial pneumonia: Characteristics of the patient-pathogen interaction. Respir Care 1989;34:116–124
7. Pugliese G (ed): Universal Precautions. Policies, Procedures, and Practices. American Hospital Publishing. Chicago, 1991
8. Corey L, Spear PG: Infections with *herpes simplex* viruses. N Engl J Med 1986;314:686–691, 749–757
9. Gerberding JL: Reducing occupational risk of HIV infection. Hosp Pract, June 15, 1991:103–118
10. Craven DE, Connolly MG, Lichtenberg DA et al: Contamination of mechanical ventilators with tubing changes every 24 or 48 hours. N Engl J Med 1982;306:1505–1509
11. Dreyfuss D, Djedaini K, Weber P et al: Prospective study of nosocomial pneumonia and of patient and circuit colonization during mechanical ventilation with circuit changes every 48 hours versus no change. Am Rev Respir Dis 1991;143:738–743
12. Driks MR, Craven DE, Celli BR et al: Nosocomial pneumonia in intubated patients given sucralfate as compared to antacids or histamine type 2 blockers. The role of gastric colonization. N Engl J Med 1987;317:1376–1382
13. Pugin J, Auckenthaler R, Lew DP, Suter PM: Oropharyngeal decontamination decreases incidence of ventilator-associated pneumonia. A randomized, placebo-controlled, double-blind clinical trial. JAMA 1991;265:2704–2710
14. Weinstein RA: Selective intestinal decontamination—an infection control measure whose time has come? Ann Intern Med 1989;110:853–855

Chapter 98

Pulmonary Rehabilitation

Andrew L. Ries

CHAPTER OUTLINE

DEFINITION AND OVERVIEW

Comprehensive rehabilitation programs for patients with chronic pulmonary diseases are well established as a means of enhancing standard medical therapy in order to control and alleviate symptoms and to optimize the patient's functional capacity.[1–9] The primary goal of these programs is to restore the patient to the highest possible level of independent function. This goal may be accomplished by helping patients to become more knowledgeable about their disease, more actively involved in their own health care, and more independent in performing daily care activities and therefore less dependent on family, friends, health professionals, and expensive medical resources.

Standard medical therapy is important in alleviating symptoms of chronic respiratory disease, particularly the distressing symptom of breathlessness (dyspnea).[2] However, many patients and physicians are left to cope with the problems of a chronic, largely irreversible disease process. A common attitude is that "nothing more can be done." Survival in patients with chronic obstructive pulmonary disease (COPD) is clearly related to age and degree of pulmonary impairment as measured by forced expiratory volume in 1 second (FEV_1). In addition, however, the patient's exercise tolerance and perceived physical disability may also be important predictors of mortality.[10]

In 1974 the American College of Chest Physicians' Committee on Pulmonary Rehabilitation adopted the following definition[1]:

> Pulmonary rehabilitation may be defined as an art of medical practice wherein an individually tailored, multidisciplinary program is formulated which through accurate diagnosis, therapy, emotional support, and education, stabilizes or reverses both the physio- and psychopathology of pulmonary diseases and attempts to return the patient to the highest possible functional capacity allowed by his pulmonary handicap and overall life situation.

This definition highlights three important features of successful rehabilitation programs:

1. *Individual*: Patients with disabling COPD require individual assessment of their needs, individual attention, and a program designed to meet realistic individual goals.

2. *Multidisciplinary*: Pulmonary rehabilitation programs provide access to information from a variety of health care disciplines, which is integrated by experienced staff into a comprehensive, cohesive program designed to meet the needs of each patient.
3. *Attention to Physio- and Psychopathology*: To be successful, pulmonary rehabilitation programs must pay attention to psychological and emotional problems as well as help to optimize medical therapy to improve lung function.

Successful pulmonary rehabilitation programs are typically provided by a multidisciplinary team of health care professionals, which may include physicians, respiratory care practitioners, nurses, physical therapists, exercise physiologists, psychologists, pharmacists, or other individuals with the appropriate interest and expertise. Specific team makeup depends on the resources and expertise available. Responsibilities of team members generally cross disciplines, but the necessary skills have been delineated.[11]

Within this general framework, successful pulmonary rehabilitation programs have been established in various settings and formats (e.g., inpatient or outpatient, hospital or practice based).[4,7,8,12–16] Both inpatient and outpatient programs have distinct advantages and disadvantages: inpatient management, particularly in the early phases, may be best for patients with more severe disease,[7,12,17] but outpatient programs may be more appropriate for better functioning or working patients.

The key to success in any program is a dedicated and enthusiastic staff, which is familiar with the problems of pulmonary patients and can relate well to and motivate them. Since many of the patients are elderly, program staff should be particularly sensitive to the needs and problems of older individuals.[18]

Although pulmonary rehabilitation programs have been developed primarily for patients with COPD, these programs may also be useful for patients with other pulmonary diseases.[19]

PATIENT SELECTION AND EVALUATION

An important factor in the success of pulmonary rehabilitation is the selection of patients. Appropriate patients are those with symptomatic lung disease producing perceived impairment or disability and who are motivated to be actively involved in their own care to improve their health status.[1,20] Patients with mild disease may need education about appropriate respiratory care practices to prevent future complications but may not yet perceive their problem as severe enough to warrant a comprehensive care program. On the other hand, patients with severe disease may be too limited to benefit significantly. Resting hypercapnia alone should not be considered an indication of too severe lung disease; Foster et al.[21] reported that hypercapnic patients achieved the same benefits from pulmonary rehabilitation as eucapnic ones.

Other factors are also important in evaluating patients. The role of the rehabilitation program is to support the patient and the physician, not to assume responsibility for primary medical care. Pulmonary rehabilitation is not first-line therapy for chronic pulmonary disease and should be started only after patients have been stabilized on standard medical therapy. The assessment and treatment plan can then be based on the patient's optimal level of function. Patients also should not have other disabling or unstable conditions that would limit their ability to participate and to concentrate fully on rehabilitation activities. Such conditions may include, but are not limited to, unstable heart disease, psychiatric illness, or concurrent evaluation for a potentially serious health problem.

The initial step in evaluating patients for pulmonary rehabilitation is an interview, which should thoroughly review the patient's medical history and assess psychosocial problems and needs.[1] Communication and cooperation with the primary care physician is also important. Care and attention in this initial evaluation will result in setting appropriate individual goals compatible with both the patient's and the physician's expectations and the program's objectives.

Psychosocial Assessment

Successful rehabilitation requires attention not only to physical problems but also to psychological, emotional, and social ones common to patients with chronic lung disease as they struggle to deal with symptoms that are often poorly understood.[22–26] Commonly, such patients become depressed, frightened, anxious, and more dependent on others to care for their needs. Psychological status is an important determinant of pulmonary symptoms reported by patients.[27]

Progressive dyspnea is a frightening symptom and may lead to a vicious fear-dyspnea cycle: with progressive disease, less exertion results in more dyspnea, which produces more fear and anxiety which, in turn, leads to more dyspnea. Ultimately, the patient avoids any physical activity associated with these unpleasant symptoms. In the extreme, patients may set up a stationary "command post" from which they rarely venture forth except to seek relief in physicians' offices and hospitals. In addition, Jensen[28] reported that high stress and low social support were better predictors of subsequent hospitalizations than severity of illness in patients with obstructive lung disease.

In order to deal with these problems, the initial evaluation should include an assessment of the patient's psychological state (e.g., depression or other psychological test findings) and close attention to psychosocial clues during screening interviews (e.g., family and social support, activities of daily living, employment potential).[23] Cognitive impairment that may limit the patient's ability to participate should be recognized. Spouses, family members, and close friends may provide valuable insight and should be included in the screening process and program whenever possible. Psychosocial assessment of patients with chronic respiratory disease is discussed more fully in Chapter 60.

Pulmonary Function and Exercise Evaluation

The complexity of the diagnostic testing performed depends on the individual patient and on the facilities available. Pulmonary function testing helps to characterize and quantify impairment from the patient's lung disease. Spirometry and lung volume measurements are most useful and can be supplemented with other tests as needed.

Exercise testing is generally necessary to assess the patient's exercise tolerance and to evaluate possible blood gas changes with exercise (i.e., hypoxemia or hypercapnia). It may also help to uncover other, co-existing diseases common in older patients (e.g., heart disease). The exercise test can also be used to establish a safe and appropriate prescription for subsequent training.[31,32]

Maximal exercise tolerance of patients with moderate to severe ventilatory dysfunction is limited largely by their breathing capacity. Simple pulmonary function parameters (e.g., FEV_1 and maximum voluntary ventilation [MVV]) can be used to estimate a patient's maximum exercise ventilation. However, pulmonary function measurements only provide a rough estimate of a patient's maximum work capacity; the exercise tolerance of pulmonary patients will depend considerably on the individual's perception and tolerance of the subjective symptom of breathlessness (dyspnea).[32] Therefore, it is important to have patients exercise to assess each patient's current level of function and symptom tolerance.

Exercise testing is most easily carried out by using the type of exercise to be used in training (e.g., treadmill testing for a walking program). Work load, heart rate, electrocardiogram, and arterial oxygenation should be measured and/or monitored and an ECG obtained during testing. Other measurements such as minute ventilation or expired gas analysis, which are needed to calculate variables such as O_2 consumption ($\dot{V}O_2$), may be made depending on the interest and expertise of the referring physicians, program staff, and laboratory personnel but are probably not necessary for all programs. Exercise testing protocols should also take into account the considerable variations in test results in stable pulmonary patients and the normal improvement that may be seen on repeat testing, particularly in patients who are unused to physical activity.[33]

Measurement of arterial blood gases at rest and during exercise is important because of the frequently unexpected and unpredictable occurrence of exercise-induced hypoxemia.[34] Blood gas sampling during exercise adds a significant degree of complexity to testing. Noninvasive techniques, such as cutaneous oximetry, are useful for continuous monitoring but have limited accuracy for precise assessment of arterial oxygenation (95 percent confidence limit equal to $\pm$ 4 to 5 percent variation in O_2 saturation of arterial blood [SaO_2]).[35]

PROGRAM STRUCTURE AND CONTENT

Although pulmonary rehabilitation programs differ in structure and content, comprehensive ones typically include several key components: general education (for patients and family); respiratory and chest physiotherapy instruction; psychosocial support; and exercise conditioning (Table 98-1). It is difficult to assess the relative contributions of individual components that are so interrelated. For example, many consider exercise conditioning to be the central feature of pulmonary rehabilitation. However, during an exercise training program provided by knowledgeable and enthusiastic staff, patients also receive considerable education and psychosocial support.

General Education

Success of pulmonary rehabilitation is dependent on the understanding and active involvement both of patients and of those who are important for their social support. Education has been recommended and included as an integral component[6,36]; even patients with severe disease can gain a better understanding of their disease.[37] Standardized testing instruments for knowledge assessment have been developed and validated.[38] However, it is not clear whether knowledge alone will lead to improved health status, since it may be difficult to change attitudes and behavior. A variety of teaching formats have been used. Patients require specific, individualized strategies, and instruction should be designed to fit each patient's learning ability.

Howland and co-workers[39] performed a controlled study of the effect of education alone on health status in patients with COPD in two matched communities. In one community patients were identified, assessed, and offered an education program (41 percent completed the program); in the other community, patients were only identified, assessed, and notified of the findings (80 percent completed pre- and post-program evaluations). After 1 year the health education program was found to have had no significant impact on health status, as measured by symptom status, physical function,

Table 98-1. Components of a Comprehensive Pulmonary Rehabilitation Program

- Patient evaluation
  - Medical evaluation
  - Psychosocial assessment
  - Physiologic testing
    - Pulmonary function
    - Exercise
    - Arterial blood gas analysis
  - Goal setting
- Program content
  - General education
  - Respiratory and chest physiotherapy instruction
  - Psychosocial support
  - Exercise training

mental health, or social function. Only health locus of control was significantly different after the intervention, indicating that patients who received the education program were more likely to believe that they could control their own health. These findings suggest that, although education alone may improve patients' knowledge of disease, it may not produce significant change in their health status.

Ashikaga et al.[40] evaluated a community-based education program, which included didactic material, demonstration of self-help skills, and group discussions dealing with psychosocial aspects of COPD. As compared with control participants who received written material only, the experimental subjects demonstrated a significant improvement in their knowledge of disease. However, the control subjects showed significant improvement in their perceived chance of improvement and reduction in social disability. These findings suggest that positive information presented to control patients, without counseling or open discussion, may have resulted in a false expectation of improvement, which emphasizes the importance of providing time for counseling patients in the proper interpretation of educational material presented.

Respiratory and Chest Physiotherapy Instruction

Many patients with COPD use, abuse, and are confused about respiratory and chest physiotherapy techniques. As part of a comprehensive rehabilitation program, each patient's need for respiratory care techniques should be assessed and instruction provided in their proper use. Such techniques may include chest physiotherapy maneuvers to enhance mucociliary clearance and control excess secretions, breathing training techniques to relieve and control dyspnea and improve ventilatory function, and proper use of respiratory care equipment including nebulizers, metered dose inhalers, and O_2.[6,41]

Bronchial Hygiene

Patients with chronic lung disease have abnormal lung clearance mechanisms, which make them more susceptible to problems with retained secretions and infections. Therefore, rehabilitation programs typically teach appropriate coughing and chest physiotherapy techniques for secretion control. These are important for patients with excess mucus production during exacerbations and as routine preventive measures for patients with chronic sputum production.

Several studies have reported benefits from the techniques taught, which typically include controlled coughing, postural drainage, and chest vibration and/or percussion.[18,41–45] The efficacy of individual techniques is difficult to determine; available evidence suggests that postural drainage and controlled coughing (or the forced expiration technique[46]) may be the most effective.[44,47] Administration of nebulized saline or bronchodilators may increase secretion clearance.[48] These techniques are most effective in patients with a large amount of sputum (e.g., more than 30 mL/d), whether from chronic or acute conditions. The benefits in patients without excess sputum is less clear. Also, these techniques may induce bronchoconstriction in patients with reactive airways. Whether the chest physical therapy techniques add significantly to effective coughing alone is not clear. Use of mucolytic agents to reduce the viscosity of secretions is of questionable benefit; in several studies these agents have not appeared to be any more effective than placebo.[18] In addition, intermittent positive pressure breathing (IPPB) has been evaluated systematically for this purpose and found to be ineffective.[49,50]

Breathing Retraining Techniques

Pulmonary rehabilitation programs typically teach breathing techniques such as diaphragmatic and pursed lip breathing aimed at helping patients to relieve and control breathlessness, improve the ventilatory pattern (by slowing respiratory rate and/or increasing tidal volume), prevent dynamic airway compression, improve respiratory synchrony of abdominal and thoracic musculature, and improve gas exchange.[2,3,41,43,51–53]

A review of clinical studies evaluating the effects of breathing training techniques points out that improvement in clinical symptoms (e.g., dyspnea) is a more consistent finding than measurable changes in physiologic parameters.[52] Also, as pointed out by Miller,[53] it is difficult to distinguish the separate contributions of each of the various methods since they are frequently taught together and integrated with other aspects of rehabilitation such as patient education and psychosocial support.

The most consistent physiologic change observed after breathing training in patients with COPD is an increase in tidal volume and a decrease in respiratory rate. Motley demonstrated improved gas exchange associated with controlled, slow deep breathing in 35 patients with COPD.[54] He noted an increase in SaO_2 in 33 patients, along with a decrease in $PaCO_2$ and slight improvement in steady-state diffusing capacity with the controlled breathing technique. Other studies have reported improvement in ventilatory efficiency with a technique of paced slow breathing.[55,56] However, this technique does not appear to be associated with the same degree of symptomatic relief commonly experienced with pursed lip breathing.

Diaphragmatic Breathing

The diaphragmatic breathing technique was described by Barach and co-workers[57,58] and Miller[53] as a maneuver in which the patient attempts to coordinate abdominal wall expansion with inspiration and to slow expiration through pursed lips.[52] The primary aim is to slow respiratory rate and increase tidal volume.

Miller[59] found a significant increase in diaphragmatic excursion after 6 to 8 weeks of diaphragmatic breathing training in a group of 24 patients with stable COPD. This was associated with a significant increase (34 percent) in resting tidal volume and decrease (42 percent) in respiratory rate without change in total ventilation at rest or with exercise. This improved ventilatory efficiency resulted in improved gas exchange with increased SaO_2, decreased $PaCO_2$, and increased exercise tolerance with less dyspnea.

Sinclair,[60] in a study of the effects of diaphragmatic breathing accompanied by relaxation therapy over several weeks in 22 patients with COPD, found no change in measurements of pulmonary function but an increase in diaphragmatic excursion; 14 of these patients, however, noted symptomatic improvement. Similar results were reported by Becklake et al.,[61] who noted subjective improvement from diaphragmatic breathing and relaxation therapy in 8 of 10 patients, who, however, showed no significant changes in measurements of pulmonary function.

In a pilot study Williams et al.[62] examined spirometry, 12-minute walking distance, and ratings of perceived exertion in eight patients with COPD after 3 weeks of placebo physiotherapy and 3 weeks of diaphragmatic breathing training. They found no change in any of the measured parameters. Sackner et al.[63] studied the effects of diaphragmatic breathing on the distribution of ventilation in 11 patients with COPD and found no change in indices of distribution calculated from the nitrogen-washout curve or from xenon ventilation lung scans.

Pursed Lip Breathing

Pursed lip breathing is the other technique typically taught with diaphragmatic breathing for patients with COPD.[52,53,57] This type of breathing was observed by Laennec as early as 1830 and was advocated as a physical exercise for pulmonary patients in the early part of the twentieth century.[64] It is a maneuver, often performed naturally by patients, in which the lips are used to narrow the airway during expiration. The aims are to slow the expiratory phase and to maintain positive pressure in the airways to "keep the airway open" and improve ventilatory efficiency.

Mueller et al.[65] found that pursed lip breathing led to an increase in tidal volume and decrease in respiratory rate in patients with COPD both at rest and during exercise. This led to an improvement in ventilatory efficiency, that is, to a decrease in the expired minute ventilation ($\dot{V}_E$) needed for a given $\dot{V}O_2$ level, and 7 of 12 patients also experienced symptomatic relief of dyspnea.

Thoman et al.[66] studied pursed lip breathing in 21 patients with COPD and reported improved ventilation to poorly ventilated areas of the lung as compared with normal breathing.[66] In addition, both pursed lip and controlled rate breathing produced a significant change in respiratory pattern, with an increase in tidal volume and a decrease in respiratory rate in each of seven patients studied.

Tiep and co-workers compared pursed lips breathing with general relaxation in 12 patients with COPD.[67] During pursed lip breathing patients watched the digital readout of an ear oximeter. These authors found significantly higher SaO_2 and tidal volume and lower respiratory rate during pursed lip breathing, with no change in $\dot{V}_E$.

Oxygen

Supplemental O_2 therapy is beneficial for patients with significant resting arterial hypoxemia from either acute or chronic lung disease.[68,69] As discussed in Chapter 63, long-term continuous O_2 therapy has been clearly shown to improve survival and reduce morbidity in hypoxemic patients with COPD.[2,70–72] In fact, this is the only treatment that has been proved to prolong survival in these patients. Possible benefits of supplemental O_2 for nonhypoxemic patients or for patients with hypoxemia only under certain conditions (e.g., exercise or sleep) are less clearly defined.[31,69,70]

The effects on exercise tolerance of O_2 administered routinely to patients with COPD have been variable. In a study of 27 COPD patients participating in a pulmonary rehabilitation program, Longo et al.[73] found no significant improvement in breathlessness or exercise tolerance from O_2 at 2 or 4 L/min as compared with compressed air. There was slight improvement, however, in the subset of patients with exercise-induced hypoxemia. On the other hand, Vyas et al.[74] reported a significant increase in maximum work rate and O_2 uptake in 12 COPD patients when breathing 40 percent O_2 as compared with room air, administered in a double-blind fashion. Zack and Palange,[75] in a study of COPD patients entering a pulmonary rehabilitation program reported a 28 percent increase in maximum exercise work load for patients breathing O_2 at 4 L/min as compared with room air.[75]

Davidson et al.[76] found improvement in rated dyspnea, endurance walking time, and 6-minute walking distance with 4 L/min of O_2 regardless of the degree of hypoxemia present at rest or with exercise. In addition, the benefit from supplemental O_2 was not cancelled by the effort required to carry a portable O_2 cylinder. Bradley et al.[77] compared maximum exercise tolerance and exercise endurance when breathing room air, compressed air, and supplemental O_2 at 5 L/min in 26 patients with COPD. They reported improvement in exercise endurance but not maximum work rate on supplemental O_2 as compared with either room or compressed air. Thus, it appears that supplemental O_2 administered routinely to patients with COPD may result in improvement in exercise endurance but variable changes in maximal exercise tolerance. The potential benefits may depend on the amount of O_2 administered.

Although continuous O_2 therapy for hypoxemic patients is feasible and safe, maintaining patients on O_2 presents a number of problems.[69,78] This is particularly difficult for physically disabled and older patients who may need assistance in handling, using, and caring safely for such equipment. Therefore, in pulmonary rehabilitation it is important to assess each patient's O_2 needs and provide instruction in the most appropriate techniques (see Ch. 99).

Psychosocial Support

An essential component of a comprehensive pulmonary rehabilitation program is the psychosocial support provided to combat symptoms that reflect progressive feelings of hopelessness and inability to cope with the disease.[2,6,22–26] Depression is common.[24,79] Patients may show symptoms of anxiety (particularly fear of dyspnea), denial, anger, and isolation and become sedentary and dependent on family members, friends, and medical services to provide for their needs, and they may become overly concerned with other physical problems and psychosomatic symptoms. Sexual dysfunction and fear of sexual activities are common, often unspoken, consequences of chronic lung disease; patients can be helped by appropriate counseling from knowledgeable and supportive staff.[80–82] Patients may also demonstrate cognitive and neuropsychological dysfunction, possibly related to or exacerbated by the effects of hypoxemia on the brain.

Psychosocial support is best provided by warm and enthusiastic staff who are able to communicate effectively with patients and to devote the time and effort necessary to understand and motivate them. Important family members and friends should be included in program activities so that they can understand and cope better with the patient's disease. Support groups and group therapy sessions are also effective. Patients with moderately severe psychological disorders may benefit from individual counseling and psychotherapy. Psychotropic drugs should generally be reserved for patients with severe levels of psychological dysfunction.

In a randomized controlled trial of exercise training in 39 patients with COPD and coal workers' pneumoconiosis, Cockcroft et al.[83] found significant improvement in two tests administered to evaluate psychological variables in both the experimental and control groups. This emphasizes the problem of distinguishing the effects of various components of a comprehensive pulmonary rehabilitation program, since patients may demonstrate improved psychological performance from even minimal attention and intervention, such as participation in a clinical study as a control subject.

Jensen measured stress and social support in 59 patients with COPD and randomly assigned 30 "high-risk" patients to either a pulmonary rehabilitation, a self-help support, or a control group. He reported that the high-risk control patients were hospitalized significantly more frequently than either low-risk or high-risk patients in the rehabilitation and self-help groups.[28] These findings emphasize the important influence of psychosocial status on hospitalization rates in these patients and the beneficial effect of rehabilitation services in reducing the frequency of hospitalization.

Agle et al.[84] evaluated physiologic and psychologic status in 24 patients before and after a comprehensive inpatient pulmonary rehabilitation program. They found that success in rehabilitation was correlated with the psychological and not the physiologic measurements. Good responders tended to have less severe psychological symptoms (depression, anxiety, body preoccupation) initially and to show improvement at 1 year. In particular, positive changes were related to desensitization to fear of dyspnea and to increased autonomy in symptom control. By contrast, poor responders had more baseline psychologic dysfunction and showed little change after the program.

Relaxation Training

Because dyspnea in chronic lung disease is closely associated with accompanying fear and anxiety, techniques of relaxation training have been incorporated into pulmonary rehabilitation programs. Renfroe[85] evaluated progressive muscle relaxation training in 10 patients with COPD in comparison with a control group, who were told to relax but not given specific instructions. In relaxation training patients are instructed to sequentially tense and then relax 16 different muscle groups. After the relaxation sessions, the experimental group demonstrated significantly greater reduction in measurements of dyspnea and anxiety than did control subjects. Also, change in dyspnea was significantly correlated with change in anxiety. These findings suggest that relaxation training can significantly improve symptoms of both dyspnea and anxiety in these patients.

Exercise

Exercise is generally considered to be an important component of pulmonary rehabilitation.[1,6,86,87] Available evidence indicates that accepted benefits from exercise reconditioning in COPD patients include increases in endurance, maximum O_2 consumption ($\dot{V}O_2max$), and skill in task performance.[87,88] However, the optimal methods of training and the mechanisms of the improvements seen have not yet been clearly defined for pulmonary patients.[31]

Of all the components provided in a comprehensive pulmonary rehabilitation program, exercise is probably the most difficult in terms of personnel, equipment, and expertise. One should be careful in automatically applying principles derived in normal subjects or cardiac patients to patients with chronic lung disease because of differences in limitations to exercise performance and principles and problems of training.[7,31,89–91]

A variety of approaches have been used in exercise training for the patient with chronic lung disease. To be successful, the program should be designed to fit the individual patient's physical abilities, interests, resources, and environment. For general application, techniques should be simple and inexpensive.[18] As in normal subjects and in other patient populations, benefits from exercise training are largely specific to the muscles and tasks involved in the training—patients tend to do best on activities and exercises for which they are trained.[92]

There is considerable evidence of both physiologically and psychologically favorable responses to exercise training in patients with chronic lung disease.[2,3,31,88] Patients may increase their maximum capacity and/or endurance for exercise and physical activity even though lung function does not usually change. Exercise training also provides an ideal opportunity for patients to learn their capacity for physical work and to use and practice methods for controlling dyspnea (e.g., breathing and relaxation techniques).

The exercise program needs to be safe and appropriate for each patient's interest, environment, and level of function and should be based on the results of initial exercise testing. Training should utilize methods easily adapted to the home setting. Walking programs are particularly useful for physically limited patients and have the added benefit of encouraging patients to expand their social horizons. In inclement weather patients can frequently walk indoors (e.g., in shopping malls). Other types of exercise (e.g., cycling, swimming) may also be effective. Patients should be encouraged to incorporate regular exercise into activities they enjoy (e.g., golf, gardening). Since many patients with COPD have limited exercise tolerance, emphasis during training should be placed on increasing endurance, which will allow patients to become more functional within their physical limits. Increase in exercise level is also frequently possible as patients gain experience and confidence with their exercise program.

Prescription

Although selection of training targets based on percentages of maximum heart rate or $\dot{V}O_2max$ are well established in normal subjects or other patient populations, selection of an appropriate training prescription for patients with chronic lung disease is not clearly defined. Exercise tolerance in patients with advanced COPD is typically limited by maximum ventilation and the perception of breathlessness (dyspnea). Such patients frequently do not reach limits of cardiac or peripheral muscle performance.

There has been much controversy about the selection of appropriate intensity targets for training patients with chronic lung disease. Use of a target heart rate, as in normal subjects and cardiac patients, has been advocated by some authors,[5] although it is recognized that such targets may not be reliable for patients with more severe disease.[86] Wasserman et al.[93] reported that about two-thirds of patients with moderate to severe COPD will develop significant metabolic acidosis during exercise. For these patients exercise training above this level (the anaerobic threshold) would result in physiologic benefits related to reduction in the exercise metabolic acidosis; however, patients who do not develop metabolic acidosis during exercise would not be expected to demonstrate these physiologic changes from training. Wasserman et al.[93] question the value of exercise training for these patients; but this view ignores the other possible effects and benefits of training.

It has also been reported that many patients with advanced chronic lung disease can be trained at high percentages of maximum exercise tolerance, which may approach or even exceed the maximum level reached on the initial exercise test.[94] Patients with mild lung disease may be trained at submaximal levels that are higher than the usual 60 to 70 percent of maximum expected in normal persons or cardiac patients. In a study of intensive exercise training in 59 inpatients with moderate to severe COPD, Carter et al.[95] trained patients at levels near their ventilatory limits and reported mean peak exercise ventilation of 94 to 100 percent of measured MVV, at baseline, after training, and 3 months later. Patients demonstrated improved maximum exercise level and ventilation with training. These findings suggest that even patients with advanced disease can be trained successfully at or near maximal levels.

Some pulmonary rehabilitation programs therefore define exercise targets and progression during training by symptom tolerance rather than by targets based on heart rate, work level, or other physiologic measurements.[75,86] Ratings of perceived symptoms (e.g., breathlessness) help in teaching patients to exercise to "target" levels of breathing discomfort.[96] Therefore, after the initial exercise test to assess a patient's maximal exercise tolerance, a typical approach would be to begin training at a level that the patient can sustain with reasonable comfort for several minutes. This is an adequate starting point for training that emphasizes increasing endurance. Increase in time or level of exercise may then be made according to the patient's symptom tolerance.

Exercise-Induced Hypoxemia

A major problem in planning a safe exercise program for patients with COPD is the potential occurrence of exercise-induced hypoxemia. Patients who may or may not be hypoxemic at rest may develop changes in arterial oxygenation that cannot be predicted reliably from resting measurements of pulmonary function or gas exchange.[34] Normal individuals do not develop hypoxemia with exercise, and patients with mild COPD may demonstrate no change or an improvement in PaO_2 during exercise. However, PaO_2 may increase, decrease, or remain unchanged with exercise in patients with moderate to severe COPD. Therefore, it is important to measure arterial oxygenation at rest and during exercise to detect significant exercise-induced hypoxemia and to decide how much O_2 is necessary for safe training. With the availability of convenient portable systems for ambulatory O_2 delivery, hypoxemia is not a contraindication to exercise training.

Other Types of Exercise

Upper Extremity Training

Exercise programs for patients with COPD have typically emphasized lower extremity training (e.g., walking or cycling). Other types of exercise may also be beneficial for the many physically limited pulmonary patients who have difficulty performing even simple activities of daily living. For instance, many patients with COPD report disabling dyspnea for daily activities involving the upper extremities (e.g., lifting or grooming) at work levels much lower than for the lower extremities.[97–99] Upper extremity exercise is accompanied by a higher ventilatory demand for a given level of work than occurs with lower extremity exercise.[100,101] Also, since exercise training is generally specific to the muscles and tasks involved in training,[102–106] upper extremity exercises may be important in helping pulmonary patients with common daily activities.[98]

Ries et al.[98] evaluated two upper extremity home training programs in 45 patients with COPD who were participating concurrently in a multidisciplinary pulmonary rehabilitation program. As compared with control subjects who did not perform upper extremity training, patients in both experimental groups demonstrated improved upper extremity performance in tests most specific to the training provided. However, there were no significant changes in tests of ventilatory muscle performance or simulated activities of daily living.

Celli et al.[97] evaluated thoracic and abdominal respiratory synchrony and transdiaphragmatic pressure during unsupported arm and leg cycle exercise in 12 patients with severe COPD. They found that endurance for arm exercise was significantly less than for leg exercise even though heart rate and O_2 uptake were lower. Also, in the five patients with the most severe COPD, arm exercise was limited by dyspnea and was accompanied by dyssynchronous thoracoabdominal breathing. By contrast, in the other seven patients arm exercise was limited by muscle fatigue, and respiratory dyssynchrony did not develop. Respiratory dyssynchrony did not develop in any patient during leg exercise. Maximal transdiaphragmatic pressure decreased similarly in both groups after both arm and leg exercise. Celli et al.[97] suggest that the added burden on the accessory respiratory muscles during upper extremity exercise leads to an increased ventilatory muscle burden, early fatigue, and dyssynchronous breathing, which contributes to the dyspnea observed during such activity. However, this result does not appear to be due solely to diaphragmatic fatigue.

In a subsequent study Criner and Celli[107] compared unsupported and supported arm exercise in 11 patients with severe COPD. They found that exercise endurance was significantly shorter for unsupported than for supported arm exercise even though heart rate, ventilation, and O_2 uptake were lower. In examining transdiaphragmatic pressures, these authors noted that unsupported arm exercise was associated with a different breathing pattern, in which more of the ventilatory load was shifted from the inspiratory rib cage muscles to the diaphragm and muscles of expiration.

Ventilatory Muscle Training

The potential role of ventilatory muscle fatigue as a cause of respiratory failure and ventilatory limitation in patients with COPD has stimulated attempts to train the ventilatory muscles.[108–110] Both isocapnic hyperventilation[111,112] and inspiratory resistive loading[113] have been shown to improve the function of these muscles both in normal subjects and in patients with lung disease. In normal individuals, however, because respiratory muscles do not limit exercise tolerance, specific respiratory muscle training is unlikely to be of clinical benefit. However, in pulmonary patients, who may be limited by respiratory muscle function, there may be a role for such training.

Much of the work in this area has focused on patients with COPD. Improvement in the exercise performance of such patients from ventilatory muscle training alone has not been demonstrated consistently, and the potential role of such training if incorporated routinely into pulmonary rehabilitation programs has not been clearly established.[109] For instance, Pardy et al.[113] reported improved exercise performance from ventilatory muscle training only in a subset of COPD patients who demonstrated evidence of inspiratory muscle fatigue during exercise. However, at present there is no simple method to select patients most likely to benefit from this type of training.

Some of the problems with early studies of inspiratory resistive muscle training are that the inspiratory load was not monitored or controlled and that appropriate control groups were not used.[110] Later studies, which controlled for the training load, have reported more encouraging but still variable results. Larson et al.[114] conducted a randomized study of inspiratory resistive training with the load set at either 15 or 30 percent of the patient's maximum inspiratory pressure (PImax). They reported significant improvement in inspiratory muscle strength and endurance as well as in the 12-minute walk distance for patients training at the higher targets. Harver et al.[115] randomly assigned patients to inspiratory resistive training either with minimal load or with added loads, using a device that provided visual feedback of targeted training levels (constant mouth pressure). As compared with control subjects, experimental subjects demonstrated a significant decrease in rated dyspnea after 8 weeks of training. Measurements of PImax increased significantly in experimental subjects but not above the levels in control subjects, who improved slightly.

Goldstein et al.[116] conducted a controlled study of inspiratory resistive training at 30 percent of PImax in patients participating concurrently in a pulmonary rehabilitation program. Following training plus rehabilitation, experimental subjects demonstrated a significant increase in inspiratory muscle endurance (versus a slight, nonsignificant increase in control subjects). Pulmonary function measurements (including PImax) did not change in either group, and the 6-minute walk distance increased similarly for both groups.

Thus, although ventilatory muscle training may result in improved ventilatory muscle function or symptoms for some patients with COPD, it is not yet clear that this modality is appropriate for general application. More research is needed to better select patients for this type of training and to determine whether improved ventilatory muscle performance will translate into improvement in exercise tolerance, activities of daily living, or other features of life quality for these patients.[110]

Benefits of Exercise Training—Controlled Studies

Many studies have reported benefits of exercise conditioning in patients with COPD.[117] Because training programs may also include other elements important to the rehabilitation effort, it is difficult to determine which effects may be specifically attributed to exercise training. However, several controlled clinical trials of exercise conditioning and rehabilitation have been performed, which do demonstrate the effectiveness of exercise training in COPD patients.

Cockcroft et al.[118] randomly assigned 39 men with both COPD and coal workers' pneumoconiosis to a 6-week exercise training program (19 patients) or to an untreated control group (20 patients).[118] The exercise program included gymnasium activities on cycle ergometers and rowing machines, swimming, and walking. After the program patients were instructed to continue walking and stair climbing exercises at home. Patients in the control group received no exercise advice, but after 4 months they were allowed to enter the 6-week exercise program. Of the 34 patients who completed the study (18 treatment, 16 control), those in the exercise group experienced subjective benefits, with a decrease in reported symptoms and a 23 percent increase in the 12-minute walk distance ($P < .05$) after 2 months. Patients in the control group reported little change in subjective symptoms and increased their 12-minute walk distance by only 8 percent (*P* not significant). After 4 months the 12-minute walk distance was not significantly different between groups, primarily because of continued improvement in the control subjects. The treatment group maintained most of their improvement after 7 months of follow-up. FEV_1 did not change in either group during the study, whereas forced vital capacity (FVC) increased slightly in both.

Patients in this study also completed two questionnaires designed to assess psychological variables.[83] It is noteworthy that both groups showed significant improvement in these psychological tests, which were not significantly different between groups, although changes in the exercise group were slightly greater. The changes in the psychological tests were not correlated with changes in the 12-minute walk distance. These findings suggest that improvement in exercise tolerance was not solely related to changes in psychological factors, but they also imply that participation in a study with added attention may in itself improve the psychological state of patients with COPD.

McGavin et al.[119] randomly allocated 28 patients with COPD to a 3-month unsupervised home exercise program involving stair climbing or to a nonexercise control group. Four exercise patients did not complete the study (two who failed to comply, one who died, and one who became ill) leaving 12 in each group. Significantly more patients in the exercise group noted subjective improvement in sense of well-being, breathlessness, cough, and sputum. There was also a significant increase in exercise performance in the trained patients versus the control patients. The 12-minute walk distance increased 6 percent in the exercise group and decreased 2 percent in the control group. The improvement in the patients who exercised was accompanied by a significant increase in stride length, indicating improvement in the mechanical efficiency of walking. On the maximal cycle ergometer test, maximum work load increased by 23 percent in the exercise group ($P < .05$) versus a 4 percent decrease in the control group (*P* not significant), whereas $\dot{V}O_2max$ increased by 16 percent (*P* not significant) in trained patients versus a 12 percent decrease in control subjects ($P < .05$).

Sinclair and Ingram assigned 17 patients with COPD who lived within their city to an exercise training program and used 16 patients who lived outside the city as a nonexercise control group.[120] Exercise training consisted of a daily 12-minute walking distance test and supervised stair climbing exercise. Training was begun in the hospital and continued at home with weekly supervision. Patients were followed for up to 12 months. The exercise group demonstrated improvement in the 12-minute walk distance, which was maintained at 12 months, and subjective improvements in well-being, dyspnea, and daily activities. The nonequivalent control group did not show these changes. Improvement in exercise performance in the trained patients was associated with a decrease in number of steps and increase in stride length, indicating improvement in the mechanical efficiency of walking.

Ambrosino et al.[121] randomly assigned 23 patients to a medical and rehabilitative therapy group and 28 patients to medical therapy alone for 1 month. Rehabilitative therapy included breathing control techniques of relaxation and slow breathing, diaphragmatic breathing, and pursed lip breathing. Even though patients were not given specific exercise training, the experimental group demonstrated improvement in maximal exercise tolerance on a cycle ergometer, as well as improved efficiency of their ventilatory pattern, with a decrease in respiratory rate and an increase in tidal volume. These changes were not present in the control group.

Busch and McClements[122] randomly allocated 20 patients with advanced COPD to a home-based exercise program or to a control group, who were visited by a physical therapist but not instructed in exercise. After 18 weeks they found a significant difference between groups in physical work capacity on an incremental cycle ergometer test; this difference was due to a 3 percent increase in the exercise group versus a 28 percent decrease in the control group. These differences were not present in a home exercise test performed at 6-week intervals or in symptom scores of dyspnea. However, in their analysis the authors excluded three patients in the exercise group who were noncompliant with training and three patients in the control group, one who died and two who began exercising on their own. In the remaining patients, the exercise group appeared to have lower baseline exercise tolerance. This exclusion allows analysis of the effects of exercise training but highlights the problems of trying to separate individual components of a rehabilitation program when patients may change behavior because of other interventions (e.g., begin exercising after enrolling in the study and being visited by a physical therapist). Nevertheless, these results emphasize the importance of a control group in such studies because treated patients with COPD who change little over time may, in fact, be significantly better than untreated patients, whose function often declines.

Booker[123] randomly allocated 128 patients with COPD to one of three groups: control, exercise, or physiotherapy (exercise plus breathing control techniques). Over 12 months of follow-up, patients in both experimental groups demonstrated significant improvement in measures included on a daily activities questionnaire and less mood disturbance. There was no statistically significant change in the 6-minute walk distance in any of the three groups. However, Booker points out the possible limitation of using a timed walking test to evaluate the results of such programs, since patients with COPD are typically taught to take more time with activities in order to achieve more with less distress. These changes would not be reflected in a timed exercise test, which measures maximum distance covered in a set time.

Chester et al.[124] compared the effects of exercise training in 21 COPD patients and 8 control patients who were not randomly selected. The trained patients demonstrated significant improvement in total treadmill work, associated with a decrease in O_2 consumption and minute ventilation at comparable levels of work. Control patients showed no increase in work tolerance. There were no changes in either group in resting pulmonary function or in rest and exercise measures of gas exchange and hemodynamics. The authors concluded that the improved work tolerance was importantly related to improved efficiency of walking and desensitization to the sensation of dyspnea.

OUTCOMES

The typical multidisciplinary, comprehensive pulmonary rehabilitation program includes a variety of treatment modalities, which may be individualized according to the needs of each patient and the resources and expertise available in a particular program. In examining the benefits of pulmonary rehabilitation, therefore, it is important to consider more general outcomes that may result from participation in such a program (Table 98-2). It is difficult to distinguish the relative contributions of specific components that are so integrally related. For example, almost any treatment (e.g., education or exercise) provided by well trained and enthusiastic personnel will inevitably also provide important elements of psychosocial support and motivation for these sick and disabled patients. Also, benefits may differ for individual patients with different specific goals. Many of the published clinical studies involve small numbers of patients and, as a result, analyses that examine group means may miss significant benefits for individual patients.[53]

Hospitalizations and Use of Medical Resources

Comprehensive pulmonary rehabilitation programs have been shown to produce cost-effective benefits for patients with COPD. Several studies have included analysis of hospitalization and medical resource utilization before and after participation in a program. Given the high costs of acute care hospitalization for these frequently sick patients, the potential savings from a reduction in hospital days alone is significant.

Lertzman and Cherniack[6] reported an average decrease of 20 hospital days per year attributable to pulmonary rehabilitation, which resulted in an estimated savings of $2000 per patient based on a 1976 Canadian hospital cost of $100 per day. Petty et al.[8] reported a 38 percent reduction in total hospital days (from 868 to 542) among 85 patients with COPD, who were evaluated 1 year after entry into a pulmonary rehabilitation program in comparison with the year prior to entry. In a randomized controlled study, Jensen[28] reported that pulmonary rehabilitation led to significantly fewer hospitalizations over 6 months of follow-up in COPD patients with high-risk markers for psychosocial problems. In an evaluation of an inpatient pulmonary rehabilitation program, Agle et al.[84] reported 30 hospital admissions among 24 patients in the year prior to rehabilitation, compared with only 5 admissions in the subsequent year.

Several reports have examined follow-up data for longer than the first year after rehabilitation. Hudson et al.[125] reported a survey of hospitalizations for pulmonary disease in 64 patients who participated in a comprehensive pulmonary rehabilitation program and who had known follow-up after 4 years (44 alive, 20 dead). In the 44 patients alive 4 years after the program, days of hospitalization in the year prior to the program (529) were reduced by 73 percent (145 days) in year 1, 49 percent (270 days) in year 2, 47 percent (278 days) in year 3, and 61 percent (207 days) in year 4. This benefit was most striking in the 14 of the 44 patients who had been hospitalized in the year prior to the program; their hospitalization days per patient decreased from 38 in the year before to 10 in the year after rehabilitation. The 64 patients, including the 20 who died, had a total of 631 days of hospitalization in the year prior to the rehabilitation program versus 309 days (a 52 percent reduction) in the first year and 350 days (a 45 percent reduction) in the second year after the program.

Johnson et al.[17] reported a 55 percent decrease in hospitalization days in the year after versus the year before an inpatient pulmonary rehabilitation program that included 96 patients with severe COPD (mean FEV_1, 0.87 L). The data suggested a mean decrease of 23 hospital days per year in these patients. This group has also reported a cost-benefit analysis of long-term follow-up of 193 patients who underwent inpatient pulmonary rehabilitation.[126] They estimated an average reduction of 21 hospital days per surviving patient per year. Despite the cost of inpatient rehabilitation ($9000 in 1982), they estimated a net cost saving of $11,200 per patient over 2.8 years of follow-up due to reduced hospitalization.

Hodgkin and coworkers[4,5] have reported an average reduction from 19 hospital days in the year prior to rehabilitation to slightly more than 6 days in the first year after the program in 80 patients. In addition, the improvement was maintained for the 8 years of follow-up for which data were analyzed and was seen in both survivors and nonsurvivors over the period of follow-up.[4,5]

In a study comparing 252 COPD patients who participated in a comprehensive pulmonary rehabilitation program with 50 nonrehabilitation patients selected from an outpatient clinic, Haas and Cardon[14] reported that 8 percent of the rehabilitated patients and 17 percent of control patients were placed in nursing homes after 5 years. In addition, 19 percent

Table 98-2. Results of Pulmonary Rehabilitation

Results of Pulmonary Rehabilitation
Decrease in
Hospitalizations and use of medical resources
Respiratory symptoms (e.g., dyspnea)
Psychological symptoms (e.g., fear, depression)
Improvement in
Quality of life
Exercise tolerance—endurance, maximal level
Knowledge about lung disease
Ability to perform daily activities
Return to work
No change in lung function
?Change in survival

of the rehabilitation group versus only 5 percent of the control group were able to care for themselves at that time.

Quality of Life and Symptoms

After rehabilitation many patients have an improved quality of life, showing a reduction in respiratory symptoms, increase in exercise tolerance and level of physical activity, greater independence and ability to perform activities of daily living, and improvement in psychological function, with less anxiety and depression and increased feelings of hope, control, and self-esteem.[8] Therefore, to evaluate the effectiveness of pulmonary rehabilitation, it would be important to incorporate measurements that reflect changes in quality of life. Several investigators have developed and validated instruments for such use in patients with chronic lung diseases.[25,127,128]

Bebout et al.[13] administered a quality of life questionnaire to 75 patients with COPD an average of 92 months (a minimum of 24 months) after a comprehensive rehabilitation program. Among the 43 patients who responded at follow-up, more than 50 percent reported improvement in their dyspnea classification, ability to go outside, frequency of difficult breathing episodes, and self-assurance.

In a long-term study of multidisciplinary pulmonary rehabilitation in 31 consecutive patients, Guyatt et al.[129] included measures of quality of life in the chronic respiratory disease questionnaire. Of the 31 patients, 24 demonstrated improvement in quality of life 2 weeks after rehabilitation, and over 6 months of follow-up, the improved quality of life was sustained in 11 of these 24.

In a study of 197 outpatients in a pulmonary rehabilitation program in a community hospital, Mall and Medeiros[15] found that 77 percent of patients with worse than class 1 dyspnea improved their dyspnea classification.

In a randomized controlled study of the influence of behavioral factors on the effectiveness of exercise in patients with COPD, Atkins et al.[127] administered extensive psychosocial outcome parameters, including an established scale to measure quality of well-being. After 3 months of exercise and behavioral intervention (without formal pulmonary rehabilitation) and an additional 3 months of follow-up, they found that in comparison with an untreated control group, three different experimental groups demonstrated significantly greater positive changes in the parameters measuring quality of well-being. Using these data to estimate and compare the cost-effectiveness of intervention stategies in producing a well year of life, the investigators concluded that even this modest treatment program resulted in significant cost benefits for these patients.

Although there are only a few experimental studies that systematically examine quality of life changes resulting from pulmonary rehabilitation, the symptomatic benefits reported by patients and their physicians are significant and are a major factor contributing to the enthusiasm these persons have for such programs. Improving patient symptoms and quality of life is certainly an important outcome of medical care. Future research is needed in this area.

Pulmonary Function Tests

Pulmonary rehabilitation programs have not resulted in any consistent improvement in lung function measurements in patients with COPD who have been receiving good medical therapy, including bronchodilator medications, prior to beginning the program.[5,8] In one randomized clinical trial of medical and rehabilitative therapy versus medical therapy alone, Ambrosino et al. reported a significant increase in FEV_1 and PaO_2 with a decrease in $PaCO_2$ in the experimental group only.[121] Similar but nonsignificant trends were seen in the control group. However, since patients were enrolled in this study prior to any therapy, these findings cannot be attributed to the rehabilitation components. Most other studies, however, have reported no significant change in FEV_1 or arterial blood gas measurements and variable changes in FVC after either pulmonary rehabilitation or exercise training programs.[118–120, 124, 130]

Survival

It is clear that survival for patients with recognized COPD is reduced considerably in comparison with normal populations (approximately 50 percent survival at 5 years, 25 percent at 10 years[131]). This poor survival is largely a result of the diseases being typically recognized and diagnosed at an advanced stage. Studies that have examined the survival of patients with COPD after pulmonary rehabilitation have shown variable results. There are no prospective randomly controlled studies currently in the literature that provide convincing evidence one way or another about this question.

In a retrospective study of 75 patients with COPD and a mean follow-up of 92 months, Bebout et al.[13] reported improved survival after a comprehensive pulmonary rehabilitation program as compared with that reported in other published studies. However, patients in this study had less severe disease than in the comparison studies. In patients with less severe disease (FEV_1 greater than 1.24 L), survival at 2 to 7 years was significantly greater than that reported in the literature for the natural history of COPD.

In a prospective study of 182 consecutive patients who participated in a comprehensive outpatient pulmonary rehabilitation program, Sahn et al.[132] reported 41 percent survival at 5 years and 17 percent at 10 years. However, this program was conducted at altitude, a factor that would reduce survival for patients with COPD. When data at 2.5 years of follow-up were compared with those from a study of the natural history of COPD for patients at altitude,[133] survival was found to be significantly improved (67 percent versus 50 percent).

In a study comparing 252 rehabilitated patients with 50 control patients selected from an outpatient clinic, Haas and

Cardon[14] reported 5-year mortality rates from respiratory failure of 22 percent in the rehabilitated patients and 42 percent in controls.

Occupational Changes

Vocational rehabilitation may be difficult once the patient has stopped work because of severe, disabling disease.[6] In addition, COPD typically presents in the older ages, when patients are more likely to be retired and less inclined to return to gainful employment. For the younger, working patient, the optimal time for rehabilitation, then, is before disability occurs. Patients with less severe disease may be able to return to work and increase their performance of vocational and recreational activities. In addition to the level of pulmonary impairment, an individual's potential for and success in vocational rehabilitation will depend on other factors, including age, intelligence, motivation, education, capacity for retraining, the physical demands of a particular job, and support and understanding from an employer.[134,135]

In an evaluation of 182 consecutive patients enrolled in a pulmonary rehabilitation program, Petty et al.[136] found that 32 percent had been working at least part time on entry into the program. As compared with the nonworking patients, working patients were significantly younger and had better exercise tolerance despite no differences in measurements of pulmonary function or arterial blood gases. These observations emphasize the importance of variables other than the degree of pulmonary impairment per se in determining an individual's ability to maintain gainful employment.

In a separate study Petty et al.[8] reported that among 85 patients with COPD evaluated 1 year after participation in a pulmonary rehabilitation program, 21 patients were employed at least part-time during the whole year and 35 additional patients were employed during at least part of the year, and 8 patients returned to work after more than 1 year of unemployment.

Haas and Cardon[14] found that 25 percent of 252 patients with COPD who participated in a pulmonary rehabilitation program that included vocational counseling and rehabilitation were able to engage in full-time work 5 years after the program. In comparison, only 3 percent of 50 control patients selected from an outpatient clinic were working 5 years later.

In a controlled clinical trial, Lustig et al.[137] randomly allocated 45 patients with COPD to three groups: (1) pulmonary rehabilitation; (2) psychotherapy alone; and (3) no treatment. They found that as compared with the no treatment group, patients in both the pulmonary rehabilitation and the psychotherapy group showed improvement in measurements of psychological function. However, although all patients were given vocational counseling, significantly more of the pulmonary rehabilitation group subsequently engaged in vocational activities. Of the 15 patients in each group, 11 rehabilitation patients but only 4 psychotherapy and 3 no treatment patients were employed 6 weeks later.

Kass et al.[135] reported on the work status of 147 patients followed up at a mean of 31 months after admission to a pulmonary rehabilitation program. They found that 21 percent were still working, 23 percent had worked for at least 6 months but were no longer working, 24 percent had not worked after rehabilitation, and 32 percent had died. They reported that physiologic measurements (e.g., FEV_1) correlated better with vocational status than measured psychologic factors. In a subsequent study, results of the Minnesota Multiphasic Personality Inventory (MMPI) were used to predict vocational adjustment in these patients.[138] Patients who worked more than 6 months were more gregarious, self-confident, and more likely to use denial. By contrast, patients who did not work were more anxious, self-doubting, and irritable.

Long-Term Follow-Up

Few studies of pulmonary rehabilitation programs have systematically followed patients for more than a few months. In the short term, patients frequently demonstrate a dramatic improvement in symptoms, tolerance for exercise and physical activities, and quality of life; however, in some patients the beneficial effects appear to decrease over the longer term. Therefore, in evaluating and structuring pulmonary rehabilitation programs, it is important to consider longer-term outcomes and to consider whether repeat sessions for reinforcement and maintenance would be worthwhile additions to these programs.

Guyatt et al.[129] followed 31 consecutive patients enrolled in a multidisciplinary inpatient pulmonary rehabilitation program for 6 months. Primary outcome measures included a chronic respiratory disease questionnaire to measure quality of life and a 6-minute walk test to assess exercise tolerance. Of the 28 patients who completed the program, 24 demonstrated improvement in quality of life 2 weeks later. After 6 months, however, improved quality of life was sustained in 11 patients but had declined in 13 patients. With respect to exercise training, 13 of the 28 patients who completed the program stopped exercising within 1 month of discharge. For 17 patients who performed the 6-minute walk test during 6 months of follow-up, the distance walked improved significantly at 2 weeks and then declined somewhat but remained significantly greater than baseline.

In a randomized trial of exercise training in 39 patients, Cockcroft et al.[118] reported significant increase in the 12-minute walk distance in trained patients as compared with control patients at 2 months of follow-up. Most of this improvement was maintained in the exercise program participants for up to 7 months. However, the difference between them and control subjects was not significant at 4 months owing to an increase in exercise performance of the control group.

Fishman and Petty[130] re-evaluated 30 patients with COPD 1 year after participation in a pulmonary rehabilitation program. They found significant improvement in MVV (without change in FEV_1), walking exercise tolerance, and patient ratings of affective distress. However, as these authors point out, it is difficult to assess the overall impact of the program without reference to an untreated control group since, many of the measured variables expected to worsen over 1 year "did not change."

Tydeman et al. enrolled 24 patients with COPD in a supervised exercise training program.[139] After these patients reached maximum improvement with supervised training, they continued to exercise at home but were randomly allocated to continued weekly supervised sessions or to no supervision. Of the 24 patients, 16 completed the trial. The length of time to reach peak performance on the variety of exercise tasks used ranged from 26 to 51 weeks (mean, 36 weeks). For the 12-minute walk test, the patients demonstrated a 42 percent increase, most of which occurred over the first 4 weeks of training. On re-evaluation at up to 6 months after the random allocation, both groups of patients maintained the improvement in exercise performance with daily home walking regardless of whether they had regular supervision. These findings suggest that for motivated patients who complete the training program and maintain home exercise, the benefits of exercise training can be maintained without frequent supervision.

Therefore it is difficult to evaluate long-term outcomes of pulmonary rehabilitation programs or components without appropriate control for the expected progression of disease and changes in function over time. Longer-term reinforcement sessions may be important if the short-term benefits are to be maintained; however, such reinforcement may not be necessary for some highly motivated patients.

References

1. American Thoracic Society: Pulmonary rehabilitation. Am Rev Respir Dis 1981;124:663–666
2. American Thoracic Society: Standards for the diagnosis and care of patients with chronic obstructive pulmonary disease (COPD) and asthma. Am Rev Respir Dis 1987;136:225–244
3. Cotes JE, Bishop JM, Capel LH et al: Disabling chest disease: Prevention and care: A report of the Royal College of Physicians by the College Committee on Thoracic Medicine. J R Coll Physicians Lond 1981;15:69–87
4. Hodgkin JE, Zorn EG, Connors GL (eds): Pulmonary Rehabilitation—Guidelines to Success. Butterworth, Boston, 1984
5. Hodgkin JE: Pulmonary rehabilitation: Structure, components, and benefits. J Cardiopulmonary Rehabil 1988;11:423–434
6. Lertzman MM, Cherniack RM: Rehabilitation of patients with chronic obstructive pulmonary disease. Am Rev Respir Dis 1976;114:1145–1165
7. Moser KM, Bokinsky GE, Savage RT et al: Results of a comprehensive rehabilitation program: Physiologic and functional effects on patients with chronic obstructive pulmonary disease. Arch Intern Med 1980;140:1596–1601
8. Petty TL, Nett LM, Finigan MM et al: A comprehensive care program for chronic airway obstruction: Methods and preliminary evaluation of symptomatic and functional improvement. Ann Intern Med 1969;70:1109–1120
9. Ries AL: Pulmonary rehabilitation. pp. 1325–1331. In Fishman AP (ed): Pulmonary Diseases and Disorders. 2nd Ed. McGraw-Hill, New York, 1988
10. Anthonisen NR, Wright EC, Hodgkin JE: Prognosis in chronic obstructive pulmonary disease. Am Rev Respir Dis 1986;133:14–20
11. Kirilloff LH, Carpenter V, Kerby GR et al: Skills of the health team involved in out-of-hospital care for patients with COPD. Am Rev Respir Dis 1986;133:948–949
12. Kimbel P, Kaplan AS, Alkalay I, Lester D: An inhospital program for rehabilitation of patients with chronic obstructive pulmonary disease. Chest, Suppl. 1971;60:6S–10S
13. Bebout DE, Hodgkin JE, Zorn EG et al: Clinical and physiological outcomes of a university-hospital pulmonary rehabilitation program. Respir Care 1983;28:1468–1473
14. Haas A, Cardon H: Rehabilitation in chronic obstructive pulmonary disease: A 5 year study of 252 male patients. Med Clin North Am 1969;53:593–606
15. Mall RW, Medeiros M: Objective evaluation of results of a pulmonary rehabilitation program in a community hospital. Chest 1988;94:1156–1160
16. White B, Andrews JL Jr, Mogan JJ, Downes-Vogel P: Pulmonary rehabilitation in an ambulatory group practice setting. Med Clin North Am 1979;63:379–390
17. Johnson HR, Tanzi F, Balchum OJ et al: Inpatient comprehensive pulmonary rehabilitation in severe COPD. Respir Ther 1980;May/June:15–19
18. Paine R, Make BJ: Pulmonary rehabilitation for the elderly. Clin Geriatr Med 1986;2:313–335
19. Foster S, Saadeh P, Thomas HM: Pulmonary rehabilitation in lung diseases other than COPD. Am Rev Respir Dis, suppl. 1989;39:A332
20. Connors GA, Hodgkin JE, Asmus RM: A careful assessment is crucial to successful pulmonary rehabilitation. J Cardiopulmonary Rehabil 1988;11:435–438
21. Foster S, Lopez D, Thomas HM: Pulmonary rehabilitation in COPD patients with elevated PCO_2. Am Rev Respir Dis 1988;138:1519–1523
22. Agle DP, Baum GL: Psychological aspects of chronic obstructive pulmonary disease. Med Clin North Am 1977;61:749–758
23. Dudley DL, Glaser EM, Jorgenson BN, Logan DL: Psychosocial concomitants to rehabilitation in chronic obstructive pulmonary disease: Part 1. Psychosocial and psychological considerations; Part 2. Psychosocial treatment; Part 3. Dealing with psychiatric disease (as distinguished from psychosocial or psychophysiologic problems). Chest 1980;77:413–420; 544–551; 677–684
24. McSweeney AJ, Grant I, Heaton RK et al: Life quality of patients with chronic obstructive pulmonary disease. Arch Intern Med 1982;142:473–478
25. Prigatano GP, Wright EC, Levin D: Quality of life and its predictors in patients with mild hypoxemia and chronic obstructive pulmonary disease. Arch Intern Med 1984;144:1613–1619
26. Sandhu HS: Psychosocial issues in chronic obstructive pulmonary disease. Clin Chest Med 1986;7:629–642
27. Dales RE, Spitzer WO, Schechter MT, Suissa S: The influence of psychological status on respiratory symptom reporting. Am Rev Respir Dis 1989;139:1459–1463
28. Jensen PS: Risk, protective factors, and supportive interventions in chronic airway obstruction. Arch Gen Psychiatry 1983;40:1203–1207
29. Clausen JL, Zarins LP (eds): Pulmonary Function Testing Guidelines and Controversies: Equipment, Methods, and Normal Values. Academic Press, New York, 1982
30. Wilson AF: Pulmonary Function Testing Indications and Interpretations. Grune & Stratton, Orlando, FL, 1985
31. Belman MJ, Wasserman K: Exercise training and testing in patients with chronic obstructive pulmonary disease. Basics RD 1981;10:1–6
32. Ries AL: The role of exercise testing in pulmonary diagnosis. Clin Chest Med 1987;8:81–89
33. Mungall IPF, Hainsworth R: Assessment of respiratory function in patients with chronic obstructive airways disease. Thorax 1979;34:254–258
34. Ries AL, Farrow JT, Clausen JL: Pulmonary function tests cannot predict exercise-induced hypoxemia in chronic obstructive pulmonary disease. Chest 1988;93:454–459
35. Ries AL, Farrow JT, Clausen JL: Accuracy of two ear oxi-

meters at rest and during exercise in pulmonary patients. Am Rev Respir Dis 1985;132:685–689
36. Gilmartin ME: Patient and family education. Clin Chest Med 1986;7:619–627
37. Neish CM, Hopp JW: The role of education in pulmonary rehabilitation. J Cardiopulmonary Rehabil 1988;11:439–441
38. Hopp JW, Lee JW, Hills R: Development and validation of a pulmonary rehabilitation knowledge test. J Cardiopulmonary Rehabil 1989;7:273–280
39. Howland J, Nelson EC, Barlow PB et al: Chronic obstructive airway disease: Impact of health education. Chest 1986;90:233–238
40. Ashikaga T, Vacek PM, Lewis SO: Evaluation of a community-based education program for individuals with chronic obstructive pulmonary disease. J Rehabil 1980;46:23–27
41. Rochester DF, Goldberg SK: Techniques of respiratory physical therapy. Am Rev Respir Dis, suppl. 1980; 122:133–146
42. Kirilloff LH, Owens GR, Rogers RM, Mazzocco MC: Does chest physical therapy work? Chest 1985;88:436–444
43. Moser KM, Archibald C, Hansen P et al: Shortness of Breath–A Guide to Better Living and Breathing. 3rd Ed. CV Mosby, St. Louis, 1983
44. Sutton PP, Parker RA, Webber BA et al: Assessment of the forced expiration technique, postural drainage and directed coughing in chest physiotherapy. Eur J Respir Dis 1983;64:62–68
45. Sutton PP, Pavia D, Bateman JRM, Clarke SW: Chest physiotherapy: A review. Eur J Respir Dis 1982;63:188–201
46. Pryor JA, Webber BA, Hodson ME, Batten JC: Evaluation of the forced expiration technique as an adjunct to postural drainage in treatment of cystic fibrosis. Br Med J 1979;2:417–418
47. Sutton PP: Chest physiotherapy: Time for reappraisal. Br J Dis Chest 1988;82:127–137
48. Sutton PP, Gemmell HG, Innes N et al: Use of nebulised saline and nebulised terbutaline as an adjunct to chest physiotherapy. Thorax 1988;43:57–60
49. The Intermittent Positive Pressure Breathing Trial Group: Intermittent positive pressure breathing therapy of chronic obstructive pulmonary disease. Ann Intern Med 1983;99:612–620
50. Lefcoe NM, Paterson NAM: Adjunct therapy in chronic obstructive pulmonary disease. Am J Med 1973;54:343–350
51. Campbell EJM, Friend J: Action of breathing exercises in pulmonary emphysema. Lancet 1955;1:325–329
52. Faling LJ. Pulmonary rehabilitation—physical modalities. Clin Chest Med 1986;7:599–618
53. Miller WF: Physical therapeutic measures in the treatment of chronic bronchopulmonary disorders: Methods for breathing training. Am J Med 1958;24:929–940
54. Motley HL: The effects of slow deep breathing on the blood gas exchange in emphysema. Am Rev Respir Dis 1963;88:484–492
55. Paul G, Eldridge F, Mitchell J, Fiene T: Some effects of slowing respiration rate in chronic emphysema and bronchitis. J Appl Physiol 1966;1:877–882
56. Sergysels R, Willeput R, Lenders D et al: Low frequency breathing at rest and during exercise in severe chronic obstructive bronchitis. Thorax 1979;34:536–539
57. Barach AL: Breathing exercises in pulmonary emphysema and allied chronic respiratory disease. Arch Phys Med Rehabil 1955;36:379–390
58. Barach AL, Bickerman HA, Beck G: Advances in the treatment of non-tuberculous pulmonary disease. Bull NY Acad Med 1952;28:353–384
59. Miller WF: A physiologic evaluation of the effects of diaphragmatic breathing training in patients with chronic pulmonary emphysema. Am J Med 1954;17:471–477
60. Sinclair JD: The effect of breathing exercises in pulmonary emphysema. Thorax 1955;10:246–249
61. Becklake MR, McGregor M, Goldman HI, Braudo JL: A study of the effects of physiotherapy in chronic hypertrophic emphysema using lung function tests. Chest 1954;26:180–191
62. Williams IP, Smith CM, McGavin CR: Diaphragmatic breathing training and walking performance in chronic airways obstruction. Br J Dis Chest 1982;76:164–166
63. Sackner MA, Silva G, Banks JM et al: Distribution of ventilation during diaphragmatic breathing in obstructive lung disease. Am Rev Respir Dis 1974;109:331–337
64. Barach AL: Physiologic advantages of grunting, groaning, and pursed-lip breathing: Adaptive symptoms related to the development of continuous positive pressure breathing. Bull NY Acad Med 1973;49:666–673
65. Mueller RE, Petty TL, Filley GF: Ventilation and arterial blood gas changes induced by pursed lips breathing. J Appl Physiol 1970;28:784–789
66. Thoman RL, Stoker GL, Ross JC: The efficacy of pursed-lips breathing in patients with chronic obstructive pulmonary disease. Am Rev Respir Dis 1966;93:100–106
67. Tiep BL, Burns M, Kao D et al: Pursed lips breathing training using ear oximetry. Chest 1986;90:218–221
68. Block AJ: Low flow oxygen therapy: Treatment of the ambulant outpatient. Am Rev Respir Dis 1974;110:71–83
69. Fulmer JD, Snider GL: ACCP-NHLBI national conference on oxygen therapy. Chest 1984;86:234–247
70. Anthonisen NR: Long-term oxygen therapy. Ann Intern Med 1983;99:519–527
71. Medical Research Council Working Party: Long-term domiciliary oxygen therapy in chronic hypoxic cor pulmonale complicating chronic bronchitis and emphysema. Lancet 1981;1:681–686
72. Nocturnal Oxygen Therapy Trial Group: Continuous or nocturnal oxygen therapy in hypoxemic chronic obstructive lung disease: A clinical trial. Ann Intern Med 1980;93:391–398
73. Longo AM, Moser KM, Luchsinger PC: The role of oxygen therapy in rehabilitation of patients with chronic obstructive pulmonary disease. Am Rev Respir Dis 1971;103:690–697
74. Vyas MN, Banister EW, Morton JW, Grzybowski S: Response to exercise in patients with chronic airway obstruction: II. Effects of breathing 40 per cent oxygen. Am Rev Respir Dis 1971;103:401–412
75. Zack MB, Palange AV: Oxygen supplemented exercise of ventilatory and nonventilatory muscles in pulmonary rehabilitation. Chest 1985;88:669–675
76. Davidson AC, Leach R, George RJD, Geddes DM: Supplemental oxygen and exercise ability in chronic obstructive airways disease. Thorax 1988;43:965–971
77. Bradley BL, Garner AE, Billiu D et al: Oxygen-assisted exercise in chronic obstructive lung disease: The effect on exercise capacity and arterial blood gas tensions. Am Rev Respir Dis 1978;118:239–243
78. Tiep BL: Oxygen therapy for the mobile patient. J Cardiopulmonary Rehabil 1988;11:442–448
79. Light RW, Merrill EJ, Despars JA et al: Prevalence of depression and anxiety in patients with COPD: Relationship to functional capacity. Chest 1985;87:35–38
80. Curgian LM, Gronkiewicz CA: Enhancing sexual performance in COPD. Nurse Pract 1988;13:34–38
81. Fletcher EC, Martin RJ: Sexual dysfunction and erectile impotence in chronic obstructive pulmonary disease. Chest 1982;81:413–421
82. Timms RM: Sexual dysfunction and chronic obstructive pulmonary disease. Chest 1982;81:398–400
83. Cockcroft A, Berry G, Brown EB, Exall C: Psychological changes during a controlled trial of rehabilitation in chronic respiratory disability. Thorax 1982;37:413–416
84. Agle DP, Baum GL, Chester EH, Wendt M: Multidiscipline treatment of chronic pulmonary insufficiency: 1. Psychologic aspects of rehabilitation. Psychosom Med 1973;35:41–49
85. Renfroe KL: Effect of progressive relaxation on dyspnea and state anxiety in patients with chronic obstructive pulmonary disease. Heart Lung 1988;17:408–413
86. Belman MJ: Exercise in chronic obstructive pulmonary disease. Clin Chest Med 1986;7:585–597

87. Shephard RJ: On the design and effectiveness of training regimens in chronic obstructive lung disease. Bull Eur Physiopathol Respir 1977;13:457–469
88. Hughes RL, Davison R: Limitations of exercise reconditioning in COLD. Chest 1983;83:241–249
89. Belman MJ, Kendregan BA: Exercise training fails to increase skeletal muscle enzymes in patients with chronic obstructive pulmonary disease. Am Rev Respir Dis 1981;123:256–261
90. Brown HV, Wasserman K: Exercise performance in chronic obstructive pulmonary diseases. Med Clin North Am 1981;65:525–547
91. Casaburi R, Wasserman K: Exercise training in pulmonary rehabilitation. N Engl J Med 1986;314:1509–1511
92. Paez PN, Phillipson EA, Masangkay M, Sproule BJ: The physiologic basis of training patients with emphysema. Am Rev Respir Dis 1967;95:944–953
93. Wasserman K, Sue DY, Casaburi R, Moricca RB: Selection criteria for exercise training in pulmonary rehabilitation. Eur Respir J, suppl. 7, 1989;2:604S–610S
94. Ries AL, Archibald CJ: Endurance exercise training at maximal targets in patients with chronic obstructive pulmonary disease. J Cardiopulmonary Rehabil 1987;7:594–601
95. Carter R, Nicotra B, Clark L et al: Exercise conditioning in the rehabilitation of patients with chronic obstructive pulmonary disease. Arch Phys Med Rehabil 1988;69:118–122
96. Borg GAV: Psychophysical bases of perceived exertion. Med Sci Sports Exerc 1982;14:377–381
97. Celli BR, Rassulo J, Make BJ: Dyssynchronous breathing during arm but not leg exercise in patients with chronic airflow obstruction. N Engl J Med 1986;314:1485–1490
98. Ries AL, Ellis B, Hawkins RW: Upper extremity exercise training in chronic obstructive pulmonary disease. Chest 1988;93:688–692
99. Tangri S, Woolf CR: The breathing pattern in chronic obstructive lung disease during the performance of some common daily activities. Chest 1973;63:126–127
100. Reybrouck T, Heigenhauser GF, Faulkner JA: Limitations to maximum oxygen uptake in arm, leg, and combined arm-leg ergometry. J Appl Physiol 1975;38:774–779
101. Vokac Z, Bell H, Bautz-Holter E, Rodahl K: Oxygen uptake/heart rate relationship in leg and arm exercise, sitting and standing. J Appl Physiol 1975;39:54–59
102. Davies CTM, Sargeant AJ: Effects of training on the physiological responses to one- and two-leg work. J Appl Physiol 1975;38:377–381
103. Gergley TJ, McArdle WD, DeJesus P et al: Specificity of arm training on aerobic power during swimming and running. Med Sci Sports Exerc 1984;16:349–354
104. Magel JR, McArdle WD, Toner M, Delio DJ: Metabolic and cardiovascular adjustment to arm training. J Appl Physiol 1978;45:75–79
105. Saltin B, Nazar K, Costill DL et al: The nature of the training response; peripheral and central adaptations to one-legged exercise. Acta Physiol Scand 1976;96:289–305
106. Stamford BA, Cuddihee RW, Moffatt RJ, Rowland R: Task specific changes in maximal oxygen uptake resulting from arm versus leg training. Ergonomics 1978;21:1–9
107. Criner GJ, Celli BR: Effect of unsupported arm exercise on ventilatory muscle recruitment in patients with severe chronic airflow obstruction. Am Rev Respir Dis 1988;138:856–861
108. Celli BR: Respiratory muscle function. Clin Chest Med 1986;7:567–584
109. Pardy RL, Reid WD, Belman MJ: Respiratory muscle training. Clin Chest Med 1988;9:287–296
110. Grassino A: Inspiratory muscle training in COPD patients. Eur Respir J, suppl. 7, 1989;2:581S–586S
111. Belman MJ, Mittman C, Weir R: Ventilatory muscle training improves exercise capacity in chronic obstructive pulmonary disease patients. Am Rev Respir Dis 1980;121:273–280
112. Leith DE, Bradley M: Ventilatory muscle strength and endurance training. J Appl Physiol 1976;41:508–516
113. Pardy RL, Rivington RN, Despas PJ, Macklem PT: The effects of inspiratory muscle training on exercise performance in chronic airflow limitation. Am Rev Respir Dis 1981;123:426–433
114. Larson JL, Kim MJ, Sharp JT, Larson DA: Inspiratory muscle training with a pressure threshold breathing device in patients with chronic obstructive pulmonary disease. Am Rev Respir Dis 1988;138:689–696
115. Harver A, Mahler DA, Daubenspeck JA: Targeted inspiratory muscle training improves respiratory muscle function and reduces dyspnea in patients with chronic obstructive pulmonary disease. Ann Intern Med 1989;111:117–124
116. Goldstein R, De Rosie J, Long S et al: Applicability of a threshold loading device for inspiratory muscle testing and training in patients with COLD. Chest 1989;96:564–571
117. Holle RHO, Williams DV, Vandree JC et al: Increased muscle efficiency and sustained benefits in an outpatient community hospital-based pulmonary rehabilitation program. Chest 1988;94:1161–1168
118. Cockcroft AE, Saunders MT, Berry G: Randomised controlled trial of rehabilitation in chronic respiratory disability. Thorax 1981;36:200–203
119. McGavin CR, Gupta SP, Lloyd EL, McHardy JR: Physical rehabilitation or chronic bronchitis: Results of a controlled trial of exercises in the home. Thorax 1977;32:307–311
120. Sinclair DJM, Ingram CG: Controlled trial of supervised exercise training in chronic bronchitis. Br Med J 1980;280:519–521
121. Ambrosino N, Paggiaro PL, Macchi M et al: A study of short-term effect of rehabilitative therapy in chronic obstructive pulmonary disease. Respiration 1981;41:40–44
122. Busch AJ, McClements JD: Effects of a supervised home exercise program on patients with severe chronic obstructive pulmonary disease. Phys Ther 1988;68:469–474
123. Booker HA: Exercise training and breathing control in patients with chronic airflow limitation. Physiotherapy 1984;70:258–260
124. Chester EH, Belman MJ, Bahler RC et al: Multidisciplinary treatment of chronic pulmonary insufficiency: 3. The effect of physical training on cardiopulmonary performance in patients with chronic obstructive pulmonary disease. Chest 1977;72:695–702
125. Hudson LD, Tyler ML, Petty TL: Hospitalization needs during an outpatient rehabilitation program for severe chronic airway obstruction. Chest 1976;70:606–610
126. Johnson NR, De Florio GP, Einstein H: Cost/benefit outcomes of pulmonary rehabilitation in severe chronic obstructive pulmonary disease, abstracted. Am Rev Respir Dis 1983;127:111
127. Atkins CJ, Kaplan RM, Timms RM et al: Behavioral exercise programs in the management of chronic obstructive pulmonary disease. J Consult Clin Psychol 1984;52:591–603
128. Kaplan RM, Atkins CJ, Timms R: Validity of a quality of well-being scale as an outcome measure in chronic obstructive pulmonary disease. J Chronic Dis 1984;37:85–95
129. Guyatt GH, Berman LB, Townsend M: Long-term outcome after respiratory rehabilitation. Can Med Assoc J 1987;137:1089–1095
130. Fishman DB, Petty TL: Physical, symptomatic, and psychological improvement in patients receiving comprehensive care for chronic airway obstruction. J Chronic Dis 1971;24:775–785
131. Traver GA, Cline MG, Burrows B: Predictors of mortality in chronic obstructive pulmonary disease: A 15-year follow-up study. Am Rev Respir Dis 1979;119:895–902
132. Sahn SA, Nett LM, Petty TL: Ten-year follow-up of a comprehensive rehabilitation program for severe COPD. Chest 1980;77:311–314
133. Renzetti AD Jr, McClement JH, Litt BD: The Veterans Administration cooperative study of pulmonary function: III. Mortality in relation to respiratory function in chronic obstructive pulmonary disease. Am J Med 1966;41:115–129
134. Daughton DM, Fix AJ, Kass I et al: Physiological-intellectual components of rehabilitation success in patients with chronic

obstructive pulmonary disease (COPD). J Chronic Dis 1979;32:405–409

135. Kass I, Dyksterhuis JE, Rubin H, Patil KD: Correlation of psychophysiologic variables with vocational rehabilitation outcome in patients with chronic obstructive pulmonary disease. Chest 1975;67:433–440
136. Petty TL, MacIlroy ER, Swigert MA, Brink GA: Chronic airway obstruction, respiratory insufficiency, and gainful employment. Arch Environ Health 1970;21:71–78
137. Lustig FM, Haas A, Castillo R: Clinical and rehabilitation regime in patients with chronic obstructive pulmonary disease. Arch Phys Med Rehabil 1972;53:315–322
138. Fix AJ, Daughton D, Kass I et al: Personality traits affecting vocational rehabilitation success in patients with chronic obstructive pulmonary disease. Psychol Rep 1978;43:939–944
139. Tydeman DE, Chandler AR, Graveling BM et al: An investigation into the effects of exercise tolerance training on patients with chronic airways obstruction. Physiotherapy 1984;70:261–264

Chapter 99

Long-Term Oxygen Therapy

Kent L. Christopher

CHAPTER OUTLINE

SCIENTIFIC FOUNDATIONS OF LONG-TERM OXYGEN THERAPY

The history of O_2 therapy spans three centuries. Scheele first produced O_2 by heating dry silver carbonate (Ag_2CO_3) in 1771, but Joseph Priestley is usually credited with the discovery of O_2 in 1774. Priestley's insight into the potential therapeutic role of O_2 is reflected in his writings. He once stated, "The greater strength and vinacity of the flame of the candle in this pure air . . . might be particularly salutary to the lungs in certain morbid cases." Later, Lavoisier reproduced Priestley's experiments and called the new gas "oxygeine," or "acid maker." The first therapeutic application of O_2 took place in 1800, when Thomas Beddoes began treating patients at the Pneumatic Institute in Bristol, England.

Over a century passed before the concept of O_2 therapy re-emerged. The nasal catheter was developed in 1907, and the O_2 mask was described in 1918. In 1922 Barach[1] introduced a modified O_2 tent for treatment of patients hospitalized with pneumonia. Finally during the 1950s Barach[2] from the United States and Cotes and Gilson[3] from the United Kingdom began using small compressed cylinders to administer O_2 during ambulation. This birth of the idea of ambulatory home O_2 therapy was complemented by technological advances in delivery devices. For example, the nasal catheter evolved into a more comfortable and practical nasal cannula (Fig. 99-1), and liquid transfilling O_2 sources became available.

During the 1960s investigators from Denver, Colorado,[4–6] and Birmingham, England,[7] began evaluating the physiologic benefits of long-term home O_2 therapy. Improvement in exercise tolerance and erythrocytosis were noted, and results in a few patients suggested that pulmonary artery pressures and pulmonary vascular resistance might be reduced. However, as late as the 1970s the appropriate duration of home O_2 use was unclear. As described in Chapter 63, the combined results of the Nocturnal Oxygen Therapy Trial (NOTT)[8] and the British Medical Research Council (MRC) trial[9] showed that survival was greatest with *continuous ambulatory O_2*.

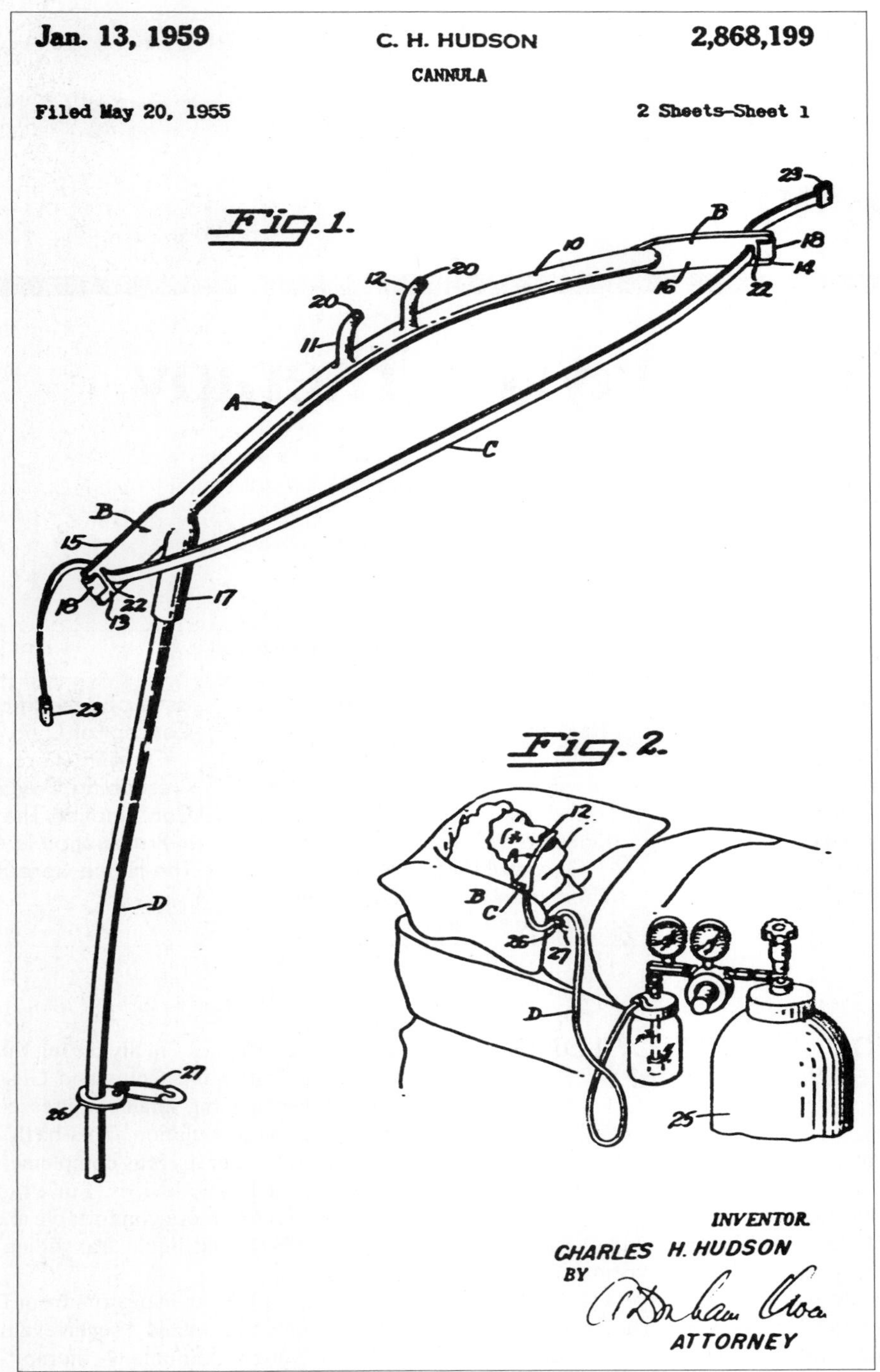

Figure 99-1. The design of the nasal cannula has not changed significantly since it was first patented in 1959. (This illustration is from U.S. Patent 2,868,199 issued in 1959 to C.H. Hudson.)

OXYGEN DELIVERY SYSTEMS

A variety of stationary and portable O_2 sources and several delivery devices are used to administer O_2 in the home. The availability of equipment varies from one area of the world to another, largely on the basis of economic, governmental, and logistic considerations. Petty[10] has recently reviewed the availability of home O_2 around the world.

Stationary Oxygen Sources

There are three commercially available sources of home O_2: compressed gas cylinders, O_2 concentrators or enrichers, and liquid O_2 reservoirs.

Compressed Gas Cylinders

In some countries home O_2 is unavailable. However, in countries where it is prescribed, the most common source is the compressed gas cylinder. Since gaseous O_2 was initially "bottled" in 1888, its processing and distribution have come under strict regulatory control. For example, in the United States the Department of Transportation (through the Interstate Commerce Commission) has responsibility for the manufacturing, hydrostatic testing, marketing and transportation of cylinders of O_2 and all other compressed gases. Pressure relief devices must be incorporated into the design of the high-pressure cylinders, and a complex array of diameter- and pin-index safety systems provides for attachment of regulators to the correct cylinders. The National Fire and Protection Agency sets regulations governing the safe handling and storage of compressed gas cylinders in the home. Because O_2 is a drug, the Food and Drug Administration requires that medical grade O_2 meet or exceed 99 percent purity.

Cylinders for O_2 are available in the United States in a variety of sizes (Table 99-1) and in three different materials of construction. The seamless carbon steel cylinder designated by the Department of Transportation as DOT 3A is not heat treated. The DOT 3AA is a heat-treated seamless cylinder constructed of a harder, more durable steel. The DOT-AL is a lightweight seamless aluminum cylinder, which has only been available in a portable size.

Table 99-1. Commonly Used Compressed Gas Cylinders

Cylinder Size	Dimensions (in.)	Weight (lb)	Oxygen Capacity (L)	Duration (h) at 2 L/min
B	3 × 15	4.25	150	1.25
D	4 × 17	10	400	3.50
E	4 × 29	12	680	5.50
M	7 × 45	70	3625	30.2
H	9 × 55	130	6700	55.0

(From Goodman,[121] with permission.)

Even though liquid O_2 was starting to become available in the 1960s, large H or K compressed gas cylinders were commonly used as the stationary sources. Figure 99-2A shows a patient receiving home O_2 from an H cylinder. As a stationary O_2 source, the unit is large, awkward, and extremely heavy. Other disadvantages are that it is unsightly and must be secured to keep it from falling and causing injury. The contents of O_2 cylinders are pressurized up to 2200 psi when full, and they can become "projectile missiles" if the integrity of the container is disrupted. Finally, the duration of the gas supply is much shorter than with a liquid source, and frequent deliveries by the home care company (with their associated cost) are required when the patient receives continuous O_2.

One major advantage of the compressed gas stationary source is that it is more readily available around the world than either the concentrator or the liquid reservoir. Unlike the concentrator, it does not require a source of electrical energy, and in contrast to liquid reservoirs, extensive capitalization of specialized transfilling equipment is unnecessary. Stationary compressed gas cylinders have the highest flow capabilities of any source for home use—up to 15 L/min.

Oxygen Concentrators

The O_2 concentrator, the second stationary source of O_2, has been commercially available since 1974. It is electrically powered and uses a filtering mechanism to purify entrained ambient air. The most common design of the O_2 concentrator employs molecular sieve beds made of granular zeolite crystals. These crystals contain a network of small (5Å diameter) holes, which allow O_2 and trace amounts of argon to pass through as the gases are pressurized to 10 to 30 psi. The delivered O_2 concentration tends to fall slightly with increasing flow rate but is generally in the high 90 percent range. The maximum flow is less than that obtained with either compressed gas cylinders or liquid systems, rarely exceeding 5 L/min. A compressed gas cylinder is necessary as a standby O_2 source in the event of mechanical failure of the concentrator or interruption of the power supply.

Another design of concentrator, called an O_2 enricher, differs from the sieve bed concentrator in that O_2 is concentrated by passing ambient air across a 1-μm thick plastic membrane. Water vapor and O_2 pass through the membrane to deliver O_2 at a concentration of approximately 40 percent at three times the ambient relative humidity. Although the enricher offers humidification, the obvious disadvantage is the low delivered O_2 concentration.

The various commercially available concentrators are shown in Table 99-2. Concentrators have gained high acceptance because they are the most cost-effective stationary delivery device. The cost of delivering bulk O_2 is avoided, maintenance requirements are low, and concentrators are more visually appealing than compressed gas cylinders. One disadvantage is that they are electrically powered and a con-

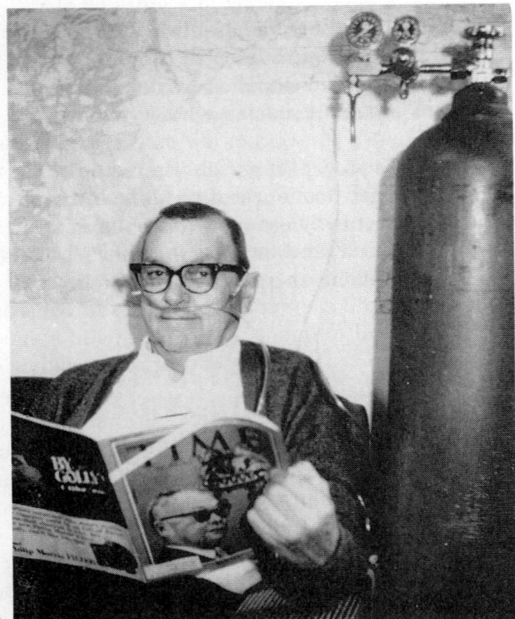

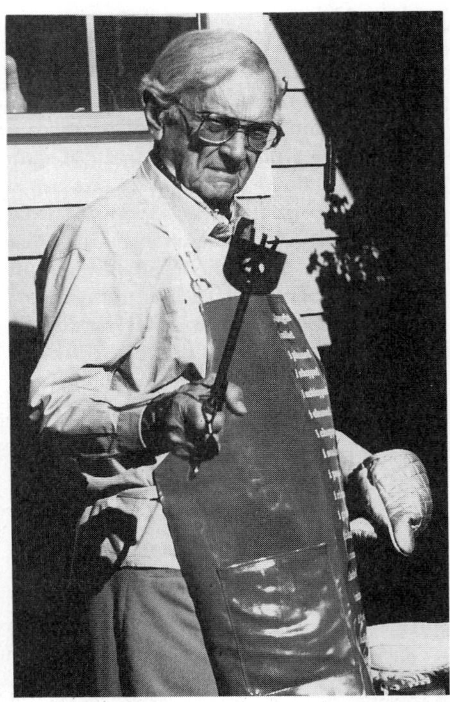

Figure 99-2. (**A**) This photograph from the 1960s shows a patient receiving home O_2 therapy with a large H cylinder. The technology for compressed gas cylinders has not changed since the 1960s. (**B**) In this photograph of the same patient taken 25 years later, he is using a portable liquid source and a transtracheal catheter that is concealed from view.

stant, reliable source of electricity is necessary. Third party payers and national health care systems do not cover these electrical costs; the annual increase in the electrical bill for 24 h/d use is about \$120 to \$240 in the United States. Furthermore, the noise and heat generated by the compressors within the concentrators can be a constant annoyance to some patients and to others in the room.

Liquid Oxygen Reservoirs

Gaseous O_2 condenses to liquid when manufacturers lower its temperature to −297.3°F or below. Large trucks deliver the liquid O_2 to the patient's home, where the stationary liquid reservoir is "transfilled" from the larger vessel within the truck (Figure 99-3). The design of the stationary liquid reservoir is similar to that of a thermos bottle, with a vacuum between an inner and outer shell. Some O_2 spontaneously enters the gaseous phase above the liquid and escapes through a controlled temperature environment provided by a coil of metal tubing. Finally, gaseous O_2 is delivered to the patient at a controlled rate via a flowmeter. Several commercially available stationary liquid O_2 sources are described in Table 99-3.

The stationary liquid O_2 delivery systems have two major advantages. First, liquid O_2 is much more "compact" than O_2 in the gaseous state. In fact, 1 lb of liquid will generate 342 L of the gas. Home care providers can make fewer deliveries since the contents of stationary liquid systems last much longer than those of compressed gas cylinders. The second major advantage of the liquid delivery system is that it is the only stationary source that can be used in the home to transfill portable units. As compared with compressed gas cylinder pressures of up to 2200 psi, liquid sources have a driving pressure about 100-fold lower (20 to 25 psi). Because of this relatively low pressure, patients can be safely taught to transfill their portable unit on an as-needed basis (Fig. 99-4). The stationary liquid system is visually more appealing than the compressed gas cyclinder and does not produce either noise or heat, as does the concentrator.

A major disadvantage of liquid O_2 is that home care providers encounter high capitalization costs for suitably equipped delivery trucks. The stationary and portable delivery sources are also expensive. Although bulk liquid O_2 is inexpensive to the supplier, the costs involved in delivering the O_2 to the home can be substantial. Consequently, liquid O_2 is unavailable in many rural or small communities in the United States and is totally unavailable in many countries. Another disadvantage of liquid O_2 is that, even though flows up to 8 L/min are possible, both the stationary and portable units can occasionally "freeze" at these flows. As a result, either the O_2 supply may be interrupted or the bulk O_2 may freely escape from the vessel into the atmosphere. Although the stationary and portable units are virtually silent while being used in routine O_2 delivery to the patient, O_2 escaping during the portable transfilling process can be

Table 99-2. Currently Available Oxygen Concentrators

Model	Weight (lb)	Power Consumption (W)	Concentration (+ or − 3%)	Maximum Flow (L/min)
Briox Technology				
Briox 4 plus	55	280	93% at 3 L/min	3
Briox 6 plus	60	340	93% at 3 L/min	3
John Bunn Co.				
Bunn Natural	29	250	90% at 5 L/min	5
Bunn 3001	43	280	90% at 3 L/min	3
Bunn 5001	50	375	95% at 3 L/min	3
Devilbiss				
Devo 44	44	390	95% at 1–3 L/min 90% at 4 L/min 82% at 5 L/min	5
Devo MC29	29	420	95% at 1 L/min 93% at 2 L/min 90% at 3 L/min	3
Erie Medical				
Eriette	57	420	95% at 2 L/min	2
Healthdyne				
BX-3000	54	340	90% at .5–4 L/min 85% at 5 L/min	5
Hudson 6400	59	330	93% at 3 L/min	3
Inspiron				
3500	54	350	94% at 1–2 L/min 92% at 3 L/min 90% at 4 L/min	4
Invacare				
Mobilaire II	64	320	95% at 1–2 L/min 93% at 3 L/min	3
MADA/Resp O_2	44	400	95% at 1–2 L/min 90% at 3 L/min	3
Mountain Medical				
Aspen	42	200	93% at 1–2 L/min	2
Sage	48	420	95% at 1–2 L/min 93% at 3 L/min	3
Summit	59	430	95% at 1–3 L/min 93% at 4 L/min 85% at 5 L/min	5
Econo$_2$	114	395	95% at 1–4 L/min 90% at 5 L/min	5
OECO				
OE Junior[a]	58	200	40% at 1–6 L/min	6
High Humidity[a]	110	225	40% at 1–6 L/min	6
Penox				
Mini ox	52	325	95% at 2 L/min	2
BX-5000	55	345	90% at 0.5–4 L/min	5
Puritan Bennett				
Companion PB-590	59	400	95% at 1–4 L/min 90% at 5 L/min	5
Companion 492	49	350	95% at 1–3 L/min 92% at 4 L/min	4
Companion 492A	57	400	95% at 1–3 L/min 92% at 4 L/min	4
Roman Labs				
Freedom O_2 DC-100	29	118	93% at 2 L/min	2
Freedom O_2 AC-300	34	235	93% at 3 L/min	3
Emperor O_2	49	440	95% at 1–4.5 L/min 93% at 5 L/min	5

[a] Oxygen enrichers.

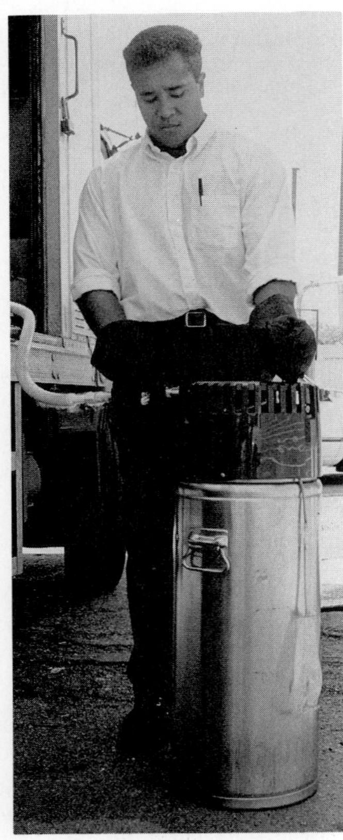

Figure 99-3. Periodically the home care provider comes to the home to transfill the stationary liquid O_2 source from a delivery truck equipped with a large liquid supply.

noisy. A reported but rare complication of liquid O_2 therapy is a thermal burn, which can result when the transfilling process is not performed properly. Another disadvantage of the liquid source is that evaporative loss of O_2 occurs and can be up to 0.055 lb/h. The design of the modern liquid stationary reservoirs has minimized this loss, and no appreciable evaporation occurs while the unit is delivering a flow of O_2. Some loss does occur with the portable transfilling process and while either unit sits unused.

Portable Oxygen Sources

The compressed gas cylinders, concentrators, and liquid reservoirs described previously are stationary O_2 sources in that they are usually "parked" somewhere in the home environment. While receiving O_2 from the stationary source, patients are literally tethered to the unit by the 25- to 50-ft O_2 extension tubing (Fig. 99-5). Consequently, truly compliant patients are greatly restricted in their ability to ambulate from one room to another within their home. To venture outside the 25- to 50-ft radius, patients for whom "continuous" O_2 has been prescribed must either resort to

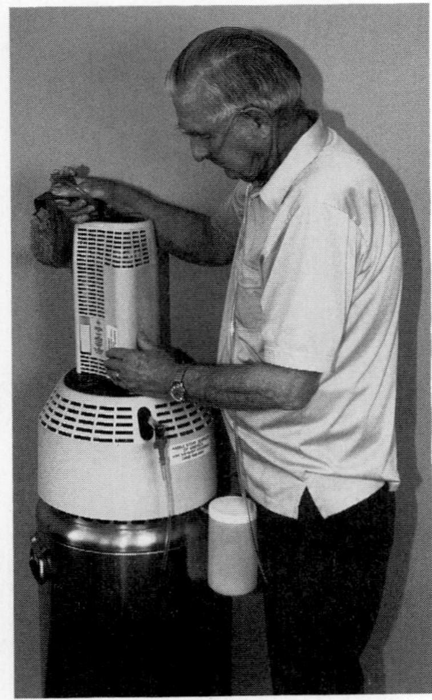

Figure 99-4. This patient has been taught to safely transfill the small portable liquid unit from the larger stationary source.

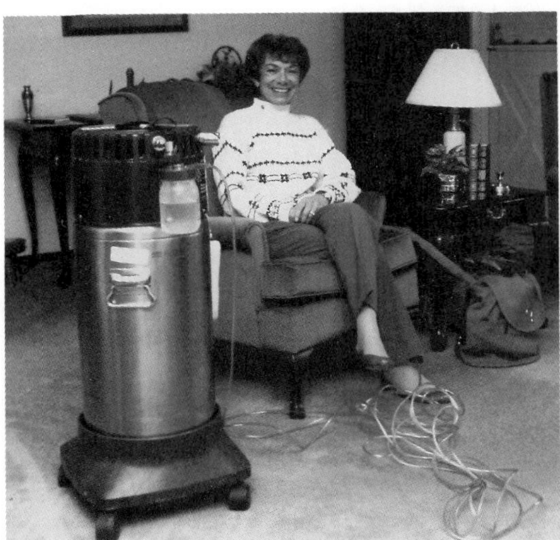

Figure 99-5. While in the home, this patient receiving continuous transtracheal O_2 is "tethered" to the stationary source by the 25-foot extension hose. Injuries (e.g., hip fractures) can occur by tripping over the awkward extension tubing.

Table 99-3. Liquid Oxygen Systems

Manufacturer	Stationary Units			Portable Units		
	Weight (lb)	Flow Range (L/min)	Duration (d) at 2 L/min	Weight (lb)	Flow Range (L/min)	Duration (d) at 2 L/min
Bunn	130	1–8	7–11	11	0.5–8	8–9
Pulsair Inc.						
Grandeair	140	0.25–12	11			
Stationair	99	0.25–12	7			
Travelair II				13.8	0.25–6	13
Travelair I				9.3	0.25–6	6.9
Wanderair II D				6.5	0.125–2	3.3
Pulsair OMS I				7.6	0.25–6	3.3
Pulsair OMS II				10.0	0.25–6	6.9
Cryogenics						
Liberator 45	163	0.25–6	12			
Liberator 30	122	0.25–6	8			
Liberator 20	86	0.25–6	5			
Stroller				9.6	0.25–6	7.5
Sprint				6.9	0.25–6	4.3
Inspiron	130	1–8	7–11	11	0.5–8	8–9
Lincare						
OR 212	70	0–15	3.38			
OR 313	116	0–15	8.3			
Standard use walker				7.5	1–5	4
Extended use walker				10.0	1–5	8
Mark 4 W50 walker				8.0	0.25–6	8
Penox						
Large base unit	151	0–8	12			
Standard base	116	0–8	8			
Mini base	89	0–8	5			
Lightweight				5	0.25–5	2.75
1 Portable				6.5	0.25–5	3
2 Portable				8.5	1–5	6
3 Portable				12	1–5	11
Puritan-Bennett						
Companion 21	92	0.25–6	6			
Companion 31	125	0.25–6	8			
Companion 41	160	0.25–6	11			
Companion 1000				7.5	0.25–6	8.5

noncompliance and remove their O_2 device or be transferred to another O_2 source. Third party payers and national health care systems generally do not cover more than one stationary O_2 unit. Therefore, portable sources have been used in home O_2 therapy.

A practical definition of a portable unit is one that allows the patient to receive O_2 while away from the stationary source. Compressed gas, concentrator, and liquid O_2 portable units are commercially available. From a clinical perspective, there are degrees of portability. At one end of the spectrum, some units are *transportable* in that they allow patients to receive O_2 while being transported from one place to another. These sources are heavy, bulky, and awkward and are either difficult or impossible for the patient to carry. At the other end of the spectrum, *ambulatory* O_2 sources are lightweight, streamlined, and capable of being carried by the patient during ambulation.

Compressed Gas Cylinders

Portable compressed gas cylinders are simply smaller versions of the H or K tanks, and their salient features have been presented previously. The E cylinder (Table 99-1) is the most commonly used portable companion to the concentrator and stationary compressed gas source. The advantage of this cylinder is that it is readily available and inexpensive to supply to a patient who requires 2 L/min or less and only occasionally leaves the home for a couple of hours at a time. If the patient is quite active outside the home, the quantity of cylinders required may make this portable O_2 source less attractive from an economic standpoint. The major disadvantage of the E cylinder is that it is not a truly "ambulatory" unit as previously defined. A full cylinder can weigh up to 18 lb and must be pushed or pulled with a cart (Fig. 99-6). The maximal duration of the tank's

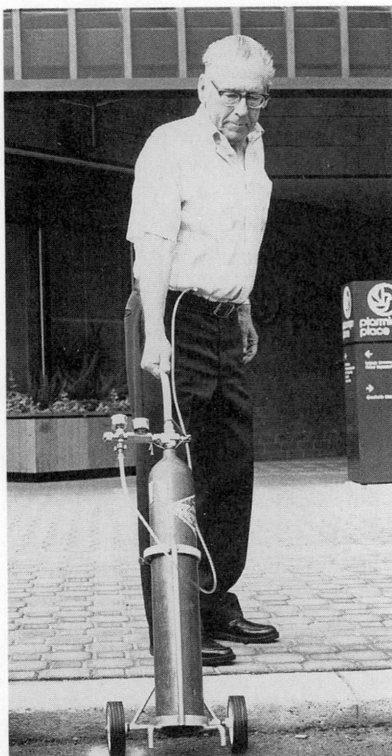

Figure 99-6. Portable E cylinders are heavy and awkward and have a relatively short duration of use. They are not true ambulatory devices because they cannot be carried by the ambulatory patient.

supply is less than 6 hours at the standard 2 L/min flow rate, and much shorter use can be anticipated with higher flow requirements. Lighter construction with seamless aluminum (DOT-AL) makes the E cylinder more portable, but it is still impractical to carry. Of the commercially available compressed gas cylinders, seamless aluminum D and B tanks have the best potential for use in ambulatory O_2 therapy. However, the duration of the cylinder contents can be short (e.g., 1 to 3.5 hours) with a standard 2 L/min flow.

Oxygen Concentrators

Stationary O_2 concentrators of the future may be able to transfill portable tanks in the home. Lightweight ambulatory concentrators will probably be developed that have an energy source capable of generating many hours of O_2 use. Presently, only a transportable O_2 concentrator is available. One commercial unit weighs 34 lb but is in the form of a suitcase and can deliver up to 3 L/min (Fig. 99-7). Direct current application allows a 2 L/min model to be powered by a standard 12-volt battery during automobile travel.

Liquid Oxygen Reservoirs

The portable liquid O_2 reservoirs (Table 99-3) are similar to the stationary units in that they represent an equally efficient method of storing a large O_2 supply in a compact vessel. In contrast to the small compressed gas cylinders, some portable liquid reservoirs may provide the average 2 L/min patient with up to 8 hours of O_2 therapy. Most portable liquid O_2 sources are truly "ambulatory" units since they are light enough (10 lb or less) to be carried by most patients. Because it can be transfilled in the home (Fig. 99-4), coupled with its lighter weight and longer-lasting O_2 supply, the liquid O_2 reservoir is the best ambulatory source for the active patient. More technical discussions of O_2 delivery systems can be found elsewhere.[11,12]

OXYGEN DELIVERY DEVICES

Standard Nasal Cannula

The standard nasal cannula is the most commonly used delivery device for both in-hospital and home use. A major advantage of this device is that it is simple to use and requires little patient instruction. The nasal cannula is inexpensive because of the high volume of its in-hospital and home use as well as its simple polyvinylchloride (PVC) construction. Complications and sequelae reported with long-term use of the nasal cannula are shown in Table 99-4. It is often uncomfortable owing to irritation over the ears and under the nose, and patients can develop a contact dermatitis from the PVC. Improvement may occur by changing to a cannula made of a biocompatible silicone product. Complaints of a dry nose or throat are common, particularly in arid climates or with high flow rates. Recurrent or severe epistaxis can present a management problem, and patients occasionally develop an associated perforation of the nasal septum. Although this is not a true complication, some persons find the nasal cannula unsightly and therefore resist travel outside the home. Of note, results of the NOTT study[8] showed that patients assigned to the "continuous" group used the nasal O_2 for only a mean of 17.7 hours rather than the 24 hours

Table 99-4. Complications and Sequelae of the Nasal Cannula

Sequelae
Nasal crusting and blockage
Postnasal drip
Pharyngitis sicca
Impaired sense of smell and taste
Hoarseness
Complications
Ulceration of columella nasi
Ulceration of ears
Contact dermatitis of face
Recurrent epistaxis
Septal perforation
Acute sinusitis
Acute otitis or serous otitis
Tear duct blockage (epiphora)
Cellulitis (bacterial and fungal)

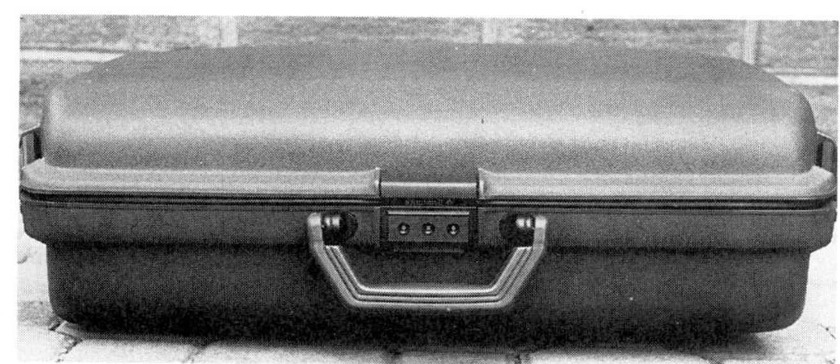

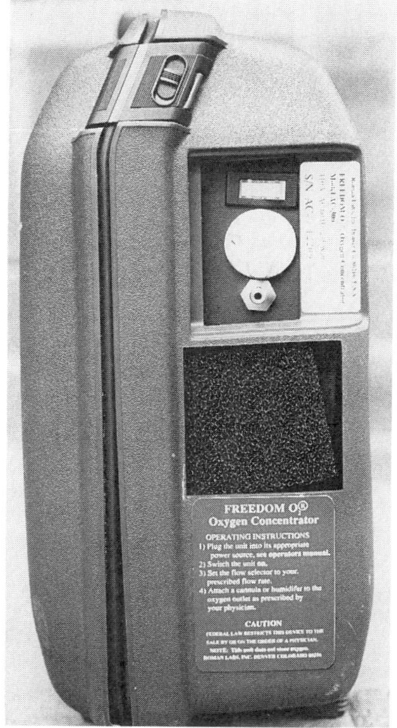

Figure 99-7. (**A & B**) The Freedom O_2 concentrator (Roman Labs Inc., Englewood, CO) is in the form of a suitcase and is transportable. The AC-300 model can deliver up to 3 L/min. Model DC-100 can be used with a 12-volt automobile battery but has a limit of 2 L/min.

called for in the study design. These data suggest an inherent compliance problem with nasal O_2.

The O_2 masks discussed in Chapter 75 are rarely used in the home for a variety of reasons. In addition to their discomfort, masks do not lend themselves to activities of daily living such as eating and speaking. The high O_2 flow requirements associated with masks also make them impractical for home use. Occasionally a patient with a laryngectomy or tracheostomy may require supplemental O_2 along with a source of humidification. "Trach collars" or T-piece adaptors and associated tubing and humidifiers can be used in the same manner described for the hospitalized patient in Chapter 75. Compressed gas cylinders or liquid reservoirs are the likely choices for an O_2 source with these delivery devices, and, furthermore, can also be interfaced with volume-cycled machines to deliver home mechanical ventilation to the patient with a trachotomy, as described in Chapter 101.

Oxygen Conserving Devices and Techniques

Other O_2 delivery devices have evolved as a result of the special needs of the ambulatory O_2 patient. For example, in the home, unlike the hospital setting, patients receiving O_2 have the opportunity to remain active. In fact, a primary goal of home O_2 therapy is to offer the patient maximum mobility. One way to accomplish this is to conserve O_2 and maximize the duration of the portable O_2 supply. Devices for conserving O_2 include reservoir cannulas and pendants, demand O_2 delivery devices, and transtracheal O_2 catheters.

Reservoir Devices

Reservoir devices[13–27] store exhaled O_2 in valveless expandable chambers under the nostrils (Fig. 99-8), or via large-bore tubing in a single valveless expandable chamber having the design of a pendant across the chest (Fig. 99-9). During subsequent inhalation through the nostrils, the O_2 is evacuated from the reservoir. Conservation of O_2 is achieved, since the constant flow of O_2 from the source can be reduced. Reservoir devices are conceptually similar in function to partial rebreathing masks, described in Chapter 75. The major advantage of both the nasal and pendant reservoir is that O_2 flow requirements can be reduced. Tiep and associates have extensively evaluated these reservoir devices and reported savings of 50 to 75 percent.[13–18] A disadvantage of the reservoir concept as presently available is that both inspiration and expiration must occur through the nostrils. Patients with chronic airflow obstruction often exhale through the mouth with pursed lip breathing, and the efficiency of both reservoir devices has been shown to be reduced in this setting. A pendant that allows for pursed lip breathing has been described,[17] but the nasal reservoir is

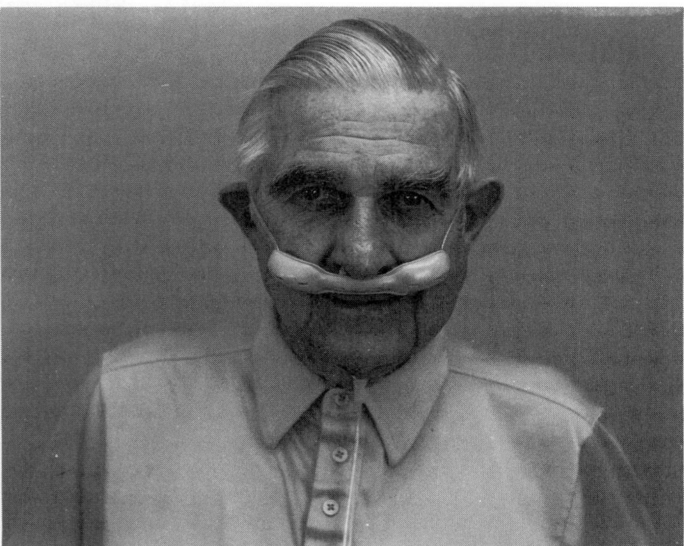

Figure 99-8. The Oxymizer Reservoir Cannula (Chad Therapeutics Inc., Chatsworth, CA).

large and noticeable on the face and patients often object to its appearance.[18] Some individuals find the large-bore tubing of the pendant both cosmetically objectionable and uncomfortable because of its weight.[18]

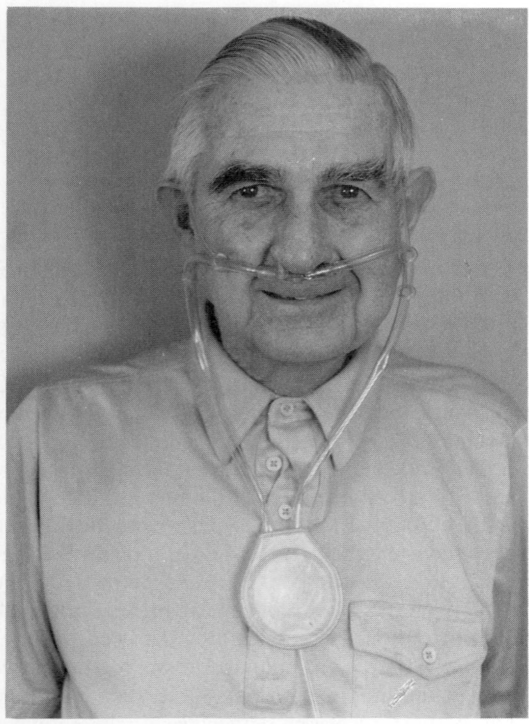

Figure 99-9. The Oxymizer Pendant (Chad Therapeutics Inc., Chatsworth, CA).

Demand Oxygen Delivery Devices

A demand O_2 delivery system (DODS) is an electronic device that senses the initiation of an inspiratory effort and delivers O_2 only during the inspiratory phase. Adequate O_2 saturation can be maintained while conserving the O_2 that would generally be wasted on exhalation with continuous flow devices. The onset of inspiration is commonly sensed by a pressure transducer, but there are a variety of methods for determining how the O_2 pulse is delivered.

The commercially available DODS devices are listed in Table 99-5. Pulsair Inc. manufactures a portable unit that is physically incorporated into the liquid O_2 unit. As the transducer senses an inspiratory effort, a fixed volume of O_2 is delivered. With each breath, approximately 16.5 mL is administered for each 1 L/min nasal cannula equivalent flow setting. In other words, if the unit were set at 2 L/min, the patient would receive approximately 33 mL of O_2 with each inspiration. Pulsair Inc. manufactures a second model intended for use with the stationary source, which, unlike the portable DODS, can be used with either liquid or compressed gaseous O_2. The stationary DODS also has an "apnea" or "failure to cycle" alarm with a variable time delay setting. In contrast to the concept of setting a constant volume to be given with each breath, Chad Therapeutics has designed a portable DODS that delivers the same volume with each breath but can be adjusted to administer a bolus at intervals ranging from one of every four breaths (1 setting) to each of every four breaths (4 setting). An apnea alarm is not provided, and the unit has been used with both liquid and compressed gas portable sources.

An example of an entirely different principle of operation is the DODS manufactured by Puritan-Bennett, which continuously computes the respiratory rate. On the basis of this

Table 99-5. Demand Oxygen Delivery Systems

	Puritan-Bennett Corp.		Chad Therapeutics	Pulsair Inc.		John Bunn Co.	
	Companion 5	Companion 6	Oxymatic	OMS-20 OMS-50	Pulsair OMS-1 Pulsair OMS-2	Portamate	Omni
Range of reported oxygen savings	50–60%	50–60%	7:1	60–70%	60–70%	50–60%	50–60%
Delivers a constant O_2 volume per minute—pulse volume depends on respiratory rate	Yes	Yes	No	No	No	No	No
Consistent O_2 pulse volume with each breath—volume is adjustable	No	No	No	Yes	Yes	No	No
Consistent O_2 pulse volume with each breath—breaths per delivery adjustable (e.g., 4:1)	No	No	Yes	No	No	No	No
DODS incorporated into portable oxygen source	No	No	No	No	Yes	No	No
Used with compressed gas (CG), liquid (L), or both (B)	B	B	B	B	L	B	B
Delivery source is portable (P), stationary (S), or both (B)	B	S	P	B	P	B	B
Apnea or failure to cycle alarm	Yes	Yes	No	Yes	No	No	Yes
Low battery alarm	Yes	Yes	Yes	Yes	Yes	No	Yes
Battery duration	3 h	3 h	2–4 wk	38 h	26 h	8–12 h	8–12 h
Weight of DODS	26 oz	26 oz	11 oz	15 oz	7–10 lb	1 lb	1 lb

information, the O_2 delivery is adjusted so that flow begins with inspiration and approximately 40 percent of the continuous flow equivalent is administered. The unit has an apnea alarm and defaults to continuous flow as a safety feature. The DODS can be used with either a stationary or a portable source, but with portable sources the battery lasts only 3 hours. The John Bunn Co. also offers a unit that calculates the respiratory rate and adjusts the O_2 delivery accordingly.

The major advantage of the DODS is O_2 conservation, which should offer the ambulatory patient greater mobility outside the home with longer-lasting (and potentially lighter weight) portable O_2 sources. Reduction in bulk O_2 use may also have some economic impact on either the third party payer or the home care provider. A factor that offsets the cost savings achieved with bulk O_2 conservation is the additional cost of the DODS, which currently is borne by the home care provider. In the United States, Medicare or other third party payers generally do not provide additional reimbursement for such technology.

A disadvantage of portable liquid O_2 sources with built-in DODS units is that they are limited to use by patients having access to compatible transfilling stationary sources. "Stand alone" DODS units have the advantage of being used with a variety of both liquid and compressed gas stationary and portable sources. However, ambulatory patients must juggle both the DODs and the portable source. The impracticalities of a heavy DODS unit or short battery life offset the benefits of O_2 conservation. Apnea or failure-to-cycle alarms are an asset for stationary sources, particularly when patients receive pulse O_2 during sleep. The attentive home care practitioner may even help to identify an occasional unsuspected sleep apnea patient when the alarm persists in the absence of identifiable mechanical failure of the unit. Failure-to-cycle alarms are less important with portable unit use; in fact, many patients using a portable DODS unit are kept aware that it is functioning by either the sound the device generates when it cycles or the nasal sensation caused by the pulse delivery. By contrast, an occasional patient will find a particular device objectionable because of the noise or the nasal irritation resulting from the pulse delivery. Some newer models have a silent event light, which reassures the patient that the unit is pulsing.

The O_2 savings reported with DODS vary among investigators and among commercially available products.[28–48] Results also depend on whether patients were studied during brief periods of rest, exercise, or sleep. Overall, claims of O_2 savings with these systems range from about 50 to as much as 87 percent. However, studies have generally not measured the actual monthly bulk O_2 savings or objectively quantified the duration of portable use outside the home.

Another proposed advantage of the DODS is that reduced O_2 needs make a humidifier unnecessary. In fact, a humidifier is not recommended because condensate may adversely affect the electronics of the system and the dead space within the humidifier may alter the performance of the transducer. Although the standard 8 ft of O_2 hose routinely supplied with the nasal cannula is usually not an issue, individual DODS units may not function reliably if excessive lengths of connecting tubing are employed.

Transtracheal Oxygen Therapy

The history of transtracheal O_2 therapy[49–112] dates from 1982 when Heimlich[49] published the first report on this modality. In his study a customized 14-gauge breakaway needle was used to insert a 16-gauge Teflon intravenous catheter at the second tracheal interspace in 14 hospitalized patients. The catheter was secured in place with a reversed pediatric tracheostomy tube and tied around the neck with umbilical tape. Immediately following the procedure, patients received O_2 through the "Microtrach" via a modified intravenous infusion tubing at flow rates that were generally less than 1 L/min. Shortly thereafter, Hoffman[50,64] and Bloom[53] from the United States, Banner and Govan[63] from England, and Leger and Robert[51] from France also began reporting experience with transtracheal O_2 therapy.

In 1986, since the specific indications for transtracheal O_2 therapy had not been defined, my associates and I initially determined that we could easily justify evaluating this new technology in a group of end-stage patients who were refractory to the standard nasal cannula.[56] By definition, this small group of patients was refractory because arterial oxygenation was inadequate on the maximum tolerated nasal cannula flow. Both nasal cannula and mask therapy were required in some. Results showed adequate oxygenation on transtracheal O_2 therapy at flows that were compatible with home liquid O_2 sources (2 to 6 L/min) and there was a mean reduction in flow requirement of 72 percent.[56]

Over the next few years we came to realize that transtracheal O_2 therapy had its greatest therapeutic value in the management of selected patients with chronic hypoxemia who were treated early in the course of their illness.[55,57,68,70,73] All the published experience with transtracheal O_2 currently available is cited at the end of this chapter.[49–112] The potential benefits of transtracheal O_2 therapy are shown in Table 99-6. When 50 patients seeking transtracheal O_2 therapy were prospectively asked to identify and rank their reasons for wanting this alternative form of O_2 delivery, they rated improved comfort and mobility as first and second, respectively.[77] Patients usually find the transtracheal catheter much more comfortable than the nasal cannula. Improved mobility can result from the reduction in the resting O_2 flow requirement of approximately 50 percent reported by many investigators. As with other O_2-conserving devices, lower flows with transtracheal delivery offer the patient a longer duration of the portable supply and an opportunity for increased activity away from the home. Improved mobility may also result from the reduced dyspnea reported with transtracheal O_2 therapy, and a recent study shows improved exercise capacity.[103] In addition, reduced inspired ventilatory requirements with transtracheal O_2 delivery[90,92,97,99] may decrease the work of breathing[100] and increase tolerance for activity. Finally, patients concerned about their appearance can hide the transtracheal catheter and O_2 source from view, and the duration of the portable source can be further extended by combining transtracheal[60,67,101,102] with pulse delivery (Fig. 99-10). The net result of the above benefits is that patients truly use their transtracheal O_2 for the prescribed 24 hours per day rather than the 18 hours[8] reported with the nasal cannula. There is potential for further reduction of erythrocytosis[56,73] and cor pulmonale[56] in certain individuals. By extrapolation from the MRC[9] and NOTT data,[8] survival might be increased beyond what was seen with the "continuous" nasal O_2 group, but this hypothesis has yet to be tested.

Several types of transtracheal O_2 catheters are currently commercially available. One design has been marketed in the United States since 1985 and is now available in some

Table 99-6. Potential Benefits, Specific Indications, Contraindications and Precautions with Transtracheal Oxygen Therapy

Potential benefits as compared with the nasal cannula
- 24-h/d compliance
- Improved mobility
  - Improved exercise tolerance
  - Extended portable tank range
- Improved comfort
- Avoidance of complications of nasal cannula
- Effective in refractory hypoxemia
- Cosmetically more acceptable
- Reduced dyspnea

Specific indications
- Need for improved mobility
- Suboptimal compliance related to the nasal cannula
- Complications from the nasal cannula
- Cor pulmonale or erythrocytosis with nasal cannula
- Refractory hypoxemia
- Patient preference

Contraindications
- Mental or physical incompetence
- Acute (uncompensated) hypercapnia
- Severe anxiety neurosis
- Pleura herniated over puncture site
- Upper airway obstruction

Precautions indicated
- Poor mechanical reserve
- Profound hypoxemia
- Chronic (compensated) hypercapnia
- Obese neck or other anatomic abnormality
- Mild to moderate anxiety
- Bronchial hyperreactivity
- Copious or viscous sputum
- Serious cardiac arrhythmia
- Bleeding disorder

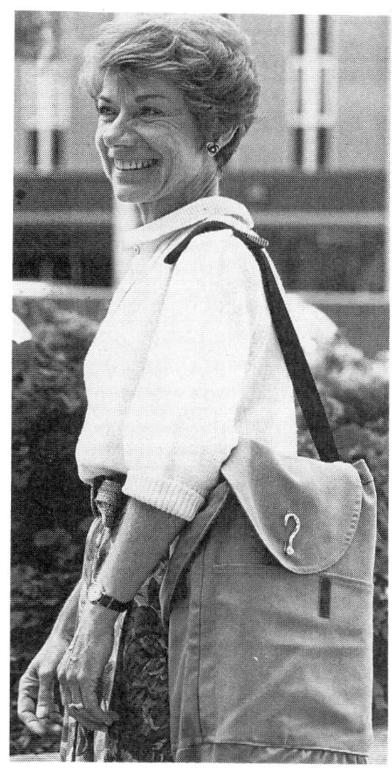

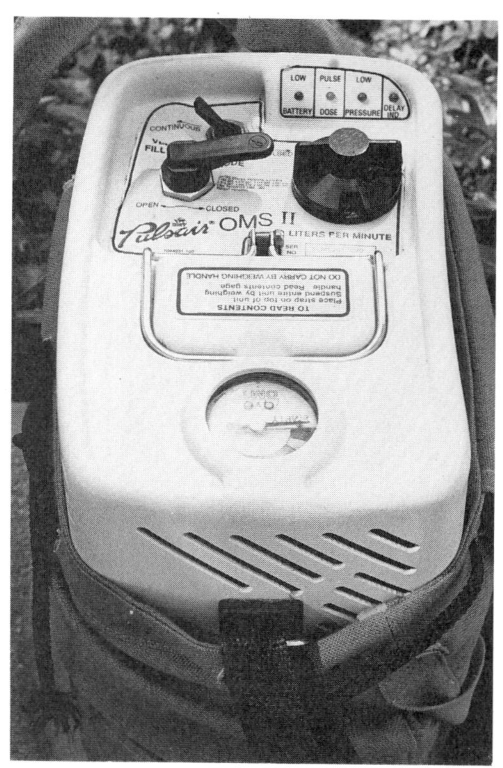

Figure 99-10. (**A**) This patient with emphysema has been receiving transtracheal O_2 since August 1986. She has learned to completely conceal her catheter, O_2 hose, and liquid source. (**B**) The patient extends the duration of her portable O_2 by combining transtracheal technology with a pulse device (Pulsair OMS I, Pulsair Inc., Ft. Pierce, FL).

other countries, including parts of Europe. A stenting device and two types of number 9 french catheters are manufactured by Transtracheal Systems (Englewood, CO). The stent is a nonfunctioning catheter that is placed by a needle–wire guide–tissue dilator method similar to the Seldinger technique for placement of a vascular catheter.[55,73] O_2 is not delivered through the trachea for 1 week in order to minimize subcutaneous emphysema, discomfort, and excessive cough. After 1 week of ''stenting'' the tract, the device is removed over a wire guide, and a functioning SCOOP-1 transtracheal catheter is inserted. The SCOOP-1 catheter is cleaned in place for an additional 5 to 7 weeks until the tract has epithelialized and the patient can learn to periodically remove the catheter for cleaning (Fig. 99-11). The SCOOP-1 catheter has a single distal port and is considered a low-flow catheter, which is recommended for the vast majority of patients who require resting transtracheal flows of 2 L/min or less. Once the tract is mature, a high-flow SCOOP-2 catheter design, with a distal port and multiple side ports, is available to accommodate the needs of the rare patient who requires resting transtracheal flows greater than 2 L/min.

Another catheter design is marketed in Europe by SMAD (SMAD Laboratoires Pharmaceutics, L'Arbresle, France). The number 8 french Oxycath is also inserted percutaneously into the trachea by a modified Seldinger technique.[61] Although a stent is not used, O_2 flow through the catheter is delayed for the reasons described above. The Oxycath is similar to the SCOOP-2 catheter in the characteristics of the plastic, the internal diameter, and the presence of side holes, but differs in the flange design, overall length, and the absence of a distal port. Patients also learn to clean the Oxycath in place while the tract is becoming epithelialized. As with the SCOOP catheters, the Oxycath and its mature tract are large enough to allow patients to easily remove and reinsert the catheter during this cleaning process. A third catheter design is available in the United States through Cook (Cook Critical Care, Bloomington, IN). In the operating room,[72] the ITOC catheter is surgically tunneled under the skin from the lower thorax to the neck in a fashion similar to placement of a Hickman intravenous catheter. The tip of the device is then placed high within the cervical trachea by a modified Seldinger technique, and the catheter is permanently sutured into place. The ITOC is similar to the SCOOP and Oxycath with respect to diameter but otherwise differs greatly from the other two, particularly in terms of placement and catheter care. To date, more experience has been reported in the literature with the SCOOP[55–58,60,61,65,67,71,73–82,84–90,97,100,102–108,110–112] than with either the Oxycath[61] or the ITOC device.[66,69,72]

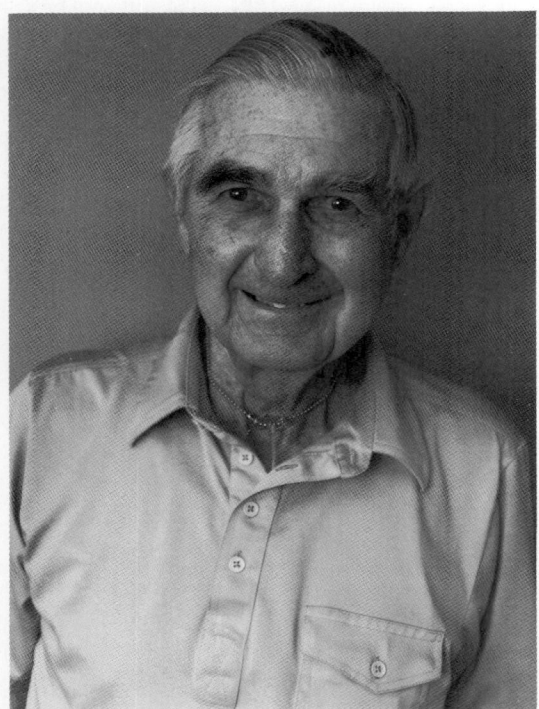

Figure 99-11. This patient has a mature tracheocutaneous fistula and removes the transtracheal catheter on a daily basis for cleaning.

Finally, a catheter called the Microtrach has recently been placed on the market by Ballard Medical (Salt Lake City, UT). This is significantly different from the modified 16-gauge Teflon intravenous catheter previously evaluated by Heimlich[49,54,59,91] as a custom device. The Ballard Microtrach is similar to the SCOOP and Oxycath designs in terms of composition, internal diameter, length, and method of insertion. It primarily differs in that transtracheal O_2 is administered immediately after insertion and the catheter is only cleaned in place and is replaced every month by exchange over a wire guide. At the time of writing there have not been publications in the medical literature on experience with the Ballard Microtrach.

My clinical experience is biased toward one insertion technique and one catheter design. However, experience has also led me to the conclusion that the key to successfully treating patients is to offer them a complete program for care rather than to focus entirely on the transtracheal catheter insertion technique and the theoretical concepts of various catheter designs. The transtracheal O_2 program must be instituted through a team effort. The members of the team should include a physician and either a respiratory therapist or a nurse who is specifically trained in administering transtracheal O_2 therapy. The home care provider should also be involved, and the patient and significant other should feel that they are part of the team.

The transtracheal O_2 program that my colleagues and I have described[55–57,62,68,70,73] has four clinically defined phases of care (Table 99-7). Phase I consists of patient orientation, evaluation, and selection as well as preparation for the transtracheal procedure. Potential patients and their significant others are encouraged to attend an orientation session, which uses educational videotapes and includes a question and answer period led by a trained clinician and an actual patient who is receiving transtracheal O_2. Efforts are made to help individuals develop a realistic understanding of this therapy. Interested patients then undergo an evaluation involving a few tests as well as history, physical examination, and a review process that is conducted by the physician. The goal is to properly select patients by making certain that they meet both the general indications for home O_2 and the specific indications for transtracheal O_2 therapy. Patients in whom contraindications are identified are excluded. Precautions regarding transtracheal O_2 therapy are listed in Table 99-6. This phase is completed when the patient has been prepared for the procedure.

In Phase II the transtracheal stent is inserted under local anesthesia. Most patients are treated on an outpatient basis. The goal of this phase is to create a quality tract while keeping the patient comfortable and stable. In Phase III the stent is removed over a wire guide, and a functioning transtracheal catheter is inserted. Proper O_2 flow rates during rest and exertion are determined and the clinician carefully instructs both the patient and significant other how to properly clean the catheter in place using instilled saline and a cleaning rod. The clinician has the patient come back within the next 3 to 7 days for removal of the catheter over a wire guide for cleaning and to evaluate secretions. During the remainder of the 4 to 6 weeks required for tract maturity, the patient can be asked to return as needed for external cleaning of the catheter and secretion management. In Phase IV, which begins when the tracheocutaneous fistula is fully mature, patients are taught to remove the catheter for cleaning on a regular basis. Catheter cleaning can be scheduled according to the patient's individual needs. The routine can vary from twice daily removal to daily cleaning of the catheter in place with removal for cleaning only once every few weeks.

My associates and I have reported our experience with the sequelae and complications encountered in this program for transtracheal O_2 therapy; results are presented in Table 99-8. Some groups have reported more difficulty administering transtracheal O_2[71,82,84,87,105,108] than others.[49–70,72–81,85,86,88–91,93–104,106,107,109–112] As with any procedure or therapy, the incidence of problems depends somewhat on how investigators define both minor and major sequelae and complications. I suspect that the difficulty encountered depends largely on how well trained the group is initially and how

Table 99-7. Four Clinically Defined Phases of a Program for Transtracheal Oxygen Therapy

Phase I	Orientation, evaluation, selection and preparation
Phase II	Transtracheal procedure and stent week
Phase III	Transtracheal oxygen therapy—immature tract
Phase IV	Transtracheal oxygen therapy—mature tract

Table 99-8. Potential Sequelae and Complications of Transtracheal Oxygen

Frequent transient sequelae
Tenderness at puncture site
Mild increase in cough
Increase in sputum
Mild hemoptysis
Infrequent sequelae (*usually avoidable*)
Cephalad catheter (*catheter design is important*)
Symptomatic mucus balls (*proper adherence to catheter care protocols*)
Hoarseness (*avoidance of a cricothyroid puncture*)
Tract closure (*patient education*)
Contact or candidal dermatitis (*avoidance of topical antibiotics and irritants*)
Potential complications
Extravasated air
Subcutaneous emphysema (1%)
Pneumomediastinum (rare)
Pneumothorax (rare)
Infection
Tracheal chondritis (5–10%)
Cellulitis (1%)
Abscess (rare)
Bleeding >10 mL (rare)
Acute respiratory failure, bronchospasm (1%)
Keloid formation (5%)

committed the group is to keeping up with changes and improvements in protocols. Success is also a function of the number of patients treated by a group of investigators. In general, transtracheal O_2 therapy has been found to be safe and complications tend to be minor. More serious complications are likely to be reported as transtracheal O_2 therapy becomes more widely used.[82,87,108] As with any medical technology, patients can get into trouble if caregivers are inadequately trained, careless technique is employed, or clinicians improperly breach established protocols. Another potential disadvantage of this form of O_2 delivery is that some Medicare carriers and third party payers may still be unfamiliar with it, and reimbursement problems have arisen.

PRESCRIBING LONG-TERM OXYGEN THERAPY

The reader should now have an in-depth understanding of the physiologic concepts involved in the process of respiration (Ch. 1) and the factors that determine O_2 need (Ch. 2). Pathophysiologic events resulting in hypoxemia (Ch. 29) and the adverse effects of inadequate blood oxygenation should be clear. Furthermore, the general principles involved in the treatment of chronic hypoxemia were discussed in Chapter 63. This chapter has presented the various systems available for long-term delivery of O_2 to patients in the home. Based on that information, the reader should now be able to define the stationary and portable O_2 sources as well as the delivery device that best meet the specific needs of the individual patient. This technical information is an integral part of the design of a proper O_2 prescription. In order to complete the home O_2 prescription, a number of general and specific clinical issues must be addressed.

Indications

The indications for O_2 therapy have been discussed in Chapter 63. The criteria for qualifying for long-term O_2 in the NOTT study[8] were so well thought out that physicians generally accept them as indications for prescribing long-term O_2 therapy. Furthermore, the U.S. Health Care Financing Administration (HCFA) generally accepts these criteria for reimbursement for Medicare patients. Other third party payers in the United States have tended to follow suit.

Disorders Qualifying for Home Oxygen

The efficacy of long-term home O_2 therapy has only been thoroughly studied in patients with chronic obstructive pulmonary disease (COPD), which is primarily due to chronic bronchitis and emphysema.[8,9] However, clinical experience and extrapolation from previous studies suggest that patients with other diseases resulting in chronic hypoxemia may benefit as well. Examples of such disorders are cystic fibrosis, bronchiectasis, interstitial lung disease, kyphoscoliosis, obesity, primary alveolar hypoventilation, lung or chest wall resection, neuromuscular disorders, sleep disorders of breathing, primary pulmonary hypertension, and left ventricular failure.

Documentation of Long-Term Oxygen Need

Continuous home O_2 is recommended if patients have chronic hypoxemia with a PaO_2 while breathing ambient air of less than 56 mmHg. Although this absolute cutoff is somewhat arbitrary, patients with a PaO_2 below 56 mmHg have values that are in the steep portion of the oxyhemoglobin dissociation curve, where small decreases in PaO_2 result in large (and significant) decreases in oxyhemoglobin saturation and arterial O_2 content. As discussed in Chapter 63, patients with an ambient air PaO_2 in the 56 to 59 mmHg range may qualify for a continuous home O_2 if they have evidence of end-organ failure as demonstrated by the presence of cor pulmonale or erythrocytosis.

A potential pitfall of using only a PaO_2 or arterial saturation (SaO_2) value to evaluate supplemental O_2 need is that it may not accurately reflect the ability of the patient's lungs to extract O_2 while breathing ambient air. For example, Table 99-9 shows three different arterial blood gas measurements that were theoretically obtained in one individual with severe COPD. The PaO_2 results range from 48 to 60 mmHg. The degree of impairment in transporting O_2 from air into the arterial circulation (alveolar-arterial PO_2 difference [$P(A\text{-}a)O_2$]) is exactly the same under each condition. The

Table 99-9. Arterial Blood Gas and Oximetry Results Determined Three Times on the Same Occasion from a Hypothetical Patient, Assuming Three Different Levels of Alveolar Ventilation

	Sample 1	Sample 2	Sample 3
PaO_2 (mmHg)	48	54	60
SaO_2 (%)	83	89	93
$PaCO_2$ (mmHg)	52	47	42
Arterial pH	7.38	7.43	7.48
$P(A\text{-}a)O_2$ (mmHg)	42	42	42

differences in PaO_2 are due entirely to differences in alveolar ventilation as reflected by $PaCO_2$. Under current Medicare guidelines for reimbursement, continuous home O_2 would be authorized under the first two examples but denied in the third, even though all three results were obtained on the *same* patient.

The altitude at which a patient resides should be taken into consideration when prescribing home O_2. For example, a patient tested in Denver, Colorado (elevation 5280 ft above sea level) with a PaO_2 of 56 mmHg while breathing ambient air will be significantly more hypoxemic when home in Evergreen, Colorado (elevation 7278 ft above sea level), 30 miles away. By contrast, a patient from Colby, Kansas (elevation 2180 ft above sea level) who has a PaO_2 of 54 mm Hg on ambient air on referral to Denver will probably not require O_2 on returning home.

The SaO_2 value can also be used to assess O_2 delivery. Although pulse oximetry may be efficacious in monitoring or titrating the SaO_2 of patients already receiving O_2 therapy, this technology is not recommended as documentation for long-term O_2 need (see Ch. 63). The reader has previously reviewed the potential effects of multiple factors (other than PaO_2) on SaO_2 through alterations in the oxyhemoglobin dissociation curve. Noninvasive pulse oximetry has additional pitfalls that can lead to inaccurate results, including the presence of carboxyhemoglobin, dark skin complexion, jaundice, or alterations in cutaneous perfusion due to Raynaud's phenomenon, hemodynamic instability, or exercise.

Since continuous O_2 therapy improves survival, patients with chronic hypoxemia should receive O_2 for the remainder of their lives. The commitment to home O_2 involves a major change in the patient's life-style and a significant expense. Therefore, it is appropriate to be certain that the hypoxemia is persistent over time and cannot be corrected with maximal medical therapy. For example, 1043 patients screened for the NOTT study[8] had arterial blood gas values when breathing ambient air that showed hypoxemia. Following 3 weeks of treatment with "intensive bronchodilator therapy," repeat arterial blood gas measurements obtained at a time when patients were "free of exacerbations" showed that the hypoxemia resolved in 45 percent of the subjects, making supplemental O_2 therapy unnecessary in those individuals.

Short-Term versus Long-Term Oxygen Therapy

Largely owing to present-day financial constraints, patients are tending to be discharged from the hospital earlier and earlier in the course of their illnesses. In the case of patients who are hypoxemic at the time of discharge, it seems reasonable to send them home on short-term continuous O_2 therapy for a few weeks until they become medically stable on maximal therapy. If they continue to demonstrate hypoxemia, then a commitment to long-term O_2 therapy can be made. Although some authors have suggested that patients need not receive supplemental O_2 during this observation period of up to 3 months,[113,114] there is some risk of morbidity and mortality, and it seems prudent to offer short-term supplemental O_2 during the observation period.

Issue of Recertification

Since the middle 1980s, issues about Medicare reimbursement in the United States have been discussed.[115–117] Once chronic hypoxemia has been demonstrated, additional blood gases or pulse oximetry measurements may be very helpful in adjusting the administration of O_2 and other medications. However, additional measurements of ambient air blood O_2 tensions for recertification purposes should be discouraged.[117] In support of this point, O'Donohue[118] has recently published data suggesting that administration of O_2 may be reparative to patients with documented chronic hypoxemia. Upon repeating ambient air arterial blood gas measurements after a 6-month period in which transtracheal O_2 therapy was the primary treatment variable, he found that 20 percent of patients no longer qualified for home O_2 because their PaO_2 values while breathing ambient air had increased to levels above 55 mmHg. Through retrospective analysis of a study by Weitzenblum et al.,[119] he found that a similar phenomenon occurred in some patients receiving long-term O_2 by nasal cannula. Since increases after 3 months in ambient air PaO_2 values may be due to the beneficial effects of O_2 therapy, mandatory recertification by criteria based on ambient air blood gas values may unintentionally result in withdrawal of an effective therapy.

Concept of Long-Term Intermittent Home Oxygen Therapy

Based on the reader's current understanding of hypoxemia and treatment concepts, it should be clear that there is no place for empirical O_2 therapy for dyspnea in the absence of hypoxemia. Likewise, there is no medical justification for O_2 therapy on an as-needed basis. However, long-term intermittent as opposed to continuous O_2 therapy may be administered in the home to individuals who are hypoxemic only under conditions of sleep and exercise. Owing to technological constraints, arterial blood gas measurements are generally not practical during studies of sleep and exercise, and one must rely on pulse oximetry data. What constitutes a "significant" duration and degree of desaturation from a clinical and a certification standpoint is somewhat arbitrary. HCFA currently accepts any decrease in ambient air SaO_2 to less than 89 percent during sleep or exercise as documentation of need. Although short-term medical benefits of O_2 during exercise and sleep can be demonstrated, whether there are definite long-term benefits is unclear.

Prescribing Oxygen Flow

Clearly, the presence of hypoxemia should be carefully demonstrated. It is also important to document that hypoxemia is relieved with O_2 administration. Pulse oximetry (or arterial blood gases) should be used to confirm that supplemental O_2 administered at rest increases the SaO_2 to 90 percent or above (or the PaO_2 to greater than 60 mmHg). The resting O_2 flow required to achieve that value should be noted on the prescription. Since patients will uniformly require increased O_2 flow during activity, pulse oximetry should be used to objectively titrate flow during ambulation and that flow should also be noted in the prescription. In some individuals it might also be important to evaluate O_2 requirement during sleep and to define that flow in the O_2 prescription as well.

It is well known that patients with hypoxemia and chronic hypercapnia who receive supplemental O_2 may demonstrate an increase in $PaCO_2$ and a concomitant decrease in pH. However, as discussed in Chapter 63 and illustrated in Figure 63-3, the changes in $PaCO_2$ and pH are related to O_2 flow and the magnitude of the subsequent PaO_2 elevation.[120] Vast clinical experience around the world suggests that only minor and clinically insignificant hypercapnia results when supplemental O_2 is judiciously used to elevate PaO_2 to a range between 55 and 75 mmHg. The real medical concern would be if supplemental O_2 were withheld because of fear of hypercapnia; the deleterious effects of untreated hypoxemia are quite clear.[9] As a final point on this issue, patients with hypercapnia should have O_2 therapy monitored by resting arterial blood measurements rather than by oximetry so that $PaCO_2$ and pH can also be evaluated.

Confirmation That the Oxygen Prescription Is Adequate

Pulse oximetry or arterial blood gas measurements can confirm that the O_2 flows are adequate through intermittent spot checks. As with other prescribed medications, the appropriate dose or flow requirement for O_2 may change over time. Variations are generally due to alterations in the patient's clinical condition. In addition to actual measurements of blood O_2, changes in blood hematocrit or peripheral edema may signal alterations in end-organ failure due to hypoxemia.

Patients are often quite variable in their acceptance of continuous O_2, and compliance may be influenced by how well the delivery source and device are matched to the patient's needs. Therefore, the clinician must periodically inquire about compliance on supplemental O_2. Increased efforts in patient education or changes in the O_2 source and/or delivery device may be necessary to maximize patient compliance and thereby improve both the quality and duration of life.

The Home Care Provider

The home care provider must play an integral role in long-term O_2 therapy. This health care professional must interface with the hospital respiratory care practitioner, discharge planner, and physician to make certain that the transition from hospital to home is a smooth one. The home care respiratory care practitioner periodically evaluates and educates the patient and the family; home care providers must also periodically check to make certain that the O_2 delivery equipment is functioning properly. Owing both to cost constraints of capitalization of equipment and to logistic problems encountered in rural areas, individual home care companies may not be able to provide all types of O_2 equipment to all patients. However, the physician, the hospital-based respiratory care practitioner (or nurse), and the home care provider all have the common goal of offering the highest quality of care to the O_2-dependent patient.

References

1. Barach AL: The therapeutic use of oxygen. JAMA 1922;79:693–698
2. Petty TL, Nett LM: The history of long-term oxygen therapy. Respir Care 1983;28:859–865
3. Cotes JE, Gilson JC: Effect of oxygen in exercise ability in chronic respiratory insufficiency: Use of portable apparatus. Lancet 1956;1:822–826
4. Levine BE, Bigelow DB, Hamstra RD et al: The role of long-term continuous oxygen administration in patients with chronic airway obstruction with hypoxemia. Ann Intern Med 1967;66:639–650
5. Petty TL, Finigan MM: Clinical evaluation of prolonged ambulatory oxygen therapy in chronic airway obstruction. Am J Med 1968;45:242–252
6. Neff TA, Petty TL: Long-term continuous oxygen therapy in chronic airway obstruction: Mortality in relationship to cor pulmonale, hypoxemia and hypercapnia. Ann Intern Med 1970;72:621–626
7. Abraham AS, Cole RB, Bishop JM: Reversal of pulmonary hypertension by prolonged oxygen administration to patients with chronic bronchitis. Circ Res 1968;23:147–157
8. Nocturnal Oxygen Therapy Trial Group: Continuous or nocturnal oxygen therapy in hypoxemic chronic obstructive lung disease. A clinical trial. Ann Intern Med 1980;93:391–398
9. Report of the Medical Research Council Working Party: Long term domiciliary oxygen therapy in chronic hypoxic cor pulmonale complicating chronic bronchitis and emphysema. Lancet 1981;1:681–685

10. Petty TL: Home oxygen therapy around the world. pp. 660–668. In Christopher KL (guest ed): Problems in Respiratory Care: The Current Status of Oxygen Therapy. JB Lippincott, Philadelphia, 1990
11. Lucas J: Selecting the optimal oxygen system. pp. 59–93. In Lucas J, Golish JA, Sleeper G, O'Ryan JA (eds): Home Respiratory Care. Appleton & Lange, East Norwalk, CT, 1988
12. McPherson SP: Respiratory Therapy Equipment. 3rd Ed. CV Mosby, St. Louis, 1985
13. Tiep BL, Nicotra B, Carter R et al: A new oxygen saving nasal cannula. Am Rev Respir Dis 1983;127(4, pt 2):86
14. Tiep BL, Nicotra B, Carter R et al: Evaluation of a low flow oxygen conserving nasal cannula. Am Rev Respir Dis 1984;130:500–502
15. Tiep BL, Nicotra B, Carter R et al: Evaluation of an oxygen-conserving nasal cannula. Respir Care 1985;30:19–25
16. Tiep BL, Belman MJ, Mittman C et al: A new pendant storage oxygen-conserving nasal cannula. Chest 1985;87:381–383
17. Tiep BL, Burns M, Hererra J: A new pendant oxygen-conserving cannula which allows pursed lips breathing. Chest 1989;95:857–860
18. Tiep BL: Long-term oxygen therapy. Clin Chest Med 1990;11:505–522
19. Soffer M, Tashkin DP, Shapiro BJ et al: Conservation of oxygen supply using a reservoir nasal cannula in hypoxemic patients at rest and during exercise. Chest 1985;88:663–668
20. Moore-Gillon JC, George RJ, Geddes DM: An oxygen conserving nasal cannula. Thorax 1985;40:817–819
21. Gould GA, Hayhurst MD, Scott W, Flenley DC: Clinical assessment of oxygen conserving devices in chronic bronchitis and emphysema. Thorax 1985;40:820–824
22. Hayhurst MD, Fourie ATJ, Begg MR: A new low-flow oxygen-conserving cannula. S Afr Med J 1987;71:251–252
23. Hussey JD, Massey LA, Lakshminarayan S: Evaluation of the effect of a reservoir cannula on oxygen saturation during rest and exercise in patients with COPD, abstracted. Respir Care 1985;30:888
24. Leger P, Perrin F, Robert D: Evaluation of three oxygen saving devices. Am Rev Respir Dis 1985;131:A100
25. Gonzales S, Huntington D, Remo R, Light RW: Efficacy of the oxymizer pendant in reducing oxygen requirements of hypoxemic patients. Respir Care 1986;31:681–688
26. Carter R, Williams JS, Berry J et al: Evaluation of the pendant oxygen conserving nasal cannula during exercise. Chest 1986;89:806–810
27. Claiborne RA, Paynter DE, Dutt AK: Evaluation of the use of an oxygen conservation device in long term oxygen therapy. Am Rev Respir Dis 1987;136:1095–1098
28. Pflug AE, Cheney FW, Butler J: Evaluation of an intermittent oxygen flow system. Am Rev Respir Dis 1972;105:449–452
29. Robert D, Perrin F, Leger P: Oxygen savings device for COPD patients under oxygen therapy. Am Rev Respir Dis 1983;85(4, pt 2):111
30. Robert D, Leger P, Perrin F: Evaluation of an intermittent flow oxygen system. Bull Eur Physiopathol Respir 1986;22:315–318
31. Mecikalski M, Shigeoka JW: A demand valve conserves oxygen in subjects with chronic obstructive pulmonary disease. Chest 1984;86:667–670
32. Rinow ME, Saltzman AR: Effectiveness of a new oxygen demand valve in chronic hypoxemia. Chest 1984;86:312A
33. Crabb K, Kerby GR, Pingleton SK, Bracken K: Evaluation of an intermittent flow system for delivery of oxygen via nasal cannula in patients with stable cardiopulmonary disease, abstracted. Chest 1984;86:312
34. Floreani A, Kerby GR, Whitman RA, Shippy MB. Evaluation of a demand flow oxygen delivery device, abstracted. Chest 1986;89:484s
35. Senn S, Wanger J, Fernandez E, Cherniack RM. Efficacy of a pulsed oxygen delivery device during exercise in patients with chronic respiratory disease. Chest 1989;96:467–472
36. Bower JS, Brook CJ, Zimmer K, Davis D: Performance of a demand oxygen saver system during rest, exercise, and sleep in hypoxemic patients. Chest 1988;94:77–80
37. Romberger DJ, Kerby GR, Hanson FN et al: Comparison of continuous and pulse flow oxygen in hospital patients. Am Rev Respir Dis 1988;137:158A
38. Brook CJ, Bower FS, Davis DM et al: Performance of a demand oxygen saver system during rest, exercise and sleep in hypoxemic patients. Am Rev Respir Dis 1986;33:209A
39. Auerbach D, Flick MR, Block AJ: A new oxygen cannula system using intermittent-demand nasal flow. Chest 1978;74:39–44
40. Anderson WM, Ryerson G, Block AJ: Evaluation of an intermittent demand nasal oxygen flow system with a fluidic valve, abstracted. Chest 1984;86:313
41. Altman FM, Block AJ: Evaluation of a fluidic intermittent flow system for the delivery of nasal oxygen, abstracted. Am Rev Respir Dis 1981;112:105
42. Franco MA, Llompart JA, Teague R et al: Pulse dose oxygen delivery system, abstracted. Respir Care 1984;29:1034A
43. Tiep BL, Nicotra MB, Carter R et al: Low-concentration oxygen therapy via a demand oxygen delivery system. Chest 1985;87:636–638
44. Moore LP, Hillard DW, Block AJ: Product validation for the intermittent demand oxygen system (Oxymatic), abstracted. Am Rev Respir Dis 1986;133(4, pt 2):210
45. Tiep BL, Carter R, Nicotra MB et al: Demand oxygen delivery during exercise. Chest 1987;91:15–20
46. Tremper JC, Campbell SC, Kelly SJ et al: Reliability of the electronic oxygen conserver, abstracted. Am Rev Respir Dis 1987;135(4, pt 2):194
47. Carter R, Tashkin D, Djahed B et al: Demand oxygen delivery for patients with restrictive lung disease, abstracted. Chest 1987;92:154
48. Carter R, Tashkin D, Djahed B et al: Demand oxygen delivery for patients with restrictive lung disease. Chest 1989;96:1307–1311
49. Heimlich, HJ: Respiratory rehabilitation with transtracheal oxygen system. Ann Otol Rhinol Laryngol 1982;91:643–647
50. Kirilloff LH, Dauber JH, Ferson PF, Openbrier DR: Nasal cannula and transtracheal delivery of oxygen, abstracted. Chest 1984;86:313
51. Leger P, Gerard M, Mercatello A, Robert D: Transtracheal catheter for oxygen therapy of patients requiring high oxygen flow, abstracted. Respiration, suppl. 1, 1984;46:103
52. Hoddes E, Spofford BT, Christopher KL et al: Treatment of obstructive sleep apnea syndrome with transtracheal gas delivery, abstracted. Sleep Res 1985;14:164
53. Bloom BS, Daniel J, Kissick WL et al: Transtracheal portable oxygen in chronic pulmonary disease, abstracted. Am Rev Respir Dis 1985;131(4, pt 2):A112
54. Heimlich HJ, Carr GC: Transtracheal catheter technique for pulmonary rehabilitation. Ann Otol Rhinol Laryngol 1985;94:502–504
55. Spofford BT, Christopher KL: The ITOT manual for transtracheal oxygen therapy. Institute for Transtracheal Oxygen Therapy, Denver, 1986
56. Christopher KL, Spofford BT, Brannin PK, Petty TL: Transtracheal oxygen therapy for refractory hypoxemia. JAMA 1986;256:494–497
57. Christopher KL, Spofford BT, Brannin PK, Petty TL. The safety, efficacy and efficiency of a new transtracheal procedure and catheter, abstracted. Am Rev Respir Dis 1986;133:A209
58. Spofford BT, Christopher KL, Hoddes ES: Transtracheal oxygen for obstructive sleep apnea, abstracted. Chest 1986;89:485S
59. Heimlich HJ, Carr GC: Transtracheal oxygen for chronic lung disease, abstracted. Chest 1986;89:484S
60. Christopher KL, Spofford BT, Hoddes E et al: Pulse transtracheal oxygen therapy, abstracted. Chest 1986;89:486S

61. Leger P, Gerard M, Robert D: Home use of transtracheal catheter for long term oxygen therapy of 30 chronic respiratory insufficiency patients, abstracted. Chest 1986;89:486S
62. Spofford BT, Christopher KL: Tight control of oxygenation, abstracted. Chest 1986;89:486S
63. Banner NR, Govan JR: Long term transtracheal oxygen delivery through microcatheter in patients with hypoxemia due to chronic obstructive airways disease. Br Med J 1986;293:111–114
64. Hoffman LA, Dauber JH, Ferson PF et al: Patient response to transtracheal oxygen delivery. Am Rev Respir Dis 1987;135:153–156
65. Wesmiller SW, Hoffman LA, Dauber JH et al: Exercise tolerance during nasal cannula and transtracheal catheter oxygen administration, abstracted. Am Rev Respir Dis 1987;135:A280
66. Cary JM, Johnson LP, Davido JL: The transtracheal oxygen catheter: A new and efficient system for long term oxygen needs, abstracted. Am Rev Respir Dis 1987;135:A410
67. Petrun MD, McCarty DC, Spofford BT, Christopher KL: Pulse oxygen delivery via transtracheal catheter, abstracted. Chest 1987;92:154S
68. Christopher KL, Spofford BT: Transtracheal oxygen therapy. Pulmonary and Critical Care Update. American College of Chest Physicians 1987;lesson 28:1–7
69. Cary JM, Johnson LP, Davido JL: Successful continuous oxygen therapy using an intra-tracheal catheter, abstracted. Chest 1987;92:153S
70. Spofford B, Christopher K, McCarty D, Goodman J: Transtracheal oxygen therapy: A guide for the respiratory therapist. Respir Care 1987;32:345–352
71. Stoller J, Stelmach K, Ahmad M: Type and frequency of complications of transtracheal oxygen therapy with the SCOOP system, abstracted. Chest 1987;92:155S
72. Johnson LP, Cary JM: The implanted intratracheal oxygen catheter. Surg Gynecol Obstet 1987;165:75–76
73. Christopher KL, Spofford BT, Petrun MD et al: A program for transtracheal oxygen delivery: Assessment of safety and efficacy. Ann Intern Med 1987;107:802–808
74. Wesmiller SW, Hoffman LA, Dauber JH et al: Twelve minute walk distance during nasal cannula and transtracheal oxygen delivery, abstracted. Am Rev Respir Dis 1988;137:A156
75. Hoffman LA, Dauber JH, Wesmiller SW et al: Nasal cannula and transtracheal oxygen: A comparison of patients response following six months use of each technique, abstracted. Am Rev Respir Dis 1988;137:A156
76. Hansen LA, Scanlon PD, Staats BA et al: Transtracheal oxygen catheters do not reduce oxygen requirements for most patients, abstracted. Am Rev Respir Dis 1988;137:A157
77. Spofford BT, Christopher KL, Petty TL et al: Why do patients want transtracheal oxygen? abstracted. Am Rev Respir Dis 1988;137:A157
78. Dewan NA, Dell CW, O'Donohue WJ et al: Smell and taste function in patients with transtracheal oxygen therapy, abstracted. Am Rev Respir Dis 1988;137:A445
79. Bell CW, O'Donohue WJ, Dewan N, Anderson B: Exercise tolerance improves following implementation of transtracheal oxygen therapy, abstracted. Am Rev Respir Dis 1988;137:A515
80. Elmer JC, Farney RJ, Walker JM et al: The comparison of transtracheal oxygen with other therapies for obstructive sleep apnea, abstracted. Am Rev Respir Dis 1988;137:A311
81. Rollins DR, Hoak A, Heggestad J, Shyrock S: Improved exercise tolerance documented in transtracheal oxygen therapy patients enrolled in a pulmonary conditioning program, abstracted. Am Rev Respir Dis 1988;137:A481
82. Couser J, Martinez F, Make B: Respiratory tract infection as a possible complication in patients using transtracheal oxygen, abstracted. Chest 1988;94:32S
83. Frye K, Shukla L, Selecky P: A new device for transtracheal oxygen therapy in patients with cuffless tracheostomy tubes, abstracted. Chest 1988;94:32S
84. Hansen LA, Staats BA, Scanlon PD et al: Transtracheal oxygen therapy: Long term follow-up, abstracted. Chest 1988;94:32S
85. Tiep BL, Christopher KL, Spofford BT et al: Pulsed transtracheal oxygen, abstracted. Chest 1988;94:91S
86. Simpson RL, Spofford BT, Goodman JR et al: SCOOP transtracheal oxygen: tract problems, abstracted. Respir Care 1988;33:921
87. Fletcher EC, Nickeson D, Costarangos-Galarza C: Endotracheal mass resulting from a transtracheal oxygen catheter. Chest 1988;93:438–439
88. Christopher KL: At-home administration of oxygen. pp 9–18. In Kacmarek RM, Stroller JK (eds): Current Respiratory Care. DC Decker, Toronto, 1988
89. Bell CW, O'Donohue WJ, Dewan NA et al: Effects of transtracheal oxygen therapy on exercise capacity. J Cardiopulmon Rehabil 1988;11:449–452
90. Couser JI, Make BJ: Transtracheal oxygen decreases inspired minute ventilation. Am Rev Respir Dis 1989;139:627–631
91. Heimlich HJ, Gerson CC: The Micro-Trach: A seven-year experience with transtracheal oxygen therapy. Chest 1989;95:1008–1012
92. Bergofsky EH, Hurewitz AN: Airway insufflation: Physiologic effects on acute and chronic gas exchange in humans. Am Rev Respir Dis 1989;140:885–890
93. Johnson RC, Kollef MH, Browning R: Transtracheal oxygen and the perception of dyspnea, abstracted. Am Rev Respir Dis 1989;139:A9
94. Bloom BS, Daniel JM, Wiseman M et al: Transtracheal oxygen delivery and patients with chronic obstructive pulmonary disease. Respir Med 1989;83:281–288
95. Caras WE, Perry ME, Blue PW et al: Ventilatory effects of transtracheal oxygenation (tto), abstracted. Am Rev Respir Dis 1989;139:A445
96. Evans RB, Hanes S, Kennedy W: Transtracheal oxygen improves FEV_1 and weight, abstracted. Chest 1989;96:230S
97. Christopher KL, Murry I, Simpson R et al: Transtracheal augmentation of ventilation, abstracted. Chest 1989;96:174S
98. Cannizzaro GF, Zanoli P, Pivirotto F, Pesce L: Transtracheal catheter don't seem to represent a path for bacterial colonization, abstracted. Chest 1989;96:283S
99. Schaten MA, Christopher KL, Goodman S et al: High-flow transtracheal oxygen: A promixing technique for the management of hypercarbic respiratory failure, abstracted. Chest 1990;98:22S
100. Benditt JO, Rassulo J, Celli BR: Work of breathing during direct tracheal O_2 administration in patients with severe chronic lung disease. Am Rev Respir Dis 1990;141:A883
101. Tiep BL, Christopher KL, Spofford BT et al: Pulsed nasal and transtracheal oxygen delivery. Chest 1990;97:364–368
102. Yaeger ES, Christopher KL, Goodman S et al: Transtracheal and nasal oxygen: and assessment of pulse and continuous flow, abstracted. Chest 1990;98:21S
103. Wesmiller SW, Hoffman LA, Sciurba FC et al: Exercise tolerance during nasal cannula and transtracheal oxygen delivery. Am Rev Respir Dis 1990;141:789–791
104. Chauncey JB, Aldrich MS: Preliminary findings in the treatment of obstructive sleep apnea with transtracheal oxygen. Sleep 1990;13:167–174
105. Adamo JP, Mehta AC, Stelmach K et al: The Cleveland Clinic's experience with transtracheal oxygen therapy. Respir Care 1990;35:153–160
106. Sciurba FC, Hoffman LA, Wesmiller SW et al: Compensation of spirometric measurements during delivery of transtracheal oxygen. Am Rev Respir Dis 1990;141:A880
107. Winn RE, Kollef MH: Use of transtracheal catheter for treatment of hypoxic respiratory failure when mechanical ventilation was refused. Crit Care Med 1990;18:1498
108. Burton G, Wagshul FA, Kime W, Henderson D: Fatal mucus-ball obstruction of the central airway in a transtracheal oxygen therapy patient, abstracted. Respir Care 1990;35:1143

109. Walsh DA, Govan JR: Long term continuous domiciliary oxygen therapy by transtracheal catheter. Thorax 1990;45:478–481
110. Hoffman LA, Johnson JT, Wesmiller SW et al: Transtracheal delivery of oxygen: Efficacy and safety for long-term continuous therapy. Ann Otol Rhinol Laryngol 1991;100:108–115
111. Dewan NA, Bell CW, O'Donohue WJ et al: Sequelae and complications during long-term follow-up of transtracheal oxygen therapy (TTO_2), abstracted. Am Rev Respir Dis, suppl. 1991;143:A78
112. Hoffman LA, Johnson JT, Wesmiller SW et al: Transtracheal delivery of oxygen: efficacy and safety for long-term therapy, abstracted. Am Rev Respir Dis, suppl. 1991;143:A79
113. Levi-Valensi P, Aubry P, Rida Z et al: Selection of patients for long-term oxygen therapy (lto). Eur Respir J, suppl. 7, 1989;2:624s–629s
114. Levi-Valensi P, Weitzenblum E, Pedinielli J et al: Three-month follow-up of arterial blood gas determination in candidates for long-term oxygen therapy. Am Rev Respir Dis 1986;133:547–551
115. Conference on Home Oxygen Therapy: Problems in prescribing and supplying oxygen for Medicare patients. Am Rev Respir Dis 1986;134:340–341
116. Second Conference on Long-Term Oxygen Therapy: Further recommendations for prescribing and supplying long-term oxygen therapy. Am Rev Respir Dis 1988;138:745
117. Consensus Conference Report: New problems in supply, reimbursement and certification of medical necessity for long-term oxygen therapy. Am Rev Respir Dis 1990;142:721–724
118. O'Donohue WJ: Effect of oxygen therapy on increasing arterial oxygen tension in hypoxemic patients with stable chronic obstructive pulmonary disease while breathing ambient air. Chest 1991;100:968–972
119. Weitzenblum E, Sautegeau A, Ehrhart M et al: Long-term oxygen therapy can reverse the progression of pulmonary hypertension in patients with chronic obstructive pulmonary disease. Am Rev Respir Dis 1985;131:493–498
120. Nolte D: Nutzen und Gefahren der Sauerstofftherapie bei chronischer Ateminsuffiezienz. Wien Med Wochenschr 1976;126:325–329
121. Goodman JR: Delivery sources for home oxygen therapy. p. 563. In Christopher KL (ed): Problems in Respiratory Care: The Current Status of Oxygen Therapy. JB Lippincott, Philadelphia, 1990

Chapter 100

Travel for Patients with Chronic Respiratory Disease

Kent L. Christopher

CHAPTER OUTLINE

One of the most distressing symptoms described by patients with chronic lung disease is the sensation of profound shortness of breath with exertion. Patients who experience this extremely unpleasant sensation often respond by further reducing their activities of daily living. Ironically, the subsequent reduction in activity results in additional physiologic compromise as well as a heightened fear of any form of exertion. It is hoped that these individuals with chronic respiratory disease will continue to remain active and venture outside the home.

When a healthy person thinks of travel, transportation to distant and exotic places by trains, planes, and automobiles generally comes to mind. However, for a patient with severe disabling lung disease, travel may simply represent walking to the mailbox to pick up the daily mail or shopping at the grocery store. Even this degree of limited activity can be a frightening experience for some patients. Pulmonary rehabilitation programs can play a major role by increasing functional capacity and giving the patient confidence to travel outside the home. In addition, pulmonary rehabilitation programs often incorporate some form of organized, medically supervised travel experience. This chapter first addresses general considerations for travel for patients with chronic respiratory disease and then focuses on special issues that relate to traveling with supplemental O_2.

GENERAL CONSIDERATIONS

Patients with chronic respiratory disease who venture outside the home must do more planning than healthy individuals. These patients often must follow a complicated regimen of medications, and flexibility in drug administration may be necessary during travel. For example, to prevent a frustrating search for a rest room while traveling, diuretics should be given early or withheld until a more practical time. Furthermore, a hand-held, compressor-driven nebulizer may be used in the home, but a metered dose inhaler is more practical during travel. In addition, some spacer devices may be easier to carry in the pocket or purse than others. If a compressor is necessary during travel, light weight, compact, and even battery-operated nebulizers are commercially available. The physician must keep these issues in mind when writing prescriptions and educating patients about the proper use of medications. Patients may also have special needs that facilitate travel but require some form of special authorization or prescription, such as a handicapped parking permit, prescription for a walker or wheelchair, or authorization for O_2 during flight.

A prescription is limited to the states in which a valid medical license is held, and individuals traveling outside those states must take along an adequate supply of medications.

Since patients with chronic respiratory disease are prone to decompensation due to infections, increased airflow obstruction, and cor pulmonale, it may be good planning to give patients additional prescriptions to fill and carry with them on the trip. These extra medications might include a course of a broad-spectrum antibiotic (such as ampicillin or cefaclor), a diuretic, and a potassium supplement or a course of oral corticosteroids. If patients are experiencing difficulty when traveling out of town, they should be encouraged to call their physician long distance (just as they would if they were at home). A physician who concludes that sufficient information has been obtained over the phone to warrant treatment can instruct the patient to take the "extra" medications and avoid an unnecessary trip to an unfamiliar doctor or emergency department.

Patients should carry a formal list of their medications and dosages. No matter what the means of transportation, individuals should also be instructed to keep a few days' supply of medication on their person at all times. Even for a relatively short trip, the entire supply of medications should not be checked with the baggage, as baggage can be lost, damaged, or misplaced. If a major trip is planned, the patient should be given a letter of introduction that can be used if out-of-town medical attention is necessary. The letter may prove invaluable during an emergency if it describes the patient's diagnoses, pertinent laboratory results, treatment plan, and, when applicable, discussions and conclusions regarding the patient's wishes regarding intubation, mechanical ventilation, and resuscitation. Finally, the physician may be able to supply the patient with the names of other qualified doctors in practice at the travel destination. If the physician does not personally know someone in that area, the directories supplied by organizations such as the American College of Chest Physicians or The American Thoracic Society may give some leads. Finally, the names of board-certified pulmonologists can be requested from the medical staff office of local hospitals.

Though some individuals with chronic respiratory disease are capable of traveling independently by automobile and a variety of other means of transportation, patients with more advanced disease should travel with a companion. The ideal companion is a spouse or immediate family member with an empathy for the patient and an understanding of the patient's physical limitations as well as medical and psychological needs. The companion should encourage disabled elderly individuals to establish routines (or even ritualistic behavior) to allow them to both prepare for and cope with trips as simple as a visit to the doctor or the grandchildren. After some experience with more routine trips, the companion can become very accomplished at predicting the extra time needed to make appointments and can become skilled at finding close parking and access to elevators and escalators.

DAY-TO-DAY TRAVEL BY PUBLIC TRANSPORTATION AND AUTOMOBILES

Day-to-day public transportation by bus, train, ferry, subway, or trolley is often appealing to the young, healthy individual. However, the physical constraints and demands of mass transit may outweigh the economic and logistic advantages for the patient with advanced pulmonary disease. Elderly disabled patients may occasionally use a taxi, and it is essential that the taxi drivers remain courteous and calm in the face of the increased demands placed on them by the disabled. However, given an option, most patients with severe chronic respiratory disease prefer to rely on transportation by family and friends rather than public transportation. In this case, the driver often becomes the "companion" described previously. Although patients are often surprisingly adaptable for short trips, the characteristics of the automobile chosen for transportation may be an important issue. For example, elderly patients with lung, heart, or rheumatologic disorders may find it difficult to get in and out of either a compact car or a four-wheel drive vehicle that is relatively high off the ground. Furthermore, individuals with severe dyspnea can be very sensitive to extremes of temperature, and an automobile with a controlled temperature environment will be greatly appreciated.

Overall, automobiles have become the standard means of day-to-day transportation, and it is remarkable that many patients continue to drive safely in spite of their severe pulmonary disease. However, physicians and other health care providers may rarely encounter patients with a severe physical or cognitive disability who continue to drive automobiles in spite of obvious limitations. If it is concluded that driving an automobile would be potentially dangerous to the driver or others, the patient must be confronted about the issue. If the patient is unreceptive, it may be productive to include family or friends in the discussion. Clinicians can be torn between patient confidentiality and public safety. On a state-by-state basis, there are resources available (including the department of motor vehicles) that can assist in resolving this important issue. If it is concluded that the patient will not drive, family and friends may offer transportation and the clinician may draw on other resources by directing the patient to a variety of social services.

TRAVELING FOR RECREATIONAL ACTIVITIES

Patients with severe pulmonary disability will often conclude that their disease is not going to get the best of them when it comes to use of various means of transportation for enjoyment. Figure 100-1A depicts a patient receiving continuous O_2 whose spirit was undaunted when it came to the challenge of horseback riding. She also learned that an electric golf cart and continuous transtracheal O_2 (Fig. 100-1B) allowed her to continue to play golf in spite of severe pulmonary disease.

As a result of the efforts of organized support groups such as Emphysema Anonymous, better breather clubs, and a variety of pulmonary rehabilitation programs, patients with chronic respiratory disease can engage in group travel for recreational purposes. Early on, these support groups had a very difficult time convincing the management of corpora-

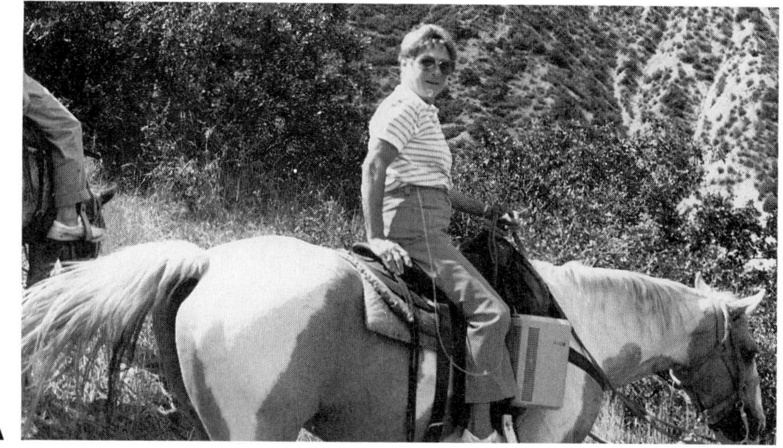

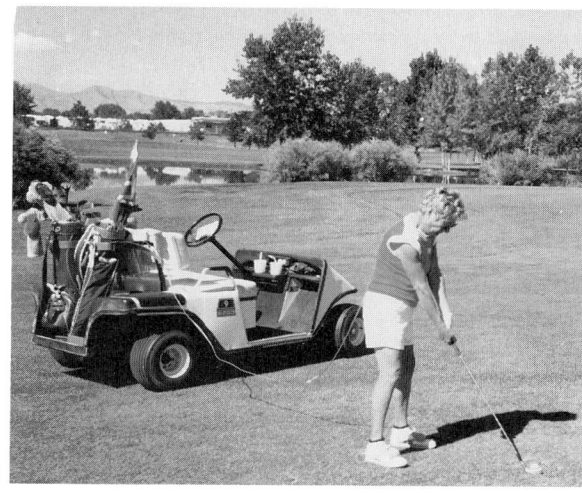

Figure 100-1. A patient who receives supplemental O_2 via transtracheal catheter **(A)** rides horseback in the Rocky Mountains and **(B)** uses an electric golf cart so that she can continue to play golf.

tions to allow a number of patients with advanced pulmonary disease to use their travel services. With perseverance, patience, extensive communication, and medical documentation, the support groups were able to convince key management personnel that there was an acceptably low liability in allowing this population of patients to travel using their transportation services. Over the years, many of these patient-oriented organizations have developed expertise in planning and conducting trips by bus, train, aircraft, and even cruise ship.[1] It usually takes a number of weeks or months to properly plan an "expedition," especially when supplemental O_2 is needed. The patient's spouse or close family member or friend is encouraged to accompany the patient and often has as much fun. Medical personnel specifically trained to advise and manage this population of patients (such as respiratory care practitioners, nurses, or pulmonary physicians) usually accompany the group. Observing the patients' enjoyment on these trips has often been so satisfying that the professionals will eagerly volunteer to participate in future trips. Overall, the transportation lines have found this to be a rewarding experience as well. Figure 100-2A shows patients from Ohio and medical staff from Florida taking a stroll aboard a cruise ship bound for Mexico. A tour group of patients with chronic respiratory disease and their companions can be seen in Figure 100-2B as they board a bus in Grand Cayman with the assistance of trained medical personnel.

Experienced organizations that sponsor group travel for patients with chronic pulmonary disease can be very helpful in offering suggestions for a particular trip, such as appropriate dress for the climate, tips on what to bring, prophylaxis for seasickness, and necessary travel documents. They can also help arrange nonstop flights to and from the destination as well as convenient shuttles and assistance with baggage. To assist in the planning, patients should supply information regarding special requirements due to physical limitations or dietary constraints. It is usually necessary for the attending physician to send the sponsoring organization a completed form that gives diagnoses, defines prescribed medication and treatment, and presents results of most re-

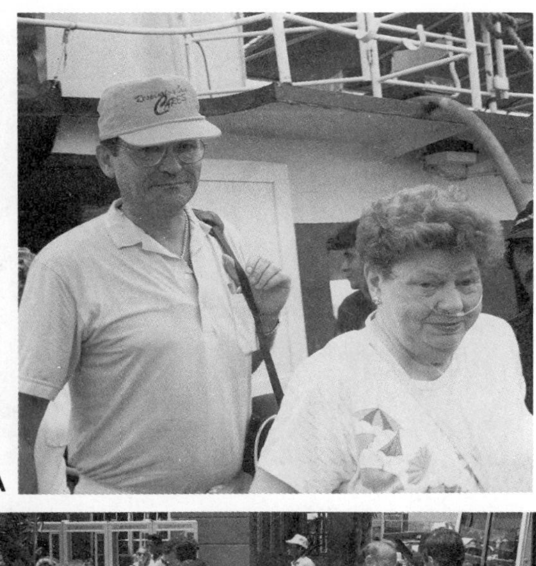

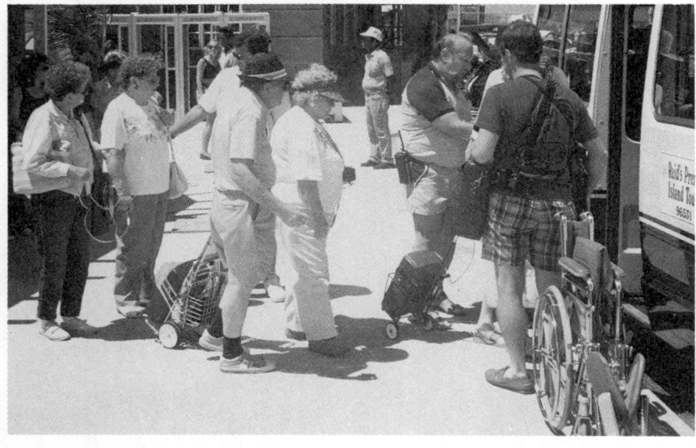

Figure 100-2. **(A)** A patient from Ohio who receives continuous O_2 is assisted by a respiratory care practitioner aboard a cruise ship bound for Cozumel, Mexico. **(B)** A tour group boards a bus in Grand Cayman with the assistance of trained medical personnel. (Photographs courtesy of David W. Robbins, DC, RRT from Robbins and Associates, Coral Gables, FL)

cent pertinent medical tests. A statement that the patient is medically stable and fit for travel is often required. Travel services can be very helpful in assigning extra staff to meet group needs as well as assigning accommodations that are physically convenient, such as aisle seats that are near exits and rest rooms and cabins or hotel rooms to which access does not require excessive walking or stair climbing.

AIR TRAVEL

Patients with chronic respiratory disease who wish to travel by commercial aircraft must do considerable planning before the flight.[2–6] Patients will generally need someone to drop them off at the airport to avoid the long walks carrying luggage from the parking lot. Arrangements with the airlines may need to include transportation from the check-in counter to the gate by either wheelchair or electric cart. If a layover is unavoidable, arrangements for assistance in transportation to connecting flights need to be made, and ample time must be allotted to avoid missing a flight. Most patients are offered the opportunity for early boarding and extra assistance by the flight attendants. As mentioned previously, patients are advised to take an extra supply of all their medications and carry them onto the aircraft. Advance aisle seat selection next to the companion and close to the exit and the rest room is advised. As with any mode of travel that requires prolonged sitting, patients are encouraged to stand and walk briefly in the aisle to prevent thromboembolism (as physical capabilities and flight conditions permit). If there are dietary constraints, special menus must be arranged in advance. Finally, on request most airlines offer wheelchair or electric cart escort on arrival from the gate to the baggage claim area.

Air travel merits some additional discussion in view of the potential deleterious effects of the high altitude encountered during flight.[2–8] Commercial air travel exposes passengers to reduced barometric pressure and thus a reduced ambient

PO_2. Modern aircraft often cruise 30,000 to 40,000 ft above sea level. At an altitude of 40,000 ft the P_IO_2 is only 29 mmHg. The cabins of the aircraft are pressurized to compensate for this dramatically reduced barometric pressure and resultant PaO_2. However, most aircraft maintain a cabin pressure that is less than sea level. The cabin pressures in commercial jet aircraft simulate an altitude between 5000 ft (as in Denver, CO) and 8000 ft (as in Vail, CO). Healthy passengers tend not to suffer any major untoward effects at cruising altitudes. Patients receiving chronic home O_2 who also routinely receive supplemental O_2 during flight can generally compensate by a planned increase in O_2 flow. However, patients who function adequately with a marginal room air PaO_2 at sea level may be at risk for experiencing clinical compromise as a result of hypoxemia during flight.

In an effort to address this issue, a number of studies have been conducted to evaluate the effect of flight on patients with chronic respiratory disease.[9–15] Two important studies were designed to predict blood O_2 levels during flight in this group of pulmonary patients. It was intended that with this knowledge one could predict who might theoretically benefit from supplemental O_2 during flight in commercial jet aircraft. One study[14] measured arterial blood gases during a flight in an unpressurized airplane that simulated cabin pressures typical of commercial air travel. In this group of 13 patients with chronic respiratory disease, the mean PaO_2 decreased from 68 mmHg at sea level to 51 mmHg at a flight altitude of 1650 m. It is interesting that the patients did not experience symptoms attributable to hypoxemia. Furthermore, investigators did not find that the patients had clinically significant decompensation with this degree of transient hypoxemia. In that same study, PaO_2 measured while breathing room air at sea level several weeks before the flight did not correlate with the blood gases measured at altitude. However, arterial blood gas levels measured 2 hours before the flight with either room air or a hypoxic gas mixture (17.2 percent O_2) did correlate with arterial blood gas levels obtained at altitude. In other study designs patients have been placed in a hypobaric chamber in an effort to simulate conditions during flight. Finally, a regression equation and nomogram were derived in a study[10] done at sea level to estimate PaO_2 at altitudes between 5000 and 10,000 ft in normocapnic patients with chronic airway obstruction.

Even though there is concern that patients with marginal oxygenation on the ground may become transiently more hypoxemic during air travel, the actual clinical impact of short-term hypoxemia in this setting is unknown. A review of the medical literature[16] confirms the general consensus that air travel is relatively safe. True in-flight medical emergencies are rare relative to the high volume of traffic. Air travel is even surprisingly safe as a means of transporting ill patients.[17] There is no evidence to suggest that patients with chronic respiratory disease have a high rate of in-flight hypoxemia-related medical emergencies. Pending future insights, I have some strategies that the reader may wish to consider regarding administration of O_2 during air travel. Certainly, patients with mild to moderate chronic respiratory disease who experience few (if any) symptoms and have normal oxygenation at rest do not need supplemental O_2 during flight. Likewise, patients with advanced disease who require continuous home O_2 (as discussed in Ch. 99) should receive supplemental O_2 on the aircraft (for example, an arbitrary flow of twice the resting requirements on the ground). The cost, inconvenience, and general unavailability of the previously described altitude simulation tests exclude these options as practical clinical tools. Nomograms have merit but do not currently accommodate a patient who has baseline ground tests at an altitude above sea level. Until studies have been done to adequately address the issue, I recommend that a patient who has a marginal resting PaO_2 while breathing room air (e.g., an arbitrary PaO_2 of 56 to 65 mmHg at sea level) should be considered for the administration of supplemental O_2 during flight.

Another dilemma arises when the patient described above has a marginal PaO_2 at home but will spend a number of days or weeks at a travel destination that is at a much higher altitude. Similarly, patients who require continuous O_2 where they reside at altitude may not require continuous O_2 when they travel closer to sea level. Whenever there is doubt, supplemental O_2 should probably be administered. However, because both pulse oximetry and arterial blood gas levels are readily available in most communities in the United States, it is recommended that patients plan to undergo an objective evaluation for O_2 need on arrival. In fact, resources for medical testing and support can be identified in advance of a scheduled trip.

TRAVELING WITH OXYGEN

Patients with chronic hypoxemia related to severe chronic obstructive pulmonary disease (COPD) were treated with supplemental O_2 as long ago as the late 1960s. Initially, there was a great concern about the safety of placing an O_2 tank in an automobile. After gaining some experience with the concept, it was concluded that it is safe for patients to take their supplemental O_2 source with them in the car. During routine short trips in a standard vehicle, patients can easily place their portable source on the floor of the back seat and receive supplemental O_2 while they sit wherever they wish. Home care providers can advise the patient regarding the appropriate stationary and portable O_2 system for longer trips and instruct the patient on how to safely secure the O_2 source within the vehicle. Recommendations will be based on liter flow requirements, duration of the trip, availability of O_2 refills, needs for a portable unit, size and characteristics of the vehicle used for transportation, needs for supplemental O_2 during overnight stays in motels or hotels, and the availability of assistance in getting the O_2 source in and out of the room. Figure 100-3A shows a transtracheal O_2 patient with her husband as they stand next to the motor home that they are using to tour the United States and Canada. Figure 100-3B shows the stationary liquid system attached to the vehicle. The liquid O_2 is piped into the motor home, and she is able to receive continuous O_2 from the stationary source while in the vehicle, even during sleep. Portable units can be transfilled from the stationary source and used while venturing out of the mobile home.

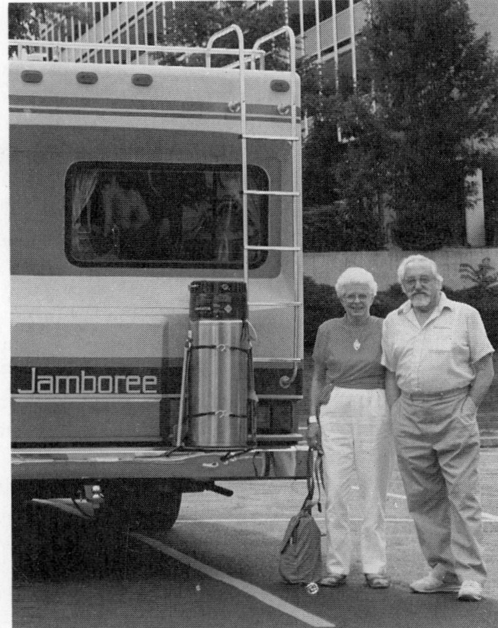

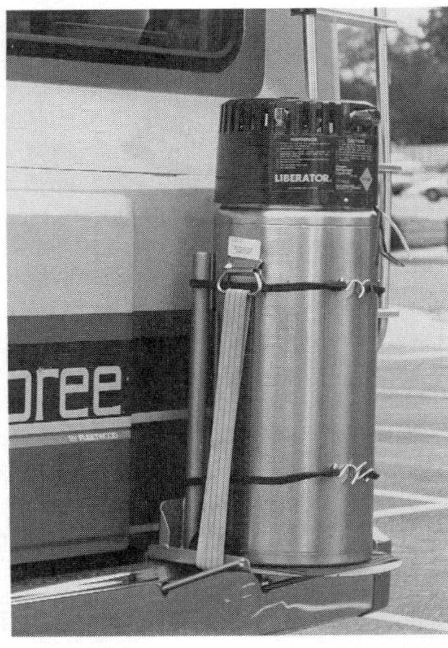

Figure 100-3. **(A)** A patient who receives continuous transtracheal O_2 and her husband stand next to the mobile home that will take them across the United States and Canada. **(B)** The stationary liquid O_2 system is attached to the rear of the vehicle.

With a less elaborate system, the patient in Figure 100-4 demonstrates how he has secured a stationary liquid O_2 source to the back of his van. With transtracheal O_2 his flow requirements are low, and he can use his portable unit while sleeping in a motel at night. As described in Chapter 99, concentrators in the form of a suitcase can be adapted to the dc car battery source to provide O_2 on the road, and an ac power source can be used outside the car. A number of small E or D cylinders stored in the trunk can be used during ambulation. If patients are traveling long distances, particularly out of state, they must make arrangements for refilling their O_2 source. Individuals who have O_2 supplied through a national home care provider can get lists of suppliers across the country. For Medicare patients in the United States, reimbursement under the ''six-point plan'' has adversely affected ability to travel. For example, there is no reimbursement structure to allow a patient to switch from a liquid O_2 source to a suitcase concentrator for a few days out of the month, and multiple home care providers supplying O_2 in liquid or compressed gas form during travel are not eager to split the fixed monthly reimbursement allotted by Medicare.

Air travel for the O_2-dependent patient can be quite complex. There are a few airlines that refuse to accept such patients. Most commercial airlines require at least a 48-hour advance notice for the flight. A written statement from the physician is usually necessary, and the physician may need to discuss the patient's medical condition and O_2 needs with the flight surgeon or airline nurse. The written document can usually be on the physician's letterhead or a prescription pad and must state the patient's diagnosis and indicate that the individual is medically stable and cleared for flight. The prescribed flow rate for O_2 should be noted, and the preferred O_2 delivery device should be specified (for example, cannula, transtracheal O_2 catheter, or mask). Airlines generally supply either a cannula or simple mask, and flight attendants are often totally unfamiliar with alternative delivery devices.

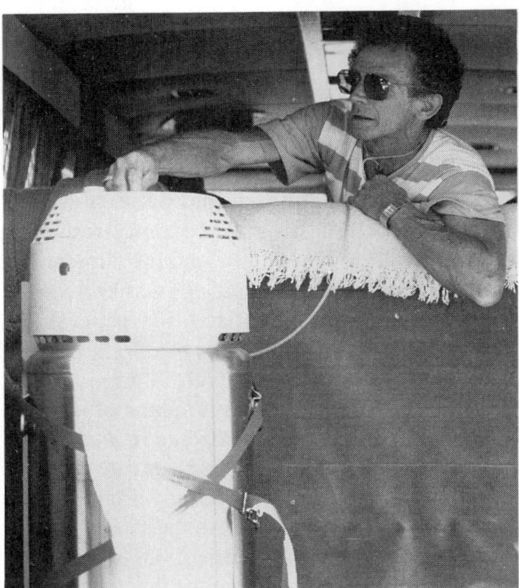

Figure 100-4. A stationary liquid O_2 source is safely secured in the back of this patient's van.

A comment from physicians stating that patients will be responsible for supplying and using their own cannula transtracheal catheter (when only masks are available) or may help.

Uniformly, commercial airlines in the United States will not allow patients to board with their O_2 source, as dictated by Federal Aviation Administration (FAA) regulations. However, patients are responsible for supplying their own O_2 to and from the aircraft. They must also arrange for any O_2 that might be necessary during a layover or transfer to a connecting flight. This policy can create major inconveniences and logistic dilemmas. Figure 100-5A shows the embarrassment of a patient being "frisked" on his way to the gate. According to airline regulations, he was using his own metal-containing liquid O_2 source when the metal detector gave the alarm. A friend had to accompany him to the aircraft to take his portable unit home. When on the plane, he switched to the small compressed gas cylinder (Fig. 100-5B) and connected it to his transtracheal catheter. The patient sat next to his wife during the flight (Fig. 100-5C). Through advance arrangements, a home care provider at his destination brought a portable liquid O_2 source and gave it to him as he left the plane (Fig. 100-5D). Although many home care companies offer this service at no charge, the airlines always charge the patient an additional fee, generally about $50 per flight, for in-flight O_2. If a connecting flight is necessary, even with the same airline, an additional charge is encountered. After accompanying O_2-dependent patients on a number of flights with a variety of airlines, I have concluded that regulators can occasionally be faulty and need to be replaced during flight. Airlines can underestimate the patient's bulk O_2 needs and flight attendants generally need to be more knowledgeable about the O_2 equipment and the special needs of this group of passengers. In spite of these comments, it

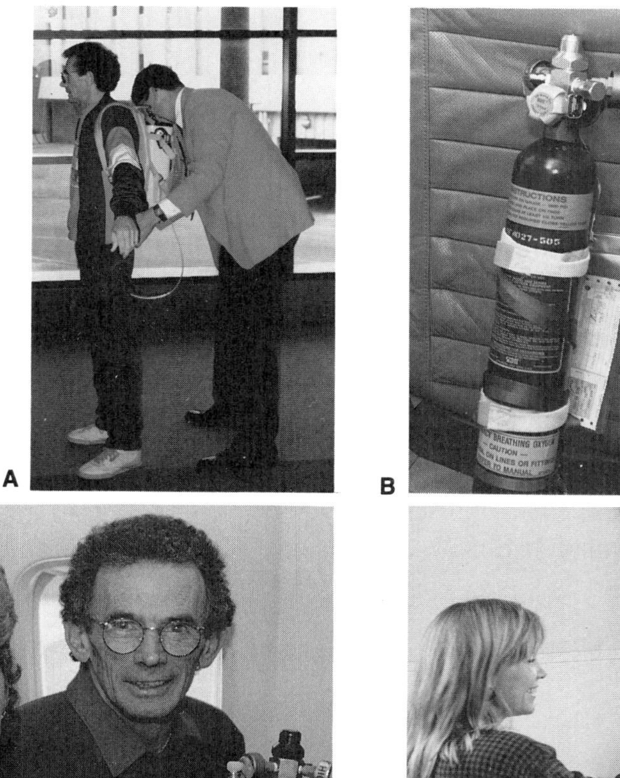

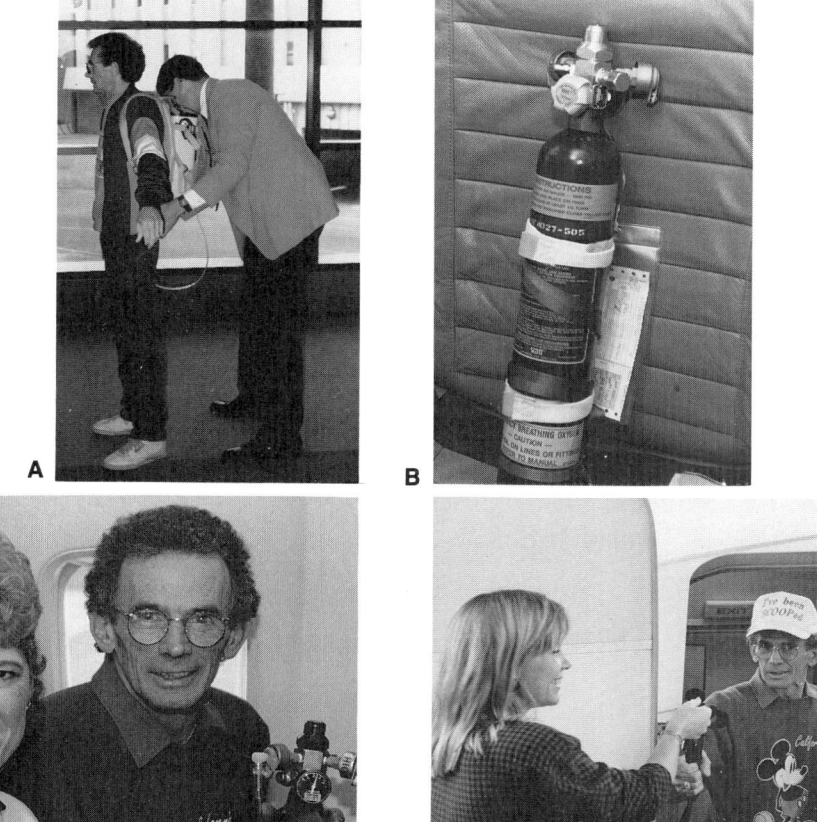

Figure 100-5. **(A)** A patient using a metal-containing portable O_2 source is "frisked" on his way to the gate. **(B)** When on the plane, the airline provides him with a small compressed gas O_2 cylinder. **(C)** His wife accompanies him during flight and **(D)** a homecare provider meets him with O_2 as he leaves the plane after landing at his destination.

must be emphasized that patients generally tolerate flights well. However, to optimize the flight experience for the O_2-dependent, it is imperative that physician, respiratory care practitioner, and patient organizations address these issues with individual airlines and the FAA.

Individual patients requiring supplemental O_2 can also travel by bus, train, or cruise ship. As with air travel, extensive planning and organization are often necessary. Travel out of the country can be done, but is even more complex. Figure 100-6A shows a transtracheal O_2 patient and his wife as they attend the formal "captain's night" aboard a cruise ship on the Atlantic Ocean. The O_2 suitcase used for ambulation aboard ship contains compressed gas cylinders, as shown in Figure 100-6B. As liquid O_2 is not commonly available outside the United States and Canada, this system was found to be the most practical on his extensive travels. The system was used for sightseeing by bus (Fig. 100-6C) as this patient went from castles in Denmark (Fig. 100-7A) to the Tivoli Gardens in Copenhagen (Fig. 100-7B) and visited the windmills in Holland and the Russian Museum in Leningrad (not shown). Arrangements were made with O_2 distributors to stockpile portable compressed gas

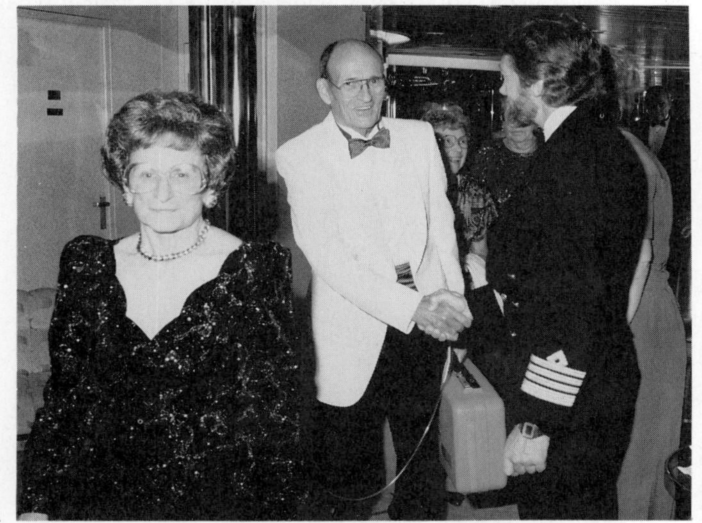

A

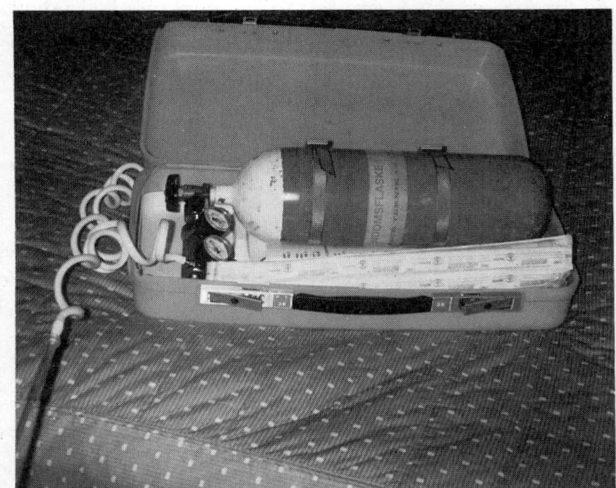

B

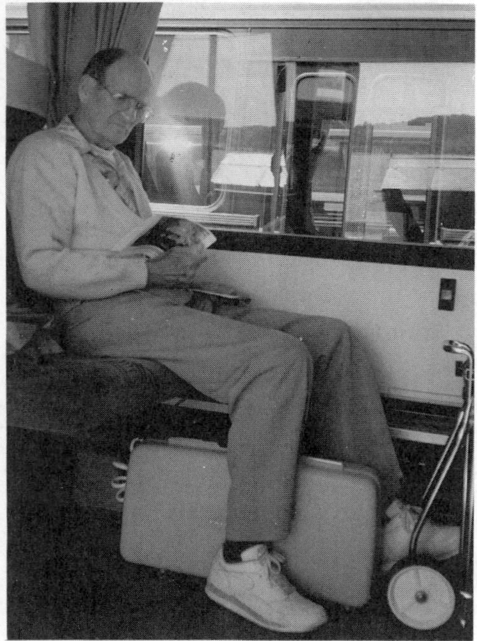

C

Figure 100-6. **(A)** A transtracheal O_2 patient carries his supplemental O_2 source as both he and his wife greet the captain aboard a cruise ship on the Atlantic Ocean. **(B)** The red suitcase conceals a small compressed gas O_2 cylinder. **(C)** The system can also be used in numerous countries while traveling by bus.

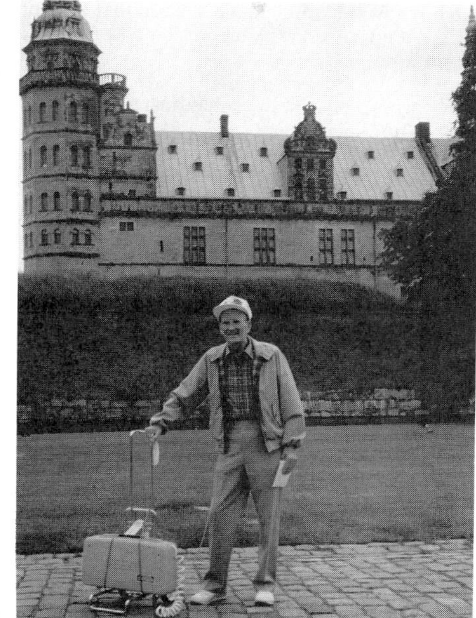

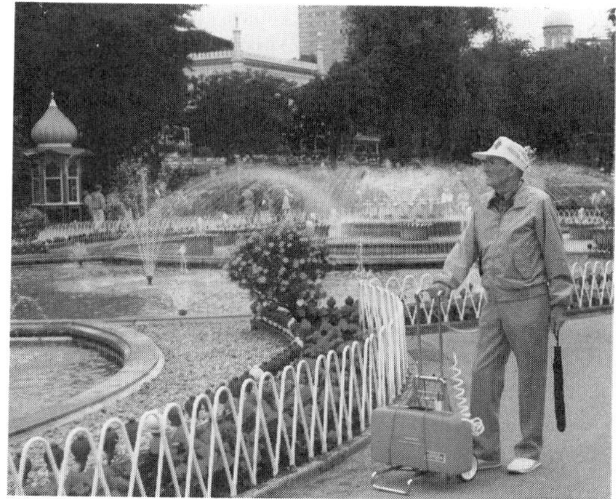

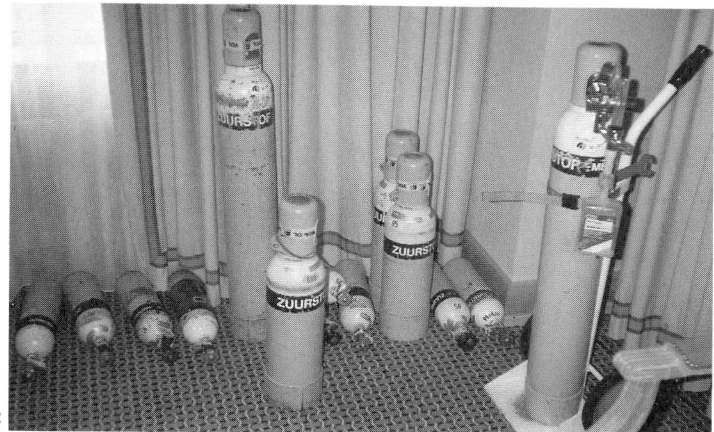

Figure 100-7. This adventurous patient is able to receive continuous supplemental O_2 while he travels from **(A)** castles in Denmark to **(B)** the Tivoli Gardens in Copenhagen. **(C)** To ensure that he has an adequate supply of the easily depleted compressed gas O_2 cylinders, the patient must make arrangements with O_2 suppliers to "stockpile" cylinders in various hotel rooms along his journey.

cylinders in various hotel rooms (Fig. 100-7C). The suitcase concentrator presented in Chapter 99 (Fig. 99-7) was used while in the ship's cabin.

In this modern age individuals must experience some form of travel in order to achieve a higher quality of life. Patients with chronic pulmonary disease are no exception. Travel may be as simple as a short trip by automobile to visit grandchildren on an important holiday; by contrast, travel can be as complex as a trip across Europe while receiving continuous O_2 therapy. My hat is off to any individual suffering from chronic lung disease who is willing to venture outside the home to explore new horizons. As clinicians trained in the care of these patients, we must do everything we can to make exploration of those new horizons possible.

References

1. Burns MR: Cruising with COPD. Am J Nurs 1987:479–482
2. Gong H: Advising pulmonary patients about commercial air travel. J Respir Dis 1990;11:484–499
3. Richards PR: The effects of air travel on passengers with cardiovascular and respiratory diseases. Practitioner 1973;210:232–241
4. Gong H: Air travel and patients with chronic obstructive pulmonary disease, editorial. Ann Intern Med 1984;100:595–597
5. Wachtel TJ: Medical hazards of air travel for older people. Geriatrics 1983;38:78–81
6. Gong H: Advising patients with pulmonary diseases on air travel. Ann Intern Med 1989;111:349–357
7. Aldrete JA, Aldrete LE: Oxygen concentrations in commercial aircraft flights. South Med J 1983;76:12–14

8. Cottrell JJ: Altitude exposures during aircraft flight—flying higher. Chest 1988;92:81–84
9. Gong H, Tashkin DP, Lee EY, Simmons MS: Hypoxia-altitude simulation test. Am Rev Respir Dis 1984;130:980–986
10. Matthys H, Volz H, Ernst H et al: Kardiopulmonale Belastung von Flugpassagieren mit obstruktiven Ventilationsstörungen. Schweiz Med Wochenschr 1974;104:1786–1789
11. Tomashefski JF, Shillito FH, Billings CE, Ashe WF: Effects of moderate altitude on patients with pulmonary and cardiac impairment. West J Med 1964;101:358–362
12. Shillito FH, Tomashefski JF, Ashe WF: The exposure of ambulatory patients to moderate altitudes. Aerospace Med 1963;34:850–857
13. Hartmann B, Unger M, Debelic M, Hilpert P: Blutgaswerte und Atemwegswiderstand bei Gesunden und Patienten mit obstruktiven Atemwegserkrankungen vor und nach Hohenadaptation. Respiration 1974;31:7–20
14. Schwartz JS, Bencowitz HZ, Moser KM: Air travel hypoxemia with chronic obstructive pulmonary disease. Ann Intern Med 1984;100:473–477
15. Dillard TA, Berg BW, Rajagopal KR et al: Hypoxemia during air travel in patients with chronic obstructive pulmonary disease. Ann Intern Med 1989;111:362–367
16. AMA Commission on Emergency Medical Services: Medical aspects of transportation aboard commercial aircraft. JAMA 1982;247:1007–1011
17. Cowan MN: Transporting ill patients by aircraft. Consultant 1979:67–73

Chapter 101

Long-Term Mechanical Ventilation Outside the Hospital

Mary E. Gilmartin

CHAPTER OUTLINE

The use of mechanical ventilation has traditionally been confined to the acute care environment, but in recent years many patients have been maintained outside the hospital on ventilatory support. Involvement with the discharge process and home care of ventilator-assisted patients can either be a very rewarding or a very frustrating experience for allied health professionals. Successful cases of ventilator-assisted individuals require a great deal of organization and cooperation between the physician, allied health professionals, patient, family, and third party payers, an in-depth knowledge of the psychosocial aspects of patient care, and skill in teaching nonmedical people.

This chapter discusses the selection of appropriate candidates for ventilatory support outside the hospital and the most appropriate site for continued care, the recent experience with long-term ventilation, the team approach to discharge planning and home care, and types of ventilators used in the home.

For a more comprehensive discussion of the process of home ventilator care the reader is referred to recent reviews.[1–24]

HISTORY OF MECHANICAL VENTILATION OUTSIDE THE HOSPITAL

The home use of mechanical ventilators dates back to the worldwide poliomyelitis (polio) epidemics prior to the discovery of the Salk and Sabin vaccines in the 1950s. Compared with the technology available today, the application of mechanical ventilation in the polio era was very simple. The tank respirator, or iron lung, developed in 1928 by Drinker,[25] increased survival during the acute phase of infection and was used for long-term ventilation if there was irreversible damage. The iron lung was initially manufactured by the Warren E. Collins Co. in Massachusetts and then by John H. Emerson, also of Massachusetts.[26,27] Another device, the chest cuirass or ''turtle shell,'' was available at the same time, but its application was limited by design problems, and it was more widely used during the later epidemics.[28] The pneumowrap (''poncho,'' ''raincoat'') was developed during the polio epidemic of the 1950s.[29] Since home mechanical ventilation was noninvasive, it was relatively simple as compared with current problems we have with positive pressure ventilation. Reimbursement was not an issue since the equipment was provided by the hospital or manufacturer. Regional centers for the care of polio patients were developed (funding was available through the March of Dimes), and a few of these centers (Rancho Los Amigos and Goldwater Hospital) remain open today.[20]

Advances in trauma care and the capability of resuscitating victims of spinal cord injury at the accident scene have led to the use of ventilatory support in the home for patients with such injuries. The development and specialization of regional spinal cord centers has enabled many patients to survive the chronic effects of spinal cord injury and lead productive lives in their homes. This has coincided with advances in positive pressure ventilation. Since the early 1970s the development of small, portable, and increasingly sophisticated ventilators has allowed many patients to be not only at home but out in the workplace and to engage in social activities away from home.

Since the early 1980s the media has been involved in publicizing the plight of many ventilator-assisted children and adults. The Katie Beckett case, which was brought to the attention of President Ronald Reagan, resulted in the inception of the Katie Beckett waiver. Many children had been essentially living in acute care hospitals because of lack of funding for home care, and the waiver provided the necessary funding for medical care, equipment, and caregiver support in the home. The late Senator Jacob Javits, who had amyotrophic lateral sclerosis, continued to function in the work environment even though he required continuous ventilatory support. He gave renewed hope to those suffering from similar neuromuscular disease.

Today we have the technological resources to provide home ventilatory support for children and adults, but problems arise with regard to the financial and emotional costs that society is willing and able to support. We are also faced daily with the ethical dilemma of deciding who will benefit the most from long-term ventilatory support.

MEDICAL ASPECTS OF PATIENT SELECTION

Deciding which patient is a good candidate for home ventilatory support depends on many factors, the most important of which is the medical condition that necessitates long-term mechanical ventilation (Table 101-1). Other aspects of patient selection, such as the effects of coexisting disease and the medical stability of the patient, also have implications for the ability of the patient to function outside the

Table 101-1. Conditions That May Necessitate Long-Term Mechanical Ventilation

Neuromuscular Disorders
- Central nervous system
  - Central hypoventilation syndromes
  - Ondine's curse
  - Arnold-Chiari malformation
- Spinal cord
  - Traumatic injuries
  - Thoracic myelomeningocele
  - Syringomyelia
- Anterior horn cell (lower motor neuron)
  - Poliomyelitis
  - Spinal muscle atrophy (Werdnig-Hoffmann)
  - Amyotrophic lateral sclerosis[a]
- Muscle
  - Muscular dystrophy (Duchenne's, limb girdle, myotonic dystrophy)
  - Congenital myopathies
- Peripheral nerve
  - Phrenic neuropathies
  - Diaphragmatic paralysis: idiopathic; postsurgical
  - Guillain-Barré syndrome

Chest Wall and Diaphragmatic Defects
- Kyphoscoliosis
- Postsurgical (thoracoplasty)
- Diaphragmatic hernia

Primary Pulmonary Disorders
- Tracheomalacia
- Bronchiectasis
- Bronchopulmonary dysplasia
- Chronic aspiration
- Chronic bronchitis, emphysema[a]
- Cystic fibrosis[a]
- Interstitial lung disease (multiple causes)[a]
- Adult respiratory distress syndrome[a]

[a] Less appropriate disorders for home mechanical ventilation.
(From Gilmartin,[72] with permission.)

hospital setting. The determination of the need for ventilatory support is reviewed in Chapter 81.

Appropriate Diagnoses for Home Ventilation

As noted in Table 101-1, many of the conditions that can lead to ventilator dependence are neuromuscular or skeletal in origin and may affect both children and adults. Severe neuromuscular or skeletal deformity may impair respiratory muscle function as a result of generalized muscle weakness, diaphragm paralysis, or thoracic bellows deformity and may in turn result in failure of the ventilatory pump and inadequate spontaneous ventilation.[19,30] Since some of these neuromuscular disorders, such as muscular dystrophy, spinal muscle atrophy, and kyphoscoliosis, are slowly progressive over time, decisions about long-term ventilation can be made electively rather than emergently. Other disorders, such as traumatic injuries of the spinal cord, postsurgical diaphragmatic paralysis, and Guillain-Barré syndrome, will require immediate ventilatory support. Some patients with cervical spine injuries may regain some use of their ventilatory muscles when the acute effects of the injury are past, and most patients with Guillain-Barré syndrome will have full recovery. Central hypoventilation may be congenital or acquired and may be further subdivided into idiopathic or anatomic. Ondine's curse is an example of idiopathic central hypoventilation in which the individual loses the ability to breathe automatically; breathing in patients with this disorder becomes a purely voluntary function, so that they require assisted ventilation during sleep.[19,30] The Arnold-Chiari malformation is an anatomic abnormality in which the medulla and the inferior-posterior portion of the cerebellar hemispheres herniate through the foramen magnum. Acquired forms of central hypoventilation may be the result of infection, vascular accidents, or trauma.

Patients who have had poliomyelitis requiring assisted ventilation during the acute phase may develop respiratory failure necessitating ventilatory support later in life. The late effects of polio (postpolio syndrome) are experienced by many polio survivors in which there is progression of muscle weakness and atrophy. Although the exact mechanism is unclear, the syndrome does not seem to be due to reactivation of the poliovirus, but rather to further failure of the remaining anterior horn cells or to loss of motor neurons secondary to the aging process.[31]

Many children who require mechanical ventilation for neuromuscular disorders may actually develop chronic lung disease due to repeated infections associated with prolonged mechanical ventilation and tracheostomy. These children may also develop pulmonary hypertension and cor pulmonale secondary to inadequate ventilation and/or periods of hypoxemia.[19] Children with pulmonary and airway disease are increasingly often becoming candidates for long-term ventilatory support.[13] Schreiner et al.[32] reported that most children on home ventilation either had bronchopulmonary dysplasia or tracheomalacia.

Inappropriate Diagnoses for Home Ventilation

Use of long-term ventilation for patients who have primary pulmonary disease generates much more controversy and is less appropriate than its use in the conditions discussed above (Table 101-1). The primary pulmonary disorders are progressive, and by the time mechanical ventilation is needed they are far advanced and the patient has concomitant pulmonary hypertension and cor pulmonale. The clinical status of such patients can deteriorate rapidly secondary to airflow obstruction, infection, and heart failure. Patients with cystic fibrosis already have received multiple antibiotics for infections which has produced resistance in the causative organisms; placing these patients on a ventilator via a tracheostomy does little to decrease their copious secretions and recurrent infections.

Patients who have interstitial lung disease are not candidates for long-term ventilation because of the severity of their disease. They generally have hypoxemia and dyspnea that is refractory to medical management, and mechanical ventilation may actually increase their work of breathing.[19,30]

Patients with intrinsic lung and airway disease are much more difficult to manage at home because of their complicated respiratory status. The need for changes in ventilatory and O_2 requirements can be monitored, intravenous antibiotics can be administered, and other drug regimens can be used in the home but at an extremely high monetary and emotional cost, and most third party payers will not cover this level of care outside the hospital.

Implications of Coexisting Diseases

The patient's primary disease may be amenable to long-term ventilation, but if other underlying diseases that increase disability or affect prognosis are present, mechanical ventilation will probably not be feasible outside the hospital. For example, a patient with coronary artery disease or cardiomyopathy may be very stable in the intensive care unit (ICU), but when progressive rehabilitation begins, cardiac dysfunction becomes apparent. For some of these patients cardiac medications may be helpful, but for others the side effects of the medications may lead to other problems. When home care is contemplated, a cardiac evaluation should be considered, especially in the elderly patient. A Holter monitor and cardiac echo, or gated blood pool scan will give much needed information regarding the feasibility of rehabilitation.

Patients with underlying terminal cancer should not be considered for home ventilatory care because of the time and expense needed to prepare the patient and family for home care. Even with full-time professional caregivers in the home, the family must also understand the care procedures in the event that the caregivers are not available. Since discharge planning can be a lengthy process, an anticipated patient survival of only a few days or weeks makes home care difficult to justify.

Patients with an unstable psychiatric history should not be considered for home care. They would most likely be incapable of making reasonable judgments or decisions about their care needs and are at high risk for physical or mechanical problems.

Patient Stability and Medical Readiness for Discharge

A physician who has reached the opinion that a patient is a candidate for home care or a skilled nursing facility must then ascertain whether the patient meets the medical criteria for discharge (Table 101-2). It is not appropriate for a patient to be sent home when not medically or emotionally ready. High O_2 concentrations and high levels of positive end-expiratory pressure (PEEP) imply that the patient is still critically ill and may require intense medical interventions in the home.[19,30] Also, providing higher O_2 concentrations and PEEP levels in the home requires more adaptations to the ventilator and circuit, with consequent increased potential for malfunctions. Use of intermittent mandatory ventilation (IMV) in the home may increase the work of breathing and require separate circuits to provide adequate flow for the patient's spontaneous breathing, thereby increasing the potential for error.[33]

Infants and children need adequate nutrition for growth and development and to increase their potential for weaning from mechanical support.[34] An infant's failure to thrive may be indicative of irreversible damage, and placement in the home may not be in the best interest of the infant or the family.

Table 101-2. Long-Term Mechanical Ventilation: Patient Stability and Medical Readiness for Discharge

Control or absence of sustained dyspnea
Acceptable arterial blood gases with $FiO_2 < 0.40$
Stable ventilator parameters $FiO_2 < 0.40$ Assist/control or pressure-limited mode (pediatrics) Limited use of PEEP Minimal fluctuations in airway resistance or compliance Stable "free time" periods
Optimal metabolic and acid-base status
Absence of acute infectious processes
Absence of life-threatening cardiac dysfunction or arrhythmias
Stability of other organ systems
Ability to clear secretions and protect airways
Adequate nutrition
Progression of growth and development in children
If artificial airway, tracheostomy rather than oral or nasal airway
Ability to handle daily stressors
Management at home expected to be stable without the need for readmission within at least 1 month

(From Gilmartin,[72] with permission.)

OTHER ASPECTS OF PATIENT SELECTION

The medical aspects of patient selection are only part of the process leading to successful care outside the hospital. Equally important is the individualization and uniqueness of the patients that are cared for in everyday practice. Since many factors may play a role in successful outcomes, it is important to look at all the factors that would make a patient an ideal candidate; this ideal candidate can serve as a model for selecting an acceptable candidate. Table 101-3 lists important characteristics to be considered in the selection process, many of which can be determined through psychological testing and a thorough history.[35] Patients' ability to cope with stressors in their lives is a good indicator of how they will cope with the stress of long-term mechanical ventilation. They must be optimistic about their future and think that returning home and continuing with their lives is important. Motivation is necessary to get through the process of medical treatment and preparation for discharge. Patients must take part in the plan of care and the decision making; allowing others to make the decisions will increase the risk of failure. Because of changes or problems that may occur in their physical condition, caregiver support, and equipment, patients need to be able to call on all available internal and external resources and adapt to changes fairly easily. Most patients and families who have successfully withstood the stress of rehabilitation, discharge planning, and home care have had a good sense of humor and could retrospectively look at all of their mishaps with amusement. Patients must also have the ability to direct others, especially if they are not able to provide their own care and need to rely on family or unskilled caregivers.

The ideal patient also has an extremely close and supportive family and other social supports. Successful home care patients are not treated as sick persons, but as integral members of the family with family responsibilities. Maintaining much of their prior role in the family is integral to patient feelings of self-worth.

A college education is an ideal background since the patient needs to understand the many concepts of medical and physical care as well as the mechanical aspects. However, health care professionals must understand the many factors that interfere with learning, even in the college-educated person, such as denial, emotional instability, health beliefs, and physical condition.[36]

A patient with adequate financial resources (i.e., an insurance policy that covers the majority of home care costs, along with personal assets) will have much less worry about equipment, home modifications, caretakers, and daily survival than patients without financial resources. A patient with a stable neuromuscular condition is also an ideal candidate, as discussed above. The patient who has significant

Table 101-3. Patient Characteristics That May Determine Success in Home Ventilator Care

Characteristic	Ideal	Acceptable	Unacceptable
Individual coping styles	Optimistic Motivated Resourceful Flexible Adaptable Sense of humor Directive	Optimistic Motivated Sense of humor	None
Support systems	Close family and social supports	Social supports	Lack of family and social supports
Education	College degree Ability to learn	Able to learn Mechanically astute	Altered mental status Unable to learn
Financial resources	Adequate personal assets Optimal health insurance coverage	Adequate health insurance coverage	Lack of personal assets Lack of health insurance
Medical condition	Stable neuromuscular disease Significant "free time" off the ventilator No other medical illnesses	Stable neuromuscular or obstructive airway disease Limited or no "free time" off the ventilator	Medically unstable
Self-care ability	Ability to provide self-care and/or direct others	Able to provide self care	Unable to care for self or direct others

(From Gilmartin,[72] with permission.)

"free time" off the ventilator is ideal because this may mean lower equipment needs and fewer potential problems associated with interruptions in power or equipment malfunctions.

Since most people would not fit the ideal category, we must decide on criteria for the acceptable patient. These patients still need to feel optimistic and be motivated to progress toward the goal of going home and functioning independently. A sense of humor is still important, since many more frustrations may be encountered. Acceptable patients may be rigid rather than flexible or adaptable to change, which may make them very anxious when problems arise.

These patients may not have family support but will have close friends or strong community support. They will be able to ask for help and accept the aid offered to them. Even if they do not have any formal education, they will have the ability to learn and will feel less threatened by home care when they understand the mechanics of the equipment. The health care team can bolster patients' self-confidence through recognition of their mechanical aptitude. The acceptable patient will need adequate third party payment even if it is through a state medicaid program. Patients who lack personal financial assets need to be self-sufficient in their care since adequate caregiver support may not be funded. Patients with very stable primary pulmonary disease rather than neuromuscular disease may be acceptable, even if they require full-time ventilatory support.

The third group of patients consists of those who are unacceptable for home care. As noted in Table 101-3, these patients do not have any coping skills or have an altered mental status. They do not have family support, or they live in an area without any community services. These patients do not have any financial support or health insurance and do not qualify for state-funded programs. Other unacceptable patients are those who have had very unstable disease and are unable to provide self-care or to direct others. Placing this type of patient in the home would greatly increase the chances of fatal complications. Additionally, if the goal of discharge planning is to have safe, competent, and cost-effective home care, this type of patient does not qualify.

Determining the patient's acceptability for home care will help decrease the frustrations and failures in discharge planning and decrease the exorbitant medical costs of hospital care. These determinations need to be made early in the hospitalization or even before ventilatory support is initiated.

EXPERIENCE WITH HOME MECHANICAL VENTILATION

Experience in the United States and Canada

Since the early 1980s there have been numerous reports of patients discharged to home with ventilatory support.[1-4,6,8,24,37] Many of these reports discuss only small numbers of patients who were successfully discharged to home and only briefly discuss the complexities of discharge planning and home care, while others look at larger numbers of patients cared for in the home and the long-term outcome as well as the course over time.[4,11,14,17,18,22,23,38,39] In general, most of the reports have shown that patients with neuromuscular disease are much better candidates than those with pulmonary disease. Even though patients with neuromuscular disease may have more physical care needs than those with chronic obstructive pulmonary disease (COPD), they have fewer problems with airflow variability, concomitant cardiac disease, respiratory care needs, dyspnea, and progressive loss of lung function. Many patients with COPD also experience much more anxiety and disabling fear because of the above problems.

Czorniak et al.[40] reviewed the clinical course of 14 patients with COPD and 21 patients with neuromuscular disorders who were followed at home for an average of 31 months (range, 5 to 66 months) after hospital discharge. The COPD patients averaged 2.7 hospital admissions per year, with an average time in the hospital of 54 days per year, whereas the neuromuscular patients only averaged 0.7 admissions and 9.8 hospital days per year. Seven of the neuromuscular patients did not have any readmissions. Over half of the readmissions for both groups of patients were for respiratory problems, which included the need for increased ventilatory support (29 percent), pneumonia (10 percent), and bronchitis (9 percent). Airway problems related to the tracheostomy accounted for 14 percent of the readmissions. Some of the readmissions for nonpulmonary causes were related to surgical procedures, seizure disorders, or fractures and, rarely, power failure and ventilator malfunction.

Table 101-4 shows the characteristics of patients discharged between 1981 and 1989 from Boston University Medical Center and National Jewish Center for Immunology and Respiratory Medicine.[41] Even though survival for patients with neuromuscular disorders was longer than for those for COPD, many of the COPD patients were able to continue with an active life and be self-sufficient in a number of their care needs. In informal discussions with many of these patients and their family members, they expressed pleasure in the opportunity to be back in the home even though they were more restricted in performing prior activities. They also believed that a positive attitude about what they could perform made it much easier to accept the presence of a life-support device in the home.

Table 101-4. Outcomes of 80 Ventilator-Assisted Patients in Boston/Denver Series (1981–1989)

	COPD	Neuromuscular
Admissions	35	43
Age		
mean	61.4 ± 1.2	51.2 ± 16.1
range	46–78	22–81
Outcome		
Home care	24	39
Chronic hospital	3	4
Died in hospital	8	0
Independence[a]		
Maximal	7	15
Moderate	12	9
Minimal	15	11
None	1	8
Free time off the home ventilator		
<2 hours	15	8
2–7 hours	8	3
8–15 hours	10	12
16–24 hours	2	20

[a] Maximal, performs own care independently; moderate, performs most of own care except for showering and meal preparation; minimal, can wash, dress, and eat at bedside once materials are set up; none, needs complete assistance with almost all personal care.

(From Make and Gilmartin,[41] with permission.)

Experience in Europe

Many of the problems that we face in the United States are not issues in Europe because of the difference in health care payment provisions. In France the care is coordinated, medically supervised, and funded through regional associations.[42] Many patients in France are electively placed on mechanical ventilation as they are gradually deteriorating, rather than acutely decompensating, with the rationale that periodic rest of the respiratory muscles will prevent acute respiratory failure.[43] Pierson[42] has observed that if elective ventilation were initiated in the United States in less acutely ill patients, at least 10,000 patients would be receiving ventilatory assistance.

Robert and associates[21] have followed a large group of ventilator-assisted patients in the home; their data have shown 90 percent survival of 41 postpolio patients over 18 years but less than a 20 percent survival of 10 patients with bronchiectasis over 4 years. Their data show a 22 percent survival for 50 COPD patients over 8 years.[21] Dull and Sadoul[44] followed eight patients with COPD for over 1.5 years; they demonstrated that there was a reduction in $PaCO_2$ but no decrease in hospitalizations after institution of mechanical ventilation.

There are very few reports from other European countries regarding long-term ventilatory support, although in England it has been used for years in selected patients, and some hospitals have established home ventilation programs.[45] A study in Germany on six patients with neuromuscular disorders and three with COPD showed that noninvasive intermittent ventilatory support with a nasal mask significantly increased maximal inspiratory pressures and reduced the demand on the inspiratory muscles by increasing muscular strength.[46] In Italy a 1990 study of six patients, three with COPD and three with neuromuscular disorders, who received positive pressure ventilation via tracheostomy, showed a significant improvement in blood gases and a decrease in hospitalization.[47]

Elective Use of Mechanical Ventilation

Most patients in the United States are placed on a mechanical ventilator for acute respiratory failure, but as noted above, in France this is done electively with many patients.

Since elective ventilation is instituted when a patient is relatively stable, the hospitalization period is much shorter and less critical care is required than with a patient in acute respiratory failure. Thus, the cost of such care will be greatly reduced. With the availability of noninvasive positive pressure ventilation via nasal mask or mouthpiece, as well as the continued use of negative pressure ventilation, the need for backup equipment is less, and additional supplies for tracheostomy care and suctioning are not needed.

Most patients with neuromuscular disease have the time to make decisions about their future needs regarding ventilatory assistance. As the disease progresses, the available options should be discussed with the patient or, in the case of young children, with the parents prior to the onset of respiratory failure. These people should have the opportunity to meet with other ventilator-assisted patients and families and be realistically told about the pros and cons of long-term ventilatory support. They need to understand that if the disease is a progressive one, eventually full-time ventilatory assistance will be needed.

Data were collected at Boston University Medical Center from 1981 to 1988 on 39 patients with neuromuscular disorders, 14 of whom were initially treated with negative pressure ventilation or a pneumobelt. Four of these patients changed to nasal positive pressure ventilation mainly for comfort and ease of application, and six patients progressed to positive pressure ventilation via a tracheostomy. Recently at this center, night-time ventilation via nasal mask was initiated in four patients with neuromuscular disorders; one of these patients uses a mouthpiece during the day for intermittent ventilation. Many of the patients in the Boston program did not know about the long-term effects of their disorders and therefore entered the hospital in acute respiratory failure requiring a prolonged hospitalization.

There are many ethical issues surrounding long-term ventilatory support. Many of these issues are related to the financial implications and the high costs of medical care, while others are related to perceived quality of life and the dilemma of prolonging life when there is no hope for cure. The emotional cost may also be too high; the parents of a ventilator-assisted child worry about how they will be able to continue caring for the child as they age or who will provide the care when they die. They also worry about where the money will come from for long-term care. In today's society reimbursement is not available for home care or skilled nursing facilities for many patients on a ventilator. It is for all these reasons that the patient and family need a realistic picture of the future and should be given the opportunity to make their own decisions. We need to understand that many patients will not be able to make a decision or will change their minds at the last minute. If this happens, we cannot abandon them but need to continue to provide support and help them maintain their dignity throughout a terrible ordeal. This chapter cannot deal with all of the ethical dilemmas associated with long-term ventilation, whether electively or acutely initiated, but we must look at each person as an individual and try not to let our values interfere with the patient's decision or the care that we provide.

PLACEMENT ALTERNATIVES OUTSIDE THE HOSPITAL

Home

For most patients home is the preferred discharge destination. The psychological benefit of a return to family and familiar surroundings is the major stimulus in discharging a patient to home, though in many communities it may be the only alternative to acute care hospitals.[48] A patient cannot be discharged to home if there are inadequate physical and financial support services or if the patient is medically unstable.

Skilled Nursing Facilities

A skilled nursing facility may be an extended care facility, a chronic care hospital, a convalescent center, or a nursing home.[20,48] In past years the use of these facilities for long-term ventilator patients was impossible because of lack of reimbursement, inadequate staffing, lack of trained staff, and the expense of buying or renting the equipment. Some facilities have developed specialized units for ventilator patients with the help of physicians and allied health professionals. They have been able to obtain adequate reimbursement from third party payers for the necessary level of care, and they have an agreement with a local hospital to take patients who require acute care. One such facility is Jewish Memorial Hospital in Boston. Pulmonary physicians from Boston University Medical Center coordinate the program with the rehabilitation team at the facility. These physicians make daily rounds and are on call for problems that may arise. The nurses received special training from the physicians and respiratory therapists at the hospital.

Other states may not be so fortunate in having chronic facilities available. In Colorado some nursing homes will take ventilator patients but only if they qualify for Medicaid or have private insurance. These few facilities are funded through the state's hospital backup program. They do not have respiratory therapists on staff but have coverage through a local durable medical equipment (DME) company. The staff caring for these patients generally consists of licensed practical nurses and nursing assistants, with registered nurse support only in a supervisory capacity.

Some hospitals may already own a nursing home and can use part of it for ventilator patients. This is advantageous for those patients who cannot be discharged home or do not qualify for skilled nursing facilities. The daily cost to the hospital will be much less than if the patient were kept in the ICU, step down unit, or medical-surgical unit.

Specialized Respiratory Care Centers

Some specialized respiratory care facilities are centers that managed polio survivors during the previous epidemics, but as the incidence of polio declined, these units have undertaken the care of long-term ventilator patients.[20,48]

More recently, the Health Care Financing Administration requested professional assistance in defining criteria for the establishment of demonstration units for ventilator-assisted patients in hospitals.[49] Though these regional centers are not for long-term placement of ventilator patients, they may provide important data regarding the actual costs of caring for these patients and determine if mortality and morbidity are changed in specialized units outside the ICU.

Congregate Living Centers

Congregate living centers are located in residential settings and are more like private homes.[20,48] "New Start Homes" in California are centers developed by a nurse for ventilator-assisted patients. There is professional caregiver support around the clock, but the residents are encouraged to make their own decisions and to have certain responsibilities regarding the household functions. Such centers usually have a van, and residents participate in shopping and cooking. Patients have their own rooms, which gives them the privacy that a skilled nursing facility cannot provide. These California facilities required a special grant to continue operation.

MULTIDISCIPLINARY TEAM APPROACH TO DISCHARGE PLANNING AND HOME CARE

Hospital Team

Discharge planning for a potential home care candidate may be accomplished by only a physician, nurse, and therapist or with the help of the other allied professionals. Whoever is involved, the key to successful discharge is coordination of the services provided by many different individuals. Figure 101-1 charts the structure of the hospital and home care team.

The physician, as a key player on the team, must see the worth of the discharge planning process, needs to have an interest in the rehabilitation process and home care, and should not be motivated by the desire to remove the patient from the hospital service. The physician is the leader of the team and advises the other team members as to the patient's medical stability.[20]

Nurses provide care on a 24-hour basis and are responsible for teaching the patient and family self-care techniques related to personal care as well as respiratory care prior to hospital discharge. The nurse is constantly striving to advance the patient and family toward independence. Since many hospitals use the primary nurse model, the nurse also may coordinate the services of rehabilitation, respiratory therapy, and other providers in the patient's daily care plan. This daily schedule aids the patient in establishing a routine and prevents fatigue by incorporating rest periods throughout the day.

The respiratory therapist has a key role in ensuring adequate ventilation and monitoring the patient's response to therapy. The therapist also has many teaching responsibilities with the patient and caregivers. Generally, the therapist will teach the patient about the ventilator, the accessory equipment, emergency measures, and aerosol therapy. The therapist will usually coordinate the equipment list with the home care company and have the patient use the equipment prior to discharge. The therapist is also the resource person for assisting other team members to understand the equipment and to reinforce the education provided by the therapist. The therapist should also be familiar with current trends in home care and equipment safety.

The rehabilitation services consist of physical and occu-

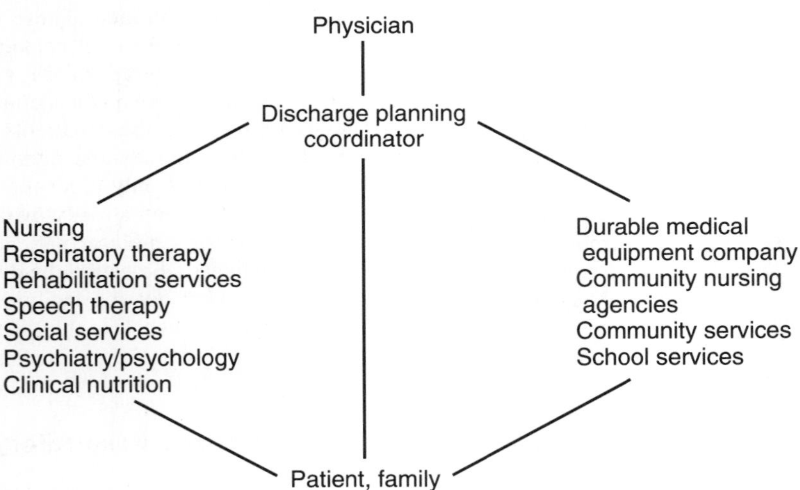

Figure 101-1. Multidisciplinary team for hospital and home care of ventilator-assisted individuals. (From Gilmartin,[72] with permission.)

Table 101-5. Communication Alternatives for Ventilator-Assisted Patients

Cuff deflation (or uncuffed tracheostomy tube)
"Talking" tracheostomy tube
Electrolarynx
Neck placement
Intra-oral placement
Pneumatic voice device
Lip speaking
Writing
Sign language
Communication boards
Alphabet keyboards with printed messages
Preprogrammed computers with voice synthesizers

(From Gilmartin,[72] with permission.)

pational therapy and in some institutions recreational therapy. These services are essential in determining the patient's rehabilitation potential in terms of muscle strength and endurance and ability to perform activities of daily living. They also will determine the need for assistive devices such as wheelchairs, walkers, arm supports, bathing aids, and safety devices for the bathroom. They may also participate in the home evaluation and work with the patient on homemaking activities.

A speech therapist may work with the ventilator-assisted patient in determining the best communication alternative if normal speech is not possible. Table 101-5 lists some of the communication alternatives available to ventilator-assisted individuals. The ability to communicate is essential in the rehabilitation of these patients. The speech therapist also plays a key role in assessing patients' swallowing ability and their potential for aspiration.[50]

The social worker participates in evaluating potential patients for a home care program and in determining their ability to cope with the stress of discharge planning and home care. The social worker also aids the team in determining insurance coverage and/or the patient's ability to pay directly or qualify for additional financial coverage. The social worker will partake in determining the need for psychiatric consultation. Psychiatric services may be needed in addition to the social worker if more intensive therapy is needed or if psychotropic medications are indicated. The psychologist assesses the need for psychological testing to determine cognitive impairment.

The nutritionist plays a major role in determining the nutritional status of patients at admission and as they progress through the discharge planning process and also assists patients in developing good dietary habits and planning a suitable diet for individual needs.

In many hospitals the link between all the above services and the home care team is a discharge planner or case manager. This person may either be a nurse or respiratory therapist and should have the following qualifications: (1) ability to work with the staff, patient, family, and community services; (2) thorough knowledge of respiratory care; (3) experience in discharge planning; (4) understanding of home care reimbursement and regulations; (5) collaborative and trusting relationship with the primary physician; and (6) experience with home care.[20] The coordinator would also be available for follow-up with the patient after discharge.

Home Care Team

The home care team may only include the primary physician, patient, family and DME company, or as in the case of children, it may include such extensive services as home nursing agencies, community services, school services, and privately funded caregivers. The physician still has the same function as the inpatient physician but needs to rely on the home caregivers for their input and ongoing assessment.

The DME company provides all the equipment and supplies that the patient will need in the home. Respiratory therapists are also provided, since third party payers will not directly reimburse for respiratory therapy service. The DME company is responsible for ongoing quality control of the equipment and timely preventive maintenance and repairs. The respiratory therapist may see the patient daily when first discharged and then weekly or monthly depending on the patient. There is always a therapist on call for emergencies. The therapist may also be involved with discharge planning and teaching prior to discharge and is responsible for continued education of the patient and family after discharge.

The nursing agency may be a nonprofit or for-profit company. The services that the patient receives at home are dependent on reimbursement and not always on the patient's needs. The patient may only need intermittent nursing visits for assessment, teaching, or nursing tasks that cannot be performed by the patient or family, or, as with children or severely disabled adults 24-hour skilled nursing may be required. Many nursing agencies have the capabilities of providing both types of service. The nursing agency can provide unskilled caregivers for personal care and homemaking, but the patient and family must be able to provide the more complex tasks of suctioning, tracheostomy care, and ventilator care. Other services such as physical, occupational, speech, and social services may also be provided by the nursing agency.

Community services may consist of transportation to and from a routine doctor's appointment or to school. Emergency medical services are needed whenever patients are home on ventilatory support; they may be provided through the local hospital or the fire or police department, which should also be informed whenever a patient is discharged home on life support equipment. Their services may also include an emergency communication system that is installed in a patient's home, especially if the patient lives alone. The community may also have a service that will provide daily meals for the patient, although generally this is only one meal a day. Other services may include day care or volunteers, who may be extremely helpful in providing relief to caregivers.

Today, as more children are discharged to home, the need for school accommodations is extremely important. Many children are now mainstreamed into the regular school system because of their parents' efforts, but because these children require expertise in their care needs, teachers, school nurses, and counselors need special instructions in dealing with them. Often nurses caring for pediatric patients at home will also go to school with them to provide care.

The patient and family are key members of the team because without their desire for the patient to be at home and cooperation in providing care, home care will be a failure. Many patients may actually be able to perform all their own care or to direct family or other unskilled caregivers in doing so, but they need the continued support of the physician or home care coordinator. If the family is providing all the care, the availability of respite care is extremely important.

PREPARATION OF THE PATIENT AND FAMILY FOR HOME

Education

Table 101-6 lists many of the skills that patients and families will need to be self-sufficient at home. Not all patients will need all these skills, and some will need additional instruction, depending on individual problems. A master checklist should be developed listing many of these basic skills that must be taught; other skills can be written on the list for individual patients. It is imperative to document when teaching of each task was begun and when the patient and caregivers performed it independently.[20] This checklist will help each of the home care team members to advance the patient toward self-care. If the patient has difficulties in learning certain tasks, it should be discussed at team meetings. Consistency is very important in teaching patients, and all members of the team need to make sure they are not giving the patient mixed messages. Patients and families also learn by observing their care, and the home care team may inadvertently teach bad techniques by not performing a procedure properly.[36] The team must decide who will teach the various skills that the patient and family need, thereby lessening the confusion for the patient and ensuring that all the skills will be taught. Reinforcement and positive feedback can be provided by all team members. The patient and family should not be inundated with all the material at once, but teaching should be provided on a timely basis, allowing for adequate practice and progressing from the simple to the more complex tasks. In a 1990 study of patient perception of teaching home ventilator care, the patients expressed the view that teaching should be done at the bedside with only one or two family members present and that instruction should be provided by the team member in short sessions by the demonstration technique.[51] The patients also considered learning the skills to be much more important than learning about their lung disease.

Table 101-6. Long-Term Mechanical Ventilation: Skills Needed by Patient and/or Caregivers Prior to Discharge

- Self-Care Techniques
  - Airway management
    - Tracheostomy and stoma care
    - Cuff care
    - Tracheal suctioning
    - Changing the tracheostomy tube
    - Changing the tracheostomy ties
  - Chest physical therapy techniques
    - Percussion
    - Vibration
    - Coughing
  - Medication administration
    - Oral
    - Inhaled
  - Bed to chair transfers
  - Feeding tube care
  - Indwelling catheter care
  - Implantable IV line care
  - Bowel care
  - Switching from ventilator to weaning device
- Equipment Maintenance
  - Ventilator
  - Humidifier
  - Suction machines
  - Battery and charger
  - Oxygen administration
  - Manual resuscitator
  - Troubleshooting for problems
  - Cleaning and disinfection
- Emergency Measures
  - Ventilator failure
  - Power failure
  - Dislodged tracheostomy tube
  - Obstructed airway
  - Cuff leaks
  - Shortness of breath
  - Ventilator circuitry problems
  - Infection
  - Falls
  - Bleeding
  - Cardiac arrest

(From Gilmartin,[72] with permission.)

Rehabilitation

Teaching is one part of the rehabilitation process, but increasing the patient's functional potential is equally important. Patients with a neuromuscular impairment may not be able to increase strength and endurance but can be assisted in preserving the strength that they have and preventing further contractures by daily stretching. Aids for mobility and physical functioning, such as arm supports, splints, and bracing can help to increase the quality of life of many physically impaired persons. Many of the principles of pulmonary rehabilitation can be incorporated into the care plan of patients with COPD. Short- and long-term goals are a very important part of the rehabilitation process—patients need to see improvement, and realistic short-term goals give them the impetus to continue toward their long-term goal of going home. Like all people, patients and families need to know that they are doing a good job, and listing their accomplishments increases their motivation and makes them more optimistic about the future.[52] As with education, the patient should progress from the simple to the more complex tasks; this would relate to the level of energy expenditure for each task. As patients begin to exercise and move about, their ventilatory and O_2 requirements need to be assessed. An extensive review of pulmonary rehabilitation is presented in Chapter 98.

Depending on the patient's ventilatory needs, a portable ventilator can be mounted on a wheelchair or cart so that the patient can increase ambulation and move away from the bed. If the patient cannot ambulate, a decision is needed about the type of wheelchair that will be required. A motorized wheelchair may seem to be a wonderful idea, but if there is no access into the home or even from room to room, the chair will only be an expensive "white elephant."

Children's needs are very different since if they are doing well, their mobility requirements will change frequently. The caregivers need to be versatile in providing them with some mobility. Just as children outgrow shoes, they also outgrow their equipment, their ventilator settings, and their tracheostomy tubes, and therefore they need frequent evaluation.

Children's normal developmental care needs must also be evaluated frequently. Their rehabilitation will include speech therapy, play therapy, and education, depending on the age of the child. A child who has never been out of the hospital does not know about any of the things that most people take for granted. What a delight to see a child's expression the first time that child feels a cool breeze, sits out in the sun, touches a tree, or sees a lake.

Selection of Caregivers

Prior to discharge a decision needs to be made about who will be providing the patient's care. In adults this may be fairly simple; patients who are capable will provide most of their own care. A family member may assist with the care of a patient who is not capable, but if the patient is 75 years old with a spouse of the same age, neither may be capable of providing all the care. It must be determined how much skilled care (e.g., intravenous care, airway management, tube feedings, or monitoring of progressive weaning attempts) will be needed, or whether the patient will only need unskilled care for bathing, dressing, meal preparation, and other homemaking activities. Other critical factors in caregiver selection will be the patient's medical condition and the specifications for funding by the third party payer. Many patients with neuromuscular disorders may be involved with centers for independent living in their community and have personal care attendants funded through the agency. These caregivers are hired and trained independently by the patient, which generally places no restrictions on the complex tasks that they may perform. When home health aides are provided through a home health agency, there are many restrictions on the complexity of the care that may be provided. This would limit the ability of many patients to be at home, since they may be able to do the simpler tasks by themselves but need help with more complex care and not have the means to hire registered nurses. Because of these problems it is important to determine early in the discharge planning process the patient's current insurance coverage and whether the patient will qualify for additional funding; a child may qualify for a waiver, but the application process may take months. Also, the local nursing agency will provide information on the services they can realistically provide given their personnel constraints and the patient's third party coverage.

Assessment of the Home

Prior to discharge, members of the hospital team and personnel of the DME company should visit the patient's home and assess the potential barriers to the patient's ability to function in the home environment. Which team members visit the home is dependent on the patient's functional status; a patient who requires many adaptive devices, including a wheelchair, will need the input of the physical and occupational therapist as well as the nurse and respiratory therapist. Table 101-7 lists the general components of a home assessment. When a child is discharged to home, the team may also need to look at the school or play areas that the child will be using. In general, there should be adequate space for the patient, equipment, storage of supplies, and privacy. The electrical system needs particular attention, especially if the house is old and the wiring or grounded outlets are inadequate to handle the added load imposed by the respiratory equipment. Optimally, the ventilator and accessory equipment should have their own circuit.[53] Home modifications are out-of-pocket costs to the patient, and esthetically the home should remain a home, not a hospital.

Table 101-7. Long-Term Mechanical Ventilation: Assessment of the Home

Accessibility
In and out of home
Bathroom
Kitchen
Between rooms
Wheelchair mobility
Doorway width
Thresholds
Stairways
Carpeting
Equipment
Electrical amperage
Grounded outlets
Space
Environment
Temperature
Lighting
Living space

(From Gilmartin,[72] with permission.)

Obstacles to Discharge

Discharging ventilator-assisted patient to home may be one of the most complex activities that health care professionals are faced with and requires a great deal of expertise in discharge planning, psychosocial adaptations to illness, and understanding of home health care regulations.[54] Lack of communication between the physician and the allied health team is one of the initial obstacles; patients are still medically unstable, and their safety cannot be guaranteed in the home. The physician may tell the patient and family that a patient will be home in 1 or 2 weeks without discussing with the team members the patient's and family's progress in learning the required care.

Inadequate coordination between the hospital team and the home care team is another obstacle. Equipment may not have been ordered or not be available, the patient may not have had time to use the equipment, or the type of caretaker needed by the patient may not be available.

Another major obstacle to discharge is fear and ambivalence about leaving the protective hospital environment. Patients and families may react to this by becoming more dependent, becoming angry and anxious, having an increase in somatic complaints, missing teaching sessions, or not making the necessary home arrangements, or the family may visit less.[35] These reactions need to be anticipated by the hospital team and prevented when possible. Frequent family meetings help to alleviate the stress and assure the patient and family that the team recognizes the stress that they are under. Assuring patients of continued support after discharge is also helpful, since they may feel that hospital personnel are abandoning them. Trips away from the bedside and hospital will help patients gain confidence in their own caretaking abilities while they will be returning for the support they have been receiving. Meeting the home care team and being reassured that the home care team will continue with the outline of care provided in the hospital are helpful to patients.

Lack of adequate reimbursement is another major obstacle to discharge of ventilator-assisted patients.

MECHANICAL VENTILATORS AND ACCESSORY EQUIPMENT USED IN THE HOME

Positive Pressure Ventilation

The positive pressure ventilators used in the home are smaller, more portable, less sophisticated, and have fewer features and alarms than those used in the critical care environment. Even though less sophisticated than hospital ventilators, the home ventilator models developed since the mid-1980s are all microprocessor-controlled. Figures 101-2 through 101-6 identify most of these ventilators. Table 101-8 lists the ventilators with each of their individual features, and other reviews discuss them in greater depth.[55,56]

Generally, the three modes of ventilation used in the home are assist-control, synchronized intermittent mandatory ventilation (SIMV), and pressure-limited ventilation. For adults assist-control mode is the preferred choice, since the work of breathing is minimal. Kacmarek et al.[33] have shown that the work of spontaneous breathing in the SIMV mode is greatly increased because gas must be drawn through the piston chamber and air-intake valve and there is no continuous flow or demand valve. Greater patient effort is also required to maintain flow through bubble-type humidifiers

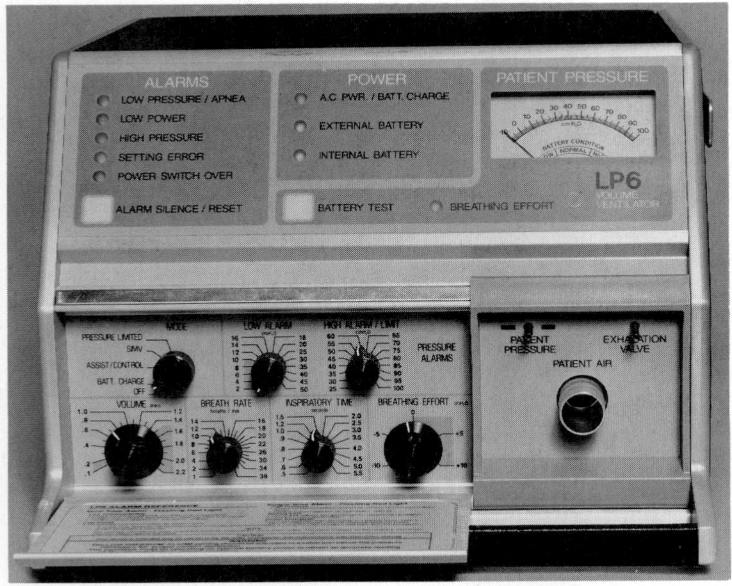

Figure 101-2. LP-6 ventilator. (Courtesy of Aequitron Medical Inc., Minneapolis, MN.)

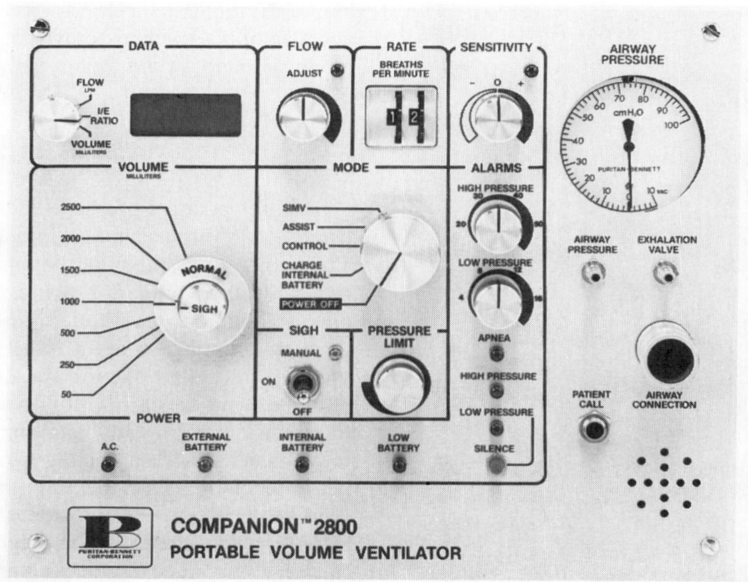

Figure 101-3. Companion 2800. (Courtesy of Puritan-Bennett Corp., Overland Park, KS.)

than through a blow-by or wick-style humidifier.[56,57] If the SIMV mode is considered, a one-way valve proximal to the humidifier with a continuous flow of gas should be used, and if a cascade humidifier is used, the tower should be removed. The patient's safety must always be considered when altering ventilator circuits, since modifications may add to the complexity of the device and increase the potential for untoward complications. When using the SIMV mode on selected patients, selection of a high ventilator rate (above 10 breaths per minute), replacement of the air-intake filter with a lower resistance bacteria filter, and removal of the tower from the humidifier will decrease the work of breathing.[57]

Home ventilation assistance for infants and children is more complex than for adults. The ventilators specifically designed for infants are not considered "user friendly," are more costly to operate, are not readily portable, have a limited minute volume capability, and their tidal volume delivery can vary tremendously.[58] With ventilators designed for home care, conventional volume-cycled ventilation cannot be used. The focus must change to a volume-cycled, pres-

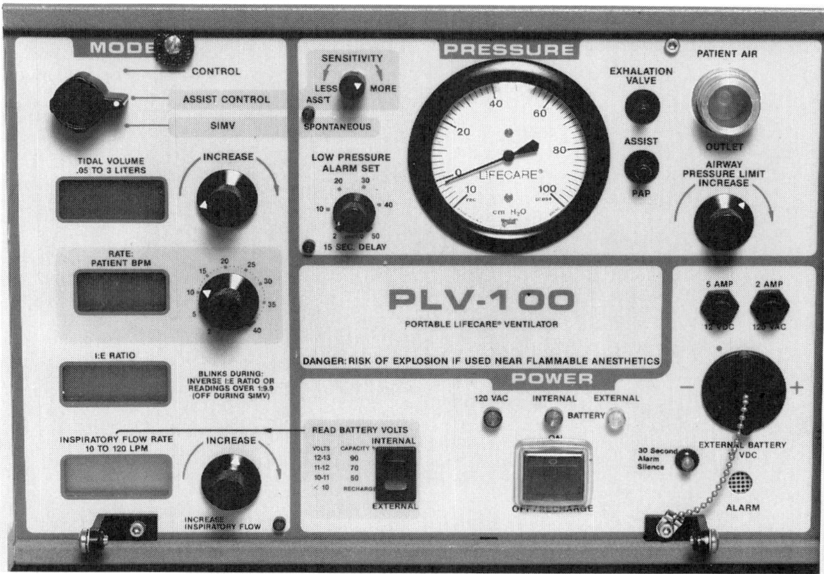

Figure 101-4. PLV-100. (Courtesy of LIFECARE, Lafayette, CO.)

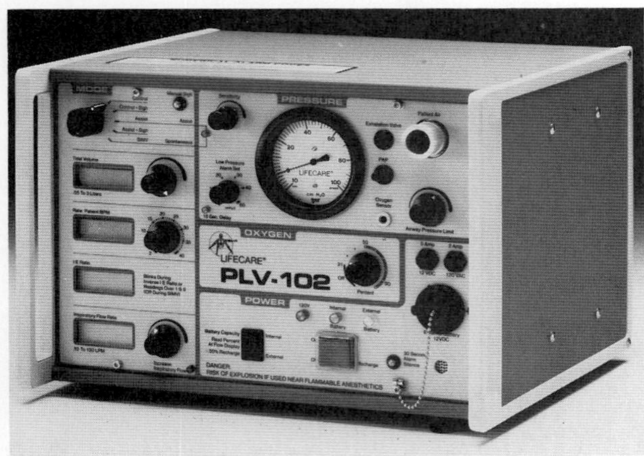

Figure 101-5. PLV-102. (Courtesy of LIFECARE, Lafayette, CO.)

sure-oriented approach, because exhaled volumes are not accurate when a cuffless tracheostomy tube is used.[58] Generally, system pressures of about 20 to 25 cmH_2O and inspiratory times of about 0.8 to 1.0 seconds are necessary to provide appropriate tidal volumes for infants.[58] If the SIMV mode is used, the rate may need to be set slightly higher than that of the pediatric ventilator because of the increased work of breathing and mechanical dead space.[58] The increased mechanical dead space results from the use of adult circuits and the positioning of the exhalation valve away from the infant's neck.[58]

Since many infants who are placed on ventilators may actually show some improvement in lung function, their ventilatory needs change and the leak around the tracheal tube increases as they grow; routine monitoring of oxygenation and ventilation must be performed at least monthly. The type and size of the tracheostomy tube must also be evaluated on a regular basis as the infant grows.

Methods of Delivery

In adults positive pressure ventilation can be provided via tracheostomy, nasal mask, mouthpiece or full face mask. Tracheostomy is the most common method since many patients receive ventilation acutely via an endotracheal tube and are unable to be weaned. The advantages of ventilation through a tracheostomy are (1) provision of accurate tidal volume, unless an uncuffed tracheostomy tube is used; (2) reduced dead space; (3) ability to communicate; (4) potentially normal eating and drinking; and (5) less restriction of movement. The disadvantages are related to the invasiveness, which increases the potential for infection and tracheal damage. The tube needs periodic replacement and daily care, and the tracheal stoma also needs daily care. The use of a tracheostomy tube requires additional equipment and supplies in the home, which adds to the expense of home ventilator care. Psychologically, the patient needs to deal with the change in self-image imposed by the tube in the neck.[57]

The use of nasal masks to provide positive pressure ventilation has recently sparked the interest of health care professionals. Nasal continuous positive airway pressure (CPAP) masks, and more recently custom-made masks, have provided the ability to apply noninvasive nighttime mechanical ventilation to many patients with neuromuscular or skeletal disorders.[12,15,57,59–61] Since this method of ventilation may be electively initiated in a patient with deteriorating respiratory function, hospitalization and overall expenses are greatly decreased. Patients may only need a 2- or 3-day admission for adjustment of the mask, regulation of adequate

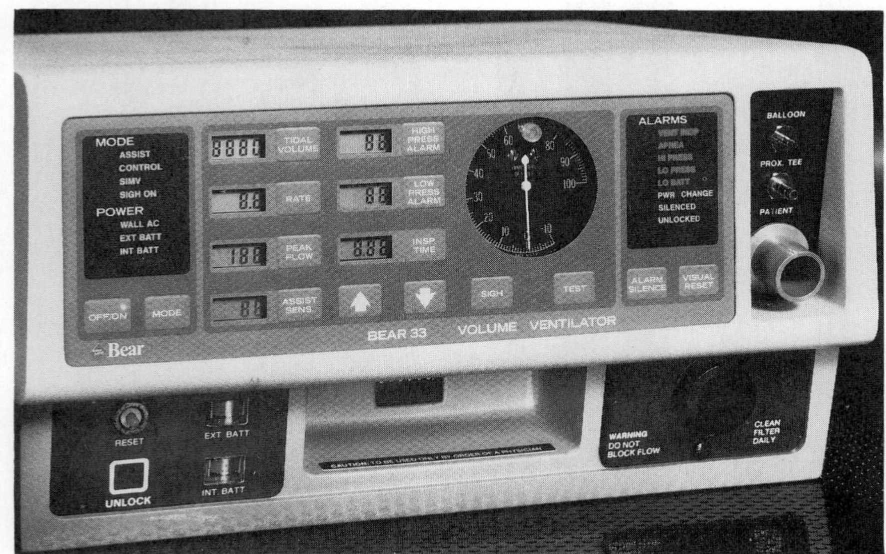

Figure 101-6. Bear 33. (Courtesy of Bear Medical Systems, Inc., Riverside, CA.)

Table 101-8. Home Care Positive-Pressure Ventilators

	Modes	VT (mL)	Rate (breaths/min)	I/E Ratio	Alarms	Power Sources	O_2	Alarm Silencer/Reset	Panel Lock
Aequitron Medical Inc. (Minneapolis, MN)									
LP6	Assist/control, SIMV pressure-limited	100–2200	1–38	Variable	Ventilator malfunction Low pressure High pressure Low power Apnea I/E ratio (inverse, setting error) Power switchover	AC, DC, internal battery	Bleed-in, reservoir	Yes/1 min	—
Puritan Bennett Corp. (Overland Park, KS)									
Companion 2800	Control, assist/control, SIMV, sigh	50–2800	1–69	Variable	Ventilator malfunction Low pressure High pressure Low power Apnea I/E ratio (inverse) Power switchover Inspiratory flow	AC, DC, internal battery	Bleed-in, accumulator	Yes/1 min	—
LIFECARE (Lafayette, CO)									
PVV	Control	50–3000	8–30	Fixed 1:1	Low pressure High pressure Low power Power failure	AC, DC, internal battery	Bleed-in	No	—
PLV-100	Control, assist/control SIMV	50–3000	2–40	Variable	Ventilator malfunction Low pressure High pressure Low power Power failure Apnea I/E ratio (inverse) Inspiratory flow Reverse battery cable connection	AC, DC, internal battery	Bleed-in	Yes	—
PLV-102	Control, assist/control SIMV, sigh	50–3000	2–40	Variable	Ventilator malfunction Low pressure High pressure Low power Power failure Apnea I/E ratio (inverse) Power switchover Inspiratory flow Reverse battery cable connection	AC, DC, internal battery	Bleed-in, blender, O_2 change	Yes/30 sec	—
Bear Medical Systems, Inc. (Riverside, CA)									
Bear 33	Control, assist/control SIMV, sigh	100–2200	2–40	Variable	Ventilator inoperation Low pressure High pressure Power failure Apnea Power switchover Inspiratory flow (I/E ratio)	AC, DC, internal battery	Bleed-in, accumulator	Yes/1 min	Yes/15 sec
L'Air Liquide (Paris, France)									
Monnal D (L.D.)[a]	Control, assist/control	Variable	8–40	Variable	Power failure Minimum pressure	220 volts			

VT, tidal volume; I/E ratio, inspiratory/expiratory ratio.

[a] Flow rate (air) compressor-driven equals 0–20 L/min; other features include a safety pressure of 0–80 cmH_2O, a nebulizer, bacterial filter, and humidifier (L.D. model).

ventilation, and teaching. Other advantages of the mask are that it allows normal cough and humidification and requires less accessory equipment. Its disadvantages are the potential for skin abrasions, mouth leak, gastric distension, and nasal congestion.[12,57] An airtight seal may also be difficult to obtain with a standard nasal mask, which would necessitate a custom-made mask. Since nasal ventilation is mainly for nighttime ventilatory support, the need for other methods of ventilation must be discussed with the patient as respiratory status deteriorates.

The other method of providing ventilatory support is via a mouthpiece, which can be a simple one that the patient holds with lips and teeth or one with a lip seal held in place with straps. If the mouthpiece is used during sleep, a nose clip is needed to prevent leaking. Custom-made mouthpieces have also been made. This method of ventilation has been used for years by patients with polio.[62] Its advantages and disadvantages are similar to those of nasal ventilation, with the additional disadvantage of speech difficulty if the straps and a mouth seal are needed.[57,62] Full face mask ventilation has also been used but has disadvantages similar to those of positive pressure via nasal mask or mouthpiece, with an additional risk of aspiration and the disadvantage of the inability to speak at all while the mask is in place.

The assist-control mode is used for noninvasive ventilation with the sensitivity set at a level requiring very little effort to initiate the breath. The ability to adjust the flow rate separately may be helpful in preventing gastric distension. A regular ventilator circuit and exhalation valve are used, and usually a humidifier is not needed since the normal method of humidification is not altered.

Oxygen Delivery with Portable Positive Pressure Ventilators

Since none of the small home care ventilators except the Life-Care PLV-102 incorporate a blender, the consistency of O_2 delivery may vary considerably. Some of the models have an optional accumulator or reservoir, which is attached at the point of gas entry into the ventilator. This unit will improve the consistency of the delivered inspired O_2 fraction ($F_{I}O_2$). Another method of delivering O_2 to the patient is the use of a bleed-in system, whereby O_2 is incorporated into the ventilator circuit. The circuit and humidifier act as a reservoir between ventilator breaths, but if the SIMV mode is used, the patient will reduce this reservoir of O_2 during spontaneous ventilation. This may reduce the delivered $F_{I}O_2$, which in turn may increase the patient's respiratory rate, and the patient may actually have periods of hypoxemia. During assisted ventilation if the patient's ventilation increases the delivered $F_{I}O_2$ will decrease. Since bleeding in O_2 is the simplest method of O_2 delivery, usually requiring very small increments of O_2 flow, it is better to have a slightly higher $F_{I}O_2$ to allow for changes in respiratory rate.

Another method of O_2 delivery is the use of a Venturi device on the air intake valve. The problem with this method is the need for a higher O_2 flow, depending on the required $F_{I}O_2$, and the device can become dislodged from the ventilator without this being detected by the caregivers. Patients who require a very accurate $F_{I}O_2$ will need a ventilator that uses an accumulator or blender.

Negative Pressure Ventilation

As noted earlier in the chapter, negative pressure ventilation has been available since the early 1900s. A negative pressure ventilator consists of a generator and a chamber; the generator powers the unit, and the chamber surrounds the patient's chest and abdomen. The iron lung is the only ventilator that incorporates both generator and chamber in one unit. Other devices such as the cuirass or chest shell, pulmowrap, and Porta-Lung (made by W.W. "Sunny" Weingarten, Denver, CO) require a separate negative pressure generator.[55–57] Table 101-9 lists specifications of some of the negative pressure generators.

The iron lung is very durable and easy to operate, but it is cumbersome and stationary, and the provision of patient care is difficult. The Porta-Lung, a modification of the iron lung, is lightweight and more portable but is not suitable for a large person. The cuirass or chest shell is much easier to use, but adequate ventilation may not be achieved even with a custom-fitted shell. Other disadvantages of the shells are irritation or chafing where the rim comes in contact with the skin.

The pulmowrap may provide adequate ventilation, since the grid rests over the chest and abdomen with the negative pressure applied to the pulmowrap. Its disadvantage is the difficulty of getting the immobilized patient into it; the patient needs to lie supine and the bed needs to be flat. It also can cause back, shoulder, and arm pain. Major leaks may occur at the hips where the belt is attached, which is more of a problem in very thin patients. A pneumosuit, which is similar to the pulmowrap, includes leggings, which lessen the problem with leaks; it is easier to get into, especially for patients with COPD.

Other problems with negative pressure devices are the potential for obstructive sleep apnea and patients' complaints of feeling cold, and if clothing is worn, it may potentially be sucked into the hose, interfering with the operation of the ventilator. Eating and drinking may be contraindicated because of the potential for aspiration.[56,57]

Other Ventilatory Assist Devices

Use of positive and negative pressure ventilation is the most common approach to treating respiratory failure, but many patients have been treated successfully, on either a short or long-term basis, with other assistive devices. These are the pneumobelt and rocking bed, both of which have been used since the 1950s to provide ventilation for patients with neuromuscular disease, most notably polio.

The pneumobelt consists of an inflatable bladder inside a corset; the corset is fitted around the abdomen with the bladder connected to a positive pressure device. As the bladder

Table 101-9. Negative Pressure Ventilators

	Mode	Pressure Range (cm H_2O)	Rate	I/E Ratio	Alarms	Power Source
J. H. Emerson Company (Cambridge, MA)						
Emerson 33-CRE	Control	0–50	0–30 to 40 (variable)	Variable	None	AC only
Emerson 33-CRX	Control	0–60	0–40	Variable	None	AC only
Emerson 33-CRA	Assist (no backup rate)	0–40 to 50	Determined by patient, needs inspiratory effort of 0.5–1.0 cm H_2O, measured through a "cannula"	Variable	None	AC only
Puritan Bennett Corp. (Overland Park, KS)						
Maxivent (Thompson)[a]	Control	Negative 0–70 Positive 0–80	8–24	Fixed 1:2	Low pressure Machine failure Power failure	AC only
LIFECARE (Lafayette, CO)						
170C	Control	Negative 0–60 Positive 0–60	10–40	Fixed 1:1.5	Power loss	AC or DC

[a] Also has setting for alarm silence; resets in 1 min.

is inflated, the abdominal wall is compressed, the diaphragm is elevated, and expiration occurs.[57] When the bladder deflates, the abdominal pressure is relieved, and inspiration occurs passively as the diaphragm descends. The patient needs to be upright, since the diaphragm descends with the aid of gravity.[56,57,63,64]

The rocking bed consists of a platform with a mattress, on top of a motor with leg supports. The pitch of the bed and the rate of rocking can be altered—the maximum arc is 60 degrees total, and the rate can vary from 8 to 34 per minute.[57] The factors that influence changes in lung volume are the compliance of the lungs, rib cage, diaphragm, and abdominal wall, the effective length of the abdominal column, and the angle of the trunk to horizontal.[56,57,65]

Accessory Equipment in the Home

Table 101-10 lists the accessory equipment needed by the patient with an artificial airway, distinguishing between equipment that is absolutely needed by all patients and that which may be needed by individual patients. The recommendation for the backup ventilator was one of the outcomes of the consensus conference held in 1988 in Denver.[66]

Miscellaneous Equipment

Table 101-11 lists the miscellaneous equipment that may be needed in the home. This is individualized for every patient, and all members of the discharge planning team may be involved in its selection. Disposable supplies used in the home are also individualized for every patient.[3,54,57]

COSTS OF HOME VENTILATOR CARE

Earlier in this chapter, under nonmedical aspects of patient selection, it was noted that the patient needed adequate finances or insurance coverage to be maintained at home. Without one or both of these factors, home care cannot be a viable option. Many insurance policies will cover hospital care but will have minimal or nonexistent home care cov-

Table 101-10. Accessory Ventilator Equipment for Patients with Artificial Airways in the Home

Absolute necessity
Manual resuscitator bag
Humidifier
Suction machine
Electrical
Battery
Backup ventilator[a]
Battery[a]
Battery charger[a]
Ventilator cable to battery[a]
Secondary ventilator alarms
Individual need
O_2
Hygroscopic condenser-humidifier
Water traps
Compressors
Medication delivery
Aerosol
Generator
Remote alarms

[a] Needed for any patient who cannot wean for 4 consecutive hours or who lives in a rural area.

(From Gilmartin,[72] with permission.)

Table 101-11. Miscellaneous Equipment That May Be Needed in the Home

To enhance patient mobility
Wheelchair: manual/motorized
Walker
Ventilator/battery tray for wheelchair
Ramps
Lifting device
To enhance self-care
Commode
Elevated toilet seat
Safety bars
Electric bed
Environmental control units (ECU)
Patient assist devices: long-handled brushes
To enhance the environment
Flashlights/battery-powered lamps
Call lights
Electrical power strip with circuit breaker
Telephone communication systems

erage, even if it can be shown that home care will be a less expensive alternative. The American Association for Respiratory Care (AARC) estimated the mean cost of home care for ventilator-assisted patients to be $1766 per month in 1984, as compared with $22,569 for hospital care.[67] A study by LaFond et al.[68] showed the average cost of home care in 1987 to be $2976 per month. Figure 101-7 shows the various components of home care costs.[69] Creese and Fielden demonstrated that home care produced a 33 percent reduction in costs as compared with hospital care for 14 ventilator-assisted patients with polio in England.[70] Other investigators have also shown substantial savings in providing home care.[2,3,4,71]

The need for nursing care in the home is the single factor most responsible for the variation in home care costs for each patient. The cost of skilled nursing care ranges from $25 to $40 per hour. This range is based on geographic location and privately hired versus agency nurses. Home care equipment costs are also high, and equipment may be rented rather than purchased to ensure continued maintenance and home monitoring. At this time Medicare will only reimburse for rental of ventilators. The high costs of the equipment may also reflect the lack of reimbursement for respiratory therapy services in the home; the cost of the services needs to be built into the monthly rental to ensure ongoing quality assurance. Reimbursement for respiratory therapy services has been an ongoing issue in Congress since the early 1980s. Discharging stable patients who are capable of providing their own care or only need help from the family will greatly reduce the costs of home care.

PSYCHOSOCIAL CONSIDERATIONS IN HOME VENTILATOR CARE

Medical follow-up of a ventilator patient after discharge is only one aspect of care, and for many stable patients it may be a very minor part. For many patients and their families, psychological support is a major part of care after discharge from the hospital.[52] Psychosocial problems related to acute care are discussed in Chapter 104. Some of the factors that create problems with discharge and home care are listed in Table 101-12; problems related to discharge planning have been discussed under Obstacles to Discharge.

After discharge the illness and dependency on a machine become a reality. Some patients may magically think that they will be back to normal once they return to their home environment, and when it does not happen depression sets in. If the patient and family are providing all the care, they may feel overwhelmed by the "burden." Generally, the first month at home may be the most difficult for patients and

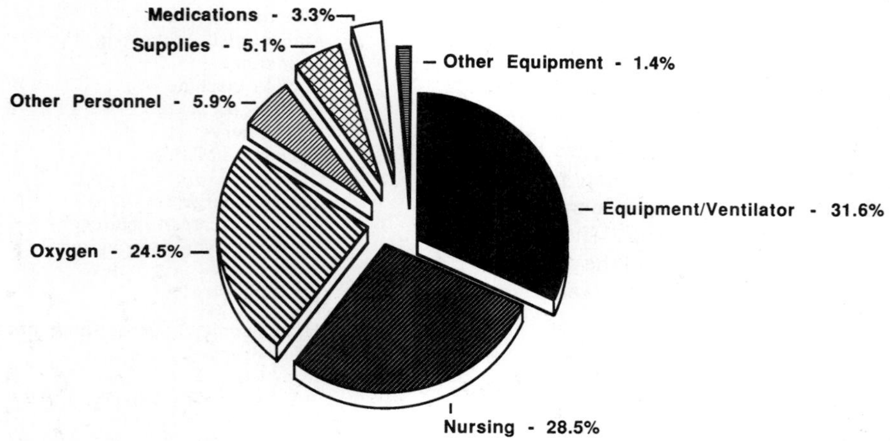

Figure 101-7. Average payments for home care for ventilator-assisted individuals in 1987 reported by the Boston University program. (From Make and Gilmartin,[69] with permission.)

Table 101-12. Long-Term Mechanical Ventilation: Patient Psychosocial Concommitants to Discharge Planning and Home Care

Change from protective environment
Change from hospital to family caregivers
Ambivalence/guilt
Impact of the illness
Demands on the family
Loss of privacy
Sibling rivalry
Loss of recreational, social, family time
Worry about the future

families who provide all their own care. They are establishing routines, gaining confidence, and trying to remember everything that was taught. Frequent visits by DME company personnel, reassurance, and review of skills they have been taught will help. Realistic discussions prior to discharge and meeting with other patients and families who have been through the same problems will also help. When a patient can progress from being "ill" to being disabled, the transition will be much smoother. Risk-taking is an essential part of gaining independence as long as these risks do not result from denial and are not maladaptive behaviors.[35]

Another problem faced by the patient and family, especially if other caretakers are in the home, is the loss of privacy. The family may feel that they are being constantly observed and are not able to continue with normal family life. When the patient is a child, sibling rivalry may become a problem—the healthy children may feel that the disabled child gets all the attention, and they may begin to misbehave in response to this. The parents may feel that they are shortchanging the other children because the care of the disabled child takes so much of their physical and emotional energy. The entire family is affected by the loss of recreational, social, and family time. The unanticipated monetary costs, constant fear of losing financial support because of limited insurance coverage, fear of losing their own health, and worry about the future take their toll on the family. The family may feel extremely angry toward the patient and yet feel guilty about this anger.

How can we help patients and families deal with these issues? We need to recognize that these issues are realities, discuss them openly, and help the family think of strategies to alleviate or prevent problems. Many times just knowing that their responses are normal and experienced by others is very helpful. Providing counseling and respite care may help to alleviate some of the problems, but respite care cannot be promised if there is no mechanism for providing it. Networking with other families and support groups will be helpful even if it can only be by telephone.

The ability to express feelings is helpful, although with children this may not always be possible. With adult patients, confronting them about their behavior if they are acting inappropriately or are being demanding is very important. Children may think that they can escape the consequences of inappropriate behavior when they are disabled, but they need to be disciplined just as the healthy siblings would be. Families who try to maintain a sense of normal family life tend to do better. Patients who are integrated into the normal family functioning will have a sense of worth and feel that they still have a role in the family.

Successful home care is dependent on adequate communication between the patient, family, and health care providers, on adaptive coping skills that were present before the illness, and on maintaining individual identity within the family structure, as well as on a sense of family identity and finally, on a strong social support network.[35]

References

1. Banaszak EF, Travers H, Frazier M et al: Home ventilator care. Respir Care 1981;26:1262–1268
2. Burr BH, Buyer B, Todres ID et al: Home care for children on respirators. N Engl J Med 1983;309:1319–1323
3. Feldman J, Tuteur PG: Mechanical ventilation: From hospital intensive care to home. Heart Lung 1982;11:162–165
4. Fischer DA, Prentice WS: Feasibility of home care for certain respiratory-dependent restrictive or obstructive lung disease patients. Chest 1982;82:739–743
5. Garay SM, Turino GM, Goldring RM: Sustained reversal of chronic hypercapnia in patients with alveolar hypoventilation syndromes: Long-term maintenance with noninvasive nocturnal mechanical ventilation. Am J Med 1981;70:269–274
6. Gilmartin M, Make B: Home care of ventilator-dependent persons. Respir Care 1983;28:1490–1497
7. Gilmartin M, Make BJ: Mechanical ventilation in the home. Curr Rev Respir Ther 1985;7:139–143
8. Giovannoni R: Chronic ventilator care: From hospital to home. Respir Ther 1984;14:29–33
9. Goldberg AI, Kettrick R, Buzdygan D et al: Home ventilation program for infants and children. Crit Care Med 1980;8:238–243
10. Hoeppner VH, Cockcroft DW, Dosman JA et al: Night-time ventilation improves respiratory failure in secondary kyphoscoliosis. Am Rev Respir Dis 1984;129:240–243
11. Indihar FJ, Walker NE: Experience with a prolonged respiratory care unit revisited. Chest 1984;86:616–620
12. Kerby GR, Mayer LS, Pingleton SK: Nocturnal positive pressure ventilation via nasal mask. Am Rev Respir Dis 1987; 137:738–740
13. Kettrick RG, Donar ME: Ventilator-assisted infants and children. Probl Respir Care 1988;1(2):269–278
14. Kopacz MA, Moriarty-Wright R: Multidisciplinary approach for the patient on a home ventilator. Heart Lung 1984;13:255–262
15. Leger P, Jennequin J, Gerard M, Robert D: Home positive pressure ventilation via nasal mask for patients with neuromuscular weakness or restrictive lung or chest wall disease. Respir Care 1989;34:73–77
16. Make B, Gilmartin M, Brody JS, Snider GL: Rehabilitation of ventilator-dependent persons with lung disease: The concept and initial experience. Chest 1984;86:358–365
17. Make BJ: Long-term management of ventilator-assisted individuals. The Boston University experience. Respir Care 1986;31:303–310
18. Make BJ, Gilmartin M: Rehabilitation of ventilator-assisted individuals. Clin Chest Med 1986;7:679–691
19. O'Donohue WJ, Giovannoni RM, Goldberg AI et al: Long-term mechanical ventilation: Guidelines for management in the home and alternate community sites. Chest, suppl. 1986;90:1S–37S
20. Prentice WS: Transition from hospital to home. Prob Respir Care 1988;1(2):174–191

21. Robert D, Gérard M, Leger P et al: Domiciliary mechanical ventilation by tracheostomy for chronic respiratory failure. Rev Fr Mal Respir 1983;11:923–936
22. Sivak ED, Cordasco EM, Gipson WT et al: Home care ventilation: The Cleveland Clinic experience from 1977 to 1985. Respir Care 1986;31:294–302
23. Splaingard ML, Frates RC Jr, Harrison GM et al: Home positive pressure ventilation: Twenty years' experience. Chest 1983;84:376–382
24. Goldberg AI: Mechanical ventilation and respiratory care in the home in the 1990's: Some personal observations. Respir Care 1990;35:247–259
25. Drinker P, Shaw LA: An apparatus for the prolonged administration of artificial ventilation. J Clin Invest 1929;7:229
26. Drinker PA, McKhann CF: The iron lung, first practical means of respiratory support. JAMA 1986;255:1476–1480
27. Gorham J: A medical triumph: The iron lung. Respir Ther 1979;Jan/Feb:71–73
28. Collier CR, Affeldt JE: Ventilatory efficiency of the cuirass respirator in totally paralyzed chronic poliomyelitis patients. J Appl Physiol 1954;6:531–538
29. Hill NS: Clinical application of body ventilators. Chest 1986;90:897–905
30. O'Donohue WJ, Branson RD, Hoppough JM, Make BJ: Criteria for establishing units for chronic ventilator-dependent patients in hospitals. Respir Care 1988;33:1044–1046
31. Cosgrove JL, Alexander MA, Mitts EL et al: Late effects of poliomyelitis. Arch Phys Med Rehabil 1987;68:4–7
32. Schreiner MS, Downes JJ, Kettrick RG et al: Chronic respiratory failure in infants. JAMA 1987;258:3398–3404
33. Kacmarek RM, Stanek KS, McMahon K et al: Improved work of breathing during synchronized intermittent mandatory ventilation (SIMV) via home care ventilators. Am Rev Respir Dis 1988;137(4, pt 2):64
34. Donar ME: Community care: Pediatric home mechanical ventilation. Holistic Nurse Pract 1988;2:68–80
35. LaFond L, Horner J: Psychological issues related to long-term ventilatory support. Probl Respir Care 1988;1(2):241–256
36. Gilmartin M: Patient and family education. Clin Chest Med 1986;7:619–627
37. Frates RC, Splaingard ML, Smith DO et al: Outcome of home mechanical ventilation in children. J Pediatr 1985;106:850
38. Splaingard ML, Frates RC, Jefferson LS et al: Home negative pressure ventilation: Report of 20 years experience in patients with neuromuscular disease. Arch Phys Med Rehabil 1985;66:239–242
39. Review. Home ventilation: Status in Ontario. Ont Med Rev 1986;Jan:14–16
40. Czorniak MA, Gilmartin ME, Make BJ: Home mechanical ventilation: Clinical course of patients with neuromuscular disease (NMD) and chronic obstructive pulmonary disease (COPD). Am Rev Respir Dis 1987;135(4, pt 2):A194
41. Make BJ, Gilmartin ME: Mechanical ventilation in the home. Crit Care Clin 1990;6:785–796
42. Pierson DJ: Home respiratory care in different countries. Eur Respir J, suppl. 7, 1989;2:630S–636S
43. Robert D, Fournier G, Thomas L et al: Indications de la ventilation chronique à domicile par trachéotomie de l'insuffisance chronique non paralytique. Rev Fr Mal Respir 1979;7:353–355
44. Dull WL, Sadoul P: Home ventilators in patients with severe lung disease, abstracted. Am Rev Respir Dis, suppl. 1981;123:74
45. Goldberg AI, Faure EAM: Home care for life supported persons in England: The responaut approach. Chest 1984;86:910–914
46. Laier-Groeneveld G, Criée CP, Hüttemann Y: Noninvasive intermittent ventilation—indication by respiratory muscle function. Respir Care 1990;35:35
47. Zaniboni S, Zacaria S, Ferrario P et al: Short and mid-term effects of home mechanical ventilation in hypoxemic hypercapnic respiratory failure. Respir Care 1990;35:35
48. Prentice WS: Placement alternatives for long-term ventilator care. Respir Care 1986;31:288–293
49. O'Donohue WJ Jr: Patient selection and discharge criteria for home ventilator care. Probl Respir Care 1988;1(2):167–174
50. Weisinger W, Goldsmith T: Artificial ventilation. Its import on communication and swallowing problems. Probl Respir Care 1988;1(2):204–216
51. Thompson CL, Richmond M: Teaching home care for ventilator-dependent patients: The patients' perception. Heart Lung 1990;19:79–83
52. Gilmartin M: Mechanical ventilation in the home: An overview. Probl Respir Care 1988;1(2):155–166
53. Wilhelm L, Plummer A: Role of the home care practitioner. Probl Respir Care. 1988;1(2):279–292
54. Johnson DL, Giovannoni RM, Driscoll SA: Ventilator-assisted Patient Care: Planning for Hospital Discharge and Home Care. Aspen, Rockville, MD, 1986
55. McPherson SP: Respiratory Home Care Equipment. Kendall/Hunt, Dubuque, IA, 1988
56. Kacmarek RM, Spearman CB: Equipment used for ventilatory support in the home. Respir Care 1986;31:311–328
57. O'Donnell C, Gilmartin ME: Home mechanical ventilators and accessory equipment. Probl Respir Care 1988;1(2):217–240
58. Kacmarek RM, Thompson SE: Respiratory care of the ventilator-assisted infant in the home. Respir Care 1986;31:605–614
59. Bach JR, Alba A, Mosher R: Intermittent positive pressure ventilation via nasal access in the management of respiratory insufficiency. Chest 1987;92:168–170
60. Ellis ER, McCavley VB, Mellis C, Sullivan C: Treatment of alveolar hypoventilation in a six year old girl with intermittent positive pressure ventilation through a nose mask. Am Rev Respir Dis 1987;136:188–191
61. Braun NM: Nocturnal ventilation—a new method, editorial. Am Rev Respir Dis 1987;135:523
62. Bach JR, Alba AS, Bohatuik G: Mouth intermittent positive pressure ventilation in the management of post polio respiratory insufficiency. Chest 1987;91:859–864
63. Adamson JP, Stein JD: Application of abdominal pressure for artificial respiration. JAMA 1959;169:1613–1617
64. Miller JH, Thomas E, Wilmont CB: Pneumobelt use among high quadriplegic population. Arch Phys Med Rehabil 1988;69:369–372
65. Coville P, Shugg C, Ferris BF: Effects of body tilting on respiratory mechanics. J Appl Physiol 1956;9:19–24
66. Plummer AL, O'Donohue WJ, Petty TL et al: Consensus conference on problems in home mechanical ventilation. Am Rev Respir Dis 1989;140:555–560
67. AARTimes: Association holds press conference on ventilator survey. AARTimes 1984;8(April):28–31
68. LaFond L, Make BJ, Gilmartin ME: Home care costs for ventilator-assisted individuals, abstracted. Am Rev Respir Dis 1988;137(4, pt 2):62
69. Make BJ, Gilmartin ME: Care of the ventilator-assisted individual in the home and alternate sites. pp. 669–690. Hodgkin JE, Burton G, Ward J eds. Respiratory Care: A Guide to Clinical Practice. 3rd Ed. JB Lippincott, Philadelphia, 1991
70. Creese AL, Fielden R: Hospital or home care for the severely disabled: A cost comparison. Br J Prev Soc Med 1977;31:116–121
71. Sivak ED, Cordasco EM, Gipson WT: Pulmonary mechanical ventilation at home: A reasonable and less expensive alternative. Respir Care 1983;28:42–49
72. Gilmartin ME: Long term mechanical ventilation. Patient selection and discharge planning. Respir Care 1991;36:205–216

Chapter 102

Smoking Cessation

Louise M. Nett
David J. Pierson

CHAPTER OUTLINE

Smoking is the most important modifiable cause of death in the United States—one out of six deaths is related to smoking, and each year 390,000 Americans die from tobacco-related disease.

Every year 1 million Americans improve their health by stopping smoking. Most smokers quit on their own, and only 10 to 20 percent seek help from programs. Smokers learn something with each attempt to quit and this helps to improve their success. People who are unable to quit on their own, however, seek help from programs. Community assist programs for cessation of smoking are many and varied; most commonly used are those offered by the American Cancer Society and American Lung Association. Many commercial programs are listed in the yellow pages of the telephone directory. The basis of these programs is group support, education, and behavior modification. Their length and content vary, which makes it quite difficult to compare one with the other. Most programs report success in different ways. A major problem in assessing program success is the lack both of uniformity and of biologic verification of smoking cessation.[1] Smokers tend to overestimate their success when only a verbal report is issued.

Nicotine dependency treatment refers to medical treatment of tobacco addiction, which follows the medical model used in other diseases. Diagnosis is determined by extensive history, physical examination, and laboratory tests. Patients with the medical diagnosis of nicotine dependency are treated with pharmacologic strategies, education, and home and office follow-up. Medical evaluation and treatment of smokers are experiencing a growth phase since the release of nicotine polacrilex (Nicorette) gum in 1984, and especially with the introduction of transdermal nicotine patches in 1991.

Other approaches to cessation of smoking are hypnosis, acupuncture, rapid smoking, aversive therapy, and nicotine fading. Smoking cessation methods and techniques are reviewed in a comprehensive book on the subject,[1] as well as in recent comprehensive reviews.[2,3] Although none of these techniques are significantly useful alone, they may be of some value when combined with other techniques. At this time the literature is inconclusive regarding the effectiveness of these techniques when used in isolation.

MOTIVATION TO QUIT

Quitting without Help

The Adult Use of Tobacco Survey indicates that 90 percent of successful quitters use individual methods of smoking cessation rather than organized programs[4]—most smokers simply go "cold turkey."[5] Success rates for smokers who quit on their own are often higher than for smokers who use a cessation program. Smokers who fail on their own may then choose to attend a group cessation program. Heavy smokers, smokers who have made previous attempts to quit, and women are more likely to use formal stop smoking programs. These groups of individuals usually have more difficulty quitting.[6]

Smokers who succeed in quitting generally are male, white, older, and better educated and have made fewer previous quitting attempts. Success is also correlated with the time at which the first cigarette is smoked in the morning, as well as with heavy smokers with symptoms.[7] Smokers who delay the first cigarette of the day for more than 30 minutes are less addicted and more likely to be successful in quitting.[8] Less addicted smokers are more successful at quitting than highly addicted smokers. Smokers with symptoms find it hard to deny that smoking is having adverse effects on their health; this provides a strong motivation to quit.[9]

Motivating Factors

Personal reasons to quit smoking are important motivating factors. Smokers who want to quit are more successful than those less motivated.[10] The main reasons are health, example of others, aesthetics, and mastery. Many smokers also recognize the antisocial aspect of smoking.[11] In the 1960s about half of the males in the United States smoked; today less than one-third smoke. The trend is away from smoking. Most smokers now moderate their smoking when around nonsmokers because of social disapproval. Health-conscious smokers who have changed to low-fat diets, started exercising, and wear seat belts should realize that the most important health improvement is to stop smoking.

Health professionals have successfully used biologic tests to motivate smokers to quit and remain abstinent. Spirometry and exhaled carbon monoxide testing have proved useful motivating events.[12–14] Health professionals can review the results of such tests with the patient while pointing out the effect of smoking on test results. If spirometry results are normal, this often provides reassurance to the patient that it is not too late to quit. Spirometry should be performed on all smokers. Patients with decreased vital capacity and/or forced expiratory volume in the first second (FEV_1) are at risk for cardiopulmonary disease. A white laboratory coat worn by the health professional can enhance the effectiveness of advice to quit smoking.[15]

Exhaled CO levels are always abnormal in an inhaling cigarette smoker. The usual value for a one-pack-per-day smoker is 25 to 30 ppm. Instantaneous biofeedback of the patient's own value make this an important medical test, and ready availability of portable testing devices increases the potential for wide application of this tool.

Readiness to Quit

Readiness to quit may be enhanced when patients are hospitalized. There can be little denial at this time of the health risks of smoking, and it may be an ideal time for intervention. Of cardiac patients who receive advice to quit after an acute event, 45 percent do so; however, when advice to quit is coupled with 2 hours of education in relapse prevention, the success rate increases to 71 percent.[16]

Health professionals can assist patients who are ready to quit. Once the decision to quit has been made, a quit date should be selected. Preparation for quitting includes instruction in behavior change and how to break old habits. This is the time to evaluate for nicotine dependence and to educate in coping skills for relapse prevention.

Social Pressure to Quit

Smoking restrictions at the workplace and in public help in motivating some smokers to quit. The decision to quit is occasionally moved ahead to the date of a workplace smoking ban.[17,18] Hospitals and health care centers should set an example by maintaining their facilities as nonsmoking environments. Signs prohibiting smoking because of its risk to patients and staff can serve as a means of educating visitors to the health center. This not so subtle message about smoking and its consequences to health is reinforced with every visit.

BENEFITS OF SMOKING CESSATION

The benefits of ceasing tobacco use are many.[2,3,19] Smokers will experience a reduction in symptoms, decreased risk of complications (including death), improved vigor, and improved senses of smell and taste with cessation of tobacco use. Smoking cessation results in a decreased risk of mortality from coronary artery disease, and the degree of risk reduction is determined by the length of time after cessation, the amount smoked, and the duration of smoking before cessation.[20]

Cough and sputum production are irritating symptoms, which will improve within 1 month of cessation of cigarette use.[19,21] Improvement in these symptoms corresponds to healing of the respiratory mucous membrane when exposure to the irritating components of tobacco smoke is eliminated. Figure 102-1 illustrates dramatically the differences in the ciliated epithelium of the smoker and the nonsmoker.[22] Showing photographs such as those in Figure 102-1 to smokers, while providing reassurance that the changes are potentially reversible, may assist in motivating them to quit.

Improvement in pulmonary function tests has also been reported with cessation of cigarette smoking.[23,24] Snoring prevalence is high in smokers but declines in exsmokers. Heavy smokers may also have mild obstructive sleep apnea[25]; the benefits of quitting for this population are obvious. Smokers who are considered for nocturnal continuous positive airway pressure (CPAP) devices may show an interest in stopping smoking if this association is discussed with them.

The benefits of smoking cessation for patients with

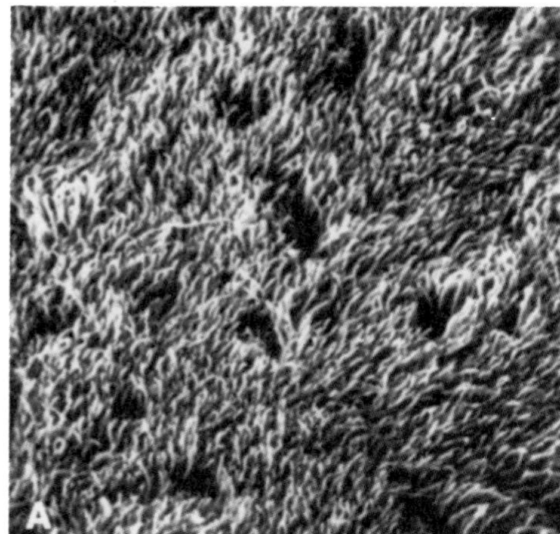

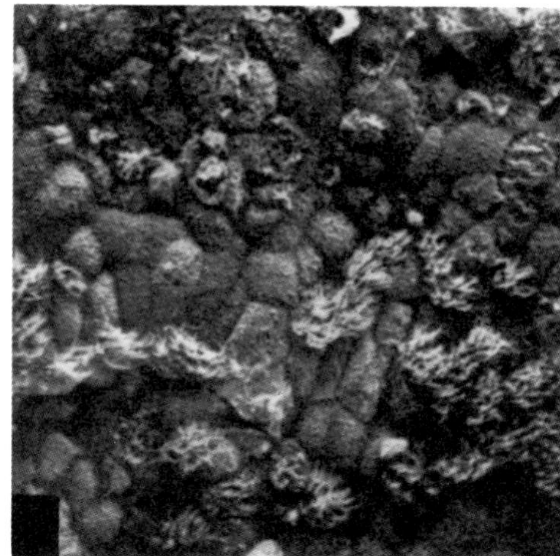

Figure 102-1. Low-power scanning electron micrographs of biopsies of human bronchial mucosa. (**A**) Biopsy from a healthy nonsmoker. Note the continuous "shag carpet" of cilia, with scattered indentations indicating the location of mucus-producing cells. (**B**) Biopsy from a "healthy" smoker. There is a marked reduction in ciliated cells and a striking proliferation of (nonciliated) mucus-producing cells. (From Regland et al.,[22] with permission.)

asthma, ulcers, peripheral vascular disease, and memory loss should be reviewed. Cerebral perfusion is improved in elderly patients who stop smoking.[26] Many elderly people believe it is too late to quit; pointing out this little known benefit may stimulate some of these persons to make a new attempt. Parents of asthmatic children, especially the mothers, should be taught that their smoking affects the child. Reports indicate that the child is more likely to develop asthma and will need more medication if the mother smokes.[27,28]

SMOKING CESSATION METHODS

Medical Intervention

The health team can develop treatment programs for smokers. When these programs incorporate multiple modalities, success is improved. Programs should include physicians and nonphysicians and should use multiple individual group sessions. The patient should receive the message, and education in the process of quitting, from all team members. Face-to-face intervention and support with nicotine replacement therapy improves success rates.[29]

The National Cancer Institute advises physicians to use a four-step process to aide smokers in quitting,[30] the key components of which are (1) ask, (2) advise, (3) assist, (4) arrange. This minimal intervention strategy should be used with all patients who smoke, and the health team should develop a system for implementing it. The office receptionist or hospital admission clerk should identify all smokers by asking the question. A routine technique for reporting that the question was asked should be developed; for example, a simple color-coded dot on the outside of the patient's chart can alert the team to the smoker. The physician is the key person to advise the patient to quit smoking. The team can agree on supportive information to tell or give to the patient in order to reinforce the physician's advice. That a patient smokes should set in motion a comprehensive treatment program delivered by the entire health team. Arranging for continued follow-up is important in preventing relapse.

Training physicians in smoking cessation techniques does increase their involvement in counseling patients about smoking.[31–33] Physicians and health professionals who receive special education for intervention are usually more enthusiastic about treatment of smokers. There is a general perception that smokers have already been advised to quit: in fact, only half usually have received advice to quit, and few receive instruction in how to quit. Stopping smoking is like any other behavior change and for the nicotine-dependent patient is often an involved process. In preparation for quitting it is important to assess the smoker's motivation to quit, confidence in ability to quit, readiness to quit, and reasons to quit. Also relevant to success are social support from friends and family. Evaluation for nicotine dependence by history of current cigarette use and past attempts to quit is useful. A brief history will give health professionals useful data to assist the smoker as the patient makes the next quit effort (Fig. 102-2).

In-Hospital Intervention

The leading health problems in the United States are related to tobacco consumption, mainly cigarette use.[35] There are 30 million hospital admissions each year. Using the national prevalence of smoking data, one can assume that at least 30 percent of all hospitalized patients are smokers on

History, Motivation, and Self-Efficacy Form

Full Name: ______________________ Date: ______________________

1. How motivated are you to quit smoking?

Not motivated									Extremely motivated
1	2	3	4	5	6	7	8	9	10

2. How confident are you that you will be smoke-free 1 year from now?

Not confident									Extremely confident
1	2	3	4	5	6	7	8	9	10

3. How ready are you to quit at this time?

Not at all ready									Very ready
1	2	3	4	5	6	7	8	9	10

4. How much support do you have for quitting?

None									Lots of support
1	2	3	4	5	6	7	8	9	10

5. Who else smokes in your home? ______________________

6. What could make you go back to smoking when you quit for awhile? ______________________

____

7. How are you preparing to quit? ______________________

____

8. How many times have you quit in the past? ________

How long were you quit each time? _____1 _____2 _____3 _____4

Why did you go back to smoking? ______________________

____

9. How much did you suffer during past quit attempts?

Severe misery									No problem
1	2	3	4	5	6	7	8	9	10

10. How sad are you to be losing your "old friend" the cigarette?

Very sad									Not sad
1	2	3	4	5	6	7	8	9	10

11. What cigarette do you now smoke? ______________________

What was your other brand in the past? ______________________

12. How much do you smoke now each day? ______________________

In the past did you smoke _____ more? _____ the same? _____ less?

13. Do you smoke within 30 minutes of arising? _____ yes _____ no

14. What is your main reason to quit? ______________________

____

15. Do you think your health is affected by continued smoking?

Not at all									Makes it worse
1	2	3	4	5	6	7	8	9	10

Figure 102-2. Example of a simple form that health professionals can use to assess a patient's degree of nicotine dependence and stated motivations for quitting.

admission to the hospital. This gives health professionals the opportunity to assist 10 million smokers while they are hospitalized.

The American Association for Respiratory Care (AARC) is encouraging the development of in-hospital programs for bedside treatment of nicotine dependence. The basis of such a program is outlined in a publication that is a joint project of the National Heart, Lung and Blood Institute and AARC.[36] The booklet describes four levels of involvement: at level 1 respiratory care practitioners and other clinicians discuss the benefits of smoking cessation with all patients; at level 2 clinicians give individualized counseling at the bedside to all patients interested in quitting; at level 3 patients in all departments of the hospital are offered education and counseling; and at level 4 attempts are made to reach out to the community by offering group support classes and counseling.

A Treatment Protocol

A comprehensive treatment protocol for nicotine dependence includes evaluation, education, therapy, and follow-up, as well as pharmacologic support. Evaluation of the hospitalized smoker includes evaluation of nicotine dependence. The Diagnostic and Statistical Manual of Mental Disorders lists nicotine dependence (305.10) and nicotine withdrawal (292.00) as disorders.[37] Dependent smokers continue to use tobacco even though they know it can worsen physical health; have tried to quit and failed; and experience at least four of the following cardinal withdrawal symptoms on cessation:

1. Craving for tobacco
2. Irritability, frustration, or anger
3. Anxiety or restlessness
4. Difficulty concentrating
5. Decreased heart rate
6. Increased appetite or weight gain

Respiratory care practitioners can assist the physician by documenting the history of addiction and withdrawal. A daily report of withdrawal symptoms on the patient's medical record further documents the problem (Fig. 102-3).

Nicotine replacement therapy improves the quit success rate in dependent smokers who are motivated to quit. Replacement nicotine in a gum base has been used effectively in treatment programs.[38–40] Preliminary data from studies using transdermal nicotine patches indicate that this route of administration can be effective as well.[41,42] As with any medication program, the value of the medication is based on patient understanding, participation, and correct usage. Like insulin replacement therapy, nicotine replacement therapy must achieve adequate blood levels to relieve withdrawal symptoms, and also like insulin therapy, it requires that the patient participate in a comprehensive behavioral program. Medication alone is not successful but enhances the success of a complete program.

A program initiated while the smoker is an inpatient should include a follow-up component. Some programs follow patients up through cardiac or pulmonary rehabilitation programs. The least expensive but effective techniques for follow-up are phone calls and letters.

Smoking Cessation Classes

The majority of stop smoking programs include education about smoking as a habit/addiction, behavior change, the importance of social support, and coping techniques to prevent relapse. The intensity and depth of the information given varies with the type of program and the skills of the group leader. It is difficult to compare the success rates between programs because of the many variables of the available programs.

The length of the program may have an impact on success. Individuals who are willing to stay with a program for up to 3 months may be more motivated to quit, but success may relate to participants' subsequent determination to remain abstinent. Programs of short duration may appeal to a different category of smoker. The 2-week programs may not offer long enough support to prevent relapse.

Programs usually report success in the short term. Relapse continues through the first year after cessation. There is some continued attrition up to 2 years, but the standard follow-up is 1 year. The majority of programs assess success by phone or mail follow-up, and few undertake biologic verification. When CO level, cotinine, or thiocyanate testing is used to verify success, about 20 percent of smokers overestimate their success at smoking cessation. Some researchers refer to this as "nicotine amnesia."

Behavior Modification

Many smokers with disease who continue to smoke are dependent on nicotine. All smokers are habituated to cigarettes, and their habituation is reinforced 100 to 200 times per day, since the average smoker inhales 7 to 10 puffs per cigarette. This "second nature" habit will be hard to break. Replacing cigarettes with a nonhazardous substance may help a smoker to change behavior. Nontoxic substitutes for cigarettes include toothpicks, swizzle sticks, sugarless lollipops, and objects to twiddle with, such as rubber bands and paper clips.

Behavior change is facilitated by better understanding the behavior. Keeping a daily diary or self-monitoring the habit is useful in decreasing the behavior. Smokers who fill out a daily form noting time at which the need of a cigarette is felt routinely cut consumption.

Nicotine fading or reduction is useful in inducing smokers to change brands. This weaning from brand loyalty is the first step in change. Smokers tend to identify with their own brand and find less pleasure in a new brand of cigarettes. Reducing the amount of nicotine by changing to low-nicotine cigarettes is not always possible, as smokers who switch to low-nicotine cigarettes usually inhale longer and more deeply to extract their usual level of nicotine no matter what brand is used.[43] Smokers who are able to reduce the amount of nicotine by smoking less may be more successful at quit-

Withdrawal Symptom Flow Sheet

Name Plate

Date: ______________________

____

Special Notes:

Date/Session	/1	/2	/3	/4	/5	/6	/7	/8
Carbon monoxide								
VC								
FEV_1								
Number of nicorettes								
Withdrawal symptoms Use nicotine withdrawal score sheet to tabulate score from 1 to 5								
Craving for nicotine								
Irritable, angry, frustrated								
Anxiety								
Difficulty concentrating								
Restlessness								
Change in heart rate								
Increased appetite								
Other								
Constipation								
Insomnia								
Headaches								
Teary-weepy								

Figure 102-3. Daily record of withdrawal symptoms and other manifestations during abstinence from nicotine and cigarette smoking.

ting. Tapering to a lower dosage may have therapeutic implications. Most smokers can reduce their consumption by one-third without suffering withdrawal symptoms. It makes sense that smokers who are accustomed to a lower level of nicotine will have more success at cessation.

RELAPSE PREVENTION

Relapse prevention skill training should start when the smoking cessation program begins, rather than being delayed until the end of the program. Smokers need to identify high-risk situations that may lead to a return to smoking. Coping strategies that the smoker believes will be helpful should be explored.[44] Cognitive and behavioral techniques should be realistic in relation to the patient's own life-style and personality. Role playing may enhance the selection of a realistic coping technique; smokers who plan to "tough it out" are often counted among those who relapse.

Marlatt and Gordon[45] have explored reasons for relapse. Negative emotional states rather than urges and temptations cause a return to smoking. Smokers who view smoking as a black and white, either/or phenomenon have a rigid approach to smoking cessation. Smokers who believe one cigarette (a lapse) is a very serious event and are unable to be self-forgiving usually relapse.[45] Although breaking abstinence by having one cigarette may lead the smoker to feel all is lost, this concrete thinking disregards smoking cessation as a process and focuses on it as an event. Marlatt and Gordon call this the *abstinent violation effect*. This unforgiving attitude is too harsh and will cause many smokers to say "I just couldn't do it, it's too hard to quit." Quitting takes practice, and the process of quitting takes time.

References

1. Schwartz JL: Review and evaluation of smoking cessation methods—the United States and Canada, 1978–1985. NIH Publication No. 87-2940, National Cancer Institute, Division of Cancer Prevention and Control, Washington, D.C., 1987
2. Fisher EB, Haire-Joshu D, Morgan GD et al: Smoking and smoking cessation. Am Rev Respir Dis 1990;142:702–720
3. Sees KL: Cigarette smoking, nicotine dependence, and treatment. West J Med 1990;152:578–584
4. Centers for Disease Control: Tobacco use in 1986: Methods and basic tabulations from adult use of tobacco survey. U.S. Department of Health & Human Services, Rockville, MD, 1989
5. Fiore M, Novotny TE, Pierce JP et al: Methods used to quit smoking in the United States. JAMA, 1990;263:2760–2765
6. The Health Consequences of Smoking: Nicotine Addiction. A Report of the Surgeon General. Publication No. 88-8406, U.S. Department of Health & Human Services, Rockville, MD, 1988
7. Kabat GC, Wynder EL: Determinants of quitting smoking. Am J Publ Health 1987;77:1301–1305
8. Kozlowski LT, Wilkinson DP, Skinner W et al: Comparing tobacco cigarette dependence with other drug dependencies. JAMA 1989;261:898–901
9. Burt A, Thornley P, Illingworth D et al: Stopping smoking after myocardial infarction. Lancet 1974;1:304–306
10. McFall RM, Hommen CL Jr: Motivation, structure and self monitoring: Role of non-specific factors in smoking reduction. Consulting Clin Psychol 1971;1:80–86
11. Ferguson T: The Smoker's Book of Health: How to Keep Yourself Healthier and Reduce Your Smoking Risks. GP Putnam's Sons Publishers, New York, 1987
12. Petty TL, Pierson DJ, Dick NP et al: Follow up evaluation of a prevalence study for chronic obstructive bronchitis and chronic airways obstruction. Am Rev Respir Dis 1976;114:881–890
13. Hepper NGG, Drage CW, Davies SF et al: Chronic obstructive pulmonary disease: A community-oriented program including professional education and screening by a voluntary health agency. Am Rev Respir Dis 1980;121:97–104
14. Risser NL, Belcher DW: Adding spirometry, carbon monoxide and pulmonary symptoms results to smoking cessation counseling. J Gen Intern Med 1990;5:16–22
15. Raw M: Persuading people to stop smoking. Behav Res Ther 1976;14:97–101
16. Barr-Taylor C, Houston-Miller N, Killen JD, DeBusk RF: Smoking cessation after acute myocardial infarction—the effects of a nurse-managed intervention. Ann Intern Med 1990;113:118–123
17. Andrews J: Reducing smoking in the hospital. Chest 1983;84:206–209
18. Becker DM, Conner HF, Waranch HR et al: The impact of total ban on smoking in Johns Hopkins Children's Center. JAMA 1989;262:799–802
19. Tobin MJ, Suffredini AF, Grenvik A: Short-term effects of smoking cessation. Respir Care 1984;29:641–649
20. Department of Health and Human Services: The Health Consequences of Smoking: Cardiovascular Disease. A Report of the Surgeon General. Rockville, MD, 1983
21. Buist AS, Sexton GJ, Nagy JM, Ross BB: The effect of smoking cessation and modification on lung functions. Am Rev Respir Dis 1976;114:115–122
22. Regland B, Cajander S, Wiman L-G, Falkmer S: Scanning electron microscopy of the bronchial mucosa in some lung diseases using bronchoscopy specimens. Scand J Respir Dis 1976; 57:171–182
23. Paxton R, Scott S: Non-smoking reinforced by improvements in lung function. Addict Behav 1981;6:313–315
24. McCarthy DS, Douglas BC, Cherniack RM: Effect of modification of the smoking habit on lung function. Am Rev Respir Dis 1976;114:103–113
25. Berry RB, Block AJ: Positive nasal airway pressure eliminates snoring as well as obstructive sleep apnea. Chest 1984;85:15–20
26. Rogers RL, Meyer JS, Judd BW, Martel KF: Abstention from cigarette smoking improves cerebral perfusion among elderly chronic smokers. JAMA 1985;253:2970–2974
27. Murray AB, Morrison BJ: Passive smoking and the seasonal difference of severity of asthma in children. Chest 1988;94:701–708
28. Weitzman M, Gortmaker S, Walker DK, Sobol A: Maternal smoking and childhood asthma. Pediatrics 1990;85:505–511
29. Kottke TE, Battista RN, DeFriese GH, Brekke ML: Attributes of successful smoking cessation interventions in medical practice—a meta-analysis of 39 controlled trials. JAMA 1988;259:2883–2889
30. U.S. Department of Health and Human Services: How To Help Your Patients Stop Smoking. NIH Publication No. 89-3064. Public Health Service, National Institutes of Health, National Cancer Institute, Bethesda, MD, 1989
31. Cummings SR, Coates TJ, Richard RJ et al: Training physicians in counseling about smoking cessation—a randomized trial of the Quit for Life Program. Ann Intern Med 1989;110:640–647
32. Kottke TE, Brekke ML, Solberg LI, Hughes JR: A randomized trial to increase smoking intervention by physicians—doctors helping smokers, Round I. JAMA 1989;261:2101–2106
33. Wilson DM, Lindsay EA, Best JA et al: A smoking cessation intervention program for family physicians. Can Med Assoc J 1987;137:613–619
34. Anda RF, Remington PL, Sienko DG, Davis RM: Are physi-

cians advising smokers to quit? The patient's perspective. JAMA 1987;257:1916–1919
35. The Health Consequences of Smoking: 25 Years of Programs. A Report of the Surgeon General. US Department of Health and Human Services, Public Health Service, Rockville, MD, 1989
36. U.S. Department of Health and Human Services: How You Can Help Patients Stop Smoking—Opportunities for Respiratory Care Practitioners. NIH Publication No. 89-2961. Public Health Service, National Institutes of Health, National Heart, Lung and Blood Institute, Bethesda, MD, 1989
37. American Psychiatric Association: Diagnostic and Statistical Manual of Mental Disorders. 3rd Ed. Revised. American Psychiatric Association, Washington, DC, 1987
38. Schneider NG, Jarvik ME, Forsythe AB et al: Nicotine gum in smoking cessation: A placebo-controlled, double-blind trial. Addict Behav 1983;8:253–261
39. Hjalmarson AI: Effect of nicotine chewing gum in smoking cessation. JAMA 1984;252:2835–2838
40. Tonnesen P, Fryd V, Hansen M et al: Two and four mg nicotine chewing gum and group counseling in smoking cessation: An open randomized controlled trial with a 22-month follow-up. Addict Behav 1988;13:17–27
41. Transdermal Nicotine Study Group: Transdermal nicotine for smoking cessation. Six-month results from two multicenter controlled clinical trials. JAMA 1991;266:3133–3138
42. Hurt RD, Langer GG, Offord KP et al: Nicotine-replacement therapy with use of a transdermal nicotine patch—a randomized double-blind placebo-controlled trial. Mayo Clin Proc 1990;65:1529–1537
43. Henningfield JE: Nicotine—An Old Fashioned Addiction. Chelsea House Publishers, New York, 1985
44. Stevens VJ, Hollis JF: Preventing Smoking Relapse Using an Individually Tailored Skills-Training Technique. Consult Clin Psychol 1989;57:420–424
45. Marlatt GA, Gordon JR: Relapse Prevention. Guilford Press, New York, 1985

Chapter 103

Ethical Issues in Respiratory Care

Thomas A. Raffin

CHAPTER OUTLINE

In the 1980s great attention began to be paid to biomedical ethics. One of the reasons for this sudden focus was the impact of the 1976 Karen Ann Quinlan case, which established in the state of New Jersey that patients with essentially no chance to regain a reasonable quality of life could be withdrawn from extraordinary life support.[1] In 1983 the President's Commission for the Study of Ethical Problems in Medicine and Biomedical and Behavioral Research published its extensive and groundbreaking report to the nation.[2] At the same time physicians, lawyers, scholars, ethicists, and ethics committees began to study biomedical ethics and the ethical dilemmas that confront medicine.[3–8] Because of the enormous growth in biomedical technology and the capabilities of modern medicine, we are suddenly faced with novel and highly complex ethical quandaries wherever we turn: the use of human fetal tissue, gene therapy in humans, genetic alteration of nonhuman species, and newer approaches to in vitro fertilization. As we try to respond to these advances in medicine, we still have conflicts over older and exceedingly complex ethical problems: use of animals in education and research, abortion, relieving suffering of irreversibly impaired patients with powerful analgesics that might hasten their deaths, and withdrawing food and water from patients in chronic persistent vegetative states.

Besides all these ethical problems, modern medicine throughout the world is beginning to outstrip the ability of society to pay for technologic innovations. This is nowhere more apparent than in the United States. There is a growing call for health care providers to become "economic gatekeepers" to decrease the spiraling costs of health care. In the United States health care providers, payers, and the public realize that our health care system is impaired, in need of fiscal control, weakened by entrepreneurial special interests, and without effective leadership from the executive or Legislative branch of government, or organized medicine.

With the marked attention on ethics in general and biomedical ethics in particular, the time seems ripe for solving our dilemmas with honesty, integrity, and responsibility. This means that all health care providers from neurosurgeons to respiratory therapists, all payors from the federal government to the small insurance company that might cancel a policy because the insured has cancer, and all consumers must come together and participate in the development of an ethical, cost-effective health care system.

The respiratory care professional is intimately involved in providing care for patients and working on the health care team when difficult ethical issues arise, such as withholding and withdrawing life support from patients. This chapter identifies general ethical principles that must be understood in order to provide ethical respiratory care. Recent legal precedents in the United States are discussed briefly. Since organ transplantation is increasing in a dramatic fashion both in the United States and elsewhere throughout the world, it is important to understand the ethical problems that organ transplantation presents. Finally, the major thrust of this chapter is to investigate the ethics and practicalities of the range of options in withholding and withdrawing life support, from the institution of basic life support to the withdrawal of advanced life support.

GENERAL ETHICAL PRINCIPLES

Fundamental ethical principles are discussed exhaustively in various books on biomedical ethics.[6–8] There are four fundamental ethical principles that must be understood if clinicians are to provide the highest quality of health care. The first principle is *beneficence*, which means to do good or, in medicine, to restore health and relieve suffering. Health care providers have regarded these goals as fundamental to the practice of medicine since the time of Hippocrates. Conflicting with the principle of beneficence is the tendency since the 1950s of certain health care practitioners and manufacturers to build into health care costs inappropriately high margins of profit. Examples include excessive profits on the part of corporations producing medical supplies, equipment, and drugs; overutilization of diagnostic and therapeutic modalities, including endoscopy and surgery; and yearly earnings of health care professionals significantly in excess of $500,000. These high costs have overtaxed society's ability to pay for health care and have proved destructive to the American health care system.

The second fundamental ethical principle is that of *nonmaleficence*, which means to do no harm (*primum non nocere*). This is an exceedingly important ethical principle and means that a health care provider should not deliver a therapy if the odds are greater that it will harm than that it will benefit the patient. A good example of a violation of this ethical principle occurs when a health care practitioner provides a nonindicated therapy to a patient that results in morbidity or mortality. For respiratory care clinicians this might mean providing nonindicated respiratory care that results in harm or injury. Such an act is in direct violation of the principle of nonmaleficence. Unfortunately, it is common for health care providers to violate this principle because of the great complexity and tremendous range of newly available diagnostic and therapeutic modalities. Another (hypothetical) example of such a violation is the following: a patient asks a physician for an antibiotic to treat a viral cold. The physician, knowing that the patient will not be benefited by an antibiotic, nevertheless bows to the patient's pressure and prescribes a commonly used one; and 10 days later the patient has a violent reaction to the antibiotic and subsequently becomes critically ill and dies. This type of example, which thankfully occurs rarely, gives us insight into how easily the principle of nonmaleficence can be violated.

The third fundamental ethical principle is *autonomy*, which means in the United States that legally competent adults who are not trying to commit suicide are in charge of their own health care. This is probably the most important ethical principle. For example, a person who has been found to have a curable cancer but who, instead of seeking modern therapy decides to pray for recovery of health, has the right to do this under the U.S. Constitution. It is vital in the practice of modern medicine to provide informed consent to patients so that they know the risks and benefits of a diagnostic or therapeutic procedure and therefore, through their autonomy, can make a decision as to whether to undergo that procedure. It is incumbent on the health care provider to be honest and to make sure that communication has been truthful.[9] In the case of respiratory care practitioners, it is important to understand that, when either providing a diagnostic test or treating a patient, the patient should have already given informed consent and agreed to the plan. If an adult patient is not legally competent to give informed consent, then a relative or other surrogate decision maker should be involved. It is important to point out that minors do not have autonomy under law to make health care decisions. Additionally, the courts in the United States believe that they have more responsibility than parents in making key health care decisions for minors. For example, if parents discover that their child has acute leukemia and they want to take the child to be treated with unproven apricot pit (laetrile) therapy instead of standard-of-practice therapy for leukemia, the court will intercede and take the child away from the parents to make sure that the child receives standard-of-practice care. Recent decisions concerning children whose parents are religiously opposed to standard-of-practice health care underscore this legal point.

The fourth fundamental ethical principle is *justice*, which supports the fair allocation of medical resources. There is no question that at present in the United States we do not have just allocation of medical resources. Disadvantaged Americans suffer greater morbidity from major illnesses and die younger than the middle class. Additionally, federal and state governments pass regulations and statutes that provide unjust care for the poor and disadvantaged. For example, not to allow the poor to receive transplantations or abortions while allowing the middle class these procedures is not consonant with a just system of health care.

These four fundamental ethical principles interact in a dynamic and often antagonistic fashion when a specific biomedical ethical issue is analyzed. Depending on one's point of view, an individual can use one or more of these principles to support an argument even though another person may use the same ethical principle to support a diametrically opposed position. One example of how these fundamental principles come into conflict can be seen in the present debate over the management of human immunodeficiency virus (HIV) infections: preventing infection in persons unknowingly exposed to HIV may conflict with respecting the autonomy of infected persons and the confidentiality of their HIV test.

LEGAL PRECEDENTS

Many state courts and legislatures have rendered decisions that have helped to build the legal framework concerning biomedical ethical issues. A court decision in one particular state does not make law for any other state. For example, the Quinlan case, which was decided in New Jersey, is not precedent law used in legal decision making in the State of California.[1] In 1990 the United States Supreme Court upheld the right of a state (Missouri) to determine what level of data is necessary to prove that a patient in a chronic persistent vegetative state wanted nutrition and hydration withdrawn (Cruzan case).[10] The majority of the Supreme Court supported the right of American citizens to decide what type of health care they will accept. Although the state of Missouri did not believe that enough proof had been presented to allow withdrawal of nutrition and hydration from Nancy Cruzan, after new testimony had been produced, they agreed. Nancy Cruzan's nasogastric tube feedings were discontinued and she died in December of 1990.

The right of legally competent adult Americans to make decisions concerning their own health care is based on a "right to privacy" that is based on interpretation from the American Constitution. There is no written section of the Constitution that gives legal autonomy to Americans to decide whether they wish to receive indicated medical therapy.

During the 1980s California courts were extremely active in hearing cases that concerned withholding or withdrawal of life support. In fact, there was a great deal of all types of litigation in California, including some litigation prejudicial to respiratory care practitioners. In the 1983 California case of *Barber v. Superior Court*, murder charges were lodged against two physicians who with the informed consent of the family withdrew intravenous nourishment and hydration from an irreversibly comatose patient.[11] The Superior Court dismissed the charges and presented the concept known as *proportionality*, to be used in decision making when considering withdrawal of life support. The court defined proportional treatment as that which, in the view of the patient (or the surrogate), has at least a reasonable chance of providing benefits to the patient that outweigh the burdens attendant to the treatment. The court relied on the precedent of the Quinlan decision,[1] which examined whether there was a reasonable possibility for the patient to return to a cognitive and sapient life as distinguished from continuing to exist in a biologically vegetative state. The California court wrote that a benefit exists when life-sustaining treatment contemplates, at the very least, a remission of symptoms, which would enable the patient to return to a normal functioning, integrated existence.

The right of competent adult patients with incurable but not imminently fatal diseases to refuse treatment over the objection of physicians and hospitals was affirmed in the California case of *Bartling v. Superior Court*.[12] The patient, Bartling, and his family desired his removal from a ventilator since his prognosis was poor. The physicians and hospital refused, but the Superior Court ruled in favor of Bartling (following his death). A 1986 decision in California, *Bouvia v. Superior Court,* established the right to refuse both nourishment and hydration.[13] Since that decision more than 15 states have supported the right of patients to have nourishment and hydration ended when they are in a chronic, persistent vegetative state.

The ruling in a 1986 Massachusetts case, *Brophy v. New England Sinai Hospital,* supported the withholding of nutrition and hydration from a patient who was in a chronic, persistent vegetative state. The Massachusetts court took this position because the evidence revealed that the patient would never regain cognitive behavior, the ability to communicate, or the capability to interact purposefully with his environment.[14]

In 1988 the state of California ruled in the Drabick case that mentally incapacitated patients are entitled to have appropriate decisions made on their behalf by surrogate decision makers.[15] In this case the family wanted food and water withdrawn from the patient, Drabick, who was in a chronic, persistent vegetative state. This plan was supported and carried out. However, this biomedical ethical issue still remains quite controversial and arose again in the Cruzan case, mentioned above.

In addition to court cases throughout the United States, the type of situation discussed above has led to a move to develop individual state documents that will serve as living wills. Generic living wills are available from the Society for the Right to Die or Concern for Dying. If a living will has not been approved by a specific state legislature, it is not legally binding. However, these documents still are of much value to families, loved ones, friends, and health care team members such as respiratory care clinicians in determining what the patient would have wanted if not legally incompetent. As of 1991, more than 42 states have legislated living will documents. In 1984 the California state legislature developed the California Durable Power of Attorney for Health Care, a legally protected procedure whereby people can indicate treatment preferences in various situations and designate an "attorney in fact," who is empowered to make medical decisions should patients become unable to decide for themselves.[16] The first state law providing for a durable power of attorney for health care was passed in Pennsylvania in 1982. Not only is it important for adult Americans to have a will that will significantly assist surviving family members, but it is also extremely important to complete a living will (if possible, one that has been developed by a specific state law). The living will is of great value to family members or surrogate decision makers because it assists them in making incredibly difficult decisions and helping them to avoid extreme guilt if a decision is made to withhold or withdraw life support.[17]

ORGAN TRANSPLANTATION

The development of organ transplantation has been a remarkable story in modern scientific medicine. Transplantation of kidneys, hearts, and bone marrow is commonplace, and heart-lung, bilateral lung, and unilateral lung transplantation is now becoming established as an effective therapy for selected patients.[18] Because of the development of organ transplantation, death was redefined so that physicians who removed organs from patients who were on life support would not be accused of murder. This is a good example of how significant advances in technology have changed ethical and legal concepts.

Death is defined as the total and irreversible loss of brain function.[2] To determine brain death, one must demonstrate irreversible loss of cerebral hemispheric and brain stem function, including ventilatory reflexes. Brain death cannot be declared in patients whose central nervous systems are depressed by hypothermia or drugs. It is not mandatory to perform electroencephalography or cerebral blood flow studies in patients to confirm brain death. Family or surrogate approval is not required before brain death is determined because clinical diagnosis is a medical issue, but it is mandatory that family or surrogate approval be given before retrieval of organs for transplantation.

Since one of the major limitations to widespread transplantation in the United States is scarcity of donor organs, it is important to make sure that health care providers discuss this issue with family members or surrogates of patients who are brain dead or near brain dead and might be ideal organ donors. There is some reluctance on the part of health care providers to discuss these issues with families, but just as it is crucial to obtain informed consent from patients or their families or surrogates, it is necessary to discuss these issues in an honest, sensitive, and open way. In fact, several states have adopted legislation that requires discussion of transplantation with the surrogates of patients who are probably brain dead. In these states, physicians who hold such discussions are not subject to legal liability.

It is incumbent on all clinicians to do their best to identify potential transplant donors and to recommend to the health care team that the question of transplantation be addressed with the family or surrogates of the brain dead patient.

WITHHOLDING AND WITHDRAWING LIFE SUPPORT

Key Principles

Four key principles must be understood when considering withholding and withdrawing life support: (1) establish the source of authority; (2) achieve effective communication with patients and families; (3) determine patient desires early in the care-giving process; and (4) recognize patient rights. The most important principle is to understand that the patient is the true source of authority when considering the initiation or withdrawal of life support. Even though physicians must identify options available to patients, it is vital to recognize that true authority over the patient never resides with the physician. Patients alone, or their legal surrogates, have the right to control what happens to them. A variety of ethical dilemmas in respiratory and critical care situations develop as a result of overt or tacit violations of this principle. Physicians are actually consultants who evaluate their patient's problems, present reasonable options for treatment in understandable language, and facilitate decision making. Except in medical emergencies, doctors should only proceed with treatments after those with the true authority have clearly decided what they want.

One of the most important professional skills in the delivery of health care is the ability to communicate effectively with patients, families, or legal surrogates. This is also extremely important in the delivery of health care by respiratory care clinicians. In respiratory care situations, fear, stress, intimidation, and lack of familiarity with the setting can overwhelm even sophisticated patients and families. Health care professionals are responsible not merely for attempting to communicate but also for ensuring that effective communication takes place.

Obviously, some physicians and respiratory care practitioners communicate better than others; thus, when they are made aware of communication problems by patients, families, or other members of the health care team, they should probably work to correct them and when necessary enlist a proven facilitator, social worker, chaplain, or psychotherapist to assist in communication. Communication in respiratory care emergencies can be extremely difficult for health care professionals for a variety of reasons: (1) each instance is stressful and emotionally wrenching; (2) the accumulation of many such cases exacts a high price from health care professionals in terms of fatigue, emotional distance, and personal fear of death, guilt, insecurity, and anxiety; and (3) effective communication in catastrophic situations requires time, a scarce commodity, among physicians and other respiratory care personnel. Facilitators can be extremely valuable to the health care team when there is not enough time or there is some difficulty with communication.

In order to optimize communication, several guidelines should be kept in mind. (1) Create an environment that assists communication. Rushed or chaotic settings such as those in a hospital corridor can impair effective decision making. (2) Because stress often impairs reasoning ability, keep communication simple, and it will be more helpful. (3) Encourage patients, families, or surrogates to ask questions and express their feelings.

It is important to present information in a language and at a level of detail that helps patients or surrogates to understand and make difficult decisions. It is not useful to speak honestly about a situation if one is intimidating people with an esoteric vocabulary, unnecessary details, or an inappropriate emotional tone. It is illuminating to ask patients, families, or surrogates to summarize what they have been told in order to check the accuracy of one's communication. Not only will this help clinicians to gauge how effective their communication has been, but it will also provide them with the opportunity to correct misunderstandings.

Physicians and health care teams are obligated to ascertain, whenever possible, the views of each patient or representative on the balance between quality and mere prolongation of life—the concept of proportionality. Health care professionals must avoid making assumptions in this area, especially with patients of different religious or ethnic backgrounds. The balance between the possible extension of life and the reduction of quality of life resulting from any management decision must be described and discussed with each patient. Absolute candor about the level of discomfort associated with any anticipated treatment is essential, but emotional coldness or brutal abruptness should be avoided.

It is important to remember there is no evidence that one accomplishes anything by painting an unduly optimistic picture. By presenting such a prognosis, a health care professional may unintentionally appear untrustworthy at a time when the patient's ability to trust the doctor is particularly critical. It is wise to explore specific treatment options for probable complications as early as possible to avoid unnecessary guilt among surrogates who are forced to decide for incompetent patients.

It is important that respiratory care clinicians and other members of the health care team understand what rights patients have. The American Hospital Association has developed a code of patient's rights, which in many states is required by law to be posted in appropriate places in every hospital.[19] This code includes the rights to receive considerate and respectful care; to receive information about the illness, the course of treatment, and the prospects for recovery in terms that the patient can understand; to receive as much information about any proposed treatment or procedure as the patient may need to give informed consent or to refuse a course of treatment (except in emergencies, this information should include a description of the procedure or the treatment, the medically important risks involved in this treatment, alternative courses of treatment or nontreatment and the risks involved in each, and the name of the person who will carry out the treatment or procedure); to participate actively in decisions regarding medical care (to the extent permitted by law, this includes the right to refuse treatment); and to have all patients' rights apply to the person who may have legal responsibility to make decisions about medical care on behalf of the patient.

Initiation of Basic Life Support

Basic life support measures such as provision of food, water, and supplementary O_2 are among the most difficult to forego in medical practice because they are so easy to provide. Because of this, health care professionals may provide these basics of care almost as a reflex without fully considering whether they are performing a truly caring act.

Health care teams including respiratory care practitioners should not routinely provide basic life support measures without a careful decision making process that takes into account several major points. First, every medical intervention should serve what patients or their surrogates consider to be in the best interest of the patient. Second, it is wise to include close family members in the decision making process whenever possible. This enlists the family on the side of the eventual treatment course, minimizing the possibility of extraordinarily difficult conflicts at times of great stress. Third, physicians should anticipate the likely medical course and elicit clearly, in advance, the specific choices the patient wishes to make for each possible situation.

Fourth, once any medical intervention is begun during grave illness, withdrawing it in order to avoid an agonizing dying process requires a direct action resulting in death. However necessary, humane, and appropriate such an action may be, the persons who must make such decisions and those carrying them out are inevitably left with disturbing feelings. If the desire to persist in treatment seems inappropriate, a direct, logical challenge by the professional will often fail, whereas a nonjudgmental exploration of underlying feelings can result in sound decision making.

Institution of Advanced Life Support

Cardiopulmonary resuscitation (CPR) raises many ethical questions. A patient in cardiac or pulmonary arrest presents health care team members and respiratory care professionals with a medical emergency that requires a set of automatic responses if function is to be restored before severe organ damage or death occurs. Unless the health care professionals involved in the CPR are aware of the patient's previously expressed wishes about CPR, the team must act first and evaluate later.

A 1983 study of all the resuscitations at a major medical center in one year showed that only 14 percent of those who received CPR survived to leave the hospital.[20] Only 19 percent of all patients had discussed the procedure with their physicians, and in only 33 percent of the cases had the family been consulted about resuscitation, even though more than 95 percent of the physicians claimed to believe such consultations appropriate. In a related study involving do-not-resuscitate orders, 22 percent of patients and 86 percent of families were involved in decisions not to resuscitate.[21] The families identified the attending physician to be the best source of help with their decisions. Other useful factors included the presence of coma or brain death, indicating a hopeless prognosis; support and reassurance from physicians and nurses that the decision was appropriate; assurances from staff that care and comfort would be maintained; and previous conversations with the patient about resuscitation. In a more recent study (1989), the success rate of cardiopulmonary resuscitation in elderly patients was evaluated by retrospective review of the charts of 503 consecutive patients aged 70 and over who received CPR in five Boston health care institutions.[22] Of these 503 patients, 112 (22 percent) survived initially, but only 19 (3.8 percent) survived to hospital discharge.

These studies highlight the ethical dilemma presented by CPR. Given the invasive and, at times, brutal nature of the procedure, it is hard to reconcile the relatively small chance of a successful outcome with the loss of a more dignified death, particularly in the setting of chronic, severely debilitating, or terminal conditions. In considering the ethical dilemmas surrounding CPR, several important points should be taken into account by the clinicians on the health care team. First, since CPR might occur during the hospitalization of an elderly, chronically ill, or terminally ill person, there is little ethical justification for not discussing it in advance and determining whether the patient might want a do-not-resuscitate order written. This also applies to similar patients who remain at home or in nursing homes. Second, the code status of patients should be identified early and efficiently conveyed to families or surrogates and all health care providers. Third, prominent signs in front of medical charts or records are useful.

It is common for severely ill patients to choose CPR as opposed to supporting a do-not-resuscitate order. When one is looking down from the precipice into the unknown of death, the vision can be frightening. Therefore, it is not unexpected for most patients to want CPR when they talk with health care team members. However, a second question needs to be asked, namely, whether the patients would agree with discontinuing extraordinary life support on which they might be placed after surviving CPR if the health care team believes 72 hours later that there is, in essence, no chance to regain a reasonable quality of life. Most patients, when considering this possibility, will give their permission to physicians to withdraw life support and allow them to die a peaceful and dignified death. Therefore, there are two questions that must be discussed with patients concerning CPR: Does the patient want CPR, and if the answer is yes, what are the patient's instructions if placed on extraordinary life support with, in essence, no chance for significant recovery.

Withdrawal of Advanced Life Support

One of the most difficult duties for health care professionals is to work with families and/or surrogates making the decision to withdraw advanced life support. In the ideal situation, in which discussions were previously held with the patient, the guidelines for the withdrawal of life support would already have been well defined for health care team members, families, or surrogates. In reality, such clear definition is much more the exception than the rule. The following are suggestions for health care team members:

1. Be familiar with the published literature concerning the likelihood of medical benefit from further treatment, such as APACHE (Acute Physiologic Assessment and Chronic Health Evaluation) II, which provides valuable prognostic guidelines.[23,24]
2. It is important to determine whether the patient is legally competent. Evaluation of the patient's mental status is vital to decision making, and psychiatric consultation should be sought when competence cannot be clearly identified. In the Bartling case it was determined through the courts that the patient was legally competent to decide he wanted life support withdrawn even though he was on mechanical ventilation.[12]
3. Seek unanimity among members of the health care team. Problems may arise when any professional feels excluded from the decision-making process. Because nurses provide most of the intensive care, they often have information about patients and families that is available only to those who spend many hours at the bedside. Additionally, respiratory care providers have their own sets of insights into patient care and family dynamics.
4. Do not rush decision making with families. These negotiations must be regarded as delicate processes with their own timing. Facilitation by nonphysician experts, especially chaplains, is often invaluable. The health care team should work with the family toward unanimous decisions regarding the life support of incompetent patients.
5. Establish time-limited goals based on clinical judgment and information, such as the APACHE II data. After learning that a health care team recommends withdrawal of life support, families are often overwhelmed with confusion and guilt and may resist the advice. They can be helped in decision making if concrete temporal milestones can be identified that herald improvement or failure. For example, a physician might make the following statement to the adult children of a man who has been on a ventilator with respiratory and renal failure for 4 weeks: If we see no signs that your father has improved over the next 72 hours, we believe you should consider withdrawing life support. We believe that your father is suffering and has essentially no chance to regain any reasonable quality of life and that to withdraw life support would allow him a more peaceful and dignified death.
6. An effective way for physicians to tell a patient's family that life support should be withdrawn is a statement such as: It is my best judgment, and that of the other members of the health care team, that your relative has essentially no chance to regain a reasonable quality of life. We believe that life support should be withdrawn, which means that your relative will probably die. There are two important components to this statement—first, it is realistically qualified in a way that implies the decision must be shared. Second, it is made clear that death is the probable result of the recommended course. Without this knowledge there can be no true informed consent, and potential liability (both emotional and legal) is present.
7. Grief-stricken or guilty family members may attempt to relieve their distress at the patient's expense by pressing for disproportionate treatment. Such insistence usually dissolves once the underlying feelings are acknowledged and understood.

8. Professionals should avoid involving themselves with cases that are inconsistent with their ethical principles. The tension and resentment inevitably arising under such circumstances may compromise clinical judgment. If such involvement cannot be avoided, frequent ventilation of feelings with understanding colleagues will make optimal care more likely.
9. If patients are judged incompetent and no written or oral communication about withdrawal or treatment exists, the problem is more difficult. The most satisfactory resolution of such cases occurs when professionals and families explore the quality-of-life values previously held by the patient. Once family members have agreed the patient would not have wanted to go on, consent to withdraw treatment usually follows. If no one knows the patient well enough to provide written information about the patient's quality-of-life values, professionals can establish a group composed of physicians, nurses, respiratory care practitioners, family or friends, and two patient advocates (at least one of whom represents an organized religion, preferably that of the patient). This group identifies what is believed to be the most thoughtful "substituted judgment." Decisions should be made by family, friends, and health care providers and facilitators. Only rarely is legal assistance necessary. However, health care team members must be familiar with their own state's laws and regulations.

Withdrawal of Basic Life Support

The withdrawal of basic life support, such as hydration or nutrition by intravenous lines or feeding tubes, is ethically controversial and complex, as has been described above. A number of states have already heard cases concerning the withdrawal of food and water from patients in chronic, persistent vegetative states and have ruled that, in appropriate situations, this is a reasonable act.[10,14,15]

The key to resolving ethical problems in this area lies in clarifying the patient's interests. In the presence of informed consent and sensitive psychosocial management of decision making, most painful ambiguities can be resolved.

References

1. In re Quinlan, 70 N.J. 10, 355 A.2d 647; 79 ALR 3d 205 (1976)
2. President's Commissions for the Study of Ethical Problems in Medicine and Biomedical and Behavioral Research: Deciding to Forego Life-Sustaining Treatment. U.S. Government Printing Office, Washington, DC, 1983
3. Thomas JA, Hamm TE Jr, Perkins PL, Raffin TA, and Stanford University Medical Center Committee on Ethics: Special report: Animal research at Stanford University: Principles, policies, and practices. N Engl J Med 1988;318:1630–1632
4. Greely HT, Hamm T, Johnson R et al and Stanford University Medical Center Committee on Ethics: The ethical use of human fetal tissue in medicine. N Engl J Med 1989;320:1093–1096
5. Ruark JE, Raffin TA and Stanford University Medical Center Committee on Ethics: Initiating and withdrawing life support: Principles and practices in adult medicine. N Engl J Med 1988;318:25–30
6. Raffin TA, Shurkin J, Sinkler WS: Intensive Care: Facing the Critical Choices. WH Freeman, New York, 1988
7. Brody H: Ethical Decisions in Medicine. Little Brown, Boston, 1976
8. Young EWD: Alpha and Omega: Ethics at the Frontiers of Life and Death. Addison Wesley, Reading, MA, 1988
9. Bok S: Lying: Moral Choice in Public and Private Life. Pantheon, New York, 1978
10. Loh B, Ruse F, Dornbrand L: Family decision making on trial: Who decides for incompetent patients? N Engl J Med 1990;322:1228–1232
11. *Barber v. Superior Court*, 147 Cal. App. 3d 1006 (1983)
12. *Bartling v. Superior Court*, 179 Cal. App. 3d 1127 (1984)
13. *Bouvia v. Superior Court*, 179 Cal. App. 3d 1127 (1986)
14. *Brophy v. New England Sinai Hospital*, 497 N.E.2d 626 (Mass. 1986)
15. Conservatorship of Drabick, 200 Cal. App. 3d 185 (1988)
16. Gilfix M, Raffin TA: Withholding or withdrawing extraordinary life support: Optimizing rights and limiting liability. West J Med 1984;141:387–394
17. Raffin TA: Value of the living will. Chest 1986;90:444–446
18. Stevens JH, Raffin TA, Baldwin JC: The current status of human lung transplantation. Surg Gynecol Obstet 1989;169:179–185
19. Title 22, Section 70707, California Administrative Code
20. Bedell SE, Delbanco TL, Cook EF, Epstein FH: Survival after cardiopulmonary resuscitation in the hospital. N Engl J Med 1983;309:569–576
21. Bedell SE, Pelle D, Maher PL, Cleary PD: Do-not-resuscitate orders for critically ill patients in the hospital: How are they used and what is their impact? JAMA 1986;75:402–408
22. Murphy DJ, Murray AM, Robinsone BE, Campion EW: Outcomes of cardiopulmonary resuscitation in the elderly. Ann Intern Med 1989;111:199–205
23. Raffin TA: ICU survival of patients with systemic illness. Am Rev Respir Dis 1989;140:S28–S35
24. Knaus WA, Wagner DP, Lynn J: Short-term mortality predictions for critically ill hospitalized adults: Science and ethics. Science 1991;254:389–394

Chapter 104

Psychosocial Aspects of Critical Care*

Lynn Grose McHugh
Kimberly G. Clark
David J. Pierson

CHAPTER OUTLINE

The intensive care unit (ICU) brings together two important and increasingly influential forces in health care—the rapidly expanding use of high-technology equipment and techniques and a growing recognition of the importance of the psychosocial aspects of health care. Critical care is one of the most visible examples of the tremendous impact that innovations in technology have had on the nature and limits of medical care. These innovations also raise a number of new psychosocial and bioethical issues, as well as questions and problems for patients, families, and staff. Our ability to keep people alive is far more advanced than our ability to rehabilitate them and return them to a fulfilling and productive place in society. Increasing automation has brought a sense of depersonalization to the care of the critically ill. Machines rather than staff seem to dominate the critical care environment. However, there have also been positive impacts. As the physiologic aspects of patient care become more automated, staff can give more attention to the psychological aspects of critical care.

The importance of psychosocial issues in health care is evidenced by the rapid growth of such interrelated fields as behavioral medicine, health psychology, medical sociology, and psychosocial nursing. Increased attention to the psychosocial aspects of critical care has greatly increased our understanding of human behavior in response to illness. The development of empirically based models of behaviors, cognitions, and emotions has led to a better understanding of the complex relationship between stress and coping and has

*Text adapted from Clark and Boltwood,[1] with permission.

emphasized the remarkable adaptive capacities of the individual.[1]

The psychosocial dimension of health care is a combination of behavioral, emotional, physical, and social factors affecting an individual's interaction with the environment (see Ch. 60). A systems approach provides a way to understand how these many variables interrelate and interact and their impact on the critical care patient, family, and staff. A collaborative practice has evolved among many groups of practitioners, all who contribute to the patient's care. These groups include nurses, respiratory care practitioners, physicians, social workers, pharmacists, physical therapists, occupational therapists, nutritionists, and ethicists. Clearly there is a need for regular, consistent communication.

A patient may be admitted to the ICU for one of many reasons. Whether the admission is the result of an unexpected accident or part of a larger problem such as alcoholism or mental illness, the ICU assumes special importance because it often represents the patient's first contact in a complex relationship with the health care system that may continue for several months. For these reasons it is important to examine the patient, the family, and the staff as they function and interact under the tension of life-threatening illness in the highly technological, fast-paced atmosphere of a critical care setting. This chapter, adapted in part from Clark and Boltwood,[1] considers each of these elements in turn.

THE PATIENT

Types of Psychosocial Stress

There are several types of psychological stress that the critically ill patient may encounter, including depersonalization and dehumanization, sensory overload, sensory deprivation, loss of privacy, psychological immobility, and physical immobility[3] (Table 104-1).

Depersonalization and Dehumanization

When first entering the ICU, the patients are usually in a state of shock. Roberts[4] observed that the initial emotional reaction may occur "at the time of the physiological crisis or whenever the person becomes consciously aware of his or her illness." Depersonalization is subjectively experienced as profound numbness, strangeness, and unreality. Depersonalized patients will think, react, and act, but their initial experience will be that of a detached spectator who is observing another person's performance.

The patient who experiences depersonalization may also

Table 104-1. Types of Psychological Stress in Critical Care Patients

Stress	Characteristics	Management Strategies
Depersonalization	Feelings of numbness, strangeness, and unreality	Focus on patient as a person, instead of as a patient with an illness Use patient's preferred name
Dehumanization	Situation in which patient is so divested of usual human capacities and functions as to feel "less than a person"	Inform patient of tests and procedures well in advance, with frequent reminders Allow patient and family to participate in decisions about as many aspects of care as possible
Sensory overload	Situation in which patient receives multiple stimuli of varying types, timing, intensity, and duration and is unable to escape them	Keep lighting as low as possible at night Reduce bedside noise levels by turning alarms down or resetting them to alarm only at nursing station Minimize traffic around bedside Group patients requiring similar levels of staff attention together to minimize disturbances at nearby bedsides Provide earplugs if patient wishes them
Sensory deprivation	Patient experiences a reduced number of meaningful stimuli, a lack of familiar stimuli, and a misinterpretation of stimuli	Explain various aspects of environment to patient: staff names and duties; purposes and operation of call lights and monitors; location of nursing station, bed, windows, family room, etc. Orient patient to outside world: clocks, calendars, radio, television, telephone Provide personal items, such as photographs and cards, in patient's view Provide repeated, consistent orientation to place and time Allow for frequent visits by family and friends
Loss of privacy	Loss of control of private domain, privacy retreat, and personal space	Allow recovery time for patient between examinations and procedures Remove unnecessary equipment from bedside Allow patient to have private time for self and family and friends
Psychological immobility	Condition in which patient is physically well enough to function occupationally and socially but becomes an invalid because of fears, symptoms, or attitudes	Explain reasons for monitors and alarms Identify and explain unfamiliar equipment Enhance patient's self-esteem through descriptions of progress and accomplishments Provide progress boards with graphs and other depictions of patient's progress

feel dehumanized. Dehumanization occurs when the patient is divested of human capacities and functions to the point of feeling less than a person. This experience takes place most often in situations in which one person or group is responsible for making the daily decisions about the comfort and welfare of others.

Depersonalization and dehumanization occur in several situations, for example, when the patient is perceived as a diagnosis rather than as an individual and becomes stereotyped by the staff on the basis of that diagnosis; when equipment and care techniques are valued above the person's individuality; when a patient is routinely examined by large staff groups without advance notice; and when an objective and detached discussion of the patient by the staff is held in the patient's presence.

Management

To foster personalization and humanization, the focus must be on the patient as a person instead of as a patient with an illness. A trusting relationship between staff and the patient can be established by using staff members' names in the introduction and by using the patient's preferred name. While gaining pertinent personal patient data, the staff should engage the patient in nonmedically related conversation. The staff should also inform the patient well in advance of tests and procedures. The patient and family need to participate in decisions regarding as many aspects of care as possible and to personalize, establish, and maintain the patient's territory.[4]

Sensory Overload

Changes in the nature and amount of stimuli can produce physiologic, cognitive, and behavioral changes.[5] These reactions range from mild changes, such as increases in blood pressure and heart rate, to multiple psychotic reactions such as gross disorientation and hallucinations.

In an ICU patients' control over sensory input is severely limited. They are unable to regulate the type, timing, intensity, or duration of the multiple stimuli in the environment and have little or no ability to escape them. Stimuli that are available are often foreign, unclear, misunderstood, and unnatural—for example, they do not follow the normal circadian cycles by which most of us live. These stimuli are very threatening when experienced in combination with patients' lack of control and fear about their physical condition. Sensory overload can become a very real danger for critical care patients.

Contributing Elements

The ICU environment is designed to provide constant monitoring and observation of the patient, and this invariably results in sensory overload from many directions. Lights are on 24 hours a day, staff members are always near the patient's bedside, and the conversations of others can constantly be overheard. Equipment is designed for the convenience of staff, not patients. Monitors, ventilators, infusion pumps, and other electronic devices emit constant noise, punctuated by startling and frequent alarms. In addition to the cacophony of an individual patient's own machinery, that patient is surrounded by other patients and medical teams with their own complement of sensory stimuli, further adding to the sensory overload.

In the critical care setting sensory overload is often associated with sleep deprivation, and this is responsible for many disorientation problems.[6] The constant lighting, noise, and monitoring in the ICU, combined with patient anxiety, provide an environment in which it is difficult or impossible to obtain the uninterrupted sleep that all patients need.

Management

The ICU staff should assess the environment in terms of all the patient's senses. In making this assessment it is important to ask the patient which stimuli make sleep difficult, as well as to obtain information on prehospitalization sleep patterns. Lighting levels should be kept as low as possible during the night. When more lighting is needed, the patient can be given eye patches. Noise levels can sometimes be reduced by adjusting alarms to go off at the nursing station rather than at the bedside. Minimizing traffic around the patient also helps. Whenever possible, patients requiring similar levels of attention should be grouped together in order to minimize the disturbances created by attention at nearby bedsides. Providing patients with earplugs can block noise that cannot otherwise be eliminated.

Sensory Deprivation

In the ICU sensory deprivation is not due simply to a reduction in stimulation of the patient's senses. More importantly, it is related to a reduction in meaningful stimuli, the lack of familiar stimuli, and the misinterpretation of stimuli.

The patient's mobility is severely limited because of confinement to bed 24 hours per day. Injury, restraints, dressings, pharmacologic paralysis, and the use of various machines and other apparatus further restrict movement. This limitation also reduces the patient's visual field. Auditory stimulation is restricted by the constant background noise of equipment and activity. What can be heard and seen is often misunderstood because of the patient's inability to make visual associations and to comprehend the medical jargon used by staff. Restriction of mobility produces the same effects on the patient's tactile perceptions.[5]

A history of mental illness, alcohol or drug abuse, or cognitive deficits can also predispose the patient to sensory problems. The elderly are at special risk and have been known to spend days in critical care settings before it is discovered that they are in need of missing eyeglasses or hearing aids.

Sensory deprivation needs to be examined in the broader context of the social and environmental isolation experienced by the patient. The patient is removed from all familiar objects and individuals. Visits from family and friends are usually restricted in frequency and duration for medical and administrative reasons. The patient's environment is cold, impersonal, confusing, and threatening. The large number of previously unknown people providing care makes it difficult to develop meaningful supportive relationships with the staff. Masks, gowns, gloves, and uniforms also contribute to the depersonalization of those people surrounding the patient.

Effects of Sensory Deprivation

As with sensory overload, the effects of sensory deprivation range from mild cognitive, affective, and behavior disturbances to frank delirium. Delirium due to the stress of the critical care setting is characterized by disorientation, illusions (misperception of an actual stimulus), hallucinations (perception of a stimulus that is not present), memory disturbances, impaired thinking, and variability of behavior and affect. Fluctuations in mental status are a hallmark of delirium. Its onset can be acute or gradual, and symptoms frequently wax and wane. In some instances overall behavior is slowed, but it is more often agitated. Affect can include depression and/or anxiety. Patients may be aware of and very frightened by symptoms of delirium and at times may try to hide or deny anything that might show that they are "going crazy."

Management

The nature and function of various aspects of the environment should be explained to patients upon their admission to the ICU. These practices are of equal importance for both responsive and unresponsive patients. The process should begin with staff introductions and descriptions of staff functions. The purpose and function of such equipment as call lights and monitors should be reviewed with patients, and when possible, patients should be given an orientation to the unit, such as the location of the nursing station, other patients, and the family room. Patients should also be given an idea of how the unit relates to the rest of the hospital and the "outside" world (e.g., views from windows). Items that help to orient patients and link them with the outside world, such as clocks, calendars, radios, television sets, and telephones, should be provided. Photographs, cards, and other personal items are important for both patients and staff to personalize patients and their immediate environment. Regardless of patients' level of responsiveness, visitors play an important role in providing stimulation, orientation, and reassurance. Finally, patients may need consistent, repeated orientation because of sedation requirements.

If patients become delirious, a first priority must be to ensure physical protection from injury. Second, medical reasons for a change in mental status such as sepsis, metabolic imbalance, or trauma must be ruled out. The clinician must carefully assess elderly patients, who may experience dementia and delirium simultaneously. For patients who are aware of and frightened by their delirium, a calm reassuring voice is as important as its informational content. Both patients and family members should be assured that this is a common occurrence and does not predict future mental health. Clinicians should not try to reason or bargain with patients. Because complex explanations serve only to further confuse cognitively impaired patients, information should be kept simple.

Loss of Privacy

Bakker and Bakker-Rabdau[7] have described three different types of territories in which a person will try to exercise control. These include a private domain, an actual space seen as owned by the person; the privacy retreat, which is an area in which to escape the attention of others; and personal space, the distance between the person and others that is determined by the intimacy of their relationship.

ICU patients may feel loss of control in each territory. The private domain (i.e., the bed and surrounding area) consists of a very small space, made even smaller by the use of extra equipment or side rails on the bed. A place for private retreat is virtually nonexistent: patients are under constant surveillance and subject to unannounced intrusions by staff or visitors. Determination of personal space is also out of patients' control, as scores of staff persons pick, probe, and prod their bodies on a regular basis.

Management

Privacy is difficult to achieve in an ICU even in the best of circumstances. However, feelings of intrusion may be diminished if patients are allowed increased recovery time between tests and examinations and if they are fully aware of the schedule for procedures. All unnecessary equipment should be removed from the sight of patients, and all staff should be made aware that patients must have privacy.[8] Finally, patients need private time for themselves or with family and friends.

Psychological Immobility

According to Roberts,[4] psychological immobility exists when a patient is "physically well enough to function occupationally and socially but has fears, symptoms or attitudes which make him an invalid." Psychological immobility can be prevented by manipulating environmental factors, enhancing self-image, and addressing the role disturbance that the patient may be experiencing.

The environment can contribute to psychological immobility when unfamiliar noises are associated with the patient's physical movement. For example, an alarm may emit a loud noise when a patient moves because a cardiac monitor lead becomes disconnected. If potentially threatening noises are explained and minimized and unfamiliar objects are explained or removed, the patient's environment becomes more familiar. There is then less chance that the strange environment will frighten the patient into psychological immobility.

Self-image can be enhanced by identifying patients' accomplishments, by encouraging them to focus on functioning as whole persons rather than as ailing organs, and by realistically defining the physical limitations created by the illness or injury. As patients recover, the introduction of progress boards describing activity levels and exercise progression can promote self-image, enabling patients to visualize their accomplishments through the use of graphs.

Role disturbance occurs when a health problem threatens a patient's place in society. For example, a man who has been hospitalized for a massive myocardial infarction and cannot return to his normal occupation of welder faces the loss of his job, his position as breadwinner for his family, and his sense of being a functioning member of society. To ameliorate the effects of these losses, the exploration of alternative roles and new areas of productiveness must be encouraged.

Coping Mechanisms

Coping can be broadly defined as response to a perceived threat.[9] The coping process may proceed in different modes as well as having several different functions, and no single strategy is best. Instead, coping should be evaluated in terms of the effectiveness with which tasks are accomplished and the associated physiologic and psychological cost to the patient.

When facing a physiologic crisis, patients may decide to cope in several ways, including remaining in a dependent sick role, denying the existence of the problem, or realistically integrating the current illness and future limitations into a new life. The patient can practice denial, as by sleeping excessively to escape facing the problem, or surrender and remain dependent, as by passively submitting to what is perceived to be a hopeless situation. Patients may also take actions aimed at strengthening their resources against harm, such as postoperative use of an incentive spirometer to prevent atelectasis. Patients can cope by choosing one of the above avenues or by additional strategies.

According to Strain,[3] who is a leader in this field, the ideal process for coping with critical illness includes regression to near total dependence on others, maintenance of adequate defense mechanisms against the stress caused by illness, development of trust in the medical staff, and access to the services of an empathetic and flexible critical care team.

Psychological Reactions in Critical Care Patients

Common psychological reactions are anxiety, depression, denial, anger, and dependency (Table 104-2). These reactions vary according to the illness or injury, the type of ICU, and the length of the patient's stay in that setting.[8]

Anxiety

The most common psychological reaction in the critical care setting is anxiety. This reaction may include threats to biologic integrity as well as threats to self-esteem. One outcome of this anxious response is an increase in the number of nightmares reported by ICU patients. These nightmare episodes usually include dreams about being held prisoner and dreams about death. Strategies that help reduce anxiety include orienting patients frequently to their surroundings, planning their care, and allowing them to make choices regarding baths and activities.[10]

Depression

Patients manifest depression by feelings of hopelessness, loneliness, and powerlessness. Threats to their sense of autonomy, self-esteem, independence, strength, and integrity may foster a sense of hopelessness. Patients may also feel hopeless if their ability to function is impaired or if they are separated from those they love.[8] Measures to relieve depression are designed to foster hope, eliminate loneliness, and restore power.

Denial

Denial is the conscious or unconscious rejection of part or all of the meaning of an event in order to allay fear, anxiety, or other unpleasant effects.[11] Features of denial include minimizing or repudiating the problem, disassociating oneself from the problem, and externalizing blame. When denial is manifested by minimizing problems, patients may insist that potentially serious symptoms, such as chest pains, are due to minor ailments such as indigestion. Repudiation is an extreme form of minimization in which patients completely disregard dangerous symptoms. Disassociation occurs when patients refuse to believe that a diseased organ or injured body part belongs to them. For example, use of the words "the old ticker" instead of "my heart" is a clue that a patient may be using denial as a defense mechanism. Externalization is evident when patients blame staff, family members, or unrelated circumstances for their health problems.

Denial is not necessarily harmful in and of itself. This reaction serves the useful function of providing the time to mobilize inner resources before confronting reality. In most cases time will resolve the issue of denial, and the most appropriate response of the staff may be to wait for this to happen. Occasionally, however, denial results in behavior that is harmful to patients, and it is necessary to take measures to reduce the denial. After making the assessment that denial is being harmfully manifested, clinicians should point out the incongruity between patients' symptoms and their perception of the events. In order to protect patients' integrity, the reason behind their actions must be pursued. This is most effectively done in a gentle, persistent manner.[10] If the denial presents a major threat to life, as with a ventilator-dependent patient who repeatedly attempts extubation, direct confrontation becomes necessary.

Anger

Anger and hostility can be psychological defense mechanisms that serve to mask anxiety. Factors leading to the development of anger or hostility include frustration, loss of self-esteem, and unmet needs for status and prestige.[4]

Table 104-2. Characteristics and Management of Psychological Reactions in Critical Care Patients

Reaction	Manifestations	Management Strategies
Anxiety	Nightmares	Orient patient frequently to surroundings Allow for choices in daily care Provide liberal visiting hours by loved ones
Depression	Hopelessness	Provide patient with attainable goals Help maintain optimistic belief in self
	Loneliness	Provide information on patient's condition Share details of illness Teach patient about healing Involve family in patient care Talk to, not around, patient
	Powerlessness	Allow patient to express feelings Allow patient to choose personal items to have in sight Allow for choices in daily care
Denial	Inappropriate cheerfulness	Gentle, persistent discussions
	Unwillingness to accept illness or injury	Direct confrontation
Anger	Escape and withdrawal by sleeping	Encourage patient to talk in open, frank forum, without fear of reprisal
	Guilt	Help patient differentiate between authentic and assumed areas of patient's responsibility; promote forgiveness
	Scapegoating	Establish short-term behavior contracts for severe anger
	Passive-aggressive behavior	Request psychiatric services
Dependency	Undercomplaining	Consistent, confident reassurances
	Helplessness	Frequent, brief, unsolicited visits to the bedside Patient teaching to help patients express emotions and ask for help
	Excessive demands for attention	Provide clear, objective limits Behavioral contracts that specify behavioral expectations for patient and staff

Patients may have several reasons for becoming angry while in the ICU. Resentment of their dependent status and of the situation that led to their hospitalization may foster anger. Anger may also result from conflicts over the issue of authority and can lead to patient rebellion against a particularly autocratic staff member. Memories of prior unpleasant hospital experiences may be transferred and generalized to the current situation and lead to repressed or overt hostility.

Anger is expressed both internally and externally. The patient may turn feelings inward because it is socially unacceptable to outwardly display anger.[4] Examples of internalization of anger are escape and withdrawal, as when patients sleep excessively because expressing anger is culturally taboo; feelings of guilt, especially when patients perceive that they have abandoned their responsibilities by being ill or injured; and passive resistance, as when patients refuse to communicate or participate in their health care, asking, "What difference does it make how I feel?"

Patients who externalize their anger do so by scapegoating—that is, by displacing their wrath at the situation onto the staff or family. Perceived threats to one's self-image are often countered by sarcasm, verbal attack, or rudeness. Passive-aggressive behavior is probably the most frustrating form of anger to manage. Patients with this behavior are outwardly compliant but behaviorally disruptive. Examples include patients who criticize staff members behind their backs rather than confronting them with a problem and patients who purposely defecate in bed rather than requesting a bedpan. Strategies to channel anger include allowing patients to express anger and helping them to realize that such feelings are normal.

Dependency

Much of the dependency displayed by patients in ICUs is appropriate in light of their medical condition. Critical care unit patients are often undercomplainers, either because the discomfort experienced is counterbalanced by the care and personal attention received or because preoccupation with the illness itself is such that the surroundings may not be noticed. The patient is entirely dependent on ICU staff members, so to complain or criticize is to risk their good will. In addition, patients may be too ill to complain or may be receiving drugs (e.g., muscle relaxants) that render them incapable of doing so.

Dependent behaviors are frequently intensified when patients experience a combination of fear and feelings of powerlessness and lack of control over themselves and their environment.[12] The degree of dependency present in the patient's premorbid self-image, life-style, and coping styles is also a contributing factor. As might be expected, patients who have been dependent in the past are likely to react to the stress of hospitalization with dependent behavior. Interestingly, however, individuals who are used to having a great deal of control over their environment also frequently react to sudden loss of control by becoming very dependent. The patient's communication skills constitute another factor in that those who are unable to express their fears or to ask for reassurance often display strong dependency needs.

Dependent behavior is usually expressed in the form of helplessness and/or excessive demands for attention. Dependent patients often seem to be unable to do anything for themselves, making constant requests for assistance with even the most trivial matters. There may be repeated requests for information and reassurance. Dependent patients are often hypervigilant and react to minor changes in their environment or health status with excessive anxiety. Management approaches should address the patient's fear and lack of control.[13]

Problems and Interventions in Specific Situations

Ventilator Dependency

Patients who are attached to a ventilator are in a particularly difficult psychological situation because they are totally dependent on a machine that will never let them forget it is there[14] (Table 104-3). The hisses, alarms, and tubing are constant reminders that inability to breathe can result from a malfunction. The ventilator noise is monotonous, yet rhythmic, and causes anxiety, sensory overload, social isolation, and sleep deprivation.[12] The inability to verbally communicate with staff and family secondary to the endotracheal tube causes severe emotional stress.[15]

Some patients are given neuromuscular blocking agents to paralyze the body and thus allow for smoother operation of the ventilator.[16] Such necessary medical interventions result in fully conscious patients who cannot communicate effectively with anyone and are entirely dependent on others for every conceivable need. Anxiolytics and analgesics must be administered along with paralytic agents, rendering patients amnestic but also confused. The same anxiety-ridden situation exists for confused, combative, or sedated patients who automatically attempt extubation in order to be relieved of the noxious equipment in their throats.[17] These situations may necessitate the use of restraints, which not only creates total dependency but intensifies feelings of disfigurement. Patients not previously familiar with mechanical ventilation, such as those suffering from trauma, may be fearful yet hopeful for ventilator removal; on the other hand, patients with severe chronic obstructive pulmonary disease (COPD) or with the acquired immunodeficiency syndrome (AIDS) may be more familiar with the ventilator but also less hopeful and in more despair over the potential outcome.[12] During suctioning procedures the sense of choking and suffocation is intense and can create fear and anticipatory dread in the patient, particularly if the patient's condition leaves little or no reserve.

Table 104-3. Psychosocial Difficulties in Ventilator-Dependent Patients

Problem	Possible Solutions
Communication problems	Take time to talk Use alphabet, sign board, magic slate, colored pens Electronic larynx
Dependence/loss of control	Allow patient choice when possible Keep patient informed about progress Inform patient beforehand about procedures and their rationale (e.g., use of suctioning, restraints, neuromuscular blocking agents) Call device
Fear of death or disability	Inform and orient patient as to safety features and alarms on ventilator Inform patient of ventilator setting changes before they are made Assess patient's concerns and permit emotional expression with support and empathy Keep management controversies away from bedside Inform patient when it is time for suctioning and indicate how long the procedure will last
Isolation or fear of strangers	Establish continuity of care each change of shift Allow and encourage visitation whenever possible
Sensory alteration	Use calendar, clock, family visits, etc., to keep patient oriented Orient patient repeatedly when necessary "Routinize" care to approximate day-night diurnal cycle as much as possible

(Adapted from Gale and O'Shanick,[12] with permission.)

Patients with respiratory failure suffer the most anxiety at the time of weaning from the ventilator, especially if they have been receiving mechanical ventilation for weeks to months. Despite all the attendant discomforts of being attached to a ventilator, the machine nonetheless keeps the patient alive. Threatened with separation from the ventilator and fearful of suffocation, the patient may react with panic that will make successful weaning difficult. The psychophysiologic complexity of the situation increases if the patient becomes depressed at having failed the weaning process. Since both anxiety and depression affect respiratory drive, the patient may descend into a negative spiral, which will indefinitely postpone ability to breathe independently.

Ideally, patients should be warned in advance of the possibility of mechanical ventilation. A better situation for a patient is to awaken from anesthesia and learn that a ventilator was not needed than to regain consciousness and discover that one cannot breathe on one's own. When unexpected ventilator dependency occurs because of sudden trauma or illness, the anxiety is difficult to relieve. Most relaxation techniques are inapplicable because they involve controlled breathing. However, relaxation and security can be achieved by addressing the two main sources of the patient's stress—fear of the machine or of human failure and inability to communicate verbally.[16] A team approach is critically important in caring for the ventilator-dependent critically ill patient. This interdisciplinary approach requires good communication and close cooperation among different services so that the patient receives care that is integrated from shift to shift and consistent. Table 104-3 lists common psychological reactions to ventilator dependence, with appropriate interventions to minimize these reactions.[12]

Disfigurement

Distortion of body image occurs when a patient is threatened with the possibility or reality of amputation or mutilation (Table 104-4). This loss of a body part or function may result in loss of security or self-esteem due to alteration in the appearance and/or functioning of the body.

Lee[18] contends that emotional reactions to disfigurement may be conceptualized into specific stages. First is the impact phase, which occurs at the time of the traumatic incident or whenever patients become consciously aware of the injury. During this stage patients are in a state of shock and experience a sense of unreality. The second stage is retreat, during which time the meaning of the disfigurement becomes overwhelming, and patients use avoidance or denial to cope with reality. The retreat stage allows time for patients to reorganize and strengthen their forces in preparation for the third phase, acknowledgment.

During the acknowledgment stage a patient mourns the loss of body image, which Lee[18] states "is a product of his total intra- and interpersonal life experience and directly influences the individuality, sociality, and potentiality of the human being. Disfigurement has limited his freedom and his sense of uniqueness has become negative." The need to mourn is gradually replaced by the decision to try new approaches to living and marks the beginning of the reconstruction phase. In this final stage the patient must integrate the altered body image, reorganize social values, and adjust to new technical devices or procedures.

Adaptation to alteration in the body's structure and function depends on the nature of the threat. For instance, patients who suddenly find themselves paraplegics must adapt differently from those who lose a hand. Other factors that influence patient adaptation include the value that the patient attaches to the injured or mutilated part, coping ability as determined by the patient's history of response to past crises, the response to the disfigurement from family and friends, and the resources available to patient and family as the changes occur.[4]

For supportive care to be successful, the staff must first learn patients' perceptions of what happened to them. If a patient's account is incorrect, staff members can reorient the patient by giving an account of the accident and the location and extent of the injury. The clinician should be sensitive and responsive to the patient's emotional status and encourage mourning regarding the disfigurement. Staff should also realistically inform patients that recovery is progressing by focusing on the positive aspects of the altered body image. Additional support can be gained by introducing patients to people who have similar problems.

Cardiac Arrest

Patients who survive cardiac arrest often demonstrate an increase in apprehension at being left alone, as well as an increase in nightmares[8] (Table 104-5). Talking with these patients in short, frequent visits in the hours and days following cardiac arrest is helpful if the patients are allowed to express their feelings about the event in order to neutralize anxiety that would otherwise be repressed or defended against. Particularly fearful patients should be reminded of the constant monitoring by the machines and the proximity of the staff. If appropriate, patients can be provided with statistics that optimistically predict survival rates for the underlying disease or can be informed of current advances in medical research that may provide a future cure. Prior to discharge, the staff can make sure that family members and friends who are most likely to be in the company of the patient have training in cardiopulmonary resuscitation.[19] If appropriate, patients can be encouraged to join cardiac rehabilitation programs or support groups that bring them together with others who have experienced cardiac arrest. Most patients experience only short-term apprehension and, with the exception

Table 104-4. Psychosocial Difficulties Related to Disfigurement in Critically Ill Patients

Phase	Reaction	Strategies for Support
Impact	State of shock; sense of unreality	Explore patient's perceptions of what happened Reorient patient with description of accident and location and extent of injury
Retreat	Feelings of being overwhelmed; use of avoidance or denial to cope with reality	Be sensitive and responsive to patient's emotional status
Acknowledgment	Mourning loss of body image	Encourage mourning with respect to the disfigurement
Reconstruction	Integration of altered body image; reorganization of social values; adjustment to new technical devices or procedures	Begin establishment of mutual support groups by introducing patient to others who have similar injuries or illnesses

Table 104-5. Psychosocial Difficulties and Support Strategies Following Cardiac Arrest

Difficulties
Apprehension about being left alone
Increase in nightmares
Fear of recurrent arrest
Strategies for support
Allow patient to express feelings about the event
Remind patient about continuous monitoring systems and proximity of staff
Teach family members techniques of cardiopulmonary resuscitation
Encourage participation in cardiac rehabilitation programs and survivor support groups

of those with a history of prior emotional disturbances, the long-term capacity of survivors to adjust is high.[8]

Transfer Out of the Intensive Care Unit

Factors Contributing to Patient Anxiety

The ICU patient experiences transfer anxiety when moved from a familiar, relatively secure situation to a less familiar environment (Table 104-6). This situation occurs frequently, especially with patients who have been in the ICU for several months, as is often the case with the adult respiratory distress syndrome (ARDS). Such patients feel separated from both machines and staff that maintained close personal surveillance over their care. Transfer anxiety can result, too, from patients' lack of control over the determination of when they will be moved from the critical care unit. The anxiety occurs when patients are abruptly changed from a passive dependent state to an independent state in which they have no control.

Table 104-6. Transfer Anxiety about Leaving the ICU: Potential Reasons and Strategies for Support

Reasons for anxiety
Movement from familiar to unfamiliar environment, especially if patient has been critically ill for several months
Separation from both machines and staff that maintained close surveillance
Lack of control over timing and move
Change from dependent role to a more independent one
Feelings of rejection when told that a "sicker" patient needs the ICU bed
Strategies for support
Define the process of "graduation" from the ICU at the time of admission
Inform patient well in advance of the planned transfer out of the ICU, with appropriate reminders
Introduce floor staff to the patient in advance of the planned transfer
Move patient during daylight hours
Place patient close to the nursing station or close to the room door

With the suddenness of the transfer from the critical care unit, patients may not have the time necessary to understand the positive reasons for this change in environment and may thus feel rejected. Such rejection may be exacerbated when patients who still view themselves as seriously ill are told that their beds are needed by other critically ill persons. Furthermore, patients may perceive the move from a close-surveillance private room to a low-supervision ward environment as a "demotion."

Transfer from the ICU at night is another reason for anxiety. The transferred patient does not have the opportunity to become familiar with the new environment, which will be darkened, with a new roommate, who is probably asleep, or with the nurse, since fewer are on staff at night. For visually impaired or elderly patients, nighttime transfer may result in so much mental confusion and physiologic stress that readmission to the critical care unit may be necessary.

Anxiety-related psychological changes include emotional lability, self-preoccupation, emotional responses inappropriate to the situation, frequent mention of death, regression, inadequate or inaccurate recall in the absence of precipitating physical factors, paranoia, delusions, hallucinations, and repetitious verbal chatter accompanied by changes in voice tone and speech. Patients may also unconsciously use defense mechanisms such as rationalization, denial, or projection.[20]

Because physiologic alterations can produce negative psychological effects and vice versa, it is often very difficult to sort out the initial causative event in a transfer anxiety reaction. The complicated interplay in these stress-related reactions makes intervention a major challenge for the clinician.

Strategies for Minimizing Transfer Anxiety

Interventions to minimize transfer anxiety are most effective when practiced from the onset of a patient's stay in the ICU (Table 104-6). Upon initial admission, the conditions necessary for graduation from the critical care setting (e.g., weaned from the ventilator, chest tubes pulled, activity levels increased to a predetermined degree) should be defined. Staff should provide continuous reports on medical status and inform patients well in advance of the date of planned transfer. Patients should be assured in a positive manner that the transfer is a cause for celebration rather than a threat to recovery. They are less likely to feel abandoned if the floor nurse meets them in the ICU before the actual transfer takes place. One can gradually remove objects from a patient's environment that reinforce the sense of being critically ill. Moving patients during daylight hours, preferably to an intermediate care unit that can easily be visited by members of the ICU, will further facilitate a comfortable transfer. Patients may also prefer to have a bed next to the door and close to the nurses' station, especially if they have been in the ICU for a long time. The high quantity of traffic in the hallway and close to the nurses' station can actually be reassuring to the patient.

In one study unprepared patients transferring from the ICU experienced a 70 percent rate of cardiovascular complications, and 32 percent had elevated urinary catecholamine excretion; among those patients prepared in advance for transfer, there were no cardiovascular complications, and increased urinary catecholamine excretion was noted in only 2 percent.[16]

THE FAMILY

Effects of Critical Care Admission on the Family

Hospitalization of a family member in an ICU represents a sudden crisis without time for preparation. This type of crisis is intense, demanding, and chaotic for all involved; at the same time, it often marks the beginning of a long-term "career" for patient and family. The experiences and responses of the family in the critical care setting set the tone for what is to follow.

In some ways the same accomplishments that have contributed so much to the improvement of mortality and morbidity rates in critical care (factors such as large multidisciplinary staffs, high-technology equipment, and regionalized trauma centers) present special kinds of stress for the patient's family. These factors can be described as the psychosocial costs of improved health care.

The development of regionalized tertiary care centers often results in immediate transportation of the patient to a facility many miles from home and family. These distances often split family members in terms both of mutual support and of carrying out role responsibilities whether as parent, financial provider, or social support provider.[21] Removal of the patient from the family constellation results in sudden role changes as other family members are forced to take on duties previously carried out by the patient. Loss of income from the provider, costs associated with travel and staying near the hospital, and staggering medical expenses often create an instant financial crisis for the family.

The ICU is frightening, unfamiliar territory for most family members, who find the object of their concern surrounded by strange equipment, unusual sounds, and unfamiliar smells. Although the technical intricacies of this setting are unclear, they combine with the frantic pace of the unit's personnel to give the family a clear message that the patient is critically ill. Moreover, the patient is seen surrounded by multiple caregivers, whose individual roles are often bewilderingly uncertain. Their use of medical terminology may intimidate and confuse rather than educate and comfort. The family may find it difficult to figure out who is in charge and how important decisions are made. If families obtain slightly different information from different staff members, it is easy for them to conclude that important decisions are being made in a disorganized, haphazard fashion.

Assessment of the Family

Every family brings a unique history, with its own strengths and weaknesses, to the critical care unit. This history has an important bearing on how the family will react to and cope with the crisis it faces. A comprehensive assessment is essential to maximize the family's coping abilities and to work with both the family and the patient. A model outline for the assessment of families of critical care patients is presented in Table 104-7.

Table 104-7. Model Outline for Assessment of Families of Critical Care Patients

Demographic information
Family constellation
Interpersonal support network/resources
Baseline social and emotional functioning
Recent family stressors/problems
Financial resources
Cultural factors related to illness/injury, health, and medical treatment
General health beliefs and previous history with medical institutions
Ongoing family responsibilities
Special needs/problems identified by the family
Understanding of patient's illness/injury
Understanding of patient's current condition, prognosis, and proposed treatment plan
Current levels of behavioral, cognitive, and affective function of individual family members

As previously stated, ongoing family responsibilities increase as family members take on the essential tasks normally performed by the patient. Furthermore, as discussed in Chapter 60, members of each family have cultural beliefs, expectations, and experiences that affect the way in which they interpret and cope with what is happening to and around them. Many sincere attempts to support families fail because of failure to understand the family's perception of events.

Crisis Intervention

A crisis occurs when a group or individual identifies a stressful event that threatens a perceived need and that cannot be controlled by the usual problem-solving skills. The identified stressful event for the family of a critically ill patient is usually the patient's hospitalization and/or the realization that the patient is in a life-threatening condition. The perceived need is the contribution that the patient makes to the family. The usual problem-solving skills are coping mechanisms that have successfully reduced stresses in the past but that are currently not working. The family's ability to cope depends on the strength of its members' relationships to one another, the familial role of the patient, the abruptness of the illness or injury, the predictability of the patient's prognosis, the family's resources (financial, spiritual, etc), and the family's previous encounters with similar crises.

Characteristics of Family Crisis

Under severe stress, the family will experience fluctuating levels of anxiety, confusion, and helplessness. Members' attention is narrowly focused on the condition of the patient, and they are less able to process information, organize daily living activities, and resolve intrafamily conflicts. A sense of urgency and emotional hypertension pervades all forms of communication.

Epperson has identified the phases that family members may go through as they adapt to a crisis.[22] These phases, illustrated conceptually in Figure 104-1, usually occur sequentially, as shown in the figure, although certain family members may experience aspects of more than one phase at a given time, and others may return to earlier phases before finally entering the recovery phase.

A period of *high anxiety* usually occurs first and is characterized by physical agitation, muscle tension, and physiologic reactions such as nausea or fainting. The *denial* phase is a time of psychological preparation and contains elements of hope that the patient will quickly return to good health. During the *anger* phase, blame may be directed at the patient or another family member, or the family may unite in their expressions of anger with the medical staff or with life in general.[23]

The phase of *remorse* includes feelings of guilt and sorrow, expressed in statements of regret at not being able to prevent the illness or injury. The *grief* phase, when the sense of loss is almost overwhelming, is of a duration and intensity that depends on the patient's condition, the length of hospitalization, family solidarity, and the degree of remorse experienced by the family. *Reconciliation* is the phase during which the family begins to mobilize its resources after realizing that a tragedy has, in fact, occurred but that the family can and will survive. This final phase does not connote acceptance, however, in that the family is not free of discomfort and unhappiness.

Table 104-8. Strategies for Assisting Families in Recovery Following Catastrophic Illness or Injury

Crisis Stage	Helping Strategies
High anxiety	Provide brief, accurate information about the critically ill patient Provide frequent information updates Discuss benefits of life-saving technologies
Denial	Respect family's need for psychological protection Be reality-based about information provided
Anger	Allow expression of the emotion Allow family to focus on *real* source of anger
Remorse	Allow family members to relieve themselves of the burden of guilt by discussing what they in reality could have done to prevent illness or injury
Grief	Encourage family members to release their sorrow over threatened loss of a loved one Offer quiet support
Reconciliation	Help family to develop a useful plan of action Define resources that are appropriately available

Effective Family Intervention Techniques

The goal of crisis intervention is to re-establish equilibrium. In the critical care setting family members need help to define the crisis and perceive it from their perspective. If they see the situation as a crisis but have resources to deal with it or if they do not see it as a crisis at all, staff attempts at intervention will be resented. Although families under sudden, severe stress will differ in the sequence and rate of passage from one distinct phase of crisis to another, there remain identifiable ways in which families can be assisted in the recovery process[22] (Table 104-8).

As is true of any intervention mode that uses stages to describe emotional states, a family can skirt around or eliminate certain phases. Different individuals within the family will proceed at different rates and in varying directions in their process of adapting to the crisis. Intervention techniques should thus be designed to meet the unique needs expressed by the family both as a whole and individually.

Meeting the Needs of Families

The needs of families range from philosophic to concrete. In a survey of needs conducted by Molter, families listed hope as their greatest need, followed by honest information from the staff and a sense that the staff is concerned about the patient.[24] Concrete needs such as the availability of a private physical space are also a high priority. Atkinson et al.[25] have developed the following categories of a family's needs: being in attendance with the patient, receiving information on the condition of the patient, feeling useful, having the opportunity to express feelings about the situation, and receiving emotional support.

When the patient is hospitalized, the waiting room of the

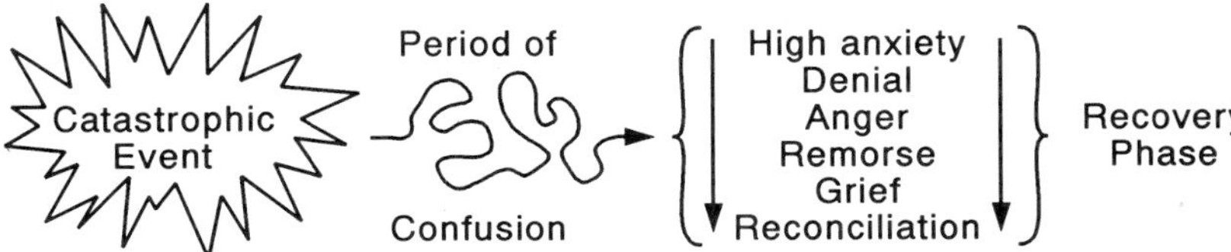

Figure 104-1. A family's response to crisis, such as the sudden critical illness of one of its members, typically consists of several distinct phases. After an initial period of confusion, the family progresses through the six phases shown. More than one phase may exist simultaneously, and some family members may return to earlier phases before finally recovering from the crisis.

critical care unit often becomes a 24-hour home for the family, and all other routine activities cease. At this time the basic aspects of self-care, such as eating and sleeping, are often neglected. Helping the family to recognize that these activities are important and making sure that family members are continuing these basic activities is a first step in helping them begin to cope adequately with the crisis.[26]

As the time that the patient has been in critical condition stretches from hours to days, the frustration that the family members feel in not being able to "fix" the patient becomes increasingly apparent. Staff members can help the family deal with these feelings of helplessness and lack of control by working to identify important active tasks into which their energies can be usefully channeled. By dealing with issues such as medical insurance, taking care of normal family responsibilities, and working on tasks that the patient is currently unable to deal with, family members can take an active role in resolving secondary health care problems.

The family also needs to be given explicit "permission" to spend time away from the hospital. By defining one of their major tasks as caring for themselves, scheduling time away from the hospital can be seen as a positive activity. Working with the family to develop a realistic visiting schedule helps to reduce time spent "wringing their hands" in the waiting room and also helps the staff to schedule time when the patient is available for visits.

Emotional support for families can also come from the families of other patients. Many times ad hoc interfamily support groups form spontaneously in ICU waiting rooms, and such informal alliances can provide substantial support for families in crisis.

Communication Problems with the Family

Receiving information is an important form of support for the family and is an essential factor in helping families deal with the crisis at hand. Clear and consistent communication of information to the family is of the utmost importance; however, the structure and function of the ICU tend to make this task difficult.

The health care delivery system with which the family deals in the critical care environment is in many ways the antithesis of the model of the family doctor whom the family may have known and trusted for years. In the ICU the family usually finds the patient's life in the hands of strangers. Even when families begin to familiarize themselves with certain staff members, there is the chance that the patient will be transferred to another service or unit and these individuals will be replaced by new strangers. As a result, the center of decision making is often difficult to locate, which is confusing and frustrating to family members.

Resolution of Communication Problems

A systematic, comprehensive routine for providing patient information to families is important. From the time of admission, honesty and a caring attitude toward the relatives is essential.[24] The complexity and detail of the information should depend on the family's level of understanding. Attempts to withhold information, aside from being unethical, usually result in erosion of trust in the staff. Since family members in a crisis will only retain a small portion of the data provided to them, information must be repeated frequently in small doses. Having family members repeat the information aloud allows the staff to assess the degree to which it has been assimilated and interpreted, to correct errors, and to provide clarifications.

Whether in verbal or visual form, families need clear information about the elements of treatment, its rationale, and that it may change over time. Explaining the rationale for the patient's treatment can help families to avoid false beliefs and expectations. For example, the notion that sick individuals are best treated with complete rest is common among people with little experience in modern health care settings. Without understanding the basis for treatment, the sight of an ill patient being made to sit up and exercise can frighten and confuse families.

The families of ICU patients often engage in a type of information seeking that can be called "number chasing." They cling to reports of vital signs and laboratory results as indicators of the patient's condition, particularly when the prognosis is unclear. Misinterpretation of these data can lead to further misconceptions about the patient's status and may lead to conflict if the staff tries to withhold this information. The best approach in this case is to explain to the family that they will not find reliable reassurance in sheer numbers. Staff members can emphasize that they will continue to be honest and that they understand how difficult it is for the family to deal with the continual anxiety of an uncertain prognosis.

Family Conferences

Family conferences offer another way to facilitate communication and reduce conflict between family and staff. They also provide a good opportunity to assess family coping strategies, to deal with interfamily conflict, and to analyze the family's level of understanding of the patient's condition, prognosis, and treatment. Family conferences are most helpful if they are held on a regular basis. When a patient's condition worsens, staff will find it helpful to rehearse the information that is to be relayed before contacting the family. The meeting should be held where the family can sit down in uninterrupted privacy rather than in a crowded hallway.

As with the patient, telling the family the truth is vitally important. Staff members should inform the family briefly but as clearly as possible about the current situation. Information should be given in such a way as to encourage further dialogue, allowing family members time to ask questions and to comprehend what they have just heard. The staff should not be afraid of silences in the conversation but should use them to observe and assess emotional reactions.

Transfer Out of the Intensive Care Unit

The patient's transfer from the ICU is another anxiety-provoking time for the family. After patients have experi-

Table 104-9. Social Support Systems

Types and Sources	Purposes	Examples
Tangible support Family Friends Government funds Social service agencies Private foundations	Reduce negative impact of critical illness on family members Accomplish hospitalization-related tasks Assist family members with usual responsibilities to free them to deal with crisis Take on responsibilities of hospitalized person and family	Arrange help for child care and other domestic responsibilities Assist with housing Help with transportation Provide referrals to appropriate hospital personnel or community assistance programs Maintain up-to-date resource list of support groups and agencies
Psychological support Close family and friends	Help family to cope with crisis Validate stress that family feels Let family know that strong emotional reactions are normal Help to reduce feelings of despair and hopelessness	Listen to families Provide nurturing acceptance Provide cognitive and behavioral strategies for reducing anxiety precipitated by feelings of helplessness Give love and attention to the family Write note to staff about those qualities that make the patient unique and important in their lives
Neighbors; co-workers	Lighten emotional loads	Watch empty house Relieve job responsibilities
Clergy	Reinforce faith and increase spiritual strength	Provide for frequent visits
Nurses; respiratory care practitioners; physicians	Be available 24 hours a day	Listen and give emotional support
Social workers; psychologists; psychiatrists; psychiatric nurses	Provide direct psychological support Special training to assist people in crisis Seen by family as "safe" persons in whom to confide	Provide appropriate strategies to help family cope with stress
Family support groups	Increases likelihood that family members will be able to discuss anxieties and receive validation for their feelings	Provide regular meetings Correct misconceptions Provide information Help mobilize resources within group

enced intensive nursing and respiratory care in the ICU, their families may worry that they may receive inadequate attention in the ward. Transfer also means having to become acquainted with new personnel, to whom they must entrust care of the patient. Families are often more anxious than patients at the time of transfer, especially when they get less information than patients do. A conference at the time of transfer can inform and reassure the family. Anxiety can be further reduced by allowing the family to accompany the patient to the ward and to meet pertinent staff.

Social Support Systems

The need for support is the most commonly voiced concern of families of critical care patients. Although the importance of social support for seriously ill patients and their families is universally acknowledged, there is no consensual definition of precisely what social support is and how it operates.[27] Families of critical care patients need both tangible and psychological support[28] (Table 104-9). Once this support is established, anxieties and feelings of helplessness can be reduced.[29]

PATIENT-FAMILY INTERACTIONS

Visiting Hours

Preparing the Family for Visiting the ICU

Staff personnel need to prepare family members before they visit the patient to alleviate fears about the visit and to ensure that the visit will go as smoothly as possible. Family members should be told what they will see when they go into the patient's room. This description should include an explanation of the machinery at the bedside, the types of tubes and lines that will be connected to the patient, and what the patient's general appearance will be. A description of the patient's level of consciousness is also important. The family should be encouraged to talk to and touch the patient. Families often worry that they will "wear out" the patient by visiting too long. Staff can assure them that they are not responsible for determining patient distress and are an important source of support for the patient.[30]

Eventually, family members will develop their own set of cues as to how the patient is doing, based on the amount and location of equipment, the behavior and affect of the staff, and the patient's responses. The staff needs to explore this process with the family and correct misperceptions when necessary.

Visits by Children

Staff and family sometimes try to discourage visits by children to patients in the ICU. They incorrectly believe that such visits will expose children to experiences with which they will be unable to cope. However, refusal to let a child who wants to visit do so may lead the imagination to be worse than reality. Children often assume, if they are not allowed to visit a family member, that the patient is dead.

The best way to decide whether a child should visit a patient in the ICU is to ask the child directly. If the child wants to visit and the patient so desires, the visit should be allowed. If the child does not want to visit, the issue should not be forced.

The patient's disfigurement, intubation, or lack of consciousness do not in themselves preclude a child's visit as long as the child can recognize the patient in some way. Like all visitors, children should be told, at their level of understanding, whom and what they will see when they enter the ICU. Following the visit, children should be helped to process the experience. Questions should be answered and possible misconceptions corrected.[21]

Strategies That Enhance Patient-Family Communication

Once the family knows the patient's condition, the questions they ask most frequently are, When do I get to see the patient? What should I say? and How should I act? In looking for the right thing to say, families are caught between conflicting concerns about what is best for the patient and their own fears and anxieties. As a result, they often express themselves with a combination of sympathy and avoidance that leaves patients with an unsettling mixture of negative and positive responses to their condition.[31] An example of this situation is one in which two relatives may be trauma victims in a motor vehicle accident and one dies. Sometimes family members are reluctant to tell the living but critically ill patient about the death. Staff members have a privileged position in helping the families and patients to communicate more effectively.[32]

Honest communication should be emphasized. More damage is done by trying to conceal emotions, concerns, and observations than by openly expressing them in a caring and supportive context. If family members are not in tune with what the patient wants to discuss, communication closes down. The patient soon learns not to relate any negative emotions for fear of upsetting visitors and losing their support. Visitor patterns of avoidance can lead to patient and family presenting each other with false fronts of optimism and nonchalance that conceal multiple anxieties. In this case, both patient and family are robbed of one of the therapeutic values of expressing their concerns, which is the normalization of internal fears and anxieties that comes from open, honest discussion of their feelings.

THE STAFF

Unlike patients and their families, ICU staff members are there by their own choice. The critical care environment offers an intense and intellectually exciting experience that allows staff not only the ability to work very closely with patients and other staff members but also to provide care that has a direct and very visible impact. When success comes, the experience can be spectacular and gratifying. The exhilaration of a major "save" and the immediate bonding with the patient that can take place in a crisis situation are of a level of intensity rarely seen in other health care settings. Working in an ICU also provides attractive patient/staff ratios, the challenge of using skills in a high-technology setting, the opportunity for close teamwork, and the prestige, respect, and recognition of peers and the general public.[33]

Psychological Costs of Working in the Critical Care Environment

Individual personality traits such as competitiveness and compulsive single-mindedness, which were functional attributes during professional training, may be liabilities when

Table 104-10. Maladaptive Coping Strategies Employed by Critical Care Staff to Reduce Stress

Adaptation	Purpose	Examples
Emotional withdrawal from patient, family, or staff	Increase emotional distance between caregiver and patient and/or family	Nurse always cares for comatose patients Physician gives orders brusquely Social worker spends inordinate amount of time investigating community resources
Depersonalization	Increase emotional distance	Communication with patient and family is technical and abbreviated Patients are referred to by bed number or diagnosis ("the closed head injury in bed 3") Cynical eponyms or remarks about patients ("gomer," "crock," "alkie")
Denial	Attempt to cope with frustrating problems	Failure to recognize insensitive or inadequate patient care Ignoring or not acknowledging an important issue

Table 104-11. Work-Related Stress in Critical Care: Sources and Possible Coping Strategies

Source of Stress	Result	Coping Strategies
Physical work environment Poor lighting Excessive noise levels Overcrowding Supply shortages	Frustration Decreased staff efficiency Poor staff morale	Allow staff input into changes (e.g., lighting, color schemes, physical layout of work areas) Provide "quiet place" or lounge for staff
Excessive work loads; frequent and unpredictable patient census changes	Decreased coping ability Chronic distress Impaired overall efficiency of critical care unit	Creative utilization and scheduling of staff Extensive orientation of new staff to standards and procedures Provision of "perks" in the workplace (e.g., administrative time, continuing education, conferences, teaching assignments, research, committee participation)
High-technology, past-paced environment	Blaming others Questioning abilities of co-workers	Clear guidelines for clinical care, decision making, and conflict resolution Clear guidelines for operational procedures (who does what, where, when, why) Systematic orientation programs to introduce and carefully integrate new staff
Family-induced stress Varying cultural and socioeconomic backgrounds Anxious family members Balancing care of patient and family	Emotionally taxing Feelings of falling short of family's expectations	Focus on patient first, then family Set clear goals and limits and explain rationale to visitors Provide training and consultation to staff about cultural and psychological needs of family
Patient-induced stress (as a result of caring for critically ill patients and the taxing nature of such care)	Feelings of inadequacy Difficulty coping when patients are vulnerable, suffering, or fearful	Administrative awareness of the stressfulness of environment on staff Need for congruence of administrative and staff goals Promotion of visits by recovered ICU patients Provide environment for peer support through support groups or informal conversation Maintain life-style with attention to physical health and balance of recreation and work
Stresses related to caring for the dying patient	Frustration that cure is not possible Staff conflict over efficacy of treatment and value or ethics of research Internal conflict with respect to cure versus care and comfort Intermittent brief periods of silliness	Pre-employment screening for those with inordinate fear of death or inadequate coping skills Develop support groups Consult with mental health professionals for care consultations with individuals and groups
Stress related to the dying patient who is familiar, completely alert, and appreciative	Depression Frustration	Allow caregivers to go through death and dying stages Develop self-awareness about one's own reaction to death
Stress related to the young dying patient, especially if the same age as caregiver	Hyperdiligent concern Internalization of self-reproach Increased intensity of response to death	Have organized meetings to address group and individual morale issues with respect to dealing with painful feelings in response to the death

trying to cope effectively with the chronically stressful setting of intensive care. Health care professionals, accustomed to receiving positive reinforcement for excessive work hours and high visibility performance, may maintain a hectic work pace that erodes patient care and self-care.[34]

Such a pace may mean that the patient receives less personal attention or that the family is forgotten in the waiting room. More likely, however, the greatest cost will be to the care provider. By maintaining the appearance of calm and control under any circumstance, critical care staff may inadvertently learn to deny their own emotions, even while dealing daily with human loss, disfigurement, and death. This may in turn lead to episodes of emotional distress or depression, alcohol or drug abuse, stress-related illness, or social isolation.

Maladaptive Coping Strategies Used in Response to Stress

Professional pressures allow those who work in a critical care setting limited opportunity to recognize the extreme stress with which they are faced and little guidance as to how to cope. Withdrawing emotionally from patient, family, and peer pressures frequently becomes easier than remaining in the grip of frustration and sorrow.[35] By blocking the ability to feel or share emotions, the staff person can function at a superficial level of comfort. Clinicians working in the ICU can develop several types of maladaptive coping, which although inherently protective from a stressful environment, are negative in their impact on both patients and other staff (Table 104-10).

Sources of Work-Related Stress and Strategies to Reduce Stress

There are several sources of work-related stress in the ICU, including inadequate physical work environment, excessive work loads, a high-technology fast-paced environment, family-induced stress, patient-induced stress, and stress related to caring for the dying patient.[36] These stressors place heavy demands on staff members and may result in decreased ability to cope. In order to prevent eventual "burn-out" from a combination of these stressors, several strategies are available[37] (Table 104-11).

References

1. Clark K, Boltwood M: Psychosocial aspects of critical care. pp. 93–121. In Zschoche DA (ed): Mosby's Comprehensive Review of Critical Care. CV Mosby, St. Louis, 1986
2. Adler NE, Cohen F, Stone GC: Themes and professional prospects in health psychology. pp. 573–590. In Stone GC, Cohen F, Adler NE (eds): Health Psychology: A Handbook. Jossey-Bass, San Francisco, 1979
3. Strain JJ: Psychological reactions to acute medical illness and critical care. Crit Care Med 1978;6:39–44
4. Roberts SL: Behavioral Concepts and the Critically Ill Patient. Prentice-Hall, Englewood Cliffs, NJ, 1976
5. Lindsley D: Sensory Deprivation. Harvard University Press, Cambridge, MA, 1965
6. Dement WC: Some Must Watch While Some Must Sleep. San Francisco Book Co., San Francisco, 1972
7. Bakker CB, Bakker-Rabdau MK: Basic characteristics of human territoriality. pp. 11–32. In No Trespassing! Explorations in Human Territoriality. Chandler & Sharpe, San Francisco, 1973
8. Cassem NH, Hackett TP: The setting of intensive care. pp. 319–341. In Hackett TP, Cassem NH (eds): Massachusetts General Hospital Handbook of General Hospital Psychiatry. CV Mosby, St. Louis, 1978
9. Cohen F, Lazuras RS: Coping with the stresses of illness. pp. 217–254. In Stone GC, Cohen F, Adler NE (eds): Health Psychology: A Handbook. Jossey-Bass, San Francisco, 1979
10. Cassem NH: Psychiatric problems of the critically ill patients. pp. 1404–1413. In Shoemaker WE, Ayres S, Grenvik A et al. (eds): Textbook of Critical Care. 2nd Ed. WB Saunders, Philadelphia, 1989
11. Hackett TP, Cassem NH, Wishnie HA: The coronary care unit: An appraisal of its psychologic hazards. N Engl J Med 1968;279:1365–1370
12. Gale J, O'Shanick GJ: Psychiatric aspects of respirator treatment and pulmonary intensive care. Adv Pychosom Med 1985;14:93–108
13. Simons RD, McFadd A, Frank HA et al: Behavioral contracting in a burn care facility: A strategy for patient participation. J Trauma 1978;18:257–260
14. Clark K: Psychosocial aspects of prolonged ventilator dependency. Respir Care 1986;31:329–333
15. Wallace-Barnhill G: Psychological problems for patients, families and health professionals. pp. 1414–1420. In Shoemaker WC, Ayres S, Grenvik A et al (eds): Textbook of Critical Care. 2nd Ed. WB Saunders, Philadelphia, 1989
16. Kornfeld DS: The intensive care unit in adults: Coronary care and general medical/surgical. Adv Psychosom Med 1980;10:1–29
17. Linn LJ: Psychosocial needs of patients with acute respiratory failure. pp. 131–140. In Sutterly DC, Connelly GF (eds): Coping with Stress: A Nursing Perspective. Aspen Systems, Rockville, MD, 1982
18. Lee JM: Emotional reactions to trauma. Nurs Clin North Am 1970;5:577–587
19. Sigsbee M, Geden EA: Effects of anxiety on family members of patients with cardiac disease learning cardiopulmonary resuscitation. Heart Lung 1990;19:662–665
20. Murray RL: Assessment of psychologic status in the surgical ICU patient. Nurs Clin North Am 1975;10:69–81
21. Titler MG, Cohen MZ, Craft MJ: Impact of adult critical care hospitalization: Perceptions of patients, spouses, children, and nurses. Heart Lung 1991;20:174–182
22. Epperson MM: Families in sudden crisis: Process and intervention in a critical care center. Soc Work Health Care 1977;2:265–273
23. Leavitt MB: Family recovery after vascular surgery. Heart Lung 1990;19:486–490
24. Molter NC: Need of relatives of critically ill patients: A descriptive study. Heart Lung 1979;8:332–339
25. Atkinson JH, Stewart N, Gardner D: The family meeting in critical care settings. J Trauma 1980;20:43–46
26. Mirr MP: Factors affecting decisions made by family members of patients with severe head injury. Heart Lung 1991;20:228–235
27. DiMatteo MR, Hays R: Social support and serious illness. pp. 117–148. In Gottlieb BH (ed): Social Networks and Social Support. Sage Publications, Beverly Hills, 1981
28. Caplan R: Patient provider and organization: Hypothesized determinants of adherence. pp. 75–110. In Cohen SJ (ed): New Directions in Patient Compliance. DC Heath, Lexington, MA, 1979
29. Abramson LY, Seligman MEP, Teasdale JD: Learned helplessness in humans: Critique and reformulation. J Abnorm Psychol 1978;87:49–74
30. Simpson T: The family as a source of support for the critically ill adult. AACN Clin Issues Crit Care Nurs 1991;2:229–235
31. Wortman CB, Dunkel-Schetler C: Interpersonal relationships and cancer: A theoretical analysis. J Soc Issues 1979;35:120–155
32. Simpson T: Needs and concerns of families of critically ill adults. Focus Crit Care 1989;16:388–397
33. Bailey JT, Steffen SM, Grout JW: The stress audit: Identifying the stressors of ICU nursing. J Nurs Educ 1980;19:15–25
34. DiMatteo MR, Freedman HS: Social Psychology and Medicine. Oelgeschlager, Cambridge, MA, 1982, pp. 311–339
35. Artinian NT: Stress experience of spouses of patients having coronary artery bypass during hospitalization and 6 weeks after discharge. Heart Lung. 1991;20:52–59
36. McCue JD: The effects of stress on patients and their medical practice. N Engl J Med 1982;306:458–463
37. Schwartz-Lookinland S: Stress and coping in the ICU: Implications for nursing practice. pp. 1432–1436. In Shoemaker WC, Ayres S, Grenvik A et al (eds): Textbook of Critical Care. 2nd Ed. WB Saunders, Philadelphia, 1989

Chapter 105

Sexuality in Respiratory Care

Paul A. Selecky

CHAPTER OUTLINE

Sexuality is an integral part of human personality, and thus to some degree influences everything we think, feel, and do. Our training as health professionals teaches us to focus on the *total patient*. We become knowledgeable in normal and abnormal respiratory structure and function and skillful in diagnostic and therapeutic procedures. At the same time, we learn to provide professional services to the patient as a person, not just to a set of lungs or a blood gas abnormality. This concept of caring for the total patient includes the patient's sexuality, which makes it an appropriate subject in a textbook on respiratory care.

SEX VERSUS SEXUALITY

It is important that we define sex and sexuality to avoid confusion. The term *sex* conjures up different meanings, but here it refers to the physical and often genital aspects of our genders. The term *sexuality* defines a broader focus including not only our physical nature but our emotions and intellect as well. This latter term is therefore a better descriptor of us as total persons—an aspect of our nature that influences how we look, think, and feel or, as it were, our body, mind, and soul.

Simply put, we are physically either male or female. As complex beings, however, each of us has a mixture of classically masculine and feminine traits in varying degrees that influence what we think and feel. It can be said that each of our human interactions is influenced in some way by our sexuality. Some interactions are very personal and intimate, some are genital; however even slight interaction is touched with an element of sexuality. Sexuality, therefore, is not just something that we do; sexuality is something that we are.

As health professionals it is important to realize that our sexuality also affects professional relationships with both patients and co-workers. Our sexuality is such an integral part of our lives that we often take it for granted. Nonetheless, our sexuality helps shape our self-image, as well as how we are perceived by others.

The special role of health professionals places us immediately in the patient's personal life, often creating an "instant intimacy" that would not otherwise occur. We present ourselves to patients as authorities in respiratory care who have come to minister to their respiratory needs. Our human sexuality impinges on these relationships as it does all others, but the unbalanced nature of this professional relationship makes it unique and at times can lead to sexual interactions that could compromise the goals and purposes of that relationship. The purpose of this chapter is to describe the impact of sexuality on the health professional's relationship with patients, in positive situations and also in situations that may damage this relationship.

SEXUALITY OF THE CAREGIVER

In order for us to better understand the impact of sexuality on professional relationships, it is important that we first understand ourselves as sexual persons. Our physical identities as male or female are clearly defined, but any other attempt at describing our sexual selves is fraught with confusion and frustration. That is the beauty of the human personality, each of us being unique in how we feel as men or women and as persons.

As mentioned above, our sexuality influences everything we think, feel, and do. Our self-concept as sexual persons is obviously rooted in our physical gender, but our self-identity as adult men or women has been influenced by our life experiences. Our personality traits, value systems, and feelings about right versus wrong and normal versus abnormal behavior have all evolved over time and continue to evolve. They are a product of our family life; our religious beliefs, our education, and the society in which we live. We therefore approach our caregiver roles as men or women with complex sets of feelings that mold us into personal perceptions of ourselves as sexual beings and of how others view us. Our interactions with others are thus influenced by whether we are single, married, divorced, or widowed, our physical attractiveness, our experiences with committed relationships and physical and emotional intimacies, our sexual preference and many other variables—in short, who we are as sexual persons.

As health professionals, we must understand our sexual feelings and desires, sexual fears, sexual comfort level, and sexual knowledge base. It is important that our professional education has included the *facts* about human sexuality, but it is more important that we understand our *attitudes* about this integral part of our own person and our patients. Our focus is the scientific field of respiratory care, but our professional skills in this arena must be plied in the context of the total human experience. It is this classical mixing of the art and science of medicine that makes clinical medicine so exciting and so demanding.

SEXUALITY OF THE PATIENT

The importance of understanding one's sexuality as a health professional applies to one's patients as well. All of us, whether patient or professional, have a perception of ourselves as sexual beings and experience the impact of sexuality on our relationships. This realization does not go away when we become patients, and it is often heightened. For example, everyone has had the experience of undergoing a physical examination or diagnostic test as a patient, feeling somewhat vulnerable at being in a state of undress in front of a relative stranger, be it physician, nurse, respiratory care clinician, radiology technician or other health care professional. We have suppressed our uneasiness and embarrassment in order to accomplish the objective of undergoing the examination, but our sexual feelings were clearly there. It was a tolerable experience but readily illustrates the importance of our recognizing the sexuality of the patients we encounter.

Simplistically, we do not treat just the bronchospasm of asthma. We also attempt to relieve the physical and emotional distress of persons who are single, married, divorced, or widowed and who have varying degrees of concern about the impact of their respiratory illness on their lives in general and as sexual beings.

It is also important to realize the direct impact of a disease process on sexual functioning. Chronic lung diseases can take their toll on patients' physical and emotional states. Sexuality is likely of little concern to patients who are confronting a life-threatening illness, but this issue often rises to the surface if the disease and its impact become prolonged or chronic. The patients wonder about the impact of the lung disease on their physical attractiveness and on their ability to perform as lovers. They fear that lovemaking may flare their respiratory symptoms. They also balk at the role of being dependent on others, often becoming depressed and losing interest in their own well-being and interactions with others. They may feel less masculine or less feminine. They also may suffer side effects of their medications and treatments that sap their sexual energy and physical ability in lovemaking.

For many patients these problems are compounded by the natural process of aging. It is clear that sexuality lasts a lifetime, but it rises and falls in our level of consciousness and changes in response to our life's experiences. It does not disappear, although it is altered and sometimes diminished by aging. This may be interpreted falsely by the patient as being the result of illness.

The primary focus of the clinician is the patient, but changes in sexuality often affect the patient's sexual partner and other intimates. The patient is a sexual being and also may be a husband, wife, or lover, whose illness may be affecting others more than is apparent. Our duty as clinicians is to patients and their needs, but it is the wise clinician who includes a patient's sexual partner in working to understand and cope with the disease process. The sexual partner may be filled with concerns, as this illness often affects the partner's life as well. The partner likewise fears that lovemaking may cause the patient's breathing problems to flare, may be struggling with the change of the patient's role in their intimate relationship, and may need help in communicating these feelings to the patient.

SEXUALITY AND THE CAREGIVER-PATIENT RELATIONSHIP

Sexuality impinges to a varying degree on all our professional relationships as caregivers. This may be minimal, as during brief patient encounters that occur when delivering respiratory treatments, or it may be more involved as the product of an ongoing professional relationship, such as might develop in a pulmonary rehabilitation setting. Many professionals entered the health care field because of a combined interest in people and the world of science. It is important, however, that we examine the uniqueness of our relationship with patients that makes it different from other relationships in our lives.

The purpose of our interaction with the patient is to develop a professional relationship, obtain objective clinical data, and proceed with appropriate therapy.[1] It has been described as a *fiduciary* relationship, a term usually used by the legal profession. "Nevertheless," writes psychologist Shirley Feldman-Summers, "most people who offer medical, mental health, and legal services can readily understand what is implied by that term—that is, it refers to a special relationship in which one person accepts the trust and confidence of another to act in the latter's best interest."[2] The clinician-patient relationship is built on trust and power, with the health professional (the fiduciary) holding the authority in the relationship, the patient remaining dependent and vulnerable. The professional is granted instant access to the patient's private and personal life. Moreover—and this is unique to the medical profession—the health professional views patients' bodies in a manner that otherwise might not be allowed except in an intimate setting. We are charged with protecting the privacy of that professional relationship. Psychologist Eugene Kennedy points out in his book on sexual counseling that we are really presenting our patients with the *gift* of ourselves as competent, mature, and understanding individuals.[3]

Surprisingly little information is provided in the literature on how to preserve and protect this fiduciary relationship from sexual intrusion, except in the medicolegal arena or the ongoing relationship of therapist-client in counseling and psychotherapy. As has been discussed, sexuality affects this relationship and should be addressed.

Our function as caregivers requires us to respect the patient's privacy, as illustrated readily by our response to the professional privilege of performing a physical examination on the patient. It is important that we remember our own sense of vulnerability on the patient side of the relationship. Clinicians should take care to examine the patient with proper draping of the body, particularly the genital area and buttocks and the breasts in women. When appropriate, curtains should be drawn around the patient's bed or the door should be at least partly closed to block the peering eyes of the casual passerby. We can provide greater comfort to patients by "talking them through" the examination, describing our actions with each step, as we examine the upper airway, lungs, heart, extremities, or any part of the body, and particularly when examining the patient's chest from the back out of direct view.

In addition to using proper physical examination techniques, clinicians should always respect the patient's "personal space." Touch is an important part of the healing profession and is obviously necessary during the physical examination. At other times, however, the patient may feel your touch to be intrusive. Hugging a small asthmatic child who is afraid or lonely or gently holding the hand of a familiar patient who is in need of comfort may seem appropriate at times. A random arm around the shoulder, however, especially with patients of the clinician's own age, may make them feel uncomfortable and give the impression that the proper boundaries of the relationship have been overstepped. Caregivers are often guided by their own sense of comfort in these circumstances but must be aware of the patient's comfort zone as well.

How we speak to patients also portrays a message about how we respect the patients' sexuality. It may seem appropriate to address patients on a first-name basis when they are of similar age to or younger than the caregiver, perhaps asking the patient for permission to use their first name when unsure. On the other hand, most caregivers find it more comfortable to address older patients by their last names unless advised differently by the patient. Pseudofamiliar and often demeaning terms such as "sweetie" or "honey" should be avoided, although caregivers may find themselves on the unpleasant receiving end of these labels at times.

Clinicians can further enhance the patient's trust by maintaining the confidentiality of the relationship, particularly as it applies to the patient's sexuality. Health professionals are candidly aware of the impersonal and sometimes callous manner in which our colleagues sometimes refer to patients, such as "the COPDer in 734" or "the CABG on the vent in CCU 5," and we should strive to maintain respectful professional demeanor. Similarly, nothing is more inappropriate than to whisper during shift change what one has just learned about a certain patient's sexual preference. The clinician has a duty to respect patients' privacy and to avoid judging them just because their sexual orientation and/or behavior is different from the clinician's own. This personal information likely plays little role in the immediate professional responsibilities of the clinician.

Health professionals are challenged to be warm and caring in their interactions with patients but also to remain scientifically objective. This combination is a paradox and is impossible to achieve. All caregiver-patient interactions are relational and cannot be exclusively objective.[3] The impact of sexuality on this relationship may be minimal or even nonerotic at times, but some relationships can stir the sexual feelings of the caregiver and/or the patient. This is only natural, and it would be blindness to ignore it. Patients can clearly be sexually attracted to the caregiver and vice versa—many individuals are very attractive to the eye and to the emotions. It is important that caregivers learn to recognize their sexual feelings for patients, if any, and to put these feelings into the proper perspective of the professional relationship.

We should strive neither to be totally loving and caring nor to be totally objective but to maintain an appropriate balance between those two goals. When our warm and caring nature interferes with our objectivity, however, we are failing in our fiduciary relationship to the patient. Sexual feelings for the patient, unchecked by maintaining a professional distance, can generate guilt and anxiety in the caregiver and cause the motives for maintaining the relationship to become muddled. All of us have sexual needs and desires that are a part of our being, but it is our responsibility to identify and understand these feelings in order to better serve the patient and to maintain the patient's trust and confidence. This requires self-discipline.

SEXUAL INTERACTIONS BETWEEN CAREGIVER AND PATIENT

Suppose that a patient asks a caregiver for a date or "comes on" to the caregiver sexually. Suppose that a long-term pulmonary rehabilitation patient says "I think I love you." What does one say? How does one respond? If we believe that sexuality impinges in some way on all our relationships, it is easy to understand how patients or caregivers may want to express their sexual desires.

We need only examine the fiduciary nature of the caregiver-patient relationship to understand how such a situation can occur. The patient is often in a vulnerable position, looking to the caregiver for help, at times like a child to a parent. In fact, abuses of this relationship in the form of sexual intercourse between the patient and the caregiver have been described as being similar to incest.[4,5]

Sexual interaction in a professional relationship often springs from the process of *transference*, first identified by Freud as a behavioral phenomenon by which patients displace previously experienced behavior and emotions onto the caregiver.[1,3] This occurs readily in psychiatry but can occur in all professional relationships. The patient develops feelings for the caregiver that previously had been directed toward others in their lives, often a parent. These are not necessarily sexual but can be.

A particularly vulnerable patient may confuse these past feelings as truly being directed toward the caregiver. This is more likely in patients who have low self-esteem and an increased need for approval and dependency. Their thoughts and actions may also be marred by impaired judgment, perhaps exacerbated by the stresses of the illness.[2] The caregiver, by the nature of the relationship, is providing warmth and support, giving the patient personal attention, and conveying the message that the patient is worthwhile, all of which feed the patient's attraction to the caregiver. This transference phenomenon is not inherently pathologic but must be recognized by the caregiver. It may need to be addressed at times in order to avoid having the patient overstep the boundaries of the relationship, thereby causing embarrassment and likely harming the relationship.

Countertransference is the caregiver's response to the patient's transference. This likewise is not necessarily pathologic but must be identified and understood by the caregiver. It is natural to respond positively to a patient's admiration, but it is important to remember that the patient is responding to the relationship, not to the caregiver, however flattering it might be to assume the latter.

At times, such interactions between caregiver and patient may be helpful to the relationship, as when discussing common interests (sports, travel, gardening), which can create a common bond. On the other hand, there are professional pitfalls in the transference phenomenon, exhibited by the seductive patient or caregiver, as discussed below.[1]

The combination of a psychologically vulnerable patient and unstable caregiver can be disastrous, often leading to destruction of the relationship, or worse, ethics violations and risk of litigation. Such outcomes are fortunately uncommon but have been described in a variety of fiduciary relationships, involving not only health professionals but also lawyers, clergy, social workers, educators, and others held in a position of trust.[2]

The incidence of sexual or romantic relationships in this setting has been studied in psychiatry. In a 1986 questionnaire survey, 7 percent of male psychiatrists and 3 percent of female psychiatrists reported having physical sexual contact with their patients. This is likely an underestimate of the practice, as only 24 percent of the 5574 psychiatrists polled responded to the questionnaire. Most who engaged in sexual contact were male psychiatrists who interacted with their female patients, largely because of love or pleasure.[6] Some reported that their motive was to be therapeutic to the patient. Concern for this problem has led to official ethics statements by professional psychiatric groups.[7,8]

The consequences of an intimate sexual interaction between patient and caregiver appear obvious and focus on the violation of the trust that is at the heart of this fiduciary relationship. Whether it is a health professional, lawyer, or teacher who engages in a romantic and/or sexual relationship with a patient, client, or student, it changes the relationship and is often harmful to one or both. Fiduciaries may wish to continue such relationships because of their own sexual needs rather than for the primary reasons the relationship began. This creates confusion on the part of patients, who often are already suffering from psychological problems. At the very least, patients eventually decide that their trust has been abused and that exploitation has occurred, often leading to a decreased willingness to trust others in the future.[2] A similarity with incest has been mentioned above; the patients develop similar symptoms, such as shame and guilt that they have been victimized. Their families and friends likewise respond similarly, with disbelief and embarrassment.[5] Others have classified such action as a form of rape.[9] As Kardener has stated concerning the field of psychiatry: "It is psychologically a frighteningly high price the patient must pay, since good lovers are much easier to find than good caretakers."[10]

Nearly all professionals as far back as Hippocrates agree that the caregiver should avoid sexual involvement with a patient.[4,11] Such involvement is never an act between consenting adults because of the asymmetric nature of the relationship.[3] Regardless of whether consent has been given, exploitation can still take place because the caregiver is aware of the patient's vulnerabilities. At the very least, such sexual involvement creates an unnecessary risk for psychological harm to the patient. In summary, as Engel has pointed out, your sexual partner might occasionally and transiently become your patient, as when you treat your husband, wife, or lover—but your patient should never become one's sexual partner.[12]

When does the professional relationship end? When is it appropriate for a caregiver to become romantically or sexually involved with a former patient? The answers are not clear in many situations. The Canadian Psychiatric Association has clearly stated: "Termination of therapy in itself is no justification for sexualizing the relationship."[8] Some psychiatric hospitals, however, permit social relationships between staff and former patients 1 year after discharge.[13]

The majority of these viewpoints are expressed in the context of the uniquely vulnerable psychiatrist-patient relationship and are difficult to translate to the field of respiratory care. It appears that each situation must be judged on its own merit, with the realization that long-lasting and successful romantic relationships and perhaps marriages have more than likely developed between respiratory care professionals and former patients over the years. Regardless of this, it would be prudent to consider the impact of patient *transference* and caregiver *countertransference* on a former patient's invitation to dinner before accepting such an invitation.

SEXUAL ISSUES IN RESPIRATORY CARE

In addition to the day to day impact of sexuality on professional relationships, special issues may arise. These may result from the need of a particular patient who has chosen the caregiver as a source of sexual information or to help resolve a problem. At other times sexual issues may mar the relationship.

Seductive Behavior

Seductive behavior by the patient or caregiver may be communicating any of a variety of needs. These may be physical sexual needs, or the behavior may be an expression of loneliness and the need for love and/or attention, sometimes only the latter. In all instances, such behavior is potentially disruptive and must be addressed.

It may be quite natural for a caregiver to be sexually attracted to a patient, but it is inappropriate and unethical to act out those feelings. Caregivers must examine why such a sexual attraction is occurring or persisting. What do these feelings tell the caregivers about themselves? What personal needs might they be reflecting? They may be the result of feelings of isolation, longing for nurturing, or unfulfilled sexual needs or perhaps may be symptoms of a more deeply rooted emotional problem.

Such sexual feelings generally cloud the professional nature of the relationship and must be addressed either personally or with the help of counseling. An immediate solution may be to transfer the care of the patient to another caregiver. It may also be appropriate to discuss these feelings with co-workers, who may be having a similar reaction to the patient.

Seductive behavior by patients may be motivated by similar needs. Such behavior is often attributed to female patients, who may dress seductively, wearing progressively skimpier clothing with successive visits by the caregiver. The patient may wear seductive undergarments, asking her caregiver to express an opinion on the style, or occasionally may disrobe more than is necessary for an examination. Male patients may exhibit seductive behavior toward their caregivers as well. These patients may be responding to their need to control the relationship, finding reward in manipulating the caregiver's feelings. On the other hand, acting as a tease may be the patient's usual style of interacting with others. Such behavior may also be the symptom of a hysterical personality.[3]

Regardless of the motivation, seductive behavior should be addressed by the caregiver.[1] Although it may be only teasing or a transient flirtation, the behavior may make the caregiver uncomfortable. It is also important to remember that the behavior is most often aimed at the relationship, not at the caregiver, however tantalizing the caregiver might find it to play along.

As mentioned in connection with caregivers' feelings toward patients, caregivers could avoid the situation by transferring such patients' care to others, but scientific inquisitiveness and desire to help may urge them to discuss the behavior openly with the patient. Lewis and Usdin recommend addressing the aggressively seductive patient with a comment such as: "At times you make me feel that you are interested in something more than my being a [therapist/nurse] doctor," or similarly, "Somehow I sense that you want something more from me than being your [therapist/nurse] doctor, and I am uncomfortable with that feeling."[14] This may provide an opportunity for the patient to explore the needs that underlie that behavior and allow the caregiver to offer advice, such as directing the patient to a professional resource. Some caregivers choose to address the behavior in a less direct manner by casually mentioning a spouse or children (some invent them for the occasion) in order to inform the patient that they are not "available."

Seductive behavior by the patient may be an expression of loneliness or fear of rejection. In sexual matters the *why* is generally more important than the *what*.[3] Why is the patient behaving this way? Why is the patient behaving this way toward the specific clinician? We must listen to both the "words and the music" that the patient is expressing.

It is important to preserve the patient's respect and self-esteem in responding, acknowledging the patient's sexuality and perhaps pointing out that the patient is an attractive person but that such behavior makes the clinician uncomfortable. It may be easier to focus on the behavior and how it affects oneself, rather than focusing on the patient. Realize that the patient may be unwilling or unable to explore this subject any further and may in fact deny the behavior or become angry at one's suggestion. Regardless, it may be prudent to discuss this interaction with a superior or other professionals on the health care team.

Sexual Counseling

Health professionals may find themselves thrust into the role of sexual counselors when patients bring up questions and concerns that do not seem directly related to the illness that is being treated. On the other hand, the patient's respiratory symptoms may in fact be having a direct negative impact on their sexual functioning, and they may ask for the clinician's help. These encounters are more likely to occur in the setting of a pulmonary rehabilitation program, and in fact this subject is often included in the health education provided to the patient.

Most health professionals have had only limited training in counseling patients about sexual concerns and may feel uncomfortable and unprepared. The questions may be raised nonetheless and should be addressed, not ignored or shunted to some other caregiver. Many questions are an expression of patients' fears and concerns about the impact of the illness on their physical attractiveness and ability to perform as lovers. They may need reassurance, which the caregiver can give by being "sex-positive" rather than by ignoring or playing down such concerns (verbal communication from LP Alperstein, 1990). We should perhaps consider that patients are paying us compliments by asking such questions, indicating that we are approachable and good listeners.

In most instances the questions can be addressed from one's own fund of knowledge, often drawing from one's experiences but avoiding any discussion of one's personal life. Even if a clinician does not know the answer to the question, it is beneficial to acknowledge the patient's concerns and attempt to find an answer. Any lack of confidence on the part of the clinician may be bolstered by spending time studying the subject from available resources.[3,15–18] A number of patient education publications are also available that can help in this regard.[9–21]

Patients should be made aware that severity of lung disease does not necessarily correlate with ability to function sexually; the data are contradictory.[22–24] It is also important for them to know the impact of normal aging on sexual functioning.[15,18] Medications may impair sexual functioning and/or desire, an effect more commonly seen with sedatives, tranquilizers, and antihypertensives, which can cause or aggravate male impotence.[16,17] The caregiver should be familiar with resource persons within the medical community to whom the patient can be referred.

The pulmonary rehabilitation setting is ideal for openly addressing the impact of lung disease on the patient's sexuality. Many programs introduce the subject as a part of their entrance interview, creating an atmosphere that enables the patient to discuss these often sensitive issues. The spouse or other sexual partner is also invited to participate in the discussion. Sexuality is also an appropriate discussion topic for patient support groups.[25] Formal educational presentations can be made to groups of patients, such as the Better Breathers Clubs of the American Lung Association. Audiovisual programs are available to help educate patients and professionals.[26–29] It is important that we be useful to our patients, which includes addressing their sexual questions and concerns.

Sexual Harassment

Sexual harassment has been defined by the Equal Employment Opportunity Commission as "unwelcome sexual advances, requests for sexual favors, and other verbal or physical conduct of a sexual nature."[30] This can come from patients, co-workers, supervisors, or others on the health care team.

Sexual advances by patients may be verbal or physical, subtle or direct—patients who linger or lean unnecessarily when touched by the breast of the clinician during treatment, who "accidentally" expose their genitals, or who openly make sexual and sometimes vulgar remarks. The motive of many patients is usually easily interpreted as aggressive acting out. The behavior of some may disguise underlying emotional needs. These patients may feel sickly and unattractive and be fearful about their own sexuality, and they are testing to see how the clinician will respond—whether with attraction or disgust.

At times it may be wiser and easier for clinicians to ignore a patient's remarks so as not to reinforce the action or indicate that the patient is successfully manipulating them. On the other hand, one's own self-respect may necessitate responding by telling patients that their comments are unacceptable. Sexual touches or other physical advances are more difficult to ignore and should be addressed by telling the patient not to take such liberties, moving away, or pulling the patient's hands away if necessary. Professional demeanor should be maintained in all situations; the clinician should never strike the patient in retaliation. Patients who appear to be exposing their bodies unnecessarily should be told politely but plainly to cover up. Demented or brain-injured patients may need to be reminded or covered up directly by the caregiver.

Sexual harassment becomes unlawful when submission to the advance is a condition of employment, promotion, or job assignment or when such behavior interferes with the caregiver's job performance.[31] Long before it becomes unlawful, however, it can have a negative impact on the health care setting. The incidence depends on the definition of sexual harassment, but a recent survey among nurses indicated a significant problem, the typical perpetrators being male patients, physicians, co-workers, supervisors, and a variety of others in that order.[31] Reported harassments included all levels of interactions, from suggestive stares or comments to inappropriate touching and, rarely, attempted or actual rape. Characteristically the victims were younger women with less professional nursing experience. Marital status and race were not significant discriminators. Although such questionnaire surveys are often marred by a biased response, sexual harassment in health care settings can be a problem and should be addressed by educational and remedial efforts, which might include providing assertiveness training to the staff.

Sexual Abuse

Children and the elderly can be victims of neglect and abuse, including sexual abuse. Diagnosis and treatment generally fall within the province of the physician and social and legal agencies, but all professionals providing services to children and the elderly are legally required by most states to report suspected incidents of abuse and neglect. Legal immunity is provided for making such reports. Most jurisdictions may impose a civil or criminal penalty for failure to report.[32] It is our obligation, therefore, as respiratory care professionals to become involved in reporting and protecting any children or elderly persons who might be suffering such abuses.

Child sexual abuse is a major problem, estimates indicating that 100,000 to 500,000 suffer sexual molestation yearly, with significantly more cases going unreported. By definition, sexual abuse is the sexual exploitation of a child for the gratification of an adult. It ranges from exhibitionism to fondling and/or intercourse and includes the use of a child in pornography. The perpetrators are commonly men, but sexual abuse by women has been reported in 5 to 20 percent of cases.[33] Child molesters may be family members or others outside the home who provide child care. The medical literature describes the psychodynamics and social circumstances that are thought to result in such abuse.[33,34]

Clinicians may detect a potential victim of sexual abuse during the course of providing respiratory care. This may be the result of a frank disclosure by the victim, or suspicion may be raised by the victim's behavior or physical findings. *Behavioral signs* suggesting possible sexual abuse depend on the age and emotional maturity of the child, the nature and the duration of the abuse, and the child's relationship to the offender. Children may display an unexpected familiarity with sexual matters or show pseudomature personality development. They may make sexual comments or use sexual language not usually attributed to children of their age. Small children may engage in highly sexualized play with other children or may be found to be masturbating frequently. Because of the negative impact of the abuse on children, they may be socially withdrawn and appear frightened of adults. They may exhibit poor self-esteem and express feelings of shame or guilt. Enuresis (urinary incontinence) and encopresis (fecal incontinence) may be other behavioral signs, although they are not exclusive to victims of sexual abuse. *Physical signs* that may indicate sexual abuse include bruises or bleeding of the genitalia or perianal area, difficulty in walking or sitting, torn or bloody underclothing, and the presence of sexually transmitted diseases.

When a child describes a possible sexual abuse or demonstrates behavior or physical signs that raise suspicion of abuse, it is the responsibility of the health professional to notify appropriate resources. This might start with the clinician's immediate superior and perhaps the leader of the child's health care team. An interview conducted by a trained professional, perhaps the patient's physician, should then follow. If suspicions persist after the interview, the requirements of the local jurisdiction should then be followed. Requirements vary somewhat but generally include designation of a social or legal agency to conduct an investigation and provide for treatment as needed. The laws that require the reporting of sexual abuse include reporting suspicion of other physical abuse, physical neglect, and emotional cruelty, as well as situations in which the child is deprived of adequate "nurturance, health, education and safety," as described by the American Medical Association's Council on Scientific Affairs.[32]

Elderly patients may also be subjects of sexual abuse.[35] Physical signs might include trauma to the perineal area and buttocks (e.g., cigarette burns), often superimposed on other findings of physical abuse. Victims are usually widows who are advanced in years and have mental and/or physical impairments that make them dependent on others for their care and/or sustenance. Such patients may describe living in isolated cramped quarters or being deprived of needed medication or functional aids such as a walker, eyeglasses, or a hearing aid. On the other hand, the victim may remain silent when questioned, for fear of retaliation by the abuser, and refuse further evaluation. If the patient is in imminent danger, steps must be taken to provide protection from the abuser. Many states have enacted laws requiring reporting mechanisms and the provision of protective services when abuse and/or neglect of the elderly is suspected. It is important that all health professionals be familiar with the requirements in their local jurisdictions.

Sexual Bias

At times health professionals may sense a sexual bias in themselves or in their patients that interferes with their professional relationship and the delivery of care. This is illustrated in the care of patients with the acquired immunodeficiency syndrome (AIDS), most of whom at this time are homosexual men. Some health professionals have expressed an aversion to caring for AIDS patients, often because of the fear of contagion. In several studies some clinicians have reported feeling uncomfortable about treating AIDS patients who are homosexuals, stating that this feeling interferes with their being able to provide professional and compassionate care.[36]

The homosexual AIDS patient commonly senses that aversion, which can stifle his efforts to talk about his fears and further intensify the helplessness that accompanies this life-threatening illness. The health professional should be watchful for such biases and guard against them. Open discussion with others on the health care team may air and resolve some of these feelings. Our responsibility as health professionals is to minister to the needs of all patients under our care, regardless of whether they are young or old, attractive or homely, or appreciative of or resistant to our efforts, and regardless of their personal sexual preferences and/or behavior. Anything less is unacceptable.

Male-male interactions can generate obstacles to compassionate patient care in nonhomosexual settings as well.[37] Female-female interactions in the health care arena are not often affected by sexual bias. Communication between male patient and male health professional may be inadequate. A man may feel uncomfortable in the dependent role of patient and struggle to maintain control of the relationship. The boundaries of the respective roles of patient and caregiver therefore become fuzzy, and the patient may then find it difficult to express concerns about his lung disease or to specifically discuss its impact on his sexual functioning or desire.

It is important to understand that male-male professional relationships can lead to development of strong feelings of closeness and affection. When a man develops such feelings for another man, health professional or patient, he may become uncomfortable if he has not had warm and caring emotions for a male at other times in his life. These feelings may generate fears of innate homosexuality and block further communication.

On the other hand, the patient may feel such attachment to his male physician, nurse, or respiratory clinician, especially in a long-term or life-threatening situation, that he feels the need to express these feelings. This may come as a shock to the male health professional who is not accustomed to such intimate disclosures from other men, causing him to push the patient away as a defensive mechanism. In such instances the caregiver needs to examine his feelings about his own sexuality and come to grips with this bias.

Cystic Fibrosis

Cystic fibrosis (CF) is the most common of the fatal inherited diseases of whites, occurring in about 1 in 2000 live births, and is transmitted as an autosomal recessive trait.[38] The classic findings consist of a triad of suppurative pulmonary disease, pancreatic insufficiency, and an elevated chloride concentration in sweat. The impact is described in greater detail in Chapter 42 but is included here because the disease causes infertility in over 98 percent of men as a result of azoospermia.[38,39] The reproductive tract in female CF patients is anatomically normal, but their fertility is often decreased for secondary reasons, usually attributed to their chronic illness and malnutrition, which can lead to anovulatory menstrual cycles. In addition, the vaginal mucus can be thick, impacting the cervix and thus causing a mechanical obstruction to sperm. Successful pregnancies have occurred nonetheless, although often fraught with complications for mother and fetus.

Modern respiratory care and the use of antibiotics have increased median survival in CF patients to the mid-twenties, so that a number are reaching adulthood and making decisions about marriage and parenthood. Health professionals involved in their care should be familiar with the impact of this disease on fertility and be prepared to provide information on sexual matters to the patients and to help them in their decision making.[39] Such pregnancy decisions are complicated by the woman's fear of the increased risk (2.5 percent) of transmitting CF to her children; the risk can be as high as 50 percent if the father carries the recessive gene.[38,39]

Sexual functioning of CF patients may also be impaired as a result of the impact of the chronic disease process on their psychosexual development.[40] Single female CF patients have been described as dating later in life and less often and feeling less attractive and having less sexual desire than their healthy counterparts. Single male CF patients appear to have fewer problems in sexual functioning than female CF patients. Other data suggest that there may be significant individual differences, some CF patients functioning quite well sexually even in the face of severe disease.[24] Physically healthy married couples frequently have sexual problems, and CF patients are no exception. Pessimistic generalizations about the sexual functioning of CF patients in marriage are thus unwarranted.

EDUCATION IN HUMAN SEXUALITY

Interactions between health professionals and patients, like all human interactions, are influenced by emotions, including feelings about sexuality. Despite the seemingly explosive sexual revolution with its attendant flood of knowledge and discussion about human sexuality, many individuals continue to have significant gaps in their education. This lack of information, often compounded by misinformation, results in a negative attitude about sex and sexuality, which can hamper the health professional in the care of patients. Many students entering the professional field of respiratory care have reasonably accurate factual information about sex. Like many individuals, however, their education concerning the impact of sexuality on their interactions with others is limited. The same observations can be made concerning patients and their families.

Health professionals are in a unique position to enhance the understanding of sex and sexuality by broadening their education on this subject and then functioning as educators of patients. In addition, it is perhaps more important than having accurate knowledge of the *facts* about sex and its abuses for health professionals to work to identify their own sexual *attitudes*, both toward themselves and toward others.

One cannot begin to understand patients' feelings or begin to discuss sexual issues with them without identifying one's own feelings about sex. As Kennedy has written, "feelings about sex need to be distinguished from sexual feelings."[3] Ideally, we should be "sex-positive" in our attitudes, but negative feelings are often present and should not be denied. The health professional is thrust into the role of an authority, with the patient being dependent. Negative sexual attitudes of the health professional, conscious or subconscious, can thus have an undue impact on the relationship with the patient.

A mental self-examination is the first step in human sexuality education for the health professional. Our patients expect us to be knowledgeable in respiratory care and often assume that this applies to the whole human experience. Patients not only expect us to know about the impact of lung disease on respiratory function but also assume that we understand the patients' sexual feelings, especially in long-term relationships, such as occur in pulmonary rehabilitation or home care. We may be expected to help resolve the sexual feelings of patients who feel unattractive and unwanted or the sexual feelings of dying patients who may clamor for reassurance and support as they are losing not only their lives but their loves as well.

Formal education in the field of sex and sexuality and its impact on respiratory care should be a part of training programs for all health professionals. In its absence, available educational resources should be sought by the student and practicing clinician.[15–17] Education in human sexuality should also be provided to patients and their families as well as to the general public. As mentioned above, the pulmonary rehabilitation program is an ideal setting for such educational efforts. At the very least, patient education materials should be made readily available where patients and their families congregate, as in clinic and physicians' waiting rooms, hospital lobbies, and the health education section of public libraries.[19–21]

Unfortunately, little has been written about educating professionals on the impact of sexuality on the caregiver-patient interaction except to be aware of its abuses. The latter are serious violations of the basic trust that the patient has placed in the professional relationship and should be dealt with directly. The most productive approach is to prevent these abuses from occurring. This has been addressed in the field of psychiatry, in which physicians and allied health professionals are being taught to identify both the vulnerable therapist and vulnerable patient.[13] Health professionals in other fields should follow psychiatry's lead by introducing education in sexuality to the orientation of new staff and reinforcing it by continuing professional education efforts on at least an annual basis.

Those who develop the policies and procedures of respiratory care departments should recognize the impact of sexuality on the health professional relationship and provide established guidelines and practices for resolving or preventing sexual problems. Supervisory personnel should be trained to identify the potentially vulnerable health professional who may be having personal struggles with low self-esteem, sexual inadequacy, loneliness, or perhaps emotional instability. Others unfortunately may be truly exploitative by nature.[13] Such individuals may benefit from counseling and should be given job assignments that do not further stress this vulnerability.

Supervisors should raise issues of sexual feelings with the staff from time to time, perhaps during shift meetings, especially if comments have been made about certain patients or members of the staff. Educators should do the same for their students as they go through clinical training. Such discussions might be guided by a trained counselor or social worker if the supervisor or educator feels ill prepared. An atmosphere of open discussion should be created to allow the health professional and student to discuss their concerns regarding the impact of sexuality on patient care.

Many of the sexual situations discussed above have arisen in respiratory care departments throughout the country but are often erroneously kept secret by the staff and not addressed openly by supervisory personnel. This attitude and practice have no place in the health care arena.

References

1. Zinn WM: Transference phenomena in medical practice: Being whom the patient needs. Ann Intern Med 1990;113:293–298
2. Feldman-Summers S: Sexual contact in fiduciary relationships. pp. 193–209. In Gabbard GO (ed): Sexual Exploitation in Professional Relationships. American Psychiatric Association Press, Washington, DC, 1989
3. Kennedy E: Sexual Counseling. A Practical Guide for Those Who Help Others. Continuum Publishing, 1989, pp. 25, 34–39, 63–72, 173–180
4. Carr M, Robinson GE: Fatal attraction: The ethical and clinical dilemma of patient-therapist sex. Can J Psychiatry 1990;35:122–127
5. Gabbard GO (ed): Sexual Exploitation in Professional Relationships. American Psychiatric Association Press, Washington, DC, 1989, p. xi
6. Gartrell N, Herman J, Olarte S, et al: Psychiatrist-patient sexual contact: Results of a national survey. I: Prevalence. Am J Psychiatry 1986;143:1126–1131
7. American Psychiatric Association: The Principles of Medical Ethics with Annotations Especially Applicable to Psychiatry. American Psychiatric Association Press, Washington, DC, 1985
8. Sreenivasan U: Sexual exploitation of patients: The position of the Canadian Psychiatric Association. Can J Psychiatry 1989;34:234–237
9. Rapp MS: Sexual misconduct. Can Med Assoc J 1987;137:193–194
10. Kardener S: Sex and the physician-patient relationship. Am J Psychiatry 1974;131:1134–1136
11. Herman JL, Gartrell N, Olarte S et al: Psychiatrist-patient sexual contact: Results of a national survey. II: Psychiatrists' attitudes. Am J Psychiatry 1987;144:164–169
12. Engel HG: Physicians' sexual feelings toward patients. Med Aspects Hum Sexuality 1987;May:41–48; Letters, 1987;Oct:47–57
13. Averill SC, Beale D, Benfer B et al: Preventing staff-patient sexual relationships. Bull Menninger Clin 1989;53:384–393
14. Lewis JM, Usdin G: Disease, illness, and the interview. p. 18. In Usdin G, Lewis JM (eds): Psychiatry in General Medical Practice. McGraw-Hill, New York, 1979
15. Selecky PA: Sexuality and the COPD patient. pp. 215–226. In Hodgkin JE, Petty TL (eds): Chronic Obstructive Pulmonary Disease. WB Saunders, Philadelphia, 1987
16. Kolodny RC, Masters WH, Johnson VE: Textbook of Sexual Medicine. Little Brown, Boston, 1979
17. Lief HI (ed): Sexual Problems in Medical Practice. American Medical Association, Monroe, WI, 1981
18. Croft LH: Sexuality in Later Life: A Counselling Guide for Physicians. John Wright, Boston, 1982
19. Selecky PA: Sexuality and Chronic Breathing Problems. American Lung Association of Orange County, Santa Ana, CA, 1989
20. Eckert RC, Bartsch K, Dowell D et al: Being Close. National Jewish Hospital/National Asthma Center, Denver, 1984
21. Butler RN, Lewis MI: Love and Sex After Sixty: A Guide for Men and Women for Their Later Years. Perennial, New York, 1976
22. Fox LS: Physiological correlates of sexual performance capacity in the male pulmonary patient, Lecture. American Thoracic Society, Annual Scientific Meeting, Los Angeles, May 18, 1982. Am Rev Respir Dis, suppl. 1982;25:34
23. Fletcher EC, Martin RJ: Sexual dysfunction and erectile impotence in chronic obstructive pulmonary disease. Chest 1982;81:413–421
24. Levine SB, Stern RC: Sexual function in cystic fibrosis. Chest 1982;81:422–428
25. Hahn K: Sexuality and COPD. Rehabil Nurs 1989;14:191–195
26. Kravetz HM: A Visit with Harry (slide-tape program). Howard M. Kravetz, MD, Prescott, AZ, 1981
27. Kravetz HM: A Visit with Helen (slide-tape program). Howard M. Kravetz, MD, Prescott, AZ, 1982
28. University of Nebraska, Lincoln: Sexuality and Aging, videotape. Nebraska Projects, Lincoln, NE, 1987
29. Kravetz HM, Weiss M, Meadows R: Sexual Counseling for the Male Pulmonary Patient, slide-tape program. Howard M. Kravetz, MD, Prescott, AZ, 1980
30. Ledgerwood DE, Johnson-Dietz S: The EECO's foray into sex-

ual harassment: Interpreting the new guidelines for employer liability. Labor Law J 1980;31:741–744
31. Grieco A: Scope and nature of sexual harassment in nursing. J Sex Res 1987;23:261–266
32. American Medical Association, Council on Scientific Affairs: AMA diagnostic and treatment guidelines concerning child abuse and neglect. JAMA 1985;254:796–800
33. Fuller KA: Child molestation and pedophilia. JAMA 1989;261:602–606
34. Green AH: Child maltreatment and its victims. Psychiatr Clin North Am 1988;11:591–610
35. Kallman H: Detecting abuse in the elderly. Med Aspects Hum Sexuality 1987;Mar:89–99
36. Baron DA, Hueholt TM: Physicians' and healthcare workers' reactions to caring for AIDS patients. Med Aspects Hum Sexuality 1987;Dec:42–48
37. Myers MF: The male physician/male patient relationship. Med Aspects Hum Sexuality 1988;Sept:51–58
38. Davis PB, diSant'Agnese PA: Diagnosis and treatment of cystic fibrosis. Chest 1984;85:802–809
39. Brown MA, Taussig LM: Fertility, birth control and pregnancy in adult patients with cystic fibrosis. Pulmon Perspect 5 (1): 1988
40. Coffman CB, Levine SB, Althof SE, Stern RC: Sexual adaptation among single young adults with cystic fibrosis. Chest 1984;86:412–418

Appendix

Guide to Conversion of Units

The units of measure used throughout this book are those in common use in the United States. The following tables (Tables A-1 and A-2) and graphs (Fig. A-1) are provided to enable the reader to convert from English measure and other nonstandardized units to those of *le Système International d'Unites* (SI units).[1-4]

Table A-1. Conversion Factors for Units Commonly Used in Medicine

Physical Quantity	Conventional Unit	SI Unit	Conversion Factor[a]
Length	inch (in.)	meter (m)	0.025 4
	foot (ft)	m	0.304 8
Area	in.^{2}	m^2	6.452×10^{-4}
	ft^2	m^2	0.092 90
Volume	dL (= 100 mL)	L	0.01
	ft^3	m^3	0.028 32
	ft^3	L	28.32
	fluid ounce → mL		29.57
Amount of substance	mg/dL	mmol/L	10/molecular weight
	mEq/L	mmol/L	valence
	mL of gas at STPD	mmol	0.044 62
Force (weight)	pound (lb)	newton (N)	4.448
	dyne	N	0.000 01
	kilogram-force	N	9.807
	pound → kilogram-force		0.453 6
	ounce → gram-force		28.35
Pressure	cmH_2O	kilopascal (kPa)	0.098 06
	mmHg (torr)	kPa	0.133 3
	pounds/in.^{2} (psi)	kPa	6.895
	psi → cmH_2O		70.31
	cmH_2O → torr		0.7355
	standard atmosphere	kPa	101.3
	millibar (mbar)	kPa	0.100 0
Work, energy	kg·m	joule (J)	9.807
	L·cmH_2O	J	0.098 06
	calorie (cal)	J	4.185
	kilocalorie (kcal)	J	4 185
	British thermal unit (BTU)	J	1055
Power	$kg\cdot m\cdot min^{-1}$	watt (W)	0.163 4
Surface tension	dyn/cm	N/m	0.001
Compliance	L/cmH_2O	L/kPa	10.20
Resistance	$cmH_2O\cdot s\cdot L^{-1}$	$kPa\cdot s\cdot L^{-1}$	0.098 06
	$cmH_2O\cdot min\cdot L^{-1}$	$kPa\cdot s\cdot L^{-1}$	5.884
Gas transport (ideal gas, STPD)	$mL\cdot s^{-1}\cdot cmH_2O^{-1}$	$mmol\cdot s^{-1}\cdot kPa^{-1}$	0.455 0
Temperature	°C	°K	°K = °C + 273.15
	°F → °C		°C = (°F − 32)/1.8
	°C → °F		°F = (1.8·°C) + 32

STPD, standard temperature and pressure, dry.

[a] To convert from conventional to SI unit, multiply conventional unit by conversion factor. To convert in the opposite direction, divide by conversion factor. Examples: 10 torr = 10 × 0.133 3 kPa = 1.333 kPa, 1 L = 1 L/0.10 = 10 dL.

(From Chatburn,[1] with permission.)

Table A-2. Examples of Conversions Commonly Used in Respiratory Physiology and Respiratory Care

Physical Quantity	Known Unit	Desired Unit	Example of Conversion Calculation
Force (or mass)	lb	kg	$150\ \text{lb} \times \frac{0.4536\ \text{kg}}{1\ \text{lb}} = 68\ \text{kg}$
	kg	lb	$68\ \text{kg} \times \frac{1\ \text{lb}}{0.4536\ \text{kg}} = 150\ \text{lb}$
Pressure	torr	kPa	$35\ \text{torr} \times \frac{0.1333\ \text{kPa}}{1\ \text{torr}} = 4.7\ \text{kPa}$
	kPa	torr	$4.7\ \text{kPa} \times \frac{1\ \text{torr}}{0.1333\ \text{kPa}} = 35\ \text{torr}$
	psi	torr	$1.0\ \text{psi} \times \frac{70.31\ \text{cmH}_2\text{O}}{1\ \text{psi}} \times \frac{0.7355\ \text{torr}}{1\ \text{cmH}_2\text{O}} = 52\ \text{torr}$
	torr	psi	$51.72\ \text{torr} \times \frac{1\ \text{cmH}_2\text{O}}{0.7355\ \text{torr}} \times \frac{1\ \text{psi}}{70.31\ \text{cmH}_2\text{O}} = 1.0\ \text{psi}$
Work	L·cmH$_2$O	kg·m	$20\ \text{L·cmH}_2\text{O} \times \frac{0.09806\ \text{J}}{1\ \text{L·cmH}_2\text{O}} \times \frac{1\ \text{kg·m}}{9.807\ \text{J}} = 0.2\ \text{kg·m}$
	J	L·cmH$_2$O	$2\ \text{J} \times \frac{1\ \text{kg·m}}{9.807\text{J}} \times \frac{1\ \text{L·cmH}_2\text{O}}{0.01\ \text{kg·m}} = 20\ \text{L·cmH}_2\text{O}$
Power	kg·m·min^{-1}	W	$2.5\ \text{kg·m·min}^{-1} \times \frac{0.1634\ \text{W}}{1\ \text{kg·m·min}^{-1}} = 0.41\ \text{W}$
Compliance	ml/cmH$_2$O	L/kPa	$100\ \text{mL·cmH}_2\text{O} \times \frac{1\ \text{L}}{1000\ \text{mL}} \times \frac{10.20\ \text{L·kPa}^{-1}}{1\ \text{L·cmH}_2\text{O}^{-1}} = 1.02\ \text{L·kPa}^{-1}$
Resistance	cmH$_2$O·s·L^{-1}	kPa·s·L^{-1}	$55\ \text{cmH}_2\text{O·s·L}^{-1} \times \frac{0.090806\ \text{kPa·L}^{-1}}{1\ \text{cmH}_2\text{O·s·L}^{-1}} = 5.4\ \text{kPa·s·L}^{-1}$

Note: Retain all digits during computation to avoid roundoff error. However, the least precise measurement used in a calculation determines the number of significant digits in the answer. Thus, the final product or quotient should be written with the same number of significant figures as the term with the fewest significant figures, as shown in the examples above. The least ambiguous method of indicating the number of significant figures is to write the number in scientific notation. For example, the number 30 may have either one or two significant figures, but written as 3.0×10^1, it is understood that there are two significant figures. For more information about scientific notation, significant figures, and rounding off, see Lough MD, Chatburn RL, Shrock WA, Handbook of Respiratory Care. Yearbook Medical Publishers, Chicago, 1985, pp. 170–173.

(From Chatburn,[1] with permission.)

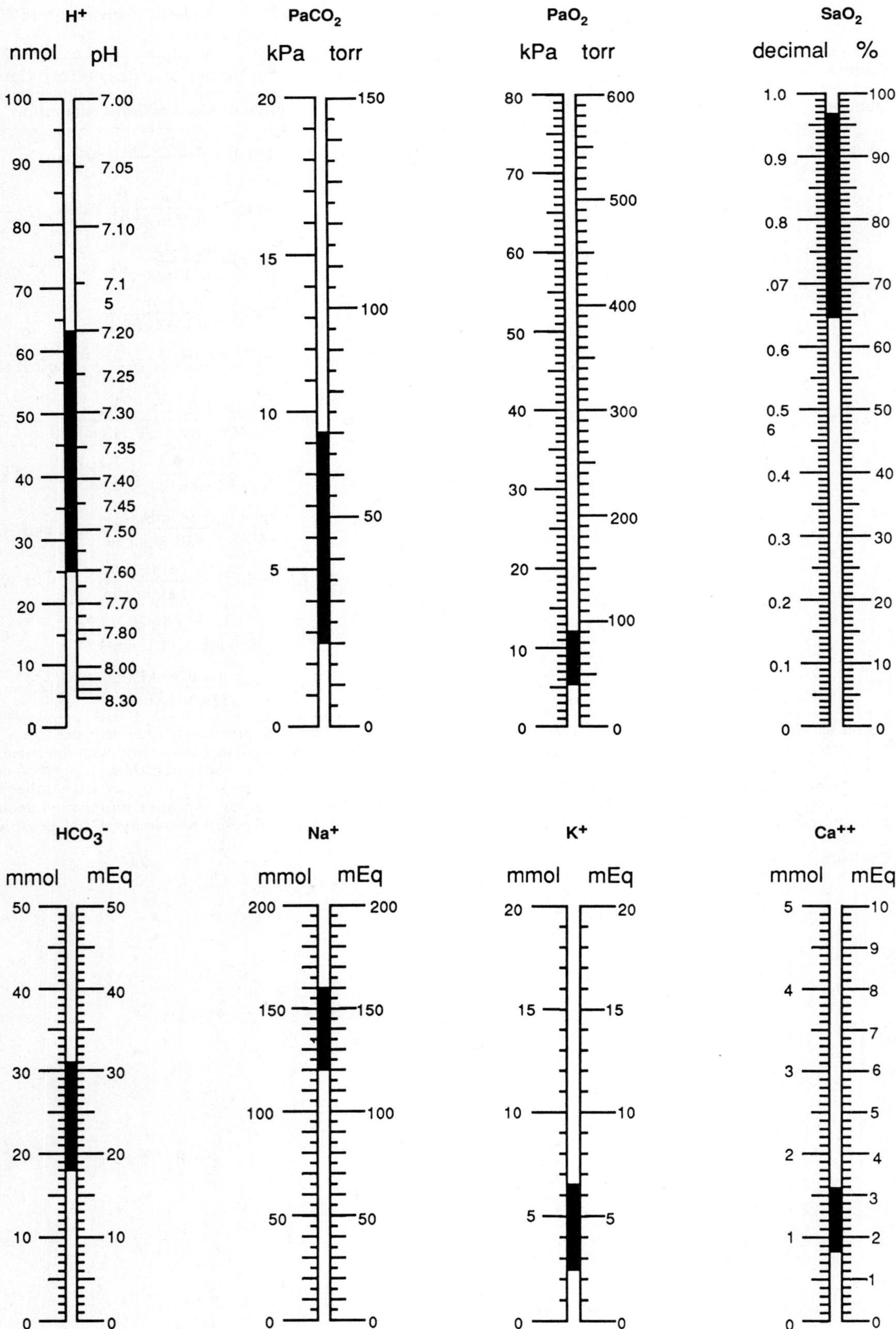

Figure A-1. Nomograms for converting units associated with blood gas analysis. Solid bar indicates range between critical values. (From Lundberg et al.,[4] with permission.)

References

1. Chatburn RL: Measurement, physical quantities, and le Systeme Interntional d'Unites (SI units). Respir Care 1988;33:861–873
2. Young DS: Implementation of SI units for clinical laboratory data. Style specifications and conversion tables. Ann Intern Med 1987;106:114–129
3. Council on Scientific Affairs: SI units for clinical laboratory data. JAMA 1985;253:2553–2554
4. Lundberg GD, Iverson C, Radulescu G: Now read this: The SI units are here. JAMA 1986;255:2329–2339

Index

Page numbers followed by f *indicate figures; those followed by* t *indicate tables.*

B

C

D

E

G

I

J

K

M

O

W

X

Z